Third Edition

SEAFOOD
and
FRESHWATER TOXINS

PHARMACOLOGY, PHYSIOLOGY, AND DETECTION

EDITED BY Luis M. Botana

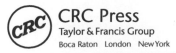

CRC Press
Taylor & Francis Group
Boca Raton   London   New York

CRC Press is an imprint of the
Taylor & Francis Group, an **informa** business

CRC Press
Taylor & Francis Group
6000 Broken Sound Parkway NW, Suite 300
Boca Raton, FL 33487-2742

First issued in paperback 2019

ISBN-13: 978-1-4665-0514-8 (hbk)
ISBN-13: 978-0-367-37880-6 (pbk)

Library of Congress Cataloging-in-Publication Data

Seafood and freshwater toxins : pharmacology, physiology, and detection / editor, Luis M. Botana. -- Third edition.
    p. ; cm.
    Includes bibliographical references and index.
    Summary: "This book provides an overview of the current state of knowledge from several perspectives. Incorporating toxicology, chemistry, ecology, and economics, the book covers the biological aspects of the bloom and the effects and actions of each toxin, with emphasis on human response. It discusses the use of animals, receptors, antibodies, and aptamers as tools for method development. It highlights the legal and economic perspectives of toxic incidence in industrial activity and international regulation and monitoring programs"--Provided by publisher.
    ISBN 978-1-4665-0514-8 (hardback : alk. paper)
    I. Botana, Luis M., editor of compilation.
    [DNLM: 1. Marine Toxins--analysis. 2. Marine Toxins--pharmacology. 3. Marine Toxins--poisoning. 4. Food Contamination. 5. Seafood--poisoning. 6. Water Pollution--adverse effects. QW 630.5.M3]

    QP632.M37
    615.9'45--dc23

2013049467

Visit the Taylor & Francis Web site at
http://www.taylorandfrancis.com

and the CRC Press Web site at
http://www.crcpress.com

Contents

Part I   General Considerations

Part II   Impact

Part III   Technology

Part IV   Nonneurotoxic Lipophilic Toxins

Preface

When the first edition of this title was published, I felt the need to gather all the information regarding pharmacology and toxicology of marine toxins. At the time, the available information was limited, as evidenced by the second edition, which has shown how fast the discovery and identification of new toxins are progressing.

The publication of a third edition of this book about marine and freshwater toxins indicates not only that scientists and technicians demand this type of information, but also that there are new topics to discuss. And this is so because the last few years have brought about many changes in this field. These changes were mainly due to the advance of analytical technology, most notably mass spectrometry, that allowed the identification of small amounts of toxins, tracking of old samples back in time, and the realization that most of the toxins are present everywhere, making it a global problem. If the second edition provided a clear picture of the increase in the number of toxin groups and analogs in each group, this edition is mostly influenced by the changes in regulatory aspects, climate change evidences, new technologies, and toxicology. What we know now is that the chemical diversity of toxins is very high, that their profile is changing as a consequence of human or climatic interference, and that many new technologies can be used to cultivate the algae, identify the toxins, and isolate and quantify them. There is much information about the potential use of marine compounds as lead structures for drug development, and yet we do not know why they are being synthesized by the microorganisms that produce them.

We still have the same old problems: scarcity of available compounds, although new players have entered the marine toxin standard arena, and unclear toxicological information, which was an actual limitation for the European Food Safety working group. Therefore, there is still much to be done.

The book chapters cover several aspects of toxins. Part I includes an overview and covers general issues related to their detection, ecology, diversity, and climate change. Part II refers to impact, in terms of epidemiology, toxicology, economy, and surveillance. Part III is focused on technology available for the detection (biosensors and functional assays, mass spectrometry, nanotechnology and biotechnology, and standards) of toxins. Finally, Parts IV to VII give detailed descriptions of the chemical diversity of the groups and their biological sources, their modes of action, and the use of marine and freshwater toxins as lead structures in drug development.

Acknowledgments

All the contributing authors are leading experts in their fields. I would like to acknowledge the time and effort that they have put into this work. Without their collaboration, this book would never have been possible.

I also thank all the readers of this book. They allowed the publication of this third edition and helped consolidate the title as a reference in the field.

Editor

Luis M. Botana is a professor of pharmacology at the Veterinary School, University of Santiago de Compostela, Lugo, Spain. He did his postdoctoral work as a Fogarty Fellow at the Johns Hopkins University (1990–1992). He served as director of the European Community Reference Laboratory for Marine Biotoxins (2005–2009) and as director of the Department of Pharmacology of the USC (2004–2012).

Dr. Botana's research group is a world leader in toxicology, mechanistic and pharmacological use of marine and freshwater toxins, and methodological developments for the detection of marine toxins. He has published more than 250 papers, directed 35 PhD theses, acquired 25 patents, and edited several books. He can be considered a reference in the field!

Dr. Botana has served as director or has participated in several international projects, such as DETECTOX, CIGUATOOLS, ATLANTOX, PHARMATLANTIC, BIOCOP, MICROAQUA, SPIES-DETOX, BEADS, BAMMBO, and PHARMASEA. His research has aimed at the use of marine toxins as leads for drugs to treat cancer, Alzheimer's disease, transplant rejection, and allergies. He has also developed in vitro functional methods for all toxin groups by means of several technological approaches.

Contributors

Waldo Acevedo-Castillo
School of Science
Institute of Chemistry
Pontificial Catholic University of Valparaíso
Valparaíso, Chile

Amparo Alfonso
Faculty of Veterinary Science
Department of Pharmacology
University of Santiago de Compostela
Lugo, Spain

Carmen Alfonso
Laboratorio CIFGA S.A.
Lugo, Spain

Eva Alonso
Faculty of Veterinary Medicine
Department of Pharmacology
University of Santiago de Compostela
Lugo, Spain

Mercedes Álvarez
Laboratorio CIFGA S.A.
Lugo, Spain

Álvaro Antelo
Laboratorio CIFGA S.A.
Lugo, Spain

Rómulo Aráoz
Laboratoire de Neurobiologie et Développement
Institut de Neurobiologie Alfred Fessard
Centre National de la Recherche Scientifique
Gif-sur-Yvette, France

Vaishali P. Bane
Mass Spectrometry Research Centre (MSRC)
PROTEOBIO Research Groups
and
Department of Chemistry
Cork Institute of Technology
Cork, Ireland

Manuel Bañobre-López
International Iberian Nanotechnology
   Laboratory
Braga, Portugal

Evelyne Benoit
Laboratoire de Neurobiologie et Développement
Institut de Neurobiologie Alfred Fessard
Centre National de la Recherche Scientifique
Gif-sur-Yvette, France

Gary Bignami
Bignami Consulting
Honolulu, Hawaii

Luis M. Botana
Faculty of Veterinary Medicine
Department of Pharmacology
University of Santiago de Compostela
Lugo, Spain

Andreas Brust
Institute for Molecular Bioscience
The University of Queensland
Brisbane, Queensland, Australia

Ana G. Cabado
Spanish National Association of SeaFood
   Producers-Technological Centre
ANFACO-CECOPESCA
Vigo, Spain

Eva Cagide
Laboratorio CIFGA S.A.
Lugo, Spain

Katrina Campbell
Institute for Global Food Security
School of Biological Sciences
Queen's University Belfast
Belfast, Northern Ireland

María-José Chapela
Spanish National Association of SeaFood
    Producers-Technological Centre
ANFACO-CECOPESCA
Vigo, Spain

Y. Chisti
School of Engineering
Massey University
Palmerston North, New Zealand

Justine Dauphard
Mass Spectrometry Research Centre (MSRC)
PROTEOBIO Research Groups
and
Department of Chemistry
Cork Institute of Technology
Cork, Ireland

Antonio M.G. de Diego
Institute for Ear Research
University College London
London, United Kingdom

Giorgia del Favero
Department of Life Sciences
University of Trieste
Trieste, Italy

Gregory J. Doucette
Center for Coastal Environmental Health &
    Biomolecular Research
NOAA/National Ocean Service
Charleston, South Carolina

Christopher T. Elliott
Institute for Global Food Security
Queen's University Belfast
Belfast, Ireland

Begoña Espiña
International Iberian Nanotechnology
    Laboratory
Braga, Portugal

Paula Fajardo
Spanish National Association of SeaFood
    Producers-Technological Centre
ANFACO-CECOPESCA
Vigo, Spain

Ricardo Felix
Department of Cell Biology
Center for Research and Advanced Studies of the
    National Polytechnic Institute
Mexico City, Mexico

Martiña Ferreira
Spanish National Association of SeaFood
    Producers-Technological Centre
ANFACO-CECOPESCA
Vigo, Spain

María Fraga
Faculty of Veterinary Science
Department of Pharmacology
University of Santiago de Compostela
Lugo, Spain

Paulo P. Freitas
International Iberian Nanotechnology
    Laboratory
Braga, Portugal

Ambrose Furey
Mass Spectrometry Research Centre (MSRC)
PROTEOBIO Research Groups
and
Department of Chemistry
Cork Institute of Technology
Cork, Ireland

Haruhiko Fuwa
Graduate School of Life Sciences
Tohoku University
Sendai, Japan

J. Gallardo-Rodríguez
Department of Chemical Engineering
University of Almería
Almería, Spain

Luis Gandía
Facultad de Medicina
Departamento de Farmacología y Terapéutica
Instituto Teófilo Hernando
Universidad Autónoma de Madrid
Madrid, Spain

María A. Gandini
Department of Cell Biology
Center for Research and Advanced Studies of the
    National Polytechnic Institute
Mexico City, Mexico

Antonio G. García
Facultad de Medicina
Departamento de Farmacología y Terapéutica
Instituto Teófilo Hernando
Universidad Autónoma de Madrid
and
Instituto de Investigación Sanitaria
Servicio de Farmacología Clínica
Hospital Universitario de la Princesa
Madrid, Spain

F. García-Camacho
Department of Chemical Engineering
University of Almería
Almería, Spain

Alejandro Garrido
Spanish National Association of SeaFood
    Producers-Technological Centre
ANFACO-CECOPESCA
Vigo, Spain

Arjen Gerssen
Business Unit Contaminants and Toxins
RIKILT Wageningen UR
Wageningen, the Netherlands

Juan Jesús Gestal Otero
School of Medicine and Odontology
Department of Psychiatry, Radiology
    and Public Health
University of Santiago de Compostela
Santiago de Compostela, Spain

Philipp Hess
Institut Français de Recherche pour l'Exploitation
    de la Mer
Laboratoire Phycotoxines
Nantes, France

Michael J. Holmes
Queensland Department of Science, Information
    Technology, Innovation and the Arts
Brisbane, Queensland, Australia

Bogdan I. Iorga
Institut de Chimie des Substances Naturelles
    LabEx
LERMIT Centre National de la Recherche
    Scientifique
Gif-sur-Yvette, France

Thierry Jauffrais
Phycotoxins Laboratory
Ifremer, French Research Institute for
    Exploitation of the Sea
and
Sea, Molecules and Health Laboratory
Nantes University
Nantes, France

Panagiota Katikou
National Reference Laboratory on Marine
    Biotoxins
Institute of Food Hygiene of Thessaloniki
Ministry of Rural Development and Food
Thessaloniki, Greece

Jane Kilcoyne
Biotoxin Chemistry
Marine Institute
Galway, Ireland

Bernd Krock
Ecological Chemistry
Alfred Wegener Institute for Polar and Marine
    Research
Bremerhaven, Germany

Jorge Lago
Spanish National Association of SeaFood
    Producers-Technological Centre
ANFACO-CECOPESCA
Vigo, Spain

Pedro Leão
Interdisciplinary Center of Marine and
    Environmental Research (CIIMAR/CIMAR)
University of Porto
Porto, Portugal

Mary Lehane
Mass Spectrometry Research Centre (MSRC)
PROTEOBIO Research Groups
and
Department of Chemistry
Cork Institute of Technology
Cork, Ireland

Richard J. Lewis
Institute for Molecular Bioscience
The University of Queensland
Brisbane, Queensland, Australia

Patricio Leyton
School of Science
Institute of Chemistry
Pontificial Catholic University of Valparaíso
Valparaíso, Chile

Ignacio López-González
Department of Developmental Genetics and
  Molecular Physiology
Institute of Biotechnology
National Autonomous University of Mexico
Cuernavaca, México

L. López-Rosales
Department of Chemical Engineering
University of Almería
Almería, Spain

M. Carmen Louzao
Faculty of Veterinary Medicine
Department of Pharmacology
University of Santiago de Compostela
Lugo, Spain

Verónica C. Martins
International Iberian Nanotechnology
  Laboratory
Braga, Portugal

Pearse McCarron
National Research Council of Canada
Measurement Science and Standards
Halifax, Nova Scotia, Canada

Christopher O. Miles
Section for Chemistry and Toxicology
Norwegian Veterinary Institute
Oslo, Norway

Jordi Molgó
Laboratoire de Neurobiologie et Développement
Institut de Neurobiologie Alfred Fessard
Centre National de la Recherche Scientifique
Gif-sur-Yvette, France

E. Molina-Grima
Department of Chemical Engineering
University of Almería
Almería, Spain

Rex Munday
Ruakura Research Centre
AgResearch Ltd
Hamilton, New Zealand

John O'Halloran
School of Biological, Earth and Environmental
  Sciences
University College Cork
Cork, Ireland

Richard O'Kennedy
School of Biotechnology
Dublin City University
Dublin, Ireland

Alberto Otero
Spanish National Association of SeaFood
  Producers-Technological Centre
ANFACO-CECOPESCA
Vigo, Spain

Paz Otero
Faculty of Veterinary Medicine
Department of Pharmacology
University of Santiago de Compostela
Lugo, Spain

Fernando Padín
Facultad de Medicina
Departamento de Farmacología y Terapéutica
Instituto Teófilo Hernando
Universidad Autónoma de Madrid
Madrid, Spain

Marco Pelin
Department of Life Sciences
University of Trieste
Trieste, Italy

Frank van Pelt
Department of Pharmacology and Therapeutics
University College Cork
Cork, Ireland

Mark Poli
U.S. Army Medical Research Institute of
  Infectious Diseases
Fort Detrick, Maryland

Clare H. Redshaw
European Centre for Environment and Human
Health
University of Exeter Medical School
Truro, United Kingdom

and

School of Geography, Earth and Environmental
Sciences
University of Plymouth
Plymouth, United Kingdom

Juan G. Reyes
School of Science
Institute of Chemistry
Pontifical Catholic University of Valparaíso
Valparaíso, Chile

José Rivas
International Iberian Nanotechnology
Laboratory
Braga, Portugal

Laura Pérez Rodríguez
Faculty of Veterinary Science
Department of Pharmacology
University of Santiago de Compostela
Lugo, Spain

Paula Rodríguez
Faculty of Veterinary Science
Department of Pharmacology
University of Santiago de Compostela
Lugo, Spain

Juan A. Rubiolo
Faculty of Veterinary Science
Department of Pharmacology
University of Santiago de Compostela
Lugo, Spain

Rafael Salas
Marine Environment and Food Safety
Phytoplankton Department
Marine Institute
Galway, Ireland

Claudia Sánchez-Cárdenas
Department of Developmental Genetics and
Molecular Physiology
Institute of Biotechnology
National Autonomous University of Mexico
Cuernavaca, México

A. Sánchez-Mirón
Department of Chemical Engineering
University of Almería
Almería, Spain

Joe Silke
Marine Environment and Food Safety Services
Marine Institute
Galway, Ireland

Paul T. Smith
University of Western Sydney
Richmond, New South Wales, Australia

Edwina Stack
Global Biotherapeutics Technologies
Pfizer R&D
Dublin, Ireland

Supanoi Subsinserm
Chemical Laboratory System Development
Fish Inspection and Quality Control Division
Department of Fisheries
Bangkok, Thailand

Toshiyuki Suzuki
Research Center for Biochemistry and Food
Technology
National Research Institute of Fisheries Science
Yokohama, Japan

Eva Ternon
Nice Institute of Chemistry
University of Nice-Sophia Antipolis
Nice, France

Olivier P. Thomas
Nice Institute of Chemistry
University of Nice-Sophia Antipolis
Nice, France

Urban Tillmann
Ecological Chemistry
Alfred Wegener Institute for Polar and Marine
Research
Bremerhaven, Germany

Araceli Tobío
Faculty of Veterinary Science
Department of Pharmacology
University of Santiago de Compostela
Lugo, Spain

Claudia L. Treviño
Department of Developmental Genetics and
    Molecular Physiology
Institute of Biotechnology
National Autonomous University of Mexico
Cuernavaca, México

Marcela B. Treviño
Math and Sciences Department
Edison State College
Fort Myers, Florida

Aurelia Tubaro
Department of Life Sciences
University of Trieste
Trieste, Italy

Andrew Turner
Food Safety Group
Centre for Environment, Fisheries and
    Aquaculture Science
Weymouth, Dorset, United Kingdom

Michael J. Twiner
Department of Natural Sciences
University of Michigan–Dearborn
Dearborn, Michigan

Carmen Vale
Faculty of Veterinary Science
Department of Pharmacology
University of Santiago de Compostela
Lugo, Spain

Paulo Vale
Portuguese Institute for Sea and Atmosphere
    (IPMA)
Sea and Marine Resources Department
    (DMRM)
Lisboa, Portugal

Vitor Vasconcelos
Interdisciplinary Center of Marine and
    Environmental Research (CIIMAR/CIMAR)
and
Faculty of Sciences
Department of Biology
Porto University
Porto, Portugal

Irina Vetter
Institute for Molecular Bioscience
The University of Queensland
Brisbane, Queensland, Australia

Juan Manuel Vieites
Spanish National Association of SeaFood
    Producers-Technological Centre
ANFACO-CECOPESCA
Vigo, Spain

Natalia Vilariño
Faculty of Veterinary Science
Department of Pharmacology
University of Santiago de Compostela
Lugo, Spain

Aristidis Vlamis
National Reference Laboratory on Marine
    Biotoxins
Institute of Food Hygiene of Thessaloniki
Ministry of Rural Development and Food
Thessaloniki, Greece

Mari Yotsu-Yamashita
Graduate School of Agricultural Science
Tohoku University
Sendai, Japan

Arash Zamyadi
Department of Civil Engineering
University of Toronto
Toronto, Ontario, Canada

Katharina Zimmermann
Institute for Molecular Bioscience
The University of Queensland
Brisbane, Queensland, Australia

Part I

General Considerations

1

Dinoflagellate Toxins: An Overview

Michael J. Holmes, Andreas Brust, and Richard J. Lewis

CONTENTS

1.1 Introduction

Dinoflagellates are microscopic, mostly unicellular algae (protists) that live in freshwater and marine waters. They have a fossil record stretching back only to the Mesozoic; however, biochemical evidence suggests that ancestors of dinoflagellates swam in early Cambrian seas some 500 million years ago (Moldowan and Talyzina 1998, Fensome et al. 1999). The majority of the approximately 2000 extant species are marine and have a free-living stage that is predominantly planktonic (Taylor et al. 2008). They are important primary producers being second only to the diatoms among the micro-phytoplankton in the 10–200 μm size range. Approximately half of the extant species are classified as photosynthetic, although the importance of mixotrophy is being increasingly recognized for many species previously presumed to be faculatively photosynthetic (Burkholder et al. 2008). In addition to planktonic species, there are also many in which the free-living form attaches or lives on benthic substrates. There has been a considerable increase in the study of these benthic species in recent years because of the high proportion that produce toxins.

Dinoflagellates contribute the majority of toxin-producing marine microalgal species. However, only a relatively small number of dinoflagellate species produce bioactive molecules that are toxic to other organisms. The majority of these are photosynthetic or mixotrophic species that produce "toxins" that can act directly to harm aquatic life or accumulate through food chains to cause poisoning of other aquatic organisms, birds, and humans. The last three decades have seen an increased emphasis on harmful algal bloom research with an ever-increasing number of potentially toxin-producing species being discovered. Anderson and Lobel (1987) first noted that the proportion of toxic dinoflagellate species is greater among free-living benthic species than planktonic forms. This generalization is still valid, although many recently described species have not been tested for toxicity. This is partly because toxicity testing, especially on vertebrates, has been curtailed by increasingly stringent ethical guidelines. Although there are good reasons for limiting animal testing and developing alternatives for routine analysis of well-characterized toxins, there are advantages that whole animal responses provide in detecting previously unknown toxins or bioactive compounds with new mechanisms of action. At present, the mouse bioassay is still used for routine testing for paralytic shellfish poisoning (PSP) toxins as there are no alternative validated methods that are accepted to measure the composite toxic potency in shellfish (Van Dolah et al. 2012). However, this will likely change in the near future for such a well-characterized suite of toxins with many analogs commercially available for calibrating chemical, biochemical, and cell-based detection methods.

Where it is permitted, mouse bioassay allows characterization of unknown mammalian toxin(s) based upon careful observation of the signs displayed and quantification of the toxin amount based upon time to death (required for purification of the toxin, usually with the goal of elucidating the toxin structure). One mouse unit (MU) is usually considered equivalent to an LD_{50} dose, expressed either per 20 g or kg of mouse. Determination of the presence of a toxin is usually based upon a maximum amount of extract injected that is lethal to mice at 1 g dried extract weight per kg mouse body weight (i.e., 1 g/kg or 20 mg extract per 20 g mouse) (Holmes and Lewis 2002). Nonspecific lethality (e.g., from nontoxic lipids) can occur at even lower doses, and therefore, the presence of toxicity, especially of crude extracts, has to be interpreted with careful observation of the signs displayed by animals (Takagi et al. 1984, Lewis and Sellin 1992). Caution is therefore necessary to interpret toxicity at doses higher than 1 g/kg.

In this review, we discuss the marine dinoflagellates known to produce toxins, especially those species that produce toxins that accumulate through food chains to cause human poisoning. Describing a compound as a "toxin" can depend upon the perspective of the investigator as the toxicity of a bioactive compound can vary manyfold depending upon the susceptibility of the target species and route of administration (Munday 2006). Many compounds produced by dinoflagellates are toxic to test organisms that they would not usually come in contact with outside a laboratory or experimental context (Sournia 1995, Holmes and Lewis 2002). Another problem in reviewing toxin-producing dinoflagellates is the frequent name changes that have occurred for many species. This greatly complicates the literature for many researchers whose primary focus is on the toxins and other bioactive compounds, rather than their biological origin. For example, the reevaluation of detailed thecal plate morphology and increasing reliance upon genetic relationships to define species is producing a legacy of confusing taxonomic designations not easy for even experienced researchers to follow (Scholin 1998, Anderson et al. 2012a). This difficulty is partly because the species concept is not easy to apply to dinoflagellates (Taylor 1985, Fensome et al. 1993, Lundholm and Moestrup 2006, Taylor et al. 2008). Historically they have been defined in terms of "morphospecies," but this concept may not always be sufficient to delineate cryptic species (genospecies) or alternatively may reflect morphological plasticity that cannot be reconciled with genetic differences. There are arguments and counterarguments for stabilizing taxonomic nomenclature with conservative morphological traits (Anderson et al. 2012b). Many toxinologists no doubt find the increasing reliance upon genomics for species identification frustrating, especially when trying to work with field material. However, to ignore these morphologically cryptic differences also risks missing important underlying ecological or toxinological patterns. Even in the absence of taxonomic uncertainty, there are many examples of strain—and biogeographical—differences in toxin production by dinoflagellate (Costas et al. 1995, Scholin 1998, Anderson et al. 2012b). Caution is therefore necessary as toxin production cannot always be globally attributed to particular species or species assemblages.

Holmes and Lewis (2002) compiled a list of 62 toxin-producing dinoflagellate species that was arranged to be most useful to toxinologists. Research over the past decade has seen the identification of species that produce toxins that increase considerably and the clarification of the dinoflagellate origin of a number of marine toxins. While we fully expect that new dinoflagellate species and new bioactive compounds will continue to be discovered, Anderson et al. (2012b) boldly suggest that all major toxin-associated syndromes are now fully described. This review summarizes the predominant poisonings of dinoflagellate origin and lists those species responsible for causing them. For completeness, a number of dinoflagellate toxins currently not associated with human health problems are discussed as well as species responsible for killing fish.

1.2 Harmful Impacts from Dinoflagellate Toxins

1.2.1 Paralytic Shellfish Poisoning Caused by Toxins Originating from the Dinoflagellates *Alexandrium* spp., *Gymnodinium catenatum,* and *Pyrodinium bahamense*

PSP is generally caused by eating shellfish, especially bivalves, which have been contaminated with saxitoxin and its analogs (Figure 1.1). It is a global, coastal phenomenon being found on all continents and from cold to tropical waters. Shellfish accumulate these PSP toxins when they filter feed on toxic species of planktonic dinoflagellates belonging to *Alexandrium* spp., *Gymnodinium catenatum,* or *Pyrodinium bahamense*. The PSP toxins are collectively known as "saxitoxins" or paralytic shellfish toxins, with 57 analogs so far identified, of which 38 are produced by dinoflagellates (Rossini and Hess 2010, Wiese et al. 2010). The parent compound, saxitoxin, is the most potent of these analogs and was named after the toxic butter clams *Saxidomus giganteus* from which it was first isolated. The majority of saxitoxin analogs are highly water soluble and chemically stable under mild acidic conditions, but decay rapidly under alkaline conditions. In addition to dinoflagellates, a number of freshwater and brackish species of cyanobacteria are known to produce these toxins (Deeds et al. 2008, Wiese et al. 2010).

Saxitoxin is a highly potent compound that binds to site-1 of voltage-gated sodium channels inhibiting nerve signaling and muscle contraction (reviewed by Llewellyn 2009). It has the same mechanism of action as tetrodotoxin, first isolated from pufferfish, and the two toxins interact competitively at an overlapping binding site to inhibit sodium ion conduction through this channel. Human symptoms of PSP appear within minutes to ~2 h after consumption of contaminated seafood. The initial symptoms are often gastrointestinal but these are soon followed by neurological symptoms that can eventually lead to respiratory paralysis (hence the name of the disease) and death. The minimum lethal dose (LD_{50}) of saxitoxin injected i.p. in mice is ~10 µg/kg, although the relevant oral toxicity is much lower (260 µg/kg, Aune 2008). Any shellfish containing 0.8 µg or more of paralytic shellfish toxins (saxitoxin equivalents) per gram of edible tissue is considered unfit for human consumption (the Philippines set a lower limit of 0.4 µg/g in 1988 to protect children who may be reliant upon shellfish for food but this was revised to 0.6 µg/g in 2010) (Holmes and Lewis 2002). The lethal effects of these toxins are fast acting, killing mice within 20 min of injection of a minimum lethal dose (~1 LD_{50}). Saxitoxin (and ricin) are the only naturally occurring compounds listed under the most controlled group of chemicals, Schedule 1A of the Chemical Weapons Convention (Organization for the Prohibition of Chemical Weapons, http://www.opcw.org/chemical-weapons-convention/annex-on-chemicals/b-schedules-of-chemicals/schedule-1/).

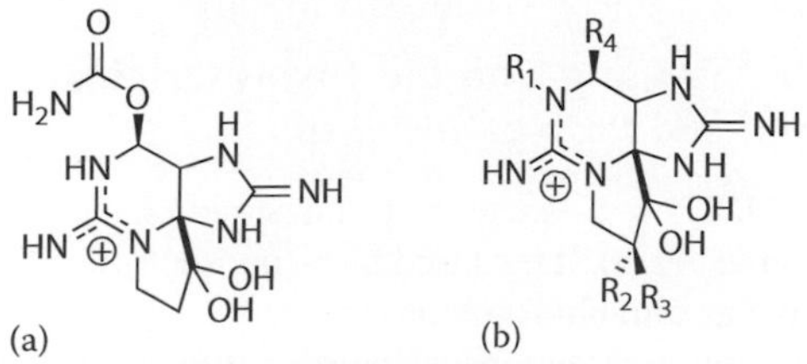

FIGURE 1.1 Saxitoxin (a) and position of side chains (R1–R4) of its analogs (b) that cause PSP. (From Rossini, G.P. and Hess, P., *EXS*, 100, 65, 2010; Wiese, M. et al., *Mar. Drugs*, 8, 2185, 2010.)

While bivalve shellfish are the major vectors for human poisoning, gastropods, crustaceans, and plankton-eating fishes (clupeids) have also caused PSP (Deeds et al. 2008). Recently, saxitoxins were also the cause of human poisoning in Florida from the consumption of pufferfish (Quilliam et al. 2004). Such fishes have long been associated with tetrodotoxin poisoning in the Pacific. However, in Florida, pufferfish species not previously associated with toxicity were found to contain considerable concentrations of saxitoxins (Deeds et al. 2008). The origin of these pufferfish toxins is thought to be the planktonic dinoflagellate *P. bahamense* (Landsberg et al. 2006). *P. bahamense* is a tropical, euryhaline species that continues to be a major cause of seafood toxicity throughout Southeast Asia and has caused many fatalities (Hallegraeff and Maclean 1989, Usup et al. 2012). The first confirmed toxic bloom of *P. bahamense* occurred in Papua New Guinea as recently as 1972 (Maclean 1977, 1989). *Pyrodinium* is a monospecific genus with two varieties described: *P. bahamense* var. *compressum* from the Pacific and *P. bahamense* var. *bahamense* from the Atlantic and Caribbean (Steidinger and Tangen 1997). While *P. bahamense* var. *compressum* has caused poisonings throughout Southeast Asia and the Pacific coast of Central America, *P. bahamense* var. *bahamense* was thought to be nontoxic (Steidinger and Tangen 1997). This biogeographical model for separation of toxin-producing varieties was shattered by the pufferfish poisonings in Florida (Landsberg et al. 2006). Western Pacific isolates of *P. bahamense* produce mainly gonyautoxin-5, saxitoxin, and/or neosaxitoxin (Oshima 1989, Usup et al. 1994).

G. catenatum is a chain-forming, planktonic dinoflagellate distributed across all continents except Antarctica (Lundholm and Moestrup 2006). It is the only species of *Gymnodinium* known to produce PSP toxins. It has a broad temperature distribution being found in waters of more than 42° south latitude (e.g., Tasmania) to less than 2° north of the equator in Singapore (Hallegraeff and Fraga 1998, Holmes et al. 2002). The discovery of lipophilic, hydroxybenzoate analogs of the saxitoxins from *G. catenatum* in recent years has increased the number and complexity of known saxitoxin analogs (Negri et al. 2003, Vale 2010). These analogs are now thought to dominate the toxin profile of many strains of *G. catenatum* (in terms of mole percentage or mol%) (Negri et al. 2007). However, overall toxicity does not necessarily equate to the linear sum of the toxicities of individual analogs in mixtures of toxins (Llewellyn 2006). Until the discovery of the hydroxybenzoate analogs, the toxin profiles of most *G. catenatum* strains were considered to be dominated by the less-toxic N-sulfocarbamoyl toxins (Negri et al. 2001), although strains with profiles dominated by the more potent carbamoyl forms were also known to occur (Holmes et al. 2002).

The majority of PSP contamination of shellfish around the world is caused by species of the planktonic dinoflagellate belonging to the genus *Alexandrium*. This is a much studied and broadly distributed group that has undergone a number of taxonomic revisions, and they have been described in the literature under the synonyms *Goniodoma, Protogonyaulax, Gonyaulax,* and *Gessnerium* (Balech 1995). These are among the most difficult groups of toxic dinoflagellate species for identification (Anderson et al. 2012a). John et al. (2003) listed 29 species of *Alexandrium* and suggested that 9 produce PSP toxins, whereas Holmes and Lewis (2002) listed 12 putative PSP-producing *Alexandrium* spp. The revised list (Table 1.1) contains 11 species with *A. angustitabulatum* and *A. lusitanicum* now considered to be conspecific with *A. minimum* (Lilly et al. 2005, Moestrup et al. 2009) and *A. peruvianum* recently found to produce paralytic shellfish toxins (Borkman et al. 2012). Deeds et al. (2008) provide an overview of the variety of PSP-toxin profiles produced by the various *Alexandrium* spp., and the reviews of Anderson et al. (2012a,b) explore the strain and genotypic variation within this genus.

1.2.2 Diarrhetic Shellfish Poisoning with the Toxins Originating from *Dinophysis* spp. and *Prorocentrum* spp.

Diarrhetic shellfish poisoning (DSP) is a severe gastrointestinal disease that was first identified from Japan in the 1970s (Yasumoto et al. 1978). It is caused by eating shellfish that have been contaminated by okadaic acid and analogs known as dinophysistoxins (Figure 1.2). These are lipophilic, polyether toxins that act by inhibiting serine/threonine protein phosphatases (Bialojan and Takai 1988) to cause inflammation of the intestinal tract and diarrhea (Terao et al. 1986). There are more than 20 known analogs of okadaic acid, but most are considerably less potent inhibitors of protein phosphatases than okadaic acid

TABLE 1.1

Alexandrium spp. Reported to Produce PSP Toxins

Number	Species	Reference for PSP Toxin Production
1	*A. acatenella* (Whedon & Kofoid) Balech	As *G. acatenella,* Prakash and Taylor (1966)
2	*A. andersonii* Balech	Ciminiello et al. (2000)
3	*A. affine* (Inoue & Fukuyo) Balech	Reported as low toxicity or nontoxic, Anderson et al. (2012a)
4	*A. catenella* (Whedon & Kofoid) Balech	As *G. catenella,* Burke et al. (1960)
5	*A. cohorticula* (Whedon & Kofoid) Balech	Fukuyo et al. (1989) and Taylor et al. (1995) suggest caution because of similarity to *A. tamiyavanichi*
6	*A. fundyense* Balech	Anderson et al. (1990)
7	*A. minutum* Halim	Oshima et al. (1989)
8	*A. ostenfeldii* (Paulsen) Balech & Tangen	Balech and Tangen (1985), Hansen et al. (1992)
9	*A. peruvianum* (Balech & de Mendiola) Balech & Tangen	Lim et al. (2005)
10	*A. tamarense* (Lebour) Balech	As *G. tamarensis,* Shimizu et al. (1975)
11	*A. tamiyavanichi* Balech	As *P. cohorticula,* Kodama et al. (1988)

Notes: For additional comments, see Deeds et al. 2008 and Anderson et al. 2012a. *Alexandrium leei* may also be a weak producer of PSP toxins (Nguyen-Ngoc 2004).

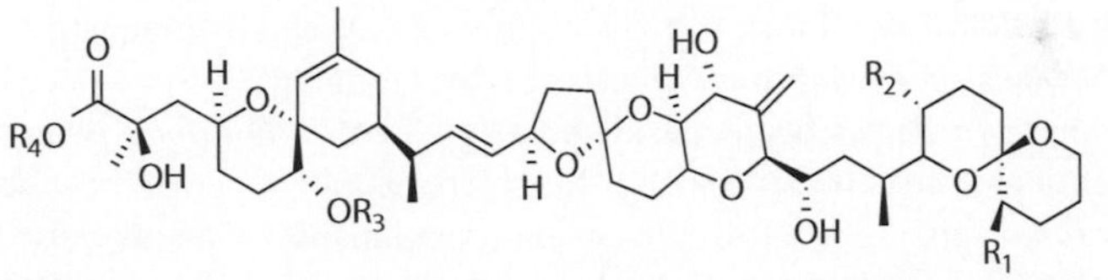

FIGURE 1.2 DSP is caused by okadaic acid and analogs known as dinophysistoxins. (From Yanagi, T. et al., *Agric. Biol. Chem.*, 53, 525, 1989; Nishiwaki, S. et al., *Carcinogenesis*, 11, 1837, 1990; Sasaki, K. et al., *Biochem. J.*, 298, 259, 1994.)

(Yanagi et al. 1989, Nishiwaki et al. 1990, Sasaki et al. 1994). The potency of these analogs is markedly affected by modifications to the carboxyl group or the four hydroxyls (Nishiwaki et al. 1990). Okadaic acid and dinophysistoxin-1 have similar i.p. toxicities (LD_{50}) in mice of approximately 200 and 160 µg/kg (Aune 2008). Unlike PSP, DSP is rarely life threatening and because of the diffuse nature of the gastrointestinal symptoms it induces, it can be easily confused with illnesses caused by inappropriate food storage or preparation. Symptoms can last up to 3 days (Tubaro et al. 2008). DSP toxins are sometimes classified into three groups based upon structural similarities: (1) okadaic acid/dinophysistoxin analogs, (2) pectenotoxins, and (3) yessotoxins (YTXs). However, no human poisonings from pectenotoxins or YTXs have been confirmed, and in animal studies, they do not induce diarrhea and are much less toxic when introduced orally than via injection (Suzuki and Quilliam 2011). Therefore, even though pectenotoxins can be produced by the same *Dinophysis* spp. that produce okadaic acid (Pizarro et al. 2008), we do not consider YTXs and pectenotoxins as DSP toxins and discuss them separately in Section 1.2.7.1. The name dinophysistoxin was derived from the genus *Dinophysis* from which 35-methyl okadaic acid (dinophysistoxin-1) was first identified (Murata et al. 1982), whereas okadaic acid was first isolated from a marine sponge, *Halichondria okadai* (Tachibana et al. 1981).

Shellfish contaminated by DSP toxins are considered unfit for human consumption if they accumulate more than 0.16 µg okadaic acid equivalents per gram of shellfish meat (Opinion of the Scientific Panel on Contaminants in the Food Chain on a request from the European Commission on marine biotoxins in shellfish–okadaic acid and analogs, 2008). These toxins can also be transferred through the invertebrate food chain as Torgersen et al. (2005) report a DSP outbreak caused by eating crabs that had been contaminated from preying upon mussels containing DSP toxins. The majority of DSP contamination of shellfish is caused from bivalves filter feeding on toxic species of planktonic dinoflagellates of the

TABLE 1.2

Dinophysis and *Phalacroma* spp. Reported to Produce Analogs of Okadaic Acid and/or Pectenotoxins

Number	Species	Reference for Toxin Production
1	*D. acuminata* Claparède & Lachmann	Lee et al. (1989)
2	*D. acuta* Ehrenberg	Lee et al. (1989)
3	*D. caudata* Saville-Kent	Holmes et al. (1999)
4	*D. fortii* Pavillard	Yasumoto et al. (1980)
5	*D. infundibulus* Schiller	Suzuki et al. (2009)
6	*D. miles* Cleve	Marasigan et al. (2001)
7	*D. norvegica* Claparède & Lachmann	Lee et al. (1989)
8	*D. ovum* Schütt	Raho et al. (2008)
9	*D. sacculus* Stein	Giacobbe et al. (2000)
10	*D. tripos* Gourret	Lee et al. (1989)
11	*P. mitra* Schütt	As *D. mitra*, Lee et al. (1989)
12	*P. rotundatum* (Claparède & Lachmann) Kofoid & Michener	As *D. rotundata*, Lee et al. (1989)

Source: Modified from Reguera, B. et al., *Harmful Algae*, 14, 87, 2012.

genus *Dinophysis*. In a review of harmful *Dinophysis* spp., Reguera et al. (2012) listed 10 species of *Dinophysis* that produce okadaic acid or dinophysistoxins (and/or pectenotoxins) as well as 2 species of the related genus *Phalacroma* (Table 1.2). This number is a small minority of the 104 species of *Dinophysis* and 41 species of *Phalacroma* considered by Gómez (2005) to occur across the world's oceans. *Phalacroma* has sometimes been considered a synonym of *Dinophysis,* but molecular analysis of a large group of Dinophysiales by Jensen and Daugbjerg (2009) supported the separation of the two genera. Most *Phalacroma* spp. are heterotrophic oceanic organisms, whereas most *Dinophysis* spp. are photosynthetic and/or mixotrophic coastal organisms (Hallegraeff and Lucas 1988). However, many *Dinophysis* spp. considered to be photosynthetic may derive their chloroplasts through predation (kleptoplasty) of other phytoplankton (Jacobson and Anderson 1994, Nagai et al. 2008, Nishitani et al. 2008b).

The recent ability to culture *Dinophysis* spp. using prey organisms (Park et al. 2006, Nishitani et al. 2008a, Hackett et al. 2009) has facilitated physiological studies of toxin production (Kamiyama and Suzuki 2009, Fux et al. 2011, Nagai et al. 2011). The alternative method for detecting toxin production was to concentrate cells from the wild for analysis. This includes isolating sufficient individual cells for extraction by hand under a microscope using a capillary pipette (Lee et al. 1989, Holmes et al. 1999) or collecting cells from near monospecific blooms using a plankton net. Okadaic acid and dinophysistoxin-1 were recently detected from as few as 32 micropipetted cells, although this was from relatively high cellular concentrations of okadaic acid and dinophysistoxins-1 in *D. fortii* (Suzuki et al. 2009). The sensitivity of analytical detection methods, especially those based on liquid chromatography–mass spectrometry, has increased markedly in recent years, and it is likely that toxin detection will soon be possible from single cells.

Seven species of *Dinophysis*, *D. acuminata, D. acuta, D. caudata, D. fortii, D. miles, D. ovum,* and *D. sacculus,* have been associated with DSP events (Reguera et al. 2012). To our knowledge, the remaining species listed as DSP toxin producers in Table 1.2 have not yet been associated with human poisoning. DSP toxins are also produced by a number of benthic species of *Prorocentrum* (reviewed by Holmes and Lewis 2002) and recently the first planktonic species of Prorocentrum to produce okadaic acid was discovered, *P. texanum* (Henrichs et al. 2013). The genus *Prorocentrum* includes more than 50 species (Gómez 2005) with most being planktonic, but there are also many benthic/tycoplanktonic species. The majority of the planktonic species are nontoxic, whereas a number of benthic species produce DSP toxins (covered in more detail in Section 1.2.6.2). However, only *P. lima* has so far been implicated in DSP contamination of shellfish (Lawrence et al. 2000). *P. lima* is a benthic dinoflagellate but turbulence can resuspend cells in the water column for a short time, and presumably these resuspended cells can be filtered out of the water by shellfish. In the study reported by Lawrence et al. (2000), *P. lima* cells were found growing as epiphytes on the biofouling of mussel socks in Nova Scotia, Canada.

Although humans are the only species known to be poisoned by DSP toxins through ingestion of food (shellfish), there is no obvious reason why a broader range of species might not be affected. The recent detection of low levels of okadaic acid from bottlenose dolphins (*Tursiops truncatus*) suggests the potential for such poisonings to occur in at least some marine mammals (Fire et al. 2011). It is also interesting to speculate on the potential for herbivorous marine mammals such as dugong (*Dugong dugon*) to be exposed to these toxins, through consumption of seagrass supporting epiphytic *Prorocentrum* spp. producing DSP toxins. This would be analogous to poisoning of manatees from the incidental ingestion of planktonic, toxic *Karenia brevis* dinoflagellates while feeding on seagrass during *K. brevis* blooms (O'Shea et al. 1991). Further research is needed to examine the potential of DSP-producing dinoflagellates to grow epiphytically on seagrasses.

1.2.3 Neurotoxic Shellfish Poisoning with the Toxins Originating from *Karenia* spp.

Neurotoxic shellfish poisoning (NSP) is a neurological disease caused by eating shellfish contaminated with lipid-soluble, polyether toxins called brevetoxins (abbreviated BTX or PbTX). This disease is mostly known from the Gulf of Mexico, especially the west coast of Florida, but in recent years, NSP has also occurred repeatedly in New Zealand. *K. brevis* is the dinoflagellate responsible for NSP in North America and is the best studied of all the 12 known *Karenia* spp. (Davis 1948, Brand et al. 2012). A number of raphidophyte species also produce BTXs (Landsberg 2002, Furey et al. 2007).

NSP is generally not a life-threatening illness with symptoms appearing 30 min to 3 h after eating contaminated shellfish and resolving within a few days. Initial symptoms typically include abdominal pain, nausea, vomiting, and diarrhea accompanied by paresthesia of the lips, face, and extremities. No human mortalities are known. However, when blooms of *K. brevis* are carried into coastal zones, wind and wave action can rupture cells and aerosolize the toxins, and onshore winds can cause respiratory distress in coastal populations (Cheng et al. 2005, 2010).

Many BTX analogs have been isolated from *K. brevis* or shellfish; all based around two structural backbones (named A and B) of relatively rigid polyether rings producing ladderlike structures (Figure 1.3) (Baden and Adams 2000). These toxins share many structural similarities with the ciguatoxins (CTXs), and both groups are depolarizing toxins that bind to site-5 of voltage-gated sodium channels (Lombet et al. 1987). Like saxitoxin and tetrodotoxin, BTXs and CTXs are competitive inhibitors but activate

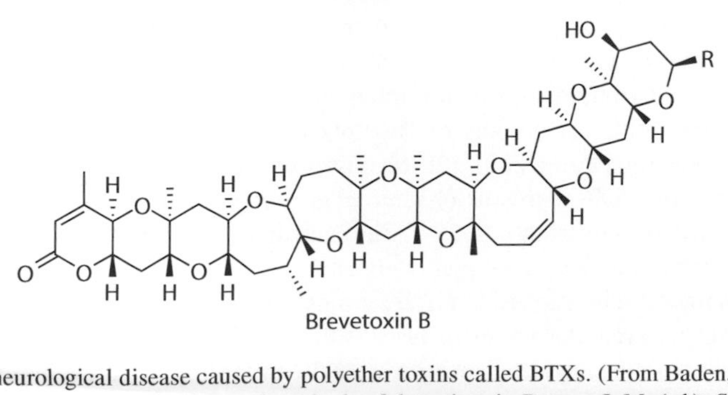

Brevetoxin A

Brevetoxin B

FIGURE 1.3 NSP, a neurological disease caused by polyether toxins called BTXs. (From Baden, D.C. and Adams, D.J., Brevetoxins: Chemistry, mechanism of action and methods of detection, in Botana, L.M. (ed.), *Seafood and Freshwater Toxins*, Marcel Dekker Inc., New York, pp. 505–532, 2000.)

rather than block sodium channels. This activation produces initial nerve stimulation seen even at low concentrations, followed by a depolarization-induced block that is prominent at higher concentrations.

The most toxic BTXs extracted from *K. brevis* are BTX-2 and BTX-3, with i.p. LD_{50} to mice of approximately 200 and 170 µg/kg and oral toxicities of 6600 and 520 µg/kg, respectively (Baden and Mende 1982). Compared to many other dinoflagellate toxins, the BTXs are not particularly toxic to mammals, with potencies comparable to the DSP toxins. However, the BTXs are far more potent towards fish (Baden and Mende 1982, Lewis 1992), explaining the prevalence of fish kills associated with *K. brevis* blooms. The regulatory level in the United States for consumption of shellfish is 20 MUs of BTXs (MU)/100 g shellfish meat, equal to about 0.08 µg BTX-2 equivalents per gram shellfish meat (Aune 2008). However, shellfish can metabolize the toxins (Dickey et al. 1999, Ishida et al. 2004, Abraham et al. 2012) with the taurine conjugate (BTX-B1) apparently the most toxic to mice at 50 µg/kg (Ishida et al. 1995).

K. brevis was formerly known as *G. breve* and *Ptychodiscus brevis* (hence the PbTX abbreviation used in some of the literature for BTXs). *Karenia* are small, planktonic, photosynthetic dinoflagellates with the genus only recognized since Daugbjerg et al. (2000) established it from groups of polyphyletic species previously lumped together in *Gymnodinium* and *Gyrodinium*. A major distinguishing characteristic of *Karenia* spp. is the presence of fucoxanthin as the major accessory pigment instead of peridinin found in most dinoflagellate species (Daugbjerg et al. 2000).

BTX analogs or related toxins have also been detected in other *Karenia* spp. based upon ELISA screening or an association with NSP events in New Zealand and South Africa. In New Zealand, this includes *K. bicuneiformis* (cited as *K. bidigitata*) (Haywood et al. 2004), *K. brevisulcata* (as *G. brevisulcatum*) (Chang 1999, 2011), *K. concordia* (as *K.* cf. *brevis*) (Chang and Ryan 2004, Chang et al. 2006, Chang 2011), *K. papillionacea* (Haywood et al. 2004), and *K. selliformis* (Haywood et al. 2004). Similarly, *K. cristata* from South Africa was linked with causing respiratory distress (Botes et al. 2003). In New Zealand, the presence of BTXs was proven by the isolation and structural elucidation of BTX-B1, BTX-B2, and BTX-B3 from green-lipped mussels (Ishida et al. 1995, Morohashi et al. 1995, Murata et al. 1998). Many new *Karenia* spp. have been discovered over the last decade including many associated with fish kills (reviewed by Brand et al. 2012). It remains to be seen how many of these are ultimately shown to be capable of producing BTXs that are toxic to mammals.

While NSP is a nonfatal human illness caused by eating shellfish contaminated with toxins produced by species of *Karenia*, the majority of known species in the genus produce toxins that kill fish, birds, and marine mammals (Brand et al. 2012). However, at least in some fish species, BTXs can also bioaccumulate into the muscle (flesh) of fish analogous to the CTXs (Naar et al. 2007), although they are far less toxic than the CTXs (Lewis 1992).

1.2.4 Azaspiracid Shellfish Poisoning Caused by Toxins Originating from *Azadinium* spp. and *Amphidoma languida*

Azaspiracid shellfish poisoning (AZP) is the most recent shellfish poisoning disease characterized. It was originally discovered in 1995 in Europe after people became ill with DSP-like symptoms from eating Irish mussels that had been screened for DSP and cleared for consumption (Satake et al. 1998b,c). The cause of these poisonings was a class of polyether toxins with unique spiro-ring assemblies named azaspiracids (AZAs) (Figure 1.4). To date, 24 AZA analogs have been described, including a number thought to be produced from bioconversion in shellfish (Rehmann et al. 2008, Furey et al. 2010). Although AZA produce similar symptoms to DSP toxins, they do not inhibit protein phosphatases (Twiner et al. 2005). However, Furey et al. (2010) raised concerns about the consumption of shellfish with co-occurring DSP and AZP toxins as okadaic acid is a tumor promoter (Suganuma et al. 1988) and AZA are tumor initiators (Ito 2008). AZA-1 inhibits endocytosis of plasma membrane proteins but the molecular target of AZA is not yet known (Bellocci et al. 2010). The minimum i.p. lethal doses to mice of the predominant AZA analogs found in Irish mussels are ~200, 110, and 140 µg/kg for AZA-1, AZA-2, and AZA-3, respectively (Satake et al. 1998c, Ofuji et al. 1999), comparable with the major DSP toxins. The maximum recommended level of AZA in shellfish for human consumption is 0.03 µg AZA-1 equivalents per gram shellfish meat (Furey et al. 2010).

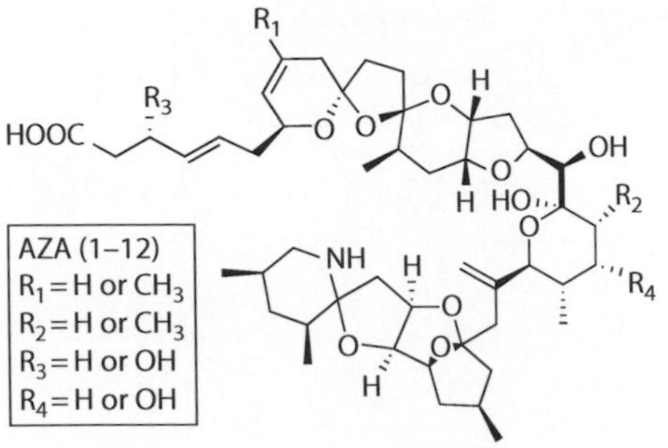

FIGURE 1.4 AZP is caused by a class of polyether toxins with unique spiro-ring assemblies named AZAs. To date, 12 AZA analogs have been described. A further 12 are thought to be produced from bioconversion in shellfish by the oxidation of methyl groups to carboxylic acids, with the site of oxidation not known. (From Rehmann, N. et al., *Rapid Commun. Mass Spec.*, 22, 549, 2008; Furey, A. et al., *Toxicon*, 56, 173, 2010.)

The AZA has been found to be extensively distributed in European shellfish, although all human poisonings to date have only originated from Irish mussels (Furey et al. 2010). However, AZA has also been detected in the coastal waters of Japan (from a sponge) and in scallops and mussels from Chile (Ueoka et al. 2009, López-Rivera et al. 2010). The origin of AZA was originally suggested to be the heterotrophic dinoflagellate *Protoperidinium crassipes* (James et al. 2003) but is now thought to be species belonging to a new genus called *Azadinium* (Tillmann et al. 2009, Jauffrais et al. 2012) and more recently the related genera *Amphidoma* (Krock et al. 2012, Tillmann et al. 2012). The naming of the causative dinoflagellate, *Azadinium*, after the toxin it produces is a departure from most previous harmful algal bloom syndromes where the toxin names are more often derived from the source organism or the food chain vectors that lead to poisoning. *Azadinium spinosum* was the first species shown to produce AZA and is a small, planktonic, photosynthetic dinoflagellate (Krock et al. 2009, Tillmann et al. 2009, Jauffrais et al. 2012). AZA may also be produced by other species of *Azadinium* including *A. poporum* from the North Sea and an isolate named *A.* cf. *poporum* from Korea and a related genus *Amphidoma languida* from Ireland (Krock et al. 2012). The original attribution of AZA production to *Protoperidinium* (James et al. 2003) is thought to be explained by *P. crassipes* accumulating AZA toxins by preying upon the source dinoflagellate(s) (Tillmann et al. 2009, Furey et al. 2010). A putatively nontoxic *Azadinium* sp. *A. obesum* has also been recently described (Tillmann et al. 2010).

1.2.5 Ciguatera Caused by *Gambierdiscus* spp.

Ciguatera is an ichthysarcotoxism caused by eating usually edible species of marine fish whose flesh has been contaminated with CTXs (Lewis 2001). Described initially from the Caribbean by Peter Martyr in 1555 (Gudger 1930), it is the most prevalent nonbacterial illness associated with seafood consumption worldwide. In most cases, the fish that cause ciguatera are carnivorous species caught from warmer (generally tropical) waters and are often associated with coral reefs. As coral reef fishes tend to attract premium prices and are shipped to restaurants and food outlets all around the world, ciguatera is increasingly occurring outside of its historical distribution. Ciguatera can be a debilitating disease but it is rarely fatal. Initial symptoms vary depending upon the geographical distribution of the CTXs contaminating fish but include both neurological (paresthesias) and gastrointestinal symptoms and appear within 0.5–12 h after eating contaminated fish (Bagnis et al. 1979, Lawrence et al. 1980). One of the most diagnostic symptoms is a reversal of temperature perception where cold items produce a burning sensation typical of cold allodynia (Gillespie et al. 1986), which is caused by activation of specific cold pain neural pathways (Vetter et al. 2012). Recovery from ciguatera poisoning generally occurs within about 2 weeks but in some cases can persist for months or years. A previous exposure to ciguatera does not infer immunity but can render the sufferer more sensitive to any subsequent poisoning (Gillespie et al. 1986). In addition to poisoning humans, there is also

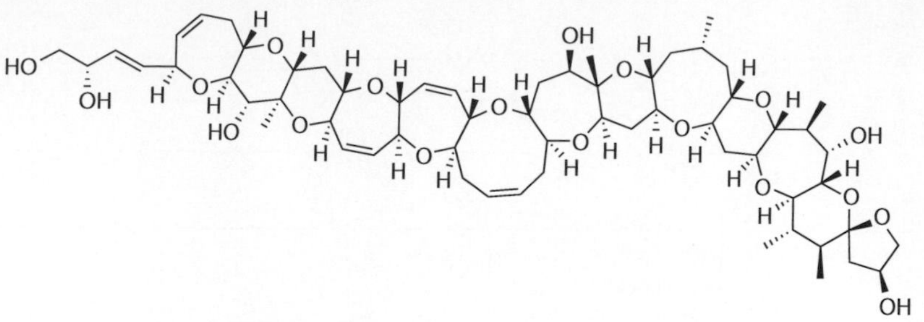

FIGURE 1.5 CTXs are lipophilic, polyether toxins with rigid structures similar to the BTXs (Figure 1.3). Different structural forms of CTXs occur in the Pacific, Indian, and Atlantic Oceans. (From Murata, M. et al., *J. Am. Chem. Soc.*, 111, 8929, 1989; Lewis, R.J. et al., *Toxicon*, 29, 1115, 1991; Lewis, R.J. et al., *J. Am. Chem. Soc.*, 120, 5914, 1998; Hamilton, B. et al., *Toxicon*, 40, 1347, 2002a; Hamilton, B. et al., *Toxicon*, 40, 685, 2002b; Boada, L.D. et al., *Toxicon*, 56, 1516, 2010.)

evidence that Hawaiian monk seals are exposed to CTXs through their diet but the impact on the health of these animals has not been determined (Bottein et al. 2011).

Ciguatoxic fish occur sporadically and are generally unpredictable in both their timing and location. It is therefore not possible to test a "representative" sample of fish to determine the toxin potential of the remaining untested fish, even for a batch of fish caught on the same day from the same reef. This limits the scope for effective public health management of ciguatera and contrasts with the various shellfish diseases already discussed that are effectively managed through routine testing of representative shellfish samples.

The CTXs are lipophilic, polyether toxins with rigid, ladderlike structures similar to the BTXs (Figure 1.5). They activate voltage-gated sodium channels causing initial stimulation and then depolarization block of excitable tissues (Lombet et al. 1987). CTX-1, the major toxin extracted from ciguateric fishes from the Pacific Ocean (PCTX-1), is the most potent CTX known, with an i.p. LD_{50} in mice of approximately 0.5 µg/kg (Murata et al. 1989, Lewis et al. 1991). Different structural forms of CTXs occur in the Pacific, Indian, and Atlantic Oceans (Murata et al. 1989, Lewis et al. 1991, 1998, Hamilton et al. 2002a,b, Boada et al. 2010). These structural differences affect their toxicities and are thought to contribute to the different symptomologies that occur from fish caught in the different oceans and seas (Lewis 2000). The actual structures of the Indian Ocean CTXs (ICTXs) are not known due to difficulties isolating this form of CTX (Hamilton et al. 2002b).

Unlike shellfish poisonings that accumulate their toxin load directly by filter feeding on the toxic dinoflagellates, ciguatera involves the food chain transfer of toxins from the dinoflagellate source, through herbivorous fishes or invertebrates into carnivorous fishes. This food chain transfer of toxins was first suggested by Mills (1956) and Randall (1958) long before the dinoflagellate origin was found. It wasn't until a joint Japanese–French expedition to the Gambier Islands that the benthic dinoflagellate *G. toxicus* was discovered and first linked to ciguatera (Yasumoto et al. 1977a,b). The genus is named after the Gambier Islands, a ciguatera endemic region in French Polynesia from which the species was first discovered and its being discoid (anterior–posteriorly compressed) shape (Adachi and Fukuyo 1979). It is now almost certain that the original type described by Adachi and Fukuyo (1979) represented a mix of morphologically similar species (Litaker et al. 2009). To resolve this, Litaker et al. (2009) redesignated the epitype for *G. toxicus* (in Chinain et al. 1999) and Figure 1.1 from the original description in Adachi and Fukuyo (1979) as the lectotype. To date, nine anterior–posteriorly compressed (discus shaped) species have been described as well as two globular species (Table 1.3).

Gambierdiscus spp. are benthic dinoflagellates that are mostly found as epiphytes in oligotrophic waters on a range of biotic and abiotic substrates including macroalgae, turf algae, detritus, and sand. They are photosynthetic or mixotrophic (Faust 1998) and can attach firmly to substrates using mucous strands or "webs" (Yasumoto et al. 1977b). However, along with many other benthic dinoflagellate species, they can briefly swim or be resuspended into the plankton by turbulence, that is, be tycoplanktonic. The toxins they produce are biotransferred into the food chains of fishes through herbivorous fishes or invertebrates (reviewed by Lewis and Holmes 1993, Cruz-Rivera and Villareal 2006). There appears to be biogeographical differences in the suite of *Gambierdiscus* spp. found in the various oceans and seas (Litaker et al. 2010).

TABLE 1.3

List of All Known *Gambierdiscus* spp. with References to CTX Production from Species with Confirmed Identification (Consistent with Identification Mostly after Chinain et al. 1999 and Litaker et al. 2009)

Number	Anterior–Posteriorly Compressed *Gambierdiscus* spp.	Reference for CTX Production[a]
1	*G. toxicus* Chinain, Faust, Holmes, Litaker (Adachi & Fukuyo)	—
2	*G. belizeanus* Faust	Chinain et al. (2010)
3	*G. australes* Faust & Chinain	Chinain et al. (1999)
4	*G. pacificus* Chinain & Faust	Chinain et al. (1999), Caillaud et al. (2011)
5	*G. polynesiensis* Chinain & Faust	Chinain et al. (1999, 2010)
6	*G. caribaeus* Vandersea, Litaker, Faust, Kibler, Holland, & Tester	Roeder et al. (2010)
7	*G. carolinianus* Litaker, Vandersea, Faust, Kibler, Holland, & Tester	—
8	*G. carpenteri* Kibler, Litaker, Faust, Holland, Vandersea, & Tester	—
9	*G. excentricus* Fraga	Fraga et al. (2011)
	Globular-shaped *Gambierdiscus* spp.	
10	*G. yasumotoi* Holmes	—
11	*G. ruetzleri* Faust, Litaker, Vandersea, Kibler, Holland, & Tester	—

Note: An additional putative species, *Gambierdiscus* ribotype 2 has been recently indicated (Kibler 2012).
[a] Based upon use of methods that clearly differentiate CTXs from maitotoxins, or experience with authentic CTXs that provide confidence in the ability to differentiate CTXs from maitotoxins.

If *Alexandrium* spp. are the most difficult group of toxic dinoflagellates with respect to their taxonomy (Anderson et al. 2012a), then the literature with respect to toxin production by the *Gambierdiscus* spp. complex is some of the most difficult to understand. This is because many early attempts to characterize CTX production from *Gambierdiscus* cultures used methods that could not distinguish any CTXs produced from the considerable amounts of maitotoxin typically produced by these dinoflagellates (Holmes and Lewis 2002). The name maitotoxin is derived from "Maito," the Tahitian name for the bristletooth surgeonfish *Ctenochaetus striatus*, from which the toxin was first detected (Yasumoto et al. 1976). Maitotoxins are large, extremely potent, hydrophilic polyether toxins that to date have not been shown to accumulate in fishes through the food chain and are unlikely to contribute to human poisoning (Lewis and Holmes 1993). The exception to this generalization may be poisonings arising from consumption of the viscera of herbivorous reef fishes such as surgeonfishes (Yasumoto et al. 1976), although theoretically this could also be a mechanism for intoxication by a cocktail of toxins produced by many other benthic dinoflagellate toxins, including okadaic acid analogs (Section 1.2.6.2) and palytoxin (PTX) analogs (Section 1.2.6.1). "Fatty" fish viscera are often considered a desirable food item in island nations without ready access to other animal fats. However, even in the case of consumption of reef fish viscera, Lewis (2001) questioned whether there was evidence for maitotoxins causing human poisoning based upon the absence of differential symptomology.

The structure of only one maitotoxin (Figure 1.6) has so far been determined (Murata et al. 1993), although different forms have been shown to be produced by different isolates and these can vary up to about three times in size (Holmes et al. 1990, Holmes and Lewis 1994). Maitotoxins are some of the most potent marine toxins known with i.p. LD_{50} in mice of 0.05 μg/kg; however, they are considerably less potent orally (Kelly et al. 1986, Murata et al. 1993). There is evidence that maitotoxins may have a toxic effect on some fish species (Davin et al. 1986), in which case, they may play a role in funneling CTXs into the marine food chain by increasing the risk of predation by carnivorous fish (reviewed by

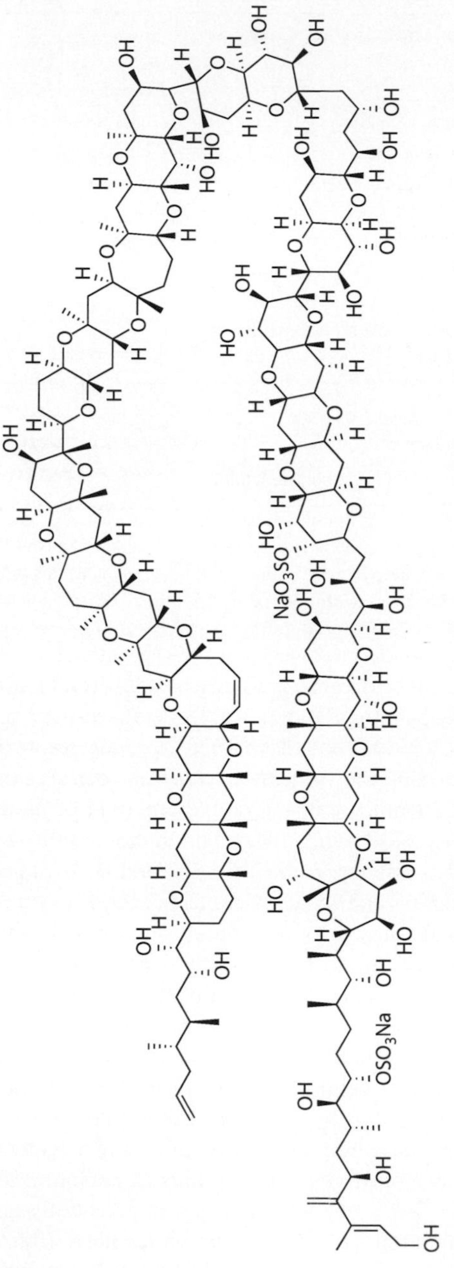

FIGURE 1.6 Maitotoxins are large, potent, sulfated, hydrophilic polyether toxins. (From Murata, M. et al., *J. Am. Chem. Soc.*, 115, 2060, 1993.)

Lewis and Holmes 1993). CTXs may also exacerbate this by exerting a toxic effect on fishes (Capra et al. 1988, Lewis 1992). The mechanism of action of maitotoxin appears to involve the activation of calcium-permeable nonselective cation channels (Trevino et al. 2008).

Murata et al. (1990) and Satake et al. (1993) provided the definitive structural proof for production of CTXs from *Gambierdiscus* (attributed to *G. toxicus* at a time when the dinoflagellate was considered a monospecific genus). Earlier reports also refer to these toxins as gambiertoxins, but this term has since been abandoned in favor of CTXs or CTX analogs. The term gambiertoxins reflected a cautious approach to the identification of the toxins isolated because the major CTXs found in Pacific Ocean (PCTX-1) and Atlantic Ocean/Caribbean Sea fishes (CCTX-1) have not been detected from *Gambierdiscus* spp. Instead, less polar analogs such as PCTX-4A (Figure 1.5) have been identified as the precursor of the major CTX found in Pacific Ocean fishes (PCTX-1) (Murata et al. 1990). PCTX-4A is also known as "scaritoxin" as it has been extracted from ciguateric parrotfish from the genus *Scarus* (Satake et al. 1997a). Lewis and Holmes (1993) suggested a model whereby the CTX analog produced by *Gambierdiscus* (PCTX-4A) could be biotransformed/metabolized through the food chain into PCTX-1. The CTX analog PCTX-3C has also been identified as a major toxin from both *Gambierdiscus* (*G. polynesiensis*) and ciguateric fish (the latter as 2,3-dihydroxyPCTX-3C and 51-hydroxyPCTX-3C) (Satake et al. 1993, 1998a, Chinain et al. 2010). Yogi et al. (2011) have recently identified 12 CTX analogs from *Gambierdiscus* including trace amounts of the diastereomers PCTX-2 and PCTX-3 (54-deoxy-PCTX-1 and 52-epi-54-deoxy-PCTX-1) that had previously been identified from ciguateric fishes (Lewis et al. 1991). The most potent producer of CTXs appears to be *G. polynesiensis* (Chinain et al. 2010), although in nature, up to four *Gambierdiscus* spp. have been found on a single macroalgal substrate (Vandersea et al. 2012). Two general correlations have been observed in relation to *Gambierdiscus* toxicity (Litaker et al. 2010), species with inherently slower growth rates appear to have higher CTX concentrations per cell (Chinain et al. 2010), and total toxicity (mainly reflecting maitotoxin production) is inversely correlated with the latitude of the cells they were isolated from (Bomber et al. 1989).

Holmes et al. (1991) reported the strain-dependent production of CTXs from only a minority of *Gambierdiscus* clonal cultures at a time when the genus was considered monotypic. However, the recent discovery of many new, morphologically similar species begs the question whether CTX production is the result of species and/or strain dependence. Sperr and Doucette (1996) suggested that CTX production could be increased when *Gambierdiscus* was grown at high nitrogen to phosphorus ratios. This result needs following up, although Lartigue et al. (2009) could not find any difference when *Gambierdiscus* was grown under different nitrogen regimes. The redesignation of *G. toxicus* by Litaker et al. (2009) to an apparently nonciguatoxic type in Chinain et al. (1999) has had the unfortunate result of making the type species not now known to produce CTXs (Parsons et al. 2012). This suggests that only 6 of the 11 or 12 known species of *Gambierdiscus* have so far been shown to produce CTXs (Table 1.3). The recent description of CTX from *G. toxicus* isolated from Vietnam by Roeder et al. (2010) needs further clarification as the species identification may not have taken into account the recent redescription of *G. toxicus* by Litaker et al. (2009). Roeder et al. (2010) did find that salinity influenced the ratio of CTXs produced by *Gambierdiscus*.

Toxins other than CTXs and CTX analogs have also been occasionally implicated in causing ciguatera. For example, fish contaminated with palytoxin (PTX) have caused human illness and death (Noguchi et al. 1987, Kodama et al. 1989). However, Lewis and Holmes (1993) suggested that PTX poisoning should not be regarded as part of the ciguatera syndrome even though mild PTX poisoning could be mistaken for ciguatera. PTX analogs are produced by benthic dinoflagellates belonging to the genus *Ostreopsis*, which often co-occur with *Gambierdiscus* spp. so potentially the toxins could enter similar marine food chains as the CTXs (Section 1.2.6). Okadaic acid analogs (DSP toxins) have also been suggested to have a role in ciguatera (Gamboa et al. 1992). These toxins are also produced by benthic dinoflagellates belonging to the genus *Prorocentrum* (Section 1.2.6.2), so could also be transferred through marine food chains. However, we remain unaware of any evidence demonstrating the accumulation of okadaic acid in the flesh of fishes in sufficient concentrations to cause human poisoning. There are also reports of the cyanobacteria *Trichodesmium* producing CTX-like compounds (Hahn and Capra 1992, Endean et al. 1993, Kerbrat et al. 2010).

1.2.6 Toxins Produced by Benthic Dinoflagellates Including *Ostreopsis* spp., *Prorocentrum* spp., *Coolia* spp., and *Amphidinium* spp.

1.2.6.1 Ostreopsis *spp.*

Ostreopsis spp. are often found as part of an assemblage of benthic dinoflagellate species on similar substrates to those supporting species of *Gambierdiscus*. Nine species have so far been described (Table 1.4), five of which are thought to produce toxins, while the remaining four species are yet to be analyzed (Holmes and Lewis 2002, Parsons et al. 2012). However, phylogenetic analyses of *O. lenticularis* and *O. labens* clustered together in a single clade suggesting that these species designations may require revision (Penna et al. 2010, Parsons et al. 2012). *O. siamensis*, *O.* cf. *ovata,* and *O. mascarenensis* have been implicated in production of PTX analogs named, ostreocins, ovatoxins, and mascarenotoxins, respectively (reviewed by Parsons et al. 2012). PTX (Figure 1.7) is a large, water-soluble polyalcohol and one of the most potent marine toxins known with an i.p. LD_{50} in mice of approximately 0.3 µg/kg (Riobó et al. 2008). It is second only to maitotoxin in size and potency of the known nonproteinaceous, marine toxins. PTX was originally isolated from the zoanthid *Palythoa toxica*, collected from a Hawaiian tide pool through the cultural knowledge of native Hawaiians (Moore and Scheuer 1971). The tide pool was taboo to native Hawaiians because of the toxicity associated with the "moss" (*Palythoa*) growing in it (Ciminiello et al. 2010b). PTX binds to the N^+/K^+-ATPase (sodium pump) and converts it into a nonselective cationic pore leading to cell depolarization (reviewed by Vale 2008).

PTX analogs have since been detected in many marine organisms including a number of zoanthids species, fish, crustaceans, molluscs, sea anemone, sea urchins, seaweed, and species of *Ostreopsis* (Munday 2008a). Human poisonings have occurred from consumption of crabs and fish with the latter sometimes referred to as ciguatera. However, a number of these PTX poisonings have occurred from consumption of toxic clupeid fishes, for example, plankton-eating herrings and sardines, and this disease is distinct from ciguatera and referred to as clupeotoxism (Onuma et al. 1999). In humans, PTX causes gastrointestinal symptoms and paresthesia of the extremities with respiratory distress and cyanosis preceding death in fatal cases (Munday 2008a). The mortality rate for clupeotoxism is much higher than for ciguatera. There is evidence that the PTX analogs detected in at least some of these contaminated fishes have been derived from fish feeding on species of *Ostreopsis*, including *O. siamensis* (Onuma et al. 1999, Taniyama et al. 2003). An additional planktonic food chain for transfer of PTXs has been suggested based upon production of PTX analogs by the marine cyanobacteria *Trichodesmium* (Kerbrat et al. 2011).

O. ovata is the smallest of the known species of *Ostreopsis* and was generally thought to be nontoxic or weakly toxic (Holmes and Lewis 2002), until mass human health problems occurred in the northern Mediterranean Sea attributed to blooms of this dinoflagellate (Parsons et al. 2012). *Ostreopsis* cf. *ovata* has been forming summer blooms in the northern Mediterranean since the late 1990s associated with mortalities of benthic organisms, but in the summer of 2005, hundreds of people required medical

TABLE 1.4

List of All Known *Ostreopsis* spp. with References to Those Species Known to Produce Toxins

Number	Species	Reference for Toxicity
1	*O. ovata* Fukuyo	Nakajima et al. (1981), Ciminiello et al. (2006)
2	*O. siamensis* Schmidt	Usami et al. (1995)
3	*O. lenticularis* Fukuyo	Tosteson et al. (1986) but see caution about species identification by Parsons et al. (2012)
4	*O. heptagona* Norris, Bomber & Balech	Norris et al. (1985)
5	*O. belizeanus* Faust	—
6	*O. caribbeanus* Faust	—
7	*O. labens* Faust & Morton	—
8	*O. marinus* Faust	—
9	*O. mascarenensis* Quod	Lenoir et al. (2004)

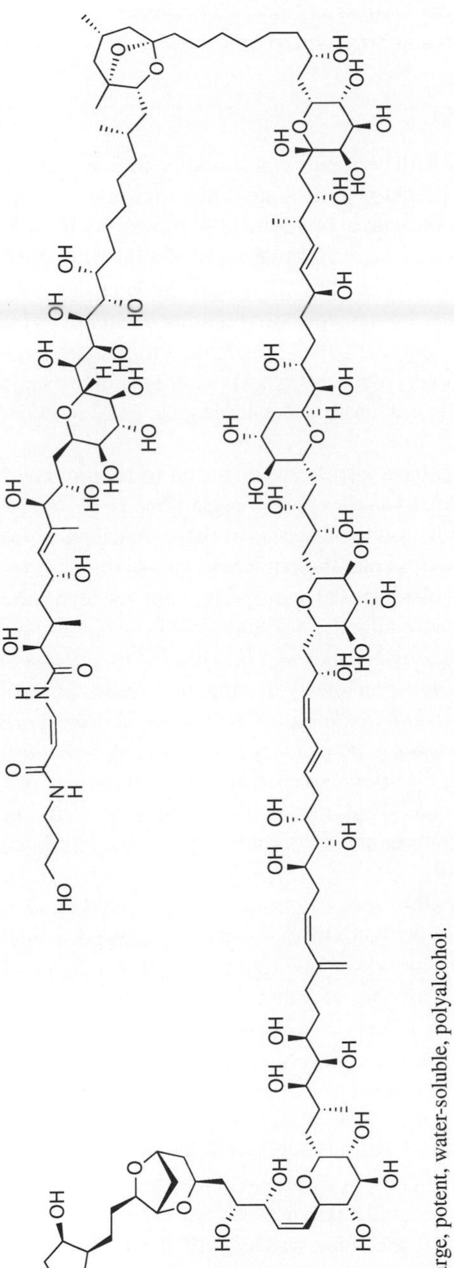

FIGURE 1.7 PTX is a large, potent, water-soluble, polyalcohol.

attention after exposure to marine aerosols during a large bloom of this species (Ciminiello et al. 2010b). Cultures of these Mediterranean isolates have since been shown to produce a range of PTX analogs named ovatoxins and mascarenotoxins (Ciminiello et al. 2010a, Rossi et al. 2010, Parsons et al. 2012). Prior to these human intoxications in the Mediterranean, *O. ovata* had only been reported as producing a weakly toxic water-soluble fraction from Okinawan cells (Nakajima et al. 1981). Additionally, *O. ovata* from the Caribbean (Tindall et al. 1990) and Singapore (Holmes et al. 1998) were reported as being nontoxic.

1.2.6.2 Prorocentrum *spp.*

Prorocentrum is a large genus with both planktonic and benthic representatives. The latter can be resuspended by turbulence into the plankton to become tycoplanktonic. Gómez (2005) listed 56 species in the genus. However, new species continue to be discovered especially from benthic substrates. A number of the benthic species produce okadaic acid and analogs of okadaic acid (DSP toxins), but this does not necessarily indicate that the toxins produced by these species enter marine food chains and accumulate to concentrations sufficient to cause human poisoning (Holmes and Lewis 2002). Probably the most studied of these benthic *Prorocentrum* spp. is *P. lima*, which has a broad geographical distribution from tropical to cool temperate waters. Shellfish have been experimentally shown capable of accumulating DSP toxins from *P. lima* indicating that this is a feasible mechanism for causing DSP (Pillet and Houvenaghel 1995, Lawrence et al. 2000).

Okadaic acid and its analogs have also been suggested to accumulate in fish via marine food chains from benthic *Prorocentrum* spp. to cause ciguatera (Gamboa et al. 1992). As many of these species are found growing as epiphytes on the same substrates as those that support *Gambierdiscus* (Section 1.2.5), it is feasible that *Prorocentrum* toxins enter the same food chains that lead to ciguatera poisoning. However, this remains a hypothesis since okadaic acid analogs have not yet been shown to accumulate into fish flesh at concentrations sufficient to cause human poisoning, that is, about 200 µg/kg (Holmes and Lewis 2002).

To the best of our knowledge, seven species of benthic *Prorocentrum* have so far been proven to produce okadaic acid analogs (Table 1.5). However, many more benthic species remain to be tested, including *P. bimaculatum, P. caribbaeum, P. clipeus, P. consutum, P. foraminosum, P. formosum, P. fukuyoi, P. glenanicum, P. levis, P. panamense, P. pseudopanamense, P. reticulatum, P. ruetzlerianum, P. sabulosum, P. sculptile, P. tropicalis, P. tsawwassenense,* and *P. vietnamensis.* Uncharacterized toxins have been reported from *P. cassubicum* (Tindall et al. 1989) and *P. mexicanum* (Tindall et al. 1984). In addition, a range of macrocyclic compounds and other polyketides have been isolated from *Prorocentrum* spp. (reviewed by Hu et al. 2010).

P. borbonicum is a toxic, benthic species isolated from the Indian Ocean that produces borbotoxins (Ten-Hage et al. 2000b). These borbotoxins have been suggested to include PTX analogs (Ten-Hage et al. 2002), which if proven could indicate another potential source for the toxins that cause clupeotoxism. As well as toxic species, a number of nontoxic, benthic *Prorocentrum* spp. are known including *P. emarginatum, P. elegans,* and *P. norrisanum* (Morton et al. 2000).

Planktonic species of *Prorocentrum* are common bloom-forming dinoflagellates with a number of species associated with harmful events. Two planktonic *Prorocentrum* spp. have been associated with production of ichthyotoxins: *P. minimum* (Grzebyk et al. 1997) and *P. concavum* (Quod et al. 1995). *P. arabianum* was also thought to be an ichthyotoxic, bloom-forming species, but Mohammad-Noor et al. (2007) suggest that this species is synonymous with *P. concavum. P. concavum* has also been described as a benthic dinoflagellate (Fukuyo 1981), indicating the tycoplanktonic nature of this species. A new planktonic species, *P. texanum*, was recently discovered and found to produce okadaic acid (Henrichs et al. 2013).

1.2.6.3 Coolia *spp.*

Five benthic species of *Coolia* are known (in order of discovery): *C. monotis, C. tropicalis, C. aerolata, C. canariensis,* and *C. malayensis.* They form part of benthic dinoflagellate assemblages often found on a range of substrates with *Gambierdiscus, Ostreopsis, Prorocentrum,* and *Amphidinium.* Cooliatoxin (i.p. LD_{50} in mice of 1 mg/kg) is the only toxin so far isolated from *Coolia* and putatively attributed to

TABLE 1.5

List of All Known Benthic *Prorocentrum* spp. That Produce Okadaic Acid Analogs
(DSP Toxins)

Number	Species	Reference for Production of Okadaic Acid Analogs
1	*P. arenarium* Faust	Ten-Hage et al. (2000a)
2	*P. belizeanum* Faust	Morton et al. (1998)
3	*P. faustiae* Morton	Morton (1998)
4	*P. hoffmannianum* Faust	Aikman et al. (1993)
5	*P. lima* (Ehrenberg) Dodge (Faust)	Murakami et al. (1982)
6	*P. maculosum* Faust	Dickey et al. (1990) but misidentified as *P. concavum* (Zhou and Fritz 1993)
7	*P. rhathymum* Loeblich, Sherley, & Schmidt	An et al. (2010), Caillaud et al. (2010)

cultured *C. monotis* isolated from Australia when the genus was monotypic (Holmes et al. 1995). Rhodes and Thomas (1997) subsequently reported *C. monotis* extracts from New Zealand were toxic to invertebrate larvae. However, a number of studies have failed to detect toxicity from this species (Pagliara and Caroppo 2012, Mohammad-Noor et al. 2013). Holmes and Lewis (2002) reported that the morphology of the cells they extracted for cooliatoxin was relatively large and possibly more spherical than the original description of *C. monotis*. It is now thought that this toxin-producing species was likely *C. tropicalis* (Mohammad-Noor et al. 2013). To date, there is no evidence for the accumulation of this toxin through marine food chains to cause human poisoning (Holmes et al. 1995).

1.2.6.4 Amphidinium *spp.*

The dinoflagellate genus *Amphidinium* is a polyphyletic genus and one of the most diverse of all benthic dinoflagellate genera that include symbiotic, benthic, and planktonic species (Daugbjerg et al. 2000, Hoppenrath et al. 2012). Increasing numbers of phylogenetic studies are starting to produce a much greater understanding of this group and the erection of many new genera formerly classified in *Amphidinium* such as *Ankistrodinium* (Hoppenrath et al. 2012), *Testudodinium* (Horiguchi et al. 2012), and *Apicoporus* (Sparmann et al. 2008). Ichthyotoxic, bioactive compounds (such as the amphipathic, linear polyketides called amphidinols, Figure 1.8) have been reported from *Amphidinium,* but to our knowledge, these have not been implicated in human or wildlife poisonings. However, these species have been of major interest to marine chemists and pharmacologists with the isolation of numerous bioactive macrocycles (reviewed by Kobayashi and Kubota 2007).

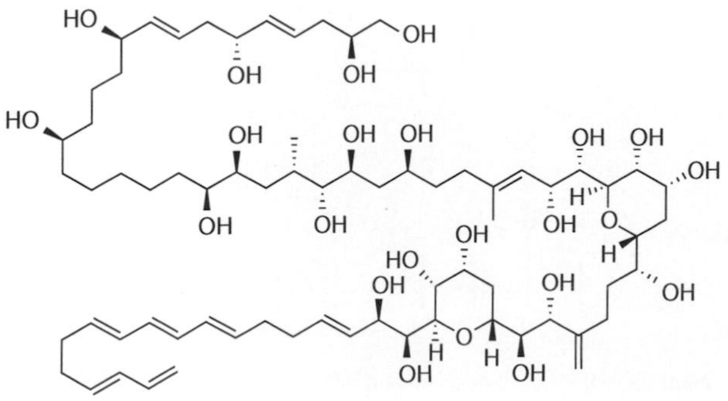

FIGURE 1.8 Amphidinols (amphidinol 3 shown here) from *Amphidinium* sp. have not been implicated in human poisonings.

1.2.7 Other Dinoflagellate "Toxins" Not Clearly Affecting Human Health Issues

1.2.7.1 Pectenotoxins and Yessotoxins

Pectenotoxins are lipophilic toxins with similar structures to okadaic acid except that the carboxyl moiety is in the form of a macrocyclic lactone (Figure 1.9). They often co-occur in shellfish with okadaic acid analogs that cause DSP, and for some time, they were considered part of the DSP syndrome (Section 1.2.2). However, pectenotoxins do not cause diarrhea in animal studies and they are far less toxic to mice orally than by i.p. injection (Miles et al. 2004). No human intoxications are known.

Pectenotoxins are usually abbreviated PTX, but this abbreviation is also commonly used for palytoxin (Section 1.2.7). Pectenotoxins were first isolated and named from the Japanese scallop, *Patinopecten yessoensis* (Yasumoto et al. 1985). They are cytotoxic compounds that have hepatotoxic actions when injected i.p. (Terao et al. 1986, Vilariño and Espiña 2008). Pectenotoxin-1 (PTX-1), PTX-2, PTX-3, and PTX-11 are the most toxic analogs when injected i.p. into mice with LD_{50}'s between 219 and 411 µg/kg; however, oral toxicities are generally greater than 5 mg/kg (reviewed by Munday 2008b). Pectenotoxins can be bioconverted to their seco-acid forms through metabolism in shellfish (Miles et al. 2004, Suzuki 2008). It is not surprising that pectenotoxins often co-occur with DSP toxins in shellfish as both are produced by species of dinophysoid dinoflagellates. To date, pectenotoxins have been isolated from *D. acuta, D. acuminata, D. caudata, D. fortii, D. infundibulus, D. norvegica,* and *Phalacroma rotundatum* (as *D. rotundata*) (Lee et al. 1989, Fernández et al. 2006, Suzuki 2008, Suzuki et al. 2009).

YTXs (Figure 1.10) are lipophilic, sulfated, ladder-shaped polycyclic ether toxins with similar structures to the BTXs and CTXs (Paz et al. 2008, Ciminiello and Fattorusso 2008). Like the pectenotoxins, YTXs

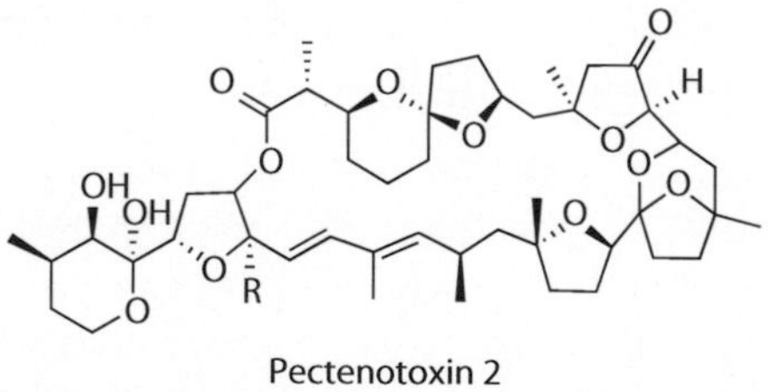

Pectenotoxin 2

FIGURE 1.9 Pectenotoxins are lipophilic toxins with similar structures to okadaic acid. (From Lee, J.S. et al., *J. Appl. Phycol.*, 1, 147, 1989; Fernández, M.L. et al., *Toxicon*, 48, 477, 2006; Suzuki, T., Chemistry, metabolism, and chemical detection methods of pectenotoxins, in: Botana, L.M. (ed.), *Seafood and Freshwater Toxins, Pharmacology, Physiology, and Detection*, CRC Press, Boca Raton, FL, pp. 343–359, 2008; Suzuki, T. et al., *Harmful Algae*, 8, 233, 2009.)

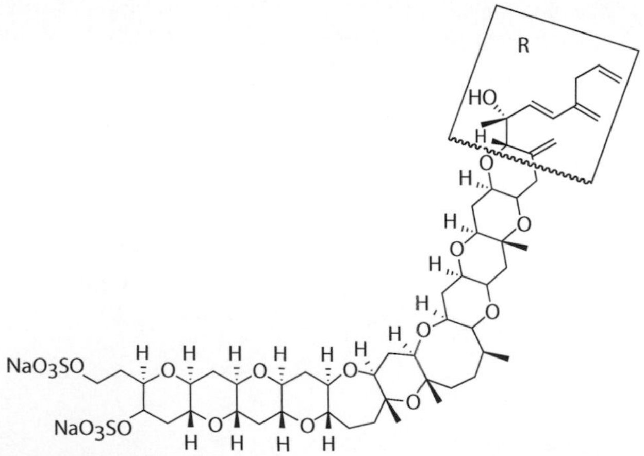

FIGURE 1.10 YTXs are lipophilic, sulfated, ladder-shaped polycyclic ether toxins with similar structures to the BTXs and CTXs. Analogs are distinguished by changes in the square, adjacent to the K-ring. (From Paz, B. et al., *Mar. Drugs*, 6, 73, 2008; Ciminiello, P. and Fattorusso, E., Chemistry, metabolism, and chemical analysis, in: Botana, L.M. (ed.), *Seafood and Freshwater Toxins Pharmacology, Physiology and Detection*, CRC Press, Boca Raton, FL, pp. 287–314, 2008.)

were first isolated from the Japanese scallop, *Patinopecten yessoensis* (Murata et al. 1987). YTXs also often co-occur in shellfish contaminated with DSP toxins although in this case they have different dinoflagellate origins. Both pectenotoxins and YTXs give positive results when tested by the conventional mouse bioassay for DSP, one reason why the mouse bioassay is no longer the favored method for detection of DSP toxins. YTXs do not induce diarrhea in animal studies, and no human intoxications are known. YTX and homo-YTX are the most toxic analogs known with i.p. LD_{50} in mice of ~100 µg/kg (Ogino et al. 1997, reviewed by Paz et al. 2008). However, they are not lethal to mice orally at 1 mg/kg (Tubaro et al. 2003). YTXs are cytotoxic but their primary mechanism of action is not known (Franchini et al. 2010, Tubaro et al. 2010).

YTXs have multiple dinoflagellate origins, having been isolated from the photosynthetic, planktonic species *Protoceratium reticulatum* (Satake et al. 1997b), *Lingulodinium polyedrum* (Tubaro et al. 1998), and *Gonyaulax spinifera* (Rhodes et al. 2006).

1.2.7.2 Macrocyclic Imines: Spirolides, Gymnodimine, and Pinnatoxins

Spirolides, gymnodimine, and pinnatoxins are lipophilic, fast-acting toxins with six- or seven-membered imino rings that have a dinoflagellate origin (Cembella and Krock 2008). The toxins are thought to act through antagonism of nicotinic acetylcholine receptors causing respiratory depression (Munday et al. 2004, Bourne et al. 2010, Hellyer et al. 2011). Spirolides (Figure 1.11) were first identified in the early 1990s based upon unusual toxicity of shellfish extracts screened by mouse bioassay (Hu et al. 1995). The most toxic analogs have i.p. LD_{50}'s in mice of between 7 and 8 µg/kg; however, oral toxicity administered by gavage is at least an order of magnitude lower and as yet there are no proven reports of human poisoning (Munday et al. 2012). Since their discovery in shellfish from the Atlantic coast of Canada, spirolides have been reported in the United States, Scotland, Norway, Spain, France, Italy, Denmark, and Chile (Otero et al. 2012 and references therein). Spirolides are produced by planktonic species of *Alexandrium* with *A. ostenfeldii* considered the primary producer (Cembella et al. 1999, Cembella and Krock 2008), but *A. peruvianum* has also been shown to produce these toxins (Tomas et al. 2012). Both of these species can also produce PSP toxins (Hansen et al. 1992, Lim et al. 2005; Section 1.2.1), and *A. peruvianum* has also been shown to produce gymnodimine (Van Wagoner et al. 2011).

Gymnodimines (Figure 1.12) are some of the smallest cyclic imine toxins and where first detected from New Zealand oysters by mouse bioassay (Seki et al. 1995). Gymnodimines were responsible for producing false-positive results in mouse bioassays used for screening shellfish for NSP toxins (Section 1.2.3). The most potent analog has an LD_{50} for i.p. injection in mice of 96 µg/kg; however, oral toxicity when administered by gavage is considerably lower, and when administered orally with food, toxicity was not detectable at 7.5 mg/kg (Munday et al. 2004). There are as yet no proven cases of human poisoning from gymnodimines. Gymnodimines were initially attributed to the planktonic dinoflagellate *G.* cf. *mikimotoi* (Seki et al. 1995), but it was later realized to be a new species, *Karenia selliformis* (Haywood et al. 2004). Gymnodimines have also been recently attributed to *A. peruvianum* (Van Wagoner et al. 2011, Borkman et al. 2012).

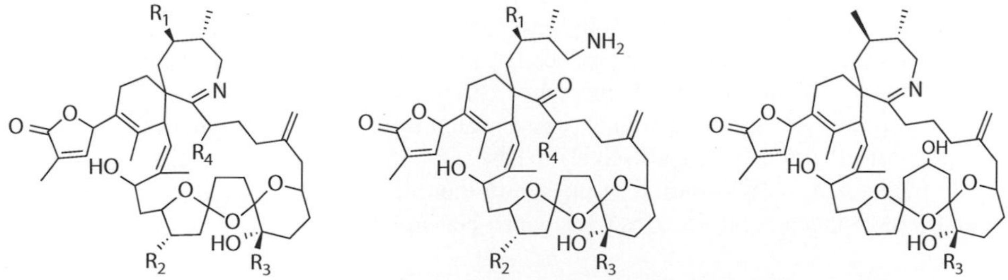

FIGURE 1.11 Spirolides (SPX) are produced by planktonic species of *Alexandrium* with *A. ostenfeldii* considered the primary source. There are several studies on mass spectrometric (MS) and nuclear magnetic resonance (NMR) methods that have been used for structure elucidation of SPX. Based on their chemical structure, SPXs are divided into three classes. (From Cembella, A.D. et al., *Nat. Toxins*, 7, 197, 1999; Cembella, A. and Krock, B., Cyclic imine toxins: Chemistry, biogeography, biosynthesis, and pharmacology, in: Botana, L.M. (ed.), *Seafood and Freshwater Toxins Pharmacology, Physiology and Detection*, CRC Press, Boca Raton, FL, pp. 561–580, 2008.)

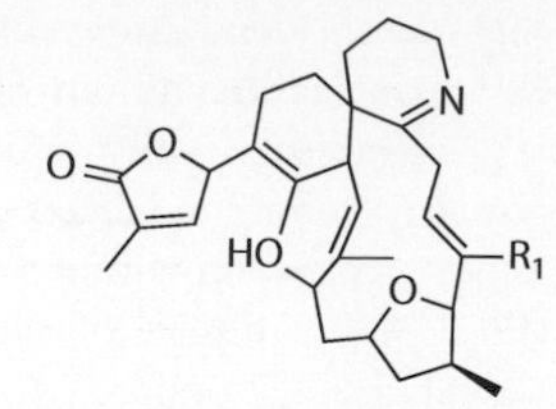

FIGURE 1.12 Gymnodimines: one of the smallest cyclic imine toxins from *K. selliformis*. (From Haywood, A.J. et al., *J. Phycol.*, 40, 165, 2004.)

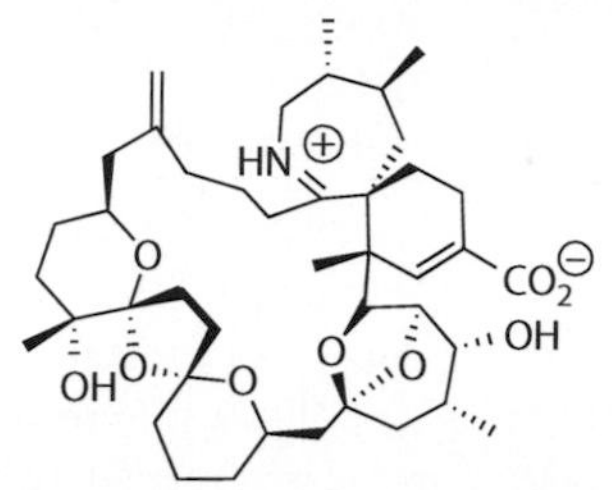

FIGURE 1.13 Pinnatoxins produced by the small, photosynthetic, planktonic, peridinoid dinoflagellate *V. rugosum*. (From Rhodes, L. et al., *Phycologia*, 50, 624, 2011; Smith, K.F. et al., *Harmful Algae*, 10, 702, 2011.)

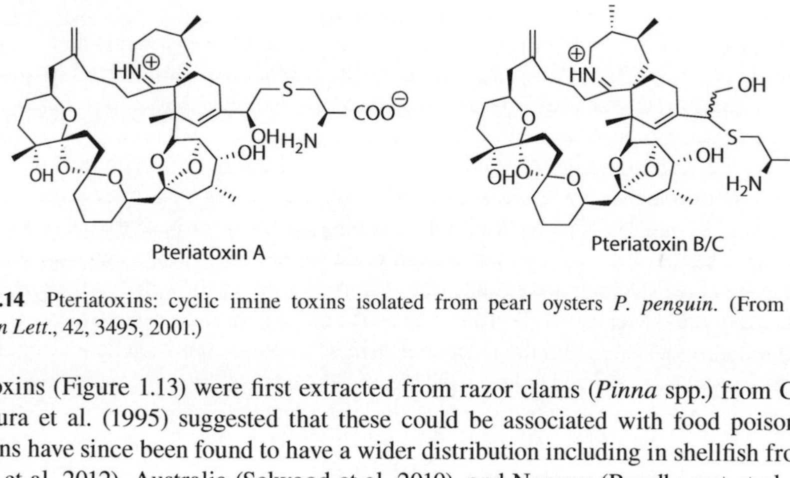

Pteriatoxin A

Pteriatoxin B/C

FIGURE 1.14 Pteriatoxins: cyclic imine toxins isolated from pearl oysters *P. penguin*. (From Takada, N. et al., *Tetrahedron Lett.*, 42, 3495, 2001.)

Pinnatoxins (Figure 1.13) were first extracted from razor clams (*Pinna* spp.) from China and Japan, and Uemura et al. (1995) suggested that these could be associated with food poisoning in humans. Pinnatoxins have since been found to have a wider distribution including in shellfish from New Zealand (McNabb et al. 2012), Australia (Selwood et al. 2010), and Norway (Rundberget et al. 2011). However, McNabb et al. (2012) concluded that at least in New Zealand, there was no evidence to link pinnatoxins with human intoxications. Pinnatoxins are produced by the small, photosynthetic, planktonic, peridinoid dinoflagellate *Vulcanodinium rugosum* (Rhodes et al. 2011, Smith et al. 2011).

Pteriatoxins (Figure 1.14) are cyclic imine toxins isolated from pearl oysters *Pteria penguin* in Japan (Takada et al. 2001). Pteriatoxins are also likely to have a dinoflagellate origin based upon their similar structures to pinnatoxins, only differing in the substitution of a glycine residue at carbon-33. We are unaware of any association of pteriatoxins with human poisoning.

1.2.8 Dinoflagellate Species Associated with Fish Kills

Many dinoflagellate species are associated with fish kills with the majority belonging to small gymnodinoid species. One of the best studied of these is *Karenia brevis* that produces BTXs (Figure 1.3) that cause recurring fish kills in the Gulf of Mexico, a phenomenon first reported by Ingersoll (1882) (Section 1.2.3). However, most of the 12 known species of *Karenia* are now thought to produce toxins that kill fish

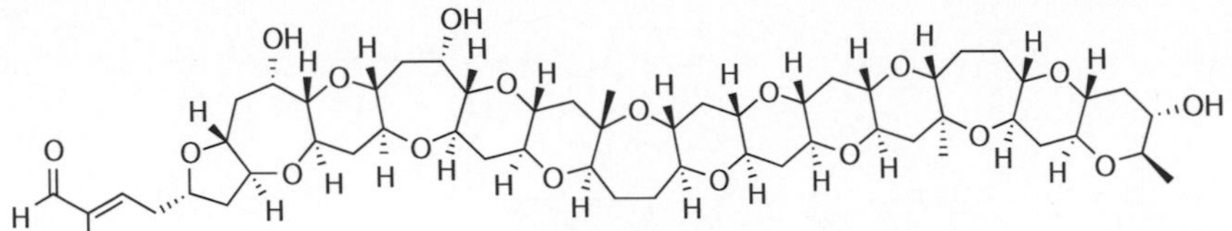

FIGURE 1.15 Gymnocins: isolated from *K. mikimotoi*. (From Satake, M. et al., *Tetrahedron Lett.*, 43, 5829, 2002; Satake, M. et al., *Tetrahedron Lett.*, 46, 3537, 2005.)

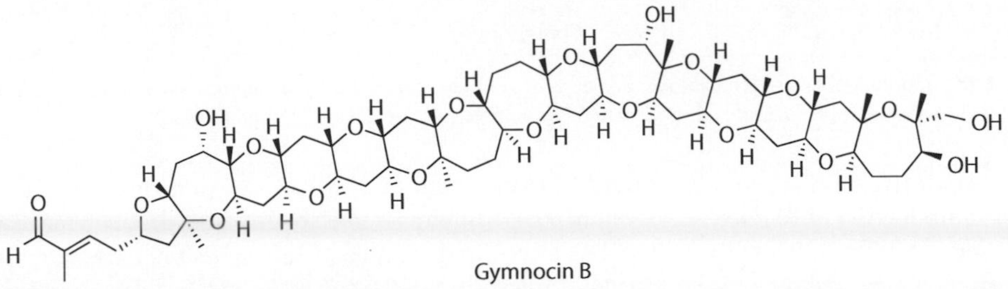

and other marine organisms, and *Karenia* blooms have been associated with fish kills on all continents except Antarctica (reviewed by Brand et al. 2012). *K. brevisulcata* has caused extensive fish mortalities in New Zealand and produces a suite of lipid-soluble and water-soluble toxins, the latter known as brevisulcatic acids (Holland et al. 2012). The cyclic polyether structure of one these potent lipid-soluble toxins (brevisulcenal-F) was recently determined (Hamamoto et al. 2012). *K. mikimotoi* has caused fish deaths in many parts of the world with Brand et al. (2012) reporting anecdotal evidence for blooms occurring off Ireland in the late 1800s. This species produces cytotoxic, cyclic polyether toxins that were named gymnocins after its previous genus name (*Gymnodinium mikimotoi*). Two gymnocins (Figure 1.15) have been isolated from *K. mikimotoi* (Satake et al. 2002, 2005). However, the toxins produced by many *Karenia* spp. remain to be elucidated.

Karlotoxins (Figure 1.16) are potent fish-killing toxins produced by *Karlodinium veneficum* that are similar in structure to the amphidinols produced by *Amphidinium* (Van Wagoner et al. 2008, 2010, Peng et al. 2010). *K. veneficum* is a small mixotrophic dinoflagellate formerly known as *Gyrodinium estuariale*, *Gymnodinium galatheanum*, *G. veneficum*, and *K. micrum* (Bergholtz et al. 2006). This dinoflagellate is thought to cause extensive fish kills around the world (Place et al. 2012).

Goniodomins (Figure 1.17) are polyether macrolides responsible for killing fish that are produced by *Alexandrium monilatum* (formerly *Gonyaulax monilata*) (Howell 1953, Anderson et al. 2012a)

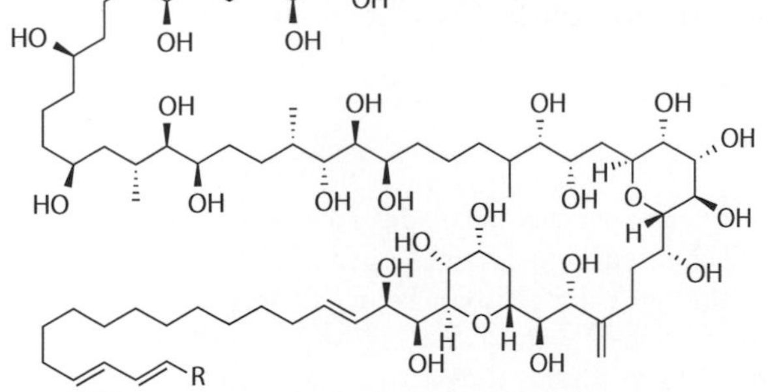

Karlotoxin 1 (R = H)
Karlotoxin 2 (R = Cl)

FIGURE 1.16 Karlotoxins produced by *K. veneficum* are similar in structure to the amphidinols produced by *Amphidinium*. (From Van Wagoner, R.M. et al., *Tetrahedron Lett.*, 49, 6457, 2008; Van Wagoner, R.M. et al., *J. Nat. Prod.*, 73, 1360, 2010; Peng, J. et al., *J. Am. Chem. Soc.*, 132, 3277, 2010.)

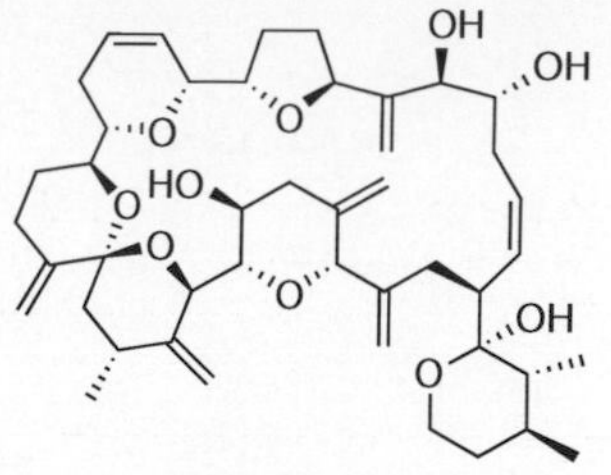

Goniodomin A

FIGURE 1.17 Goniodomins are ichthyotoxic polyether macrolides produced by *A. monilatum* (formerly *G. monilata*) (Howell 1953, Anderson et al. 2012a) and *A. hiranoi* (*G. pseudogoniaulax*) (Murakami et al. 1988).

and *A. hiranoi* (*Goniodoma pseudogoniaulax*) (Murakami et al. 1988). *Alexandrium* spp. are better known for production of PSP toxins (Section 1.2.1) although some species also produce macrocyclic imines (Section 1.2.7.2). Recently, *A. leei* was also found capable of killing fish in laboratory studies but the toxin(s) have yet to be characterized (Tang et al. 2007).

One of the most controversial groups of fish-killing microalgae is the *Pfiesteria*-like dinoflagellates. The extent to which *Pfiesteria* and *Pfiesteria*-like dinoflagellates cause human poisoning remains to be determined and is part of the controversy surrounding this group (Swinker et al. 2002, Burkholder and Marshall 2012 and references therein, see also Schrader [2010]). *Pfiesteria* are small heterotrophic, micropredatory species with *P. piscicida* being the first described (Burkholder et al. 1992, Steidinger et al. 1996). *Pfiesteria piscicida* has been associated with large fish kills on the east coast of the United States (Burkholder and Marshall 2012), although sometimes in association with other fish-killing microalgae, including *Karlodinium veneficum* and other *Pfiesteria*-like dinoflagellates (Marshall et al. 1999, Berry et al. 2002, Litaker et al. 2003, Place et al. 2012). A partial structure consistent with experimental data has been proposed by Moeller et al. (2007) for a labile, metal-complexing toxin isolated from *P. piscicida* that acts via metal-mediated free radical production. This toxin structure is unlike the polyketide ichthyotoxins produced by most other fish-killing dinoflagellates (Berry et al. 2002). A second fish-killing species of *Pfiesteria*, *P. (Pseudopfiesteria) shumwayae,* has also been described (Glasgow et al. 2001, Litaker et al. 2005, Burkholder and Marshall 2012) as well as the micro-predatory *Pfiesteria*-like dinoflagellates *Stoeckeria algicida* (Jeong et al. 2005), *Cryptoperidiniopsis brodyi* (Steidinger et al. 2006), and *Luciella masanensis* and *L. atlantis* (Mason et al. 2007).

A range of other dinoflagellate species have been associated with fish kills in the wild or with producing fish-killing activity in laboratory studies, but as yet the toxins have not been characterized or structurally elucidated. These include *Cochlodinium* spp. especially *C. polykrikoides* (Kim 1998, Tang and Gobler 2009, reviewed by Kudela and Gobler [2012]) and *Takayama pulchella* (*G. pulchellum*) (Steidinger et al. 1998, de Salas et al. 2003).

1.3 Conclusions

Dinoflagellates form a minor component of the biodiversity of marine microalgae but are responsible for numerous harmful algal blooms and are the major source of toxins that accumulate through marine food chains to cause human poisoning. These poisonings include PSP, NSP, DSP, AZP, ciguatera, clupeotoxism, and possibly toxicosis associated with *Pfiesteria* toxin. Dinoflagellates also produce toxins that kill fish and other aquatic life. The broad suite of bioactive chemicals produced by dinoflagellates has made them a focus for study by many scientific disciplines across medicine, chemistry, and biology. Anderson et al. (2012b) have recently suggested that major toxin syndromes associated with human poisoning may already be fully described. Whether time proves Anderson et al. (2012b) correct or not, we confidently expect that new bioactive compounds will continue to be discovered from dinoflagellates especially as many new species are discovered each year.

REFERENCES

Abraham A, Wang Y, El Said KR, Plakas SM (2012) Characterization of brevetoxin metabolism in *Karenia brevis* bloom-exposed clams (*Mercenaria* sp.) by LC-MS/MS. *Toxicon* 60: 1030–1040.

Adachi R, Fukuyo Y (1979) The thecal structure of a marine toxic dinoflagellate *Gambierdiscus toxicus* gen. et sp. nov. collected in a ciguatera-endemic area. *Bull. Jpn. Soc. Sci. Fish.* 45: 67–71.

Aikman KE, Tindall DR, Morton SL (1993) Physiology and potency of the dinoflagellate *Prorocentrum hoffmannianum* (Faust) during one complete growth cycle. In: Smadya TJ, Shimuzu Y (eds.) *Toxic Phytoplankton in the Sea*. Elsevier, Amsterdam, the Netherlands, pp. 463–468.

An T, Winshell J, Scorzetti G, Fell JW, Rein KS (2010) Identification of okadaic acid production in the marine dinoflagellate *Prorocentrum rhathymum* from Florida Bay. *Toxicon* 55: 653–657.

Anderson DM, Alpermann TJ, Cembella AD, Collos Y, Masseret E, Monstressor M (2012a) The globally distributed genus *Alexandrium*: Multifaceted roles in marine ecosystems and impacts on human health. *Harmful Algae* 14: 10–35.

Anderson DM, Cembella AD, Haellegraeff GM (2012b) Progress in understanding harmful algal blooms: Paradigm shifts and new technologies for research, monitoring, and management. *Annu. Rev. Mar. Sci.* 4: 143–176.

Anderson DM, Kulis DM, Sullivan JJ, Hall S (1990) Toxin composition variation in one isolate of the dinoflagellate *Alexandrium fundyense*. *Toxicon* 28: 885–893.

Anderson DM, Lobel PS (1987) The continuing enigma of ciguatera. *Biol. Bull.* 172: 89–107.

Aune T (2008) Risk assessment of marine toxins. In: Botana LM (ed.) *Seafood and Freshwater Toxins, Pharmacology, Physiology and Detection*. CRC Press, Boca Raton, FL, pp. 3–20.

Baden DC, Adams DJ (2000) Brevetoxins: Chemistry, mechanism of action and methods of detection. In: Botana LM (ed.) *Seafood and Freshwater Toxins*. Marcel Dekker Inc., New York, pp. 505–532.

Baden DC, Mende TJ (1982) Toxicity of two toxins from the Florida red tide marine dinoflagellate, *Ptychodiscus brevis*. *Toxicon* 20: 457–461.

Bagnis R, Kuberski T, Laughier S (1979) Clinical observations on 3,09 cases of ciguatera (fish poisoning) in the South Pacific. *Am. J. Trop. Med. Hyg.* 28: 1067–1073.

Balech E (1995) The genus *Alexandrium* Halim (Dinoflagellata). Sherkin Island Marine Station Special Publications, Cork, 151pp.

Balech R, Tangen K (1985) Morphology and taxonomy of toxic species in the *tamarensis* group (Dinophyceae): *Alexandrium excavatum* (Braarud) comb. nov. and *Alexandrium ostenfeldii* (Paulsen) comb. nov. *Sarsia* 70: 333–343.

Bellocci M, Sala GL, Callegari F, Rossini GP (2010) Azaspiracid-1 inhibits endocytosis of plasma membrane proteins in epithelial cells. *Toxicol. Sci.* 117: 109–121.

Bergholtz T, Daugbjerg N, Moestrup Ø, Fernándeez-Tejedor M (2006) On the identity of *Karlodinium veneficum* and description of *Karlodinium armiger* sp. nov. (Dinophyceae), based on light and electron microscopy, nuclear-encoded LSU rDNA, and pigment composition. *J. Phycol.* 42: 170–193.

Berry JP, Reece KS, Rein KS, Baden DG, Haas LW, Ribeiro WL, Shields JD, Snyder RV, Vogelbein WK, Gawley RE (2002) Are *Pfiesteria* species toxicogenic? Evidence against production of ichthyotoxins by *Pfiesteria shumwayae*. *Proc. Natl. Acad. Sci. USA* 99: 10970–10975.

Bialojan C, Takai A (1988) Inhibitory effect of a marine-sponge toxin, okadaic acid, on protein phosphatases. *Biochem. J.* 256: 283–290.

Boada LD, Zumbado M, Luzardo OP, Almeida-Gonzáez M, Plakas SM, Granade HR, Abraham A, Jester ELE, Dickey RW (2010) Ciguatera fish poisoning on the West Africa Coast: An emerging risk in the Canary Islands (Spain). *Toxicon* 56: 1516–1519.

Bomber JW, Tindall DR, Miller DM (1989) Genetic variability in toxin potencies among seventeen clones of *Gambierdiscus toxicus*. *J. Phycol.* 25: 617–625.

Borkman DG, Smayda TJ, Tomas CR, York R, Strangman W, Wright JLC (2012) Toxic *Alexandrium peruvianum* (Balech and de Mendiola) Balech and Tangen in Narragansett Bay, Rhode Island. *Harmful Algae* 19: 92–100.

Botes L, Sym SD, Pitcher GC (2003) *Karenia cristata* sp. nov. and *Karenia bicuneiformis* sp. nov. (Gymnodiniales, Dinophyceae): Two new *Karenia* species of the South African coast. *Phycologia* 42: 563–571.

Bottein M-YD, Kashinsky L, Wang Z, Littnan C, Ramsdell JS (2011) Identification of ciguatoxins in Hawaiian monk seals *Monachus schauinslandi* from the northwestern and main Hawaiian Islands. *Environ. Sci. Technol.* 45: 5403–5409.

Bourne Y, Radić Z, Aráoz R, Talley TT, Benoit E, Servent D, Taylor P, Molgó J, Marchot P (2010) Structural determinants in phycotoxins abd AChBP conferring high affinity binding and nicotinic ACHR antagonism. *Proc. Natl. Acad. Sci. USA* 107: 6076–6081.

Brand LE, Campbell L, Bresnan E (2012) *Karenia*: The biology and ecology of a toxic genus. *Harmful Algae* 14: 156–178.

Burke JM, Marchisotto J, McLaughlin JJA, Provasoli L (1960) Analysis of the toxin produced by *Gonyaulax catenella* in axenic culture. *Ann. NY Acad. Sci.* 90: 837–842.

Burkholder JM, Gilbert PM, Skelton HM (2008) Mixotrophy, a major mode of nutrition for harmful algal species in eutrophic waters. *Harmful Algae* 8: 77–93.

Burkholder JM, Marshall HG (2012) Toxigenic *Pfiesteria* species—Updates on biology, ecology, toxins, and impacts. *Harmful Algae* 14: 196–230.

Burkholder JM, Noga EJ, Hobbs CH, Glasgow HB, Smith SA (1992) New "Phantom" dinoflagellate is the causative agent of major estuarine fish kills. *Nature* 358: 407–410.

Caillaud A, de la Iglesia P, Barber E, Eixarch H, Mohamma-Noor N, Yasumoto T, Diogène J (2011) Monitoring of dissolved ciguatoxin and maitotoxin using solid-phase adsorption toxin tracking devices: Application to *Gambierdiscus pacificus* in culture. *Harmful Algae* 10: 433–446.

Caillaud A, de la Iglesia P, Campàs M, Elandaloussi L, Fernández M, Mohammad-Noor N, Andree K, Diogène J (2010) Evidence of okadaic acid production in a cultured strain of the marine dinoflagellate *Prorocentrum rhathymum* from Malaysia. *Toxicon* 55: 633–637.

Capra MF, Cameron J, Flowers AE, Combe IF, Blanton CG, Hahn S (1988) The effects of ciguatoxins in teleosts. In: Choat et al. (eds.) *6th International Coral Reef Symposium Executive Committee*, Townsville, Queensland, Australia, vol. 3, pp. 37–41.

Cembella A, Krock B (2008) Cyclic imine toxins: Chemistry, biogeography, biosynthesis, and pharmacology. In: Botana LM (ed.) *Seafood and Freshwater Toxins Pharmacology, Physiology and Detection*. CRC Press, Boca Raton, FL, pp. 561–580.

Cembella AD, Lewis NI, Quilliam MA (1999) Spirolide composition of micro-extracted pooled cells isolated from natural plankton assemblages and from cultures of the dinoflagellate *Alexandrium ostenfeldii*. *Nat. Toxins* 7: 197–206.

Chang FH (1999) *Gymnodinium brevisulcatum* sp. nov. (Gymnodiniales, Dinophyceae), a new species isolated from the 1998 summer toxic bloom in Wellington Harbour, New Zealand. *Phycologia* 38: 337–384.

Chang FH (2011) Toxic effects of three closely-related dinoflagellates, *Karenia concordia*, *K. brevisulcata* and *K. mikimotoi* (Gymnodiniales, Dinophyceae) on other microalgal species. *Harmful Algae* 10: 181–187.

Chang FH, Bourdelais AJ, Baden DG, Gall M, Hulston D, Webb V (2006) *Karenia concordia* (Dinophyceae) as a brevetoxin-producer and comparison with two closely related species *K. brevisulcata* and *K. mikimotoi*. In: *12th International Conference on Harmful Algae, Programme and Abstracts*, Copenhagen, Denmark, September 4–8, p. 51.

Chang FH, Ryan KG (2004) *Karenia concordia* sp. nov. (Gymnodiniales, Dinophyceae), a new nonthecate dinoflagellate isolated from the New Zealand northeast coast during the 2002 harmful algal bloom events. *Phycologia* 43: 552–562.

Cheng YS, Villareal TA, Zhou Y, Gao J, Pierce R, Naar J, Baden DG (2005) Characterization of red tide aerosol on the Texas coast. *Harmful Algae* 4: 87–94.

Cheng YS, Zhou Y, Pierce RH, Henry M, Baden DG (2010) Characterization of red tide aerosol and the temporal profile of aerosol concentration. *Toxicon* 55: 992–929.

Chinain M, Darius HT, Ung A, Cruchet P, Wang Z et al. (2010) Growth and toxin production in the ciguatera-causing dinoflagellate *Gambierdiscus polynesiensis* (Dinophyceae) in culture. *Toxicon* 56: 739–750.

Chinain M, Faust MA, Pauillac S (1999) Morphology and molecular analyses of three species of *Gambierdiscus* (Dinophyceae): *G. pacificus* sp. nov., *G. australes* sp. nov., and *G. polynesiensis* sp. nov. *J. Phycol.* 35: 1282–1296.

Ciminiello P, Dell'Aversano C, Dello Iacovo E, Fattorusso E, Forino M, Grauso L, Tartaglione L, Guerrini F, Pistocchi R (2010a) Complex palytoxin-like profile of *Ostreopsis ovata*. Identification of four new ovatoxins by high resolution liquid chromatography/mass spectrometry. *Rapid Commun. Mass Spectrom.* 24: 2735–2744.

Ciminiello P, Dell'Aversano C, Fattorussa E, Forino M (2010b). Palytoxins: A still haunting Hawaiian curse. *Phytochem. Rev.* 9: 491–500.

Ciminiello P, Dell'Aversano C, Fattorusso E, Forino M, Magno GS, Tartaglione L, Grillo C, Melchiorre N (2006) The Genoa 2005 outbreak. Determination of putative palytoxin in Mediterranean *Ostreopsis ovata* by a new liquid chromatography mass spectrometry method. *Anal. Chem.* 78: 6153–6159.

Ciminiello P, Fattorusso E (2008) Chemistry, metabolism, and chemical analysis. In: Botana LM (ed.) *Seafood and Freshwater Toxins Pharmacology, Physiology and Detection.* CRC Press, Boca Raton, FL, pp. 287–314.

Ciminiello P, Fattorusso E, Forino M, Montressor M (2000) Saxitoxin and neosaxitoxin as toxic principles of *Alexandrium andersoni* (Dinophyceae) from the Gulf of Naples, Italy. *Toxicon* 38: 1871–1877.

Costas E, Zardoya R, Baustista J, Garrido A, Rojo C, López-Rodas (1995) Morphospecies vs. genospecies in toxic marine dinoflagellates: An analysis of *Gymnodinium catenatum/Gyrodinium impudicum* and *Alexandrium minutum/A. lusitanicum* using antibodies, lectens, and gene sequences. *J. Phycol.* 31: 801–807.

Cruz-Rivera E, Villareal TA (2006) Macroalgal palatability and the flux of ciguatera toxins through marine food webs. *Harmful Algae* 5: 487–525.

Daugbjerg N, Hansen G, Larsen J, Moestrup Ø (2000) Phylogeny of some of the major genera of dinoflagellates based on ultrastructure and partial LSU rDNA sequence data, including the erection of three new genera of unarmoured dinoflagellates. *Phycologia* 39: 302–317.

Davin WT, Kohler CC, Tindall DR (1986) Effects of ciguatera toxins on the bluehead. *Trans. Am. Fish. Soc.* 115: 908–912.

Davis C (1948) *Gymnodinium breve*: A cause of discolored water and animal mortality in the Gulf of Mexico. *Bot. Gaz.* 109: 358–360.

Deeds JR, Landsberg JH, Etheridge SM, Pitcher GC, Longan SW (2008) Non-traditional vectors for paralytic shellfish poisoning. *Mar. Drugs* 6: 308–348.

Dickey RW, Bobzin SC, Faulkner DJ, Bencsath FA, Andrzejewski D (1990) Identification of okadaic acid from a Caribbean dinoflagellate *Prorocentrum concavum*. *Toxicon* 28: 371–377.

Dickey RW, Jester E, Granade R, Mowdy D, Moncreiff C, Rebarchik D, Robl M, Musser S, Poli M (1999) Monitoring brevetoxins during a *Gymnodinium breve* red tide: Comparison of sodium channel specific cytotoxicity assay and mouse bioassay for determination of neurotoxic shellfish toxins in shellfish extracts. *Nat. Toxins* 7: 157–165.

Endean R, Monks SA, Griffith JK, Llewellyn LE (1993) Apparent relationships between toxins elaborated by the cyanobacterium *Trichodesmium erythraeum* and those present in the Spanish mackerel *Scomberomorus commersoni*. *Toxicon* 31: 1155–1165.

Faust MA (1998) Mixotrophy in tropical benthic dinoflagellates. In: Reguera B, Blanco J, Fernandéz L, Wyatts T (eds.) *Harmful Algae*. Xunta de Galacia and International Oceanographic Commission of UNESCO, Santiago de Compostela, pp. 390–393.

Fensome RA, Saldarriaga JF, Taylor FJR (1999) Dinoflagellate phylogeny revisited: Reconciling morphological and molecular based phylogenies. *GRANA* 38: 66–80.

Fensome RA, Taylor FJR, Norris G, Sarjeant WAS, Wharton DI, Williams GL (1993) A classification of living and fossil dinoflagellates. *Micropaleontology*, Special Publication No. 7, 351pp.

Fernández ML, Reguera B, González-Gil S, Míguez A (2006) Pectenotoxin-2 in single cell isolates of *Dinophysis caudata* and *Dinophysis acuta* from the Galicean Rías (NW Spain). *Toxicon* 48: 477–490.

Fire SE, Wang Z, Byrd M, Whitehead HR (2011) Co-occurrence of multiple classes of harmful algal toxins in bottlenose dolphins (*Tursiops truncatus*) stranding during an unusual mortality event in Texas, USA. *Harmful Algae* 10: 330–336.

Fraga S, Rodriguez F, Caillaud A, Diogene J, Nicolas R, Zapata M (2011) *Gambierdiscus excentricus* sp. nov. (Dinophyceae), a benthic toxic dinoflagellate from the Canary Islands (NE Atlantic Ocean). *Harmful Algae* 11: 10–22.

Franchini A, Malagoli D, Ottaviani E (2010) Targets and effects of yessotoxin, okadaic acid and palytoxin: A differential review. *Mar. Drugs* 8: 658–677.

Fukuyo Y (1981) Taxonomical study on benthic dinoflagellates collected in coral reefs. *Bull. Jpn. Soc. Sci. Fish.* 47: 967–978.

Fukuyo Y, Yoshida K, Ogata T, Ishimaru T, Kodama M, Pholpunthin P, Wiessang S, Phanichyakarn V, Piyakarnchana T (1989) Suspected causative dinoflagellates of paralytic shellfish poisoning in the Gulf of Thailand. In: Okaichi T, Anderson DM, Nemoto T (eds.) *Red Tides: Biology, Environmental Science and Toxicology*. Elsevier, New York, pp. 403–406.

Furey A, García J, O'Callaghan K, Lehane M, Amandi MJ, James KJ (2007) Brevetoxins: Structure, toxicology, and origin. In: Botana LM (ed.) *Phycotoxins: Chemistry and Biochemistry*. Blackwell, Oxford, U.K., pp. 19–46.

Furey A, O'Doherty S, O'Callaghan K, Lehane M, James KJ (2010) Azaspiracid poisoning (AZP) toxins in shellfish: Toxicological and health considerations. *Toxicon* 56: 173–190.

Fux E, Smith J, Tong M, Guzmán L, Anderson DM (2011) Toxin profiles of five geographical isolates of *Dinophysis* spp. from North and South America. *Toxicon* 57: 275–287.

Gamboa PM, Park DL, Fremy J-M (1992) Extraction and purification of toxic fractions from barracuda (*Sphyraena barracuda*) implicated in ciguatera poisoning. In: Tosteson TR (ed.) *Proceedings of the Third International Conference on Ciguatera Fish Poisoning,* La Parguera, Puerto Rico, Polysciences Publications, Laval, Quebec, Canada, pp. 13–24.

Giacobbe MG, Peena A, Ceredi A, Milandri A, Poletti R, Yang X (2000) Toxicity and ribosomal DNA of the dinoflagellate *Dinophysis sacculus* (Dinophyta). *Phycologia* 39: 177–182.

Gillespie NC, Lewis RJ, Pearn JH, Bourke ATC, Holmes MJ, Bourke JB, Shields WJ (1986) Ciguatera in Australia: Occurrence, clinical features, pathophysiology and management. *Med. J. Aust.* 145: 584–590.

Glasgow HB, Burkhlder JM, Morton SL, Springer J (2001) A second species of ichthyotoxic *Pfiesteria* (Dinamoebales, Dinophyceae). *Phycologia* 40: 234–245.

Gómez F (2005) A list of free-living dinoflagellate species in the world's oceans. *Acta Bot. Croat.* 64: 129–212.

Grzebyk D, Denardou A, Berland B, Pouchus YF (1997) Evidence of a new toxin in the red-tide dinoflagellate *Prorocentrum minimum*. *J. Plankton Res.* 19: 1111–1124.

Gudger EW (1930) Poisonous fishes and fish poisoning, with special reference to ciguatera in the West Indies. *Am. J. Trop. Med.* 10: 43–55.

Hackett JD, Tong M, Kulis DM, Fux E, Hess P, Bire R, Anderson DM (2009) DSP production de novo in cultures of *Dinophysis acuminata* (Dinophyceae) from North America. *Harmful Algae* 8: 873–879.

Hahn ST, Capra M (1992) The cyanobacterium *Oscillatoria erythraea*—A potential source of toxin in the ciguatera food chain. *Food Addit. Contam.* 9: 351–355.

Hallegraeff GM, Fraga S (1998) Bloom dynamics of the toxic dinoflagellate *Gymnodinium catenatum*, with emphasis on Tasmanian and Spanish coastal waters. In: Anderson DM, Cembella AD, Hallegraeff GM (eds.) *Physiological Ecology of Harmful Algal Blooms*. Springer, Berlin, Germany, pp. 59–80.

Hallegraeff GM, Lucas IAN (1988) The marine dinoflagellate genus *Dinophysis* (Dinophyceae): Photosynthetic, neritic and non-photosynthetic, oceanic species. *Phycologia* 27: 25–42.

Hallegraeff GM, Maclean JL (eds.) (1989) *ICLARM Conference Proceedings 21 on Biology, Epidemiology and Management of Pyrodinium Red Tides*. Fisheries Department, Ministry of Development, Brunei Darussalam, and International Center for Living Aquatic Resources Management, Manilla, Philippines, 286pp.

Hamamoto Y, Tachibana K, Holland PT, Shi F, Beuzenberg V, Itoh Y, Satake M (2012) Brevisulcenal-F: A polycyclic ether toxin associated with massive fish-kills in New Zealand. *J. Am. Chem. Soc.* 134: 4963–4968.

Hamilton B, Hurbungs M, Jones A, Lewis RJ (2002a) Multiple ciguatoxins present in Indian Ocean reef fish. *Toxicon* 40: 1347–1353.

Hamilton B, Hurbungs M, Vernoux JP, Jones A, Lewis RJ (2002b) Isolation and characterization of Indian Ocean ciguatoxin. *Toxicon* 40: 685–693.

Hansen PJ, Cembella AD, Moestrup Ø (1992) The marine dinoflagellate *Alexandrium ostenfeldii*: Paralytic shellfish toxin concentration, composition, and toxicity to a tintinnid ciliate. *J. Phycol.* 28: 597–603.

Haywood AJ, Steidinger KA, Truby EW, Berquist PR, Berquist PL, Adamsom J, MacKenzie L (2004) Comparative morphology and molecular phylogenetic analysis of three new species of the genus *Karenia* (Dinophyceae) from New Zealand. *J. Phycol.* 40: 165–179.

Hellyer SD, Selwood AI, Rhodes L, Kerr DS (2011) Marine algal pinnatoxins E and F cause neuromuscular block in an in vitro hemidiaphragm preparation. *Toxicon* 58: 693–699.

Henrichs DW, Scott PS, Steidinger KA, Errera RM, Abraham A, Campbell L (2013) Morphology and phylogeny of *Prorocentrum texanum* sp. nov. (Dinophyceae): A new toxic dinoflagellate from the Gulf of Mexico coastal waters exhibiting two distinct morphologies. *J. Phycol.* 49: 143–155.

Holland PT, Shi F, Satake M, Hamamoto Y, Ito E, Beuzenberg V, McNabb P et al. (2012) Novel toxins produced by the dinoflagellate *Karenia brevisulcata*. *Harmful Algae* 13: 47–57.

Holmes MJ, Bolch CJS, Green DH, Cembella AD, Teo SLM (2002) Singapore isolates of the dinoflagellate *Gymnodinium catenatum* (Dinophyceae) produce a unique profile of paralytic shellfish poisoning toxins. *J. Phycol.* 38: 96–106.

Holmes MJ, Lee FC, Teo SLM, Khoo HW (1998) A survey of benthic dinoflagellates on Singapore reefs. In: Reguera B, Blanco J, Fernández ML, Wyatt T (eds.) *Harmful Algae*. Xunta de Galacia and International Oceanographic Commission of UNESCO, Santiago de Compostela, pp. 50–51.

Holmes MJ, Lewis R (2002) Toxin-producing dinoflagellates. In: Ménez A (ed.) *Perspectives in Molecular Toxinology*. John Wiley & Sons Ltd., Chichester, U.K., pp. 39–65.

Holmes MJ, Lewis RJ (1994) Purification and characterisation of large and small maitotoxins from cultured *Gambierdiscus toxicus*. *Nat. Toxins* 2: 64–72.

Holmes MJ, Lewis RJ, Gillespie NC (1990) Toxicity of Australian and French Polynesian strains of *Gambierdiscus toxicus* (Dinophyceae) grown in culture: Characterization of a new type of maitotoxin. *Toxicon* 28: 1159–1172.

Holmes MJ, Lewis RJ, Jones A, Wong Hoy A (1995) Cooliatoxin, the first toxin from *Coolia monotis* (Dinophyceae). *Nat. Toxins* 3: 355–362.

Holmes MJ, Lewis RJ, Poli MA, Gillespie NC (1991) Strain dependent production of ciguatoxin precursors (gambiertoxins) by *Gambierdiscus toxicus* (Dinophyceae) in culture. *Toxicon* 29: 761–775.

Holmes MJ, Teo, SLM, Lee FC, Khoo HW (1999) Persistent low concentrations of diarrhetic shellfish toxins in green mussels *Perna viridis* from the Johor Strait, Singapore: First record of diarrhetic shellfish toxins from South East Asia. *Mar. Ecol. Prog. Ser.* 181: 257–268.

Hoppenrath T, Murray S, Sparmann SF, Leandser BS (2012) Morphology and molecular phylogeny of *Ankistrodinium* gen. nov. (Dinophyceae), a new genus of marine sand-dwelling dinoflagellates formerly classified within *Amphidinium*. *J. Phycol.* 48: 1143–1152.

Horiguchi T, Tamura M, Katsumata K, Yamaguchi A (2012) *Testudodinium* gen. nov. (Dinophyceae), a new genus of sand-dwelling dinoflagellates formerly classified in the genus *Amphidinium*. *Phycol. Res.* 60: 137–149.

Howell JF (1953) *Gonyaulax monilata* sp. nov., the causative dinoflagellate of a red tide on the east coast of Florida in August–September, 1951. *Trans. Am. Microsc. Soc.* 72: 153–156.

Hu T, Curtis JM, Oshima Y, Quilliam MA, Walter JA, Watson-Wright WM, Wright JLC (1995) Spirolides B and D, two novel macrocycles isolated from the digestive glands of shellfish. *J. Chem. Soc., Chem. Commun.* 2159–2161.

Hu W, Xu J, Sinkkonen J, Wu J (2010) Polyketides from marine dinoflagellates of the genus *Prorocentrum*, biosynthetic origin and bioactivity of their okadaic acid analogues. *Mini-Rev. Med. Chem.* 10: 51–61.

Ingersoll E (1882) On the fish mortality in the Gulf of Mexico. *Proc. US Natl. Mus.* 4: 74–80.

Ishida H, Nozawa A, Nukuya H, Rhodes L, McNabb P, Holland PT, Tsuiji K (2004) Confirmation of brevetoxin metabolism in cockle, *Austrovenus stutchburyi*, and greenshell mussels, *Perna canaliculus*, associated with New Zealand neurotoxic shellfish poisoning, by controlled exposure to *Karenia brevis*. *Toxicon* 43: 701–712.

Ishida H, Nozawa A, Totoribe K, Muramatsu N, Nukaya H, Tsuji K, Yamaguchi K, Yasumoto T, Kaspar H, Berkett N, Kosuge T (1995) Brevetoxin B1, a new polyether marine toxin from the New Zealand shellfish, *Austrovenus stutchburyi*. *Tetrahedron Lett.* 36: 725–728.

Ito E (2008) Toxicology of Azaspiracid-1: Acute and chronic poisoning, tumorigenicity and chemical structure relationship to toxicity in a mouse bioassay. In: Botana LM (ed.) *Seafood and Freshwater Toxins: Pharmacology, Physiology and Detection*. CRC Press, Taylor & Francis, New York, pp. 775–784.

Jacobson DM, Anderson RA (1994) The discovery of mixotrophy in photosynthetic species of *Dinophysis* (Dinophyceae): Light and electron microscopical observations of food vacuoles in *Dinophysis acuminata*, *D. norvegica* and two heterotrophic dinophysoid dinoflagellates. *Phycologia* 33: 97–110.

James KJ, Moroney C, Roden C, Satake M, Yasumoto T, Lehane M, Furey A (2003) Ubiquitous "benign" alga emerges as the cause of shellfish contamination responsible for the human toxic syndrome, azaspiracid poisoning. *Toxicon* 41: 145–154.

Jauffrais T, Herrenknecht C, Séchet V, Sibat V, Tillmann U, Krock B, Kilkoyne J, Miles CO, McCarron P, Amzil Z, Hess P (2012) Quantitative analysis of azaspiracids in *Azadinium spinosum* cultures. *Anal. Bioanal. Chem.* 403: 833–846.

Jensen MH, Daugbjerg N (2009) Molecular phylogeny of selected species of the order Dinophysiales (Dinophyceae)-testing the hypothesis of a dinophysoid radiation. *J. Phycol.* 45: 1136–1152.

Jeong HJ, Kim JS, Park JY, Kim JH, Kim S, Lee I, Lee SH, Ha JH, Yih WH (2005) *Stoeckeria algicida* n. gen., n. sp. (dinophyceae) from the coastal waters off southern Korea: Morphology and small subunit ribosomal DNA sequence. *J. Eukary. Micro.* 52: 382–390.

John U, Fensome RA, Medlin LK (2003) The application of a molecular clock based on molecular sequences and the fossil record to explain biogeographic distributions within the *Alexandrium tamarense* "species complex." *Mar. Biol. Evol.* 20: 1015–1027.

Kamiyama T, Suzuki T (2009) Production of dinophysistoxin-1 and pectenotoxin-2 by a culture of *Dinophysis acuminata* (Dinophyceae). *Harmful Algae* 8: 312–317.

Kelly BA, Jollow DJ, Felton ET, Voegtline MS, Higerd TB (1986) Response of mice to *Gambierdiscus toxicus* toxin. *Marine Fish. Rev.* 48: 35–37.

Kerbrat AS, Amzil Z, Pawlowietz R, Golubic S, Sibat M, Darius HT, Chinain M, Laurent D (2011) First evidence of palytoxin and 42-hydroxy-palytoxin in the marine cyanobacterium *Trichodesmium. Mar. Drugs* 9: 543–560.

Kerbrat AS, Darius HT, Pauillac S, Chinain M, Laurent D (2010) Detection of ciguatoxin-like and paralysing toxins in Trichodesmium spp. from New Caledonia lagoon. *Mar. Poll. Bull.* 61: 360–366.

Kibler SR, Litaker RW, Holland WC, Vandersea MW, Tester PA (2012) Growth of eight *Gambierdiscus* (Dinophyceae) species: Effects of temperature, salinity and irradiance. *Harmful Algae* 19: 1–14.

Kim HG (1998) *Cochlodinium polykrikoides* blooms in Korean coastal waters and their mitigation. In: Reguera B, Blanco J, Fernández ML, Wyatt T (eds.) *Harmful Algae.* Xunta de Galicia and Intergovernmental Oceanographic Commission of UNESCO, Santiago de Compostela, Spain, pp. 227–228.

Kobayashi J, Kubota T (2007) Bioactive macrolides and polyketides from marine dinoflagellates of the genus *Amphidinium. J. Nat. Prod.* 70: 451–460.

Kodama AM, Hokama Y, Yasumoto T, Fukui M, Manea SJ, Sutherland N (1989) Clinical (mackerel). *Toxicon* 27: 1051–1053.

Kodama M, Ogata T, Fukuyo Y, Ishimaru T, Wisessand S, Saitanu K, Panichyakarn V, Piyakarnchana T (1988) *Protogonyaulax cohorticula*, a toxic dinoflagellate found in the Gulf of Thailand. *Toxicon* 26: 707–712.

Krock B, Tillmann U, John U, Cembella A (2009) Characterization of azaspiracids in plankton size-fractions and isolation of an azaspiracid-producing dinoflagellate from the North Sea. *Harmful Algae* 8: 254–263.

Krock B, Tillmann U, Vosz D, Koch B, Salas R, Witt M, Potvin É, Jeong HJ (2012) New azaspiracids in Amphidomataceae (Dinophyceae). *Toxicon* 60: 830–839.

Kudela RM, Gobler CJ (2012) Harmful dinoflagellate blooms caused by *Cochlodinium* sp.: Global expansion and ecological strategies facilitating bloom formation. *Harmful Algae* 14: 71–86.

Landsberg JH (2002) The effects of harmful algal blooms on aquatic organisms. *Rev. Fish. Sci.* 10: 113–390.

Landsberg JH, Hall S, Johannessen JN, White KD, Conrad SM et al. (2006) Saxitoxin puffer fish poisoning in the United States with the first report of *Pyrodinium bahamense* as the putative toxin source. *Environ. Health Persp.* 114: 1502–1507.

Lartigue J, Jester ELE, Dickey RW, Villareal TA (2009) Nitrogen source effects on the growth and toxicity of two strains of the ciguatera-causing dinoflagellate *Gambierdiscus toxicus. Harmful Algae* 8: 781–791.

Lawrence DN, Enriquez MB, Lumish RM, Maceo A (1980) Ciguatera fish poisoning in Miami. *J. Am. Med. Assoc.* 244: 254–258.

Lawrence JE, Grant J, Quilliam MA, Bauder AG, Cembella AD (2000) Colonization and growth of the toxic dinoflagellate *Prorocentrum lima* and associated fouling macroalgae on mussels in suspended culture. *Mar. Ecol. Prog. Ser.* 201: 147–154.

Lee JS, Igarashi T, Fraga S, Dahl E, Hovgaard P, Yasumoto T (1989) Determination of diarrhetic shellfish toxins in various dinoflagellate species. *J. Appl. Phycol.* 1: 147–152.

Lenoir S, Ten-Hage L, Turquet J, Quod JP, Bernard C, Hennison MC (2004) First evidence of palytoxin analogues from an *Ostreopsis mascarenensis* (Dinophyceae) benthic bloom in Southwestern Indian ocean. *J. Phycol.* 40: 1042–1051.

Lewis RJ (1992) Ciguatoxins are potent ichthyotoxins. *Toxicon* 30: 207–211.

Lewis RJ (2000) Ciguatera management. *SPC Live Reef Fish Information Bulletin #7*, pp. 11–13.

Lewis RJ (2001) The changing face of ciguatera. *Toxicon* 39: 97–106.

Lewis RJ, Holmes MJ (1993) Origin and transfer of toxins involved in ciguatera. *Comp. Biochem. Physiol.* 106C: 615–628.

Lewis RJ, Sellin M (1992) Multiple ciguatoxins in the flesh of fish. *Toxicon* 30: 915–919.

Lewis RJ, Sellin M, Poli MA, Norton RS, MacLeod JK, Sheil MM (1991) Purification and characterization of ciguatoxins from moray eel (*Lycodontis javanicus*, Muraenidae). *Toxicon* 29: 1115–1127.

Lewis RJ, Vernoux JP, Brereton IM (1998) Structure of Caribbean ciguatoxin isolated from *Caranx latus. J. Am. Chem. Soc.* 120: 5914–5920.

Lilly EL, Halanych KM, Anderson DM (2005) Phylogeny, biogeography, and species boundaries within the *Alexandrium minutum* group. *Harmful Algae* 4: 1004–1020.

Lim PT, Usup G, Leaw CP, Ogata T (2005) First report of *Alexandrium taylori* and *Alexandrium peruvianum* (Dinophyceae) in Malaysian waters. *Harmful Algae* 4: 391–400.

Litaker RW, Steidinger KA, Mason PL, Landsberg JH, Shields JD et al. (2005) The reclassification of *Pfiesteria shumwayae* (Dinophyceae): *Pseudopfiesteria*, gen. nov. *J. Phycol*. 41: 643–651.

Litaker RW, Vandersea MW, Faust MA, Kibler SR, Chinain M, Holmes MJ, Holland WC, Tester PA (2009) Taxonomy of *Gambierdiscus* including four new species, *Gambierdiscus caribaeus*, *Gambierdiscus carolinianus*, *Gambierdiscus carpenteri* and *Gambierdiscus ruetzleri* (Gonyaucales, Dinophyceae). *Phycologia* 48: 344–390.

Litaker RW, Vandersea MA, Faust MA, Kibler SR, Nau AW, Holland WC, Chinain M, Holmes MJ, Tester PA (2010) Global distribution of ciguatera causing dinoflagellates in the genus *Gambierdiscus*. *Toxicon* 56: 711–730.

Litaker RW, Vandersea MW, Kibler SR, Reece KS, Stokes NA, Steidinger KA, Millie DF, Bendis BJ, Pigg RJ, Tester PA (2003) Identification of *Pfiesteria piscicida* (Dinophyceae) and *Pfiesteria*-like organisms using internal transcribed spacer-specific PCR assays. *J. Phycol*. 39: 754–761.

Llewellyn LE (2006) The behavior of mixtures of mixtures of paralytic shellfish toxins in competitive binding assays. *Chem. Res. Toxicol*. 19: 661–667.

Llewellyn LE (2009) Sodium channel inhibiting marine toxins. *Prog. Mol. Subcell. Biol*. 46: 67–97.

Lombet A, Bidard JN, Lazdunski M (1987) Ciguatoxin and brevetoxins share a common receptor site on the neuronal voltage-dependent Na^+ channel. *FEBS Lett*. 219: 355–359.

López-Rivera AOCK, Moriarty M, O'Driscoll D, Hamilton B, Lehane M, James KJ, Furey A (2010) First evidence of azaspiracids (AZAs): A family of lipophilic polyether marine toxins in scallops (*Argopecten purpuratus*) and mussels (*Mytilus chilensis*) collected in two regions of Chile. *Toxicon* 55: 692–701.

Lundholm N, Moestrup Ø (2006) The biogeography of harmful algae. In: Granéli E, Turner JT (eds.) *Ecology of Harmful Algae*. Springer, Berlin, Germany, pp. 23–35.

Maclean JL (1977) Observations on *Pyrodinium bahamense* Plate, a toxic dinoflagellate in Papua New Guinea. *Agric. J*. 24: 131–138.

Maclean JL (1989) An overview of *Pyrodinium* red tides in the western Pacific. In: Hallegraeff GM, Maclean JL (eds.) *ICLARM Conference Proceedings 21 on Biology, Epidemiology and Management of Pyrodinium Red Tides*. Fisheries Department, Ministry of Development, Brunei Darussalam, and International Center for Living Aquatic Resources Management, Manilla, Philippines, pp. 1–7.

Marasigan A, Sato S, Fukuyo Y, Kodama M (2001) Accumulation of a high level of diarrhetic shellfish toxins in the green mussel *Perna viridis* during a bloom of *Dinophysis caudata* and *Dinophysis miles* in Saipan Bay, Panay Island, the Philippines. *Fish. Sci*. 67: 994–996.

Marshall HG, Seaborn D, Wolny J (1999) Monitoring result for *Pfiesteria piscicida* and *Pfiesteria*-like organisms from Virginia waters in 1998. *Virginia J. Sci*. 50: 287–298.

Mason PL, Litaker RW, Jeong HJ, Ha JH, Reece KS et al. (2007) Description of a new genus of *Pfiesteria*-like dinoflagellate, *Luciella* gen. nov. (Dinophyceae), including two new species: *Luciella masanensis* sp. nov. and *Luciella atlantis* sp. nov. *J. Phycol*. 43: 798–810.

McNabb PS, McCoubrey DJ, Rhodes L, Smith K, Selwood AI, van Ginkel R, MacKenzie AL, Munday R, Holland PT (2012) New perspectives in biotoxin detection in Rangaunu Harbour, New Zealand arising from the discovery of pinnatoxins. *Harmful Algae* 13: 34–39.

Miles CO, Wilkins AL, Munday R, Dines MH, Hawkes AD et al. (2004) Isolation of pectenotoxin-2 from *Dinophysis acuta* and its conversion to pectenotoxin-2 seco acid, and preliminary assessment of their acute toxicities. *Toxicon* 43: 1–9.

Mills AR (1956) Poisonous fish in the South Pacific. *J. Trop. Med. Hyg*. 59: 99–103.

Moeller PDR, Beauchesne KR, Huncik KM, Davis WC, Christopher SJ, Riggs-Gelasco P, Gelasco AK (2007) Metal complexes and free radical toxins produced by *Pfiesteria piscicida*. *Environ. Sci. Technol*. 41: 1166–1172.

Moestrup Ø, Akselman R, Cronberg G, Elbraechter M, Fraga S et al. (eds.) (2009 onwards). IOC-UNESCO taxonomic reference list of Harmful Micro Algae. Available online at http://www.marinespecies.org/HAB, accessed on 2012-10-11.

Mohammad-Noor N, Moestrup Ø, Daugbjerg N (2007) Light, electron microscopy and DNA sequences of the dinoflagellate *Prorocentrum concavum* (syn. *P. arabianum*) with special emphasis on the periflagellar area. *Phycologia* 46: 549–564.

Mohammad-Noor N, Moestrup Ø, Lundholm N, Fraga S, Holmes MJ, Saleh E (2013) Autecology and phylogeny of *Coolia tropicalis* and *Coolia malayensis* (Dinophyceae), with emphasis on taxonomy of *C. tropicalis* based on light microscopy, scanning electron microscopy and LSU rDNA. *J. Phycol*. 49: 536–545.

Moldowan JM, Talyzina NM (1998) Biogeochemical evidence for dinoflagellate ancestors in the early Cambrian. *Nature* 281: 1168–1170.

Moore RE, Scheuer PJ (1971) Palytoxin—New marine toxin from a coelenterate. *Science* 172: 495–498.

Morohashi A, Satake M, Murata K, Naoki H, Kaspar HF, Yasumoto T (1995) Brevetoxin B3, a new breve-toxin analog isolated from the Greenshell mussel *Perna canaliculus* involved in Neurotoxic Shellfish Poisoning in New Zealand. *Tetrahedron Lett.* 36: 8995–8998.

Morton SL (1998) Morphology and toxicity of *Prorocentrum faustiae* sp. nov., a toxic species of non-plank-tonic dinoflagellate from Heron Island, Australia. *Bot. Mar.* 41: 565–569.

Morton SL, Moeller PDR, Young KA, Lanoue B (1998) Okadaic acid production from the marine dinofla-gellate *Prorocentrum belizeanum* Faust isolated from the Belizean coral reef ecosystem. *Toxicon* 36: 201–206.

Morton SL, Petitpain DL, Busman M, Moeller PDR (2000) Production of okadaic acid and Dinophysis toxins by different species of *Prorocentrum*. In: Hallegraeff G (convener) Conference Abstracts and Participants, *9th International Conference on Harmful Algal Blooms*, Hobart, Tasmania, Australia, p. 183.

Munday R (2006) Toxicological requirements for risk assessment of shellfish contaminants: A review. *Afr. J. Mar. Sci.* 28: 447–449.

Munday R (2008a) Occurrence and toxicology of palytoxins. In: Botana LM (ed.) *Seafood and Freshwater Toxins, Pharmacology, Physiology, and Detection*. CRC Press, Boca Raton, FL, pp. 693–713.

Munday R (2008b) Toxicology of pectenotoxins. In: Botana LM (ed.) *Seafood and Freshwater Toxins, Pharmacology, Physiology, and Detection*. CRC Press, Boca Raton, FL, pp. 371–380.

Munday R, Quilliam MA, LeBlanc P, Lewis N, Gallant P, Sperker SA, Ewart HS, MacKinnon SL (2012) Investigations into the toxicology of spirolides, a group of marine phycotoxins. *Toxins* 4: 1–14.

Munday R, Towers NR, MacKenzie L, Beuzenberg V, Holland PT, Miles CO (2004) Acute toxicity of gymn-odimine to mice. *Toxicon* 44: 173–178.

Murakami M, Makabe K, Yanaguchi K, Konosu S, Walchli MR (1988) Goniodomin A, a novel polyether mac-rolide from the dinoflagellate *Goniodoma pseudogoniaulax*. *Tetrahedron Lett.* 29: 1149–1152.

Murakami Y, Oshima Y, Yasumoto T (1982) Identification of okadaic acid as a toxic component of a marine dinoflagellate *Prorocentrum lima*. *Bull. Jpn. Soc. Sci. Fish.* 48: 69–72.

Murata M, Kumagai M, Lee JS, Yasumoto T (1987) Isolation and structure of yessotoxin, a novel polyether compound implicated in diarrhetic shellfish poisoning. *Tetrahedron Lett.* 28: 5869–5872.

Murata M, Legrand AM, Ishibashi Y, Fukui M, Yasumoto T (1990) Structures and configurations of ciguatoxin from the moray eel *Gymnothorax javanicus* and its likely precursor from the dinoflagellate *Gambierdiscus toxicus*. *J. Am. Chem. Soc.* 112: 4380–4386.

Murata M, Legrand AM, Ishibashi Y, Yasumoto T (1989) Structures of ciguatoxin and its congener. *J. Am. Chem. Soc.* 111: 8929–8931.

Murata M, Naoki H, Iwashita T, Matsunaga S, Sasaki M, Yokoyama A, Yasumoto T (1993) Structure of mai-totoxin. *J. Am. Chem. Soc.* 115: 2060–2062.

Murata K, Satake M, Naoki H, Kaspar HF, Yasumoto T (1998) Isolation and structure of a new brevetoxin ana-log, brevetoxin B2, from Greenshell Mussels from New Zealand. *Tetrahedron* 54: 735–742.

Murata M, Shimatani M, Sugitani H, Oshima Y, Yasumoto T (1982) Isolation and structural elucidation of the causative toxin of the diarrhetic shellfish poisoning. *Bull. Jpn. Soc. Sci. Fish.* 48: 549–552.

Naar JP, Flewelling LJ, Lenz A, Abbott JP, Granholm A et al. (2007) Brevetoxins, like ciguatoxins, are potent ichthyotoxic neurotoxins that accumulate in fish. *Toxicon* 50: 707–723.

Nagai S, Nishitani G, Tomaru Y, Sakiyama S, Kamiyama T (2008) Predation by the toxic dinoflagellate *Dinophysis fortii* on the ciliate *Myrionecta rubra* and observation of sequestration of ciliate chloroplasts. *J. Phycol.* 44: 909–922.

Nagai S, Suzuki T, Nishikawa T, Kamiyama T (2011) Differences in the production and excretion kinetics of okadaic acid, dinophysistoxin-1, and pectenotoxin-2 between cultures of *Dinophysis acuminata* and *Dinophysis fortii* isolated from western Japan. *J. Phycol.* 47: 1326–1337.

Nakajima I, Oshima Y, Yasumoto T (1981) Toxicity of benthic dinoflagellates in Okinawa. *Bull. Jpn. Soc. Sci. Fish.* 47: 1029–1033.

Negri A, Bolch CJS, Blackburn S, Dickman M, Llewewellyn LE, Méndez S (2001) Paralytic shellfish toxins in *Gymnodinium catenatum* strains from six countries. In: Hallegraeff GM, Blackburn SI, Bolch CJ, Lewis RJ (eds.) *Harmful Algal Blooms 2000*. Intergovernmental Oceanographic Commission of UNESCO, Paris, France, pp. 210–213.

Negri A, Bolch CJS, Geier S, Green DH, Park T-G, Blackburn SI (2007) Widespread presence of hydrophobic paralytic shellfish toxins in *Gymnodinium catenatum*. *Harmful Algae* 6: 774–780.

Negri A, Stirling D, Quilliam M, Blackburn S, Bolch C, Burton I, Eaglesham G, Thomas K, Walter J, Willis R (2003) Three novel hydroxybenzoate saxitoxin analogues isolated from the dinoflagellate *Gymnodinium catenatum*. *Chem. Res. Toxicol*. 16: 1029–1033.

Nguyen-Ngoc L (2004) An autecological study of the potentially toxic dinoflagellate *Alexandrium affine* isolated from Vietnamese waters. *Harmful Algae* 3: 117–129.

Nishitani G, Nagai S, Sakiyama S, Kamiyama T (2008a) Successful cultivation of the toxic dinoflagellate *Dinophysis caudata* (Dinophyceae). *Plankton Benthos Res*. 3: 78–85.

Nishitani G, Nagai S, Takano Y, Sakiyama S, Baba K, Kamiyama (2008b) Growth characteristics and phylogenetic analysis of the marine dinoflagellate *Dinophysis infundibulus* (Dinophyceae). *Aquat. Microb. Ecol*. 52: 209–221.

Nishiwaki S, Fujiki H, Suganumi M, Furuya-Suguri H, Matsushima R et al. (1990) Structure–activity relationship within a series of okadaic acid derivatives. *Carcinogenesis* 11: 1837–1841.

Noguchi T, Hwang DF, Arakawa O, Daigo K, Sato S, Ozari H, Kawai N, Ito M, Hashimoto K (1987) Palytoxin as the causative agent in the parrotfish poisoning. In: Gopalakrishnakone P, Tan CK (eds.) *Progress in Venom and Toxin Research*. National University of Singapore, Singapore, pp. 325–335.

Norris DR, Bomber JW, Balech E (1985) Benthic dinoflagellates associated with ciguatera from the Florida Keys. I. *Ostreopsis heptagona* sp. nov. In: Anderson DM, White AW, Baden DG (eds.) *Toxic Dinoflagellates*. Elsevier, New York, pp. 39–44.

Ofuji K, Satake M, McMahon T, Silke J, James KJ, Naoki H, Oshima Y, Yasumoto T (1999) Two analogs of azaspiracid isolated from mussels *Mytilus edulis*, involved in human intoxication in Ireland. *Nat. Toxins* 7: 99–102.

Ogino H, Kumagi M, Yasumoto T (1997) Toxicologic evaluation of yessotoxin. *Nat. Toxins* 5: 255–259.

Onuma Y, Satake M, Ukena T, Roux J, Chanteau S, Rasolofornirna N, Ratsimaloto M, Naoki H, Yasumoto T (1999) Identification of palytoxin as the cause of clupeotoxism. *Toxicon* 37: 66–65.

O'Shea TJ, Rathbun GB, Bonde RK, Buergelt CD, Odell DK (1991) An epizootic of Florida manatees associated with a dinoflagellate bloom. *Mar. Mammal Sci*. 7: 165–179.

Oshima Y (1989) Toxins in *Pyrodinium bahamense* var. *compressum* and infested marine organisms. In: Hallegraeff GM, Maclean JL (eds.) *ICLARM Conference Proceedings 21 on Biology, Epidemiology and Management of Pyrodinium Red Tides*. Fisheries Department, Ministry of Development, Brunei Darussalam, and International Center for Living Aquatic Resources Management, Manila, Philippines, pp. 73–79.

Oshima Y, Hirota M, Yasumoto T, Hallegraeff GM, Blackburn SI, Steffensen DA (1989) Production of paralytic shellfish toxins by the dinoflagellate *Alexandrium minutum* Halim from Australia. *Bull. Jpn. Soc. Sci. Fish*. 55: 925.

Otero P, Alfonso A, Rodríguez P, Rubiolo JA, Cifuentes JM, Bermúdez R, Vieytes MR, Boatan LM (2012) Pharmacokinetic and toxicological data of spirolides after oral and intraperitoneal administration. *Food Chem. Toxicol*. 50: 232–237.

Pagliara P, Caroppo C (2012) Toxicity assessment of *Amphidinium carterae, Coolia* cfr. *monotis* and *Ostreopsis* cfr. *ovata* (Dinophyta) isolated from the northern Ionian Sea (Mediterranean Sea). *Toxicon* 60: 1203–1214.

Park MG, Kim S, Kim HS, Myung G, Kang YG, Yih W (2006) First successful culture of the marine dinoflagellate *Dinophysis acuminata*. *Aquat. Microb. Ecol*. 45: 101–106.

Parsons ML, Aligizaki K, Bottein M-YD, Fraga S, Morton SL, Penna A, Rhodes L (2012) *Gambierdiscus* and *Ostreopsis*: Reassessment of the state of knowledge of their taxonomy, geography, ecophysiology, and toxicology. *Harmful Algae* 14: 107–129.

Paz B, Daranas AH, Norte M, Riobó P, Franco JM, Fernández JM (2008) Yessotoxins, a group of marine polyether toxins: An overview. *Mar. Drugs* 6: 73–102.

Peng J, Place AR, Yoshida W, Clemens A, Hamann MT (2010) Structure and absolute configuration of karlotoxin-2, an ichthyotoxin from the marine dinoflagellate *Karlodinium veneficum*. *J. Am. Chem. Soc*. 132: 3277–3279.

Penna A, Fraga S, Battocchi C, Casabianca S, Riobó P, Giacobbe MG, Vernesi C (2010) A phylogeography study of the toxic benthic genus *Ostreopsis* Schmidt. *J. Biogeogr*. 37: 830–841.

Pillet S, Houvenaghel G (1995) Influence of experimental toxification by DSP producing microalgae, *Prorocentrum lima*, on clearance rate in blue mussels Mytilus edulis. In: Lassus P, Arzul G, Erard E, Gentien P, Marcaillou C (eds.) *Harmful Marine Algal Blooms*. Lavoisier-Intercept Ltd., Paris, France, pp. 481–486.

Pizarro G, Escalera L, González-Gil S, Franco JM, Reguera B (2008) Growth, behaviour and cell toxin quota of *Dinophysis acuta* during a daily cycle. *Mar. Ecol. Prog. Ser.* 353: 89–105.

Place AR, Bowers HA, Bachvaroff TR, Adolf JE, Deeds JR, Sheng J (2012) *Karlodinium veneficum*—The little dinoflagellate with a big bite. *Harmful Algae* 14: 179–195.

Prakash A, Taylor FJR (1966) A "red water" bloom of *Gonyaulax acatenella* in the Strait of Georgia and its relation to paralytic shellfish toxicity. *J. Fish. Bd. Can.* 23: 1265–1270.

Quilliam M, Wechsler D, Marcus S, Ruck B, Wekell M, Hawryluk T (2004) Detection and identification of paralytic shellfish poisoning toxins in Florida pufferfish responsible for incidents of neurologic illness. In: Steidinger KA, Landsberg JH, Tomas CR, Vargo GA (eds.) *Harmful Algae 2002.* Florida Fish and Wildlife Commission, Florida Institute of Oceanography, and International Oceanographic Commission of UNESCO. St. Petersburg, pp. 116–118.

Quod JP, Turquet J, Diogene G, Fessard V (1995) Screening of extracts of dinoflagellates from coral reefs (Reunion Island, SW Indian Ocean), and their biological activities. In: Lassus P, Arzul G, Erard E, Gentien P, Marcaillou C (eds.) *Harmful Marine Algal Blooms.* Lavoisier, New York, pp. 815–820.

Raho N, Pizarro G, Escalera L, Reguera B, Marín I (2008) Morphology, toxin composition and molecular analysis of *Dinophysis ovum* Schütt, a dinoflagellate of the "*Dinophysis acuminata*" complex. *Harmful Algae* 7: 839–848.

Randall JE (1958) A review of ciguatera, tropical fish poisoning, with a tentative explanation of its cause. *Bull. Mar. Sci.* 8: 236–267.

Rehmann N, Hess P, Quilliam MA (2008) Discovery of new analogs of the marine biotoxin azaspiracid in blue mussels *Mytilus edulis* by ultra-performance liquid chromatography/tandem mass spectrometry. *Rapid Commun. Mass Spectrom.* 22: 549–558.

Reguera B, Velo-Suárez L, Raine R, Park MG (2012) Harmful *Dinophysis* species: A review. *Harmful Algae* 14: 87–106.

Rhodes L, McNabb P, de Salas M, Briggs L, Beuzenberg V, Gladstone M (2006) Yessotoxin production by *Gonyaulax spinifera*. *Harmful Algae* 5: 148–155.

Rhodes L, Smith K, Selwood A, McNabb P, Munday R, Suda S, Molenaar S, Hallegraeff GM (2011) Dinoflagellate *Vulcanodinium rugosum* identified as the causative organism of pinnatoxins in Australia, New Zealand and Japan. *Phycologia* 50: 624–628.

Rhodes LL, Thomas A (1997) *Coolia monotis* (Dinophyceae): A toxic epiphytic microalgal species found in New Zealand. *New Zealand J. Mar. Freshwater Res.* 31: 139–141.

Riobó P, Paz B, Franco JM, Vazquez JA, Murado MA, Cacho E (2008) Mouse bioassay for palytoxin. Specific symptoms and dose-response against dose-death time relationships. *Food Chem. Toxicol.* 46: 2639–2647.

Roeder K, Erler K, Kibler S, Tester P, The HV, Nguyen-Ngoc L, Gerdts G, Luckas B (2010) Characteristic profiles of ciguatera toxins in different strains of *Gambierdiscus* spp. *Toxicon* 56: 731–738.

Rossi R, Castellano V, Scalo E, Serpe L, Zingone A, Soprano V (2010) New palytoxin-like molecules in Mediterranean *Ostreopsis* cf. *ovata* (Dinoflagellates) and in *Palythoa tuberculosa* detected by liquid chromatography-electrospray ionization time-of-flight mass spectrometry. *Toxicon* 56: 1382–1387.

Rossini GP, Hess P (2010) Phycotoxins: Chemistry, mechanisms of action and shellfish poisoning. *EXS* 100: 65–122.

Rundberget T, Bunaes Aasen JA, Selwood AI, Miles CO (2011) Pinnatoxins and spirolides in Norwegian blue mussels and seawater. *Toxicon* 58: 700–711.

de Salas MF, Bolch CJS, Botes L, Nash G, Wright SW, Hallegraeff GM (2003) *Takayama* gen. nov. (Gymnodiniales, Dinophyceae), a new genus of unarmoured dinoflagellates with sigmoid apical grooves, including the description of two new species. *J. Phycol.* 39: 1233–1246.

Sasaki K, Murata M, Yasumoto T, Mieskes G, Takai A (1994) Affinity of okadaic acid to type-1 and type-2A protein phosphatases is markedly reduced by oxidation of its 27-hydroxyl group. *Biochem. J.* 298: 259–262.

Satake M, Fukui M, Legrand AM, Cruchet P, Yasumoto T (1998a) Isolation and structures of new ciguatoxin analogs, 2,3-DihydroxyCTX3C and 51-HydroxyCTX3C, accumulated in tropical reef fish. *Tetrahedron Lett.* 39: 1197–1198.

Satake M, Ishibashi Y, Legrand A-M, Yasumoto T (1997a) Isolation and structure of ciguatoxin-4a, a new ciguatoxin precursor, from cultures of dinoflagellate *Gambierdiscus toxicus* and Parrotfish *Scarus gibbus*. *Biosci. Biotechnol. Biochem.* 60: 2103–2105.

Satake M, MacKenzie L, Yasumoto T (1997b) Identification of *Protoceratium reticulatum* as the biogenic origin of yessotoxin. *Nat. Toxins* 5: 164–167.

Satake M, Murata M, Yasumoto T (1993) The structure of CTX-3C, a ciguatoxin congener isolated from cultured *Gambierdiscus toxicus*. *Tetrahedron Lett*. 34: 1975–1978.

Satake M, Ofugi K, James KJ, Furey A, Yasumoto T (1998b) New toxic event caused by Irish mussels. In: Reguera B et al. (eds.) *Proceedings of the VIII International Conference on Harmful Algae*, (June 1999, Vigo, Spain), pp. 468–469. Xunta de Galacia and IOC of UNESCO.

Satake M, Ofuji K, Naoki H, James KJ, Furey A, McMahon T, Silke J, Yasumoto T (1998c) Azaspiracid, a new marine toxin having unique spiro ring assemblies, isolated from Irish mussels, *Mytilus edulis*. *J. Am. Chem. Soc*. 120: 9967–9968.

Satake M, Shoji M, Oshima Y, Naoki H, Fujita T, Yasumoto T (2002) Gymnocin-A, a cytotoxic polyether from the notorious red tide dinoflagellate, *Gymnodinium mikimotoi*. *Tetrahedron Lett*. 43: 5829–5832.

Satake M, Tanaka Y, Ishikura Y, Oshima Y, Naoki H, Yasumoto T (2005) Gymnocin-B with the largest contiguous polyether rinds from the red tide dinoflagellate, *Karenia* (formerly *Gymnodinium*) *mikimotoi*. *Tetrahedron Lett*. 46: 3537–3540.

Scholin CA (1998) Morphological, genetic, and biogeographical relationships of the toxic dinoflagellates *Alexandrium tamarense*, *A. catenella* and *A. fundyense*. In Anderson DM, Cembella AM, Hallegraeff GM (eds.) *Physiological Ecology of Harmful Algal Blooms*. Springer, Berlin, Germany, pp. 13–27.

Schrader A (2010) Responding to *Pfiesteria piscicida* (the fish killer): Phantomatic ontologies, indeterminacy, and responsibility in toxic microbiology. *Soc. Studies Sci*. 40: 275–306.

Seki T, Satake M, MacKenzie L, Kaspar H, Yasumoto T (1995) Gymnodimine, a new marine toxin of unprecedented structure isolated from New Zealand oysters and the dinoflagellate, *Gymnodinium* sp. *Tetrahedron Lett*. 36: 7093–7096.

Selwood AI, Miles CO, Wilkins Al, van Ginkel R, Munday R, Rise F, McNabb P (2010) Isolation and structural determination, and acute toxicity of novel pinnatoxins E, F and G. *J. Agric. Food Chem*. 58: 6532–6542.

Shimizu Y, Alam M, Oshima Y, Fallon WE (1975) Presence of four toxins in red tide infested clams and *Gonyaulax tamarensis* cells. *Biochem. Biophys. Res. Commun*. 66: 731–737.

Smith KF, Rhodes LL, Suda S, Selwwod AI (2011) A dinoflagellate producer of pinnatoxin G, isolated from sub-tropical Japanese waters. *Harmful Algae* 10: 702–705.

Sournia A (1995) Red tide and toxic marine phytoplankton of the world ocean: An inquiry into biodiversity. In: Lassus P, Arzul G, Erard E, Gentien P, Marcaillou C (eds.) *Harmful Marine Algal Blooms*. Lavoisier, New York, pp. 103–112.

Sparmann SF, Leander BS, Hoppenrath M (2008) Comparative morphology and molecular phylogeny of *Apicoporus* n. gen: A new genus of marine benthic dinoflagellate formerly classified with *Amphidinium*. *Protist* 159: 383–399.

Sperr AE, Doucette GJ (1996) Variation in growth rate and ciguatera toxin production among geographically distinct clones of *Gambierdiscus toxicus*. In: Yasumoto T, Oshima Y, Fukuyo Y (eds.) *Harmful and Toxic Algal Blooms*. UNESCO, Paris, France, pp. 309–312.

Steidinger KA, Burkholder JM, Glasgow HB, Hobbs CW, Truby E, Garrett J, Noga EJ, Smith SA (1996) *Pfiesteria piscicida* gen. et sp. nov. (Pfiesteriaceae, fam. nov.), a new toxic dinoflagellate with a complex life cycle and behavior. *J. Phycol*. 32: 157–164.

Steidinger KA, Landsberg JH, Mason PL, Vogelbein WK, Tester PA, Litaker RW (2006) *Crytoperidiniopsis brodyi* gen. et sp. nov. (Dinophyceae), a small lightly armored dinoflagellate in the Pfiesteriaceae. *J. Phycol*. 42: 951–961.

Steidinger KA, Landsberh JH, Truby EW, Roberts BS (1998) First report of *Gymnodinium pulchellum* (Dinophyceae) in North America and associated fish kills in the Indian River, Florida. *J. Phycol*. 34: 431–437.

Steidinger KA, Tangen K (1997) Dinoflagellates. In: Tomas C (ed.) *Identifying Marine Phytoplankton*. Academic Press, San Diego, CA, pp. 387–584.

Suganuma M, Fujiki H, Suguri H, Yoshizawa S, Hirota M, Ojika M, Wakamatsu K, Yamada K, Sugimura T (1988) Okadaic acid: An additional non-phorbol-12-tetradecanoate-13-acetate-type tumor promoter. *Proc. Natl. Acad. Sci*. 85: 1768–1771.

Suzuki T (2008) Chemistry, metabolism, and chemical detection methods of pectenotoxins. In: Botana LM (ed.) *Seafood and Freshwater Toxins, Pharmacology, Physiology, and Detection*. CRC Press, Boca Raton, FL, pp. 343–359.

Suzuki T, Miyazono A, Baba K, Sugawara R, Kamiyama T (2009) LC-MS/MS analysis of okadaic acid analogues and other lipophilic toxins in single-cell isolates of several *Dinophysis* species collected in Hokkaido Japan. *Harmful Algae* 8: 233–238.

Suzuki T, Quilliam MA (2011) LC-MS/MS analysis of diarrhetic shellfish poisoning (DSP) toxins, okadaic acid and dinophysistoxin analogues, and other lipophilic toxins. *Anal. Sci.* 27: 571–584.

Swinker M, Tester P, Attix DK, Schmechel D (2002) Humman health effects of exposure to *Pfiesteria piscicida*: A review. *Microbes Infection* 4: 751–762.

Tachibana K, Scheuer PJ, Tsukitani Y, Kikuchi H, Van Engen D, Clardy J, Gopichand Y, Schmitz FJ (1981). Okadaic acid, a cytotoxic polyether from two marine sponges of the genus *Halichondria*. *J. Am. Chem. Soc.* 103: 2469–2471.

Takada N, Umemura N, Suenaga K, Uemura D (2001) Structural determination of pteriatoxins A, B and C, extremely potent toxins from the bivalve *Pteria penguin*. *Tetrahedron Lett.* 42: 3495–3497.

Takagi T, Hayashi K, Itabashi Y (1984) Toxic effect of free unsaturated fatty acids in the mouse assay of diarrhetic shellfish toxin by intraperitoneal injection. *Bull. Jpn. Soc. Sci. Fish.* 50: 1413–1418.

Tang YZ, Gobler CJ (2009) Characterization of the toxicity of *Cochlodinium polykrikoides* isolates from northeast US estuaries to finfish and shellfish. *Harmful Algae* 8: 454–462.

Tang YZ, Kong L, Holmes MJ (2007) Dinoflagellate *Alexandrium leei* (Dinophyceae) from Singapore coastal waters produces a water-soluble ichthyotoxin. *Mar. Biol.* 150: 541–549.

Taniyama S, Arakawa O, Terada M, Nishio S, Takatani T, Mahmud Y, Noguchi T (2003) *Ostreopsis* sp., a possible origin of palytoxin (PTX) in parrotfish *Scarus ovifrons*. *Toxicon* 42: 29–33.

Taylor FJR (1985) The taxonomy and relationships of red tide dinoflagellate. In: Anderson DM, White AW, Baden DG (eds.) *Toxic Dinoflagellates*. Elsevier, New York, pp. 11–26.

Taylor FJR, Fukuto Y, Larsen J (1995) Taxonomy of harmful dinoflagellates. In: Hallegraeff GM, Anderson DM, Cembella A (eds.) *Manual on Harmful Marine Microalgae*. IOC Manuals and Guides No. 33, UNESCO, Paris, France, pp. 283–317.

Taylor FJR, Hoppenrath M, Saldarriaga JF (2008) Dinoflagellate diversity and distribution. *Biodivers. Conserv.* 17: 407–418.

Ten-Hage L, Delaunay N, Pichon V, Couté A, Puiseux-Dao S, Turquet J (2000a) Okadaic acid production from the marine dinoflagellate *Prorocentrum arenarium* Faust (Dinophyceae) isolated from the Europa Island coral reef ecosystem. *Toxicon* 38: 1043–1054.

Ten-Hage L, Robillot C, Turquet J, Le Gall F, Le Caer J-P, Bultel V, Guyot M, Mogó J (2002) Effects of toxic extracts and purified borbotoxins from *Prorocentrum borbonicum* (Dinophyceae) on vertebrate neuromuscular junctions. *Toxicon* 40: 137–148.

Ten-Hage L, Turquet J, Quod J-P, Puiseux-Dao S, Coute A (2000b) *Prorocentrum borbonicum* sp. nov. (Dinophyceae), a new toxic benthic dinoflagellate from the southwestern Indian Ocean. *Phycologia* 39: 296–301.

Terao K, Ito E, Yanagi T, Yasumoto T (1986) Histopathological studies on experimental marine toxin poisoning. I. Ultrastructural changes in the small intestine and liver of suckling mice induced by dinophysistoxin-1 and pectenotoxin-1. *Toxicon* 24: 1141–1151.

Tillmann U, Elbrächter M, John U, Krock B, Cembella A (2010) *Azadinium obesum* (Dinophyceae), a new nontoxic species in the genus that can produce azaspiracid toxins. *Phycologia* 49: 169–182.

Tillmann U, Elbrächter M, Krock B, John U, Cembella A. (2009) *Azadinium spinosum* gen. et sp. nov. (Dinophyceae) identified as a primary producer of azaspiracid toxins. *Eur. J. Phycol.* 44: 63–79.

Tillmann U, Salas R, Gottschling M, Krock B, O'Driscoll D, Elbrächter M (2012) *Amphidoma languida* sp. nov. (Dinophyceae) reveals a close relationship between *Amphidoma* and *Azadinium*. *Protist* 163: 701–719.

Tindall DR, Dickey RW, Carlson RD, Morey-Gaines G (1984) Ciguatoxigenic dinoflagellates from the Caribbean Sea. In: Ragelis EP (ed.) *Seafood Toxins*. ACS Symposium Series No. 262, American Chemical Society, Washington, DC, pp. 225–240.

Tindall DR, Miller DM, Bomber JW (1989) Culture and toxicity of dinoflagellates from ciguatera endemic regions of the worlds. *Toxicon* 27: 83.

Tindall DR, Miller DM, Tindall PM (1990) Toxicity of *Ostreopsis lenticularis* from the British and United States Virgin Islands. In: Granéli E, Sundström L, Edler L, Anderson DM (eds.) *Toxic Marine Phytoplankton*. Elsevier, New York, pp. 424–429.

Tomas CR, van Wagoner R, Tatters AO, White KD, Hall S, Wright JLC (2012) *Alexandrium peruvianum* (Balech and Mendiola) Balech and Tangen a new toxic species for coastal North Carolina. *Harmful Algae* 17: 54–63.

Torgersen T, Aasen J, Aune T (2005) Diarrhetic shellfish poisoning by okadaic acid esters from brown crabs (*Cancer pagurus*) in Norway. *Toxicon* 46: 572–578.

Tosteson TR, Ballantine DL, Tosteson CG, Bardales AT, Durst HD, Higerd TB (1986) Comparative toxicity of *Gambierdiscus toxicus*, *Ostreopsis* cf. *lenticularis*, and associated microflora. *Mar. Fish. Rev.* 48: 57–59.

Trevino CL, Escobar L, Vaca L, Morales-Tlalpan V, Ocampo AY, Darszon A (2008) Maitotoxin: A unique pharmacological tool for elucidating Ca^{2+}-dependent mechanism. In: Botana LM (ed.) *Seafood and Freshwater Toxins, Pharmacology, Physiology and Detection*. CRC Press, Boca Raton, FL, pp. 503–616.

Tubaro A, Dell'Ovo V, Florio C (2010) Yessotoxins: A toxicological review. *Toxicon* 56: 163–172.

Tubaro A, Sidari L, Della Loggia R, Yasumoto T (1998) Occurrence of homoyessotoxin in phytoplankton and mussels from Northern Adriatic Sea. In: Reguera B, Blanco J, Fernábdez ML, Wyatt T (eds.) *Harmful Algae*. Xunta de Galacia and International Oceanographic Commission of UNESCO, Santiago de Compstela, Spain, pp. 470–472.

Tubaro A, Sosa S, Bornancin A, Hungerford J (2008) Pharmacology and toxicology of diarrhetic shellfish toxins. In: Botana LM (ed.) *Seafood and Freshwater Toxins Pharmacology, Physiology, and Detection*. CRC Press, Boca Raton, FL, pp. 229–253.

Tubaro A, Sosa S, Carbonatto M, Altinier G, Vita F, Melato M, Satake M, Yasumoto T (2003) Oral and intra-peritoneal acute toxicity studies of yessotoxin and homoyessotoxins in mice. *Toxicon* 41: 783–792.

Twiner MJ, Hess P, Dechraoui MY, McMahon T, Samons MS, Satake M, Yasumoto T, Ramsdell JS, Doucette GJ (2005) Cytotoxic and cytoskeletal effects of azaspiracid-1 on mammalian cell lines. *Toxicon* 45: 891–900.

Uemura D, Chou T, Haino T, Nagatsu A, Fukuzawa S, Zheng SZ, Chen HS (1995) Pinnatoxin A: A toxic amphoteric macrocycle from the Okinawan bivalve *Pinna muricata*. *J. Am. Chem. Soc.* 117: 1155–1156.

Ueoka R, Ito A, Izumikawa M, Maeda S, Takagi M, Shin-ya K, Yoshida M, van Soest RWM, Matsunaga S (2009) Isolation of azaspiracids-2 from a marine sponge *Echinoclathria* sp. as a potent cytotoxin. *Toxicon* 53: 680–684.

Usami M, Satake M, Ishida S, Inoue A, Kan Y (1995) Palytoxin analogs from the dinoflagellate *Ostreopsis siamensis*. *J. Am Chem. Soc.* 117: 5389–5390.

Usup G, Ahmad A, Matsuoka K, Lim PT, Leaw CP (2012) Biology, ecology and bloom dynamics of the toxic marine dinoflagellate *Pyrodinium bahamense*. *Harmful Algae* 14: 301–312.

Usup G, Kulis DM, Anderson DM (1994) Growth and toxin production of the toxic dinoflagellate *Pyrodinium bahamense* var. *compressum* in laboratory cultures. *Nat. Toxins* 2: 254–262.

Vale C (2008) Palytoxins: Pharmacology and biological detection methods. In: Botana LM (ed.) *Seafood and Freshwater Toxins, Pharmacology, Physiology, and Detection*. CRC Press, Boca Raton, FL, pp. 675–691.

Vale P (2010) New saxitoxin analogues in the marine environment: Developments in toxin chemistry, detection and transformation during the 2000s. *Phytochem. Rev.* 9: 525–535.

Vandersea MW, Kibler SR, Holland WC, Tester PA, Schultz TF, Faust MA, Holmes MJ, Chinain M, Litaker RW (2012) Development of semi-quantitative PCR assays for the detection and enumeration of *Gambierdiscus* species (Gonyaulacales, Dinophyceae). *J. Phycol.* 48: 902–915.

Van Dolah FM, Fire SE, Leighfield TA, Mikulski CM, Doucette GJ (2012) Determination of paralytic shellfish toxins in shellfish receptor binding assay: Collaborative study. *J. AOAC* 95: 795–812.

Van Wagoner RM, Deeds JR, Satake M, Ribeiro AA, Place AR, Wright JLC (2008) Isolation and character-ization of karlotoxin 1, a new amphipathic toxin from *Karlodinium veneficum*. *Tetrahedron Lett.* 49: 6457–6461.

Van Wagoner RM, Deeds JR, Tatters AO, Place AR, Tomas CR, Wright JLC (2010) Structure and relative potency of several karlotoxins from *Karlodinium veneficum*. *J. Nat. Prod.* 73: 1360–1365.

Van Wagoner RM, Misner I, Tomas CR, Wright JLC (2011) Occurrence of 12 methylgymnodimine in a spiro-lide producing dinoflagellate *Alexandrium peruvianum* and the biogenic implications. *Tetrahedron Lett.* 52: 4243–4246.

Vetter I, Touska F, Hess A, Hinsbey R, Sattler S et al. (2012) Ciguatoxins activate specific cold pain pathways to elicit burning pain from cooling. *EMBO J.* 31: 3795–3808.

Vilariño N, Espiña B (2008) Pharmacology of pectenotoxins. In: Botana LM (ed.) *Seafood and Freshwater Toxins Pharmacology, Physiology and Detection*. CRC Press, Boca Raton, FL, pp. 361–369.

Wiese M, D'Agostino PM, Mihali TK, Moffitt MC, Neilan BA (2010) Neurotoxic alkaloids: Saxitoxin and its analogs. *Mar. Drugs* 8: 2185–2211.

Yanagi T, Murata M, Torigoe K, Yasumoto T (1989) Biological activities of semisynthetic analogs of dinophy-sistoxin-3, the major diarrhetic shellfish toxin. *Agric. Biol. Chem.* 53: 525–529.

Yasumoto T, Bagnis R, Thevenin S, Garcon M (1977a) A survey of comparative toxicity in the food chain of ciguatera. *Bull. Jpn. Soc. Sci. Fish.* 43: 1015–1019.

Yasumoto T, Bagnis R, Vernoux JP (1976) Toxicity of the surgeonfishes-II. Properties of the principal water soluble toxin. *Bull. Jpn. Soc. Sci. Fish.* 42: 359–365.

Yasumoto T, Murata M, Oshima Y, Sano M, Matsumoto GK, Clardy J (1985) Diarrhetic shellfish toxins. *Tetrahedron* 41: 1019–1025.

Yasumoto T, Nakajima I, Bagnis R, Adachi R (1977b) Finding of a dinoflagellate as a likely culprit for ciguatera. *Bull. Jpn. Soc. Sci. Fish.* 43: 1021–1026.

Yasumoto T, Oshima Y, Sugawara W, Fukuyo Y, Oguri H, Igarashi T, Fujita N (1980) Identification of *Dinophysis fortii* as the causative organism of diarrhetic shellfish poisoning. *Bull. Jpn. Soc. Sci. Fish.* 46: 1405–1411.

Yasumoto T, Oshima Y, Yamaguchi M (1978) Occurrence of a new type of shellfish poisoning in the Tohoku district. *Bull. Jpn. Soc. Sci. Fish.* 44: 1249–1255.

Yogi K, Oshiro N, Inafuku Y, Hirama M, Yasumoto T (2011) Detailed LC-MS/MS analysis of ciguatoxins revealing distinct regional and species characteristics in fish and causative alga from the Pacific. *Anal. Chem.* 83: 8886–8891.

Zhou J, Fritz L (1993) Ultrastructure of two toxic marine dinoflagellates, *Prorocentrum lima* and *Prorocentrum maculosum*. *Phycologia* 32: 444–450.

2

Guide to Phycotoxin Monitoring of Bivalve Mollusk-Harvesting Areas

Luis M. Botana

CONTENTS

2.1 Introduction

The sea has been the source of more than 21,000 structurally diverse bioactive natural compounds originated from marine species since 1970,[7] and dinoflagellates were a major source of these compounds.[28] There are about 2000 species of dinoflagellates, half of which perform photosynthesis and about 100 are producers of marine toxins.[40,60,69] Marine toxins, which are secondary metabolites of great potency and undefined biological role,[9,43] accumulate at staggering concentrations in mollusks as a consequence of their fast filter-feeding biology since mollusks feed with dinoflagellates. This accumulation of toxins in the digestive tract of the mollusks, called hepatopancreas, has been recognized as a food safety risk ever since the first intoxications in humans were described.[66,83]

Consequently to this risk, all producing countries must quantify, before putting the molluskan product in the market, the presence of the toxins that could pose a human risk. There are several legislations that regulate the procedural control of the market in order to avoid the toxins to reach the consumers. Depending on the type of commercial product, each country has adapted its legislation to its market. But globalization of markets has triggered a new phenomenon, where local risks are no longer restricted to consumers from the area, as many other markets can be reached by exports of local farming. Therefore, the presence of toxins in one reduced area or may cause intoxications in consumers in another continent. Consequently, control in border inspection laboratories is a fundamental aspect of international trading. Another chapter in this book (Chapter 8) covers the economical significance of international seafood commerce.

The European Union (EU) is the largest consumer of seafood products and therefore a major importer of products from third countries. As a consequence, many third countries implement, in their legislation and control programs, a monitoring surveillance that complies with EU legislation. Another chapter in this book (Chapter 10) shows the system in Asia, using Thailand as a good example of a third country adapting its system to export to Europe. There are several models with regard to international inspections, the European, which is supervised by the Food Veterinary Office (FVO) (http://ec.europa.eu/food/fvo/index_en.cfm), the FDA (http://www.fda.gov/ICECI/Inspections/default.htm), and others (Russia, Korea, Japan, etc.). Since the inspections carried out by the European FVO are available on the web, they provide an international guide as to what is required in terms of equivalency or compliance. A system is equivalent when it provides a similar level of consumer protection, although using a system that may differ philosophically quite a lot; on the other hand, a system is compliant when the exporter partner is implementing the requirements that the importer side demands. An example of equivalency is the United States and the EU: both systems are different, yet commercial trading is in hand. An example of compliance by implementation is Thailand, which has adapted its regulation to fit European regulations.

This chapter will focus mostly on the European system, as the EU is the largest importer of seafood products, and many exporter countries have implemented the European system, which is also mandatory in all countries in Europe.

2.2 Legislation

Official control is clarified in Regulation 882/2004.[18] This regulation, on the introductory remark 17, states that

> "Laboratories involved in the analysis of official samples should work in accordance with internationally approved procedures or criteria based performance standards and use methods of analysis that have as far as possible been validated. Such laboratories should in particular have equipment that enables the correct determination of standards such as maximum residue levels fixed by Community law"

Introductory remarks 18, 19, and 20 explain the need of National Reference Laboratories in European countries, and in countries trading with the EU

> "The designation of Community and national reference laboratories should contribute to a high quality and uniformity of analytical results. This objective can be achieved by activities such as the application of validated analytical methods, ensuring that reference materials are available, the organisation of comparative testing and the training of staff from laboratories. The activities of reference laboratories should cover all the areas of feed and food law and animal health, in particular those areas where there is a need for precise analytical and diagnostic results. For a number of activities related to official controls, the European Committee for Standardisation (CEN) has developed European Standards (EN Standards) appropriate for the purpose of this Regulation. These EN Standards relate in particular to the operation and assessment of testing laboratories and to the operation and accreditation of control bodies. International standards have also been drawn up by the International Organisation for Standardisation (ISO) and the International Union of Pure and Applied Chemistry (IUPAC). These standards might, in certain well defined cases, be appropriate for the purposes of this Regulation, taking into account that performance criteria are laid down in feed and food law in order to ensure flexibility and cost effectiveness."

Article 5 of this Regulation states that competent authorities should designate accredited laboratories for food safety control, and specifically article 12 clarifies the type of accreditation, which is "EN ISO/IEC 17025 on 'General requirements for the competence of testing and calibration laboratories'; EN 45002 on

'General criteria for the assessment of testing laboratories'; EN 45003 on 'Calibration and testing laboratory accreditation system-General requirements for operation and recognition.'"

Basically, most of the countries have this system in place, with a competent authority to coordinate, and a few accredited laboratories for all routine food safety controls. Although the system is clear, sometimes it becomes very difficult to implement it for several reasons: (1) some third countries are too small and do not have an accreditation body and (2) there are not enough laboratories in the country to run yearly proficiency tests. The lack of enough laboratories to perform proficiency tests (also referred to as external quality assessment) is a problem of statistical nature, as a minimum of laboratories are needed to perform statistical analysis of the results, and sometimes there is only one laboratory in the whole country, or not enough to do comparisons in terms of proficiency. Therefore, it is a common solution to do international proficiency tests, organized by specific laboratories of commercial nature (i.e., RIQAS, QUASIMEME, and AOAC), official (i.e., IRMM in the EU and FDA in the United States), by National Reference Laboratories, or by (in the case of the EU) the EU Reference Laboratory for marine biotoxins, which is located in Spain (http://www.aesan.msssi.gob.es/en/CRLMB/web/home.shtml). In some other cases, several countries participate in proficiency exercises organized by one of them; this approach is sometimes utilized in, for example, South America.

2.3 Production

2.3.1 Classified Production Areas

Once the country initiates the process to engage international trading, it must have, within the control system, defined production areas. A production area is a body of water adequately identified by means of satellite marks (GPS), regional maps, and any other means (buoys or anchored floating devices) to allow a precise identification of the boundaries of the water surface where seafood captures take place. Production areas should be defined for all live bivalve mollusks: live echinoderms, live tunicates, and live marine gastropods intended for human consumption, as stated in Regulation 853/2004.[19] The competent authority is responsible for the definition of production areas and their surveillance; hence, the presence of toxic phytoplanktons should trigger a reaction by the authorities to close those production areas with toxins for as long as necessary to ensure consumer food safety. Regulation 853 allows relaying, which is the transfer of seafood from a toxic area to an area without dinoflagellates so that the product is detoxified (see Scheme 2.1).

2.3.2 Nonclassified Production Areas

Some species, given their habitat, cannot be collected from specific classified production areas, as they are located in fishing areas in an open ocean. This is the case for gasteropods, that is, conch (*Strombus gigas*) in Jamaica, or pectinidae, that is, scallops (*Patinopecten* spp.) in Scotland. The circumstances of gasteropods and scallops are very different. Gasteropods are not filter-feeding animals and their accumulation of toxins must be slow, whereas scallops are slow-filter feeding and they take much longer than mussels to both accumulate and release the toxins. This open ocean or nonclassified production area situation and their specific cases are covered in Regulation 505/2010[24] that clarifies that the official controls on pectinidae and live marine gastropods, which are not filter feeders, harvested outside classified production areas are to be carried out in fish auctions, dispatch centers, and processing establishments. Nonetheless, gasteropods are now known to be a source of a new type of intoxication caused by toxins, which are not produced by dinoflagellates, namely, tetrodotoxins, as recently evidenced in *Charonia lampas* in Spain[64] and in several potential vectors in Portugal.[68] Tetrodotoxin-producing fish families (Tetraodontidae, Molidae, Diodontidae, and Canthigasteridae), known to cause human intoxications,[4] are required by Regulation 853 (Annex III, Section VIII, Chapter V, E.1) not to be placed on the market. Since tetrodotoxin from gasteropods is not included in European legislation as a causative source of toxicity in seafood, this is obviously a serious cause of concern.

As for tetrodotoxin, another fish toxin that originates in dinoglagellates is the ciguatoxin group. Regulation 853 (Annex III, Section VIII, Chapter V, E.2) requires the absence of ciguatoxin and other muscle-paralyzing

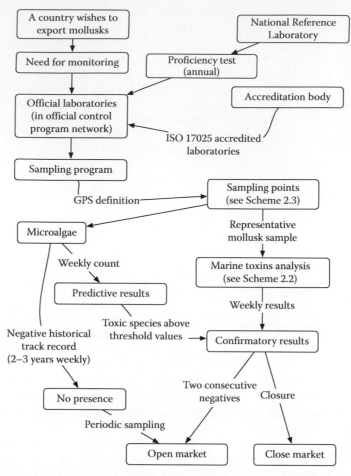

SCHEME 2.1   Programs and conditions to open a market to bivalves.

toxins (brevetoxin), but since there is no specific limit this legal requirement is very difficult to implement. Ciguatoxin has been reported as a causative source of toxicity in Europe,[46] hence again a specific legislation is much needed, in a similar fashion as the US system, where FDA requires maximum specific levels of 0.01 ppb P-CTX-1 equivalents for Pacific ciguatoxin and 0.1 ppb C-CTX-1 equivalent for Caribbean ciguatoxin in reef fish associated with these toxins, namely, barracuda (*Sphyraenidae*), amberjack (*Seriola*), grouper (*Serranidae*), snapper (*Lutjanidae*), po'ou (*Chelinus* spp.), jack (*Carangidae* spp.), travelly (*Caranx* spp.), wrasse (*Labridae* spp.), surgeon fish (*Acanthuridae* spp.), moray eel (*Muraenidae* spp.), roi (*Cephalopholis* spp.), and parrot fish (*Scaridae* spp.) (http://www.fda.gov/downloads/Food/GuidanceRegulation/UCM252395.pdf).

2.4   Sampling in Production Areas

A sampling program is conceived to identify risks related to marine toxins and takes measures to elude their presence on the food chain. Therefore, two types of controls are usually in place, and they are both demanded by legislation, phytoplankton count and monitoring, and analysis of product meat.

2.4.1   Phytoplankton Monitoring

One relevant aspect of a monitoring program is the periodic sampling of the phytoplankton (see Scheme 2.2). The goal of this control is to use the presence of phytoplankton as a predictive measure to ensure

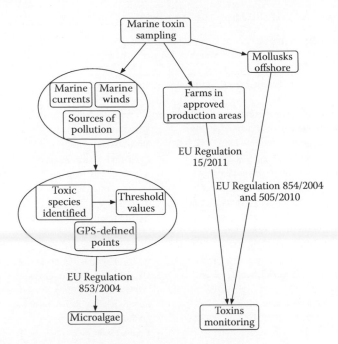

SCHEME 2.2   Parameters that should be controlled in a monitoring program.

that the commercial product is not toxin and has a few days in advance before the algae reach the extraction areas. Therefore, a phytoplankton sampling point should be located in an area of predictive nature, which is usually the one closest to the incoming direction of the water currents. Although this concept is easy to understand, the implementation is far from straightforward. The reason is that sometimes currents around a coastal platform are circular around the production area, sometimes the area is very dependent on tides, and in other occasions the wind counteracts the currents and modifies the displacement of the toxic bloom. As a matter of fact, very few countries are able to have good predictive systems. The frequency of the sampling should be weekly, but a slower pace is allowed if enough studies demonstrate the lack of risk. These studies should be carried out for a period of time, which, depending on the area, should be at least 3 years. All these aspects are covered in Regulation 854/2004.[20]

Given the ecology of some microalgae, the water column to be sampled is very important, as depending on the depths the number of dinoflagellates (or diatoms in the case of domoic acid) may change quite notably. Some laboratories take samples at more than one depth, while others utilize a value that is the average of a sample taken thorough several meters of water depth. How the method is used is a matter of knowing the characteristics of the area of sampling. Once the values of cell counts are increased, precautionary measures, or closures of the areas, should be implemented in the working plan of the authorities and producers. For this, very reliable communication systems between authorities and producers should be defined on the working plan. Depending on the country, the system is different, from automatic linked networks, to communication by fax, telephone, or SMS.

One important technical issue is which species should be monitored, and this will depend greatly on a good knowledge of the ecology of the coastal area; also, threshold values for algae count, above which specific measures are taken, should be defined on the working program. Given the complexity of the taxonomy of microalgae, and for this reason, most of the monitoring programs are linked to oceanographic institutes or university researchers that provide a scientific insight regarding species relevant to the area. Table 2.1 lists the most common genus toxic microalgae, and a complete and up-to-date review is available in this book (Chapter 20).

2.4.2 Meat Monitoring

Although the monitoring of phytoplankton is important, in the end the important aspect for authorities is that the commercial product should be free of toxins. For this, a weekly extraction of the product should

TABLE 2.1

Common Toxic Microalgae

Genus (and Some Examples)	Toxin
Karenia (*K. selliformis, K. bidigitatum, K. mikimotoi, K. brevisulcata*)	Brevetoxins, Cyclic imines
Chatonella (*Ch. antiqua, Ch. marina*)	Brevetoxins
Heterosigma (*H. akashiwo*)	Brevetoxins
Fibrocapsa (*F. japonica*)	Brevetoxins
Gambierdiscus (*G. toxicus, G. pacificus, G. belizeanus, G. australes, G. plynesiensis, G. yasumotoi*)	Ciguatoxins, maitotoxins
Protoceratium (*P. reticulatum* (=*Gonyaulax grindleyi*))	Yessotoxins
Alexandrium[42] (*A. ostenfeldii, A. peruvianum, A. minutum, A. tamarense, A. catenella*)	Saxitoxins, gonyautoxins, cyclic imines (*A. ostenfeldii, A. peruvianum*)[42]
Gymnodinium (*G. catenatum, G. mikimotoi* (=*Karenia mikimotoi*))	Saxitoxins, gonyautoxins, cyclic imines (Gymnodimine (*G. mikimotoi*))
Prorocentrum (*P. lima, P. maculosum, P. micans, P. mexicanum*)	Okadaic acid, dinophysistoxins, cyclic imines (prorocentrolides)
Ostreopsis[14,17,76] (*O. lenticularis, O. ovata, O. siamensis, O. mascareniensis*)	Palytoxins, ostreocins, ovatoxins,[14,17,76] mascarenotoxins
Coolia (*C. monitis*)	Coolia toxins
Amphidinium (*A. carterae*)	Ciguatoxins
Lingulodinium (*L. polyedra* (=*Gonyaulax polyedra*))	Yessotoxins
Gonyaulax (*G. spinifera*)	Yessotoxins
Pseudo nitzschia (*P. australis, P. multiseries, P. seriata*)	Domoic acid
Dinophysis (*D. tripos, D. rotundata, D. sacculus, D. fortii, D. caudata, D. acuminata, D. acuta, D. norvegica, D. mitra*)	Okadaic acid, dinophysistoxins, pectenotoxins
Pyrodinium (*P. bahamense*)	Saxitoxin, gonyautoxins
Phalacroma (*P. rotundata*)	Okadaic acid, dinophysistoxins
Azadinium[34,37] (*A. spinosum*)	Azaspiracids
Vulcanodinium[62] (*V. rugosum*)	Cyclic imines (pinnatoxin)
Amphora (*A. coffeaeformis*)	Domoic acid
Nitzschia (*N. navis-varingica*)	Domoic acid

Note: Unless indicated, taken from reviews for non-DSP,[40] DSP,[60] ASP,[36] cyclic imines,[16] and palytoxin[35]-producing organisms.

be taken from a representative and fixed point in the production area. The weekly control must be done at least during extraction periods when harvesting is allowed (harvesting season), but some countries perform controls all year. As for phytoplankton, risk assessment studies should be performed if the frequency is lower than weekly, so that enough evidence exists to support a fortnightly of even lower frequency. A reasonable study time frame should be at least 3 years.

One risky aspect of marine toxins, in some geographical areas, is that the presence of dinoflagellates may not be a warning sign, and mollusks may become toxic with no clear increase of microalgae counts. On the other side, the warning sign of algae count may not be enough if the income of the bloom is too fast. This is actually rather common in some areas, where from the initial increase in algae numbers to actual presence of toxic meat may elapse only 2 or 3 days; hence, a weekly frequency would not be sufficient to alert and prevent the presence of toxins in the marketed product. The amount of sample to be taken is also important, in order to have enough material left for counteranalysis in case of conflict. It is surprising that the number of cases where no sample is left for counteranalysis after an intoxication was reported in the Rapid Alert Systems (RAS) in Europe or after an alert in third countries.

Another approach taken by some producers or authorities is to have a sentinel, or indicator, specie that accumulate the toxin much faster than the commercial product being extracted, as is the case of mussels in a cage to predict the potential toxicity in clams or scallops, which have a slower toxic accumulation. In any way, the sampling point should be fixed, preferably by GPS coordinates. For each production area, there should be one or more sampling points, depending on the geography of the area, the size, etc. The definition of a sampling point should be the consequence of a study to define previously the condition of the area. A reasonable time frame for the study is 3 years. Sentinel species are also used when the commercial product is very valuable and scarce or is difficult to obtain for a frequent sampling program. It is important to highlight that toxicity should not be present on the commercial product, so that if the indicator species becomes toxic, but the commercial extracted product is not, the area may remain open until the commercial product becomes toxic above the legally defined levels.

Once the toxin is detected above the legal limits, the production area should be closed, and not reopened until "at least two consecutive results below the regulatory limit separated at least 48 hours" are provided[20] (Chapter I, Annex II, C.2).

2.5 Toxin Control

It is Regulation 853, Annex III, Section VII, Chapter V[19] that defines the toxin levels allowed in live bivalve mollusks, before they reach the market: for paralytic shellfish poison (PSP), 800 µg/kg; for amnesic shellfish poison (ASP), 20 mg of domoic acid per kilogram; for okadaic acid, dinophysistoxins, and pectenotoxins together, 160 µg of okadaic acid equivalents per kilogram; for yessotoxins, 3.75 mg of yessotoxin equivalent per kilogram; and for azaspiracids, 160 µg of azaspiracid equivalents per kilogram. It must be highlighted that toxin results should be referred to amounts (micrograms or milligrams) per kilogram of product flesh. Although these toxin limits were the subject of many technical debates, regarding not only the limits but also which toxins should be legally regulated or not (i.e., Canada does not regulate yesstoxins, and some authors claim that cyclic imines may be a risk), a rather complete study was carried out by a working group within the European Food Safety Agency. This working group concluded that toxin limits should be modified and that the mouse bioassay was no longer acceptable. Nevertheless, the lack of sufficient scientific information has prevented the EFSA working group from taking solid conclusions, and basically more information needed was the main conclusion for each of the toxin groups.[47–58] Among the conclusions taken on the working group, the sensitivity of the mouse bioassay was questioned, as reflects the fact that legal levels of the toxins were defined precisely to match the threshold sensitivity of mice. Another important consequence of this working group was to suggest lower toxin levels for some of the toxins, which were below the sensitivity of the bioassay. The European Commission did use the conclusions of the working group to change the reference method from the bioassay to the analytical identification of toxin analogs by mass spectrometry (LC-MS), as indicated in Regulation 15/2011,[61] but toxin levels remained unchanged. After Regulation 15/2011, bioassay and LC-MS will coexist for 3 years, starting in 2011, and after December 2014 LC-MS will be the reference method (see Scheme 2.3).

Since the criteria of the EFSA working group were based on food safety and risk assessment, it is surprising that the toxin levels remained unchanged and still matched the sensitivity of the bioassay when they could be modified to follow EFSA recommendations regarding food safety. Table 2.2 shows that the consumers are not adequately protected with current limits, with the exception of yessotoxin, the risk being higher for saxitoxin and analogs, then azaspiracids, domoic acid, okadaic acid, and pectenotoxins, in this order. Probably the most striking observation of the EFSA working group was that current legislation is defined for a daily consumption of 100 g mollusk flesh, while the available consumption surveys indicate that this value is too low and unrealistic to assess an acute risk, and a daily intake of 400 g would be preferable to cover and protect above 95% of the consumers.[58] This is supported by the observation that the percentage of samples compliant with the EU current limit by exceeding the concentration compatible with ARfD (see Table 2.2) is 32% for okadaic acid and analogs and 25% for saxitoxin and analogs.[50]

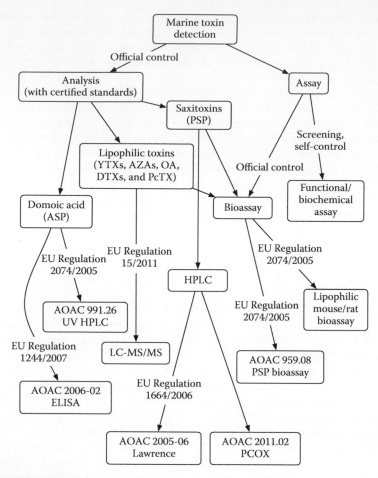

SCHEME 2.3 Legal Regulations for toxins and detection methods. *Note*: YTX levels were increased to 3.75 mg/kg while editing this chapter (Regulation 786/2013).

TABLE 2.2

EFSA Working Group Conclusions on Exposure Levels

Toxin Group	Current Limit (µg/kg Meat)	Exposure with 400 g Meat Intake (µg/Person)	Maximum µg Toxin with 400 g with ARfD Set by EFSA: ARfD (µg/kg b.w.)/Max Concentration (µg/kg Meat)	Ratio (B/A)
AZA	160 (A)	64	0.3/45 (B)	0.28[a]
PTX	160 (A)	64	0.2/30 (B)	0.19[a]
YTX	1 mg (A)	400	25/3.75 mg (B)	3.75[b]
STX	800 (A)	320	0.5/75 (B)	0.09[a]
DA	20 mg (A)	8	30/4.5 mg (B)	0.23[a]

Source: Panel, E.C., *EFSA J.*, 1306, 1, 2009.

Note: Level of protection expressed by ratio B/A:

[a] B/A < 1: current limit protects less than 95% of the population.

[b] B/A > 1: current limit protects more than 95% of the population.

It is very important to highlight the fact that in the end the ultimate responsibility for what reaches the market is the commercial agent (food business operators), so end products must be guaranteed for food safety. For this reason, many commercial agents perform their own checks before the product reaches commercial channels. All methodology and legislation applies to these products (see Chapters 3, 13, and 14 for methodology).

2.5.1 Exceptions

Although toxin levels are determined after extraction and before the product reaches the market, there is one matter for concern that has never been adequately addressed—it is the increase in concentration of the toxins after some products are cooked or steamed for industrial canning or other uses. Since cooking means water loss, the concentration of toxins might be rather high, and products that were extracted within legal toxin limits may become toxic after cooking. The increase in toxin concentration has been reported to be up to twofold.[31] The EFSA working group addressed this issue[47] with a recommendation to include this problem in official control systems.

Another exceptional case is the extraction of scallops with high levels of domoic acid. Scallops have a slow kinetic in both uptake and release of the toxin. The depuration is as low as 0.007/day.[6] As a matter of fact, scallops may become toxic for years when they accumulate domoic acid as a consequence of *Pseudo nitzschia* blooms.[41] Consequently, and to avoid very prolonged periods of closures, there is one regulation[27] that allows the extraction of scallops with toxin limits above 20 mg/kg, but below 250 mg/kg, and to remove the hepatopancreas, where most of the toxin is accumulated, before the product is placed on the market. The product should never contain more than 20 mg/kg in gonads and adductor muscle, while edible parts should not contain more than 4.6 mg/kg, and only approved establishments are allowed for this selective extraction of hepatopancreas of the species allowed, *Pecten jacobeus* and *Pecten maximus*. A similar exception rules for Mediterranean cockle from Spain (*Acanthocardia tuberculata*), which poses a PSP accumulation problem.[5] Regulation 96/77[26] allows extraction of this product above the legal limit of 800 µg/kg and below 3000 µg/kg, for a heat treatment to reduce toxicity, as long as the 800 µg/kg limit is respected after the treatment. The rationale supporting this exception is that heating the meat allows PSP toxin lo leach out into the cooking water and medium, including the canning process; the toxin reduction is as high as 86%.[80]

2.5.2 Bioassays

The mouse bioassay, after many years of being the reference method for marine toxins monitoring, is about to be replaced by chromatographic separation with mass spectrophotometric detection methods (LC-MS). The use of the mouse bioassay is regulated in legislation[22] and has been described in detail in several studies[8,33] and by EFSA.[49,50] It is reported that the mouse bioassay has only a 40% probability to detect okadaic acid and analogs at the current EU limit of 160 µg/kg OA. But the main advantage of the bioassay is its universal detection nature, so that any toxic activity, known or unknown, would be picked up by the method. A never fully clarified case of positive bioassays that took place in France, in Arcachon,[29] has brought about the problem of potential false-positives, and this prompted the proposal of in vitro assays[39,67] that could be used as screening alternatives to the universal detection capability of the mouse bioassay.[10,11,15,81]

The PSP bioassay remains to be the reference method for saxitoxin and analogs.[2] Although this method implies the sacrifice of animals, which is against the directive on animal protection,[25] it is still the only method that can evaluate the complete toxicity of the PSP group (saxitoxin and all its analogs) in a semi-quantitative and rather fast way. Although from a practical approach chromatographic methods as screening are replacing the use of animals in many monitoring laboratories, in the case of a legal challenge, the reference method is the bioassay. A very important precaution to take while doing the PSP bioassay is the control of pH at values around 3, as it has been reported a 10-fold increase in toxicity during acidic extraction of some analogs (C toxins to goniautoxins and goniautoxins to saxitoxins[8,77]). Since the response to the toxins is dependent on the weight, to log the animal weight and the time of death for each assay should be a standard precaution to do the calculations. Also, the use of animals that were not properly calibrated against the toxicity of a standard of saxitoxin or an equivalent amount of an analog is a common misprac-tice. Since each animal strain provides different responses to the same amount of toxin, a reference value for death time versus toxin amount for an animal strain (mouse unit) should be determined with a certain periodicity (6 months to a year) while using the same type of animals.[70]

2.5.2.1 Sample Preparation

Mollusks accumulate the toxins in the digestive tract and, therefore, this part is usually utilized for the extraction of the compounds to be injected on the bioassay. Since mollusks modify quite notably their weight depending on their reproductive cycle, and the season, the weight ratio for whole body/ hepatopancreas may change significantly, and therefore the results are prone to large variations. To avoid this, the European Network of National Reference Laboratories agreed on a harmonized protocol that defines the use of solvents, extraction procedure, and the use of whole body for most of the species, in order to reduce the very large variations on results that were obtained before, that is, by using 10 hepatopancreas or 10 whole bodies (http://www.aesan.msssi.gob.es/en/CRLMB/web/procedimientos_crlmb/ crlmb_standard_operating_procedures.shtml).

2.5.3 Instrumental Analysis

Instrumental analysis of marine toxins by HPLC and mass spectrometry is well described in specific chapters in this book. Liquid chromatography with ultraviolet detection is legally required as a reference method for domoic acid,[21] although an ELISA method has been also approved for this group.[23] Saxitoxin and analogs are required by legislation to be detected, identified, and quantified[22] using an internationally validated method.[21] At this time, two possible methods are validated for fluorescent detection (see Chapter 13 in this book), one precolumn method, developed by Lawrence,[38] then validated for certain matrices and standards,[3] and further extended to more toxins and matrices,[74,75] and another postcolumn,[65] recently validated as well.[78] The postcolumn method is an advance to improve the tedious analysis and limitations of the precolumn method.[63,73] The use of standard toxic equivalent factors for this toxin group was proposed by EFSA[52] on the ground of toxicity studies on the sodium channel and in mice using certified standards[77] (see Scheme 2.3).

The legislation considers the possibility of having new methods for screening and even official control, even though the reference method in case of legal challenge is only one. To have a new method, it is important to follow the IUPAC approach for interlaboratory validation[32] and validate the method through some approval system, such as AOAC (Association of Official Analytical Chemists) or CEN (European Committee for Normalization), which is the European equivalent to ISO (International Standardization Organization). The performance of AOAC makes validation faster and easier to reach than the slow and hard to reach CEN system (the marine toxins working group has been unoperational in CEN in several occasions due to lack of funds, and when active, the meetings took place on a yearly basis). Since CEN has as goal the normalization of methods and standards, there is the paradoxical situation where methods for marine toxins were standardized (i.e., CEN/TC 275/WG 5 HPLC method for PSP toxins (DIN EN 14526)) with limited legal value or actual demand. In any case, a validation process is rather slow and costly, and there is no guarantee of a final success, as the method must prove its robustness in the end. But this is the way to pursue the approval of a new validated method. It is a common error to consider a single laboratory validation[72] as a validation process, and this is not the case. A single laboratory validation is only acceptable to implement the use of a method in house, but must never be regarded as a path to consider a method validated. The more complex the method, the more restrictive the conditions to avoid multiple errors in uncontrolled factors, as it was recently shown[44]; hence, a single laboratory validation can never justify the validity of a method to be used in different locations (see Schemes 2.4 and 2.5).

2.5.3.1 Uncontrolled Factors

The translation of the bioassay to LC-MS[61] has several drawbacks. The unknown toxicity of many toxin analogs as compared to the reference compound creates the first problem, namely, the use of toxic equivalent factors (TEF) to report a set of analogs as one single equivalent amount of reference compound.

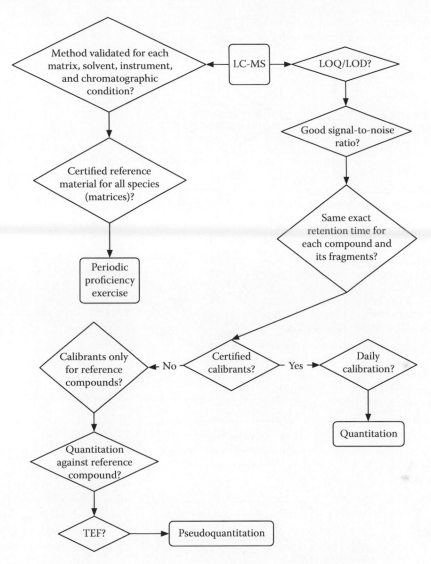

SCHEME 2.4 Decision tree based on availability of standards and TEF values for monitoring.

This problem has been addressed in depth in a review.[12] A second problem related to the use of LC-MS is the need of one standard for each analog to be quantified. Since there are not enough commercial standards for each analog, many analysts quantify several analogs with one single compound, and this has led to very large errors in quantification, up to 200%.[44] A third aspect not resolved by the use of LC-MS is that several uncontrolled factors, such as the ionization source or even the brand of the solvents used for the mobile phase, are also a source of very large fluctuations in results. A fourth source of variation is the need to convert analytical results into toxicological data. Since LC-MS is a targeted technique, where only seeked compounds are identified, any unknown toxin presence would not be acknowledged. As a consequence, the real risk of those toxins not included in the legislation (cyclic imines, tetrodotoxin, palytoxins, and ostreocins) is never studied and therefore not understood (Table 2.3). In the case of cyclic imines, which are known to bind to nicotinic receptors, some of them bind with irreversible unions,[13] and they also bind to muscarinic receptors.[82] Cyclic imines cross the blood–brain barrier very quickly; in only 2 min after its intraperitoneal injection, they are found in brain and remain detectable even 24 h post-administration,[1] and they are absorbed orally.[45] The fact that cyclic imines absorb orally, they reach

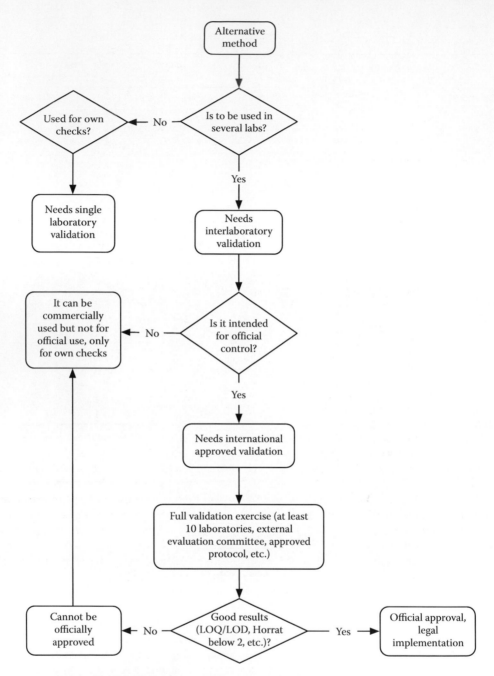

SCHEME 2.5 Decision tree for approval and validation of new methods.

the brain and are not controlled in monitoring programs because legislation does not require so, should be an actual cause for concern in the long term, as the consequences of the combination of oral absorption, irreversible binding, and nicotinic activity are not understood for these compounds. The EFSA working group did not reach a solid conclusion given the lack of information at the time of the report.[56] Nevertheless, experimental evidence supports a sharp decrease of the toxicity, at least for acute toxicity (see Chapter 7), of these compounds in the presence of food.[42]

TABLE 2.3

Advantages and Disadvantages of LC-MS versus Bioassay

	LC-MS Advantage	LC-MS Disadvantage	Bioassay Advantage	Bioassay Disadvantage
Analytical profile	Best approach	Identifies only targeted compounds	Provides amount estimation of all toxic compounds	Cannot give profile, only toxin group
Toxicity	No advantage	Problems with use of TEF[12]	Gives total toxicity	Toxicity may not be caused by toxic compounds (false-positives)
Quantification	Good for targeted compounds	Large errors due to uncontrolled factors[44]	Good for total toxicity[30]; PSP method is very reproducible	Little information on source of toxicity (based on extraction method)
Method	Several validated methods, EU RL and Refs.[71,79]	Difficult to harmonize results from each method	Several protocols, but one harmonized protocol available at EU RL web page	Difficult to harmonize results specially for lipophilic toxins
Matrix	No advantage	Result is very dependent on matrix used	The bioassay result is less dependent on the matrix used	Salt concentration may cause false-positives

2.5.3.2 Standards

Chapter 15 covers the important aspect of using and elaborating certified reference standards of marine toxins for monitoring purposes. To date, the only commercial supplier of certified standards in Europe is CIFGA (www.cifga.com), and outside Europe the NRC in Canada. A certified calibrant is that one for which the amount and stability is documented by proper studies. This is a very important aspect of the use of analytical methods to monitor the presence of very toxin compounds, in terms of food safety. If the standard used is not certified (which means a stability study and an accredited way to demonstrate the amount contained in the recipient), the errors in the final results could be very important, and this would increase notably food safety risks, most notably false-negative-biased results that allow toxic products to reach the market. As an example of products bought in our laboratory from commercial noncertified sources, we found 5 mg domoic acid to be really 7.2 mg, and 1 mg okadaic acid to be 400 µg. These variations are rather common and highlight the need of quality-certified calibrants. One very important consequence of this variation on the precise concentration of toxin, depending on the brand, is the toxicological information available.[9] The LD_{50} calculations in toxicology usually require rather large amounts, and for cost reasons, the toxins used are rarely certified materials. Given the variation of concentrations found in noncertified commercial sources, the toxicological results can differ quite notably, as it is commonly observed. The dispersion of results was already noted by the EFSA working group, and it is in fact an important aspect to keep in mind for the future.

The use of certified calibrants is so important that all accreditation systems require daily calibrations of the instruments, and even this measure cannot avoid biased results caused by uncontrolled factors.[44] Also, it is rather important the matrix effect, which any method must evaluate by means of recovery and spiking studies. To date, most of the available matrices are provided by the NRC, and they are cooked. Since the monitoring tasks are carried out with noncooked matrices, there is a bias in the validation process with respect to real samples. There will be soon noncooked matrices available, which will allow a proper calibration of the extraction procedure (see Chapter 15).

2.5.3.3 Live Bivalves versus Processed Products

European legislation has been defined for the control of live bivalves. Once the product is processed, the loss of water, and the physical change on the matrix may modify the nature of the results, and the legislation is not adequately written for this situation. Therefore, there are several causes that may provide results that are difficult to interpretate. One cause, very common, is the matrix: matrix effect has been recognized as a complex issue in marine toxin analysis; hence, it should always be addressed in any monitoring program. Most of the validations are carried out with the commercially frequent matrices, but given the wide diversity of species worldwide, it is rather common that a method is applied to a specie for which no validation was performed, and this may change the results quite notably. Therefore, in-house validations for each matrix should at least be done to identify the performance of a method in any given product.[32] The performance in the use of LC-MS as a routine method has to be carefully defined in pre-processed or processed products, as lipophilic toxins are determined from hepatopancreas, and processed products, which many times are canned in oil, may leak the compounds to the oil.[59] Also, as mentioned before, the loss of water and the consequent concentration of the compounds during cooking/canning is a fundamental source of analytical variations in processed products.

2.5.3.4 Consolidated Versions

It is rather complex to follow the modifications in European legislation. As a consequence, each of the legal requirements, such as Regulations 15/2011, 1224/2007, 1664/2006, etc., is incorporated into the last version of the Regulation they modify, in this case Regulation 2074/2005. Therefore, the easiest approach to understand the most current text of any Regulation is to download from the Commission legal website the so-called *Consolidated Version*, which incorporates all previous modifications. Consequently, the current consolidated version of Regulation 2074 shows already each previous legal change regarding methods to use; likewise, the same applies to Regulation 853 or 854.

REFERENCES

1. Alonso, E., Otero, P., Vale, C. et al. 2013. Benefit of 13-desmethyl spirolide C treatment in triple transgenic mouse model of Alzheimer disease: Beta-amyloid and neuronal markers improvement. *Curr Alzheimer Res*, 10, 279–289.
2. AOAC. 2005. AOAC official method 959.08 paralytic shellfish poison. Biological method. First action 1959. Final action. *Official Methods of Analysis of the AOAC*, Gaithersburg, Maryland, Method 49.10.01.
3. AOAC. 2005. Method 2005.06: Paralytic shellfish poisoning toxins in shellfish. Prechromatographic oxidation and liquid chromatography with fluorescence detection. *Official Methods of Analysis of the Association of Official Analytical Chemists*, Method 2005.06, First Action.
4. Awada, A., Chalhoub, V., Awada, L., and Yazbeck, P. 2010. Deep non-reactive reversible coma after a Mediterranean neurotoxic fish poisoning. *Rev Neurol* (Paris), 166, 337–340.
5. Berenguer, J. A., Gonzalez, L., Jimenez, I. et al. 1993. The effect of commercial processing on the paralytic shellfish poison (PSP) content of naturally-contaminated *Acanthocardia tuberculatum* L. *Food Addit Contam*, 10, 217–230.
6. Blanco, J., Acosta, C. P., Bermudez De La Puente, M., and Salgado, C. 2002. Depuration and anatomical distribution of the amnesic shellfish poisoning (ASP) toxin domoic acid in the king scallop Pecten maximus. *Aquat Toxicol*, 60, 111–121.
7. Blunt, J. W., Copp, B. R., Hu, W. P. et al. 2009. Marine natural products. *Nat Prod Rep*, 26, 170–244.
8. Botana, L. M. 2008. The mouse bioassay as a universal detector. In: Botana, L. M. (ed.) *Seafood and Freshwater Toxins: Pharmacology, Physiology and Detection*, 2nd edn. Boca Raton, FL: CRC Press (Taylor & Francis Group).
9. Botana, L. M. 2012. A perspective on the toxicology of marine toxins. *Chem Res Toxicol*, 25, 1800–1804.
10. Botana, L. M., Louzao, M. C., Alfonso, A. et al. (eds.) 2011. *Measurement of Algal Toxins in the Environment*. Chichester, U.K.: John Wiley & Sons Ltd.
11. Botana, L. M., Vieytes, M. R., Botana, A. M., Vale, C., and Vilariño, N. 2012. Biological methods for detection of phycotoxins: Bioassays and in vitro assays. In: Cabado, A. G. and Vieites, J. M. (eds.) *New Trends in Marine and Freshwater Toxins*. New York: Nova Science Publishers, Inc.

12. Botana, L. M., Vilariño, N., Elliott, C. T. et al. 2010. The problem of toxicity equivalent factors in developing alternative methods to animal bioassays for marine toxin detection. *Trends Anal Chem*, 29, 1316–1325.

13. Bourne, Y., Radic, Z., Araoz, R. et al. 2010. Structural determinants in phycotoxins and AChBP conferring high affinity binding and nicotinic AChR antagonism. *Proc Natl Acad Sci USA*, 107, 6076–6081.

14. Cagide, E., Louzao, M. C., Espina, B. et al. 2009. Production of functionally active palytoxin-like compounds by Mediterranean Ostreopsis cf. siamensis. *Cell Physiol Biochem*, 23, 431–440.

15. Campbell, A., Vilariño, N., Botana, L. M., and Elliott, C. T. 2011. A European perspective on progress in moving away from the mouse bioassay for marine-toxin analysis. *Trends Anal Chem*, 30, 239–253.

16. Cembella, A. and Krock, B. 2008. Cyclic imine toxins: Chemistry, biogeography, biosynthesis and pharmacology. In: Botana, L. M. (ed.) *Seafood and Freshwater Toxins: Pharmacology, Physiology and Detection*, 2nd edn. Boca Raton, FL: CRC Press (Taylor & Francis Group).

17. Ciminiello, P., Dell'aversano, C., Fattorusso, E. et al. 2008. Putative palytoxin and its new analogue, ovatoxin-a, in *Ostreopsis ovata* collected along the Ligurian coasts during the 2006 toxic outbreak. *J Am Soc Mass Spectrom*, 19, 111–120.

18. Commission, E. 2004. Commission Regulation (EC) No 882/2004 of 29 April 2004 on official controls performed to ensure the verification of compliance with feed and food law, animal health and animal welfare rules. *Off J Eur Union*, L165, 1–141.

19. Commission, E. 2004. Regulation (EC) No 853/2004 of the European Parliament and of the Council of 29 April 2004 laying down specific hygiene rules for food of animal origin. *Off J Eur Union*, L226, 22–82.

20. Commission, E. 2004. Regulation (EC) No 854/2004 of the European Parliament and of the Council of 29 April 2004 laying down specific rules for the organisation of official controls on products of animal origin intended for human consumption. *Off J Eur Union*, L226, 83–127.

21. Commission, E. 2005. Commission Regulation (EC) No 2074/2005 of 5 December 2005 laying down implementing measures for certain products under Regulation (EC) No 853/2004 of the European Parliament and of the Council and for the organisation of official controls under Regulation (EC) No 854/2004 of the European Parliament and of the Council and Regulation (EC) No 882/2004 of the European Parliament and of the Council, derogating from Regulation (EC) No 852/2004 of the European Parliament and of the Council and amending Regulations (EC) No 853/2004 and (EC) No 854/2004. *Off J Eur Union*, L338, 27–59.

22. Commission, E. 2006. Commission Regulation (EC) No 1664/2006 of 6 November 2006 amending Regulation (EC) No 2074/2005 as regards implementing measures for certain products of animal origin intended for human consumption and repealing certain implementing measures. *Off J Eur Union*, L320, 13–45.

23. Commission, E. 2007. Commission Regulation (EC) No 1244/2007 of 24 October 2007 amending Regulation (EC) No 2074/2005 as regards implementing measures for certain products of animal origin intended for human consumption and laying down specific rules on official controls for the inspection area. *Off J Eur Union*, L281, 12–18.

24. Commission, E. 2010. Commission Regulation (EU) No 505/2010 of 14 June 2010 amending Annex II to Regulation (EC) No 854/2004 of the European Parliament and of the Council laying down specific rules for the organisation of officials controls on products of animal origin intended for human consumption. *Off J Eur Comm*, L149, 1–2.

25. Communities, E. 1986. Council Directive of 24 November 1986 on the approximation of laws, regulations and administrative provisions of the Member States regarding the protection of animals used for experimental and other scientific purposes (86/609/EEC). *Off J Eur Comm*, L358, 1–29.

26. Communities, T. C. O. T. E. 1997. 96/77/EC: Commission Decision of 18 January 1996 establishing the conditions for the harvesting and processing of certain bivalve molluscs coming from areas where the paralytic shellfish poison level exceeds the limit laid down by Council Directive 91/492/EEC. *Off J Eur Comm*, L15, 46–47.

27. Communities, T. C. O. T. E. 2002. Commission decision of 15 March 2002 establishing special health checks for the harvesting and processing of certain bivalve molluscs with a level of amnesic shellfish poison (ASP) exceeding the limit laid down by Council Directive 91/492/EEC. *Off J Eur Comm*, L75, 65–66.

28. Gallardo-Rodriguez, J., Sanchez-Miron, A., Garcia-Camacho, F. et al. 2012. Bioactives from microalgal dinoflagellates. *Biotechnol Adv*, 30, 1673–1684.

29. Gueguen, M., Amiard, J. C., Arnich, N. et al. 2011. Shellfish and residual chemical contaminants: Hazards, monitoring, and health risk assessment along French coasts. *Rev Env Contamin Toxicol*, 213, 55–111.

30. Hess, P., Butter, T., Petersen, A., Silke, J., and Mcmahon, T. 2009. Performance of the EU-harmonised mouse bioassay for lipophilic toxins for the detection of azaspiracids in naturally contaminated mussel (*Mytilus edulis*) hepatopancreas tissue homogenates characterised by liquid chromatography coupled to tandem mass spectrometry. *Toxicon*, 53, 713–722.

31. Hess, P., Nguyen, L., Aasen, J. et al. 2005. Tissue distribution, effects of cooking and parameters affecting the extraction of azaspiracids from mussels, *Mytilus edulis*, prior to analysis by liquid chromatography coupled to mass spectrometry. *Toxicon*, 46, 62–71.

32. IUPAC. 1989. Guidelines for collaborative study of procedure to validate characteristics of a method of analysis. *J Assoc Off Anal Chem*, 72, 694–704.

33. James, K. J., Bishop, A. G., Carmody, E. P., and Kelly, S. S. 2000. Enteric toxic episodes. Detection methods for okadaic acid and analogues. In: Botana, L. M. (ed.) *Seafood and Freshwater Toxins: Pharmacology, Physiology and Detection*. New York: Marcel Dekker.

34. Jauffrais, T., Herrenknecht, C., Sechet, V. et al. 2012. Quantitative analysis of azaspiracids in Azadinium spinosum cultures. *Anal Bioanal Chem*, 403, 833–846.

35. Katikou, P. 2008. Palytoxin and analogues: Ecobiology and origin, chemistry, metabolism, and chemical analysis. In: Botana, L. M. (ed.) *Seafood and Freshwater Toxins: Pharmacology, Physiology and Detection*, 2nd edn. Boca Raton, FL: CRC Press (Taylor & Francis Group).

36. Kotaki, Y. 2008. Ecobiology of ammesic shellfish toxin producing diatoms. In: Botana, L. M. (ed.) *Seafood and Freshwater Toxins: Pharmacology, Physiology and Detection*, 2nd edn. Boca Raton, FL: CRC Press (Taylor & Francis Group).

37. Krock, B., Tillmann, U., John, U., and Cembella, A. 2008. LC-MS-MS aboard ship: Tandem mass spectrometry in the search for phycotoxins and novel toxigenic plankton from the North Sea. *Anal Bioanal Chem*, 392, 797–803.

38. Lawrence, J. F., Niedzwiadek, B., and Menard, C. 2005. Quantitative determination of paralytic shellfish poisoning toxins in shellfish using prechromatographic oxidation and liquid chromatography with fluorescence detection: Collaborative study. *J AOAC Int*, 88, 1714–1732.

39. Ledreux, A., Serandour, A. L., Morin, B. et al. 2012. Collaborative study for the detection of toxic compounds in shellfish extracts using cell-based assays. Part II: Application to shellfish extracts spiked with lipophilic marine toxins. *Anal Bioanal Chem*, 403, 1995–2007.

40. Mackenzie, L. 2008. Ecobiology of the brevetoxin, ciguatoxin and cyclic imine producers. In: Botana, L. M. (ed.) *Seafood and Freshwater Toxins: Pharmacology, Physiology and Detection*, 2nd edn. Boca Raton, FL: CRC Press (Taylor & Francis Group).

41. Mauriz, A. and Blanco, J. 2010. Distribution and linkage of domoic acid (amnesic shellfish poisoning toxins) in subcellular fractions of the digestive gland of the scallop Pecten maximus. *Toxicon*, 55, 606–611.

42. Munday, R., Quilliam, M. A., Leblanc, P. et al. 2012. Investigations into the toxicology of spirolides, a group of marine phycotoxins. *Toxins*, 4, 1–14.

43. Nicolaou, K. C., Frederick, M. O., and Aversa, R. J. 2008. The continuing saga of the marine polyether biotoxins. *Angew Chem*, 47, 7182–7225.

44. Otero, P., Alfonso, A., Alfonso, C. et al. 2011. Effect of uncontrolled factors in a validated liquid chromatography-tandem mass spectrometry method question its use as a reference method for marine toxins: Major causes for concern. *Anal Chem*, 83, 5903–5911.

45. Otero, P., Alfonso, A., Rodriguez, P. et al. 2012. Pharmacokinetic and toxicological data of spirolides after oral and intraperitoneal administration. *Food Chem Toxicol*, 50, 232–237.

46. Otero, P., Perez, S., Alfonso, A. et al. 2010. First toxin profile of ciguateric fish in Madeira Arquipelago (Europe). *Anal Chem*, 82, 6032–6039.

47. Panel, E. C. 2008. Influence of processing on the levels of lipophilic marine biotoxins in bivalve molluscs. Statement of the Panel on Contaminants in the Food Chain. *EFSA J*, 1016, 1–10.

48. Panel, E. C. 2008. Opinion of the Scientific Panel on Contaminants in the Food Chain on a request from the European Commission on Marine Biotoxins in Shellfish—Azaspiracids. *EFSA J*, 723, 1–52.

49. Panel, E. C. 2008. Opinion of the Scientific Panel on Contaminants in the Food Chain on a request from the European Commission on Marine Biotoxins in Shellfish—Okadaic acid and analogues. *EFSA J*, 589, 1–62.

50. Panel, E. C. 2008. Scientific opinion on marine biotoxins in shellfish—Yessotoxin group. EFSA Panel on Contaminants in the Food Chain (CONTAM). *EFSA J*, 907, 1–62.
51. Panel, E. C. 2009. Marine biotoxins in shellfish—Summary on regulated marine biotoxins. Scientific opinion of the panel on contaminants in the food chain. *EFSA J*, 1306, 1–23.
52. Panel, E. C. 2009. Opinion of the Scientific Panel on Contaminants in the Food Chain on a request from the European Commission on Marine Biotoxins in Shellfish—Saxitoxin group. *EFSA J*, 1019, 1–76.
53. Panel, E. C. 2009. Scientific opinion on marine biotoxins in shellfish—Domoic acid. EFSA Panel on Contaminants in the Food Chain (CONTAM). *EFSA J*, 1181, 1–61.
54. Panel, E. C. 2009. Scientific opinion on marine biotoxins in shellfish—Palytoxin group. EFSA Panel on Contaminants in the Food Chain (CONTAM). *EFSA J*, 7, 1393–1431.
55. Panel, E. C. 2009. Scientific opinion on marine biotoxins in shellfish—Pectenotoxin group. EFSA Panel on Contaminants in the Food Chain (CONTAM). *EFSA J*, 1109, 1–47.
56. Panel, E. C. 2010. Scientific opinion on marine biotoxins in shellfish—Cyclic imines (spirolides, gymnodimines, pinnatoxins and pteriatoxins). EFSA Panel on Contaminants in the Food Chain (CONTAM). *EFSA J*, 8, 1628–1667.
57. Panel, E. C. 2010. Scientific opinion on marine biotoxins in shellfish—Emerging toxins: Ciguatoxin-group toxins. EFSA Panel on Contaminants in the Food Chain. *EFSA J*, 8, 1627–1665.
58. Panel, E. C. 2010. Statement on further elaboration of the consumption figure of 400 g shellfish meat on the basis of new consumption data. EFSA Panel on Contaminants in the Food Chain (CONTAM). *EFSA J*, 8, 1706–1726.
59. Reboreda, A., Lago, J., Chapela, M. J. et al. 2010. Decrease of marine toxin content in bivalves by industrial processes. *Toxicon*, 55, 235–243.
60. Reguera, B. and Pizarro, G. 2008. Planktonic dinoflagellates that contain polyether toxins of the old "DSP complex." In: Botana, L. M. (ed.) *Seafood and Freshwater Toxins: Pharmacology, Physiology and Detection*, 2nd edn. Boca Raton, FL: CRC Press (Taylor & Francis Group).
61. Regulation, C. 2011. Commission Regulation (EU) No 15/2011 of 10 January 2011 amending Regulation (EC) No 2074/2005 as regards recognised testing methods for detecting marine biotoxins in live bivalve molluscs. *Off J Eur Comm*, L6, 3–4.
62. Rhodes, L., Smith, K., Selwood, A. et al. 2011. Dinoflagellate *Vulcanodinium rugosum* identified as the causative organism of pinnatoxins in Australia, New Zealand and Japan. *Phycologia*, 50, 624–628.
63. Rodriguez, P., Alfonso, A., Botana, A. M., Vieytes, M. R., and Botana, L. M. 2010. Comparative analysis of pre- and post-column oxidation methods for detection of paralytic shellfish toxins. *Toxicon*, 56, 448–457.
64. Rodriguez, P., Alfonso, A., Vale, C. et al. 2008. First toxicity report of tetrodotoxin and 5,6,11-trideoxyTTX in the trumpet shell Charonia lampas lampas in Europe. *Anal Chem*, 80, 5622–5629.
65. Rourke, W. A., Murphy, C. J., Pitcher, G. et al. 2008. Rapid postcolumn methodology for determination of paralytic shellfish toxins in shellfish tissue. *J AOAC Int*, 91, 589–597.
66. Schantz, E. J. 1979. Poisonous dinoflagellates. In: *Biochemistry and Physiology of Protozoa*. New York: Academic Press Inc.
67. Serandour, A. L., Ledreux, A., Morin, B. et al. 2012. Collaborative study for the detection of toxic compounds in shellfish extracts using cell-based assays. Part I: Screening strategy and pre-validation study with lipophilic marine toxins. *Anal Bioanal Chem*, 403, 1983–1993.
68. Silva, M., Azevedo, J., Rodriguez, P. et al. 2012. New gastropod vectors and tetrodotoxin potential expansion in temperate waters of the Atlantic Ocean. *Mar Drugs*, 10, 712–726.
69. Smayda, T. 1997. Harmful algal blooms: Their ecophysiology and general relevance to phytoplankton blooms in the sea. *Limnol Oceanogr*, 42, 1137–1153.
70. Sommer, H. and Meyer, K. F. 1937. Paralytic shellfish poisoning. *Arch Path*, 24, 560–598.
71. These, A., Klemm, C., Nausch, I., and Uhlig, S. 2011. Results of a European interlaboratory method validation study for the quantitative determination of lipophilic marine biotoxins in raw and cooked shellfish based on high-performance liquid chromatography-tandem mass spectrometry. Part I: Collaborative study. *Anal Bioanal Chem*, 399, 1245–1256.
72. Thompson, M., Ellison, S., and Wood, R. 2002. Harmonized guidelines for single-laboratory validation of methods of analysis. *Pure Appl Chem*, 74, 835–855.
73. Turner, A. D., Hatfield, R. G., Rapkova, M. et al. 2011. Comparison of AOAC 2005.06 LC official method with other methodologies for the quantitation of paralytic shellfish poisoning toxins in UK shellfish species. *Anal Bioanal Chem*, 399, 1257–1270.

74. Turner, A. D., Hatfield, R. G., Rapkova-Dhanji, M. et al. 2010. Single-laboratory validation of a refined AOAC HPLC method 2005.06 for oysters, cockles, and clams in U.K. shellfish. *J AOAC Int*, 93, 1482–1493.
75. Turner, A. D., Norton, D. M., Hatfield, R. G. et al. 2009. Refinement and extension of AOAC Method 2005.06 to include additional toxins in mussels: Single-laboratory validation. *J AOAC Int*, 92, 190–207.
76. Ukena, T., Satake, M., Usami, M. et al. 2001. Structure elucidation of ostreocin D, a palytoxin analog isolated from the dinoflagellate *Ostreopsis siamensis*. *Biosci Biotechnol Biochem*, 65, 2585–2588.
77. Vale, C., Alfonso, A., Vieytes, M. R. et al. 2008. In vitro and in vivo evaluation of paralytic shellfish poisoning toxin potency and the influence of the pH of extraction. *Anal Chem*, 80, 1770–1776.
78. Van De Riet, J., Gibbs, R. S., Muggah, P. M. et al. 2011. Liquid chromatography post-column oxidation (PCOX) method for the determination of paralytic shellfish toxins in mussels, clams, oysters, and scallops: Collaborative study. *J AOAC Int*, 94, 1154–1176.
79. Van Den Top, H. J., Gerssen, A., Mccarron, P., and Van Egmond, H. P. 2011. Quantitative determination of marine lipophilic toxins in mussels, oysters and cockles using liquid chromatography-mass spectrometry: Inter-laboratory validation study. *Food Additives Contamin*, 28, 1745–1757.
80. Vieites, J. M., Botana, L. M., Vieytes, M. R., and Leira, F. J. 1999. Canning process that diminishes paralytic shellfish poison in naturally contaminated mussels (*Mytilus galloprovincialis*). *J Food Prot*, 62, 515–519.
81. Vilarino, N., Louzao, M. C., Vieytes, M. R., and Botana, L. M. 2010. Biological methods for marine toxin detection. *Anal Bioanal Chem*, 397, 1673–1681.
82. Wandscheer, C. B., Vilarino, N., Espina, B., Louzao, M. C., and Botana, L. M. 2010. Human muscarinic acetylcholine receptors are a target of the marine toxin 13-desmethyl C spirolide. *Chem Res Toxicol*, 23, 1753–1761.
83. Yasumoto, T. 2000. Historic considerations regarding seafood safety. In: Botana, L. M. (ed.) *Seafood and Freshwater Toxins: Pharmacology, Physiology and Detection*. New York: Marcel Dekker.

3

Marker Compounds, Relative Response Factors, and Toxic Equivalent Factors

Paz Otero and Paula Rodríguez

CONTENTS

3.1 Marker Compounds and Toxic Equivalent Factors

3.1.1 General Considerations

The risk associated with the consumption of shellfish has lead the authorities worldwide to install monitoring systems that prevent toxic shellfish from reaching the markets and intoxicate the consumers. The marine toxin monitoring has become an important issue not only from a health perspective but also from the economic point of view since the presence of toxins in controlled waters gives rise to the closure of the production areas, with the consequent economic losses. It is therefore important to spend as little time as possible in the analysis and interpretation of the results using rapid and effective detection methods to avoid a distortion of the placement of commercial products in the market. For many years, the mousse bioassay (MBA) has been considered as the reference monitoring method for marine toxins (both hydrophilic and lipophilic toxins).[1] It was used for the first time to analyze paralytic shellfish poisoning (PSP) toxins from acid extracts of mussels in 1937[2] and then the protocol was standardized and validated by an intercomparative study. Today this method is considered the reference detection method for PSP toxins, and it is used in the monitoring programs all over the world.[3] The MBA for lipophilic toxins was developed by Yasumoto and has been used until now as a universal detection method for lipophilic compounds.[4] However, in the last few years, the European Legislation established to be in accordance with animal health protection all possible replacement, and reduction of animals must be taken into account when biological methods are used.[1] Moreover, the MBA began to be not considered an appropriate tool for control purposes due to the high variability in the results, the insufficient detection capability, and the limited specificity.[5] Following these premises, in the last decade, laboratories had developed analytical methods, mainly in vitro assays (cell, receptor, enzymatic inhibition, and immunoassays) and chemical methods including high performance-liquid chromatography (HPLC), with ultraviolet (UV), fluorescence (FL), and mass spectrometric (MS) detection.[6] However, despite the great effort made in the development of the sensitive and effective in vitro alternatives methods to MBA,[7–12] none of these is legally admitted for the control of marine toxins with the exception of the enzyme-linked immunoabsorption assay (ELISA) for the official control of DA in shellfish for human consumption.[13] In general, there is a clear tendency of the substitution of MBA for chromatographic techniques. In fact, in 2011, the European legislation defined the chromatographic techniques

TABLE 3.1

Legislated Toxins in the UE, Official Detection Methods, and Maximum Toxic Limits for Each Toxin Group

	Toxin Groups	Official Methods	Legislated Toxins	Limits
Hydrophilic	DA	HPLC, ELISA	<u>DA</u> and analogs (iso-DA A, D, E, F, and epi-DA)	20 mg DA/kg
	STX	HPLC, MBA	<u>STX</u> and analogs (dcSTX, GTX-1,4, GTX-2,3, GTX-5, C1,2, C3,4, NEO)	0.8 mg eq STX/kg
Lipophilic	YTXs	MBA, LC-MS/MS	<u>YTX</u>, 45-OH-DTX, homoYTX, 45-homoYTX	1 mg eq YTX/kg
	AZAs		<u>AZA-1</u>, AZA-2, AZA-3	0.16 mg eq AZA-1/kg
	OA		<u>OA</u>, DTX-1, DTX-2, DTX-3	0.16 mg eq OA/kg
	PTXs		PTX-1, <u>PTX-2</u>	

Note: The reference compound of each group is underlined.

coupled to mass spectrometry as the reference method to replace the MBA to detect the lipophilic marine toxins and in order to allow member states to adapt their method to the chemical method, a transition period of 3 years was fixed. After this period, in 2014, the biological methods should be used as a matter of routine and only during the periodic monitoring of production areas for detecting new or unknown marine toxins.[14] Today, European Union (EU) legislation recognizes different detection methods for some marine toxins but many of them are not legislated. Table 3.1 summarizes the regulated marine toxins, the official methods for their detection and the maximum limits in mollusks according to the present legal values. For a routine monitoring control, experts on biotoxins consider that it is not practical to fully determine the presence of all toxin levels in the mollusks. Only a few analogs are legislated, and most of them have to be referred to a predominant compound of the group named reference compound (RC). If no toxic adequate information about a compound is available, it is proposed that new analogs present in shellfish at less than 5% of the RC should not be regulated.[15] Thus, independently of the method employed, analytical data should be expressed as milligrams of the RC equivalents per kilogram of whole flesh. Therefore, to measure the toxicity of a sample, it is usually employed a value that shows the relative potency of each compound compared to the toxicity of the RC in the group. This ratio of toxic potencies is named the toxic relative toxicity factor or toxic equivalent factor (TEF). In the case of chromatographic methods, these values are necessary to translate the analytical result in a general toxic value. For instance, in the case of AZA group, results should be expressed as milligrams of AZA-1 equivalents per kilogram of whole flesh, using TEFs for AZA-2 and AZA-3, and the other AZA analogs are considered for low relevance.

Unlike the analytical methods that provide information on the toxic profile of a sample, the functional methods give an overall toxic value of a group of compounds. These have the advantage of being high-throughput screening methods and also detecting novel toxins while there is no need for applying TEF values. However, since false positives or negatives can occur due to the matrix effect, it is complex and difficult to develop a functional assay that embraces all lipophilic or hydrophilic toxins in a single test. Therefore, both analytical and functional methods should be combined to give complete information of a sample. As summarized in Scheme 3.1, the analytical methods need TEFs to give the toxic value of a sample and, to achieve these values, high quantities of standards of both reference compound and analogs are required to carry out toxicological studies and to define the TEF for each compound. If the toxicological data obtained by different methods allow to prove the equivalent TEF values, these could be used on the validation of a method.

3.1.2 Lipophilic Marine Toxin Detection

The LC-MS/MS technique has been used for many years for the detection of lipophilic marine toxins in different molluscan shellfish matrices such as mussel, clams, or cockles.[16–18] Most of LC-MS/MS methods were focused on the identification of new analogs in algae or shellfish or in the elucidation of the structure

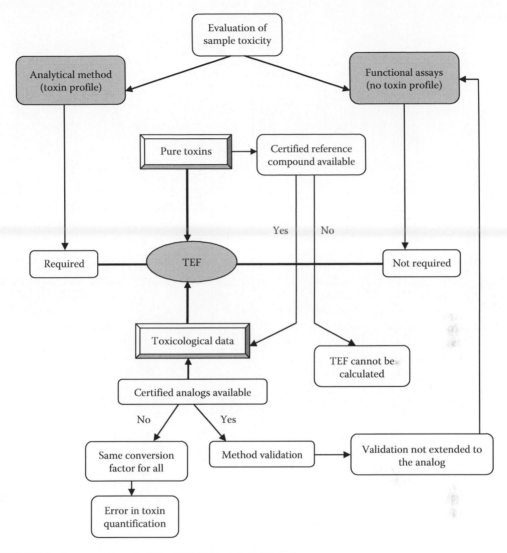

SCHEME 3.1 Necessary items to define TEF for analytical approach.

of new compounds.[19–21] Nonetheless, in the last decade, LC-MS/MS multitoxin methods have been in development with the aim of detecting the most representative compounds of the AZA, YTX, PTX, cyclic imines (CI), and OA group toxins in a short period of time. These methods use reverse phase chromatography on a C8 or C18 silica column and isocratic or gradient elution with acetonitrile (ACN)/water mobile phases containing volatile modifiers such as acetic acid, formic acid, ammonium formate, or ammonium acetate. LC-MS/MS technology has been evaluated, and it is considered to be successful by many laboratories for the control of lipophilic marine toxins. Toxins can be detected using mobile phases with a wide pH range. The first proposed multitoxin method worked under acid chromatographic conditions.[22] It uses as buffer ammonium formate and formic acid in a pH 2. This method was validated in 2005[23] and has been widely used since then for the toxin detection and identification.[17,24–26] Then, an LC-MS/MS in-house validation for the analysis of lipophilic marine toxins under basic conditions was performed.[27] In this case, toxin separation was carried out at pH 11 and it seems that better limits of detection (LODs) in mussel extracts were achieved compared to the acidic method.[24] Less extreme pH conditions were proposed using ammonium acetate as buffer (pH 6.8)[28] and using ammonium bicarbonate (pH 7.9).[29] Table 3.2 collects the most representative LC-MS/MS methodology to detect the lipophilic marine toxins worldwide.

TABLE 3.2

Summary of Multitoxin LC-MS/MS Methods to Detect the Lipophilic Marine Toxins

Chromatography	Column	Mobile Phase (A) and (B) with the Modifiers		Flow (mL/min)	i.v. (μL)	LOD/LOQ	References
Acid conditions	Hypersil Gold C18 m (2.1 × 100 mm, 1.9 μm)	(A): water (B): ACN 90%	0.1% formic acid, pH 3	0.4	3	LODs (ng/mL): GYM, SPX, PTX-2, AZA-1, AZA-2, AZA-3 (0.041–0.10); YTX, OA, DTX-1, DTX-2 (1.6–5.1)	[26]
	BDS Hypersil C8 (50 × 2.1 mm, 3 μm)	(A): water (B): ACN 95%	2 mM ammonium formate and 50 mM formic acid, pH 2.6	0.2	10	LODs (pg): OA (22.1), YTX (6.1), AZA-1 (1.1), PTX-2 (6.9), SPX-1 (1.9), GYM (14.1)	[24]
	X-Bridge C8 (50 × 2.1 mm; 3.5 μm)	(A): water (B): ACN 95%	2 mM ammonium formate and 50 mM formic acid, pH 2	0.5	5	LOQs (μg/kg): AZA-1 (8.7), GYM (6.1), OA (14.9), PTX-2 (25.6), SPX-1 (33.7); YTX (377.1)	[30]
	BDS Hypersil C8 (50 × 2.1 mm, 3 μm)	(A): water (B): ACN 95%	2 mM ammonium formate and 50 mM formic acid	0.25	5	LODs (μg/kg): OA (10), AZA-1 (0.3)	[25]
	BDS Hypersil C8 (50 × 2 mm, 3 μm)	(A): water (B): ACN 95%	2 mM ammonium formate and 50 mM formic acid	0.2	5	LODs (μg/kg): OA (15), PTX-2 (10), SPX-1 (4)	[17]
Basic conditions	X-Bridge C18 (150 × 3 mm; 5 μm)	(A): water (B): ACN 90%	6.7 mM ammonium hydroxide, pH 11	0.4	10	LODs (pg): OA (1.4), YTX (21.3), AZA-1 (5.4), PTX-2 (1.1)	[31]

	Column	Mobile phase	Buffer			LODs/LOQs	Ref.
	X-Bridge C18 (150 × 3 mm; 5 μm)	(A): water (B): ACN 90%	6.7 mM ammonium hydroxide, pH 11	0.4	10	LODs (pg): OA (9.1), YTX (2.2), AZA-1 (1.1), PTX-2 (7.4), SPX-1 (0.8 pg), GYM (3.7)	[24]
	X-Bridge C8 (50 × 2.1 mm; 3.5 μm)	(A): water (B): ACN 90%	6.7 mM ammonia, pH 11	0.5	10	LOQs (μg/kg): AZA-1 (6), GYM (13.2), OA (3.6), PTX-2 (13.4), SPX-1 (14.7); YTX (36.0)	[30]
	X-Bridge C18 (150 × 3 mm; 5 μm)	(A): water (B): ACN 90%	6.7 mM ammonium hydroxide	0.25	5	LODs (μg/kg): OA (5), AZA-1 (0.5)	[25]
Close to the neutral conditions	Gemini NX column (150 × 2 mm; 3 μm)	(A): water (B): ACN 95%	5 mM ammonium hydrogencarbonate, pH 7.9	0.2	5	LODs (ng/mL): OA (0.2), PTX-2 (0.2), AZA-1 (0.2), YTX (0.3)	[29]
	X-Bridge C8 (50 × 2.1 mm; 3.5 μm)	(A): water (B): ACN 90%	5 mM ammonium bicarbonate, pH 7.9	0.5	5	LOQs (μg/kg): AZA-1 (9.2), GYM (1.5), OA (22), PTX-2 (5.3), SPX-1 (55.7); YTX (> 300)	[30]
	X-Bridge C8 (50 × 2.1 mm; 3.5 μm)	(A): water (B): ACN 90%	5 mM ammonium acetate, pH 6.8	0.5	5	LOQs (μg/kg): AZA-1 (12.4), GYM (4.7), OA (26.9), PTX-2 (71.6), SPX-1 (8.2); YTX (>300)	[30]

Note: Methods are classified according to the liquid chromatography conditions: acid, basic, or close to neutral conditions. The limits of detection (LODs) and limits of quantification (LOQs) obtained for the lipophilic toxins are also indicated on it. ACN, acetonitrile; AZA, azaspiracid; DTX, dinophysistoxin; GYM, gymnodimine; OA, okadaic acid; PTX, petecnotoxin; SPX, spirolide; YTX, yessotoxin.

In Europe, chromatographic techniques coupled to mass spectrometry were the method of choice to replace the MBA to detect lipophilic marine toxins.[14] The mouse bioassay for lipophilic toxin detection, which has been used up to now as an exclusive reference method, was replaced by the LC-MS/MS approach with this new regulation. Currently, an approved protocol is available[32] where some LC-MS/MS conditions are fixed in order to be followed for the marine toxins official control. However, as shown in a comparative study,[33] the parameters of the LC-MS/MS methods should be defined as tightly as possible since it has been found that differences in the OA quantification of up to 200% when different reagents or number of transitions are used or when a toxin is quantified with the analog standard.

It is necessary to keep in mind that with the change in the legislation, from MBA to analytical techniques, the use of TEFs is necessary to understand the toxicity of the seafood samples before they enter the commercial channel and reach consumers. Likewise, the use of TEFs requires the knowledge of the toxicity of each analog present in a sample in order to translate analytical data into total toxicity. In the last decades, the toxicity of lipophilic marine toxins was assessed by several in vivo and in vitro assays. Most of the in vivo assays are acute toxicity assays to determine the lethal dose 50 (LD_{50}) after both oral and intraperitoneal (*i.p.*) administration.[34–37] There is a lack of information concerning the long-term risk associated to the consumption of mollusk intoxicated with some toxins. For example, the spirolide toxin group is not identified as dangerous and, in fact, they are not regulated, but studies demonstrated that the mechanism of action of these toxins is in relationship with the blockade of the muscarinic and nicotinic receptors (mAChR and the nAChR) on the nervous system.[38,39] These compounds cross the blood–brain barrier,[40] and therefore they might pose a, so far undefined, long-term risk to consumers. The toxic potency of the lipophilic marine toxins is also checked using a functional method based on the in vitro use of its specific receptor. These methods are related to the mode of action of the toxin, and their capacity to detect the different toxic compounds is usually related to their toxic potency. They use the receptor of the toxin group as a base for the assay and show a response that is proportional to the toxic potency of the group. Therefore, TEFs of toxins can be calculated by *i.p.* or oral administration of mice or by comparing effects directly through their receptors for those toxins whose mechanisms of action are known and bind to defined receptors. Opposite to *i.p.* administrations, oral toxicity studies provide information that compare better to human food poisonings because it takes into account the ratio of the absorption of the toxic molecule in the digestive system of mammalians. In addition, they have the advantage of allowing to follow the toxin kinetic in the mammal's body by analyzing the blood, urine, and feces at different times after the toxin is administrated.[34] However, given the lack of enough information available in regard to the oral route, the European Food Safety Authority (EFSA) panel proposed TEFs based on acute effects after *i.p.* administration.[5] The limited toxicological information does not allow the setting of TEFs for the oral route for any of the toxin groups. Even for the *i.p.* route, the available toxicity data are very limited for the AZA-, YTX-, and PTX-group toxins. Further toxicological data are needed for the establishment of TEFs for the oral route of administration for all toxin groups. EFSA mentions that milligram amounts of purified toxins should be produced for this purpose and that the TEF values should be revised when studies on acute oral toxicity data for the relevant analogs of each toxin group become available.[5]

Table 3.3 collects information concerning the TEFs obtained in different in vivo and in vitro studies for the main lipophilic marine toxins. Also, summarize the opinion of EFSA about the TEFs of the lipophilic marine toxins legislated.[5] TEFs have been used to convert the concentrations of the OA-, AZA-, YTX-, and PTX-group toxins respectively into OA, AZA-1, YTX, and PTX-2 equivalents in order to allow the combined toxicity of different analogs. The information available in the bibliography differs according to the toxin group and method employed. In some cases, there is not a pure amount of the toxin to perform studies or the compound target is not known, which makes difficult to design a functional method based on an in vitro assay.[41] As shown, different values of TEFs are obtained depending on whether in vivo or an in vitro assay is used. It is important to find the proper TEF for the toxic conversion, especially for the legislated toxins, when only the chromatographic techniques can be used for the food control. Since each toxin has a different mechanism of action and shows a different toxicity, it is worth studying the particular situation for each toxin. In general, AZA TEFs estimated based on in vivo studies suggest less potency differences between these three AZA analogs as compared to the in vitro data.[42] Regarding the OA group, results from recent years indicate a lower acute toxicity of DTX-2 in MBA, compared with OA and DTX-1.[35] In this case, the TEFs for DTX-1 and DTX-2 fixed by EFSA in 1 and 0.6, respectively, are based on *i.p.*

LD_{50} experiments and the TEFs obtained by PP2A inhibition assays seem that they are values coincident for many experiments, and thus these TEFs may be the correct values for these toxins. YTX is less toxic to mice after oral administration than after *i.p.* injection. No deaths were recorded in mice that were given YTX up to 50 mg/kg,[36] and no deaths or signals of toxicity were seen in mice dosed orally with homo YTX or 45-OH-YTX up to 1 mg/kg.[43] In this case, the use of TEFs calculated with *i.p.* data can include errors since an analytical result will provide a toxic value of a compound that does not show oral toxicity. For the detection of PTXs, there are not many methods that use biological components. Some functional, multi-toxin detection assays have been developed based on the induction in hepatocytes of apoptosis or cytotoxicity by several PTX toxins, like the series of studies based on the observed damage in the actin cytoskeleton and in the viability of primary cultured rat hepatocytes when different analogs of PTXs are used.[44]

It is important to highlight the role of CI toxin group in the new EU reference method. This toxin group comprises spirolides, gymnodimines, pinnatoxins, and pteriatoxins.[48] CI are a group of toxins not regulated, and are therefore not included in the official methods. An MBA is capable of detecting OA, YTXs, AZA, and CI group toxins (all toxins and analogs) that show toxicity; however, the LC-MS/MS-based methods only can detect the toxins you select in the official method. As they are not legislated toxins, EFSA do not show values of TEFs for these toxins.[5,49] CI group could be included in the multitoxin LC-MS/MS official methods because they are detected in the same chromatographic conditions than the remaining lipophilic marine toxins legislated. Therefore, it would be useful to have TEF values available in case these toxins are legislated. Table 3.3 collects the TEF value obtained with spirolides toxicity studies. The proposed TEF is referred to 13-desmethyl spirolide C because it is the most frequent analog found in mollusks. By oral route, 20-MeG referred to 13-desMeC has a TEF = 1 because the LD_{50} for both analogs is 157 µg/kg.[50] However, the TEF of 20-MeG calculated by *i.p.* injection is less than 0.44 since the LD_{50} for 13-desMeC is 27 µg/kg and 20-MeG in doses up to 63 µg/kg do not produce any death.[34] Therefore, there is a large difference in TEF values obtained with *i.p.* or oral assays. Regarding CI toxins in Europe, the highest concern for several years was for spirolides. Despite the fact that human intoxications have never been associated with the consumption of spirolides, they are very toxic compounds by *i.p.* administrations to mice and they are the most extended group of CI toxins. However, pinnatoxins (also belonging to the CI group) are appearing in the Europe coasts.[51] These toxins are produced by *Vulcanodinium*

TABLE 3.3

Toxic Equivalent Factors to be Used with the Aim to Translate Analytical Data into Total Toxicity

Toxin Group		TEF A	TEF B	TEF C
OA	OA	1		1
	DTX-1			1
	DTX-2	0.58[35]		0.6
AZAs	AZA-1		1	1
	AZA-2		8.2[42]	1.8
	AZA-3		4.5[42]	1.4
YTXs	YTX	1	1	1
	Homo YTX	1.15[36]	1[45]	1
	45-OH-YTX		0.38[12]	1
	45-OH-Homo YTX	<0.68[36]	0.064[45]	0.5
PTXs	PTX-1	1.04[46]	0.073[44]	1
	PTX-2	1	1	1
SPXs	13-desMeC	1	1	
	13,19-didesMeC	0.87[34]	0.64[47]	
	20-MeG	<0.44[34]		

Note: Values were obtained with data from different in vivo (TEF A) and in vitro (TEF B) assays. The TEF values adopted by EFSA CONTAM Panel[5] (TEF C), are based on acute toxicity following *i.p.* administration to mice.

rugosum dinoflagellate[52] and initially detected in Chinese shellfish.[53] Recently, pinnatoxins have appeared in Norwegian blue mussels[51] and *Vulcanodinium rugosum* was also found in the Mediterranean coast of France.[54] Some analogs of pinnatoxins are more toxic than spirolides by oral ingestion via food.[55] Thus, this group of toxins should begin to be considered in the lipophilic marine toxin monitoring in Europe.

In summary, the presence of new analogs, new toxins from other localizations are issues that must be taken into account when any analytical method is used. The substitution of MBA to chemical methods requires the knowledge of the toxicity of each analog present in a sample and to define how the value for the toxic conversion is calculated since different values of TEFs are obtained depending on whether oral, *i.p.* administration or an in vitro data are used. In order to use chemical methods as the only and proper reference method for lipophilic toxin detection, it becomes necessary to use the individual standards for the quantification of each toxin[33] as to use the correct TEF values, since if the TEFs are not applied properly they can greatly affect the final results.

3.1.3 Hydrophilic Marine Toxin Detection

With regard to the chemical analytical methods, only two are currently being officially used for marine toxin detection: HPLC-UV for domoic acid and analogs[56] and HPLC with FLD for saxitoxin and analogs.[57] The last one, known as the "Lawrence method," has been subjected to continuous and further refinements due to many drawbacks identified in the LC method application (i.e., coelution of peaks).[58] So, a full single laboratory validation in a wide range of species to include additional toxins (dcGTX2,3 and dcNEO) was performed.[59,60] However, this method still does not cover the full spectrum of saxitoxin analogs, and since some toxins coelute the major problem continues to be the complex interpretation and transformation of chromatographic peaks into toxic values. This issue does not appear with the domoic acid due to the limited presence of analogs in nature and matrix contaminated with this toxin (generally scallops). Thus, the DA structure allows a simple and more intuitive UV detection. Following the problems encountered in the Lawrence method, some laboratories or research centers continue working on better and simpler methods. In fact, a post-column oxidation (PCOX) LC-FLD has been validated and approved as an official method.[61,62] As an alternative to the analytical techniques, a variety of functional and biochemical methods have been described, such as phosphatase, immunochemical and enzyme-linked immunosorbent assays,[7,8,63–65] and also biosensor techniques.[8,66] A recent alternative is the receptor binding assay, which has become an official AOAC method following an extensive period of validation.[67] The functional methods, unlike analytical methods, do not need TEF since they give information of whether a sample is toxic or not.

For monitoring purpose in the PSP analysis, it is necessary to apply TEFs to translate the analytical result in a toxic value. Since these factors may differ depending on the technology/system used, the European Commission considers TEFs (Table 3.4) provided by EFSA opinions as the reference values to apply for all calculations.[5,14] As the STX is the RC in the group, all analogs detected should be expressed as a quantity of STX equivalent. Therefore, the total PSP toxicity is calculated by adding individual toxin concentrations and applying TEFs determined for each toxin (see formula). For those isomers forming the same coeluting oxidation products during the HPLC analysis (GTX1,4, GTX2,3, C1,2, and dcGTX2,3), the highest toxicity factor of two isomers is used to calculate the toxicity contribution of each toxin.[68]

$$\mu g\, STX\, 2HCl \frac{equivalents}{kg} = \left(\sum_{i=1}^{n} Cm_i \times T_i \right) \times 372.2$$

where

Cm_i is the toxin concentration (μmol/kg) of each detected analog
T_i is the specific toxicity factor of the PSP toxins according to EFSA
372.2 is the molecular weight from STX 2HCL (g/mol)

The influence of using the highest TEF of the isomeric analogs can lead to an overestimation of the final toxic value in the analytical method regarding the MBA. This is not the major reason and could also affect the matrix or the dinoflagellate producer.[70] Overestimation in the AOAC LC method makes the PSP group still require the use of bioassay for the complete detection of the full toxins.

TABLE 3.4

TEFs of STX and Analogs

Toxin	TEF_1	TEF_2
STX	1[a]	1[b]
NeoSTX	1[a]	1.1[b]
GTX1	1[a]	0.9[b]
GTX2	0.4[a]	0.3[b]
GTX3	0.6[a]	0.6[b]
GTX4	0.7[a]	0.6[b]
GTX5	0.1[a]	0.06[b]
GTX6	0.1[a]	0.06[b]
C1		0.005[b]
C2	0.1[a]	0.08[b]
C3		0.01[b]
C4	0.1[a]	0.04[b]
dcSTX	1[a]	0.7[b]
dcNeoSTX	0.1[a]	0.7[b]
dcGTX2	0.2[a]	0.16[b]
dcGTX3	0.4	0.4[b]
11-Hydroxy-STX	0.3	

[a] Data from [72], summarized in [5].
[b] Data from [69], as shown in [66].

An important problem in the official LC method is that TEFs are not defined for all PSP toxins in the group; it is due to scarcity of information on the biological activity of these toxins. Most studies report data on the acute toxicity in rats and mousse after *i.p.* administration. It is usually because the oral absorption assays leads to large variations in the results, and also the influence of many factors (i.e., animals fasted) can modify the toxin effect. Likewise, to perform these studies high and pure toxin amounts are needed and sometimes these are not available. So, the accessible TEFs provide limited information on the real toxicity.[71] Usually when no certified standards are available, toxicological data are obtained from a RC in the group (i.e., STX) and the same equivalence factor is assumed for the other analogs. But in this way mistakes in quantification will be made, especially in the analytical methods, since not all analogs have the same toxicity. In the case of PSP, toxicity varies depending on the functional groups. The most potent are NEO, GTX1, and dc-STX that have the same potency as STX. Therefore, it is very important to dispose TEF for each analog, and for that it is necessary that certified analogs are available to perform complete toxicological studies and to define TEFs accurately.

TEFs are usually calculated by *i.p.* injection in mice or by comparing effects directly through their receptors if the amount is not enough to use animals. However, there is not sufficient data evaluating simultaneously the potency of the PSP standards in vitro and by MBA. Only recently the relative toxicity factors of STX analogs were reported for those analogs available in certified form.[72,73] With the current TEFs acknowledge for some of the analogs, the use of analytical methods for STX group can only be partially implemented in the regulatory systems. This group still requires the use of bioassay for the complete detection. Only DA detection is fully implemented by HPLC, and all other toxin groups still need a method to replace the bioassay.

3.2 Relative Response Factors

The chromatography is an old instrumental technique,[74] used over a century as an analyte separation method.[75,76] In the HPLC technology, the sample is injected with a mobile phase and is eluted through a chromatographic column. In recent years, the chromatography has evolved and it has converted into an extended analysis method for all kinds of marine compounds. This is in a very specific method since both the previous extraction methods from matrix and the chromatographic procedures are carried out based on the type of toxin. Today, the identification and quantification of toxins in order to protect the human health has become the main part of the work based on HPLC by coupling detection systems that leads to sensible detection methods.[77,78] To carry out good toxin identification, it is necessary to select a proper detection system that measures the different physical–chemical properties of the molecule. The detection nature and detector type play a critical role, and thus UV, FL, or MS detection is chosen depending on the properties of the toxins. The majority of the toxins do not have characteristic chromophores groups in their structures, thus the use of UV detectors results in methods with poor sensitivity and selectivity.[79] To be able to use a FL detector, toxins should have groups susceptible of being derivatized into fluorescent products like the case of PSP toxins.[68] However, the MS uses the mass/charge (*m/z*) ratio of the eluted compounds and is applicable to any analyte. Compounds are ionized in negative or positive mode, then separated by the *m/z* ratio and finally detected and registered in the chromatograms by converting the ion flow in an electric signal. MS is the most sensitive, selective and universal detection and the most commonly technique used for the marine toxin detection employing mass analyzers as the quadrupole (Q) and triple quadrupole (TQ) mass spectrometers,[80,81] ion trap (IT),[82] time of flight (ToF),[83] or hybrid instrument (IT-ToF; Q-ToF; IT-LC/ESI-MS/MS).[84] Studies with lipophilic toxins using four analyzers showed the variability in the LODs for PTX-2 and OA, TQ-MS being the most sensitive mass analyzers.[85] In fact, TQ-MS is the most frequently detector used for routine quantitative analysis of shellfish samples.

In the chromatograms, toxins are represented graphically as a peak with a height or area specific for the same LC and MS analysis conditions. That is, each compound gives rise to a characteristic response factor in a detector for the same measurement conditions. Response factor, in chromatography and spectroscopy, is defined as the ratio between a signal produced by an analyte and the quantity of analyte that produces the signal. And it depends on the total ionization cross section and the ionizing path length.[86] The electronic configuration of the molecule plays an important role in its ionization processes as well.[86] In order to calculate the response factor of the compound, the experimental conditions (temperature, pressure, mobile phases, and MS parameters) must be fixed since the minimum change in the pH or components in the mobile phase affects the molecule response factor.

Figure 3.1 shows the OA, DTX-1, and DTX-2 chromatograms obtained by two MS methods in a QTRAP LC/MS/MS system, which integrates a hybrid quadrupole-linear IT mass spectrometer equipped with an ESI source.[33] The first MS method (Figure 3.1a) included a huge number of lipophilic toxins, a total of 10 transitions for checking the following compounds: DTX-1 (*m/z* 817.5 > 255.5, *m/z* 817.5 > 113.5), OA and DTX-2 (*m/z* 803.5 > 255.5, *m/z* 803.5 > 113.5), YTX (*m/z* 1141.4 > 1061.5, *m/z* 1141.4 > 855.4), homo YTX (*m/z* 1155.3 > 1075.3, *m/z* 1155.3 > 869.3), and 45-OH-YTX (*m/z* 1157.5 > 1077.5, 1157.5 > 855.5). The second MS method (Figure 3.1b) included only the specific transitions for the three diarrheic toxins, OA, DTX-1, and DTX-2, a total of four transitions. The amount of OA, DTX-1, and DTX-2 injected by both methods (Figure 3.1a and b) is the same, 2.5 ng of toxin by injection (500 ng/mL, 5 μL). The remaining analysis conditions and experiment procedures are shown in a comparative study reported in 2011.[33] As Figure 3.1a shows, the OA, DTX-1, and DTX-2 signals obtained by the method with a large number of toxins are around 1000 counts per second (cps). DTX-1 gave rise to a peak with an intensity of 1250 cps, and OA and DTX-2 have a signal of 1050 and 975 cps, respectively. In Figure 3.1b, the signal produced by the same amount of each compound is higher for three toxins, OA (1700 cps), DTX-2 (1250 cps), and DTX-1 (1690 cps). Therefore, the signal and area obtained analyzing by the MS method with 10 transitions were considerably lower than those obtained by a method with 4 transitions. These different signals result in different toxin amounts when they are quantifying with a calibration curve. Also, when a component in the mobile phase changes, toxins give rise to different response factors in the detector and thus variations in the toxin concentrations were obtained as well. This was checked with three mobile phases done with three ACN brands. In this study, each toxin was quantified by using the two MS methods. Figure 3.2 collects the effect of the ACN from the mobile phase on the quantification of OA, DTX-1, and DTX-2 by LC-MS/MS. As Figure 3.2a shows, when 160 ng/mL OA was injected, a range from 215 to 116 ng/mL was detected depending on the ACN brand and MS method employed. Underestimations or overestimations (from 110 to 169 ng/mL) were also observed when 160 ng/mL of DTX-1 was injected (Figure 3.2b). In the case of DTX-2 (Figure 3.2c), the system detected a range 104–186 ng/mL, despite the fact that 160 ng/mL was injected.

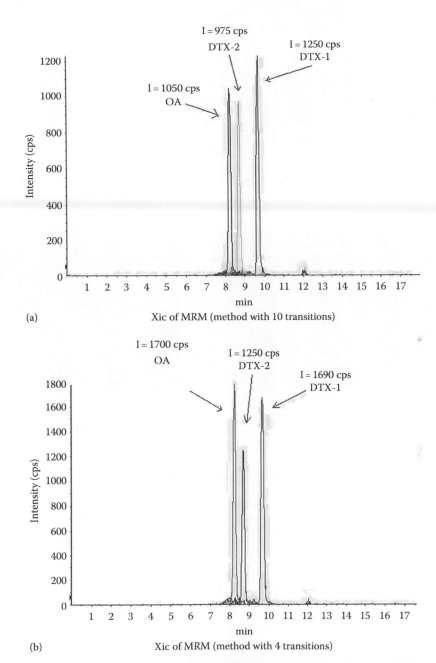

FIGURE 3.1 OA, DTX-2, and DTX-1 chromatograms in MRM negative mode obtained by LC-MS/MS analysis of the three standards diluted in methanol. The equipment used was a HPLC system, from Shimadzu (Kyoto, Japan), coupled to a QTRAP LC/MS/MS system from Applied Biosystems (the United States), which integrate a hybrid quadrupole-linear ion trap mass spectrometer equipped with an ESI source. The column used for the analysis was a BDS-Hypersil C8, 50 mm × 2 mm, 3 μm particle size. Mobile phase was composed by water (a) and ACN/water (95:5) (b), both containing 50 mM formic acid and 2 mM ammonium formate. (a) Toxins were analyzed with a MS method, which included 10 toxin transitions. (b) Toxins were analyzed with a MS method, which included 4 toxin transitions. Toxin concentration was 500 ng/mL for each standard and the inject volume was 5 μL.

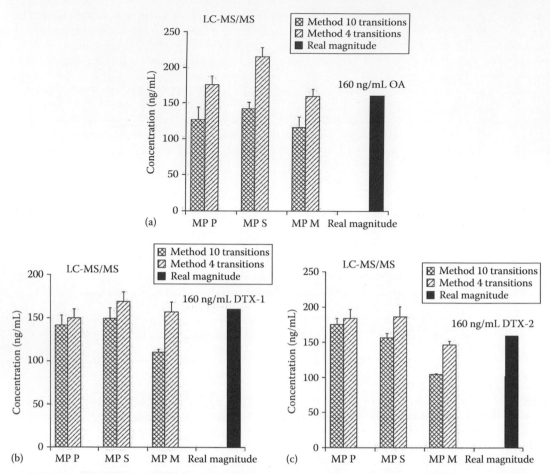

FIGURE 3.2 Effect of ACN from the mobile phase on the quantification of OA, DTX-1, and DTX-2 by LC-MS/MS. MP P: mobile phase containing ACN from Panreac. MP S: mobile phase containing ACN from Sigma. MP M: mobile phase containing ACN from Merk. Each toxin was quantified by using two MS methods: a MS method that includes 10 toxin transitions and a MS method that includes 4 toxin transitions. Each graphic represents the concentrations in methanol for (a) OA, (b) DTX-1, and (c) DTX-2. Mean ± SEM of n = 3 experiments. Black column: theoretical concentration of toxin (160 ng/mL). Open columns: toxin concentration obtained by each MS method.

Similarly, the same experiment was carried out using other equipment consisting in ultra performance liquid chromatography (UPLC) system coupled to a Xevo TQ MS mass spectrometer.[33] This is another TQ detector manufacturer. The OA, DTX-1, and DTX-2 quantification was also different depending on the ACN from the mobile phase and also different from the results shown in Figure 3.2, obtained with the LC-MS/MS equipment. Therefore, comparing analytical results using different detector does not provide the same compound response. Results using one detector differ from results obtained using another detector.[33] A compressive study using three types of spectrometers was performed to investigate the mass spectrometric behavior of AZAs.[87] In the AZA experiment, TQ, IT, and Q-ToF hybrid mass spectrometry was used. It was observed that the mass spectrometry behavior is even more dependent of the type of the mass spectrometry (IT, TQ, and Q-ToF) than the manufacturer of the mass spectrometry. Therefore, the response factor depends on the detection system and must be calculated for each compound with a particular detector.

The objective of the quantitative methods by MS is to provide an accuracy and reliable determination of the toxin amount found in sample. Up to now, toxin MS detection and quantification is usually performed in selected ion monitoring (SIM) mode or multiple reaction monitoring (MRM) using two transitions per toxin.[17] The transition with the highest intensity is used for quantification while the transition with the lowest intensity is used for confirmatory purposes. PTX, AZA, and CI toxin groups are preferably ionized with the instrument operate in positive ionization mode while OA and YTX toxins groups are ionized in negative ionization mode. In the quantitative methods based on SIM detection with one ion per compound and external calibration, only the parent ion is monitored and therefore the confirmatory character of the method is limited. However, SIM detection methods are more sensitive than MRM methods since the monitored ion intensity generally is higher. This technique is proper when toxin standards are available and have numerous advantages like the high sensibility in the quantitative analysis, especially when coupled to high-resolution separation methods like UPLC.[88,89] However, at the same time quantitative determination is hindered due to the lack of standard materials. To quantify toxins when no standards are available, sometimes the calibration curve constructed for one toxin is used for quantification of other toxins from the same group.[32,80] It is assumed that analogs from the same toxin group provide an equimolar response by MS/MS tandem detection. For example, in the case of AZA group, it is used as the marker compound of the group (AZA-1) to quantify AZA-2 and AZA-3 because three toxins have a similar chemical structure and is expected will have the same ionization behavior.[32] However, following this premise, errors up to 200% in the toxin quantification can be obtained.[33] In this case, the response factors have to be used to solve the measure values and to compensate the variations produced in the response of an instrument due to the different toxins. The term of relative response factor (RRF) is the measure of the relative response of the instrument detector to an analyte compared to an external standard. RRF is determined by the analysis of standards and is used to calculate the concentrations of analytes in samples for which no standards are available. RRF can be calculated using the following equation:

$$RRF = \frac{(Ac \times Cs)}{(As \times Cc)}$$

where
  RRF is the relative response factor
  Ac is the area of the target analyte
  As is the area of the corresponding standard
  Cs is the concentration of the corresponding standard
  Cc is the concentration of the target analyte

Figure 3.3 summarizes a typical case of toxin quantification when OA standard is available and it is used for DTX-1 and DTX-2 quantification. These results have already been shown in the comparative study[33]; however, in this chapter, we can remark the differences obtained in the toxin quantification when they were measured by two TQ detectors. As it can be observed, the DTX-1 amount can be increased up to 40% or decreased up to 21% depending on the equipment and the mobile phase used. Equally, DTX-2 amount could be overestimated up to 88% or underestimated up to 33%. Therefore, detectors do not respond equally to different compounds. The analogs do not ionize in the same way and do not have the same response. All data shown in Figure 3.3 were obtained with the same MS parameters for three toxins.[90] When one toxin is quantified with the analog standard, it is critical to maintain the same ionization parameters, even that they are not the optimum values for any of them, that is, the collision and cone energies should be equal for all compounds since when DTX-1 is measured with a collision energy of 90 and OA with 65, errors up to 10 times more from those shown in Figure 3.3 can be obtained (data not shown).

Besides the legislated toxins included in the official methods in Europe (AZAs, PTXs, YTX, and OA group toxins), there are other toxin groups from tropical waters whose occurrence is increasing globally in countries not expected for their latitudes, like ciguatoxins (CTXs). So far, this kind of toxins has been only linked to the Caribbean, Pacific, and Indic areas causing human foodborne intoxication named ciguatera fish poisoning (CFP).[91–93] In the last decade, these compounds have been detected in waters belonging to Spanish[94] and Portuguese Islands[89] in the south of Europe. The fact that these toxins begin to appear in new countries make necessary to design detection methods that detect CTXs in shellfish before they enter in the food chain. In principle, these toxins are suitably detected by LC-MS/MS techniques with chromatographic systems comprising a wide range of C8 and C18 columns[95–98] and mobile phases composed generally by ACN and water buffered with formic acid, ammonium formate,

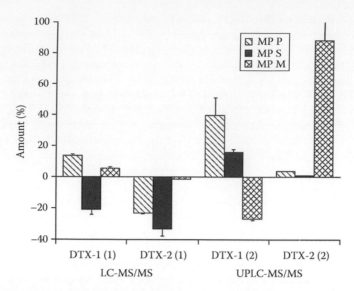

FIGURE 3.3 Quantification of DTX-1 and DTX-2 using OA calibration curve. Data obtained from LC-MS/MS and UPLC-MS/MS instrument. Terms in parenthesis (1) or (2) represent the quantification done in (1) LC-MS/MS and (2) UPLC-MS/MS toxins were dissolved in methanol. MP P: mobile phase containing ACN from Panreac. MP S: mobile phase containing ACN from Sigma. MP M: mobile phase containing ACN from Merck. Each toxin was quantified by using an MS method that includes 10 toxin transitions. Each column represents the mean ± SEM of n = 9 experiments. The line represents the amount of toxin obtained within its own calibration curve.

ammonium acetate, and trifluorocetic acid.[99] The MS detection is usually performed in positive ionization MRM mode[94,100] or only used the first quadrupole in the Q1 mode.[95,101] However, due to the nature of the molecule, in some cases, CTXs give rise to MS spectra with adducts that make the interpretation difficult. CTXs family toxins show multiple losses of water and forms sodium and ammonium adducts.[101] The ionization behavior is a characteristic pattern of ion formation for polyethers compounds. However, the intensity of ammonium, potassium, sodium adducts ions, and losses of waters can vary depending on the mobile phase and the type of CTX polyether compound. Thus, it is necessary for the correspondent standard for the correct identification. Moreover, there are a lot congeners, more than 50 have been identified,[102] and it is very frequently the presence of several CTXs with equal molecular weight in the same extract eluting in different retention times.[99] This issue makes the CTX identification by LC-MS/MS difficult. Figure 3.4 shows the chromatogram and spectrum of the two compounds of the CTX family, gambierol with molecular weight (M.W. 756.99) (Figure 3.4a) and its heptacyclic analog (M.W 612.79)[103] (Figure 3.4b). Gambierol is a marine polycyclic ether toxin, first isolated along with CTXs from the dinoflagellate *Gambierdiscus toxicus*.[104] The ionization behavior of Gambierol and CTXs in mass spectrometry techniques is comparable due to their polycyclic structure. Gambierol and its heptacyclic analog were analyzed consecutively in a LC-MS-IT-ToF system, which performs separations with IT and ToF mass spectrometers arranged in tandem. The amount analyzed of two standards, by the same MS method, was 5 µL of a concentration of 500 ng/mL in methanol. As it can be observed in Figure 3.4a, the maximum intensity for gambierol molecule is for the ion 757.461 *m/z* due to the $[M\ ^+H]^+$, which generates a peak with a height of $1.6 \times 100,000$ cps. This mass is followed in height by the ion 739.441 *m/z* due to one H_2O losses ($[M\ ^+H\ ^-H_2O]^+$) and that forms a peak with a height of $0.4 \times 100,000$ cps. In the spectrum of the heptacyclic analog of gambierol (Figure 3.4b), the $[M\ ^+H]^+$ is not the most prominent ion, as it happens in the case of gambierol. However, the maximum intensity is for the ion 595.365 *m/z* due to one H_2O water losses (peak with an intensity of $6.0 \times 1,000,000$ cps), followed by the ion 613.386 *m/z* $[M\ ^+H]^+$, which generates a peak with an intensity of $0.9 \times 1,000,000$ cps. Therefore, despite the fact that both compounds have a similar chemical structure, each compound gives rises to a spectrum whose response factor is not comparable. The response factor of each ion is very different between two molecules and this fact can lead to consequences in the quantification when no standards are available and one analog of the group is used to quantify the other analog. In case heptacyclic analog standard is not available, and

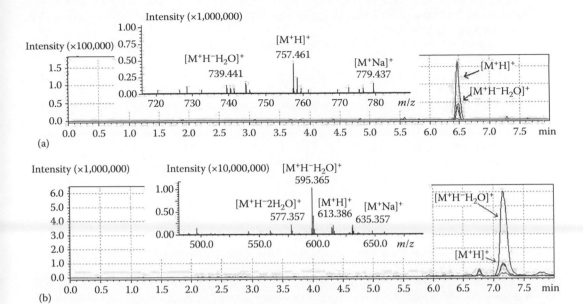

FIGURE 3.4 Chromatogram and spectrum of gambierol (a) and its heptacyclic analog (b) standards (500 ng/mL) obtained in the LC-MS-IT-ToF system from Shimadzu (Kyoto, Japan). The column used for the identifications was a Waters Acquity UPLC® BEH C$_{18}$ (100 mm × 2.1, 1.7 μm) with a mobile phase, composed by water (a) and methanol 95% (b), both containing 5 mM ammonium formate and 0.1% formic acid. The mobile phase flow rate was 0.25 mL/min and the injection volume was 5 μL. Intensity units in counts per second (cps).

gambierol standard is used to quantify it in a sample, large errors in the quantification would be obtained. For example, if the [M $^+$H$^-$H$_2$O]$^+$ monitored ion is used to quantify the gambierol and also its analog, a value of 150 times more in the heptacyclic compound amount would be obtained with the LC method shown in Figure 3.4. This means that a sample spiking with 100 ng of heptacyclic would be quantified as 15 μg of toxin. Therefore, from all lipophilic marine toxins, the availability of standards for the CTX group is especially a need in the LC-MS/MS method developing.

ACKNOWLEDGMENTS

This work was funded with the following FEDER cofunded grants: From Ministerio de Ciencia y Tecnología, Spain: AGL2009-13581-CO2-01, AGL2012-40485-CO2-01. From Xunta de Galicia, Spain: 10PXIB261254 PR. From the European Union's Seventh Framework Programme managed by REA—Research Executive Agency http://ec.europa.eu/research/rea (FP7/2007-2013) under grant agreement Nos. 211326 CP (CONffIDENCE), 265896 BAMMBO, 265409 μAQUA, and 262649 BEADS, 315285 Ciguatools and 312184 PharmaSea. From the Atlantic Area Programme (Interreg IVB Trans-national): 2009-1/117 Pharmatlantic.

REFERENCES

1. Hess, P., Grune, B., Anderson, D. B. et al., 2006. Three Rs approaches in marine biotoxin testing. The report and recommendations of a joint ECVAM/DG SANCO workshop (*ECVAM Workshop 54*). *Altern. Lab. Anim.*, 34, 193–224.
2. Sommer, H. and Meiker, K. F., 1937. Paralytic shellfish poisoning. *Arch. Pathol.*, 24, 560–598.
3. AOAC, 1990. Paralytic shellfish poison. Biological method. Final action [M]. In *Official Methods of Analysis*, Hellrich, E. B. K., ed. Association of Official Methods of Analytical Chemists, Arlington, VA, pp. 881–882.
4. Yasumoto, T., Oshima, Y., and Yamaguchi, M., 1978. Occurrence of a new type of shellfish poisoning in the Tohoku district. *Bull. Jpn. Soc. Sci. Fish*, 44, 1249–1255.

5. EFSA Panel, 2009. Scientific opinion on marine biotoxins in shellfish—Summary on regulated marine biotoxins. *EFSA J.,* 1306, 1–23.

6. Van Dolah, F. and Ramsdell, J., 2001. Review and assessment of in vitro detection methods for algal toxins. *AOAC Int.,* 84, 1617–1625.

7. Vieytes, M. R., Fontal, O. I., Leira, F., Baptista de Sousa, J. M., and Botana, L. M., 1997. A fluorescent microplate assay for diarrheic shellfish toxins. *Anal. Biochem.,* 248, 258–264.

8. Fonfría, E. S., Vilariño, N., Campbell, K. et al., 2007. Paralytic shellfish poisoning detection by surface plasmon resonance-based biosensors in shellfish matrixes. *Anal. Chem.,* 79, 6303–6311.

9. Otero, P., Alfonso, A., Alfonso, C. et al., 2011. First direct fluorescence polarization assay for the detection and quantification of spirolides in mussel samples. *Anal. Chim. Acta,* 701(2), 200–208.

10. Alfonso, C., Alfonso, A., Pazos, M. J. et al., 2007. Extraction and cleaning methods to detect yessotoxins in contaminated mussels. *Anal. Biochem.,* 363, 228–238.

11. Alfonso, C., Alfonso, A., Vieytes, M. R., Yasumoto, T., and Botana, L. M., 2005. Quantification of yessotoxin using the fluorescence polarization technique and study of the adequate extraction procedure. *Anal. Biochem.,* 344, 266–274.

12. Pazos, M. J., Alfonso, A., Vieytes, M. R., Yasumoto, T., and Botana, L. M., 2006. Study of the interaction between different phosphodiesterases and yessotoxin using a resonant mirror biosensor. *Chem. Res. Toxicol.,* 19, 794–800.

13. Commission (EC), 2007. Commission regulation (EC) No 1244/2007 of 24 October 2007 amending regulation (EC) No 1244/2007 as regards implementing measures for certain products of animal origin intended for human consumption and laying down specific rules on official controls for the inspection of meat. *Off. J. Eur. Union,* L281, 12–18.

14. Commission Regulation (EU), 15/2011, 2011. Amending Regulation (EC) No 2074/2005 as regards recognised testing methods for detecting marine biotoxins in live bivalve molluscs. *Off. J. Eur. Union,* 3–6.

15. FAO/IOC/WHO, 2011. Summary of the FAO/IOC/WHO expert consultation on biotoxins in bivalve molluscs. In *Assessment and Management of Biotoxin Risks in Bivalve Molluscs,* Food and Agriculture Organization of the United Nations, ed. FAO Fisheries and Aquaculture technical paper, Rome, Italy, pp. 271–281.

16. James, K., Furey, A., Lehane, M. et al., 2002. First evidence of an extensive northern European distribution of azaspiracid poisoning (AZP) toxins in shellfish. *Toxicon,* 40, 909–915.

17. Villar-Gonzalez, A., Rodriguez-Velasco, M. L., Ben-Gigirey, B., and Botana, L. M., 2007. Lipophilic toxin profile in Galicia (Spain): 2005 toxic episode. *Toxicon,* 49, 1129–1134.

18. Aasen, J. A., Hardstaff, W., Aune, T., and Quilliam, M. A., 2006. Discovery of fatty acid ester metabolites of spirolide toxins in mussels from Norway using liquid chromatography/tandem mass spectrometry. *Rapid Commun. Mass Spectrom.,* 20, 1531–1537.

19. Marr, J., Hu, T., Pleasance, S., Quilliam, M., and Wright, J., 1992. Detection of new 7-O-acyl derivatives of diarrhetic shellfish poisoning toxins by liquid chromatography-mass spectrometry. *Toxicon,* 30, 1621–1630.

20. Draisci, R., Lucentini, L., Giannetti, L., Boria, P., and Poletti, R., 1996. First report of pectenotoxin-2 (PTX-2) in algae (*Dinophysis fortii*) related to seafood poisoning in Europe. *Toxicon,* 34, 923–935.

21. Furey, A., Braña-Magdalena, A., Lehane, M. et al., 2002. Determination of azaspiracids in shellfish using liquid chromatography/tandem electrospray mass spectrometry. *Rapid Commun. Mass Spectrom.,* 16, 238–242.

22. Quilliam, M. A., Hess, P., and Dell'Aversano, C., 2001. In *Mycotoxins and Phycotoxins in Perspective at the Turn of the Century,* Dekoe, W., Samson, R., Egmond, H., Gilbert, J., and Sabino, M., eds. Wageningen, the Netherlands, p. 383. Proceedings of the Xth International IUPAC Symposium on Mycotoxins and Phycotoxins, Sao Paulo, Brazil, May 22–25, 2000.

23. McNabb, P., Selwood, A. I., Holland, P. T. et al., 2005. Multiresidue method for determination of algal toxins in shellfish: Single-laboratory validation and interlaboratory study. *J. AOAC Int.,* 88, 761–772.

24. Gerssen, A., Mulder, P. P., McElhinney, M. A., and de Boer, J., 2009. Liquid chromatography-tandem mass spectrometry method for the detection of marine lipophilic toxins under alkaline conditions. *J. Chromatogr. A,* 1216, 1421–1430.

25. Kilcoyne, J. and Fux, E., 2010. Strategies for the elimination of matrix effects in the liquid chromatography tandem mass spectrometry analysis of the lipophilic toxins okadaic acid and azaspiracid-1 in molluscan shellfish. *J. Chromatogr. A,* 1217, 7123–7130.

26. Blay, P., Hui, J. P., Chang, J., and Melanson, J. E., 2011. Screening for multiple classes of marine biotoxins by liquid chromatography-high-resolution mass spectrometry. *Anal. Bioanal. Chem.*, 400, 577–585.

27. Gerssen, A., van Olst, E. H., Mulder, P. P., and de Boer, J., 2010. In-house validation of a liquid chromatography tandem mass spectrometry method for the analysis of lipophilic marine toxins in shellfish using matrix-matched calibration. *Anal. Bioanal. Chem.*, 397, 3079–3088.

28. Stobo, L., Lacaze, J., Scott, A., Gallacher, S., Smith, E., and Quilliam, M., 2005. Liquid chromatography with mass spectrometry—Detection of lipophilic shellfish toxins. *J. AOAC Int.*, 88, 1371–1382.

29. These, A., Scholz, J., and Preiss-Weigert, A., 2009. Sensitive method for the determination of lipophilic marine biotoxins in extracts of mussels and processed shellfish by high-performance liquid chromatography-tandem mass spectrometry based on enrichment by solid-phase extraction. *J. Chromatogr. A*, 1216, 4529–4538.

30. Garcia-Altares, M., Diogene, J., and de la Iglesia, P., 2013. The implementation of liquid chromatography tandem mass spectrometry for the official control of lipophilic toxins in seafood: Single-laboratory validation under four chromatographic conditions. *J. Chromatogr. A*, 1275, 48–60.

31. Gerssen, A., Mulder, P. P., and de Boer, J., 2011. Screening of lipophilic marine toxins in shellfish and algae: Development of a library using liquid chromatography coupled to orbitrap mass spectrometry. *Anal. Chim. Acta*, 685(2), 176–185.

32. EU-RL, 2011. EU-Harmonised standard operating procedure for determination of Lipophilic marine biotoxins in molluscs by LC-MS/MS. Version 4, pp. 1–31.

33. Otero, P., Alfonso, A., Alfonso, C., Rodriguez, P., Vyeites, M. R., and Botana, L. M., 2011. Effect of uncontrolled factors in a validated liquid chromatography-tandem mass spectrometry method question its use as reference method for marine toxins: Major causes for concern. *Anal. Chem.*, 83, 5903–5911.

34. Otero, P., Alfonso, A., Rodriguez, P. et al., 2012. Pharmacokinetic and toxicological data of spirolides after oral and intraperitoneal administration. *Food Chem. Toxicol.*, 50, 232–237.

35. Aune, T., Larsen, S., Aasen, J. A., Rehmann, N., Satake, M., and Hess, P., 2007. Relative toxicity of dinophysistoxin-2 (DTX-2) compared with okadaic acid, based on acute intraperitoneal toxicity in mice. *Toxicon*, 49, 1–7.

36. Tubaro, A., Sosa, S., Carbonatto, M. et al., 2003. Oral and intraperitoneal acute toxicity studies of yessotoxin and homoyessotoxins in mice. *Toxicon*, 41, 783–792.

37. Munday, R., Towers, N. R., Mackenzie, L., Beuzenberg, V., Holland, P. T., and Miles, C. O., 2004. Acute toxicity of gymnodimine to mice. *Toxicon*, 44, 173–178.

38. Wandscheer, C. B., Vilarino, N., Espina, B., Louzao, M. C., and Botana, L. M., 2010. Human muscarinic acetylcholine receptors are a target of the marine toxin 13-desmethyl C spirolide. *Chem. Res. Toxicol.*, 23, 1753–1761.

39. Bourne, Y., Radic, Z., Aráoz, R. et al., 2010. Structural determinants in phycotoxins and AChBP conferring high affinity binding and nicotinic AChR antagonism. *Proc. Natl. Acad. Sci. USA*, 107, 6076–6081.

40. Alonso, E., Otero, P., Vale, C. et al., 2013. Benefit of 13-desmethyl spirolide C treatment in triple transgenic mouse model of alzheimer disease: Beta-amyloid and neuronal markers improvement. *Curr. Alzheimer Res.*, 10, 279–289.

41. Botana, L. M., 2012. A perspective on the toxicology of marine toxins. *Chem. Res. Toxicol.*, 25, 1800–1804.

42. Twiner, M. J., El-Ladki, R., Kilcoyne, J., and Doucette, G. J., 2012. Comparative effects of the marine algal toxins azaspiracid-1, -2, and -3 on Jurkat T lymphocyte cells. *Chem. Res. Toxicol.*, 25, 747–754.

43. Munday, R., Aune, T., and Rossini, G. P., 2008. Toxicology of yessotoxins. In *Seafood and Freshwater Toxins: Pharmacology, Physiology, and Detection*, Botana, L. M., ed. CRC Press, Boca Raton, FL, pp. 581–594.

44. Espina, B., Louzao, M. C., Ares, I. R., Fonfría, E. S., Vilariño, N., Vieytes, M. R., Yasumoto, T., and Botana L. M., 2010. Impact of the pectenotoxin C-43 oxidation degree on its cytotoxic effect on rat hepatocytes. *Chem. Res. Toxicol.*, 23, 504–515.

45. Ferrari, S., Ciminiello, P., Dell'Aversano, C. et al., 2004. Structure-activity relationships of yessotoxins in cultured cells. *Chem. Res. Toxicol.*, 17, 1251–1257.

46. Yasumoto, T., Murata, M., Oshima, Y., Sano, M., Matsumoto, G. K., and Clardy, J., 1985. Diarrhetic shellfish toxins. *Tetrahedron*, 41, 1019–1025.

47. Fonfria, E. S., Vilarino, N., Molgo, J. et al., 2010. Detection of 13,19-didesmethyl C spirolide by fluorescence polarization using Torpedo electrocyte membranes. *Anal. Biochem.*, 403, 102–107.

48. MacKinnon, S. L., Cembella, A. D., Quilliam, M. A. et al., 2004. The characterization of two new spirolides isolated from danish strains of the toxigenic dinoflagellate *Alexandrium ostenfeldii*. In *Harmful Algae 2002*, Steidinger, K. A., Landsberg, J. H., Tomas, C. R., and Vargo, G. A., eds. Institute for Marine Biosciences, National Research Council of Canada, Halifax, Nova Scotia, Canada, pp. 186–188.
49. Alexander, J., Benford, D. J., Boobis, A. et al., 2010. Scientific opinion on marine biotoxins in shellfish—Cyclic imines (spirolides, gymnodimines, pinnatoxins and pteriatoxins). *EFSA J.*, 8(6), 1628–1667.
50. Munday, R., 2008. Toxicology of cyclic imines: Gymnodimine, spirolides, pinnatoxins, pteriatoxins, prorocentrolide, spiro-prorocentrimine, and symbioimines. In *Seafood and Freshwater Toxins: Pharmacology, Physiology, and Detection*, Botana, L. M., ed. CRC Press, Boca Raton, FL, pp. 581–594.
51. Rundberget, T., Aasen, J. A., Selwood, A. I., and Miles, C. O., 2011. Pinnatoxins and spirolides in Norwegian blue mussels and seawater. *Toxicon*, 58, 700–711.
52. Rhodes, L., Smith, K., Selwood, A. I. et al., 2011. Dinoflagellate *Vulcandinium rugosum* identified as the causative organism of pinnatoxins in Australia, New Zealand and Japan. *Phycologia*, 50, 624.
53. Zheng, S., Huang, F., Chen, S. et al., 1990. The isolation and bioactivities of pinnatoxin. *Chin. J. Mar. Drugs*, 9, 33–35.
54. Nézan, E. and Chomérat, N., 2011. *Vulcanodinium rugosum* gen. et sp. nov. (Dinophyceae), un nouveau dinoflagellé marin de la cote méditerranéenne française. *Cryptogamie, Algologie*, 32, 3–18.
55. Munday, R., Selwood, A. I., and Rhodes, L., 2012. Acute toxicity of pinnatoxins E, F and G to mice. *Toxicon*, 60, 995–999.
56. AOAC, 2000. Official method 991.26. Domoic acid in mussels, liquid chromatography method. In *Official Methods of Analysis of AOAC International*, Horowitz, W., Ed. AOAC International, Gaithersburg, MD.
57. Lawrence, J. F., Niedzwiadek, B., and Menard, C., 2005. Quantitative determination of paralytic shellfish poisoning toxins in shellfish using prechromatographic oxidation and liquid chromatography with fluorescence detection: Collaborative study. *J. AOAC Int.*, 88, 1714–1732.
58. Ben-Gigirey, B., Rodríguez-Velasco, M. L., Villar-González, A., and Botana, L. M., 2007. Influence of the sample toxic profile on the suitability of a high performance liquid chromatography method for official paralytic shellfish toxins control. *J. Chromatogr. A*, 78–87.
59. Turner, A. D., Norton, D. M., Hatfield, R. G. et al., 2009. Single laboratory validation of the AOAC LC method (2005.06) for mussels: Refinement and extension of the method to additional toxins. *J. AOAC Int.*, 92, 190–207.
60. Turner, A. D., Hatfield, R. G., Rapkova-Dhanji, M., Norton, D. M., Algoet, M., and Lees, D. N., 2010. Single-laboratory validation of a refined AOAC HPLC method 2005.06 for oysters, cockles, and clams in UK shellfish. *J. AOAC Int.*, 93, 1482–1493.
61. AOAC, 2011. AOAC official method 2011.02. Determination of paralytic shellfish poisoning toxins in mussels, clams, oysters and scallops. In *Post-Column Oxidation Method (PCOX): First Action 2011.* AOAC International, Gaithersburg, MD.
62. van de Riet, J. M., Gibbs, R. S., Muggah, P. M., Rouke, W. A., MacNeil, J. D., and Quilliam, M. A., 2011. Liquid chromatographic post-column oxidation (PCOX) method for the determination of paralytic shellfish toxins in mussels, clams, oysters and scallops: Collaborative study. *J. AOAC Int.*, 94, 1154–1176.
63. Chu, F. S., Hsu, K. H., Huang, X., Barrett, R., and Allison, C., 1996. Screening of paralytic shellfish poisoning toxins in naturally occurring samples with three different direct competitive enzyme-linked immunosorbent assays. *J. Agric. Food Chem.*, 44, 4043–4047.
64. Kleivdal, H., Kristiansen, S. I., Nilsen, M. V. et al., 2007. Determination of domoic acid toxins in shellfish by biosense ASP ELISA—A direct competitive enzyme-linked immunosorbent assay: Collaborative study. *J. AOAC Int.*, 90, 1011–1027.
65. Garet, E., González-Fernández, A., Lago, J., Vieites, J. M., and Cabado, A. G., 2010. Comparative evaluation of enzyme-linked immunoassay and reference methods for the detection of shellfish hydrophilic toxins in several presentations of seafood. *J. Agric. Food Chem.*, 58, 1410–1415.
66. Campbell, K., Haughey, S. A., van den Top, H. et al., 2010. Single laboratory validation of a surface plasmon resonance biosensor screening method for paralytic shellfish poisoning toxins. *Anal. Chem.*, 82, 2977–2988.
67. AOAC, 2011. AOAC official method 2011.27. In *Paralytic Shellfish Toxins (PSTs) in Shellfish, Receptor Binding Assay*. AOAC International, Gaithersburg, MD.

68. CEN, 2009. Determination of PSP toxins in shellfish-HPLC method using pre-column derivatization with peroxide or periodate oxidation. European Committee for Standardization (CEN/TC 275/WG 5 N457).

69. Oshima, Y., 1995. Postcolumn derivatization liquid chromatographic method for paralytic shellfish toxins. *J. AOAC Int.*, 78, 528–532.

70. Turner, A. D., Hatfield, R. G., Rapkova, M. et al., 2011. Comparison of AOAC 2005.06 LC official method with other methodologies for the quantitation of paralytic shellfish poisoning toxins in UK shellfish species. *Anal. Bioanal. Chem.*, 399, 1257–1270.

71. Botana, L. M., Vilarino, N., Alfonso, A. et al., 2010. The problem of toxicity equivalent factors in developing alternative methods to animal bioassays for marine-toxin detection. *Trends Anal. Chem.*, 29, 1316–1325.

72. Vale, C., Alfonso, A., Vieytes, M. R. et al., 2008. In vitro and in vivo evaluation of paralytic shellfish poisoning toxin potency and the influence of the pH of extraction. *Anal. Chem.*, 80, 1770–1776.

73. Perez, S., Vale, C., Botana, A. M., Alonso, E., Vieytes, M. R., and Botana, L. M., 2011. Determination of toxicity equivalent factors for paralytic shellfish toxins by electrophysiological measurements in cultured neurons. *Chem. Res. Toxicol.*, 24(7), 1153–1157.

74. Tswett, M., 1906. Adsorptionsanalyse und Chromatographische methode. Anwendung auf die chemie des chlorophylls. *Ber. Deutsch. Bot. Ges*, 24, 384–393.

75. Kim, Y. and Padilla, G., 1976. Purification of the ichthyotoxic component of Gymnodinium breve (red tide dinoflagellate) toxin by high pressure liquid chromatography. *Toxicon*, 14, 379–387.

76. Chanteau, S., Bagnis, R., and Yasumoto, T., 1976. Purification of ciguatoxin from the loach, Epinephelus microdon (Bleeker). *Biochimie*, 58, 1149–1151.

77. Ciminiello, P., Dell'Aversano, C., Dello Iacovo, E. et al., 2011. Palytoxin in seafood by liquid chromatography tandem mass spectrometry: Investigation of extraction efficiency and matrix effect. *Anal. Bioanal. Chem.*, 401, 1043–1050.

78. Liu, R., Liang, Y., Wu, X., Xu, D., Liu, Y., and Liu, L., 2011. First report on the detection of pectenotoxin groups in Chinese shellfish by LC-MS/MS. *Toxicon*, 57, 1000–1007.

79. Caillaud, A., de la Iglesia, P., Darius, H. T. et al., 2010. Update on methodologies available for ciguatoxin determination: Perspectives to confront the onset of ciguatera fish poisoning in Europe. *Mar. Drugs*, 8, 1838–1907.

80. These, A., Klemm, C., Nausch, I., and Uhlig, S., 2011. Results of a European interlaboratory method validation study for the quantitative determination of lipophilic marine biotoxins in raw and cooked shellfish based on high-performance liquid chromatography-tandem mass spectrometry. Part I: Collaborative study. *Anal. Bioanal. Chem.*, 399, 1245–1256.

81. Otero, P., Alfonso, A., Alfonso, C. et al., 2010. New protocol to obtain spirolides from *Alexandrium ostenfeldii* cultures with high recovery and purity. *Biomed. Chromatogr.*, 24, 878–886.

82. Rodríguez, P., Alfonso, A., Vale, C. et al., 2008. First toxicity report of tetrodotoxin and 5,6,11-trideoxyTTX in the trumpet shell Charonia lampas lampas in Europe. *Anal. Chem.*, 80, 5622–5629.

83. Meisen, I., Distler, U., Muthing, J. et al., 2009. Direct coupling of high-performance thin-layer chromatography with UV spectroscopy and IR-MALDI orthogonal TOF MS for the analysis of cyanobacterial toxins. *Anal. Chem.*, 81, 3858–3866.

84. Ferranti, P., Fabbrocino, S., Nasi, A. et al., 2009. Liquid chromatography coupled to quadruple time-of-flight tandem mass spectrometry for microcystin analysis in freshwaters: Method performances and characterisation of a novel variant of microcystin-RR. *Rapid Commun. Mass Spectrom.*, 23, 1328–1336.

85. Gerssen, A., Mulder, P., van Rhijn, H., and de Boer, J., 2008. Mass spectrometric analysis of the marine lipophilic biotoxins pectenotoxin-2 and okadaic acid by four different types of mass spectrometers. *J. Mass Spectrom.*, 43, 1140–1147.

86. Arh, G., Klasinc, L., Veber, M., and Pompe, M., 2010. Modeling of the mass spectrometric response factors in non-target analysis. *Acta Chim. Slov.*, 57, 581–585.

87. Brombacher, S., Edmonds, S., and Volver, D., 2002. Studies on azaspiracid biotoxins II. Mass spectral behavior and structural elucidation of azaspiracid analogues. *Rapid Commun. Mass Spectrom.*, 16, 2306–2316.

88. Fux, E., McMillan, D., Bire, R., and Hess, P., 2007. Development of an ultra-performance liquid chromatography-mass spectrometry method for the detection of lipophilic marine toxins. *J. Chromatogr. A*, 1157, 273–280.

89. Otero, P., Perez, S., Alfonso, A. et al., 2010. First toxin profile of ciguateric fish in Madeira Arquipelago (Europe). *Anal. Chem.*, 82, 6032–6039.

90. Otero, P., Alfons, A., Alfonso, C., Rodriguez, P., Vyeites, M. R., and Botana, L. M., 2012. Response to comments on the effect of uncontrolled factors in a validated liquid chromatography-tandem mass spectrometry method question its use as reference method for marine toxins: Major causes for concern. *Anal. Chem.*, 84(1), 481–483.

91. Pottier, I., Vernoux, J. P., and Lewis, R. J., 2001. Ciguatera fish poisoning in the Caribbean islands and Western Atlantic. *Rev. Environ. Contam. Toxicol.*, 168, 99–141.

92. Dickey, R. W., 2008. Ciguatera toxins: Chemistry, toxicology, and detection. In *Seafood and Freshwater Toxins: Pharmacology, Physiology, and Detection*, Botana, L. M. ed. Marcel Dekker, New York, pp. 479–500.

93. Dickey, R. W. and Plakas, S. M., 2009. Ciguatera: A public health perspective. *Toxicon*, 56(2), 123–136.

94. Pérez-Arellano, J. L., Luzardo, O. P., Pérez Brito, A. et al., 2005. Ciguatera fish poisoning, Canary Islands. *Emer. Infect. Diseases*, 11, 1981–1982.

95. Hamilton, B., Hurbungs, M., Jones, A., and Lewis, R. J., 2002. Multiple ciguatoxins present in Indian Ocean reef fish. *Toxicon*, 40, 1347–1353.

96. Hamilton, B., Hurbungs, M., Vernoux, J. P., Jones, A., and Lewis, R. J., 2002. Isolation and characterisation of Indian Ocean ciguatoxin. *Toxicon*, 40, 685–693.

97. Lewis, R. J., Yang, A., and Jones, A., 2009. Rapid extraction combined with LC-tandem mass spectrometry (CREM-LC/MS/MS) for the determination of ciguatoxins in ciguateric fish flesh. *Toxicon*, 54, 62–66.

98. Dechraoui, M. Y., Tiedeken, J. A., Persad, R. et al., 2005. Use of two detection methods to discriminate ciguatoxins from brevetoxins: Application to great barracuda from Florida keys. *Toxicon*, 46, 261–270.

99. Lewis, R. J. and Jones, A., 1997. Characterization of ciguatoxins and ciguatoxin congeners present in ciguateric fish by gradient reverse-phase high-performance liquid chromatography/mass spectrometry. *Toxicon*, 35, 159–168.

100. Roeder, K., Erler, K., Kibler, S. et al., 2010. Characteristic profiles of ciguatera toxins in different strains of *Gambierdiscus* spp. *Toxicon*, 56, 731–738.

101. Pottier, I., Vernoux, J. P., Jones, A., and Lewis, R. J., 2002. Analysis of toxin profiles in three different fish species causing ciguatera fish poisoning in Guadeloupe, French West Indies. *Food Addit. Contam.*, 19, 1034–1042.

102. Litaker, R. W., Vandersea, M. W., Faust, M. A. et al., 2010. Global distribution of ciguatera causing dinoflagellates in the genus *Gambierdiscus*. *Toxicon*, 56, 711–730.

103. Perez, S., Vale, C., Alonso, E. et al., 2012. Effect of gambierol and its tetracyclic and heptacyclic analogues in cultured cerebellar neurons: A structure-activity relationships study. *Chem. Res. Toxicol.*, 25, 1929–1937.

104. Satake, M., Murata, M., and Yasumoto, T., 1993. Gambierol: A new toxic polyether compound isolated from the marine dinoflagellate *Gambierdiscus* toxicus. *J. Am. Chem. Soc.*, 115, 361–362.

4

Toxins from Marine Invertebrates

Eva Ternon and Olivier P. Thomas

CONTENTS

In the marine environment, invertebrates like corals, jellyfishes, or mollusks are well known by SCUBA divers as potential toxic species. We will describe in this section the main defensive arsenal of these living beauties. Even if a review has been recently published in this topic,[1] we will rather endeavor to restrict our analysis to toxins originated from invertebrate cells even if this is sometimes challenging to confirm this origin. Indeed, it has long been recognized that most invertebrates and especially the filter filters (bivalves, cnidarians, sponges, etc.) bioaccumulate and concentrate a large diversity of microorganisms that may be the real producers of target toxins. The readers will have to refer to the corresponding sections of this book for further information on toxins of microbial origin. We have organized this section according to the taxonomic group of the toxin producers.

4.1 Cnidarians

Among marine invertebrate animals, the phylum Cnidaria is one of the oldest living groups (>500 M years). These animals are simply built with two layers of cells, ectoderm and endoderm, set within a radial symmetry and separated by a noncellular matrix, the mesohyl. They possess a single body cavity devoted to their digestive system. Marine cnidarians are mostly distributed among four classes: Anthozoa (hard corals, gorgonians, soft corals, sea pens, sea anemones, etc.), Cubozoa (box jellyfishes), Scyphozoa (jellyfishes), and Hydrozoa (hydroids and fire corals).

Cnidarians are mostly predators. This group of sessile or pelagic organisms has developed a formidable and complex device to catch prey. All cnidarians present specialized cells called nematocytes that contain nematocysts and venoms. After mechanical or chemical stimulation, an arrow-like tube is extruded from the nematocyst and the venom is injected into the target animal within 3 ms.[2] A myriad of toxins compose the venom of cnidarians,[3] and they were shown to potentially cause severe hemolytic, cytolytic, and neurotoxic effects on the target organisms.[4] These toxins can also affect humans by causing cardiotoxicity, dermatitis, local itching, swelling, erythema, paralysis, pain, and necrosis.[5]

The identification and structure characterization of these toxins are important for a complete understanding of their mode of action. However, if nematocysts, as venom apparatus, have been studied since the nineteenth century,[6] research on venoms and associated toxins is emerging with the development of appropriate biochemical techniques for their isolation and structure characterization that started during the twentieth century. The group of Richert was the first to partially purify and study two active components ("congestine" and "thalassine") from tentacle extracts of the European sea anemone *Actinia equina*.[7,8] In the 1950s, the column chromatography method had been widely developed and used to isolate proteins and peptides toxins from cnidarian venoms. However, research on the effects of purified toxins instead of the whole venom really started during the late twentieth century.[9]

Toxins isolated from cnidarians can be classified as peptidic (peptides or proteins) and nonpeptidic substances (purines, quaternary ammonium compounds, biogenic amines, and betaines).[5] The following part offers a review of the different toxins that have been described so far according to this classification. To date, only a small number of 3D structures have been described for the corresponding toxins. Structural determination was usually performed using nuclear magnetic resonance (NMR) or x-ray crystallography.

4.1.1 Peptides and Proteins

Peptides and proteins constitute the largest group of toxins found in cnidarians (Table 4.1). It is noteworthy that most of the research on toxins produced by species of the phylum Cnidaria has been carried out on sea anemones.[10] Indeed, more than 40 species have been studied for that purpose so far, allowing the identification of 166 peptides, 22 cytolysin proteins, and 3 phospholipases A2 enzymes within 9 sea anemone families.[11] On the contrary, and despite important research efforts, relatively few toxins have been isolated from the classes Cubozoa and Scyphozoa.

4.1.1.1 Peptides Acting on Sodium and/or Potassium Channels

A large number of peptides with low molecular weights have been found in sea anemones.[12] The most thoroughly characterized peptidic toxins are those affecting sodium and/or potassium channels. Both groups of toxins are made up of several groups with distinct molecular weights and structural characteristics.

Toxins affecting sodium channels were the first cnidarian peptides identified and they can be grouped into three structural classes: type 1 (mostly from the family Actiniidae) and type 2 toxins (mostly from the family Stichodactylidae) are made up of molecules containing between 45 and 50 amino acid residues, cross-linked by three disulfide bonds, and formed by a core of four-stranded antiparallel β-sheets.[13,14] Type 3 toxins are shorter peptides containing 27–32 amino acid residues with 4 disulfide bonds, and rigid β and γ turns. Only a limited number of this type has been reported (five toxins so far). Although types 1 and 2 show extensive sequence homology within each class (≥60%), only about 30%

TABLE 4.1

List of Peptidic Toxins Isolated from Cnidarian Organisms

Type	Target	Current Name	Type	Biological Group	Species	3D Structure	References
Peptides	Na+ channel toxins	Ae I	Type I	Sea anemone	*Actinia equina*		[61]
		AETX-I	Type I	Sea anemone	*Anemonia erythraea*		[62]
		ATX-I	Type I	Sea anemone	*Anemonia sulcata*	Yes (A)	[63]
		ATX-II	Type I	Sea anemone	*Anemonia viridis*		[64]
		ATX-III	Type III	Sea anemone	*Anemonia sulcata*	Yes	[65]
		ATX-V	Type I	Sea anemone	*Anemonia viridis*		[66]
		Am-3	Type I	Sea anemone	*Antheopsis maculata*		[67]
		Anthopleurin-A and -B (AP-A and -B)	Type I	Sea anemone	*Anthopleura xanthogrammica*	Yes	[68,69]
		Anthopleurin C	Type I	Sea anemone	*Anthopleura elegantissima*		[70]
		APE 1-(1–2) and APE 2-(1–2)	Type I	Sea anemone	*Anthopleura elegantissima*		[71]
		AFT-I and -II	Type I	Sea anemone	*Anthopleura fuscoviridis*		[72]
		Toxin Hk (2, 7, 8, and 16)	Type I	Sea anemone	*Anthopleura species*		[73]
		Toxins PCR (1–7)	Type I	Sea anemone	*Anthopleura xanthogrammica*		[74]
		BcIII	Type I	Sea anemone	*Bunodosoma caissarum*		[75]
		Cangitoxin (0, 2, and 3)	Type I	Sea anemone	*Bunodosoma cangicum*		[76,77]
		NeurotoxinBg-2, 3	Type I	Sea anemone	*Bunodosoma granulifera*		[78]
		Calitoxin (1, 2)	Others	Sea anemone	*Calliactis parasitica*		[79,80]
		CgNa	Type I	Sea anemone	*Condyctalis gigantea*	Yes	[62,81]
		Cp I	Type I	Sea anemone	*Condyctalis passiflora*		[82]

(continued)

TABLE 4.1 (continued)

List of Peptidic Toxins Isolated from Cnidarian Organisms

Type	Target	Current Name	Type	Biological Group	Species	3D Structure	References
		Ca I	Type II	Sea anemone	*Cryptodendrum adhaesivum*		[83]
		Halcurin	Type II	Sea anemone	*Halcurias carlgreni*		[84]
		Rm (1–5)	Type II	Sea anemone	*Heteractis crispa*		[85,86]
		Toxin Rc-1	Type I	Sea anemone	*Heteractis crispa*		[62]
		Hh x	Type II	Sea anemone	*Heterodactyla hemprichi*		[83]
	Na+ channel toxins	Neurotoxin Nv1	Type II	Sea anemone	*Nematostella vectensis*		[87,88]
		Pa-TX	Type III	Sea anemone	*Parasicyonis actinostoloides*	Yes	[89]
		Rp-II, -III	Type II	Sea anemone	*Radianthus paumotensis*		[90]
		Sh 1	Type II	Sea anemone	*Stichodactyla helianthus*	Yes	[63,91]
		Gigantoxin -2, -3	Types I and II	Sea anemone	*Stichodactyla gigantea*		[92]
		SHTX-4	Type II	Sea anemone	*Stichodactyla haddoni*		[93]
		Ta I	Type II	Sea anemone	*Thalassianthus aster*		[83]
	K+ channel toxins	ShK	Type I	Sea anemone	*Stichodactyla helianthus*	Yes	[94,95]
		BgK	Type I	Sea anemone	*Bunodosoma granulifera*	Yes	[96]
		BDS I and II	Types II and III	Sea anemone	*Anemonia viridis*	Yes (I)	[97]
		APETx1 and 2	Type III	Sea anemone	*Anthopleura elegantissima*	Yes	[98,99]
		AeK	Type I	Sea anemone	*Actinia equina*		[100]
		AETX-K	Type I	Sea anemone	*Anemonia erythraea*		[101]
		SA5 II	Type II	Sea anemone	*Anemonia viridis*		[64]
		Kalicludin (1–3)	Type II	Sea anemone	*Anemonia viridis*		[102]
		Kaliseptin	Type I	Sea anemone	*Anemonia viridis*		[102]
		Am-2	Type III	Sea anemone	*Antheopsis maculata*		[67]

Group	Toxin	Type	Organism	Species	Recombinant	Ref.
	Bc-IV	Type III	Sea anemone	*Bunodosoma caissarum*		[103]
	Bc-V	Type III	Sea anemone	*Bunodosoma caissarum*		[77]
	Toxin Bcg III	Type III	Sea anemone	*Bunodosoma cangicum*		[77]
	Polypeptide HC1	Type II	Sea anemone	*Heteractis crispa*		[104]
	Kuniz-type trypsin inhibitor IV	Type II	Sea anemone	*Heteractis crispa*	Yes	[105]
	Metridin	Type I	Sea anemone	*Metridium senile*		[106]
	HmK	Type I	Sea anemone	*Radianthus magnifica*		[107]
	SHPI-1, 2	Type II	Sea anemone	*Stichodactyla helianthus*		[108,109]
Phospholipase A2	SHTX-1/SHTX-2 and 3	Types IV and II	Sea anemone	*Stichodactyla haddoni*		[93]
	AcPLA2		Sea anemone	*Adamsia palliata*		[21]
	Cationic protein C1		Sea anemone	*Bunodosoma caissarum*		[5]
	Phospholipase A2		Sea anemone	*Condylactis gigantea*		[110]
	UcPLA2		Sea anemone	*Urticina crassicornis*		[111]
	Milleporin-1		Fire coral	*Millepora plathyphylla*		[112]
	Proteins		Fire coral	*Millepora complanata*		[113]
Cytolytic proteins	Cytolysin RTX-A; - S-II	Type I	Sea anemone	*Heteractis crispa*		[114,115]
	Equinatoxin (I, II, III, IV, V)	Actinoporin	Sea anemone	*Actinia equina*	Yes—Equinatoxin II	[28,116–118]
	Stycholysin (I, II, III)	Actinoporin	Sea anemone	*Stichodactyla heliantus*	Yes—Stycholysin II	[119]
	AvT-I, -II	Actinoporin	Sea anemone	*Actineria villosa*		[36,37,120]
	Fragaceatoxin C	Actinoporin	Sea anemone	*Actinia fragacea*	Yes	[121]
	Tenebrosin-(A, B, C)	Actinoporin	Sea anemone	*Actinia tenebrosa*		[122,123]
	Bandaporin	Actinoporin	Sea anemone	*Anthopleura asiatica*		[10]
	Actinoporin Or- (A, G)	Actinoporin	Sea anemone	*Oulactis orientalis*		[124]
	Pstx-20A	Actinoporin	Sea anemone	*Phyllodiscus semoni*		[125]
	HMg (I, II, III)	Actinoporin	Sea anemone	*Radianthus magnifica*		[126,127]
	Hemolytic toxin	Actinoporin	Sea anemone	*Radianthus magnifica*		[128]
	Cytolysin Src-I	Actinoporin	Sea anemone	*Sagartia rosea*		[129]

(continued)

TABLE 4.1 (continued)

List of Peptidic Toxins Isolated from Cnidarian Organisms

Type	Target	Current Name	Type	Biological Group	Species	3D Structure	References
		Up-1	Type III	Sea anemone	*Urticina piscivora*		[32]
		Uc-I	Type III	Sea anemone	*Urticina crassicornis*		[130]
		Urticinatoxin	Type III	Sea anemone	*Urticina crassicornis*		[111]
		PsTX-60 (A, B)	MACPF	Sea anemone	*Phyllodiscus semoni*		[33]
		AvTX-60A	MACPF	Sea anemone	*Actineria villosa*		[34]
		Hydralysin		Hydra	*Chlorohydra viridissima*		[38]
		Cytotoxins		Fire coral	*Millepora tenera*		[131]
		Cytotoxins		Fire coral	*Millepora alicornis*		[131]
		Millepora cytotoxin MCTx-1		Fire coral	*Millepora tenera*		[40]
		Proteins		Fire coral	*Millepora plathyphylla*		[132]
		Physalitoxin		Hydrozoa	*Physalia physalis*		[133]
		pCrTX-I, II, III		Box jellyfish	*Carybdea rastonii*		[134]
		CrTX-A, B		Box jellyfish	*Carybdea rastonii*		[135]
		CaTX-A, B		Box jellyfish	*Carybdea alata*		[42]
		CAH1		Box jellyfish	*Carybdea alata*		[42]
		CqTX-1		Box jellyfish	*Chiropsalmus quadrigatus*		[44]
		CfTX-1, 2		Box jellyfish	*Chironex fleckeri*		[43]
		Four major proteins	40, 45, 80, and 106 kDa	Box jellyfish	*Carukia barnesi*		[136]
		Bio-active proteins	10–30 kDa; 40–50 kDa; 120 and 170 kDa	Box jellyfish	*Chironex fleckeri*		[137–139]
		CARTOX + 1 neurotoxin + 3 cytolysins	107 kDa + 120 kDa + 220, 139, and 36 kDa	Box jellyfish	*Carybdea marsupialis*		[140,141]

Source: Rearranged from Frazao, B. et al., *Mar. Drugs*, 10, 1812, 2012.

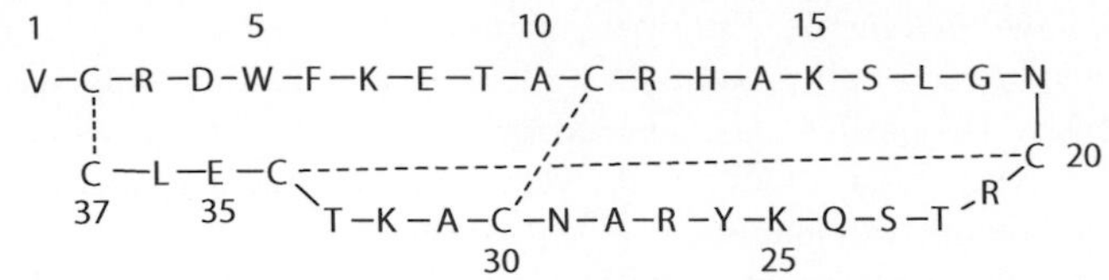

FIGURE 4.1 Chemical structure of BgK.

of homology was found between the two classes.[15] Type 3 toxins lack homology with both previous types. It is noteworthy that a sodium channel blocker has been isolated from a hexacoral, a species of the genus *Goniopora*.[16]

In the last decades, intense investigation has been performed on modulating peptides that affect the gating of potassium channels. These simple peptides with molecular weights 3–5 kDa consist of a chain of amino acid residues whose folded structure is stabilized by four disulfide bonds. According to the length of the peptides chain, four structural types of peptides, grouping 10 K$^+$ channel blockers, have been characterized across the various sea anemones species.[10,17] Type 1 peptides consist of a 35–37 amino acid chain and 3 disulfide bonds (BgK, Figure 4.1); type 2 peptides contain 58 or 59 amino acid residues and 3 disulfide bonds; type 3 peptides contain 41–42 amino acid residues and 3 disulfide bonds; and type 4 contains 28 amino acid residues and 2 disulfide bridges.

It is noteworthy that a protein toxin affecting Ca^{2+} channels has been isolated from an unidentified species of the genus *Goniopora* from the Red Sea.[18]

4.1.1.2 Phospholipase A2

All classes of the phylum Cnidaria present catalytic activity of phospholipases A2 (PLA2) enzymes, suggesting that these enzymes can be associated to the toxicity of this animal group.[5] However, this toxic role has not been already clearly demonstrated.[19] These enzymes, firstly isolated in *Aiptasia pallida*, are presynaptic neurotoxins and exist in two isozymic forms, α and β.[20]

A specific type of PLA2 enzymes is secreted by cnidarians and can be classified into various groups (I–XIV) and subgroups, according to their molecular structure.[19] Up to now, few cases of PLA2s venoms have been deeply studied and sequenced.[10] The first cnidarian PLA2 was cloned and sequenced from the sea anemone *Adamsia carciniopados*.[21]

4.1.1.3 Cytolysin Proteins

This class of toxic proteins are also called pore-forming toxins as they form pores in cell membranes.[22,23] Scientific interest for this class of compounds began in the 1970s studying sea anemone toxicity. Since then, several groups of cytolysins proteins have been discovered, among which 13 have their amino acid sequence described.[10] However, no classification is currently available as their structural characterization is far to be achieved.[24]

4.1.1.3.1 In Sea Anemones

Concerning the particular group of sea anemones, five polypeptidic groups based upon primary structure and functional properties were identified.[10,24]

Type I is composed of a group of small proteins of molecular weight (5–16 kDa).[3,25]

Type II or actinoporins are highly basic proteins of low molecular weight (18–20 kDa).[23] These water-soluble and stable proteins constitute the most studied group of cnidarian pore-forming toxins.[26] Actinoporins were named according to their ability to bind the membrane phospholipid domains of the host organism; oligomerizing and forming cation selective pores.[4] The first actinoporin was isolated from the sea anemone *Actinia equine*,[27] and named equinatoxin (Eqt). It is composed of three isotoxins (I, II, and III). Intensive efforts have been devoted to Eqt II, the most abundant equinatoxin,[28] as well as to two other major isotoxins, sticholysin (St) I and II,[29] isolated from the sea anemone *Stichodactyla helianthus*.[23] Both equinatoxins and sticholysins 3D structure have been elucidated.[30,31] Although these small proteins lack disulfide bonds, their folded structures are very stable due to an extensive BB-pleated sheet secondary structure that involves most of their peptide bonds.[1] Most of the cytolytic proteins found in the venom of sea anemones share characteristics with these two cysteineless proteins (Eqt and St).

Type III cytolysins are constituted by a heterogeneous group of proteins of higher molecular weight ranged from 28 to 45 kDa,[32] potentially lacking PLA activity. To date, these cytolytic proteins have only been isolated from species of the genus *Urticina*.[24] Contrary to actinoporins, cytolysins contain cysteine residues.

Type IV is a family of proteins possessing the membrane-attack complex/perforin (MACPF) domain. The membrane-attack complex (MAC) of the complement system and perforin (PF) form pores on the target membrane.[10] Up to now, very few toxins of this family have been isolated from sea anemones. In 2002, a new cytolytic protein of 55 kDa was discovered in the sea anemone *Phyllodiscus semoni* that presents homologies with two other proteins of the MACPF family, PsTX-60A and PsTX-60B (~60 kDa).[33] The latest proteins present a primary structure close to AvTX-60A, a Type IV toxin found in the sea anemone *Actineria villosa*.[34–37]

Type V toxins are composed of a single thiol-activated cytolysin of 80 kDa, isolated from *Metridium senile*.[29]

4.1.1.3.2 In Hydrozoa

Hydralysins constitute a novel group of pore-forming cnidarian toxins, isolated in 2003 from the green hydra *Chlorohydra viridissima*.[38] Regarding their structure and function, these toxins are different from other cnidarian toxins but similar to bacterial and fungal toxins. Homologies are encountered between the different hydralysins, such as molecular weight (27–31 kDa) and sequence.[39]

Fire coral cytotoxins are potent proteins with low molecular weight (~18 kDa). One cytotoxin-1 (MCTx-1) was isolated from *M. dichotoma* var. *tenera*, and partially sequenced.[40] MCTx-1 is an acidic protein of 222 amino acid residues that lacks PLA2 activity.

4.1.1.3.3 In Scyphozoa and Cubozoa

Very potent cytolytic proteins (~50 kDa) have been isolated from jellyfish of both Scyphozoa and Cubozoa groups.[24] However, despite many attempts and on the contrary to other cnidarians, cytolytic proteins composing jellyfish venoms have been very difficult to isolate as stable and bioactive toxins.[1,41] Additionally, the use of venoms of partially purified proteins precludes firm conclusions on the detailed structure and mechanisms of action of these cytolysins.

Using molecular biological methods,[42] the first cubozoan protein toxin (CrTx-A and CrTx-B) was sequenced from the carybdeid box jellyfish *Carybdea alata* and homologous protein toxins from three other box jellyfish species were isolated and characterized consequently (see Table 4.1).[43] Regarding their amino acid sequence, these toxins were shown to present certain common features and thus belong to a distinct and novel family of cnidarian bioactive proteins.[43,44] Finally, this family of cubozoan toxins gathers five proteins (42–46 kDa), isolated from four different species. However, no structural characterization of cubozoan proteins has been reported to date. Although 63 amino acids are conserved across the 5 homologous toxin sequences, various structure, specificities, and functions exist between carybdeids and chirodropids protein toxins.[43] The use of new biological tools is expected to bring new insights on cubozoan and scyphozoan bioactive proteins.

4.1.2 Nonpeptidic Substances

Nonpeptidic toxins have been identified, for example, in the octocoral anthozoan branch (soft coral), such as polyethers,[45] steroids, acetogenins, sesquiterpenes, and a large number of terpenoids, especially diterpenoids (order Gorgonacea),[46] as well as compounds related to pigments (i.e., zooxanthin).[47] The most potent marine cnidarian toxin was thought to be palytoxin, a complex polyether (2659–2680 Da),[48] first isolated from a species of the genus *Palythoa*.[49,50] Besides *Palythoa*, this toxin has been later found in other species such as another zoantharian of the genus *Zoanthus*,[51] as well as the sea anemone *Radianthus*

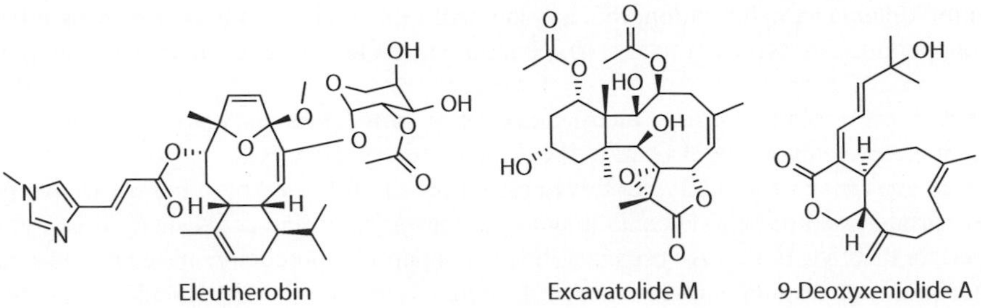

Eleutherobin   Excavatolide M   9-Deoxyxeniolide A

FIGURE 4.2 Cytotoxic diterpenoids from cnidarians.

macrodactylus.[52] Regarding its 3D structure,[48] palytoxin is one of the largest and most complex natural products known to date (elemental composition, $C_{129}H_{223}N_3O_{54}$).[45] Because of its presence in different invertebrates and because of the recent report of the group of Laurent, a microalgal origin is strongly suggested and then these compounds are clearly out of the scope of this review, dedicated to pure cnidarians toxins.[53] These complex polyethers are indeed very often produced by microalgae and especially dinoflagellates. This remark is of general concern as the origin of toxins is usually an unresolved issue. In our case, we will mainly focus on toxins that have been clearly identified from invertebrate origin.

Within this frame, diterpenoids constitute the most studied group of true nonpeptidic cnidarian toxins, with 177 articles and up to 622 compounds published to date, for the single gorgonian coral group.[46] One of the first compounds identified in this group was sarcophine.[54] Diterpenoids contain carbocyclic rings with 3–14 carbons as well as acyclic skeletons with novel branching patterns. Among terpenoids, the particular subgroup cembranoids has been discovered about 50 years ago from the Caribbean gorgonian *Eunicea mammosa* ciere.[55] Up to now, more than 300 cembranoids compounds have been identified,[56] and they were shown to exhibit a wide range of biological activities.[57]

Despite the large knowledge acquired on structural diversity of cyclic diterpenes, their classification remains confusing.[46] Gorgonians are rich sources of terpenoids that can be classified into 40 skeletal classes. Some of the most potent and cytotoxic compounds of this family are represented in Figure 4.2.

Other nonpeptidic compounds have been identified in octocorals, such as prostaglandins,[58] the muricin saponins,[59] and pseudopterosins,[60] but like diterpenoids they rather poorly affect the ion channels (Table 4.1).

4.2 Mollusks

The toxicity of bivalves and other gastropods is often associated to the bioaccumulation of poisoning toxins produced by associated microorganism and these compounds are clearly out of the scope of this review. Within the most studied class Gastropoda, we will focus on toxins of pure invertebrate origin: peptides from cone snails belonging to the family Conidae, and nonpeptidic toxins from the larger infraclass Opisthobranchia, where the shell is absent or present inside the body of the animal.

4.2.1 Peptides from Cone Snails

Marine snails belonging to the genus *Conus* are gastropods that have evolved into effective predators through the development of venom, either used for self-defense or prey capture. This venom is loaded into a hollow harpoon that the snail injects into the intended prey (fish, worms, other snails), and it consists in an arsenal of biologically active peptides, commonly referred as conopeptides.[142] These conopeptide compounds act to block voltage- and ligand-gated ion channels[143] and are specifically optimized for a target.

The genus *Conus* is represented by approximately 700 species. Every single species of cone snails contains upward of 100 different peptides, leading to a potential of 70,000 existing sequences of conopeptides.[144,145] However, due to the frequent description of new species and the availability of new techniques for venom characterization, this number will most probably be increased by a factor 10 or more.[146] Conopeptides are typically small, 10–40 amino acids long,[147] and can contain up to 5 disulfide bonds.[148]

Conopeptides are assembled from intermediate-sized propeptide molecules, 60–90 amino acids long,[149] which are proteolytically cleaved to yield the mature peptide. Conopeptide precursors show a typical pattern consisting of a highly conserved signal region, followed by a more variable pro-region and a hyper-variable mature peptide containing a few conserved amino acids such as the cysteine residues required for disulfide bonds. An organization of conopeptides precursors based on the conservation of the signal sequence throughout the process of peptide maturation was established.[150] This process involves the excision of *N*- and *C*-terminal region of the protein receptors,[150] as well as the post-translational modification of some amino acids.[151] Conopeptides have a high frequency of post-translational modifications, which generates a rich chemical diversity.

According to their amino acid sequence, two classes of conopeptides can be defined: disulfide-rich peptides and nondisulfide-rich peptides.[152] The former were named conotoxins[153] and present two or more disulfide bonds while the latter is formed by one or none disulfide bonds.[142,154] Conotoxins are further divided into unique superfamilies (A, B, C, D, I, J, L, M, O, P, S, T, V, X, and Y[144,146]; according to their cysteine framework pattern,[142] derived from the number of residues contained in each of the three loop regions CC(X4-6)C(X4-5)C(X1-5), where X4-6 represents four to six amino acids in the first loop, X4-5 represents four to five amino acids in the second loop, and X1-5 represents one to five amino acids in the third loop.[149] The cysteine general pattern of some superfamilies was recently reported.[144,146] Superfamilies: A,[155] I,[156] M,[149] O,[152] P,[157] T,[158,159] and S.[160]

Some of the peptidic superfamilies are further divided into branches, based on the number of cysteine residues. For instance, the M superfamily presents five branches, from M-1 to M-5, grouped into Mini-M (M1–M3) and Maxi-M (M4 and M5) for respectively less and more than 22 amino acids in the mature peptide.[143,145]

The current structural database only describes a small proportion of conopeptide diversity. The most studied structures belong to the A (29), O1 (20), and M (13) superfamilies.[154] Among the other superfamilies, some of them are represented by less than 5 three-dimensional structures and remaining ones have no published structures.

Ziconotide (Prialt®) is undoubtedly the most famous conotoxin known so far due to its presence in the market to treat refractory pain (Figure 4.3).[161]

4.2.2 Nonpeptidic Substances from Sea Slugs

Mollusks and sea slugs (Opistobranchia) in particular are a group of marine organisms that are well known for the production of nonpeptidic bioactive substances.[162] Some of the compounds found in nudibranchs or sea hares were clearly identified as dietary metabolites due to the feeding behavior of both organisms (respectively on sponges and some macroalgae). Although these compounds present a lower toxicity than peptidic substances, some of them can still be classified as toxins.

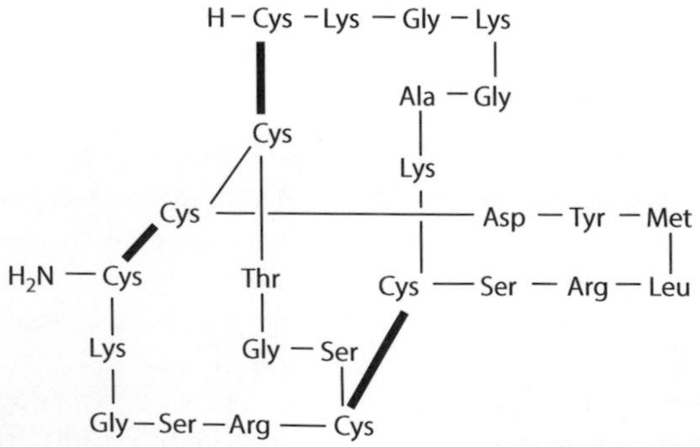

FIGURE 4.3 Structure of ziconotide, a peptidic toxin from a cone snail.

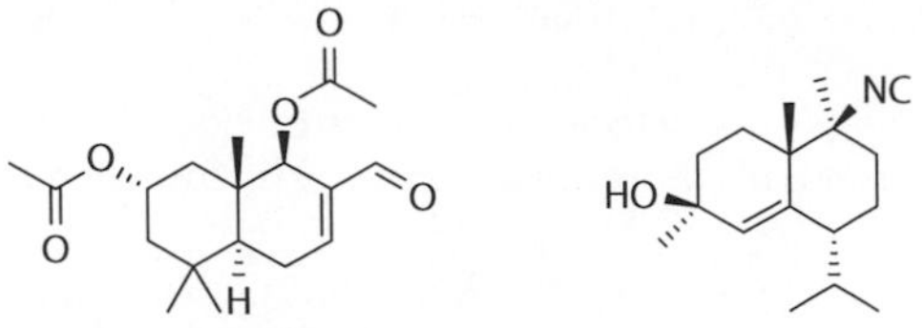

Hodgsonal

FIGURE 4.4 Examples of toxic terpenoids from nudibranchs. (From Manzo, E. et al., *J. Nat. Prod.*, 67, 1701, 2004.)

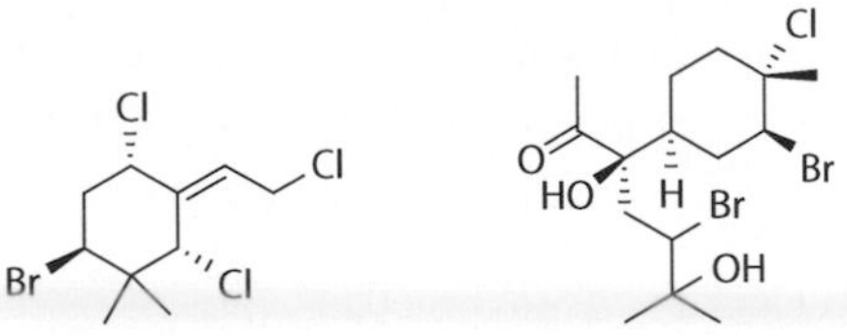

Apakaochtodene A   Aplysiadiol

FIGURE 4.5 Some examples of halogenated derivatives from sea hares. (From Brito, I. et al., *Tetrahedron*, 62, 9655, 2006.)

4.2.2.1 Terpenoids from Nudibranchs

A large chemical diversity has been isolated from nudibranchs and especially for compounds of terpenoid origin.[163] Several studies have demonstrated the dietary origin of several classes of terpenoids present in nudibranchs (Figure 4.4). These toxins would originate from sponge natural products. They would be further biochemically transformed and the derived toxins sequestered in the mantle of the organisms avoiding the palatability of the animals or even acting as chemical defenses.[164] In some terpenoids, the biosynthesis has been demonstrated to occur *de novo* and this ability may have been acquired all along the evolutionary history of these animals.[165]

Several compounds of this family exhibit strong antifouling activity, thus evidencing their role as toxins.

4.2.2.2 Halogenated Derivatives from Sea Hares

Sea hares have attracted the interest of natural product chemists and biochemists for a long time. Indeed, they are renowned producers of toxic substances that may acquire from their diet, especially macroalgae,[167] but in some cases they produce larger proteins acting like true toxins. In particular, species of the genus *Aplysia* were shown to produce a large diversity of toxic proteins present in the ink released by this mollusk.[168] However, most of the toxins found to date are halogenated derivatives originated from the algae diets of these animals and further metabolized leading to a toxic substance that is also sequestered by the animal (Figure 4.5).[169]

4.3 Worms

At least 12 phyla of worms have been identified so far. Little scientific attention has been paid to marine worms, while some phyla (Nemertea, Annelida, Nematoda, and Platyhelminthes) have been shown to produce toxins for defensive and escape strategies. Most of these toxins have been identified as peptides, proteins, but also alkaloids.

4.3.1 Peptides

The phylum Nemertea (Nemertine) is subdivided into four classes: Anopla (subclass Heteronemertine), Enopla (subclass Hoplonemertine), Paleonermeta, and Nemertea incertae sedis. In 1936, the presence of toxins in nermetines was evidenced for the very first time and they were called "amphiporine" and "nemertine."[171]

4.3.1.1 From Nemertea

Most of the nemertine toxins are produced by members of the heteronemertine group. Heteronemertines are able to produce peptide neurotoxins as well as cytolytic peptides, but no alkaloids have been isolated so far from these organisms.[172]

Two genera were shown to biosynthesize neurotoxic peptides: *Lineus* and *Cerebratulus*. The molecular weights of these small peptides are respectively 2–3 and 0.6 kDa. Neurotoxic peptides from *Cerebratulus* were named "B" toxins as they were identified after the "A" cytolytic peptides (see later section), also found in heteronemertines. Complete sequences of the two most abundant B-toxins, B-II and B-IV, have been determined.[173,174] These very basic peptides contain 55 amino acids residues cross-linked by four disulfide bridges. The B-IV toxin NMR data evidenced a helical protein with no β-sheet structure, which possesses a helical-like structure for the *C*-terminal five residues and a largely unstructured *N*-terminus.[175]

So far, cytolytic proteins have only been found in heteronemertines and paleonemertines groups.[172] At least, four homologous integumentary "A"-toxins potent cytolysins with molecular weight of 10 kDa have been found.[176,177] Isotoxin A-III has been sequenced and contains many basic amino acids as well as three disulfide bonds.[178] Structural analyses reveal the presence of approximately 60% α-helix and 10% β-sheet.[172]

4.3.1.2 From Annelids

Only very few neuropeptides and cytolytic proteins from annelids have been purified and sequenced.[1] Those basic peptides consist of α-helical segments that are folded together and stabilized by four disulfide bonds. The major neurotoxin possesses a molecular size of approximately 320 kDa.[172,179] Two potent antibacterial peptides of molecular size 2.8 kDa have been found in species of the genus *Arenicola*: the arenicins.[180] Two isoforms were sequenced and showed 21 amino acids residues and a single disulfide bond.

4.3.1.3 From Nematoda and Platyhelminthes

Cytolytic peptides were found in both phyla, with molecular weights ranging from 9 kDa (helminth peptide clonorin)[181] to 65 kDa (hookworm hemolytic peptide).[182]

4.3.2 Alkaloids

The very first toxin isolated from a worm was the hoplonemertine alkaloid anabaseine (Figure 4.4).[183] Only few toxins from worms have been examined in detail. The most abundant of these alkaloids is nemertelline, a tetrapyridyl compound (Figure 4.6).[184]

Some polychaetes secrete toxic mucus when disturbed, with alkaloids as active constituents. This is the case of the polychaete *Lumbriconereis brevicirra* that produces nereistoxin (Figure 4.7), a dimethylamine possessing a 1.2-dithiolane ring whose structure was determined by synthesis.[185,186]

Species of flatworms, arrowworms, and polychaetes have been reported to contain tetrodotoxin alkaloids.[187,188] However, these toxins were later shown to be produced by associated bacteria.[189,190]

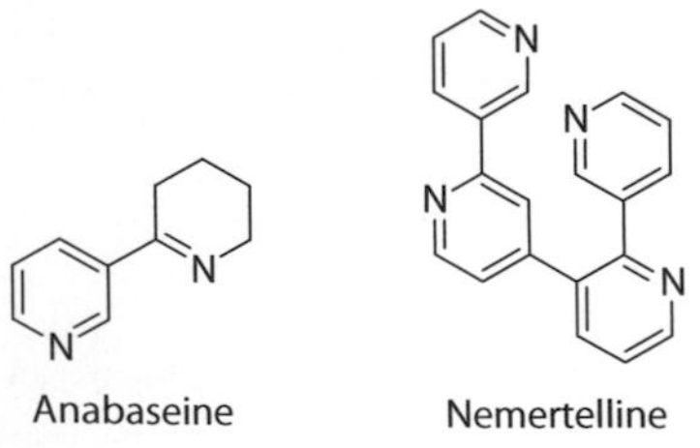

Anabaseine   Nemertelline

FIGURE 4.6 Structure of worm toxic alkaloids.

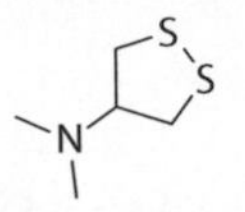

FIGURE 4.7   Structure of the annelid toxin nereistoxin.

4.4 Echinoderms

The phylum Echinodermata is composed of several classes of unique marine species. Among the most widespread classes we can cite sea stars (asteroids), brittle stars (ophiuroids), sea urchins (echinoids), crinoids, and sea cucumbers (holothurians). While ophiuroids and crinoids do not produce accepted toxins, the other three classes of echinoderms clearly contain toxic species.

4.4.1 Saponins from Sea Cucumbers and Sea Stars

Sea cucumbers (Holothuroidea) have been shown to possess only a small number of predators. The toxicity of the body wall and the presence of Cuvierian tubules seem to be the most effective antipredation mechanisms developed by these organisms.[191] It has been demonstrated that all sea cucumbers contain saponins in their body wall and viscera. Most of the saponins have a triterpenoid aglycone structure (Figure 4.8). Due to their physicochemical properties, sea cucumber saponins named holothurins exhibit a wide range of biological effects ranging from cytotoxicity to hemolytic actions. These compounds have been suggested to act as toxins against a large array of predators and their defense has been recently proven.[192] Other classes of toxic saponins, named asterosaponins, have also been identified in sea stars (Asteroidea).[193,194] Asterosaponins have also been demonstrated to exhibit a wide range of biological activities.[195]

Structurally diverse saponins have also been isolated from other marine invertebrates like sponges,[196,197] and then appear as common chemical weapons in the marine environment.

4.4.2 Peptides from Sea Urchins

Several species of sea urchins (Echinoidea) are dangerous to humans. Envenomations are caused by stings from either pedicellariae or spines.[198] The toxopneustid sea urchins have well-developed globiferous pedicellariae with bioactive substances.[199] The hollow primary spines of diadematid sea urchins are suggested to also contain bioactive substances. After purification and structure identification, these bioactive substances were proven to belong to the large protein group of lectins (19–28 kDa) and these substances could cause smooth muscle contraction and relaxation. The bioactive lectin contractin A appeared as a phopholipase A_2-like substance.

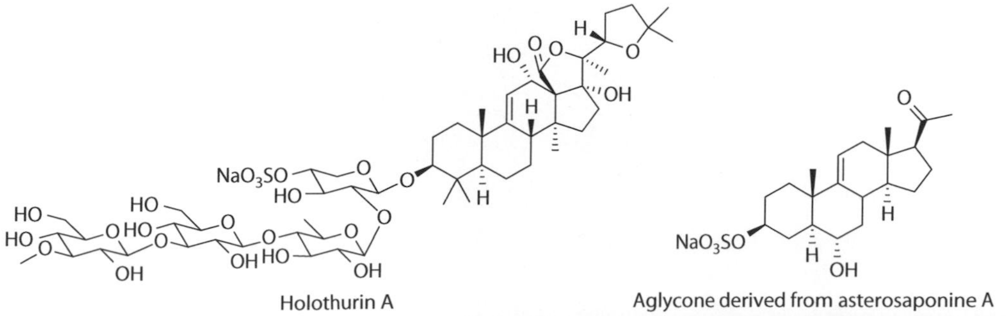

Holothurin A   Aglycone derived from asterosaponine A

FIGURE 4.8   Structure of some sea cucumber and starfish saponins.

4.5 Ascidians

A wide range of toxins with interesting pharmacological properties have been isolated from ascidians.[200] These often nitrogenated compounds include cyclic peptides but also aromatic alkaloids. The majority of these compounds are cytotoxic, and in some cases the mechanisms of action have been investigated.

4.5.1 Peptides

Two closely related family of bioactive pepides have been isolated from tunicates, namely, the didemnins and the tamandarins (Figure 4.9).[201]

Even if didemnins were only found in some tunicates like *Trididemnum solidum* and *Aplidium albicans*, a bacterial origin of these compounds was evidenced.[202] This finding is of high relevance for the pharmaceutical applications of these important compounds like aplidine that is currently under clinical trials for several applications. Invertebrate-derived natural products with complex polyketide and nonribosomal peptide structures are generally found to be of microbial origin since the molecular basis governing their biosyntheses resides exclusively in microbes.[203]

Further peptide-derived patellamides were first isolated from asicidans and they were later originated from cyanobacterial symbionts (Figure 4.9).[204]

4.5.2 Alkaloids

Ecteinascidin alkaloids were first identified in the tunicate *Ecteinascidia turbinata*. ET-743 (Yondelis®, Figure 4.10) has been recently approved as an anticancer agent to treat ovarian neoplasms and sarcoma.[205] Here also a microbial origin was quickly hypothesized due to the presence of close analogues in other marine invertebrates and a possible NRPS origin. This assumption was later confirmed using biomolecular and biochemical tools.[206]

A large array of pyridoacridine alkaloids has been isolated almost exclusively from tunicates and sponges, thus suggesting an invertebrate origin for these toxins (Figure 4.11).[207] These unique polyaromatic derivatives exhibit diverse biological activities.[208]

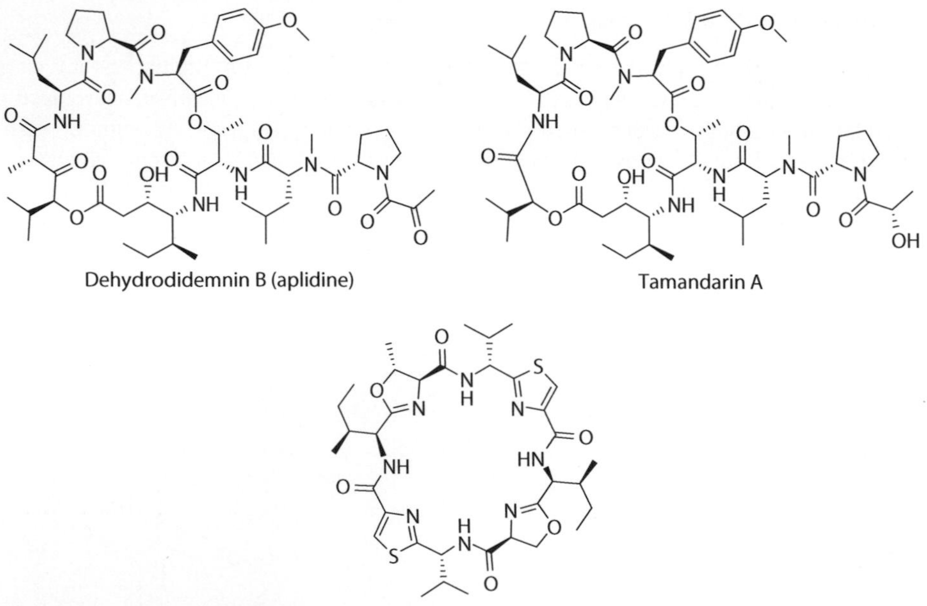

Dehydrodidemnin B (aplidine)

Tamandarin A

Patellamide A

FIGURE 4.9 Bioactive peptides isolated from ascidians.

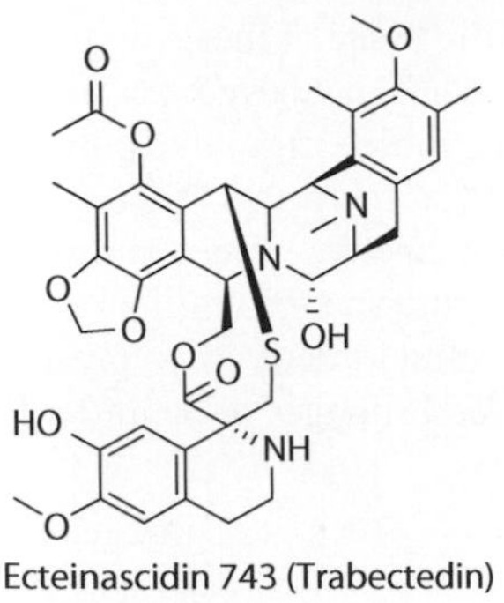

FIGURE 4.10 Structure of ET-743 isolated from a tunicate.

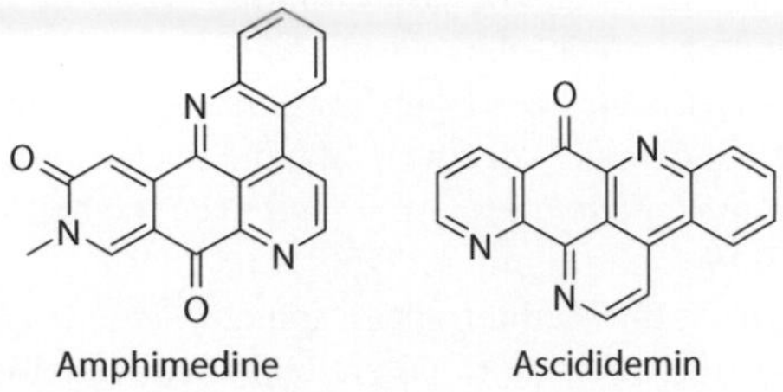

FIGURE 4.11 Bioactive pyridoacridine derivatives from tunicates.

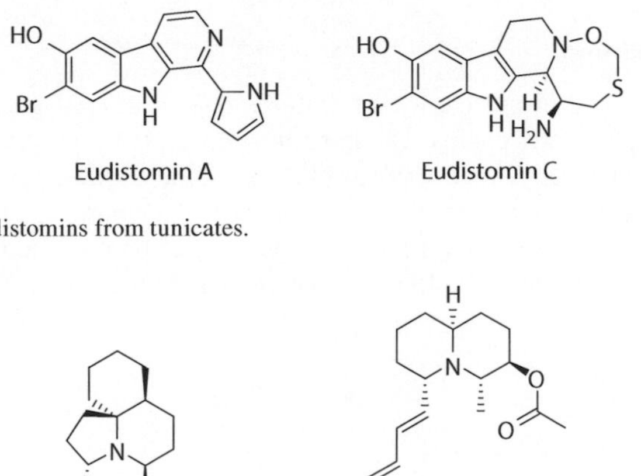

FIGURE 4.12 Bioactive eudistomins from tunicates.

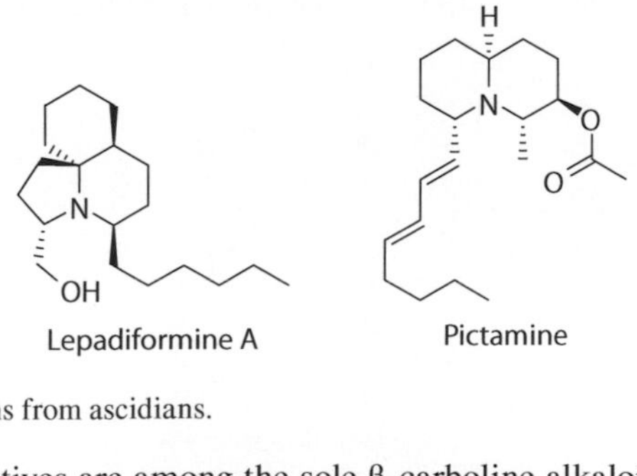

FIGURE 4.13 Nonaromatic toxins from ascidians.

Finally, eudistomine derivatives are among the sole β-carboline alkaloid isolated from marine invertebrates (Figure 4.12). They also were associated to diverse biological activities.[209]

Other nonaromatic alkaloids identified in ascidians have also been shown to exhibit potent toxic effects (Figure 4.13).[210,211]

4.6 Sponges

Marine sponges, as sessile filter-feeders, are known to produce the largest chemical diversity of secondary metabolites in the marine environment. Nevertheless, they seem devoid of true toxic weapons of peptidic and/or protein origin.[212] This outstanding chemodiversity has often been associated to the diversity of microbes hosted at the surface or in the tissue of these organisms. It will not be possible to encompass all the families of bioactive natural products that have been isolated in sponges. First, we will not detail compounds that may obviously be of microbial origin like polyethers, long polyketides but also peptides that would imply renowned microbial PKS and/or NRPS enzymatic clusters.[213] We will rather focus on compounds present in large quantities in sponge tissues and that have showed a true toxicity to mammals. In this case, we have selected two pure sponge families of highly nitrogenated compounds, mainly found in two orders: 3-alkylpyridiniums and its derivatives present in sponges of the order Haplosclerida and guanidine polyketides found in several sponges of the order Poecilosclerida.

4.6.1 3-Alkylpyridiniums

A large number of 3-alkylpiperidine derivatives have been isolated from marine sponges.[214–217] Even if some examples are found in mollusks that can originate from a sponge diet, they seem to be restricted to sponges and especially to the order Haplosclerida (mainly from the genus *Haliclona*). They were consequently accepted as chemotaxonomic markers of this order.[218,219] The chemical diversity in this group includes monomers like the niphatesines from *Haliclona* sp.,[220] dimers that can be cyclic like the cyclostelletamines from *Stelletta maxima*,[221] or linear like the pachychalines from *Pachychalina* sp.,[222] trimers like the viscosamine from *Haliclona viscose*,[223] and even the highly bioactive polymers halitoxins from sponges of the genus *Haliclona* (Figure 4.14).[224]

Poly-3-alkylpyridinium salts from the Mediterranean sponge *Reniera sarai* have been largely studied and they were shown to possess a broad range of potent biological activities, the most prominent being cytolytic, haemolytic, acetylcholinesterase inhibitory, and then can be considered as true sponge toxins even if their invertebrate origin has not been demonstrated.[225]

4.6.2 Guanidine Alkaloids

The second interesting family of sponge toxins features one or several guanidine groups linked to long and often cyclized polyacetate chains. The guanidine group is frequently found in sponge natural products and especially in a large family of polycyclic guanidine alkaloids produced by sponges.[226–231] This type of alkaloids is even recognized as chemotaxonomic markers of sponges of the family Crambeidae (order Poecilosclerida).[218] These compounds seem to be restricted to marine sponge of the order Poecilosclerida, and they are exemplified by the complex chemical architecture of ptilomycalin,

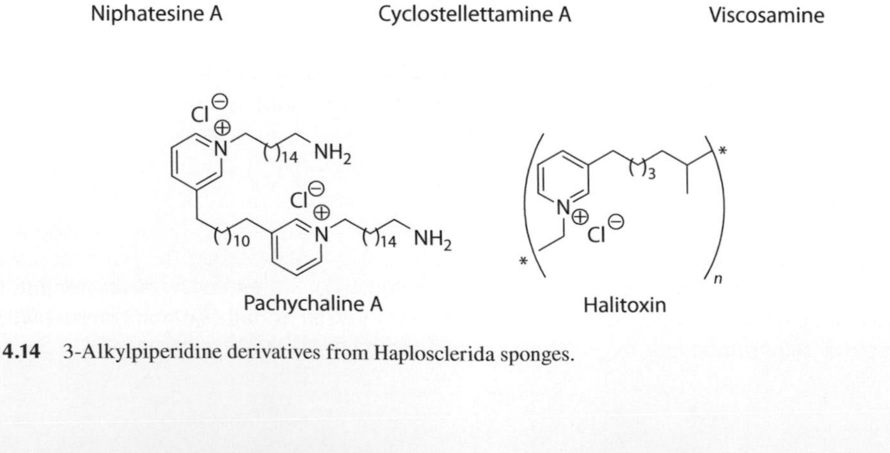

Niphatesine A   Cyclostellettamine A   Viscosamine

Pachychaline A   Halitoxin

FIGURE 4.14   3-Alkylpiperidine derivatives from Haplosclerida sponges.

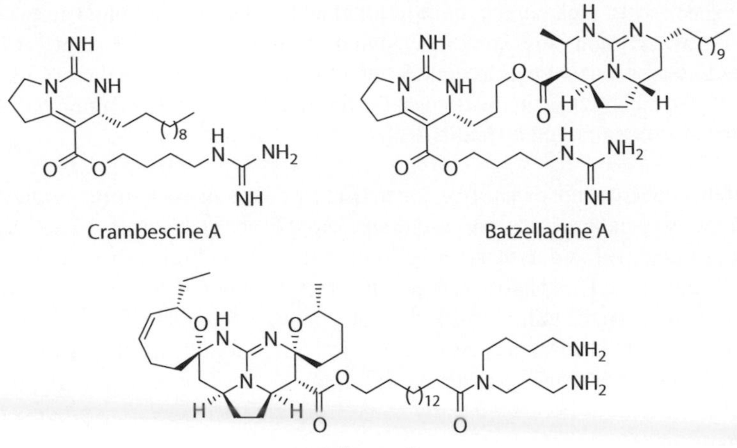

Crambescine A   Batzelladine A

Ptilomycalin

FIGURE 4.15 Bioactive guanidine alkaloids found in Poecilosclerida sponges.

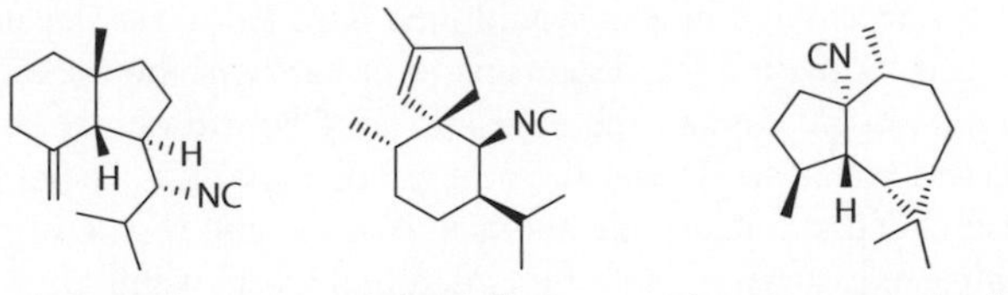

Axisonitrile-1   Axisonitrile-3   1-Isocyanoaromadendrane

FIGURE 4.16 Bioactive isocyanide terpenoids from sponges.

batzelladines, crambescidins, and crambescins that are abundantly found in the Mediterranean sponge *Crambe crambe* (Figure 4.15).[232]

Differential effects of crambescins and crambescidin 816 in voltage-gated sodium, potassium, and calcium channels were evidenced in neurons, clearly emphasizing the high toxicity of these compounds.[233]

4.6.3 Isocyanide Terpenoids

The presence of the isocyanide group is quite rare in terrestrial natural products while a large quantity of sponge secondary metabolites was found to contain this functional group.[234] Axisonitrile-1, the major component of the Mediterranean sponge *Axinella cannabina* (renamed *Acanthella cannabina*), exhibited deterrence activity on fishes (Figure 4.16).[235] The fish toxicity detected for the extract of the Mediterranean sponge *Acanthella acuta* was attributed to 1-isocyanoaromadendrane, axisonitrile-3 being also present in the extract (Figure 4.16).[236]

Even if the toxicity of these compounds for mammals remains to be clearly demonstrated, their bioactivity does not leave any doubt.

4.7 Concluding Remarks

All along this review, we clearly underlined two distinct types of toxins produced by marine invertebrates:

- Ribosomal peptides and proteins with strong toxic effects on mammals similar to the toxins produced by terrestrial toxic species like snails or scorpions. They are clearly produced by the invertebrates and stored in dedicated cells. In the marine environment, they have been evidenced in sea anemones, hydra, and jellyfishes but also cone snails, worms, and some sea urchins.

- Small-size specialized metabolites, mainly alkaloids or terpenoids found in sponges, ascidians, gorgonians, echinoderms, nudibranchs, and sea hares. Their true origin is often highly challenging to assess, but we may assume a role of invertebrate cells in the biosynthesis due to their usual high concentration in the tissues. Furthermore, some of the compounds have clearly a dietary origin as exemplified by nudibranchs and sea hares toxins.

We are aware that this review is not exhaustive due to the large diversity of natural products isolated from marine invertebrates, especially gorgonians, ascidians, sponges, or nudibranchs. The origin of the compounds is sometimes doubtful and associated microorganisms may be involved in the biosynthesis of some families of compounds. This is, for example, the case when nonribosomal peptides or polyketides are found in low quantities in the animal tissues. Strong evidences would suggest a microbial origin as NRPS and PKS gene clusters have been decoded in several microorganisms like bacteria, cyanobacteria, microalgae, or even fungi. Additionally, other complex polyethers of terpenoid origin are usually found in a large array of invertebrates but they usually come from a bioaccumulation process of microbes by these filtering organisms.

These results are of high evolutionary significance and raise the question of the emergence of small size specialized compounds. Most of the pelagic or mobile organisms have kept the first genes of the central metabolism leading to peptidic and proteinic toxins. The coevolution of these species with a large diversity of microbes in the marine environment would then have led to the development of divergent metabolic pathways developed by these microorganisms to circumvent the toxicity induced by invertebrate toxins. This adaptation could explain the appearance of nonribosomal peptide synthases and polyketide synthases in the microbial world and then the production of a second class of compounds much more specialized also called secondary metabolites. Benthic and sessile organisms like sponges and gorgonians that live in close association with this microbial world would then have required other strategies to face these toxins, adapting some gene clusters to produce nonpeptidic substances leading to other classes of biological activities like alkaloids or terpenoids. Finally, sea hares and nudibranchs that feed these benthic organisms would have adapted and modified slightly the defensive benthic toxins in order to defend themselves.

Of course, this cycle is pure assumption and deserves clear evolutionary studies at the biomolecular level but the appearance of the specialized metabolism stands in the oceans, at the interaction of marine invertebrates and microbes.

REFERENCES

1. Fusetani, N., 2009. Marine toxins: An overview, in *Marine Toxins as Research Tools*. Fusetani, N. and Kem, W., eds. Springer, Berlin, Germany, pp. 1–44.
2. Ozbek, S., Balasubramanian, P. G., and Holstein, T. W., 2009. Cnidocyst structure and the biomechanics of discharge. *Toxicon*, 54, 1038–1045.
3. Maçek, P., Belmonte, G., Pederzolli, C. et al. 1994. Mechanism of action of equinatoxin II, a cytolysin from the sea anemone *Actinia equina L.* belonging to the family of actinoporins. *Toxicology*, 87, 205–227.
4. Suput, 2009. In vivo effects of cnidarian toxins and venoms. *Toxicon*, 54, 1190–1200.
5. Martins, R. D., Alves, R. S., Martins, A. M. C. et al. 2009. Purification and characterization of the biological effects of phospholipase A2 from sea anemone *Bunodosoma caissarum*. *Toxicon*, 54, 413–420.
6. Turk, T. and Kem, W. R., 2009. The phylum Cnidaria and investigations of its toxins and venoms until 1990. *Toxicon*, 54, 1031–1037.
7. Richet, C., 1903. Des poisons contenus dans les tentacules des Actinies (congestine et thalassine). *Comptes Rendus de la Société de Biologie*, 55, 246–248.
8. Richet, C., 1903. De la thalassine, toxine cristallisée pruritogène. *Comptes Rendus de la Société de Biologie*, 55, 707–710.
9. Beress, L., Beress, R., and Wunderer, G., 1975. Purification of three polypeptides with neuroand cardiotoxic activity from the sea anemone *Anemonia sulcata*. *Toxicon*, 13, 359–364.

10. Frazao, B., Vasconcelos, V., and Antunes, A., 2012. Sea anemone (Cnidaria, Anthozoa, Actiniaria) toxins: An overview. *Mar. Drugs*, 10, 1812–1851.
11. Oliveira, J. S., Fuentes-Silva, D., and King, G. F., 2012. Development of a rational nomenclature for naming peptide and protein toxins from sea anemones. *Toxicon*, 60, 539–550.
12. Beress, L., 1982. Bioloically active compounds from coelenterates. *Pure Appl. Chem.*, 54, 1981–1994.
13. Wilcox, G. R., Fogh, R. H., and Norton, R. S., 1993. Refined structure in solution of the sea anemone neurotoxin ShI. *J. Biol. Chem.*, 268, 24707–24719.
14. Widmer, H., Billeter, M., and Wüthrich, K., 1989. Three-dimensional structure of the neurotoxin ATX Ia from *Anemonia sulcata* in aqueous solution determined by nuclear magnetic resonance spectroscopy. *Proteins: Struct. Funct. Bioinf.*, 6, 357–371.
15. Norton, R. S., 1991. Structure and structure-function relationships of sea anemone proteins that interact with the sodium channel. *Toxicon*, 29, 1051–1084.
16. Muramatsu, I., Fujiwara, M., Miura, A. et al. 1985. Effects of Goniopora toxin on crayfish giant axons. *J. Pharmacol. Exp. Ther.*, 234, 307–315.
17. Castañeda, O. and Harvey, A. L., 2009. Discovery and characterization of cnidarian peptide toxins that affect neuronal potassium ion channels. *Toxicon*, 54, 1119–1124.
18. Qar, J., Schweitz, H., Schmid, A. et al. 1986. A polypeptide toxin from the coral Goniopora. Purification and action on Ca^{2+} channels. *FEBS Lett.*, 202, 331–336.
19. Nevalainen, T. J., Peuravuori, H. J., Quinn, R. J. et al. 2004. Phospholipase A2 in Cnidaria. *Comp. Biochem. Physiol., Part B: Biochem. Mol. Biol.*, 139, 731–735.
20. Hessinger, D. A. and Lenhoff, H. M., 1973. Assay and properties of the hemolysis activity of pure venom from the nematocysts of the acontia of the sea anemone *Aiptasia pallida*. *Arch. Biochem. Biophys.*, 159, 629–638.
21. Talvinen, K. A. and Nevalainen, T. J., 2002. Cloning of a novel phospholipase A2 from the cnidarian *Adamsia carciniopados*. *Comp. Biochem. Physiol., Part B: Biochem. Mol. Biol.*, 132, 571–578.
22. Kem, W., 1988. Sea anemone toxin structure and action, in *The Biology of Nematocysts*. Hessinger, D. A. and Lenhoff, H. M., eds. Academic Press, New York, pp. 375–405.
23. Kem, W. R. and Dunn, B. M., 1988. Separation and characterization of four different amino acid sequence variants of a sea anemone (*Stichodactyla helianthus*) protein cytolysin. *Toxicon*, 26, 997–1008.
24. Anderluh, G., Sepcic, K., Turk, T. et al. 2011. Cytolytic proteins from cnidarians—An overview. *Acta Chim. Slov.*, 58, 724–729.
25. Bernheimer, A. W. and Avigad, L. S., 1976. Properties of a toxin from the sea anemone Stoichacis helianthus, including specific binding to sphingomyelin. *Proc. Natl. Acad. Sci. U S A*, 73, 467–471.
26. Norton, R. S., 2009. Structures of sea anemone toxins. *Toxicon*, 54, 1075–1088.
27. Ferlan, I. and Lebez, D., 1974. Equinatoxin, a lethal protein from Actinia equina—I. Purification and characterization. *Toxicon*, 12, 57–58.
28. Maçek, P. and Lebez, D., 1988. Isolation and characterization of three lethal and hemolytic toxins from the sea anemone *Actinia equina L. Toxicon*, 26, 441–451.
29. Anderluh, G. and Maçek, P., 2002. Cytolytic peptide and protein toxins from sea anemones (Anthozoa: Actiniaria). *Toxicon*, 40, 111–124.
30. Hinds, M. G., Zhang, W., Anderluh, G. et al. 2002. Solution structure of the eukaryotic pore-forming cytolysin equinatoxin II: Implications for pore formation. *J. Mol. Biol.*, 315, 1219–1229.
31. Mancheno, J. M., Martin-Benito, J., Martinez-Ripoll, M. et al. 2003. Crystal and electron microscopy structures of sticholysin II actinoporin reveal insights into the mechanism of membrane pore formation. *Structure*, 11, 1319–1328.
32. Cline, E. I., Wiebe, L. I., Young, J. D. et al. 1995. Toxic effects of the novel protein UPI from the sea anemone *Urticina piscivora*. *Pharmacol. Res.*, 32, 309–314.
33. Nagai, H., Oshiro, N., Takuwa-Kuroda, K. et al. 2002. Novel proteinaceous toxins from the nematocyst venom of the Okinawan sea anemone *Phyllodiscus semoni Kwietniewski*. *Biochem. Biophys. Res. Commun.*, 294, 760–763.
34. Oshiro, N., Kobayashi, C., Iwanaga, S. et al. 2004. A new membrane-attack complex/perforin (MACPF) domain lethal toxin from the nematocyst venom of the Okinawan sea anemone *Actineria villosa*. *Toxicon*, 43, 225–228.
35. Satoh, H., Oshiro, N., Iwanaga, S. et al. 2007. Characterization of PsTX-60B, a new membrane-attack complex/perforin (MACPF) family toxin, from the venomous sea anemone *Phyllodiscus semoni*. *Toxicon*, 49, 1208–1210.

36. Uechi, G.-i., Toma, H., Arakawa, T. et al. 2005. Biochemical and physiological analyses of a hemolytic toxin isolated from a sea anemone *Actineria villosa*. *Toxicon*, 45, 761–766.
37. Uechi, G.-i., Toma, H., Arakawa, T. et al. 2010. Molecular characterization on the genome structure of hemolysin toxin isoforms isolated from sea anemone *Actineria villosa* and *Phyllodiscus semoni*. *Toxicon*, 56, 1470–1476.
38. Zhang, M., Fishman, Y., Sher, D. et al. 2003. Hydralysin, a novel animal group-selective paralytic and cytolytic protein from a noncnidocystic origin in hydra. *Biochemistry*, 42, 8939–8944.
39. Sher, D., Fishman, Y., Zhang, M. et al. 2005. Hydralysins, a new category of ß-pore-forming toxins in cnidaria. *J. Biol. Chem.*, 280, 22847–22855.
40. Iguchi, A., Iwanaga, S., and Nagai, H., 2008. Isolation and characterization of a novel protein toxin from fire coral. *Biochem. Biophys. Res. Commun.*, 365, 107–112.
41. Brinkman, D. L. and Burnell, J. N., 2009. Biochemical and molecular characterisation of cubozoan protein toxins. *Toxicon*, 54, 1162–1173.
42. Nagai, H., Takuwa, K., Nakao, M. et al. 2000. Isolation and characterization of a novel protein toxin from the Hawaiian box jellyfish (Sea Wasp) *Carybdea alata*. *Biochem. Biophys. Res. Commun.*, 275, 589–594.
43. Brinkman, D. and Burnell, J., 2007. Identification, cloning and sequencing of two major venom proteins from the box jellyfish, *Chironex fleckeri*. *Toxicon*, 50, 850–860.
44. Nagai, H., Takuwa-Kuroda, K., Nakao, M. et al. 2002. A novel protein toxin from the deadly box jellyfish (Sea Wasp, Habu-kurage) *Chiropsalmus quadrigatus*. *Biosci. Biotechnol. Biochem.*, 66, 97–102.
45. Wu, C. H., 2009. Palytoxin: Membrane mechanisms of action. *Toxicon*, 54, 1183–1189.
46. Berrue, F. and Kerr, R. G., 2009. Diterpenes from gorgonian corals. *Nat. Prod. Rep.*, 26, 681–710.
47. Cariello, L. and Tota, B., 1974. Inhibition of succinic oxidase activity of beef heart mitochondria by a new fluorescent metabolite, zoanthoxantin. *Cell. Mol. Life Sci.*, 30, 244–245.
48. Moore, R. E. and Bartolini, G., 1981. Structure of palytoxin. *J. Am. Chem. Soc.*, 103, 2491–2494.
49. Hashimoto, Y., Fusetani, N., and Kimura, S., 1969. Aluterin: A toxin of filefish, *Aluteria scripta*, probably originating from a zoantharian *Palythoa tuberculosa*. *Bull. Jpn. Soc. Sci. Fish.*, 35, 1086–1093.
50. Moore, R. E. and Scheuer, P. J., 1971. Palytoxin: A new marine toxin from a coelenterate. *Science*, 172, 495–498.
51. Gleibs, S., Mebs, D., and Werding, B., 1995. Studies on the origin and distribution of palytoxin in a Caribbean coral reef. *Toxicon*, 33, 1531–1537.
52. Mahnir, V. M., Kozlovskaya, E. P., and Kalinovsky, A. I., 1992. Sea anemone *Radianthus macrodactylus*— A new source of palytoxin. *Toxicon*, 30, 1449–1456.
53. Kerbrat, A. S., Amzil, Z., Pawlowiez, R. et al. 2011. First evidence of palytoxin and 42-hydroxy-palytoxin in the marine cyanobacterium trichodesmium. *Mar. Drugs*, 9, 543–560.
54. Neeman, I., Fishelson, L., and Kashman, Y., 1974. Sarcophine—A new toxin from the soft coral *Sarcophiton glaucum* (Alcyonaria). *Toxicon*, 12, 593–598.
55. Ciereszko, L. S., Sifford, D. H., and Weinheimer, A. J., 1960. Chemistry of coelenterates. I. Occurrence of terpenoid compounds in gorgonians. *Ann. NY Acad. Sci.*, 90, 917–919.
56. Ferchmin, P. A., Pagan, O. R., Ulrich, H. et al. 2009. Actions of octocoral and tobacco cembranoids on nicotinic receptors. *Toxicon*, 54, 1174–1182.
57. Coll, J. C., 1992. ChemInform abstract: The chemistry and chemical ecology of octocorals (Coelenterata, Anthozoa, Octocorallia). *ChemInform*, 23, 37.
58. Weinheimer, A. J. and Spraggins, R. L., 1969. The occurrence of two new prostaglandin derivatives (15-epi-PGA2 and its acetate, methyl ester) in the *gorgonian Plexaura* homomalla chemistry of coelenterates. XV. *Tetrahedron Lett.*, 10, 5185–5188.
59. Bandurraga, M. M. and Fenical, W., 1985. Isolation of the muricins: Evidence of a chemical adaptation against fouling in the marine octocoral *Muricea fruticosa* (gorgonacea). *Tetrahedron*, 41, 1057–1065.
60. Look, S. A., Fenical, W., Jacobs, R. S. et al. 1986. The pseudopterosins: Anti-inflammatory and analgesic natural products from the sea whip *Pseudopterogorgia elisabethae*. *Proc. Natl. Acad. Sci. U S A*, 83, 6238–6240.
61. Lin, X.-y., Ishida, M., Nagashima, Y. et al. 1996. A polypeptide toxin in the sea anemone *Actinia equina* homologous with other sea anemone sodium channel toxins: Isolation and amino acid sequence. *Toxicon*, 34, 57–65.
62. Shiomi, K., Lin, X.-y., Nagashima, Y. et al. 1996. Isolation and amino-acid sequence of a polypeptide toxin from the sea anemone *Radianthus crispus*. *Fish. Sci.*, 62, 629–633.

63. Wunderer, G. and Eulitz, M., 1978. Amino-acid sequence of toxin I from *Anemonia sulcata*. *Eur. J. Biochem.*, 89, 11–17.

64. Wunderer, G., Béress, L., Machleidt, W. et al. 1976. Broad-specificity inhibitors from sea anemones, in *Methods Enzymology*. Laszlo, L., ed. Academic Press, New York, pp. 881–888.

65. Martinez, G., Kopeyan, C., Schweitz, H. et al. 1977. Toxin III from *Anemonia sulcata*: Primary structure. *FEBS Lett.*, 84, 247–252.

66. Scheffler, J.-J., Tsugita, A., Linden, G. et al. 1982. The amino acid sequence of toxin V from *Anemonia sulcata*. *Biochem. Biophys. Res. Commun.*, 107, 272–278.

67. Honma, T., Hasegawa, Y., Ishida, M. et al. 2005. Isolation and molecular cloning of novel peptide toxins from the sea anemone *Antheopsis maculata*. *Toxicon*, 45, 33–41.

68. Tanaka, M., Haniu, M., Yasunoby, K. T. et al. 1977. Amino acid sequence of the *Anthopleura xanthogrammica* heart stimulant, anthopleurin-B. *Biochemistry*, 16, 204–208.

69. Reimer, N. S., Yasunobu, C. L., Yasunoby, K. T. et al. 1985. Amino acid sequence of the *Anthopleura xanthogrammica* heart stimulant, anthopleurin-B. *J. Biol. Chem.*, 260, 8690–8693.

70. Norton, T. R., 1981. Cardiotonic polypeptides from *Anthopleura xanthogrammica* (Brandt) and *A. elegantissima* (Brandt). *Fed. Proc.*, 40, 21–25.

71. Bruhn, T., Schaller, C., Schulze, C. et al. 2001. Isolation and characterisation of five neurotoxic and cardiotoxic polypeptides from the sea anemone *Anthopleura elegantissima*. *Toxicon*, 39, 693–702.

72. Sunahara, S., Muramoto, K., Tenma, K. et al. 1987. Amino acid sequence of two sea anemone toxins from *Anthopleura fuscoviridis*. *Toxicon*, 25, 211–219.

73. Wang, L., Ou, J., Peng, L. et al. 2004. Functional expression and characterization of four novel neurotoxins from sea anemone *Anthopleura* sp. *Biochem. Biophys. Res. Commun.*, 313, 163–170.

74. Kelso, G. J. and Blumenthal, K. M., 1998. Identification and characterization of novel sodium channel toxins from the sea anemone *Anthopleura xanthogrammica*. *Toxicon*, 36, 41–51.

75. Malpezzi, E. L. A., de Freitas, J., Muramoto, K. et al. 1993. Characterization of peptides in sea anemone venom collected by a novel procedure. *Toxicon*, 31, 853–864.

76. Cunha, R. B., Santana, A. N. C., Amaral, P. C. et al. 2005. Primary structure, behavioral and electroencephalographic effects of an epileptogenic peptide from the sea anemone *Bunodosoma cangicum*. *Toxicon*, 45, 207–217.

77. Zaharenko, A. J., Ferreira Jr., W. A., Oliveira, J. S. et al. 2008. Proteomics of the neurotoxic fraction from the sea anemone *Bunodosoma cangicum* venom: Novel peptides belonging to new classes of toxins. *Comp. Biochem. Physiol., Part D: Genom. Proteom.*, 3, 219–225.

78. Loret, E. P., del Valle, R. M., Mansuelle, P. et al. 1994. Positively charged amino acid residues located similarly in sea anemone and scorpion toxins. *J. Biol. Chem.*, 269, 16785–16788.

79. Cariello, L., De Santis, A., Fiore, F. et al. 1989. Calitoxin, a neurotoxic peptide from the sea anemone *Calliactis parasitica*: Amino-acid sequence and electrophysiological properties. *Biochemistry*, 28, 2484–2489.

80. Spagnuolo, A., Zanetti, L., Cariello, L. et al. 1994. Isolation and characterization of two genes encoding calitoxins, neurotoxic peptides from *Calliactis parasitica* (Cnidaria). *Gene*, 138, 187–191.

81. Ständker, L., Béress, L., Garateix, A. et al. 2006. A new toxin from the sea anemone *Condylactis gigantea* with effect on sodium channel inactivation. *Toxicon*, 48, 211–220.

82. Wanke, E., Zaharenko, A. J., Redaelli, E. et al. 2009. Actions of sea anemone type 1 neurotoxins on voltage-gated sodium channel isoforms. *Toxicon*, 54, 1102–1111.

83. Maeda, M., Honma, T., and Shiomi, K., 2010. Isolation and cDNA cloning of type 2 sodium channel peptide toxins from three species of sea anemones (*Cryptodendrum adhaesivum*, *Heterodactyla hemprichii* and *Thalassianthus aster*) belonging to the family Thalassianthidae. *Comp. Biochem. Physiol., Part B: Biochem. Mol. Biol.*, 157, 389–393.

84. Ishida, M., Yokoyama, A., Shimakura, K. et al. 1997. Halcurin, a polypeptide toxin from the sea anemone *Halcurias* sp., with a structural resemblance to type 1 and 2 toxins. *Toxicon*, 35, 537–544.

85. Zykova, T. A. and Kozlovskaia, E. P., 1989. Amino acid sequence of a neurotoxin from the anemone *Radianthus macrodactylus*. *Bioorg. Khim.*, 15, 1301–1306.

86. Zykova, T. A. and Kozlovskaia, E. P., 1989. Disulfide bonds in neurotoxin-III from the sea anemone *Radianthus macrodactylus*. *Bioorg. Khim.*, 15, 904–907.

87. Moran, Y., Weinberger, H., Sullivan, J. C. et al. 2008. Concerted evolution of sea anemone neurotoxin genes is revealed through analysis of the *Nematostella vectensis* Genome. *Mol. Biol. Evol.*, 25, 737–747.

88. Putnam, N. H., Srivastava, M., Hellsten, U. et al. 2007. Sea anemone genome reveals ancestral eumetazoan gene repertoire and genomic organization. *Science*, 317, 86–94.
89. Nishida, S., Fujita, S., Warashina, A. et al. 1985. Amino acid sequence of a sea anemone toxin from *Parasicyonis actinostoloides*. *Eur. J. Biochem.*, 150, 171–173.
90. Schweitz, H., Bidard, J. N., Frelin, C. et al. 1985. Purification, sequence, and pharmacological properties of sea anemone toxins from *Radianthus paumotensis*. A new class of sea anemone toxins acting on the sodium channel. *Biochemistry*, 24, 3554–3561.
91. Kem, W. R., Parten, B., Pennington, M. W. et al. 1989. Isolation, characterization, and amino acid sequence of a polypeptide neurotoxin occurring in the sea anemone *Stichodactyla helianthus*. *Biochemistry*, 28, 3483–3489.
92. Shiomi, K., Honma, T., Ide, M. et al. 2003. An epidermal growth factor-like toxin and two sodium channel toxins from the sea anemone *Stichodactyla gigantea*. *Toxicon*, 41, 229–236.
93. Honma, T., Kawahata, S., Ishida, M. et al. 2008. Novel peptide toxins from the sea anemone *Stichodactyla haddoni*. *Peptides*, 29, 536–544.
94. Castañeda, O., Sotolongo, V., Amor, A. M. et al. 1995. Characterization of a potassium channel toxin from the Caribbean sea anemone *Stichodactyla helianthus*. *Toxicon*, 33, 603–613.
95. Rodríguez, A. A., Cassoli, J. S., Sa, F. et al. 2012. Peptide fingerprinting of the neurotoxic fractions isolated from the secretions of sea anemones *Stichodactyla helianthus* and *Bunodosoma granulifera*. New members of the APETx-like family identified by a 454 pyrosequencing approach. *Peptides*, 34, 26–38.
96. Aneiros, A., García, I., Martínez, J. et al. 1993. A potassium channel toxin from the secretion of the sea anemone *Bunodosoma granulifera*: Isolation, amino acid sequence and biological activity. *Biochim. Biophys. Acta-Gen. Subj.*, 1157, 86–92.
97. Diochot, S., Schweitz, H., Béress, L. et al. 1998. Sea anemone peptides with a specific blocking activity against the fast inactivating potassium channel Kv3.4. *J. Biol. Chem.*, 273, 6744–6749.
98. Chagot, B., Diochot, S., Pimentel, C. et al. 2005. Solution structure of APETx1 from the sea anemone *Anthopleura elegantissima*: A new fold for an HERG toxin. *Proteins: Struct. Funct. Bioinf.*, 59, 380–386.
99. Diochot, S., Loret, E., Bruhn, T. et al. 2003. APETx1, a new toxin from the sea anemone *Anthopleura elegantissima*, blocks voltage-gated human ether-a-go-go–related gene potassium channels. *Mol. Pharmacol.*, 64, 59–69.
100. Minagawa, S., Ishida, M., Nagashima, Y. et al. 1998. Primary structure of a potassium channel toxin from the sea anemone *Actinia equina*. *FEBS Lett.*, 427, 149–151.
101. Hasegawa, Y., Honma, T., Nagai, H. et al. 2006. Isolation and cDNA cloning of a potassium channel peptide toxin from the sea anemone *Anemonia erythraea*. *Toxicon*, 48, 536–542.
102. Schweitz, H., Bruhn, T., Guillemare, E. et al. 1995. Kalicludines and kalispetine. Two different classes of sea anemone toxins for voltage sensitive K+ channels. *J. Biol. Chem.*, 270, 25121–25126.
103. Oliveira, J. S., Zaharenko, A. J., Ferreira, Jr., W. A. et al. 2006. BcIV, a new paralyzing peptide obtained from the venom of the sea anemone *Bunodosoma caissarum*. A comparison with the Na+ channel toxin BcIII. *Biochim. Biophys. Acta, Proteins Proteomics*, 1764, 1592–1600.
104. Andreev, Y. A., kozlov, S. A., Koshelev, S. G. et al. 2008. Analgesic compound from sea anemone *Heteractis crispa* is the first polypeptide inhibitor of vanilloid receptor 1 TRPV1). *J. Biol. Chem.*, 283, 23914–23921.
105. Zykova, T. A., Vinokurov, L. M., Markova, L. F. et al. 1985. Amino-acid sequence of trypsin inhibitor IV from *Radianthus macrodactylus*. *Bioorg. Khim.*, 11, 293–301.
106. Krebs, H. C. and Habermehl, G. G., 1987. Isolation and structural determintion of a hemolytic active peptide from the sea anemone *Metridium senile*. *Naturwissenschaften*, 74, 395–396.
107. Gendeh, G. S., Young, L. C., de Medeiros, C. L. et al. 1997. A new potassium channel toxin from the sea anemone *Heteractis magnifica*: Isolation, cDNA cloning and functional expression. *Biochemistry*, 36, 11461–11471.
108. Delfín, J., Martínez, I., Antuch, W. et al. 1996. Purification, characterization and immobilization of proteinase inhibitors from *Stichodactyla helianthus*. *Toxicon*, 34, 1367–1376.
109. Diaz, J., Morera, V., Delfin, J. et al. 1998. Purification and partial characterization of a novel proteinase inhibitor from the sea anemone *Stichodactyla helianthus*. *Toxicon*, 36, 1275–1276.
110. Romero, L., Marcussi, S., Marchi-Salvador, D. P. et al. 2010. Enzymatic and structural characterization of a basic phospholipase A2 from the sea anemone *Condylactis gigantea*. *Biochimie*, 92, 1063–1071.
111. Razpotnik, A., Križaj, I., Šribar, J. et al. 2010. A new phospholipase A2 isolated from the sea anemone *Urticina crassicornis*—Its primary structure and phylogenetic classification. *FEBS J.*, 277, 2641–2653.

112. Radwan, F. F. Y. and Aboul-Dahab, H. M., 2004. Milleporin-1, a new phospholipase A2 active protein from the fire coral *Millepora platyphylla* nematocysts. *Comp. Biochem. Physiol. C Toxicol. Pharmacol.*, 139, 267–272.

113. Ibarra-Alvarado, C., Alejandro García, J., Aguilar, M. B. et al. 2007. Biochemical and pharmacological characterization of toxins obtained from the fire coral *Millepora complanata*. *Comp. Biochem. Physiol., Part C: Toxicol. Pharmacol.*, 146, 511–518.

114. Il'ina, A., Lipkin, A., Barsova, E. et al. 2006. Amino acid sequence of RTX-A's isoform actinoporin from the sea anemone, *Radianthus macrodactylus*. *Toxicon*, 47, 517–520.

115. Klyshko, E. V., Issaeva, M. P., Monastyrnaya, M. M. et al. 2004. Isolation, properties and partial amino acid sequence of a new actinoporin from the sea anemone *Radianthus macrodactylus*. *Toxicon*, 44, 315–324.

116. Anderluh, G., Križaj, I., Štrukelj, B. et al. 1999. Equinatoxins, pore-forming proteins from the sea anemone *Actinia equina*, belong to a multigene family. *Toxicon*, 37, 1391–1401.

117. Anderluh, G., Pungerčar, J., Štrukelj, B. et al. 1996. Cloning, sequencing, and expression of equinatoxin II. *Biochem. Biophys. Res. Commun.*, 220, 437–442.

118. Pungerčar, J., Anderluh, G., Maček, P. et al. 1997. Sequence analysis of the cDNA encoding the precursor of equinatoxin V, a newly discovered hemolysin from the sea anemone *Actinia equina*. *Biochim. Biophys. Acta.*, 1341, 105–107.

119. Huerta, V., Morera, V., Guanche, Y. et al. 2001. Primary structure of two cytolysin isoforms from *Stichodactyla helianthus* differing in their hemolytic activity. *Toxicon*, 39, 1253–1256.

120. Uechi, G.-i., Toma, H., Arakawa, T. et al. 2005. Molecular cloning and functional expression of hemolysin from the sea anemone *Actineria villosa*. *Protein Exp. Purif.*, 40, 379–384.

121. Bellomio, A., Morante, K., Barlič, A. et al. 2009. Purification, cloning and characterization of fragaceatoxin C, a novel actinoporin from the sea anemone *Actinia fragacea*. *Toxicon*, 54, 869–880.

122. Norton, R. S., Bobek, G., Ivanov, J. O. et al. 1990. Purification and characterisation of proteins with cardiac stimulatory and haemolytic activity from the anemone *Actinia tenebrosa*. *Toxicon*, 28, 29–41.

123. Simpson, R. J., Reid, G. E., Moritz, R. L. et al. 1990. Complete amino acid sequence of tenebrosin-C, a cardiac stimulatory and haemolytic protein from the sea anemone *Actinia tenebrosa*. *Eur. J. Biochem.*, 190, 319–328.

124. Il'ina, A. P., Monastyrnaia, M. M., Isaeva, M. P. et al. 2005. Primary structures of actinoporins from sea anemone *Oulactis orientalis*. *Bioorg. Khim.*, 31, 357–362.

125. Nagai, H., Oshiro, N., Takuwa-Kuroda, K. et al. 2002. A new polypeptide toxin from the nematocyst venom of an Okinawan sea anemone *Phyllodiscus semoni*. *Biosci. Biotechnol. Biochem.*, 66, 2621–2625.

126. Khoo, K. S., Kam, W. K., Khoo, H. E. et al. 1993. Purification and partial characterization of two cytolysins from a tropical sea anemone, *Heteractis magnifica*. *Toxicon*, 31, 1567–1579.

127. Wang, Y., Chua, K. L., and Khoo, H. E., 2000. A new cytolysin from the sea anemone, *Heteractis magnifica*: Isolation, cDNA cloning and functional expression. *Biochim. Biophys. Acta.*, 1478, 9–18.

128. Črnigoj Kristan, K., Viero, G., Dalla Serra, M. et al. 2009. Molecular mechanism of pore formation by actinoporins. *Toxicon*, 54, 1125–1134.

129. Jiang, X.-Y., Yang, W.-l., Chen, H.-P. et al. 2002. Cloning and characterization of an acidic cytolysin cDNA from sea anemone *Sagartia rosea*. *Toxicon*, 40, 1563–1569.

130. Razpotnik, A., Križaj, I., Kem, W. R. et al. 2009. A new cytolytic protein from the sea anemone *Urticina crassicornis* that binds to cholesterol- and sphingomyelin-rich membranes. *Toxicon*, 53, 762–769.

131. Wittle, L. W., TScura, E. D., and Middlebrook, R. E., 1974. Stinging coral (*Millepora tenera*) toxin: A comparison of crude extracts with isolated nematocyst extracts. *Toxicon*, 12, 481–486.

132. Shiomi, K., Hosaka, M., Yanaike, N. et al. 1989. Partial characterization of venoms from two species of fire corals *Millepora platyphylla* and *Millepora dichotoma*. *Nippon Suisan Gakkaishi*, 55, 357–362.

133. Tamkun, M. M. and Hessinger, D. A., 1981. Isolation and partial characterization of a hemolytic and toxic protein from the nematocyst venom of the Portuguese man-of-war, *Physalia physalis*. *BBA, Protein Structure*, 667, 87–98.

134. Azuma, H., Ishikawa, M., Nakajima, T. et al. 1986. Calcium-dependent contractile response of arterial smooth muscle to a jellyfish toxin (pCrTX: *Carybdea rastonii*). *Br. J. Pharmacol.*, 88, 549–559.

135. Nagai, H., Takuwa, K., Nakao, M. et al. 2000. Novel proteinaceous toxins from the box jellyfish (Sea Wasp) *Carybdea rastoni*. *Biochem. Biophys. Res. Commun.*, 275, 582–588.

136. Wiltshire, C. J., Sutherland, S. K., Fenner, P. J. et al. 2000. Optimization and preliminary characterization of venom isolated from 3 medically important jellyfish: The box (*Chironex fleckeri*), Irukandji (*Carukia barnesi*), and blubber (*Catostylus mosaicus*) jellyfish. *Wildern. Environ. Med.*, 11, 241–250.

137. Othman, I. and Burnett, J. W., 1990. Techniques applicable for purifying *Chironex fleckeri* (box-jellyfish) venom. *Toxicon*, 28, 821–835.
138. Endean, R., Monks, S. A., and Cameron, A. M., 1993. Toxins from the box-jellyfish *Chironex fleckeri*. *Toxicon*, 31, 397–410.
139. Naguib, A. M. F., Bansal, J., Calton, G. J. et al. 1988. Purification of *Chironex fleckeri* venom components using Chironex immunoaffinity chromatography. *Toxicon*, 26, 387–394.
140. Rottini, G., Gusmani, L., Parovel, E. et al. 1995. Purification and properties of a cytolytic toxin in venom of the jellyfish *Carybdea marsupialis*. *Toxicon*, 33, 315–326.
141. Sánchez-Rodríguez, J., Torrens, E., and Segura-Puertas, L., 2006. Partial purification and characterization of a novel neurotoxin and three cytolysins from box jellyfish (*Carybdea marsupialis*) nematocyst venom. *Arch. Toxicol.*, 80, 163–168.
142. Kaas, Q., Westermann, J.-C., Halai, R. et al. 2008. ConoServer, a database for conopeptide sequences and structures. *Bioinformatics*, 24, 445–446.
143. Becker, S. and Terlau, H., 2008. Toxins from cone snails: Properties, applications and biotechnological production. *Appl. Microbiol. Biotechnol.*, 79, 1–9.
144. Olivera, B. M., 2006. Conus peptides: Biodiversity-based discovery and exogenomics. *J. Biol. Chem.*, 281, 31173–31177.
145. Jacob, R. and McDougal, O., 2010. The M-superfamily of conotoxins: A review. *Cell. Mol. Life Sci.*, 67, 17–27.
146. Puillandre, N., Koua, D., Favreau, P. et al. 2012. Molecular phylogeny, classification and evolution of conopeptides. *J. Mol. Evol.*, 74, 297–309.
147. Myers, R. A., Cruz, L. J., Rivier, J. E. et al. 1993. Conus peptides as chemical probes for receptors and ion channels. *Chem. Rev.*, 93, 1923–1936.
148. Craik, D. J. and Adams, D. J., 2007. Chemical modification of conotoxins to improve stability and activity. *ACS Chem. Biol.*, 2, 457–468.
149. Corpuz, P. G., Jacobsen, R. B., Jimenez, E. C. et al. 2005. Definition of the M-conotoxin superfamily: Characterization of novel peptides from Molluscivorous *Conus* venoms. *Biochemistry*, 44, 8176–8186.
150. Woodward, S. R., Cruz, L. J., Olivera, B. M. et al. 1990. Constant and hypervariable regions in conotoxin propeptides. *EMBO J.*, 9, 1015–1020.
151. Craig, A. G., Bandyopadhyay, P., and Olivera, B. M., 1999. Post-translationally modified neuropeptides from Conus venoms. *Eur. J. Biochem.*, 264, 271–275.
152. Terlau, H. and Olivera, B. M., 2004. Conus venoms: A rich source of novel ion channel-targeted peptides. *Physiol. Rev.*, 84, 41–68.
153. Olivera, B., Rivier, J., Clark, C. et al. 1990. Diversity of Conus neuropeptides. *Science*, 249, 257–263.
154. Kaas, Q., Westermann, J.-C., and Craik, D. J., 2010. Conopeptide characterization and classifications: An analysis using ConoServer. *Toxicon*, 55, 1491–1509.
155. Santos, A. D., McIntosh, J. M., Hillyard, D. R. et al. 2004. The A-superfamily of conotoxins: Structural and functional divergence. *J. Biol. Chem.*, 279, 17596–17606.
156. Buczek, O., Bulaj, G., and Olivera, B. M., 2005. Conotoxins and the posttranslational modification of secreted gene products. *Cell. Mol. Life Sci.*, 62, 3067–3079.
157. Lirazan, M. B., Hooper, D., Corpuz, G. P. et al. 2000. The spasmodic peptide defines a new conotoxin superfamily. *Biochemistry*, 39, 1583–1588.
158. McIntosh, J. M., Corpuz, G. O., Layer, R. T. et al. 2000. Isolation and characterization of a novel conus peptide with apparent antinociceptive activity. *J. Biol. Chem.*, 275, 32391–32397.
159. Walker, C. S., Steel, D., Jacobsen, R. B. et al. 1999. The T-superfamily of conotoxins. *J. Biol. Chem.*, 274, 30664–30671.
160. Teichert, R. W., Jimenez, E. C., and Olivera, B. M., 2005. αS-Conotoxin RVIIIA: A structurally unique conotoxin that broadly targets nicotinic acetylcholine receptors. *Biochemistry*, 44, 7897–7902.
161. Essack, M., Bajic, V. B., and Archer, J. A. C., 2012. Conotoxins that confer therapeutic possibilities. *Mar. Drugs*, 10, 1244–1265.
162. Cimino, G. and Gavagnin, M., 2006. Molluscs: From chemo-ecological study to biotechnological application, in *Progress Molecular Subcellular Biology*, Vol. 43, Springer-Verlag, New York.
163. Ishibashi, M., Yamaguchi, Y., and Hirano, Y. J., 2006. Bioactive natural products from nudibranchs, in *Biomaterials from Aquatic and Terrestrial Organisms*. Fingermann, M. and Nagabhushanam, R., eds. Science Publishers, Inc., Enfield, NH, pp. 513–535.

164. Cimino, G. and Ghiselin, M. T., 1999. Chemical defense and evolutionary trends in biosynthetic capacity among dorid nudibranchs (Mollusca: Gastropoda: Opisthobranchia). *Chemoecology*, 9, 187–207.

165. Kubanek, J., Graziani, E. I., and Andersen, R. J., 1997. Investigations of terpenoid biosynthesis by the dorid nudibranch *Cadlina luteomarginata*. *J. Org. Chem.*, 62, 7239–7246.

166. Manzo, E., Ciavatta, M. L., Gavagnin, M. et al. 2004. Isocyanide terpene metabolites of *Phyllidiella pustulosa*, a nudibranch from the South China Sea. *J. Nat. Prod.*, 67, 1701–1704.

167. Barsby, T., 2006. Drug discovery and sea hares: Bigger is better. *Trends Biotechnol.*, 24, 1–3.

168. O'Keefe, B. R., 2001. Biologically active proteins from natural product extracts. *J. Nat. Prod.*, 64, 1373–1381.

169. David, W. G. and Valerie, J. P., 2001. Chemical defenses in the sea hare *Aplysia parvula*: Importance of diet and sequestration of algal secondary metabolites. *Mar. Ecol. Prog. Ser.*, 215, 261–274.

170. Brito, I., Dias, T., Diaz-Marrero, A. R. et al. 2006. Aplysiadiol from *Aplysia dactylomela* suggested a key intermediate for a unified biogenesis of regular and irregular marine algal bisabolene-type metabolites. *Tetrahedron*, 62, 9655–9660.

171. Bacq, Z. M., 1936. Les poisons des nemertiens. *Bull. Acad. R. Belg. Clin. Sci.*, 22, 1072–1079.

172. Kem, W. R., 2013. Worm peptides, in *Handbook of Biologically Active Peptides*. 2nd edn. Kastin, A. J., ed. Elsevier, San Diego, CA, pp. 483–488.

173. Blumenthal, K. M. and Kem, W. R., 1976. Structure and action of heteronemertine polypeptide toxins. Primary structure of *Cerebratulus lacteus* toxin B-IV. *J. Biol. Chem.*, 251, 6025–6029.

174. Blumenthal, K. M., Keim, P. S., Heinrikson, R. L. et al. 1981. Amino acid sequence of *Cerebratulus* toxin B-II and revised structure of toxin B-IV. *J. Biol. Chem.*, 256, 9063–9067.

175. Barnham, K. J., Dyke, T. R., Kem, W. R. et al. 1997. Structure of neurotoxin B-IV from the marine Worm *Cerebratulus lacteus*: A helical hairpin cross-linked by disulphide bonding. *J. Mol. Biol.*, 268, 886–902.

176. Kem, W. R., 1994. Structure and membrane actions of a marine worm protein cytolysin, *Cerebratulus* toxin A-III. *Toxicology*, 87, 189–203.

177. Kem, W. R. and Blumenthal, K. M., 1978. Purification and characterization of the cytotoxic *Cerebratulus* A toxins. *J. Biol. Chem.*, 253, 5752–5757.

178. Blumenthal, K. M. and Kem, W. R., 1980. Structure and action of heteronemertine polypeptide toxins. Primary structure of *Cerebratulus lacteus* toxin A-III. *J. Biol. Chem.*, 255, 8266–8272.

179. Bon, C., Saliou, B., Thieffry, M. et al. 1985. Partial purification of α-glycerotoxin, a presynaptic neurotoxin from the venom glands of the polychaete annelid glycera convoluta. *Neurochem. Int.*, 7, 63–75.

180. Ovchinnikova, T. V., Aleshina, G. M., Balandin, S. V. et al. 2004. Purification and primary structure of two isoforms of arenicin, a novel antimicrobial peptide from marine polychaeta *Arenicola marina*. *FEBS Lett.*, 577, 209–214.

181. Dzik, J. M., 2006. Molecules released by helminth parasites involved in host colonization. *Acta Biochim. Pol.*, 53, 33–64.

182. Don, T. A., Jones, M. K., Smyth, D. et al. 2004. A pore-forming haemolysin from the hookworm, *Ancylostoma caninum*. *Int. J. Parasitol.*, 34, 1029–1035.

183. Kem, W. R., Abbott, B. C., and Coates, R. M., 1971. Isolation and structure of a hoplonemertine toxin. *Toxicon*, 9, 15–22.

184. Kem, W., Soti, F., Wildeboer, K. et al. 2006. The nemertine toxin anabaseine and its derivative DMXBA (GTS-21): Chemical and pharmacological properties. *Mar. Drugs*, 4, 255–273.

185. Okaichi, T. and Hashimoto, T., 1962. The structure of nereistoxin. *Agric. Biol. Chem.*, 26, 224–227.

186. Hagiwara, H., Numata, M., Konishi, K. et al. 1965. Synthesis of nereistoxin and related compounds. *Chem. Pharm. Bull.*, 13, 253–260.

187. Ritson-Williams, R. R., Yotsu-Yamashita, M., and Paul, V., 2006. Ecological functions of tetrodotoxin in a deadly polyclad flatworm. *Proc. Natl. Acad. Sci.*, 2006, 3176–3179.

188. Yasumoto, T., Nagai, H., Yasumura, D. et al. 1986. Interspecific distribution and possible origin of tetrodotoxin. *Ann. NY Acad. Sci.*, 479, 44–51.

189. Carroll, S., McEvoy, E. G., and Gibson, R., 2003. The production of tetrodotoxin-like substances by nemertean worms in conjunction with bacteria. *J. Exp. Mar. Biol. Ecol.*, 288, 51–63.

190. Thuesen, E. V. and Kogure, K., 1989. Bacterial production of tetrodotoxin in four species of *Chaetognatha*. *Biol. Bull. Mar. Biol. Lab.*, 176, 191–194.

191. Van Dyck, S., Flammang, P., Meriaux, C. et al. 2010. Localization of secondary metabolites in marine invertebrates: Contribution of MALDI MSI for the study of saponins in cuvierian tubules of *H. forskali*. *PLoS One*, 5, e13923.

192. Van Dyck, S., Caulier, G., Todesco, M. et al. 2011. The triterpene glycosides of *Holothuria forskali*: Usefulness and efficiency as a chemical defense mechanism against predatory fish. *J. Exp. Biol.*, 214, 1347–1356.

193. Kicha, A. A., Kalinovsky, A. I., Ivanchina, N. V. et al. 2000. Polyhydroxylated steroidal saponins from Asteroidea (Starfish). *Proc. Phytochem. Soc. Eur.*, 45, 65–72.

194. Minale, L., Riccio, R., and Zollo, F., 1993. Steroidal oligoglycosides and polyhydroxysteroids from echinoderms. *Prog. Chem. Org. Nat. Prod.*, 62, 75–308.

195. Fusetani, N., Kato, Y., Hashimoto, K. et al. 1984. Biological activities of asterosaponins with special reference to structure–activity relationships. *J. Nat. Prod.*, 47, 997–1002.

196. Kalinin, V. I., Ivanchina, N. V., Krasokhin, V. B. et al. 2012. Glycosides from marine sponges (Porifera, Demospongiae): Structures, taxonomical distribution, biological activities and biological roles. *Mar. Drugs*, 10, 1671–1710.

197. Ivanchina, N. V., Kicha, A. A., and Stonik, V. A., 2011. Steroid glycosides from marine organisms. *Steroids*, 76, 425–454.

198. Nakagawa, H., Tanigawa, T., Tomita, K. et al. 2003. Recent studies on the pathological effects of purified sea urchin toxins. *Toxin Rev.*, 22, 633–649.

199. Edo, K., Sakai, H., Nakagawa, H. et al. 2012. Immunomodulatory activity of a pedicellarial venom lectin from the toxopneustid sea urchin, *Toxopneustes pileolus*. *Toxin Rev.*, 31, 54–60.

200. Watters, D. J. and van den Brenk, A. L., 1993. Toxins from ascidians. *Toxicon*, 31, 1349–1372.

201. Lee, J., Currano, J. N., Carroll, P. J. et al. 2012. Didemnins, tamandarins and related natural products. *Nat. Prod. Rep.*, 29, 404–424.

202. Xu, Y., Kersten, R. D., Nam, S.-J. et al. 2012. Bacterial biosynthesis and maturation of the didemnin anti-cancer agents. *J. Am. Chem. Soc.*, 134, 8625–8632.

203. Lane, A. L. and Moore, B. S., 2011. A sea of biosynthesis: Marine natural products meet the molecular age. *Nat. Prod. Rep.*, 28, 411–428.

204. Donia, M. S., Hathaway, B. J., Sudek, S. et al. 2006. Natural combinatorial peptide libraries in cyanobacterial symbionts of marine ascidians. *Nat. Chem. Biol.*, 2, 729–735.

205. Vincenzi, B., Napolitano, A., Frezza, A. M. et al. 2010. Wide-spectrum characterization of trabectedin: Biology, clinical activity and future perspectives. *Pharmacogenomics*, 11, 865–878.

206. Rath, C. M., Janto, B., Earl, J. et al. 2011. Meta-omic characterization of the marine invertebrate microbial consortium that produces the chemotherapeutic natural product ET-743. *ACS Chem. Biol.*, 6, 1244–1256.

207. Molinski, T. F., 1993. Marine pyridoacridine alkaloids: Structure, synthesis, and biological chemistry. *Chem. Rev.*, 93, 1825–1838.

208. Marshall, K. M. and Barrows, L. R., 2004. Biological activities of pyridoacridines. *Nat. Prod. Rep.*, 21, 731–751.

209. Rinehart, K. L., Kobayashi, J., Harbour, G. C. et al. 1987. Eudistomins A-Q,.beta.-carbolines from the antiviral Caribbean tunicate *Eudistoma olivaceum*. *J. Am. Chem. Soc.*, 109, 3378–3387.

210. Sauviat, M.-P., Vercauteren, J., Grimaud, N. et al. 2006. Sensitivity of cardiac background inward rectifying K+ outward current (IK1) to the alkaloids lepadiformines A, B, and C. *J. Nat. Prod.*, 69, 558–562.

211. Tsuneki, H., You, Y., Toyooka, N. et al. 2005. Marine alkaloids (-)-pictamine and (-)-lepadin B block neuronal nicotinic acetylcholine receptors. *Biol. Pharm. Bull.*, 28, 611–614.

212. Genta-Jouve, G. and Thomas, O. P., 2012. Chapter four—Sponge chemical diversity: From biosynthetic pathways to ecological roles, in *Advances Marine Biology*. Mikel A., Becerro, M. J. U. M. M., and Xavier, T., eds. Academic Press, New York, pp. 183–230.

213. Gulavita, N. K., Wright, A. E., McCarthy, P. J. et al. 1996. Cytotoxic peptides from marine sponges. *J. Nat. Toxins*, 5, 225–234.

214. Timm, C., Mordhorst, T., and Köck, M., 2010. Synthesis of 3-alkylpyridinium alkaloids from the arctic sponge *Haliclona viscosa*. *Mar. Drugs*, 8, 483–497.

215. Timm, C., Volk, C., Sasse, F. et al. 2008. The first cyclic monomeric 3-alkylpyridinium alkaloid from natural sources: Identification, synthesis, and biological activity. *Org. Biomol. Chem.*, 6, 4036–4040.

216. Sepcic, K. and Turk, T., 2006. 3-Alkylpyridinium compounds as potential non-toxic antifouling agents. *Prog. Mol. Subcell. Biol.*, 42, 105–124.

217. Sepcic, K., 2000. Bioactive alkylpyridinium compounds from marine sponges. *Toxin Rev.*, 19, 139–160.
218. Erpenbeck, D. and van Soest, R. W. M., 2007. Status and perspective of sponge chemosystematics. *Mar. Biotechnol.*, 9, 2–19.
219. Andersen, R. J., van Soest, R. W. M., and Kong, F., 1996. 3-Alkylpiperidine alkaloids isolated from marine sponges in the order Haplosclerida, in *Alkaloids: Chemical and Biological Perspectives*. Pelletier, S. W., ed. Pergamon, New York, pp. 301–355.
220. Kobayashi, J. i., Murayama, T., Kosuge, S. et al. 1990. Niphatesines A-D, new antineoplastic pyridine alkaloids from the Okinawan marine sponge *Niphates* sp. *J. Chem. Soc., Perkin Trans.*, 1, 3301–3303.
221. Fusetani, N., Asai, N., Matsunaga, S. et al. 1994. Bioactive marine metabolites. 59. Cyclostellettamines A-F, pyridine alkaloids which inhibit binding of methyl quinuclidinyl benzilate (QNB) to muscarinic acetylcholine receptors, from the marine sponge, *Stelletta maxima*. *Tetrahedron Lett.*, 35, 3967–3970.
222. Laville, R., Thomas, O. P., Berrue, F. et al. 2008. Pachychalines A-C: Novel 3-alkylpyridinium salts from the marine sponge *Pachychalina* sp. *Eur. J. Org. Chem.*, 121–125.
223. Volk, C. A. and Koeck, M., 2003. Viscosamine: The first naturally occurring trimeric 3-alkyl pyridinium alkaloid. *Org. Lett.*, 5, 3567–3569.
224. Schmitz, F. J., Hollenbeak, K. H., and Campbell, D. C., 1978. Marine natural products: Halitoxin, toxic complex of several marine sponges of the genus *Haliclona*. *J. Org. Chem.*, 43, 3916–3922.
225. Turk, T., Frangez, R., and Sepcic, K., 2007. Mechanisms of toxicity of 3-alkylpyridinium polymers from marine sponge *Reniera sarai*. *Mar. Drugs*, 5, 157–167.
226. Berlinck, R. G. S. and Kossuga, M. H., 2008. Guanidine alkaloids from marine invertebrates, in *Modern Alkaloids*. Fattorusso, E. and Taglialatela-Scafati, O., eds. Wiley-VCH Verlag GmbH & Co. KGaA, Weinheim, Germany, pp. 305–337.
227. Berlinck, R. G. S. and Kossuga, M. H., 2005. Natural guanidine derivatives. *Nat. Prod. Rep.*, 22, 516–550.
228. Berlinck, R. G. S., 2002. Natural guanidine derivatives. *Nat. Prod. Rep.*, 19, 617–649.
229. Berlinck, R. G. S., 1999. Natural guanidine derivatives. *Nat. Prod. Rep.*, 16, 339–365.
230. Berlinck, R. G. S., 1996. Natural guanidine derivatives. *Nat. Prod. Rep.*, 13, 377–409.
231. Berlinck, R. G. S., Burtoloso, A. C. B., Trindade-Silva, A. E. et al. 2010. The chemistry and biology of organic guanidine derivatives. *Nat. Prod. Rep.*, 27, 1871–1907.
232. Becerro, M., Uriz, M., and Turon, X., 1997. Chemically-mediated interactions in benthic organisms: The chemical ecology of *Crambe crambe* (Porifera, Poecilosclerida). *Hydrobiologia*, 355, 77–89.
233. Martin, V., Vale, C., Bondu, S. et al. 2013. Differential effects of crambescins and Crambescidin 816 in voltage-gated sodium, potassium and calcium channels in neurons. *Chem. Res. Toxicol.*, 26, 169–178.
234. Scheuer, P. J., 1992. Isocyanides and cyanides as natural products. *Acc. Chem. Res.*, 25, 433–439.
235. Cimino, G., de Rosa, S., de Stefano, S. et al. 1982. The chemical defense of four Mediterranean nudibranchs. *Comp. Biochem. Physiol., Part B: Biochem. Mol. Biol.*, 73, 471–474.
236. Braekman, J. C., Daloze, D., Deneubourg, F. et al. 1987. I-Isocyanoaromadendrane: A new isonitrile sesquiterpene from the sponge *Acanthella Acuta*. *Bull. Soc. Chim. Belg.*, 96, 539–543.

5

Emerging Toxic Cyanobacterial Issues in Freshwater Sources: Influence of Climate Change

Arash Zamyadi

CONTENTS

5.1 Introduction

Potentially toxic cyanobacteria have been increasingly detected in water sources in recent years across the planet (Chorus and Bartram, 1999; Carmichael, 2001; Svrcek and Smith, 2004; Giani et al., 2005; Agence Française de Sécurité Sanitaire des Aliments (AFSSA) and Agence Française de Sécurité Sanitaire de l'Environnement et du Travail (AFSSET), 2006; McQuaid et al., 2011). Cyanotoxins and taste and odor (T&O) compounds produced by cyanobacteria are some of the main emerging water contaminants in recent years (Carmichael et al., 2001; Zamyadi et al., 2012c).

Cyanobacteria, also known as blue-green algae, are prokaryotic photosynthetic microorganisms present in most ecosystems. They are asexual phytoplanktons with gram-negative cell walls (Agence Française de Sécurité Sanitaire des Aliments (AFSSA) and Agence Française de Sécurité Sanitaire de l'Environnement et du Travail (AFSSET), 2006; Hudnell, 2006). Their pigmentation can vary from blue-green to red. Cyanobacteria have long been recognized for their nitrogen-fixing capacity (the ability to convert atmospheric N_2 to NH_3), which contributes to global soil and water fertility. Furthermore, they are probably one of the primary organisms responsible for providing an oxygen-rich atmosphere on Earth (Chorus and Bartram, 1999; Svrcek and Smith, 2004). It is estimated that cyanobacteria have been present in the earth's life cycle for over 3.5 billion years (Hudnell, 2006). However, during the last three decades, most of the published literature covering cyanobacteria has introduced them as a potent producer of a variety of toxins responsible for intermittent but repeated widespread poisoning of wild and domestic animals, aquacultured fish, and humans (Chorus and Bartram, 1999; Carmichael et al., 2001). Many potentially toxic species of cyanobacteria (Figure 5.1) and their associated toxins have been detected.

The toxic effects of toxins produced by these species include (Table 5.1) hepatotoxicity, neurotoxicity, cytotoxicity, genotoxicity, dermatotoxicity, and endotoxicity (Svrcek and Smith, 2004). The main toxins of interest concerning human health are microcystins (MCs), anatoxin-a, cylindrospermopsin (CYN), and saxitoxins (STXs) (Duy et al., 2000; Shaw et al., 2000; Li et al., 2001; Zamyadi et al., 2010, 2012c). Meanwhile, the MC analogs are the most commonly reported of the algal toxins worldwide (Cooperative Research Centre for Water Quality and Treatment, 2006).

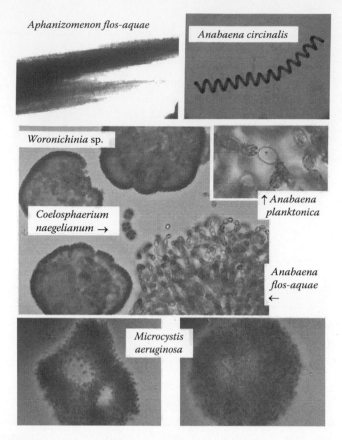

FIGURE 5.1　Microscopic photo of several cyanobacterial species detected in freshwater bodies located in the northeastern regions of the American continent.

Cyanobacteria grow and produce their toxins in surface waters throughout the world, particularly under eutrophic conditions, but also in the metalimnion of deep mesotrophic reservoirs. Many of these surface waters are used for drinking water production and recreational activities. While it is not known for certain why cyanobacteria produce toxins, it has been surmised that their toxin-synthesizing capacities are evolutionary carry-overs and/or protective discharges. Researchers have shown some cyanobacteria toxins to be potent inhibitors of aquatic invertebrate grazers (Carmichael, 1992; Chorus and Bartram, 1999; Gijsbertsen-Abrahamse et al., 2006).

The accumulation of many excessively buoyant cyanobacterial cells or colonies (scum) at the surface of water bodies is called a bloom event or proliferation (Figure 5.2). In extreme cases, such agglomeration may become very dense (Figure 5.3) and even gain a gelatinous consistency and sometimes even looks like blue-green paint or jelly (Figure 5.4) (Cooperative Research Centre for Water Quality and Treatment, 2006). The nature of cyanobacterial proliferation is very dynamic, and the bloom event will be followed by dying-off phase and release of cell-bound material including toxins and T&O compounds (Agence Française de Sécurité Sanitaire des Aliments (AFSSA) and Agence Française de Sécurité Sanitaire de l'Environnement et du Travail (AFSSET), 2006).

In bloom events, more cyanobacterial biomass indicates a higher probability of toxin presence. However, in some cases, low number of highly toxic cells produced more toxins compared to high number of less toxic cells (McQuaid et al., 2011; Zamyadi et al., 2012c). The biosynthesis of cyanotoxins is an energy-intensive process, and the toxic properties of these molecules may have nothing to do with their functions (Wilhelm et al., 2007). Cyanotoxins are largely retained within the cyanobacterial

TABLE 5.1

Known Freshwater Cyanotoxins, Their Toxicity, Cyanobacteria Species Producing the Toxins, and Water Quality Alert Levels

Cyanotoxin	LD_{50}[a] (i.p. Mouse µg/kg Body Weight)	Cyanobacteria Species Producing the Toxins	Mechanism of Toxicity
MCs in general (~60 known analogs)	45–1000	*Microcystis, Anabaena, Planktothrix, Oscillatoria,*	Hepatotoxic: protein phosphatase blockers by
MC-LR	50 (25–125)	*Nostoc, Hapalosiphon*	covalent binding and cause
MC-LA	50	*Anabaenopsis*	hemorrhaging of the liver.
MC-YR	70	*Aphanizomenon*	
MC-RR	300–600		
STXs also known as paralytic shellfish poisons in general (~30 known analogs)	10–30	*Anabaena, Aphanizomenon, Cylindrospermopsis, Lyngbya*	Neurotoxin: STXs are potent voltage-gated sodium channel antagonists, causing numbness, paralysis, and
STX			death by respiratory arrest.
C-toxin 1 and 2 (C1 and C2)			STX disrupts the nervous
Gonyautoxin 2 and 3 (GTX2 and GTX3)			system via binding to the sodium channel and inhibits the sodium ions transport.
CYN	200–2100	*Cylindrospermopsis, Aphanizomenon, Umezakia, Raphidiopsis, Anabaena*	Cytotoxic: blocks protein synthesis.
Anatoxin		*Anabaena* sp.,	Neurotoxic: acute poisoning
Anatoxin-a	200–250	*Aphanizomenon* sp.,	results in death by paralysis
Anatoxin-a(S)	20–40	*Oscillatoria* sp., *Cylindrospermopsis* sp., *Lyngbya* sp., *Schizothrix* sp.	and respiratory failure. Acute toxicity only at very high cell densities.

Sources: Catterall, W.A., *Annu. Rev. Pharmacol. Toxicol.,* 20, 15, 1980; Höger, S.J., Problems during drinking water treatment of cyanobacterial-loaded surface waters: Consequences for human health (Thesis), Gefördert durch die Deutsche Bundesstiftung Umwelt (DBU), Germany, p. 208, 2003; Svrcek, C. and Smith, D.W., *Environ. Eng. Sci.,* 3, 155, 2004; Humpage, A., *Toxins Types, Toxicokinetics and Toxicodynamics* (Chapter 16), Springer-Verlag Inc., New York, p. 34, 2008; Ellis, D., Guide d'intervention pour les propriétaires, les exploitants ou les concepteurs de stations de production d'eau potable municipales aux prises avec une problématique de fleurs d'eau de cyanobactéries, Quebec, Ministère du Développement durable, de l'Environnement et des Parcs, Direction des politiques de l'eau, Montreal Quebec, Canada, p. 46, 2009; Newcombe, G. et al., Management strategies for cyanobacteria (blue-green algae): A guide for water utilities, The Cooperative Research Centre for Water Quality and Treatment, Research Report No. 74, Adelaide, South Australia, Australia 2010; Merel, S., *Toxicon,* 55, 677, 2010.

[a] LD_{50} is the dose of toxins that is lethal to 50% of the test population.

cell during its growth phase with 10%–20% as extracellular; a sudden increase in the concentration of dissolved toxins in the water column can occur after the collapse of a bloom and consequent cell lysis (Jones and Orr, 1994; Hyenstrand et al., 2003).

Several authors (Salinger, 2005; Zamyadi, 2011; Sinha et al., 2012) concluded that both global warming and more frequent sampling could be the main reasons behind the increasing detection of cyanobacterial species in water resources. For example, Sinha et al. (2012) have reviewed the scientific publications reporting the regional occurrence of a cyanobacterial species, that is, *Cylindrospermopsis raciborskii*, from 1950 to 2010. *Cylindrospermopsis raciborskii* is a cyanobacterial species with potential to produce cytotoxin, that is, CYN, and neurotoxin, that is, STXs (Svrcek and Smith, 2004; Agence Française de Sécurité Sanitaire des Aliments (AFSSA) and Agence Française de Sécurité Sanitaire de l'Environnement et du Travail (AFSSET), 2006). Sinha et al. (2012) classified the available data on the occurrence of this cyanobacterial species into two periods, (1) prior to 1990 and (2) post 1990. A visible increase in detection of *Cylindrospermopsis*

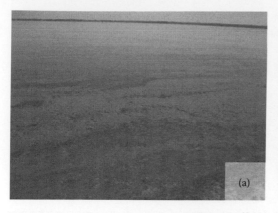
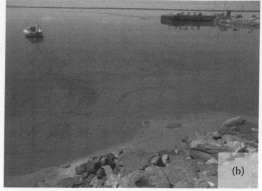

FIGURE 5.2   (a) Cyanobacterial bloom formation in the Canadian side of the Lake Champlain, located in the northeastern region of the American continent (summer 2011), and (b) mixed cyanobacterial and Chlorophyta bloom from the same water body.

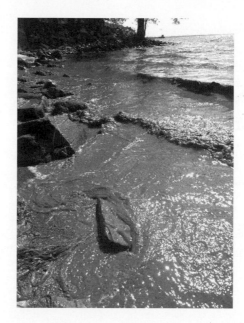

FIGURE 5.3   Very dense cyanobacterial bloom in the Canadian side of the Lake Champlain (summer 2011).

raciborskii has been observed during the second period compare to the first period. This increase is particularly important in temperate zones, for example, Europe and North America. However, Sinha et al. (2012) mentioned that the characterization of CYN by Ohtani et al. (1992) could have caused a particular attention to *Cylindrospermopsis raciborskii* surveillance and detection. However, these authors also demonstrated that the temperature in temperate regions has increased in a greater scale compared to tropical regions and earth average temperature. Considering these observations, cyanobacteria and the potential influence of global climate change are the focus of this chapter.

The extent of increase in average global temperature during the last 113 years varies from 0.2°C to 1.0°C depending on the reference document and the time period during which the reference document focused on (Salinger, 2005; Solomon et al., 2007; Sinha et al., 2012). Also, it has been observed (Intergovernmental Panel on Climate Change, 2007) that during the twentieth century, the Northern Hemisphere mean temperature has risen ~0.2°C more than the Southern Hemisphere temperature. Sinha et al. (2012) concluded that despite all variations between available studies, it is clear that the mean global temperature is increasing. Furthermore, the magnitude of variations between regional temperature increases is higher compared to the variation of global temperature increase (Hulme et al., 2001; Ventura et al., 2002; Yan et al., 2002;

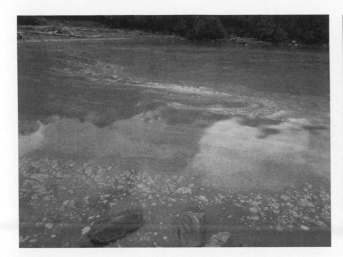
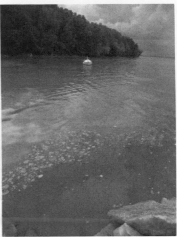

FIGURE 5.4   An extreme case of a cyanobacterial bloom with a gelatinous consistency and a blue-green color in the Canadian side of the Lake Champlain (summer 2011).

Maracchi et al., 2005; Nicholls and Collins, 2006; Brunet et al., 2007; Intergovernmental Panel on Climate Change, 2007; Sinha et al., 2012). For example, Europe's maximum temperature raise is ~3.9°C, while the African continent maximum temperature raise is below 0.8°C (Sinha et al., 2012).

Several predictive models have been developed to foresee the future of global climate change and associated increases in temperature and its consequences. It has been predicted that the mean global temperature will rise by 1.1°C–6.4°C by the end of the twenty-first century compared to 1990 (Roijackers and Lürling, 2007). Also, the highest probability for the global temperature increase during the first half of the twenty-first century is between 1°C and 2°C (Roijackers and Lürling, 2007). Hurrell (1995) demonstrated that the raise in the Northern Hemisphere temperature during the last 40 years of the twentieth century was related to the North Atlantic Oscillation (NAO). Furthermore, Briand et al. (2004) concluded that the global climate change and increase in the surface temperature of water bodies are linked to NAO-related temperature changes. Thus, the possible changes in atmospheric circulations influence the climate modeling results and temperature raise predictions. Furthermore, the regional variations in the climate change consequences are of great importance and include several unknowns.

While climate change and global warming are proven facts, several questions remain regarding the impact of these changes on cyanobacteria and their associated toxins. It is important to consider that due to the lack of historic data, particularly in temperate/Nordic regions, the assessment of climate change impacts on cyanobacterial presence and their toxin production is still in its initial phase. For instance, during summer and fall of 2006 and 2007 in Eastern Canada, a large number of water bodies, which were affected by potentially toxic cyanobacterial blooms, were reported to the provincial water authorities. The investigations by the concerned authorities confirmed the presence of toxic cyanobacteria in these water bodies. Nevertheless, during the same period, cyanobacterial bloom issues became a media subject. Hence, public awareness resulted in the reporting of this high number of water bodies. However, this number of water bodies with detected cyanobacterial presence stayed within a constant range even after the restoration of intensive cyanobacterial monitoring plan by the provincial government in this region. Furthermore, several unknown factors are involved with the variations in the intensity of these bloom events and the seasonal variation of present species. Climate change and global warning could be a potential cause behind these variations. However, long-term environmental surveillance studies are required to understand the impact of climate change on variations in freshwater toxins and to evaluate the risks associated with drinking water production and recreational activities.

Several authors suggest that climate change impacts might prolong conditions that favor toxic and nontoxic cyanobacterial blooms (Paerl and Paul, 2012; Sinha et al., 2012). Thus, establishment and succession of cyanobacteria due to climate change impacts and higher cell numbers could lead to higher toxin concentrations in freshwater sources. The objective of this chapter is to evaluate the influence of global climate change on the presence of freshwater toxins and the associated risks for different water uses. To achieve this goal, this chapter studies the known factors that influence the proliferation of cyanobacteria and their toxin production and the possible influence of climate change on each of these factors. Finally, the potential risks associated with the proliferation of toxic species for drinking water production and water recreational activities are evaluated.

5.2 Climate Change and Proliferation of Potentially Toxic Cyanobacteria and Toxin Production

The focus of this section is to review several of the known factors that influence the proliferation of potentially toxic cyanobacteria and their toxin production. Furthermore, the impact of climate change on these factors and consequently on cyanobacterial blooms and toxin production will be discussed.

Eutrophication is defined as enrichment of a water body by natural or artificial substances, for example, nitrogen and phosphorus substances, and the subsequent response of the aquatic ecosystem to this new condition. It has been demonstrated that eutrophication and increase in water temperature directly influence the frequency and duration of cyanobacterial blooms, as well as that of related issues such as toxins and T&O compounds in freshwater sources (Hudon et al., 2000; Cooperative Research Centre for Water Quality and Treatment, 2004; Paerl and Fulton, 2006; Reynolds, 2006). Furthermore, recent laboratory, field, and modeling studies show that climate change and its impact on surface water eutrophication continue to enhance the timing and proportional dominance of the potentially toxic cyanobacteria in diverse water bodies (Elliott, 2012; Paerl and Paul, 2012). Climate change effects, including global warming and consequent hydrological changes, enhance the eutrophication of water bodies. They also influence cyanobacterial metabolism, growth season and rate, and proliferation (Paerl and Paul, 2012).

One of the main contributing factors in the formation of cyanobacterial bloom are the nutrients particularly nitrogen, phosphorus, and iron, which control the biomass. Nitrogen is an important factor controlling the growth of cyanobacterial cells and their toxin production (Orr and Jones, 1998; Herrero et al., 2001). Particularly, peak toxin production by cyanobacterial cells was observed in the presence of dissolved inorganic nitrogen (most common forms: ammonium, nitrite, and nitrate) (Saker and Griffiths, 2001; Saker and Neilan, 2001; Herrero et al., 2004; Muro-Pastor et al., 2005). Due to the increasing nutrient pollution of freshwater ecosystems and high phosphorus levels in particular (over 25 µg/L), several water bodies including the drinking water resources suffer from extensive cyanobacterial blooms in the summer (Cooperative Research Centre for Water Quality and Treatment, 2004; Gregor et al., 2007). Significant changes in the native benthic community might cause the loss of nitrogen forms for key phytoplankton species. Thus, the dominance within the phytoplankton community shifts to cyanobacteria species capable of nitrogen fixation (Hoffman et al., 1995). Low nitrogen–phosphorus ratios (less than 29:1) favor the development of cyanobacterial blooms (Cooperative Research Centre for Water Quality and Treatment, 2004).

Rapid development in urbanization, agricultural activity, and industrial productivity has caused significant increase in nitrogen and phosphorus discharge to water bodies across the globe (Giani et al., 2005; Paerl and Paul, 2012). Paerl and Paul (2012) reviewed several scientific publications on the presence of cyanobacterial blooms in Lake Taihu. This lake is the third largest lake in China situated in Jiangsu Province with a rapidly growing economy and industrial production. These authors have observed a continuous increase in nitrogen and phosphorus discharge to this lake in the past 50 years due to significant population growth and industrial activity. They have concluded that these changes are responsible for the May–October shift in the lake's phytoplankton community from diatom to cyanobacteria, that is, *Microcystis* spp. Furthermore, assessing the available regional meteorological data and phytoplankton monitoring data, Paerl and Paul (2012) concluded that the increase in annual average air and water temperature in the Lake Taihu is associated with increase in phytoplankton presence in this lake. While climate change and global warming influence the proliferation of potentially toxic cyanobacteria in freshwater sources, unsustainable human activities play a key role in enhancing these bloom events.

After investigating several scientific publications, Paerl and Paul (2012) concluded that there is a strong positive correlation between annual average temperature and cyanobacterial dominance in tropical and subtropical water bodies. These authors also mentioned that some high-altitude lakes, lakes with acidic conditions (pH <6), severely nutrient-limited lakes, lakes with short water residence time, and water bodies with poorly stratified conditions are exceptions to this correlation. In addition, Paerl and Paul (2012) observed that nutrient enrichment of water bodies enhances furthermore the cyanobacterial dominance as the temperature rises. Furthermore, they have concluded that the increase in water temperature without significant increase in nutrient load and regional effects of warming enhance the presence of potentially toxic cyanobacteria.

The climate change effects with respect to air/water temperature include warmer winters, less frost and less snow cover, and longer summer heat. These effects with respect to precipitation could translate to more intense precipitation in both summer and winter, more rainfalls in early spring, fewer rainy days in summer, and a significant increase in the intensity of rain events (Carey et al., 2012; Elliott, 2012; Paerl and Paul, 2012; Reichwaldt and Ghadouani, 2012; Sinha et al., 2012). These changes in the precipitation trend result in short-term extreme runoff events but decrease the total water discharge to lakes and consequently lower water levels. It has been shown that these changes in air/water temperature and precipitation patterns favor the dominance of cyanobacteria and their toxin production.

Low turbulence leading to the reduction of turbidity to moderate levels, long residence time, and increased light intensity favors cyanobacterial dominance in water bodies (Cooperative Research Centre for Water Quality and Treatment, 2004; Hudnell, 2006). Several potentially toxic freshwater cyanobacterial species, for example, *Cylindrospermopsis*, *Microcystis*, and *Lyngbya*, form dense surface blooms in nutrient-rich water bodies that influence the light exposure of other phytoplankton and help them to continue dominating the system (Paerl and Paul, 2012). Furthermore, Kardinaal et al. (2007) have demonstrated that the length of warm season (i.e., spring and summer) and available daylight play a considerable role in the competition between toxic and nontoxic strains of cyanobacterial species.

The review of published literature using environmental collected data and analysis (Paerl and Paul, 2012) and lake modeling (Elliott, 2012) suggests that global warming causes extreme discharge of nutrients into water bodies, influences the thermal stratification, and transforms freshwater discharge, flow pattern, and hydraulic residence time. Consequently, these effects of global warming enhance proliferation and abundance of cyanobacteria compared to other phytoplankton community and production of cyanotoxins.

Paerl and Paul (2012) concluded that several general trends have been established in the expansion of cyanobacteria and cyanotoxin production due to climate change. However, the vulnerability of water bodies to toxic bloom presence and the risks associated with these blooms might vary based on site-specific condition. Several factors like hydrography and geomorphology, hydraulic residence time, variable nutrient inputs and grazing pressures, and seasonal and interannual rainfall are site-specific factors that influence the presence of toxic cyanobacteria against the general trends. Therefore, the development of site-specific risk assessment tools and local intervention/management action plans is necessary.

5.3 Risks Associated with Proliferation of Potentially Toxic Cyanobacteria

The most undesirable effects of cyanobacterial blooms in freshwater sources with regard to health risk for human being are summarized as follows (Agence Française de Sécurité Sanitaire des Aliments (AFSSA) and Agence Française de Sécurité Sanitaire de l'Environnement et du Travail (AFSSET), 2006; Li et al., 2007; Kommineni et al., 2009; Newcombe et al., 2010; Zamyadi et al., 2012b,c, 2013; Bogialli et al., 2013):

1. Human health effects due to direct contact with cyanobacterial cells during water recreational activities, for example, skin or mucous membrane problems as a result of bathing in waters affected by blooms.
2. Complication of the drinking water treatment process which includes the following:
   a. Toxic cells accumulation during treatment within water treatment plants
   b. Breakthrough of toxins and cells into treated water
   c. Sudden changes in raw water characteristics, for example, pH; disruption of treatment processes, for example, malfunction of flocculation reactions; increasing the consumption of coagulant; and generation of disinfection by-products due to organic materials involved with bloom matrix

3. Disruption of dialysis equipment by accelerated clogging if the water treatment is inadequate.

4. Production of T&O compounds such as the most commonly occurring geosmin and 2-methy-lisoborneol (MIB), which are very hard to be removed from water, that is, conventional treatment (e.g., coagulation/clarification, filtration, and oxidation using chlorine and hydrogen peroxide), is inefficient.

Results of several years of monitoring in different freshwater sources across the globe (Boyer et al., 2001; Agence Française de Sécurité Sanitaire des Aliments (AFSSA) and Agence Française de Sécurité Sanitaire de l'Environnement et du Travail (AFSSET), 2006; McQuaid et al., 2011; Zamyadi et al., 2012c, 2013; Zhao, 2012; Bogialli et al., 2013) demonstrate that water authorities and water treatment utilities need to have a proper knowledge of the presence of potentially toxic cyanobacteria and their proliferation over the source in order to evaluate the risk of toxin breakthrough into the treated water. The frequent monitoring of cyanotoxins provides high-quality documentation of high cyanotoxin concentrations at the water intake of drinking water treatment utilities, even in more temperate regions (McQuaid, 2009). Furthermore, cyanobacterial monitoring results demonstrate the multispecies composition of cyanobacteria during bloom events in certain temperate region, for example, Eastern Canada, and the change in dominant species between water bodies and between seasons (McQuaid et al., 2011; Zamyadi et al., 2012c).

5.3.1 Fate of Potentially Toxic Cyanobacteria in Drinking Water Treatment

Understanding the treatment barriers that are used for drinking water production and assessment of their limitation are essential for proper evaluation of risk of breakthrough of freshwater toxins into the treated water. In several regions including the North America, drinking water is produced from several protected and semi-protected sources, and the water treatment process does not include conventional filtration. In these cases, disinfection is applied directly to raw water. In the United States, unfiltered water serves approximately 11,000,000 customers and includes cities such as New York City (NY), Boston (MA), Portland (ME), Portland (OR), and San Francisco (CA) (S. Regli, pers. comm.). In Quebec (Canada) alone, there are 130 small and very small utilities that produce unfiltered drinking water (Ministère du Développement Durable de l'Environnement et des Parcs, 2008). Unfiltered plants typically apply single or dual disinfection, usually chlorination, ozonation, and/or ultraviolet (UV) oxidation, directly to raw water that may contain cyanobacterial cells. Pre-oxidation ahead of filtration is commonly used in water treatment for many purposes, including manganese and iron removal, optimized particle removal (including the reduction of algal cells), and filter cycle optimization (Petrusevski et al., 1995; Mouchet and Bonnelye, 1998; Chen and Yeh, 2005; von Sperling et al., 2008). Furthermore, pre/post-chlorination is a common practice for drinking water production in several regions. For example, in 97% of drinking water treatment plants in Quebec, pre-/post-chlorination is used for drinking water production (Barbeau et al., 2009). As mentioned previously, climate change effect might enhance the frequency of potentially toxic cyanobacterial blooms in freshwater sources. Therefore, water treatment plants producing unfiltered drinking water and plants relying on pre-oxidation and filtration to remove cells have to evaluate the vulnerability of their treatment process to potential breakthrough of toxic cells.

The health relevance of cyanobacteria and their associated toxins, the treatment challenges to remove these compounds, and the observed trends of growing predominance of cyanobacteria in surface water all require a comprehensive study of monitoring, treatment, and management options. Because of the human health effects of toxic cyanobacteria, authorities worldwide have introduced threshold alert levels (Table 5.2) for toxins in water used for human consumption (drinking and recreational activities). Also in some regions, for example, states of Queensland and Victoria in Australia, authorities have issued toxin threshold levels for water used for agricultural irrigation and livestock (Orr and Schneider, 2006; McFarlane and McLennan, 2008).

Once a proper understanding of a given plant and the threshold levels have been established, the monitoring regime should focus on situations and bloom events that have been identified as critical for

TABLE 5.2

Drinking Water Quality Alert Levels for Freshwater Cyanotoxins

Cyanotoxin	Health-Based Exposure Guidelines/ Recommended Alert Levels
MCs and its most known analogs	South Africa: 0.8 µg/L MC-LR
MC-LR	World Health Organization (WHO), Czech
MC-LA	Republic, China, France, Italy, Japan, Korea,
MC-YR	New Zealand, Norway, Poland: 1 µg/L MC-LR
MC-RR	Brazil, Spain: 1 µg/L MCs
	Australia: 1.3 µg/L MC-LR toxicity equivalent
	Canada (Environment Canada): 1.5 µg/L MC-LR toxicity
	Quebec (Canada): 1.5 µg/L MC-LR toxicity
STXs and the its most known analogs	Australia, Brazil, and New Zealand: 3.0 µg/L STX
STX	toxicity equivalent
C-toxin 1 and C-toxin 2 (C1 and C2)	
Gonyautoxin 2 and gonyautoxin 3 (GTX2 and GTX3)	
CYN	New Zealand: 1 µg/L
	Brazil: 15 µg/L
Anatoxin	Quebec (Canada): 3.7 µg/L
Anatoxin-a	
Anatoxin-a(S)	

Sources: Chorus, I. and Bartram, J., *Toxic Cyanobacteria in Water: A Guide to Their Public Health Consequences, Monitoring and Management*, World Health Organization (WHO), London, U.K., 1999; Svrcek, C. and Smith, D.W., *Environ. Eng. Sci.*, 3, 155, 2004; Ellis, D., Guide d'intervention pour les propriétaires, les exploitants ou les concepteurs de stations de production d'eau potable municipales aux prises avec une problématique de fleurs d'eau de cyanobactéries, Quebec, Ministère du Développement durable, de l'Environnement et des Parcs, Direction des politiques de l'eau, Montreal Quebec, Canada, p. 46, 2009; Newcombe, G. et al., Management strategies for cyanobacteria (blue-green algae): A guide for water utilities, The Cooperative Research Centre for Water Quality and Treatment, Research Report No. 74, Adelaide, South Australia, Australia, 2010.

public safety. Application of a comprehensive risk assessment and management approach that includes all steps of drinking water supply from the watershed to the consumer could provide water utilities with a most efficient tool to consistently ensure the safety of their potable water (Bartram et al., 2009). The "water safety plan" as promoted by the World Health Organization is a comprehensive risk assessment and management strategy (Bartram et al., 2009).

Furthermore, a good understanding of (1) the recorded historic occurrence of cyanobacteria and their associated toxins in water sources across the globe and (2) their impact on the intake of drinking water treatment plants and drinking water production is essential to the management of the risks associated with these emerging contaminants. A series of studies (McQuaid et al., 2011; Zamyadi et al., 2012c, 2013) that have been conducted from 2007 to 2012 in a Canadian drinking water treatment plant provides a proper example of the necessity of understanding the impact of blooms over the source on the water intake and the treatment train. The studied drinking water treatment plant draws its raw water from Missisquoi Bay (Canadian side of Lake Champlain) that is often subject to cyanobacterial proliferations. The concentration of cyanobacteria in raw water varies widely and is not generally associated with high concentrations of cyanotoxins. However, more frequent monitoring, that is, daily samplings, during these studies showed that high concentrations of cyanotoxins (over 118.7 µg/L total MCs) could be detected in raw water at the water intake of this plant. These documented cases suggest that the water utilities need to evaluate the short-term risk, that is, 6–24 h, of elevated toxin concentrations at their water intake.

The observations of cyanobacterial bloom events (McQuaid et al., 2011; Zamyadi et al., 2012d) from May to November in a temperate region, that is, province of Quebec in Canada, underline the urgent need for an all-inclusive management strategy focusing on site-specific challenges. However, despite the fact that the authorities have followed the levels of cyanotoxin on a regular basis within these studied water treatment plants and other facilities prone to cyanobacterial blooms, high concentrations of toxins had not been measured in the samples taken (Zamyadi, 2011). It is hypothesized that the sampling schedules and frequency recommended in the existing guidelines, for example, weekly sampling, did not necessarily coincide with peak periods of toxins. As Australian experiences demonstrated, regular cyanobacterial monitoring has to be conducted at high frequency, and it is essential to incorporate the event-based monitoring into the cyanobacterial management strategies (Zamyadi, 2011). The Australian water authorities' strategies in the management of cyanobacteria-related issues are exemplary. The Australians have successfully adapted intensive in vivo cyanobacterial monitoring, with all the known interferences involved, into their management plans. Furthermore, in bloom season, water bodies are monitored on a daily basis, and drinking water treatment plants are informed about the cyanobacteria presence within proximity of their water intakes.

Very little information is available on the duration and frequency of peak events of cyanobacteria and cyanotoxins in raw water, their intensity, and the subsequent impact throughout the treatment process. Figure 5.5 shows presence of toxic cyanobacterial cells at the water intake of a drinking water treatment plant (inside the plant) in Canada 2 days after the disappearance of the surface bloom event over the source. It is essential to figure out if the presence of toxic cyanobacterial cells at the water intake of water treatment facilities might lead to (1) passage of cyanotoxins in treated water and (2) significant accumulation of cyanobacterial cells in different treatment processes. In case of a potential accumulation, the risk associated with this phenomenon needs to be quantified and remedial measures identified.

Cyanobacteria and chlorophyceae were detected as dominant species during algal-related issues in 76 drinking water treatment plants across the United States (West, Midwest, South and Northeast regions) (Kommineni et al., 2009). Apart from major concerns regarding the presence and elimination of toxins and T&O compounds, these events negatively influenced the operation of the plants and performance of treatment barriers.

Recent cyanobacterial monitoring in a drinking water treatment plant in Eastern Canada documented the presence of toxic cyanobacterial scum inside the plant on several occasions (Zamyadi et al., 2012c, 2013). These results demonstrated that cyanobacterial cells could accumulate and perhaps grow in the sludge of clarifiers and in the water over the sedimentation basin. Figure 5.6 shows the accumulation of cyanobacterial cells in the water over the sedimentation tank in this plant. In one occasion in summer 2010, the cyanobacterial scum detected over the sedimentation tank was highly toxic, and 10,331 µg/L of total MCs was detected in this scum sample (Zamyadi et al., 2012c). Also, small traces of CYN (0.29 µg/L) were found in the water samples from this scum. During the same scum event, the concentration of the total MCs in the sludge bed of the clarifier was 23.92 µg/L.

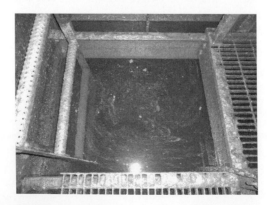

FIGURE 5.5 Presence of high cell numbers of toxic cyanobacterial cells at the water intake at a Canadian drinking water treatment plant (summer 2011).

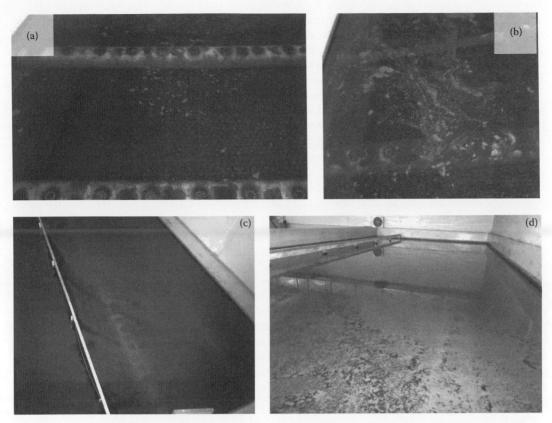

FIGURE 5.6 Accumulation of toxic cyanobacterial cells in the water over the sedimentation tank of clarifiers in a drinking water treatment plant in Eastern Canada (summer 2011), (a and b) local coverage of the surface water, and (c and d) complete coverage of the surface water.

The water from the surface of the sedimentation tank directly flows to the filtration basin. The release of cell-bound toxin in the sedimentation tank, for example, from the cells accumulated in the sludge and/or scum in the surface water, could cause the breakthrough of toxins into filtered water. Figure 5.7 shows cyanobacterial accumulation in the water over the filtration basin in a Canadian water treatment plant. The maximum total MC concentration in samples from this scum was 171 µg/L (Zamyadi et al., 2012d).

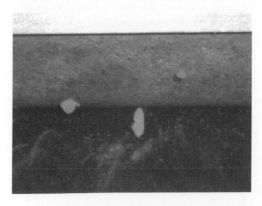

FIGURE 5.7 Accumulation of toxic cyanobacterial cells in the water over the filtration basin in a drinking water treatment plant in Eastern Canada (summer 2011).

The presence of cyanobacterial scum in filtration basin could cause filter clogging, shorter filter run times, disruption of filtration, and breakthrough of cells and toxins into the filtered water (Meriluoto and Codd, 2005; Kommineni et al., 2009; Zamyadi et al., 2013). Increase in filtered water turbidity due to breakthrough of cells could also lead to loss of credit removal for waterborne pathogens, that is, *Giardia*, *Cryptosporidium*, and virus, and greater health risk for the public.

The breakthrough of very high cell numbers, for example, over 100,000 cells/mL, into the water intake of water treatment plants intensifies the accumulation process within the identified processes. However, it has been observed that flow of low cell numbers, below 2000 cells/mL, can also lead to major accumulation of cyanobacteria inside water treatment plants (Zamyadi et al., 2012a). The variations in toxin content per cell in natural bloom samples highlight the importance of cyanobacterial monitoring even in low numbers.

The accumulation of toxic cyanobacterial cells inside a water treatment plant, particularly in the clarification and filtration basins, increases the potential concentration of toxins that might reached the post-oxidation process. The accumulation of highly toxic cells (10,331 µg/L of total MCs) in the sedimentation tank of a water treatment plant in Eastern Canada (Zamyadi et al., 2012c) led to the breakthrough of cyanotoxins into the treated water. The concentration of the total MCs in the treated water, that is, post-chlorination, of this plant on this occasion was 2.47 µg/L including 1.74 µg/L MC-LR (Zamyadi et al., 2012c). The detected total MCs and MC-LR concentration in treated water on this occasion exceeded recommended levels of these toxins in potable water by Health Canada (1.5 µg/L MC-LR) and the World Health Organization (1 µg/L MC-LR). This incident is the first documented breakthrough of cyanotoxins into treated water in a temperate region. This information demonstrates that water authorities in temperate and Nordic regions need to assess the vulnerability of their treatment facilities against the risk of freshwater toxin breakthrough into their treated water. Furthermore, Fan (2012) showed that the oxidation efficiency in removal of cell-bound toxins from natural blooms is different from removal of dissolved toxins in laboratory assays. These results confirm that the cyanotoxin oxidation kinetics models derived from dissolved toxins in laboratory conditions may not always be valid in natural conditions. Furthermore, it is important to take into consideration that while an oxidant agent might be efficient for removal of a certain type of toxins, it might not help with the removal of other toxins. For example, while chlorination is efficient form removal of MCs and STXs, it is not efficient for oxidation of anatoxins and its variants.

5.3.2 Risk Assessment and Intervention/Management Strategy

As proposed by Carrière et al. (2010), water utilities would benefit from the assessment of their treatment train vulnerability to different climate change scenarios and consequent toxin production and breakthrough. However, current rapid technological and economical advances and resulting changes in lifestyle and policy will significantly influence the humankind response to global climate change and its consequences. Therefore, Moss et al. (2010) suggested that the development of future scenarios for climate change research and assessment needs to include these recent changes in human capacity to respond to global warming.

The risk evaluation for breakthrough of freshwater toxins into treated water has to include the fate of both cell-bound and dissolved toxins during different treatment processes. Furthermore, for better management of potentially toxic cyanobacteria inside water treatment plants, it is needed to classify the processes or the phenomenon (e.g., hydraulic stress in the pumps or during the filter backwash) that leads to the release of cell-bound toxins inside the treatment facilities. Ultimately, these recent observations show the importance of (1) targeting maximum periods of proliferation to conduct the risk characterization for cyanobacteria and their associated toxins and (2) verifying if this risk can be amplified in the drinking water treatment plants. The prolonged accumulation of cells in the sludge bed and filter media in water treatment plants located in temperate regions suggests that monitoring the breakthrough and accumulation of algal cells including cyanobacteria in treatment plants considered at low risk of extreme bloom events is of interest. These observations highlight the potential vulnerability of other water intakes to potentially toxic cyanobacterial blooms and the importance of carrying out more intensive monitoring in sites considered at risk.

REFERENCES

Agence Française de Sécurité Sanitaire des Aliments (AFSSA) and Agence Française de Sécurité Sanitaire de l'Environnement et du Travail (AFSSET). (2006) Avis de relatif à l'évaluation des risques liés à la présence de cyanobactéries dans les cours d'eau destinés à la baignade et/ou à d'autres usages. AFSSA–AFSSET, France, p. 232.

Barbeau, B., Carrière, A., Prévost, M., Zamyadi, A., and Chevalier, P. (2009) Changements climatiques au Québec méridional. Analyse de la vulnérabilité des installations québécoises de production d'eau potable aux cyanobactéries toxiques. Institut National de Santé Publique du Québec, Montreal, Quebec, Canada, p. 16.

Bartram, J., Corrales, L., Davison, A., Deere, D., Drury, D., Gordon, B., Howard, G., Rinehold, A., and Stevens, M. (2009) *Water Safety Plan Manual: Step-by-Step Risk Management for Drinking-Water Suppliers*. World Health Organisation (WHO), Geneva, Switzerland.

Bogialli, S., Nigro Di Gregorio, F., Lucentini, L., Ferretti, E., Ottaviani, M., Ungaro, N., Abis, P. P., and Cannarozzi De Grazia, M. (2013) Management of a toxic cyanobacterium bloom (Planktothrix rubescens) affecting an Italian drinking water basin: A case study. *Environmental Science and Technology* 47(1), 574–583.

Boyer, G. L., Yang, X., Patchett, E. A., and Satchwell, M. F. (2001) Cyanobacteria toxins in upstate New York waters: A comparison on Onondaga Lake and Oneida Lake. *2nd Annual Onondaga Lake Conference*, Syracuse, New York.

Briand, J. F., Leboulanger, C., Humbert, J. F., Bernard, C., and Dufour, P. (2004) *Cylindrospermopsis raciborskii* (cyanobacteria) invasion at mid-latitudes: Selection, wide physiological tolerance or global warming? *Journal of Phycology* 40(2), 231–238.

Brunet, M., Jones, P. D., Sigro, J., Saladie, O., Aguilar, E., Moberg, A., Della-Marta, P. M., Lister, D., Walther, A., and Lopez, D. (2007) Temporal and spatial temperature variability and change over Spain during 1850 and 2005. *Journal of Geophysics Research* 112, D12117.

Carey, C. C., Ibelings, B. W., Hoffmann, E. P., Hamilton, D. P., and Brookes, J. D. (2012) Eco-physiological adaptations that favour freshwater cyanobacteria in a changing climate. *Water Research* 46, 1394–1407.

Carmichael, W. W. (1992) Cyanobacteria secondary metabolites—The Cyanotoxins (a review). *Journal of Applied Bacteriology* 72, 445–459.

Carmichael, W. W. (2001) *Assessment of Blue-Green Algal Toxins in Raw and Finished Drinking Water*. American Water Works Association Research Foundation, Denver, CO.

Carmichael, W. W., Azevedo, S. M. F. O., An, J. S., Molica, R. J. R., Jochimsen, E. M., Lau, S., Rinehart, K. L., Shaw, G. R., and Eaglesham, G. K. (2001) Human fatalities from cyanobacteria: Chemical and biological evidence for cyanotoxins. *Environmental Health Perspectives* 109, 663–668.

Carrière, A., Prévost, M., Zamyadi, A., Chevalier, P., and Barbeau, B. (2010) Vulnerability of Quebec drinking-water treatment plants to cyanotoxins in a climate change context. *Journal of Water and Health* 08.3, 455–465.

Catterall, W. A. (1980) Neurotoxins that act on voltage-sensitive sodium channels in excitable membranes. *Annual Review of Pharmacology and Toxicology* 20, 15–43.

Chen, J.-J. and Yeh, H.-H. (2005) The mechanisms of potassium permanganate on algae removal. *Water Research* 39(18), 4420–4428.

Chorus, I. and Bartram, J. (1999) *Toxic Cyanobacteria in Water: A Guide to Their Public Health Consequences, Monitoring and Management*. World Health Organization (WHO), London, U.K.

Cooperative Research Centre for Water Quality and Treatment. (2004) *Management Strategies for Algal Toxins*. Adelaide, South Australia, Australia.

Cooperative Research Centre for Water Quality and Treatment. (2006) *Cyanobacteria: Management and Implications for Water Quality*. Fact sheet number: FS 2. Adelaide, South Australia, Australia, p. 36.

Duy, T. N., Lam, P. K. S., Shaw, G. R., and Connell, D. W. (2000) Toxicology and risk assessment of freshwater cyanobacterial (blue-green algal) toxins in water. *Reviews of Environmental Contamination Toxicology* 163, 113–186.

Elliott, J. A. (2012) Is the future blue-green? A review of the current model predictions of how climate change could affect pelagic freshwater cyanobacteria. *Water Research* 46, 1364–1371.

Ellis, D. (2009) Guide d'intervention pour les propriétaires, les exploitants ou les concepteurs de stations de production d'eau potable municipales aux prises avec une problématique de fleurs d'eau de cyanobactéries. Quebec, Ministère du Développement durable, de l'Environnement et des Parcs, Direction des politiques de l'eau, Montreal, Quebec, Canada, p. 46.

Fan, Y. (2012) Chlorination of toxic cyanobacterial cells and their associated toxins (MSc dissertation). Department of Civil, Geological and Mining Engineering, École Polytechnique de Montréal, Montreal, Canada.

Giani, A., Bird, D. F., Prairie, Y. T., and Lawrence, J. F. (2005) Empirical study of cyanobacterial toxicity along a trophic gradient of lakes. *Canadian Journal of Fisheries and Aquatic Sciences* 62, 2100–2109.

Gijsbertsen-Abrahamse, A. J., Schmidt, W., Chorus, I., and Heijman, S. G. J. (2006) Removal of cyanotoxins by ultrafiltration and nanofiltration. *Journal of Membrane Science* 276, 252–259.

Gregor, J., Marsalek, B., and Sipkova, H. (2007) Detection and estimation of potentially toxic cyanobacteria in raw water at the drinking water treatment plant by in vivo fluorescence method. *Water Research* 41, 228–234.

Herrero, A., Muro-Pastor, A. M., and Flores, E. (2001) Nitrogen control in cyanobacteria. *Journal of Bacteriology* 183(2), 411–425.

Herrero, A., Muro-Pastor, A. M., Valladares, A., and Flores, E. (2004) Cellular differentiation and the NtcA transcription factor in filamentous cyanobacteria. *Federation of European Microbiological Societies (FEMS) Microbiology Reviews* 28(4), 469–487.

Hoffman, D. J., Rattner, B. A., Burton, G. A., and Cairns, J. (1995) *Handbook of Ecotoxicology.* CRC Press Inc, Boca Raton, FL.

Höger, S. J. (2003) Problems during drinking water treatment of cyanobacterial-loaded surface waters: Consequences for human health (Thesis). Gefördert durch die Deutsche Bundesstiftung Umwelt (DBU), Germany, p. 208.

Hudnell, K. (2006) Cyanobacterial harmful algal blooms: An increasing risk to human health and ecosystem sustainability. *New Drinking Water Regulations, An International Symposium.* Indianapolis, IN.

Hudon, C., Lalonde, S., and Gagnon, P. (2000) Ranking the effects of site exposure, plant growth form, water depth, and transparency on aquatic plant biomass. *Canadian Journal of Fisheries and Aquatic Sciences* 57, 31–42.

Hulme, M., Doherty, R., Ngara, T., New, M., and Lister, D. (2001) African climate change: 1900–2100. *Climate Research* 17(2), 145–168.

Humpage, A. (2008) Toxins types, toxicokinetics and toxicodynamics, Chapter 16. In *Cyanobacterial Harmful Algal Blooms: State of the Science and Research Needs,* Hudnell, H. K., ed., Springer-Verlag Inc., New York, p. 34.

Hurrell, J. W. (1995) Decadal trends in the North Atlantic oscillation: Regional temperatures and precipitation. *Science* 269(5224), 676–679.

Hyenstrand, P., Rohrlack, T., Beattie, K. A., Metcalf, J. S., Codd, G. A., and Christoffersen, K. (2003) Laboratory studies of dissolved radiolabelled microcystin-LR in lake water. *Water Research* 37, 3299–3306.

Intergovernmental Panel on Climate Change (IPCC). (2007) *Summary for Policymakers: A Report of Working Group I to the IPCC.* University Press, Cambridge, U.K., p. 18.

Jones, G. J. and Orr, P. T. (1994) Release and degradation of microcystin following algicide treatment of a *Microcystis aeruginosa* bloom in a recreational lake, as determined by HPLC and protein phosphatase inhibition assay. *Water Research* 28, 871–876.

Kardinaal, W. E. A., Janse, I., Kamst-van Agterveld, M., Meima, M., Snoek, J., Mur, L. R., Huisman, J., Zwart, G., and Visser, P. M. (2007) *Microcystis* genotype succession in relation to microcystin concentrations in freshwater lakes. *Aquatic Microbial Ecology* 48, 1–12.

Kommineni, S., Amante, K., Karnik, B., Sommerfeld, M., and Dempster, T. (2009) *Strategies for Controlling and Mitigating Algal Growth within Water Treatment Plants.* Water Research Foundation, Denver, CO.

Li, L., Wan, N., Gan, N. Q., Xia, B. D., and Song, L. R. (2007) Annual dynamics and origins of the odorous compounds in the pilot experimental area of Lake Dianchi, China. *Water Science and Technology* 55, 43–50.

Li, R., Carmichael, W. W., Brittain, S., Eaglesham, G. K., Shaw, G. R., Mahakhant, A., Noparatnaraporn, N., Yongmanitchai, W., Kaya, K., and Watanabe, M. M. (2001) Isolation and identification of the cyanotoxin cylindrospermopsin and deoxy-cylindrospermopsin from a Thailand strain of *Cylindrospermopsis raciborskii* (Cyanobacteria). *Toxicon* 39, 973–980.

Maracchi, G., Sirotenko, O., and Bindi, M. (2005) Impacts of present and future climate variability on agriculture and forestry in the temperate regions: Europe. *Increasing Climate Variability and Change* 70, 117–135.

McFarlane, G. and McLennan, C. (2008) *Recycled Water Supply System Western Treatment Plant.* Melbourne Water, Melbourne, Queensland, Australia.

McQuaid, N. (2009) Establishment of an early warning systems for cyanobacteria using an online multi-probe system measuring physicochemical parameters, chlorophyll and phycocyanin (Master thesis). Department of Civil, Geological and Mining Engineering, École Polytechnique de Montréal, Montreal, Quebec, Canada.

McQuaid, N., Zamyadi, A., Prévost, M., Bird, D. F., and Dorner, S. (2011) Use of *in vivo* phycocyanin fluorescence to monitor potential microcystin producing cyanobacterial biovolume in a drinking water source. *Journal of Environmental Monitoring* 13, 455–463.

Merel, S., Clément, M., and Thomas, O. (2010) Review state of the art on cyanotoxins in water and their behaviour towards chlorine. *Toxicon* 55, 677–691.

Meriluoto, J. and Codd, G. A. (2005) *TOXIC: Cyanobacterial Monitoring and Cyanotoxin Analysis*. Åbo Akademi University Press, Åbo, Finland.

Ministère du Développement Durable de l'Environnement et des Parcs (MDDEP). (2008) Portrait des stations municipales de production d'eau potable approvisionnées en eau de surface au Québec. État de la situation au printemps, Montreal, Quebec, Canada, p. 42.

Moss, R. H., Edmonds, J. A., Hibbard, K. A., Manning, M. R., Rose, S. K., van Vuuren, D. P., Carter, T. R. et al. (2010) The next generation of scenarios for climate change research and assessment. *Nature* 463, 747–756.

Mouchet, P. and Bonnelye, V. (1998) Solving algae problems: French expertise and world-wide applications. *Water Supply: Research and Technology-Aqua*, 47(3), 125–141.

Muro-Pastor, M. I., Reyes, J. C., and Florencio, F. J. (2005) Ammonium assimilation in cyanobacteria. *Photosynthesis Research* 83(2), 135–150.

Newcombe, G., House, J., Ho, L., Baker, P., and Burch, M. (2010) Management strategies for cyanobacteria (blue-green algae): A guide for water utilities. The Cooperative Research Centre for Water Quality and Treatment, Research Report No. 74. Adelaide, South Australia, Australia.

Nicholls, N. and Collins, D. (2006) Observed change in Australia over the past century. *Energy and Environment* 17, 1–12.

Ohtani, I., Moore, R. E., and Runnegar, M. T. C. (1992) Cylindrospermopsin: A potent hepatotoxin from the blue-green alga Cylindrospermopsis raciborskii. *Journal of the American Chemical Society* 114(20), 7941–7942.

Orr, P. T. and Jones, G. J. (1998) Relationship between microcystin production and cell division rates in nitrogen-limited *Microcystis aeruginosa* cultures. *Limnology and Oceanography* 43(7), 1604–1614.

Orr, P. T. and Schneider, M. P. (2006) *Toxic Cyanobacteria Risk Assessment Reservoir Vulnerability and Water Use Best Practice*. South-East Queensland Water Corporation, Brisbane, Queensland, Australia.

Paerl, H. W. and Fulton III, R. S. (2006) Ecology of harmful cyanobacteria, In: Graneli, E. and Turner, J. (eds.), *Ecology of Harmful Marine Algae*. Springer-Verlag, Berlin, Germany, pp. 95–107.

Paerl, H. W. and Paul, V. J. (2012) Climate change: Links to global expansion of harmful cyanobacteria. *Water Research* 46, 1349–1363.

Petrusevski, B., van Breeman, A. N., and Alaerts, G. J. (1995) Optimisation of coagulation conditions for direct filtration of impounded surface water. *Water Supply: Research and Technology-Aqua* 44(2), 93–102.

Reichwaldt, E. S. and Ghadouani, A. (2012) Effects of rainfall patterns on toxic cyanobacterial blooms in a changing climate: Between simplistic scenarios and complex dynamics. *Water Research* 46, 1372–1393.

Reynolds, C. S. (2006) *Ecology of Phytoplankton (Ecology, Biodiversity and Conservation)*. Cambridge University Press, Cambridge, U.K., p. 535.

Roijackers, R. M. M. and Lürling, M. F. L. L. W. (2007) *Climate Change and Bathing Water Quality*. Environmental Science Group Aquatic Ecology and Water Quality Chair, Wageningen, the Netherlands, p. 39.

Saker, M. L. and Griffiths, D. J. (2001) Occurrence of blooms of the cyanobacterium *Cylindrospermopsis raciborskii* (Woloszynska) Seenayya and Subba Raju in a North Queensland domestic water supply. *Marine and Freshwater Research* 52(6), 907–915.

Saker, M. L. and Neilan, B. A. (2001) Varied diazotrophs, morphologies, and toxicities of genetically similar isolates of *Cylindrospermopsis raciborskii* (Nostocales, Cyanophyceae) from northern Australia. *Applied Environmental Microbiology* 67(4), 1839–1845.

Salinger, M. J. (2005) Climate variability and change: Past, present and future—An overview. *Climatic Change* 70(1), 9–29.

Shaw, G. R., Seawright, A. A., Moore, M. R., and Lam, P. K. S. (2000) Cylindrospermopsin, a cyanobacterial alkaloid: Evaluation of its toxicologic activity. *Therapeutic Drug Monitoring* 22, 89–92.

Sinha, R., Pearson, L. A., Davis, T. W., Burford, M. A., Orr, P. T., and Neilan, B. A. (2012) Increased incidence of *Cylindrospermopsis raciborskii* in temperate zones: Is climate change responsible? *Water Research* 46, 1408–1419.

Solomon, S., Qin, D., Manning, M., Chen, Z., Marquis, M., Averyt, K. B., Tignor, M., and Miller, H. L. (eds.). (2007) *Climate Change 2007: The Physical Science Basis Contribution of Working Group I to the Fourth Assessment Report of the Intergovernmental Panel on Climate Change (IPCC)*. Cambridge University Press, Cambridge, U.K., p. 996.

Svrcek, C. and Smith, D. W. (2004) Cyanobacteria toxins and the current state of knowledge on water treatment options: A review. *Environmental Engineering and Science* 3(3), 155–185.

Ventura, F., Rossi, P. P., and Ardizzoni, E. (2002) Temperature and precipitation trends in Bologna (Italy) from 1952 to 1999. *Atmospheric Research* 61, 203–214.

von Sperling, E., da Silva Ferreira, A. C., and Ludolf Gomes, L. N. (2008) Comparative eutrophication development in two to nutrient concentrations and bacteria growth. *Desalination* 226, 169–174.

Watzin, M. C., Miller, E. B., Shambaugh, A. D., and Kreider, M. A. (2006) Application of the WHO alert level framework to cyanobacterial monitoring of Lake Champlain, Vermont. *Environmental Toxicology* 21(3), 278–288.

Wilhelm, S. W., Ouellette, A. J. A., and Rinta-Kanto, J. (2007) *Development of Molecular Reporters for Microcystis Activity and Toxicity*. American Water Works Association Research Foundation, Denver, CO.

Yan, Z., Jones, P., Davies, T., Moberg, A., Bergström, H., Camuffo, D., Cocheo, C., Maugeri, M., Demarée, G., and Verhoeve, T. (2002) Trends of extreme temperatures in Europe and China based on daily observations. *Climatic Change* 53(1), 355–392.

Zamyadi, A. (2011) The value of in vivo monitoring and chlorination for the control of toxic cyanobacteria in drinking water production (PhD dissertation). Department of Civil, Geological and Mining Engineering, École Polytechnique de Montréal, Montreal, Quebec, Canada.

Zamyadi, A., Dorner, S., Ndong, M., Ellis, D., Bolduc, A., Bastien, C., and Prévost, M. (2012a) Breakthrough and accumulation of toxic cyanobacteria in full scale clarification and filtration processes. *2012 American Water Works Association (AWWA) Water Quality Technology Conference (WQTC)*, Toronto, Ontario, Canada.

Zamyadi, A., Dorner, S., Sauvé, S., Ellis, D., Bolduc, A., Bastien, C., and Prévost, M. (2013) Species-dependence of cyanobacteria removal efficiency by different drinking water treatment processes. *Water Research* 47(8), 1080–1090.

Zamyadi, A., Ho, L., Newcombe, G., Bustamante, H., and Prévost, M. (2012b) Fate of toxic cyanobacterial cells and disinfection by-products formation after chlorination. *Water Research* 46(5), 1524–1535.

Zamyadi, A., Ho, L., Newcombe, G., Daly, R. I., Burch, M., Baker, P., and Prévost, M. (2010) Release and oxidation of cell-bound Saxitoxins during chlorination of *Anabaena circinalis* cells. *Environmental Science and Technology* 44(23), 9055–9061.

Zamyadi, A., MacLeod, S., Fan, Y., McQuaid, N., Dorner, S., Sauvé, S., and Prévost, M. (2012c) Toxic cyanobacterial breakthrough and accumulation in a drinking water plant: A monitoring and treatment challenge. *Water Research* 46(5), 1511–1523.

Zamyadi, A., McQuaid, N., Prévost, M., and Dorner, S. (2012d) Monitoring of potentially toxic cyanobacteria using an online multi-probe in drinking water sources. *Journal of Environmental Monitoring* 14, 579–588.

Zhao, S. (2012) Historical trends of cyanobacteria and their toxins in four eastern Canadian source waters (MSc dissertation). Department of Civil, Geological and Mining Engineering, École Polytechnique de Montréal, Montreal, Quebec, Canada.

Part II

Impact

6

Epidemiology of Marine Toxins

Juan Jesús Gestal Otero

CONTENTS

6.1 Introduction

Since ancient times, there have been references to the awareness of existing poisonings related to fish and shellfish consumption.

The first Egyptian plague ("all the water that was in the river turned to blood and the fish that were in the river died: and the river stank and the Egyptians could not drink of the water of the river; and there was blood throughout all the land of Egypt"[1]) could very well have been due to a toxic "red tide."

The ancient Chinese pharmacopoeia (2800 BC) warns against and makes recommendations on balloon fish consumption.[2] Nevertheless, we can assume that humankind knew of the red tide dangers before the written word, given the discovery of the 26-million-year-old fossil *Gonyaulax polyedra*. In 1880, Taharain[3] discovered the marine toxin closely associated with poisonings after the consumption of puffer fish, named tetrodotoxin (TTX). Since 1964, when tarichatoxin in the eggs of California newts, *Taricha torosa*, was identified as TTX,[4] it has been isolated from many marine animals.[5]

In several cultures and religions, we find prohibitions of the consumption of shellfish. The Old Testament (*Deuteronomy* 14: 9–10) says: *These ye shall eat of all that are in waters: all that have fins and scales shall ye eat: And whatsoever hath not fins and scales ye may not eat; it is unclean unto you.*

Even in pre-Colombian America, the hazards of eating shellfish extracted from the sea when it presented a red color during the day or a glow during the night were already known. To avert this danger, watchmen were placed in affected spots that would alert travelers of such hazards. According to Halstead,[6] it is the first known health quarantine in North America.

References to ciguatera-like illness, the widespread ichthyosarcotoxism,[7,8] which causes gastrointestinal, neurological, and cardiovascular disturbances, can be found in the *Chronicle of the Indies* by Peter Martyr of Anglería, in 1555, but possible even earlier references to ciguatera include the *Odyssey* by Homer (800 BC) and an outbreak in China in 600 BC. In the times of Alexander the Great (323–356 BC), soldiers were forbidden to eat fish to prevent the disease. More definitive reports occur in 1601 (Indian Ocean), in 1770 (South Pacific), in 1774 (New Caledonia) by Captain James Cook, and in 1792 in French Polynesia (FP).

The first scientific reference to human shellfish poisoning is probably the one in "Ephémérides des curieux de la nature" (1689), quoted in 1851 by Chevalier and Duchesne,[9,10] but Captain Vancouver realized the first written report of an outbreak in 1801, about an outbreak in British Columbia, which occurred in 1793.[11]

The term "ciguatera" is probably derived from *cigua*, a Spanish word borrowed from the Taino natives for a sea snail, *Cittarium pica*, a common edible turban or top-shaped speckled shell marine snail of the Caribbean, commonly consumed in the Caribbean, particularly in "cebiche," and which was associated earlier with this illness or with a similar illness produced by "red tide." This mollusk is sometimes called *siwa* in the English-speaking Caribbean. The word ciguatera was used in 1787 by biologist Antonio Parra in his description of intoxication with *C. pica*, and then by the Cuban naturalist Felipe Poey to describe similar cases.[12]

Our knowledge of ciguatera has progressed significantly since 1959 when Randall proposed that the toxin was introduced into the food chain by consuming herbivorous fish that consumed toxic microalgae and that, in turn, were consumed by larger predatory fish.[13] Remarkable advances include the identification and isolation of ciguatoxin (CTX) in 1967,[14] the discovery by Yasumoto et al.[15] from a species of the toxin-producing dinoflagellate, and the identification of the chemical structure of an important CTX and its precursor in the dinoflagellate *Gambierdiscus toxicus*.[16]

Since 1800s, we have the knowledge of the periodic red tides in the Gulf of Mexico and Florida east coast, known as "Florida red tides." During that time, the consumption of shellfish can lead to poisoning named neurotoxic shellfish poisoning (NSP), with symptoms digestive, neurological, and cardiac, and even the exposure to marine aerosols may cause a respiratory syndrome. The toxins responsible were isolated in the 1970s, and their structures were determined in the 1980s. The toxins are produced by the strains of the algal *Karenia brevis*, and they were named "brevetoxins" (PbTxs) for *Ptychodiscus brevis* toxins, because the algal *K. brevis* formerly was known as *Ptychodiscus brevis*.

In Europe, there are scientific descriptions of paralytic shellfish poisoning (PSP) outbreaks dating back to 1689.[6,7] It is worth pointing out the Wilhelmshaven case (1885) that sparked off the scientific solving of mussel poisoning, although the precise connection of the poisoning to mussels would not be established until 1927, when an outbreak took place in the central California coast, which resulted in 102 people being ill and 6 deaths. The ensuing studies led Sommer and Meyer[17,18] to the discovery that the cause was the dinoflagellate *A. catenella* and their toxins and to the beginning of in-depth studies. Halstead[6] compiled all the cases published worldwide up to 1965.

All these episodes refer to poisoning by paralyzing toxins. Awareness of the actual toxins that cause the diarrhea events is more recent. The first known diarrheic poisoning event associated to toxic mussel consumption (described all the time as "mussels that had ingested dinoflagellates") took place in the Easterscheldt area in the Netherlands in 1961.[19] That same year, there were other cases recorded in Waddensea. The next outbreak in Easterscheldt occurred in 1971 and affected 100 people. There are also references to the ingestion of blue mussels in Scandinavia (Norway) in 1968.[20] Next years, several cases were reported in the Oslofjord area. They were classified as "unidentified mussel poisoning."

In October 1976, in the Netherlands, 25 people were taken ill after eating mussels from Waddensea.[21] That year, Yasumoto et al.[22] described diarrheic shellfish poisoning (DSP) for the first time in a food poisoning outbreak due to the ingestion of mussels and scallops that took place in northeastern Japan. The same year, we[23] treated the first cases of PSP detected in Galicia (Spain), and in the summer of 1978, there were a series of diarrheic events in the Ría de Ares area. In the town of Lorbé (Oleiros, close to the city of A Coruña), we studied episodes related to mussel consumption. We ruled out microbiological causes and attributed those episodes to an unknown toxin caught by the mussels in their growing zone, as had happened with PSP in previous years.

In the following summers, we studied similar epidemiological outbreaks that, after an incubation period of a few hours, presented as diarrhea, nausea, vomiting, and abdominal pain, without fever. This was associated with the consumption of steamed mussels. Patients would recover in 1 or 3 days.

In 1981, the greatest diarrheic poisoning associated with mussel consumption occurred, affecting around 5000 people all over Spain, mostly in Madrid. Once again, the epidemiology analysis associated diarrhea with mussels. By then, Yasumoto's[24,25] works were already known. These poisoning cases by the DSP toxin in Galicia as well as in the rest of Spain run parallel to those that occurred in Japan in 1976 and 1977, and before and after in many other European, Asian, and American countries.

Yasumoto et al.[24] reported events in Japan and related them to eating mussels contaminated with the DSP toxin, pointing out that it was a lipophilic toxin referred to as DSP in later works.[25]

In Galicia, from the beginning of the 1980s, and particularly in the second half of this decade, a progressive increase in contaminations of phytoplankton origin in bivalve shellfish was observed. Since then, these toxic episodes have been regularly detected in seawater, and many of them were related to the presence of lipophilic class toxins, usually DSP toxins.[26–28]

In 1987, a new neurotoxic illness after the consumption of domoic acid (DA)–contaminated mussels harvested from cultivation beds on the eastern coast of Prince Edward Island, Canada, was described. It was named amnesic shellfish poisoning (ASP). This was the first and so far the only serious human outbreak of ASP occurred after consuming DA-contaminated mussels, which involved 150 reported cases, 19 hospitalizations, and 4 deaths.[29–31] DA was originally identified from the macro red algae, *Chondria armata*, in Southern Japan by Takemoto and Daigo, in 1958, following investigations on the antihelmintic and insecticidal activity of seaweed extracts.[32–35] After the 1987 outbreak of ASP in Canada, marine diatoms of the genus *Pseudo-nitzschia* were also shown to produce DA.[31]

In 1995, during an outbreak of diarrheal poisoning occurred in the Netherlands following the consumption of Irish mussels (*Mytilus edulis*), a new toxin group called azaspiracid (AZA) was identified.[36-39] The name aza-spir-acid comes from its chemical structure, a cyclic amine (or *aza* group), a unique tri-*spiro*-assembly and a carboxylic *acid* group.

In recent decades, there has been an increase in aquaculture activities, maritime traffic, and tourism, which favors the global spread of toxic dinoflagellates, increased algal blooms, and exposing as many people to mollusks and fish-contaminated in exotic countries.

The interests and research in these issues have increased, and new toxins are discovered. Some such as cyclic imines (spirolides, gymnodimines, pinnatoxins and pteriatoxins, procentrolides, and spiroprocentrimines), which although kill the mice, have not been associated with human poisonings.

In recent times, toxins produced by cyanobacterias ("blue-green algae") are being paid increasing interest. They can produce a myriad of toxic substances: microcystin (MCYST), cylindrospermopsin (CYN), and metabolites, and even saxitoxin, a related chemical paralytic shellfish toxin (PST).

Environmental and human health effects may occur after subacute or chronic exposure to toxins produced by freshwater cyanobacteria, through drinking or recreational use of water. There is much evidence that cyanobacterial toxins can accumulate through various trophic levels of the food webs. MCYST has accumulated in various fish and other vertebrates (such as waterfowl) as well as in freshwater invertebrates (gastropods and bivalve mollusks) and zooplankton.

6.2 Economical Relevance

The problem of toxic bivalve shellfish (mussels, clams, cockles, scallop, etc.) affects not only public health but also the tourist industry (exports, markets, advertising, and negative publicity), and it also represents a serious problem for the shellfish industry.

It has no easy solution, since the procedures used in the purification of plants are excellent for eliminating potential microbiological contamination, but have no effect on the biotoxin content.

The presence of toxic "red tides" means having to close down the shellfish fisheries in the affected areas and having to endure for long periods a situation of economic hazard for a great number of families that directly or indirectly depend on these fishing trades. Moreover, if control failures occur and there are cases of human poisoning, the discredit and mistrust created can lead to loss of markets that become hard to recover.

From the beginning of the 1980s, and particularly in the second half of the decade, a progressive increase in poisoning episodes of phytoplankton origin in bivalve shellfish was observed in Galicia. Mussel extraction was prohibited for up to 200 days/year in some areas.

Those economical aspects are studied in Chapter 8.

6.3 Limitations of Epidemiological Studies

The epidemiology of human disease caused by harmful marine phytoplankton is still at an early stage. This lack of progress in the phycotoxin disease epidemiology is attributed to a lack of clinical testing methods that has led to a large underestimation of the incidence of human poisonings due to algal toxins, especially since many of the symptoms are similar to viral and bacterial infections.

Epidemiology studies are limited to the more description of clinically identified cases and little else. More recently, the studies have included laboratory testing of ingested food.

The lack of biomarkers is a hindrance to the discovery of the real incidence, since it is possible to confirm clinical cases only in their acute stage and as long as there is some food remains available or their origin is known and a sample can be obtained. Asymptomatic cases and those where this possible cause is not considered go undiagnosed. In addition, only acute intoxications due to algal toxins are recognized, and there is very little knowledge of the human impacts due to chronic exposure to these toxins.

This is also made difficult because many people suffering from DSP do not seek medical treatment and doctors fail to diagnose it because of the many different causes of gastroenteritis. Study of DSP outbreaks depends on infrequent reports.

Biomarkers that measure exposure and effect may be qualitative and quantitative. In order to be useful, they should be detected early in human biological fluids accessible and acceptable. Ideally, biomarkers should also allow for the identification of subclinical cases. Other considerations to be borne in mind are the speed in testing, precocity in its application, and price.

In order to have the exposure markers available, it is necessary to develop the toxicological analysis of toxin levels and their metabolites in body fluids. At present, effect markers are based on the clinical picture. It is important to develop markers for subclinical physiological changes.

Studies aimed at establishing epidemiological associations between various factors and an intoxication can be carried out at two levels: The first comprises the study of the conditions that cause the explosive growth of dinoflagellates, resulting in the production of toxins and their concentration in shellfish. The second level studies the factors causing the specific toxic event in humans.

Knowing the environmental and feeding factors associated with the space distribution and occurrence of poisoning in shellfish allows us to establish risk zones of varying degrees, which together with knowing the seasonal events or cyclical phenomena will contribute to toxic episode prevention in humans.

The retrospective study of previous outbreaks and researching the possibility of future ones allow us to define risk groups and event-associated factors useful for monitoring and preventing toxic events.

6.4 Harmful Algal Blooms

Harmful algal blooms (HABs) or "red tides" are a natural occurrence in coastal countries that consist of the massive proliferation of unicellular organisms present in phytoplankton, which presents natural growing-and-decreasing cycles. Sometimes, and under favorable environmental conditions, some of these organisms (dinoflagellates) causing an explosive growth that gives the well-known coloring of water has given place to the name of "red tide," but the term "harmful algal blooms" is preferred.

Those cycles are regulated by the chemical and physical conditions of water, such as a mild temperature, a drop in the water salt content, still waters, light (long days), and concentrations of some organic and inorganic substances (nutrients), as well as biological interactions.

The bloom, as described by Mons et al.,[40] starts initially as a small population of cells in the lag phase or as cysts residing in the bottom sediment. Certain climatic and environmental conditions such as changes in salinity, increased water temperature, nutrients, and sunlight encourage germination of cysts, which on entering into a vegetative state reproduce rapidly. Bloom once triggered enters a phase of exponential growth of the population, which results in a huge increase in the same. The highest percentage of toxic cells is generally recorded in the middle of the exponential growth phase. As time passes, the blooms cause a marked decrease in nutrient and carbon dioxide content in the water and degrade environmental conditions, limiting the growth of the population. Entered, then, in a stationary phase, and water is stabilized becomes reddish fluorescent known as red tide. Environmental degradation continues and increases cell death until the population is destroyed. At this stage, many species of dinoflagellates form cysts of resistance that sink to the bottom, waiting for the next flowering.

These events can have negative environmental impacts including oxygen depletion of the water column and damage to the gills of fish. Moreover, when they are toxic species, they can cause mass mortalities of fish, birds, and marine mammals or the accumulation of toxins in the marine food web, leading to eventual human poisoning through the consumption of contaminated shellfish, coral reef fish, and finfish, or through water or aerosol exposure.[41] One of the most dramatic events involving sea mammals was the extensive mass mortalities to sea lions in California due to DA intoxication, where the main vector was anchovy (*Engraulis mordax*). Over 400 sea lions (*Zalophus californianus*) died, and many others displayed signs of neurological dysfunction during May and June 1998.[42]

Smayda estimated that only 60–80 species of about 4000 known phytoplankton are potentially toxin producing and capable of producing HABs.[43]

In recent years, one seems to have produced an increase in the worldwide occurrence of algal toxins in shellfish and several new toxin classes identified. This has resulted in adverse impacts on public health and the economy and has become a global concern.

Dinoflagellates reproduce themselves by simple or multiple partitions, and after an intense breeding activity, they encyst and settle for long periods in the bottom of the sea. The beginning and development of HABs, as well as their later disappearance, depends on the interaction of multiple biological, biochemical, hydrographical, and weather-related factors that are not yet fully known. In some regions, HABs are frequent and have become yearly events, whereas in others, they appear irregularly or occasionally.

Nevertheless, the reasons behind the apparent expansion of HABs and shellfish toxicity remain unclear. Numerous factors being implied included climate change, anthropogenic activities, eutrophication, changes in shellfish cultivation, increased global marine traffic, improved toxin detection, and better food control and toxin monitoring programs.[44]

The release of ballast waters has been shown to be responsible for transport to distant locations and invasions of exotic species, including algae, bacteria, and zooplankton. Algal cysts in ballast waters have been identified as the cause of new PSP events in the regions of Australia.[45,46]

Other recent evidence of an increased global expansion of HABs includes the first reports of palytoxin and TTX in European waters and the discovery of AZAs in Japan.[47]

In mid-July 2005, an outbreak with a total of 209 cases of respiratory illness (rhinorrhea, cough, fever, bronchoconstriction with mild breathing difficulties, wheezing, and, in a few cases, conjunctivitis) occurred in Genoa and La Spezia, in the northwest of Italy. For almost all these people, the symptoms stopped after a few hours, and only 20 people required hospitalization.[48,49] Affected people had spent time near or on the beach at the specific tracts of the coast near the cities of where the presence of *Ostreopsis ovata* algal blooms has been well documented, and a palytoxin analog was identified as the probable causative agent.[50] *Ostreopsis* spp. are widely distributed in tropical and subtropical areas, but recently, these dinoflagellates have also started to appear in the Mediterranean. In previous years, similar events were reported in other Italian regions, in Toscana (west coast of Italy), Puglia (southeast coast of Italy), and Sicily (in southern Italy), although these were less widespread and intense.[51,52]

Three years ago, Fernandez-Ortega et al. described the first European case of TTX intoxication in a patient who ingested part of a trumpet shellfish (*Charonia sauliae*) harvested from the Atlantic Ocean in Southern Europe. The mollusk was captured in the southern coast of Portugal during September 2007, that is, when the waters are warmest. The mollusk landed at the port of Huelva (south of Spain) from where it was transported in a refrigerated truck to the market of Malaga (Spain) to be sold.[53]

The appearance of HABs is due to two sets of factors: those that favor the growth of the microalgae population and those that favor their concentration.

6.4.1 Factors Influencing the Increase in Microalgae Population

- Changes in the water temperature influence the state of the dinoflagellates. Decreasing temperature induces its encystment, while increasing temperature induces its growth.[54]
- Sunlight: Essential for conditioning photosynthetic vegetative processes.
- Salinity: Its decrease, caused by freshwater flowing into the sea from rivers or by heavy rainfall, favors the presence of red tides.
- Water enriched with nutrients, organic substances: Coming from atmospheric deposition of nitrogen, from agricultural and urban sources, land drainage, or marine plants, fish, and other decomposing dead matter, can lead to increased algal blooms.[43,55]
- The increased aquaculture activities, resulting in increased nutrient that increases the eutrophication of the coast, which favors an increase in algal blooms.
- Metals and chelants: Metals decrease growth while chelants increase it.
- Substances promoting growth (vitamin B_{12}).
- Calm seas: Favor growth and the accumulation of phytoplankton.

6.4.2 Factors Influencing Concentration

Dinoflagellates gather in clusters due to hydrological concentration phenomena. These accumulation processes are influenced by mild winds that blow the surface waters toward the shore. Converging phenomena cause the concentration of dinoflagellates along the front line of two water masses of different densities. Convection movements due to the wind increase the concentration of dinoflagellates in converging lines.

When environmental conditions are not favorable, the haploid vegetative cells of very many dinoflagellate species form cysts that can resist very adverse conditions and remain viable in the sediment for long periods of over 15 years. This fact means that they can be carried viable from one zone to another where they can develop their mobile stage, going through an adverse medium in their journey.

The cyst germination is conditioned by internal factors and by external, or triggering, factors (temperature, light, and oxygenation). Dinoflagellates have maturing and latency periods. When cysts germinate and mobile cells emerge, their survival depends on their capacity to free themselves from the sediment and get into the water column (this is favored by turbulence, which is then harmful to the dinoflagellate population development that needs still waters to avoid dispersion) and the chance of finding a favorable medium in the water column. The relevance of the cyst population depends on their abundance in the sediment, capacity to germinate, and survival of the emerging mobile cells.

Bivalve shellfish filter water and retain the phytoplankton, which is not toxic to them. The degree of poisoning acquired by shellfish will depend on the toxicity per cell of the toxic phytoplankton organisms.

Toxins are secondary metabolites produced by toxic phytoplankton whose physiological and ecological functions are unknown. The amount and rate relative to toxins produced depends on intrinsic factors of the cells (genotype, age, size, cell cycle moment, and general physiological state).

6.5 Classification of Marine Toxins

There are around 60–80 toxic marine microalgae species throughout the world, with dinoflagellates accounting for 75% of all such species. Consumption of seafood contaminated by algal toxins results in various seafood poisoning syndromes: DSP, PSP, NSP, ASP, ciguatera fish poisoning (CFP), TTX and azaspiracid shellfish poisoning (AZP). Several new poisoning syndromes resulting from newly appearing dinoflagellate toxins, such as palytoxin, have been recently reported and characterized.

Different criteria can be used for classifying the marine toxins: characteristics and chemical structure, clinical syndromes, etc. In public health, we must use a classification to provide us with useful information for epidemiological research, which allows us a rapid clinical orientation of the problem and to take preventive measures. So, we classify the seafood poisoning according to the main transmission vector in shellfish poisoning (DSP, AZP, PSP, NSP, ASP, and YXT) and fish poisoning (TTX and CFP). The shellfish poisoning is categorized according to the clinical syndromes in diarrheic (DSP and AZP), neurotoxic (PSP, NSP, and ASP), and other (YXT) toxins.

Filter-feeding bivalve mollusks (mussels, clams, scallops, and oysters) are the most important vectors of shellfish toxins, but they are not the only vectors. Gastropods and crustaceans are also known to be responsible for human intoxication,[56] but its importance in the extension of transmission to humans is low because its consumption is rare. Herbivorous finfish that ingest toxic algae and fish such as puffer fish are also involved in the transmission of some toxins, but its importance is much lower.

In crustaceans, paralytic and amnesic toxins have been reported on several occasions,[57–61] and DSP toxins have been reported in Portuguese green crabs (*Carcinus maenas*)[62] and Norwegian brown crabs (*Cancer pagurus*)[63,64] in both cases causing human intoxications upon consumption.

6.6 Shellfish Poisonings

6.6.1 Diarrheic Toxins: Diarrheic Shellfish Poisoning

Three chemically different lipophilic groups of toxins have been historically associated with DSP: okadaic acid (OA) and dinophysistoxins (DTXs), pectenotoxins (PTXs), and yessotoxins (YTXs).

Diarrheic effects have only been proven for OA, DTX-1, and its C-7 acyl derivative (DTX-3), whereas YTXs only possess high toxicity by intraperitoneal injection in mice like PTXs 1–4 that cause liver necrosis when administered in the same way. Therefore, in 2002, the European Union (EU) has excluded the YTXs from the DSP group of toxins, and a separate regulation was established. The United States has no guidance for YTX.

OA and DTX: Toxins from the OA group have been known to cause the disease in humans since the late 1970s. The syndrome was named diarrheic shellfish poisoning due to the dominating symptoms.

The first DSP group toxin was isolated from mussel digestive glands and was called DTX-1.[65] Observation by spectral comparison showed that it was 35-*R*-methyl OA. Later, other OA derivatives were identified. OA had been isolated for the first time from the *Halichondria okadai* sponge in 1981[66]; later, it was also found in the *P. lima* and *Dinophysis* spp. dinoflagellates. The DTX-3 (7-*O*-acyl-35-(*R*)-methylokadaic acid) was identified in northeastern Japan during intoxication by scallops,[67] and the DTX-2 (31, demethyl-35-methylokadaic acid) was first identified in Irish mussels[68] and after that in Galician[69] and Portuguese[70] mussels.

Significant portions of the total toxin content found in bivalves consist of acylated forms of the toxins. This depends on the bivalve species, for instance, oysters accumulate most of the toxins DTXs, while in mussels, it might be about a half of the total. Since the acyl derivatives have been undetected only in the digestive gland of contaminated shellfish, it has been suggested that they are the product of the animal metabolism but not produced de novo by the microalgae.[71] Garcia et al.[72] describes for the first time a DSP intoxication episode due to consumption of mussels (*M. chilensis*) contaminated with 7-*O*-acyl-derivative dinophysistoxin-1 (named DTX-3) in San José de la Mariquina (Chilean Patagonia Fjords) in January 2004. This compound does not inhibit protein phosphatases and also does not elicit the symptoms described for DSP. The explanation for the diarrheic symptoms in the intoxicated patients would be the metabolic transformation of DTX-3 into DTX-1 in the stomach of the poisoned patients.

OA is the predominant toxin in most European countries, although DTX-2 has been reported in Ireland,[73] Spain,[70] and Portugal.

Pectenotoxins: PTXs are macrolactones that contain multiple polyether ring units and were first isolated from Japanese scallops (*Patinopecten yessoensis*).[74,75] Later, 15 homologous ones were described, PTX-2 and PTX-11 being the most toxic.

In experimental animals, they exert a strong hepatotoxic effect, but their diarrheic effect is mild and even undetectable,[76–78] and they are much less potent via the oral route. PTXs are not diarrheic in humans. It has been shown that PTX-1, PTX-2, PTX-6, and PTX-11 disrupt the filamentous actin (F-actin) cytoskeleton in NRK-52E cells, rabbit enterocytes, and neuroblastoma cells, and it is proposed that PTXs exert their toxicity by this mechanism.[79–83]

PTX-2, PTX-2sa, and 7-epi-pectenotoxin-2seco-acid (7-epi PTX2sa) are the predominant analogs in European shellfish.

There are no data indicating adverse effects in humans associated with PTXs in shellfish. PTXs exclusively arise from *Dinophysis* spp. and are always accompanied by toxins from the OA group. In 2009, the EFSA has suggested that the PTXs should be classified individually.[84]

Of all these toxins, only OA and its derivatives (DTX) cause acute gastrointestinal toxicity. The molecular mechanism responsible for the diarrhetic symptoms observed in both animals and humans after the ingestion of OA was originally proposed to involve hyperphosphorylation of proteins that control sodium secretion by intestinal cells.[85]

Apart from these acute effects, the OA group of toxins seems to have some important chronic effects. These toxins have been found to be potent tumor promoters.[86–88]

6.6.1.1 Clinical Features

Clinic begins between 30 min and 2 h after ingestion of contaminated seafood. The main symptoms in humans include diarrhea, nausea, and vomiting and abdominal pain. Symptoms are never fatal, the treatment is symptomatic, and there is a complete recovery within 3 days. The severity of symptoms varies depending on the amount of toxins ingested and generally requires no hospitalization.

The OA, the DTX-3, and DTX-1 toxins cause diarrhea in humans, but the PTX has a low diarrheic potential, but the intraperitoneal injection in rodents is toxic to the liver. It is unclear whether the PTX threaten the health of consumers of contaminated mussels.

6.6.1.2 Health Relevance

DSP is relevant from a health viewpoint not only because of its acute effects but also because of its potential chronic effects, which are not yet fully understood. Regarding chronic effects, OA and DTX-1 have been shown to be potent tumor promoters, and given that the stomach, small intestine, and colon have binding sites of OA, this could be implicated in the growth of gastrointestinal tumors.[89–93] Mutagenic[90] and immunotoxic effects due to a marked suppression of interleukin-1 production have also been described.[91]

It has been shown in experimental animals that PTX-1 is hepatotoxic and induces rapid necrosis of hepatocytes, with a pathological action similar to that of phalloidin. In rats intraperitoneally injected with PTXs, the liver finally appears granulated and the hepatocytes contain many vacuoles. All these chronic effects need to be studied in depth, and they underline the relevance and dimension of the problem and the need to avoid ingestion of this toxin.

6.6.1.3 Frequency and Distribution of DSP

The real incidence of human DSP is hard to assess, since its clinical symptoms can be mistaken for diarrhea from other causes, and it can go unrecorded owing to its benign evolution and many people suffering from DSP do not seek medical treatment. Isolated cases usually go undetected, and they only become known in countries where outbreaks have to be reported by law.

At present, the appearance of human poisoning cases is something that should not take place, and it only reflects a considerable failure in the watching and preventing process that should be operating and to which we will refer later.

Research on outbreaks in humans has only contributed to prevention, determining their origin, and the potential exposure of other groups of people to shellfish of the same origin. The main interest regarding prevention is the watching and early detection of toxic episodes in the sea that would allow the adoption of measures (forbidding shellfish extraction in the affected areas and informing people against its consumption). In countries where this watch network based on early detection is not possible, the watch on early detection of human intoxication can be useful in spotting the hazard and taking preventive measures that can avoid its spread.

6.6.1.4 Incidence

As pointed out before, the lack of biomarkers does not allow us to know the real incidence of DSP in humans, since our awareness of it is limited to notified outbreaks. In the last 30 years, the incidence of DSP events in humans has decreased and practically disappeared in developed countries where, as an answer to the problem, watch networks have been developed to detect the presence of toxic plankton species and poisoning in shellfish. This has not been the case in countries where such a watch network is not available. Nevertheless, poisoning episodes in the sea have increased, and this is partly due to a higher awareness of the disease and to setting watching schemes and also due to its spreading to new, and sometimes far apart, geographic zones, aided by international trade of seafood and the chance that cysts of exotic plankton species, producers of toxins, travel with them and settle in these new zones where they were previously unknown. Thus, the phytotoxic hazard becomes a public health problem worldwide.

Although shellfish poisoning is widely spread all over the world, affecting warm and tropical zones, Europe and Japan are the most affected areas. Some reports show that DSP events have also taken place in other parts of the world (Australia, New Zealand, Indonesia, and Argentina).[92,93]

6.6.1.4.1 Outbreaks in Europe

The first outbreaks were reported in the Easterscheldt area and the Waddensea[21] of Netherlands in 1961.[19] In 1976, another outbreak occurred in Waddensea affecting 25 people.

In Spain, the first cases were detected, as we said before, in 1978 in the Ares Estuary.[94] New events also took place in the following years, the main one occurring in 1981 with 5000 cases. Since then, DSP has been regularly detected in seawater.

In Germany, in September 1978, single cases of DSP intoxication were reported in the Husum area. In November 1986, at least eight people were affected. Since 1986, DSP has regularly been detected on the coast of German Bight, but no large outbreaks of DSP have been described.[95]

Various DSP outbreaks were reported in France during the 1980s, and they affected large numbers of people. In the Loire-Atlantique district and in Normandy, 3300 and 150 cases were detected, respectively, in 1983, and 70 and 2000, respectively, in 1984. Other DSP events were reported in 1985 (a few cases) and 1987 (2000 cases).[92] In 1990, there was an outbreak affecting 415 people due to mussels imported from the north Danish coast. It had a toxic OA load of 170 μg/100 g of meat.[96] Since the watch network was set in 1984, an increase has been observed in the toxic tides frequency as well as its spreading to other previously uncontaminated areas.

The first outbreak reported in Norway due to a *Dinophysis* spp. toxin[97] took place during a long contamination period (October 1984–April 1985), during which around 400 cases were detected among people living in the southwest coast of Norway. Coinciding with this outbreak, another one took place in October 1984, in the west coast of Sweden, where DSP events had already been taking place since 1983, affecting about 100 people.[98] In 1986–1987, a monitoring program for DSP toxins was established in Norway. In the summer of 2002, several hundred people were taken ill after eating self-harvested brown crabs (*C. pagurus*) in the southern part of Norway.[63,64]

In Portugal, since 1987, when they were spotted for the first time, DSP toxins have been detected regularly in bivalve shellfish from the northern coast including the Aveiro Estuary and the Mondego Estuary. In February 1994, an outbreak by *Donax* clams affected 18 people.[99] In the summer of 2001, another human DSP outbreak with five cases was confirmed. In 2002, an outbreak with 40 cases occurred in Northern Portugal,[100] and another outbreak in September with 32 cases after eating blue mussels, 4 cases after ingestion of razor clams (*Solen marginatus*), and 1 after ingestion of a large number of green crabs.

The first DSP event in Italy was in 1989, where affected cases were found on the north and northwest Adriatic coasts.

Since 1990, when the watch network was set up in Denmark, mussels contaminated with DSP have been detected during many summers.

In Ireland (1991–1994), since the watch program was set up, DSP has been detected in shellfish samples almost every year. The strictness and the duration of closure of shellfisheries vary according to years. The events are recorded in the summer and autumn months (June–December).

In the United Kingdom, outbreaks were reported in 1994, June (2 cases),[101] in 1997, March (49 cases),[102] and in 1997, June (55 cases)[103] all by mussels.

Since February–June 1997, an outbreak by mussels was confirmed in Croatia.[104] In 1998, several hundred cases by mussels were confirmed in Slovenia too.[105]

In January 2000, the first outbreak was detected in the Greater Thessaloniki area (Greece) affecting 120 people after eating mussels.[106]

In February 2002, an outbreak occurred in Antwerp (Belgium) with 403 cases of DSP, after consumption of boiled blue mussels imported from Denmark.[107]

In January and February, 2006, in Bizerte's Lagoon (Tunisia), DSP was detected for the first time, in cultivated mussels, in concentration superior to the limit established by EU, without human cases taking place.[108]

6.6.1.4.2 Outbreaks in Asia

The first episodes of DSP in Asia, due to the ingestion of toxic blue mussels and scallops, were those mentioned earlier. They took place in northeastern Japan in 1976 and 1977 and affected 164 people.[22,24]

New outbreaks were recorded later. Between 1976 and 1984, Kawabata reports that there were 34 outbreaks affecting 1257 people.[109] The Japanese and European shores are the most affected by toxic blooms.

On the coasts of China also, DSP's presence,[110–112] which took place between May 25 and 30, 2011, was detected. This was an important outbreak that affected more than 200 persons, after the consumption of mussels, in the cities of Ningbo and Ningde, near the coast of the East China Sea. In the mussels implicated in the poisoning event in Ningbo City, combined levels of free OA and DTX-1 were more than 25 times the EU limit.[113]

Toxic red tides have also been described in the Russian East coast (*Dinophysis acuminate, D. acuta, D. fortii*, and *D. norvergica*)[114] and the presence of DSP toxins in shellfish from India[115] although human cases have not been reported.

6.6.1.4.3 Outbreaks in America

Since 1970, outbreaks associated with DSP intoxications have occurred throughout Patagonian fjords in Chile, being kept since then its presence in the zone.[116–118]

The first reported DSP event in North America was in 1990 in Nova Scotia off the eastern coast of Canada and was due to DTX-1. It affected 16 people.[119] Other events were reported later in the same region.[120] In 1989, a red tide was detected on Long Island, New York (with a high number of *D. acuminata*). It was of low toxicity in shellfish (0.5 MU), and no human cases were reported.[121] Another outbreak by oysters was reported, in 1990, in the Gulf of Mexico.[122]

In January 1991, an outbreak affecting 120 people was detected in Chile. *D. acuta* was identified as the responsible toxin.[123] In January 1992, DSP toxins were also detected on the coast of Uruguay.[124]

The first human-documented episode of DSP occurred in Argentina was reported from the Gulfs San José and Nuevo, Patagonia, Argentina, in 2001. Another outbreak with approximately 40 cases occurred, in March 2002, in the Chubut Province, Argentina. Those affected had eaten blue mussels and clams with DSP from the North-Patagonian gulfs. This episode coincided with the presence of the *Prorocentrum lima*. In January 2010, the toxin-producing dinoflagellates *Dinophysis acuminata* and *D. caudata* (10^3 cells/L) were detected in wild clams *Mesodesma mactroides* and *Donax hanleyanus* from Mar Azul intertidal beach, during routine plankton monitoring in Buenos Aires Province coastal waters, Argentina.

6.6.1.4.4 Outbreaks in Oceania

Some reports show that DSP events have also taken place in other parts of the world (Australia, New Zealand, and Indonesia). In Australia, an outbreak of DSP associated with the consumption of pipis (*Plebidonax deltoides*) occurred in 1997, in which 102 people were affected.[125]

6.6.1.5 Epidemiology Chain

In order to systematize an epidemiological study oriented toward the prevention of DSP, we will follow the epidemiological chain pattern developed in 1931 by Stallybrass, the great scholar of epidemiology.

The dinoflagellates are the intoxication source of DSP, and the vectors are the bivalve shellfish with toxins—mainly mussels—although sometimes scallops are also involved. The subjects at risk are the people eating them, who usually live on the coast, have a low education, and are consumers of shellfish; moreover, they pick the shellfish themselves directly from the shore, thus bypassing any health control, which increases the risk.

6.6.1.5.1 Intoxication Source

Dinophysis dinoflagellates in 1989, and later *Prorocentrum* dinoflagellates and *Phalacroma rotundatum*[126,127] were identified as the organisms responsible for producing the DSP toxin.

In Western Europe, the predominant types are usually *Dinophysis* spp. (*D. acuta*, *D. acuminate*, *D. caudata*, *D. fortii*, *D. miles*, *D. norvegica*, *D. rapa*, and *D. sacculus*), while *Prorocentrum* (*P. lima*, *P. arenarium*, *P. hoffmannianum*, *P. maculosum*, *P. faustiae*, *P. levis*, and *P. belizeanum*) is more often found in Japan.[128–134]

D. acuminata and *D. acuta* species are the most widely spread in European waters.[135,136] *D. acuminata* is the main component in the greatest algal blooms on the northwestern shores in France. *D. acuta* affects the Atlantic coast of Galicia and Portugal,[137] the southwest coast of Ireland,[138] Sweden, and Norwegian fjords, and is the main agent of DSP outbreaks in Chile[137,139] and New Zealand.[140] On the European coasts, we also have *D. caudata* and *D. tripas* in the Iberian coast; *D. rotundata* in the whole coast and *D. sacculus* in the Mediterranean Sea, and the Iberian and French coast. In the Adriatic Sea (Italy), *D. fortii* has also been identified,[141] as have *D. norvergicus*[142] together with *D. acuminata*, *D. acuta*, and *P. micans* in Norway. Associated with toxic outbreaks, some other species have been detected: *Lingulodinium polyedra* in the Adriatic Sea and *Protoceratium reticulatum* in the Norwegian and the Adriatic Sea. The presence of these dinoflagellates, even in small concentrations (hundreds of cells per liter), can lead to poisoning of shellfish. Their ingestion causes poisoning in humans.

In the Galician Rías (Estuaries) of Spain, episodes of DSP appear associated mainly with a proliferation of *D. acuminata* in Ría de Ares and *D. acuminata* and *D. acuta* in Rías Bajas, although, at times, other species such as *D. caudata*, *D. tripos*, and *D. rotundata* can contribute significantly to the level of diarrheic toxins detected.

6.6.1.5.2 Vectors

Bivalve shellfish, mainly mussels and less frequently scallops, are the DSP toxin vectors. Also, there have been described cases by the consumption of scallops, razor clams (*Solen marginatus*), *Donax* clams (*D. trunculus*), green crabs (*C. maenas*), and brown crabs (*C. pagurus*) in Norway.

But the bivalve mollusks are not the only vectors for the transfer of marine phycotoxins; gasteropods (snails) and crustaceans (lobsters, horseshoe crabs, and green crabs) are also responsible for human illness and fatalities.[143]

All they acquire the toxin when there are some species of toxic dinoflagellates in the plankton to which they feed. Ninety-five percent of the toxin accumulates in the hepatopancreas of the mussel without it suffering any chemical changes, and apparently, the toxin does not alter the mussel's physiological functioning. The amount of toxin retained depends not only on the number of dinoflagellates present in the medium and its toxic load, but also on the amount of water filtered by the shellfish.

The highest levels of DSP toxins are found in blue mussels (*M. edulis*), lower levels in scallops, and very low levels in oysters.[144]

6.6.1.5.3 Vulnerability Factors

Personal features: People most at risk are those living in the seashore of countries with underdeveloped monitoring systems, with no watch network for sea toxicity events, and a low level of health education. Traditionally, they are consumers of shellfish, which they usually pick themselves from the sea without it undergoing any health control. There are no differences in sex and age.

Time distribution: Toxic episodes generally appear in summer and autumn months, although occasionally they appear in the earlier end of winter or early spring. In the Netherlands, in the years 1981, 1986, 1987, and 1989, events were recorded during September and October, and once even in December. In the Galician Estuaries (Spain), *D. acuminata* is present practically all year-round. It proliferates usually in April, although some years, this happens in late February or March, presenting maximum or minimum levels until mid- or late autumn. Usually, *D. acuta* appears associated with southern winds from September to November due to the advection from towns in the surrounding coastal area, and *D. caudata* is usually found isolated in the plankton.

Space distribution: DSP is widely spread around the world. Europe's western shores and Japan's shores are affected the most.

6.6.1.6 *Public Health Issues*

The implementation of programs monitoring for the presence of DSP-producing microalgae and the presence of DSP in shellfish can minimize public health risks.

In Europe, the Regulation EC 853/2004 of de European Parliament and of the Council, of April 2004, 29, establishes the maximum level admissible of lipophilic toxins.[145]

The Regulation EC 854/2004 of de European Parliament and of the Council, of April 2004, 29, establishes the official controls concerning live bivalve mollusks from classified production areas.[146]

Sampling plans to check for the presence of toxin-producing plankton in production and relaying waters and for biotoxins in live bivalve mollusks must take particular account of possible variations in the presence of plankton containing marine biotoxins. Sampling must comprise the following:

- Periodic sampling to detect changes in the composition of plankton-containing toxins and their geographic distribution. Results suggesting an accumulation of toxins in mollusk flesh must be followed by intensive sampling.

- Periodic toxicity tests using those mollusks from the affected area most susceptible to contamination.

The sampling frequency for toxin analysis in the mollusks is, as a general rule, to be weekly during the periods at which harvesting is allowed. This frequency may be reduced in specific areas or for specific types of mollusks, if a risk assessment on toxins or phytoplankton occurrence suggests a very low risk of toxic episodes. It is to be increased where such an assessment suggests that weekly sampling would not be sufficient. The risk assessment is to be periodically reviewed in order to assess the risk of toxins occurring in the live bivalve mollusks from these areas.

When knowledge of toxin accumulation rates is available for a group of species growing in the same area, a species with the highest rate may be used as an indicator species. This will allow the exploitation of all species in the group if toxin levels in the indicator species are below the regulatory limits. When toxin levels in the indicator species are above the regulatory limits, harvesting of the other species is only to be allowed if further analysis on the other species shows toxin levels below the limits.

With regard to the monitoring of plankton, the samples are to be representative of the water column and to provide information on the presence of toxic species as well as on population trends.

If any changes in toxic populations that may lead to toxin accumulation are detected, the sampling frequency of mollusks is to be increased or precautionary closures of the areas are to be established until results of toxin analysis are obtained.[146]

The Commission Regulation EC No. 2074/2005, of December 5, 2005, establishes the methods of analysis of the lipophilic toxins.[147]

Regulation EC 854/2004 of de European Parliament and of the Council, of April 29, 2004, establishes the official controls concerning live bivalve mollusks from classified production areas.[146] Commission Regulation (EC) No. 2074/2005[147] of December 5, 2005, Laying Down Implementing Measures for certain products under Regulation (EC) no. 853/2004 of the European Parliament and of the Council and for the organization of official controls under Regulation (EC) no. 854/2004 of the European Parliament and of the Council and Regulation (EC) no. 882/2004 of the European Parliament and of the Council, derogating from Regulation (EC) no. 852/2004 of the European Parliament and of the Council and amending Regulations (EC) no. 853/2004 and (EC) no. 854/2004, sets recognized testing methods for detecting marine biotoxins (PSP, ASP, and lipophilic toxins). Modified by Commission Regulations no. 1664/2006, no. 1244/2007, and no. 15/2011.

Commission Regulation (EU) no. 15/2011 of January 10, 2011, amending Regulation (EC) no. 2074/2005 as regards recognized testing methods for detecting marine biotoxins in live bivalve mollusks. The EU-RL liquid chromatography/mass spectrometry (LC–MS/MS) method shall be the reference method for the detection of lipophilic toxins (OA and DTXs, PTXS, YTX, and AZAs). It should be used routinely for official controls at all stages of the food chain and for self-monitoring by food business operators. Allows use of the mouse bioassay until December 31, 2014. From that date, the mouse bioassay is used only during periodic inspections of the production areas and resettlement areas to detect new or unknown marine toxins under national control programs developed by Member States. Other methods, such as LC–MS method, high-performance liquid chromatography (HPLC) with appropriate detection, immunoassays, and functional assays, such as the phosphatase inhibition assay, can be used as alternatives or supplementary to the EU-RL LC–MS/MS method under certain conditions.

If new analogs of public health significance are discovered, they should be included in the analysis. Standards must be available before chemical analysis is possible. Total toxicity shall be calculated using conversion factors based on the toxicity data available for each toxin. The performance characteristics of these methods shall be defined after validation following an internationally agreed protocol.[147]

With a view to eliminating discrepancies between the member states and harmonizing the European market, the European Commission named a reference national laboratory in each member country (LNRS) and a sole community reference laboratory (EU-RL), in order to set up and coordinate a network for exchanging information, knowledge, and experiences, and create a forum for method and toxicology agreements. The Exterior Health Laboratory in Vigo (Galicia, Spain), under the Ministry of Health and Consumption, was appointed Community Laboratory of Reference.[148]

6.6.2 Azaspiracids

The AZAs are a new group of toxins identified in 1995 during an outbreak in the Netherlands, when symptoms of DSP poisoning were observed, but with very low concentration of OA and DTX in shellfish.[36] Three years later, the toxin was isolated and named azaspiracid,[39] the first member of a novel group of marine biotoxins designated, and later structurally revised.[149]

6.6.2.1 Toxin

The AZA group includes the original algal toxins AZA-1 and -2, as well as mussel metabolites AZA-3 to -12, -17, -19, -21, and -23,[150] of which only AZA-1 and AZA-2 have been found in plankton samples,[151] while all other variants were detected in shellfish and are regarded as shellfish metabolites.[152]

6.6.2.2 Clinical Features

After an incubation period of 3–18 h, AZAs cause a clinical illness that is similar to that produced by DSP poisoning. There are no specific laboratory tests that are useful in the diagnosis of AZA poisoning. Diagnosis is based on characteristic symptoms, supported by testing of suspected seafood. There is no specific antidote, and the treatment is symptomatic and supportive only. Complete cure is achieved in 2–5 days.

In animal studies, when the AZA is administered per os, it caused the degeneration of epithelial cells and necrosis of the lamina propria in the villi of the small intestine and in lymphoid tissues such as thymus, spleen, and the Peyer's patches; fat accumulation in the liver and degeneration of hepatocytes; reduction of nongranulocytes; and damage to T- and B-cells in the spleen. Overall, AZA-1 induced a far greater degree of tissue injury and slower recovery time when compared with OA.[153,154] One study reported that AZA (tumor initiators) and DSP (tumor promoters) toxins in shellfish could cause intoxication concurrently.

6.6.2.3 Geographic Distribution

AZA poisoning has been reported in five countries, all of them in the EU and all from the consumption of mussels cultivated in Ireland. The first outbreak occurred in the Netherlands in November 1995 with eight people affected. The symptoms were similar to those of DSP, but the concentration of the major DSP toxins was very low. No known organisms producing DSP toxins were observed in water samples collected at that time. In addition, a slowly progressing paralysis was observed in the mouse assay using mussel extracts. These neurotoxic symptoms were quite different from typical DSP toxicity. Subsequently, AZA was identified, and the new toxic syndrome was called AZA shellfish poisoning.

The next outbreak occurred in Ireland, in September–October 1997, and was caused by the consumption of mussels from Arranmore Islands region on Donegal, Northwest Ireland,[155] and AZP persisted in this region for 7–8 months. Terry McMahon supplied details of the Arranmore AZA incident. About 20 individuals were affected in the outbreak, and a doctor examined 7–8 of these. Symptoms were vomiting, diarrhea, and nausea. There were no signs of any hepatotoxic effect, and no individuals subsequently presented with illnesses that could be related to the initial intoxication. Some patients reported illness following the consumption of as few as 10–12 mussels. All patients recovered completely after 2–5 days.[156,157]

Some episodes occurred later in Italy (10 cases) in September 1998, in France (about 20–30 cases) in September 1998, and in the United Kingdom (12–16 cases) in August 2000. In England, several incidents of AZA poisoning were reported in Sheffield, Warrington, Aylesbury, and the Isle of Wight. AZAs have been found in mussels (*M. edulis*) from Sognafjord, Southwest Norway,[158] and Craster in the northeast coast of England.

AZA-contaminated mussels have been found on the east coast of England and along the Norwegian west coast.[159] Reported AZA occurrences outside of northern European waters include the coast of Portugal[160] and northwest Morocco.[161] They have also been found in scallops (*P. maximum*) from Brittany, France,[162] and mussels (*M. galloprovincialis*) from Spain, Argentina,[163] Mexico,[164] Chile,[165] and recently Korea.[166] So far, shellfish from areas outside Europe have not caused yet cases of human intoxication due to AZP.[167]

6.6.2.4 Epidemiological Chain

6.6.2.4.1 Source of Intoxication

Considerable efforts were made to try to identify the biological source of AZAs, and in 2003, James et al.[151] reported *Protoperidinium crassipes* as the causative organism. However, subsequent studies indicate that the progenitor is *Azadinium spinosum*, a newly discovered dinophycae.[168]

Protoperidinium crassipes was not found to produce AZAs in culture. Furthermore, analysis of picked cells of *P. crassipes* in Norway showed no presence of AZAs.[169] As *P. crassipes* is a predator algae, it is possible that it might feed on AZA-producing phytoplankton, and to be a mere vector for the culprit species upon which it feeds.[170]

Now we know that AZA is produced by a small photosynthetic thecate dinoflagellate, subsequently named *Azadinium spinosum* (Elbrächter and Tillmann, strain 3D9),[168] which was isolated during an oceanographic survey in the North Sea, conducted by Tillman et al.[168,170,171]

6.6.2.4.2 Vectors

In all outbreaks, mussels (*M. edulis*) were the only shellfish responsible. Mussels were the shellfish with the highest toxin concentration: 4.2 µg/g. Only oysters accumulated toxins at levels (2.45 µg/g) comparable to mussels.[154] In other shellfish, the concentration detected was much lower: scallops (0.40 µg/g), cockles (0.20 µg/g), and clams (0.61 µg/g).

All reported cases were due to Irish shellfish before 2001, the year in which the EU adopted legal limits for AZA and the biotoxin monitoring program was improved. Since then, no case has been declared.

Although initially AZAs appeared only in mussels from Ireland, later they were detected in other bivalve mollusks, such as oysters (*Crassostrea gigas* and *Ostrea edulis*), scallops (*Pecten maximus*), clams (*Tapes philippinarum*), cockles (*Cardium edule*),[172] and razor clams (*Ensis siliqua*),[173,174] and in 2005 and 2006, they were for the first time detected in brown crabs (*C. pagurus*) from the west coast of Sweden and the north and northwest coast of Norway.[175]

Distribution of AZAs in mussel tissues has been studied with variable results. In one experiment, AZA-1–AZA-3 were distributed throughout tissues, with AZA-1 being predominant in the digestive glands and AZA-3 in the remaining tissues,[176] whereas in another study, AZAs were accumulated in the digestive glands only.[177]

Initially, mussel digestive glands contain most of the AZA; then AZAs migrate to other mussel tissues, leading to persistent contamination. AZA-1 is the predominant toxin in the digestive glands: AZA-3 is predominant in other tissues.

6.6.2.5 Seasonal Variation and Duration of Toxicity in Shellfish

AZA contamination of shellfish can occur in all seasons; however, it is likely to be prevalent in the summer months (mostly late summer). In one study, AZA-1–AZA-5 were found in mussels in November 1997.

A long duration of contamination has been reported with toxins remaining in the mussels for at least 6–8 months after the initial poisoning.[178,179]

6.6.2.6 Public Health Issues

EU legislation established that the maximum level of AZAs (AZA-1–AZA-3) in bivalve mollusks, echinoderms, tunicates, and marine gastropods is 160 g of AZA equivalents per kilogram (measured in the whole body or any part edible separately).[180]

However, the EU currently regulates only AZA-1–3.[181] The other analogs had initially been found at lower concentrations and were therefore not deemed to be significant, but little is known about these additional analogs, and to date, only 1–5 have been isolated and fully characterized.

6.6.3 Neurotoxic Toxins

6.6.3.1 Paralytic Shellfish Poisoning

PSP is an illness that may have serious and potentially fatal effects. It is caused by eating bivalve shellfish and other molluskan shellfish that have been contaminated by toxins produced by certain species of microscopic marine algae found in coastal waters. Lobster and crab tomalley (also called hepatopancreas, which is the soft green substance inside the body cavity) can also accumulate the toxins that cause PSP.

Saxitoxin and saxitoxin-related compounds (STXs) are responsible for the sometimes-fatal toxic seafood-related syndromes, PSP and saxitoxin puffer fish poisoning (SPFP).

6.6.3.1.1 Toxin

PSP toxins are collectively called saxitoxins (STXs). They are heat-stable and water-soluble nonproteinaceous toxins. Saxitoxin is the most toxic and also the best studied among the PSP-associated toxins. It is so named because it was originally isolated from the clam *Saxidomus giganteus*.[182]

STX and its 57 analogs can be structurally classified into several classes such as monosulfated, disulfated, decarbamoylated, and the recently discovered hydrophobic analogs each with varying levels of toxicity. Biotransformation of the PSTs into other PST analogs has been identified within marine invertebrates, humans, and bacteria.[183]

Saxitoxins are potent neurotoxins that are able to block the production of action potentials in neuronal cells. The guanidinium moiety of the saxitoxins binds onto a region of the sodium channel known as site 1 and blocks the opening of sodium channels.[184–186] The primary site of action of STXs in humans is the peripheral nervous system. The lethal dose in humans is 1–4 mg STX, or equivalent STXs, and levels up to 100 mg STX equivalents/g shellfish have been reported. However, hospitalization of affected individuals is critical to deal with respiratory paralysis, and STXs clear from the blood within 24 h leaving no organ damage or long-term effects.

6.6.3.1.2 Geographic Distribution

Blooms of dinoflagellates producing PSP occur in both Northern and Southern Hemispheres, most commonly along the cold water marine coasts in southern Chile,[187,188] Japan, Canada,[189–191] and the northern United States,[192,193] and PSP cases have been reported from as far south as Chile and as far north as Alaska.[194] Other cases have occurred in Australia,[195] Taiwan,[196] South Africa,[197] England,[198] Guatemala,[199] Costa Rica,[200] Singapore,[201,202] Spain,[23,203] México,[204] and other areas of the United States.[205,206]

6.6.3.1.3 Incidence

Since the first episodes described in the eighteenth century, many reports of PSP associated with human severe intoxication and death have become available worldwide. The first PSP event was reported in 1927 near San Francisco, CA, and was caused by a dinoflagellate, *A. catenella*, which resulted in 102 people being ill and 6 deaths.[18]

Gessner et al.,[207-209] in Alaska, performed the only two studies that allow us to know the incidence. The first was based on a retrospective review of surveillance data collected from 1973 to 1992 by the Alaska Division of Public Health. Based on overall population data from Alaska and 117 reported cases during this period, the estimated incidence was 1.2/100,000 persons per year.

The second study[210] attempted to identify more clearly the incidence among high-risk populations by using a randomized telephone survey between two coastal populations. This study found an incidence of 150 and 1,500/100,000 persons per year in Kodiak and Old Harbor, respectively, and 560 and 1,570/100,000 persons per year among persons who reported consuming shellfish collected from unregulated beaches. The incidence calculated from surveillance data from the Department of Health for the same period was 6 and 170/100,000 persons per year for Kodiak and Old Harbor, respectively. The large difference in estimated incidence between survey and surveillance data indicates that even in a state with a high awareness of PSP, surveillance data grossly underestimate true incidence.

Although STXs are detected in the coastal waters and shellfish in many European countries, human intoxications are rare. In the 1970s, there were several PSP intoxications involving 80–120 individuals, in Spain, France, Switzerland, and the United Kingdom by mussels produced in Spain, Portugal, and the United Kingdom,[210,211] but implementation of good regulatory control has effectively eliminated further major outbreaks.

In October 1976, we attended three consecutive outbreaks occurred in the north of the Arosa Estuary (in the towns of Puebla and Boiro, A Coruña, Galicia, Spain). Ten people were affected by the consumption of mussels. They were the first cases described in Spain. In addition, there were 63 cases in other Spanish provinces, 100 in France, and 31 in Switzerland, totaling 308 affected people. In the United Kingdom, the first reliably reported outbreak of PSP was on the East Coast in 1969. There were 70 human cases of illness and caused the death of numerous birds and other marine mammals in the region.[212-215] Throughout 1999–2009, the toxin PSP has maintained a low level in routine testing.

In the last 30 years, there have been outbreaks of PSP worldwide.[216] In Chile and Argentina, there have been repeated PSP outbreaks, with 21 PSP deaths reported in Chile since 1991.[217] The largest PSP outbreak occurred in 1987 in Guatemala, where 187 people were affected, of which 26 died. It has been estimated that there are 2000 human PSP intoxications per year.

In the Philippines, there have been an estimated 2000 cases of PSP between 1983 and 1998, with 115 deaths.[218] Blooms of *Pyrodinium* spp. were the main cause of these intoxications, and these blooms have spread throughout the tropical Pacific region. Climate change has been implicated with an apparent correlation between these HABs and the occurrence of El Niño Southern Oscillation events.[219]

PSP outbreaks have occurred on both the eastern and western coastlines on North America, with Alaska being particularly badly affected and toxic events have been reported for more than 130 years.[18,220]

In Alaska, PSP poisonings remain an important issue today. Since 1998, fewer than 10 cases have been reported annually. From 2005 to 2009, only two cases of PSP were reported to the Epidemiologic Service; however, mild cases may often go unreported. But an important outbreak with 21 cases was reported in May–June 2011 (8 confirmed cases and 13 probable cases). Most had eaten cockles and blue mussels and one by *littleneck clam* that they had collected on the beach.[221]

Active case finding during these investigations enabled epidemiologists to identify many people who did not seek care and would never have been reported. This suggests that the overall burden of PSP in Alaska is likely to be greatly underestimated through standard reporting. Because reporting prompts public health prevention efforts, we strongly encourage health-care providers and PSP patients to notify to Epidemiological Service immediately, even if symptoms are mild.

Large marine mammals have also been affected by PSP, and 14 humpback whales died in Cape Cod Bay in 1987 from exposure to STXs where mackerel was suspected to be the main vector.[40]

6.6.3.1.4 Epidemiology Chain

6.6.3.1.4.1 Source of Intoxication PSTs are produced in varying proportions by different dinoflagellate species and even by different isolates within a species. Dinoflagellates that produce STXs belong to three genera: *Alexandrium*, *Gymnodinium*, and *Pyrodinium*.

The species of dinoflagellates that have been reported to produce saxitoxins are *Alexandrium acatenella*, *A. andersonii*, *A. catenella*, *A. tamarense*, *A. fundyense*, *A. hiranoi*, *A. monilatum*, *A. minutum*, *A. lusitanicum*, *A. tamiyavanichii*, *A. taylori*, and *A. peruvianum*, as well as *Gymnodinium catenatum* and *Pyrodinium bahamense*.

Besides dinoflagellates, more recently, cyanobacteria have also been described to be able to produce PSP.[222] More precisely, species of the genera *Aphanizomenon flosaquae*,[223] *Anabaena circinalis*,[224] *Lyngbya wollei*,[225] *Planktothrix*,[226] and *Cylindrospermopsis raciborskii*,[227] and *Raphidiopsis* have been identified as potential producers.[228,229] In Europe, these toxins had been described in isolated strains from Italy and Germany,[230,231] in water samples from Denmark and Finland,[232,233] and in both water samples and isolated strains from Portugal[234] or France,[235] and Spain[236] in Tajo, Guadiana, and Guadalquivir rivers. In Mexico,[237] the presence of PSP and CYN was first detected in a freshwater system, Lago Catemaco, and apparent bioaccumulation of the toxins by tegogolo snails (*Pomacea patula catemacensis*), which is consumed both locally and commercially, and by finfish.[238]

STXs have been documented to occur when dinoflagellates were apparently absent.[239] Although still not definitively proven, a bacterial origin for STXs has been proposed, and bacteria may play a role in the production of STXs in certain dinoflagellate species.[240–243]

Summary:

> *In marine environments*: PSTs are primarily produced by the eukaryotic dinoflagellates, belonging to the genera *Alexandrium*, *Gymnodinium*, and *Pyrodinium*.[244–246] The toxins are passed through the marine food web via vector organisms, which accumulate the toxins by feeding on PST-producing dinoflagellates without apparent harm to themselves.[247] These include filter-feeding invertebrates such as shellfish, crustaceans, and mollusks and also other, nontraditional vectors such as gastropods and planktivorous fish.[248]
>
> *In freshwater environments*: The PSTs are produced by prokaryotic cyanobacteria belonging to the genera *Anabaena*, *Cylindrospermopsis*, *Aphanizomenon*, *Planktothrix*, *Lyngbya*, and *Rivularia*. Cyanobacterial PST-producing blooms result in the contamination of drinking and recreational water resources. In the past, high levels of toxins have been detected in the freshwater resources of many countries such as Australia, Brazil, United States, Mexico, Germany, and China.[249–254]

6.6.3.1.4.2 Vectors There are many reports that PSP can be transmitted, accumulated, and metabolized along the food chain, resulting in toxins accumulated in not only filter-feeding bivalves (butter clams, mussels, cockles, and geoducks) and herbivorous fishes, but also in organisms at higher trophic levels, such as aquatic crustaceans and even some marine mammals.[255] Because STXs are also produced by freshwater cyanobacteria, there is a potential for STXs to be transferred through the freshwater food web and pose a risk to human consumers of freshwater products (e.g., mollusks) contaminated by these toxins.[256] But to date, all documented human cases have been caused by toxic marine dinoflagellates (Figure 6.1).

Most human cases of PSP poisoning have consumed toxic bivalves, but occasionally, nontraditional vectors such as toxic gastropods and crustaceans,[257] and rarely toxic fish[143] are implicated.

In temperate zones, bivalve mollusk-associated seafood PSP cases are mainly in mussels and clams and, to a lesser extent, in oysters, scallops, and cockles. The highest toxicity level concentrations have been found in mussels *M. edulis* and *M. trossulus*, in softshell clams, *Washington butterclams*, and in the scallops *P. yessoensis* and *Placopecten magellanicus*. In other bivalves, such as northern quahogs and oysters, *Crassostrea* spp., STXs are at low levels or are absent.[258,259] Under similar conditions, the mussels accumulate PSP toxin more of the oysters.

The location of the toxin components in the various bivalve tissues and organs varies between species. Mussels concentrate 96% toxicity in the viscera that constitute 30% of total weight. In scallops,

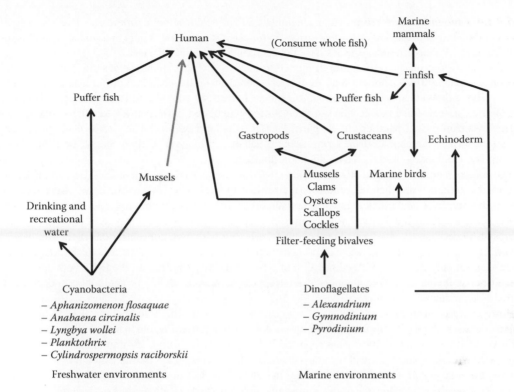

FIGURE 6.1 PSP transmission in food web. To date, all documented human cases of PSP have been caused by toxic marine dinoflagellates.

P. magellanicus and *P. yessoensis*, most of the toxins are concentrated in the digestive gland. Clams also initially accumulate in the viscera and later can be detected in siphon, and in other animal parts. This biphasic pattern is the best way to describe the kinetics of accumulation and elimination of toxins. Toxins accumulate in the viscera and reach a level two-to-five times higher than in the rest of the tissues. Less toxic tissues are tissues locomotive, foot, and adductor muscle. The removing viscera toxin occurs more rapidly than the rest of the tissues.

Bivalves retain STXs for different lengths of time and the toxic components retained vary. According to the kinetics of the elimination of toxins, the bivalves are classified[260] as moderate or fast eliminators (*M. edulis* and *Mya arenaria*); they can eliminate STXs in weeks,[261] and slow eliminators such as *Saxidomus giganteus*, *Washington butterclams*, Atlantic surfclams (*Spisula solidissima*), and the scallops (*P. magellanicus*, *P. yessoensis*) retain high levels of toxins for long periods of time (months to more than 5 years).[262–264]

6.6.3.1.4.3 Nontraditional Vectors for PSP Nonbivalve invertebrates have increasingly been documented to accumulate STXs[261] and have been implicated in PSP incidents. Among the mollusks, apart from traditional bivalve vectors, gastropods and rarely cephalopods (the octopus *Abdopus* sp.)[265] accumulate STXs apparently without any obvious ill effects.[266,267]

Molluskan gastropods including abalone, oysterdrills, volutes, whelks, periwinkles, moon snails, conch, slipper limpets, and turban shells accumulate STXs primarily acquired through predation (in many cases of toxic bivalves).[268] Because gastropods are able to bioaccumulate high concentrations of STXs, they are a significant risk to human consumers and have been the cause of multiple fatalities, particularly in the Far East.

STXs have been found in xanthid crabs and in other crab species,[269–272] crayfish, penaeid shrimp, barnacles, and lobsters.[247] In October 2000, an adult male, in East Timor, died within hours of ingesting a xanthid crab *Zosimus aeneus*.[273]

Other nonmolluskan invertebrates that accumulate STXs include annelid tubeworms *Eudistylia* sp.,[274] and echinoderm starfish *Asterias amurensis*, *Astropecten scoparius*, *A. polyacanthus*, and *Pisaster ochraceus*.[275,276] Thus far, these species have not been implicated in PSP cases.

STXs have been incidentally found in numerous species of fish (Atlantic mackerel, chub mackerel, short mackerel, *Sardinella*, southern puffer fish, checkered puffer fish, bandtail puffer fish, Pacific saury, Pacific cod, salmon shark, chum salmon, knobsnout parrotfish, starry toadfish, white-spotted puffer, map puffer, narrow-lined puffer, black-spotted puffer, reticulated puffer, starry toadfish, milk-spotted puffer, Amazon puffer, panther puffer, purple puffer, ocellated puffer, puffer, arrowhead puffer, and brown puffer), in Argentina, Brunei Darussalam, Sabah in Malaysia, United States, Iwate in Japan, Philippines, Bangladesh, Brazil, Thailand, and Cambodia.

The herring, cod, salmon, and other commercial fish species are very sensitive to toxins and die before PSP toxins in their flesh reach concentrations hazardous to human health, but since the toxins accumulate in the gut, liver, and other organs of the fish, other fish, marine mammals, and birds that eat the whole fish are endangered. In 1987, four humpback whales died in Cape Cod Bay in Massachusetts. The autopsy revealed that the whales had ingested mackerel PSP with high concentrations in their bodies.

For this reason, the fish, with the exception of puffer fish, are not usually vectors for STX(s) transfer if humans eat only the muscle. Accumulation of STXs is usually confined to the fish's gut, and certain species perish before detectable amounts of toxin appear in the muscle[277,278] or negligible concentrations of toxins accumulate in the muscle.

However, those who consume whole fish and eat the viscera are likely to become sick. In Southeast Asian countries like the Philippines, where it is customary to eat small whole fish, including the possibly toxic viscera, PSP incidents have been reported.[279,280] In 1976, in Brunei, 14 nonfatal PSP cases were associated with the consumption of the planktivorous fish *Rastrelliger* sp. during a bloom of *Pyrodinium bahamense* var. *compressum*.[281] In Indonesia, in 1983, there has been an outbreak of PSP with 191 cases and 4 deaths in humans due to the consumption of planktivorous clupeoid fish *Sardinella* spp. and *Selaroides leptolepis*. In a second incident in November 1983, 45 people became ill after consuming fish.

The transport of STXs through the food web and the vectoring and accumulation of toxins through zooplankton have been identified as important mechanisms by which toxins become available to higher trophic levels such as fish.[282–287]

6.6.3.1.5 Saxitoxin Puffer Fish Poisoning

The fish of the family Tetraodontidae (puffer fish) inhabiting marine and freshwater habitats accumulate STX in muscle in amounts capable to produce human poisoning. Kodama et al.[288] first described STX as a minor component of highly toxic (with TTX) *Takifugu pardalis* livers in Japan. Soon after, Nakamura et al.[289] confirmed the STX as a minor component in the additional Japanese species *T. poecilonotus* and *T. vermicularis*, and Nakashima et al.[290] as a major toxin in *Arothron firmamentum*. STXs were found to be the sole toxic component in a range of freshwater puffer fish, some responsible for human poisoning events, in Thailand, Bangladesh, Brazil, and Cambodia. Seven species of marine puffer fish in the Philippines were found to contain both STXs and TTX, with STXs being the dominant toxin in several species.[291]

In 2002, other cases have been described in Florida, Virginia, and New Jersey (in the United States) after consuming puffer fish *S. nephelus* originating from the northern Indian River Lagoon (IRL) on Florida's central east coast.[292]

Uneaten fish muscle samples from the New Jersey incident, surprisingly, found to contain no detectable TTX but to contain significant amounts of STX, with lesser amounts of the STX congeners B1 and dcSTX.[293] This same combination of toxins was too confirmed in meal remnants from two separate poisoning events in 2004.[294] In total, 28 cases of SPFP were reported from 2002 to 2004 all due to fish originating from the northern IRL.[295] These were the first reports of STXs both in Florida marine waters and in indigenous puffer fish in the United States.

6.6.3.1.6 Temporal Distribution

The dinoflagellates are developed at relatively high temperatures and strong sunlight, so in Europe and South Africa, cases of poisoning and death usually occur between May and November, while in North America occurring between July and September.

A study of 20 years of surveillance data in Alaska found that while the majority of cases occurred during late spring and early summer, cases occurred during all seasons of the year and during every month except November and December.[220] Similarly, a large series in eastern Canada reported outbreaks between March and November with the great majority occurring between June and September. Outbreaks in Costa Rica and México, by contrast, have occurred during October and December.

6.6.3.1.7 Importance

The threat of PSP is not only a major cause of concern for public health but is also detrimental to the economy. Outbreaks of PSTs often result in the death of marine life and livestock, the closure of contaminated fisheries, while the continual expenditure required for the maintenance and running of monitoring programs, all combine to present a major economic burden around the world.[296,297]

6.6.3.1.8 Clinical Features

The incubation period for PSP ranges from minutes to hours. On the outbreak we have studied, the incubation period varied from 0.5 to 6 h.

The symptoms of PSP include a tickling sensation of the lips, mouth, and tongue, numbness of the extremities, gastrointestinal problems, difficulty in breathing, and a sense of dissociation followed by complete paralysis. In milder cases, symptoms are tingling and numbness of lips, mouth, and tongue; unsteadiness; weakness; feeling of floating in the air; and polyuria with clear urine; adynamia in arms and legs; salivation; sweating; changes in the pronunciation of words; and dysphagia. Depending on the degree of involvement, the full restoration ranged from 1 to 3 days, with fatigue during convalescence. More severe cases may involve dyspnea, muscle weakness or frank paralysis, ataxia and respiratory insufficiency, and the very serious intoxication cases may involve respiratory arrest and cardiovascular shock or death.[188]

6.6.3.1.9 Treatment

Currently, there is no antidote for PSP. Symptomatic treatment, including respiratory support and fluid therapy, is the only treatment available. Although recovery is usually complete with symptom resolution within hours to days after onset, fatal cases have been documented.

6.6.3.1.10 Public Health Issues

The implementation of programs monitoring for the presence of both STX-producing microalgae and the presence of STXs in shellfish can minimize public health risks (see later in this chapter).

Commission Regulation (EC) no. 1664/2006 of November 6, 2006, amending Regulation (EC) no. 2074/2005 as regards Paralytic Shellfish Poison (PSP) detection method sets that the PSP content of edible parts of mollusks (the whole body or any part edible separately) must be detected in accordance with the biological testing method or any other internationally recognized method. The so-called Lawrence method may also be used as an alternative method for the detection of those toxins as published in AOAC Official Method 2005.06 (Paralytic Shellfish Poisoning Toxins in Shellfish). If the results are challenged, the reference method shall be the biological method. This will be reviewed in light of the successful completion of the harmonization of the implementing steps of the Lawrence method by the Community Reference Laboratory for marine biotoxins.

6.6.3.2 Amnesic Shellfish Poisoning

The ASP is a neurotoxic illness caused by the consumption of shellfish that have accumulated DA. The first and so far only serious human outbreak of ASP occurred after consuming DA-contaminated mussels harvested from cultivation beds on the eastern coast of Prince Edward Island, Canada, in 1987 involved 150 reported cases, 19 hospitalizations, and 4 deaths after the consumption of contaminated mussels.[29–31]

DA was originally identified from the macro red algae, *C. armata*, in Southern Japan by Takemoto and Daigo, in 1958, following investigations on the antihelmintic and insecticidal activity of seaweed extracts.[32–35] After 1987 outbreak of ASP in Canada, marine diatoms of the genus *Pseudo-nitzschia* were also shown to produce DA.

Symptoms ranged from gastrointestinal disturbances, to neurotoxic effects such as confusion, disorientation, seizures, and permanent short-term memory loss and in the most severe cases death. The neurotoxic properties of DA result in neuronal degeneration and necrosis in specific regions of the hippocampus.

6.6.3.2.1 Toxin

The chemical, which causes ASP, was subsequently identified as DA, an amino acid produced by some species of phytoplankton. DA can be bioconcentrated by shellfish and, thus, can then enter the human food chain.

DA's 10 isomers (isodomoic acids A–H and DA 5′ diastereomer) have been identified in marine samples.[298–300]

DA is produced by a number of marine organisms.[301] The isodomoic acids are minor constituents relative to DA and are not always present in shellfish contaminated with ASP. They are water soluble and do not degrade under ambient temperatures or when exposed to light in sterile saline solution,[302] but it has been shown to decompose under acidic conditions (50% DA loss in 1 week at pH 3).[303]

DA can be converted to isodomoic acids when exposed to ultraviolet light or heat.[304] Therefore, it has been suggested that DA may be the product of biosynthesis, which is subsequently converted to isodomoic acids under appropriate environmental conditions.

6.6.3.2.2 Incidence

Following the outbreak of ASP, Canada's many regulatory agencies worldwide have established biotoxin monitoring programs. After that, no new human ASP episode has been documented. Of course, it is possible that an ASP event may go unidentified particularly in underdeveloped nations and along vast stretches of coastline where monitoring coverage is sporadic or nonexistent.[305]

However, toxic blooms of DA-producing diatoms are a global issue and appear to be increasing in frequency and toxicity, thereby presenting a continued threat to human health and seafood safety.

Soon after the establishment of monitoring programs in Europe, DA was found in shellfish from Galicia, Spain,[306] Ireland,[307] Portugal,[308] Scotland,[309] and France.[310]

In Ireland, only the king scallop (*P. maximus*) exhibited high levels of toxin. Although a record high level of DA (2820 mg DA/g) was found in the digestive glands of scallops, the adductor muscle and gonad contained levels below or just over the regulatory limit of 20 mg DA/g.[311] It would therefore be a prudent and simple food safety measure to recommend the nonconsumption of the digestive glands of these shellfish to reduce the risk of exposure of humans to ASP. DA has also been found in shellfish from New Zealand, Australia, and Chile, but there have been no major toxic incidents involving humans. Further information regarding ASP and DA can be found in a recent review.[312]

6.6.3.2.3 Epidemiology Chain

6.6.3.2.3.1 Source of Toxin   *Pseudo-nitzschia* spp. is widely distributed across the world in seawaters of both warm and cold climates. Most strains of *Pseudo-nitzschia* are reported to produce DA, but only a few are implicated in the contamination of shellfish and DA poisoning. These include *P. multiseries*, *P. pseudodelicassima*, and *P. australis*.[313]

DA production varies greatly with strain. It is thought to be increased in response to environmental stresses, such as temperature change.[314] Although warmer sea temperatures (14°C–17°C) tend to be associated with increased DA production,[315] some strains have adapted to growth in cooler waters, for example, *P. seriata* produces high concentrations of DA at 4°C.[316]

6.6.3.2.3.2 Vectors   The greatest risk of DA exposure for humans and marine wildlife comes from the dietary consumption of DA-contaminated filter-feeding marine organisms such as shellfish and finfish.[317]

DA has been shown to accumulate in a wide variety of shellfish species such as types of cockles (*Cerastoderma edule*), mussels (*M. edulis*), razor clams (*Siliqua patula*), dungeness crabs and scallops (*P. maximus*), peppery furrow shell (*Scrobicularia plana*), crabs (*C. magister*), and finfish planktivorous anchovies (*E. mordax*) and mackerel (*Scomber japonicus*). DA was also found in benthic crustaceans, but the sources and the transmission ways to these crustaceans remain unknown.

Furthermore, no study has been carried out so far to determine how the accumulated toxin could affect subsequent consumers.[318,320]

Shellfish accumulate DA either by direct filtration of the plankton or by feeding directly on contaminated organisms, and thus, concentration is highest in the digestive glands compared with other tissues. But there are wide variations in tissue distribution and accumulation rate in commercially important species of shellfish. DA is found throughout all tissues in the razor clam, whereas a majority of the toxin is confined in the viscera in mussels and fish. Arevalo et al.[321] have been studied the anatomical distribution of DA in scallop (*P. maximus*). In one study, they analyzed only hepatopancreas, muscles, and gonads. In the second, they analyzed combined hepatopancreas, muscles, and gonads and other soft tissues. In the first study, 98.8% of the overall DA content (hepatopancreas, gonads, and muscles) was located in the hepatopancreas, and in the second (which included total tissue), 79.3% of the total DA content was located in the hepatopancreas; negligible amounts were found in the gonads and muscles and about 14.5% in the remaining soft tissues.

There are also marked differences in the rate of depuration of DA between shellfish species. Thus, while that 50% of the DA content was eliminated from blue mussels (*M. edulis*) within 24 h,[322] it took 86 days for a comparable proportion of DA to be eliminated from razor clams (*S. patula*).[323] Scallops and razor clams have been shown to have slower depuration rates compared to mussels.[324–326] In fact, razor clams have been shown to retain DA for up to a year. DA is also known to accumulate in fish such as anchovies and mackerel,[327] but the levels are much lower compared with those found in shellfish.

Studies on the effects of frozen storage and cooking on DA concentrations in shellfish are limited, but they suggest that these processes reduced the overall levels of DA.[328,329]

The removal rate is highly dependent on where the toxin is stored in the animal, for example, gastrointestinal toxins are removed more easily than toxins bound to tissues. In the mussel (*M. edulis*) and oysters (*Crassostrea virginica*), the bulk of the DA resides in the intestines. It has been shown that the mussels purified DA quite fast.

Razor clam (*S. patula*) debugging is not very fast. In these, they found higher levels of DA concentrated in the edible muscle tissue and other minor parts of edibles tissues. In anchovies, DA was found in the viscera and muscle of fish. DA was detected only in the viscera of dungeness crabs (*C. magister*). There are little data on retention times of toxins in crabs and carnivorous gastropods; the general trend in these organisms suggests prolonged retention.

Stewart et al.[332] noted a high possibility that indigenous bacteria could be a significant factor in eliminating DA shellfish species that readily purified. This was demonstrated with mussels *M. edulis* and clams *Mya arenaria*. Stewart et al.[332] suggested various mechanisms used by different seafood with DA, readily available in some types of mussels and clams, but probably retained in the digestive glands of either red scallops or mussels and consequently largely unavailable for bacterial use.

Mammals and birds affectation: DA detected in planktivorous anchovies in California caused the deaths of many brown pelicans, cormorants, and sea lions,[331] indicating that finfish, shellfish, and cephalopods can vector this toxin.[332,333]

In September 1991, an unexplained pelican (*Pelecanus occidentalis*) and cormorant (*Phalacrocorax penicillatus*) death in Monterey Bay, California, was attributed to a DA poisoning outbreak caused by *P. australis*, a diatom of the same family, ingested by anchovies and in turn ingested by these birds.

The DA also appeared in the west coast of the United States causing the death of pelicans and cormorants, after feeding with DA-contaminated anchovies (*E. mordax*). In that area, the diatom *P. australis* appeared to be the source organism. In the viscera of anchovies, 485 µg/g DA was found.

Anchovies are mainly carnivorous, but in the absence of other sources of energy they consume phytoplankton. McGinness et al.[334] showed that the stomachs of northern anchovy (*E. mordax*) in Monterey Bay, California (August 1992), contained nine different species of *Pseudo-nitzschia*, including four producing DA under both natural and laboratory conditions. The study showed the northern anchovies' ability to filter pennate diatoms from the near-surface seawater.

In January 1996, death claimed brown pelicans (*P. occidentalis*) in Cabo San Lucas at the tip of the peninsula of Baja California (Mexico) to the feeding of mackerel (*Scomber japonicus*) contaminated with *Pseudo-nitzschia* spp. DA producer.[335]

An event that generated worldwide publicity was when 70 sea lions were washed up onto beaches in California.[327] It was evident that they were suffering from neurological problems including seizures, and 47 animals died. DA was identified in fecal samples from these animals and in anchovies collected nearby.[42] DA was transmitted to the sea lions via planktivorous anchovies, *E. mordax*. The highest concentrations of DA in anchovies occurred in the viscera (223 µg/g), which exceeded the values in the body tissues by sevenfold. The pelicans, cormorants, loons, grebes, sea otters, and dolphins, which consumed sea foods contaminated with DA, suffered disorientation and often death.[336] More than 400 California sea lions (*Z. californianus*) died along the central California coast in May and June 1998.

James et al.[44] performed an interesting description of the poisoning of Monterey Bay, relating the strange behavior of cormorants and pelicans in the poisoning of Monterey Bay (vomiting, unusual head movements, and scratching, with many deaths)[337] with the event that happened in the summer of 1961, near Santa Cruz in California. Flocks of shearwaters began acting erratically, flying into houses and cars, pecking people, breaking windows, and vomiting. These "strange" events were reported in the local newspapers, and these clippings were included with Alfred Hitchcock's studio proposal to make the film *The Birds* based on Daphne du Maurier's novella.

In subsequent years, several similar incidents of DA contamination of seafood and mortalities to marine animals and bird occurred along the same coastline, which have been attributed to DA produced by blooms of *Pseudo-nitzschia* spp.[338]

6.6.3.2.3.3 Risk Factors Age

Among ill persons, males and the elderly had an increased risk of memory loss and hospitalization. Perl et al.[31] has suggested that the association with age was due to increased renal disease in the elderly and thus that DA is excreted through the kidneys. By contrast, Auer has suggested that increased susceptibility with age is related to the dendritic location of excitatory receptors and the increased branching of neuronal dendritic trees among the elderly.[339]

Ethnic group: Some ethnic groups may have an increased risk of toxin exposure because of different patterns of seafood consumption, for example, the practice of eating the viscera of crabs among persons of Chinese descent in Washington State.[340] Specific parts of different species may concentrate toxin, for example, the viscera of dungeness crabs or the foot of razor clams.[341] Selective consumption of these parts may increase the risk of illness.

Cooking: In the Canadian outbreak, cooking was not protective; another study, however, suggests that boiling dungeness crabs significantly reduces the visceral toxin level.

6.6.3.2.4 Geographic Distribution

DA-producing diatoms have been isolated on the east and west coasts of the United States and Canada, Europe, Australia, New Zealand, Korea, Japan, and Vietnam, and therefore, monitoring programs are becoming increasingly more common in these areas.

6.6.3.2.5 Seasonal Variations

There are seasonal variations in phytoplankton blooms with numbers increasing in spring and autumn when there is heavy rainfall and a rich nutrient availability. Light and certain temperature range are essential for the synthesis of DA. Its maximum production occurs during the stationary phase of algal growth and stimulated by the presence of extracellular bacteria.[342]

6.6.3.2.6 Clinical Features

Almost all of the information regarding clinical features derives from the Canada outbreak. The incubation period varied from 15 min to 38 h (mean, 5.5 h) after mussels' ingestion. Acute illness characterized by gastrointestinal and unusual neurological symptoms was reported in the people affected. Approximately 150 reports of this illness were received, although only 107 individuals fulfilled the clinical definition of the illness, and of these, the most common gastrointestinal symptoms were vomiting (76%), abdominal cramps (50%), and diarrhea (42%), and the most common neurological symptoms were severe headache (43%) and loss of short-term memory (25%). The illness was particularly severe in 19 individuals who were hospitalized, and 12 individuals with particularly severe symptoms (e.g., seizures, coma, profuse respiratory secretions, or unstable blood pressure) required treatment in an intensive care unit. Three patients died in hospital 11–24 days after the consumption of mussels.

The mussels that had been ingested had been contaminated with DA from a bloom of the phytoplankton *Pseudonitzschia f. multiseries* in the Port Edward Island region, where the mussels had originated.[286]

Concentrations of DA in mussels collected from the implicated region after the outbreak ranged from 1.9 to 5.2 mg/g tissue. DA was not detected in the samples of blood or cerebrospinal fluid of 17 patients that were tested. However, there was an interval of at least 2 days between the ingestion of the mussels and this analysis, which may have been long enough for DA to be excreted from the body.

6.6.3.2.7 Chronic Exposure to Low Levels of Toxin

Current monitoring programs appear to be effective at preventing acute DA poisoning in humans, but there may be impacts due to repetitive long-term low-level exposure that have yet to be identified.

In sea lions, a chronic DA toxic syndrome,[343] which is distinguishable from acute toxicosis, has been characterized. The identification of a second form of chronic toxicity reveals the potential for additional manifestations of DA-related disease in other mammalian species.

Currently, sea lions are being used as a sentinel species for predicting potential human health threats associated with deteriorating ocean conditions at the West Coast Center for Oceans and Human Health at the Northwest Fisheries Science Center in Seattle, Washington.

6.6.3.2.8 Public Health Issues

It is based on the routine monitoring of phytoplankton that can provide early warning of an adequate bloom, but it alone does not provide sufficient protection to the public health risks of ASP. Therefore, sampling of indicator species such as mussels should be complemented by phytoplankton surveys, using a variety of analytical methods to determine the accumulated levels of DA in a particular part of the coast. Undoubtedly, the rapid reliable detection of DA and estimation of the cumulative toxicity of DA isomers as well as validation of these methods for use on a global scale are of great importance.

Mussels have relatively rapid uptake and depuration rates for DA, and so it is fairly straightforward for monitoring programs to protect seafood consumers from DA contamination in this species. Anchovies and sand crabs also appear to depurate DA rapidly in synchrony with toxic *Pseudo-nitzschia* blooms with DA levels dropping to undetectable levels within a week of bloom termination.[59,344]

DA limits: After the 1987 ASP outbreak, the Canadian authorities imposed an action limit for DA in mussels of 20 mg DA/g mussel flesh, which when exceeded would result in closure of shellfish-harvesting areas. This action limit was derived from a retrospective estimation of the level of DA in mussels, which had caused illness in some consumers during the ASP outbreak (200 mg DA/g of mussel flesh) and incorporation a 10-fold safety factor.[345]

The action limit employed by Canada has been adopted elsewhere and is the limit enforced in the EU, the United States, New Zealand, and Australia for DA in a variety of shellfish species.

Commission Regulation (EC) no. 1244/2007 of October 24, 2007, amending Regulation (EC) no. 2074/2005 with respect to Amnesic Shellfish Poison (ASP) detection method sets that the total content of ASP of edible parts of mollusks (the entire body or any part edible separately) must be detected using the HPLC method or any other internationally recognized method. However, for screening purposes, the 2006.02 ASP ELISA method as published in the *AOAC Journal* of June 2006 may also be used to detect the total content of ASP of edible parts of mollusks. If the results are challenged, the reference method shall be the HPLC method.

6.6.3.3 Neurotoxic Shellfish Poisoning

NSP is a disease caused by the consumption of molluskan shellfish contaminated with toxins known as the brevetoxins (PbTxs). These toxins are secreted by algal blooms and accumulate in the bodies of shellfish. This illness is associated with exposure to PbTxs known as "Florida red tide." Exposure to the toxin can be by eating contaminated seafood or by the inhalation of aerosolized toxin.

Nowadays, NSP is a relatively rare disease due to the stringent monitoring and timely closure of toxin-contaminated shellfish beds in the Gulf of Mexico. However, it has been noted that this illness is likely to be misdiagnosed and is probably more common than previously thought, particularly among visitors and subpopulations not informed of shellfish bed closures or shellfish-harvesting bans.[346]

Clinically, it is characterized by an acute gastroenteritis with neurological symptoms following the consumption of shellfish contaminated with NSP or an apparently reversible upper respiratory syndrome after inhalation of aerosols and the dinoflagellate and their toxins.

It can be a severe acute disease with the requirement of emergency room and intensive care during the first hours or, in the most severe cases, days to prevent respiratory failure. Even with a severe acute illness, victims are usually discharged from the hospital within days; there is almost nothing known about the subchronic or chronic sequelae of an acute NSP episode.

The toxins are called brevetoxins (PbTxs). They were isolated in the 1970s,[347–349] and their structures were determined in the 1980s.[350,351] They are produced by the strains of the algal *K. brevis*. In the 1980s, they were named "brevetoxins" (PbTxs) for *P. brevis* toxins, because the algal *K. brevis* formerly was known as *Ptychodiscus brevis*.

There are over 10 different brevetoxins isolated from seawater blooms and *K. brevis* cultures in the laboratory, as well as multiple analogs and derivatives from the metabolism of shellfish and other organisms.[352–358] The most potent varieties are PbTx-1, PbTx-2, and PbTx-3.

These lipid-soluble, heat-stable brevetoxins adversely affect human health as well as ecological ecosystems. Their mode of action is by binding to the site 5 on the α-subunit of voltage-sensitive sodium channels, which control the generation of action potentials in nerve, muscle, and cardiac tissue, enhancing channel opening and inhibiting channel closure, resulting in a dose-dependent depolarization of excitable neuronal membranes, which leads to the incessant activation of the cells that cause paralysis and fatigue. These toxins harm the nervous system of an organism even at small concentrations.

6.6.3.3.1 Epidemiology Chain

6.6.3.3.1.1 Source of Intoxication   The NSP is produced by the strains of the algal *K. brevis* that periodically cause well-documented blooms, known as "Florida red tides" on the Florida west coast since the 1800s. More recently, Florida red tides have spread as far as the eastern coast of Mexico and have been entrained in the Gulf Loop, the current that brings Gulf waters to the shores of North Carolina. In 1992–1993, the largest documented outbreak of NSP occurred in New Zealand. There were over 186 cases of poisoning during a period of several weeks. The cases presented both gastrointestinal symptoms and respiratory problems due to aerosol inhalation.[359]

Other brevetoxin-producing dinoflagellate blooms have been identified in diverse geographic locations worldwide, including New Zealand, Australia, and Scotland.[360–364]

6.6.3.3.1.2 Vectors and Routes of Transmission   When *K. brevis* red tides occur, toxins are let out in the oceans and may kill or harm marine animals, as well as cause human illness from eating filter-feeding bivalves that have retained levels of these toxins, or by inhalation of aerosolized toxins carried onshore in sea spray.

Ingestion: The most common way for humans to be exposed to these toxins is by the consumption of contaminated shellfish that leads to NSP. Oysters, clams, and coquinas have been associated with NSP.[365,366]

No definitive evidence exists of any health effects to the shellfish by *K. brevis* red tides, with possible exception of scallops.[367–369] Scallops are less tolerant of brevetoxins than other bivalves. Scallop mortalities occur during *K. brevis* red tides.

Oysters and clams are clearly a danger to humans during and after *K. brevis* blooms. Other species of shellfish less widely consumed can accumulate toxins as well and, on occasion, have led to human illness. Smaller bivalves (e.g., chione clams and coquinas) can accumulate extremely high levels of brevetoxins. Whelks were implicated in an NSP event in 1996.

Chronic low-level exposure to brevetoxins and metabolites through shellfish and fish can occur, and the effects are not known.

Inhalation: The formation of aerosolized toxins occurs through lysis of the *K. brevis* cells by wave action in the tides. PbTx-2 is the most prevalent brevetoxin variety in marine aerosol. Brevetoxin aerosols have been demonstrated to travel as much as a mile inland from coastal areas during an active Florida red tide, particularly when there are strong onshore winds.[370]

Humans, as well as marine mammals, are a high-risk group to brevetoxin inhalation. Aerosolized toxins carried onshore in sea spray cause eye and throat irritation, nasal congestion, cough, wheezing, shortness of breath, and further complications in individuals with chronic inflammatory lung conditions. Exposure to the aerosolized toxins is also linked to the deaths of many marine mammals. While a link between symptoms and toxin exposure has been established, the exact causative mechanism behind the pathology has not been concluded.

The particle size of the brevetoxin aerosol was characterized during a Florida red tide bloom. They have a geometric mean of approximately 8–9 μ. This is an important information in terms of the potential for respiratory effects of brevetoxin aerosols in humans. The particle size needs to be less than 5 μ to reach the lower airway; therefore, with a geometric mean of 8–9 μ, only 10%–20% of these particles are small enough to enter the human lung.[371–375]

6.6.3.3.1.3 Affectation of Fish, Birds, and Aquatic Mammals

Ecological health effects of toxic red tides are massive mortality rates for invertebrates, fish, birds, and even some marine mammals including manatees and bottlenose dolphins. This could be either by direct exposure to the toxins themselves or from the brevetoxins in the food web.

Fish kills in the Gulf of Mexico have been reported since as far back as 1844. These fish kills associated with these red tides have been estimated up to 100 tons of fish per day during an active red tide. The fish are killed apparently through lack of muscle coordination and paralysis, convulsions, and death by respiratory failure. Fish die when they are exposed to brevetoxins dissolved in seawater, but they can survive and accumulate brevetoxins and metabolites when they feed on contaminated prey. Accumulation in or food web transfer by fish has not been regarded as a threat. However, brevetoxin transfer through fish was hypothesized by Steidinger to explain the presence of brevetoxin found in some of the dolphins from the 1987 to 1988 mortality as well as in some prey species, and a significantly increased gastrointestinal illness emergency room admissions during the active Florida red tide period was also observed.[376–379] To date, alarming levels of brevetoxins in the muscles of live fish have not been found. Internal organs of fish can be very toxic and should not be eaten.

Multiple die-offs of marine mammals have been reported in association with Florida red tide and brevetoxins.[380–382] In 1996, a prolonged Florida red tide in the Gulf of Mexico resulted in the documented deaths of 149 endangered Florida manatees.[383] The brevetoxin exposure of the manatees appears to have been prolonged inhalation of the red tide toxin aerosol and/or ingestion of contaminated seawater over several weeks. For marine organisms, these toxins can cause disorientation, losing their ability to hunt or navigate the oceans, and can also disrupt their ability to swim properly, putting them in a paralyzed position causing death. Birds die acutely with neurological and hematologic effects, too. Brevetoxin is heat stable, and thus, cooking contaminated seafood will not alter the risk of intoxication. Furthermore, the toxin is lipid-soluble rather than water-soluble, and thus, boiling or steaming contaminated food is similarly unlikely to alter the risk of intoxication.[384]

6.6.3.3.2 Clinical Features

The median latent period between ingestion of shellfish and onset of illness are 3 h (range 15 min–18 h) with a similar onset for both gastrointestinal and neurological symptoms. In the North Carolina outbreak, it was from 30 min to 3 days (median 17 h).

NSP typically causes gastrointestinal symptoms of nausea, diarrhea, and abdominal pain, as well as the neurological symptoms primarily consisting of paresthesias similar to those seen with CFP (including reports of circumoral paresthesias and hot/cold temperature reversal). Cerebellar symptoms such as vertigo and incoordination also reportedly occur. In severe cases, bradycardia, headache, dilated pupils, convulsions, and the subsequent need for respiratory support have been reported. Death from NSP (rather than from PSP or ciguatera) is rare.

In the North Carolina outbreak involving 48 persons,[385] the most common symptoms were paresthesias (81%), vertigo (60%), malaise (50%), abdominal pain (48%), nausea (44%), diarrhea (33%), weakness (31%), ataxia (27%), chills (21%), headache (15%), myalgia (13%), and vomiting (10%). Reportedly, symptoms resolve within a few days after exposure; however, no studies have been reported evaluating possible chronic health effects after acute NSP.

Exposure to aerosols containing brevetoxins may cause conjunctival irritation, rhinorrhea, and respiratory irritation, and possibly exacerbate or cause symptoms similar to reactive airways disease. Some people also report other symptoms such as dizziness, tunnel vision, and skin rashes. In the normal population, the irritation and bronchoconstriction are usually rapidly reversible by leaving the beach area or entering an air-conditioned area.[386,387] However, people with asthma are apparently particularly susceptible.

Studies in a group of very healthy nonasthmatic lifeguards have found self-reports of significantly increased respiratory symptoms after completing an 8 h work shift during an active Florida red tide,[388] but no a significant decrease in their pulmonary function was observed. Other studies have found an increase in emergency room admissions for acute and subchronic respiratory health effects (e.g., asthma, bronchitis, and pneumonia) and prolonged respiratory symptoms, and increased use of medication and doctor visits, among those who were exposed to the Florida red tide aerosols.[389,390] Asthmatics aged 12 and older had significant increases in self-reported respiratory symptoms and significant decreases in respiratory function measured by spirometry after only 1 h of acute exposure to aerosolized brevetoxins during an active Florida red tide.[391–394,432–434,460]

The exposure usually occurs on or near beaches with an active red tide bloom. Onshore winds and breaking surf result in the release of the toxins into the water and into the onshore aerosol.

Brevetoxin produces contraction of the lower airway smooth muscle by stimulation of the cholinergic nerve fiber sodium channels with acetylcholine release. In addition, there appears to induce the release of histamine from mast cells, and the combination of these actions results in adverse airway effects. Furthermore, brevetoxin exposure by the respiratory route results in systemic distribution of brevetoxin. Bossart et al.[381] postulated that the effects of aerosolized brevetoxins may be chronic not just acute. These chronic effects would begin with the initial phagocytosis by macrophages, inhibition of cathepsins, and apoptosis of these cells, followed by the phagocytosis of the debris by new macrophages, ultimately resulting in chronic neurointoxication, hemolytic anemia, and/or immunologic compromise.

Reports of airway irritant effects from Florida red tide have been documented in the Western literature since 1844.[370] Earlier accounts from Spanish explorers of an "irritating essence" predate 1600. Past explanations for Florida red tide respiratory distress have included World War I nerve gas release,[395] "fast"- and "slow"-acting toxins,[396] a phosphorylated organic molecule,[397] and green particles as fragments of a marine alga.[398]

6.6.3.3.3 Treatment

Treatment for shellfish poisoning is supportive (i.e., fluid replacement and respiratory support if necessary). In PSP, emesis may not occur; hence gastric lavage is commonly used.

Commonly used asthma medications (e.g., beta-agonists, cromolyn, and steroids), as well as antihistamines and brevenal, can prevent the respiratory effects of subsequent aerosolized brevetoxin exposure. In addition, the beta-agonists and brevenal can reverse or treat these effects if given after the brevetoxin exposure.[399–403]

6.6.3.3.4 Public Health Issues

Phytoplankton and toxins levels in the shellfish bed should be monitored and the harvest of the bed should be prohibited closed when specified toxic levels are detected. For the aerosolized red tide respiratory irritation, water and air monitoring could detect high levels in the air, and warning notices can be posted along affected coastal areas for susceptible subpopulations. Surveillance and reporting of red tide disease in humans, other mammals, and animals are important for early warning, prevention, and further understanding of these diseases. In addition, education and outreach programs to health-care providers, workers involved in the seafood and tourism industries, and the general public are important components of successful monitoring and surveillance programs.[404]

Since the mid-1970s, the Florida Department of Agriculture and Consumer Services has conducted a monitoring program of shellfish beds in the Gulf of Mexico. Beds are closed when the level of *K. brevis* exceed 5000 cells/L near or in harvesting areas. The areas remain closed until at least 2 weeks after a drop in cell counts below the action level and mouse bioassay results in shellfish below 20 MU (mouse units)/100 g. No regulatory limit exists for brevetoxin in the seawater. The regulatory limit for shellfish is 20 MU/100 g of shellfish meat, which is equivalent to 80 µg brevetoxin/100 g of shellfish meat.[405] The standardized mouse bioassay is used to test specimens for neurotoxicity.

These monitoring programs should prevent the ingestion of NSP related to contaminated shellfish consumption in most of the Florida human population but not in areas where red tide is not an annual event or where monitoring programs do not exist (e.g., North Carolina). Furthermore, such monitoring programs do not prevent the respiratory irritation associated with exposure to aerosolized red tide toxins, although they could serve as early warning devices. In Florida, where the red tides occur almost yearly, beaches are not closed to recreational or occupational activities even during active nearshore blooms.

In the case of aerosolized red tide toxin respiratory irritation, the use of particle filter masks may prevent or diminish the symptoms, and retreating to air-conditioned environment reportedly will provide relief from the airborne irritation.[406]

6.6.4 Yessotoxins

The YTXs are a group of bisulfate polyether toxins with a structure similar to brevetoxins (brevetoxin-type polyether), which were isolated from *P. yessoensis*.[407] They are produced by the dinoflagellates *P. reticulatum*[408] and by the *L. polyedrum*.[409] Their presence in shellfish was discovered due to their high acute toxicity in mice after intraperitoneal injection of lipophilic extracts. They are much less potent via the oral route, and they do not induce diarrhea. There are no reports of human intoxications caused by YTXs.[410] Until now, up to 90 YTXs analogs have been described.[411] EFSA identified YTX, 1a-homo-YTX, 45-hydroxy-YTX, and 45-hydroxy-1a-homo-YTX as the most important YTXs present in shellfish.[412]

YTXs do not induce diarrhea in rodents, but the intraperitoneal injection of either is lethal to mice. They have been shown to cause heart damage. Almost all cardiac muscle cells of mice inoculated with these toxins were swollen. On the other hand, YTXs do not cause damage in the liver, pancreas, lungs, kidneys, and adrenergic glands. All these chronic effects need to be studied in depth, and they underline the relevance and dimension of the problem and the need to avoid ingestion of these toxins.

6.6.5 Ichthyosarcotoxism

6.6.5.1 Ciguatera

CFP is an ichthyosarcotoxism, endemic in tropical and subtropical regions around the world, in Pacific and Indian Oceans, and in Caribbean area.[413–415] It is caused by the bioaccumulation of cyclic polyether lipophilic neurotoxins named as ciguatoxins (CTXs) produced primarily by an epiphytic benthic dinoflagellate species of the genus *Gambierdiscus* spp.[416] These toxins are lipid soluble and heat stable.[417] In some cases, cyanobacteria can also be involved in CTX production.[418,419] There have been more than 12 types of CTX identified to date, which are structurally similar to each other. Isoform production is strain dependent, and it is possible that certain strains produce CTX in larger quantities than others; however, they may be more difficult to isolate and culture.[420]

Maitotoxin (MTX) is yet another toxin that is believed to cause ciguatera with different symptoms. It is also produced by *G. toxicus* but in much greater amounts than CTX. It is unique in terms of its molecular size and structural complex as well as its extremely potent bioactivity.[421] MTX acts on calcium channels in a receptor-mediated process by increasing calcium flux in a number of cell types. This results in muscle contractions, altered neurotransmission, hormone release, and phospholipid metabolism.

CFP is the most common nonbacterial food-borne illness associated with the consumption of fish worldwide.[7,8,422]

Severe neurological and gastrointestinal and cardiac symptoms as well as, in some cases, chronic neurological symptoms lasting weeks to months, have been experienced by people after the consumption of coral reef fish toxic.

6.6.5.1.1 Worldwide Distribution and Incidence

Ciguatera is associated with environments tropical marine and occurs between 35° N and 35° S latitude. In the Atlantic, it is common in Florida, the Bahamas, throughout the Caribbean, particularly in Cuba, Dominican Republic, Haiti, Puerto Rico, and the Leeward Islands, including the islands Virgin. In the Pacific, it occurs in Polynesia French, the Philippines, Fiji, Samoa, Tonga, Vanuatu, Hawaii, Cook and Marshall Islands, New Caledonia, and Australia. In the Indian Ocean, ciguatera occurs commonly in Reunion, Madagascar, Mauritius, and Seychelles, and has also been reported in Sri Lanka, the Maldives, and the archipelagos Comoro and Chagos. It should be noted that fish and seafood imported from these sites can cause ciguatera anywhere in the world.

The true worldwide incidence of CFP is difficult to ascertain due to underreporting.[423–425] It is estimated to be 50,000 new cases per year.[426,427] There are no laboratory tests for the diagnosis of ciguatera in patients and the diagnosis is based on symptoms and history of consumption of suspected toxic fish.

Outbreaks of ciguatera have been reported in tropical or subtropical regions around the world, including Hong Kong,[428] Okinawa, Japan,[429] and FP,[430] Australia, and Texas and Southern California in the United States.[431] The average incidence rate in the endemic US territories is estimated to be 5–70 cases per 10,000 population.[432] CFP is particularly prevalent across the Pacific Island countries and territories (PICTs).

The Pacific region itself accounts for between 3400 and 4700 ciguateric intoxications per year, which should represent only 10%–20% of the real number of cases.[433] One of the most affected countries is Tuvalu, where the prevalence may be up to 240/10,000 population, whereas it ranges from 1 to 50/10,000 population in the other Pacific countries. In FP, the prevalence was of 35.6/10,000 population between 1992 and 2001; the incidence of CFP in FP decreased to approximately 14.5/10,000 in 2008 probably due to improvement in the public health system.[434] A similar situation is found in Cook Islands, where the CFP incidence varied from 204 to 1,058/10,000 population per year between 1994 and 2010.[435] In New Caledonia, there is generally a low prevalence of intoxication, around 10/10,000 population. The doctors rarely reported food-borne intoxications. Ciguatera poisoning is often underdiagnosed and underreported, with only 2%–10% of cases reported to health authorities. Estimates of the incidence of ciguatera in Oceania have ranged from 0.5/10,000 population/year in Hawaii to 5,850/10,000 population/year in FP.

Skinner et al.[436] studied the extent of Ciguatera in the PICTs, through a questionnaire e-mailed to the Health and Fisheries Authorities of the PICTs. There were 39,677 reported cases from 17 PICTs, with a mean annual incidence of 194 cases per 100,000 people across the region from 1998 to 2008. Compared to the reported annual incidence of 104/100,000 population from 1973 to 1983, there has been a 60% increase in the annual incidence of ciguatera between the two time periods based on PICTs that reported for both time periods. The reported cases for the recent 11-year period showed high levels of interyear variability within and between PICTs. Using the conservative estimate that the official reported ciguatera represents 20% of actual incidence,[437] the actual average overall incidence for the region would be 970/100,000 population for 1998–2008. Others have estimated that only 5%–10% of ciguatera cases are actually reported.

In Lesser Antilles, the easternmost part of the Caribbean has been an increase in incidence from 1981 through 1996–2006. In 1981, Antigua-Barbuda and Montserrat reported 6 and 42 cases per 10,000 population respectively for 34 and 59 cases per 10,000 population years in 1996–2006.

With increases in interstate fish transport, more outbreaks have occurred in areas without the risk of indigenous ciguatera such as Canada,[438] Rhode Island,[439] California,[440] and Vermont.[441] In addition, clinicians in any part of the world may see patients who present after acquiring illness during travel.[442,443] Finally, one report identified a case of ciguatera that resulted from the consumption of farm-raised salmon, raising the possibility of ciguatera occurring in novel locations.[444]

Confirmed cases of ciguatoxic poisoning outside endemic areas in temperate regions of the world have also been reported and often linked to the consumption of imported toxic fish.[445] Recent observations also suggest the expansion of the biogeographic range of *Gamberdiscus* spp. and ciguatoxic fish.[446,447]

CFP had not been described on the West Africa Coast until a 2004 outbreak in the Canary Islands. In 2008–2009, two additional outbreaks of ciguatera occurred. Individuals afflicted had consumed lesser amberjack (*Seriola rivoliana*) captured from nearby waters. Caribbean ciguatoxin-1 (C-CTX-1) was confirmed in fish samples by LC-MS/MS. Ciguatoxic fish in this region may pose a new health risk for the seafood consumer.[448]

The Canary Islands Archipelago is considered a nonendemic region for CFP.[449] In 2004, the first documented outbreak of CFP in the Canary Islands occurred. In the same year, *Gambierdiscus* spp. was found in the waters of the Canary Islands Archipelago, adjacent to the islands of Tenerife and La Gomera.[450] In 2008 and 2009, two additional outbreaks occurred. Implicated fish were captured regionally and were tested and confirmed positive for CTXs. These findings reinforce the data suggesting geographic expansion of CFP endemicity worldwide. In the first outbreak of CFP, in 2004, illnesses were linked to a single fish, a lesser amberjack (*S. rivoliana*), captured along the eastern coast of the Islands. Individuals who consumed portions of the fish presented gastrointestinal (nausea, vomiting, and diarrhea) and neurological (metallic taste, myalgia, paresthesia, and reversal of hot and cold sensations) symptoms consistent with CFP. Gastrointestinal symptoms resolved in 24–48 h, while neurological symptoms were slowly resolved over a period of months.

In 2008, public health authorities of the Canary Islands investigated a second outbreak of CFP involving 20–30 individuals. Symptoms reported were mainly gastrointestinal (nausea, vomiting, and diarrhea) occurring within a few hours after the consumption of fish identified as lesser amberjack, as in the 2004 outbreak. The amberjack involved in this event were captured off the northern coast of the Canary Islands, near the Salvagem Islands (Portugal).

In 2009, public health authorities of the Canary Islands investigated a third putative outbreak of CFP. An estimated 10–40 individuals developed gastrointestinal symptoms (nausea, vomiting, and diarrhea) after the consumption of filets of the lesser amberjack from a supermarket. As in the previous outbreaks, amberjack were captured in the area north of the Canary Islands, near the Salvagem Islands, too. The toxin confirmed in fish samples implicated in the Canary Islands outbreaks was Caribbean CTX (C-CTX-1).

There have been confirmed reports of ciguatoxic fish in other nonendemic areas such as barracuda (*Sphyraena barracuda*) and snapper (*Lutjanus* sp.) from Cameroon, West Africa; rabbitfish (putatively *Siganus* sp.) caught in Haifa Bay in the Eastern Mediterranean basin[451]; and fish reportedly carrying CTXs from Crete in 2007.[452] These CFP occurrences may be attributed to range extensions for *Gambierdiscus* into higher latitudes in response to climate change, as predicted by Tester.[453]

Human activities may be responsible in part for the transfer of toxic phytoplankton among different regions of the world, such as transport by ship ballast water. Other anthropogenic and natural perturbations in oceanic and coastal waters, including nutrient loading, changes in sea surface temperature, and habitat alteration, may impact the abundance and geographic distribution of *Gambierdiscus* spp. and ciguatoxic fish.

In recent years, there has also been an increase in inquiries for ciguatera patients who have spent their holidays in tropical regions, particularly in the Pacific Islands and the northern regions of Australia, and in the Caribbean.

The cases are infrequent in Spain, the majority are from the Dominican Republic or Cuba, both important tourist destinations for Spaniards.[454,455] In 2011, Herrero-Martínez et al.[456] describe a case of ciguatera in a traveler to Santo Domingo (Dominican Republic). This is a 44-year-old woman. The clinic began at 6 h of having consumed silk snapper (*L. vivanus*) boiled.

The ciguatera must be considered in the differential diagnosis of a gastrointestinal and neurological picture after the ingestion of fish in travelers to endemic areas, and the treatment restored with the major possible briefness.

6.6.5.1.2 Economic Importance

Ciguatera causes significant economic losses in tropical and subtropical countries. On the one hand, losses of hundreds of thousands of dollars in the marketing of fisheries, and on the other hand, it may also adversely affect the tourist industry, particularly hotels and restaurants. A single outbreak well publicized may adversely affect income not only at one or several businesses but also for an entire geographic area.

6.6.5.1.3 Epidemiologic Chain

CFP outbreaks present a public health challenge in areas where *Gambierdiscus* is endemic because, on a local scale, outbreaks are both temporally and spatially variable.[457]

6.6.5.1.3.1 Source of Intoxication The dinoflagellates of the genus *Gambierdiscus* live as an epiphyte predominantly in association with macroalgae in coral reefs in tropical and subtropical climates.[458,459] It exhibits a strong preference for algal macrophytes.[460,461] Although it can spread to new regions on pieces of floating algae, this species is not of red tides.

The suite of *Gambierdiscus* species found in the Atlantic appeared distinct from that in the Pacific. *G. belizeanus*, *G. carolinianus*, *G. ruetzleri*, and *Gambierdiscus* ribotypes 1 and 2 were isolated from the Atlantic, whereas *G. australes*, *G. pacificus*, *G. polynesiensis*, *G. toxicus*, and *G. yasumotoi* were exclusively isolated from the Pacific. In contrast, *G. carpenteri* and *G. caribaeus* were found in both the Atlantic and Pacific and likely have a global distribution.

The toxin is oil soluble, odorless, colorless, tasteless, and heat stable. As these toxins bioaccumulate, they are frequently modified to form several major, and numerous minor, chemical congeners whose toxicity can vary significantly. To date, over 50 different congeners have been identified.[462] The dominant CTXs recovered from Caribbean (C-CTX-1 and C-CTX-2) and Pacific (P-CTX-C3) fish are structurally distinct. The postulated cause for this discrepancy is a difference in the precursor toxins produced by the *Gambierdiscus* species in each region.[463–468,502]

6.6.5.1.3.2 Vectors The toxin is transferred through the food web when the algae are consumed by herbivorous fish, which are consumed by carnivorous fish, with more accumulation and concentration accompanying each step, which are in turn consumed by humans.[12,469]

Large carnivorous fishes associated with coral reefs are frequently involved, but more than 400 species have been reported in ciguatera poisoning incidents.[12] The most common high CFP risk species were groupers (*Serranids*), king mackerels (*Scombrids*), snappers (*Lutjanids*), barracudas (*Sphyaraenids*), emperors (*Lethrinids*), trevallies (*Carangids*), parrotfish (*Scarids*), and wrasses (labrids). The size (age) of the fish also plays a critical role in the potential ciguatoxic risk.[470,471] The highest concentration of toxin is found in the liver, brain, and gonads of the fish.

Sometimes it can also be transmitted through shellfish. Four cases of ciguatera have been reported for shellfish consumption in New Caledonia consistent with previous reports[472] where epidemiological, toxicological, and chemical studies carried out in Lifou (Loyalty Islands, New Caledonia) pointed out the occurrence of cyanotoxins in giant clams (*Tridacna* spp.) harvested in the surroundings of a cyanobacteria-contaminated area. Data from these analyses strongly suggested the possible link between the severe ciguatera-like poisoning events in Lifou and the occurrence of neurotoxic blooms of *Hydrocoleum* spp.

Transmission has also been shown to occur via consumption of breast milk from an affected mother to her infant and across the placenta to the embryo/fetus.[473–475]

6.6.5.1.3.3 Predisposing Factors The best documented conditions associated with *Gambierdiscus* abundance and CFP events are the following:

Stable elevated water temperatures: Distribution and abundance of the genus *Gambierdiscus* are reported to correlate positively with water temperature. Annual water temperatures between 21°C and 31°C with optimum between 25°C and 29°C favor the development of *Gambierdiscus*.[476–486] The thermal optimum for five of six *Gambierdiscus* species tested was ≥29°C. In consequence, there is growing concern that increasing temperature, associated with climate change, may increase the incidence of CFP. Tester et al.[487] carried out a literature review, and a uniform regionwide survey (1996–2006) of CFP cases was conducted. The highest CFP incidence rates were in the eastern Caribbean, where water temperatures are warmest and least variable.

Favorable environmental conditions: Abundant macrophytes, algal turfs, or biofilms to which cells can attach[487–492]; low-to-moderate turbulence[493–496]; high stable salinities[497–499] actual or attenuated light levels <10% of incident[500,501]; and sufficient or elevated nutrient inputs, some of which can be obtained directly from the macrophyte hosts. The overall palatability of the macrophytes within any given environment is another factor that may be important in governing CFP occurrences. In theory, habitats dominated by chemically or structurally defended macroalgae, which are poorly grazed, are less likely to become ciguatoxic than habitats containing a greater proportion of palatable species.[380] But this hypothesis needs to be rigorously tested.

Environmental disturbances can cause the appearance of algal blooms[502–504]: coral bleaching events; anthropogenic or natural nutrient inputs; coastal development; events such as storms, hurricanes, heavy rains, earthquakes, tidal waves, or human activities can cause reef disturbance, including coral bleaching events, dredging, and bomb testing[505] leading to an increase in ciguatera outbreaks.[506]

The magnitude of the population response, however, is critically dependent on the intensity, timing, and scale of the disturbance.[507–509] The common mechanism appears to be an alteration in the prevailing community structure, which allows an increase in the macroalgae and algal turfs favorable for *Gambierdiscus* colonization and growth.[510–513] If the disturbance fosters a sufficient increase in toxic cells, a CFP event often ensues. Many of these disturbances also coincide with periods of elevated water temperatures or nutrient inputs, which may interact synergistically with habitat changes to increase *Gambierdiscus* abundance.

The least understood aspect of CFP is how environmental conditions and inherent genetic differences among species/strains interact to control per cell CTX toxicity. It is likely these factors interact in a complex way as evidenced by the fact that *Gambierdiscus* biomass correlates well with toxicity sometimes, but not others.[514]

Depending on the species composition of a *Gambierdiscus* bloom, its toxicity can conservatively vary by more than 100-fold. This range is approximately 10-fold greater than that likely induced by environmental up- or downregulation of toxicity. Interspecific differences in toxicity may therefore play a predominant role in causing CFP events relative to environmentally modulated toxicity.

Season: There is considerable evidence that ciguatoxicity varies seasonally,[515] although not all studies show this.[516] Tosteson[517] reported a seasonal correlation between the abundance of toxic, benthic dinoflagellates and the toxicity of barracuda and incidences of CFP in Puerto Rico from 1985 to 1988. Data collected from the southwest coast of Puerto Rico from 1990 to 2000 showed a gradual loss of seasonality and a significant increase in the fraction of toxic barracuda. He argued that these changes were due to increasing periods of elevated sea surface temperatures in the Caribbean. While considerable evidence exists that ciguatoxicity does vary seasonally, not all studies reflect this.

Some suggest that there may be cultural practices that cause CFP incidences to mimic seasonal patterns,[518] especially when holiday meals include large reef fish.

CTX is known to be concentrated in the liver, roe, head, and other viscera of suspect fish, and the larger the fish, the greater its chance of being toxic.[519,520] Many of these anatomical items are popular with the Asian community, and for banquet-style meals, dishes could be prepared from large fish.

6.6.5.1.4 Clinical Features

Ciguatera disease produces a myriad of gastrointestinal, neurological, and cardiac symptoms.[521–525] Symptoms of intoxication can be quite diverse and appear dependent on a combination of the amount of toxin consumed, the suite of toxins present in the tainted fish, and an individual's susceptibility.

The gastrointestinal phase includes abdominal pain, nausea vomiting, and diarrhea. It usually begins within 6–12 h after the ingestion of contaminated seafood, but it can be quite variable ranging from less than 1 h to up to 48 h following exposure[526] and the symptoms lasting 1–2 days. It is followed by a neurological phase whose symptoms include circumoral and extremity paresthesias, and hot–cold reversal, itching on hands and feet, and others (weakness, dizziness, ataxia, arthralgia, myalgia, blurred vision, and headache).[527–529] Ciguatera is well known in New Caledonia under the name "Gratte," which means scratching owing to the itching syndrome commonly associated with the chronic stage of the disease. These neurological signs may persist for months or years after the onset. Finally, in severe cases,[530] cardiac symptoms, such as hypotension and bradycardia, as well as paralysis are present. Occasionally, death may occur.

Paradoxical dysesthesia, which manifests as numbness of extremities, troubles on contact with water, or cold allodynia, is considered almost pathognomonic for ciguatera toxin poisoning, but the cold allodynia is also reported following exposure to brevetoxin. Indeed, these neurological symptoms are much more often reported (more than 80% of cases) by patients than gastrointestinal symptoms (under 50%).[531] Cardiac and respiratory symptoms, which are usually associated with severity of disease, were not very frequent (under 15%). Although deaths have been reported,[605] they rarely occur in ciguatera poisoning.

Exacerbations of signs are described after the consumption of seafood, nontoxic fishes, eggs, or alcohol.[532]

In endemic areas, many people report experiencing poisoning and even many have suffered several episodes of poisoning throughout their life. Among the 559 patients, 210 were poisoned at least once in their life (37.8%). Fifty-six persons (26.7%) presented multiple episodes of poisoning of which the maximum was 15 episodes.

6.6.5.1.4.1 Diagnose   There is no evidence of accurate diagnostic for CTX poisoning. Presently, the diagnosis is based on symptoms and immediate history of the consumption of patient's food.

There are tests for ciguatera in fish and seafood, the most common being the bioassay mouse, but the procedures are complicated and may take more than 4 days to get results.

6.6.5.1.5 Treatment

There is no specific treatment for ciguatera. Normally, the patients are given supportive treatment therapies to reduce the symptoms (analgesics to control pain and antihistamines to reduce itching). Tract decontamination gastrointestinal activated carbon can be beneficial if done within 3 or 4 h of toxin ingestion, and the use of antiemetics can control vomiting. Volume replacement therapies are essential to counteract the fluid loss caused by vomiting and diarrhea, and the use of atropine recommended as a treatment for bradycardia. The use of mannitol has become common in the treatment of ciguatera. As for the treatment, the evidence is nowadays scanty. There is sufficient consensus in administering mannitol in the first 48–72 h, though there have been observed cases in which the beneficial effect has remained even after weeks of evolution.[533,534]

It might be useful for 3–6 months or at least up to the resolution of the symptoms to avoid such food as alcohol, nuts, fish, caffeine, pork, or chicken, the dehydration, or the accomplishment of physical intense exercise.

6.6.5.1.6 Public Health Issues

CFP represents a worrying public health issue because of its high prevalence, which can be severe and can lead to death.[535] The complexity of its epidemiology is responsible for the poor management of the risk in tropical fish markets.

The collection of CFP epidemiological data is inefficient, and the public health impact of this disease is likely significantly underestimated. This is attributable in part to reticence of the public to report the illness in endemic areas and the lack of diagnostic recognition in nonendemic areas.

It is needed for public health and fishery professionals to receive up-to-date information about regional CFP occurrences. The absence of a uniform reporting procedure for CFP cases and a universal location where data could be stored have hampered regional understanding of the scope of this important public health issue.

A standardized reporting protocol and website where CFP data can be uploaded must be developed. In addition, the CFP website will be linked to near real-time environmental data. If data on CFP episodes are uploaded as soon as they occur on a website that displays geographic locations and links to environmental variables such as sea surface temperature, this could help provide timely warnings for local residents, physicians, and public health officials of the countries affected.

It is necessary to establish a coordinated program of Fisheries Administrations and Public Health and a proactive surveillance system. A good governance strategy cannot be achieved if proactive surveillance is not conducted in parallel to any health action.[536] On a global level, the collection of epidemiological data on CFP has been inefficient. Accordingly, a large-scale database should be maintained, probably through regional organizations.

Developing a monitoring system for predicting CFP will be very important, but it has many difficulties. The toxicity varies mucho among species and strains. Currently, peaks in *Gambierdiscus* abundance precede CFP outbreaks by approximately 1 month to 1 year, but that not all increases in cell abundance result in increased CFP. Consequently, monitoring *Gambierdiscus* cell densities alone might result in numerous false alarms, which would undermine the public's confidence in the monitoring system and its effectiveness as a management tool.

Given that toxicity of *Gambierdiscus* populations is largely determined by differences among strains of the same species rather than interspecies differences; therefore, the prediction becomes much more difficult, depending on the discovery and development of molecular markers capable of distinguishing toxic from nontoxic strains. Currently, this is not possible. Alternatively, it may be necessary to develop cost-effective analytical techniques that can be used to detect toxin levels in real time.

Development of an effective monitoring system may ultimately require a hybrid approach utilizing both cell densities and direct toxin detection methods. Under this scenario, *Gambierdiscus* abundance or species composition data could be used to identify periods of potential risk, during which the more detailed analytical analyses could be employed. This approach would allow managers to reserve the more precise, but expensive analytical methods for periods of greatest potential threat.

Implementation of any regulation should aim to ban some specific species and sizes suspected to cause ciguatera from the market, such as grouper, snapper, barracuda, and surgeon fish in FP,[537] and barracuda in Miami.[538]

Laboratory tests, despite its limitations, should be conducted on random samples of risky fish that are regularly sold on the market.[539–541] Three years ago, Public Health Analytical Laboratory of the State of Queensland, Australia, had established a method for the detection and quantification of Pacific CTXs in fish flesh.[542] However, it is more time consuming and expensive.

A multidisciplinary approach should be applied. To optimize risk management physicians and veterinarians should be informed about the identification of clinical cases.[551] Fish experts and restaurateurs should be informed as well.[543] Sensitize doctors to report cases and to inform restaurateurs of the risk of CFP and the need to avoid large reef fish, especially the head and other viscera, is important.

Where governments have not acted, the combination of legal decisions and insurance industry pressure has prompted interventions such as the placement of warnings on restaurant menus in endemic areas.[544]

Public health and regulatory measures to control ciguatera should consider the relative value of a fish diet compared to the risk of ciguatera, the economic and social importance of fish harvesting to a community, the anticipated intervention when toxic fish are identified (particularly if toxic fish represent a considerable portion of the total harvest), and guidelines for the relaxation of specific restrictions (e.g., import or export restrictions) once implemented.

In the Pacific region, Lewis[545] and Bourdy et al.[546] report a number of strategies that islanders have adopted to avoid ciguatera including avoidance of high-risk species, discarding the internal organs of fish, and feeding fish to a pet and observing the reaction. Additional strategies have been employed that are less effective or ineffective, such as cooking the fish with plant materials or feeling the texture of the fish. Another report documents similar practices among the residents of the Dominican Republic.[547] It is unclear, however, how many people avoid fish because of the presence of CTX. In Puerto Rico, an area with relatively high levels of health and a diversified economy, the threat of ciguatera has been shown to lead people to avoid eating fish entirely.[548]

On a personal level, the risk of ciguatera is usually small, but the only sure way to avoid poisoning is to not eat fish or seafood from tropical reefs. This, however, is often not possible or practical. Avoiding the internal organs of fish, which often accumulate toxins, can reduce the risk, but fish evisceration does not appear to be protective,[520,549] despite concentration of toxin in specific organs, and because the toxin is heat stable, cooking also provides no protection. Other reported risk factors include exertion and eating large fish.

This process seems a priority in the actual context of an increasing CFP prevalence in the endemic areas that may continue during the near future, even if there is not any clear evidence so far of a link between CFP and climate change.[550] The involvement of cyanobacteria in CFP and the potential increase in algal blooms in the context of climate change would logically increase the global CFP risk within the next decades.

6.6.5.2 Tetrodotoxin

TTX is a marine toxin called the family Tetraodontiformes puffer fish, which was discovered by Taharain in 1880.[3] This marine toxin has been closely associated with poisonings after the consumption of puffer fish.

Since 1964, when tarichatoxin in the eggs of California newts, *T. torosa*, was identified as TTX,[551] it has been isolated from many marine animals, such as newts,[552] gobies, frogs, crabs,[553] the blue-ringed octopus,[554] star fish,[555] and various species of gastropods[556] and worms.[557,558]

Cases of poisoning are most prevalent in Asian countries, with an estimated 50 deaths annually due to TTX poisoning in Japan,[559] as well as repeated cases in Singapore, Taiwan, and Bangladesh.

Symptoms of TTX poisoning include numbness of the face and extremities, paralysis, respiratory failure, circulatory collapse, and death.

6.6.5.2.1 Toxin

TTX is a potent neurotoxin of low molecular weight. It was first isolated in 1950 by Yokoo,[560] and its structure identified in 1964 by Woodward.[561] It is considered the most lethal toxin in the marine environment.

Like the STX, the TTX inhibits nerve and muscle conduction by selectively blocking sodium channels, resulting in respiratory paralysis that causes death. Both toxins bind to the same cell site.

The lethal potency of TTX is 5,000–6,000 MU/mg, and the minimum lethal dose for humans is estimated to be approximately 10,000 MU ($\approx$2 mg).[562] Various TTX derivatives have so far been separated from puffer fish and/or some other TTX-bearing organisms.[563,564]

TTX-bearing animals have a high tolerance to TTX, which allows them to retain and accumulate. It seems that the TTX is present as an antipredator defense to protect its own eggs or external enemies, as venom, as a sex pheromone, and as an attractant for TTX-sequestering organisms.[565]

TTX-producing organisms have been found to have TTX-resistant sodium channels. In addition, some species have been found to produce TTX-binding compounds that are able to neutralize the effects of TTX.[566] In them, the aromatic amino acid commonly located in the p-loop region of domain I in TTX-sensitive sodium channels is replaced by a nonaromatic amino acid, resulting in extremely low affinity to TTX.[567]

6.6.5.2.2 Incidence

No reliable incidence data exist for TTX poisoning. The most extensive data on TTX poisoning come from Japan, where 6386 cases of puffer fish poisoning were reported during the 78-year period, 1886–1963 (59.4% were fatal).[568,569] With the exception of the period during World War II, the number of reported puffer fish poisoning episodes in Japan during 1886–1963 remained relatively constant at 100–300 per year. In addition, during the same period, no systematic decrease in the case fatality rate occurred. More recently, 495 persons became ill from puffer fish ingestion during 1977–1986.

In the period 1995–2007, there have been 724 incidents in Japan, and 1078 people were poisoned of which 212 died. The mortality from puffer fish poisoning in the entire period was 19.7%.

Other Southeast Asian countries have also reported cases of TTX poisoning. A report from the Poison Control Center in Taiwan, with a 1989 population of approximately 20,000,000, identified 20 outbreaks involving 52 patients during 1988 through 1995.[570] Similarly, in Thailand, 71 persons developed TTX poisoning from horseshoe crab, *Limulus polyphemus*, ingestion during January 1994 through May 1995.[571] In Asia, especially in China, 42 outbreaks of TTX-associated paralytic snail poisoning, involving 309 cases of illness, occurred from 1977 to 2001.[572]

6.6.5.2.3 Geographic Distribution

Cases of poisoning are more prevalent in Asian countries. In Japan, about 50 deaths occur annually due to poisoning by TTX. Other hard-hit countries are Taiwan and Thailand. The intoxication has been also reported from China (over 300 intoxicated and 16 deaths during 1977–2001), Hong Kong, Singapore, Bangladesh, Madagascar, Philippines, Malaysia, the South Pacific, and Australia. In contrast, outbreaks in other countries outside the Indo-Pacific area are rare. Isolated episodes have been reported in the United States (California), Mexico, Morocco, Malaysia, Lebanon, and Egypt. In the United States, only few cases have occurred, the most caused by imported fish from Japan or Taiwan.

The Suez Canal permits migration of fish from the Indo-Pacific Ocean to the Mediterranean Sea. This phenomenon (*Lessepsian migration*) has enabled poisonous fish species to colonize the Mediterranean Sea. *Lessepsian migration* is named after Ferdinand de Lesseps, the French engineer in charge of the canal's construction, a known phenomenon of the influx of Indo-Pacific fauna from the tropical Red Sea via the Suez Canal into the Mediterranean.

On the topic at hand, this has already happened. *L. sceleratus*, puffer fish of the family Tetraodontidae, was first collected in the Mediterranean Sea in February 2003 from Gökova Bay (southern Aegean Sea, Turkey)[573] and in November 2004 from Jaffa along the Israeli coast.[574] In Greek waters, *L. sceleratus* was first recorded from the Cretan Sea (Aegean Sea) in July 2005.[575] Since then, *L. sceleratus* has been recorded with an increasing frequency, in many areas of Aegean Sea, Greece. In 2009, Katikou et al.[576] performed the first report for the presence of toxicity in *L. sceleratus* caught in European coastal waters.

To date, 62 fish species have been recorded to invade the Mediterranean this way; and the LS is the largest one at present. Other four puffer fish species have been found in the Mediterranean, three (*Lagocephalus suezensis*, *Torquigener flavimaculosus*, and *Tylerius spinosissimus*) are small, and their potential consumption by humans is doubtful. The medium-sized (up to 40 cm) *L. spadiceus* has been known in the Mediterranean since the 1920s,[577] but no cases of consumption or poisoning have been reported.

TTX and/or possibly PSP toxins from the puffer fish *L. sceleratus* could be a new emerging risk in the European fisheries sector. In fact, in 2007, 13 Israeli patients aged 26–70 years were admitted in the Western Galilee Hospital by intoxication after consuming *L. sceleratus*. Two patients needed mechanical ventilation.[578,579]

Additionally, in 2010, Fernández-Ortega et al.[53] described the first European case of TTX intoxication in a patient who ingested part of a trumpet shellfish (*C. sauliae*) from the Atlantic Ocean in Southern Europe. Molluscum was captured in the southern coast of Portugal, during September 2007, which is when the waters are warmest. Landed in Huelva (South of Spain), it was transported in a refrigerated truck to Malaga (Spain) market, where it was purchased by the patient. The trumpet shellfish (*C. lampas sauliae*) had been implicated in some cases of TTX intoxication, indeed.

This case alerts us to the possibility that this toxin is in European coastal waters. This should be included in the differential diagnosis of similar cases in Europe, and we must be aware of their possible presence in Europe.

The recent report about the presence of TTX in the marine gastropod *C. lampas lampas* confirms that occurrence of TTX in Mediterranean Sea is a matter of concern. A potential explanation of these phenomena could be an ecological change due to the global warming effect.

6.6.5.2.4 Epidemiological Chain

6.6.5.2.4.1 Source of Intoxication Marine bacteria produce the TTX, and puffer fish and other organisms accumulate through the food chain that begins in bacteria. Marine bacterium that produced TTX was first reported in *Vibrio* sp. isolated from the intestines of a xanthid crab, *Atergatis floridus*.[580] After that, numerous TTX-producing bacteria have been isolated from various marine organisms, including *Shewanella alga* and *Alteromonas tetraodonis* isolated from a red alga *Jania* sp.[581]; *S. putrefaciens* from a TTX-bearing marine puffer *T. niphobles*[582]; *Pseudomonas* species from the marine red alga, *Jania* species, and *Pseudomonas* sp. from the skin of puffer fish, *Fugu poecilonotus*[583]; *Vibrio alginolyticus* from the starfish *A. polyacanthus*,[584] and the intestines of puffer fish, *Fugu vermicularis vermicularis*; *Alteromonas*, *Bacillus*, and *Vibrio* from the blue-ringed octopus[585]; *Vibrio*, *Aeromonas*, *Flavobacterium*, and *Pseudomonas* from the Taiwanese lined moon shell *Natica lineata*[586]; *Vibrio parahaemolyticus*, *V. alginolyticus*, *Pseudomonas*, and *Plesiomonas* from the a gastropod *N. clathrata*[587]; *V. alginolyticus* from the intestines of puffer fish *F. vermiculaaris radiatus*,[588] *Microbacterium arabinogalactanolyticum*, *Serratia marcescens*, and *V. alginolyticus* from puffer fish collected along the Hong Kong coastal waters.[589] TTX-producing bacteria have been isolated from marine and freshwater sediment.[590]

Finally, TTX-producing bacteria have been isolated from marine or freshwater sediment.[591–594] All these lead us to conclude that various species of bacteria are involved in TTX synthesis and in their introduction into the food chain.

6.6.5.2.4.2 Vectors   It was long believed that TTX was present only in the puffer fish. Mosher et al.[553] detected it in the eggs of the California newt *T. torosa* in 1964. After that, TTX was found in a wide variety of animals:

- Platyhelminthes
  - Flatworms (*Planocera* spp.)
- Nemertinea
  - Ribbonworms (*Lineus fuscoviridis*, *Tubulanus punctatus*, and *Cephalothrix linearis*)
- Mollusca
  - Gastropoda (*C. sauliae*, *Babylonia japonica*, *Tutufa lissostoma*, *Zeuxis siquijorensis*, *Niotha clathrata*, *N. lineata*, *Cymatium echo*, *Pugilina ternotoma*)
  - Cephalopoda (*Hapalochlaena maculosa*)
- Annelida: Polychaeta (*Pseudopolamilla occelata*)
- Arthropoda
  - Xanthidae crabs (*A. floridus*, *Zosimus aeneus*)
- Horseshoe crab (*Carcinoscorpius rotundicauda*)
- Chaetognatha: Arrow worms (*Parasagitta* spp., *Flaccisagitta* spp.)
- Echinodermata: Starfish (*Astropecten* spp.)
- Vertebrata
- Pisces: Goby (*Yongeichthys criniger*)
- Amphibia: Newts (*Taricha* spp., *Notophthalmus* spp., *Cynopsis* spp., *Triturus* spp.)
- Frogs (*Atelopus* spp., *Colostethus* sp., *Polypedates* sp., *Brachycephalus* spp.)

Noguchi and Arakawa[595] have proposed the nest mechanism to TTX accumulation in animals (Figure 6.2): The *Vibrio alginolyticus*, *S. alga*, *S. putrefaciens*, *Alteromonas tetraodonis*, and other marine bacteria produce TTX in parasitism or symbiosis with marine animals. The TTX can be incorporated by fish or

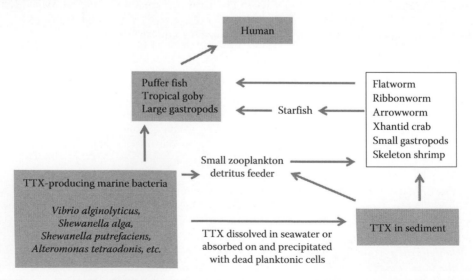

FIGURE 6.2 Mechanism to TTX accumulation in animals proposed by Noguchi and Arakawa. (From Noguchi, T. and Arakawa, O., *Mar Drugs*, 6, 220, 2008.)

large gastropods or eliminated to the seawater, being adsorbed on and precipitated with dead planktonic cells, and finally going to the marine sediment. From there, the TTX can enter the food chain passing through worms, crabs, and small gastropods, to starfish, and finally fish and large gastropods, and through these to humans.

Mechanism of transmission: The transmission to human poisoning is produced by ingestion of toxic puffer fish especially in Japan, China, and Taiwan, and less frequently by ingestion of tropical goby or by large gastropods. There have also been cases of ingestion of small gastropods, some fatal, in China and Taiwan.

In Japan, at least 22 species of marine puffer fish are toxic, all belonging to the family Tetraodontidae.[596–600] *L. wheeleri* and *L. gloveri* are generally considered nontoxic species, but sometimes have weak toxicity.[601] All species of the Ostraciontidae and Diodontidae families have no TTX, although the skin of Ostraciontidae contains a hemolytic ichthyotoxic possibly palytoxin.[602,603]

Cases of food poisoning due to ingestion of fish liver *Ostraciontidae* sometimes occurs in Japan, but the causative agent is a toxin with delayed hemolytic activity, possibly palytoxin or a similar substance, and not TTX or pahutoxin.[604]

The toxin of brackish water puffer fish species was identified as TTX,[605,606] but in the freshwater puffer fish species, PSP was detected as the main toxic principles.[607,608] Also, in some marine puffer fish (*Arothron* spp.) of the Philippines, and *Arothron firmamentum* from Japan, the main toxins are STX. Puffer fish toxicity shows remarkable individual and regional variations.

In the marine puffer fish species, toxicity is generally high in the liver and ovary followed by the intestines and skin, while in brackish water and freshwater, toxicity is higher in the skin. The muscles and testes are nontoxic or weakly toxic, except *L. lunaris* and *Chelonodon patoca*, and are regarded edible by the Japanese Ministry of Health, Labour and Welfare, including many toxic species. In *C. patoca* inhabiting brackish coastal waters and freshwater Okinawa, Amami Islands, Thailand/Bangladesh, and Cambodia, the skin has the highest toxicity.[609] In toxic marine puffer fish, liver toxicity shows very high throughout the year, except in the breeding season, during which the ovary becomes highly toxic due to the accumulation of TTX transferred from the liver.

Human intoxication from tetrodontoxin has occurred in a variety of species that live in diverse ecosystems including puffer and other tetraodontiformes fish, the blue-ringed octopus, mollusks, horseshoe crabs, and the Oregon newt. Moreover, TTX-containing fish exist in tropical waters throughout the world. For most populations, however, species that contain TTX do not constitute a significant part of the diet; gastropod mollusks, horseshoe, and other crabs are commonly eaten in Southeast Asia and, more specifically, Japan.

Small-sized brackish water and freshwater puffer fish have also occasionally caused food poisoning incidents, including fatal cases in Asian countries such as Thai, Bangladesh, and Cambodia, though the causative toxin is PSP or palytoxin-like toxin in freshwater species.[610–612]

In China and Taiwan, poisoning attributable to the ingestion of small gastropods such as *N. clathrata*, *N. vitellus*, *Oliva miniacea*, *O. Hirasei*, *Nassarius glande*, and *Z. samiplicutus* occurs frequently.[613–617] In July 2007, in Nagasaki, Japan, a food poisoning incident occurred due to the same type of small gastropod, *Alectryon glande*.

Poisoning by the ingestion of eggs of the horseshoe crab *C. rotundicauda* occasionally has registered in Thailand. The symptoms of the victims were mostly similar to those caused by TTX or PSP. The toxin of *C. rotundicauda* mainly consists of TTX and anhydroTTX,[618–620] but sometimes containing STX and neoSTX.[621] Therefore, the toxin responsible for the poisoning of the horseshoe crab is considered TTX and/or PSP.

It is possible that fatalities from eating some species of crab on Negros Island, Philippines, also resulted from TTX poisoning.

Fugu is a delicate dish prepared from *L. scleratus*, a poisonous fish that contains a potent neurotoxin TTX. Usually it is limited to Indo-Pacific Ocean, where it is responsible for many accidental deaths each year.

6.6.5.2.4.3 Risk Factors   No risk factors for TTX poisoning are known. It is likely that intoxication and its severity are dose dependent.

Age: Has not been shown to increase the risk of illness with the age. In Taiwan, the poisoning cases have been occurred in persons from 9 months to 71 years.

Temporal distribution: Cases occur during all months of the year.

Cooking and traditional methods of detoxification: The toxin is heat stable so that cooking is not protective. TTX concentrates in the viscera and roe of some animals, such as puffer fish. Presumably, removal of viscera will provide some measure of protection although cases have been reported where only the flesh of the fish was eaten. Previous exposure does not provide protection.

Many Japanese know that the puffer and especially their liver ("Kimo") are highly toxic. However, there are more than a few "Kimo" fans who dare to eat the liver in the belief that the toxin can be eliminated by their own special and traditional methods of detoxification. Consequently, food poisoning occurs frequently in Japan, caused mainly by the liver intake.

The prohibition on sale in markets and restaurants has not entirely stopped the poisoning due to the consumption of homemade "kimo," prepared with wild fish that did not pass health checks in the market.

In Taiwan and China do not eat puffer fish as often as the Japan, but there also have been many cases of poisoning. According to the register of TTX poisoning in Taiwan, there are some cases caused by the mistaken ingestion of muscles of a puffer fish species with toxic muscle, by ingesting puffer roe that had been sold as a fake of dried mullet roe called "karasumi" or by ingesting a dried dressed fish fillet produced from toxic puffer fish by a food processing company.[622–624]

6.6.5.2.5 Clinical Features

Symptom onset occurs within minutes and only rarely more than 6 h after eating a toxic animal. Perioral paresthesia is the most immediate and acral paresthesias the most common symptom. Nausea and vomiting may or may not occur. Disease may progress to dizziness, weakness, ataxia, dyspnea, diaphoresis, and death from respiratory failure. Similar to PSP, affected persons may report a floating sensation. Fukuda and Hani have divided TTX intoxication into four stages of progression:

Stage 1: Perioral and lingual numbness, with or without gastrointestinal symptoms (nausea, vomiting).

Stage 2: Numbness progresses markedly, with motor paralysis of extremities.

Stage 3: Progressive motor paralysis (aphonic, dysphagia, respiratory distress, and precordial chest pain) and bulbar muscle paralysis. The patient is still conscious.

Stage 4: Respiratory failure, hypoxia, unconsciousness and hypotension, and fixed and dilated pupils.

In 245 cases, of varying degrees of TTX poisoning, admitted to the medical service of Chon Buri Hospital between 1994 and 2006, Kanchanapongkul[625] observed that 100 were in stage 1; 74 were in stage 2; 3 were in stage 3, and 68 were in stage 4. The frequencies of symptoms and signs included the following: circumoral and lingual numbness (98%), hands and feet numbness (94.7%), weakness (59.6%), dizziness and vertigo (54.3%), nausea and vomiting (52.6%), transient hypertension (39.6%), respiratory paralysis (27.7%), fixed dilated pupils (14.7%), ophthalmoplegia (12.2%), blood pressure lower than 90/60 mmHg (5.7%), and polyuria (0.4%). The results of treatment are as follows: 239 patients (97.5%) showed complete recovery, 5 patients (2%) died, and 1 patient (0.4%) suffered anoxic brain damage. Diagnostic confirmation requires the analysis of samples of the fish and the patient's blood and urine using LC–MS.[626]

Similar to PSP, symptoms of TTX poisoning usually resolve within 1–2 days. The mortality rate is dependent on, among other things, timely access to intensive care facilities. When death results, it usually occurs within 6 h and sometimes as rapidly as 17 min, following toxin ingestion. The mortality rate from the retrospective analysis of 42 outbreaks of TTX-associated paralytic snail poisoning in Asia was 5.2% and 16% had respiratory arrest.[627] Persons who have not died within 24–48 h generally recovered completely.

6.6.5.2.6 Treatment

There is no antidote available. Treatment is supportive. When the poisoning is severe, intubation and mechanical ventilation are required. Usually, supportive care beyond 48 h is not necessary because the toxin is removed from the blood, becoming undetectable after 24 h.[628]

6.6.5.2.7 Public Health Issues

Some countries, including Japan, have enacted laws restricting the sale of certain species known to cause TTX poisoning. Japan and Taiwan have attempted to control TTX poisoning through licensing of restaurants and chefs or by establishing regulatory limits for the sale of puffer fish. As people may eat TTX from fish not served at restaurants, this approach will prevent only a portion of cases.

No regulatory limits for TTX have been established in the United States as personal importation of puffer fish is prohibited. An agreement between the US Food and Drug Administration and the Japanese Ministry of Health and Welfare has been adopted, which allows importation of *Fugu* for special occasions, provided the fish is certified safe by the Japanese government before export.

In the EU, according to the current European legislative requirements,[145–147] poisonous fish of the family Tetraodontidae and products derived from them must not be placed on the market. Despite this fact, however, one cannot exclude the possibility for accidental consumption of the species, as in the cases described earlier.

6.6.6 General Prevention

In order to systematize the prevention study, we first analyze primary prevention measures based on the sea and the market surveillance and aimed at effectively foreseeing the toxicity phenomena before it reaches the human intoxication stage. For this, a greater knowledge of the potential dinoflagellate's life cycle and influencing environmental factors is necessary. We also include here the watch for human poisoning cases to be carried out in countries where there is a possibility of setting up watching networks on the sea or in the market.

Second, we study the secondary prevention measures or measures to be adopted in a human poisoning outbreak.

Both sets of measures are fundamentally based on epidemiology watching. The weakest links in the epidemiological chain have to be identified in order to focus our attention on them.

It is not possible to act on the source of intoxication, thus avoiding the proliferation of dinoflagellates by modifying factors favorable to them. We are equally powerless in avoiding the accumulation of toxins in shellfish, or even in accelerating their detoxification. Relaying, which is moving batches of shellfish affected by biotoxins to toxin-free areas or sites where detoxification is faster, is a strategy proven successful. We can also act on the third chain link—the subjects at risk—by informing them of the hazards and providing all the means at our disposal to avoid toxic shellfish consumption. As stated earlier, dinoflagellates do not undergo organoleptic changes that would alert the consumer, and ordinary cooking does not destroy the toxins either.

In the epidemiology watch programs, it is essential to have tracers for intoxication prevention. The most widely known tracer is visualizing a red tide, which, albeit its limitations, prevents disease outbreak. Nevertheless, it is of very limited efficacy, because most of the events can take place without previous appearance of a red tide. The most efficient watch consists of determining changes in seawater warning of a potential proliferation of toxic plankton species and watching out for these species as well as the presence of toxins in shellfish.

In short, epidemiology watching is based on the early detection of a problem (presence of the marine toxins in shellfish). Each monitoring program or scheme must be adapted to the area, region, or country where it is going to be applied, bearing in mind the following:

- Incidence of the problem and its effects on the country's population and economy
- Legal infrastructure
- Available resources (human and material)
- Existing means of communication

6.6.7 Marine Biotoxin Monitoring Program

The potential monitoring of blooms requires knowledge of their ecological features. If they show signs that their increase might be due to modifiable factors (such as organic material contribution), the measures to be adopted would not be simple and would have to consider the whole fishery area as a whole.

With the data available nowadays, it seems that most blooms are controlled according to the hydrographical features of the shores, and therefore they cannot be modified, although a better understanding of them and the way they relate to phytoplankton would imply a higher capacity to predict potential events.

At present, predicting the exact appearance of blooms is not possible, hence prevention is based on setting a red tide early warning network and a self-check scheme in the purifying plant and the market, in order to determine the absence of marine toxins, at levels below those established by law. Self-detection programs are now at an advanced stage through satellite monitoring of temperature changes in seawater.

6.6.7.1 Marine Watching: Red Tide Warning Network

Sea-watching programs must be of several intensity levels, depending on the existence of toxic plankton species or conditions favoring their proliferation. There must be a perfect coordination and a fast and fluent communication network between the authorities responsible for sea watching (Fishing Administration) and for the markets (Health, Agriculture, and Food Administrations).
There are two subprograms:

1. Studies on plankton and conditions favoring its proliferation with a view to predict when toxic marine blooms are going to take place and to detect their existence (red tides) as early as possible
2. Monitoring shellfish to check the presence of toxins in authorized production areas before gathering and in purifying plants before shellfish is released on the market

In order to achieve efficient management, causing minimum disturbance to producers and allowing a safety warranty to the consumers of seafood, it is important to set zones and subzones in the shellfish farms, as well as fixed primary points shown to be most rapidly affected in the case of a toxic event, and, additionally, fixed secondary points which allow a more detailed knowledge of the affectation degree in the zones.

For sampling programs with follow-up and monitoring of toxic phytoplankton to work, better action schemes have to be set according to the species of phytoplankton causing toxicity and to the shellfish and areas affected. Those schemes have to be set before assessing the information gathered in the monitoring program on the plankton and oceanographic conditions and on the shellfish biotoxins. In Galicia (Spain), there are four action schemes set on those bases (www.intecmar.org).[629]

Scheme A (normal situation): Oceanic conditions are not favorable to the development of toxic phytoplankton species, nor are these found in significant concentrations, and there is no toxicity in bivalve shellfish.

Scheme B (alert situation), divided into three subschemes:

B1: When, in spite of favorable oceanic conditions, no potentially toxic phytoplankton species are observed in significant concentrations, and there is no toxicity in bivalve shellfish either.
B2: There are favorable oceanic conditions and the presence of potentially toxic phytoplankton species, but no toxicity in bivalve shellfish.
B3: There are favorable oceanic conditions, a significant increase in toxic population, and toxicity is detected in bivalve shellfish but in levels below the limits established by law.

Scheme C (extraction is forbidden): This is applied when toxic levels are above the law-established limits. It is divided into three subschemes:

C1: Oceanic conditions are favorable, and there is a significant increase in toxic population and in bivalve shellfish toxicity levels.

C2: Oceanic conditions are not favorable to the growth of the toxic plankton species whose population is stable or decreasing. Also, toxicity levels in the bivalve shellfish are stable or decreasing.

C3: Oceanic conditions are not favorable, and there is a significant decreasing and disappearing of toxic population, and toxicity levels are close to legal limits.

Scheme D: Oceanic conditions are not favorable to the development of toxic plankton species: potentially toxic phytoplankton species are in insignificant concentrations or absent, and toxicity stays below legal limits as a consequence of a previous event.

Bivalve shellfish samples cultivated on floating platforms must be gathered at different depths (1, 5, and 10 m), since toxicity may vary with water depth. Analysis must be carried out separately or integrated, depending on the uniformity of the degree of mussels and oceanic conditions, and accumulation of toxicity at a given depth. In natural fisheries and fish farms, samples should be as significant as possible, according to the species subjected to monitoring and the area features.

Sampling frequency varies with every action scheme:

Scheme A (all-year round): Weekly sampling of oceanic and phytoplankton conditions, as well as of biotoxins in mussels in fixed primary points, and fortnightly sampling in rock mussels.

Scheme B (alert situation):

B1: Weekly sampling of oceanic and phytoplankton conditions, as well as of biotoxins.

B2: Increasing to twice per week the sampling for biotoxins in mussels in fixed primary points.

B3: Increasing the sampling to three times per week, and when biotest results advise it, sampling of other species in fixed secondary points, susceptible to being more affected.

Scheme C (gathering is forbidden):

C1: The toxic event intensity and the existing provisions dictate the frequency and species to be sampled. Subzones (included within the same zone) bordering on a closed-down subzone are subjected to daily sampling.

C2: Gathering samples in fixed primary or secondary points to assess the degree of affectation in the zone or subzone.

C3: Sample gathering for biotoxins at least three times per week.

Scheme D: Lifting of extraction prohibition. In fixed points where toxicity remains high, though below legal limits, samples are to be gathered twice a week.

Detailed information can be seen on the Intecmar website (http://www.intecmar.org/Intecmar/Biotoxinas.aspx?sm = f).

6.6.7.2 Market Watching

Veterinary inspectors responsible for monitoring the salubrity and hygienic conditions of food carry out routine controls throughout the year. Surveillance should increase during periods when these problems tend to be present.

6.6.8 Surveillance of the Disease

Surveillance of the disease may be particularly relevant as an alternative method to primary prevention in countries that are not able to afford the cost of sustained surveillance programs in shellfish farming areas. In such circumstances, the first cases of the disease detected have to be used to adopt preventive measures and avoid further cases. At any rate, a minimum public health infrastructure should be available, such as staff with adequate training and laboratories with staff trained in standard techniques.

The education of medical and public health staff regarding diagnosis, treatment (symptomatic), and notification of suspect cases is very important for the success of a watch program.

Education of populations at risk about preventive measures, such as nonconsumption of shellfish when there are toxic red tides and never-to-eat mussels picked from cliff rocks or any shellfish picked directly on beaches, is essential and never enough. People must be well informed and updated through the most suitable means about the presence of toxic red tides, their blooming, and their disappearance.

Finally, education and cooperation with the seafood industry in everything related to poisoning risks by marine toxins as well as in primary and secondary prevention programs are necessary for the effective success of these programs.

6.6.9 Epidemiological Investigation of an Acute Outbreak of Disease

Human poisoning outbreaks may seem to be explosive, localized, and short-lived (holomiantic outbreaks), given the very short incubation period (minutes or hours), which depends on, besides toxin class, the amount of toxin swallowed (shellfish toxic load and the amount of shellfish eaten) and the exposure to a common source.

Investigations usually start from the communication of index cases to the health authorities. That reporting, which is mandatory in many countries when there is an outbreak, must be done when clinical suspicion exists, but since this is subjective, the first step will have to be to confirm the case diagnosis. Confirming the diagnosis is easier when there are toxic red tides and when physicians and populations are alerted. Isolated cases of shellfish poisoning will go undetected if they are not considered, given its unspecific symptomatology in DSP: diarrhea, nausea, vomiting, abdominal pain, and its mildness. In addition, etiology identification of clusters is even easier (episodes in which two or more cases of the same disease are interrelated).

Urgent notification to the health authorities, from the mere suspicion, is required so that they can adopt the pertinent administrative preventive measures.

During the investigation of outbreak, the three following stages are clearly marked:

1. Setting or verifying diagnosis of recorded cases and confirming the existence of an outbreak
2. Identifying the intoxication source and transmission mode
3. Identifying other people who might have been or are exposed, as well as cases that might have appeared previously: and the description of cases according to the person, place, and time variables

6.6.9.1 Outbreak Confirmation

First of all, in order to establish environmental exposure, existence of a toxic red tide, and then confirm the diagnosis in the laboratory (seafood testing), it has to be decided whether the signs and symptoms and their evolution correspond to shellfish poisoning, whether the incubation period is short (minutes to a few hours), and whether there are antecedents of shellfish or fish consumption (appropriate seafood ingestion) in its origin.

Other causes, such as toxic infection by *B. cereus* or by *V. parahaemolyticus* in DSP suspected, have to be excluded; shellfish also carries the latter. Those affected usually do not present with fever, but their incubation period is longer (12 h), and the germ can be identified in feces or food remains.

Gastroenteritis associated with a clinical picture of no fever, mussel ingestion, and a short incubation period point toward diagnosis of DSP, even more so if there is a DSP-toxic red tide at the time.

Based on the study of the Japanese outbreaks, the World Health Organization (1984) established the following symptoms in DSP disease: diarrhea (92%), nausea (80%), vomiting (79%), abdominal pain (53%), and chill (10%).

The poisoning that appears with neurological disorders is easier to identify if you have the foresight to ask for a history of recent ingestion of shellfish or exotic fish.

In order to obtain laboratory confirmation, food remains should be available (uneaten mussels) or mussel samples should be taken from the same area that the eaten mussels came from (e.g., food market, shellfish purifying plant, fish farm, and rocks).

The usual technique used is the bioassay in mice developed by Yasumoto that we described in the European Regulations, but the bioassay in mice is subject to false positives by interference of nonphyto-toxic components. There are also chemical methods such as HPLC, the most widely used method after bioassays; LC-MS; the enzyme-inhibition assays such as protein phosphatase inhibition assays, an inexpensive technique, and the immunoassays (monoclonal antibodies to OA and DTX-1, and enzyme-linked immunosorbent assay).

These techniques, and more so the bioassays, HPLC, and phosphatase inhibition, are generally used in health surveillance. Ethical and technical considerations are being focused on the development and use of health-control tests that do not require the use of animals.

6.6.9.2 Identifying Source, Transmission Mechanism, and Subjects at Risk

It is essential to know the kind of shellfish responsible for DSP or AZA intoxication and their origin, whether they were bought in the market or picked directly in fish farms or rocks, and whether there are some not yet consumed. It is also necessary to know whether they were eaten at home, in a restaurant, or in other public places.

It is also important to know whether other people have also eaten the product, searching for other cases or whether there are people who have more shellfish from the same source and have not yet consumed it. Moreover, it has to be investigated whether there have been previous cases in the area or surrounding areas.

6.6.9.3 Describing Cases according to Person, Place, and Time Variables

Regarding the person variable, information must be gathered on age, sex, and occupation: as far as the place variable is concerned, geographic distribution of the cases concerned, noting their addresses; and regarding time, it is interesting to have information on the date, time of exposure (shellfish ingestion), as well as the onset of the first symptoms and sequence of presentation. It is also advisable to collect information leading to an initial idea of the toxic load.

6.6.9.4 Administration Monitoring Measures

In the event of an outbreak, administration measures will have to be adopted forbidding shellfish gathering and setting up an area-monitoring scheme. Continuous vigilance must be exercised for the occurrence of DSP or AZA poisoning, and physicians must be warned of its existence so that they can be alert for the clinical signs of gastroenteritis. At the same time, the population will have to be made aware: industrialists, health professionals, and people in general through the mass media, warning about the hazards and advising that they must not consume the affected shellfish.

ACKNOWLEDGMENTS

I extend my thanks to Dr. Monica Perez Rios, Pharmacy PhD, for her contribution to the literature search.

REFERENCES

1. Exodus 7:v. 20–21 *The Bible*. King James Versión.
2. Kao, C.Y. 1966. Tetrodotoxin, saxitoxin and their significance in the study of excitation phenomena. *Pharmacol Rev* 18: 997–1049.
3. Hwang, D.F. and Noguchi, T. 2007. Tetrodotoxin poisoning. *Adv Food Nutr Res* 52: 142–236.
4. Mosher, H.S., Fuhrman, F.A., Buchwald, H.D., and Fischer, H.G. 1964. Tarichatoxin–tetrodotoxin: A potent neurotoxin. *Science* 144: 1100–1110.

5. Noguchi, T. and Hashimoto, Y. 1973. Isolation of tetrodotoxin from a goby *Gobius criniger*. *Toxicon* 11: 305–307.
6. Halstead, N.B. 1965. *Poisonous and Venomous Marine Animals of the World*, Vol. I, *Invertebrates*. Washington, DC: Government Printing Office.
7. Baden, D.G., Fleming, L.E., and Bean, J.A. 1995. Marine toxins. In: de Wolff, F.A., ed., *Handbook of Clinical Neurology: Intoxications of the Nervous System. II. Natural Toxins and Drugs*. Amsterdam, the Netherlands: Elsevier Science, pp. 141–175.
8. Ansdell, V.E. 2009. The pre-travel consultation counseling and advice for travelers: Food poisoning from marine toxins. In: *Travelers' Health—Yellow Book*. Atlanta, GA: Centers for Disease Control and Prevention. http://wwwn.cdc.gov/travel/yellowbook/2010/chapter-2/food-poisoningfrom- marine-toxins.aspx
9. Chevalier, A. and Duchesne, E.A. 1851. Memoire sur les empoisonnements par les huítres, les moules, les crabes, et par certains poissons de mer et de riviere. *Ann Hyg Publ (París)* 45(1): 108–147.
10. Chevalier, A. and Duchesne, E.A. 1851. Memoire sur les empoisonnements par les huítres, les moules, les crabs, et par certains poissons de mer et de riviere. *Ann Hyg Publ (París)* 45(2): 387–437.
11. Vancouver, G. 1801. *A Voyage of Discovery to the North Pacific Ocean and Round the World*. London, U.K.: John Stockdale, Vol. 4, pp. 44–47.
12. Rey, J.R. La Ciguatera. ENY-741S (IN747). Department of Entomology and Nematology, Institute of Food and Agricultural Sciences, University of Florida, Gainesville, FL, http://edis.ifas.ufl.edu/in747 (accessed October 11, 2013).
13. Randal, J.E. 1958. A review of ciguatera tropical fish poisoning with a tentative explanation of its cause. *Bull Mar Sci Gulf Carib* 8: 236–267.
14. Scheuer, P.S., Takahashi, W., Tsutsumi, J., and Yoshida, T. 1967. Ciguatoxin: Isolation and chemical nature. *Science* 155: 1267–1268.
15. Yasumoto, T., Nakajima, I., Bagnis, R. et al. 1977. Finding a dinoflagellate as a likely culprit of ciguatera. *Bull Jpn Soc Sci Fish* 43: 1021–1026.
16. Murata, M., Legrand, M.A., Ishibashi, Y., and Yasumoto, T. 1989. Structure of ciguatoxin and its congener. *J Am Chem Soc* 111: 8929–8931.
17. Meyer, K.E., Sommer, K.F., and Schoenholz, P. 1928. Mussel poisoning. *J Prev Med* 2: 365–394.
18. Sommer, K.F. and Meyer, K.E. 1937. Paralytic shellfish poisoning. *Arch Pathol* 24(5): 560–598.
19. Korringa, P. and Roskam, R.T. 1961. An unusual case of mussel poisoning. *International Council of the Exploration of the Sea (ICES)*. Council Meeting/Shellfish Committee 49, 2pp.
20. Rossebe, L., Thorson, B., and Asse, R. 1970. Etiologisk uklar matforgifnig etter konsum av blaskjell. *Norsk Vet Tidsskr* 2: 639–642.
21. Kat, M. 1979. The occurrence of *Prorocentrum* species and coincidental gastrointestinal illness of mussels consumers. In: Taylor, D. and Seliger, H.H., eds., *Toxic Dinoflagellate Blooms*. Amsterdam, the Netherlands: Elsevier, pp. 215–220.
22. Yasumoto, T., Oshima, Y., and Yamaguchi, M. 1979. Ocurrence of a new type of shellfish poisoning in Japan and chemical properties of the toxin. In: Taylor, D. and Seliger, H.H., eds., *Toxic Dinoflagellate Blooms*. Amsterdam, the Netherlands: Elsevier, pp. 495–502.
23. Gestal Otero, J.J., Hernández Cochón, J.M., Bao Fernández, O., and Martínez-Risco López, L. 1978. Brote de Mitilotoxismo en la Provincia de La Coruña. *Bol Inst Espa Océano IV* 258: 5–29.
24. Yasumoto, T., Oshima, Y., and Yamaguchi, M. 1978. Ocurrence of a new type shellfish poisoning in the Tohoku district. *Bull Jpn Soc Sci Fish* 44: 1249–1255.
25. Yasumoto, T., Oshima, Y., Sugawara, W., Fukuyo, Y., Oguri, H., Igarishi, T., and Fujita, N. 1980. Identification of *Dinophysis fortii* as the causative organism of diarrhetic shellfish poisoning. *Bull Jpn Soc Sci Fish* 46: 1405–1411.
26. Comesaña Losada, M., Leao, J.M., Gago-Martinez, A., Rodriguez Vazquez, J.A., and Quilliam, M.A. 1999. Further studies on the analysis of DSP toxin profiles in Galician mussels. *J Agric Food Chem* 47: 618–621.
27. Gago-Martinez, A., Rodriguez-Vazquez, J.A., Thibault, P., and Quilliam, M.A. 1996. Simultaneous occurrence of diarrhetic and paralytic shellfish poisoning toxins in Spanish mussels in 1993. *Nat Toxins* 4: 72–79.
28. Morono, A., Arevalo, F., Fernandez, M.L., Maneiro, J., Pazos, Y., Salgado, C., and Blanco, J. 2003. Accumulation and transformation of DSP toxins in mussels *Mytilus galloprovincialis* during a toxic episode caused by *Dinophysis acuminata*. *Aquat Toxicol* 62: 269–280.

29. Bates, S.S., Bird, C.J., de Freitas, A.S.W. et al. 1989. Pennate diatom *Nitzschia pungens* as the primary source of domoic acid, a toxin in shellfish from Eastern Prince Edward Island, Canada. *Can J Fisher Aquat Sci* 46: 1203–1215.

30. Wright, J.L.C., Boyd, R.K., Freitas, A. et al. 1989. Identification of domoic acid, a neuroexcitatory aminoacid, in toxic mussels from Eastern Prince Edward Island. *Can J Chem* 67: 481–490.

31. Perl, T.M., Bedard, L., Kosatsky, T., Hockin, J.C., Todd, E.C., and Remis, R.S. 1990. An outbreak of toxic encephalopathy caused by eating mussels contaminated with domoic acid. *N Engl J Med* 322: 1775–1780.

32. Takemoto, T. and Daigo, K. 1958. Constituents of *Chondria armata*. *Chem Pharm Bull* 6: 578–580.

33. Daigo, K. 1959. Studies on the constituents of *Chondria armata*. I. Detection of the anthelmintical constituents. *J Jpn Pharm Assoc* 79: 350–353.

34. Daigo, K. 1959. Studies on the constituents of *Chondria armata*. II. Isolation of an antihelmintical constituent. *J Pharm Soc Jpn* 79: 353–356.

35. Daigo, K. 1959. Studies on the constituents of *Chondria armata*. III. Constitution of domoic acid. *J Pharm Soc Jpn* 79: 356–360.

36. McMahon, T. and Silke, J. 1996. West coast of Ireland; winter toxicity of unknown aetiology in mussels. *Harmful Algae News* 14: 2.

37. Ito, E., Terao, K., McMahon, T., Silke, J., and Yasumoto, T. 1998. Acute pathological changes in mice caused by crude extracts of novel toxins isolated from Irish mussels. In: *Harmful Algae*. Reguera, B., Blanco, J., Fernandez, M.L., and Wyatt, T. (eds.). IOC of UNESCO and Xunta de Galicia, Santiago de Compostela, Spain, pp. 588–589.

38. Satake, M., Ofugi, K., James, K.J., Furey, A., and Yasumoto, T. 1997. New toxic event caused by Irish mussels. In: *Harmful Algae*, Reguera, B., Blanco, J., Fernandez, M.L., and Wyatt, T. (eds.). IOC of UNESCO and Xunta de Galicia, Santiago de Compostela, Spain, pp. 468–469.

39. Satake, M., Ofuji, K., Naoki, H., James, K.J., Furey, A., McMahon, T., Silke, J., and Yasumoto, T. 1998. Azaspiracid, a new marine toxin having unique spiro ring assemblies, isolated from Irish mussels, *Mytilus edulis*. *J Am Chem Soc* 120: 9967–9968.

40. Mons, M.N., Van Egmond, H.P., and Speijers, G.J.A. 1998. Paralytic shellfish poisoning: A review. RIVM Report 388802 005.

41. Van Dolah, F.M. 2000. Diversity of marine and freshwater algal toxins. In: Botana, L., ed., *Seafood Toxicology Pharmacology, Physiology and Detection*. New York: Marcel Dekker, pp. 19–43.

42. Scholin, C.A., Gulland, F., Doucette, G.J. et al. 2000. Mortality of sea lions along the central California coast linked to a toxic diatom bloom. *Nature* 403: 80–84.

43. Smayda, T.J. 1997. Harmful algal blooms: Their ecophysiology and general relevance to phytoplankton blooms in the sea. *Limnol Oceanogr* 42: 1137–1153.

44. James, K.J., Carey, B., O'Halloran, J., van Pelt, F.N.A.M., and Skrabakova, Z. 2010. Shellfish toxicity: Human health implications of marine algal toxins. *Epidemiol Infect* 138: 927–940.

45. Hallegraeff, G.M. 1993. A review of harmful algal blooms and their apparent global increase. *Phycologia* 32(2): 79–99.

46. Hallegraeff, G.M., Bolch, C.J., Bryan, J., and Koerbin, B. 1990. Microalgal spores in ship's ballast water: A danger to aquaculture. In: Graneli, E., Sundström, B., Edler, L., and Anderson, D.M., eds., *Toxic Marine Phytoplankton*. *Proceedings of the Fourth International Conference Toxic Marine Phytoplankton*, Lund, Sweden, June 26–30, 1989. New York: Elsevier, pp. 475–480.

47. Ueoka, R., Ito, A., Izumikawa, M. et al. 2009. Isolation of azaspiracid-2 from a marine sponge *Echinoclathria* sp. as a potent cytotoxin. *Toxicon* 53: 680–684.

48. Brescianini, C., Grillom, C., Melchiorre, N. et al. 2006. Ostreopsis ovata algal blooms affecting human health in Genova, Italy, 2005–2006. *Eurosurveillance* 11(9): E060907.3.

49. Durando, P., Ansaldi, F., Oreste, P. et al., and the Collaborative Group for the Ligurian Syndromic Algal Surveillance. 2007. *Ostreopsis ovata* and human health: Epidemiological and clinical features of respiratory syndrome outbreaks from a two-year syndromic surveillance, 2005–06, in north-west Italy. *Eurosurveillance* 12(23): E070607.1, June 7, 2007.

50. Ciminiello, P., Dell'Aversano, C., Fattorusso, E. et al. 2006. The Genoa 2005 outbreak. Determination of putative palytoxin in Mediterranean *Ostreopsis ovata* by a new liquid chromatography tandem mass spectrometry method. *Anal Chem* 78: 6153–6159.

51. Sansoni, G., Borghini, B., Camici, G., Casotti, M., Righini, P., and Fustighi, C. 2003. Fioriture algali di Ostreopsis ovata (Gonyaulacales: Dinophyceae): Un problema emergente. *Biol Ambient* 17(1): 17–23.
52. Gallitelli, M., Ungaro, N., Addante, L.M., Gentiloni, N., and Sabbà, C. 2005. Respiratory illness as a reaction to tropical algal blooms occurring in a temperate climate. *JAMA* 239(21): 2599–2600.
53. Fernández-Ortega, J.F., Morales-de los Santos, J.M., Herrera-Gutiérrez, M.E., Fernández-Sánchez, V., Rodríguez Loureo, P., Alfonso Rancaño, A., and Téllez-Andrade, A. 2010. Seafood intoxication by tetrodotoxin: First case in Europe. *J Emerg Med* 39(5): 612–617.
54. Moore, S.K., Trainer, V.L., Mantua, N.J. et al. 2008. Impacts of climate variability and future climate change on harmful algal blooms and human health. *Environ Health* 7(Suppl 2): S4.
55. Pearl, H.W. and Whitall, D.R. 1999. Anthropogenically-driven atmospheric nitrogen deposition, marine eutrophication and harmful algal bloom expansion: Is there a link? *Ambio* 28: 307–311.
56. Shumway, S.E. 1995. Phycotoxin-related shellfish poisoning: Bivalve molluscs are not the only vectors. *Rev Fish Sci* 3: 1–31.
57. Lawrence, J.F., Maher, M., and Watson-Wright, W. 1994. Effect of cooking on the concentration of toxins associated with paralytic shellfish poison in lobster hepatopancreas. *Toxicon* 32(1): 57–64.
58. Bretz, C.K., Manouki, T.J., and Kvitek, R.G. 2002. Emerita análoga (Stimpson) as an indicator species for paralytic shellfish poison toxicity along the California coast. *Toxicon* 40: 1189–1196.
59. Ferdin, M.E., Kvitek, R.G., Bretz, C.K., Powell, C.L., Doucette, G.J., Lefebvre, K.A., Coale, S., and Silver, M.W. 2002. Emerita analoga (Stinpson)—Possible new indicator species for the phycotoxin domoic acid in Californian coastal waters. *Toxicon* 40: 1259–1265.
60. Oikawa, H., Fujita, T., Satomi, M., Suzuki, T., Kotani, Y., and Yano, Y. 2002. Accumulation of paralytic shellfish poisoning toxins in the edible shore crab *Telmessus acutidens. Toxicon* 40: 1593–1599.
61. Costa, P., Rodrigues, S.M., Botelho, M.J., and Sampayo, M.A.M. 2003. A potential vector of domoic acid: The swimming crab *Polybius henslowii* Leach (*Decapoda-brachyura). Toxicon* 42: 135–141.
62. Vale, P. and Sampayo, M.A.M. 2002. First confirmation of human diarrhoeic poisonings by okadaic acid esters after ingestion of razor clams (*Solen marginatus*) and green grabs (*Carcinus maenas*) in Aveiro lagoon, Portugal and detection of okadaic acid esters in phytoplankton. *Toxicon* 40: 33–42.
63. Castberg, T., Torgersen, T., Aasen, J., Aune, T., and Naustvoll, L.-J. 2004. DSP toxins in *Cancer pagurus*, Linnaeus 1757, in Norwegian waters (Bracyura, Cancridae). *Sarsia* 89: 311–317.
64. Torgersen, T., Aasen, J., and Aune, T. 2005. Diarrhetic shellfish poisoning by okadaic acid esters from Brown crabs (*Cancer pagurus*) in Norway. *Toxicon* 46: 572–578.
65. Murata, M., Shimatani, M., Sugitani, H., Oshima, Y., and Yasumoto, T. 1982. Isolation and structure elucidation of the causative toxin of the diarrhetic shellfish poisoning. *Bull Jpn Soc Sci Fish* 43: 549–552.
66. Tachibana, K., Scheuer, P.J., Tsukitani, Y., Kikuchi, H., van Engen, D., Clardy, J., Gopichand, Y., and Schmitz, F.J. Okadaic acid, a cytotoxic polyether from two marine sponges of the genus *Halichondria. J Am Chem Soc* 103: 2469–2471.
67. Yasumoto, T., Murata, M., Oshima, Y., Sano, M., Matsumoto, G.K., and Clardy, J. 1985. Diarrhetic shellfish toxins. *Tetrahedron* 41: 1019–1025.
68. Hu, T., Defreitas, A.S.W., Doyle, J., Jackson, D., Marr, J., Nixon, E., Pleasance, S., Quilliam, M.A., Walter, J.A., and Wright, J.L.C. 1992. Isolation of a new diarrhetic shellfish poison from Irish mussels. *Chem Commun* 30: 39–41.
69. Blanco, J., Fernández, M.L., Marino, J., Reguera, B., Miguez, A., Maneiro, J., and Cacho, E. 1995. A preliminary model of toxin accumulation in mussels. In: Lassus, P., Arzul, P., Erard, L.E., Denn, E., Gentien, P., and Marcaillou Lebaut, C., eds., *Harmful Marine Algal Blooms*. París, France: Lavoisier Science Publishers, pp. 777–782.
70. Vale, P. and Sampayo, M.A.M. 1996. DTX-2 in Portuguese bivalves. In: Yasumoto, T., Oshima, Y., and Fukuyo Y., eds., *Harmful and Toxic Algal Blooms*. Paris, France: IOC of UNESCO, pp. 539–542.
71. Wright, J.L.C. 1995. Dealing with seafood toxins: Present approaches and future options. *Food Res Int* 28: 347–358.
72. García, C., Truan, D., Lagos, M., Santelices, J.P., Díaz, J.C., and Lagos, N. 2005. Metabolic transformation of dinophysistoxin-3 into dinophysistoxin-1 causes human intoxication by consumption of o-acyl-derivatives dinophysistoxins contaminated shellfish. *J Toxicol Sci* 30(4): 287–296.
73. Carmody, E.P., James, K., Kellt, S., and Thomas, K. 1995. Complex diarrhetic shellfish toxin profiles in Irish Mussels. In: Lassus, P., Arzul, G., Erard, L.E., Denn, E., Gentien, P., and Marcaillou Lebaut, C., eds., *Harmful Marine Algal Blooms*. París, France: Lavoisier Science Pub, pp. 273–278.

74. Yasumoto, T., Murata, M., Oshima, Y., Matsumoto, G.K., and Clardy, J. 1984. Diarrhetic shellfish poisoning. In: Ragelis, E.P., ed., *Seafood Toxins*. American Chemical Society, Symposium Series No. 262, Washington, DC: ACM, pp. 207–216.
75. Murata, M., Masaki, S., Iwashita, T., Naoki, H., and Yasumoto, T. 1986. The structure of pectenotoxin-3, a new constituent of diarrhetic shellfish toxins. *Agric Biol Chem* 50: 2693–2695.
76. Terao, H., Ito, E., Yanagi, T., and Yasumoto, T. 1986. Histopathological studies on experimental marine toxin poisoning I. Ultrastructural changes in the small intestine and liver of suckling mice induced by dinophysistoxin 1 and pectenotoxin 1. *Toxicon* 24: 1141–1151.
77. Ishige, M., Satoh, N., and Yasumoto, T. 1988. Pathological studies on the mice administered with the causative agent of diarrhetic shellfish poisoning (okadaic acid and pectenotoxin-2). *Hokkaido Inst Health* 38: 15–19.
78. Draisci, R., Lucentini, L., and Mascioni, A. 2000. Pectenotoxins and yessotoxins: Chemistry, toxicology, pharmacology, and analysis. In: Botana, L.M., ed., *Seafood Toxicity: Mode of Action, Pharmacology, and Physiology of Phycotoxins*. New York: Marcel Dekker, pp. 289–324.
79. Spector, I., Braet, F., Shochet, N.R., and Bubb, M.R. 1999. New anti-actin drugs in the study of the organization and function of the actin cytoskeleton. *Microsc Res Tech* 47: 18–37.
80. Leira, F., Cabado, A.G., Vieytes, M.R., Roman, Y., Alfonso, A., Botana, L.M., Yasumoto, T., Malaguti, C., and Rossini, G.P. 2002. Characterization of F-actin depolymerization as a major toxic event induced by pectenotoxin-6 in neuroblastoma cells. *Biochem Pharmacol* 63: 1979–1988.
81. Vale, P. and Sampayo, M.A.D. 2002. Pectenotoxin-2 seco acid, 7-epi-pectenotoxin-2 seco acid and pectenotoxin-2 in shellfish and plankton from Portugal. *Toxicon* 40: 979–987.
82. Ares, I.R., Louzao, M.C., Vieytes, M.R., Yasumoto, T., and Botana, L.M. 2005. Actin cytoskeleton of rabbit intestinal cells is a target for potent marine phycotoxins. *J Exp Biol* 208: 4345–4354.
83. Ares, I.R., Louzao, M.C., Espina, B., Vieytes, M.R., Miles, C.O., Yasumoto, T., and Botana, L.M. 2007. Lactone ring of pectenotoxins: A key factor for their activity on cytoskeletal dynamics. *Cell Physiol Biochem* 19: 283–292.
84. Alexander, J., Benford, D., Cockburn, A. et al. 2009. Marine biotoxins in shellfish—Pectenotoxin group. *EFSA J* 1109: 1–49.
85. Cohén, P., Holmes, C.F.B., and Tsukitani, Y. 1990. Okadaic acid: A new probé for the study of cellular regulation. *Trends Biochem Sci* 15: 98–102.
86. Fujiki, H., Suganuma, M., Suguri, H., Yoshizawa, S., Takagi, K., Sassa, T., Uda, N. et al. 1988. Diarrhetic shellfish toxin, dinophysistoxin-1, is a potent tumor promoter on mouse skin. *Jpn J Cáncer Res* 79: 1089–1093.
87. Ten-Hage, L., Delaunay, N., Pichon, V., Coute, A., Puiseux-Dao, S., and Turquet, J. 2000. Okadaic acid production from the marine benthic dinoflagellate *Prorocentrum arenarium Faust* (Dinophyceae) isolated from Europa Island coral reef ecosystem (SW Indian Ocean). *Toxicon* 38: 1043–1054.
88. Creppy, E.E., Traore, A., Baudrimont, I., Cascante, M., and Carratu, M.R. 2002. Recent advances in the study of epigenetic effects induced by the phycotoxin okadaic acid. *Toxicology* 181–182: 433–439.
89. Suganuma, M., Fujiki, H., Suguri, H., Yoshizawa, S., Hirota, M., Nakayasu, M., Okika, M., Wakamatsu, K., Yamada, K., and Sugimura, T. 1988. Okadaic acid: An aditional non phorbol-12-tetradecanoate-13-acetate-type promotor tumoral. *Proc Natl Acad Sci USA* 85(6): 1768–1771.
90. Aonuma, S., Ushijima, T., Nakayasu, M., Shima, H., Sugimura, T., and Nagao, M. 1991. Mutation induction by okadaic acid, a protein phosphatase inhibitor in CHL cells, but not in *S. Typhimurium*. *Mutat Res* 250: 375–381.
91. Hokama, Y., Scheuer, P.J., and Yasumoto, T. 1989. Effect of marine toxin on human peripheral blood monocytes. *J Clin Lab Anal* 3: 215–221.
92. Sundstrom, B., Edler, L., and Granéli, E. 1990. The global distribution of harmful effects of phytoplankton. In: Granéli, E., Sundstrom, B., Edler, L., and Anderson, D.M., eds., *Toxic Marine Phytoplankton*. Amsterdam, the Netherlands: Elsevier, pp. 537–541.
93. Gayoso, A.M. and Ciocco, N. 2001. Observations on *Prorocentrum lima* from North Patagonian coastal waters (Argentina) associated with a human diarrhoeic disease episode. *Harmful Algae News* 22: 4.
94. Campos, M.J., Fraga, S., Marino, J., and Sánchez, F.J. 1982. Red tide monitoring program in NW Spain. Report of 1977–1981. *International Council for the Exploration of the Sea (ICES), Council Meeting* 1982/L:2.
95. Van Egmond, H.P., Aune, T., Lassus, P., Speijers, G.J.A., and Waldock, M. 1993. Paralytic and diarrhoeic shellfish poisons: Occurrence in Europe, toxicity, analysis and regulation. *J Nat Toxins* 2(1): 41–79.

96. Hald, B., Bjergskov, T., and Emsholm, H. 1991. Monitoring and analytical programmes on phycotoxins in Denmark. In: Fremy, J.M., ed., *Proceedings of the Symposium on Marine Biotoxins*. Paris, France: Centre National d'Etudes Vétérinaires et Alimentaires de France, pp. 181–187.

97. Dahl, E. and Yndestad, M. 1985. Diarrheic shellfish poisoning (DSP) in Norway in the autumn 1984 related to the occurrence of *Dinophysis* spp. In: Anderson, D.M., White, A.W., and Badén, D.G., eds., *Toxic Dinoflagellates*. Amsterdam, the Netherlands: Elsevier, pp. 495–500.

98. Krogh, P., Edler, L., and Granéli, E. 1985. Outbreaks of diarrheic shellfish poisoning on the west coast of Sweden. In: Anderson, D.M., White, A.W., and Badén, D.G., eds., *Toxic Dinoflagellates*. Amsterdam, the Netherlands: Elsevier, pp. 501–504.

99. Vale, P. and Sampayo, M.A.M. 1999. Esters of okadaic acid and dinophysistoxin-2 in Portuguese bivalves related to human poisonings. *Toxicon* 37: 1109–1121.

100. Correia, A.M., Goncalves, G., and Saraiva, M.M. 2004. Foodborne outbreaks in the northern Portugal, 2002. *Eurosurveillance* 9(1–3): 18–20.

101. Anon. 1994. Diarrhetic shellfish poisoning associated with mussels. *CDR Weekly* 4: 101.

102. Scoging, A.C. and Bahl, M. 1998. Diarrhetic shellfish poisoning in the UK. *Lancet* 352: 117.

103. Anon. 1997. An outbreak of diarrhetic shellfish poisoning. *CDR Weekly* 7: 247.

104. Pavela-Vrančič, M., Vestrovic, V., Marasova, I., Gillman, M., Furey, A., and James, K.J. 2002. DSP toxin profile in the coastal waters of Central Adriatic Sea. *Toxicon* 40: 1601–1607.

105. Mozetic, P. and Bozic, P. 2001. DSP events in Slovenia: A need for legislative regulation. *Harmful Algae Management and Mitigation 2001*, Abstracts.

106. Economou, V., Papadopoulou, C., Brett, M., Kansouzidou, A., Charalabopoulos, K., Filioussis, G., and Seferiadis, K. 2007. Diarrheic shellfish poisoning due to toxic mussel consumption: The first recorded outbreak in Greece. *Food Addit Contam* 24(3): 297–305.

107. Martin, J.L., Hanke, A.R., and LeGresley, M.M. 2009. Long term phytoplankton monitoring, including harmful algal blooms, in the Bay of Fundy, eastern Canada. *J Sea Res* 61: 76–83.

108. Kacem, I., Hajjmen, B., and Bonaïcha, N. 2009. First evidence of okadaic acid in *Mytilus galloprovincialis* mussels, collected in a Mediterranean Lagoon, Tunisia. *Bull Environ Contam Toxicol* 82(6): 660–664.

109. Kawabata, T. 1989. Regulatory aspects of marine biotoxins in Japan. In: Natori, S., Hashimoto, K., and Ueno, Y., eds., *Mycotoxins and Phycotoxins' 88: A Collection of Invited Papers Presented at the Seventh International IUPAC Symposium on Mycotoxins and Phycotoxins*. Amsterdam, the Netherlands: Elsevier Science Pub, pp. 469–476.

110. Zhou, M., Li, J., Luckas, B. et al. 1999. A recent shellfish toxin investigation in China. *Mar Pollut Bull* 39: 331–334.

111. Mak, K.C.Y., Yu, H., Choi, M.C. et al. 2005. Okadaic acid, a causative toxin of diarrhetic shellfish poisoning, in green-lipped mussels *Perna viridis* from Hong Kong fish culture zones: Method development and monitoring. *Mar Pollut Bull* 51: 1010–1017.

112. Liu, R., Liang, Y., Wu, X., Xu, D., Liu, Y., and Liu, L. 2011. First report on the detection of pectenotoxin groups in Chinese shellfish by LC–MS/MS. *Toxicon* 57: 1000–1007.

113. Li, A., Ma, J., Cao, J., and McCarron, P. 2012. Toxins in mussels (*Mytilus galloprovincialis*) associated with diarrheic shellfish poisoning episodes in China. *Toxicon* 60: 420–425.

114. Konovalova, G.V. 1993. Toxic and potentially toxic dinoflagellates from the far east coastal waters of the USSR. In: Smayda, T.J. and Shimizu, Y., eds., *Toxic Phytoplankton Blooms in the Sea. Proceedings of the Fifth International Conference on Toxic Marine Phytoplankton*, Newport, RI, 1991. Amsterdam, the Netherlands: Elsevier, pp. 275–279.

115. Karunasagar, I., Segar, K., and Karunasagar, I. 1989. Incidence of PSP and DSP in shellfish along the coast of Karnataka state (India). In: Okachi, T., Anderson, D.M., White, A.W., and Badén, D.G., eds., *Red Tides: Biology, Environmental Science and Toxicology*. Amsterdam, the Netherlands: Elsevier, pp. 61–64.

116. Muñoz, F., Avaria, S., Sievers, H., and Prado, R. 1992. Presencia de dinoflagelados tóxicos del genero Dinophysis en el seno Aysén, *Chile Rev Biol Mar Valparaiso* 27: 187–212.

117. Uribe, J.C., García, C., Rivas, M., and Lagos, N. 2001. First report diarrheic shellfish toxins in *Magellanic Fiords*, southern Chile. *J Shellfish Res* 20: 69–74.

118. Garcia, C., Pereira, P., Valle, L., and Lagos, N. 2003. Quantitative of diarrheic shellfish poisoning toxins in Chilean mussel using pyrenyl diazomethane, as fluorescent labeling reagent. *Biol Res* 36: 1–13.

119. Quilliam, M.A., Gilgan, M.W., Pleasance, S., Defreitas, A.S.W., Douglas, D., Fritz, L., Hu, T., Marr, J.C., Smyth, C., and Wright, J.L.C. 1993. Confirmation of an incident of diarrhetic shellfish poisoning in Eastern Canadá. In: Smayda, T.J. and Shimizu, Y., eds., *Toxic Phytoplankton Blooms in the Sea. Proceedings of the Fifth International Conference on Toxic Marine Phytoplankton*, Newport, RI, 1991. Amsterdam, the Netherlands: Elsevier, pp. 547–552.

120. Gilgan, M.W., Powell, C., Van de Riet, J., Burns, B.G., Quilliam, M.A., Kennedy, K., and McKenzie, C.H. 1995. The occurrence of a serious diarrhetic shellfish poisoning episode in mussels from Newfoundland during the late autumn of 1993. In: *Four Canadian Workshops on Harmful Marine Algae*, Sydney, British Columbia, Australia, pp. 3–5.

121. Freudenthal, A.R. and Jacobs, J. 1995. Observations on *Dinophysis acuminata* and *Dinophysis norvergica* in Long Island waters: Toxicity, occurrence following diatom discolored water and co-ocurrence with *Ceratium*. In: Smayda, T.J. and Shimizu, T.J., eds., *Toxic Phytoplankton Blooms in the Sea. Proceedings of the Fifth International Conference on Toxic Marine Phytoplankton*, Newport, RI. Amsterdam, the Netherlands: Elsevier, Abstract.

122. Dickey, R.W., Fryxell, G.A., Granade, H.R., and Roelke, D. 1992. Detection of the marine toxins okadaic acid and domoic acid in shellfish and phytoplankton in the Gulf of Mexico. *Toxicon* 30: 355–359.

123. Lembeye, G., Yasumoto, T., Zhao, J., and Fernández, R. 1993. DSP outbreak in Chilean fjords. In: Smayda, T.J. and Shimizu, Y., eds., *Toxic Phytoplankton Blooms in the Sea. Proceedings of the Fifth International Conference on Toxic Marine Phytoplankton 1991*, Newport, RI. Amsterdam, the Netherlands: Elsevier, pp. 525–529.

124. Méndez, S. 1992. Update from Uruguay. An Intergovernmental Oceanographic Commission (IOC). Newsletter on toxic algae and algal blooms. *Harmful Algae News* 63: 5.

125. Quaine, J., Kraa, E., Holloway, J., White, K., McCarthy, R., Delpech, V., Trent, M., and McAnulty, J. 1997. Outbreak of gastroenteritis linked to eating pipis. New South Wales Pub. *Health Bull* 8: 103–104.

126. Caroppo, C., Congestri, R., and Bruno, M. 1999. On the presence of *Phalacroma rotundatum* in the southern Adriatic Sea (Italy). *Aquat Microb Ecol* 17: 301–310.

127. Hu, T.M., Curtis, J.M., Walter, J.A., and Wright, J.L.C. 1995. Identification of Dtx-4, a new water-soluble phosphatase inhibitor from the toxic dinoflagellate *Prorocentrum lima. J Chem Soc Chem Commun* 5: 597–599.

128. Lee, J.-S., Igarashi, T., Fraga, S., Dahl, E., Hovgaard, P., and Yasumoto, T. 1989. Determination of diarrhetic shellfish toxins in various dinoflagellates species. *J Appl Phycol* 1: 147–152.

129. Murakami, Y., Oshima, Y., and Yasumoto, T. 1982. Identification of okadaic acid as a toxic component of a marine dinoflagellate *Prorocentrum lima. Bull Jpn Soc Sci Fish* 48: 69–72.

130. Sampayo, M.A., Alvito, P., Franca, S., and Sousa, I. 1990. *Dinophysis* spp. toxicity and relation to accompanying species. In: Granéli, E., Sundström, B., Edler, L., and Anderson, D.M.M., eds., *Toxic Marine Phytoplankton*. New York: Elsevier, pp. 215–220.

131. Faust, M.A., Vandersea, M.W., Kibler, S.R., Tester, P.A., and Litaker, R.W. 2008. *Prorocentrum levis*, a new benthic species (Dinophyceae) from a Mangrove Island, Twin Cays Belize. *J Phycol* 44: 232–240.

132. Hu, T., DeFreitas, A.S.W., Curtis, J.M., Oshima, Y., Walter, J.A., and Wright, J.L.C. 1996. Isolation and structure of prorocentrolide B, a fast-acting toxin from *Prorocentrum maculosum. J Nat Prod* 59: 1010–1014.

133. Morton, S.L., Moeller, P.D.R., Young, K.A., and Lanoue, B. 1998. Okadaic acid production from the marine dinoflagellate *Prorocentrum belizeanum* faust isolated from the Belizean coral reef ecosystem. *Toxicon* 36: 201–206.

134. Zhou, J. and Fritz, L. 1994. Okadaic acid antibody localises to chloroplasts in the DSP-toxin-producing dinoflagellates *Prorocentrum lima* and *Prorocentrum maculosum. Phycologica* 33: 455–461.

135. Kat, M. 1985. *Dinophysis acuminata* blooms, the distinct cause Dutch mussel poisoning. In: Anderson, D.M., White, A.W., and Badén, D.G., eds., *Toxic Dinoflagellates*. Amsterdam, the Netherlands: Elsevier, pp. 73–77.

136. Le Baut, C., Lucas, D., and Le Deán, L. 1985. *Dinophysis acuminate* toxin status of toxicity bioassays in French. In: Anderson, D.M., White, A.W., and Badén, D.G., eds., *Toxic Dinoflagellates*. Amsterdam, the Netherlands: Elsevier, pp. 485–488.

137. Reguera, B., Bravo, I., and Fraga, S. 1990. Distribution of *Dinophysis acuta* at the time of a DSP outbreak in the rías of Pontevedra and Vigo (Galicia, NW Spain). *International Council for the Exploration of the Sea, C.M.*, 1990/ L:14, 8.

138. McMahon, T. and Silke, J. 1998. Re-occurrence of winter toxicity. *Harmful Algae News* 17: 12–16.

139. Guzmán, L. and Campodonico, I. 1975. Marea roja en la Región de Magallanes. *Publ Inst Pat Ser Mon* 9: 44.

140. MacKenzie, L., Truman, P., Satake, M. et al. 1998. Dinoflagellate blooms and associated DSP toxicity in shellfish in New Zealand. In: Reguera, B., Blanco, J., Fernádez, M.L., and Wyatt, T., eds., *Harmful Algae.* Galicia, Spain: Xunta de Galicia and Intergovernmental.

141. Tubaro, A., Sosa, S., Bussani, D., Sidari, L., Honsell, G., and Della Loggia, R. 1995. Diarrhoeic toxicity induction in mussels of the Gulf of Trieste. In: Lassus, P., Arzul, G., Erard, L.E., Denn, E., Gentien, P., and Marcaillou Lebaut, C., eds., *Harmful Marine Algal Blooms.* París, France: Lavoisier Pub, pp. 249–254.

142. Underdal, B., Yndestad, M., and Aune, T., DSP intoxications in Norway and Sweden. Autumn 1984-Spring 1985. In: Anderson, D.M., White, A.W., and Badén, D.G., eds., *Toxic Dinoflagellates.* Amsterdam, the Netherlands: Elsevier, pp. 489–494.

143. Shumway, S.E. 1995. Phycotoxin-related shellfish poisoning: Bivalve molluscs are not the only vectors. *Rev Fish Sci* 3(1): 1–31.

144. Suzuki, T. and Mitsuya, T. 2001. Comparison of dinophysistoxin-1 and esterified dinophysistoxin-1 (dinophysistoxin-3) content in the scallop Pactinopecten yessoensis and the mussel *Mytilus galloprovincialis. Toxicon* 39: 905–908.

145. Regulation EC 853/2004 of de European Parliament and of the Council, of April 29, 2004, laying down specific hygiene rules for on the hygiene of foodstuffs. Official Journal of the European Union L/226/55–82, of 29/6/2004.

146. Regulation EC 854/2004 of de European Parliament and of the Council, of April 29, 2004 laying down specific rules for the organization of official controls on products of animal origin intended for human consumption. Official Journal of the European Union L/226/83–127, of 25/6/2004.

147. Commission Regulation EC No 2074/2005 of December 5, 2005, laying down implementing measures for certain products under Regulation EC No. 853/2004 of the European Parliament and of the Council and for the organization of official controls under Regulation EC No. 854/2004 of the European Parliament and of the Council and Regulation EC No. 882/2004 of the European Parliament and of the Council, derogating from Regulation EC No. 852/2004 of the European Parliament and of the Council and amending Regulations EC No. 853/2004 and EC No. 854/2004. Official Journal of the European Union L338, 22.12.2005, pp. 27–59.

148. Council Decisión 1993/383/ EEC of June 1993, 14 on reference laboratories for the monitoring of marine biotoxins. Official Joumal of the European Union L 166. 8.7.1993, pp. 31–33.

149. Nicolaou, K.C., Koftis, T.V., Vyskocil, S., Petrovic, G., Ling, T.T., Yamada, Y.M.A., Tang, W.J., and Frederick, M.O. 2004. Structural revision and total synthesis of azaspiracid-1, part 2: Definition of the ABCD domain and total synthesis. *Angew Chem Int Ed* 43: 4318–4324.

150. Rehmann, N., Hess, P., and Quilliam, M.A. 2008. Discovery of new analogs of the marine biotoxin azaspiracid in blue mussels *Mytilus edulis* by ultra-performance liquid chromatography/tandem mass spectrometry. *Rapid Commun Mass Spectrom* 22: 549–558.

151. James, K.J., Moroney, C., Roden, C., Satake, M., Yasumoto, T., Lehane, M., and Furey, A. 2003. Ubiquitous "benign" alga emerges as the cause of shellfish contamination responsible for the human toxic syndrome, azaspiracid poisoning. *Toxicon* 41: 145–154.

152. McCarron, P., Kilcoyne, J., Miles, C.O., and Hess, P. 2009. Formation of azaspiracids-3, -4, -6, and -9 via decarboxylation of carboxyazaspiracid metabolites from shellfish. *J Agric Food Chem* 57: 160–169.

154. Ito, E., Satake, M., Ofuji, K., Kurita, N., McMahon, T. James, K.J., and Yasumoto, T. 2000. Multiple organ damage caused by a new toxin azaspiracid, isolated from mussels produced in Ireland. *Toxicon* 38: 917–930.

155. James, K.J., Hidalgo Saez, M.J., Furey, A., and Lehane, M. 2004. Azaspiracid poisoning, the food-borne illness associated with shellfish consumption. *Food Addit Contam* 21: 879–892.

156. Ofuji, K., Satake, M., McMahon, T., Silke, J., James, K.J., Naoki, H., Oshima, Y., and Yasumoto, T. 1999. Two analogs of azaspiracid isolated from mussels, *Mytilus edulis*, involved in human intoxications in Ireland. *Nat Toxins* 7: 99–102.

157. Food Safety Authority of Ireland (FSAI). 2001. Risk assessment of Azaspiracids (AZAS) in shellfish Dublín. FSAI, Dublín, Ireland, February 2001.

156. Food Safety Authority of Ireland (FSAI). 2006. Risk assessment of Azaspiracids (AZAS) in shellfish: A report of the Scientific Comité of the FSAI. FSAI, Dublín, Ireland, August 2006.

158. James, K.J., Furey, A., Lehane, M., Ramstad, H., Aune, T., Hovgaard, P., Morris, S., Higman, W., Satake, M., and Yasumoto, T. 2002. First evidence of an extensive northern European distribution of azaspiracid poisoning (AZP) toxins in shellfish. *Toxicon* 40: 909–915.

159. Lehane, M., Braña-Magdalena, A., Moroney, C., Furey, A., and James, K.J. 2002. Liquid chromatography with electrospray ion trap mass spectrometry for the determination of five azaspiracids in shellfish. *J Chromatogr A* 950: 139–147.

160. Vale, P., Bire, R., and Hess, P. 2008. Confirmation by LC-MS/MS of azaspiracids in shellfish from the Portuguese north-western coast. *Toxicon* 51(8): 1449–1456.

161. Taleb, H., Vale, P., Amanhir, R., Benhadouch, A., Sagou, R., and Chafik, A. 2006. First detection of azaspiracids in mussels in north west Africa. *J Shellfish Res* 25: 1067–1070.

162. Magdalena, A.B., Lehane, M., Krys, S., Fernández, M.L., Furey, A., and James, K.J. 2003. The first identification of azaspiracids in shellfish from France and Spain. *Toxicon* 42: 105–108.

163. Akselman, R. and Negri, R.M. 2010. Blooms of *Azadinium* cf. *spinosum* Elbrächter et Tillmann (Dinophyceae) in northern shelf waters of Argentina, Southwestern Atlantic. *Harmful Algae,* 19: 30–38.

164. Hernandez-Becerril, D.U., Escobar-Morales, S., Moreno-Gutiérrez, S.P., and Baron-Campis, S.A. 2010. Two new records of potentially toxic phytoplankton species from the Mexican Pacific. Abstract Book of the *14th International Conference on Harmful Algae.* Hersonissos-Crete, Greece, 1–5 November 2010. International Society for the Study of Harmful Algae (ISSHA) and the Hellenic Center for Marine Research (HCMR). http://www.issha.org/Welcome-to-ISSHA/Conferences/ICHA-Conferences/Past-conferences (accessed October 12, 2013).

165. López-Rivera, A., O'Callaghan, K., Moriarty, M., O'Driscoll, D., Hamilton, B., Lehane, M., James, K.J., and Furey, A. 2010. First evidence of azaspiracids (AZAs): A family of lipophilic polyether marine toxins in scallops (*Argopecten purpuratus*) and mussels (*Mytilus chilensis*) collected in two regions of Chile. *Toxicon* 55: 692–701.

166. Potvin, É., Jeong, H.J., Kang, N.S., Tillmann, U., and Krock, B. 2011. First report of the photosynthetic dinoflagellate genus *Azadinium* in the Pacific Ocean: Morphology and molecular characterization of *Azadinium* cf. *poporum. J Eukaryot Microbiol* 59: 145–156.

167. Krock, B., Tillmann, U., Vosz, D., Koch, B.P., Salas, R., Witt, M., Potvin, E., and Jeong, H.J. 2012. New azaspiracids in Amphidomataceae (Dinophyceae). *Toxicon* 60: 830–839.

168. Tillmann, U., Elbrächter, M., Krock, B., John, U., and Cembella, A. 2009. *Azadinium spinosum* gen. et sp. nov. (Dinophyceae) identified as a primary producer of azaspiracid toxins. *Eur J Phycol* 44: 63–79.

169. Miles, C.O., Wilkins, A.L., Samdal, I.A., Sandvik, M., Petersen, D., Quilliam, M.A., Naustvoll, L.J. et al. 2004. A novel pectenotoxin, PTX-12, in *Dinophysis* spp. and shellfish from Norway. *Chem Res Toxicol* 17: 1423–1433.

170. Krock, B., Tillmann, U., John, U., and Cembella, A. 2008. LC-MS-MS aboard ship: Tandem mass spectrometry in the search for phycotoxins and novel toxigenic plankton from the North Sea. *Anal Bioanal Chem* 392: 797–803.

171. Krock, B., Tillmann, U., John, U., and Cembella, A.D. 2009. Characterization of azaspiracids in plankton size-fractions and isolation of an azaspiracid-producing dinoflagellate from the North Sea. *Harmful Algae* 8: 254–263.

172. Furey, A., Moroney, C., Magdalena, A.B., Saez, M.J., Lehane, M., and James, K.J. 2003. Geographical, temporal, and species variation of the polyether toxins, azaspiracids, in shellfish. *Environ Sci Technol* 37: 3078–3084.

173. Hess, P., McMahon, T., Slattery, D., Swords, D., Dowling, G., McCarron, M., Clarke, D., Gibbons, W., Silke, J., and O'Cinneide, M. 2003. Use of LC-MS testing to identify lipophilic toxins, to establish local trends and interspecies differences and to test the comparability of LC-MS testing with the mouse bioassay: An example from the Irish Biotoxin Monitoring Programme 2001. *Molluscan Shellfish Safety, Proceedings of the Fourth International Conference on Molluscan Shellfish Safety.* Santiago de Compostella, Spain: Consellería de Pesca e Asuntos Marítimos da Xunta de Galicia, and Intergovernmental Oceanographic Commission of UNESCO, pp. 57–65.

174. Hess, P., McMahon, T., Slattery, D., Swords, D., Dowling, G., McCarron, M., Clarke, D. et al. 2001. Biotoxin chemical monitoring in Ireland 2001. In: *Proceedings of the Second Irish Marine Science Biotoxin Workshop.* Dublin, Ireland: Marine Institute, pp. 8–18.

175. Torgersen, T., Bremnes, N.B., Rundberget, T., and Aune, T. 2008. Structural confirmation and occurrence of azaspiracids in Scandinavian brown crabs (*Cancer pagurus*). *Toxicon* 51: 93–101.

176. James, K.J., Furey, A., Lehane, M., Morones, C., Fernández-Puente, P., Satake, M., and Yasumoto, T. 2002. Azaspiracid shellfish poisoning: Inusual toxin dynamics in shellfish and the increased risk of acute human intoxications. *Food Addit Contam* 19: 555–561.

177. Hess, P., Nguyen, L., Aasen, J., Keogh, M., Kilcoyne, J., McCarron, P., and Aune, T. 2005. Tissue distribution, effects of cooking and parameters affecting the extraction of azaspiracids from mussels, *Mytilus edulis*, prior to analysis by liquid chromatography coupled to mass spectrometry. *Toxicon* 46: 62–71.

178. James, K.J., Sierra, M.D., Lehane, M., Braña Magdalena, A., and Furey, A. 2003. Detection of five new hydroxyl analogues of azaspiracids in shellfish using multiple tandem mass spectrometry. *Toxicon* 41: 277–283.

179. Ofuji, K., Satake, M., and McMahon, T. 2001. Structures of azaspiracid analogs, azaspiracid-4 and azaspiracid-5 causative toxins of azaspiracid poisoning in Europe. *Biosci Biotechnol Biochem* 65(3): 740–742.

180. *European Communities Official Journal* L 075, 16/03/2002, 2002, 0064.

181. Commission Regulation (EU) No. 15/2011 of January 2011, 10th amending Regulation (EC) No. 2074/2005 as regards recognised testing methods for detecting marine biotoxins in live bivalve molluscs. L6/3–6, 2011; http://eurlex.europa.eu/LexUriServ/LexUriServ.do?uri=OJ:L:2011:006:0003:0006:EN:PDF

182. Schantz, E.J., Mold, J., Stanger, D., Shavel, J., Riel, F., Bowden, J., Lynch, J., Wyler, R., Riegel, B., and Sommer, H. 1957. Paralytic shellfish poison VI. A procedure for the isolation and purification of the poison from toxic clams and mussel tissues. *J Am Chem Soc* 79: 5230–5235.

183. Wiese, M., D'Agostino, P.M., Mihali, T.K., Moffitt, M.C., and Neilan, B.A. 2010. Neurotoxic alkaloids: Saxitoxin and its analogs. *Mar Drugs* 8: 2185–2211.

184. Lipkind, G.M. and Fozzard, H.A. 1994. A structural model of the tetrodotoxin and saxitoxin binding site of the Na^+ channel. *Biophys J* 66: 1–13.

185. Narahashi, T. 1972. Mechanism of action of tetrodotoxin and saxitoxin on excitable membranes. *Fed Proc* 31: 1124–1132.

186. Narahashi, T. 2005. Pharmacology of tetrodotoxin. *Toxin Rev* 20: 67–84.

187. Montebruno, D. 1993. Paralytic shellfish poisoning in Chile. *Med Sci Law* 33: 243–246.

188. Garcia, C., Bravo, M.C., Lagos, M., and Lagos, N. 2004. Paralytic shellfish poisoning: Post-mortem analysis of tissue and body fluid samples from human victims in the Patagonia fjords. *Toxicon* 43: 149–158.

189. Todd, E.C. 1997. Seafood-associated diseases and control in Canadá. *Rev Sci Tech* 16: 661–672.

190. Arnott, G.H. 1998. Toxic marine microalgae: A worldwide problem with major implications for seafood safety. *Adv Food Safety* 1: 24–34.

191. Todd, E., Avery, G., and Grant, G.A. 1993. An outbreak of severe paralytic shellfish poisoning in British Columbia. *Can Commun Dis Rep* 19: 99–102.

192. Whittle, K. and Gallacher, S. 2000. Marine toxins. *Br Med Bull* 56: 236–253.

193. Lip, E.K. and Rose, J.B. 1997. The role of seafood in foodborne diseases in the United States of América. *Rev Sci Tech* 16: 620–640.

194. Sobel, J. and Painter, J. 2005. Illness caused by marine toxins. *Clin Infect Dis* 41: 1290–1296.

195. Lehane, L. 2001. Paralytic shellfish poisoning: A potential public health problem. *MJA* 175: 29–31.

196. Cheng, H.S., Chua, S.O., Jung, J.S., and Yip, K.K. 1991. Creatine kinase MB elevation in paralytic shellfish poisoning. *Chest* 99: 1032–1033.

197. Popkiss, M.E.E., Horstman, D.A., and Harpur, D. 1979. Paralytic shellfish poisoning. A report of 17 cases in Cape Town. *S Afr Med J* 55: 1017–1023.

198. McCollum, J.P.K., Pearson, R.C.M., Ingham, H.R., Wood, P.C., and Dewar, H.A. 1968. An epidemic of mussel poisoning in northeast England. *Lancet* 2: 767–770.

199. Rodrigue, D.C., Etzel, R.A., Hall, S., de Porras, E., Velasquez, O.H., Tauxe, R.V., Kilbourne, E.M., and Blake, P.A. 1990. Lethal paralytic shellfish poisoning in Guatemala. *Am J Trop Med Hyg* 42: 267–271.

200. Mata, L., Abarca, G., Marranghello, L., and Viquez, R. 1990. Intoxicación paralitica por mariscos (IPM) por *Spondylus calcifer* contaminado con *Pyrodinium bahamense*, Costa Rica, 1989–1990. *Rev Biol Trop* 38: 129–136.

201. Holmes, M.J. and Teo, S.L.M. 2002. Toxic marine dinoflagellates in Singapore waters that cause seafood poisonings. *Clin Exp Pharmacol Physiol* 29: 829–836.

202. Tan, C.T.T. and Lee, E.J.D. 1986. Paralytic shellfish poisoning in Singapore. *Ann Acad Med Sing* 15: 77–79.
203. Anderson, D.M., Sullivan, J.J., and Reguera, B. 1989. Paralytic shellfish poisoning in northwest Spain: The toxicity of the dinoflagellate *Gymnodinium* catenatum. *Toxicon* 21: 665–674.
204. Castañeda, O.S., Castellanos, J.L.V., Calvan, J., Anguiano, A.S., and Nazar, A. 1991. Intoxicaciones por toxina paralizante de molusco en Oaxaca. *Salud Publica Mex* 33: 240–247.
205. Centers for Disease Control (CDC). 1991. Paralytic shellfish poisoning—Massachusetts and Alaska, 1990. *MMWR* 40: 157–161.
206. Long, R.R., Sargent, J.C., and Hammer, K. 1990. Paralytic shellfish poisoning: A case report and serial electrophysiologic observations. *Neurology* 40: 1310–1312.
207. Gessner, B.D. and Middaugh, J.P. 1995. Paralytic shellfish poisoning in Alaska: A 20-year retrospective analysis. *Am J Epidemiol* 141: 766–770.
208. Gessner, B.D. and Schloss, M. 1996. A population-based study of paralytic shellfish poisoning in Alaska. *Alaska Med* 38: 54–58, 68.
209. Gessner, B.D. and McLaughlin, J.B. 2008. Epidemiologic impact of toxic episodes: Neurotoxic toxins. In: Botana, L., ed., *Seafood and Freshwater Toxins. Pharmacology, Physiology, and Detection.* New York: Taylor & Francis Group, pp. 78–103.
210. de Carvalho, M. et al. 1998. Paralytic shellfish poisoning: Clinical and electrophysiological observations. *J Neurol* 245: 551–554.
211. Ingham, H.R., Mason, J., and Wood, P.C. 1968. Distribution of toxin in molluscan shellfish following the occurrence of mussel toxicity in northeast England. *Nature* 220: 25–27.
212. Shumway, S.E., Allen, S.M., and Boersma, P.D. 2003. Marine birds and harmful algal blooms: Sporadic victims or under-reported events? *Harmful Algae* 2: 1–17.
213. Van Dolah, F.M. 2000. Marine algal toxins: Origins, health effects, and their increased occurrence. *Environ Health Perspect* 108: 133–141.
214. Joint, I., Lewis, J., Aiken, J., Proctor, R., Moore, G., Higman, W., and Donald, M. 1997. Interannual variability of PSP outbreaks on the north east UK coast. *J Plankton Res* 19: 937–956.
215. Coulson, J.C., Potts, G.R., Deans, I.R., and Fraser, S.M. 1968. Mortality of shags and other sea birds caused by paralytic shellfish poison. *Nature* 220: 23–24.
216. Anderson, D.M., Kulis, D.M., Qi, Y., Zheng, L., Lu, S., and Lin, Y. 1996. Paralytic shellfish poisoning in Southern China. *Toxicon* 14: 579–590.
217. Lagos, N. 1998. Microalgal blooms: A global issue with negative impact in Chile. *Biol Res* 31: 375–386.
218. Jacinto, G.S., Azanza, R.V., Velasquez, I.B., and Siringan, F.P. 2006. Manila bay: Environmental challenges and opportunities. In: Wolanski, E., ed., *The Environment in Asia Pacific Harbours.* Dordrecht, the Netherlands: Springer, pp. 309–328.
219. Maclean, J.L. 1989. Indo-Pacific red tides, 1985–1988. *Mar Poll Bull* 20: 304–310.
220. Prakash, A., Medcof, J., and Tennant, A. 1971. Paralytic shellfish poisoning in Eastern Canada. *Bull Fish Res Board Can* 117: 1–88.
221. McLaughlin, J.B., Fearey, D.A., and Esposito, T.A. 2011. Paralytic shellfish poisoning. Southeast Alaska, May June 2011. *MMWR* 60(45): 1554–1556.
222. Negri, A.P. and Jones, G.J. 1995. Bioaccumulation of paralytic shellfish poisoning (PSP) toxins from the cyanobacterium *Anabaena circinalis* by the fresh-water mussel *Alathyria condola*. *Toxicon* 33: 667–678.
223. Ikawa, M., Wegener, K., Foxall, T.L., and Sasner, Jr., J.J. 1982. Comparison of the toxins of the blue-green alga *Aphanizomenon flos-aquae* with the *Gonyaulax* toxins. *Toxicon* 20: 747–752.
224. Humpage, A.R., Rositano, J., Breitag, A.H. et al. 1994. Paralytic shellfish poisons from Australian cyanobacterial blooms. *Aust J Mar Freshwat Res* 45: 761–771.
225. Carmichael, W.W., Evans, W.R., Yin, Q.Q., Bell, P., and Moczydlowski, E. 1997. Evidence for paralytic shellfish poisons in the freshwater cyanobacterium *Lyngbya wollei* (Farlow ex Gomont) comb. nov. *Appl Environ Microbiol* 63: 3104–3110.
226. Pomati, F., Sacchi, S., Rossetti, C. et al. 2000. The freshwater cyanobacterium *Planktothrix* sp. FP1: Molecular identification and detection of paralytic shellfish poisoning toxins. *J Phycol* 36: 553–562.
227. Lagos, N., Onodera, H., Zagatto, P.A., Azevedo, S.M., and Oshima, Y. 1999. The first evidence of paralytic shellfish toxins in the freshwater cyanobacterium *Cylindrospermopsis raciborskii*, isolated from Brazil. *Toxicon* 37: 1359–1373.
228. Araoz, R., Molgo, J., and de Marsac, N.T. 2010. Neurotoxic cyanobacterial toxins. *Toxicon* 56: 813–828.

229. Yunes, J.S., De la Rocha, S., Giroldo, D. et al. 2009. Release of carbohydrates and proteins by a subtropical strain of *Raphidiopsis brookii* (Cyanobacteria) able to produce saxitoxin at three nitrate concentrations. *J Phycol* 45: 585–591.
230. Pereira, P., Onodera, H., Andrinolo, D. et al. 2000. Paralytic shellfish toxins in the freshwater cyanobacterium *Aphanizomenon flos-aquae*, isolated from Montargil reservoir, Portugal. *Toxicon* 38: 1689–1702.
231. Ballot, A., Fastner, J., and Wiedner, C. 2010. Paralytic shellfish poisoning toxinproducing cyanobacterium *Aphanizomenon gracile* in northeast Germany. *Appl Environ Microbiol* 76: 1173–1180.
232. Kaas, H. and Henriksen, P. 2000. Saxitoxins (PSP toxins) in Danish lakes. *Water Res* 34: 2089–2097.
233. Rapala, J., Robertson, A., Negri, A.P. et al. 2005. First report of saxitoxin in Finnish lakes and possible associated effects on human health. *Environ Toxicol* 20: 331–340.
234. Pereira, P., Li, R.H., Carmichael, W.W., Dias, E., and Franca, S. 2004. Taxonomy and production of paralytic shellfish toxins by the freshwater cyanobacterium *Aphanizomenon gracile* LMECYA40. *Eur J Phycol* 39: 361–368.
235. Ledreux, A., Thomazeau, S., Catherine, A. et al. 2010. Evidence for saxitoxins production by the cyanobacterium *Aphanizomenon gracile* in a French recreational water body. *Harmful Algae* 10: 88–97. doi:10.1016/j.hal.2010.07.004.
236. Wörmera, L., Cirés, S., Agha, R., Verdugo, M., Hoyos, C., and Quesada, A. 2011. First detection of cyanobacterial PSP (paralytic shellfish poisoning) toxins in Spanish freshwaters. *Toxicon* 57: 918–921.
237. Berry, J.P. and Lind, O. 2010. First evidence of "paralytic shellfish toxins" and cylindrospermopsin in a Mexican freshwater system, Lago Catemaco (Veracruz), and apparent bioaccumulation of the toxins in "tegogolo" snails (Pomacea patula catemacensis). *Toxicon* 55: 930–938.
238. Berry, J.P., Jaja-Chimedza, A., Dávalos-Lind, L., and Lind, O. 2012. Apparent bioaccumulation of cylindrospermopsin and paralytic shellfish toxins by finfish in Lake Catemaco (Veracruz, Mexico). *Food Addit Contam* 29(2): 314–321.
239. Sakamoto, S., Ogata, T., Sato, S., Kodama, M., and Takeuchi, T. 1992. Causative organism of paralytic shellfish toxins other than toxic dinoflagellates. *Mar Ecol Prog Ser* 89: 229–235.
240. Kodama, M., Ogata, T., Fukuyo, Y. et al. 1988. *Protogonyaulax cohorticula*, a toxic dinoflagellate found in the Gulf of Thailand. *Toxicon* 26: 709–712.
241. Kodama, M., Ogata, T., Sato, S., and Sakamoto, S. 1990. Possible association of marine bacteria with paralytic shellfish toxicity in bivalves. *Mar Ecol Prog Ser* 61: 203–206.
242. Silva, E.S. 1990. Intracellular bacteria: The origin of dinoflagellate toxicity. *J Environ Pathol Toxicol Oncol* 10: 124–128.
243. Kodama, M., Doucette, G.J., and Green, D.H. 2006. Relationships between bacteria and harmful algae. In: *Ecology of Harmful Algae,* Granéli, E. and Turner, J.T. (eds.). Berlin, Germany: Springer-Verlag, pp. 243–255.
244. Lefebvre, K.A., Bill, B.D., Erickson, A. et al. 2008. Characterization of intracellular and extracellular saxitoxin levels in both field and cultured *Alexandrium* spp. samples from Sequim Bay, Washington. *Mar Drugs* 6: 103–116.
245. Oshima, Y., Blackburn, S.I., and Hallegraeff, G.M. 1993. Comparative study on paralytic shellfish toxin profiles of the dinoflagellate *Gymnodinium catenatum* from three different countries. *Mar Biol* 116: 471–476.
246. Usup, G., Kulis, D.M., and Anderson, D.M. 1994. Growth and toxin production of the toxic dinoflagellate *Pyrodinium bahamense* var. *compressum* in laboratory cultures. *Nat Toxins* 2: 254–262.
247. Gainey, L., Shumway, J., and Shumway, S. 1988. A compendium of the responses of bivalve molluscs to toxic dinoflagellates. *J Shellfish Res* 7: 623–628.
248. Deeds, J., Landsberg, J., Etheridge, S., Pitcher, G., and Longan, S. 2008. Non-traditional vectors for paralytic shellfish poisoning. *Mar Drugs* 6: 308–348.
249. Hoeger, S.J., Shaw, G., Hitzfeld, B.C., and Dietrich, D.R. 2004. Occurrence and elimination of cyanobacterial toxins in two Australian drinking water treatment plants. *Toxicon* 43: 639–649.
250. Molica, R.J.R., Oliveira, E.J.A., Carvalho, P.V.V.C., Costa, A.N.S.F., Cunha, M.C.C., Melo, G.L., and Azevedo, S.M.F.O. 2005. Occurrence of saxitoxins and an anatoxin-a(s)-like anticholinesterase in a Brazilian drinking water supply. *Harmful Algae* 4: 743–753.
251. Clemente, Z., Busato, R.H., Oliveira Ribeiro, C.A., Cestari, M.M., Ramsdorf, W.A., Magalhães, V.F., Wosiack, A.C., and Silva de Assis, H.C. 2010. Analyses of paralytic shellfish toxins and biomarkers in a southern Brazilian reservoir. *Toxicon* 55: 396–406.

252. Liu, Y., Chen, W., Li, D., Shen, Y., Li, G., and Liu, Y. 2006. First report of aphantoxins in China—Waterblooms of toxigenic *Aphanizomenon flos-aquae* in Lake Dianchi. *Ecotoxicol Environ Saf* 65: 84–92.
253. Codd, G.A. 1995. Cyanobacterial toxins: Occurrence, properties and biological significance. *Water Sci Technol* 32: 149–156.
254. Sivonen, K. and Jones, G. 1999. Cyanobacterial toxins. In: Chorus, I. and Bartram, J., eds., *Toxin Cyanobacteria in Water: A Guide to Their Public Health Consequences, Monitoring and Management*. London, U.K.: WHO E & FN Spon, pp. 41–111.
255. Durbin, E., Teegarden, G., Campbell, R. et al. 2002. North Atlantic right whales, *Eubalaena glacialis*, exposed to paralytic shellfish poisoning (PSP) toxins via a zooplankton vector, *Calanus finmarchicus*. *Harmful Algae* 1: 243–251.
256. Pereira, P., Dias, E., Franca, S., Pereira, E., Carolino, M., and Vasconcelos, V. 2004. Accumulation and depuration of cyanobacterial paralytic shellfish toxins by the freshwater mussel *Anodonata cygnea*. *Aquat Toxicol* 68: 339–350.
257. Shumway, S.E. 1995. Phycotoxin-related shellfish poisoning: Bivalve molluscs are not the only vectors. *Rev Fish Sci* 3: 1–31.
258. Oshima, Y., Kotaki, Y., Harada, T., and Yasumoto, T. 1984. Paralytic shellfish toxins in tropical waters. In: Ragelis, E.P., ed., *Seafood Toxins*. Washington, DC: American Chemical Society Symposium Series, pp. 161–170.
259. Bricelj, V.M. and Shumway, S.E. 1998. Paralytic shellfish toxins in bivalve molluscs: Occurrence, transfer kinetics, and biotransformation. *Rev Fish Sci* 6: 315–383.
260. Andrinolo, D., Michea, L.F., and Lagos, N. 1999. Toxic effects, pharmacokinetics and clearance of saxitoxin, a component of paralytic shellfish poison (PSP) in cats. *Toxicon* 37: 447–464.
261. Shumway, S.E., Barter, J., and Sherman-Caswell, S. 1990. Auditing the impact of toxic algal blooms on oysters. *Environ Audit* 2: 41–56.
262. Shumway, S.E. and Cembella, A.D. 1993. The impact of toxic algae on scallop culture and fisheries. *Rev Fish Sci* 1: 121–150.
263. Shumway, S.E., Sherman, S.A., Cembella, A.D., and Selvin, R. 1994. Accumulation of paralytic shellfish toxins by surfclams, *Spisula solidissima* (Dillwyn, 1897) in the Gulf of Maine: Seasonal changes, distribution between tissues, and notes on feeding habits. *Nat Toxins* 2: 236–251.
264. Beitler, M.K. and Liston, J. 1990. Uptake and distribution of PSP toxins in butter clams. In: Graneli, E., Sundstrom, B., Edler, L., and Anderson, D.M., eds., *Toxic Marine Phytoplankton*. New York: Elsevier Press, pp. 257–262.
265. Robertson, A., Stirling, D., Robillot, C., Llewellyn, L., and Negri, A. 2004. First report of saxitoxin in octopi. *Toxicon* 44: 765–771.
266. Daigo, K., Noguchi, T., Miwa, A., Kawai, N., and Hashimoto, K. 1988. Resistance of nerves from certain toxic crabs to paralytic shellfish poison and tetrodotoxin. *Toxicon* 26: 485–490.
267. Nagashima, Y., Ohgoe, H., Yamamoto, K., Shimakura, K., and Shomi, K. 1998. Resistance of non-toxic crabs to paralytic shellfish poisoning toxins. In: Reguera, B., Blanco, J., Fernandez, M.L., and Wyatt, T., eds., *Harmful Algae*. Grafisant, Santiago de Compostela, Spain: Xunta de Galicia and Intergovernmental Oceanographic Commission of UNESCO, pp. 604–606.
268. Choi, M.C., Yu, P.K.N., Hsieh, D.P.H., and Lam, P.K.S. 2006. Trophic transfer of paralytic shellfish toxins from clams (*Ruditapes philippinarum*) to gastropods (*Nassarius festivus*). *Chemosphere* 64: 1642–1649.
269. Yasumoto, T., Oshima, Y., and Konta, T. 1981. Analysis of paralytic shellfish toxins of xanthid crabs in Okinawa. *Bull Jpn Soc Sci Fish* 47: 957–959.
270. Arakawa, O., Noguchi, T., Shida, Y., and Onoue, Y. 1994. Occurrence of carbamoyl-N-hydroxy derivatives of saxitoxin and neosaxitoxin in a xanthid crab *Zosimus aeneus*. *Toxicon* 32: 175–183.
271. Arakawa, O., Nishio, S., Noguchi, T., Shida, Y., and Onoue, Y. 1995. A new saxitoxin analogue from a Xanthid crab *Atergatis floridus*. *Toxicon* 33: 1577–1584.
272. Arakawa, O., Noguchi, T., and Onoue, Y. 1995. Paralytic shellfish toxin profiles of xanthid crabs *Zosimus aeneus* and *Atergatis floridus* collected on reefs of Ishigaki Island. *Fish Sci* 61: 659–662.
273. Llewellyn, L.E., Dodd, M.J., Robertson, A., Ericson, G., de Koning, C., and Negri, A.P. 2002. Postmortem analysis of samples from a human victim of a fatal poisoning caused by the xanthid crab, *Zosimus aenus*. *Toxicon* 40: 1463–1469.
274. Jonas-Davies, J. and Liston, J. 1985. The occurrence of PSP toxins in intertidal organisms. In: Anderson, D.M., White, A.W., and Baden, D.G. eds., *Toxic Dinoflagellates*. New York: Elsevier, pp. 467–472.

275. Asakawa, M., Nishimura, F., Miyazawa, K., and Noguchi, T. 1997. Occurrence of paralytic shellfish poisons in the starfish, *Asterias amurensis* in Kure Bay, Hiroshima Prefecture, Japan. *Toxicon* 35: 1081–1087.

276. Lin, S.J., Tsai, Y.H., Lin, H.P., and Hwang, D.F. 1998. Paralytic toxins in Taiwanese starfish *Astropecten scoparius*. *Toxicon* 36: 799–803.

277. White, A.W. 1980. Recurrence of kills of Atlantic herring (*Clupea harengus harengus*) caused by dino-flagellate toxins transferred through herbivorous zooplankton. *Can J Fish Aquat Sci* 37: 2262–2265.

278. White, A.W. 2004. Paralytic shellfish toxins and finfish. In: Ragelis, E.P., ed., *Seafood Toxins*. ACS Symposium Series, Vol. 262. Washington, DC: American Chemical Society, pp. 171–180.

279. Maclean, J.L. and White, A.W. 1985. Toxic dinoflagellate blooms in Asia: A growing concern. In: Anderson, D.M., White, A.W., and Baden, D.G., eds., *Toxic Dinoflagellates*. New York: Elsevier, pp. 517–520.

280. Gonzalez, C.L., Ordonez, J.A., and Maala, A.M. 1989. Red tide: The Philippine experience. In: Okaichi, T., Anderson, D.M., and Nemoto, T., eds., *Red Tides, Biology, Environmental Science and Toxicology*. New York: Elsevier, pp. 97–100.

281. Maclean, J.L. 1979. Indo-Pacific red tides. In: Taylor, D.L. and Seliger, S.S., eds., *Toxic Dinoflagellate Blooms*. New York: Elsevier, pp. 173–178.

282. White, A.W. 1979. Dinoflagellate toxins in phytoplankton and zooplankton fractions during a Bloom of *Gonyaulax excavata*. In: Taylor, D.L. and Seliger, H.H., eds., *Toxic Dinoflagellate Blooms*. New York: Elsevier, pp. 381–384.

283. White, A.W. 1981. Marine zooplankton can accumulate and retain dinoflagellate toxins and cause fish kills. *Limnol Oceanogr* 26: 103–109.

284. Turiff, N., Runge, J.A., and Cembella, A.D. 1995. Toxin accumulation and feeding behavior of the plank-tonic copepod *Calanus finmarchicus* exposed to the red-tide dinoflagellate *Alexandrium excavatum*. *Mar Biol* 123: 55–64.

285. Teegarden, G.J. and Cembella, A.D. 1996. Grazing of toxic dinoflagellates, *Alexandrium* spp., by adult copepods of coastal Maine: Implications for the fate of paralytic shellfish toxins in marine food webs. *J Exp Mar Biol Ecol* 196: 145–176.

286. Teegarden, G.J. and Cembella, A.D. 1996. Grazing of toxic dinoflagellates, (*Alexandrium* spp.) by estua-rine copepods: Particle selection of PSP toxins in marine food webs. In: Yasumoto, T., Oshima, Y., and Fukuyo, Y., eds., *Harmful and Toxic Algal Blooms. Proceedings of the Seventh International Conference on Toxic Phytoplankton*, Sendai, Japan, July 12–16, 1995. Paris, France: IOC of UNESCO, pp. 393–396.

287. Turner, J.Y., Doucette, G.J., Powell, C.L., Kulis, D.M., Keafer, B.A., and Anderson, D.M. 2000. Accumulation of red tide toxins in larger size fractions of zooplankton assemblages from Massachusetts Bay, USA. *Mar Ecol Prog Ser* 203: 95–107.

288. Kodama, M., Ogata, T., Kawamukai, K., Oshima, Y., and Yasumoto, T. 1983. Occurrence of saxitoxin and other toxins in the liver of pufferfish *Takifugu pardalis*. *Toxicon* 21: 897–900.

289. Nakamura, M., Oshima, Y., and Yasumoto, T. 1984. Occurrence of saxitoxin in puffer fish. *Toxicon* 22: 381–385.

290. Nakashima, K., Arakawa, O., Taniyama, S., Nonaka, M., Takatani, T., Yamamori, K., Fuchi, Y., and Noguchi, T. 2004. Occurrence of saxitoxins as a major toxin in the ovary of a marine puffer *Arothron firmamentum*. *Toxicon* 43: 207–212.

291. Sato, S., Ogata, T., Borja, V., Gonzales, C., Fukuyo, Y., and Kodama, M. 2000. Frequent occurrence of paralytic shellfish poisoning toxins as dominant toxins in marine puffer from tropical water. *Toxicon* 38: 1101–1109.

292. Centers for Disease Control and Prevention (CDC). 2002. Neurologic illness associated with eating Florida puffer-fish. *MMWR* 51: 321–323.

293. Quilliam, M., Wechsler, D., Marcus, S., Ruck, B., Wekell, M., and Hawryluk, T. 2004. Detection and identification of paralytic shellfish poisoning toxins in Florida pufferfish responsible for incidents of neurologic illness. In: Steidinger, K.A., Landsberg, J.H., Tomas, C.R., and Vargo, G.A., eds., *Harmful Algae 2002. Proceedings of the Xth International Conference on Harmful Algae*. St. Petersburg, FL: Florida Fish and Wildlife Conservation Commission and Intergovernmental Oceanographic Commission of UNESCO, pp. 116–118.

294. Etheridge, S., Deeds, J., Hall, S., White, K., Flewelling, L., Abbott, J., Landsberg, J., Conrad, S., Bodager, D., and Jackow, G. 2006. Detection methods and their limitations: PSP toxins in Florida puffer fish responsible for human poisoning events in 2004. *Afr J Mar Sci* 28: 383–387.

295. Landsberg, J.H., Hall, S., Johannessen, J.N. et al. 2006. Saxitoxin puffer fish poisoning in the United States, with the first report of *Pyrodinium bahamense* as the putative toxin source. *Environ Health Perspect* 114: 1502–1507.

296. Guy, A.L. and Griffin, G. 2009. Adopting alternatives for the regulatory monitoring of shellfish for paralytic shellfish poisoning in Canada: Interface between federal regulators, science and ethics. *Regul Toxicol Pharmacol* 54: 256–263.

297. Stewart, I., Seawright, A.A., and Shaw, G.R. 2008. Cyanobacterial poisoning in livestock, wild mammals and birds—An overview. In: Hudnell, H.K., ed., *Cyanobacterial Harmful Algal Blooms: State of the Science and Research Needs*. New York: Springer, pp. 613–637.

298. Maeda, M., Kodama, T., Tanaka, T., Yoshizumi, H., Takemoto, T., Nomoto, K., and Fujita, T. 1986. Structures of isodomoic acids A, B and C, novel insecticidal amino acids from the red alga *Chondria Armata*. *Chem Pharmacol Bull* 34: 4892–4895.

299. Wright, J.L.C., Falk, M., Mcinnes, A.G., and Walter, J.A. 1990. Identification of isodomoic acid-D and 2 new geometrical-isomers of domoic acid in toxic mussels. *Can J Chem* 68: 22–25.

300. Wright, J.L.C. and Quilliam, M.A. 1995. Methods for domoic acid, the amnesic shellfish poisons. In: Hallegraeff, G., Anderson, D.M., and Cembella, A.D., eds., *Manual on Harmful Marine Microalgae*. Paris, France: UNESCO, pp. 113–133.

301. Ohfune, Y. and Tomita, M. 1982. Total synthesis of domoic acid. A revision of the original structure. *J Am Chem Soc* 104: 3511–3513.

302. Johannessen, J.N. 2000. Stability of domoic acid in saline dosing solutions. *J AOAC Int* 83: 411–412.

303. Quilliam, M.A., Sim, P.G., McCulloch, A.W., and McInnes, A.G. 1989. High-performance liquid chromatography of domoic acid, a marine neurotoxin, with application to shellfish and plankton. *Int J Environ Anal Chem* 36: 139–154.

304. Ravn, H. 1995. Amnesic shellfish poisoning (ASP). UNESCO—HAB Publication Series Volume 1. *IOC Manuals and Guides No. 31,* 15pp. http://www.jodc.go.jp/info/ioc_doc/Manual/m031v01.pdf (accessed October 12, 2013).

305. Lefebvre, K.A. and Robertson, A. 2010. Domoic acid and human exposure risks: A review. *Toxicon* 56: 218–230.

306. Miguez, A., Luisa Fernandez, M., and Fraga, S. 1998. First detection of domoic acid in Galicia (NW Spain). In: Yasumoto, T., Oshima, Y., and Fukuro, Y., eds., *Harmful and Toxic Algal Blooms*. Paris, France: Intergovernmental Oceanographic Commission of UNESCO, pp. 143–145.

307. James, K.J., Gillman, M., Lehane, M., and Gago-Martinez, A. 2000. New fluorimetric method of liquid chromatography for the determination of the neurotoxin domoic acid in seafood and marine phytoplankton. *J Chromatogr* 871: 1–6.

308. Vale, P. and Sampayo, M.A. 2001. Domoic acid in Portuguese shellfish and fish. *Toxicon* 39: 893–904.

309. Hess, P. et al. 2001. Determination and confirmation of the amnesic shellfish poisoning toxin, domoic acid in shellfish from Scotland by liquid chromatography and mass spectrometry. *J AOAC Int* 84: 1657–1667.

310. Amzil, Z. et al. 2001. Domoic acid accumulation in French shellfish in relation to toxic species of *Pseudo-nitzschia* multiseries and *P. pseudodelicatissima*. *Toxicon* 39: 1245–1251.

311. James, K.J., Gillman, M., Amandi, M.F. et al. 2005. Amnesic shellfish poisoning toxins in bivalve molluscs in Ireland. *Toxicon* 46: 852–858.

312. Pulido, O.M. 2008. Domoic acid toxicologic pathology: A review. *Mar Drugs* 6: 180–219.

313. Hay, B.E., Grant, C.M., and McCounmbrey, D.J. 2000. A review of the marine biotoxin monitoring programme for non-commercially harvested shellfish. Part 1: Technical Report. A Report for the New Zealand Ministry of Health.

314. Ramsey, U.P., Douglas, D.J., Walter, J.A., and Wright, J.L. 1998. Biosynthesis of domoic acid by the diatom *Pseudo-nitzschia* multiseries. *Nat Toxins* 6: 137–146.

315. Walz, P.M., Garrison, D.L., Graham, W.M., Cattey, M.A., Tjeerdema, R.S., and Silver, M.W. 1993. Domoic acid-producing diatom blooms in Monterey Bay, California: 1991–1993. *Nat Toxins* 2: 271–279.

316. Lundholm, N., Skov, J., Pocklington, R., and Moestrup, O. 1994. Domoic acid, the toxic amino acid responsible for amnesic shellfish poisoning, now in *Pseduonitzschia seriata* (Baccillariophyceae) in Europe. *Phycologia* 33: 475–478.

317. Kvitek, R.G., Goldberg, J.D., Smith, G.J., Doucette, G.J., and Silver, M.W. 2008. Domoic acid contamination within eight representative species from the benthic food web of Monterey Bay, California, USA. *Mar Ecol Prog Ser* 367: 35–47.

318. Wekell, J.C., Gauglitz, Jr. E.J., Barnett, H.J., Hatfield, C.L., Simons, D., and Ayres, D. 1994. Occurrence of domoic acid in Washington state razor clams (*Siliqua patula*) during 1991–1993. *Nat Toxins* 2: 197–205.

319. Horner, R.A., Garrison, D.L., and Plumley, F.G. 1997. Harmful algal blooms and red tide problems on the US west coast. *Limnol Oceanogr* 42(5): 1076–1088.

320. Rhodes, L., Scholin, C., and Garthwaite, I. 1998. *Pseudo-nitzschia* in New Zealand and the role of DNA probes and immunoassays in refining marine biotoxin monitoring programmes. *Nat Toxins* 6: 105–111.

321. Arévalo, F.F., Bermudez de la Puente, M., and Salgado, C. 1998. ASP toxicity in scallops: Individual variability and tissue distribution. In: Reguera, B., Blanco, J., Fernandez, M., and Wyatt, T., eds., *Harmful Algae, Proceedings of the VIII International Conference on Harmful Algae*, Vigo, Spain, June 1997. Vigo, Spain: Xunta de Galicia and IOC of UNESCO, pp. 499–502.

322. Novaczek, I., Madhyastha, M.S., Ablett, R.F., Donald, A., Johnson, G., Nijjar, M.S., and Sims, D.E. 1992. Depuration of domoic acid from live blue mussels *Mytilus edulis*. *Can J Fish Aquat Sci* 49: 312–318.

323. Horner, R.A., Kusske, M.B., Moynihan, B.P., Skinner, R.N., and Wekell, J.C. 1993. Retention of domoic acid by pacific razor clams, siliqua patula: Preliminary study. *J Shellfish Res* 12: 451–456.

324. Blanco, J., de la Puente, M.B., Arevalo, F., Salgado, C., and Morono, A. 2002. Depuration of mussels (*Mytilus galloprovincialis*) contaminated with domoic acid. *Aquat Living Resour* 15: 53–60.

325. Blanco, J., Acosta, C.P., Marino, C. et al. 2006. Depuration of domoic acid from different body compartments of the king scallop *Pecten maximus* grown in raft culture and natural bed. *Aquat Living Res* 19: 257–265.

326. Bogan, Y.M., Kennedy, D., Harkin, A.L., Gillespie, J., Hess, P., and Slater, J.W. 2006. Comparison of domoic acid concentration in king scallops, *Pecten maximus* from sea bed and suspended culture systems. *J shellfish Res* 25: 129–135.

327. Lefebvre, K.A., Powell, C.L., Busman, M. et al. 1999. Detection of domoic acid in northern anchovies and California sea lions associated with an unusual mortality event. *Nat Toxins* 7: 85–92.

328. Villac, M.C., Roelke, D.L., Chavez, F.P., Cifuentes, L.A., and Fryxell, G.A. 1993. *Pseudonitzschia australis* frenguelli and related species from the west coast of the USA: Occurrence and domoic acid production. *J Shellfish Res* 12: 457–465.

329. Hatfield, C.L., Gauglitz, E.J., Barnett, H.J., Lund, J.A.K., Wekell, J.C., and Eklund, M. 1995. The fate of domoic acid in Dungess crab (*Cancer magister*) as a function of processing. *J Shellfish Res* 14: 359–363.

330. Stewart, J.E., Marks, L.J., Gilgan, M.W., Pfeiffer, E., and Zwikler, B.M. 1998. Microbial utilization of the neurotoxin domoic acid: Blue mussels (*Mytilus edulis*) and soft shell clams (*Mya arenaria*) as sources of microorganisms. *Can J Microbiol* 44: 456–464.

331. Todd, E.C.D. 1993. Domoic acid and amnesic shellfish poisoning: A review. *J Food Prot* 56: 69–83.

332. Costa, P.R. and Garrido, S. 2004. Domoic acid accumulation in the sardine *Sardina pilchardus* and its relationship to *Pseudo-nitzschia* diatom ingestion. *Mar Ecol Prog Ser* 284: 261–268.

333. Busse, L.B., Venrick, E.L., Antrobus, R. et al. 2006. Domoic acid in phytoplankton and fish in San Diego, CA, USA. *Harmful Algae* 5: 91–101.

334. McGinness, K.L., Fryxell, G.A., and McEachran, J.D. 1995. *Pseudonitzschia* species found in digestive tracts of northern anchovies (*Engraulis mordax*). *Can J Zool* 73: 642–647.

335. Sierra Beltrán, A., Palafox-Uribe, M., Grajales-Montiel, J., Cruz-Villacorta, A., and Ochoa, J.L. 1997. Sea bird mortality at Cabo San Lucas, Mexico: Evidence that toxic diatom blooms are spreading. *Toxicon* 35(3): 447–453.

336. Scallet, A.C., Schmued, L.C., and Johannessen, J.N. 2005. Neurohistochemical biomarkers of marine neurotoxicant, domoic acid. *Neurotoxicol Teratol* 27: 745–752.

337. Work, T.M. et al. 1993. Epidemiology of domoic acid poisoning in brown pelicans (*Pelecanus occidentalis*) and Brandt cormorants (*Phalacrocorax penicillatus*) in California. *J Zool Wildlife Med* 24: 54–62.

338. Trainer, V.L., Hickey, B.M., and Bates, S.S. 2008. Toxic diatoms. In: Walsh, P.J. et al., eds., *Oceans and Human Health: Risks and Remedies from the Seas*. Amsterdam, the Netherlands: Elsevier, pp. 219–237.

339. Auer, R.N. 1991. Excitotoxic mechanisms, and age-related susceptibility to brain damage in ischemia, hypoglycemia and toxic mussel poisoning. *Neurotoxicology* 12: 541–546.

340. Manen, K. 1996. Establishing tolerable dungeness crab (*Cáncer magister*) and razor clam (*Siliqua patula*) domoic acid contaminant levels. *Environ Health Perspect* 104: 1230–1236.

341. Wekell, J.C., Gaugitz, Jr. E.J., Barnett, H.J., Hatfield, C.L., and Eklund, M. 1994. The occurrence of domoic acid in razor clams (*Siliqua patula*), dungeness crab (*Cáncer magister*), and anchovies (*Engraulis mordax*). *J Shellfish Res* 13: 587–593.

342. Committee on Toxicity of Chemicals in Food, Consumer Products and the Environment. 2002. Annual report, 2001. Food Standards Agency/Department of Health, London, U.K., August 2002, pp. 27–33.

343. Goldstein, T., Mazet, J.A., Zabka, T.S. et al. 2008. Novel symptomatology and changing epidemiology of domoic acid toxicosis in California sea lions (*Zalophus californianus*): An increasing risk to marine mammal health. *Proc R Soc Biol Sci Ser B* 275: 267–276.

344. Lefebvre, K.A., Silver, M.W., Coale, S.L., and Tjeerdema, R.S. 2002. Domoic acid in planktivorous fish in relation to toxic *Pseudonitzschia* cell densities. *Mar Biol* 140: 625–631.

345. Waldichuk, M. 1989. Amnesic shellfish poison. *Mar Poll Bull* 20: 359–360.

346. Watkins, S.M., Reich, A., Fleming, L.E., and Hammond, R. 2008. Neurotoxic shellfish poisoning. *Mar Drugs* 6(3): 431–455.

347. Baden, D.G., Mende, T.J., and Block, R.E. 1979. Two similar toxins from *Gymnodinium breve*. In: Taylor, D.L. and Selinger, H.H., eds., *Toxic Dinoflagellate Blooms*. Amsterdam, the Netherlands: Elsevier, p. 327.

348. Baden, D.G. and Mende, T.J. 1982. Toxicity of two toxins from the Florida red tide marine dinoflagellate, *Ptychodiscus brevis*. *Toxicon* 20: 457–461.

349. Baden, D.G., Fleming, L.E., and Bean, J.A. 1995. Marine toxins. In: Wolff, F.A., ed., *Handbook of Clinical Neurology: Intoxications of the Nervous System,* Part II, Vol. 21. New York: Elsevier, pp. 141–175.

350. Lin, Y.Y. et al. 1981. Isolation and structure of brevetoxin B from the 'red tide' dinoflagellate *Ptychodiscus brevis* (*Gymnodinium breve*). *J Am Chem Soc* 103: 6773–6775.

351. Shimizu, Y., Chou, H., Bando, H., van Duyne, G., and Clardy, J.C. 1986. Structure of brevetoxin a (GB-1 toxin), the most potent toxin in the Florida red tide organism *Gymnodinium breve* (*Ptychodiscus brevis*). *J Am Chem Soc* 108(3): 514–515.

352. Baden, D. and Fleming, L.E. 2007. *Biotoxins in Bivalve Molluscs*. Geneva, Switzerland: FAO/WHO. Brevetoxins. (ftp://ftp.fao.org/es/esn/food/biotoxin_report_en.pdf).

353. Campbell, S.K., McConnell, E.P., Bourdelais, A., Tomas, C., and Baden, D.G. 2004. The production of brevetoxin and brevetoxin-like compounds during the growth phases of *Karenia brevis*. In: Steidinger, K.A., Landsberg, J.H., Tomas, C.R., and Vargo, G.A., eds., *Harmful Algae 2002*. St. Petersburg, FL: Florida Fish and Wildlife Conservation Commission, Florida Institute of Oceanography, Intergovernmental Oceanographic Commission of UNESCO, pp. 148–149.

354. Michelliza, S., Jacocks, H., Bourdelais, A., and Baden, D.G. 2004. Synthesis, binding assays, and toxicity of new derivatives of brevetoxin b. In: Steidinger, K.A., Landsberg, J.H., Tomas, C.R., and Vargo, G.A., eds., *Harmful Algae 2002*. St. Petersburg, FL: Florida Fish and Wildlife Conservation Commission, Florida Institute of Oceanography, Intergovernmental. Oceanographic Commission of UNESCO.

355. Michelliza, S., Abraham, W.M., Jacocks, H.M., Schuster, T., and Baden, D.G. 2007. Synthesis, modeling, and biological evaluation of analogs of the semi-semisynthetic brevetoxin antagonist b-Naphthoyl-Brevetoxin. *ChemBioChem* 2007(8): 2233–2239.

356. Satake, M., Bourdelais, A., VanWagoner, R., Baden, D.G., and Wright, J.L. 2008. Brevisamide: An unprecedented monocyclic ether alkaloid from the dinoflagellate *Karenia brevis* that provides a potential model for ladder-frame initiation. *Org Lett* 10: 3465–3468.

357. Satake, M., Campbell, A., Van Wagoner, R., Bourdelais, A., Jacocks, H., Baden, D.G., and Wright, J.L. 2009. Brevisin: An aberrant polycyclic ether structure from the dinoflagellate *Karenia brevis* and its implications for polyether assembly. *J Org Chem* 74: 989–994.

358. Baden, D.G., Bourdelais, A.J., Jacocks, H., Michelliza, S., and Naar, J. 2005. Natural and derivative PbTx: Historical background, multiplicity, and effects. *Environ Health Perspect* 113: 621–625.

359. Sim, J. and Wilson, N. 1997. Surveillance of marine biotoxins, 1993–1996. *NZ Public Health Rep* 4: 9–16.

360. Hernandez-Becerril, D.U., Alonso-Rodriguez, R., Alvarez-Gongora, C. et al. 2007. Toxic and harmful marine phytoplankton and microalgae (HABs) in Mexican Coasts. *J Environ Sci Health A Tox Hazard Subst Environ Eng* 42(10): 1349–1363.

361. Haywood, A.J., Steidinger, K.A., Truby, E.W., Bergquist, P.R., Bergquist, P.L., Adamson, J., and Mackenzie, L. 2004. Comparative morphology and molecular phylogenetic analysis of 3 new species of the genus *Karenia* (Dinophyceae) from New Zealand. *J Phycol* 40(1): 165–179.

362. Kirkpatrick, B., Fleming, L.E., Squicciarini, D. et al. 2004. Literature review of Florida red tide: Implications for human health effects. *Harmful Algae* 3(2): 99–115.

363. Nozawa, A., Tsuji, K., and Ishida, H. 2003. Implication of brevetoxin B1 and PbTx-3 in neurotoxic shellfish poisoning in New Zealand by isolation and quantitative determination with liquid chromatography-tandem mass spectrometry. *Toxicon* 42(1): 91–103.
364. Steidinger, K.A. 1983. A re-evaluation of toxic dinoflagellate biology and ecology. *Prog Phycol Res* 2: 147–188.
365. Poli, M.A., Musser, S.M., Dickey, R.W. et al. 2000. Neurotoxic shellfish poisoning and brevetoxin metabolites: A case study from Florida. *Toxicon* 38: 981–993.
366. Hughes, J.M. and Merson, M.H. 1976. Fish and shellfish poisoning. *N Engl J Med* 295: 1117–1120.
367. Steidinger, K.A. and Ingle, R.M. 1972. Observations on the 1971 summer red tide in Tampa Bay. *Environ Lett* 3: 271–278.
368. Summerson, H.C. and Peterson, C.H. 1990. Recruitment failure of the Bay Scallop, *Argopecten irradians concentricus*, during the first red tide, *Pytchodiscus brevis*, outbreak recorded in North Carolina. *Estuaries* 13: 322–331.
369. Sakamoto, Y., Lockey, R.F., and Krzanowski, J.J. 1987. Shellfish and fish poisoning related to the toxic dinoflagellates. *S Med J* 80: 866–872.
370. Kirkpatrick, B., Pierce, R., Cheng, Y.S., Henry, M.S., Blum, P., Osborn, S., Nierenberg, K. et al. 2010. Inland transport of aerosolized Florida red tide toxins. *Harmful Algae* 9(2): 123–242.
371. Cheng, Y.S., Villareal, T.A., Zhou, Y. et al. 2004. Characterization of red tide aerosol on the Texas coast. In: Steidinger, K.A., Landsberg, J.H., Tomas, C.R., and Vargo, G.A., eds., *Harmful Algae 2005*. St. Petersburg, FL: Florida Fish and Wildlife Conservation Commission, Florida Institute of Oceanography, Intergovernmental Oceanographic Commission of UNESCO, pp. 499–501.
372. Cheng, Y.S., Zhou, Y., Irvin, C.M. et al. 2005. Characterization of marine aerosol for assessment of human exposure to brevetoxins. *Environ Health Perspect* 113(5): 638–643.
373. Cheng, Y.S., McDonald, J.D., Kracko, D. et al. 2005. Concentration and particle size of airborne toxic algae (brevetoxin) derived from ocean red tide events. *Environ Sci Technol* 39(10): 3443–3449.
374. Pierce, R.H., Henry, M.S., Blum, P.C., Lyons, J., Cheng, Y.S., Yazzie, D., and Zhou, Y. 2003. Brevetoxin concentrations in marine aerosol: Human exposure levels during a *Karenia brevis* harmful algal bloom. *Bull Environ Contam Toxicol* 70: 161–165.
375. Pierce, R.H. and Henry, M.S. 2008. Harmful algal toxins of the Florida red tide (*Karenia brevis*): Natural chemical stressors in South Florida coastal ecosystems. *Ecotoxicology* 17: 623–631.
376. Flewelling, L.J., Naar, J.P., and Abbott, J.P. 2005. Brevetoxicosis: Red tides and marine mammal mortalities. *Nature* 435(7043): 755–756.
377. Kirkpatrick, B., Bean, J.A., and Fleming, L.E. 2009. Gastrointestinal emergency room admissions and Florida red tide blooms. *Harmful Algae* 9: 82–86.
378. Naar, J.P., Flewelling, L.J., and Lenzi, A. 2007. Brevetoxins, like ciguatoxins, are potent ichthyotoxins that accumulate in fish. *Toxicon* 50: 707–723.
379. Perez Linares, J., Ochoa, J.L., and Gago Martinez, A. 2009. Retention and tissue damage of PSP and NSP toxins in shrimp: Is cultured shrimp a potential vector of toxins to human population? *Toxicon* 53(2): 185–195.
380. Geraci, J.R., Anderson, D.M., Timperi, R.J., St. Aubin, D.J., Early, G.A., Prescott, J.H., and Mayo, C.A. 1989. Humpback whales (*Megaoetera novaeangliae*) fatally poisoned by dinoflagellate toxin. *Can J Fish Aquat Sci* 46: 1895–1898.
381. Bossart, G.D., Baden, D.G., Ewing, R., Roberts, B., and Wright, S. 1998. Brevetoxicosis in manatees (*Trichechus manatus latirostris*) from the 1996 epizootic: Gross, histopathologic, and immunocytochemical features. *Toxicol Pathol* 26(2): 276–282.
382. O'Shea, T.J., Rathbun, G.B., Bonde, R.K., Buergelt, C.D., and Odell, D.K. 1991. An epizootic of Florida manatees associated with a dinoflagellate bloom. *Mar Mamm Sci* 7: 165–179.
383. Trainer, V.L. and Baden, D.G. 1999. High affinity binding of red tide neurotoxins to marine mammal brain. *Aquat Toxins* 46: 139–148.
384. Badén, D.G. 1989. Brevetoxins: Unique polyether dinoflagellate toxins. *FASEB J* 3: 1807–1817.
385. Morris, P.D., Campbell, D.S., Taylor, T.J., and Freeman, J.I. 1991. Clinical and epidemiological features of neurotoxic poisoning in North Carolina. *Am J Public Health* 81: 471–474.
386. Baden, D.G. 1983. Marine food-borne dinoflagellate toxins. *Int Rev Cytol* 82: 99–150.
387. Steidinger, K.A. and Baden, D.G. 1984. Toxic marine dinoflagellates. In: Spector, D.L., ed., *Dinoflagellates*. New York: Academy Press, pp. 201–261.

388. Backer, L.C., Kirkpatrick, B., and Fleming, L.E. 2005. Occupational exposure to aerosolized brevetoxins during Florida red tide events: Effects on a healthy worker population. *Environ Health Perspect* 113(5): 644–649.

389. Kirkpatrick, B., Fleming, L.E., and Backer, L.L.C. 2006. Environmental exposures to Florida red tides: Effects on emergency room respiratory diagnosis admissions. *Harmful Algae* 5: 526–533.

390. Quirino, W., Fleming, L.E., Weisman, R. et al. 2004. Follow up study of red tide associated respiratory illness. *Fla J Environ Health* 186: 18–22.

391. Cheng, Y.S., Villareal, T.A., Zhou, Y., Gao, J., Pierce, R.H., Naar, J., and Baden, D.G. 2004. Characterization of red tide aerosol on the Texas coast. In: Steidinger, K.A., Landsberg, J.H., Tomas, C.R., and Vargo, G.A., eds., *Harmful Algae 2005*. St. Petersburg, FL: Florida Fish and Wildlife Conservation Commission, Florida Institute of Oceanography, Intergovernmental Oceanographic Commission of UNESCO, pp. 499–501.

392. Fleming, L.E., Backer, L.C., and Baden, D.G. 2005. Overview of aerosolized Florida red tide toxins: Exposures and effects. *Environ Health Perspect* 113(5): 618–620.

393. Fleming, L.E., Jerez, E., Stephan, W.B., Cassedy, A., Bean, J.A., Reich, A., Kirkpatrick, B. et al. 2007. Evaluation of harmful algal bloom outreach activities. *Mar Drugs* (Special Issue on Marine Toxins) 5: 208–219.

394. Milian, A., Nierenberg, K., Fleming, L.E., Bean, J.A., Wanner, A., Reich, A., Backer, L.C., Jayroe, D., and Kirkpatrick, B. 2007. Reported respiratory symptom intensity in asthmatics during exposure to aerosolized Florida red tide toxins. *J Asthma* 44: 583–587.

395. Galtsoff, P.S. 1948. Red tide. *Spec Sci Rep US Fish Wildl Serv* 46: 1–44.

396. McFarren, E.F., Tanabe, H., Silva, F.J., Wilson, W.B., Campbell, J.E., and Lewis, K.H. 1965. The occurrence of a ciguatera-like poisons in oysters, clams, and *Gymnodinium breve* cultures. *Toxicon* 3: 111–123.

397. Martin, D.F. and Chatterjee, A.B. 1969. Isolation and characterization of a toxin from the Florida red tide organism. *Nature* 221: 9.

398. Woodcock, A.H. 1948. Note concerning human respiratory irritation associated with high concentrations of plankton and mass mortalities of marine organisms. *J Mar Res* 7: 56–62.

399. Abraham, W.M., Ahmed, A., Bourdelais, A.J., and Baden, D.G. 2003. Pathophysiologic airway responses to inhaled red tide brevetoxin in allergic sheep. *Toxicologist* 72(S-1): 115.

400. Abraham, W.M., Ahmed, A., Bourdelais, A., and Baden, D.G. 2004. Effects of novel antagonists of poly-ether brevetoxin (PbTx)-induced bronchoconstriction in allergic sheep. In: Steidinger, K.A., Landsberg, J.H., Tomas, C.R., and Vargo, G.A., eds., *Harmful Algae*. St. Petersburg, FL: Florida Fish and Wildlife Conservation Commission, Florida Institute of Oceanography, Intergovernmental Oceanographic Commission of UNESCO, pp. 496–498.

401. Abraham, W.M., Bourdelais, A.J., Ahmed, A., Serebriakov, I., and Baden, D.G. 2005. Effects of inhaled brevetoxins in allergic airways: Toxin—Allergen interactions and pharmacologic intervention. *Environ Health Perspect* 113(5): 632–637.

402. Abraham, W.M., Bourdelais, A.J., Sabater, J.R., Ahmed, A., Lee, A., Serebriakov, I., and Baden, D.G. 2005. Airway responses to aerosolized brevetoxins in an animal model of asthma. *Am J Res Crit Care Med* 171(1): 26–34.

403. Abraham, W.M. and Baden, D.G. 2006. Aerosolized Florida red toxins and human health effects. *Oceanography* 19(2): 107–109.

404. Fleming, L.E., Bean, J.A., and Baden, D.G. 1995. Epidemiology and public health. In: Hallegraeff, G.M., Anderson, D.M., and Cembella A.D., eds., *Manual on Harmful Marine Microalgae*. Paris, France: UNESCO, pp. 475–487.

405. Dickey, R., Jester, E., Granade, R., Mowdy, D., Moncreiff, C., Rebarchik, D., Robl, M., Musser, S., and Poli, M. 1999. Monitoring of brevetoxins during a *Gymnodinium* breve red tide: Comparison of a sodium channel specific cytotoxicity assay and mouse bioassay for determination of neurotoxic shellfish toxins in shellfish extracts. *Nat Toxins* 7: 157–165.

406. Music, S.I., Howell, J.T., and Brumback, L.C. 1973. Red tide: Its public health implications. *J Fla Med Assoc* 60: 27–29.

407. Murata, M., Kumagai, M., Lee, J.S., and Yasumoto, T. 1987. Isolation a structure of yessotoxin, a novel polyether compound implicated in diarrhetic shellfish poisoning. *Tetrahedron Lett* 28: 5869–5872.

408. Satake, M., Mackencie, A.L., and Yasumoto, T. 1997. Identification of *Protoceratium reticulatum* as the biogenic origin of yessotoxin. *Nat Toxins* 5: 164–167.

409. Tubaro, A., Sidari, L., Della Loggia, R., and Yasumoto, T. 1998. Ocurrence of yessotoxin-like toxins in phytoplankton and mussels from Northern Adriatic Sea. In: Reguera, B., Blanco, J., Fernandez, M.L., and Wyatt, T., eds., *Harmful Algae*. Santiago de Compostela, Spain: Xunta de Galicia and Intergovernmental Oceanographic Commission of UNESCO, pp. 470–472.
410. FAO, IOC of UNESCO, WHO. 2004. Report of the Joint FAO/IOC/WHO ad hoc Expert Consultation on biotoxins in bivalve molluscs. Oslo, Norway, September 26–30, 2004.
411. Miles, C.O., Samdal, I.A., Aasen, J.A.B. et al. 2005. Evidence for numerous analogs of yessotoxin in *Protoceratium reticulatum*. *Harmful Algae* 4: 1075–1091.
412. Alexander, J., Benford, D., Cockburn, A. et al. 2008. Marine biotoxins in shellfish—Yessotoxin group. *EFSA J* 907: 1–62.
413. Bagnis, R. 1973. *L'ichtyosarcotoxisme dans le Pacifique Sud*. Nouméa, France: Commission du Pacifique Sud, pp. 2–4.
414. Bagnis R. 1981. L'ichtyosarcotoxisme de type ciguatera: Processus biologiques connus et perspectives au seuil des années 1980. *Ann Inst Oceanogr* 57: 5–24.
415. Niaussat, P. 1982. Histoire des intoxications par les poissons des mers chaudes. *Meéd et Nutr* 28(3): 187–194.
416. Satake, M., Murata, M., and Yasumoto, T. 1993. Gambierol: A new toxic polyether compound isolated from the marine dinoflagellate *Gambierdiscus toxicus*. *J Am Chem Soc* 115(1): 361–362.
417. Baden, D.G. 1989. Brevetoxins: Unique polyether dinoflagellate toxins. *FASEB J* 3: 1807–1817.
418. Laurent, D., Kerbrat, A.S., Darius, H.T., Emmanuelle Girard, E., Golubic, S., Benoit, E., Sauviat, M.P., Chinain, M., Molgo, J., and Pauillac, S. 2008. Are cyanobacteria involved in ciguatera fish poisoning-like outbreaks in New Caledonia? *Harmful Algae* 7(6): 827–838.
419. Kerbrat, A.S., Darius, H.T., Pauillac, S., Chinain, M., and Laurent, D. 2010. Detection of ciguatoxin-like and paralysing toxins in *Trichodesmium* spp. From New Caledonia lagoon. *Mar Poll Bull* 61: 360–366.
420. Holmes, M.J., Lewis, R.J., Sellin, M., and Street, R. 1994. The origin of ciguatera in Platypus Bay, Australia. *Mem Queensl Mus* 34(3): 505–512.
421. Zheng, W., DeMattei, J.A., Wu, J.-P., Duan, J.J.-W., Cook, L.R., Oinuma, H., and Kishi, Y. 1996. Complete relative stereochemistry of maitotoxin. *J Am Chem Soc* 118: 7946–7968.
422. Friedman, M.A., Fleming, L.E., Fernandez, M. et al. 2008. Ciguatera fish poisoning: Treatment, prevention and management. *Mar Drugs* (Special Issue on Marine Toxins) 6: 456–479.
423. Lehane, L. and Lewis, R.J. 2000. Ciguatera: Recent advances but the risk remains. *Int J Food Microbiol* 61: 91–125.
424. Chateau-Degat, M.L., Huin-Blondey, M., Chinain, M. et al. 2007. Prevalence of chronic symptoms of ciguatera disease in French Polynesian adults. *Am J Trop Med Hyg* 77(5): 842–846.
425. Dickey, R.W. and Plakas, S.M. 2010. Ciguatera: A public health perspective. *Toxicon* 56: 123–136.
426. Wong, C.K.K., Hung, P., Lee, K.L., and Kam, K.M.M. 2005. Study of an outbreak of ciguatera fish poisoning in Hong Kong. *Toxicon* 46: 563–571.
427. Pauillac, S., Darius, T., and Chinain, M. 2003. Toxi-infections alimentaires. *Assoc Anc Élèves Inst Pasteur* 45(176): 148–154.
428. Wong, C.K.K., Hung, P., Lee, K.L., Mok, T., Chung, T., and Kam, K.M.M. 2008. Feature of ciguatera fish poisoning cases in Hong Kong 2004–2007. *Biomed Environ Sci* 21: 521–527.
429. Oshiro, N., Yogi, K., Asato, S., Sasaki, T., Tamanaha, K., Hirama, M., Yasumoto, T., and Inafuku, Y. 2010. Ciguatera incidence and fish toxicity in Okinawa, Japan. *Toxicon* 56(5): 656–661.
430. Chinain, M., Darius, H.T., Ung, A., Fouc, M.T., Revel, T., Cruchet, T., Pauillac, S., and Laurent, D. 2010. Ciguatera risk management in French Polynesia: The case study of Raivavae Island (*Australes Archipelago*). *Toxicon* 56: 674–690.
431. Centers for Disease Control (CDC). 2006. Ciguatera fish poisoning—Texas, 1998, and South Carolina, 2004. *MMWR* 55: 935–937.
432. Centers for Disease Control (CDC). 2009. Cluster of ciguatera fish Poisoning—North Carolina, 2007. *MMWR* 58: 283–285.
433. Laurent, D., Yeeting, B., Labrosse, P., and Gaudechoux, J.P. 2005. *Ciguatera: A Field Reference Guide* (Ciguatera: un guide pratique). Nouméa, New Caledonia: Secretariat of the Pacific Community, 91pp.
434. Château-Degat, M.L., Chinain, M., Darius, T., Dewailly, E., and Mallet, H.P. 2009. Epidemiological surveillance of ciguatera in French Polynesia. *Bull Épidémiol Hebdomadaire* 48/50: 522–525.

435. Rongo, T. and van Woesik, R. 2011. Ciguatera poisoning in Rarotonga, southern Cook Islands. *Harmful Algae* 10: 345–355.

436. Skinner, M.P., Brewer, T.D., Johnstone, R., Fleming, L.E., and Lewis, R.J. 2011. Ciguatera fish poisoning in the Pacific Islands (1998 to 2008). *PLoS* 5(12): e1416.

437. Lewis, N.D. 1986. Epidemiology and impact of Ciguatera in the Pacific—A review. *Mar Fish Rev* 48: 6–13.

438. Ho, A.M.H., Fraser, I.M., and Todd, E.C.D. 1986. Ciguatera poisoning: A report of three cases. *Ann Emerg Med* 15: 1225–1228.

439. DeFusco, D.J., O'Dowd, P., Hokama, Y., and Ott, B.R. 1993. Coma due to ciguatera poisoning in Rhode Island. *Am J Med* 95: 240–243.

440. Geller, R.J., Olson, K.R., and Senecal, P.E. 1991. Ciguatera fish poisoning in San Francisco, California, caused by imported barracuda. *West J Med* 155: 639–642.

441. Centers for Disease Control (CDC). 1986. Ciguatera fish poisoning—Vermont. *MMWR* 35: 263–264.

442. Johnson, R. and Jong, E. 1983. Ciguatera: Caribbean and Indo-Pacific fish poisoning. *West J Med* 138: 872–874.

443. Lange, W.R., Snyder, F.R., and Fudala, P.J. 1992. Travel and ciguatera fish poisoning. *Arch Intern Med* 152: 2049–2053.

444. Ebesu, J.S., Nagai, H., and Hokama, Y. 1994. The first reported case of human ciguatera possibly due to a farm cultured salmón. *Toxicon* 32: 1282–1286.

445. Farstad, D.J. and Chow, T. 2001. A brief case of ciguatera poisoning. *Wilderness Environ Med* 12: 263–269.

446. Bienfang, P.K., Parsons, M.L., Bidigare, R.R., Laws, E.A., and Moeller, P.D.R. 2008. Ciguatera fish poisoning: A synopsis from ecology to toxicity. In: Walsh, P.J., Smith, S.L., Fleming, L.E., Solo-Gabriele, H.M., and Gerwick, W.H., eds., *Oceans and Human Health: Risks and Remedies from the Seas*. Burlington, MA: Academic Press, pp. 257–270.

447. Villareal, T.A., Hanson, S., Qualia, S., Jester, E.L.E., Granade, H.R., and Dickey, R.W. 2007. Petroleum production platforms as sites for the expansion of ciguatera in the northwestern Gulf of Mexico. *Harmful Algae* 6: 253–259.

448. Boada, L.D., Zumbado, M., Luzardo, O.P., Almeida-González, M., Plakas, S.M., Granade, H.R., Abraham, A., Jester, E.L., and Dickey, R.W. 2010. Ciguatera fish poisoning on the West Africa Coast: An emerging risk in the Canary Islands (Spain). *Toxicon* 56: 1516–1519.

449. Pérez-Arellano, J., Luzardo, O., Brito, A., Cabrera, M., Zumbado, M., and Carranza, C. 2005. Ciguatera fish poisoning, Canary Islands. *Emerg Infect Dis* 11(12): 1981–1982.

450. Aligizaki, K., Nikolaidis, G., and Fraga, S. 2008. Is *Gambierdiscus* expanding to new areas? *Harmful Algae News* 36: 6–7.

451. Raikhlin-Eisenkraft, B. and Bentur, Y. 2002. Rabbitfish ("aras"): An unusual source of ciguatera poisoning. *Israel Med Assoc J* 4(1): 28–30.

452. Aligizaki, K. and Nikolaidis, G. 2008. Morphological identification of two tropical dinoflagellates of the genera *Gambierdiscus* and *Sinophysis* in the Mediterranean Sea. *J Biol Res* 9: 75–82.

453. Tester, P.A. 1994. Harmful marine phytoplankton and shellfish toxicity potential consequences of climate change. In: Wilson, M.E., Levins, R., and Spielman, A., eds., *Disease in Evolution: Global Changes and Emergence of Infectious Diseases*. New York: The New York Academy of Sciences, pp. 69–76.

454. Puente, S., Cabrera Majada, A., Lago Nunez, M., Azuara Solis, M., and González-Lahoz, J.M. 2005. Ciguatera: Ocho casos importados. *Rev Clin Esp* 205: 47–50.

455. Gascon, J., Macia, M., Oliveira, I., and Corachan, M. 2003. Intoxicación por ciguatoxina en viajeros. *Med Clin (Barc)* 120: 777–779.

456. Herrero-Martínez, J.M., Pérez-Ayala, A., Pérez-Molina, J.A., and López-Vélez, R. 2011. A case report of ciguatera fish poisoning in a traveller to Dominican Republic. *Enferm Infecc Microbiol Clin* 29(1): 70–76.

457. Brody, R.W. 1973. A study of ciguatera fish poisoning in the Virgin Islands area. CRI-T-001 CA, NOAA Sea Grant 1-35368. Caribbean Research Institute College of the Virgin Islands, St. Thomas, US Virgin Islands.

458. Yasumoto, T., Inoue, A., Bagnis, R., and Garcon, M. 1979. Ecological survey on a dinoflagellate possibly responsible for the induction of ciguatera. *Bull Jpn Soc Sci Fish* 45: 395–399.

459. Darius, H.T., Ponton, D., Revel, T., Cruchet, P., Ung, A., Tchou Fouc, M., and Chinain, M. 2007. Ciguatera risk assessment in two toxic sites of French Polynesia using the receptor-binding assay. *Toxicon* 50: 612–626.

460. Yasumoto, T., Inoue, A., Ochi, T. et al. 1980. Environmental studies on a toxic dinoflagellate responsible for ciguatera. *Bull Jpn Soc Sci Fish* 46(11): 1397–1404.
461. Ballantine, D.L., Bardales, A.T., Tosteson, T.E., and Dupont-Durst, H. 1985. Seasonal abundance of *Gambierdiscus toxicus* and *Ostreopsis* sp. in coastal waters of southwest Puerto Rico. In: Gabrie, C. and Salvat, B., eds., *Proceedings of the 5th International Coral Reef Congress*, Vol. 4. Tahiti, France: Antenne Museum-EPHE, pp. 417–422.
462. Yasumoto, T. 2001. The chemistry and biological function of natural marine toxins. *Chem Rec* 1: 228–242.
463. Vernoux, J.-P. and Lewis, R.J. 1997. Isolation and characterisation of Caribbean ciguatoxins from the horse-eye jack (*Caranx latus*). *Toxicon* 35: 889–900.
464. Lewis, R.J., Vernoux, J.P., and Brereton, I.M. 1998. Structure of Caribbean ciguatoxin isolated from *Caranx latus*. *J Am Chem Soc* 120: 5914–5920.
465. Lewis, R.J. 2001. The changing face of ciguatera. *Toxicon* 39(1): 97–106.
466. Pottier, I., Vernoux, J.-P., Jones, A., and Lewis, R.J. 2002. Characterisation of multiple Caribbean ciguatoxins and congeners in individual specimens of horse-eye jack (*Caranx latus*) by high-performance liquid chromatography/mass spectrometry. *Toxicon* 40: 929–939.
467. Pottier, I., Vernoux, J.P., Jones, A., and Lewis, R.J. 2002. Analysis of toxin profiles in three different fish species causing ciguatera fish poisoning in Guadeloupe, FrenchWest Indies. *Food Addit Contam* 19: 1034–1042.
468. Pottier, I., Hamilton, B., Jones, A., Lewis, R.J., and Vernoux, J.P. 2003. Identification of slow and fast-acting toxins in a highly ciguatoxic barracuda (*Sphyraena barracuda*) by HPLC/MS and radiolabelled ligand binding. *Toxicon* 42: 663–672.
469. Randall, J.E. 1958. A review of ciguatera, tropical fish poisoning, with a tentative explanation of its cause. *Bull Mar Sci Gulf Caribbean* 8(3): 236–267.
470. Caplan, C.E. 1998. Ciguatera fish poisoning. *Can Med Assoc J* 159: 1394.
471. Pearn, J.H. 2001. Neurology of ciguatera. *J Neurol Neurosurg Psychiatr* 70: 4–8.
472. Méjean, A., Peyraud-Thomas, C., Kerbrat, A.S., Golubic, S., Pauillac, S., Chinain, M., and Laurent, D. 2010. First identification of the neurotoxin homoanatoxin-a from mats of *Hydrocoleum lyngbyaceum* (marine cyanobacterium) possibly linked to giant clam poisoning in New Caledonia. *Toxicon* 56(5): 829–835.
473. Ruff, T.A. and Lewis, R.J. 1994. Clinical aspects of ciguatera: An overview. *Ment Queensl Mus* 34: 609–619.
474. Senecal, P.E. and Osterloh, J.D. 1991. Normal fetal outcome after maternal ciguateric toxin exposure in the second trimester. *J Toxicol Clin Toxicol* 29: 473–478.
475. Pearn, J., Harvey, P., De Ambrosis, W., Lewis, R., and McKay, R. 1982. Ciguatera and pregnancy. *Med J Aust* 1: 57–58.
476. Ballantine, D.L., Bardales, A.T., and Alvey, M.E. 1992. The culture of three dinoflagellate species associated with ciguatera. In: Calumpong, H.P. and Meñez, E.G., eds., *Proceedings of the 2nd RP-USA Phycology Symposium/Workshop*, Cebu City, Philippines. Los Baños, Laguna: National Science Foundation (U.S.)/Philippine Council for Aquatic and Marine Research & Development, pp. 261–268.
477. Bagnis, R., Legrand, A.M., and Inoue, A. 1990. Follow-up of a bloom of the toxic dinoflagellate *Gambierdiscus toxicus* on a fringing reef of Tahiti. In: Granéli, E., Sundström, B., Edler, L., and Anderson, D.M., eds., *Toxic Marine Phytoplankton*. New York: Elsevier, pp. 98–103.
478. Morton, S.L., Norris, D.R., and Bomber, J.W. 1992. Effect of temperature, salinity and light intensity on the growth and seasonality of toxic dinoflagellates associated with ciguatera. *J Exp Mar Biol Ecol* 157(1): 79–90.
479. Abbott, I.A. 1995. Hawaiian herbivorous fish: What algae are they eating, or what's left? In: Hokama, Y., Scheuer, P.J., and Yasumoto, T., eds., *Proceedings of the International Symposium on Ciguatera and Marine Natural Products*, Honolulu, HI, 1994. Honolulu, HI: Asian-Pacific Research Foundation, pp. 11–18.
480. Hokama, Y., Ebesu, J.S.M., Asuncion, D.A., and Nagai, H. 1996. Growth and cyclic studies of *Gambierdiscus toxicus* in the natural environment and in culture. In: Yasumoto, T., Oshima, Y., and Fukuyo, Y., eds., *Harmful and Toxic Algal Blooms*. Paris, France: Intergovernmental Oceanographic Commission of UNESCO, pp. 313–315.

481. Chinain, M., Germain, M., Deparis, X., Pauillac, S., and Legrand, A.M. 1999b. Seasonal abundance and toxicity of the dinoflagellate *Gambierdiscus* spp. (*Dinophyceae*), the causative agent of ciguatera in Tahiti, French Polynesia. *Mar Biol* 135(2): 259–267.

482. Hales, S., Weinstein, P., and Woodward, A. 1999. Ciguatera (fish poisoning), El Niño, and Pacific sea surface temperatures. *Ecosyst Health* 5(1): 20–25.

483. Rongo, T., Bush, M., and van Woesik, R. 2009. Did ciguatera prompt the late Holocene Polynesian voyages of discovery? *J Biogeogr* 36(8): 1423–1432.

484. Chateau-Degat, M.L., Chinain, M., Cerf, N., Gingras, S., Hubert, B., and Dewailly, E. 2005. Seawater temperature, *Gambierdiscus* spp. variability and incidence of ciguatera poisoning in French Polynesia. *Harmful Algae* 4(6): 1053–1062.

485. Bomber, J.W., Guillard, R.R.L., and Nelson, W.G. 1988. Roles of temperature, salinity, and light in seasonality, growth and toxicity of ciguatera-causing *Gambierdiscus toxicus* Adachi et Fukuyo (Dinophceae). *J Exp Mar Biol Ecol* 115(1): 53–65.

486. Tester, P.A., Feldman, R.L., Nau, A.W., Kibler, S.R., and Litaker, R.W. 2010. Ciguatera fish poisoning and sea surface temperatures in the Caribbean Sea and the West Indies. *Toxicon* 56(5): 698–710.

487. Carlson, R.D., Morey-Gaines, G., Tindall, D.R., and Dickey, R.W. 1984. Ecology of toxic dinoflagellates from the Caribbean Sea: Effects of macroalgal extracts on growth in culture. In: Ragelis, E.P., ed., *Sea Food Toxins*. Washington, DC: American Chemical Society, pp. 171–176.

488. Taylor, F.J.R. and Gustavson, M.S. 1986. An underwater survey of the organism chiefly responsible for "ciguatera" fish poisoning in the eastern Caribbean region: The benthic dinoflagellate *Gambierdiscus toxicus*. In: Stefanon, A. and Flemming, N.J., eds., *Proceedings of the 7th International Diving Science Symposium*, Padova University, Padova, Italy, pp. 95–111.

489. Grzebyk, D., Berland, B., Thomassin, B.A., Bosi, C., and Arnoux, A. 1994. Ecology of ciguateric dinoflagellates in the coral reef complex of Mayotte Island (S.W. Indian Ocean). *J Exp Mar Biol Ecol* 178(1): 51–66.

490. Asuncion, D.A., Asahina, A.Y., Muthiah, P., Hokama, Y., Higa, T., and Tananka, J. 1995. The effects of monosaccharides and natural marine products on the growth of *Gambierdiscus toxicus* in vitro. In: Hokama, Y., Scheuer, P.J., and Yasumoto, T., eds., *Proceedings of the International Symposium on Ciguatera and Marine Natural Products*, Honolulu, HI, 1994. Honolulu, HI: Asian-Pacific Research Foundation, pp. 99–107.

491. Cruz-Rivera, E. and Villareal, T.A. 2006. Macroalgal palatability and the flux of ciguatera toxins through marine foodwebs. *HarmfulAlgae* 5(5): 497–525.

492. Parsons, M.L. and Preskitt, L.B. 2007. A survey of epiphytic dinoflagellates from the coastal waters of the island of Hawai'i. *Harmful Algae* 6(5): 658–669.

493. de Sylva, D.P. 1982. A comparative survey of the populations of a Dinoflagellate, *Gambierdiscus toxicus*, in the Vicinity of St. Thomas, U.S. Virgin Islands. NOAA Contract NA 80-RAA-04083. University of Miami, Coral Gables, FL, p. 78.

494. Bomber, J.W. 1985. Ecological studies of benthic dinoflagellates associated with ciguatera from the Florida Keys. M.S. thesis, Florida Institute of Technology, Melbourne, FL, 104pp.

495. Nakahara, H., Sakami, T., Chinain, M., and Ishida, Y. 1996. The role of macroalgae in epiphytism of the toxic dinoflagellate *Gambierdiscus toxicus* (*Dinophyceae*). *Phycol Res* 44: 113–117.

496. Delgado, G., Lechuga-Devéze, C.H., Popowski, G., Troccoli, L., and Salinas, C.A. 2006. Epiphytic dinoflagellates associated with ciguatera in the northwestern coast of Cuba. *Rev Biol Trop* 54(2): 299–310.

497. Carlson, R.D. and Tindall, D.R. 1985. Distribution and periodicity of toxic dinoflagellates in the Virgin Islands. In: Anderson, D.M., White, A.W., and Baden, D.G., eds., *Toxic Dinoflagellates*. New York: Elsevier Scientific Publishing Co., pp. 271–287.

498. Taylor, F.J.R. 1985. The distribution of the dinoflagellates *Gambierdiscus toxicus* in the eastern Caribbean. In: *Proceedings of the 5th International Coral Reef Congress*, Vol. 4. Tahiti, France: Antenne Museum-EPHE, pp. 423–428.

499. Ballantine, D.L., Tosteson, T.R., and Bardales, A.T. 1988. Population dynamics and toxicity of natural populations of benthic dinoflagellates in southwestern Puerto Rico. *J Exp Mar Biol Ecol* 119(3): 201–212.

500. Bomber, J.W., Rubio, M.G., and Norris, D.R. 1989. Epiphytism of dinoflagellates associated with the disease ciguatera: Substrate specificity and nutrition. *Phycologia* 28(3): 360–368.

501. Villareal, T.A. and Morton, S.L. 2002. Use of cell-specific PAM-fluorometry to characterize host shading in the epiphytic dinoflagellate *Gambierdiscus toxicus*. *Mar Ecol* 23(2): 127–140.

502. Cooper, M.J. 1964. Ciguatera and other marine poisoning in the Gilbert Islands. *Pac Sci* 18(4): 411–440.
503. Bagnis, R. 1987. Ciguatera fish poisoning: An objective witness of the coral reef stress. In: Salvat, B., ed., *Human Impacts on Coral Reefs: Facts and Recommendations*. French Polynesia, France: Antenne Museum, pp. 241–253.
504. Rougerie, F. and Bagnis, R. 1992. Bursts of ciguatera and endo-upwelling process on coral reef. *Bull Soc Pathol Exot* 85: 464–466.
505. Ruff, T.A. 1989. Ciguatera in the Pacific: A link with military activities. *Lancet* 333(8631): 201–205.
506. Swift, A.E.B. and Swift, T.R. 1993. Ciguatera. *J Toxicol Clin Toxicol* 31: 1–29.
507. Tebano, T. 1992. Ciguatera fish poisoning and reef disturbance in South Tarawa, Kiribati. *SPC Ciguatera Info Bull* No. 2: 7. http://www.spc.int/DigitalLibrary/Doc/FAME/InfoBull/Ciguatera/2/Ciguatera2.pdf (accessed October 12, 2013).
508. Kaly, U.L. and Jones, G.P. 1994. Test of the effect of disturbance on ciguatera in Tuvalu. *Mem Queensl Mus* 34: 523- 532.
509. Briggs, A. and Leff, M. 2009. A comparison of toxic dinoflagellate densities along a gradient of human disturbance in the North Line Islands. http://stanford.sea.edu/research/Leff_Briggs_Final_Paper.pdf (accessed October 12, 2013).
510. Banner, A.H. 1974. The biological origin and transmission of ciguatoxin. In: Humm, H.J. and Lane, C.E., eds., *Bioactive Compounds from the Sea*. New York: Marcel Decker, pp. 15–36.
511. Yasumoto, T., Nakajima, I., Oshima, Y., and Bagnis, R. 1979. A new toxic dinoflagellate found in association with ciguatera. In: Taylor, D.L. and Seliger, H.H., eds., *Toxic Dinoflagellate Blooms*. New York: Elsevier, Inc., pp. 65–70.
512. Gillespie, N., Holmes, M.J., Burke, J.B., and Doley, J. 1985. Distribution and periodicity of *Gambierdiscus toxicus* in Queensland Australia. In: Anderson, D.M., White, A.W., and Baden, D.G., eds., *Toxic Dinoflagellates*. New York: Elsevier Scientific Publishing Co., pp. 183–188.
513. Kohler, S.T. and Kohler, C.C. 1992. Dead bleached coral provides new surfaces for dinoflagellates implicated in ciguatera fish poisonings. *Environ Biol Fishes* 35(4): 413–416.
514. Bagnis, R., Chanteau, S., Chungue, E., Hurtel, J.M., Yasumoto, T., and Inoue, A. 1980. Origins of ciguatera fish poisoning: A new dinoflagellate, *Gambierdiscus toxicus* Adachi and Fukuyo, definitively involved as a causal agent. *Toxicon* 18(2): 199–208.
515. Tester, P.A., Feldman, R.L., Nau, A.W., Faust, M.A., and Litaker, R.W. 2009. Ciguatera fish poisoning in the Caribbean. *Smith Contrib Mar Sci* 38: 301–311.
516. de Fouw, J.C., van Egmond, H.P., and Speijers, G.J.A. 2001. Ciguatera fish poisoning: A review. http://www.rivm.nl/bibliotheek/rapporten/388802021.pdf (accessed October 12, 2013).
517. Tosteson, T.R. 2004. Caribbean ciguatera: A changing paradigm. *Rev Biol Trop* 52: 109–113.
518. Morrison, K., Prieto, P.A., Domínguez, A.C., Waltner-Toews, D., and FitzGibbon, J. 2008. Ciguatera fish poisoning in La Habana, Cuba: A study of local social-ecological resilience. *EcoHealth* 5(3): 346–359.
519. Gillespie, N.C., Lewis, R.J., Pearn J.H. et al. 1986. Ciguatera in Australia. Occurrence, clinical features, pathophysiology and management. *Med J Aust* 145: 584–590.
520. Fenner, P.J., Lewis, R.J., Williamson, J.A., and Williams, M.L. 1997. A Queensland family with ciguatera after eating coral trout. *Med J Aust* 166: 473–475.
521. Bagnis, R., Kuberski, T., and Laugier, S. 1979. Clinical observations on 3,009 cases of ciguatera (fish poisoning) in the South Pacific. *Am J Trop Med Hyg* 28(6): 1067–1073.
522. Bourée, P., Quod, J.P., and Turquet, J. 2002. L'ichtyosarcotoxisme de type ciguatera. *Rev Fr Lab Doss Sci* 342: 65–70.
523. Legrand, A.M. and Bagnis, R. 1991. La ciguatera, un phénomène d'écotoxicologie des récifs coralliens. *Ann Inst Pasteur/Actual* 4: 255.
524. Lewis, R.J. 2006. Ciguatera: Australian perspectives on a global problem. *Toxicon* 48: 799–809.
525. Baumann, F., Bourrat, M.B., and Pauillac, S. 2010. Prevalence, symptoms and chronicity of ciguatera in New Caledonia: Results from an adult population survey conducted in Noumea during 2005. *Toxicon* 56(5): 662–667.
526. Isbister, G.K. and Kiernan, M.C. 2005. Neurotoxic marine poisoning. *Lancet Neurol* 4: 219–228.
527. Cameron, J. and Capra, M.F. 1993. The basis of the paradoxical disturbance of temperature perception in ciguatera poisoning. *Clin Toxicol* 31: 571–579.
528. DASS. Situation sanitaire en Nouvelle-Calédonie 2008. Les maladies non transmisibles: la ciguatera. http://www.gouv.nc/portal/page/portal/dass/librairie/fichiers/11140135.PDF (accessed October 12, 2013).

529. Glaziou, P. and Legrand, A.M. 1994. The epidemiology of ciguatera fish poisoning. *Toxicon* 32: 863–873.

530. Gatti, C., Oelher, E., and Legrand, A.M. 2008. Severe seafood poisoning in French Polynesia: A retrospective analysis of 129 medical files. *Toxicon* 51: 746–753.

531. Allsop, J.L., Martini, L., Lebris, H., Pollard, J., Walsh, J., and Hodgkinson, S. 1986. Les manifestations neurologiques de la ciguatera. Trois cas avec étude neurophysiologique et examen d'une biopsie nerveuse. *Rev Neurol* 142: 590–597.

532. Pottier, I., Vernoux, J.P., and Lewis, R.J. 2001. Ciguatera fish poisoning in the Caribbean Islands and Western Atlantic. *Rev Environ Contam Toxicol* 168: 99–141.

533. Mitchell, G. 2005. Treatment of a mild chronic case of ciguatera fish poisoning with intravenous mannitol, a case study. *Pac Health Dialog* 12: 155–157.

534. Perez, C.M., Vasquez, P.A., and Perret, C.F. 2001. Treatment of ciguatera poisoning with gabapentin. *N Engl J Med* 344: 692–693.

535. Hamilton, B., Whittle, N., Shaw, G., Eagleshamb, G., Moore, M.R., and Lewis, R.J. 2010. Human fatality associated with Pacific ciguatoxin contaminated fish. *Toxicon* 56(5): 668–673.

536. Goater, S., Derne, B., and Weinstein, P. 2010. Critical issues in the development of health information systems in supporting environmental health: A case study of ciguatera. *Environ Health Perspect* 119(5): 585–590.

537. Bagnis, R., Speigel, A., N'Guyen, L., and Plichart, R. 1990. Public health, epidemiological and socioeconomic patterns of ciguatera in Tahiti. In: Tosteson, T.R., ed., *Proceedings of the 3rd International Conference on Ciguatera Fish Poisoning*. Morin-Heights Quebec, Canada: Polyscience, pp. 157–168.

538. Lawrence, D.N., Enriquez, M.B., Lumish, R.M., and Maceo, A. 1980. Ciguatera fish poisoning in Miami. *JAMA* 244: 254–258.

539. Kimura, L.Y., Abad, M.A., and Hokama, Y. 1982. Evaluation of the radioimmunoassay (RÍA) for detection of ciguatoxin (CTX) in fish tissues. *J Fish Biol* 21: 671–680.

540. Hokama, Y. 1985. A rapid, simplified enzyme immunoassay stick test for the detection of ciguatoxin and related polyethers from fish tissues. *Toxicon* 23: 939–946.

541. Hokama, Y., Asahina, A.Y., Shang, E.S., Hong, T.W., and Shirai, J.L. 1993. Evaluation of the Hawaiian reef fishes with the solid phase immunobead assay. *J Clin Lab Anal* 7: 26–30.

542. Stewart, I., Lewis, R.J., Eaglesham, G.K., Graham, G.C., Poole, S., and Craig, S.B. 2010. Emerging tropical diseases in Australia. Part 2. Ciguatera fish poisoning. *Ann Trop Med Parasitol* 104(7): 557–571.

543. Morey, J.S., Ryan, J.C., Dechraoui, M.Y.B., Rezvani, A.H., Levin, E.D., Gordon, C.J., Ramsdell, J.S., and Van Dolah, F.M. 2008. Liver genomic responses to ciguatoxin: Evidence for activation of phase I and phase II detoxification pathways following an acute hypothermic response in mice. *Toxicol Sci* 103: 298–310.

544. Nellis, D.W. and Barnard, G.W. 1986. Ciguatera: A legal and social overview. *Mar Fish Rev* 48: 2–5.

545. Lewis, N.D. 1986. Disease and development: Ciguatera fish poisoning. *Soc Sci Med* 23: 983–993.

546. Bourdy, G., Cabalion, P., Amade, P., and Laurent, D. 1992. Traditional remedies used in the western Pacific for the treatment of ciguatera poisoning. *J Ethnopharmacol* 36: 163–174.

547. De Blanchard, M.D.A.C. 1996. Report on outbreaks of ciguatera in the Dominican Republic. Epidemiological aspects related to public health and the laboratory. In: *Proceedings of the Workshop Conference on Seafood Intoxications: Pan American Implications of Natural Toxins in Seafood*. Miami, FL: University of Miami, INPAAZ Country Reports Section, pp. 59–74.

548. Holt, R.J., Miro, G., and Del Valle, A. 1984. An analysis of poison control center reports of ciguatera toxicity in Puerto Rico for one year. *Clin Toxicol* 22: 177–185.

549. Monis, J.G., Lewin, P., Hargrett, N.T., Smith, W., Blake, P.A., and Schneider, R. 1982. Clinical features of ciguatera fish poisoning. A study of the disease in the US Virgin Islands. *Arch Intern Med* 142: 1090–1092.

550. Llewellyn, L. 2010. Revisiting the association between sea surface temperature and the epidemiology of fish poisoning in the south Pacific: Reassessing the link between ciguatera and climate change. *Toxicon* 56: 691–697.

551. Mosher, H.S. and Fuhrman, F.A. 1984. Occurrence and origin of tetrodotoxin. In: Ragelis, E.P., ed., *Seafood Toxins*. Washington, DC: American Chemical Society, pp. 333–344.

552. Mosher, H.S., Fuhrman, F.A., Buchwald, H.D., and Fischer, H.G. 1965. Tarichatoxin–tetrodotoxin: A potent neurotoxin. *Science* 144: 1100–1110.

553. Noguchi, T., Uzu, A., Koyama, K., Maruyama, J., and Hashimoto, K. 1983. Occurrence of tetrodotoxin as the major toxin in a xanthid crab, *Atergatis floridus*. *Bull Jpn Soc Sci fish* 49: 1887–1892.

554. Sheumack, D.D., Howden, M.E., Spence, I., and Quinn, R.J. 1978. Maculotoxin: A neurotoxin from the venom glands of the octopus *Hapalochlaena maculosa* identified as tetrodotoxin. *Science* 199: 188–191.

555. Noguchi, T., Narita, H., Maruyama, J., and Hashimoto, K. 1982. Tetrodotoxin in the starfish *Astropecten polyacanthus*, in association with toxification of a trumpet shell, "boshubora", Charonia sauliae. *Bull Jpn Soc Sci Fish* 48: 1173–1177.

556. Narita, H., Noguchi, T., Maruyama, J., Ueda, Y., Hashimoto, K., Watanabe, Y., and Hida, K. 1981. Occurrence of tetrodotoxin in a trumpet shell, "boshubora" *Charonia sauliae. Bull Jpn Soc Sci Fish* 47: 935–941.

557. Miyazawa, K., Jeon, J.K., Maruyama, J., Noguchi, T., Ito, K., and Hashimoto, K. 1986. Occurrence of a paralytic toxicity in the flatworms *Planocera* multitentaculata (Platyhelminthys). *Toxicon* 24: 645–650.

558. Miyazawa, K., Higashiyama, M., Ito, K., Noguchi, T., Arakawa, O., Shida, Y., and Hashimoto, K. 1988. Tetrodotoxin in two species of ribbon worms (Nemertini), *Lineus fuscoviridis* and *Tubulanus punctatus. Toxicon* 26: 867–874.

559. Narahashi, T. 2008. Tetrodotoxin—A brief history. *Proc Jpn Acad Ser B Phys Biol Sci* 84(5): 147–154.

560. Yokoo, A. 1950. Chemical studies on pufferfish toxin (3)—Separation of spheroidine. *Nippon Kagaku Zasshi* 71: 590–592.

561. Woodward, R.B. 1964. The structure of tetrodotoxin. *Pure Appl Chem* 9: 49–74.

562. Noguchi, T. and Ebesu, J.S.M. 2001. Puffer poisoning: Epidemiology and treatment. *J Toxicol Toxin Rev* 20: 1–10.

563. Jang, J.H. and Yotsu-Yamashita, M. 2007. 6,11-Dideoxytetrodotoxin from the puffer fish, *Fugu pardalis. Toxicon* 50: 947–951.

564. Yotsu-Yamashita, M. 2001. Chemistry of puffer fish toxin. *J Toxicol Toxin Rev* 20: 51–66.

565. Williams, B.L. 2010. Behavioral and chemical ecology of marine organisms with respect to tetrodotoxin. *Mar Drugs* 8: 381–398.

566. Shiomi, K., Yamaguchi, S., Kikuchi, T., Yamamori, K., and Matsui, T. 1992. Occurrence of tetrodotxin binding high molecular weight substances in the body fluid of shore crab (*Hemigrapsus sanguineus*). *Toxicon* 30: 1529–1537.

567. Maruta, S., Yamaoka, K., and Yotsu-Yamashita, M. 2008. Two critical residues in p-loop regions of puffer fish Na$^+$ channels on TTX-sensitivity. *Toxicon* 51: 381–387.

568. Sims, J.K. and Ostman, D.C. 1986. Puffer fish poisoning: Emergency diagnosis and management of mild human tetrodotoxication. *Ann Emerg Med* 15: 1094–1098.

569. Nowadnick, J. 1976. Puffers: A taste of death. *Sea Frontiers* 22: 350–359.

570. Yang, C.C., Liao, S.C., and Deng, J.E. 1996. Tetrodotoxin poisoning in Taiwan: An analysis of poison center data. *Vet Human Toxicol* 38: 282–286.

571. Kanchanapongkul, J. and Krittayapoositpot, P. 1995. An epidemic of tetrodotoxin poisoning following ingestion of the horseshoe crab *Carcinoscorpius rotundicauda. Southeast Asian J Trop Med Public Health* 26: 364–367.

572. Shui, L.M., Chen, K., Wang, J.Y., Mei, H.Z., Wang, A.Z., Lu, Y.H., and Hwang, D.E. 2003. Tetrodotoxin-associated snail poisoning in Zhoushan: A 25-year retrospective analysis. *J Food Prot* 66: 110–114.

573. Akyol, O., Ünal, V., Ceyhan, T., and Bilecenoglu, M. 2005. First record of the silverside blaasop, *Lagocephalus sceleratus* (Gmelin, 1789), in the Mediterranean Sea. *J Fish Biol* 66: 1183–1186.

574. Golani, D. and Levy, Y. 2005. New records and rare occurrences of fish species from the Mediterranean coast of Israel. *Zool Middle East* 36: 27–32.

575. Kasapidis, P., Peristeraki, P., Tserpes, G., and Magoulas, A. 2007. First record of the Lessepsian migrant *Lagocephalus sceleratus* (Gmelin 1789) (Osteichthyes: Tetraodontidae) in the Cretan Sea (Aegean, Greece). *Aquat Invasions* 2: 71–73.

576. Katikou, P., Georgantelis, D., Sinouris, N., Petsi, A., and Fotaras, T. 2009. First report on toxicity assessment of the Lessepsian migrant pufferfish *Lagocephalus sceleratus* (Gmelin, 1789) from European waters (Aegean Sea, Greece). *Toxicon* 54(1): 50–55.

577. Sanzo, L. 1930. Plectognati. Ricerche biologiche su materiali raccolti dal Prof. L. Sanzo nella Campagna Idrografica net Mar Rosso della R.N. Ammiraglio Magnaghi 1923–1924. *Memorie Comitato Talassografico Italiano* 167: 1–111.

578. Bentur, Y., Ashkar, J., Lurie, Y. et al. 2008. Lessepsian migration and tetrodotoxin poisoning due to *Lagocephalus sceleratus* in the eastern Mediterranean. *Toxicon* 52: 964–968.

579. Eisenman, A., Rusetski, V., Sharivker, D., Yona, Z., and Golani, D. 2008. Case report. An odd pilgrim in the Holy Land. *Am J Emerg Med* 26(3): 383.e3–383.e6.

580. Noguchi, T., Jeon, J.K., Arakawa, O. et al. 1986. Occurrence of tetrodotoxin and anhydrotetrodotoxin in *Vibrio* sp. isolated from the intestines of a xanthid crab, *Atergatis floridus*. *J Biochem (Tokyo)* 99: 311–314.

581. Yasumoto, T., Yasumura, D., Yotsu, M., Michishita, T., Endo, A., and Kotaki, Y. 1986. Bacterial production of tetrodotoxin and anhydrotetrodotoxin. *Agric Biol Chem* 50: 793–795.

582. Matsui, T., Taketsugu, S., Sato, H., Yamamori, K., Kodama, K., Ishi, A., Hirose, H., and Shimizu, C. 1990. Toxification of cultured puffer fish by the administration of tetrodotoxin producing bacteria. *Nippon Suisan Gakkaishi* 56: 705.

583. Yotsu, M., Yamazaki, T., Meguro, Y., Endo, A., Murata, M., Naoki, H., and Yasumoto, T. 1987. Production of tetrodotoxin and its derivatives by *Pseudomonas* sp. isolated from the skin of a puffer fish. *Toxicon* 25: 225–228.

584. Narita, H., Matsubara, S., Miwa, N., Akahane, S., Murakami, M., Goto, T., Nara, M. et al. 1987. *Vibrio alginolyticus*, a tetrodotoxin producing bacterium isolated from the starfish *Astropecten polyacanthus*. *Nippon Suisan Gakkaishi* 53: 617–621.

585. Hwang, D.F., Arakawa, O., Saito, T., Noguchi, T., Simidu, U., Tsukamoto, K., Shida, Y., and Hashimoto, K. 1989. Tetrodotoxin producing bacteria from the blue-ringed octopus *Octopus maculosus*. *Mar Biol* 100: 327–332.

586. Hwang, D.F., Cheng, C.A., Chen, H.C., Jeng, S.S., Noguchi, T., Ohwada, K., and Hashimoto, K. 1994. Microflora and tetrodotoxin producing bacteria in the lined moon shell *Natica lineate*. *Fish Sci* 60: 567–571.

587. Cheng, C.A., Hwang, D.F., Tsai, Y.H., Chen, H.C., Jeng, S.S., Noguchi, T., Ohwada, K., and Hasimoto, K. 1995. Microflora and tetrodotoxin-producing bacteria in a gastropod, *Niotha clathrata*. *Food Chem Toxicol* 33: 929–934.

588. Lee, M.J., Jeong, D.Y., Kim, W.S., Kim, H.D., Kim, C.H., Park, W.W., Park, Y.H., Kim, K.S., Kim, H.M., and Kim, D.S. 2000. A tetrodotoxin-producing Vibrio strain, LM-1, from the puffer fish *Fugu vermicularis radiatus*. *Appl Environ Microbiol* 66: 1698–1701

589. Yu, C.F., Yu, P.H., Chan, P.L., Yan, Q., and Wong, P.K. 2004. Two novel species of tetrodotoxin-producing bacteria isolated from toxic marine puffer fishes. *Toxicon* 44: 641–647.

590. Wu, Z., Xie, L., Xia, G., Zhang, J., Nie, Y., Hu, J., Wang, S., and Zhang, R. 2005. A new tetrodotoxin-producing actinomycete, *Nocardiopsis dassonvillei*, isolated from the ovaries of puffer fish *Fugu rubripes*. *Toxicon* 45: 851–859.

591. Do, H., Kogure, K., and Simidu, U. 1990. Identification of deep-sea sediment bacteria which produce tetrodotoxin. *Appl Environ Microbiol* 56: 1162–1163.

592. Do, H., Kogure, K., Imada, C., Noguchi, T., Ohwada, K., and Simidu, U. 1991. Tetrodotoxin production of actimomycetes isolated from marine sediment. *J Appl Bacteriol* 70: 464–468.

593. Do, H., Hamasaki, K., Ohwada, K., Simidu, U., Noguchi, T., Shida, Y., and Kogure, K. 1993. Presence of tetrodotoxin and tetrodotoxin-producing bacteria in freshwater sediments. *Appl Environ Microbiol* 59: 3934–3937.

594. Kogure, K., Do, H.K., Thuesen, E.V., Nanba, K., Ohwase, K., and Simidu, U. 1988. Accumulation of tetrodotoxin in marine sediments. *Mar Ecol Prog Ser* 45: 303–305.

595. Noguchi, T. and Arakawa, O. 2008. Tetrodotoxin. Distribution and accumulation in aquatic organisms, and cases of human intoxication. *Mar Drugs* 6: 220–242.

596. Tani, I. 1945. *Studies on Japanese Pufffish in Association with Poisoning due to Ingestion of Them.* Tokyo, Japan: Teikoku Tosho, p. 103.

597. Environmental Health Bureau, Ministry of Health and Welfare. 1984. *Pufferfishes Available in Japan— An Illustrated Guide to Their Identification.* Tokyo, Japan: Chuo-Hokishuppan, p. 79.

598. Kanoh, S. 1988. Distribution of tetrodotoxin in vertebrates. In: Hashimoto, K., ed., *Recent Advances in Tetrodotoxin Research.* Tokyo, Japan: Koseisha-Koseikaku, pp. 32–44.

599. Fuchi, Y., Narimatsu, H., Nakama, S. et al. 1991. Tissue distribution of toxicity in a pufferfish, *Arothron firmamentum* ("hoshifugu"). *J Food Hyg Soc Jpn* 32: 520–524.

600. Khora, S.S., Isa, J., and Yasumoto, T. 1991. Toxicity of puffers from Okinawa. *Jpn Nippon Suisan Gakkaishi* 57: 163–167.

601. Hwang, D.F., Kao, C.Y., Yang, H.C., Jeng, S.S., Noguchi, T., and Hashimoto, K. 1992. Toxicity of puffer in Taiwan. *Nippon Suisan Gakkaishi* 58: 1541–1547.

602. Boylan, D.B. and Scheuer, P.J. 1967. Pahutoxin: A fish poison. *Science* 155: 52.

603. Thomson, D.A. 1968. Drugs from the sea. In: Freudenthal, H.D., ed., *Marine Technology Society*. Washington, DC: Marine Technology Society, p. 203.

604. Taniyama, S. 2002. Toxicity and toxin profile of marine boxfish. In: *Studies on Parrotfish Poisoning and Similar Incidents Caused by Other Fishes*, PhD thesis, Nagasaki University, Nagasaki, Japan, pp. 73–80.

605. Mahmud, Y., Yamamori, K., and Noguchi, T. 1999. Occurrence of TTX in a brackishwater puffer "midorifugu" *Tetraodon nigroviridis*, collected from Thailand. *J Food Hyg Soc Jpn* 40: 363–367.

606. Mahmud, Y., Yamamori, K., and Noguchi, T. 1999. Toxicity and tetrodotoxin as the toxic principle of a brackishwater puffer *Tetraodon steindachneri*, collected from Thailand. *J Food Hyg Soc Jpn* 40: 391–395.

607. Kungsuwan, A., Arakawa, O., Promdet, M., and Onoue, Y. 1997. Occurrence of paralytic shellfish poisons in Thai freshwater puffers. *Toxicon* 35: 1341–1346.

608. Sato, S., Kodama, M., Ogata, T., Saitanu, K., Furuya, M., Hirayama, K., and Kakinuma, K. 1997. Saxitoxin as toxic principle of a freshwater puffer, *Tetraodon fangi*, in Thailand. *Toxicon* 35: 137–140.

609. Mahmud, Y., Tanu, M.B., Takatani, T., Asayama, E., Arakawa, O., and Noguchi, T. 2001. *Chelonodon patoca*, a highly toxic marine puffer in Japan. *J Nat Toxins* 10: 69–74.

610. Ngy, L., Tada, K., Yu, C.F., Takatani, T., and Arakawa, O. 2008. Occurrence of paralytic shellfish toxins in Cambodian Mekong pufferfish *Tetraodon turgidus*: Selective toxin accumulation in the skin. *Toxicon* 51: 280–288.

611. Laobhripatr, S., Limpakarnjanarat, K., Sangwonloy, O. et al. 1990. Food poisoning due to consumption of the freshwater puffer *Tetraodon fangi* in Thailand. *Toxicon* 28: 1372–1375.

612. Mahmud, Y., Arakawa, O., and Noguchi T. 2000. An epidemic survey on freshwater puffer poisoning in Bangladesh. *J Nat Toxins* 9: 319–326.

613. Hwang, D.F., Cheng, C.A., Tsai, Y.H., Shih, D.Y.C., Ko, H.C., Yang, R.Z., and Jeng, S.S. 1995. Identification of tetrodotoxin and paralytic shellfish toxins in marine gastropods implicated in food poisoning. *Fish Sci* 61: 675–679.

614. Hwang, D.F., Shiu, Y.C., Hwang, P.A., and Lu, Y.H. 2002. Tetrodotoxin in gastropods snails implicated in food poisoning in northern Taiwan. *J Food Sci* 65: 1341–1344.

615. Hwang, P.A., Tsai, Y.H., Lu, Y.H., and Hwang, D.F. 2003. Paralytic toxins in three new gastropod *Olividae* species implicated in food poisoning in southern Taiwan. *Toxicon* 41: 529–533.

616. Hwang, P.A., Tsai, Y.H., Deng, J.F., Cheng, C.A., Ho, P.H., and Hwang, D.F. 2005. Identification of tetrodotoxin in a marine gastropod *Nassarius glans* responsible for human morbidity and mortality in Taiwan. *J Food Prot* 68: 1696–1701.

617. Shiu, Y.C., Lu, Y.H., Tsai, Y.H., and Hwang, D.F. 2003. Occurrence of tetrodotoxin in the causative gastropod *Polinices didyma* and another gastropod *Natica lineata* collected from western Taiwan. *J Food Drug Anal* 11: 159–163.

618. Kungsuwan, A., Nagashima, Y., Noguchi, T., Shida, Y., Suvapeepan, S., Suwansakornkul, P., and Hashimoto, K. 1987. Tetrodotoxin in the horseshoe crab *Carcinoscorpius rotundicauda* inhabiting Thailand. *Nippon Suisan Gakkaishi* 53: 261–266.

619. Tanu, M.B. and Noguchi, T. 1999. Tetrodotoxin as a toxin principle in the horseshoe crab *Carcinoscorpius rotundicauda* collected from Bangladesh. *J Food Hyg Soc Jpn* 40: 426–431.

620. Ngy, L., Yu, C.F., Takatani, T., and Arakawa, O. 2007. Toxicity assessment for the horseshoe crab *Carcinoscorpius rotundicauda* collected from Cambodia. *Toxicon* 49: 843–847.

621. Fusetani, N., Endo, H., Hashimoto, K., and Kodama, M. 1983. Occurrence and properties of toxins in the horseshoe crab *Carcinoscorpius rotundicauda*. *Toxicon* 21: 165–168.

622. Du, S.S., Fu, Y.M., Shih, Y.C., Chang, P.C., Chou, S.S., Lue, Y.H., and Hwang, D.F. 1999. First report on suspected food poisoning with ingestion of dried seasoned fish fillet. *J Food Drug Anal* 7: 163–167.

623. Hsieh, Y.W., Hwang, P.A., Pan, H.H., Chen, J.B., and Hwang, D.F. 2003. Identification of tetrodotoxin and fish species in an adulterated dried mullet roe implicated in food poisoning. *J Food Sci* 68: 142–146.

624. Hwang, D.F., Hwang, P.A., Tsai, Y.H., and Lu, Y.H. Identification of tetrodotoxin and fish species in dried dressed fish fillets implicated in food poisoning. *J Food Prot* 65: 389–392.

625. Kanchanapongkul, J. 2008. Tetrodotoxin poisoning following ingestion of the toxic eggs of the horseshoe crab *Carcinoscorpius rotundicauda*, a case series from 1994 through 2006. *Southeast Asian J Trop Med Public Health* 39(2): 303–306.

626. O'Leary, M.A., Schneider, J.J., and Isbister, G.K. 2004. Use of high performance liquid chromatography to measure tetrodotoxin in serum and urine of poisoned patients. *Toxicon* 44: 549–553.

627. Centers for Disease Control (CDC). 1996. Tetrodotoxin poisoning associated with eating puffer fish transported from Japan—California, 1996. *MMWR* 45: 389–391.
628. Holland, P.T. 2008. Analysis of marine toxins—Techniques, method validation, calibration standards and screening methods. In: Botana, L.M., ed., *Seafood and Freshwater Toxins: Pharmacology, Physiology, and Detection*, 2nd edn. New York: CRC Press, pp. 21–50.
629. Consellería de Pesca, Marisqueo y Acuicultura. Orden de 14 de noviembre de 1995 por la que se regula el programa de actuaciones para el control de biotoxinas marinas en moluscos bivalvos y otros organismos procedentes de la pesca, el marisqueo y la acuicultura. Diario Oficial de Galicia no 221, de 17 de noviembre, pp. 8454–8467.

7

Toxicology of Seafood Toxins: A Critical Review

Rex Munday

CONTENTS

7.1 Introduction

Since earliest times, human food has been contaminated with bioactive substances. These may be derived from plants, such as solanine in green potatoes or the cyanide in cassava, or from fungi, bacteria, and other microorganisms. More recently, chemicals have been deliberately added to food as flavors, colors, preservatives, and other substances designed to improve the appearance or organoleptic properties of food or to extend its shelf life, while the use of chemical pesticides has inevitably led to contamination of foodstuffs with trace amounts of these substances. Humans have learned to avoid eating green potatoes and to process cassava to reduce its content of cyanide, but other additives and contaminants are impossible to avoid, thus possibly posing a risk to health.

Risk may be defined as "The probability that an adverse effect will be induced in an individual through contact with a particular substance." Risk is a function of the dose of the substance and its intrinsic toxicity. That is to say that a small dose of a highly toxic contaminant will cause harm, while a large dose of a substance of low intrinsic toxicity will give an equivalent effect. For risk assessment, therefore, it is necessary to determine the levels of additives and contaminants in food and to establish their toxic potential.

A basic principle of toxicology is that for any poison, there is a dose below which it will have no perceptible adverse effect on the consumer. This is defined as the no observable adverse effect level (NOAEL). Such a tenet is justified by the fact that animals have evolved in the presence of many toxins and have developed very effective defenses against them. It is only when these defenses are overwhelmed that toxic effects occur. A second parameter encountered in toxicological evaluations is the lowest observable adverse effect level (LOAEL), the lowest dose at which statistically and/or biologically significant adverse effects are observed. The relationship between the NOAEL and LOAEL depends on the slope of the dose–response curve.

Two scenarios of toxic effects may be envisioned. Firstly, there are acute effects, induced by a single exposure to a toxic compound. For assessment of such risk, acute toxicity studies are required, in which progressively increasing single doses of the test compound are administered to animals, usually mice or rats, in order to establish the median lethal dose (LD_{50}), defined as the dose required to kill 50% of the tested population. The Organisation for Economic Co-operation and Development (OECD) has published guidelines on the assessment of acute toxicity (Guidelines 420, 423, and 425). A previous acute toxicity guideline (Guideline 401) was deleted in 2001, and data obtained by this method are no longer acceptable to regulatory authorities. The most recent guideline is the "up-and-down" procedure, Guideline 425, which has the advantage of minimizing the number of animals required for estimating the LD_{50} of a compound while providing confidence intervals of this estimate. This technique has shown good correlation with other methods of acute toxicity determination.[1] By administration of doses below the LD_{50}, it is possible to establish the NOAEL and LOAEL for acute exposure to the test substance. In some publications, the minimum lethal dose (MLD) of a substance is given as an indication of its acute toxicity. This is the lowest dose at which death is observed in a group of animals given the test substance. The MLD bears no consistent relationship to the LD_{50} and is an imprecise parameter that is strongly dependent on the number of animals in each group and the interval between the doses employed. Even worse, acute toxicity is sometimes expressed as "lethality" or "lethal dose," a nonspecific term that could indicate an MLD, an LD_{50}, or an LD_{100}, the last named indicating a dose sufficient to kill all of a group of animals.

Secondly, there are chronic effects, induced by repeated exposure to a toxic compound. Again, OECD Guidelines (Guidelines 407, 408, 452, 453) are available for the conduct of short-term (28- and 90-day) and chronic toxicity (up to 2 years) studies in rodents. In addition, studies on possible effects on reproduction, together with assessment of potential carcinogenicity and teratogenicity, are required for a full risk assessment. With regard to carcinogenicity, in vitro or short-term in vivo mutagenicity studies are valuable indicators of neoplastic potential.[2]

From acute toxicity data, by application of a safety factor (also referred to as an uncertainty factor), it is possible to obtain an estimate of the acute reference dose (ARfD) of the substance for humans. The ARfD is defined as "An estimate of the amount of a substance in food and/or drinking water, normally expressed on a milligram per kilogram body weight basis, that can be ingested in a period of 24 h or less without appreciable health risk to the consumer."[3] From repeated-exposure studies, also after application of a safety factor, the tolerable daily intake (TDI, also known as the acceptable daily intake or, in the United States, the reference dose) for humans can be estimated. The TDI is defined as "An estimate of the amount of a substance in food and/or drinking water, normally expressed on a milligram per kilogram body weight basis, that can be ingested daily over a lifetime without appreciable health risk to the consumer."[4]

For such studies, several important points need to be considered. Firstly, the route of administration must be the same as that encountered in the human situation, that is, oral. Many data are available on the toxicity of food contaminants by intraperitoneal injection, but such data are of limited value for risk assessment. Injected compounds are rapidly and extensively absorbed from the peritoneal cavity, whereas the gastrointestinal tract is designed to minimize absorption of many harmful substances. Intraperitoneal toxicity will therefore give a high estimate of the toxicity of substances that require absorption for expression of toxicity and, at best, can be considered as a "worst-case scenario." In future studies, priority should be given to oral toxicity studies, but here again there are pitfalls to be avoided. It has been argued[5] that gavage, in which a solution of the test substance is delivered to the stomach of an animal via a tube inserted into the esophagus, may give an artifactually high estimate of toxicity in acute studies. Rodent stomach contents are semisolid, quite unlike the liquid material that is present in the human stomach. After gavage, the solution containing the test substance will not mix with the rodent's stomach contents but will flow around the semisolid mass to be delivered directly to the duodenum, where rapid absorption may occur. This does not happen when humans eat food contaminants, since the food, with its associated toxins, becomes mixed with the liquid stomach contents and thus diluted. The contaminant will then be delivered slowly to the duodenum, at a lower concentration than that associated with gavage in rodents. Gavage is also associated with other problems, and its use and reliability is dependent upon the skill of the operator.[6,7] It has been reported that test materials may be deposited in the lungs of more than 30% of mice after gavage,[8] which may not only induce pulmonary lesions but also toxic changes in other organs, since toxic substances are readily absorbed from the lungs. Pulmonary delivery may be due to excessively rapid delivery, causing reflux up the esophagus and into the trachea,[9] or by the use of large volumes.[10] A dose of no more than 10 mL/kg body weight, equivalent to no more than 200 μL for a 20 g mouse, is recommended.[10]

The human situation can be more accurately replicated in rodents by administration by voluntary feeding, in which the test substance is mixed with a small amount of food and given to the animals. In this way, the spiked food, and its content of contaminant, mixes with the food within the rodent stomach, thus simulating the human situation. There is no problem with administering toxins to rats in this way, since these animals readily accept novel foodstuffs. Vanilla-flavored wafers[11] and chocolate[12] have been recommended for oral delivery of xenobiotics to rats, although these animals will eagerly consume many other foodstuffs, such as egg, meat, and shellfish flesh. Mice, however, are more difficult. The use of bacon-flavored pills as an alternative to gavage for mice has been suggested,[13] but this approach would be of no use for acute toxicity studies, since the animals were found to take up to 30 min to consume the pill. Acute toxicity studies require delivery of the whole amount of the test substance within seconds. Mice fasted overnight will rapidly eat a small piece of mousefood, either dry or moistened with water. In some cases, however, the animals appear to be able to detect the presence of harmful materials in dry mousefood, and the use of moistened food, provided as a thick paste, is preferable. Alternatively, other foods may be employed. It has been found that mice, after a period of training, will readily eat cream cheese or a mixture of low-fat peanut butter (53%), casein (10%), and sucrose (37%). The latter food has the advantage of containing the same proportions of fat, protein, and carbohydrate as those commonly found in the human diet, but in studies on the acute toxicity of pinnatoxin F, no differences in response were observed among animals given this substance on mousefood or in cream cheese or the peanut butter mix.[14] The advantage of the last-named two vehicles is that when the animals have grown accustomed to them, they are rapidly and enthusiastically eaten by both fasted and fed mice. Other authors have reported difficulties in obtaining rapid ingestion of contaminated food by mice,[15] and the need for training must be stressed, due to the suspicion with which mice regard unfamiliar foodstuffs. Training is best accomplished in a group-housing situation, in which mice are offered the uncontaminated new food each day. Some mice will take small amounts of the food, and when they discover that this is associated with no adverse effects, they will eat large quantities when given the opportunity. More cautious mice, seeing the enthusiastic ingestion of the new food by their cage-mates, will join in, and with very few exceptions, the whole group will readily eat the new food after a week's training, and a 200 mg portion will be consumed in 30–60 s.

The use of gavage in long-term studies must also be evaluated. The OECD recommends that gavage should be used in chronic toxicity studies only when this route and method of administration represents potential human exposure, as with pharmaceuticals. In all other instances, administration via the diet or drinking water is recommended.[16] Significant differences have been observed between gavage and feeding in the pharmacokinetics and pharmacodynamics of chemicals,[17] and their chronic toxicity is often higher by gavage than when administered in food or water.[18–21]

The question also arises as to whether rodents should be fasted before administration of the test substances in acute toxicity trials or whether fed animals should be employed. This again may make a significant difference to the estimation of toxicity. By gavage, fasted mice are generally more susceptible to toxins than fed animals, most likely due to more rapid delivery to the duodenum due to the smaller amount of food in the stomach. While fasted mice may be more relevant to the human situation for foodstuffs consumed for breakfast, it could be argued that at other times of the day, the fed animal is more relevant to the human than the fasted.

Sex, strain, and age (as reflected by body weight) have been shown to influence susceptibility in acute toxicity studies. While it is to be expected that different laboratories will employ different sexes and strains of mice, and animals of different ages, it is important that these characteristics are specified in toxicological reports. With regard to age, acute toxicity tests employ healthy young adult rodents. In extrapolating from animals to the human situation, however, it must be remembered that very young and very old individuals may be at particular risk of intoxication by harmful chemicals, due to deficiencies in rates of detoxification and/or excretion.[22–24]

Also of importance is the characterization of the material that is being tested. It is important that the identity and purity of a test material is confirmed in the testing laboratory before conducting toxicological tests, and this should be stated in publications.

Food additives and pesticide residues rank highly in consumer perception of risk, but these compounds have generally undergone extensive toxicological evaluation so that scientifically sound limits for levels in food can be set. The same cannot be said, however, of many of the contaminants from microorganisms, particularly those derived from aquatic microalgae and diatoms. Contaminants in seafood cause illness in thousands of people every year. In extreme cases, death may ensue. Proper risk assessment of such contaminants is urgently needed in order to reduce the incidence of poisoning in consumers of seafood. For this purpose, it is essential that the toxicological assessments are conducted in such a way that relevant regulatory limits for the contaminants can be determined.

In this chapter, the toxicology of seafood toxins is reviewed, and an attempt has been made to highlight the deficiencies in the toxicological data that preclude proper risk assessment of such substances.

7.2 Azaspiracids

7.2.1 Production and Distribution of Azaspiracids

The lipophilic polyether azaspiracids (AZAs) are synthesized by the dinoflagellate *Azadinium spinosum*.[25,26] In culture, this organism produces AZA-1, AZA-2, and an unidentified isomer of AZA-2.[27] When taken up by molluscs, however, these compounds undergo metabolism, and many more AZA derivatives are found in seafood.[28] Three such metabolites (AZA-3, AZA-4, and AZA-5) have been fully characterized.[29,30] AZA-3 is formed from AZA-1 by demethylation, while AZA-4 and AZA-5 are hydroxylated derivatives of AZA-3. The last-named compounds occur only at low levels in shellfish, and AZA-1, AZA-2, and AZA-3 are believed to be the compounds of highest toxicological significance.[31] The structures of these compounds, and of other AZA metabolites, are given by Rehmann et al.[28] AZAs were first identified in mussels from Killary Harbour, Ireland. Subsequent studies have shown, however, that these substances are of widespread distribution, being found in shellfish from England, Scotland, Norway, the Netherlands, France, Spain, Portugal, Italy, Morocco, Canada, Chile, and Korea.[25,32,33] AZAs have also been found in crabs from Norway and Sweden.[34]

7.2.2 Toxicity of Azaspiracids to Experimental Animals

The toxicology of AZAs has been reviewed.[35]

7.2.2.1 Acute Toxicities of Azaspiracids by Intraperitoneal Injection

No LD_{50}s for AZAs are available. Data on the "lethalities" of several AZA derivatives, extracted from mussels, by intraperitoneal injection in mice are shown in Table 7.1.

Of the compounds tested, AZA-2 and AZA-3 appear to be the most acutely toxic, followed by AZA-1. AZA-4 is less toxic, while comparison with AZA-5 is not possible, since the lethal dose of this substance was simply quoted as "less than 1 mg/kg." No data on the symptoms of intoxication by the pure AZAs at lethal doses are available.

A partially purified extract of mussels implicated in the Irish poisoning incident, coded "KT3," was dosed to mice by intraperitoneal injection. Mice became inactive within 10 min of injection, and deaths occurred within a 24 h period. At necropsy, the liver was found to be enlarged and pale in color, while marked decreases in the weights of thymus and spleen were recorded. Histological examination revealed centrilobular hepatocytic hypertrophy, together with fat deposition. Marked pyknosis of peripheral parenchymal cells in the pancreas and hemorrhagic erosions in the stomach were also observed.[37]

7.2.2.2 Acute Toxicities of Azaspiracids by Oral Administration

Oral administration of KT3, the crude extract of toxic mussels, caused marked gastrointestinal changes in mice. Secretion of fluid from the ileum was observed, accompanied by necrosis of villous epithelial cells. Edema in the lamina propria was also recorded.[37]

Ito[35] administered AZA-1, extracted from mussels and of unspecified purity, by gavage to groups of mice of different ages, at doses of between 250 and 600 μg/kg. Both mice receiving 300 μg/kg died, while only three out of six mice died at a dose of 600 μg/kg. In a later experiment by the same group, however, using authenticated synthetic AZA-1, the lethal dose was estimated at >700 μg/kg.[38] No deaths occurred at 300 μg/kg after oral administration of a certified sample of AZA-1,[15] while a later study indicated an LD_{50} of 775 μg/kg for this material.[39]

Increased liver weights, associated with hepatic lipidosis, were observed in mice killed 24 h after an oral dose of mussel-derived AZA-1 at 500 μg/kg. Single-cell necrosis of hepatocytes was also recorded. Mice given 500–900 μg/kg AZA-1 showed necrosis of lymphocytes in the thymus, spleen, and Peyer's patches of the small intestine, although no histological alterations were observed in the kidney, heart, pancreas, or lungs. After oral administration of 600–700 μg/kg of AZA-1, progressive damage to the villi and lamina propria of the small intestine was observed,[40] similar to the changes in these tissues recorded with okadaic acid and the dinophysistoxins.[35] Small amounts of watery material appeared in the small intestine 4 h after a dose of 300 μg/kg, although no diarrhea was observed.[40]

TABLE 7.1

Acute Toxicities of AZAs by Intraperitoneal Injection in Mice

Compound	Strain of Mouse	Sex of Mouse	State of Alimentation	Parameter	Acute Toxicity (μg/kg Body Weight)	Reference
AZA-1	ddY	Male	?	"Lethality"	200	[36]
AZA-2	ddY	Male	?	"Lethality"	~110	[29]
AZA-3	ddY	Male	?	"Lethality"	~140	[29]
AZA-4	ddY	Male	?	"Lethality"	~470	[29]
AZA-5	ddY	Male	?	"Lethality"	<1000	[29]

Note: "?" indicates that this information was not provided in the cited reference.

Mice dosed orally with synthetic AZA-1 at 500–900 µg/kg again showed liver enlargement with fat deposition. In the intestine, however, no fluid accumulation was recorded, and the severity of the damage to villi and the lamina propria appeared to be lower than that seen with the AZA-1 isolated from mussels.[38] In a later study, using certified AZA-1, only mild exfoliation of epithelial cells and slight edema and hyperemia of the lamina propria were observed in the duodenum of mice after an oral dose of 300 µg/kg. No lesions were recorded in other parts of the gastrointestinal tract or in the brain, heart, lungs, thymus, liver, spleen, or kidneys of the treated animals, and the duodenal damage was fully healed 7 days after dosing.[15] Dilatation of the upper and middle small intestine was observed in mice dosed orally with certified AZA-1 at 420–780 µg/kg, and the contents were abnormally fluid. The livers of these animals were pale, but no histological changes were recorded in this organ.[39]

The acute toxicity of AZA-1 and the severity of the histological changes in the gastrointestinal tract induced by this substance were not increased by simultaneous administration of okadaic acid.[39]

7.2.2.3 Repeated-Dose Studies with Azaspiracid

Ten mice that survived single oral doses of mussel-derived AZA-1 at 300–450 µg/kg were given a second dose of 250 or 300 µg/kg 2 days later, and the animals were killed at various time intervals thereafter. Changes in lymphoid tissues resolved after 10 days, and the liver became normal after 15 days. Infiltration of cells into the pulmonary alveolar wall was reported 8 weeks after the second dose,[41] although this observation is surprising, since no histological changes were recorded in the lung after acute administration of AZA-1.[40] Lesions in the gastrointestinal mucosa persisted for 3 months after AZA-1 administration, an effect ascribed to bacterial infection.[35]

In a second experiment, groups of mice were dosed by gavage with mussel-derived AZA-1 at 1, 5, 20, or 50 µg/kg twice a week, over a period of up to 20 weeks.[41] At the highest dose, all mice died or were killed *in extremis* within 40 doses, and at the 20 µg/kg dose, 30% of the mice died. In these animals, interstitial inflammation and congestion was observed in the lungs, together with occasional focal necrosis and slight inflammation in the liver. In the small intestine, shortened villi, edema, and atrophy of the lamina propria were observed. No effects were recorded at the 1 and 5 µg/kg dose levels, and no diarrhea was reported in the animals at any dose level. The mice that survived 40 doses were subsequently left untreated for up to 3 months. Four lung tumors were observed in these mice, and in order to further investigate the possible carcinogenicity of AZA-1, an additional experiment was conducted, involving administration of AZA-1 to mice at dose levels of between 5 and 20 µg/kg, once or twice per week, for a total of between 20 and 40 doses. The majority of these mice were killed after 8 months. No tumors were seen at this time. The remaining 20 mice were kept for a further 4 months, when 9 tumors (7 lung tumors and 2 malignant lymphomas) were found.[35] The tumor incidence in the mice dosed with AZA-1 was not, however, significantly different from that in the control animals.[31]

7.2.3 Effects of Azaspiracids in Humans

Several incidents of human intoxication have been reported, mostly due to mussels sourced from Ireland.[42,43] The symptoms of intoxication are the same as those observed in diarrhetic shellfish poisoning (DSP), consisting of nausea, vomiting, diarrhea, and stomach cramps.[44] No deaths attributable to AZA ingestion have been reported.

7.2.4 Metabolism and Disposition of Azaspiracids

After oral administration to mice, AZA-1 was detected in the heart, lungs, liver, spleen, kidneys, brain, and gastrointestinal tract of the animals. Among the internal organs, the kidneys and spleen contained the highest concentrations after 24 h, while only trace amounts were present in the brain. At this time, less than 2% of the administered dose remained in the internal organs; after 7 days, the amount remaining was less than 1% of the dose.[15] When AZA-1 and okadaic acid were simultaneously administered by gavage to mice, the degree of absorption of both compounds was decreased,[39] while the absorption of yessotoxin (YTX) was unchanged when administered simultaneously with AZA-1.[45]

No information on the in vivo metabolism of AZAs is available. The incubation of AZA-1 with rat liver post-mitochondrial supernatant led to the formation of oxygenated products, as detected by mass spectrometry, although the metabolites were not characterized. There was also evidence that AZA-1 underwent glucuronidation under these conditions.[46]

7.2.5 Mechanism of Toxicity of Azaspiracids

The mechanism or mechanisms whereby AZAs exert their toxic effects are unknown. With regard to diarrheagenicity, the inhibition of protein phosphatases (which may, or may not, be involved in the diarrhetic effect of okadaic acid [Section 7.7]) cannot be a factor, since mussel homogenates containing AZAs did not inhibit the activity of protein phosphatase-1[47] and AZA-1 had no effect on protein phosphatase 2 activity at a concentration of 83 nM in a system in which the median effective dose (ED_{50}) of okadaic acid was 1.5 nM.[48] Unlike many other shellfish toxins, AZA-1 has no effect on voltage-gated sodium channels.[49]

7.2.6 Mutagenicity of Azaspiracids

No information on the possible mutagenic effects of AZAs is available.

7.2.7 Regulation of Azaspiracids

The current European limit is set at 160 μg of AZA-1 equivalents/kg shellfish meat,[31] and this level was also recommended by the Codex Committee on Fish and Fishery Products (CCFFP).[50] However, based on the very limited human data, the European Food Safety Authority (EFSA) Panel on Contaminants in the Food Chain (The EFSA CONTAM Panel) established an ARfD of 0.2 μg AZA-1 equivalents/kg. The Panel noted that a 400 g portion of shellfish meat containing AZAs at the regulatory limit would result in an intake of 1 μg of AZA-1 equivalents/kg body weight for a 60 kg adult, exceeding the ARfD by a factor of 5, and concluded that in order that the ARfD should not be exceeded, shellfish meat should contain no more than 30 μg AZA-1 equivalents/kg.[31]

7.2.8 Conclusions

The toxicological information on AZAs is inadequate. No LD_{50}s of AZA are available either by oral administration or by injection. Published data on toxicity by intraperitoneal injection were reported as "lethalities," an ambiguous term. Furthermore, it appears that these data are based on results from only a very small number of animals.[36] Although these figures have been used by regulatory authorities in calculating toxic equivalency factors (TEFs) for AZA derivatives, they must be regarded as approximations only, and this route of administration is not relevant to the human situation. Very limited data on the oral toxicity of AZAs are available. The determination of LD_{50}s by oral administration, using validated methodologies and certified samples of the test materials, is required in order to provide authentic TEFs.

There are possible problems with the purity of the AZA-1 employed in some of the published studies. The toxicity of fully authenticated AZA-1 appeared to be lower than the material of unspecified purity that was isolated from mussels, and the greatest effects on fluid accumulation in the small intestine were induced by a crude extract of mussels, suggesting that other components of this extract had important effects on the gastrointestinal tract. There is also conflict in reports with regard to the sites of histological change following oral administration of AZA-1. Ito et al.[40] reported pathological changes in the liver, thymus, and spleen of mice after a single dose of mussel-derived AZA-1, while the certified material employed by Aasen et al.[15] and Aune et al.[39] induced no changes in these organs.

While the pulmonary tumors seen in the repeat-dosing experiment with AZA-1 are widely cited as indicating a carcinogenic effect of this substance, the carcinogenicity of AZA-1 cannot be considered to be proven. The CD-1 mice used in the experiments by Ito[35] have a high spontaneous incidence of lung tumors, as do many other strains of laboratory mouse.[51,52] In their review of the use of the mouse in carcinogenicity testing, Grasso and Crampton[53] concluded that "the induction of pulmonary tumors in the mouse has limited relevance in terms of human carcinogenic hazard." In any future studies designed to assess the possible pulmonary carcinogenicity of AZAs, the use of rats would be preferable, since these animals have a low spontaneous incidence of lung cancer.[52] The evaluation of the mutagenic potential of AZA in the Ames test would be valuable as a first step in evaluating the possible carcinogenicity of AZAs.

7.3 Brevetoxins

7.3.1 Production and Distribution of Brevetoxins

Brevetoxins (BTXs) are produced by dinoflagellates of the genus *Karenia*.[54,55] Although *Karenia* species are of worldwide distribution,[56] adverse effects on human health due to BTXs have been reported only from the Gulf of Mexico, North Carolina, and Texas in the United States and from the Hauraki Gulf of New Zealand.[55,56]

BTXs are divided into two types (A and B), according to the structure of their polyether backbone. BTXs of the A type comprise BTX-1, BTX-7, and BTX-10. The last-named compounds are formed from BTX-1 by reduction of the double bond and the aldehyde group of the 4-carbon chain on the J-ring. Type B compounds comprise BTX-2, BTX-3, BTX-5, BTX-6, BTX-8, and BTX-9, which again differ in the structure of the terminal 4-carbon chain.

The chemistry of the BTXs is further complicated by the fact that the compounds produced by the microalgae undergo metabolism when ingested by shellfish. BTX-B5 results from oxidation of the terminal aldehyde group of BTX-2 to a carboxylic acid. BTX-B1 is formed from this compound by conjugation with taurine. The conjugation of BTX-2 with glutathione, with reduction of the aldehyde group, followed by metabolism of the conjugate by peptidases, yields the cysteine conjugate desoxy-BTX-B2. The oxidation of this compound to a sulfoxide forms BTX-B2, which undergoes conjugation with fatty acids to yield BTX-B4.[54,57,58] BTX-B3 is formed through the opening of the D-ring of BTX-3, followed by the esterification of the alcohol so formed with fatty acids and oxidation of the terminal aldehyde group. The structures of all these compounds are given by Ramsdell.[54]

7.3.2 Toxicity of Brevetoxins to Experimental Animals

7.3.2.1 Acute Toxicities of Brevetoxins by Intraperitoneal Injection

Data on the acute toxicities of BTX derivatives by intraperitoneal injection are summarized in Table 7.2.

Estimates of the LD_{50} of BTX-2 by intraperitoneal injection in mice range from 200 to 350 µg/kg. The reduction of the aldehyde function of BTX-2 to the corresponding alcohol, yielding BTX-3, has little effect on toxicity, with LD_{50} values between 170 and 250 µg/kg being reported. Similarly, the oxidation of the aldehyde function of BTX-2 to a carboxylic acid, to form BTX-B5, causes little change in acute intraperitoneal toxicity. In contrast, the epoxidation of the C27–29 double bond of BTX-2, forming BTX-6, markedly decreases toxicity, with no deaths being reported at a dose of 3000 µg/kg. The taurine conjugate at C42 of oxidized BTX-2 (BTX-B1) was shown to be substantially more toxic than BTX-2 and BTX-3, with an MLD of only 50 µg/kg. The cysteine conjugate at the C50 olefinic group of BTX-3 (*S*-deoxy-BTX-B2) and the sulfoxide of this compound (BTX-B2) are of similar toxicity to BTX-2 and BTX-3, with LD_{50} values of 211–400 µg/kg being reported. The conjugation of the cysteine amide function of BTX-B2 with a fatty acid, however, increases toxicity. A mixture of the *N*-palmitoyl and *N*-myristoyl conjugates of BTX-B2 (BTX-B4) was shown to be lethal at a dose of around 100 µg/kg, while the LD_{50} of a fully characterized sample of *N*-palmitoyl BTX-B2 was only 13 µg/kg, the lowest value for any of the BTX derivatives so far characterized. No acute toxicity data are available for BTX-1, BTX-4, BTX-5, BTX-7, BTX-8, BTX-9, and BTX-10.

Abdominal breathing, with higher than normal respiration rates, was observed soon after injection of BTX derivatives. At lethal doses, mice subsequently became immobile, and their respiration rates

TABLE 7.2

Acute Toxicities of BTX Derivatives by Intraperitoneal Injection in Mice

Compound	Strain of Mouse	Sex of Mouse	State of Alimentation	Parameter	Acute Toxicity (µg/kg Body Weight)[a]	Reference
BTX-2	Swiss	Female	Fasted	LD_{50}	200 (150–270)	[59]
BTX-2	Balb-c	Female	Fed	LD_{50}	350	[60]
BTX-3	CD-1	Female	?	MLD	187	[61]
BTX-3	Swiss	Female	Fasted	LD_{50}	170 (140–210)	[59]
BTX-3	Swiss	Female	Fed	LD_{50}	250 (176–328)	[62]
BTX-6	?	?	?	MLD	>3000	[60]
BTX-B1	?	?	?	MLD	50	[63]
BTX-B2	ddY	Male	?	MLD	306	[64]
BTX-B2	Swiss	Female	Fed	LD_{50}	400 (283–525)[b]	[62]
S-Desoxy-BTX-B2	Swiss	Female	Fed	LD_{50}	211 (200–250)	[62]
N-Palmitoyl-BTX-B2	Swiss	Female	Fed	LD_{50}	13 (8–21)	[65]
BTX-B4	?	?	?	"Lethality"	~100	[66]
BTX-B5	?	?	?	MLD	300–500	[67]

Note: "?" indicates that this information was not provided in the cited reference.

[a] Figures in brackets indicate 95% confidence limits.
[b] Confidence limits corrected from Selwood et al.[62]

progressively declined until breathing ceased completely. Shortly before death, respiration was very slow and gasping. Exophthalmia was observed, and the hind legs of the animals became extended. At high doses of BTX-2 and BTX-B2, death generally occurred within 1 h after injection,[64,66] but at doses close to the LD_{50}, the time to death was much longer.[62] Death times with fatty acid conjugates were prolonged, even at high doses. The time to death with BTX-B4 was reported to be between 6 and 24 h,[66] while the shortest time to death observed with *N*-palmitoyl BTX-B2 was 14 h.[65] At sublethal doses, respiration rates again declined, and the mice became hunched and immobile, with limb paralysis. Breathing rates subsequently increased, however, and the behavior and appearance of the animals normalized after 3–5 h.[62] Reversible hypothermia has also been observed in mice receiving sublethal doses of BTX-3 intraperitoneally.[61]

7.3.2.2 Acute Toxicity of Brevetoxins by Oral Administration

Very little data are available on the oral toxicity of BTX derivatives, but BTX-2 was reported to be more than 30 times less toxic by gavage than by intraperitoneal injection. In contrast, BTX-3 was only ~2.5 times less toxic orally than by injection.[59] Mice killed 8, 24, or 48 h after sublethal oral doses of BTX-2 or BTX-6 showed no histological changes in the heart, lung, kidneys, or intestines. Hemosiderosis was noted in the spleen and liver of animals dosed with BTX-6, but not in those receiving BTX-2.[60]

7.3.2.3 Repeated-Dose Studies on Brevetoxins

No studies on the effects of repeated oral doses of BTX derivatives have been reported, although subchronic inhalation experiments have been performed. The exposure of rats to aerosolized BTX-3 through nose-only inhalation for 5 or 22 days was not associated with any clinical signs of toxicity. A slight increase in the number of pulmonary alveolar macrophages was observed, but there was no evidence of cytotoxicity or inflammation in the lungs. Antibody production by splenic lymphocytes was significantly depressed. No histological lesions were observed in the nose, liver, or bone marrow, and in these studies, no neuronal damage or loss was detected in sections of the hippocampus or cerebellar cortex.[68,69] Later work, however, showed neuronal damage in a specific area of the cerebrum, the retrosplenial cortex, in mice exposed to BTX-3 by inhalation on 2 consecutive days.[70]

7.3.3 Effects of Brevetoxins in Humans

BTXs are responsible for neurotoxic shellfish poisoning (NSP). The consumption of shellfish contaminated with these substances leads to both gastrointestinal symptoms (nausea, vomiting, and diarrhea) and neurological effects, including paresthesia, reversal of temperature sensation, ataxia, and disorientation. In severe cases, partial limb paralysis occurs, together with respiratory distress, which, in some cases, requires artificial ventilation.[55,71] Even in individuals suffering severe illness, the symptoms resolve within a few days, and no deaths from NSP have been reported.

Harmful effects in humans through ingestion of BTX-contaminated seafood are relatively uncommon, but more widespread exposure of humans to BTXs occurs through inhalation. *Karenia brevis* is a fragile, unarmored dinoflagellate that readily breaks under the action of waves. With an inshore wind, beachgoers and persons living close to the beach may be exposed to aerosols containing BTXs, in which BTX-2 and BTX-3 predominate.[72] Such exposure leads to irritation of the conjunctiva and of the respiratory tract, as reflected by nonproductive cough, dyspnea, rhinorrhea, and sneezing.[73] The respiratory effects are particularly pronounced in asthmatics.[71,74]

7.3.4 Metabolism and Disposition of Brevetoxins

The metabolism of BTX derivatives has been extensively studied in vitro. BTX-2 underwent oxidation, reduction, and conjugation when incubated with purified rat cytochrome P450s (CYPs). It was reduced to BTX-3 and subsequently to BTX-9, oxidized to BTX-B5 and BTX-6, and conjugated with glutathione. The latter was degraded to *S*-desoxy-BTX-B2.[75] Purified human CYPs and human liver microsomes also mediated the reduction of BTX-2 to BTX-3 and BTX-9. BTX-5 and 41,43-dihydro-BTX-B5 were also formed.[76] There was also evidence of opening of the terminal lactone ring in BTX-1 and BTX-2 incubated with rat hepatocytes or rat liver microsomes.[77]

Results of metabolic studies in animals and in humans are largely in accord with the in vitro studies. The major urinary metabolites of BTX-2 after intraperitoneal injection in rats were the cysteine sulfoxide conjugate (BTX-B2) and *S*-desoxy-BTX-B2.[78] BTX-2, BTX-3, 41,43-dihydro-BTX-B5, and 27,28-epoxy-BTX-3 were found in the urine of individuals consuming shellfish contaminated with BTXs, and the formation of a methylsulfoxy derivative of BTX-3 was also suggested.[79,80]

BTX-3 is rapidly cleared from the blood of rats following intravenous injection, distributing to muscle, liver, and intestine.[81] This compound is rapidly absorbed from the lungs and from the gastrointestinal tract and again is distributed among various organs, including the brain, indicating that this substance can cross the blood–brain barrier.[82–84] BTX-3 is also able to cross the placenta, and substantial amounts of this substance were found in mouse fetuses soon after intratracheal administration to the dam.[85]

By intravenous or intratracheal administration, BTX-3 was mainly eliminated via the feces.[81,83] After intraperitoneal or oral administration, however, BTX-2 and BTX-3 are excreted largely via the urine.[78,84] The formation of the polar cysteine conjugates with BTX-2 facilitated the rapid excretion of this substance, which was eliminated faster than BTX-3, which is less readily conjugated by thiols.[78] Both BTX-2 and BTX-3 remain in rat tissues for prolonged periods (6–8 days) after dosing, whether given by injection or by gavage.[78,81,84]

7.3.5 Mechanism of Toxicity of Brevetoxins

There is evidence that BTXs exert their toxic effects through activation of site 5 of the α-subunit of voltage-gated sodium channels.[54] Such activation leads to increased sodium permeability and depolarization of the cell membrane. BTX-2 and BTX-3 have been shown to inhibit neuromuscular transmission in the rat phrenic nerve–hemidiaphragm preparation,[86,87] due to blockade of nerve impulses to the muscle. The effect of BTX derivatives on neuromuscular transmission is consistent with the respiratory paralysis seen in mice after lethal doses of these substances.

Some information is available on the correlation between the acute toxicities of BTXs to mice and their activities toward sodium channels, as measured by toxicity to neuroblastoma cells in the presence

TABLE 7.3

Comparison of Acute Toxicities of BTX Derivatives with their Activity toward Sodium Channels In Vitro

Compound	Relative Acute Toxicity by Intraperitoneal Injection[a]	Relative Toxicity to Neuroblastoma Cells[b]	Relative Receptor Binding, Rat Brain Membrane[b]	Relative Receptor Binding, HEKμ1 Cells[b]	Relative Receptor Binding, HEKhH1a Cells[b]
BTX-3	1.0	1.0	1.0	1.0	1.0
BTX-B2	0.53	0.32, 0.38	0.09, 0.13	0.12	0.06
S-Desoxy-BTX-2	1.0	0.13	0.11	0.14	0.07
N-Palmitoyl-BTX-B2	16.2	12.7	1.1	ND	ND

Note: ND, not determined.

[a] The LD_{50} of BTX-3 was taken as 210 μg/kg (the mean of data from Dechraoui Bottein et al.[65] and Baden and Mende[59]). The LD_{50}s of BTX-B2, *S*-desoxy-BTX-2, and *N*-palmitoyl BTX-B2 are from Dechraoui Bottein et al.[65] and Selwood et al.[62]

[b] Data from Dechraoui Bottein et al.[65,88]

of ouabain and veratridine or by receptor-binding assays (Table 7.3). In general, there is little correlation between toxicity in vivo and effects in vitro, but it is interesting to note that the results of the neuroblastoma assay with *N*-palmitoyl BTX-B2 were in agreement with the high toxicity of this substance to mice.

7.3.6 Mutagenicity of Brevetoxins

Neither BTX-2 nor BTX-6 was mutagenic in the Ames test with tester strains TA 98 and TA 100, with or without metabolic activation.[89] BTX-2 induced chromosomal aberrations in Chinese hamster ovary cells in vitro, while BTX-2, BTX-3, and BTX-9 were shown to cause DNA strand breaks in isolated human lymphocytes.[90] Similarly, BTX-2, BTX-3, and BTX-6 caused DNA breaks in Jurkat E6-1 cells,[91] and DNA damage was also observed in the hepatocytes of rats dosed intratracheally with BTX-2.[89] BTX-2 and BTX-6 formed covalent DNA adducts when incubated with rat lung cells in vitro and in lung cells of rats after intratracheal administration.[92]

7.3.7 Regulation of Brevetoxins

No regulations exist for BTXs in Europe. The regulatory limit is set at 0.8 mg BTX-2 equivalents/kg shellfish meat in the United States, New Zealand, and Australia,[93] and this level was supported by the CCFFP.[50] In 2010, the EFSA CONTAM Panel concluded that insufficient data were available for setting an ARfD for BTXs.[93]

7.3.8 Conclusions

Humans may be exposed to BTXs through both ingestion and inhalation. Exposure through inhalation involves mainly BTX-2 and BTX-3, and while some studies on repeated inhalation by rodents indicate only minor effects, the possibility of neuronal damage, as reported by Yan et al.,[70] requires further investigation. The damage to the retrosplenial cortex of mice that was shown in this study may be significant. This area of the brain is involved in learning and memory,[70] and since BTX-3 can be transferred across the placenta, the possibility of developmental and learning deficiencies, as described in animals exposed to domoic acid *in utero* (Section 7.6), must be considered.

The BTXs are slowly eliminated from the body, raising the possibility that accumulation could occur in individuals who are regularly exposed to these substances. Analyses of tissue levels of BTXs after repeated doses of these substances by inhalation or by oral administration in animals would shed light on this possibility.

The exposure of humans to BTXs by ingestion mainly involves metabolites produced in shellfish, some of which are more toxic than BTX-2 and BTX-3. Future work should focus on the most toxic metabolites, with a need for oral toxicity data in animals and identification of target organs. Hematological investigations are also required, since the splenic and hepatic hemosiderosis seen in animals dosed orally with BTX-6 suggests that some BTX derivatives may induce hemolytic anemia.

While the action of BTX derivatives on voltage-gated sodium channels has been extensively investigated, it would appear that at the present time, neither receptor-binding assays nor cytotoxicity determinations are able to accurately predict the in vivo toxicity of these substances.

The evidence for genotoxicity of BTXs is inconclusive. While BTX-2, BTX-3, and BTX-6 caused DNA breaks in cells in vitro, the levels employed in these experiments also induced apoptosis. The DNA damage that was observed may thus reflect cell death rather than genotoxicity. BTX-2 was negative in the Ames test, as was BTX-6. The negative result with the latter compound is interesting, since BTX-6 contains an epoxide moiety, a functional group often associated with mutagenic and carcinogenic activity. Of more concern is the in vivo data on DNA fragmentation and adduct formation after intratracheal administration. Further work in this area is needed.

7.4 Ciguatoxins, Maitotoxins, Gambierol, and Gambieric Acids

7.4.1 Production and Distribution of Ciguatoxins and Derivatives

In 1977, Yasumoto et al.[94] isolated a dinoflagellate from the Gambier Islands, French Polynesia, which they suggested was responsible for ciguatera fish poisoning (CFP), a type of food poisoning that is endemic in this area. They tentatively placed this organism in the genus *Diplopsalis*, but it was subsequently shown by Adachi and Fukuyo[95] to represent a new genus and was named *Gambierdiscus toxicus* in 1979. Since that time, many publications on toxic species of *Gambierdiscus* have been published, referring to the organism as *G. toxicus*. However, recent detailed studies by Litaker et al.[96] on the taxonomy of *Gambierdiscus* suggest that toxic species within this genus may not necessarily be identical to the organism described by Adachi and Fukuyo. Members of the genus *Gambierdiscus* have now been found in many other parts of the world, including Japan, Korea, Singapore, Australia, Papua New Guinea, Central and South America, the islands of the Caribbean, Mauritius, the Seychelles, the Canary Islands, and Crete.[97–99]

Gambierdiscus species produce a range of polyether toxins, the most extensively studied of which are the ciguatoxins. The structures of the compounds that are produced by this organism vary with location, and in order to distinguish among them, a prefix is added to the name—P for compounds from the Pacific, C for compounds from the Caribbean, and I for those from the Indian Ocean. The toxins produced by the microalgae pass up the food chain, and many ciguatoxins have been isolated from finfish. Some of these compounds undergo metabolism after ingestion by fish, so that the latter may contain not only the toxins found in the dinoflagellates but also derivatives of these substances. As of 2011, 23 ciguatoxin derivatives from the Pacific had been identified,[100] and the structures of the Caribbean ciguatoxin C-CTX-1 and its epimer C-CTX-2 had been determined.[101,102] Several ciguatoxins have been detected in fish caught in the Indian Ocean, although these have not yet been fully characterized.[103] The structures of many of the compounds isolated from *Gambierdiscus* and from fish are given by Yasumoto[104] and by Dickey.[105]

Gambierdiscus species also synthesize gambieric acids,[106] gambierol,[107] and maitotoxins.[108,109] A compound designated ciguaterin was found in ciguatoxic fish from Japanese waters.[110] The structure of this substance is unknown, but the production of amino acids after acid hydrolysis indicated the presence of a peptide function.[111]

7.4.2 Toxicity of Ciguatoxins and Derivatives to Experimental Animals

7.4.2.1 Acute Toxicities of Ciguatoxins and Derivatives by Intraperitoneal Injection

The toxicities of ciguatoxin and related compounds to mice by intraperitoneal injection are summarized in Table 7.4.

TABLE 7.4

Acute Toxicities of Ciguatoxins and Related Compounds by Intraperitoneal Injection in Mice

Compound	Mouse Strain	Mouse Sex	State of Alimentation	Parameter	Acute Toxicity (μg/kg Body Weight)	Reference
P-CTX-1	Quackenbush	Male and female	?	LD_{50}	0.25	[112]
P-CTX-1	Swiss	?	?	LD_{50}	0.4	[113]
P-CTX-1	?	?	?	LD_{50}	0.45	[114]
P-CTX-1	?	?	?	"Lethal potency"	0.35	[115]
P-CTX-1	Swiss	Male and female	?	LD_{50}	0.33	[116]
P-CTX-2	Quackenbush	Male and female	?	LD_{50}	2.3	[112]
P-CTX-3	Quackenbush	Male and female	?	LD_{50}	0.9	[112]
P-CTX-3C	?	?	?	"Lethality"	1.3	[117]
P-CTX-3C	Swiss	Male and female	?	LD_{50}	2.5	[116]
2,3-Dihydroxy-P-CTX-3	?	?	?	"Lethality"	~1.8	[118]
51-Hydroxy-P-CTX-3	?	?	?	"Lethality"	0.27	[118]
51-Hydroxy-P-CTX-3, F ring opened	?	?	?	MLD	>667[a]	[119]
51-Hydroxy-P-CTX-3, 8-membered F ring	?	?	?	MLD	>667[a]	[119]
P-CTX-4A	?	?	?	"Lethality"	~2	[120]
P-CTX-4B	?	?	?	"Lethal potency"	~4	[115]
P-CTX-4B	Swiss	Male and female	?	LD_{50}	10	[116]
C-CTX-1	Quackenbush	Male and female	Fed	LD_{50}	3.6	[101]
C-CTX-2	Quackenbush	Male and female	Fed	LD_{50}	~1	[101]
Maitotoxin	?	Female	?	"Lethal dose"	15,000–20,000	[121]
Maitotoxin	?	?	?	MLD	5	[122]
Maitotoxin	?	?	?	"Lethality"	0.13	[123]
Maitotoxin	ddY	Male	?	LD_{50}	0.05	[124]
Maitotoxin-2	Quackenbush	?	?	LD_{50}	0.08	[109]
Mono-desulfo-maitotoxin	ddY	Male	?	LD_{50}	0.6	[125]
Di-desulfo-maitotoxin	ddY	Male	?	LD_{50}	15	[125]
Gambierol	?	?	?	LD_{50}	50	[107]
Gambierol	ICR	Male	?	"Lethal dose"	~80	[126]
Gambierol	ddY	Male	?	MLD	50–75	[127]
Gambieric acid A	?	?	?	MLD	>1000[a]	[106]
Gambieric acid B	?	?	?	MLD	>1000[a]	[106]

Note: "?" indicates that this information was not provided in the cited reference.

[a] No deaths occurred at this dose.

P-CTX-4A, P-CTX-4B, and P-CTX-3C from Pacific *Gambierdiscus* species are highly toxic to mice, with LD_{50}s between 2 and 10 µg/kg. The fish metabolites P-CTX-1 and 51-hydroxy-P-CTX-3 are even more toxic, with estimates of LD_{50}s ranging from 0.25 to 0.45 µg/kg. P-CTX-2 and P-CTX-3, other fish metabolites from the Pacific, were less toxic than P-CTX-1 and 51-hydroxy-P-CTX-3, as were C-CTX-1 and C-CTX-2 from fish caught in the Caribbean.

The symptoms of intoxication by ciguatoxins in mice after intraperitoneal injection include diarrhea, lacrimation, hypersalivation, loss of activity, hypothermia, hind limb paralysis, and respiratory distress.[97,101,112] At lethal doses, death is due to respiratory failure. The ciguatoxins are slow-acting poisons, with death occurring up to 24 h after dosing.[116] Mice surviving longer than 24 h recover completely.[101]

Intraperitoneal injection of P-CTX-1 or P-CTX-4C caused single-cell necrosis in the cardiac ventricular septa, together with hypertrophy of myocytes and of the endothelial lining cells of cardiac capillaries. Hepatic congestion, with thrombi in hepatic veins, was also observed. The diarrhea induced by the ciguatoxins after intraperitoneal injection was not associated with significant morphological changes in the duodenum, jejunum, or ileum, but epithelial damage was recorded in the upper part of the colon, with excessive secretion of mucus.[128,129]

Reports on the toxicity of maitotoxin are rather confusing. In 1971, Yasumoto et al.[130] described a water-soluble material from surgeonfish. In 1976, this material was named "maitotoxin," which was slightly toxic to mice, causing death at a dose of 15–20 mg/kg. Acid hydrolysis of this substance yielded fatty acids, a sphingosine-like base, hexoses, and amino acids.[121] A year later, a substance "regarded as maitotoxin" was isolated from the dinoflagellate that was later named *G. toxicus*.[94] It was subsequently reported that the degradation products from the "maitotoxin" from surgeonfish were probably formed from contaminants, and the material from the dinoflagellate was shown to be of much higher toxicity, killing mice at a dose of 5 µg/kg.[122] In 1988, Yokoyama et al.[123] reported on the isolation of "pure" maitotoxin, with an LD_{50} in mice of 0.13 µg/kg. Further purification appears to have been achieved by 1994, however, when Murata et al.[124] reported on the structure of maitotoxin, revising the LD_{50} of this substance to 0.05 µg/kg. It would appear from the toxicity data that the water-soluble material obtained from surgeonfish in 1971 and 1976 contained little or no maitotoxin. Even the material isolated in 1978, assuming that it contained no other toxic species, would have contained only 1% maitotoxin, based on an LD_{50} of the pure substance of 0.05 µg/kg. Fully characterized samples of mono- and di-desulfo-maitotoxin were shown to be less toxic than the parent compound by factors of 12 and 300, respectively,[125] while a second maitotoxin derivative (maitotoxin-2), isolated from a *Gambierdiscus* species, was of similar toxicity to maitotoxin itself.[109]

The symptoms of intoxication seen with maitotoxin are similar to those with the ciguatoxins, although the time to death appears to be shorter than that recorded with the latter compounds.[131] A single intraperitoneal injection of maitotoxin caused gastric and intestinal distension, with moderate ascites, accompanied by focal necrosis of the gastric mucosa and edema of the submucosa. Marked degeneration of thymic lymphocytes was also recorded.[132]

Gambierol was shown to be less toxic than the ciguatoxin derivatives. This substance is a relatively fast-acting toxin, with deaths occurring at up to 3 h after dosing. Hypersalivation was a pronounced feature of the toxicity of this substance.[126]

The gambieric acids are of low toxicity, with no effects being recorded at an intraperitoneal dose of 1000 µg/kg.

Ciguaterin was shown to be a powerful emetic in cats, but it had no effect in mice or rats, and did not induce the characteristic symptoms of ciguatera.[110]

7.4.2.2 Acute Toxicities of Ciguatoxins and Derivatives by Oral Administration

Although relatively little information is available on the acute oral toxicity of the ciguatoxins, it would appear that toxicity by gavage is not grossly dissimilar to that by injection. The oral LD_{50} of P-CTX-1 was reported[133] as 0.22 µg/kg, while mice died after gavage with P-CTX-1, P-CTX-2, or P-CTX-3 at only twice the intraperitoneal LD_{50}.[112] The symptoms of intoxication following oral administration of ciguatoxins were similar to those recorded after intraperitoneal injection, although no diarrhea was induced via the oral route.[129]

Similarly, the toxicity of gambierol by gavage was reported to be similar to that by intraperitoneal injection, although LD_{50}s were not determined. The symptoms of intoxication by both routes were the same. A single oral dose of gambierol led to congestion of the heart, lungs, liver, and kidneys, and edema and separation of myocardial fibers were observed. At lethal doses, dilatation of the stomach and intestines was recorded, together with ulceration of the gastric mucosa.[126]

7.4.2.3 Repeated-Dose Studies on Ciguatoxins and Derivatives

There is evidence that the toxicity of P-CTX-1 is cumulative. No deaths were recorded in mice injected with this substance at 0.26 µg/kg, but after a second dose at the same level 3 days after the first, 50% of a group of mice died.[134] Furthermore, while no pathological changes were observed in the hearts of mice after a single oral or intraperitoneal dose of 0.1 µg/kg P-CTX-1 or P-CTX-4C, when this dose was given daily for 15 days, cardiac changes similar to those seen after lethal doses of these substances were observed. These changes were largely reversible after cessation of dosing.[135] Furthermore, less frequent administration for longer periods gave similar results. Weekly oral administration of P-CTX-1 at 0.1 µg/kg for 18 weeks or 0.05 µg/kg for 40 weeks led to pronounced cardiac changes.[136]

Repeated intraperitoneal injections of maitotoxin caused marked atrophy of the spleen and thymus, with decreased numbers of lymphocytes in these organs and in the blood. Cytoplasmic vacuolation was observed in the zona fasciculata of the adrenals, and the stomachs of the animals were dilated, with multiple ulcers. The histological changes in the spleen, thymus, and adrenals were prevented by the administration of cobaltous chloride to the animals in their drinking water, and the splenic and thymic changes were not seen in adrenalectomized animals.[137]

7.4.3 Effects of Ciguatoxins and Derivatives in Humans

Ciguatera is endemic in many tropical and subtropical areas, and thousands of people are affected by CFP each year.[138] Until recently, outbreaks in other parts of the world have been restricted to individuals who had traveled in, or who had eaten fish exported from, endemic areas. In 2004, however, ciguatera was confirmed after consumption of fish caught in the Canary Islands.[139] More incidents of intoxication have been reported in this area since that time, and the presence of ciguatoxins in fish from this location has been confirmed.[140] Ciguatoxins have also been identified in fish from the Madeira Archipelago, and poisoning with symptoms consistent with ciguatera has been reported in these islands.[141] Ciguatoxins were suggested to be responsible for poisoning after consumption of rabbitfish from the Eastern Mediterranean,[142] and there is evidence for the presence of ciguatoxins in fish in this area.[143]

The symptoms of intoxication are many and varied and include both gastrointestinal (diarrhea, nausea, and vomiting) and neurologic (paresthesia, dysesthesia, arthralgia, myalgia, headache, and muscular weakness).[97,138,144] In severe cases, paralysis and death through respiratory failure occurs, although the mortality rate in CFP is low.[144] The adverse effects of CFP may persist for years and may reoccur after exercise or weight loss, possibly due to the release of stored ciguatoxins from adipose tissue. Alcohol or high-protein foods may increase the severity of CFP symptoms.[144]

Little information on diagnostic enzyme levels or histological changes in victims of CFP are available. Barkin[145] reported a high incidence of elevated blood urea nitrogen in individuals consuming a ciguateric fish, suggesting renal damage. No histological changes were observed, however, in the kidneys of an individual who died from CFP, although hepatic necrosis was recorded in this person.[146] Nakano[147] reported elevated levels of creatine phosphokinase in the blood of seven men affected with ciguatera. Biopsy revealed necrosis of skeletal muscle fibers. Similarly, an individual showing the characteristic signs of CFP showed elevated plasma creatine phosphokinase activity, with evidence of myoglobinuria,[148] and elevated creatine phosphokinase, associated with severe muscle pain, was identified in an outbreak of CFP caused by consumption of a fish caught in the Caribbean.[149]

It appears that ciguatoxins can cross the placenta. A woman who ate a ciguateric fish 2 days before the expected birth date of her child noticed a pronounced increase in fetal movement. The baby was born with left-sided facial palsy and possible myotonia of the small muscles of the hands, but the child appeared normal at 6 weeks of age.[150] Increased fetal movements were also observed after consumption of a ciguateric fish by a woman 16 weeks pregnant. At term, she gave birth to a healthy baby, which developed normally over the subsequent 10-month observation period.[151] Minor toxic changes were observed in infants suckled by mothers suffering ciguatera poisoning, suggesting that ciguatoxins may be secreted in breast milk.[152,153] This is unproven, however, since no analyses of the milk were undertaken.

No antidotes for CFP exist, and there are no drugs or traditional remedies that have conclusively been proven to be effective for its treatment.[154]

7.4.4 Metabolism and Disposition of Ciguatoxins and Derivatives

P-CTX-1 was rapidly absorbed when dosed to rats either by intraperitoneal injection or by gavage and was distributed to the liver, muscle, and brain of the animals. Four days after dosing, the brain contained the highest concentration, and muscle the highest total amount. Excretion was largely via the feces, with smaller amounts in urine. Several metabolites were detected, but were not characterized. The terminal half-life was estimated at 4 days.[155]

It was estimated that at least 10% of ingested ciguatoxin remained in the liver of a man who died 6 days after ingestion of a ciguateric fish.[156] No other tissues from this individual were analyzed.

7.4.5 Mechanism of Toxicity of Ciguatoxins and Derivatives

Ciguatoxins, maitotoxins, and gambierol all cause death in mice through respiratory paralysis, suggesting that these substances exert their lethal effects through a common mechanism, possibly via effects on cation channels.

Ciguatoxins are potent activators of voltage-gated sodium channels, binding to site 5, the same site as that bound by the BTXs,[144,157] which leads to increased sodium permeability and depolarization of the cell membrane. Like BTX, P-CTX-1 blocks neuromuscular transmission in the rat phrenic nerve–hemidiaphragm preparation,[133] and such an effect is consistent with the respiratory paralysis seen in mice after lethal doses of ciguatoxins.

Maitotoxin and gambierol have little or no effect on voltage-gated sodium channels,[158,159] but they do interact with other cation channels. There is evidence that maitotoxin activates a nonselective voltage-independent cation channel, leading to an increase in the intracellular concentrations of both sodium and calcium, resulting in membrane depolarization.[160] The effects of this substance on lymphoid tissue have been attributed to stimulation of cortisol release from the adrenals through maitotoxin-stimulated calcium influx into this organ, and it was suggested that the protective effects of cobaltous chloride were due to blockade of calcium channels by this substance.[137] Gambierol has been reported to inhibit voltage-gated potassium channels.[158,159]

While effects on cation channels may explain the lethal effects of ciguatoxin and derivatives in animals, it has been argued that effects on such channels *per se* cannot explain the wide range of toxic symptoms induced by the ciguatoxins in humans. It has been suggested that channel activation may lead to a cascade of events resulting in increased production of nitric oxide. The latter, by reaction with superoxide, forms the highly reactive oxidizing agent peroxynitrite' and oxidative stress, leading to the formation of pro-inflammatory cytokines, may be involved in some of the toxic changes induced by the ciguatoxins.[161,162]

7.4.6 Mutagenicity of Ciguatoxin and Derivatives

No information on the mutagenic potential of ciguatoxins or its derivatives appears to be available.

7.4.7 Regulation of Ciguatoxins and Derivatives

The EFSA CONTAM Panel reported on ciguatoxins in 2010.[163] They did not consider other possible contributors to CFP, such as gambierol and maitotoxin. TEFs were suggested, based on toxicity to animals by intraperitoneal injection. The Panel noted that insufficient data were available for establishing an ARfD or a TDI for ciguatoxins but, based on human data, proposed a regulatory limit of 0.01 µg of P-CTX-1 equivalents per kilogram of fish.

7.4.8 Conclusions

CFP is a major human health problem. Its incidence has recently increased in the Pacific and is expected to continue to increase in this area due to continued reef degradation and global warming.[164] The recent observations of CFP in the Atlantic and possibly also in the Mediterranean indicate that the distribution of this disease is widening, in accord with the spread of *Gambierdiscus* species into new areas.

The suggested regulatory limit for ciguatoxins uses TEFs based on intraperitoneal injection. The establishment of LD_{50}s for the various ciguatoxin derivatives by the oral route would be valuable, so that relevant TEFs can be determined for these substances.

Long-term feeding studies are required in order to permit the establishment of a TDI. This is particularly important for the ciguatoxins, since there is evidence that they accumulate in the tissues of both experimental animals and humans and that their toxic effects increase with the duration of exposure. The regulatory limit, which is based on acute, not chronic, effects, may therefore be set too low.

The mutagenicity of ciguatoxins or other toxins possibly involved in CFP has not been studied. An Ames test on these substances would be valuable. Furthermore, since ciguatoxins have been shown to cross the placental barrier, studies on the possible teratogenic effects of these substances and their long-term effects on offspring are called for.

The possible involvement of other toxins, particularly maitotoxin, in CFP needs investigation. Although maitotoxin is exceptionally toxic by intraperitoneal injection, its possible involvement in CFP has largely been ignored or dismissed. It has repeatedly been stated in the literature that maitotoxins are unlikely to be involved, based on a stated low oral toxicity of maitotoxin and its inability to accumulate in the flesh of fish. Neither of these premises appear to be well founded. There appears to be no published data on the oral toxicity of maitotoxin in the literature. The statement that "the relatively low oral potency of the maitotoxins is likely to limit its role in human intoxication"[165] was referenced to Kelley et al.[166] and to Yasumoto (1979, unpublished result). The statement that "maitotoxins.... are 100 times less toxic [than ciguatoxin] when taken orally"[167] was referenced to Yokoyama et al.[123] Neither the paper by Kelley et al. nor that by Yokoyama et al. mentions the oral toxicity of maitotoxin, while results by Yasumoto in 1979 could only have involved experiments with the semipurified material from *Gambierdiscus*, which was lethal to mice at an intraperitoneal dose of 5 µg/kg. Since it was later shown that pure maitotoxin is lethal at 0.05 µg/kg, the material available in 1979 could have contained but little maitotoxin. The statement that "maitotoxin has been found in the gut contents of surgeonfishes but there is little evidence that maitotoxin is accumulated in the flesh of these or other fishes"[168] is referenced to the 1976 paper by Yasumoto et al.,[121] which describes the substance from surgeonfish that caused death in mice at a dose of 15–20 mg/kg and was degraded to fatty acids, a sphingosine-like base, hexoses, and amino acids. Whatever this material was, it was certainly not maitotoxin, and the cited paper makes no mention of the distribution of toxins among fish tissues.

The involvement of gambierol in CFP does not appear to have been considered. Although less toxic than the ciguatoxins, an LD_{50} of 50–80 µg/kg still indicates a highly toxic substance, and the accumulation of this substance in fish could contribute to toxicity. It is very unlikely that the relatively nontoxic gambieric acids and ciguaterin contribute to CFP.

The involvement of palytoxin, or of the palytoxin congeners synthesized by *Ostreopsis* species, in the etiology of CFP has been suggested.[98,148] Both *Gambierdiscus* and *Ostreopsis* spp. are found in areas in which fish causing CFP have been caught,[98] and the observation of increased plasma creatine phosphokinase levels, skeletal muscle necrosis, and myoglobinuria in victims of CFP[147,148] is of interest, since myotoxicity is a common finding in palytoxin intoxication in humans (Section 7.8). Further research in this area is required.

7.5 Cyclic Imines

7.5.1 Production and Distribution of Cyclic Imines

The cyclic imine group of marine toxins consists of gymnodimines, spirolides, pinnatoxins, pteriatoxins, prorocentrolide, spiro-prorocentrimine, and symbioimines.

Gymnodimines A, B, and C were isolated and characterized from a New Zealand strain of the dinoflagellate *Karenia selliformis* (formerly *Gymnodinium* cf. *mikimotoi*),[169–171] while 12-methyl gymnodimine was identified in an American strain of *Alexandrium peruvianum*.[172]

Spirolides are produced by *Alexandrium ostenfeldii*[173] and *A. peruvianum*,[172,174] and spirolides A, B, C, D, H, and I have been isolated from these organisms, together with 13-desmethyl spirolide C, 27-hydroxy-13-desmethyl spirolide C, 27-hydroxy-13,19-didesmethyl spirolide C, 27-oxo-13,19-didesmethyl spirolide C, and 13-desmethyl spirolide D.[175–179] After ingestion by shellfish, spirolides undergo metabolism, and spirolides E and F have been found in Canadian shellfish,[180] and a complex mixture of fatty acid esters of 20-methyl spirolide G was isolated from Norwegian mussels.[181]

The dinoflagellate *Vulcanodinium rugosum* is responsible for the production of pinnatoxins.[182,183] Again, pinnatoxins appear to undergo metabolism in shellfish, with fatty acid esters of pinnatoxins A and G being found in mussels from Eastern Canada.[184]

Prorocentrolide A was isolated from cultures of *Prorocentrum lima*,[185] while prorocentrolide B was shown to be present in cultures of *Prorocentrum maculosum*.[186] Pteriatoxins A, B, and C were isolated from the pearl oyster *Pteria penguin* from Japan,[187] but the organism responsible for the production of these compounds has not yet been identified. Spiro-prorocentrimine was reported to be present in an unidentified benthic *Prorocentrum* species from Taiwan,[188] while symbioimine was isolated from a *Symbiodinium* species living symbiotically in a marine flatworm.[189]

Cyclic imines are of worldwide distribution. Gymnodimine A was first reported in shellfish from New Zealand in 1995.[169] Since then, this substance and its congeners have been found in shellfish and/or marine microalgae from Tunisia,[190] Canada,[191] China,[192] Croatia,[193] Australia,[194] South Africa,[195] Chile,[196] and the United States.[172] Spirolides were first reported in Canadian shellfish[197] but have now been discovered in seafood in Italy,[198] Spain,[199] France,[200] Ireland,[174] Scotland,[201] Croatia,[193] Norway,[202] Denmark,[173] New Zealand,[203] Chile,[204] and the United States.[205] Until 2010, pinnatoxins had been shown to be present only in Japanese shellfish, but in that year, these substances were detected in Pacific oysters from Australia[206] and have subsequently been found in shellfish from New Zealand,[207] Europe,[183] Canada,[184] and Norway.[208] Pteriatoxins, prorocentrolide, spiro-prorocentrimine, and symbioimines were isolated from shellfish from Southeast Asia[187–189] and as yet do not appear to have been found in any other location.

7.5.2 Toxicity of Cyclic Imines to Experimental Animals

The toxicology of cyclic imines has been reviewed.[203]

7.5.2.1 *Acute Toxicities of Gymnodimine and Gymnodamine by Intraperitoneal Injection*

The acute toxicities of gymnodimines and its reduction product, gymnodamine, by intraperitoneal injection are shown in Table 7.5.

Early reports indicated that gymnodimine was of relatively low toxicity by intraperitoneal injection, but later studies using fully authenticated material showed much higher toxicity, with LD_{50}s of ~100 µg/kg being reported. Gymnodimine B is considerably less toxic than gymnodimine A by intraperitoneal injection, and gymnodamine, in which the imino group of gymnodimine is reduced to a secondary amine, has been shown to be of very low toxicity, with no deaths occurring at an intraperitoneal dose of 4040 µg/kg, the highest dose tested.

The clinical signs of intoxication by gymnodimine A are highly characteristic. Following intraperitoneal injection, mice became lethargic and moved with a rolling gait. At lethal doses, mice became completely immobile, with their hind legs paralyzed and partly extended. They were unresponsive to stimuli

TABLE 7.5

Acute Toxicities of Gymnodimines A and B and of Gymnodamine by Intraperitoneal Injection in Mice

Compound	Strain of Mouse	Sex of Mouse	State of Alimentation	Parameter	Acute Toxicity (µg/kg Body Weight)[a]	References
Gymnodimine A	?	?	?	MLD	450	[169,209]
Gymnodimine A	?	?	?	MLD	700	[210]
Gymnodimine A	Swiss albino	Female	Fed	LD$_{50}$	96 (79–118)	[211]
Gymnodimine A	Swiss Webster	Male	?	LD$_{50}$	100	[212]
Gymnodimine B	Swiss Webster	Male	?	LD$_{50}$	800	[212]
Gymnodamine	?	?	?	MLD	>4040	[210]

Note: "?" indicates that this information was not provided in the cited reference.

[a] Figures in brackets indicate 95% confidence limits.

at this time. Subsequently, the respiration rate of the mice progressively decreased, with pronounced abdominal breathing, until respiration ceased completely. Running movements, accompanied by exophthalmia, were seen immediately before death, and the hind legs of the animals became fully extended. Death occurred no later than 15 min after injection of gymnodimine A. At toxic, but sublethal, doses of this substance, immobility, abdominal breathing, and decreased respiration rates were observed, but the mice subsequently recovered, and their appearance and behavior became normal within 30 min after dosing and remained normal for the subsequent 21-day observation period.[211]

The short-acting cholinesterase inhibitors, neostigmine and physostigmine, protected against gymnodimine toxicity. No deaths occurred in mice injected with these substances immediately before challenge with gymnodimine A at 192 µg/kg, a dose that was lethal to all the control animals.[211]

7.5.2.2 Acute Toxicity of Gymnodimine by Oral Administration

The LD$_{50}$ of gymnodimine A by gavage was higher than that by intraperitoneal injection (Table 7.6), but the symptoms of intoxication were the same as those recorded after intraperitoneal injection. Gymnodimine A was even less toxic by feeding, with no effects being recorded after a dose of 7500 µg/kg.

7.5.2.3 Acute Toxicities of Spirolides by Intraperitoneal Injection

The acute toxicities of spirolide derivatives by intraperitoneal injection are shown in Table 7.7.

Studies in one laboratory[213] showed very high toxicity of certified and accurately quantitated samples of spirolide C, 13-desmethyl spirolide C, and 20-methyl spirolide G, with LD$_{50}$ values of 8.0, 6.9, and 8.0 µg/kg, respectively. In other experiments, however, which employed commercially available material,[214] significantly lower toxicities of 13-desmethyl C and 20-methyl spirolide G (LD$_{50}$s of 27.9 and >63.5 µg/kg, respectively) were reported. Fasting had no effect on the intraperitoneal toxicity of 13-desmethyl spirolide C.[213]

TABLE 7.6

Acute Toxicity of Gymnodimine A by Oral Administration to Mice

Compound	Strain of Mouse	Sex of Mouse	State of Alimentation	Method of Administration	Parameter	Acute Toxicity (µg/kg Body Weight)[a]
Gymnodimine A	Swiss albino	Female	Fed	Gavage	LD$_{50}$	755 (600–945)[a]
Gymnodimine A	Swiss albino	Female	Fasted	Feeding method 1[b]	LD$_{50}$	>7500[c]

[a] Figures in brackets indicate 95% confidence limits. Data from Munday et al.[211]

[b] Feeding method 1: gymnodimine was fed absorbed on dry mousefood.

[c] No effects were observed at this dose.

TABLE 7.7

Acute Toxicities of Spirolides by Intraperitoneal Injection in Mice

Compound	Strain of Mouse	Sex of Mouse	State of Alimentation	Parameter	Acute Toxicity (µg/kg Body Weight)[a]	Reference
Spirolide A	Swiss albino	Female	Fed	LD_{50}	37 (35–44)	[213]
Spirolide B	Swiss albino	Female	Fed	LD_{50}	99	[213]
Spirolide B	?	?	?	LD_{100}	250	[197]
Dihydrospirolide B	?	?	?	MLD	>1000[b]	[180]
Spirolide C	Swiss albino	Female	Fed	LD_{50}	8.0 (4.6–16.0)	[213]
13-Desmethyl spirolide C	Swiss albino	Female	Fed	LD_{50}	6.9 (5.0–8.0)	[213]
13-Desmethyl spirolide C	Swiss albino	Female	Fasted	LD_{50}	6.9 (5.0–8.0)	[213]
13-Desmethyl spirolide C	Swiss albino	?	?	LD_{50}	27.9	[214]
27-Hydroxy-13-desmethyl spirolide C	?	?	?	MLD	>27	[178]
27-oxo-13,19-Didesmethyl spirolide C	?	?	?	MLD	>35	[178]
13,19-Didesmethyl spirolide C	Swiss albino	?	?	LD_{50}	32	[214]
13,19-Didesmethyl spirolide C	?	?	?	MLD	30	[176]
Spirolide D	?	?	?	LD_{100}	250	[197]
Spirolide E	?	?	?	MLD	>1000[b]	[180]
Spirolide F	?	?	?	MLD	>1000[b]	[180]
20-Methyl spirolide G	Swiss albino	Female	Fed	LD_{50}	8.0 (3.9–14.0)	[213]
20-Methyl spirolide G	Swiss albino	?	?	MLD	>63.5	[214]
Spirolide H	Swiss albino	Female	Fed	MLD	>2000	[175]

Note: "?" indicates that this information was not provided in the cited reference.

[a] Figures in brackets indicate 95% confidence limits.

[b] No effects were observed at this dose.

Spirolides A and B and 13,19-didesmethyl spirolide C are less toxic than the previously mentioned compounds. 27-Hydroxy-13-desmethyl spirolide C and 27-oxo-13,19-didesmethyl spirolide C appear to be of similar toxicity, though no definitive LD_{50}s for these compounds are presently available.

Spirolides E, F, and H and dihydrospirolide B are much less toxic. Spirolides E and F, in which the imine ring is opened, and dihydrospirolide B, in which the imine group is reduced to a secondary amine, were without effect at a dose of 1000 µg/kg, while only transient effects were induced in mice dosed intraperitoneally with spirolide H at 2000 µg/kg.

The symptoms of intoxication by spirolides are very similar to those observed with gymnodimine. At lethal doses, death occurred between 3 and 20 min after dosing.[213]

At toxic, but sublethal, doses of the spirolides, mice became immobile, with rapid, shallow abdominal breathing, and their hind legs became extended. Recovery occurred within 1 h, and the appearance and behavior of the mice remained normal throughout the subsequent observation period.[213]

7.5.2.4 Acute Toxicities of Spirolides by Oral Administration

The spirolides are less toxic by gavage than by intraperitoneal injection, and in this case, fasting was associated with an increase in toxicity. These substances are even less toxic by feeding, and again fasted mice were more susceptible to their toxic effects than fed animals. The method of feeding, whether by the use of cream cheese or dry or moist mousefood, had no significant effect on the LD_{50} of 13-desmethyl C (Table 7.8). The time to death was longer in mice receiving the spirolides by oral administration than in those injected with these substances, with deaths occurring at up to 35 min after toxin administration.[213]

TABLE 7.8

Acute Toxicities of Spirolides by Oral Administration to Mice

Compound	Strain of Mouse	Sex of Mouse	State of Alimentation	Method of Administration[a]	Parameter	Acute Toxicity (μg/kg Body Weight)[b]
Spirolide A	Swiss albino	Female	Fed	Gavage	LD_{50}	550 (436–690)
Spirolide A	Swiss albino	Female	Fasted	Gavage	LD_{50}	240 (188–298)
Spirolide A	Swiss albino	Female	Fed	Feeding method 2	LD_{50}	1300 (1250–1580)
Spirolide A	Swiss albino	Female	Fasted	Feeding method 2	LD_{50}	1200 (1047–3690)
Spirolide B	Swiss albino	Female	Fasted	Gavage	LD_{50}	440 (320–500)
Spirolide C	Swiss albino	Female	Fasted	Gavage	LD_{50}	53 (50–63)
Spirolide C	Swiss albino	Female	Fed	Feeding method 2	LD_{50}	780
Spirolide C	Swiss albino	Female	Fasted	Feeding method 2	LD_{50}	500 (353–657)
13-Desmethyl spirolide C	Swiss albino	Female	Fed	Gavage	LD_{50}	160 (123–198)
13-Desmethyl spirolide C	Swiss albino	Female	Fasted	Gavage	LD_{50}	130 (87–166)
13-Desmethyl spirolide C	Swiss albino	Female	Fed	Feeding method 2	LD_{50}	1000 (861–1290)
13-Desmethyl spirolide C	Swiss albino	Female	Fasted	Feeding method 2	LD_{50}	500 (381–707)
13-Desmethyl spirolide C	Swiss albino	Female	Fasted	Feeding method 1	LD_{50}	630 (547–829)
13-Desmethyl spirolide C	Swiss albino	Female	Fasted	Feeding method 3	LD_{50}	590 (500–625)
20-Methyl spirolide G	Swiss albino	Female	Fed	Gavage	LD_{50}	160
20-Methyl spirolide G	Swiss albino	Female	Fasted	Gavage	LD_{50}	88 (27–120)
20-Methyl spirolide G	Swiss albino	Female	Fasted	Feeding method 2	LD_{50}	500 (381–707)

[a] Feeding method 1: The test substance was fed absorbed on dry mousefood. Feeding method 2: The test substance was fed mixed with cream cheese. Feeding method 3: The test substance was fed mixed with moist mousefood.
[b] Figures in brackets indicate 95% confidence limits. All data from Munday et al.[213]

7.5.2.5 Acute Toxicities of Pinnatoxins by Intraperitoneal Injection

The acute toxicities of pinnatoxin derivatives by intraperitoneal injection are summarized in Table 7.9.

The LD_{99} of natural pinnatoxin A was estimated at 135 and 180 μg/kg, while the synthetic epimer, (−) pinnatoxin A, showed no effects at a dose of ~5000 μg/kg. A mixture of pinnatoxins B and C was highly toxic to mice, with a reported LD_{99} of 22 μg/kg. Pinnatoxin F is of similar toxicity. Pinnatoxins E and G are less toxic, with LD_{50} values between 45 and 57 μg/kg, while pinnatoxin D appears to be of much lower toxic potential. The acute intraperitoneal toxicities of pinnatoxins E, F, and G in fasted mice were not significantly different from those in fed animals.

The symptoms of intoxication by pinnatoxins by intraperitoneal injection closely resembled those of gymnodimine and the spirolides, although death times at lethal doses (30–50 min) and recovery times after sublethal doses (2–3 h) were longer with the pinnatoxins than with the other cyclic imines.[14]

7.5.2.6 Acute Toxicities of Pinnatoxins by Oral Administration

Pinnatoxins are less toxic by gavage than by intraperitoneal injection (Table 7.10), although wide variations were observed among the different compounds in the degree of disparity.

TABLE 7.9

Acute Toxicities of Pinnatoxins by Intraperitoneal Injection in Mice

Compound	Strain of Mouse	Sex of Mouse	State of Alimentation	Parameter	Acute Toxicity (µg/kg Body Weight)[a]	Reference
(+)-Pinnatoxin A	?	?	?	LD_{99}	180	[215]
(+)-Pinnatoxin A	?	?	?	LD_{99}	135	[216]
(−)-Pinnatoxin A	?	?	?	MLD	>5000[b]	[216]
Pinnatoxins B and C[c]	?	?	?	LD_{99}	22	[217]
Pinnatoxin D	?	?	?	LD_{99}	400	[218]
Pinnatoxin E	Swiss albino	Female	Fed	LD_{50}	45.0 (35.0–66.0)	[206]
Pinnatoxin E	Swiss albino	Female	Fed	LD_{50}	57.0 (39.7–75.3)	[14]
Pinnatoxin E	Swiss albino	Female	Fasted	LD_{50}	48.0 (33.5–63.5)	[14]
Pinnatoxin F	Swiss albino	Female	Fed	LD_{50}	16.0 (12.0–23.0)	[206]
Pinnatoxin F	Swiss albino	Female	Fed	LD_{50}	12.7 (9.5–14.6)	[14]
Pinnatoxin F	Swiss albino	Female	Fasted	LD_{50}	14.9 (12.6–15.8)	[14]
Pinnatoxin G	Swiss albino	Female	Fed	LD_{50}	50.0 (35.0–66.0)	[206]
Pinnatoxin G	Swiss albino	Female	Fed	LD_{50}	48.0 (36.3–68.1)	[14]
Pinnatoxin G	Swiss albino	Female	Fasted	LD_{50}	42.7 (40.0–50.0)	[14]

Note: "?" indicates that this information was not provided in the cited reference.

[a] Figures in brackets indicate 95% confidence limits.

[b] No effects were observed at this dose.

[c] 1:1 mixture of B and C. These compounds are stereoisomers.

TABLE 7.10

Acute Toxicities of Pinnatoxins by Oral Administration to Mice

Compound	Strain of Mouse	Sex of Mouse	State of Alimentation	Method of Administration[a]	Parameter	Acute Toxicity (µg/kg Body Weight)[b]
Pinnatoxin E	Swiss albino	Female	Fed	Gavage	LD_{50}	2800 (2380–3000)
Pinnatoxin F	Swiss albino	Female	Fed	Gavage	LD_{50}	25.0 (19.1–35.1)
Pinnatoxin F	Swiss albino	Female	Fasted	Gavage	LD_{50}	29.9 (25.0–32.0)
Pinnatoxin F	Swiss albino	Female	Fed	Feeding method 2	LD_{50}	50.0 (39.4–62.8)
Pinnatoxin F	Swiss albino	Female	Fasted	Feeding method 2	LD_{50}	77
Pinnatoxin F	Swiss albino	Female	Fed	Feeding method 4	LD_{50}	50.0 (37.9–71.5)
Pinnatoxin F	Swiss albino	Female	Fasted	Feeding method 4	LD_{50}	50.0 (39.4–62.8)
Pinnatoxin F	Swiss albino	Female	Fed	Feeding method 1	LD_{50}	50.0 (37.9–71.5)
Pinnatoxin G	Swiss albino	Female	Fed	Gavage	LD_{50}	150 (105–199)
Pinnatoxin G	Swiss albino	Female	Fed	Feeding method 2	LD_{50}	400 (380–470)

[a] Feeding method 1: The test substance was fed absorbed on dry mousefood. Feeding method 2: The test substance was fed mixed with cream cheese. Feeding method 3: The test substance was fed in a peanut butter mix (53% peanut butter, 10% casein, 37% sucrose).

[b] Figures in brackets indicate 95% confidence limits. All data from Munday et al.[14]

Pinnatoxin E was 49 times less toxic by gavage than by injection, a disparity similar to that observed with gymnodimine A and the spirolides. In contrast, the LD_{50}s of pinnatoxin F and pinnatoxin G were only two to three times higher by gavage than by intraperitoneal injection. In all cases, the time to death (~1.3 h) was longer than that recorded after intraperitoneal injection. The LD_{50}s of pinnatoxins F and G were higher when administered by feeding than by gavage, but again the differences were much smaller than those recorded with other cyclic imines, differing by factors of only 2.0 and 2.7, respectively. The vehicle employed for administration by feeding had no significant effect on the LD_{50}s of the former substance.[14]

7.5.2.7 Acute Toxicities of Pteriatoxins, Prorocentrolide, and Spiro-Prorocentrimine by Intraperitoneal Injection

The acute toxicities of pteriatoxins, prorocentrolide, and spiro-prorocentrimine by intraperitoneal injection are shown in Table 7.11. No information on the symptoms of intoxication by these compounds is available, although they are reported to be fast-acting toxins, like the other cyclic imines.[186] No information on their toxicity by other routes of administration is available.

7.5.3 Effects of Cyclic Imines in Humans

No reports of human illness followed the incident of gymnodimine contamination of shellfish in New Zealand in 1994.[219] Gymnodimine was subsequently shown to be present in many species of New Zealand shellfish analyzed over a period of years, although such shellfish were consumed with no reports of adverse effects.[220]

In Canada, during times when shellfish were contaminated with spirolides, there were reports of rather nonspecific symptoms of illness, such as gastric distress and tachycardia, but such reports were not conclusively attributable to shellfish consumption.[221] Positive mouse bioassay results have been recorded in Canadian shellfish each year since 1994, which were later shown to be associated with the presence of spirolides.[222] There were, however, no reports of illness in consumers.

It has often been stated in the literature that pinnatoxins in shellfish are responsible for human episodes of poisoning, citing the paper of Uemura,[215] but such statements reflect a misunderstanding of the situation. Outbreaks of human intoxication in Japan, associated with consumption of *Pinna pectinata*, were later attributed to contamination of the shellfish by *Vibrio* species.[223] Furthermore, the human intoxication associated with consumption of *Pinna attenuata* in China in 1980 and 1989 was not linked to the presence of pinnatoxins, and recent observations indicate that regular consumption of oysters definitively shown to contain pinnatoxins D, E, and F in New Zealand caused no adverse effects.[207] There have been no reports of adverse effects of pteriatoxins, prorocentrolide, spiro-prorocentrimine, or symbioimines in humans.

7.5.4 Metabolism and Disposition of Cyclic Imines

No information is available on the disposition in animals of any of the cyclic imines apart from 13-desmethyl spirolide C and 13,19-didesmethyl spirolide C. These substances are rapidly absorbed after oral administration to animals. Removal from the blood was also rapid, with the amounts of these substances being below the limit of quantitation by LC-MS 1 h after dosing. At this time, both substances were detectable in the urine, and both were present in the feces of mice after 24 h.[214]

The incubation of 13-desmethyl spirolide C with human liver microsomes in vitro led to the formation of nine oxidized metabolites, including 13,19-didesmethyl-19-carboxy spirolide C, 13,19-didesmethyl-19-hydroxymethyl spirolide C, and 13-desmethyl-17-hydroxy spirolide C,[224] but no metabolites resulting from the degradation of the imine ring were detected.

No information on the in vivo metabolism of any of the cyclic imines is available.

TABLE 7.11

Acute Toxicities of Pteriatoxins, Prorocentrolide, and Spiro-Prorocentrimine by Intraperitoneal Injection in Mice

Compound	Strain of Mouse	Sex of Mouse	State of Alimentation	Parameter	Acute Toxicity (μg/kg Body Weight)	Reference
Pteriatoxin A	?	?	?	LD_{99}	100	[187]
Pteriatoxins B and C[a]	?	?	?	LD_{99}	8	[187]
Prorocentrolide	?	?	?	"Lethality"	400	[185]
Spiro-prorocentrimine	?	?	?	LD_{99}	2500	[188]

Note: "?" indicates that this information was not provided in the cited reference.

[a] 1:1 mixture of B and C. These compounds are stereoisomers.

7.5.5 Mechanism of Toxicity of Cyclic Imines

In 2004, it was noted that the symptoms of intoxication by gymnodimine were similar to those of tubocurarine, a competitive nondepolarizing neuromuscular blocking agent that binds reversibly to postjunctional nicotinic receptors, thus blocking the transmitter action of acetylcholine.[211] By raising the acetylcholine concentration in the synaptic cleft through administration of the acetylcholinesterase inhibitors neostigmine or physostigmine, the binding of tubocurarine to the receptors is decreased, and its toxicity is diminished. Neostigmine and physostigmine similarly protected against the acute effects of gymnodimine, indicating a similar action at the neuromuscular junction to that of tubocurarine.[211]

Subsequent studies in vitro have confirmed blockade of muscle and neuronal nicotinic acetylcholine receptors by gymnodimine, with specificity toward particular receptor subtypes.[212,225] The characteristics of the receptor blockade elicited by gymnodimine A were closely similar to those induced by tubocurarine.[212] Similar effects have been recorded with 13-desmethyl spirolide C,[225] 13,19-didesmethyl spirolide C,[226] and pinnatoxins A and G.[227] Neuromuscular transmission in the mouse phrenic hemidiaphragm preparation was blocked by gymnodimine,[212] by pinnatoxin F, and by a mixture of pinnatoxin E and F[228] at nanomolar concentrations. The interaction of 13-desmethyl spirolide C with muscarinic acetylcholine receptors has also been reported,[229] although a later study showed no significant effect of this substance or of gymnodimine on muscarinic receptors.[230] The observed asphyxic death of animals receiving lethal doses of cyclic imines is consistent with the inhibition of neuromuscular transmission, leading to paralysis of the diaphragm.

The cyclic imine moiety in this group of compounds is important for toxicity, and reduction of the imine, or the opening of the ring, greatly decreases toxicity. However, while the presence of the cyclic imine function may be a necessary condition for toxicity, it is not sufficient, as shown by the relatively low acute toxicity of spirolide H. As with acute toxicity, the importance of the cyclic imine function in receptor binding has been demonstrated,[225] and this was confirmed by the observation that simple synthetic spiroimines also block nicotinic acetylcholine receptors.[231] Furthermore, opening of the imine-containing ring of pinnatoxin G, to form an amino-ketone (a compound analogous to spirolides E and F), abolished the effect on nicotinic receptors.[227] 13-Desmethyl spirolide C was shown to have a higher affinity for nicotinic acetylcholine receptors than gymnodimine,[230,232] which is in accord with the relative toxicities of these substances. In contrast, however, the affinity of 13,19-didesmethyl spirolide C was higher than that of the more toxic 13-desmethyl spirolide C,[226] indicating that binding affinity in vitro is not a reliable indicator of toxicity in vivo.

7.5.6 Regulation of Cyclic Imines

Cyclic imines are not regulated at present.[233]

7.5.7 Conclusions

Many cyclic imines show high toxicity when injected intraperitoneally in mice. The imine function is a necessary, but not sufficient, condition for toxicity, and the toxic potential of these compounds is modified by changes in the ring systems or alterations in ring substituents. The cyclic imines cause death by asphyxia, and there is good evidence that this is caused by the inhibition of neuromuscular transmission by these substances through their interaction with acetylcholine receptors.

As with many seafood contaminants, the toxicities of gymnodimine, spirolides A and C, 13-desmethyl spirolide C, and 20-methyl spirolide G by gavage are much lower than those by intraperitoneal injection. Such differences may reflect slower or less extensive absorption from the gastrointestinal tract. Pinnatoxin E is also less toxic by gavage than by injection, and this may again be attributable to differences in absorption. The lactone ring, which is patent in pinnatoxins A–D and pinnatoxin F, is opened to form a hydroxy carboxylic acid in pinnatoxin E, which would be expected to lead to an increase in hydrophilicity and decreased absorption from the gastrointestinal tract. The toxicities of gymnodimine, spirolides A and C, 13-desmethyl spirolide C, and 20-methyl spirolide G are even lower when voluntarily consumed by mice. Administration by this route, which ensures mixture of the test substance with the contents of the mouse stomach, thus avoiding rapid delivery of the test material to the absorptive areas of the small intestine and mimicking the situation in humans, is recommended by the Codex Alimentarius Commission as the preferred method of dosing seafood toxins.[50]

The relative toxicities of pinnatoxins F and G by the different routes of administration were quite different from those of the other cyclic imines. These substances were, respectively, only two and three times less toxic by gavage than by injection and only four and eight times less toxic by voluntary consumption. The high oral toxicity of these substances raises concern as to possible adverse effects in humans. It is likely, however, that pinnatoxin derivatives, including pinnatoxins F and G, have been present in microalgae and in seafood in many parts of the world for many years, yet they have never been associated with any harmful effects in consumers. It is possible that levels in seafood have never been high enough to trigger a toxic response in humans, and a systematic study of the pinnatoxin levels in seafood that are eaten by humans without adverse effects would be valuable in the risk assessment of these compounds.

The same argument applies to other cyclic imines, since none have been shown to cause intoxication in humans. Again, levels in seafood may never have reached toxic levels. It is also possible, however, that there are differences between mice and humans with regard to absorption and detoxification of cyclic imines or there are interspecies differences in the susceptibility of nicotinic receptors to this class of compound. In view of the importance of the cyclic imine function in these substances for expression of toxic effects, the identification of metabolic pathways leading to its destruction would be of great value.

No chronic toxicity studies have been performed on any of the cyclic imines. Since these substances, particularly the spirolides, are regularly consumed by humans, such studies are urgently required. An estimate of mutagenic potential, as indicated by the Ames test, is also needed.

7.6 Domoic Acid and Derivatives

7.6.1 Production and Distribution of Domoic Acid and Derivatives

Domoic acid is a toxic glutamate analogue, which was first isolated from the red macroalga *Chondria armata*.[234] Domoic acid is also produced by many species of *Pseudo-nitzschia*, which are of worldwide distribution.[235] The consumption of domoic acid-containing diatoms by filter-feeding molluscs and by planktivorous krill and finfish leads to accumulation of the toxin in these animals, and from these, domoic acid progresses further up the food chain, and this substance has been detected in the tissues of many aquatic animals.[235]

Several structural isomers of domoic acid (isodomoic acids A–H) and a stereoisomer (5′-*epi*-domoic acid) have been isolated from microalgae, diatoms, and/or shellfish.[236–241] These substances have been reported to be present in Canadian mussels, clams, and anchovies at much lower concentrations than domoic acid itself.[242]

7.6.2 Toxicity of Domoic Acid and Derivatives to Experimental Animals

The toxic effects of domoic acid in animals have been reviewed.[243–245]

7.6.2.1 Acute Toxicity of Domoic Acid and Derivatives by Intraperitoneal Injection

Data on the acute toxicity of domoic acid by intraperitoneal injection are summarized in Table 7.12.

In adult animals, the lethal dose of domoic acid in mice, rats, and monkeys by intraperitoneal injection is of the order of 4–6 mg/kg, with estimates of the NOAEL ranging from 0.6 to 1.0 mg/kg, indicating a steep dose–response curve. The acute toxicity of domoic acid in newborn rats is, however, much higher than that in adults, with an LD_{50} of only 0.25 mg/kg in 2-day old pups. While susceptibility was lower in 10-day old animals, the MLD was still ~7 times lower than in adults.[253]

Characteristic behavioral changes have been described in rodents after the administration of domoic acid by intraperitoneal injection. The animals initially became lethargic, progressing to a state of

TABLE 7.12

Acute Toxicity of Domoic Acid to Animals by Intraperitoneal Injection

Species	Strain	Age	LD$_{50}$ (mg/kg)	LOAEL (mg/kg)	NOAEL (mg/kg)	References
Mouse	CF1	Adult	6.2	1.2	0.6	[246]
Mouse	ICR	Adult	>4.0	0.25	—	[247]
Mouse	CD1	Adult	3.6 (3.2–4.0)[a]			[248,249]
Mouse	ddY	Adult	~4.0	—	—	[249]
Mouse	Swiss	Adult	6.0 (4.2–7.9)[a]			[250,251]
Rat	Sprague–Dawley	Adult	—	—	0.65	[251]
Rat	Sprague–Dawley	Adult	4.0–7.5	2.0	1.0	[246,252]
Rat	Long–Evans	2 Days	0.25	—	—	[253]
Rat	Long–Evans	5 Days	—	0.05	—	[253]
Rat	Long–Evans	10 Days	0.70	0.05	—	[253]
Cynomolgus monkey	—	Adult	<4.0[b]	—	—	[254]
Marmoset	—	Adult	3.5–4.0	—	—	[255]

[a] Figures in brackets indicate 95% confidence limits.
[b] One monkey given 4.0 mg/kg died.

immobility, often associated with forelimb rigidity. Subsequently, the animals began vigorous scratching, with the hind leg being brought forward behind the ear. In some cases, the scratching was intensive enough to draw blood. Other stereotypic responses included circular movements and head weaving. These were followed by the onset of rearing and twisting movements, with loss of postural control. In the final stages of intoxication, tremors, particularly of the front paws, with spontaneous seizures, were observed, often culminating in death.[252,256] The severity of the behavioral changes is dose related, and their onset occurs sooner at higher dose levels. Tasker et al.[256] devised a 7-point scale for scoring domoic acid-induced behavioral changes, which is very useful for comparing the relative toxicity of domoic acid derivatives and other excitotoxic compounds.[257]

Similar behavioral changes have been observed in monkeys after intraperitoneal injection of domoic acid. Furthermore, in these animals, domoic acid was shown to be a powerful emetic.[254]

Domoic acid is neurotoxic, and the pathological changes induced by this substance in the brains of animals have been extensively reviewed.[258] Although many areas of the brain suffer damage, the hippocampus is the primary target site, in which degenerative changes in neurons have consistently been reported. The severity of the lesions depends upon the dose level, the route of administration, and the extent of seizure level,[246] and their development is time dependent. Brain damage was not observed in mice 30 min after intraperitoneal administration of domoic acid,[246] although hippocampal damage was clearly evident 4 h after injection.[259]

Although by far the most attention has been focused on the cerebral lesions induced by domoic acid, toxic changes in several other tissues and organs have been reported. Necrosis of cells of the inner nuclear layer and vacuolation of cells of the outer plexiform layer of the retina have been observed in rodents and monkeys dosed intraperitoneally with domoic acid,[246,252,254] and myocardial necrosis with inflammatory cell infiltration has been observed in rats dosed with this substance by intraperitoneal injection or by direct infusion into the hippocampus.[260] Gastric and duodenal ulcers were recorded in mice dosed intraperitoneally with pure domoic acid or with an extract of toxic mussels. Pulmonary hemorrhage has also been described.[261,262]

Neonatal animals are much more susceptible to the behavioral and long-term effects of domoic acid than adults. Behavioral changes were observed in rat pups injected intraperitoneally with domoic acid, with an ED$_{50}$ of only 0.15 mg/kg at postnatal day 5. With increasing age, the susceptibility of the animals to the toxic effects of domoic acid diminished, and at postnatal day 22, the ED$_{50}$ was seven times greater than that at postnatal day 5. Aging also increases susceptibility. Rats aged 22–29 months were more sensitive to the toxic effects of intraperitoneally injected domoic acid than 2–3-month-old animals.[263]

There is evidence that animals receiving a single sublethal dose of domoic acid suffer long-term behavioral defects. Mice dosed intraperitoneally with domoic acid at 2.0 mg/kg showed impaired spatial learning 1 h after administration of the toxin, and this change was maintained throughout the subsequent 14-day observation period.[264] Injection of domoic acid at doses sufficient to cause seizures led to recurrent spontaneous seizures over a period of 6 months.[265]

Isodomoic acids A, B, and C are much less toxic to mice than domoic acid itself. Intraperitoneal injection of domoic acid at 5 mg/kg led to the expected toxic changes in mice, but only minor behavioral changes were seen with isodomoic acids A and B at 5 mg/kg or with isodomoic acid C at 20 mg/kg.[250]

7.6.2.2 Acute Toxicity of Domoic Acid by Oral Administration

Domoic acid is much less toxic to rodents by oral administration than by intraperitoneal injection (Table 7.13).

Precise LD_{50} values have not been established, but from the available data, the LD_{50} in rodents would appear to be of the order of 80 mg/kg. An important fact to note is that while the acute toxicity of injected domoic acid in rats and mice is similar to that in monkeys, there are gross differences in toxicity through oral administration, with the NOAEL in monkeys being 56–120 times lower than that in rodents. It should also be noted that the acute toxicity of domoic acid in monkeys may be even higher than that indicated in Table 7.13, since vomiting occurred after oral administration of domoic acid to these animals, so that a significant amount of the administered toxin may have been lost.[266]

Retinal and cardiac changes, similar to those recorded after injection of domoic acid in rodents and monkeys, have been observed in sea lions and sea otters after dietary exposure to the toxin.[268-270]

7.6.2.3 Acute Toxicity of Domoic Acid by Intravenous Injection

The toxicity of domoic acid by intravenous injection in rats and monkeys is considerably higher than that by intraperitoneal administration, although the symptoms of intoxication were similar by both routes of administration.[254,271]

In rats, the severity of neuronal degeneration in the hippocampus continued to progress after intravenous administration of domoic acid, reaching a plateau at 5–14 days.[272]

7.6.2.4 Repeated-Dose Studies on Domoic Acid

Two studies on the effects of repeated oral doses of domoic acid have been reported, one in rats and one in monkeys. In the rat study, animals were dosed by gavage with domoic acid at 0.1 or 5.0 mg/kg/day for 64 days. No behavioral changes were observed, and no hematological or clinical biochemical abnormalities were recorded at the end of the dosing period. There were no organ weight changes, and no lesions were observed by light microscopy in the brain, eyes, lungs, liver, spleen, pancreas, kidneys, adrenals, thyroid, pituitary, or gastrointestinal tract of the animals.[273] However, further examination of a subset of these rats by electron microscopy revealed neuronal damage in the hippocampus of rats dosed at 5.0 mg/kg/day,

TABLE 7.13

Acute Toxicity of Domoic Acid to Animals by Oral Administration

Species	Strain	Age	LD_{50} (mg/kg)	LOAEL (mg/kg)	NOAEL (mg/kg)	Reference
Mouse	CF1	Adult	71–83	35	28	[246]
Rat	Sprague–Dawley	Adult	80–82	70	60	[246]
Rat	Sprague–Dawley	Adult	>80	—	—	[266]
Cynomolgus monkey	—	Adult	>6.6[a]	—	0.5	[266]
Cynomolgus monkey	—	Adult	>10[a]	—	0.5	[267]

[a] Severe toxic effects at this dose, but no deaths.

although no brain pathology was seen in the animals receiving domoic acid at 0.1 mg/kg/day.[258] In the primate study, three cynomolgus monkeys were dosed with domoic acid at 0.5 mg/kg for 15 days and then at 0.75 mg/kg for a further 15 days. After this time, blood samples were taken for analysis of diagnostic markers, and the monkeys were killed and necropsied. All major organs were weighed and samples taken for histology. No significant changes in any parameter were recorded, and no lesions were observed by light microscopy. Unfortunately, no examination of the brains of these animals by electron microscopy was undertaken.[274]

At a dose of 5 or 20 µg/kg, dosed subcutaneously each day over postnatal days 8–14, rat pups showed no symptoms of toxicity, and their weight gains were unaffected. However, loss of hippocampal neurons occurred,[275] and hippocampal development was compromised.[276] When tested as adolescents or adults, these animals showed behavioral abnormalities and deficits in learning ability and memory.[277–284] Furthermore, a decrease in seizure threshold was observed as late as 160 days after domoic acid administration.[285]

7.6.2.5 Effects of Domoic Acid in Animals Exposed In Utero

No brain lesions were detected in newborn pups after intravenous administration of domoic acid to pregnant mice at gestational day 13, but by postnatal day 14, severe neuronal damage was observed in the hippocampus. The severity of the hippocampal changes continued to increase until the end of the observation period, at postnatal day 30.[286] When tested at 11 weeks of age, male, but not female, mice from dams given intraperitoneal injections of domoic acid at various stages of gestation showed severe impairment of learning and memory.[287] In rats, prenatal exposure to domoic acid led to persistent behavioral changes at up to 13 weeks in both males and females.[288,289]

7.6.3 Effects of Domoic Acid in Humans

In November–December 1987, a serious outbreak of food poisoning was observed in individuals who had eaten cultivated mussels from Cardigan Bay, Prince Edward Island, Canada. Gastrointestinal disorders (vomiting, stomach cramps, diarrhea, and bleeding) were commonly reported, but in some individuals, these symptoms were accompanied by pronounced and unusual neurological effects, including confusion, disorientation, seizures, and, in extreme cases, status epilepticus and coma. A case was defined as an individual showing one or more gastrointestinal symptoms within 24 h of consuming the mussels or neurological symptoms within 48 h of consumption. One hundred and seven persons met these criteria. Of these, 19 individuals required hospital treatment, of whom 12 needed intensive care because of seizures, coma, excessive pulmonary secretions, or unstable blood pressure. Of the 16 hospitalized patients for which medical records were available, 12 were over 65 years of age. The 4 individuals under 65 all had preexisting illnesses—diabetes (2 individuals), renal disease (3 individuals), and hypertension (1 individual). Three individuals, who were all over 70 years of age, died within days after ingestion of the mussels.[290,291] Histological examination of the brains of these individuals revealed neuronal necrosis and astrocytosis, particularly in the hippocampus and amygdaloid nucleus. Lesions were also observed in the anterior claustrum, nucleus accumbens, and thalamus.[290] A fourth individual, 84 years old, died of an acute myocardial infarction 3 months after eating the mussels. A fifth man showed long-term memory loss and developed temporal lobe epilepsy 1 year after mussel consumption. He died 2 years later. At necropsy, severe bilateral hippocampal sclerosis was observed.[292] The disease was named "excitotoxic amnesic shellfish poisoning,"[267] later abbreviated to "amnesic shellfish poisoning" (ASP).

From the analysis of leftover mussels and patient recall of the amount that had been eaten, it was possible to provide a rough estimate of the amount of domoic acid that caused poisoning in the Canadian outbreak. The estimate for one unaffected person was 0.2–0.3 mg/kg, while at 0.9–2.0 mg/kg, symptoms of poisoning were mainly gastrointestinal. The estimated intake in persons with clinical signs was 0.9–4.2 mg/kg, while two individuals with a domoic acid intake of 4.1 and 4.2 mg/kg suffered long-term neurological change.[293]

A follow-up study of 14 individuals who had been severely affected in the Canadian outbreak showed continuing memory defects.[290] Since the hippocampus is critical for memory function,[294] irreversible damage to this tissue would provide a plausible explanation of the reported memory loss in these persons.

The 1987 Canadian outbreak is the only authenticated example of ASP. High levels of domoic acid were found in razor clams and Dungeness crabs from Washington State and Oregon in 1991.[295] A number of individuals suffered gastrointestinal disturbances at this time, but the involvement of domoic acid in this incident was never confirmed.[293]

7.6.4 Metabolism and Disposition of Domoic Acid

It is estimated that only 1.8% of an oral dose of domoic acid is absorbed from the gastrointestinal tract of the rat.[273] The extent of absorption by monkeys, however, is more than twice that of rats.[274]

At neutral pH, domoic acid exists in a highly hydrophilic negatively charged state. Therefore, unless uptake is facilitated by a carrier, domoic acid will not readily cross the blood–brain barrier. There is no evidence for such a carrier,[296] and only small amounts of this substance are taken up into the brain, as shown with an *in situ* brain perfusion technique[297] and in experiments with radiolabeled domoic acid.[296]

The elimination of intravenous domoic acid is rapid, and plasma half-lives of 21.0 and 114.5 min have been reported in rats and monkeys, respectively.[271] The serum level of domoic acid was shown to be close to zero by 2 h after i.v. injection in rats,[271] and 95%–99% of an intraperitoneal dose was cleared from the plasma in 4 h in both rats and mice.[247,298]

In nonlactating animals, the elimination of domoic acid appears to be exclusively via the kidneys.[299] The importance of renal excretion was confirmed by the observation that plasma levels of domoic acid were seven-fold higher in nephrectomized rats than in control animals 1 h after an intravenous dose of the toxin.[296] In lactating rats, domoic acid is secreted in the milk, albeit at levels insufficient to cause acute effects in pups.[300]

Following intravenous administration to pregnant rats, domoic acid crosses the placenta and accumulates in the amniotic fluid. Domoic acid was also detected in the brains of the fetuses.[301]

7.6.5 Mechanism of Toxicity of Domoic Acid

There is good evidence that the cerebral toxicity of domoic acid reflects an excitotoxic response. In the brain, domoic acid activates α-amino-3-hydroxy-5-methyl-4-isoxazolepropionic acid and kainic acid receptors in neurons. The activation of the latter receptors results in elevated intracellular calcium levels, which lead to decreased ATP synthesis in mitochondria,[302] and generation of reactive oxygen and reactive nitrogen species.[303–305] The latter species are highly cytotoxic and may be responsible for the cell death seen in the cerebral neurons.

It has been suggested that the cardiotoxicity of domoic acid is similarly attributable to glutamate receptor subtypes in the heart,[269] but recent findings argue against this hypothesis. Cardiac necrosis can be introduced in rats by intraperitoneal injection of domoic acid at 2 mg/kg or by the infusion of 20,000 times less toxin into the hippocampus. Domoic acid was detected, albeit at low concentrations, in the hearts of rats dosed by intraperitoneal injection, but none was found in the hearts of rats receiving the test material by intra-hippocampal infusion. But both treatment protocols induced cardiac lesions of similar intensity, and both were associated with adverse effects on cardiac mitochondrial respiratory control and on enzymes of the mitochondrial respiratory chain. These results indicate that domoic acid is not directly cardiotoxic, and it was suggested that the cardiac lesions provoked by this substance reflect cardiac ischemia following seizure induction.[260]

7.6.6 Mutagenicity of Domoic Acid

Domoic acid was not genotoxic in V79 Chinese hamster lung fibroblasts, with or without metabolic activation with hepatocytes.[306] In contrast, domoic acid was reported to cause DNA damage in Caco-2 human colorectal adenocarcinoma cells.[307] No conventional mutagenicity studies have been conducted with this substance.

7.6.7 Regulation of Domoic Acid

After the Canadian incident, regulatory limits for the domoic acid content of shellfish were set. On the basis of the observed effects in humans, a LOAEL of 50 mg was estimated, equivalent to 0.714 mg/kg for a 70 kg adult. A safety factor of ~12 was applied, and assuming the consumption of 200 g of shellfish in a single meal, a regulatory limit of 20 mg/kg domoic acid in shellfish meat was derived.[308] This limit was subsequently accepted by the United States Food and Drug Administration (USFDA),[295] the Codex Alimentarius Commission,[50] and the European Union (EU)[309] and was confirmed by the Food and Agriculture Organization (FAO)/Intergovernmental Oceanographic Commission (IOC)/World Health Organization (WHO) Expert Panel in 2004.[310]

The regulatory limit for domoic acid was subsequently reevaluated by the EFSA CONTAM Panel in 2009.[293] Again based on effects in humans, the Panel estimated a LOAEL of 0.9 mg/kg and applied a safety factor of 3. A further factor of 10 was applied to account for variations in response among humans, thereby giving an ARfD of 30 µg/kg. In accord with new estimates of the intake of shellfish meat by high consumers,[311] the Panel assumed an intake of 400 g. In order for a 60 kg adult to avoid exceeding the ARfD, shellfish should contain no more than 4.5 mg/kg of domoic acid, and this value was recommended as the regulatory limit, more than four times lower than the previously accepted limit. Since domoic acid may be converted to *epi*-domoic acid during storage, this regulatory limit applies to the sum of domoic acid and its enantiomer. Because of the low levels of isodomoic acids in shellfish and their relatively low toxicity to animals, the Panel concluded that the regulation of these substances was not required. The Panel noted that the toxicological data were insufficient to establish a TDI.

7.6.8 Conclusions

It is estimated that more than 50,000 people consumed mussels contaminated with domoic acid from Cardigan Bay in 1987. But only 107 of these were diagnosed as suffering intoxication by this substance. There is no reason to assume that unaffected individuals consumed fewer mussels than those that were harmed or that the mussels that they ate contained less domoic acid. It would appear, therefore, that additional factors influence human response to domoic acid. It is also clear from animal studies that factors such as species, age, route of administration, and health status can have a major impact on the susceptibility to the toxic effects of domoic acid. There are several possible reasons for such differences.

Domoic acid is a neurotoxin, but for exertion of its effects on the brain, it must first be absorbed and then cross the blood–brain barrier. The uptake of domoic acid into the brain will be decreased if the toxin is degraded to a harmless metabolite or if it is rapidly excreted. An increased degree of absorption or a decreased rate of metabolism or excretion would therefore increase cerebral uptake, as would an increase in the permeability of the blood–brain barrier. The possibility also exists that there are differences in neuronal susceptibility to domoic acid among species or with age.

Domoic acid is a tricarboxylic acid, with pK_a values for the three carboxylic acid groups between 1.85 and 4.75.[312] At neutral pH, therefore, domoic acid will be extensively ionized and therefore not readily absorbed from the intestine. Like other acids, however, domoic acid will be subject to absorption from the stomach, under the relatively acidic conditions pertaining in this organ.[313] Since the degree of ionization will decrease with decreasing pH, absorption will occur most readily in animals with the lowest gastric pH. This consideration may explain the difference in susceptibility between monkeys (and possibly humans) and rodents after oral administration of domoic acid. The pH of the stomach of fasting cynomolgus monkeys is 1.9–2.2, much the same as that in humans.[314] In contrast, the pH of the rodent stomach is ~4.[315] Gastric pH may therefore explain the higher degree of domoic acid absorption by monkeys than by rodents and contribute to the relatively high oral toxicity of this substance to monkeys and to humans. It is also possible that ingestion of domoic acid or contaminated mussels on an empty stomach would result in higher toxicity than if consumed when the stomach contained other food, since stomach pH rises after a meal.

Deaths occurred in the Canadian outbreak in individuals over the age of 70. Increased passage across the blood–brain barrier may have contributed to the high toxicity of domoic acid in these individuals, since the permeability of the barrier increases during the normal aging process in humans.[24] Severe effects in younger people occurred only in individuals with concurrent disease, and defects in the blood–brain barrier could have contributed to the high toxicity of domoic acid in individuals with hypertension or diabetes, since the patency of the barrier is compromised in both these conditions.[316–318] The high toxicity of domoic acid in the elderly could also reflect the decline in renal function with age,[22] leading to prolonged retention of domoic acid in the plasma, and such an effect could have contributed to toxicity in individuals with preexisting renal disease. Age-related changes in the permeability of the blood–brain barrier do not appear to play a role in the relatively high susceptibility of old rats, since the ratio between brain and serum levels of domoic acid in young rats was not significantly different from that in old.[263] Impaired renal excretion has been suggested to account for the high sensitivity of old rodents, since the serum and cerebral levels of domoic acid were significantly higher in old rats than in young when given equal doses.[263] Differences in neuronal sensitivity do not appear to play a role in the relative sensitivity of old rats, since although these were more sensitive than young rats when dosed intraperitoneally, no differences in response were observed when domoic acid was infused into the hippocampus.[263]

Neonatal animals are much more susceptible to domoic acid than adults. The possibility of an immature and relatively leaky blood–brain barrier in newborns and fetuses has been discussed. Most functions of the blood–brain barrier are fully developed in the fetus and neonate, although permeability to small hydrophilic molecules is greater in the developing brain than in the adult,[319] suggesting that domoic acid could achieve higher levels in the brain of young animals. However, if the increased potency of domoic acid in neonates was due to increased permeability of the barrier, it would be expected that the serum concentration of the toxin required to cause a toxic effect would be lower in neonates than in older animals. This was not the case.[320] Impaired renal excretion may contribute to the high sensitivity of young animals. At a given dose, newborn rats maintain higher serum levels of domoic acid than adults,[253] and the rate of glomerular filtration has been shown to be lower in newborn rats and humans than in adults.[23] Recent studies[321] have demonstrated prolonged retention of domoic acid in rat fetuses, which could lead to increased susceptibility to the toxic effects of this substance.

The establishment of a regulatory limit for acute exposure to domoic acid is more complex than for many other seafood contaminants. Rodents appear to be a poor model for assessing the toxicity of domoic acid, since the lethal dose of this substance in these animals is much higher than that in humans or nonhuman primates, possibly reflecting differences in stomach pH, as discussed earlier. The current regulatory limit was established largely on the basis of effects in humans during the Canadian outbreak, with only a small number of individuals and with serious doubts as to the accuracy of the estimates of the actual amount of domoic acid consumed. However, the fact that there have been no further confirmed cases of domoic acid intoxication since the establishment of the initial (20 mg/kg) regulatory limit suggests that this limit is appropriate to avoid acute toxic effects from this substance. The new recommended limit by EFSA, at less than one-quarter of the original limit, which was based on a more rigorous safety factor and a more conservative estimate of the highest level of shellfish consumption by humans, would, if accepted by regulatory authorities, provide a greater margin of safety.

As noted by regulatory authorities, the data available on domoic acid toxicology are presently inadequate to set a TDI for this substance. Chronic toxicity studies are clearly required in order to provide the necessary information. Tests for genotoxic effects, using established procedures, are also needed.

Of more concern is the very high susceptibility of neonates to domoic acid. While babies are unlikely to consume contaminated mussels, there is the possibility of transmission via milk. Although the levels in rat milk were shown to be insufficient to cause acute effects in the pups, studies on the degree of transfer of domoic acid into the milk of primates after oral administration would be very valuable in determining whether an additional safety factor is required. It has been suggested[322] that such a safety factor should be employed in situations where long-term effects are seen in offspring when the substance is administered at doses that produce no observable adverse effects on the mother.

A further concern is the possibility of long-term neurological damage after exposure to domoic acid *in utero*. This has clearly been demonstrated in rodents after injection of domoic acid, and studies are needed to establish if this also occurs after oral administration. With regard to long-term effects in humans, it has been mentioned in conference proceedings[323,324] that a long-term epidemiological study on Native Americans is under way in the Pacific Northwest. Indigenous groups may be at risk of harmful effects from domoic acid because of their traditional high intake of shellfish, which, in this area, are often contaminated with this toxin. The results from this study will provide valuable data for clearly identifying the potential risk to human health of domoic acid.

7.7 Okadaic Acid and Derivatives

7.7.1 Production and Distribution of Okadaic Acid and Derivatives

Okadaic acid and derivatives are produced by dinoflagellates of the genera *Prorocentrum* and *Dinophysis*, which are of worldwide distribution.[325] These organisms produce a large number of polyether toxins, including okadaic acid itself, the isomeric dinophysistoxin-2 (DTX-2), dinophysistoxin-1 (DTX-1, 35-methyl-okadaic acid), and 19-*epi*-okadaic acid. Many esters formed from okadaic acid and the dinophysistoxins by conjugation of the terminal carboxylic acid group with poly-hydroxylated, sulfated, or unsaturated alcohols have also been isolated from these organisms.[326]

When ingested by shellfish, a proportion of the toxins present in the dinoflagellates are acylated at the C-7 hydroxyl group with long-chain fatty acids, forming derivatives collectively known as DTX-3.[327]

7.7.2 Toxicity of Okadaic Acid and Derivatives to Animals

7.7.2.1 Acute Toxicities of Okadaic Acid and Derivatives by Intraperitoneal Injection

The acute toxicities of okadaic acid and derivatives to mice by intraperitoneal injection are shown in Table 7.14.

Estimates of the LD_{50} of okadaic acid itself in mice range from 192 to 225 µg/kg. DTX-1 is of similar toxicity, while DTX-2 and DTX-3 are somewhat less toxic. The acylation of the 7-hydroxyl group with palmitic or linoleic acid greatly decreases toxicity, but the polyunsaturated 7-*O*-docosahexaenoyl-okadaic acid is 10 times more toxic than the saturated or di-unsaturated esters. The esterification of the terminal carboxyl group of okadaic acid with a trihydroxylated trisulfated alcohol to form DTX-4 is associated with a threefold decrease in toxicity compared with the parent compound. Significant variations in survival times have been recorded among different strains of mice injected with lethal doses of okadaic acid.[336]

After intraperitoneal injection of okadaic acid in mice, rapid distension of the duodenum and upper jejunum was observed, associated with fluid accumulation in the lumen.[330,337] There was severe damage to the epithelium of villi in the duodenum and upper jejunum, with separation and desquamation of epithelial cells from the lamina propria, although little effect was seen in the crypts. Pronounced edema of the lamina

TABLE 7.14

Acute Toxicities of Okadaic Acid and Derivatives to Mice by Intraperitoneal Injection

Compound	Strain of Mouse	Sex of Mouse	State of Alimentation	Parameter	Acute Toxicity (µg/kg Body Weight)[a]	Reference
Okadaic acid	CD-1	Female	?	LD_{50}	204	[328]
Okadaic acid	HLA:(SW)BR	Female	?	LD_{50}	210	[329]
Okadaic acid	CD-1	Female	Fed	LD_{50}	225 (176–275)	[330]
Okadaic acid	?	?	?	LD_{50}	192	[331]
Okadaic acid	ddY	Male	?	MLD	200	[332]
DTX-1	?	?	?	MLD	160	[333]
DTX-2	CD-1	Female	?	LD_{50}	352	[328]
DTX-3	?	?	?	MLD	500	[334]
DTX-4	?	?	?	LD_{50}	610	[335]
7-*O*-Palmitoyl-okadaic acid	ddY	Male	?	MLD	5550	[332]
7-*O*-Linoleoyl-okadaic acid	ddY	Male	?	MLD	5550	[332]
7-*O*-Docosahexaenoyl-okadaic acid	ddY	Male	?	MLD	550	[332]

Note: "?" indicates that this information was not provided in the cited reference.

[a] Figures in brackets indicate 95% confidence limits.

propria was observed, which was attributed to the increased permeability of vessels of the intestinal villi.[337] Erosion of the intestinal epithelium was recorded in animals injected with okadaic acid and DTX-1, while little effect on the gastrointestinal tract was observed in animals receiving the same dose of DTX-3.[338,339] Recovery from the epithelial damage began within 2 h after dosing and was virtually complete after 48 h.[338]

Massive hemorrhage and congestion in the liver of mice receiving lethal intraperitoneal doses of okadaic acid, DTX-1, and DTX-3 have been described,[338] although other authors have reported relatively minor hepatic effects (isolated necrosis, lipidosis, or vacuolation of hepatocytes) after injection of okadaic acid.[330]

7.7.2.2 Acute Toxicities of Okadaic Acid and Derivatives by Oral Administration

Relatively little information on the acute oral toxicities of okadaic acid and derivatives is available, and the data that are available are inconsistent (Table 7.15).

The LD_{50} of okadaic acid by gavage was reported as 400[340] and 880 µg/kg,[39] while Tubaro et al.[330] observed no deaths at 1000 µg/kg. Even within the same laboratory, wide variations in estimates of the LD_{50} occur. Le Hégarat et al.[341] found 100% mortality in mice dosed with okadaic acid at 300 µg/kg in one experiment, but none at 610 µg/kg in a subsequent one. It was not noted if the two experiments were conducted with the same or with different batches of the toxin. The reason or reasons for these discrepancies, which stand in sharp contrast to the uniformity of the estimates of the toxicity of okadaic acid by intraperitoneal injection, are unknown.

Toxic changes induced in the gastrointestinal tract of mice by oral administration of okadaic acid and its derivatives are very similar to those recorded after intraperitoneal injection,[330,338–340] although some epithelial damage was also observed in the cecum and large intestine, albeit less severe than that seen in the small intestine.[340] Oral administration of okadaic acid also causes edema and mucosal erosion in the stomach of mice, accompanied by acute inflammatory changes in the submucosa.[330,340,343] Oral administration of okadaic acid to rats induced similar changes to those seen in mice.[344]

No liver damage was observed in mice and rats dosed orally with okadaic acid at 750–4000 µg/kg.[339,344] In contrast, hepatic lipidosis and focal necrosis were reported in mice dosed orally with DTX-3 at 750 µg/kg.[339] Alveolar edema and hemorrhage were reported in the lungs of mice gavaged with okadaic acid at 150 µg/kg.[340]

7.7.2.3 Repeated-Dose Studies with Okadaic Acid and Derivatives

Only one repeated-dose study has been reported.[345] In this experiment, five mice were dosed with okadaic acid by gavage at 1000 µg/kg/day for 7 days. Diarrhea was observed in all of the mice. In three

TABLE 7.15

Acute Toxicities of Okadaic Acid and Derivatives to Mice by Gavage

Compound	Strain of Mouse	Sex of Mouse	State of Alimentation	Parameter	Acute Toxicity (µg/kg Body Weight)	Reference
Okadaic acid	ICR	Male	?	"Lethal dose"	400	[340]
Okadaic acid	Swiss	Female	Fed	LD_{50}	230–425[a]	[341]
Okadaic acid	Swiss	Female	Fed	LD_{50}	>610[b]	[341]
Okadaic acid	CD-1	Female	Fed	LD_{50}	1000–2000[c]	[330]
Okadaic acid	NMRI	Female	Fed	LD_{50}	880	[39]
DTX-1	ddY	Male	Fasted	LD_{50}	200–300[d]	[342]
DTX-3	ICR	Male	?	MLD	750	[338]

Note: "?" indicates that this information was not provided in the cited reference.

[a] No deaths at 230 µg/kg. All mice died at 425 µg/kg.

[b] No deaths at this dose.

[c] No deaths at 1000 µg/kg. Four out of five mice died at 2000 µg/kg.

[d] No deaths at 200 µg/kg. All mice died at 300 µg/kg.

animals, this ceased within a few hours, but in two of the mice, the diarrhea was profuse and persistent, and these animals died after the fifth dose of the test compound. The surviving mice lost body weight, associated with decreased food consumption. These were killed on the eighth day of the experiment. At necropsy, dark areas were seen on the liver surface, and the small intestine was full of fluid. No hematological changes were recorded, although increased plasma activities of aspartate aminotransferase (AST) and alanine aminotransferase (ALT), indicative of liver damage, were observed. Histology showed ulceration and submucosal inflammation of the forestomach, although no pathological changes were observed in the small intestine. Atrophic changes in the liver, lymphoid tissue, and pancreas were also observed, which were attributed to weight loss in the animals.

7.7.2.4 Tumor Promotion by Okadaic Acid and Derivatives

Repeated applications of okadaic acid or DTX-1 to mouse skin were shown to promote tumor formation following initiation with 7,12-dimethylbenz[*a*]anthracene (DMBA).[346,347] Okadaic acid, when administered via the drinking water, also acted as a tumor promoter in the rat glandular stomach after initiation with *N*-methyl-*N'*-nitro-*N*-nitrosoguanidine (MNNG).[348] In neither instance was okadaic acid or DTX-1 an initiator of cancer.

7.7.3 Effects of Okadaic Acid and Derivatives in Humans

Okadaic acid and its derivatives are responsible for Diarrhetic Shellfish Poisoning (DSP). DSP was first reported in Japan in the late 1970s,[349] but since that time, it has been recorded in many other parts of the world, including Europe, Scandinavia, North and South America, and New Zealand.[42,350] The predominant symptoms associated with DSP are nausea, vomiting, diarrhea, and abdominal pain, observed soon after ingestion of contaminated shellfish. Symptoms generally resolve within 2–3 days, and no deaths associated with DSP have been reported.

It has been suggested[351] that okadaic acid and derivatives could be a major risk factor for colorectal cancer. This concept was based on epidemiological studies reported by López-Rodas et al.[352] and Cordier et al.[353] In the first of these studies, a positive association was observed between consumption of shellfish by a Spanish population and incidence of colorectal cancer. It should be noted, however, that there was also a highly significant correlation between shellfish consumption and consumption of meat, the latter being a well-recognized factor in the induction of colorectal cancer.[354] In the study by Cordier et al., the cancer incidence in various coastal areas of France was surveyed, and possible correlations between this and the incidence and duration of shellfish harvesting closures due to the presence of okadaic acid were investigated. In men, after taking into account alcohol consumption as a confounding factor, a significant association between harvest closures and incidence of colonic cancer was observed. No such association was seen in women. No measurements of shellfish intake were made in the different areas, and toxin levels in the shellfish that were consumed were not assayed.

7.7.4 Metabolism and Disposition of Okadaic Acid and Derivatives

Seventy five percent of an oral dose of tritium-labeled okadaic acid was accounted for in the tissues, gut contents, and excreta of mice after 24 h. The test material was present in all 12 tissues examined, but the highest concentrations were found in the urine and intestinal contents. A relatively small amount was found in the feces at this time,[355] suggesting that okadaic acid undergoes enterohepatic circulation after oral dosing, consistent with previous observations following intramuscular injection of this substance.[356] Such circulation appears to be persistent, since okadaic acid was detectable in the heart, lungs, liver, and kidneys of mice for up to 2 weeks after dosing and in the small and large intestine for 4 weeks.[340] After intraperitoneal injection, 33% of the administered okadaic acid was found in the gastrointestinal tract 3 h after injection. Substantial amounts of okadaic acid remained in the liver after 22 h, again consistent with enterohepatic circulation.[357] Okadaic acid crosses the placenta, and substantial amounts were found in fetal tissues after oral administration to pregnant mice.[358]

The metabolism of okadaic acid does not appear to be have been studied in vivo, but the incubation of okadaic acid with recombinant human CYP3A4 and CYP3A5 or with human liver microsomes yielded the oxidized metabolites 11-hydroxy-okadaic acid, 43-hydroxy-okadaic acid, 36-hydroxy-okadaic acid, and 43-oxo-okadaic acid.[359,360]

In vitro, esters of okadaic acid are saponified by esterases and lipases.[361,362] Only DTX-1 was detected in the feces of individuals who consumed mussels containing DTX-3, indicating that such hydrolysis can also occur within the human gastrointestinal tract.[363]

7.7.5 Mechanism of Toxicity of Okadaic Acid and Derivatives

In 1988, Bialojan and Takai[364] reported that okadaic acid inhibited purified serine/threonine phosphatases PP1 and PP2A in vitro at nanomolar concentrations. Later studies showed that okadaic acid was also a potent inhibitor of PP4 and PP5.[365] Protein phosphatases are signal-transducing enzymes that play major roles in many cellular processes.[366,367] In 1990, Cohen et al.[368] suggested that okadaic acid "probably" causes diarrhea by stimulating the phosphorylation of proteins controlling sodium secretion by intestinal cells. This statement has been repeated many times in the literature, often with omission of the word "probably," and it is often stated that the inhibition of protein phosphatases is responsible not only for the diarrheagenic effects of okadaic acid but also for its acute toxic effects and its tumor-promoting activity. There is conflicting evidence for this hypothesis, however, and the possible role of protein phosphatase inhibition in the toxic effects of okadaic acid and derivatives requires reevaluation.

7.7.5.1 *Protein Phosphatase Inhibition and Diarrhea*

There is no correlation between the diarrheagenic activity of okadaic acid derivatives and their relative inhibitory activity toward protein phosphatases.[129] The idea that okadaic acid causes diarrhea by acting on proteins controlling sodium secretion[368] was disproved by later work showing that okadaic acid has no significant effect on ion currents in intestinal cell monolayers. It does, however, disrupt tight junctions between the cells, leading to increased paracellular permeability.[369] Evidence for increased intestinal paracellular permeability was also found in vivo,[370] and it was suggested that such an effect would lead to fluid accumulation in the intestine and hence to diarrhea. Although okadaic acid is known to enhance the phosphorylation of myosin light chain, a biochemical event that can lead to an increase in paracellular permeability, Tripuraneni et al.[369] provided evidence that this is not the mechanism whereby okadaic acid disrupts tight junctions. Rossini and Hess[371] suggested that the effects of okadaic acid on tight junctions could reflect the destruction of E-cadherin, the protein responsible for cell–cell adhesion of intestinal epithelial cells. The destruction of E-cadherin by okadaic acid has been observed in vitro,[372] though whether this process involves the inhibition of protein phosphatases is unclear. Little information on this topic is available, but it has been shown that changes in PP2A activity did not influence the utilization of E-cadherin in the formation of tight junctions in Madin–Darby canine kidney cells in vitro.[373]

In fact, diarrhea could simply result from the structural damage induced by okadaic acid in the intestine. Secretion of fluid occurs in the crypts, while absorption is mediated by the cells at the tips of the villi.[374] The crypts are largely undamaged by okadaic acid, so secretion will continue unabated, but loss of cells at the tips of villi will prevent fluid absorption, thus resulting in fluid accumulation in the intestinal lumen, and hence diarrhea.

7.7.5.2 *Protein Phosphatase Inhibition and Acute Toxicity*

The observation that DTX-2 is a weaker inhibitor of PP2A than okadaic acid and is less toxic to mice by intraperitoneal injection is consistent with the involvement of protein phosphatases in the acute toxicity of this substance.[328] Similarly, the relatively nontoxic 7-*O*-palmitoyl derivative is a weak inhibitor of PP1 and PP2A.[375,376] However, 7-*O*-acetylation of okadaic acid with a polyunsaturated fatty acid also greatly diminished activity toward the protein phosphatases,[376] yet 7-*O*-docosahexaenoyl-okadaic acid is highly toxic to mice. Similarly, DTX-4 is ~500 times less effective as a protein phosphatase inhibitor than okadaic acid,[361] but it is only three times less toxic to mice when injected intraperitoneally. It could be argued that the relatively high acute toxicity of DTX-4 reflects saponification within the peritoneal cavity, yielding okadaic acid. While such a process may occur after oral administration through the action of esterases or lipases within the intestine, as discussed earlier, saponification of injected DTX-4 is unlikely under the neutral conditions pertaining in the peritoneum and in the absence of the hydrolytic enzymes. While the inhibition of protein phosphatases by okadaic acid has been demonstrated with the purified enzymes and in cells in vitro, such inhibition has never been shown in vivo. An association between the relative acute toxicities of okadaic acid and derivatives to animals and their ability to inhibit protein phosphatases in vivo needs to be demonstrated in order to support the hypothesis that enzyme inhibition is responsible for the acute toxicity of these substances.

7.7.5.3 Protein Phosphatase Inhibition and Tumor Promotion

The initial studies by Fujiki and co-workers on tumor promotion by okadaic acid and DTX-1 were followed by a series of experiments on the promoting activity of other protein phosphatase inhibitors. It was shown that repeated application of the protein phosphatase inhibitor calyculin A, isolated from the marine sponge *Discodermia calyx*, has similar promoting activity to that of okadaic acid in DMBA-initiated skin carcinogenesis,[377] while repeated intraperitoneal injections of microcystin-LR or nodularin, also inhibitors of these enzymes, promoted tumor formation in the liver of rats following initiation with diethylnitrosamine.[378,379] These findings led to the conclusion that the inhibition of protein phosphatases is a key factor in the mechanism of action of certain tumor promoters, classified as the "okadaic acid type promoters," as distinct from promoters of the 12-*O*-tetradecanoylphorbol-13-acetate (TPA) type, and that promoting activity could be predicted on the basis of inhibitory effects on these enzymes.

In 1995, however, the Fujiki group tested tautomycin, another inhibitor of PP1 and PP2A, for tumor promotion in mouse skin initiated by DMBA and in the rat glandular stomach initiated by MNNG. Unlike the other protein phosphatase inhibitors, tautomycin had no effect on the incidence or multiplicity of skin tumors induced by DMBA. Furthermore, tautomycin actually protected against MNNG-induced cancer of the glandular stomach, rather than increasing the carcinogenicity as expected. It was therefore concluded that the inhibition of protein phosphatases is not a sufficient condition for tumor promotion.[380]

Later studies showed the importance of irritant potential for tumor promotion in the skin of mice. Okadaic acid, DTX-1, and calyculin A were shown to be highly irritant when applied to the mouse ear, but tautomycin was not.[347,377,381] Similarly, edema, inflammation, and mucosal erosion were recorded in the stomach of mice after oral administration of okadaic acid or calyculin A, while no such effect was seen with tautomycin.[343]

The importance of irritation in tumor promotion is consistent with the suggestion that pro-inflammatory cytokines, notably TNF-α, are of critical importance in tumor promotion.[382,383] Okadaic acid increased *TNF*-α gene expression in mouse skin and induced TNF-α release from cultured cells in vitro,[384] as do many other irritant materials, including the "classical" tumor promoter TPA.[383,385–387] In contrast, tautomycin has no effect on cytokine production, and the inability of this substance to act as a tumor promoter was attributed to its inability to induce TNF-α.[380] It is possible that irritation and TNF-α induction are downstream effects of protein phosphatase inhibition, although this appears unlikely in view of tumor promotion by other irritant materials, such as TPA, lyngbyatoxin, and palytoxin,[388,389] which have not been reported to inhibit protein phosphatases in the same way as okadaic acid and its derivatives.

7.7.6 Mutagenicity of Okadaic Acid and Derivatives

Studies on the mutagenicity and genotoxicity of okadaic acid have given contradictory results. No mutations were observed in the standard Ames test with *Salmonella typhimurium* strains TA98 and TA100, either in the presence or absence of metabolic activation by rat liver S9 post-mitochondrial supernatant.[390] No micronucleus formation was observed in the bone marrow of mice following an intraperitoneal dose of okadaic acid of 66.7 μg/kg,[391] but micronucleus formation has been recorded in several cell lines in vitro.[341,392–395] DNA adduct formation[396] and DNA damage have also been described in some cell lines in vitro[397–399] but not in others.[399–401] Some results are of questionable significance because of the absence of a dose–response relationship,[341,392,395] and the reported effects of metabolic activation are often contradictory. In some studies, a requirement for metabolic activation by S9 was described,[393] while other experiments showed a protective effect of S9.[395,399] The effect of S9 appears to be dependent upon the cell line, since this increased the oxidative DNA damage induced by okadaic acid in SHSY5Y cells but prevented such damage in leukocytes.[398]

7.7.7 Regulation of Okadaic Acid and Derivatives

The EFSA CONTAM Panel published a report on DSPs in 2008.[402] Based on human data, the Panel proposed an ARfD of 0.3 μg/kg of okadaic acid equivalents. Based on an intake of shellfish meat of 400 g, the regulatory limit would be set at 45 μg/kg okadaic acid equivalents/kg of shellfish meat, which is significantly lower than the present European regulatory limit of 160 μg/kg shellfish meat. The TEFs recommended by the Panel for okadaic acid, DTX-1, and DTX-2 were 1.0, 1.0, and 0.6, respectively. These are based on relative acute toxicity by intraperitoneal injection.

7.7.8 Conclusions

In view of the slow excretion of okadaic acid from the body, the possibility of accumulation in tissues, leading to increased toxicity with repeated exposure, must be considered. A chronic toxicity study would evaluate this possibility and would also provide data to permit the allocation of a TDI of this substance.

In view of the fact that okadaic acid is able to cross the placenta, experiments on the possibility teratogenicity of this substance and its potential to induce developmental changes in offspring are required.

The DSPs are tumor promoters, but the significance of this to the human situation is difficult to assess. Many compounds that have been shown to be tumor promoters in rodents are regularly consumed by humans (Section 7.13), and it would appear unlikely that the DSPs would significantly increase the total exposure of humans to tumor promoters. The DSPs were not tumor initiators in vivo, and the results of experiments on the mutagenicity of these substances, which could indicate risk of a carcinogenic action, show a degree of inconsistency. In vitro, effects are strongly dependent on the cell line employed, while in vivo data are negative[391] or inconclusive.[341] The reported epidemiological studies are also far from conclusive.

The generally held belief that the toxic effects of the DSPs are due to their ability to inhibit protein phosphatases is by no means proven. The role of protein phosphatase inhibition in acute toxicity has not been defined. Diarrhea may be due to physical damage to the intestinal epithelium and tumor promotion to irritancy.

The TEFs for DSPs are presently based upon toxicity by intraperitoneal injection. The evaluation of the relative toxicities of okadaic acid and its derivatives by the oral route would permit a more relevant estimate of such factors.

7.8 Palytoxin and Derivatives

7.8.1 Production and Distribution of Palytoxin and Derivatives

In 1971, a toxic material, named "palytoxin," was isolated from a *Palythoa* species (later named *Palythoa toxica*) from Hawaii.[403] Subsequent studies on the structure of palytoxin showed that it consisted of two isomeric components, of molecular formula $C_{129}H_{223}N_3O_{54}$, which were identified as 5- or 6-membered hemiketals. The hemiketals exist in equilibrium, with the 6-membered isomer being favored.[404,405] Palytoxin has also been isolated from *Palythoa mammillosa* from the Caribbean,[406] from *Palythoa vestita* from Hawaii,[407] *Palythoa* aff. *margaritae* from Japan,[408] and *Palythoa caribaeorum* from the Caribbean.[409] A related material of molecular formula $C_{129}H_{221}N_3O_{53}$ was isolated from an unnamed species of *Palythoa* from Tahiti.[410] Four minor palytoxins, homopalytoxin, bishomopalytoxin, neopaly-toxin, and deoxypalytoxin, have been found in *Palythoa tuberculosa*,[411] while 42-hydroxypalytoxin was isolated from Hawaiian *P. toxica* and *P. tuberculosa*.[412]

A compound similar to the palytoxins isolated from *Palythoa* species was detected in the sea anemone *Radianthus macrodactylus* from the Seychelles,[413] and two palytoxin analogues were reported in extracts of a red alga, *Chondria armata*.[414] These compounds have not been characterized.

Palytoxin derivatives are also produced by dinoflagellates of the genus *Ostreopsis*, which has a wide global distribution in temperate and tropical waters, a distribution that appears to be increasing with time.[98,415] A compound named ostreocin D was isolated from a Japanese strain of *Ostreopsis siamensis* in 1995,[416] which was later characterized as 42-hydroxy-3,26-didemethyl-19,44-dideoxypalytoxin.[417,418] This strain of *Ostreopsis* did not produce palytoxin itself. A New Zealand strain of *O. siamensis* contained a palytoxin-like material that was distinguishable from palytoxin and ostreocin D by LC-MS,[419] but which has not yet been characterized. *Ostreopsis mascarenensis* produces compounds, named mascarenotoxins, with many of the characteristics of palytoxin. The molecular weights of these substances are significantly (>100 Da) lower than those of zoanthid-derived palytoxins or ostreocin D,[420] but again the structures of these substances have not yet been determined. A compound named ovatoxin-a from cultures of Mediterranean *Ostreopsis* cf. *ovata* was reported by Ciminiello et al. in 2008.[421] This substance was later characterized as 42-hydroxy-17,44,64-trideoxypalytoxin.[422] Further four ovatoxins (b–e) have been isolated from *O.* cf. *ovata* from this same area[421,423,424] and another derivative, ovatoxin-f, has recently been reported.[425] Ovatoxins a–e have also been isolated from *O.* cf. *ovata* from Brazil,[426] and isomers of ovatoxins a, b, d, and e were found in a Japanese strain of this organism.[427] Although the molecular formulae of ovatoxins b–f are known,[424,425,428] their structures have not yet been elucidated.

Palytoxin and 42-hydroxypalytoxin have recently been reported to be present in a marine cyanobacterium of the genus *Trichodesmium* from New Caledonia.[429] The production of palytoxin by bacteria has also been suggested,[430] and several genera of bacteria, isolated from toxic *Palythoa* species, have been shown to contain palytoxin-like substances.[431,432] These substances disappeared after repeated subculturing of the bacteria, however,[431] suggesting that they may have been absorbed from the zoanthid, rather than synthesized by the bacteria. Palytoxin is similarly found in many other organisms that live in close association with zoanthid colonies.[433,434]

Palytoxin-like materials have been identified in polychaete worms and starfish that feed on zoanthids.[434,435] *P. tuberculosa* was found in the gut contents of the filefish, *Alutera scripta*, in Japan, and a compound named aluterin was isolated from its viscera. On the basis of the similarity of the toxic symptoms induced by aluterin and by authentic palytoxin, the former substance was suggested to be a palytoxin derivative.[436] Several species of butterfly fish (*Chaetodon* spp.), which are also known to feed on *Palythoa*, have been shown to contain palytoxin, predominantly in the intestines, liver, and flesh.[434]

Palytoxin derivatives would also be expected to be present in fish feeding on *Ostreopsis* species. A toxin chromatographically indistinguishable from palytoxin was isolated from the sardine *Herklotsichthys quadrimaculatus* from Madagascar. The mass spectrum was dissimilar to that of palytoxin, however, suggesting that the material was a palytoxin analogue.[437] It was suggested that the toxin accumulated in sardines following consumption of an *Ostreopsis* sp. Similarly, the presence of palytoxin or palytoxin analogues in the parrotfish *Scarus ovifrons* in Japan[438] was attributed to the consumption of *O. siamensis* by the fish.[439] Palytoxin-like material has also been detected in mackerel (*Decapterus macrosoma*) from the Philippines.[148] A toxic substance extracted from the triggerfish *Melichthys vidua* from Micronesia was indistinguishable from palytoxin on the basis of chromatographic properties, and the symptoms of intoxication were again similar to those of authentic palytoxin.[440] Palytoxin-like material was also present in an *Epinephelus* sp. in Japan,[441] in a puffer fish (*Tetraodon* sp.) from Bangladesh,[442] and in several species of reef fish in Hawaii.[443–445] Although relatively low levels of palytoxin are found in the flesh of triggerfish and parrotfish, very high levels (up to 71 mg/kg) were reported in the flesh of butterfly fish.[434]

Palytoxin and palytoxin-like substances have been isolated from several Asian crabs, including *Lophozozymus pictor*,[446,447] *Demania alcalai*,[446] and *Demania reynaudii*.[448] The source of palytoxin in crabs is not known, but endogenous production is unlikely, since, when kept in captivity, the toxicity of palytoxin-containing crabs decreased with time.[449] In crabs, levels in the whole animal may be extraordinarily high. A single specimen of *D. alcalai*, weighing 129 g, contained 11 mg of palytoxin, equivalent to 85 mg/kg in the whole animal. While the highest concentrations of palytoxin are found in the gills and viscera of crabs, levels of 2.4 mg/kg have been found in cheliped flesh.[446]

Oysters and scallops fed a New Zealand strain of *O. siamensis* contained palytoxin-like material, although none was present in mussels fed this dinoflagellate.[419] Palytoxin-like material was also identified in field samples of mussels and clams from the North Aegean Sea, which was correlated with the occurrence of *Ostreopsis* spp. in the water column.[450] Blooms of *O.* cf. *ovata* in the Mediterranean were also associated with the accumulation of both palytoxin and ovatoxin-a in mussels and sea urchins,[451] and palytoxin-like substances have also been found in octopuses from the Tyrrhenian Sea.[452]

In 1990, a compound named ostreotoxin was reported to be present in extracts of *Ostreopsis lenticularis* from the Caribbean.[453] This compound has not been characterized, and it is not known if it bears any relationship to the palytoxin derivatives isolated from *O. ovata*.

7.8.2 Toxicity of Palytoxin and Derivatives to Experimental Animals

The toxicology of palytoxin and derivatives in animals has been reviewed.[454,455]

7.8.2.1 Acute Toxicities of Palytoxin and Derivatives by Intraperitoneal Injection

Estimates of the acute toxicities of palytoxin and derivatives to mice by intraperitoneal injection are summarized in Table 7.16.

The results of the various toxicity experiments are generally quite consistent, with LD_{50}s of 0.3–0.7 µg/kg being reported in most instances, although the estimate of Ito et al.[456] is somewhat higher than the others. The early report by Kaul et al.[457] indicating a 10-fold lower LD_{50} may reflect a calculation error and should be regarded with suspicion. Ostreocin D was shown to be of similar toxicity to palytoxin.[416] Ovatoxin-a is also toxic, with 100% mortality at an intraperitoneal dose of 7.0 µg/kg,[422] although no LD_{50} data are available for this substance.

Ataxia and paralysis, particularly of the hind limbs, are seen in mice soon after the administration of toxic doses of palytoxin. Death occurs through respiratory failure, which is preceded by gasping respiration, cyanosis, and exophthalmia. Increased plasma levels of creatine phosphokinase have been recorded in mice given a sublethal intraperitoneal dose of palytoxin,[439] while increases in creatine phosphokinase,

TABLE 7.16

Acute Toxicities of Palytoxin and Derivatives to Mice by Intraperitoneal Injection

Compound	Strain of Mouse	Sex of Mouse	State of Alimentation	Parameter	Acute Toxicity (µg/kg Body Weight)	Reference
Palytoxin	ICR	Male	?	LD_{50}	1.0–1.5	[456]
Palytoxin	?	?	?	LD_{50}	0.5	[416]
Palytoxin	?	?	?	LD_{50}	0.4	[403]
Palytoxin	Swiss-Webster	Male	?	LD_{50}	0.05–0.10	[457]
Palytoxin	NMRI	Male	?	LD_{50}	0.31 (0.26–0.37)[a]	[458]
Palytoxin	?	?	?	"Toxicity"	0.6	[459]
Palytoxin	Swiss	Female	Fed	LD_{50}	0.72 (0.64–0.80)[a]	[419]
42-Hydroxy-3,26-didemethyl-19,44-dideoxypalytoxin (ostreocin D)	?	?	?	LD_{50}	0.75	[416]
42-Hydroxy-17,44,64-trideoxypalytoxin (ovatoxin-a)	?	Female	?	LD_{100}	≤7.0[b]	[422]

Note: "?" indicates that this information was not provided in the cited reference.

[a] Figures in brackets indicate 95% confidence limits.

[b] Three mice dosed at 7.0 µg/kg died. No lower doses were tested.

lactate dehydrogenase, AST, and ALT were observed in the plasma of mice dosed orally with this substance[460] or with 42-hydroxypalytoxin.[461] No hemoglobinemia was recorded in mice dosed orally with the latter substance.[461]

Peritoneal adhesions, accompanied by ascites and dilatation of the small intestine, were seen in mice injected with palytoxin,[456] and hyperemia was recorded in the nonglandular stomach of mice dosed orally with this substance.[460]

By light microscopy, single-cell necrosis was observed in the hearts of mice dosed intraperitoneally with palytoxin.[462] No histological changes were recorded in the heart or soleus muscle of mice dosed orally with palytoxin[460] or in those receiving 42-hydroxypalytoxin by the same route.[461] Inflammation of the nonglandular stomach was recorded with both these compounds, while renal tubular dilatation, hepatocellular vacuolation, and depletion of secretory material within pancreatic acini were observed with palytoxin,[460] but not with 42-hydroxypalytoxin.[461]

7.8.2.2 Acute Toxicities of Palytoxin and Derivatives by Oral Administration

Two estimates of the acute toxicity of palytoxin by gavage are available, one in fasted and one in fed mice (Table 7.17). The two estimates, which indicate that palytoxin is around 1000 times less toxic to mice by gavage than by intraperitoneal injection, are not statistically significantly different. 42-Hydroxypalytoxin was shown to be of similar toxicity to palytoxin by gavage. By feeding, palytoxin is even less toxic, with no effects being recorded at 2500 µg/kg, the highest dose tested (Table 7.17).

7.8.2.3 Repeated-Dose Studies with Palytoxin and Derivatives

In a repeated-dose experiment, mice received 5, 10, 15, or 29 daily intraperitoneal doses of palytoxin at 0.25 µg/kg. Thymic weights progressively decreased in the treated animals, and necrosis of thymic lymphocytes was recorded after 29 doses of the test substance. Necrosis of splenic lymphocytes was also observed. These changes were reversible, and lymphocyte numbers returned to normal within 1 month after the last of 29 doses.[463]

7.8.2.4 Tumor Promotion by Palytoxin

Palytoxin is a promoter of mouse skin carcinogenesis initiated by DMBA, but is not itself an initiator. It is a powerful irritant on mouse skin.[389]

7.8.3 Effects of Palytoxin and Derivatives in Humans

The toxicity of palytoxin and derivatives to humans has been reviewed.[464,465] Toxic effects through ingestion, inhalation, and skin or eye contact have been described.

Poisonings after consumption of several species of crabs and fish have been attributed to palytoxin, although leftover meals were not always analyzed. The commonest symptoms in such cases were

TABLE 7.17

Acute Toxicities of Palytoxin and Derivatives to Mice by Oral Administration

Compound	Strain of Mouse	Sex of Mouse	State of Alimentation	Method of Administration	Parameter	Acute Toxicity (µg/kg Body Weight)	Reference
Palytoxin	Swiss	Female	Fed	Gavage	LD_{50}	510 (311–809)[a]	[5]
Palytoxin	CD-1	Female	Fasted	Gavage	LD_{50}	767 (549–1039)[a]	[460]
Palytoxin	Swiss	Female	Fed	Feeding	MLD	>2500[b]	[5]
42-Hydroxypalytoxin	CD-1	Female	Fasted	Gavage	LD_{50}	651 (384–1018)[a]	[461]

[a] Figures in brackets indicate 95% confidence limits.

[b] No effects seen at this dose.

myalgia, myoglobinuria, respiratory problems, and cyanosis. Increases in creatine phosphokinase, AST, ALT, and lactate dehydrogenase have been reported in affected individuals. Death may occur through respiratory arrest. It should be noted, however, that, as of the year 2000, no more than 12 deaths had been attributed to palytoxin intoxication throughout the world.[443]

During blooms of *Ostreopsis* spp., beachgoers in Italy, Spain, France, Croatia, Tunisia, Greece, and Algeria suffered respiratory and other problems after inhalation of seawater droplets containing *Ostreopsis* cells or cell fragments.[466–468] Common symptoms were cough, dyspnea, sore throat, headache, rhinorrhea, lacrimation, and conjunctivitis, which were attributed to the local effects of the palytoxin derivatives derived from the dinoflagellates. Toxic effects have also been seen after inhalation of steam from home aquaria, following attempts to kill toxic *Palythoa* species with boiling water.[464,469]

Myalgia and increased plasma activities of creatine phosphokinase and lactate dehydrogenase were recorded in a man who cut his fingers when handling toxic zoanthids,[470] and keratoconjunctivitis was induced after an individual wiped his eye after handling such animals.[471] The irritant effects of palytoxin on the eye have long been recognized in Hawaii.[430]

7.8.4 Metabolism and Disposition of Palytoxin and Derivatives

No information on the metabolism and disposition of palytoxin and derivatives appears to be available.

7.8.5 Mechanism of Toxicity of Palytoxin and Derivatives

Palytoxin is highly toxic to isolated cells in vitro.[472] It causes lysis of erythrocyte suspensions at picomolar concentrations, a property that has been exploited in a sensitive assay for this substance.[473] Palytoxin has also been shown to bind to membranal Na^+/K^+-ATPase, converting the ion pump into a nonspecific ion channel, thereby permitting the uncontrolled transport of ions across the plasma membrane. There is evidence that such disruption of ionic equilibria is responsible for the toxic effects of palytoxin in vitro.[474]

It has often been assumed that such in vitro results can directly be extrapolated to the situation in vivo, with statements in the literature such as "palytoxin and ostreocin D are acutely toxic in experimental animals by interference with the Na^+/K^+-ATPase ion pump."[475] There is absolutely no justification for such an assumption, since there is no evidence for a pathway leading from effects on the Na^+/K^+-ATPase ion pump to death of the animal. Interestingly, although 42-hydroxypalytoxin caused hemolysis at picomolar concentrations in vitro, an effect known to be caused by disruption of transmembranal ion movements, lethal doses of this substance caused no intravascular hemolysis in mice,[461] suggesting that after absorption, palytoxin is not in a form capable of interacting with the Na^+/K^+-ATPase ion pump.

In view of the clinical signs of palytoxin intoxication, with death by respiratory arrest, effects on neuromuscular transmission could account for its lethal effects. Inhibition of neuromuscular transmission by palytoxin has been observed in the rat phrenic nerve-diaphragm preparation in vitro.[406]

7.8.6 Mutagenicity of Palytoxin

Palytoxin was negative in the Ames mutagenicity test using *S. typhimurium* strains TA98, TA100, TA102, and TA1537 with or without microsomal activation.[476]

7.8.7 Regulation of Palytoxin and Derivatives

Palytoxin and its derivatives are not regulated at present. In their 2009 review of palytoxin, however, the EFSA CONTAM Panel recommended that palytoxin should be regulated, with a limit of 30 µg/kg shellfish meat.[475] The panel paid particular attention to a report by Ito and Yasumoto[477] that purported to show absorption of palytoxin across the buccal mucosa of mice, with consequent harmful effects in tissues, particularly in the lung. Because of a perceived increase in the likelihood of palytoxin absorption in humans, they applied an additional safety factor of 10 in the risk assessment. In the experiment by Ito and Yasumoto, toxic effects were recorded when a solution of palytoxin was administered sublingually to mice at a dose of between 172 and 223 μg/kg. This method of administration is not relevant to the human situation, however, since palytoxin will not be ingested as a solution but as a mixture with food. When administered admixed with food, no effects were seen with a palytoxin dose of 2500 μg/kg,[5] suggesting that palytoxin does not undergo significant buccal absorption in mice when administered via a relevant route. Furthermore, the Panel did not consider the likelihood of a molecule with the physicochemical properties of palytoxin being able to cross the buccal mucosa of humans. There is a wealth of information on the structural requirements for buccal absorption of chemicals, reflecting current interest in administering therapeutic drugs by this route.[478,479] Lipophilic compounds are much more readily absorbed across the buccal mucosa than water-soluble substances. Furthermore, the absorption of hydrophilic compounds is greatly influenced by molecular volume, and the degree of absorption rapidly decreases with compounds of molecular weight greater than 100 Da.[480–483] The likelihood of absorption of the highly hydrophilic palytoxin, with a molecular weight of 2680 Da, is therefore remote. As discussed previously,[455] it is likely that the effects described by Ito and Yasumoto are not attributable to buccal absorption but to inhalation of a small proportion (~0.5%) of the administered palytoxin, thus causing the observed pulmonary lesions.

7.8.8 Conclusions

At present, human intoxication by palytoxin and derivatives has been attributable only to consumption of a few species of fish and crabs. This situation may change, however, if *Ostreopsis* species continue to spread and bloom, and careful monitoring of seafood for palytoxin derivatives will be required.

Muscle damage, as reflected by myalgia and myoglobinemia in humans and by elevated activities of plasma enzymes, particularly creatine phosphokinase and lactate dehydrogenase, in both animals and humans, has been reported in palytoxin intoxication. Damage to skeletal muscle is a relatively uncommon effect of toxic chemicals, and an understanding of the mechanism of action of palytoxin in this regard would be of interest.

Death appears to be attributable to respiratory failure, as seen with several other agents that inhibit neuromuscular transmission. Palytoxin has been shown to inhibit neuromuscular transmission in vitro, but further work is needed to establish the mechanism by which this occurs.

Daily intraperitoneal injections of palytoxin at doses approaching 50% of the LD_{50} caused only minor reversible changes in mouse tissues, suggesting that palytoxin does not accumulate after repeated exposure. No data on the subacute toxicity of palytoxin or its derivatives by the oral route are presently available. Such data will be required for establishing a TDI for these substances.

Palytoxin is not an initiator of skin carcinogenesis and is negative in the Ames mutagenicity tests. It is a tumor promoter in mouse skin, but this may simply reflect the irritancy of this material, as in the case of okadaic acid (Section 7.7). Irritancy could also account for the respiratory effects of inhaled palytoxin derivatives from *Ostreopsis* and for the damage caused through contact with the eye. Similarly, the peritoneal adhesions seen after injection of palytoxin and the gastric hyperemia observed after oral administration may again be attributed to local irritation.

Careful consideration needs to be given to the possible regulation of palytoxin. While such regulation may possibly be deemed prudent, the limit proposed by the EFSA CONTAM Panel may well be unnecessarily low, due to the additional safety factor imposed in response to the irrelevant dosing regimen concerning buccal absorption.

7.9 Pectenotoxins

7.9.1 Production and Distribution of Pectenotoxins

Members of the pectenotoxin (PTX) family of macrocyclic polyethers are found in shellfish in many parts of the world, including Spain, Portugal, Italy, the United Kingdom, Ireland, Croatia, Russia, Norway, Japan, Korea, China, Chile, Australia, and New Zealand.[192,484–486] The primary source of these substances is dinoflagellates of the genus *Dinophysis*. More than 20 analogues have been described, some of which are synthesized by the algae, some are formed through metabolism after uptake by shell-fish, while others appear to be artifacts produced during extraction.[484]

7.9.2 Toxicity of Pectenotoxins to Experimental Animals

7.9.2.1 Acute Toxicities of Pectenotoxins by Intraperitoneal Injection

Data on the acute toxicities of PTX derivatives to mice by intraperitoneal injection are summarized in Table 7.18.

PTX-1, PTX-2, PTX-3, and PTX-11 are of similar toxicity to mice, with lethal doses between 219 and 411 μg/kg. PTX-4 and PTX-6 are less toxic, while PTX-7, PTX-8, PTX-9, PTX-2 seco acid, and 7-*epi*-PTX-2 seco acid are less toxic still, with no deaths being recorded with these compounds at an intraperitoneal dose of 5000 μg/kg.

Mice injected with lethal doses of PTX-2 became hunched and lethargic soon after dosing. Respiration became labored, with abdominal breathing, and respiration rates progressively decreased. Cyanosis was observed shortly before death, which generally occurred between 4 and 10 h after dosing.[488,489] Serum activities of ALT, AST, and sorbitol dehydrogenase were significantly increased in mice injected with PTX-2 at 100 μg/kg or above, indicative of hepatic damage.[489]

Dose-related vacuolation of periportal hepatocytes was observed in mice injected with PTX-1. Electron microscopy suggested that the vacuoles resulted from invagination of the hepatocytic plasma membrane, and after 24 h, most hepatocytes containing multiple vacuoles had become necrotic. No changes were observed in the intestines, kidneys, or hearts of the mice.[337]

Hepatic hemorrhage and vacuolation were observed in mice injected with lethal doses of PTX-6. Renal congestion, accompanied by accumulation of tubular debris, was also seen, along with erosion of gastric and intestinal epithelia.[494]

No histological changes attributable to treatment were observed in the liver, kidneys, spleen, lungs, heart, adrenals, thyroid, trachea, ovary, uterus, tongue, thymus, brain, pancreas, or urinary bladder of mice killed 24 h after an intraperitoneal dose of 5000 μg/kg of PTX-2-seco acid or 7-*epi*-PTX-2 seco acid.[493]

TABLE 7.18

Acute Toxicities of PTX Derivatives in Mice by Intraperitoneal Injection

Compound	Strain of Mouse	Sex of Mouse	State of Alimentation	Parameter	Acute Toxicity (μg/kg Body Weight)[a]	References
PTX-1	?	?	?	MLD	250	[334]
PTX-2	?	?	?	MLD	260	[334]
PTX-2	?	?	?	MLD	230	[487]
PTX-2	Swiss albino	Female	Fed	LD_{50}	219 (183–257)[a]	[488]
PTX-2	ICR	Male	Fed	LD_{50}	411	[489]
PTX-3	?	?	?	MLD	350	[490]
PTX-4	?	?	?	MLD	770	[487]
PTX-6	?	?	?	MLD	500	[487]
PTX-7	?	?	?	MLD	>5000	[491]
PTX-8	?	?	?	MLD	>5000	[491]
PTX-9	?	?	?	MLD	>5000	[491]
PTX-11	Swiss albino	Female	Fed	LD_{50}	244 (214–277)[a]	[492]
PTX-2 seco acid	Swiss albino	Female	Fed	MLD	>5000	[488,493]
7-*epi*-PTX-2 seco acid	Swiss albino	Female	Fed	MLD	>5000	[493]

Note: "?" indicates that this information was not provided in the cited reference.

[a] Figures in brackets indicate 95% confidence limits.

7.9.2.2 Acute Toxicities of Pectenotoxins by Oral Administration

Relatively little information on the acute oral toxicity of the PTXs is available. An early report[342] gave an LD_{50} of PTX-2 of ~200 µg/kg, but this result is questionable, since the incidence of death in this experiment was not dose related. A more recent study[488] showed no deaths with PTX-2 when dosed by gavage at 5000 µg/kg. PTX-2 seco acid and PTX-11 were similarly of low oral toxicity in mice.[488,492]

Cytoplasmic vacuolation was observed in a few epithelial cells at the tips of villi of the small intestine of a mouse dosed by gavage with PTX-2 at 250 µg/kg, and more severe villous lesions were seen at higher doses.[495] Slight intestinal injuries, involving degeneration of the tips of villi, were recorded in mice dosed orally with PTX-6.[494]

In a preliminary experiment, Burgess et al.[496] found necrosis of villi and mucosal and submucosal hemorrhage in the duodena of mice dosed with a mixture of 35% PTX-2 seco acid and 65% 7-*epi*-PTX-2 seco acid extracted from Australian shellfish. In subsequent experiments, however, using different shellfish extracts, no such changes were observed, even though these extracts contained similar amounts of the seco acids. It was concluded[497] that the intestinal damage seen in the first experiment was due to the presence of okadaic acid esters in the extract, as shown in the shellfish responsible for the effects in humans seen in New South Wales in 1997 (see the following text).

7.9.2.3 Induction of Diarrhea by Pectenotoxins

Algae of the genus *Dinophysis* produce not only PTXs but also okadaic acid and its derivatives. Therefore, algal extracts and extracts of shellfish consuming *Dinophysis* inevitably contain both groups of toxins. The separation of the PTXs and DSPs is not an easy matter, particularly since the C_8-diol ester of okadaic acid is co-extracted with the PTXs and co-elutes on high-performance liquid chromatography (HPLC) with PTX-2.[488] Since the diarrheagenic activity of okadaic acid and its derivatives is well known, assessment of the ability of PTXs to induce diarrhea requires that the samples employed are proven to be free of contaminating DSPs. This has not always been the case in reported experiments with the PTXs.

Ishige et al.[495] dosed PTX-2 of unspecified purity by gavage to mice at 250 µg/kg (one mouse), 1000 µg/kg (five mice), 2000 µg/kg, and 2500 µg/kg (one mouse each). Fluid accumulation in the intestine of the mouse dosed at 250 µg/kg was observed, and diarrhea occurred in one of the five mice dosed at 1000 µg/kg and in both the mice receiving the two highest doses. Ito et al.[494] used intestinal weight as an indicator of diarrheagenicity and showed that the weight of the intestine of a single mouse dosed with PTX-2 (unspecified purity) at 500 µg/kg was higher 2 h after dosing than that of a mouse 1.0 or 1.5 h after the same dose, although no control data were given for the 2 h time point. In contrast, no diarrhea was observed in mice dosed with fully authenticated PTX-2 at 5000 µg/kg,[488] and no diarrhea was observed in mice dosed at 5000 µg/kg with pure PTX-2 seco acid or PTX-11.[488,492]

7.9.3 Effects of Pectenotoxins in Humans

There is no evidence that PTXs have caused toxic effects in humans. It was suggested[498] that the diarrhetic illness seen in 1997 after consumption of pipis harvested in New South Wales (Australia) was attributable to PTX seco acids, since PTX-2 seco acid was detected in the shellfish involved in the poisoning incident. It was subsequently shown, however, that these shellfish contained substantial amounts of okadaic acid esters, and these substances are now believed to be responsible for the observed diarrhetic effect, not the PTX derivatives.[497]

7.9.4 Metabolism and Disposition of Pectenotoxins

After oral administration of a mixture of PTX-2 and PTX-2 seco acid to mice, most of the toxins remained within the gastrointestinal tract and were excreted in the feces. Traces of the PTXs were detected in the livers of the animals after 6 h, and 11% was present in the tissues of the gastrointestinal tract. None was excreted in the urine, and none was present in the tissues of the animals after 24 h. There was a wider tissue distribution of PTXs following intraperitoneal injection, but again all the toxin was eliminated in the feces, with none in urine, indicating highly effective biliary excretion. Total recovery of the toxins was low in these experiments, suggesting inefficient extraction of the PTXs or conversion of the toxins to unidentified metabolites.[497]

7.9.5 Mechanism of Toxicity of Pectenotoxins

PTXs interact with F-actin, causing changes in the structure of the cellular cytoskeleton, and there is evidence that such interaction is involved in the toxicity of these substances to cells in vitro.[371,499] Interestingly, the PTXs that show high acute toxicity in vivo (PTX-1, PTX-2, PTX-6, and PTX-11) have all been shown to interact with actin in primary hepatocytes or neuroblastoma cells in vitro, while little or no effect was seen with the relatively nontoxic PTX-9 and PTX-2 seco acid.[500–502] Whether interactions with actin are involved in the toxicity of PTXs in vivo, and the pathway or pathways whereby such interactions could cause tissue damage or death, is presently unknown.

7.9.6 Mutagenicity of Pectenotoxins

No information on the potential mutagenicity of PTXs is available.

7.9.7 Regulation of Pectenotoxins

The PTXs were considered by the EFSA CONTAM Panel in 2009.[503] An ARfD of 0.8 µg PTX-2 equivalents was suggested, based on the observation of Ishige[495] of minor intestinal effects in mice with PTX-2 at a dose of 250 µg/kg. This would correspond to an upper limit of 120 µg PTX-2 equivalents/kg of shellfish meat, assuming a portion size of 400 g.

7.9.8 Conclusions

It is surprising that the EFSA CONTAM Panel elected to base their assessment on the 1988 publication by Ishige et al.,[495] which showed toxic effects in a single mouse dosed orally with PTX-2 of unspecified purity. The effects seen in this study involved fluid accumulation in the intestine and damage to intestinal villi. Since such changes are seen with okadaic acid derivatives, and since PTXs coexist with these substances, from which they are difficult to separate, this result must be viewed with caution, particularly since a dose of 5000 µg/kg of a certified sample of PTX-2 caused no toxic effects in mice. It is possible, therefore, that the regulatory limit suggested by the Panel is set too low. Indeed, in their review of shellfish toxins in 2006,[50] the Codex Alimentarius Commission recommended that no action level for PTXs should be set in the Codex standard and that they should not be regulated.

PTXs are toxic by intraperitoneal injection, with the major target organ being the liver. They are much less toxic orally, possibly reflecting a low level of uptake from the gastrointestinal tract. Further work on the oral toxicity of certified pure PTXs is required to give a final answer as to whether these materials can cause intestinal damage or diarrhea and to permit further discussion on the need to impose regulations on their presence in seafood.

7.10 Saxitoxin and Derivatives

7.10.1 Production and Distribution of Saxitoxin and Derivatives

Paralytic shellfish poisoning (PSP) has been recognized for many years. It is caused by a group of guanidinium derivatives, the parent compound of which is saxitoxin (STX). In the sea, dinoflagellates within the genus *Alexandrium* are the most important producers of the PSP toxins, although *Gymnodinium catenatum* and *Pyrodinium bahamense* also synthesize these substances.[504] Organisms producing STXs are of worldwide distribution and PSP outbreaks have occurred in many parts of the world.[505]

Fifty-seven analogues of STX have been described up to 2010.[506] The STXs are divided into several subgroups, the most important of which are the carbamoyl derivatives, including STX, neosaxitoxin (neoSTX), and gonyautoxins 1–4 (GTX-1–4); the mono-sulfated derivatives C1–C4, GTX-5, and GTX-6; and the decarbamoyl derivatives, decarbamoyl saxitoxin (dcSTX), decarbamoyl neosaxitoxin (dcneoSTX), and the decarbamoyl gonyautoxins (dcGTX-1–4). The structures of these substances, and of compounds in the other subgroups, are given by Wiese et al.[506]

7.10.2 Toxicity of Saxitoxin and Derivatives to Experimental Animals

7.10.2.1 *Acute Toxicity of Saxitoxin by Intraperitoneal Injection*

Estimates of the LD_{50} of STX in rats and mice by intraperitoneal injection are given in Table 7.19.

The various estimates of the LD_{50} of STX in mice are remarkably consistent at ~10 µg/kg, with females being slightly more susceptible than males. Toxicity in adult rats was similar to that in mice, but neonatal and weanling rats were significantly more susceptible to the toxic effects of STX than adults.

The symptoms of intoxication by STX are very similar to those observed with BTXs, cyclic imines, palytoxin, and tetrodotoxin (TTX) (Sections 7.3, 7.5, 7.8, and 7.11). At lethal doses, respiration rates progressively decline, and gasping respiration, together with running movements, are seen immediately before death. STX is a fast-acting toxin, with death generally occurring within 15–20 min after injection of a lethal dose.[507,511] The dose–response curve for injected STX is very steep, with an estimated LD_0 of 6.5 µg/kg and an LD_{99} of 13 µg.[507] Animals may be kept alive by application of artificial ventilation, and such animals subsequently make a full recovery.[512] At sublethal doses, animals become immobile, with decreased respiration rates, but subsequently recover, with no evidence of any long-term adverse effects.[511] In animals dying from PSP intoxication, softening and edema of the brain have been observed, together with areas of hemorrhage in the lungs and adrenals.[513]

A mouse bioassay for STX was described by Sommer and Mayer in 1937,[514] and this was later adopted as an approved AOAC assay.[515] In this protocol, STX is dosed intraperitoneally to groups of mice at a dose that gives a death time of between 5 and 7 min. From the median death time, the number of Mouse Units (MUs) in the sample can be read off from the table established by Sommer, with 1 MU being defined as the amount of STX that kills an 18–22 g mouse in 15 min.[516] Knowing the concentration of STX in the sample injected, the weight of toxin corresponding to 1 MU can be calculated. This assay is reported to be influenced by the strain of mouse employed,[507,517] by the pH of the solution injected,[507,516] and by the presence of sodium salts.[507,516] For STX itself, the weight corresponding to 1 MU has been estimated at between 0.150 and 0.274 µg.[518]

Little information on the LD_{50}s of STX derivatives is available, but relative toxicities have been estimated using the STX mouse bioassay, again determining the amount of toxin required to cause death in 5–7 min. Assuming that the dose–death time relationships for the derivatives are the same as that for STX itself, the number of MUs in the sample can be determined using Sommer's table.

TABLE 7.19

Acute Toxicity of Saxitoxin by Intraperitoneal Injection in Mice and Rats

Species	Strain	Age	Sex	State of Alimentation	LD_{50} (µg/kg Body Weight)[a]	Reference
Mouse	FDA albino	?	Male	?	10.0 (9.7–10.5)	[507]
Mouse	FDA albino	?	Female	?	8.0 (7.6–8.6)	[507]
Mouse	Swiss-Webster	?	?	Fed	11.6 (11.2–12.1)	[508]
Mouse	?	?	?	?	10.3	[509]
Mouse	ddY	?	Male	?	7.6 (7.2–8.1)	[510]
Rat	Osborne–Mendel	24 h	Male and female	Fasted	5.5 (4.7–6.5)	[511]
Rat	Osborne–Mendel	21 days	Male and female	Fasted	8.3 (7.7–9.0)	[511]
Rat	Osborne–Mendel	60–70 days	Male and female	Fasted	10.0 (8.5–11.8)	[511]

Note: "?" indicates that this information was not provided in the cited reference.

[a] Figures in brackets indicate 95% confidence intervals.

Various estimates of the relative toxicities of STX derivatives in the mouse bioassay have been published, and these were considered by the EFSA CONTAM Panel in their assessment of STX group biotoxins.[518] Taking the most recent data and giving more weight to estimate employing certified standards, the Panel estimated that STX, neoSTX, dcSTX, and GTX-1 are of equal toxicity, while dcneoSTX and GTX-2, GTX-3, and GTX-4 are 40%–70% as toxic as STX. GTX-5 and GTX-6 and the C toxins were estimated to be only one-tenth as toxic as STX. On the basis of these data, TEFs for the STX derivatives were proposed by the Panel.

7.10.2.2 Acute Toxicity of Saxitoxin by Oral Administration

The acute toxicity of STX in mice and rats is lower when administered by gavage than by injection, with estimates of the LD_{50} varying between 209 and 588 μg/kg. STX toxicity was again higher in young rats than in older animals (Table 7.20). No information on the acute oral toxicities of STX derivatives are presently available.

7.10.2.3 Repeated-Dose Studies with Saxitoxin

It has been reported that administration by gavage of one-third of the LD_{50} dose of STX to rats decreased the toxicity of a subsequent dose given 14 days later.[519] In contrast, mice surviving an initial intraperitoneal dose of an extract of STX-containing shellfish were reported to be more susceptible to a second dose administered 12–24 h later.[514]

7.10.3 Effects of Saxitoxin and Derivatives in Humans

Early symptoms of PSP intoxication in humans include a tingling sensation or numbness around the lips, which gradually spreads to the face and neck. Headache, nausea, vomiting, and diarrhea follow, with increasing muscular paralysis and respiratory distress. In severe cases, there is a high risk of death from asphyxiation unless artificial respiration is instituted. The time to onset of symptoms is dose dependent and can occur as soon as 30 min after consumption of contaminated shellfish.[42]

Estimates of the quantity of STX and its derivatives that are required to cause toxic effects in humans vary over a wide range, as reviewed by the EFSA CONTAM. Panel.[518] Various reports indicate that between 0.3 and 90 μg/kg of STX equivalents can be consumed by humans without adverse effects, while severe illness has been reported at 5.6–2058 μg/kg of STX equivalents. The factors that may lead to such discrepancies include differences in sampling time of contaminated seafood, the effects of cooking, and variations in analytical methods.[518] It has been suggested that regular consumption of PSPs by humans increases tolerance,[519] while toxicity may be greater when the contaminated seafood is eaten on an empty stomach.[517] In one case,[517] consumption of alcohol appeared to increase toxicity, although other studies have shown no adverse effect of alcohol consumption[520] or even a beneficial effect.[521]

TABLE 7.20

Acute Toxicity of Saxitoxin in Mice and Rats by Gavage

Species	Strain	Age	Sex	State of Alimentation	LD_{50} (μg/kg Body Weight)[a]	Reference
Mouse	FDA albino	?	Male	?	263 (251–267)	[507]
Mouse	ddY	?	Male	?	209 (173–255)	[510]
Rat	Osborne–Mendel	24 h	Male and female	Fasted	64 (51–80)	[511]
Rat	Osborne–Mendel	21 days	Male and female	Fasted	270 (204–356)	[511]
Rat	Osborne–Mendel	60–70 days	Male and female	Fasted	531 (490–576)	[511]
Rat	Sprague–Dawley	?	?	?	588	[519]

Note: "?" indicates that this information was not provided in the cited reference.

[a] Figures in brackets indicate 95% confidence intervals.

7.10.4 Metabolism and Disposition of Saxitoxin and Derivatives

Since symptoms of intoxication occur soon after exposure to STXs in both humans and animals, absorption must be rapid. The observation[522] that an individual noticed tingling in the lip and tongue while chewing a raw clam has been taken to indicate that absorption may occur from the buccal cavity. As pointed out, however, this does not necessarily indicate absorption from the mouth, but may simply reflect local effects on the labial and lingual epithelia.[523] STX is not absorbed from the stomach of cats[524] but is readily absorbed from the intestine of both cats and rabbits.[524,525] Studies in vitro have shown that the absorption of a mixture of GTX-2 and GTX-3 occurs via both transcellular and paracellular pathways.[526–528]

After absorption, STX and its derivatives are distributed among various organs, including the brain, indicating that these substances can cross the blood–brain barrier.[529–532] Elimination is mainly via the urine, with 58% elimination by this route after 24 h in rats following intravenous injection. Elimination of the remainder was slow, however, and STX was still detectable in the urine 6 days after administration, indicating that this substance persists in tissues for a prolonged period after dosing. An oxidized metabolite was detected in the urine, but was not characterized.[533] Similar results were found with saxitoxinol, in which the ketone group of the guanidinium moiety is reduced to an alcohol, which, although not a natural product, has been used as a model compound in the study of STX toxicokinetics. After 4 h, 60% of intravenously injected saxitoxinol had been excreted in the urine, although subsequent elimination was slow, and 28% of the dose remained in tissues after 6 days. No saxitoxinol was eliminated via the feces,[531] and it was suggested that enterohepatic circulation of this substance occurs. Several metabolites of saxitoxinol have been detected in rat tissues, but none were characterized.[532]

Mixtures of GTX-2 and GTX-3 and of C-1 and C-2 were not metabolized by rat or mouse hepatic microsomal or cytosolic fractions in vitro,[534] and no metabolism of the GTXs was observed in a cytosolic fraction of cat liver.[524] In a human liver microsomal fraction, however, the oxidation of GTX-2 and GTX-3 to GTX-1 and GTX-4 has been observed, together with glucuronidation at one of the hydroxyl groups on C-12.[535,536]

Comparison of the amounts of STX and derivatives in toxic shellfish with the amounts of these substances in the tissues and urine of individuals dying after consumption of such shellfish has confirmed that metabolism occurs in humans. Higher levels of neoSTX and GTX-1 and GTX-4 were found in the victims than those that were present in the shellfish, indicating that *N*-oxidation had occurred after ingestion. There is also evidence that decarbamoylation and desulfation occur in humans,[529,537,538] and it was suggested that at least some of these transformations take place in the intestine.[537] The possibility that desulfation of STX derivatives could also occur under the conditions pertaining in the human stomach has been considered. Such a reaction has been observed in vitro, although the reaction conditions were rather severe, involving high concentrations of acid at elevated temperatures.[539,540] Under conditions more relevant to the human situation, however, only 15% of GTX-5 was converted to STX after a 5 h incubation period,[510] indicating that this process is unlikely to be of major importance in vivo.

7.10.5 Mechanism of Toxicity of Saxitoxin and Derivatives

There is good evidence that STX and derivatives exert their toxic effects in animals through their interaction with site 1 of the α-subunit of voltage-gated sodium channels, resulting in blockade of ion conduction and generation of action potentials. This leads to progressive loss of neuromuscular function and ultimately muscular paralysis.[371] The mechanism of channel blockade has been extensively studied, and the crucial involvement of the guanidinium moiety and the two C-12 hydroxyl groups has been identified.[541,542]

The effect of STX and derivatives on neuromuscular transmission in vitro is consistent with death by respiratory paralysis in vivo. It is interesting to note that the diaphragm is particularly vulnerable to the paralyzing action of STX, and this muscle showed no response to electrical stimulation after a lethal dose of this substance.[543,544]

The relative abilities of STX and certain of its derivatives to bind to sodium channels and inhibit their activity have been investigated in a number of studies and have been compared with their

TABLE 7.21

Relative Acute Toxicities of Saxitoxin and Derivatives in Mice (Mouse Bioassay) and Relative Reactivities toward Sodium Channels In Vitro

Compound	Relative Toxicity In Vivo[a]	Relative Activity toward Sodium Channels In Vitro						
		Assay Method 1[b]	Assay Method 2[b]	Assay Method 3[b]	Assay Method 4[b]	Assay Method 5[b]	Assay Method 6[b]	Assay Method 7[b]
STX	1.0	1.0	1.0	1.0	1.0	1.0	1.0	1.0
neoSTX	1.0	—	0.69	4.5	1.0	3.6, 3.7	0.82	1.02
GTX-1	1.0	—	—	—	—	0.28	—	—
GTX-1 and GTX-4	—	—	0.98	—	—	—	0.53	0.50
GTX-2	0.4	0.2		0.22		0.15, 0.16		
GTX-2 and GTX-3	—	—	0.32	—	—	—	0.38	0.28
GTX-3	0.6	0.42	—	1.4	—	0.96		
GTX-4	0.7	—	—	—	—			
GTX-5	0.1	—	0.031, 0.039	—	—	0.024	0.09	0.09
GTX-6	0.1	—	—	—	—	—		
dcSTX	1.0	—	0.097, 0.29	—	0.2	0.44	0.84	1.00
dcneoSTX	0.4	—	—	—	0.004	—	0.48	0.44
dcGTX-2	0.2	—	—	—	—	—		
dcGTX-3	0.4	—	—	—	—	—		
C-1	—	—	—	—	—	0.0017, 0.0028		
C-2	0.1	—	—	—	—	0.029		
C-3	—	—	—	—	—	0.002		
C-4	0.1	—	—	—	—	—		

[a] Intraperitoneal, according to the protocol of the mouse bioassay. Modified from Table 14 of Ref. [518].

[b] Assay method 1: Relative blockade of sodium channels in the squid giant axon.[545] Assay method 2: Relative binding to sodium receptors of the rat cerebral cortex.[546,547] Assay method 3: Relative blockade of impulses in frog sciatic nerve.[548] Assay method 4: Relative blockade of sodium current in frog skeletal muscle fiber.[549,550] Assay method 5: Relative blockade of sodium channels from rat muscle plasma membrane.[551,552] Assay method 6: Blockade of veratridine-induced changes in membrane potential in cultured neurons.[553] Assay method 7: Inhibition of voltage-dependent sodium currents in primary cultures of cerebellar neurons.[554]

relative toxicities, as summarized in Table 7.21. There is no consistent relationship between the acute toxicities of STX derivatives, as measured by the mouse bioassay, and their activities toward sodium channels in vitro, and there is considerable variation among the results from the different sodium channel assays. While a positive relationship exists between effects on sodium channels and toxicity in the case of GTX-5 and the C toxins, other results, such as those with GTX-1, dcSTX, and dcneoSTX, do not correlate.

7.10.6 Regulation of Saxitoxin and Derivatives

Many countries regulate PSP toxins, most commonly with a regulatory limit of 80 µg of STX equivalents per 100 g of shellfish meat.[505] This limit was confirmed at the twenty-eighth Session of the CCFFP in 2006.[50] Regulations were reviewed by the EFSA CONTAM Panel in 2009.[518] On the basis of the human data, the Panel established a LOAEL of 1.5 µg/kg of STX equivalents, and the application of a threefold safety factor led to the establishment of an ARfD of 0.5 µg/kg STX equivalents. Assuming a shellfish intake of 400 g, the intake of PSPs at the presently accepted regulatory limit would be 5.3 µg/kg, which is considerably higher than the ARfD established by the Panel, who concluded that "there is a concern for health for the consumer" at the present regulatory limit.

7.10.7 Conclusions

Although the death rate from PSP is decreasing, with more widespread availability of apparatus for artificial ventilation, the contamination of seafood with STX and its derivatives remains a major problem. It is of concern that the TEFs that are used for calculating "STX equivalents" are based on intraperitoneal toxicity rather than toxicity by oral administration. Furthermore, derivation of comparative data obtained in the mouse bioassay assumes that the relationship between dose and death times for STX analogues is the same as that for STX itself. There is no evidence in support of this assumption. Only death times between 5 and 7 min are used in the determination of TEFs, and this assay would therefore overestimate the toxicity of an analogue that killed mice more rapidly than STX but would underestimate the toxicity of relatively slow-acting analogues. The relationship between this assay and the LD_{50} of STX derivatives, which is determined without reference to time of death, has not been investigated, and acute toxicity studies on STX derivatives are urgently required. The need for robust oral toxicity data on STX and derivatives has been emphasized,[518] and as pointed out by Botana et al.,[555] oral toxicity studies should be conducted according to validated methods, such as those published by the OECD.

The slow elimination of STX in animals raises the possibility of accumulation of this substance in the tissues of individuals who regularly consume seafood containing PSPs. Chronic toxicity studies in animals are required in order to evaluate the risk of repeated consumption of STX and derivatives.

Data on the levels of toxins in seafood that have caused intoxication in consumers, or which have been ingested with impunity, are of great value in risk assessment. However, in the case of PSP, a huge range of estimates of toxic and nontoxic levels of PSP toxins have been published in the literature, making evaluation difficult. Further studies in this area, using modern analytical methods for STX and its derivatives and ensuring that the samples analyzed are representative of the material consumed, would be of great value in validating regulatory limits for these substances.

7.11 Tetrodotoxin and Derivatives

7.11.1 Production and Distribution of Tetrodotoxin

The distribution of tetrodotoxin (TTX) in animals is remarkably diverse, being found in fish, gastropods, crabs, marine flatworms, ribbon worms, arrow worms, annelid worms, starfish, a sea slug, an octopus, newts, and frogs.[556–561] TTX has also been found in cultures of the dinoflagellate *Alexandrium tamarense*.[562] By far the most widely studied source of TTX is fish of the order Tetraodontiformes, the most familiar of which is the puffer fish.

Many derivatives of TTX have also been isolated from animals.[556,557,563,564] These include epimers (4-*epi*-TTX, 6-*epi*-TTX), oxidized compounds (11-oxo-TTX, tetrodonic acid), deoxygenated compounds (5-deoxy-TTX, 11-deoxy-TTX, 4-*epi*-11-deoxy-TTX, 1-hydroxy-5,11-dideoxy-TTX, 5,6,11-trideoxy-TTX, 4-*epi*-5,6,11-trideoxy-TTX, 8-*epi*-5,6,11-trideoxy-TTX, 1-hydroxy-8-*epi*-5,6,11-trideoxy-TTX), compounds with deletion of the methylene group at C-11 (11-*nor*-TTX-6(R)-ol, 11-*nor*-TTX-6(S)-ol, 11-*nor*-TTX-6,6-diol), anhydro derivatives (4,9-anhydro-TTX, 4,9-anhydro-6-*epi*-TTX, 4,9-anhydro-11-deoxy-TTX, 4,9-anhydro-8-*epi*-5,6,11-trideoxy-TTX, 1-hydroxy-4,4a-anhydro-8-*epi*-5,6,11-trideoxy-TTX), a compound modified at the C-11 hydroxymethyl group (chiriquitoxin), and a thiol conjugate (4-*S*-cysteinyl-TTX). The structures of these compounds are given by Kudo et al.[557]

The origin of TTX in marine animals, whether from endogenous or exogenous sources, has been the subject of much debate. Matsumura[565] showed that the level of TTX in puffer fish embryos increased for 4 days post-fertilization and suggested that this indicated endogenous production of the toxin. But other studies have shown that the toxicity of larvae disappeared completely within 20 days of hatching,[566] indicating that even if TTX is produced in the embryos, the ability to synthesize this substance is lost after hatching. It is now generally accepted that marine animals accumulate TTX from exogenous sources. This conclusion is supported by the fact that cultured puffer fish, raised in net cages in the sea or in tanks on land, contain little or no TTX.[567–569]

It has been suggested that TTX in marine animals originates from bacteria, and many bacteria isolated from the skin and internal organs of puffer fish have been shown to synthesize TTX in culture.[570–576] TTX-producing bacteria have also been found in the gastrointestinal tract of a starfish,[577] in gastropods,[578,579] in marine sediments,[580–582] and in a red calcareous alga of the genus *Jania*.[583] Early studies on the production of TTX by bacteria were challenged on the grounds that materials present in the culture medium gave false positives for TTX when assayed by HPLC or GC-MS,[584,585] but later studies, using multiple assay methods, have confirmed the ability of many species of bacteria to synthesize not only TTX but also 4-*epi*-TTX and anhydro-TTX.[576,586,587]

The question then arises as to whether the TTX is derived from commensal bacteria or from food containing bacterial-derived TTX. An argument for commensal production is the observation that cultured puffer fish became toxic when housed with wild, TTX-containing, puffer fish,[586] although it is possible that the cultured fish obtained TTX not through colonization by bacteria but through ingestion of TTX-containing skin or excreta from the wild fish. Sato et al.[588] found the same TTX-producing bacterium in the intestines of both cultured fish and wild fish, yet the cultured fish were not toxic. Furthermore, the commensal bacteria from puffer fish produce only very small amounts of TTX, and it is hard to see how the low rate of synthesis of TTX by these organisms could lead to the very high levels found in the tissues of the fish. It has been suggested[574] that a specific promoter is required for the rapid production of TTX in fish or that unculturable microorganisms play a role in TTX formation, but this question remains unresolved.

Conversely, there is good evidence for uptake of TTX by fish via their diet. Cultured puffer fish fed TTX-containing liver from wild puffer fish for 30 days,[589] or pure crystalline TTX for the same period,[590] accumulated up to 50% of the administered dose of toxin, mainly in the liver and skin. Subsequent feeding of a control diet for 210 days led to a decrease in hepatic levels of TTX, but an increase in the concentration of TTX in the skin, indicating transfer of the toxin from liver to skin.[589]

Interestingly, fish that do not normally contain TTX did not accumulate this substance when fed diets containing the toxin,[560,591] suggesting that TTX-containing fish have a specific mechanism for uptake and accumulation.[568] Such a mechanism is consistent with the observation that liver slices from puffer fish incubated in a TTX-containing medium readily took up the toxin, while slices from the livers of fish that do not accumulate TTX did not.[592] There is also evidence that fish that do not contain TTX are able to metabolize the toxin. This may be the case with the nontoxic puffer fish *Takifugu xanthopterus*, in which TTX is undetectable but which contains nontoxic TTX derivatives related to tetrodonic acid.[593]

The origin of TTX in gastropods is also a matter of debate. It has been argued that TTX in these animals is accumulated via food,[558,560] but TTX-producing bacteria have also been found in TTX-containing gastropods.[579]

The situation with regard to amphibians is perhaps even more confusing. It has been argued that since the level of TTX increases in the skin of captive newts fed a toxin-free diet[594] and that skin levels are regained after provocation of TTX release from this tissue by electrical stimulation,[595] there is *de novo* synthesis of this substance in these animals. But only skin levels were measured in these experiments, and it is therefore possible that redistribution of TTX from internal organs to skin occurred, as has been shown to occur in puffer fish.[589] In a more recent study on captive red-spotted newts, *Notophthalmus viridescens*, TTX levels in the whole animal were shown to decrease over time.[596] Similarly, the Japanese newt *Cynops pyrrhogaster* lost toxicity when raised on nontoxic diets.[597] Furthermore, labeled putative precursors of TTX were not incorporated into the toxin when administered to newts,[598,599] and frogs raised in captivity contained no TTX in their skin.[600] In view of this evidence, it is unlikely that TTX is of endogenous origin in amphibians, and a commensal bacterial or food source must be considered. There was no evidence for the presence of bacteria in the liver, gonads, or eggs of *Taricha granulosa* or in their surface-sterilized skin,[601] although TTX-producing bacteria were present in the gut of these animals.[599] Captive newts accumulate TTX when the toxin is given in food,[597] but TTX-containing food sources of amphibians in the wild have not been identified. Amphibians that accumulate TTX are resistant to its toxic effects, and it would again appear that only certain amphibians have the ability to accumulate this substance.

7.11.2 Toxicity of Tetrodotoxin to Experimental Animals

7.11.2.1 *Acute Toxicities of Tetrodotoxin and Derivatives by Intraperitoneal Injection*

The acute toxicities of TTX and derivatives by intraperitoneal injection are summarized in Table 7.22.

TTX itself is highly toxic, with consistent estimates of the LD_{50} by intraperitoneal injection of between 8.5 and 10.7 µg/kg. The dose–response relationship is exceptionally steep, with an MLD of 8 µg/kg and an LD_{100} of only 12 µg/kg being reported. The oxidation of the alcohol group at C-11 to an aldehyde, forming 11-oxo-TTX, or replacement of one of the protons on the C-11 hydroxymethyl group by a glycine moiety, giving chiriquitoxin, has little effect on toxicity. The stereochemistry of TTX is clearly important for toxicity, since the epimers at either the 4- or 6-position are significantly less toxic than the parent compound. Removal of one or more oxygen atoms from TTX decreases toxicity, as does dehydration to form 4,9-anhydro-TTX or removal of the methylene group at C-11 to give 11-*nor*-TTX-ol. 4-*S*-Cysteinyl-TTX and 4-*S*-glutathionyl-TTX, which are believed to be formed by the reaction of the respective thiols with 4,9-anhydro-TTX,[616] are of very low toxicity. There is no evidence for a strain effect on the acute toxicity of TTX in mice,[602] although male mice are reported to be more sensitive than females.[605]

Muscular weakness, as indicated by splaying of the hind legs, is seen in mice soon after injection of TTX. This progresses to complete paralysis, with gasping respiration. Death is due to respiratory failure.[602,617] At lethal doses, death occurs within a matter of minutes,[567,603,618] but mice surviving for 30 min or more recover completely.[619]

TABLE 7.22

Acute Toxicities of TTX and Derivatives by Intraperitoneal Injection in Mice

Compound	Strain of Mouse	Sex of Mouse	State of Alimentation	Parameter	Acute Toxicity (µg/kg Body Weight)	Reference
TTX	CF1	Male and female	?	MLD	~8	[602]
TTX	CF1	Male and female	?	LD_{50}	10.0	[602]
TTX	CF1	Male and female	?	LD_{100}	12	[602]
TTX	ddY	?	?	LD_{50}	8.5	[603]
TTX	Swiss Webster	Male	Fed	LD_{100}	10	[604]
TTX	Kunming	Male and female	?	LD_{50}	10.7	[605]
11-oxo-TTX	ddY	Male	?	LD_{99}	16	[606]
4-*epi*-TTX	ddY	Male	?	LD_{50}	64[a]	[607]
6-*epi*-TTX	?	?	?	LD_{50}	60	[608]
5-Deoxy-TTX	ddY	Male	?	MLD	>320	[609]
11-Deoxy-TTX	?	?	?	LD_{50}	71	[608]
6,11-Dideoxy-TTX	ddY	Male	?	LD_{50}	~420	[610]
8,11-Dideoxy-TTX	ddY	Male	?	MLD	>700	[611]
5,6,11-Trideoxy-TTX	?	?	?	MLD	750	[612]
4,9-Anhydro-TTX	ddY	Male	?	LD_{50}	490[a]	[607]
11-*nor*-TTX-6(*S*)-ol	?	?	?	LD_{50}	54	[613]
11-*nor*-TTX-6(*R*)-ol	?	?	?	LD_{99}	70	[614]
Chiriquitoxin	ddY	Male	?	LD_{50}	14[a]	[615]
4-*S*-Cysteinyl-TTX	ddY	Male	?	MLD	>140	[616]
4-*S*-Glutathionyl-TTX	ddY	Male	?	MLD	>860	[616]

Note: "?" indicates that this information was not provided in the cited reference.

[a] The toxicities of these compounds were reported as "MUs" calibrated against a graph of death time versus TTX dose. These figures are based on the assumption that the death time–dose relationships for the TTX derivatives are the same as that for TTX itself. It must be recognized that there is no evidence in support of this assumption.

TABLE 7.23

Acute Toxicity of TTX by Oral Administration in Mice

Strain of Mouse	Sex of Mouse	State of Alimentation	Parameter	Acute Toxicity ($\mu g/kg$ Body Weight)[a]	Reference
ddY	Male	?	LD_{50}	332	[621]
Kunming	Male and female	?	LD_{50}	532	[605]
BALB/c	Female	Fed	LD_{100}	600	[618]

Note: "?" indicates that this information was not provided in the cited reference.

Enlargement of the gall bladder was observed in mice given a lethal dose of a crude extract of puffer fish ovary. Congestion of the brain, heart, liver, gall bladder, lung, and kidneys was also observed, together with mitochondrial damage in neuronal synapses.[620]

7.11.2.2 Acute Toxicity of Tetrodotoxin by Oral Administration

There is very little information available on the acute toxicity of TTX by oral administration (Table 7.23). Estimates of 332 and 532 $\mu g/kg$ for the LD_{50} of this substance by gavage have been published, while the LD_{100} was estimated at 600 $\mu g/kg$. The symptoms of intoxication after oral administration were the same as those observed after injection, although the time to death was extended.[618]

7.11.2.3 Acute Toxicities of Tetrodotoxin and Derivatives by Intravenous Injection

TTX appears to be of similar toxicity when administered by intravenous injection as when given intraperitoneally, with an LD_{50} of 8.2 $\mu g/kg$ being reported. Tetrodonic acid is of very low toxicity, causing no deaths after intravenous injection at 300 mg/kg.[622]

7.11.2.4 Repeated-Dose Studies with Tetrodotoxin

Several studies on the effects of repeated intraperitoneal injections of crude extracts of the Tunisian puffer fish *Lagocephalus lagocephalus* in rats have been reported. After 10 daily doses of the extracts, serum activities of ALT, AST, alkaline phosphatase, lactate dehydrogenase, and γ-glutamyl transferase were significantly decreased,[623] while serum creatinine and urea levels were slightly increased.[624] Lipid peroxidation, as reflected by an increase in thiobarbituric acid-reactive substances, was observed in the liver, kidneys, brain, and erythrocytes of the animals,[623,625] while a number of circulating erythrocytes and blood hemoglobin levels were decreased.[625] Serum activities of AST and ALT were significantly increased in rats fed puffer fish extracts for 2 days, but decreased when fed the extracts for 2 months.[626,627] Focal necrosis of hepatocytes was reported,[626] although whether this result related to the animals fed for 2 days or those fed for 2 months was not clear. There was evidence of hemolysis in the latter animals.[627]

7.11.3 Effects of Tetrodotoxin in Humans

Incidents of human poisoning by TTX from fish, crabs, and/or gastropods have been reported in Japan,[558] China,[628] Taiwan,[629] Hong Kong[630] Thailand,[631] Vietnam,[632] Cambodia,[633] Malaysia,[634] Singapore,[635] the Philippines,[636] Australia,[637] Fiji,[638] Hawaii,[639] Madagascar,[640] Bangladesh,[641] Israel,[642] Egypt,[643] Lebanon,[644] the United States,[645] Mexico,[646] Italy,[647] and Spain.[648]

Symptoms of intoxication generally appear within minutes of consumption of TTX-containing food. Initial signs are perioral paresthesia and numbness of extremities, which, in severe cases, progresses to dyspnea, cyanosis, and paralysis.[649] As in animals, death is due to respiratory failure, which may occur within minutes. The prognosis for recovery is good for individuals surviving for 24 h.[560]

It is widely stated that the lethal dose of TTX for an adult human is 1–2 mg,[560,597,650,651] but it is not clear from the literature how this figure was derived. Over the years, many people have died from TTX poisoning. In Japan alone, there were 2688 deaths from puffer fish poisoning between 1927 and 1949,[652] and there were 760 incidents between 1965 and 2010, with 216 deaths.[558] The percentage mortality decreased over the latter period, presumably due to more effective emergency treatment, and the number of incidents is also decreasing, since 80% of the puffer fish sold on the Japanese market is now from cultured stock.[560] Many deaths continue to occur in less developed countries, however, often because of a lack of knowledge of the dangers associated with puffer fish consumption. There have also been problems in Europe[647] and the United States[645] with improper labeling of imported puffer fish.

One rather unusual incident was the death of a young man who accepted a dare to eat an Oregon rough-skinned newt.[653] In another case, a child ate part of the tail of a pet newt of the same species without serious effects, and both the child and the newt survived.[654]

7.11.4 Mechanism of Toxicity of Tetrodotoxin

TTX, like STX, binds at site 1 of the voltage-gated sodium channel,[655] leading to the inhibition of neuromuscular transmission. In general, there is a good correlation between the affinity of TTX derivatives for the sodium channel and their acute toxicity to mice,[656–658] although the report that 11-oxo-TTX binds four to five times more strongly to the sodium channel than TTX in vitro[659] is not in accord with the equipotency of these compounds in vivo. Interestingly, although the relatively nontoxic 4,9-anhydro-TTX was a weaker blocker of six of the seven isoforms of the channel that were tested, it was more effective than TTX in blocking the $Na_{v1.6}$ channel,[660] indicating isoform specificity among the TTX derivatives.

7.11.5 Mutagenicity of Tetrodotoxin

TTX showed no evidence of mutagenicity in the Ames test, in an in vitro lymphocyte chromosome aberration test, in the mouse bone marrow micronucleus test or in the unscheduled DNA synthesis test in rat liver.[661]

7.11.6 Regulation of Tetrodotoxin

While TTX is regulated in some Asian countries, there are no European regulations on permitted levels of TTX in food. However, European regulations prohibit the sale of fish of the puffer fish family.[662]

7.11.7 Conclusions

Deaths induced by puffer fish appear to be largely due to TTX itself, since the equally toxic 11-oxo-TTX is a minor analogue in these animals.[663] In contrast, 11-oxo-TTX may play a major role in the toxicity of certain crabs, in which it is present at higher concentration than TTX.[664] The third highly toxic TTX derivative, chiriquitoxin, is found only in newts, which are not generally consumed by humans.

Death through respiratory paralysis and the observed correlation between toxicity and activity toward the voltage-gated sodium channel are consistent with the inhibition of neuromuscular transmission as the mechanism of TTX toxicity.

The results of experiments on repeated administration of an extract of puffer fish to rats either by injection or by feeding suggest the possibility of long-term effects of TTX, such as hepatic and renal damage and hemolysis, although the observed decreases in plasma enzyme activities after long-term administration are hard to interpret. Unfortunately, the level of TTX in the extract employed in these studies was not reported, and there was only minimal histological examination of tissues. Further studies on the chronic toxicity of TTX are required.

TTX is present in certain gastropods. While these animals may be consumed locally, they are generally not widely traded in seafood markets. Of more concern would be the presence of TTX in commercially important bivalve molluscs. While TTX was not detected in blue mussels gathered from the coast of Portugal,[561] this toxin was found in the scallop *Patinopecten yessoensis* in Japan,[665] and recent work has shown trace amounts of TTX in pipis from New Zealand.[666] Careful monitoring of bivalve molluscs in areas known to contain TTX-containing animals is required, in order to evaluate the possibility of adverse effects on human health through consumption of this very toxic substance.

The source of TTX in animals remains unresolved. The accumulation of TTX from the diet, whether from bacteria or from other sources, is an attractive hypothesis, but levels in bacteria and marine sediments are low. Animals accumulate milligram quantities of TTX in their tissues, and before the dietary hypothesis can be accepted, it will be necessary to show that such quantities can be derived from the dietary sources that are available to the animals.

If the quoted lethal dose for humans is correct, humans are much more susceptible to TTX than mice. For a 60 kg individual, a dose of 2 mg would equate to 33.3 µg/kg. The oral LD_{50} of TTX in mice has been estimated at 332 or 532 µg/kg, while the LD_{100} was reported to be 600 µg/kg. The latter figure indicates a steep dose–response curve, so the MLD for a mouse would not be expected to be greatly below 300 µg/kg, nearly 10 times higher than the stated lethal dose for humans. As discussed previously (Section 7.1), much greater variations in response are to be expected in humans than in mice, but an estimate of the MLD in the latter animals would be of interest. Furthermore, the analysis of levels of TTX in seafood consumed with impunity by humans would be of great value in risk assessment.

7.12 Yessotoxin and Derivatives

7.12.1 Production and Distribution of Yessotoxin and Derivatives

The disulfated polyether YTX was first reported in extracts of the scallop *Patinopecten yessoensis* in Japan in 1987.[667] Since then, YTX has been identified in shellfish in Norway, Chile, New Zealand, the United Kingdom, Canada, Russia, France, Italy, Spain, Croatia, Korea, China, and the United States.[192,486,668–672] YTX is produced by the microalgae *Protoceratium reticulatum*,[673] *Lingulodinium polyedrum*,[674] and *Gonyaulax spinifera*.[675]

More than 90 YTX derivatives have been detected in shellfish and/or extracts of *P. reticulatum*,[676–678] the majority of which have not been characterized or evaluated for toxicity. From a regulatory standpoint, YTX itself, homo-YTX, 45-hydroxy-YTX, and 45-hydroxyhomo-YTX are considered to be the most important compounds.[679]

7.12.2 Toxicity of Yessotoxin and Derivatives to Experimental Animals

The toxicology of YTX and derivatives in animals has been reviewed.[668,680]

7.12.2.1 Acute Toxicities of Yessotoxin and Derivatives by Intraperitoneal Injection

Estimates of the LD_{50} of YTX by intraperitoneal injection (Table 7.24) vary over a wide range, with the lowest at less than 100 µg/kg and the highest at 500–750 µg/kg.

The reason or reasons for this variation are presently unclear. The effect of sex and strain of mice has been investigated using three strains of both sexes.[682] Female mice of all the strains were more susceptible to YTX toxicity than males, but in no case was the difference statistically significant. Female mice of the Swiss and NMRI strains were significantly more susceptible than females of the ICR strain, but no significant differences were seen among male mice of any of the strains. In another study,[668] no significant differences in YTX toxicity were seen between female Swiss and C57 Black mice. Differences in sex and strain thus appear to be insufficient to account for the large differences in estimates of YTX toxicity. The purity of the test substance may be an important factor. While stable in methanolic solution at −20°C, YTX decomposes to compounds of unknown toxicity when stored in the dry state.[691] If the toxicities of the decomposition products are lower than YTX itself, the use of old samples of this material would give a spuriously low estimate of acute toxicity.

The comparison of the toxicities of YTX derivatives with that of the parent compound is difficult, since in most cases, toxicity has been expressed as "lethality" rather than as an LD_{50}. It is clear, however, that 45-hydroxyhomo-YTX, 1- and 4-desulfocarboxy-homo-YTX, the 1,3-enone isomer of heptanor-41-oxo-YTX, and the trihydroxylated amide of 9-methyl-41a-homo-YTX are significantly less toxic than YTX itself, with no effects being recorded at intraperitoneal doses of 500–5000 µg/kg.

TABLE 7.24

Acute Toxicities of YTX and Derivatives to Mice by Intraperitoneal Injection

Compound	Strain of Mouse	Sex of Mouse	State of Alimentation	Parameter	Acute Toxicity (µg/kg Body Weight)[a]	Reference
YTX	ddY	Male	?	LD_{50}	80–100	[342]
YTX	?	Female	?	LD_{50}	<100[b]	[681]
YTX	Swiss albino	Female	Fed	LD_{50}	112 (96–131)	[668]
YTX	C57 Black	Female	Fed	LD_{50}	136 (112–166)	[668]
YTX	ICR (CD-1)	Male	Fed	LD_{50}	462 (353–603)	[682]
YTX	ICR (CD-1)	Female	Fed	LD_{50}	380 (357–407)	[682]
YTX	Swiss (CFW-1)	Male	Fed	LD_{50}	328 (294–375)	[682]
YTX	Swiss (CFW-1)	Female	Fed	LD_{50}	269 (221–330)	[682]
YTX	NMRI	Male	Fed	LD_{50}	412 (337–505)	[682]
YTX	NMRI	Female	Fed	LD_{50}	314 (285–346)	[682]
YTX	NMRI	Female	?	LD_{50}	500–750	[683]
YTX	CD	Female	?	LD_{50}	512 (312–618)	[330]
YTX	ICR	Male	?	LD_{50}	286[c]	[684]
Homo-YTX	CD	Female	?	LD_{50}	444 (315–830)	[330]
45-Hydroxy-YTX	?	?	?	"Lethality"	~500	[685]
45-Hydroxy-homo-YTX	CD	Female	?	MLD	>750	[330]
Carboxy-YTX	ddY	Male	?	"Toxicity"	~500	[686]
Carboxy-homo-YTX	?	?	?	"Lethality"	~500	[687]
45,46,47-Tri-*nor*-YTX	?	?	?	"Lethality"	~220	[685]
1-Desulfo-YTX	?	?	?	"Lethality"	~500	[688]
Di-desulfo-YTX	ICR	Male	?	LD_{50}	301	[684]
1-Desulfocarboxy-homo-YTX	?	Female	?	MLD	>500	[681]
4-Desulfocarboxy-homo-YTX	?	Female	?	MLD	>500	[681]
1,3-Enone isomer of heptanor-41-oxo-YTX	Swiss albino	Female	Fed	MLD	>5000	[689]
Trihydroxylated amide of 9-methyl-41a-homo-YTX	Swiss albino	Female	Fed	MLD	>5000	[690]

Note: "?" indicates that this information was not provided in the cited reference.

[a] Figures in brackets indicate 95% confidence limits.

[b] Two out of three mice died at a dose of 100 µg/kg.

[c] This figure is the LD_{50} at 3 h after dosing. Since deaths from YTX intoxication occur at times greater than 3 h, the true LD_{50} is likely to be lower than that indicated.

At high doses of YTX, deaths occur within an hour after injection.[330,342] At lower doses, mice may survive up to 10 h after YTX administration.[668] The lethal effects of YTX appear to involve respiratory failure, with dyspnea and cyanosis being observed shortly before death.[668]

By light microscopy, no changes were observed in the lungs, thymus, liver, pancreas, kidneys, adrenals, uterus, ovaries, skeletal muscle, brain, spinal cord, spleen, stomach, jejunum, colon, or rectum of mice injected with lethal doses of YTX.[330,683] In one experiment,[683] a few small intracellular vacuoles were observed in the cardiomyocytes of mice injected with YTX, associated with slight intercellular edema in the heart. The significance of this observation is dubious, however, since similar changes were seen in a control mouse in this experiment, and in a later study, no effects on the heart were seen by light microscopy in mice injected with YTX.[330] Damage to Purkinje cells in the cerebellum of mice was observed after a lethal dose of YTX,[692] while animals injected with a lethal or sublethal dose showed an inflammatory response in the duodenum and a decrease in the number of thymocytes in the thymic cortex.[693] Hepatic and pancreatic lipidosis was observed in mice after intraperitoneal injection of di-desulfo-YTX.[684]

Electron microscopy revealed ultrastructural changes in the hearts of mice injected with YTX. At a dose of 500 μg/kg, YTX caused swelling and degeneration of endothelial cells of capillaries, and cardiomyocytes in the vicinity of capillaries were swollen.[684] Similar, though less pronounced, effects were seen in a later study in mice dosed intraperitoneally with YTX at 1 mg/kg.[683]

7.12.2.2 Acute Toxicity of Yessotoxin by Oral Administration

YTX is much less toxic by oral administration than by intraperitoneal injection, with no deaths being recorded at doses up to 54 mg/kg.[680]

No ultrastructural changes were seen in the hearts of mice dosed with 500 μg/kg YTX by gavage,[684] but in mice killed 24 h after oral administration at 2.5, 5, or 10 mg/kg YTX, swelling of pericapillary myocytes, leading to separation of organelles, was observed.[683] Cytoplasmic protrusions of cardiac muscle cells into the pericapillary space, rounded mitochondria, and myofibrillar alterations were recorded 24 h after an oral dose of 1 or 2 mg/kg YTX or of 1 mg/kg homo-YTX or 45-hydroxyhomo-YTX.[330] In a later study, however, no ultrastructural changes were seen in the hearts of mice dosed orally with YTX at 1 or 5 mg/kg.[45] No ultrastructural changes were seen in the skeletal muscle of mice dosed orally with YTX at 1 or 2 mg/kg.[694]

7.12.2.3 Repeated-Dose Studies on Yessotoxin and Derivatives

No signs of toxicity were recorded in mice dosed for 7 days with YTX at 2 mg/kg/day or with homo-YTX or 45-hydroxyhomo-YTX at 1 mg/kg/day. Body weight gains were comparable to those of control animals, and no macroscopic abnormalities were observed at necropsy. Organ weights were within the normal range. Plasma levels of ALT, AST, lactate dehydrogenase, and creatine phosphokinase were normal. No histological changes were observed in the heart, liver, lungs, kidneys, spleen, thymus, pancreas, skeletal muscle, gastrointestinal tract, pancreas, brain, spinal cord, uterus, or ovaries of the mice.[345] A study involving a dose of 1 mg/kg/day YTX for 7 days gave similar results, and no ultrastructural changes were seen in the liver, kidneys, or cerebellum of these mice.[695] However, ultrastructural changes in the heart, similar to those seen after acute administration of YTX, were seen with YTX at both 1 and 2 mg/kg/day and with homo-YTX or 45-hydroxyhomo-YTX at 1 mg/kg/day.[345,695] These changes persisted for 30 days after the last dose of YTX but were imperceptible after 90 days.[695] In contrast, no ultrastructural alterations were seen in the hearts of mice dosed orally with YTX at up to 5 mg/kg, seven times over a 3-week period.[696]

7.12.3 Effects of Yessotoxins in Humans

No toxic effects resulting from YTX consumption by humans have been reported.

7.12.4 Metabolism and Disposition of Yessotoxin

One day after the final dose of seven daily oral doses of YTX at 1 mg/kg, the plasma concentration of this compound was 3.12 ng/mL.[695] Assuming a blood volume of 1.4 mL for a 20 g mouse, the total amount in the circulation would be 4.4 ng. This is equivalent to 0.02% of the amount administered per day, suggesting that YTX is poorly absorbed and/or rapidly excreted. A recent study by Aasen et al.[45] confirmed the low oral availability of YTX. One day after a dose of 1 or 5 mg/kg, the highest levels of YTX were found in the ileum and colon, and the total fraction of YTX in the internal organs accounted for less than 0.1% of the administered dose. No YTX was detected in the brain or heart.

As discussed previously (Section 7.1), a combination of toxins may cause more severe effects than either in isolation, particularly if the patency of the gastrointestinal tract is compromised, since this could increase the extent of absorption of toxins after oral administration. This possibility has been examined with YTX and AZA-1.[45] When YTX was administered to mice at the same time as AZA (the latter at a dose sufficient to cause epithelial damage in the small intestine), the amount absorbed remained unchanged. It is unlikely, therefore, that the oral toxicity of YTX would be increased in the presence of toxic levels of AZA.

7.12.5 Mechanism of Toxicity of Yessotoxin

The mechanism or mechanisms whereby YTX causes toxic effects in animals are presently unknown. In cultured cells in vitro, YTX has been shown to activate phosphodiesterases, to perturb calcium metabolism, and to cause disruption of E-cadherin,[697,698] although the association, if any, between such effects in vitro and toxicity in vivo has not been demonstrated.[371] Interestingly, the disruptive effect of YTX on E-cadherin in vitro was not replicated in vivo. Indeed, YTX actually stabilized E-cadherin in the colon of mice dosed orally with this substance.[699]

7.12.6 Regulation of Yessotoxin and Derivatives

The present regulatory limit for the sum of YTX, homo-YTX, 45-hydroxy-YTX, and 45-hydroxyhomo-YTX is 1 mg/kg shellfish flesh. The YTXs were considered by the EFSA CONTAM Panel in 2008,[679] who proposed a NOAEL of 5 mg/kg, based on oral toxicity studies in mice. Because of uncertainty as to whether the ultrastructural changes seen in mouse hearts should be considered as an adverse effect, the Panel applied an extra safety factor of 2 in addition to the default factor of 100, thereby establishing an ARfD of YTX and derivatives of 25 μg/kg. For a 60 kg individual, this equates to an intake of 1.5 mg of YTX equivalents. Using a portion size of 400 g, this figure would translate to a limit of 3.75 mg/kg shellfish flesh.

In 2004, the Joint FAO/WHO/IOC ad hoc Expert Consultation agreed on a NOAEL of 5 mg/kg for YTX and derivatives but found it unnecessary to apply the extra twofold safety factor. Based on a portion size of 400 g, their recommendation for the regulatory limit was 7.5 mg/kg shellfish flesh.[310] In 2006, the Codex Alimentarius Commission recommended that no action level for YTXs should be set in the Codex standard and that they should not be regulated.[50]

7.12.7 Conclusions

While YTX is toxic by intraperitoneal injection, it is relatively harmless via oral administration, probably reflecting low absorption by the latter route. There is no evidence that YTX or its derivatives have ever caused harm to humans, and there have been suggestions that the regulatory limit should be raised or that regulation should be abolished.

Concern remains, however, as to the significance of the ultrastructural changes in the heart seen after administration of YTX to mice. In order to provide further information as to the relevance of these changes, a study involving higher levels of YTX than those used in earlier studies is required, possibly at a level as high as 50 mg/kg, a dose that has been shown to cause no deaths in mice. At this level, which is 50 times higher than the lowest dose reported to cause ultrastructural changes in the heart, histologically recognizable cardiac lesions would be expected if the ultrastructural changes were indicative of incipient myocyte damage. The absence of such changes at high doses would suggest that the observed ultrastructural alterations are of little importance and would support arguments for the deregulation of YTX.

7.13 Discussion

As discussed previously, the risk to human health of a food contaminant is a function of its intrinsic toxicity and of the quantity that is consumed. Much progress has been made in analytical methods for seafood contaminants, both in terms of precision and accuracy, so that the quantity of such substances in food can be determined with confidence. In contrast, data on the intrinsic toxicity of many seafood contaminants are inadequate for proper risk assessment.

TABLE 7.25

Comparative Acute Toxicities of Seafood Toxins in Mice via Intraperitoneal Injection and Oral Administration[a]

Compound	LD_{50} via Intraperitoneal Injection ($\mu g/kg$)	LD_{50} via Gavage ($\mu g/kg$)	LD_{50} via Feeding ($\mu g/kg$)	Ratio of $LD_{50}s$, Gavage/i.p. Injection	Ratio of $LD_{50}s$, Feeding/i.p. Injection
Pinnatoxin F	14.4	25	50	1.7	3.5
BTX-3	210	520	ND	2.5	—
Pinnatoxin G	49	150	400	3.1	8.2
Okadaic acid	206	~1000	ND	~5	—
Gymnodimine	96	755	>7500[b]	7.8	>78
Domoic acid	5.0	80	ND	16	—
PTX-2	315	>5000[b]	ND	>16	—
Desmethyl spirolide C	6.9	160	1000	23.2	145
BTX-2	275	6,600	ND	24	—
STX	9.5	236	ND	25	—
TTX	9.6	432	ND	45	—
YTX	300	>54000[b]	ND	>180	—
Palytoxin	0.6	640	>2500[b]	1070	>4170

[a] Figures taken from previous tables and text.
[b] No effects seen at this dose.

For seafood contaminants, the route of exposure in humans is via food, and intrinsic toxicity should therefore be determined in animals via oral administration. But for nearly every class of toxin, the majority of information that is presently available relates to toxicity following intraperitoneal injection. This is of very limited use in risk assessment, since, as shown by the examples given in Table 7.25, the toxicity of a substance by intraperitoneal injection cannot be used to predict its oral toxicity, either by gavage or by voluntary feeding. In all cases for which comparative data are available, toxicity to mice by gavage is lower than that by intraperitoneal injection, and toxicity is lower still when the toxin is ingested voluntarily. There is, however, no consistent relationship between toxicity by intraperitoneal injection and by oral administration. The ratios between these parameters for the different toxins vary over a wide range, with values of more than 1000 for palytoxin, but only 1.7–3.5 for pinnatoxin F.

Further work on the oral toxicity of seafood toxins is required, and the Codex Alimentarius Commission has recommended that voluntary feeding should take priority over gavage in the evaluation of seafood toxins.[50] It should be noted, however, that while the oral route is essential for risk assessment of seafood contaminants, some algal-derived toxins, such as BTXs and ovatoxins, cause adverse effects in humans via inhalation. In this situation, inhalation studies are clearly the most appropriate for risk assessment, since the absorption and disposition of toxic substances through the lung are quite different to those via the intestine.

In many cases, the material tested in toxicological studies has not been sufficiently characterized. The gross differences in acute toxicity recorded for YTX and some cyclic imines may reflect differences in purity, and the diarrhetic effect reported for PTXs may well be due to contamination by okadaic acid derivatives. Seafood toxins vary in their stability in storage, and the use of materials that have undergone decay will obviously confound toxicological assessments. Particular care should be taken with commercial samples. From personal experience, such products may contain little of the specified substance, despite label claims of purity. The use of certified standards is ideal, and such standards for a number of seafood toxins are available. These are expensive, however, and an alternative approach is to use noncertified material that has been calibrated against certified standards immediately before use. It is important that the purity of a test material is confirmed in the testing laboratory before conducting toxicological tests and the purity of the test material should be stated in publications.[700]

While sufficient data on acute oral toxicity are available for some substances in order to permit estimation of an ARfD, in very few instances are sufficient toxicological data available for the determination of a TDI.

Because many people consume seafood on a regular basis, appropriate experiments to determine TDIs for contaminants are urgently required. Such experiments will be expensive, and since limited resources are available, it is important that these studies are focused on those contaminants that are of highest potential risk to human health. Other substances, such as YTX and PTX, which are of low oral toxicity and which have never been associated with cases of human intoxication, should be given low priority.

Another factor in risk assessment is that toxicity is assessed by experiments in animal studies, in which young, healthy rodents are employed. In contrast, human consumers vary in age and in health status. While infants and children generally appear to be well protected by the use of current safety factors,[701] the same may not be true of the elderly. Older individuals may suffer a variety of illnesses, together with impairment of renal and hepatic function, which may influence the distribution of harmful substances and their rates of detoxification and elimination. Certainly age and concurrent disease were factors in the toxic effects recorded in individuals consuming seafood contaminated with domoic acid. Furthermore, unlike experimental animals, humans eat a wide range of foodstuffs, some of which, such as heavily spiced food, may cause damage to the stomach epithelium[702] and thus could possibly increase gastric absorption of toxins. Similar effects on the stomach are seen with alcohol and certain pharmaceuticals.[703–705] The possible variation in response between animals and humans is addressed by the use of safety factors in the risk assessment, and the criteria that should be used when applying such factors have been extensively discussed.[706–708] However, the routinely used 100-fold safety factor, which although first suggested nearly 60 years ago,[709] still provides a pragmatic solution to the extrapolation of toxicity data derived from animal experiments to assessment of risk to human health.[710]

New classes of toxin may be recognized in the future, and approaches to this situation were discussed at the Joint FAO/IOC/WHO ad hoc Expert Consultation in 2004.[310] In the case of an outbreak of illness in humans not associated with known toxins, the Expert Consultation recommended that every effort should be made to identify the symptoms and clinical changes in affected individuals, in order to give information on the target site of the new toxin. Samples of the seafood eaten during the outbreak should be collected for chemical analysis. It was also recommended that initial evaluation of new toxins should be via the oral route. The major toxins should then be separated and identified and subjected to toxicological evaluation, again by oral administration, in order to establish ARfDs and TDIs.

Isolation methods for seafood toxins have traditionally used bioactivity (usually mouse toxicity) to guide the isolation process. In this way, the "major" toxin, which is primarily responsible for toxicity, is the first to be characterized. But in many microalgae and shellfish, not only the major toxin is present but also analogues, some of which may significantly contribute to overall toxicity. In order to allow for the combined toxicity of the major toxin and its analogues, the concept of "TEFs" has been introduced, in which the toxicity of the analogues is expressed as a proportion of that of the major toxin. Unfortunately, because of the paucity of data on oral toxicity, TEFs have largely been determined on the basis of acute toxicity by intraperitoneal injection[711] or from the results of functional assays in vitro.[555] But for valid estimates of TEFs by these procedures, one must be sure that toxicity by intraperitoneal injection or the response observed in functional assays accurately reflects toxicity under the conditions pertaining in humans, that is, oral ingestion. This is by no means always the case, and as discussed previously,[555] oral toxicity determinations, using validated methods, are required for analogues, in order that accurate TEFs can be established.

With the progress made over the past few years in separation and analytical techniques, many more analogues of known seafood toxins are being detected in microalgal extracts, many of which are present at extremely low levels. While possibly of academic interest, such minor components are highly unlikely to pose a risk to human health, and such studies do not contribute to risk assessment.[700] It has been proposed[310] that any analogue present at a concentration of 5% or less of that of the parent toxin should not be regulated against.

In literature reports on seafood toxicology, there is a tendency to extrapolate biochemical changes seen in vitro to toxic effects in vivo, as exemplified by the attribution of the toxic effects of okadaic acid to protein phosphatase inhibition and the toxic effects of palytoxin to effects on the Na^+/K^+-ATPase. Such *post hoc ergo propter hoc* arguments are a logical fallacy. While in vitro studies may identify biochemical changes caused by a toxin, before such changes can be held responsible for in vivo effects, it is necessary to demonstrate that the same changes are induced in vivo (or in a relevant *ex vivo* model) and to provide a plausible pathway from the in vitro change to the symptoms of intoxication in animals and the pathological changes that are induced. The exposure of an isolated cell to a toxin in tissue culture is quite different to the situation in vivo, in which the gut acts as a barrier to the absorption of many toxic compounds and in which detoxification and excretory processes occur. A good example is YTX, which shows harmful effects in vitro at nanomolar concentrations,[668] yet has no perceptible effect when administered orally at high doses to mice.

Okadaic acid and palytoxin have been shown to act as tumor promoters, and it could be argued that an additional safety factor should be employed for these substances in order to take account of this effect. However, many substances to which humans are regularly exposed, such as detergents, fatty acid esters, citrus oils, saccharin, and medium-chain hydrocarbons, have been shown to be tumor promoters in animals,[712–716] suggesting that the seafood contaminants are unlikely to significantly increase human exposure to promoters. Furthermore, there is no epidemiological evidence that exposure to tumor promoters leads to an increase in cancer incidence.[717] Since a common property of tumor promoters is their ability to induce inflammation via irritation,[718–720] the promoting activity of okadaic acid and palytoxin may simply be due to their irritant effect, which is unlikely to be expressed following exposure to small amounts of these substances in food. An extra safety factor for okadaic acid and palytoxin therefore appears to be unnecessary.

The symptoms of intoxication by poisonous substances often offer a clue as to their mode of action. In this context, it is interesting to note that the symptoms of intoxication by several seafood toxins, such as cyclic imines, palytoxin, STXs, and TTX, are the same, involving immobility, cyanosis, and dyspnea, with death through respiratory paralysis. All these compounds have been shown to exert effects on ion channels, leading to blockade of neuromuscular transmission, and paralysis of the diaphragm and intercostal muscles would be consistent with death through respiratory failure. Interestingly, many other natural toxins from plants, reptiles, amphibians, spiders, gastropods, and bacteria, such as tubocurarine,[721] aconitine and derivatives,[722,723] grayanotoxin,[723] bungarotoxin,[724,725] crotoxin,[725] taipoxin,[726] notexin,[726] conotoxins,[727,728] raventoxins,[729] huwentoxin,[730,731] lophotoxin,[732] botulinus toxin,[733] and the venoms of the Egyptian cobra,[734] coral snakes,[735,736] sea snakes,[737] death adders,[738] the poison dart frog *Phyllobates bicolor,*[739] and the polychaete worm, *Lumbrineris heteropoda,*[740] all inhibit neuromuscular transmission and induce death by respiratory paralysis. While the toxins from these sources are of grossly dissimilar structure, they all have the same biochemical effect, suggesting convergent evolution of a toxic mechanism that targets a vulnerable situation in animals—the absolute requirement for muscular activity for oxygenation of tissues. The lack of such a requirement in crustaceans, shellfish, amphibians, and finfish could account for the remarkable resistance of many of these creatures to substances causing rapid death by asphyxia in mammals.

In conclusion, while much information on the toxicology of seafood contaminants is available, there is much work still to be done. With the recognized increase in the incidence of harmful algal blooms throughout the world, the migration of harmful algal species into new areas, and the discovery of new toxigenic species of alga,[42,371,741,742] continued vigilance is needed, and robust risk assessment is required in order to protect human health while at the same time not unnecessarily disadvantaging the seafood industry by the imposition of unrealistic regulatory limits.

ACKNOWLEDGMENTS

This work was funded by the New Zealand Ministry of Business, Innovation and Employment. The most helpful comments of Dr. Lesley Rhodes are gratefully acknowledged.

REFERENCES

1. OECD, 2008. Guidelines for the Testing of Chemicals. *Guideline 425. Acute Oral Toxicity—Up-and-Down Procedure*. OECD, Paris, France.
2. Committee on Mutagenicity of Chemicals in Food Consumer Products and the Environment (COM), 2000. *Guidance on a Strategy for Testing of Chemicals for Mutagenicity*, UK Department of Health, London, U.K.
3. Pesticide residues in food, 2002. Report of the Joint Meeting of the FAO Panel of Experts on Pesticide Residues in Food and the Environment and the WHO Core Assessment Group on Pesticide Residues. http://www.fao.org/ag/AGP/AGPP/Pesticid/JMPR/Download/2002_rep/2002JMPRReport2.pdf
4. Benford, D., 2000. *The Acceptable Daily Intake. A Tool for Ensuring Food Safety*. International Life Sciences Institute Concise Monograph Series. ILSI Europe, Brussels, Belgium.

5. Munday, R., 2006. Toxicological requirements for risk assessment of shellfish contaminants: A review. *Afr. J. Mar. Sci.*, 28, 447–449.
6. Rao, G. N., Peace, T. A., and Hoskins, D. E., 2001. Training could prevent deaths due to rodent gavage procedure. *Contemp. Top. Lab. Anim. Sci.*, 40, 7–8.
7. Damsch, S., Eichenbaum, G., Tonelli, A. et al., 2011. Gavage-related reflux in rats: Identification, pathogenesis, and toxicological implications. *Toxicol. Pathol.*, 39, 348–360.
8. Craig, M. A. and Elliott, J. F., 1999. Mice fed radiolabeled protein by gavage show sporadic passage of large quantities of intact material into the blood, an artifact not associated with voluntary feeding. *Contemp. Top. Lab. Anim. Sci.*, 38, 18–23.
9. Wheatley, J. L., 2002. A gavage dosing apparatus with flexible catheter provides a less stressful gavage technique in the rat. *Lab. Anim.*, 31, 53–56.
10. Brown, A. P., Dinger, N., and Levine, B. S., 2000. Stress produced by gavage administration in the rat. *Contemp. Top. Lab. Anim. Sci.*, 39, 17–21.
11. Ferguson, S. A. and Boctor, S. Y., 2009. Use of food wafers for multiple daily oral treatments in young rats. *J. Am. Ass. Lab. Anim. Sci.*, 48, 292–295.
12. Huang-Brown, K. M. and Guhad, F. A., 2002. Chocolate, an effective means of oral drug delivery in rats. *Lab. Anim.*, 31, 34–36.
13. Walker, M. K., Boberg, J. R., Walsh, M. T. et al., 2012. A less stressful alternative to oral gavage for pharmacological and toxicological studies in mice. *Toxicol. Appl. Pharmacol.*, 260, 65–69.
14. Munday, R., Selwood, A. I., and Rhodes, L., 2012. Acute toxicity of pinnatoxins E, F and G to mice. *Toxicon*, 60, 995–999.
15. Aasen, J. A. B., Espenes, A., Hess, P., and Aune, T., 2010. Sub-lethal dosing of azaspiracid-1 in female NMRI mice. *Toxicon*, 56, 1419–1425.
16. OECD, 2009. Guidelines for the Testing of Chemicals. *Guideline 452. Chronic Toxicity Studies*. OECD, Paris, France.
17. Kapetanovic, I. M., Krishnaraj, R., Martin-Jimenez, T., Yuan, L., van Breemen, R. B., and Lyubimov, A., 2006. Effects of oral dosing paradigms (gavage versus diet) on pharmacokinetics and pharmacodynamics. *Chem.-Biol. Interact.*, 164, 68–75.
18. Dieter, M. P., Goehl, T. J., Jameson, C. W., Elwell, M. R., Hildebrandt, P. K., and Yuan, J. H., 1993. Comparison of the toxicity of citral in F344 rats and B6C3F$_1$ mice when administered by microencapsulation in feed or by corn-oil gavage. *Food Chem. Toxicol.*, 31, 463–474.
19. Larson, J. L., Wolf, D. C., and Butterworth, B. E., 1995. Induced regenerative cell proliferation in livers and kidneys of male F-344 rats given chloroform in corn oil by gavage or ad libitum in drinking water. *Toxicology*, 95, 73–86.
20. Lijinsky, W., Saavedra, J. E., and Kovatch, R. M., 1989. Carcinogenesis in rats by nitrosodialkylureas containing methyl and ethyl groups given by gavage and in drinking water. *J. Toxicol. Environ. Health*, 28, 27–38.
21. Miljkovic, A., Pfohl-Leszkowicz, A., Dobrota, M., and Mantle, P. G., 2003. Comparative responses to mode of oral administration and dose of ochratoxin A or nephrotoxic extract of *Penicillium polonicum* in rats. *Exp. Toxicol. Pathol.*, 54, 305–312.
22. Klotz, U., 2009. Pharmacokinetics and drug metabolism in the elderly. *Drug Metab. Rev.*, 41, 67–76.
23. Renwick, A. G., 1998. Toxicokinetics in infants and children in relation to the ADI and TDI. *Food Addit. Contam.*, 15, 17–35.
24. Farrall, A. J. and Wardlaw, J. M., 2009. Blood–brain barrier: Ageing and microvascular disease—Systematic review and meta-analysis. *Neurobiol. Aging*, 30, 337–352.
25. Tillmann, U., Elbrächter, M., Krock, B., John, U., and Cembella, A., 2009. *Azadinium spinosum* gen. et sp. nov. (Dinophyceae) identified as a primary producer of azaspiracid toxins. *Eur. J. Phycol.*, 44, 63–79.
26. Krock, B., Tillmann, U., Voss, D. et al., 2012. New azaspiracids in Amphidomataceae (Dinophyceae). *Toxicon*, 60, 830–839.
27. Krock, B., Tillmann, U., John, U., and Cembella, A. D., 2009. Characterization of azaspiracids in plankton size-fractions and isolation of an azaspiracid-producing dinoflagellate from the North Sea. *Harmful Algae*, 8, 254–263.
28. Rehmann, N., Hess, P., and Quilliam, M. A., 2008. Discovery of new analogs of the marine biotoxin azaspiracid in blue mussels (*Mytilus edulis*) by ultra-performance liquid chromatography/tandem mass spectrometry. *Rap. Comm. Mass Spec.*, 22, 549–558.

29. Ofuji, K., Satake, M., McMahon, T. et al., 1999. Two analogs of azaspiracid isolated from mussels, *Mytilus edulis*, involved in human intoxication in Ireland. *Nat. Toxins*, 7, 99–102.

30. Ofuji, K., Satake, M., McMahon, T. et al., 2001. Structures of azaspiracid analogs, azaspiracid-4 and azaspiracid-5, causative toxins of azaspiracid poisoning in Europe. *Biosci. Biotechnol. Biochem.*, 65, 740–742.

31. EFSA Panel on Contaminants in the Food Chain, 2008. Marine biotoxins in shellfish—Azaspiracid group. *EFSA J.*, 723, 52 pp.

32. López-Rivera, A., O'Callaghan, K., Moriarty, M. et al., 2010. First evidence of azaspiracids (AZAs): A family of lipophilic polyether marine toxins in scallops (*Argopecten purpuratus*) and mussels (*Mytilus chilensis*) collected in two regions of Chile. *Toxicon*, 55, 692–701.

33. Potvin, E., Jeong, H. J., Kang, N. S., Tillmann, U., and Krock, B., 2012. First report of the photosynthetic genus, *Azadinium* in the Pacific Ocean: Morphology and molecular characterization of *Azadinium* cf. *poporum*. *J. Eukaryot. Microbiol.*, 59, 145–156.

34. Torgersen, T., Bremnes, N. B., Rundberget, T., and Aune, T., 2008. Structural confirmation and occurrence of azaspiracids in Scandinavian brown crabs (*Cancer pagurus*). *Toxicon*, 51, 93–101.

35. Ito, E., 2008. Toxicology of azaspiracid-1: Acute and chronic poisoning, tumorigenicity, and chemical structure relationship to toxicity in a mouse model, in *Seafood and Freshwater Toxins. Pharmacology, Physiology, and Detection*, 2nd edn., Botana, L. M., ed. CRC Press, Boca Raton, FL, pp. 775–784.

36. Satake, M., Ofuji, K., Naoki, H. et al., 1998. Azaspiracid, a new marine toxin having unique spiro ring assemblies, isolated from Irish mussels, *Mytilus edulis*. *J. Am. Chem. Soc.*, 120, 9967–9968.

37. Ito, E., Terao, K., MacMahon, T., Silke, J., and Yasumoto, T., 1998. Acute pathological changes in mice caused by crude extracts of novel toxins isolated from Irish mussels, in *Harmful Algae*, Reguera, B., Blanco, J., Fernández, M. L., and Wyatt, T., eds. Xunta de Galicia and Intergovernmental Oceanographic Commission of UNESCO, Santiago de Compostela, Spain, pp. 588–589.

38. Ito, E., Frederick, M. O., Koftis, T. V. et al., 2006. Structure toxicity relationships of synthetic azaspiracid-1 and analogs in mice. *Harmful Algae*, 5, 586–591.

39. Aune, T., Espenes, A., Aasen, J. A. B., Quilliam, M. A., Hess, P., and Larsen, S., 2012. Study of possible combined toxic effects of azaspiracid-1 and okadaic acid in mice via the oral route. *Toxicon*, 60, 895–906.

40. Ito, E., Satake, M., Ofuji, K. et al., 2000. Multiple organ damage caused by a new toxin azaspiracid, isolated from mussels produced in Ireland. *Toxicon*, 38, 917–930.

41. Ito, E., Satake, M., Ofuji, K. et al., 2002. Chronic effects in mice caused by oral administration of sublethal doses of azaspiracid, a new marine toxin isolated from mussels. *Toxicon*, 40, 193–203.

42. James, K. J., Carey, B., O'Halloran, J. O., van Pelt, F. N. A. M., and Škrabáková, Z., 2010. Shellfish toxicity: Human health implications of marine algal toxins. *Epidemiol. Infect.*, 138, 927–940.

43. Klontz, K. C., Abraham, A., Plakas, S. M., and Dickey, R. W., 2009. Mussel-associated azaspiracid intoxication in the United States. *Ann. Int. Med.*, 150, 361.

44. Twiner, M. J., Rehmann, N., Hess, P., and Doucette, G. J., 2008. Azaspiracid shellfish poisoning: A review on the chemistry, ecology, and toxicology with emphasis on human health impacts. *Marine Drugs*, 6, 39–72.

45. Aasen, J. A. B., Espenes, A., Miles, C. O., Samdal, I. A., Hess, P., and Aune, T., 2011. Combined oral toxicity of azaspiracid-1 and yessotoxin in female NMRI mice. *Toxicon*, 57, 909–917.

46. Kittler, K., Preiss-Weigert, A., and These, A., 2010. Identification strategy using combined mass spectrometric techniques for elucidation of Phase I and Phase II in vitro metabolites of lipophilic marine biotoxins. *Anal. Chem.*, 82, 9329–9335.

47. Flanagan, A. F., Callanan, K. R., Donlon, J., Palmer, R., Forde, A., and Kane, M., 2001. A cytotoxicity assay for the detection and differentiation of two families of shellfish toxins. *Toxicon*, 39, 1021–1027.

48. Twiner, M. J., Hess, P., Bottein Dechraoui, M.-Y. et al., 2005. Cytotoxic and cytoskeletal effects of azaspiracid-1 on mammalian cell lines. *Toxicon*, 45, 891–900.

49. Kulagina, N. V., Twiner, M. J., Hess, P. et al., 2006. Azaspiracid-1 inhibits bioelectrical activity of spinal cord neuronal networks. *Toxicon*, 47, 766–773.

50. Codex Alimentarius Commission, 2006. *Codex Committee on Fish and Fishery Products*, Twenty-Eighth Session, Beijing, China, September 18–22, 2006. ftp://ftp.fao.org/codex/Meetings/CCFFP/ccffp28/fp2806ae.pdf

51. Giknis, M. L. A. and Clifford, C. B., 2000. Spontaneous neoplastic lesions in the Crl:CD-1®(ICR)BR mouse. Charles River Laboratories, Wilmington, MA. http://www.criver.com/sitecollectiondocuments/rm_rm_r_lesions_crl_cd_icr_br_mouse.pdf

52. Derelanko, M. J., 2002. Carcinogenesis, in *Handbook of Toxicology*, Derelanko, M. J. and Hollinger, M. A., eds. CRC Press, Boca Raton, FL, pp. 621–647.
53. Grasso, P. and Crampton, R. F., 1972. The value of the mouse in carcinogenicity testing. *Food Cosmet. Toxicol.*, 10, 418–426.
54. Ramsdell, J. S., 2008. The molecular and integrative basis to brevetoxin toxicity, in *Seafood and Freshwater Toxins. Pharmacology, Physiology, and Detection*, 2nd edn., Botana, L. M., ed. CRC Press, Boca Raton, FL, pp. 519–550.
55. Watkins, S. M., Reich, A., Fleming, L. E., and Hammond, R., 2008. Neurotoxic shellfish poisoning. *Marine Drugs*, 6, 431–455.
56. Brand, L. E., Campbell, L., and Bresnan, E., 2012. *Karenia*: The biology and ecology of a toxic genus. *Harmful Algae*, 14, 156–178.
57. Plakas, S. M., Wang, Z., El Said, K. R. et al., 2004. Brevetoxin metabolism and elimination in the Eastern oyster (*Crassostrea virginica*) after controlled exposures to *Karenia brevis*. *Toxicon*, 44, 677–685.
58. Wang, Z., Plakas, S. M., El Said, K. R., Jester, E. L. E., Granade, H. R., and Dickey, R. W., 2004. LC/MS analysis of brevetoxin metabolites in the Eastern oyster (*Crassostrea virginica*). *Toxicon*, 43, 455–465.
59. Baden, D. G. and Mende, T. J., 1982. Toxicity of two toxins from the Florida red tide marine dinoflagellate, *Ptychodiscus brevis*. *Toxicon*, 20, 457–461.
60. Walsh, P. J., Bookman, R. J., Zaias, J. et al., 2003. Toxicogenomic effects of marine brevetoxins in liver and brain of mouse. *Comp. Biochem. Physiol.*, 136B, 173–182.
61. Gordon, C. J., Kimm-Brinson, K. L., Padnos, B., and Ramsdell, J. S., 2001. Acute and delayed thermoregulatory response of mice exposed to brevetoxin. *Toxicon*, 39, 1367–1374.
62. Selwood, A. I., van Ginkel, R., Wilkins, A. L. et al., 2008. Semisynthesis of *S*-deoxybrevetoxin-B2 and brevetoxin-B2, and assessment of their acute toxicities. *Chem. Res. Toxicol.*, 21, 944–950.
63. Ishida, H., Nozawa, A., Totoribe, K. et al., 1995. Brevetoxin B_1, a new polyether marine toxin from the New Zealand shellfish, *Austrovenus stuchburyi*. *Tetrahedron Lett.*, 36, 725–728.
64. Murata, K., Satake, M., Naoki, H., Kaspar, H. F., and Yasumoto, T., 1998. Isolation and structure of a new brevetoxin analog, brevetoxin B2, from Greenshell mussels from New Zealand. *Tetrahedron*, 54, 735–742.
65. Dechraoui Bottein, M.-Y., Fuquay, J. M., Munday, R. et al., 2010. Bioassay methods for detection of *N*-palmitoylbrevetoxin-B2 (BTX-B4). *Toxicon*, 55, 497–506.
66. Morohashi, A., Satake, M., Naoki, H., Kaspar, H. F., Oshima, Y., and Yasumoto, T., 1999. Brevetoxin B4 isolated from Greenshell mussels *Perna canaliculus*, the major toxin involved in neurotoxic shellfish poisoning in New Zealand. *Nat. Toxins*, 7, 45–48.
67. Ishida, H., Nozawa, A., Hamano, H. et al., 2004. Brevetoxin B5, a new brevetoxin analog isolated from cockle *Austrovenus stutchburyi* in New Zealand, the marker for monitoring shellfish neurotoxicity. *Tetrahedron Lett.*, 45, 29–33.
68. Benson, J. M., Hahn, F. F., March, T. H. et al., 2004. Inhalation toxicity of brevetoxin 3 in rats exposed for 5 days. *J. Toxicol. Environ. Health*, 67A, 1443–1456.
69. Benson, J. M., Hahn, F. F., March, T. H. et al., 2005. Inhalation toxicity of brevetoxin 3 in rats exposed for twenty-two days. *Environ. Health Perspect.*, 113, 626–631.
70. Yan, X., Benson, J. M., Gomez, A. P., Baden, D. G., and Murray, T. F., 2006. Brevetoxin-induced neural insult in the retrosplenial cortex of mouse brain. *Inhal. Toxicol.*, 18, 1109–1116.
71. Fleming, L. E., Kirkpatrick, B., Backer, L. C. et al., 2011. Review of Florida red tide and human health effects. *Harmful Algae*, 10, 224–233.
72. Pierce, R. H., Henry, M. S., Blum, P. C. et al., 2011. Compositional changes in neurotoxins and their oxidative derivatives from the dinoflagellate, *Karenia brevis,* in seawater and marine aerosol. *J. Plankton Res.*, 33, 343–348.
73. Kirkpatrick, B., Fleming, L. E., Squicciarini, D. et al., 2004. Literature review of Florida red tide: Implications for human health effects. *Harmful Algae*, 3, 99–115.
74. Fleming, L. E., Bean, J. A., Kirkpatrick, B. et al., 2009. Exposure and effect assessment of aerosolized red tide toxins (brevetoxins) and asthma. *Environ. Health Perspect.*, 117, 1095–1100.
75. Radwan, F. F. Y. and Ramsdell, J. S., 2006. Characterization of *in vitro* oxidative and conjugative metabolic pathways for brevetoxin (PbTx-2). *Toxicol. Sci.*, 89, 57–65.
76. Guo, F., An, T., and Rein, K. S., 2010. Human metabolites of brevetoxin PbTx-2: Identification and confirmation of structure. *Toxicon*, 56, 648–651.

77. Wang, W., Hua, Y., Wang, G., and Cole, R., 2005. Characterization of rat liver microsomal and hepatocytal metabolites of brevetoxins by liquid chromatography–electrospray tandem mass spectrometry. *Anal. Bioanal. Chem.*, 383, 67–75.

78. Radwan, F. F. Y., Wang, Z., and Ramsdell, J. S., 2005. Identification of a rapid detoxification mechanism for brevetoxin in rats. *Toxicol. Sci.*, 85, 839–846.

79. Poli, M. A., Musser, S. M., Dickey, R. W., Eilers, P. P., and Hall, S., 2000. Neurotoxic shellfish poisoning and brevetoxin metabolites: A case study from Florida. *Toxicon*, 38, 981–993.

80. Abraham, A., Plakas, S. M., Flewelling, L. J. et al., 2008. Biomarkers of neurotoxic shellfish poisoning. *Toxicon*, 52, 237–245.

81. Poli, M. A., Templeton, C. B., Thompson, W. L., and Hewetson, J. F., 1990. Distribution and elimination of brevetoxin PbTx-3 in rats. *Toxicon*, 28, 903–910.

82. Benson, J. M., Tischler, D. L., and Baden, D. G., 1999. Uptake, tissue distribution, and excretion of brevetoxin 3 administered to rats by intratracheal instillation. *J. Toxicol. Environ. Health*, 57A, 345–355.

83. Tibbetts, B. M., Baden, D. G., and Benson, J. M., 2006. Uptake, tissue distribution, and excretion of brevetoxin-3 administered to mice by intratracheal instillation. *J. Toxicol. Environ. Health*, 69A, 1325–1335.

84. Cattet, M. and Geraci, J. R., 1993. Distribution and elimination of ingested brevetoxin (PbTx-3) in rats. *Toxicon*, 31, 1483–1486.

85. Benson, J. M., Gomez, A. P., Statom, G. L. et al., 2006. Placental transport of brevetoxin-3 in CD-1 mice. *Toxicon*, 48, 1018–1026.

86. Baden, D. G., Bikhazi, G., Decker, S. J., Foldes, F. F., and Leung, I., 1984. Neuromuscular blocking action of two brevetoxins from the Florida red tide organism *Ptychodiscus brevis*. *Toxicon*, 22, 75–84.

87. Tsai, M.-C., Chou, H.-N., and Chen, M.-L., 1991. Effect of brevetoxin-B on the neuromuscular transmission of the mouse diaphragm. *J. Formosan Med. Assoc.*, 90, 431–436.

88. Dechraoui Bottein, M.-Y., Wang, Z., and Ramsdell, J. S., 2007. Intrinsic potency of synthetically prepared brevetoxin cysteine metabolites BTX-B2 and desoxyBTX-B2. *Toxicon*, 50, 825–834.

89. Leighfield, T. A., Muha, N., and Ramsdell, J. S., 2009. Brevetoxin B is a clastogen in rats, but lacks mutagenic potential in the SP-98/100 Ames test. *Toxicon*, 54, 851–856.

90. Sayer, A. N., Hu, Q., Bourdelais, A. J., Baden, D. G., and Gibson, J. E., 2006. The inhibition of CHO-K1-BH4 cell proliferation and induction of chromosomal aberrations by brevetoxins in vitro. *Food Chem. Toxicol.*, 44, 1082–1091.

91. Murrell, R. and Gibson, J., 2009. Brevetoxins 2, 3, 6, and 9 show variability in potency and cause significant induction of DNA damage and apoptosis in Jurkat E6-1 cells. *Arch. Toxicol.*, 83, 1009–1019.

92. Radwan, F. F. Y. and Ramsdell, J. S., 2008. Brevetoxin forms covalent DNA adducts in rat lung following intratracheal exposure. *Environ. Health Perspect.*, 116, 930–936.

93. EFSA Panel on Contaminants in the Food Chain, 2010. Scientific opinion on marine biotoxins in shellfish—Emerging toxins: Brevetoxin group. *EFSA J.*, 1677, 29.

94. Yasumoto, T., Nakajima, I., Bagnis, R., and Adachi, R., 1977. Finding of a dinoflagellate as a likely culprit of ciguatera. *Bull. Jap. Soc. Sci. Fish.*, 43, 1021–1026.

95. Adachi, R. and Fukuyo, Y., 1979. The thecal structure of a marine toxic dinoflagellate *Gambierdiscus toxicus* gen. et sp. nov. collected in a ciguatera-endemic area. *Bull. Jap. Soc. Sci. Fish.*, 45, 67–71.

96. Litaker, R. W., Vandersea, M. W., Faust, M. A. et al., 2008. Taxonomy of *Gambierdiscus* including four new species, *Gambierdiscus caribaeus*, *Gambierdiscus carolinianus*, *Gambierdiscus carpenteri* and *Gambierdiscus ruetzleri* (Gonyaulacales, Dinophyceae). *Phycologia*, 48, 344–390.

97. Litaker, R. W., Vandersea, M. W., Faust, M. A. et al., 2010. Global distribution of ciguatera causing dinoflagellates in the genus *Gambierdiscus*. *Toxicon*, 56, 711–730.

98. Parsons, M. L., Aligizaki, K., Dechraoui Bottein, M.-Y. et al., 2012. *Gambierdiscus* and *Ostreopsis*: Reassessment of the state of knowledge of their taxonomy, geography, ecophysiology, and toxicology. *Harmful Algae*, 14, 107–129.

99. Baek, S. H., 2012. Occurrence of the toxic benthic dinoflagellate *Gambierdiscus* spp. in the uninhabited Baekdo Islands off southern coast and Seopsom Island in the vicinity of Seogwipo, Jeju Province, Korea. *Ocean Polar Res.*, 34, 65–71.

100. Yogi, K., Oshiro, N., Inafuku, Y., Hirama, M., and Yasumoto, T., 2011. Detailed LC-MS/MS analysis of ciguatoxins revealing distinct regional and species characteristics in fish and causative alga from the Pacific. *Anal. Chem.*, 83, 8886–8891.

101. Vernoux, J.-P. and Lewis, R. J., 1997. Isolation and characterisation of Caribbean ciguatoxins from the horse-eye jack (*Caranx latus*). *Toxicon*, 35, 889–900.

102. Pottier, I., Vernoux, J.-P., Jones, A., and Lewis, R. J., 2002. Characterisation of multiple Caribbean ciguatoxins and congeners in individual specimens of horse-eye jack (*Caranx latus*) by high-performance liquid chromatography/mass spectrometry. *Toxicon*, 40, 929–939.

103. Hamilton, B., Hurbungs, M., Jones, A., and Lewis, R. J., 2002. Multiple ciguatoxins present in Indian Ocean reef fish. *Toxicon*, 40, 1347–1353.

104. Yasumoto, T., 2001. The chemistry and biological function of natural marine toxins. *Chem. Rec.*, 1, 228–242.

105. Dickey, R. W., 2008. Ciguatera toxins: Chemistry, toxicology, and detection, in *Seafood and Freshwater Toxins. Pharmacology, Physiology, and Detection*, 2nd edn., Botana, L. M., ed. CRC Press, Boca Raton, FL, pp. 479–500.

106. Nagai, H., Murata, M., Torigoe, K., Satake, M., and Yasumoto, T., 1992. Gambieric acids, new potent antifungal substances with unprecedented polyether structures from a marine dinoflagellate *Gambierdiscus toxicus*. *J. Org. Chem.*, 57, 5448–5453.

107. Satake, M., Murata, M., and Yasumoto, T., 1993. Gambierol: A new toxic polyether compound isolated from the marine dinoflagellate *Gambierdiscus toxicus*. *J. Am. Chem. Soc.*, 115, 361–362.

108. Murata, M. and Yasumoto, T., 2000. The structure elucidation and biological activities of high molecular weight algal toxins: Maitotoxin, prymnesins and zooxanthellatoxins. *Nat. Prod. Rep.*, 17, 293–314.

109. Holmes, M. J. and Lewis, R. J., 1994. Purification and characterisation of large and small maitotoxins from cultured *Gambierdiscus toxicus*. *Nat. Toxins*, 2, 64–72.

110. Hashimoto, Y., Yasumoto, T., Kamiya, H., and Yoshida, T., 1969. Occurrence of ciguatoxin and ciguaterin in ciguatoxic fishes in the Ryukyu and Amami Island. *Bull. Jap. Soc. Sci. Fish.*, 35, 327–332.

111. Kamiya, H. and Hashimoto, Y., 1973. Purification of ciguaterin from the liver of the red snapper *Lutjanus bohar. Bull. Jap. Soc. Sci. Fish.*, 39, 1183–1187.

112. Lewis, R. J., Sellin, M., Poli, M. A., Norton, R. S., MacLeod, J. K., and Sheil, M. M., 1991. Purification and characterization of ciguatoxins from moray eel (*Lycodontis javanicus*, Muraenidae). *Toxicon*, 29, 1115–1127.

113. Legrand, A. M., Litaudon, M., Genthon, J. N., Bagnis, R., and Yasumoto, T., 1989. Isolation and some properties of ciguatoxin. *J. Appl. Phycol.*, 1, 183–188.

114. Tachibana, K., Nukina, M., Joh, Y.-G., and Scheuer, P. J., 1987. Recent developments in the molecular structure of ciguatoxin. *Biol. Bull.*, 172, 122–127.

115. Murata, M., Legrand, A. M., Ishibashi, Y., Fukui, M., and Yasumoto, T., 1990. Structures and configurations of ciguatoxin from the moray eel *Gymnothorax javanicus* and its likely precursor from the dinoflagellate *Gambierdiscus toxicus*. *J. Am. Chem. Soc.*, 112, 4380–4386.

116. Dechraoui, M.-Y., Naar, J., Pauillac, S., and Legrand, A.-M., 1999. Ciguatoxins and brevetoxins, neurotoxic polyether compounds active on sodium channels. *Toxicon*, 37, 125–143.

117. Satake, M., Murata, M., and Yasumoto, T., 1993. The structure of CTX3C, a ciguatoxin congener isolated from cultured *Gambierdiscus toxicus*. *Tetrahedron Lett.*, 34, 1975–1978.

118. Satake, M., Fukui, M., Legrand, A.-M., Cruchet, P., and Yasumoto, T., 1998. Isolation and structures of new ciguatoxin analogs, 2,3-dihydroxyCTX3C and 51-hydroxyCTX3C, accumulated in tropical reef fish. *Tetrahedron Lett.*, 39, 1197–1198.

119. Inoue, M., Lee, N., Miyazaki, K., Usuki, T., Matsuoka, S., and Hirama, M., 2008. Critical importance of the nine-membered F ring of ciguatoxin for potent bioactivity: Total synthesis and biological evaluation of F-ring-modified analogues. *Angew. Chem. Int. Ed.*, 47, 8611–8614.

120. Satake, M., Ishibashi, Y., Legrand, A.-M., and Yasumoto, T., 1997. Isolation and structure of ciguatoxin-4A, a new ciguatoxin precursor, from cultures of dinoflagellate *Gambierdiscus toxicus* and parrotfish *Scarus gibbus*. *Biosci. Biotechnol. Biochem.*, 60, 2103–2105.

121. Yasumoto, T., Bagnis, R., and Vernoux, J. P., 1976. Toxicity of the surgeonfishes—II. Properties of the principal water-soluble toxin. *Bull. Jap. Soc. Sci. Fish.*, 42, 359–365.

122. Yasumoto, T., Nakajima, I., Oshima, Y., and Bagnis, R., 1979. A new toxic dinoflagellate found in association with ciguatera, in *Toxic Dinoflagellate Blooms. Proceedings of the Second International Conference on Toxic Dinoflagellate Blooms*, Key Biscayne, FL, Taylor, D. I. and Seliger, H. H., eds. Elsevier, New York.

123. Yokoyama, A., Murata, M., Oshima, Y., Iwashita, T., and Yasumoto, T., 1988. Some chemical properties of maitotoxin, a putative calcium channel agonist isolated from a marine dinoflagellate. *J. Biochem. (Tokyo)*, 104, 184–187.

124. Murata, M., Naoki, H., Matsunaga, S., Satake, M., and Yasumoto, T., 1994. Structure and partial stereo-chemical assignments for maitotoxin, the most toxic and largest natural non-biopolymer. *J. Am. Chem. Soc.*, 116, 7098–7107.

125. Murata, M., Gusovsky, F., Sasaki, M., Yokoyama, A., Yasumoto, T., and Daly, J. W., 1991. Effect of maitotoxin analogues on calcium influx and phosphoinositide breakdown in cultured cells. *Toxicon*, 29, 1085–1096.

126. Ito, E., Suzuki-Toyota, F., Toshimori, K. et al., 2003. Pathological effects on mice by gambierol, possibly one of the ciguatera toxins. *Toxicon*, 42, 733–740.

127. Fuwa, H., Kainuma, N., Tachibana, K., Tsukano, C., Satake, M., and Sasaki, M., 2004. Diverted total synthesis and biological evaluation of gambierol analogues: Elucidation of crucial elements for potent toxicity. *Chem. Eur. J.*, 10, 4894–4909.

128. Terao, K., Ito, E., Oarada, M., Ishibashi, Y., Legrand, A.-M., and Yasumoto, T., 1991. Light and electron microscopic studies of pathologic changes induced in mice by ciguatoxin poisoning. *Toxicon*, 29, 633–643.

129. Ito, E., Yasumoto, T., and Terao, K., 1996. Morphological observations of diarrhea in mice caused by experimental ciguatoxicosis. *Toxicon*, 34, 111–122.

130. Yasumoto, T., Hashimoto, Y., Bagnis, R., Randall, J. E., and Banner, A. H., 1971. Toxicity of the surgeon-fishes. *Bull. Jap. Soc. Sci. Fish.*, 37, 724–734.

131. Holmes, M. J., Lewis, R. J., and Gillespie, N. C., 1990. Toxicity of Australian and French Polynesian strains of *Gambierdiscus toxicus* (Dinophyceae) grown in culture: Characterization of a new type of maitotoxin. *Toxicon*, 28, 1159–1172.

132. Terao, K., Ito, E., Sakamaki, Y., Igarashi, K., Yokoyama, A., and Yasumoto, T., 1988. Histopathological studies of experimental marine toxin poisoning. II. The acute effects of maitotoxin on the stomach, heart and lymphoid tissues in mice and rats. *Toxicon*, 26, 395–402.

133. Lewis, R. J., Wong Hoy, A. W., and Sellin, M., 1993. Ciguatera and mannitol: *In vivo* and *in vitro* assessment in mice. *Toxicon*, 31, 1039–1050.

134. Dechraoui Bottein, M.-Y., Rezvani, A. H., Gordon, C. J., Levin, E. D., and Ramsdell, J. S., 2008. Repeat exposure to ciguatoxin leads to enhanced and sustained thermoregulatory, pain threshold and motor activity responses in mice: Relationship to blood ciguatoxin concentrations. *Toxicology*, 246, 55–62.

135. Terao, K., Ito, E., and Yasumoto, T., 1992. Light and electron microscopic studies of the murine heart after repeated administrations of ciguatoxin or ciguatoxin-4c. *Nat. Toxins*, 1, 19–26.

136. Terao, K., Ito, E., Ohkusu, M., and Yasumoto, T., 1994. Pathological changes in murine hearts induced by intermittent administration of ciguatoxin. *Memoirs Qld. Museum*, 34, 621–623.

137. Terao, K., Ito, E., Kakinuma, Y. et al., 1989. Histopathological studies on experimental marine toxin poisoning—4. Pathogenesis of experimental maitotoxin poisoning. *Toxicon*, 27, 979–988.

138. Friedman, M., Fleming, L., Fernandez, M. et al., 2008. Ciguatera fish poisoning: Treatment, prevention and management. *Marine Drugs*, 6, 456–479.

139. Pérez-Arellano, J.-L., Luzardo, O. P., Brito, A. P. et al., 2005. Ciguatera fish poisoning, Canary Islands. *Emerg. Infect. Dis.*, 11, 1981–1982.

140. Boada, L. D., Zumbado, M., Luzardo, O. P. et al., 2010. Ciguatera fish poisoning on the West Africa coast: An emerging risk in the Canary Islands (Spain). *Toxicon*, 56, 1516–1519.

141. Otero, P., Pérez, S., Alfonso, A. et al., 2010. First toxin profile of ciguateric fish in Madeira Arquipelago (Europe). *Anal. Chem.*, 82, 6032–6039.

142. Raikhlin-Eisenkraft, B. and Bentur, Y., 2002. Rabbitfish ("Aras"): An unusual source of ciguatera poisoning. *Isr. Med. Ass. J.*, 4, 28–30.

143. Bentur, Y. and Spanier, E., 2007. Ciguatoxin-like substances in edible fish on the eastern Mediterranean. *Clin. Toxicol.*, 45, 695–700.

144. Nicholson, G. and Lewis, R., 2006. Ciguatoxins: Cyclic polyether modulators of voltage-gated ion channel function. *Marine Drugs*, 4, 82–118.

145. Barkin, R. M., 1974. Ciguatera poisoning: A common source outbreak. *South. Med. J.*, 67, 13–16.

146. Bagnis, R., 1970. Concerning a fatal case of ciguatera poisoning in the Tuamotu Islands. *Clin. Toxicol.*, 3, 579–583.

147. Nakano, K. K., 1983. Ciguatera poisoning: An outbreak on Midway Island. Clinical, electrophysiological and muscle biopsy findings. *J. Neurol. Orthopaed. Surg.*, 4, 11–16.

148. Kodama, A. M., Hokama, Y., Yasumoto, T., Fukui, M., Manea, S. J., and Sutherland, N., 1989. Clinical and laboratory findings implicating palytoxin as cause of ciguatera poisoning due to *Decapterus macrosoma* (mackerel). *Toxicon*, 27, 1051–1053.

149. Schlaich, C., Hagelstein, J.-G., Burchard, G.-D., and Schmiedel, S., 2012. Outbreak of ciguatera fish poisoning on a cargo ship in the Port of Hamburg. *J. Travel Med.*, 19, 238–242.

150. Pearn, J., Harvey, P., De Ambrosis, W., Lewis, R. J., and McKay, R., 1982. Ciguatera and pregnancy. *Med. J. Aust.*, 136, 57–58.

151. Senecal, P.-E. and Osterloh, J. D., 1991. Normal fetal outcome after maternal ciguateric toxin exposure in the second trimester. *Clin. Toxicol.*, 29, 473–478.

152. Blythe, D. G. and de Sylva, D. P., 1990. Mothers milk turns toxic following fish feast. *J. Am. Med. Assoc.*, 264, 2074.

153. Karalis, T., Gupta, L., Chu, M., Campbell, B. A., Capra, M. F., and Maywood, P. A., 2000. Three clusters of ciguatera poisoning: Clinical manifestations and public health implications. *Med. J. Aust.*, 172, 160–162.

154. Kumar-Roiné, S., Darius, H. T., Matsui, M. et al., 2011. A review of traditional remedies of ciguatera fish poisoning in the Pacific. *Phytother. Res.*, 25, 947–958.

155. Dechraoui Bottein, M.-Y., Wang, Z., and Ramsdell, J. S., 2011. Toxicokinetics of the ciguatoxin P-CTX-1 in rats after intraperitoneal or oral administration. *Toxicology*, 284, 1–6.

156. Hamilton, B., Whittle, N., Shaw, G., Eaglesham, G., and Moore, M. R., 2010. Human fatality associated with Pacific ciguatoxin contaminated fish. *Toxicon*, 56, 668–673.

157. Dickey, R. W. and Plakas, S. M., 2010. Ciguatera: A public health perspective. *Toxicon*, 56, 123–136.

158. Cuypers, E., Abdel-Mottaleb, Y., Kopljar, I. et al., 2008. Gambierol, a toxin produced by the dinoflagellate *Gambierdiscus toxicus*, is a potent blocker of voltage-gated potassium channels. *Toxicon*, 51, 974–983.

159. Kopljar, I., Labro, A. J., Cuypers, E. et al., 2009. A polyether biotoxin binding site on the lipid-exposed face of the pore domain of Kv channels revealed by the marine toxin gambierol. *Proc. Natl. Acad. Sci. USA*, 106, 9896–9901.

160. Trevino, C. L., Escobar, L., Vaca, L., Morales-Tlalpan, V., Ocampo, A. Y., and Darszon, A., 2008. Maitotoxin: A unique pharmacological tool for elucidating Ca^{2+}-dependent mechanisms, in *Seafood and Freshwater Toxins. Pharmacology, Physiology, and Detection*, 2nd edn., Botana, L. M., ed. CRC Press, Boca Raton, FL, pp. 503–513.

161. Kumar-Roiné, S., Matsui, M., Chinain, M., Laurent, D., and Pauillac, S., 2008. Modulation of inducible nitric oxide synthase gene expression in RAW 264.7 murine macrophages by Pacific ciguatoxin. *Nitric Oxide*, 19, 21–28.

162. Matsui, M., Kumar-Roine, S., Darius, H. T., Chinain, M., Laurent, D., and Pauillac, S., 2010. Pacific ciguatoxin 1B-induced modulation of inflammatory mediators in a murine macrophage cell line. *Toxicon*, 56, 776–784.

163. EFSA Panel on Contaminants in the Food Chain, 2010. Scientific opinion on marine biotoxins in shellfish—Emerging toxins: Ciguatoxin group. *EFSA J.*, 1627, 38.

164. Skinner, M. P., Brewer, T. D., Johnstone, R., Fleming, L. E., and Lewis, R. J., 2011. Ciguatera fish poisoning in the Pacific Islands (1998–2008). *PLoS Negl. Trop. Dis.*, 5, e1416.

165. Lewis, R. J. and Holmes, M. J., 1993. Origin and transfer of toxins involved in ciguatera. *Comp. Biochem. Physiol.*, 106C, 615–628.

166. Kelley, B. A., Jollow, D. J., Felton, E. T., Voegtline, M. S., and Higerd, T. B., 1986. Response of mice to *Gambierdiscus toxicus* toxin. *Marine Fish. Rev.*, 48(4), 35–37.

167. Laurent, D., Yeeting, B., Labrosse, P., and Gaudechoux, J.-P., 2005. *Ciguatera: A Field Reference Guide*. Secretariat of the Pacific Community, Noumea, New Caledonia.

168. Holmes, M. J. and Lewis, R. J., 1994. The origin of ciguatoxin. *Memoirs Qld. Museum*, 34, 497–504.

169. Seki, T., Satake, M., Mackenzie, L., Kaspar, H. F., and Yasumoto, T., 1995. Gymnodimine, a new marine toxin of unprecedented structure isolated from New Zealand oysters and the dinoflagellate, *Gymnodinium sp. Tetrahedron Lett.*, 36, 7093–7096.

170. Miles, C. O., Wilkins, A. L., Stirling, D. J., and MacKenzie, A. L., 2000. New analogue of gymnodimine from a *Gymnodinium* species. *J. Agric. Food Chem.*, 48, 1373–1376.

171. Miles, C. O., Wilkins, A. L., Stirling, D. J., and MacKenzie, A. L., 2003. Gymnodimine C, an isomer of gymnodimine B, from *Karenia selliformis*. *J. Agric. Food Chem.*, 51, 4838–4840.

172. Van Wagoner, R. M., Misner, I., Tomas, C. R., and Wright, J. L. C., 2011. Occurrence of 12-methylgymnodimine in a spirolide-producing dinoflagellate *Alexandrium peruvianum* and the biogenetic implications. *Tetrahedron Lett.*, 52, 4243–4246.

173. Cembella, A. D., Lewis, N. I., and Quilliam, M. A., 2000. The marine dinoflagellate *Alexandrium osten-feldii* (Dinophyceae) as the causative organism of spirolide shellfish toxins. *Phycologia*, 39, 67–74.

174. Touzet, N., Franco, J. M., and Raine, R., 2008. Morphogenetic diversity and biotoxin composition of *Alexandrium* (Dinophyceae) in Irish coastal waters. *Harmful Algae*, 7, 782–797.

175. Roach, J. S., LeBlanc, P., Lewis, N. I., Munday, R., Quilliam, M. A., and MacKinnon, S. L., 2009. Characterization of a dispiroketal spirolide subclass from *Alexandrium ostenfeldii*. *J. Nat. Prod.*, 72, 1237–1240.

176. MacKinnon, S. L., Walter, J. A., Quilliam, M. A. et al., 2006. Spirolides isolated from Danish strains of the toxigenic dinoflagellate *Alexandrium ostenfeldii*. *J. Nat. Prod.*, 69, 983–987.

177. Cembella, A. D., Lewis, N. I., and Quilliam, M. A., 1999. Spirolide composition of micro-extracted pooled cells isolated from natural plankton assemblages and from cultures of the dinoflagellate *Alexandrium ostenfeldii*. *Nat. Toxins*, 7, 197–206.

178. Ciminiello, P., Dell'Aversano, C., Iacovo, E. D. et al., 2010. Characterization of 27-hydroxy-13-desmethyl spirolide C and 27-oxo-13,19-didesmethyl spirolide C. Further insights into the complex Adriatic *Alexandrium ostenfeldii* toxin profile. *Toxicon*, 56, 1327–1333.

179. Ciminiello, P., Dell'Aversano, C., Fattorusso, E. et al., 2010. Complex toxin profile of *Mytilus gallopro-vincialis* from the Adriatic sea revealed by LC–MS. *Toxicon*, 55, 280–288.

180. Hu, T., Curtis, J. M., Walter, J. A., and Wright, J. L. C., 1996. Characterization of biologically inactive spirolides E and F: Identification of the spirolide pharmacophore. *Tetrahedron Lett.*, 37, 7671–7674.

181. Aasen, J. A. B., Hardstaff, W., Aune, T., and Quilliam, M. A., 2006. Discovery of fatty acid ester metabo-lites of spirolide toxins in mussels from Norway using liquid chromatography/tandem mass spectrom-etry. *Rap. Commun. Mass Spec.*, 20, 1531–1537.

182. Rhodes, L., Smith, K., Selwood, A. et al., 2011. Dinoflagellate *Vulcanodinium rugosum* identified as the causative organism of pinnatoxins in Australia, New Zealand and Japan. *Phycologia*, 50, 624–628.

183. Nézan, E. and Chomérat, N., 2011. *Vulcanodinium rugosum* gen. et sp. nov. (Dinophyceae), un nouveau dinoflagellé marin de la côte méditerranéenne française. *Cryptogamie Algologie*, 32, 3–18.

184. McCarron, P., Rourke, W. A., Hardstaff, W., Pooley, B., and Quilliam, M. A., 2012. Identification of pinnatoxins and discovery of their fatty acid ester metabolites in mussels (*Mytilus edulis*) from Eastern Canada. *J. Agric. Food Chem.*, 60, 1437–1446.

185. Torigoe, K., Murata, M., Yasumoto, T., and Iwashita, T., 1988. Prorocentrolide, a toxic nitrogenous mac-rocycle from a marine dinoflagellate, *Prorocentrum lima*. *J. Am. Chem. Soc.*, 110, 7876–7877.

186. Hu, T., deFreitas, A. S. W., Curtis, J. M., Oshima, Y., Walter, J. A., and Wright, J. L. C., 1996. Isolation and struc-ture of prorocentrolide B, a fast-acting toxin from *Prorocentrum maculosum*. *J. Nat. Prod.*, 59, 1010–1014.

187. Takada, N., Umemura, N., Suenaga, K., and Uemura, D., 2001. Structural determination of pteriatoxins A, B and C, extremely potent toxins from the bivalve *Pteria penguin*. *Tetrahedron Lett.*, 42, 3495–3497.

188. Lu, C.-K., Lee, G.-H., Huang, R., and Chou, H.-N., 2001. Spiro-prorocentrimine, a novel macrocyclic lactone from a benthic *Prorocentrum* sp. of Taiwan. *Tetrahedron Lett.*, 42, 1713–1716.

189. Kita, M., Kondo, M., Koyama, T. et al., 2004. Symbioimine exhibiting inhibitory effect of osteoclast differ-entiation, from the symbiotic marine dinoflagellate *Symbiodinium* sp. *J. Am. Chem. Soc.*, 126, 4794–4795.

190. Biré, R., Krys, S., Frémy, J.-M., Dragacci, S., Stirling, D., and Kharrat, R., 2002. First evidence on ocurrence of gymnodimine in clams from Tunisia. *J. Nat. Toxins*, 11, 269–275.

191. Defence Research and Development Canada, 2004. Science for a secure Canada: Building capacity. Part 1: Annual report 2003–2004. http://publications.gc.ca/collections/collection_2011/dn-nd/D66-1-2004-1-eng.pdf

192. Liu, R., Liang, Y., Wu, X., Xu, D., Liu, Y., and Liu, L., 2011. First report on the detection of pectenotoxin groups in Chinese shellfish by LC-MS/MS. *Toxicon*, 57, 1000–1007.

193. Gladan, Z. N., Ujevic, I., Milandri, A. et al., 2011. Lipophilic toxin profile in *Mytilus galloprovincialis* during episodes of diarrhetic shellfish poisoning (DSP) in the N.E. Adriatic Sea in 2006. *Molecules*, 16, 888–899.

194. Takahashi, E., Yu, Q., Eaglesham, G. et al., 2007. Occurrence and seasonal variations of algal toxins in water, phytoplankton and shellfish from North Stradbroke Island, Queensland, Australia. *Marine Environ. Res.*, 64, 429–442.

195. Krock, B., Pitcher, G. C., Ntuli, J., and Cembella, A. D., 2009. Confirmed identification of gymnodimine in oysters from the west coast of South Africa by liquid chromatography-tandem mass spectrometry. *Afr. J. Marine Sci.*, 31, 113–118.

196. Trefault, N., Krock, B., Delherbe, N., Cembella, A., and Vásquez, M., 2011. Latitudinal transects in the southeastern Pacific Ocean reveal a diverse but patchy distribution of phycotoxins. *Toxicon*, 58, 389–397.

197. Hu, T., Curtis, J. M., Oshima, Y. et al., 1995. Spirolides B and D, two novel macrocycles isolated from the digestive glands of shellfish. *Chem. Commun.*, 2159–2161.

198. Ciminiello, P., Dell'Aversano, C., Fattorusso, E. et al., 2006. Toxin profile of *Alexandrium ostenfeldii* (Dinophyceae) from the Northern Adriatic Sea revealed by liquid chromatography–mass spectrometry. *Toxicon*, 47, 597–604.

199. Villar González, A., Rodríguez-Velasco, M. L., Ben-Gigirey, B., and Botana, L. M., 2006. First evidence of spirolides in Spanish shellfish. *Toxicon*, 48, 1068–1074.

200. Amzil, Z., Sibat, M., Royer, F., Masson, N., and Abadie, E., 2007. Report on the first detection of pectenotoxin-2, spirolide-A and their derivatives in French shellfish. *Marine Drugs*, 5, 168–179.

201. Hummert, C., Rühl, A., Reinhardt, K., Gerdts, G., and Luckas, B., 2002. Simultaneous analysis of different algal toxins by LC-MS. *Chromatographia*, 55, 673–680.

202. Aasen, J., MacKinnon, S. L., LeBlanc, P. et al., 2005. Detection and identification of spirolides in Norwegian shellfish and plankton. *Chem. Res. Toxicol.*, 18, 509–515.

203. Munday, R., 2008. Toxicology of cyclic imines: Gymnodimine, spirolides, pinnatoxins, pteriatoxins, prorocentrolide, spiro-prorocentrimine, and symbioimines, in *Seafood and Freshwater Toxins. Pharmacology, Physiology and Detection*, 2nd edn., Botana, L. M., ed. CRC Press, Boca Raton, FL, pp. 581–594.

204. Álvarez, G., Uribe, E., Ávalos, P., Mariño, C., and Blanco, J., 2010. First identification of azaspiracid and spirolides in *Mesodesma donacium* and *Mulinia edulis* from Northern Chile. *Toxicon*, 55, 638–641.

205. Gribble, K. E., Keafer, B. A., Quilliam, M. A. et al., 2005. Distribution and toxicity of *Alexandrium ostenfeldii* (Dinophyceae) in the Gulf of Maine, USA. *Deep Sea Res. II*, 52, 2745–2763.

206. Selwood, A. I., Miles, C. O., Wilkins, A. L. et al., 2010. Isolation, structural determination and acute toxicity of pinnatoxins E, F and G. *J. Agric. Food Chem.*, 58, 6532–6542.

207. McNabb, P. S., McCoubrey, D. J., Rhodes, L. et al., 2012. New perspectives on biotoxin detection in Rangaunu Harbour, New Zealand arising from the discovery of pinnatoxins. *Harmful Algae*, 13, 34–39.

208. Rundberget, T., Aasen, J. A. B., Selwood, A. I., and Miles, C. O., 2011. Pinnatoxins and spirolides in Norwegian blue mussels and seawater. *Toxicon*, 58, 700–711.

209. Seki, T., Satake, M., MacKenzie, L., Kaspar, H. F., and Yasumoto, T., 1996. Gymnodimine, a novel toxic imine isolated from the Foveaux Strait oysters and *Gymnodinium* sp., in *Harmful and Toxic Algal Blooms*, Yasumoto, T., Oshima, Y., and Fukuyo, Y., eds. Intergovernmental Oceanographic Commission of UNESCO, Paris, France, pp. 495–498.

210. Stewart, M., Blunt, J. W., Munro, M. H. G., Robinson, W. T., and Hannah, D. J., 1997. The absolute stereochemistry of the New Zealand shellfish toxin gymnodimine. *Tetrahedron Lett.*, 38, 4889–4890.

211. Munday, R., Towers, N. R., Mackenzie, L., Beuzenberg, V., Holland, P. T., and Miles, C. O., 2004. Acute toxicity of gymnodimine to mice. *Toxicon*, 44, 173–178.

212. Kharrat, R., Servent, D., Girard, E. et al., 2008. The marine phycotoxin gymnodimine targets muscular and neuronal nicotinic acetylcholine receptor subtypes with high affinity. *J. Neurochem.*, 107, 952–963.

213. Munday, R., Quilliam, M. A., LeBlanc, P. et al., 2012. Investigations into the toxicology of spirolides, a group of marine phycotoxins. *Toxins*, 4, 1–14.

214. Otero, P., Alfonso, A., Rodríguez, P. et al., 2012. Pharmacokinetic and toxicological data of spirolides after oral and intraperitoneal administration. *Food Chem. Toxicol.*, 50, 232–237.

215. Uemura, D., Chou, T., Haino, T. et al., 1995. Pinnatoxin A: A toxic amphoteric macrocycle from the Okinawan bivalve *Pinna muricata*. *J. Am. Chem. Soc.*, 117, 1155–1156.

216. McCauley, J. A., Nagasawa, K., Lander, P. A., Mischke, S. G., Semones, M. A., and Kishi, Y., 1998. Total synthesis of pinnatoxin A. *J. Am. Chem. Soc.*, 120, 7647–7648.

217. Takada, N., Umemura, N., Suenaga, K. et al., 2001. Pinnatoxins B and C, the most toxic components in the pinnatoxin series from the Okinawan bivalve *Pinna muricata*. *Tetrahedron Lett.*, 42, 3491–3494.

218. Chou, T., Haino, T., Kuramoto, M., and Uemura, D., 1996. Isolation and structure of pinnatoxin D, a new shellfish poison from the Okinawan bivalve *Pinna muricata*. *Tetrahedron Lett.*, 37, 4027–4030.

219. Mackenzie, L., Haywood, A., Adamson, J. et al., 1996. Gymnodimine contamination of shellfish in New Zealand, in *Harmful and Toxic Algal Blooms*, Yasumoto, T., Oshima, Y., and Fukuyo, Y., eds. Intergovernmental Oceanographic Commission of UNESCO, Paris, France, pp. 97–100.

220. Stirling, D. J., 2001. Survey of historical New Zealand shellfish samples for accumulation of gymnodimine. *N. Z. J. Marine Freshw. Res.*, 35, 851–857.

221. Richard, D., Arsenault, E., Cembella, A., and Quilliam, M., 2001. Investigations into the toxicology and pharmacology of spirolides, a novel group of shellfish toxins, in *Harmful Algal Blooms 2000. 9th International Conference on Harmful Microalgae*, Hallegraeff, G. M., Blackburn, S. I., Bolch, C. J., and Lewis, R. J., eds. Intergovernmental Oceanographic Commission of UNESCO, Paris, France, pp. 383–386.

222. Cembella, A. D., Bauder, A. G., Lewis, N. I., and Quilliam, M., 2001. Population dynamics and spirolide composition of the toxigenic dinoflagellate *Alexandrium ostenfeldii* in coastal embayments of Nova Scotia, in *Harmful Algal Blooms 2000. 9th International Conference on Harmful Microalgae*, Hallegraeff, G. M., Blackburn, S. I., Bolch, C. J., and Lewis, R. J., eds. Intergovernmental Oceanographic Commission of UNESCO, Paris, France, pp. 173–176.

223. Otofuji, T., Ogo, A., Koishi, J. et al., 1981. Food poisoning caused by *Atrina pectinata* in the Ariake Sea. *Food Sanit. Res.*, 31, 76–83.

224. Hui, J. P. M., Grossert, S. J., Cutler, M. J., and Melanson, J. E., 2012. Strategic identification of *in vitro* metabolites of 13-desmethyl spirolide C using liquid chromatography/high-resolution mass spectrometry. *Rapid Commun Mass Spectrom.*, 26, 345–354.

225. Bourne, Y., Radić, Z., Aráoz, R. et al., 2010. Structural determinants in phycotoxins and AChBP conferring high affinity binding and nicotinic AChR antagonism. *Proc. Natl. Acad. Sci. USA*, 107, 6076–6081.

226. Fonfría, E. S., Vilariño, N., Molgó, J. et al., 2010. Detection of 13,19-didesmethyl C spirolide by fluorescence polarization using *Torpedo* electrocyte membranes. *Anal. Biochem.*, 403, 102–107.

227. Araoz, R., Servent, D., Molgó, J. et al., 2011. Total synthesis of pinnatoxins A and G and revision of the mode of action of pinnatoxin A. *J. Am. Chem. Soc.*, 133, 10499–10511.

228. Hellyer, S. D., Selwood, A. I., Rhodes, L., and Kerr, D. S., 2011. Marine algal pinnatoxins E and F cause neuromuscular block in an *in vitro* hemidiaphragm preparation. *Toxicon*, 58, 693–699.

229. Wandscheer, C. B., Vilariño, N., Espiña, B., Louzao, M. C., and Botana, L. M., 2010. Human muscarinic acetylcholine receptors are a target of the marine toxin 13-desmethyl C spirolide. *Chem. Res. Toxicol.*, 23, 1753–1761.

230. Hauser, T. A., Hepler, C. D., Kombo, D. C. et al., 2012. Comparison of acetylcholine receptor interactions of the marine toxins, 13-desmethylspirolide C and gymnodimine. *Neuropharmacology*, 62, 2239–2250.

231. Duroure, L., Jousseaume, T., Aráoz, R. et al., 2011. 6,6-Spiroimine analogs of (-)-gymnodimine A: Synthesis and biological evaluation on nicotinic acetylcholine receptors. *Org. Biomol. Chem.*, 9, 8112–8118.

232. Vilariño, N., Fonfría, E. S., Molgó, J., Aráoz, R., and Botana, L. M., 2009. Detection of gymnodimine-A and 13-desmethyl C spirolide phycotoxins by fluorescence polarization. *Anal. Chem.*, 81, 2708–2714.

233. EFSA Panel on Contaminants in the Food Chain, 2010. Scientific opinion on marine biotoxins in shellfish—Cyclic imines (spirolides, gymnodimines, pinnatoxins and pteriatoxins). *EFSA J.*, 1628, 39.

234. Takemoto, T. and Daigo, K., 1958. Constituents of *Chondria armata. Chem. Pharm. Bull.*, 6, 578–580.

235. Trainer, V. L., Bates, S. S., Lundholm, N. et al., 2012. *Pseudo-nitzschia* physiological ecology, phylogeny, toxicity, monitoring and impacts on ecosystem health. *Harmful Algae*, 14, 271–300.

236. Holland, P. T., Selwood, A. I., Mountfort, D. O. et al., 2005. Isodomoic acid C, an unusual amnesic shellfish poisoning toxin from *Pseudo-nitzschia australis. Chem. Res. Toxicol.*, 18, 814–816.

237. Wright, J. L. C., Falk, M., McInnes, A. G., and Walter, J. A., 1990. Identification of isodomoic acid D and two new geometrical isomers of domoic acid in toxic mussels. *Can. J. Chem.*, 68, 22–25.

238. Kotaki, Y., Furio, E. F., Satake, M. et al., 2005. Production of isodomoic acids A and B as major toxin components of a pennate diatom *Nitzschia navis-varingica. Toxicon*, 46, 946–953.

239. Walter, J. A., Falk, M., and Wright, J. L. C., 1994. Chemistry of the shellfish toxin domoic acid: Characterization of related compounds. *Can. J. Chem.*, 72, 430–436.

240. Zaman, L., Arakawa, O., Shimosu, A. et al., 1997. Two new isomers of domoic acid from a red alga, *Chondria armata. Toxicon*, 35, 205–212.

241. Maeda, M., Kodama, T., Tanaka, T. et al., 1986. Structures of isodomoic acids A, B and C, novel insecticidal amino acids from the red alga *Chondria armata. Chem. Pharm. Bull.*, 34, 4892–4895.

242. Zhao, J.-Y., Thibault, P., and Quilliam, M. A., 1997. Analysis of domoic acid isomers in seafood by capillary electrophoresis. *Electrophoresis*, 18, 268–276.

243. Jeffery, B., Barlow, T., Moizer, K., Paul, S., and Boyle, C., 2004. Amnesic shellfish poison. *Food Chem. Toxicol.*, 42, 545–557.

244. Todd, E. C. D., 1993. Domoic acid and amnesic shellfish poisoning—A review. *J. Food Protect.*, 56, 69–83.

245. Doucette, T. A. and Tasker, R. A., 2008. Domoic acid: Detection methods, pharmacology, and toxicology, in *Seafood and Freshwater Toxins. Pharmacology, Physiology, and Detection*, 2nd edn., Botana, L. M., ed. CRC Press, Boca Raton, FL, pp. 397–429.
246. Iverson, F., Truelove, J., Nera, E., Tryphonas, L., Campbell, J., and Lok, E., 1989. Domoic acid poisoning and mussel-associated intoxication: Preliminary investigations into the response of mice and rats to toxic mussel extract. *Food Chem. Toxicol.*, 27, 377–384.
247. Peng, Y. G. and Ramsdell, J. S., 1996. Brain Fos induction is a sensitive biomarker for the lowest observed neuroexcitatory effects of domoic acid. *Toxicol. Sci.*, 31, 162–168.
248. Grimmelt, B., Nijjar, M. S., Brown, J. et al., 1990. Relationship between domoic acid levels in the blue mussel (*Mytilus edulis*) and toxicity in mice. *Toxicon*, 28, 501–508.
249. Nagatomo, I., Akasaki, Y., Uchida, M. et al., 1999. Kainic and domoic acids differentially affect NADPH-diaphorase neurons in the mouse hippocampal formation. *Brain Res. Bull.*, 48, 277–282.
250. Munday, R., Holland, P. T., McNabb, P., Selwood, A. I., and Rhodes, L. L., 2008. Comparative toxicity to mice of domoic acid and isodomoic acids A, B and C. *Toxicon*, 52, 954–956.
251. Sobotka, T. J., Brown, R., Quander, D. Y. et al., 1996. Domoic acid: Neurobehavioral and neurohistological effects of low-dose exposure in adult rats. *Neurotoxicol. Teratol.*, 18, 659–670.
252. Tryphonas, L., Truelove, J., Nera, E., and Iverson, F., 1990. Acute neurotoxicity of domoic acid in the rat. *Toxicol. Pathol.*, 18, 1–9.
253. Xi, D., Peng, Y.-G., and Ramsdell, J. S., 1997. Domoic acid is a potent neurotoxin to neonatal rats. *Nat. Toxins*, 5, 74–79.
254. Tryphonas, L., Truelove, J., and Iverson, F., 1990. Acute parenteral neurotoxicity of domoic acid in Cynomolgus monkeys (*M. fascicularis*). *Toxicol. Pathol.*, 18, 297–303.
255. Perez-Mendes, P., Cinini, S. M., Medeiros, M. A., Tufik, S., and Mello, L. E., 2005. Behavioral and histopathological analysis of domoic acid administration in marmosets. *Epilepsia*, 46, 148–151.
256. Tasker, R. A. R., Connell, B. J., and Strain, S. M., 1991. Pharmacology of systemically administered domoic acid in mice. *Can. J. Physiol. Pharmacol.*, 69, 378–382.
257. Tasker, R. A. R. and Strain, S. M., 1998. Synergism between NMDA and domoic acid in a murine model of behavioural neurotoxicity. *NeuroToxicology*, 19, 593–598.
258. Pulido, O., 2008. Domoic acid toxicologic pathology: A review. *Marine Drugs*, 6, 180–219.
259. Strain, S. M. and Tasker, R. A. R., 1991. Hippocampal damage produced by systemic injections of domoic acid in mice. *Neuroscience*, 44, 343–352.
260. Vranyac-Tramoundanus, A., Harrison, J. C., Sawant, P. M., Kerr, D. S., and Sammut, I. A., 2011. Ischemic cardiomyopathy following seizure induction by domoic acid. *Am. J. Path.*, 179, 141–154.
261. Glavin, G. B., Bose, R., and Pinsky, C., 1989. Kynurenic acid protects against gastroduodenal ulceration in mice injected with extracts from poisonous Atlantic shellfish. *Prog. Neuro-Psychopharmacol. Biol. Psychiat.*, 13, 569–572.
262. Glavin, G. B., Pinsky, C., and Bose, R., 1990. Domoic acid-induced neurovisceral toxic syndrome: Characterization of an animal model and putative antidotes. *Brain Res. Bull.*, 24, 701–703.
263. Hesp, B. R., Clarkson, A. N., Sawant, P. M., and Kerr, D. S., 2007. Domoic acid preconditioning and seizure induction in young and aged rats. *Epilepsy Res.*, 76, 103–112.
264. Petrie, B. F., Pinsky, C., Standish, N. M., Bose, R., and Glavin, G. B., 1992. Parenteral domoic acid impairs spatial learning in mice. *Pharmacol. Biochem. Behav.*, 41, 211–214.
265. Muha, N. and Ramsdell, J. S., 2011. Domoic acid induced seizures progress to a chronic state of epilepsy in rats. *Toxicon*, 57, 168–171.
266. Tryphonas, L., Truelove, J., Todd, E., Nera, E., and Iverson, F., 1990. Experimental oral toxicity of domoic acid in Cynomolgus monkeys (*Macaca fascicularis*) and rats: Preliminary investigations. *Food Chem. Toxicol.*, 28, 707–715.
267. Tryphonas, L., Truelove, J., Iverson, F., Todd, E. C., and Nera, E. A., 1990. Neuropathology of experimental domoic acid poisoning in non-human primates and rats. *Can. Dis. Wkly Rep.*, 16(Suppl. 1E), 75–81.
268. Silvagni, P. A., Lowenstine, L. J., Spraker, T., Lipscomb, T. P., and Gulland, F. M. D., 2005. Pathology of domoic acid toxicity in California sea lions (*Zalophus californianus*). *Vet. Path.*, 42, 184–191.
269. Zabka, T. S., Goldstein, T., Cross, C. et al., 2009. Characterization of a degenerative cardiomyopathy associated with domoic acid toxicity in California sea lions (*Zalophus californianus*). *Vet. Path.*, 46, 105–119.

270. Kreuder, C., Miller, M. A., Lowenstine, L. J. et al., 2005. Evaluation of cardiac lesion and risk factors associated with myocarditis and dilated cardiomyopathy in southern sea otters (*Enhydra lutris nereis*). *Am. J. Vet. Res.*, 66, 289–299.

271. Truelove, J. and Iverson, F., 1994. Serum domoic acid clearance and clinical observations in the Cynomolgus monkey and Sprague-Dawley rat following a single IV dose. *Bull. Environ. Contam. Toxicol.*, 52, 479–486.

272. Ananth, C., Dheen, S. T., Gopalakrishnakone, P., and Kaur, C., 2003. Distribution of NADPH-diaphorase and expression of nNOS, N-methyl-D-aspartate receptor (NMDAR1) and non-NMDA glutamate receptor (GlutR2) genes in the neurons of the hippocampus after domoic acid-induced lesions in adult rats. *Hippocampus*, 13, 260–272.

273. Truelove, J., Mueller, R., Pulido, O., and Iverson, F., 1996. Subchronic toxicity study of domoic acid in the rat. *Food Chem. Toxicol.*, 34, 525–529.

274. Truelove, J., Mueller, R., Pulido, O., Martin, L., Fernie, S., and Iverson, F., 1997. 30-Day oral toxicity study of domoic acid in Cynomolgus monkeys: Lack of overt toxicity at doses approaching the acute toxic dose. *Nat. Toxins*, 5, 111–114.

275. Gill, D. A., Ramsay, S. L., and Tasker, R. A., 2010. Selective reductions in subpopulations of GABAergic neurons in a developmental rat model of epilepsy. *Brain Res.*, 1331, 114–123.

276. Bernard, P. B., MacDonald, D. S., Gill, D. A., Ryan, C. L., and Tasker, R. A., 2007. Hippocampal mossy fiber sprouting and elevated trkB receptor expression following systemic administration of low dose domoic acid during neonatal development. *Hippocampus*, 17, 1121–1133.

277. Adams, A. L., Doucette, T. A., and Ryan, C. L., 2008. Altered pre-pulse inhibition in adult rats treated neonatally with domoic acid. *Amino Acids*, 35, 157–160.

278. Gill, D. A., Bastlund, J. F., Anderson, N. J., and Tasker, R. A., 2009. Reductions in paradoxical sleep time in adult rats treated neonatally with low dose domoic acid. *Behav. Brain Res.*, 205, 564–567.

279. Perry, M. A., Ryan, C. L., and Tasker, R. A., 2009. Effects of low dose neonatal domoic acid administration on behavioural and physiological response to mild stress in adult rats. *Physiol. Behav.*, 98, 53–59.

280. Burt, M. A., Ryan, C. L., and Doucette, T. A., 2008. Low dose domoic acid in neonatal rats abolishes nicotine induced conditioned place preference during late adolescence. *Amino Acids*, 35, 247–249.

281. Tasker, R. A. R., Perry, M. A., Doucette, T. A., and Ryan, C. L., 2005. NMDA receptor involvement in the effects of low dose domoic acid in neonatal rats. *Amino Acids*, 28, 193–196.

282. Adams, A. L., Doucette, T. A., James, R., and Ryan, C. L., 2009. Persistent changes in learning and memory in rats following neonatal treatment with domoic acid. *Physiol. Behav.*, 96, 505–512.

283. Doucette, T. A., Ryan, C. L., and Tasker, R. A., 2007. Gender-based changes in cognition and emotionality in a new rat model of epilepsy. *Amino Acids*, 32, 317–322.

284. Doucette, T. A., Bernard, P. B., Yuill, P. C., Tasker, R. A., and Ryan, C. L., 2003. Low doses of non-NMDA glutamate receptor agonists alter neurobehavioural development in the rat. *Neurotoxicol. Teratol.*, 25, 473–479.

285. Gill, D. A., Bastlund, J. F., Watson, W. P., Ryan, C. L., Reynolds, D. S., and Tasker, R. A., 2010. Neonatal exposure to low-dose domoic acid lowers seizure threshold in adult rats. *Neuroscience*, 169, 1789–1799.

286. Dakshinamurti, K., Sharma, S. K., Sundaram, M., and Watanabe, T., 1993. Hippocampal changes in developing postnatal mice following intrauterine exposure to domoic acid. *J. Neurosci.*, 13, 4486–4495.

287. Tanemura, K., Igarashi, K., Matsugami, T., Aisaki, K.-I., Kitajima, S., and Kanno, J. I., 2009. Intrauterine environment-genome interaction and children's development (2); brain structure impairment and behavioral disturbance induced in male mice offspring by a single intraperitoneal administration of domoic acid. *J. Toxicol. Sci.*, 34, SP279–SP286.

288. Levin, E. D., Pang, W. G., Harrison, J., Williams, P., Petro, A., and Ramsdell, J. S., 2006. Persistent neurobehavioral effects of early postnatal domoic acid exposure in rats. *Neurotoxicol. Teratol.*, 28, 673–680.

289. Levin, E. D., Pizarro, K., Pang, W. G., Harrison, J., and Ramsdell, J. S., 2005. Persisting behavioral consequences of prenatal domoic acid exposure in rats. *Neurotoxicol. Teratol.*, 27, 719–725.

290. Teitelbaum, J. S., Zatorre, R. J., Carpenter, S. et al., 1990. Neurologic sequelae of domoic acid intoxication due to the ingestion of contaminated mussels. *New Engl. J. Med.*, 322, 1781–1787.

291. Perl, T. M., Bédard, L., Kosatsky, T., Hockin, J. C., Todd, E. C. D., and Remis, R. S., 1990. An outbreak of toxic encephalopathy caused by eating mussels contaminated with domoic acid. *New Engl. J. Med.*, 322, 1775–1780.

292. Cendes, F., Andermann, F., Carpenter, S., Zatorre, R. J., and Cashman, N. R., 1995. Temporal lobe epilepsy caused by domoic acid intoxication: Evidence for glutamate receptor–mediated excitotoxicity in humans. *Ann. Neurol.*, 37, 123–126.

293. EFSA Panel on Contaminants in the Food Chain, 2009. Marine biotoxins in shellfish—Domoic acid. *EFSA J.*, 1181, 61 pp.

294. Squire, L. and Zola-Morgan, S., 1991. The medial temporal lobe memory system. *Science*, 253, 1380–1386.

295. FDA, 2001. *Fish and Fisheries Products Hazards and Controls Guidance*, 3rd edn. Appendix 5. http://www.fda.gov/Food/GuidanceComplianceRegulatoryInformation/GuidanceDocuments/Seafood/FishandFisheriesProductsHazardsandControlsGuide/ucm120108.htm

296. Preston, E. and Hynie, I., 1991. Transfer constants for blood-brain barrier permeation of the neuroexcitatory shellfish toxin, domoic acid. *Can. J. Neurol. Sci.*, 18, 39–44.

297. Smith, Q. R., 2000. Transport of glutamate and other amino acids at the blood-brain barrier. *J. Nutr.*, 130, 1016S–1022S.

298. Maucher, J. M. and Ramsdell, J. S., 2005. Ultrasensitive detection of domoic acid in mouse blood by competitive ELISA using blood collection cards. *Toxicon*, 45, 607–613.

299. Suzuki, C. A. M. and Hierlihy, S. L., 1993. Renal clearance of domoic acid in the rat. *Food Chem. Toxicol.*, 31, 701–706.

300. Maucher, J. M. and Ramsdell, J. S., 2005. Domoic acid transfer to milk: Evaluation of a potential route of neonatal exposure. *Environ. Health Perspect.*, 113, 461–464.

301. Maucher, J. M. and Ramsdell, J. S., 2007. Maternal-fetal transfer of domoic acid in rats at two gestational time points. *Environ. Health Perspect.*, 115, 1743–1746.

302. Nijjar, M. S. and Nijjar, S. S., 2000. Domoic acid-induced neurodegeneration resulting in memory loss is mediated by Ca^{2+} overload and inhibition of Ca^{2+} + calmodulin-stimulated adenylate cyclase in rat brain. *Int. J. Mol. Med.*, 6, 377–389.

303. Ananth, C., Gopalakrishnakone, P., and Charanjit, C., 2004. Domoic acid-induced neurotoxicity in the hippocampus of adult rats. *Neurotox. Res.*, 6, 105–117.

304. Bose, R., Schnell, C. L., Pinsky, C., and Zitko, V., 1992. Effects of excitotoxins on free radical indices in mouse brain. *Toxicol. Lett.*, 60, 211–219.

305. Boldyrev, A., Bulygina, E., and Makhro, A., 2004. Glutamate receptors modulate oxidative stress in neuronal cells. A mini-review. *Neurotox. Res.*, 6, 581–587.

306. Rogers, C. G. and Boyes, B. G., 1989. Evaluation of the genotoxicity of domoic acid in a hepatocyte-mediated assay with V79 Chinese hamster lung cells. *Mutat. Res. Lett.*, 226, 191–195.

307. Carvalho Pinto-Silva, C. R., Moukha, S., Matias, W. G., and Creppy, E. E., 2008. Domoic acid induces direct DNA damage and apoptosis in Caco-2 cells: Recent advances. *Environ. Toxicol.*, 23, 657–663.

308. Wekell, J. C., Hurst, J., and Lefebvre, K. A., 2004. The origin of the regulatory limits for PSP and ASP toxins in shellfish. *J. Shellfish Res.*, 23, 927–930.

309. European Parliament, 2004. Regulation (EC) No 853/2004 of the European Parliament and of the Council. Laying down specific hygiene rules for on the hygiene of foodstuffs. *Official Journal of the European Union*, L 139/55.

310. Report of the joint FAO/IOC/WHO ad hoc expert consultation on biotoxins in Bivalve Molluscs. Oslo, Norway, September 26–30, 2004. ftp://ftp.fao.org/es/esn/food/biotoxin_report_en.pdf

311. EFSA Panel on Contaminants in the Food Chain, 2010. Statement on further elaboration of the consumption figure of 400 g shellfish meat on the basis of new consumption data. *EFSA J.*, 1706, 20 pp.

312. Walter, J. A., Leek, D. M., and Falk, M., 1992. NMR study of the protonation of domoic acid. *Can. J. Chem.*, 70, 1156–1161.

313. Schwenk, M., 1987. Drug transport in intestine, liver and kidney. *Arch. Toxicol.*, 60, 37–42.

314. Chen, E., Mahar Doan, K., Portelli, S., Coatney, R., Vaden, V., and Shi, W., 2008. Gastric pH and gastric residence time in fasted and fed conscious Cynomolgus monkeys using the Bravo® pH system. *Pharmaceut. Res.*, 25, 123–134.

315. McConnell, E. L., Basit, A. W., and Murdan, S., 2008. Measurements of rat and mouse gastrointestinal pH, fluid and lymphoid tissue, and implications for in-vivo experiments. *J. Pharm. Pharmacol.*, 60, 63–70.

316. Mooradian, A. D., 1988. Effect of aging on the blood-brain barrier. *Neurobiol. Aging*, 9, 31–39.

317. Mayhan, W. G., 1990. Disruption of blood-brain barrier during acute hypertension in adult and aged rats. *Am. J. Physiol.*, 258, H1735–H1738.

318. Huber, J. D., VanGilder, R. L., and Houser, K. A., 2006. Streptozotocin-induced diabetes progressively increases blood-brain barrier permeability in specific brain regions in rats. *Am. J. Physiol.*, 291, H2660–H2668.

319. Saunders, N. R., Habgood, M. D., and Dziegielewska, K. M., 1999. Barrier mechanisms in the brain, II. Immature brain. *Clin. Exp. Pharmacol. Physiol.*, 26, 85–91.

320. Doucette, T. A., Strain, S. M., Allen, G. V., Ryan, C. L., and Tasker, R. A. R., 2000. Comparative behavioural toxicity of domoic acid and kainic acid in neonatal rats. *Neurotoxicol. Teratol.*, 22, 863–869.

321. Fuquay, J. M., Muha, N., Wang, Z., and Ramsdell, J. S., 2012. Toxicokinetics of domoic acid in the fetal rat. *Toxicology*, 294, 36–41.

322. Renwick, A. G., Dorne, J. L., and Walton, K., 2000. An analysis of the need for an additional uncertainty factor for infants and children. *Regulat. Toxicol. Pharmacol.*, 31, 286–296.

323. Grattan, L., Roberts, S., Trainer, V. et al., 2009. Domoic acid neurotoxicity in American Indians: Baseline characteristics of the coastal cohort. *Neurotoxicol. Teratol.*, 31, 239.

324. Grattan, L. M., Roberts, S., Trainer, V. et al., 2007. Domoic acid neurotoxicity in native Americans in the Pacific Northwest: Human health project methods and update, in *Fourth Symposium on Harmful Algae in the U.S.* http://www.whoi.edu/fileserver.do?id=34443&pt=2&p=28786

325. Reguera, B., Velo-Suárez, L., Raine, R., and Park, M. G., 2012. Harmful *Dinophysis* species: A review. *Harmful Algae*, 14, 87–106.

326. Hu, W., Xu, J., Sinkkonen, J., and Wu, J., 2010. Polyketides from marine dinoflagellates of the genus *Prorocentrum*, biosynthetic origin and bioactivity of their okadaic acid analogues. *Mini-Reviews Med. Chem.*, 10, 51–61.

327. Suzuki, T., Ota, H., and Yamasaki, M., 1999. Direct evidence of transformation of dinophysistoxin-1 to 7-*O*-acyl-dinophysistoxin-1 (dinophysistoxin-3) in the scallop *Patinopecten yessoensis*. *Toxicon*, 37, 187–198.

328. Aune, T., Larsen, S., Aasen, J. A. B., Rehmann, N., Satake, M., and Hess, P., 2007. Relative toxicity of dinophysistoxin-2 (DTX-2) compared with okadaic acid, based on acute intraperitoneal toxicity in mice. *Toxicon*, 49, 1–7.

329. Dickey, R. W., Bobzin, S. C., Faulkner, D. J., Bencsath, F. A., and Andrzejewski, D., 1990. Identification of okadaic acid from a Caribbean dinoflagellate, *Prorocentrum concavum*. *Toxicon*, 28, 371–377.

330. Tubaro, A., Sosa, S., Carbonatto, M. et al., 2003. Oral and intraperitoneal acute toxicity studies of yessotoxin and homoyessotoxins in mice. *Toxicon*, 41, 783–792.

331. Tachibana, K., Scheuer, P. J., Tsukitani, Y. et al., 1981. Okadaic acid, a cytotoxic polyether from two marine sponges of the genus *Halichondria*. *J. Am. Chem. Soc.*, 103, 2469–2471.

332. Yanagi, T., Murata, M., Torigoe, K., and Yasumoto, T., 1989. Biological activities of semisynthetic analogs of dinophysistoxin-3, the major diarrhetic shellfish toxin. *Agric. Biol. Chem.*, 53, 525–529.

333. Murata, M., Shimatani, M., Sugitani, H., Oshima, Y., and Yasumoto, T., 1982. Isolation and structural elucidation of the causative toxin of the diarrhetic shellfish poisoning. *Bull. Jap. Soc. Sci. Fish.*, 48, 549–552.

334. Yasumoto, T., Murata, M., Oshima, Y., Sano, M., Matsumoto, G. K., and Clardy, J., 1985. Diarrhetic shellfish toxins. *Tetrahedron* 41, 1019–1025.

335. Hu, T., Curtis, J. M., Walter, J. A., and Wright, J. L. C., 1995. Identification of DTX-4, a new water-soluble phosphatase inhibitor from the toxic dinoflagellate *Prorocentrum lima*. *Chem. Commun.*, 597–599.

336. Suzuki, H., 2012. Susceptibility of different mice strains to okadaic acid, a diarrhetic shellfish poisoning toxin. *Food Addit. Contam.*, 29, 1307–1310.

337. Terao, K., Ito, E., Yanagi, T., and Yasumoto, T., 1986. Histopathological studies on experimental marine toxin poisoning. I. Ultrastructural changes in the small intestine and liver of suckling mice induced by dinophysistoxin-1 and pectenotoxin-1. *Toxicon*, 24, 1141–1151.

338. Ito, E. and Terao, K., 1994. Injury and recovery process of intestine caused by okadaic acid and related compounds. *Nat. Toxins*, 2, 371–377.

339. Terao, K., Ito, E., Ohkusu, M., and Yasumoto, T., 1993. A comparative study of the effects of DSP-toxins on mice and rats, in *Toxic Phytoplankton Blooms in the Sea*, Smayda, T. J. and Shimizu, Y., eds. Elsevier, New York, pp. 581–586.

340. Ito, E., Yasumoto, T., Takai, A., Imanishi, S., and Harada, K., 2002. Investigation of the distribution and excretion of okadaic acid in mice using immunostaining method. *Toxicon*, 40, 159–165.

341. Le Hégarat, L., Jacquin, A.-G., Bazin, E., and Fessard, V., 2006. Genotoxicity of the marine toxin okadaic acid, in human Caco-2 cells and in mice gut cells. *Environ. Toxicol.*, 21, 55–64.

342. Ogino, H., Kumagai, M., and Yasumoto, T., 1997. Toxicologic evaluation of yessotoxin. *Nat. Toxins*, 5, 255–259.
343. Yuasa, H., Yoshida, K., Iwata, H., Nakanishi, H., Suganuma, M., and Tatematsu, M., 1994. Increase of labeling indices in gastrointestinal mucosae of mice and rats by compounds of the okadaic acid type. *J. Cancer Res. Clin. Oncol.*, 120, 208–212.
344. Berven, G., Sætre, F., Halvorsen, K., and Seglen, P. O., 2001. Effects of the diarrhetic shellfish toxin, okadaic acid, on cytoskeletal elements, viability and functionality of rat liver and intestinal cells. *Toxicon*, 39, 349–362.
345. Tubaro, A., Sosa, S., Altinier, G. et al., 2004. Short-term oral toxicity of homoyessotoxins, yessotoxin and okadaic acid in mice. *Toxicon*, 43, 439–445.
346. Suganuma, M., Fujiki, H., Suguri, H. et al., 1988. Okadaic acid: An additional non-phorbol-12-tetradecanoate-13-acetate-type tumor promoter. *Proc. Natl. Acad. Sci. USA*, 85, 1768–1771.
347. Fujiki, H., Suganuma, M., Suguri, H. et al., 1988. Diarrhetic shellfish toxin, dinophysistoxin-1, is a potent tumor promoter on mouse skin. *Jap. J. Cancer Res.*, 79, 1089–1093.
348. Suganuma, M., Tatematsu, M., Yatsunami, J. et al., 1992. An alternative theory of tissue specificity by tumor promotion of okadaic acid in glandular stomach of SD rats. *Carcinogenesis*, 13, 1841–1845.
349. Yasumoto, T., Oshima, Y., and Yamaguchi, M., 1978. Occurrence of a new type of shellfish poisoning in the Tohoku district. *Bull. Jap. Soc. Sci. Fish.*, 44, 1249–1255.
350. Picot, C., Nguyen, T. A., Roudot, A. C., and Parent-Massin, D., 2011. A preliminary risk assessment of human exposure to phycotoxins in shellfish: A review. *Hum. Ecol. Risk Assess.*, 17, 328–366.
351. Manerio, E., Rodas, V. L., Costas, E., and Hernandez, J. M., 2008. Shellfish consumption: A major risk factor for colorectal cancer. *Med. Hypoth.*, 70, 409–412.
352. López-Rodas, V., Maneiro, E., Martinez, J., Navarro, M., and Costas, E., 2006. Harmful algal blooms, red tides and human health: Diarrhetic shellfish poisoning and colorectal cancer. *An. Real Acad. Nac. Farm.*, 72, 391–408.
353. Cordier, S., Monfort, C., Miossec, L., Richardson, S., and Belin, C., 2000. Ecological analysis of digestive cancer mortality related to contamination by diarrhetic shellfish poisoning toxins along the coasts of France. *Environ. Res.*, 84, 145–150.
354. World Cancer Research Fund/American Institute for Cancer Research, 2007. *Food, Nutrition, Physical Activity, and the Prevention of Cancer: A Global Perspective*. AICR, Washington, DC.
355. Matias, W. G., Traore, A., and Creppy, E. E., 1999. Variations in the distribution of okadaic acid in organs and biological fluids of mice related to diarrhoeic syndrome. *Hum. Exp. Toxicol.*, 18, 345–350.
356. Matias, W. G. and Creppy, E. E., 1996. Evidence for enterohepatic circulation of okadaic acid in mice. *Toxic Subst. Mech.*, 15, 405–414.
357. Fujiki, H. and Suganuma, M., 1993. Tumor promotion by inhibitors of protein phosphatases 1 and 2A: The okadaic acid class of compounds. *Adv. Cancer Res.*, 61, 143–194.
358. Matias, W. and Creppy, E., 1996. Transplacental passage of [^{3}H]-okadaic acid in pregnant mice measured by radioactivity and high-performance liquid chromatography. *Hum. Exp. Toxicol.*, 15, 226–230.
359. Guo, F., An, T., and Rein, K. S., 2010. The algal hepatoxoxin okadaic acid is a substrate for human cytochromes CYP3A4 and CYP3A5. *Toxicon*, 55, 325–332.
360. Liu, L., Guo, F., Crain, S., Quilliam, M. A., and Wang, X., 2012. The structures of three metabolites of the algal hepatotoxin okadaic acid produced by oxidation with human cytochrome P450. *Bioorg. Med. Chem.*, 20, 3742–3745.
361. Hu, T., Curtis, J. M., Walter, J. A., McLachlan, J. L., and Wright, J. L. C., 1995. Two new water-soluble DSP toxin derivatives from the dinoflagellate *Prorocentrum maculosum*: Possible storage and excretion products. *Tetrahedron Lett.*, 36, 9273–9276.
362. Doucet, E., Ross, N. N., and Quilliam, M. A., 2007. Enzymatic hydrolysis of esterified diarrhetic shellfish poisoning toxins and pectenotoxins. *Anal. Bioanal. Chem.*, 389, 335–342.
363. García, C., Truan, D., Lagos, M., Santelices, J. P., Díaz, J. C., and Lagos, N., 2005. Metabolic transformation of dinophysistoxin-3 into dinophysistoxin-1 causes human intoxication by consumption of *O*-acyl-derivatives dinophysistoxins contaminated shellfish. *J. Toxicol. Sci.*, 30, 287–296.
364. Bialojan, C. and Takai, A., 1988. Inhibitory effect of a marine-sponge toxin, okadaic acid, on protein phosphatases. Specificity and kinetics. *Biochem. J.*, 256, 283–290.
365. Honkanen, R. E. and Golden, T., 2002. Regulators of serine/threonine protein phosphatases at the dawn of a clinical era? *Curr. Med. Chem.*, 9, 2055–2075.

366. Barford, D., 1995. Protein phosphatases. *Curr. Opin. Struct. Biol.*, 5, 728–734.

367. Holmes, C. F. B. and Boland, M. P., 1993. Inhibitors of protein phosphatase-1 and -2A; two of the major serine/threonine protein phosphatases involved in cellular regulation. *Curr. Opin. Struct. Biol.*, 3, 934–943.

368. Cohen, P., Holmes, C. F. B., and Tsukitani, Y., 1990. Okadaic acid: A new probe for the study of cellular regulation. *Trends Biochem. Sci.*, 15, 98–102.

369. Tripuraneni, J., Koutsouris, A., Pestic, L., De Lanerolle, P., and Hecht, G., 1997. The toxin of diarrheic shellfish poisoning, okadaic acid, increases intestinal epithelial paracellular permeability. *Gastroenterology*, 112, 100–108.

370. Hosokawa, M., Tsukada, H., Saitou, T. et al., 1998. Effects of okadaic acid on rat colon. *Dig. Dis. Sci.*, 43, 2526–2535.

371. Rossini, G. P. and Hess, P., 2010. Phycotoxins: Chemistry, mechanisms of action and shellfish poisoning, in *Molecular, Clinical and Environmental Toxicology. Volume 2: Clinical Toxicology*, Luch, A., ed. Birkhäuser, Basel, Switzerland, pp. 65–122.

372. Malaguti, C. and Rossini, G. P., 2002. Recovery of cellular E-cadherin precedes replenishment of estrogen receptor and estrogen-dependent proliferation of breast cancer cells rescued from a death stimulus. *J. Cell. Physiol.*, 192, 171–181.

373. Nunbhakdi-Craig, V., Machleidt, T., Ogris, E., Bellotto, D., White, C. L., and Sontag, E., 2002. Protein phosphatase 2A associates with and regulates atypical PKC and the epithelial tight junction complex. *J. Cell. Biol.*, 158, 967–978.

374. Ewe, K., 1988. Intestinal transport in constipation and diarrhoea. *Pharmacology*, 36(Suppl. I), 73–84.

375. Takai, A., Murata, M., Torigoe, K., Isobe, M., Mieskes, G., and Yasumoto, T., 1992. Inhibitory effect of okadaic acid derivatives on protein phosphatases. A study on structure-affinity relationship. *Biochem. J.*, 284, 539–544.

376. Nishiwaki, S., Fujiki, H., Suganuma, M. et al., 1990. Structure-activity relationship within a series of okadaic acid derivatives. *Carcinogenesis*, 11, 1837–1841.

377. Suganuma, M., Fujiki, H., Furuya-Suguri, H. et al., 1990. Calyculin A, an inhibitor of protein phosphatases, a potent tumor promoter on CD-1 mouse skin. *Cancer Res.*, 50, 3521–3525.

378. Ohta, T., Sueoka, E., Iida, N. et al., 1994. Nodularin, a potent inhibitor of protein phosphatases 1 and 2A, is a new environmental carcinogen in male F344 rat liver. *Cancer Res.*, 54, 6402–6406.

379. Nishiwaki-Matsushima, R., Ohta, T., Nishiwaki, S. et al., 1992. Liver tumor promotion by the cyanobacterial cyclic peptide toxin microcystin-LR. *J. Cancer Res. Clin. Oncol.*, 118, 420–424.

380. Suganuma, M., Okabe, S., Sueoka, E. et al., 1995. Tautomycin: An inhibitor of protein phosphatases 1 and 2A but not a tumor promoter on mouse skin and in rat glandular stomach. *J. Cancer Res. Clin. Oncol.*, 121, 621–627.

381. Fujiki, H., Suganuma, M., Suguri, H. et al., 1987. Induction of ornithine decarboxylase activity in mouse skin by a possible tumor promoter, okadaic acid. *Proc. Jpn. Acad. Ser. B*, 63, 51–53.

382. Fujiki, H. and Suganuma, M., 1999. Unique features of the okadaic acid activity class of tumor promoters. *J. Cancer Res. Clin. Oncol.*, 125, 150–155.

383. Suganuma, M., Okabe, S., Marino, M. W., Sakai, A., Sueoka, E., and Fujiki, H., 1999. Essential role of tumor necrosis factor α (TNF-α) in tumor promotion as revealed by TNF-α-deficient mice. *Cancer Res.*, 59, 4516–4518.

384. Fujiki, H., Sueoka, E., Komori, A., and Suganuma, M., 1997. Tumor promotion and TNF-α gene expression by the okadaic acid class tumor promoters. *Environ. Carcinogen. Ecotox. Rev.*, C15, 1–40.

385. Fujiki, H., Suganuma, M., Okabe, S. et al., 2000. A new concept of tumor promotion by tumor necrosis factor-α, and cancer preventive agents (−)-epigallocatechin gallate and green tea—A review. *Cancer Detect. Prev.*, 24, 91–99.

386. Corsini, E. and Galli, C. L., 1998. Cytokines and irritant contact dermatitis. *Toxicol. Lett.*, 102–103, 277–282.

387. Lewis, R. W., McCall, J. C., Botham, P. A., and Kimber, I., 1993. Investigation of TNF-α release as a measure of skin irritancy. *Toxicol. In Vitro*, 7, 393–395.

388. Fujiki, H., Suganuma, M., Hakii, H. et al., 1984. A two-stage mouse skin carcinogenesis study of lyngbyatoxin A. *J. Cancer Res. Clin. Oncol.*, 108, 174–176.

389. Fujiki, H., Suganuma, M., Nakayasu, M. et al., 1986. Palytoxin is a non-12-*O*-tetradecanoylphorbol-13-acetate type tumor promotor in two-stage mouse skin carcinogenesis. *Carcinogenesis*, 7, 707–710.

390. Aonuma, S., Ushijima, T., Nakayasu, M., Shima, H., Sugimura, T., and Nagao, M., 1991. Mutation induction by okadaic acid, a protein phosphatase inhibitor, in CHL cells, but not in *S. typhimurium*. *Mutat. Res.*, 250, 375–381.

391. Peuch, L., 2000. Etude de l'acide okadaïque, une phycotoxine marine: développement de techniques analytiques et évaluation du potentiel genotoxique. PhD thesis, University of Paris, Paris, France, cited by Le Hégarat et al., reference 341.

392. Carvalho Pinto-Silva, C. R., Catia, R., Moukha, S., Matias, W., and Creppy, E., 2006. Comparative study of domoic acid and okadaic acid induced–chromosomal abnormalities in the CACO-2 cell line. *Int. J. Environ. Res. Public Health*, 3, 4–10.

393. Le Hégarat, L., Fessard, V., Poul, J. M., Dragacci, S., and Sanders, P., 2004. Marine toxin okadaic acid induces aneuploidy in CHO-K1 cells in presence of rat liver postmitochondrial fraction, revealed by cytokinesis-block micronucleus assay coupled to FISH. *Environ. Toxicol.*, 19, 123–128.

394. Le Hégarat, L., Puech, L., Fessard, V., Poul, J. M., and Dragacci, S., 2003. Aneugenic potential of okadaic acid revealed by the micronucleus assay combined with the FISH technique in CHO-K1 cells. *Mutagenesis*, 18, 293–298.

395. Valdiglesias, V., Laffon, B., Pásaro, E., and Méndez, J., 2011. Evaluation of okadaic acid-induced genotoxicity in human cells using the micronucleus test and γH2AX analysis. *J. Toxicol. Environ. Health, Part A*, 74, 980–992.

396. Fessard, V., Grosse, Y., Pfohl-Leszkowicz, A., and Puiseux-Dao, S., 1996. Okadaic acid treatment induces DNA adduct formation in BHK21 C13 fibroblasts and HESV keratinocytes. *Mutat. Res.*, 361, 133–141.

397. Traoré, A., Baudrimont, I., Ambaliou, S., Dano, S. D., and Creppy, E. E., 2001. DNA breaks and cell cycle arrest induced by okadaic acid in Caco-2 cells, a human colonic epithelial cell line. *Arch. Toxicol.*, 75, 110–117.

398. Valdiglesias, V., Laffon, B., Pásaro, E., Cemeli, E., Anderson, D., and Méndez, J., 2011. Induction of oxidative DNA damage by the marine toxin okadaic acid depends on human cell type. *Toxicon*, 57, 882–888.

399. Valdiglesias, V., Méndez, J., Pásaro, E., Cemeli, E., Anderson, D., and Laffon, B., 2010. Assessment of okadaic acid effects on cytotoxicity, DNA damage and DNA repair in human cells. *Mutat. Res.*, 689, 74–79.

400. Le Hégarat, L., Nesslany, F., Mourot, A., Marzin, D., and Fessard, V., 2004. Lack of DNA damage induction by okadaic acid, a marine toxin, in the CHO-Hprt and the in vitro UDS assays. *Mutat. Res.*, 564, 139–147.

401. Souid-Mensi, G., Moukha, S., Mobio, T. A., Maaroufi, K., and Creppy, E. E., 2008. The cytotoxicity and genotoxicity of okadaic acid are cell-line dependent. *Toxicon*, 51, 1338–1344.

402. EFSA Panel on Contaminants in the Food Chain, 2008. Marine biotoxins in shellfish—Okadaic acid and analogues. *EFSA J.*, 589, 62 pp.

403. Moore, R. E. and Scheuer, P. J., 1971. Palytoxin: A new marine toxin from a coelenterate. *Science*, 172, 495–498.

404. Uemura, D., Ueda, K., and Hirata, Y., 1981. Further studies on palytoxin. II. Structure of palytoxin. *Tetrahedron Lett.*, 22, 2781–2784.

405. Cha, J. K., Christ, W. J., Finan, J. M. et al., 1982. Stereochemistry of palytoxin. 4. Complete structure. *J. Am. Chem. Soc.*, 104, 7369–7371.

406. Attaway, D. H. and Ciereszko, L. S., 1974. Isolation and partial characterization of Caribbean palytoxin, in *Proceedings of the 2nd International Coral Reef Symposium*, Cameron, A. M., Cambell, B. M., Cribb, A. B. et al., eds. Brisbane, Queensland, Australia, pp. 497–504.

407. Quinn, R. J., Kashiwagi, M., Moore, R. E., and Norton, T. R., 1974. Anticancer activity of zoanthids and the associated toxin, palytoxin, against Ehrlich ascites tumor and P-388 lymphocytic leukemia in mice. *J. Pharm. Sci.*, 63, 257–260.

408. Oku, N., Sata, N. U., Matsunaga, S., Uchida, H., and Fusetani, N., 2004. Identification of palytoxin as a principle which causes morphological changes in rat 3Y1 cells in the zoanthid *Palythoa* aff. *margaritae*. *Toxicon*, 43, 21–25.

409. Béress, L., Zwick, J., Kolkenbrock, H. J., Kaul, P. N., and Wassermann, O., 1983. A method for the isolation of the Caribbean palytoxin (C-PTX) from the coelenterate (zoanthid) *Palythoa caribaeorum*. *Toxicon*, 21, 285–290.

410. Moore, R. E. and Bartolini, G., 1981. Structure of palytoxin. *J. Am. Chem. Soc.*, 103, 2491–2494.

411. Uemura, D., Hirata, Y., Iwashita, T., and Naoki, H., 1985. Studies on palytoxins. *Tetrahedron*, 41, 1007–1017.

412. Ciminiello, P., Dell'Aversano, C., Dello Iacovo, E. et al., 2009. Stereostructure and biological activity of 42-hydroxy-palytoxin: A new palytoxin analogue from Hawaiian *Palythoa* subspecies. *Chem. Res. Toxicol.*, 22, 1851–1859.

413. Mahnir, V. M., Kozlovskaya, E. P., and Kalinovsky, A. I., 1992. Sea anemone *Radianthus macrodactylus*—A new source of palytoxin. *Toxicon*, 30, 1449–1456.

414. Maeda, M., Kodama, T., Tanaka, T. et al., 1985. Structures of insecticidal substances isolated from red alga, *Chondria armata*, in *Proceedings of the 27th Symposium on the Chemistry of Natural Products*, Tanaka, O., ed. Hiroshima, Japan, pp. 616–623.

415. Rhodes, L., 2011. World-wide occurrence of the toxic dinoflagellate genus *Ostreopsis* Schmidt. *Toxicon*, 57, 400–407.

416. Usami, M., Satake, M., Ishida, S., Inoue, A., Kan, Y., and Yasumoto, T., 1995. Palytoxin analogs from the dinoflagellate *Ostreopsis siamensis*. *J. Am. Chem. Soc.*, 117, 5389–5390.

417. Ukena, T., Satake, M., Usami, M. et al., 2001. Structure elucidation of ostreocin D, a palytoxin analog isolated from the dinoflagellate *Ostreopsis siamensis*. *Biosci. Biotechnol. Biochem.*, 65, 2585–2588.

418. Ukena, T., Satake, M., Usami, M. et al., 2002. Structural confirmation of ostreocin-D by application of negative-ion fast-atom bombardment collision-induced dissociation tandem mass spectrometric methods. *Rapid Commun. Mass Spectrom.*, 16, 2387–2393.

419. Rhodes, L., Towers, N., Briggs, L., Munday, R., and Adamson, J., 2002. Uptake of palytoxin-like compounds by shellfish fed *Ostreopsis siamensis* (Dinophyceae). *N. Z. J. Marine Freshw. Res.*, 36, 631–636.

420. Lenoir, S., Ten-Hage, L., Turquet, J., Quod, J.-P., Bernard, C., and Hennion, M.-C., 2004. First evidence of palytoxin analogues from an *Ostreopsis mascarenensis* (Dinophyceae) benthic bloom in southwestern Indian Ocean. *J. Phycol.*, 40, 1042–1051.

421. Ciminiello, P., Dell'Aversano, C., Fattorusso, E. et al., 2008. Putative palytoxin and its new analogue, ovatoxin-a, in *Ostreopsis ovata* collected along the Ligurian coasts during the 2006 toxic outbreak. *J. Am. Soc. Mass Spec.*, 19, 111–120.

422. Ciminiello, P., Dell'Aversano, C., Dello Iacovo, E. et al., 2011. Isolation and structure elucidation of ovatoxin-a, the major toxin produced by *Ostreopsis ovata*. *J. Am. Chem. Soc.*, 134, 1869–1875.

423. Honsell, G., De Bortoli, M., Boscolo, S. et al., 2011. Harmful dinoflagellate *Ostreopsis* cf. *ovata* Fukuyo: Detection of ovatoxins in field samples and cell immunolocalization using antipalytoxin antibodies. *Environ. Sci. Technol.*, 45, 7051–7059.

424. Rossi, R., Castellano, V., Scalco, E., Serpe, L., Zingone, A., and Soprano, V., 2010. New palytoxin-like molecules in Mediterranean *Ostreopsis* cf. *ovata* (dinoflagellates) and in *Palythoa tuberculosa* detected by liquid chromatography-electrospray ionization time-of-flight mass spectrometry. *Toxicon*, 56, 1381–1387.

425. Ciminiello, P., Dell'Aversano, C., Iacovo, E. D. et al., 2012. Unique toxin profile of a Mediterranean *Ostreopsis* cf. *ovata* strain: HR LC-MS^n characterization of ovatoxin-f, a new palytoxin congener. *Chem. Res. Toxicol.*, 25, 1243–1252.

426. Nascimento, S. M., Corrêa, E. V., Menezes, M., Varela, D., Paredes, J., and Morris, S., 2012. Growth and toxin profile of *Ostreopsis* cf. *ovata* (Dinophyta) from Rio de Janeiro, Brazil. *Harmful Algae*, 13, 1–9.

427. Suzuki, T., Watanabe, R., Uchida, H. et al., 2012. LC-MS/MS analysis of novel ovatoxin isomers in several *Ostreopsis* strains collected in Japan. *Harmful Algae*, 20, 81–91.

428. Ciminiello, P., Dell'Aversano, C., Iacovo, E. D., Fattorusso, E., Forino, M., and Tartaglione, L., 2011. LC-MS of palytoxin and its analogues: State of the art and future perspectives. *Toxicon*, 57, 376–389.

429. Kerbrat, A. S., Amzil, Z., Pawlowiez, R. et al., 2011. First evidence of palytoxin and 42-hydroxy-palytoxin in the marine cyanobacterium *Trichodesmium*. *Marine Drugs*, 9, 543–560.

430. Moore, R. E., Helfrich, P., and Patterson, G. M. L., 1982. The deadly seaweed of Hana. *Oceanus*, 25, 54–63.

431. Frolova, G. M., Kuznetsova, T. A., Mikhailov, V. V., and Elyakov, G. B., 2000. An enzyme linked immunosorbent assay for detecting palytoxin-producing bacteria. *Russ. J. Bioorg. Chem.*, 26, 285–289.

432. Seemann, P., Gernert, C., Schmitt, S., Mebs, D., and Hentschel, U., 2009. Detection of hemolytic bacteria from *Palythoa caribaeorum* (Cnidaria, Zoantharia) using a novel palytoxin-screening assay. *Antonie van Leeuwenhoek*, 96, 405–411.

433. Mebs, D., 1998. Occurrence and sequestration of toxins in food chains. *Toxicon*, 36, 1519–1522.

434. Gleibs, S. and Mebs, D., 1999. Distribution and sequestration of palytoxin in coral reef animals. *Toxicon*, 37, 1521–1527.

435. Gleibs, S., Mebs, D., and Werding, B., 1995. Studies on the origin and distribution of palytoxin in a Caribbean coral reef. *Toxicon*, 33, 1531–1537.

436. Hashimoto, Y., Fusetani, N., and Kimura, S., 1969. Aluterin: A toxin of filefish, *Alutera scripta*, probably originating from a Zoantharian, *Palythoa tuberculosa*. *Bull. Jap. Soc. Sci. Fish.*, 35, 1086–1093.

437. Onuma, Y., Satake, M., Ukena, T. et al., 1999. Identification of putative palytoxin as the cause of clupeotoxism. *Toxicon*, 37, 55–65.

438. Noguchi, T., Hwang, D.-F., Arakawa, O. et al., 1987. Palytoxin as the causative agent in the parrotfish poisoning, in *Proceedings, First Asia-Pacific Congress on Animal, Plant and Microbial Toxins*, Gopalakrishnakone, P. and Tan, C. K., eds. Singapore, pp. 325–335.

439. Taniyama, S., Arakawa, O., Terada, M. et al., 2003. *Ostreopsis* sp., a possible origin of palytoxin (PTX) in parrotfish *Scarus ovifrons*. *Toxicon*, 42, 29–33.

440. Fukui, M., Murata, M., Inoue, A., Gawel, M., and Yasumoto, T., 1987. Occurrence of palytoxin in the trigger fish *Melichtys vidua*. *Toxicon*, 25, 1121–1124.

441. Taniyama, S., Mahmud, Y., Terada, M., Takatani, T., Arakawa, O., and Noguchi, T., 2002. Occurrence of a food poisoning incident by palytoxin from a serranid *Epinephelus* sp. in Japan. *J. Nat. Toxins*, 11, 277–282.

442. Taniyama, S., Mahmud, Y., Tanu, M. B., Takatani, T., Arakawa, O., and Noguchi, T., 2001. Delayed haemolytic activity by the freshwater puffer *Tetraodon* sp. toxin. *Toxicon*, 39, 725–727.

443. Wachi, K. M., Hokama, Y., Haga, L. S. et al., 2000. Evidence for palytoxin as one of the sheep erythrocyte lytic in lytic factors in crude extracts of ciguateric and non-ciguateric reef fish tissue. *J. Nat. Toxins*, 9, 139–146.

444. Wachi, K. M. and Hokama, Y., 2001. Diversity of marine biotoxins in the near-shore ocean area: Presence of a palytoxin-like entity at Barber's Point Harbor, Oahu. *J. Nat. Toxins*, 10, 317–333.

445. Hokama, Y., Nishimura, K. L., Takenaka, W. E., and Ebesu, J. S. M., 1997. Latex antibody test (LAT) for detection of marine toxins in ciguateric fish. *J. Nat. Toxins*, 6, 35–50.

446. Yasumoto, T., Yasumura, D., Ohizumi, Y., Takahashi, M., Alcala, A. C., and Alcala, L. C., 1986. Palytoxin in two species of xanthid crab from the Philippines. *Agric. Biol. Chem.*, 50, 163–167.

447. Lau, C. O., Tan, C. H., Khoo, H. E. et al., 1995. *Lophozozymus pictor* toxin: A fluorescent structural isomer of palytoxin. *Toxicon*, 33, 1373–1377.

448. Alcala, A. C., Alcala, L. C., Garth, J. S., Yasumura, D., and Yasumoto, T., 1988. Human fatality due to ingestion of the crab *Demania reynaudii* that contained a palytoxin-like toxin. *Toxicon*, 26, 105–107.

449. Chia, D. G. B., Lau, C. O., Ng, P. K. L., and Tan, C. H., 1993. Localization of toxins in the poisonous mosaic crab, *Lophozozymus pictor* (Fabricius, 1798) (Brachyura, Xanthidae). *Toxicon*, 31, 901–904.

450. Aligizaki, K., Katikou, P., Nikolaidis, G., and Panou, A., 2008. First episode of shellfish contamination by palytoxin-like compounds from *Ostreopsis* species (Aegean Sea, Greece). *Toxicon*, 51, 418–427.

451. Amzil, Z., Sibat, M., Chomerat, N. et al., 2012. Ovatoxin-a and palytoxin accumulation in seafood in relation to *Ostreopsis* cf. *ovata* blooms on the French Mediterranean coast. *Marine Drugs*, 10, 477–496.

452. Aligizaki, K., Katikou, P., Milandri, A., and Diogène, J., 2011. Occurrence of palytoxin-group toxins in seafood and future strategies to complement the present state of the art. *Toxicon*, 57, 390–399.

453. Tindall, D. R., Miller, D. M., and Tindall, P. M., 1990. Toxicity of *Ostreopsis lenticularis* from the British and United States Virgin Islands, in *Toxic Marine Phytoplankton*, Graneli, E., Sundstrom, B., Edler, L., and Anderson, D. M., eds. Elsevier, New York, pp. 424–429.

454. Munday, R., 2008. Occurrence and toxicology of palytoxins, in *Seafood and Freshwater Toxins. Pharmacology, Physiology and Detection*, 2nd edn. Botana, L. M., ed. CRC Press, Boca Raton, FL, pp. 693–713.

455. Munday, R., 2011. Palytoxin toxicology: Animal studies. *Toxicon*, 57, 470–477.

456. Ito, E., Ohkusu, M., and Yasumoto, T., 1996. Intestinal injuries caused by experimental palytoxicosis in mice. *Toxicon*, 34, 643–652.

457. Kaul, P. N., Farmer, M. R., and Ciereszko, L. S., 1974. Pharmacology of palytoxin: The most potent marine toxin known. *Proc. West. Pharmacol. Soc.*, 17, 294–301.

458. Riobó, P., Paz, B., Franco, J. M., Vázquez, J. A., Murado, M. A., and Cacho, E., 2008. Mouse bioassay for palytoxin. Specific symptoms and dose-response against dose-death time relationships. *Food Chem. Toxicol.*, 46, 2639–2647.

459. Kimura, S. and Hashimoto, Y., 1973. Purification of the toxin in a zoanthid *Palythoa tuberculosa*. *Publ. Seto Marine Biol. Lab.*, 20, 713–718.

460. Sosa, S., Del Favero, G., De Bortoli, M. et al., 2009. Palytoxin toxicity after acute oral administration in mice. *Toxicol. Lett.*, 191, 253–259.

461. Tubaro, A., Del Favero, G., Beltramo, D. et al., 2011. Acute oral toxicity in mice of a new palytoxin analog: 42-Hydroxy-palytoxin. *Toxicon*, 57, 755–763.

462. Terao, K. K., Ito, E., and Yasumoto, T., 1992. Light and electron microscopic observation of experimental palytoxin poisoning in mice. *Bull. Soc. Path. Ex.*, 85, 494–496.

463. Ito, E., Ohkusu, M., Terao, K., and Yasumoto, T., 1997. Effects of repeated injections of palytoxin on lymphoid tissues in mice. *Toxicon*, 35, 679–688.

464. Deeds, J. R. and Schwartz, M. D., 2010. Human risk associated with palytoxin exposure. *Toxicon*, 56, 150–162.

465. Tubaro, A., Durando, P., Del Favero, G. et al., 2011. Case definitions for human poisonings postulated to palytoxins exposure. *Toxicon*, 57, 478–495.

466. Tichadou, L., Glaizal, M., Armengaud, A. et al., 2010. Health impact of unicellular algae of the *Ostreopsis* genus blooms in the Mediterranean Sea: Experience of the French Mediterranean coast surveillance network from 2006 to 2009. *Clin. Toxicol.*, 48, 839–844.

467. Mangialajo, L., Ganzin, N., Accoroni, S. et al., 2011. Trends in *Ostreopsis* proliferation along the northern Mediterranean coasts. *Toxicon*, 57, 408–420.

468. Pfannkuchen, M., Godrijan, J., Marić Pfannkuchen, D. et al., 2012. Toxin-producing *Ostreopsis* cf. *ovata* are likely to bloom undetected along coastal areas. *Environ. Sci. Technol.*, 46, 5574–5582.

469. Snoeks, L. and Veenstra, J., 2012. Een gezin met koorts na reiniging van zeeaquarium. *Ned. Tijdschr. Geneeskunde*, 156, 526–528.

470. Hoffmann, K., Hermanns-Clausen, M., Buhl, C. et al., 2008. A case of palytoxin poisoning due to contact with zoanthid corals through a skin injury. *Toxicon*, 51, 1535–1537.

471. Moshirfar, M., Khalifa, Y. M., Espandar, L., and Mifflin, M. D., 2010. Aquarium coral keratoconjunctivitis. *Arch. Ophthalmol.*, 128, 1360–1362.

472. Bellocci, M., Sala, G. L., and Prandi, S., 2011. The cytolytic and cytotoxic activities of palytoxin. *Toxicon*, 57, 449–459.

473. Bignami, G. S., 1993. A rapid and sensitive hemolysis neutralization assay for palytoxin. *Toxicon*, 31, 817–820.

474. Rossini, G. P. and Bigiani, A., 2011. Palytoxin action on the Na^+,K^+-ATPase and the disruption of ion equilibria in biological systems. *Toxicon*, 57, 429–439.

475. EFSA Panel on Contaminants in the Food Chain, 2009. Scientific opinion on marine biotoxins in shellfish—Palytoxin group. *EFSA J.*, 1393, 38 pp.

476. Pagnon, J., Karunasinghe, N., and Ferguson, L. R., 2008, Genetic Toxicology Report. Ames bacterial mutagenicity tests, palytoxin. Technical Report, University of Auckland, Auckland, New Zealand, 2008.

477. Ito, E. and Yasumoto, T., 2009. Toxicological studies on palytoxin and ostreocin-D administered to mice by three different routes. *Toxicon*, 54, 244–251.

478. Rathbone, M. J., Drummond, B. K., and Tucker, I. G., 1994. The oral cavity as a site for systemic drug delivery. *Adv. Drug Deliv. Rev.*, 13, 1–22.

479. Shojaei, A. H., 1998. Buccal mucosa as a route for systemic drug delivery: A review. *J. Pharm. Pharmaceut. Sci.*, 1, 15–30.

480. Harris, D. and Robinson, J. R., 1992. Drug delivery via the mucous membranes of the oral cavity. *J. Pharm. Sci.*, 81, 1–10.

481. Siegel, I. A., Izutsu, K. T., and Watson, E., 1981. Mechanisms of non-electrolyte penetration across dog and rabbit oral mucosa *in vitro. Arch. Oral Biol.*, 26, 357–361.

482. Batheja, P., Thakur, R., and Michniak, B., 2007. Basic biopharmaceutics of buccal and sublingual absorption, in *Enhancement in Drug Delivery*, Touitou, E. and Barry, B. W., eds. Taylor & Francis Group, Boca Raton, FL, pp. 175–202.

483. Kokate, A., Li, X., Williams, P. J., Singh, P., and Jasti, B. R., 2009. *In silico* prediction of drug permeability across buccal mucosa. *Pharm. Res.*, 26, 1130–1139.

484. Munday, R., 2008. Toxicology of the pectenotoxins, in *Seafood and Freshwater Toxins. Pharmacology, Physiolology, and Detection*, 2nd edn., Botana, L. M., ed. CRC Press, Boca Raton, FL, pp. 371–380.

485. Blanco, J., Álvarez, G., and Uribe, E., 2007. Identification of pectenotoxins in plankton, filter feeders, and isolated cells of a *Dinophysis acuminata* with an atypical toxin profile, from Chile. *Toxicon*, 49, 710–716.

486. Lee, K. J., Mok, J. S., Song, K. C., Yu, H., Jung, J. H., and Kim, J. H., 2011. Geographical and annual variation in lipophilic shellfish toxins from oysters and mussels along the south coast of Korea. *J. Food Protect.*, 74, 2127–2133.

487. Yasumoto, T., Murata, M., Lee, J.-S., and Torigoe, K., 1988. Polyether toxins produced by dinoflagellates, in *Seventh International IUPAC Symposium on Mycotoxins and Phycotoxins '88*, Natori, S., Hashimoto, K., and Ueno, Y., eds. Tokyo, Japan, pp. 375–382.

488. Miles, C. O., Wilkins, A. L., Munday, R. et al., 2004. Isolation of pectenotoxin-2 from *Dinophysis acuta* and its conversion to pectenotoxin-2 seco acid, and preliminary assessment of their acute toxicities. *Toxicon*, 43, 1–9.

489. Yoon, M. I. and Kim, Y. C., 1997. Acute toxicity of pectenotoxin 2 and its effects on hepatic metabolizing enzyme system in mice. *Korean J. Toxicol.*, 13, 183–186.

490. Murata, M., Sano, M., Iwashita, T., Naoki, H., and Yasumoto, T., 1986. The structure of pectenotoxin-3, a new constituent of diarrhetic shellfish toxins. *Agric. Biol. Chem.*, 50, 2693–2695.

491. Sasaki, K., Wright, J. L. C., and Yasumoto, T., 1998. Identification and characterization of pectenotoxin (PTX) 4 and PTX7 as spiroketal stereoisomers of two previously reported pectenotoxins. *J. Org. Chem.*, 63, 2475–2480.

492. Suzuki, T., Walter, J. A., LeBlanc, P. et al., 2006. Identification of pectenotoxin-11 as 34S-hydroxypectenotoxin-2, a new pectenotoxin analogue in the toxic dinoflagellate *Dinophysis acuta* from New Zealand. *Chem. Res. Toxicol.*, 19, 310–318.

493. Miles, C. O., Wilkins, A. L., Munday, J. S. et al., 2006. Production of 7-*epi*-pectenotoxin-2 seco acid and assessment of its acute toxicity in mice. *J. Agric. Food Chem.*, 54, 1530–1534.

494. Ito, E., Suzuki, T., Oshima, Y., and Yasumoto, T., 2008. Studies of diarrhetic activity on pectenotoxin-6 in the mouse and rat. *Toxicon*, 51, 707–716.

495. Ishige, M., Satoh, N., and Yasumoto, T., 1988. Pathological studies on the mice administrated with the causative agent of diarrhetic shellfish poisoning (okadaic acid and pectenotoxin-2). Report, Hokkaido Institute of Public Health, Number 38, pp. 15–18.

496. Burgess, V., Seawright, A., Eaglesham, G., Shaw, G., and Moore, M., 2002. The acute oral toxicity of the shellfish toxins pectenotoxin-2 seco acid and 7-*epi*-pectenotoxin-2 seco acid in mice, in *4th International Conference on Molluscan Shellfish Safety*, Villalba, A., Reguera, B., Romalde, J. L., and Beiras, R., eds., Santiago de Compostela, Galicia, Spain.

497. Burgess, V. A., 2003. Toxicology investigations with the pectenotoxin-2 seco acids, PhD thesis, Griffith University, Nathan, Queensland, Australia. http://www4.gu.edu.au:8080/adt-root/public/adt-QGU20030905.090222/

498. Burgess, V. and Shaw, G., 2001. Pectenotoxins—An issue for public health. A review of their comparative toxicology and metabolism. *Environ. Int.*, 27, 275–283.

499. Chae, H.-D., Choi, T.-S., Kim, B.-M., Jung, J. H., Bang, Y.-J., and Shin, D. Y., 2005. Oocyte-based screening of cytokinesis inhibitors and identification of pectenotoxin-2 that induces Bim/Bax-mediated apoptosis in p53-deficient tumors. *Oncogene*, 24, 4813–4819.

500. Espiña, B., Louzao, M. C., Ares, I. R. et al., 2008. Cytoskeletal toxicity of pectenotoxins in hepatic cells. *Br. J. Pharmacol.*, 155, 934–944.

501. Espiña, B., Louzao, M. C., Ares, I. R. et al., 2010. Impact of the pectenotoxin C-43 oxidation degree on its cytotoxic effect on rat hepatocytes. *Chem. Res. Toxicol.*, 23, 504–515.

502. Ares, I. R., Louzao, M. C., Espiña, B. et al., 2007. Lactone ring of pectenotoxins: A key factor for their activity on cytoskeletal dynamics. *Cell. Physiol. Biochem.*, 19, 283–292.

503. EFSA Panel on Contaminants in the Food Chain, 2009. Marine biotoxins in shellfish—Pectenotoxin group. *EFSA J.*, 1109, 47 pp.

504. Anderson, D. M., Alpermann, T. J., Cembella, A. D., Collos, Y., Masseret, E., and Montresor, M., 2012. The globally distributed genus *Alexandrium*: Multifaceted roles in marine ecosystems and impacts on human health. *Harmful Algae*, 14, 10–35.

505. Food and Agriculture Organization of the United Nations. 2004. *Marine Biotoxins*. FAO Food and Nutrition Paper 80, Rome, Italy.

506. Wiese, M., D'Agostino, P. M., Mihali, T. K., Moffitt, M. C., and Neilan, B. A., 2010. Neurotoxic alkaloids: Saxitoxin and its analogs. *Marine Drugs*, 8, 2185–2211.

507. Wiberg, G. S. and Stephenson, N. R., 1960. Toxicologic studies on paralytic shellfish poison. *Toxicol. Appl. Pharmacol.*, 2, 607–615.

508. Davio, S. R., 1985. Neutralization of saxitoxin by anti-saxitoxin rabbit serum. *Toxicon*, 23, 669–675.

509. Evans, M. H., 1970. Two toxins from a poisonous sample of mussels *Mytilus edulis*. *Br. J. Pharmacol.*, 40, 847–865.

510. Harada, T., Oshima, Y., and Yasumoto, T., 1984. Assessment of potential activation of gonyautoxin V in the stomach of mice and rats. *Toxicon*, 22, 476–478.

511. Watts, J. S., Reilly, J., DaCosta, F. M., and Krop, S., 1966. Acute toxicity of paralytic shellfish poison in rats of different ages. *Toxicol. Appl. Pharmacol.*, 8, 286–294.

512. Kellaway, C. H., 1935. The action of mussel poison on the nervous system. *Aust. J. Exp. Biol. Med.*, 13, 79–94.

513. Covell, W. P. and Whedon, W. F., 1937. Effects of the paralytic shell-fish poison on nerve cells. *Arch. Pathol.*, 24, 411–418.

514. Sommer, H. and Meyer, K. F., 1937. Paralytic shell-fish poisoning. *Arch. Pathol.*, 24, 560–598.

515. AOAC Official Method 959.08. Paralytic shellfish poison. Biological method. in *Official Methods of Analysis of AOAC International 18th edn.* Horwitz, W. and Latimer, G. W., eds. AOAC International, Gaithersburg, MD, pp. 79–82.

516. Schantz, E. J., McFarren, E. F., Schafer, M. L., and Lewis, K. H., 1958. Purified shellfish poison for bioassay standardization. *J. Ass. Off. Anal. Chem.*, 41, 160–168.

517. Prakash, A., Medcof, J. C., and Tennant, A. D., 1971. Paralytic shellfish poisoning in Eastern Canada. Bulletin 177, Fisheries Research Board of Canada, Ottawa, Ontario, Canada.

518. EFSA Panel on Contaminants in the Food Chain, 2009. Marine biotoxins in shellfish—Saxitoxin group. *EFSA J.*, 1019, 76 pp.

519. McFarren, E. F., Schafer, M. L., Campbell, J. E., Lewis, K. H., Jensen, E. T., and Schantz, E. J., 1961. Public health significance of paralytic shellfish poison. *Adv. Food Res.*, 10, 135–179.

520. Popkiss, M. E. E., Horstman, D. A., and Harpur, D., 1979. Paralytic shellfish poisoning: A report of 17 cases in Cape Town. *South Afr. Med. J.*, 55, 1017–1023.

521. Gessner, B. D. and Middaugh, J. P., 1995. Paralytic shellfish poisoning in Alaska: A 20-year retrospective analysis. *Am. J. Epidemiol.*, 141, 766–770.

522. Bond, R. M. and Medcof, J. C., 1958. Epidemic shellfish poisoning in New Brunswick, 1957. *Can. Med. Assoc. J.*, 79, 19–24.

523. Kao, C. Y., 1966. Tetrodotoxin, saxitoxin and their significance in the study of excitation phenomena. *Pharmacol. Rev.*, 18, 997–1049.

524. Andrinolo, D., Iglesias, V., García, C., and Lagos, N., 2002. Toxicokinetics and toxicodynamics of gony-autoxins after an oral toxin dose in cats. *Toxicon*, 40, 699–709.

525. Prinzmetal, M., Sommer, H., and Leake, C. D., 1932. The pharmacological action of "mussel poison". *J. Pharmacol. Exp. Ther.*, 46, 63–73.

526. Mardones, P., Andrinolo, D., Csendes, A., and Lagos, N., 2004. Permeability of human jejunal segments to gonyautoxins measured by the Ussing chamber technique. *Toxicon*, 44, 521–528.

527. Torres, R., Pizarro, L., Csendes, A., García, C., and Lagos, N., 2007. GTX 2/3 epimers permeate the intestine through a paracellular pathway. *J. Toxicol. Sci.*, 32, 241–248.

528. Andrinolo, D., Gomes, P., Fraga, S., Soares-da-Silva, P., and Lagos, N., 2002. Transport of the organic cations gonyautoxin 2/3 epimers, a paralytic shellfish poison toxin, through the human and rat intestinal epitheliums. *Toxicon*, 40, 1389–1397.

529. García, C., del Carmen Bravo, M., Lagos, M., and Lagos, N., 2004. Paralytic shellfish poisoning: Post-mortem analysis of tissue and body fluid samples from human victims in the Patagonia fjords. *Toxicon*, 43, 149–158.

530. Cianca, R. C. C., Pallares, M. A., Barbosa, R. D., Adan, L. V., Martins, J. M. L., and Gago-Martínez, A., 2007. Application of precolumn oxidation HPLC method with fluorescence detection to evaluate saxitoxin levels in discrete brain regions of rats. *Toxicon*, 49, 89–99.

531. Hines, H. B., Naseem, S. M., and Wannemacher, R. W., 1993. [³H]-Saxitoxinol metabolism and elimination in the rat. *Toxicon*, 31, 905–908.

532. Naseem, S. M., 1996. Toxicokinetics of [³H]saxitoxinol in peripheral and central nervous system of rats. *Toxicol. Appl. Pharmacol.*, 141, 49–58.

533. Stafford, R. G. and Hines, H. B., 1995. Urinary elimination of saxitoxin after intravenous injection. *Toxicon*, 33, 1501–1510.

534. Hong, H.-Z., Lam, P. K. S., and Hsieh, D. P. H., 2003. Interactions of paralytic shellfish toxins with xenobiotic-metabolizing and antioxidant enzymes in rodents. *Toxicon*, 42, 425–431.

535. García, C., Rodriguez-Navarro, A., Díaz, J. C., Torres, R., and Lagos, N., 2009. Evidence of *in vitro* glucuronidation and enzymatic transformation of paralytic shellfish toxins by healthy human liver micro-somes fraction. *Toxicon*, 53, 206–213.

536. García, C., Barriga, A., Díaz, J. C., Lagos, M., and Lagos, N., 2010. Route of metabolization and detoxication of paralytic shellfish toxins in humans. *Toxicon*, 55, 135–144.

537. Llewellyn, L. E., Dodd, M. J., Robertson, A., Ericson, G., de Koning, C., and Negri, A. P., 2002. Postmortem analysis of samples from a human victim of a fatal poisoning caused by the xanthid crab, *Zosimus aeneus*. *Toxicon*, 40, 1463–1469.

538. Rodrigues, S. M., de Carvalho, M., Mestre, T. et al., 2012. Paralytic shellfish poisoning due to ingestion of *Gymnodinium catenatum* contaminated cockles—Application of the AOAC HPLC Official Method. *Toxicon*, 59, 558–566.

539. Hall, S., Reichardt, P. B., and Nevé, R. A., 1980. Toxins extracted from an Alaskan isolate of *Protogonyaulax* sp. *Biochem. Biophys. Res. Commun.*, 97, 649–653.

540. Laycock, M. V., Kralovec, J., and Richards, R., 1995. Some in vitro chemical interconversions of paralytic shellfish poisoning (PSP) toxins useful in the preparation of analytical standards. *J. Marine Biotechnol.*, 3, 121–125.

541. Strichartz, G., Rando, T., Hall, S. et al., 1986. On the mechanism by which saxitoxin binds to and blocks sodium channels. *Ann. N. Y. Acad. Sci.*, 479, 96–112.

542. Lipkind, G. M. and Fozzard, H. A., 1994. A structural model of the tetrodotoxin and saxitoxin binding site of the Na$^+$ channel. *Biophys. J.*, 66, 1–13.

543. Evans, M. H., 1965. Cause of death in experimental paralytic shellfish poisoning (PSP). *Br. J. Exp. Path.*, 46, 245–253.

544. Cheymol, J. and Thach, T., 1969. Action paralysante neuromusculaire de la saxitoxine chez le rat. *Thérapie*, 24, 191–198.

545. Kao, C. Y., Kao, P. N., James-Kracke, M. R., Koehn, F. E., Wichmann, C. F., and Schnoes, H. K., 1985. Actions of epimers of 12-(OH)-reduced saxitoxin and of 11-(OSO$_3$)-saxitoxin on squid axon. *Toxicon*, 23, 647–655.

546. Usup, G., Leaw, C.-P., Cheah, M.-Y., Ahmad, A., and Ng, B.-K., 2004. Analysis of paralytic shellfish poisoning toxin congeners by a sodium channel receptor binding assay. *Toxicon*, 44, 37–43.

547. Llewellyn, L. E., 2006. The behavior of mixtures of paralytic shellfish toxins in competitive binding assays. *Chem. Res. Toxicol.*, 19, 661–667.

548. Strichartz, G., 1984. Sructural determinants of the affinity of saxitoxin for neuronal sodium channels. Electrophysiological studies on frog peripheral nerve. *J. Gen. Physiol.*, 84, 281–305.

549. Yang, L., Kao, C. Y., and Oshima, Y., 1992. Actions of decarbamoyloxysaxitoxin and decarbamoylneosaxitoxin on the frog skeletal muscle fiber. *Toxicon*, 30, 645–652.

550. Kao, C. Y. and Walker, S. E., 1982. Active groups of saxitoxin and tetrodotoxin as deduced from actions of saxitoxin analogues on frog muscle and squid axon. *J. Physiol.*, 323, 619–637.

551. Moczydlowski, E., Hall, S., Garber, S. S., Strichartz, G. S., and Miller, C., 1984. Voltage-dependent blockade of muscle Na$^+$ channels by guanidinium toxins. Effect of toxin charge. *J. Gen. Physiol.*, 84, 687–704.

552. Guo, X., Uehara, A., Ravindran, A., Bryant, S. H., Hall, S., and Moczydlowski, E., 1987. Kinetic basis for insensitivity to tetrodotoxin and saxitoxin in sodium channels of canine heart and denervated rat skeletal muscle. *Biochemistry*, 26, 7546–7556.

553. Vale, C., Alfonso, A., Vieytes, M. R. et al., 2008. In vitro and in vivo evaluation of paralytic shellfish poisoning toxin potency and the influence of the pH of extraction. *Anal. Chem.*, 80, 1770–1776.

554. Perez, S., Vale, C., Botana, A. M., Alonso, E., Vieytes, M. R., and Botana, L. M., 2011. Determination of toxicity equivalent factors for paralytic shellfish toxins by electrophysiological measurements in cultured neurons. *Chem. Res. Toxicol.*, 24, 1153–1157.

555. Botana, L. M., Vilariño, N., Alfonso, A. et al., 2010. The problem of toxicity equivalent factors in developing alternative methods to animal bioassays for marine-toxin detection. *Trends Anal. Chem.*, 29, 1316–1325.

556. Miyazawa, K. and Noguchi, T., 2001. Distribution and origin of tetrodotoxin. *Toxin Rev.*, 20, 11–33.

557. Kudo, Y., Yasumoto, T., Konoki, K., Cho, Y., and Yotsu-Yamashita, M., 2012. Isolation and structural determination of the first 8-*epi*-type tetrodotoxin analogs from the newt, *Cynops ensicauda popei*, and comparison of tetrodotoxin analogs profiles of this newt and the puffer fish, *Fugu poecilonotus*. *Marine Drugs*, 10, 655–667.

558. Noguchi, T., Onuki, K., and Arakawa, O., 2011. Tetrodotoxin poisoning due to pufferfish and gastropods, and their intoxication mechanism. *ISRN Toxicology*, 2011, Article ID 276939.

559. McNabb, P., Selwood, A. I., Munday, R. et al., 2010. Detection of tetrodotoxin from the grey side-gilled sea slug—*Pleurobranchaea maculata*, and associated dog neurotoxicosis on beaches adjacent to the Hauraki Gulf, Auckland, New Zealand. *Toxicon*, 56, 466–473.

560. Hwang, D.-F. and Noguchi, T., 2007. Tetrodotoxin poisoning. *Adv. Food Nutr. Res.*, 52, 141–236.

561. Silva, M., Azevedo, J., Rodriguez, P., Alfonso, A., Botana, L. M., and Vasconcelos, V., 2012. New gastropod vectors and tetrodotoxin potential expansion in temperate waters of the Atlantic Ocean. *Marine Drugs*, 10, 712–726.

562. Kodama, M., Sato, S., Sakamoto, S., and Ogata, T., 1996. Occurrence of tetrodotoxin in *Alexandrium tamarense*, a causative dinoflagellate of paralytic shellfish poisoning. *Toxicon*, 34, 1101–1105.

563. Daly, J. W., 2004. Marine toxins and nonmarine toxins: Convergence or symbiotic organisms? *J. Nat. Prod.*, 67, 1211–1215.

564. Jang, J. and Yotsu-Yamashita, M., 2006. Distribution of tetrodotoxin, saxitoxin, and their analogs among tissues of the puffer fish *Fugu pardalis*. *Toxicon*, 48, 980–987.

565. Matsumura, K., 1998. Production of tetrodotoxin in puffer fish embryos. *Environ. Toxicol. Pharmacol.*, 6, 217–219.

566. Matsui, T., Sato, H., Hamada, S., and Shimizu, C., 1982. Comparison of the toxicity of the cultured and wild puffer fish *Fugu niphobles*. *Bull. Jap. Soc. Sci. Fish.*, 48, 253.

567. Ji, Y., Liu, Y., Gong, Q.-L., Zhou, L., and Wang, Z.-P., 2011. Toxicity of cultured puffer fish and seasonal variations in China. *Aquacult. Res.*, 42, 1186–1195.

568. Noguchi, T., Arakawa, O., and Takatani, T., 2006. Toxicity of pufferfish *Takifugu rubripes* cultured in netcages at sea or aquaria on land. *Comp. Biochem. Physiol. Part D*, 1, 153–157.

569. Matsumura, K., 1996. Tetrodotoxin concentrations in cultured puffer fish, *Fugu rubripes*. *J. Agric. Food Chem.*, 44, 1–2.

570. Campbell, S., Harada, R. M., DeFelice, S. V., Bienfang, P. K., and Li, Q. X., 2009. Bacterial production of tetrodotoxin in the pufferfish *Arothron hispidus*. *Nat. Prod. Res.*, 23, 1630–1640.

571. Wang, J., Fan, Y., and Yao, Z., 2010. Isolation of a *Lysinibacillus fusiformis* strain with tetrodotoxin-producing ability from puffer fish *Fugu obscurus* and the characterization of this strain. *Toxicon*, 56, 640–643.

572. Yu, V. C.-H., Yu, P. H.-F., Ho, K.-C., and Lee, F. W.-F., 2011. Isolation and identification of a new tetrodotoxin-producing bacterial species, *Raoultella terrigena*, from Hong Kong marine puffer fish *Takifugu niphobles*. *Marine Drugs*, 9, 2384–2396.

573. Yang, G., Xu, J., Liang, S., Ren, D., Yan, X., and Bao, B., 2010. A novel TTX-producing *Aeromonas* isolated from the ovary of *Takifugu obscurus*. *Toxicon*, 56, 324–329.

574. Chau, R., Kalaitzis, J. A., and Neilan, B. A., 2011. On the origins and biosynthesis of tetrodotoxin. *Aquat. Toxicol.*, 104, 61–72.

575. Williams, B. L., 2010. Behavioral and chemical ecology of marine organisms with respect to tetrodotoxin. *Marine Drugs*, 8, 381–398.

576. Lee, M.-J., Jeong, D.-Y., Kim, W.-S. et al., 2000. A tetrodotoxin-producing *Vibrio* strain, LM-1, from the puffer fish *Fugu vermicularis radiatus*. *Appl. Environ. Microbiol.*, 66, 1698–1701.

577. Narita, H., Matsubara, S., Miwa, N. et al., 1987. *Vibrio alginolyticus*, a TTX-producing bacterium isolated from the starfish *Astropecten polyacanthus*. *Nippon Suisan Gakkaishi*, 53, 617–621.

578. Wang, X.-J., Yu, R.-C., Luo, X., Zhou, M.-J., and Lin, X.-T., 2008. Toxin-screening and identification of bacteria isolated from highly toxic marine gastropod *Nassarius semiplicatus*. *Toxicon*, 52, 55–61.

579. Cheng, C. A., Hwang, D. F., Tsai, Y. H. et al., 1995. Microflora and tetrodotoxin-producing bacteria in a gastropod, *Niotha clathrata*. *Food Chem. Toxicol.*, 33, 929–934.

580. Do, H. K., Kogure, K., and Simidu, U., 1990. Identification of deep-sea-sediment bacteria which produce tetrodotoxin. *Appl. Environ. Microbiol.*, 56, 1162–1163.

581. Do, H. K., Kogure, K., Imada, C., Noguchi, T., Ohwada, K., and Simidu, U., 1991. Tetrodotoxin production of actinomycetes isolated from marine sediment. *J. Appl. Bacteriol.*, 70, 464–468.

582. Kogure, K., Do, H. K., Thuesen, E. V., Nanba, K., Ohwada, K., and Simidu, U., 1988. Accumulation of tetrodotoxin in marine sediment. *Marine Ecol. Prog. Ser.*, 45, 303–305.

583. Yasumoto, T., Yasumura, D., Yotsu, M., Michishita, T., Endo, A., and Kotaki, Y., 1986. Bacterial production of tetrodotoxin and anhydrotetrodotoxin. *Agric. Biol. Chem.*, 50, 793–795.

584. Matsumura, K., 1995. Reexamination of tetrodotoxin production by bacteria. *Appl. Environ. Microbiol.*, 61, 3468–3470.

585. Matsumura, K., 2001. No ability to produce tetrodotoxin in bacteria. *Appl. Environ. Microbiol.*, 67, 2393–2394.

586. Yotsu, M., Yamazaki, T., Meguro, Y. et al., 1987. Production of tetrodotoxin and its derivatives by *Pseudomonas* sp. isolated from the skin of a pufferfish. *Toxicon*, 25, 225–228.

587. Auawithoothij, W. and Noomhorm, A., 2012. *Shewanella putrefaciens*, a major microbial species related to tetrodotoxin (TTX)-accumulation of puffer fish *Lagocephalus lunaris*. *J. Appl. Microbiol.*, 113, 459–465.

588. Sato, S., Komaru, K., Ogata, T., and Kodama, M., 1990. Occurrence of tetrodotoxin in cultured puffer. *Nippon Suisan Gakkaishi*, 56, 1129–1131.

589. Kono, M., Matsui, T., Furukawa, K., Yotsu-Yamashita, M., and Yamamori, K., 2008. Accumulation of tetrodotoxin and 4,9-anhydrotetrodotoxin in cultured juvenile kusafugu *Fugu niphobles* by dietary administration of natural toxic komonfugu *Fugu poecilonotus* liver. *Toxicon*, 51, 1269–1273.

590. Yamamori, K., Kono, M., Furukawa, K., and Matsui, T., 2004. The toxification of juvenile cultured kasafugu *Takifugu niphobles* by oral administration of crystalline tetrodotoxin. *Shokuhin Eiseigaku Zasshi*, 45, 73–75.

591. Noguchi, T., Arakawa, O., and Takatani, T., 2006. TTX accumulation in pufferfish. *Comp. Biochem. Physiol. Part D*, 1, 145–152.

592. Nagashima, Y., Toyoda, M., Hasobe, M., Shimakura, K., and Shiomi, K., 2003. In vitro accumulation of tetrodotoxin in pufferfish liver tissue slices. *Toxicon*, 41, 569–574.

593. Nagashima, Y., Tanaka, N., Shimakura, K., Shiomi, K., and Shida, Y., 2001. Occurrence of tetrodotoxin-related substances in the nontoxic puffer *Takifugu xanthopterus*. *Toxicon*, 39, 415–418.

594. Hanifin, C. T., Brodie III, E. D., and Brodie Jr, E. D., 2002. Tetrodotoxin levels of the rough-skin newt, *Taricha granulosa*, increase in long-term captivity. *Toxicon*, 40, 1149–1153.

595. Cardall, B. L., Brodie Jr, E. D., Brodie III, E. D., and Hanifin, C. T., 2004. Secretion and regeneration of tetrodotoxin in the rough-skin newt (*Taricha granulosa*). *Toxicon*, 44, 933–938.

596. Yotsu-Yamashita, M., Gilhen, J., Russell, R. W. et al., 2012. Variability of tetrodotoxin and of its analogues in the red-spotted newt, *Notophthalmus viridescens* (Amphibia: Urodela: Salamandridae). *Toxicon*, 59, 257–264.

597. Noguchi, T. and Arakawa, O., 2008. Tetrodotoxin—Distribution and accumulation in aquatic organisms, and cases of human intoxication. *Marine Drugs*, 6, 220–242.

598. Shimizu, Y. and Kobayashi, M., 1983. Apparent lack of tetrodotoxin biosynthesis in captured *Taricha torosa* and *Taricha granulosa*. *Chem. Pharm. Bull.*, 31, 3625–3631.

599. Shimizu, Y., 1986. Chemistry and biochemistry of saxitoxin analogues and tetrodotoxin. *Ann. N. Y. Acad. Sci.*, 479, 24–31.

600. Daly, J. W., Padgett, W. L., Saunders, R. L., and Cover, J. F., 1997. Absence of tetrodotoxins in a captive-raised riparian frog, *Atelopus varius*. *Toxicon*, 35, 705–709.

601. Lehman, E. M., Brodie Jr, E. D., and Brodie III, E. D., 2004. No evidence for an endosymbiotic bacterial origin of tetrodotoxin in the newt *Taricha granulosa*. *Toxicon*, 44, 243–249.

602. Kao, C. Y. and Fuhrman, F. A., 1963. Pharmacological studies on tarichatoxin, a potent neurotoxin. *J. Pharmacol. Exp. Ther.*, 40, 31–40.

603. Kawasaki, H., Nagata, T., and Kanoh, S., 1973. An experience on the biological assay of the toxicity of imported fugu (Tetrodon). *J. Food Hyg. Soc. Japan*, 14, 186–190.

604. Rivera, V. R., Poli, M. A., and Bignami, G. S., 1995. Prophylaxis and treatment with a monoclonal antibody of tetrodotoxin poisoning in mice. *Toxicon*, 33, 1231–1237.

605. Xu, Q., Kai, H., Lisha, G., and Zhang, H., 2003. Toxicity of tetrodotoxin towards mice and rabbits. *J. Hyg. Res. (China)*, 32, 371–374.

606. Yotsu-Yamashita, M. and Mebs, D., 2003. Occurrence of 11-oxotetrodotoxin in the red-spotted newt, *Notophthalmus viridescens*, and further studies on the levels of tetrodotoxin and its analogues in the newt's efts. *Toxicon*, 41, 893–897.

607. Nakamura, M. and Yasumoto, T., 1985. Tetrodotoxin derivatives in puffer fish. *Toxicon*, 23, 271–276.

608. Yasumoto, T., Yotsu, M., Murata, M., and Naoki, H., 1988. New tetrodotoxin analogues from the newt *Cynops ensicauda*. *J. Am. Chem. Soc.*, 110, 2344–2345.

609. Yotsu-Yamashita, M., Schimmele, B., and Yasumoto, T., 1999. Isolation and structural assignment of 5-deoxytetrodotoxin from the puffer fish *Fugu poecilonotus*. *Biosci. Biotechnol. Biochem.*, 63, 961–963.

610. Jang, J.-H. and Yotsu-Yamashita, M., 2007. 6,11-Dideoxytetrodotoxin from the puffer fish, *Fugu pardalis*. *Toxicon*, 50, 947–951.

611. Yotsu-Yamashita, M., Urabe, D., Asai, M., Nishikawa, T., and Isobe, M., 2003. Biological activity of 8,11-dideoxytetrodotoxin: Lethality to mice and the inhibitory activity to cytotoxicity of ouabain and veratridine in mouse neuroblastoma cells, Neuro-2a. *Toxicon*, 42, 557–560.

612. Yotsu-Yamashita, M., Yamagishi, Y., and Yasumoto, T., 1995. 5,6,11-Trideoxytetrodotoxin from the puffer fish, *Fugu poecilonotus*. *Tetrahedron Lett.*, 36, 9329–9332.

613. Yotsu, M., Hayashi, Y., Khora, S. S., Sato, S., and Yasumoto, T., 1992. Isolation and structural assignment of 11-nortetrodotoxin-6(*S*)-ol from puffer *Arothron nigropunctatus*. *Biosci. Biotechnol. Biochem.*, 56, 370–371.

614. Endo, A., Khora, S. S., Murata, M., Naoki, H., and Yasumoto, T., 1988. Isolation of 11-*nor*tetrodotoxin-6(*R*)-ol and other tetrodotoxin derivatives from the puffer *Fugu niphobles*. *Tetrahedron Lett.*, 29, 4127–4128.

615. Yotsu-Yamashita, M. and Tateki, E., 2010. First report on toxins in the Panamanian toads *Atelopus limosus*, *A. glyphus* and *A. certus*. *Toxicon*, 55, 153–156.

616. Yotsu-Yamashita, M., Goto, A., and Nakagawa, T., 2005. Identification of 4-*S*-cysteinyltetrodotoxin from the liver of the puffer fish, *Fugu pardalis*, and formation of thiol adducts of tetrodotoxin from 4,9-anhydrotetrodotoxin. *Chem. Res. Toxicol.*, 18, 865–871.

617. Noguchi, T. and Mahmud, Y., 2001. Current methodologies for detection of tetrodotoxin. *Toxin Rev.*, 20, 35–50.

618. Xu, Q.-H., Zhao, X.-N., Wei, C.-H., and Rong, K.-T., 2005. Immunologic protection of anti-tetrodotoxin vaccines against lethal activities of oral tetrodotoxin challenge in mice. *Int. Immunopharmacol.*, 5, 1213–1224.

619. Pavelka, L. A., Kim, Y. H., and Mosher, H. S., 1977. Tetrodotoxin and tetrodotoxin-like compounds from the eggs of the Costa Rican frog, *Atelopus chiriquiensis*. *Toxicon*, 15, 135–139.

620. Endo, R., 1996. Histopathological and electron microscopic changes in mice treated with puffer fish toxin. *J. Toxicol. Sci.*, 21(Suppl. I), 1–14.

621. Sakai, F., Sato, A., and Uraguchi, K., 1961. Über die Atemlähmung durch Tetrodotoxin. *Naunyn-Schmiedeberg's Arch. Exp. Path. Pharmakol.*, 240, 313–321.

622. Tsuda, K., Ikuma, S., Kawamura, M. et al., 1964. Tetrodotoxin. VII. On the structures of tetrodotoxin and its derivatives. *Chem. Pharm. Bull.*, 12, 1357–1374.

623. Saoudi, M., Messarah, M., Boumendjel, A. et al., 2011. Extracted tetrodotoxin from puffer fish *Lagocephalus lagocephalus* induced hepatotoxicity and nephrotoxicity to Wistar rats. *Afr. J. Biotechnol.*, 10, 8140–8145.

624. Saoudi, M., Allagui, M. S., Abdelmouleh, A., Jamoussi, K., and El Feki, A., 2010. Protective effects of aqueous extract of *Artemisia campestris* against puffer fish *Lagocephalus lagocephalus* extract-induced oxidative damage in rats. *Exp. Toxicol. Path.*, 62, 601–605.

625. Saoudi, M., Abdelmouleh, A., Jamoussi, K., Kammoun, A., and El Feki, A., 2008. Hematological toxicity associated with tissue extract from poisonous fish *Lagocephalus lagocephalus*—Influence on erythrocyte function in Wistar rats. *J. Food Sci.*, 73, H155–H159.

626. Saoudi, M., Abdelmouleh, A., Ellouze, F., Jamoussi, K., and El Feki, A., 2008. Oxidative stress and hepatotoxicity in rats induced by poisonous pufferfish (*Lagocephalus lagocephalus*) meat. *J. Venom. Anim. Incl. Trop. Dis.*, 15, 424–443.

627. Saoudi, M., Ben Rabeh, F., Jamoussi, K., Abdelmouleh, A., Belbahri, L., and El Feki, A., 2007. Biochemical and physiological responses in Wistar rat after administration of puffer fish (*Lagocephalus lagocephalus*) flesh. *J. Food Agric. Environ.*, 5, 107–111.

628. Wang, J. and Fan, Y., 2010. Isolation and characterization of a *Bacillus* species capable of producing tetrodotoxin from the puffer fish *Fugu obscurus*. *World J. Microbiol. Biotechnol.*, 26, 1755–1760.

629. Tsai, Y.-H., Ho, P.-H., Hwang, C.-C., Hwang, P.-A., Cheng, C.-A., and Hwang, D.-F., 2006. Tetrodotoxin in several species of xanthid crabs in southern Taiwan. *Food Chem.*, 95, 205–212.

630. Lau, F. L., Wong, C. K., and Yip, S. H., 1995. Puffer fish poisoning. *J. Acc. Emerg. Med.*, 12, 214–215.

631. Chulanetra, M., Sookrung, N., Srimanote, P. et al., 2011. Toxic marine puffer fish in Thailand seas and tetrodotoxin they contained. *Toxins*, 3, 1249–1262.

632. Viet Dao, H., Takata, Y., Sato, S., Fukuyo, Y., and Kodama, M., 2009. Frequent occurrence of the tetrodotoxin-bearing horseshoe crab *Carcinoscorpius rotundicauda* in Vietnam. *Fish. Sci.*, 75, 435–438.

633. Ngy, L., Yu, C.-F., Taniyama, S., Takatani, T., and Arakawa, O., 2009. Co-occurrence of tetrodotoxin and saxitoxin in Cambodian marine pufferfish *Takifugu oblongus*. *Afr. J. Marine Sci.*, 31, 349–354.

634. Simon, K. D., Mazlan, A. G., and Usup, G., 2009. Toxicity of puffer fishes (*Lagocephalus wheeleri* Abe, Tabeta and Kitahama, 1984 and *Lagocephalus sceleratus* Gmelin, 1789) from the east coast waters of peninsular Malaysia. *J. Biol. Sci.*, 9, 482–487.

635. Chew, S. K., Goh, C. H., Wang, K. W., Mah, P. K., and Tan, B. Y., 1983. Puffer fish (tetrodotoxin) poisoning: Clinical report and role of anti-cholinesterase drugs in therapy. *Singapore Med. J.*, 24, 168–171.

636. Asakawa, M., Gomez-Delan, G., Tsuruda, S. et al., 2010. Toxicity assessment of the xanthid crab *Demania cultripes* from Cebu Island, Philippines. *J. Toxicol.*, Article ID 172367.

637. Isbister, G. K., Son, J., Wang, F. et al., 2002. Puffer fish poisoning: A potentially life-threatening condition. *Med. J. Aust.*, 177, 650–653.

638. Sorokin, M., 1973. Puffer fish poisoning. *Med. J. Aust.*, 1, 957.

639. Sims, J. K. and Ostman, D. C., 1986. Puffer fish poisoning: Emergency diagnosis and management of mild human tetrodotoxication. *Ann. Emerg. Med.*, 15, 1094–1098.

640. Ravaonindrina, N., Andriamaso, T. H., and Rasolofonirina, N., 2001. Intoxication après consommation de poisson globe à Madagascar: À propos de 4 cas. *Arch. Inst. Pasteur de Madagascar*, 67, 61–64.

641. Homaira, N., Rahman, M., Luby, S. P. et al., 2010. Multiple outbreaks of puffer fish intoxication in Bangladesh, 2008. *Am. J. Trop. Med. Hyg.*, 83, 440–444.

642. Bentur, Y., Ashkar, J., Lurie, Y. et al., 2008. Lessepsian migration and tetrodotoxin poisoning due to *Lagocephalus sceleratus* in the eastern Mediterranean. *Toxicon*, 52, 964–968.

643. Zaki, M. A. and Mossa, A.-E. A., 2005. Red Sea puffer fish poisoning: Emergency diagnosis and management of human intoxication. *Egypt. J. Aquat. Res.*, 31, 370–378.

644. Chamandi, C. S., Kallab, K., Mattar, H., and Nader, E., 2009. Human poisoning after ingestion of puffer fish caught from Mediterranean Sea. *Middle East J. Anesthesiol.*, 20, 285–288.

645. Cohen, N. J., Deeds, J. R., Wong, E. S. et al., 2009. Public health response to puffer fish (tetrodotoxin) poisoning from mislabeled product. *J. Food Protect.*, 72, 810–817.

646. Nuñez-Vázquez, E. J., Yotsu-Yamashita, M., Sierra-Beltrán, A. P., Yasumoto, T., and Ochoa, J. L., 2000. Toxicities and distribution of tetrodotoxin in the tissues of puffer fish found in the coast of the Baja California Peninsula, Mexico. *Toxicon*, 38, 729–734.

647. Pocchiari, F., 1977. Trade of misbranded frozen fish: Medical and public health implications. *Ann. Ist. Super. Sanità*, 13, 767–772.

648. Fernández-Ortega, J. F., de los Santos, J. M. M., Herrera-Gutiérrez, M. E. et al., 2010. Seafood intoxication by tetrodotoxin: First case in Europe. *J. Emerg. Med.*, 39, 612–617.

649. Kaku, N. and Meier, J., 1995. Clinical toxicology of fugu poisoning, in *Handbook of Clinical Toxicology of Animal Venoms and Poisons*, Meier, J. and White, J., eds. CRC Press, Boca Raton, FL, pp. 75–83.

650. Noguchi, T. and Ebesu, J. S. M., 2001. Puffer poisoning: Epidemiology and treatment. *Toxin Rev.*, 20, 1–10.

651. Saoudi, M., Abdelmouleh, A., and El Feki, A., 2010. Tetrodotoxin: A potent marine toxin. *Toxin Rev.*, 29, 60–70.

652. Lange, W. R., 1990. Puffer fish poisoning. *Am. Fam. Physician*, 42, 1029–1033.

653. Bradley, S. G. and Klika, L. J., 1981. A fatal poisoning from the Oregon rough-skinned newt (*Taricha granulosa*). *J. Am. Med. Assoc.*, 246, 247.

654. King, B. R., Hamilton, R. J., and Kassutto, Z., 2000. "Tail of newt": An unusual ingestion. *Pediatr. Emerg. Care*, 16, 268–269.

655. Narashi, T., 1988. Mechanism of tetrodotoxin and saxitoxin action, in *Handbook of Natural Toxins. Volume 3. Marine Toxins and Venoms*, Tu, A. T., ed. Marcel Dekkar, New York, pp. 185–210.

656. Yotsu-Yamashita, M., Sugimoto, A., Takai, A., and Yasumoto, T., 1999. Effects of specific modifications of several hydroxyls of tetrodotoxin on its affinity to rat brain membrane. *J. Pharmacol. Exp. Ther.*, 289, 1688–1696.

657. Kao, C. Y. and Yasumoto, T., 1985. Actions of 4-*epi*tetrodotoxin and anhydrotetrodotoxin on the squid axon. *Toxicon*, 23, 725–729.

658. Kao, C. Y., Yeoh, P. N., Goldfinger, M. D., Fuhrman, F. A., and Mosher, H. S., 1981. Chiriquitoxin, a new tool for mapping ionic channels. *J. Pharmacol. Exp. Ther.*, 217, 416–429.

659. Wu, B. Q., Yang, L., Kao, C. Y., Levinson, S. R., Yotsu-Yamashita, M., and Yasumoto, T., 1996. 11-oxo-Tetrodotoxin and a specifically labelled ³H-tetrodotoxin. *Toxicon*, 34, 407–416.

660. Rosker, C., Lohberger, B., Hofer, D., Steinecker, B., Quasthoff, S., and Schreibmayer, W., 2007. The TTX metabolite 4,9-anhydro-TTX is a highly specific blocker of the $Nav_{1.6}$ voltage-dependent sodium channel. *Am. J. Physiol.*, 293, C783–C789.

661. Guzmán, A., Fernández de Henestrosa, A. R., Marín, A.-P. et al., 2007. Evaluation of the genotoxic potential of the natural neurotoxin tetrodotoxin (TTX) in a battery of *in vitro* and *in vivo* genotoxicity assays. *Mutat. Res.*, 634, 14–24.

662. Paredes, I., Rietjens, I. M. C. M., Vieites, J. M., and Cabado, A. G., 2011. Update of risk assessments of main marine biotoxins in the European Union. *Toxicon*, 58, 336–354.

663. Khora, S. S. and Yasumoto, T., 1989. Isolation of 11-oxotetrodotoxin from the puffer *Arothron nigro-punctatus*. *Tetrahedron Lett.*, 30, 4393–4394.

664. Arakawa, O., Noguchi, T., Shida, Y., and Onoue, Y., 1994. Occurrence of 11-oxotetrodotoxin and 11-*nor*tetro-dotoxin-6(*R*)-ol in a xanthid crab *Atergatis floridus* collected at Kojima, Ishigaki Island. *Fish. Sci.*, 60, 769–771.

665. Kodama, M., Sato, S., and Ogata, T., 1993. *Alexandrium tamarense* as a source of tetrodotoxin in the scallop *Patinopecten yessoensis*, in *Toxic Phytoplankton Blooms in the Sea*, Smayda, T. J. and Shimizu, Y., eds. Elsevier, New York, pp. 401–406.

666. McNabb, P., Cawthron Institute, Nelson, New Zealand. 2012. Personal communication.

667. Murata, M., Kumagai, M., Lee, J. S., and Yasumoto, T., 1987. Isolation and structure of yessotoxin, a novel polyether compound implicated in diarrhetic shellfish poisoning. *Tetrahedron Lett.*, 28, 5869–5872.

668. Munday, R., Aune, T., and Rossini, G. P., 2008. Toxicology of the yessotoxins, in *Seafood and Freshwater Toxins. Pharmacology, Physiology, and Detection*, 2nd edn., Botana, L. M., ed. CRC Press, Boca Raton, FL, pp. 329–339.

669. Espenes, A., Aasen, J., Hetland, D. et al., 2004. Toxicity of yessotoxin in mice after repeated oral expo-sure, in *5th International Conference on Molluscan Shellfish Safety*, Henshilwood, K., Deegan, B., McMahon, T. et al., eds., Galway, Ireland, pp. 419–423.

670. Amzil, Z., Sibat, M., Royer, F., and Savar, V., 2008. First report on azaspiracid and yessotoxin groups detection in French shellfish. *Toxicon*, 52, 39–48.

671. Howard, M. D. A., Silver, M., and Kudela, R. M., 2008. Yessotoxin detected in mussel (*Mytilus califor-nicus*) and phytoplankton samples from the U.S. west coast. *Harmful Algae*, 7, 646–652.

672. Gladan, Ž. N., Ujević, I., Milandri, A. et al., 2010. Is yessotoxin the main phycotoxin in Croatian waters? *Marine Drugs*, 8, 460–470.

673. Satake, M., MacKenzie, L., and Yasumoto, T., 1997. Identification of *Protoceratium reticulatum* as the biogenetic origin of yessotoxin. *Nat. Toxins*, 5, 164–167.

674. Paz, B., Riobó, P., Luisa Fernández, M., Fraga, S., and Franco, J. M., 2004. Production and release of yessotoxins by the dinoflagellates *Protoceratium reticulatum* and *Lingulodinium polyedrum* in culture. *Toxicon*, 44, 251–258.

675. Rhodes, L., McNabb, P., de Salas, M., Briggs, L., Beuzenberg, V., and Gladstone, M., 2006. Yessotoxin production by *Gonyaulax spinifera*. *Harmful Algae*, 5, 148–155.

676. Miles, C. O., Samdal, I. A., Aasen, J. A. G. et al., 2005. Evidence for numerous analogs of yessotoxin in *Protoceratium reticulatum*. *Harmful Algae*, 4, 1075–1091.

677. Domínguez, H. J., Souto, M. L., Norte, M., Daranas, A. H., and Fernández, J. J., 2010. Adriatoxin-B, the first C_{13} terminal truncated YTX analogue obtained from dinoflagellates. *Toxicon*, 55, 1484–1490.

678. Ciminiello, P., Fattorusso, E., Forino, M., Magno, S., Poletti, R., and Viviani, R., 1998. Isolation of adria-toxin, a new analogue of yessotoxin from mussels of the Adriatic sea. *Tetrahedron Lett.*, 39, 8897–8900.

679. EFSA Panel on Contaminants in the Food Chain, 2008. Marine biotoxins in shellfish—Yessotoxin group. *EFSA J.*, 907, 62 pp.

680. Tubaro, A., Dell'Ovo, V., Sosa, S., and Florio, C., 2010. Yessotoxins: A toxicological overview. *Toxicon*, 56, 163–172.

681. Ciminiello, P., Dell'Aversano, C., Fattorusso, E. et al., 2007. Desulfoyessotoxins from Adriatic mussels: A new problem for seafood safety control. *Chem. Res. Toxicol.*, 20, 95–98.

682. Aune, T., Aasen, J. A. B., Miles, C. O., and Larsen, S., 2008. Effect of mouse strain and gender on LD_{50} of yessotoxin. *Toxicon*, 52, 535–540.

683. Aune, T., Sørby, R., Yasumoto, T., Ramstad, H., and Landsverk, T., 2002. Comparison of oral and intra-peritoneal toxicity of yessotoxin towards mice. *Toxicon*, 40, 77–82.

684. Terao, K., Ito, E., Oarada, M., Murata, M., and Yasumoto, T., 1990. Histopathological studies on experi-mental marine toxin poisoning—5. The effects in mice of yessotoxin isolated from *Patinopecten yes-soensis* and of a desulfated derivative. *Toxicon*, 28, 1095–1104.

685. Satake, M., Terasawa, K., Kadowaki, Y., and Yasumoto, T., 1996. Relative configuration of yessotoxin and isolation of two new analogs from toxic scallops. *Tetrahedron Lett.*, 37, 5955–5958.

686. Ciminiello, P., Fattorusso, E., Forino, M., Poletti, R., and Viviani, R., 2000. A new analogue of yesso-toxin, carboxyyessotoxin, isolated from Adriatic sea mussels. *Eur. J. Org. Chem.*, 2000, 291–295.

687. Ciminiello, P., Fattorusso, E., Forino, M., Poletti, R., and Viviani, R., 2000. Structure determination of carboxyhomoyessotoxin, a new yessotoxin analogue isolated from Adriatic mussels. *Chem. Res. Toxicol.*, 13, 770–774.

688. Daiguji, M., Satake, M., Ramstad, H., Aune, T., Naoki, H., and Yasumoto, T., 1998. Structure and fluoro-metric HPLC determination of 1-desulfoyessotoxin, a new yessotoxin analog isolated from mussels from Norway. *Nat. Toxins*, 6, 235–239.

689. Miles, C. O., Wilkins, A. L., Hawkes, A. D. et al., 2004. Isolation of a 1,3-enone isomer of heptanor-41-oxoyessotoxin from *Protoceratium reticulatum* cultures. *Toxicon*, 44, 325–336.

690. Miles, C. O., Wilkins, A. L., Hawkes, A. D. et al., 2005. Polyhydroxylated amide analogs of yessotoxin from *Protoceratium reticulatum*. *Toxicon*, 45, 61–71.

691. Loader, J. I., Hawkes, A. D., Beuzenberg, V. et al., 2007. Convenient large-scale purification of yesso-toxin from *Protoceratium reticulatum* culture and isolation of a novel furanoyessotoxin. *J. Agric. Food Chem.*, 55, 11093–11100.

692. Franchini, A., Marchesini, E., Poletti, R., and Ottaviani, E., 2004. Acute toxic effect of the algal yesso-toxin on Purkinje cells from the cerebellum of Swiss CD1 mice. *Toxicon*, 43, 347–352.

693. Franchini, A., Marchesini, E., Poletti, R., and Ottaviani, E., 2004. Lethal and sub-lethal yessotoxin dose-induced morpho-functional alterations in intraperitoneal injected Swiss CD1 mice. *Toxicon*, 44, 83–90.

694. Tubaro, A., Bandi, E., Sosa, S. et al., 2008. Effects of yessotoxin (YTX) on the skeletal muscle: An update. *Food Addit. Contam.*, 25, 1095–1100.

695. Tubaro, A., Giangaspero, A., Ardizzone, M. et al., 2008. Ultrastructural damage to heart tissue from repeated oral exposure to yessotoxin resolves in 3 months. *Toxicon*, 51, 1225–1235.

696. Arevalo, F., Pazos, Y., Correa, J. et al., 2004, First reported case of yessotoxins in mussels in the Galican Rias during a bloom of *Lingulodinium polyedrum* Stein (Dodge), in *5th International Conference on Molluscan Shellfish Safety*, Henshilwood, K., Deegan, B., McMahon, T. et al., eds., Galway, Ireland, pp. 184–189.

697. Alfonso, A. and Alfonso, C., 2008. Pharmacology and mechanism of action: Biological detection, in *Seafood and Freshwater Toxins. Pharmacology, Physiolology, and Detection*, 2nd edn., Botana, L. M., ed. CRC Press, Boca Raton, FL, pp. 315–327.

698. Ronzitti, G., Callegari, F., Malaguti, C., and Rossini, G. P., 2004. Selective disruption of the E-cadherin-catenin system by an algal toxin. *Br. J. Cancer*, 90, 1100–1107.

699. Callegari, F., Sosa, S., Ferrari, S. et al., 2006. Oral administration of yessotoxin stabilizes E-cadherin in mouse colon. *Toxicology*, 227, 145–155.

700. Botana, L. M., 2012. A perspective on the toxicology of marine toxins. *Chem. Res. Toxicol.*, 25, 1800–1804.

701. Dourson, M., Charnley, G., and Scheuplein, R., 2002. Differential sensitivity of children and adults to chemical toxicity. II. Risk and regulation. *Regulat. Toxicol. Pharmacol.*, 35, 448–467.

702. Schneider, M. A., DeLuca, V., and Gray, S. J., 1956. The effect of spice ingestion upon the stomach. *Am. J. Gastroenterol.*, 26, 722–732.

703. Domschke, S. and Domschke, W., 1984. Gastroduodenal damage due to drugs, alcohol and smoking. *Clin. Gastroenterol.*, 13, 405–436.

704. MacMath, T. L., 1990. Alcohol and gastrointestinal bleeding. *Emerg. Med. Clin. North Am.*, 8, 859–872.

705. Rainsford, K. D., 1982. An analysis of the gastro-intestinal side-effects of non-steroidal anti-inflammatory drugs, with particular reference to comparative studies in man and laboratory species. *Rheumatol. Int.*, 2, 1–10.

706. Renwick, A. G., 2000. The use of safety or uncertainty factors in the setting of acute reference doses. *Food Addit. Contam.*, 17, 627–635.

707. Renwick, A. G., 1995. The use of an additional safety or uncertainly factor for nature of toxicity in the estimation of acceptable daily intake and tolerable daily intake values. *Regulat. Toxicol. Pharmacol.*, 22, 250–261.

708. Steel, D., 2011. Extrapolation, uncertainty factors, and the precautionary principle. *Studies Hist. Phil. Biol. Biomed. Sci.*, 42, 356–364.

709. Lehman, A. J. and Fitzhugh, O. G., 1954. Quarterly report to the Editor on topics of current interest. 100-Fold margin of safety. *Quart. Bull. Ass. Food Drug. Off. US,* 18, 33–35.

710. Renwick, A. G., 1991. Safety factors and establishment of acceptable daily intakes. *Food Addit. Contam.*, 8, 135–150.

711. EFSA Panel on Contaminants in the Food Chain, 2009. Marine biotoxins in shellfish—Summary on regulated marine biotoxins. *EFSA J.*, 1306, 23 pp.

712. Boutwell, R. K., 1974. The function and mechanism of promoters of carcinogenesis. *CRC Crit. Rev. Toxicol.*, 2, 419–443.

713. Nessel, C. S., Freeman, J. J., Forgash, R. C., and McKee, R. H., 1999. The role of dermal irritation in the skin promoting activity of petroleum middle distillates. *Toxicol. Sci.*, 49, 48–55.

714. Setälä, K., Setälä, H., and Holsti, P., 1954. A new and physicochemically well-defined group of tumor-promoting (cocarcinogenic) agents for mouse skin. *Science*, 120, 1075–1076.

715. Roe, F. J. C. and Peirce, W. E. H., 1960. Tumor promotion by citrus oils: Tumors of the skin and urethral orifice in mice. *J. Natl. Cancer Inst.*, 24, 1389–1403.

716. Boyland, E., 1987. Estimation of acceptable levels of tumour promoters. *Br. J. Ind. Med.*, 44, 422–423.

717. Weisburger, J. H. and Williams, G. M., 1983. The distinct health risk analyses required for genotoxic carcinogens and promoting agents. *Environ. Health Perspect.*, 50, 233–245.

718. Kuraishy, A., Karin, M., and Grivennikov, S. I., 2011. Tumor promotion via injury- and death-induced inflammation. *Immunity*, 35, 467–477.

719. Slaga, T. J., 1980. Antiinflammatory steroids: Potent inhibitors of tumor promotion, in *Carcinogenesis, Volume 5: Modifiers of Chemical Carcinogenesis*, Slaga, T. J., ed. Raven Press, New York, pp. 111–126.

720. Fürstenberger, G., Csuk-Glänzer, B. I., Marks, F., and Keppler, D., 1994. Phorbol ester-induced leukotriene biosynthesis and tumor promotion in mouse epidermis. *Carcinogenesis*, 15, 2823–2827.

721. Taylor, P., 1996. Agents acting at the neuromuscular junction and autonomic ganglia, in *Goodman & Gilson's: The Pharmacological Basis of Therapeutics*, 9th edn., Hardman, J. G., Limbird, L. E., Molinoff, P. B., Ruddon, R. W., and Gilman, A. G., eds. McGraw-Hill, New York, pp. 177–197.

722. Friese, J., Gleitz, J., Gutser, U. T. et al., 1997. *Aconitum* sp. alkaloids: The modulation of voltage-dependent Na$^+$ channels, toxicity and antinociceptive properties. *Eur. J. Pharmacol.*, 337, 165–174.

723. Mebs, D. and Hucho, F., 1990. Toxins acting on ion channels and synapses, in *Handbook of Toxinology*, Schier, W. T. and Mebs, D., eds. Marcel Dekker, New York, pp. 493–598.

724. Kuch, U., Molles, B. E., Omori-Satoh, T., Chanhome, L., Samejima, Y., and Mebs, D., 2003. Identification of alpha-bungarotoxin (A31) as the major postsynaptic neurotoxin, and complete nucleotide identity of a genomic DNA of *Bungarus candidus* from Java with exons of the *Bungarus multicinctus* alpha-bungarotoxin (A31) gene. *Toxicon*, 42, 381–390.

725. Hawgood, B. J., 1989. How similar are the actions of crotoxin and β-bungarotoxin? *Acta Physiol. Pharmacol. Latinoamer.*, 39, 397–406.

726. Thesleff, S., 1977. Neurotoxins which block transmitter release from nerve terminals. *Naunyn-Schmiedeberg's Arch. Pharmacol.*, 297, S5–S7.

727. Marshall, I. G. and Harvey, A. L., 1990. Selective neuromuscular blocking properties of α-conotoxins *in vivo*. *Toxicon*, 28, 231–234.

728. Cruz, L. J., Gray, W. R., and Olivera, B. M., 1978. Purification and properties of a myotoxin from *Conus geographus* venom. *Arch. Biochem. Biophys.*, 190, 539–548.

729. Zeng, X.-Z., Xiao, Q.-B., and Liang, S.-P., 2003. Purification and characterization of raventoxin-I and raventoxin-III, two neurotoxic peptides from the venom of the spider *Macrothele raveni*. *Toxicon*, 41, 651–656.

730. Zhou, P.-A., Xie, X.-J., Li, M. et al., 1997. Blockade of neuromuscular transmission by huwentoxin-I, purified from the venom of the Chinese bird spider *Selenocosmia huwena*. *Toxicon*, 35, 39–45.

731. Liang, S., Qin, Y., Zhang, D., Pan, X., Chen, X., and Xie, J., 1993. Biological characterization of spider (*Selenocosmia huwena*) crude venom. *Zoological Res.*, 14, 65–71.

732. Culver, P. and Jacobs, R. S., 1981. Lophotoxin: A neuromuscular acting toxin from the sea whip (*Lophogorgia rigida*). *Toxicon*, 19, 825–830.

733. Davis, L., 2003. Botulism. *Curr. Treat. Options Neurol.*, 5, 23–31.

734. Guieu, R., Rosso, J.-P., and Rochat, H., 1994. Anticholinesterases and experimental envenomation by *Naja*. *Comp. Biochem. Physiol.*, 109C, 265–268.

735. Vital Brazil, O., 1987. Coral snake venoms: Mode of action and pathophysiology of experimental envenomation. *Rev. Inst. Med. Trop. São Paulo*, 29, 119–126.

736. Camargo, T. M., de Roodt, A. R., da Cruz-Höfling, M. A., and Rodrigues-Simioni, L., 2011. The neuro-muscular activity of *Micrurus pyrrhocryptus* venom and its neutralization by commercial and specific coral snake antivenoms. *J. Venom Res.*, 2, 24–31.
737. Tu, A. T., 1987. Biotoxicology of sea snake venoms. *Ann. Emerg. Med.*, 16, 1023–1028.
738. Wickramaratna, J. C. and Hodgson, W. C. A pharmacological examination of venoms from three species of death adder (*Acanthopis antarcticus*, *Acanthopis praelongis* and *Acanthopis pyrrhus*). *Toxicon*, 39, 209–216.
739. Märki, F. and Witkop, B., 1963. The venom of the Colombian arrow poison frog *Phyllobates bicolor*. *Experientia*, 19, 329–338.
740. Schopp, R. T. and DeClue, J. W., 1980. Paralytic properties of 4-N,N-dimethylamino-1,2-dithiolane (nereistoxin). *Arch. Int. Pharmacodyn. Ther.*, 248, 166–176.
741. Anderson, D. M., Cembella, A. D., and Hallegraeff, G. M., 2012. Progress in understanding harmful algal blooms: Paradigm shifts ar.d new technologies for research, monitoring, and management. *Ann. Rev. Marine Sci.*, 4, 143–176.
742. Miraglia, M., Marvin, H. J. P., Kleter, G. A. et al., 2009. Climate change and food safety: An emerging issue with special focus on Europe. *Food Chem. Toxicol.*, 47, 1009–1021.

8

World Production of Bivalve Mollusks and Socioeconomic Facts Related to the Impact of Marine Biotoxins

Martiña Ferreira, Jorge Lago, Juan Manuel Vieites, and Ana G. Cabado

CONTENTS

Trade of bivalve mollusks is an economic activity of crucial importance in many coastal areas in the world, particularly in developing countries, which continue to account for the bulk of world exports of fish and fishery products, including bivalves.[1] Global bivalve production is shown in Figure 8.1. Overall, bivalve production has increased from 5.3 million tonnes in 1990 to 14.6 million tonnes in 2010. Nevertheless, this increase is due to the fast growth of aquaculture production, which increased from 3.3 million tonnes, equivalent to 62% of total bivalve production, to 12.9 million tonnes in 2010, that is, 88% of total bivalve production. The value of aquaculture products has increased accordingly, from 3,500 to 13,000 million USD in 2010. Meanwhile, captures have slightly decreased from 2.0 to 1.7 million tonnes in the same period.[2]

Aquaculture is defined by the Food and Agriculture Organization of the United Nations (FAO) as "the farming of aquatic organisms including fish, mollusks, crustaceans, and aquatic plants. Farming implies some form of intervention in the rearing process to enhance production, such as regular stocking, feeding, and protection from predators. Farming also implies individual or corporate ownership of the stock being cultivated." [3] Aquaculture production refers to the outputs intended for consumption, excluding harvest for ornamental purposes.[4] Aquaculture is the fastest expanding animal food-producing sector, and it is expected that total production from both capture and aquaculture will exceed that of beef, pork, or poultry in the next decade.[1]

The expansion of bivalve aquaculture has been particularly remarkable in Asia, where bivalve production has nearly doubled in the last 20 years, from 6.1 million tonnes in 1990 to 11.6 million tonnes in 2010. China is by far the first producer of aquaculture bivalves worldwide, with 10.3 million tonnes produced in 2010; Japan, South Korea, and Thailand are also important producers. America bivalve aquaculture has also undergone a strong increase, from 162,000 to 520,000 tonnes between 1990 and 2010. This is due mainly to the expansion of mussel culture in Chile, although Canada, the United States, and Brazil also account for remarkable increases. Bivalve aquaculture production has remained relatively

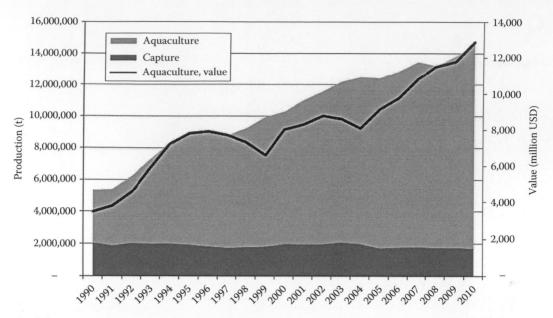

FIGURE 8.1 World production of bivalves from 1990 and 2010 and total value of bivalve aquaculture production. (From FAO, FAO Fisheries & Aquaculture—Global Statistics Collection, 2012.)

stable in Europe although a slight decrease, from 710,000 to 633,000 tonnes, has been recorded. Oceania production has increased from 84,000 to 116,000 tonnes, whereas African bivalve aquaculture production is incidental, with quantities in most years smaller than 2,000 tonnes.[2]

Clams, cockles, and ark shells are the most important bivalve group, with 5.5 million tonnes produced in 2010, followed by oysters with 4.6 million tonnes in the same period. Scallops account for more than 2.5 million tonnes, and mussels for 1.9 million tonnes produced in 2010.[2]

Toxic episodes caused by the presence of marine biotoxins, produced by some phytoplankton species, have a direct impact on the production and commercialization of marine bivalves worldwide, not only on shellfish harvesters and the aquaculture industry but also on coastal economies and on human health. This is particularly true in countries where monitoring programs for the detection of marine biotoxins have been developed and, consequently, a more strict control of the safety of seafood products exists, including specific regulations on the maximum permitted levels of marine biotoxins. This issue will be described in this section with examples of the impact of marine biotoxins in the trade of different groups of marine bivalves, together with the main facts and figures of the production of bivalve mollusks from aquaculture and captures from wild populations.

8.1 Production Data of the Main Groups of Bivalves

8.1.1 Clams, Cockles, and Ark Shells

Clams (a wide number of species included in the order Veneroida), cockles (Fam. Cardiidae), and ark shells (Fam. Arcidae) constitute the economically most important group of bivalves. Worldwide production surpassed 5.5 million tonnes in 2010, a twofold increase with regard to 1997, and this increase is due to the expansion of aquaculture, since wild captures have slightly decreased in the same period (Table 8.1). Consequently, aquaculture, which in 1997 represented 69% of the production of this group of bivalves, currently accounts for 88%. Asia, where aquaculture underwent a threefold increase from 1.7 to 4.6 million tonnes between 1997 and 2010, is the main producer of clams, cockles, and ark shells, despite a decrease of wild captures.[2]

Japan, Indonesia, South Korea, Thailand, and Turkey are the most important producers of wild clams, cockles, or ark shells in Asia. Japan accounted for 71,000 tonnes in 2010, which involves a strong decrease in comparison with the 106,000 tonnes captured in 1997. The Japanese carpet shell (*Ruditapes*

TABLE 8.1

World Production of Clams, Cockles, and Ark Shells from Aquaculture and Wild Captures (Tonnes)

	1997	1998	1999	2000	2001	2002	2003	2004	2005	2006	2007	2008	2009	2010
Aquaculture														
Africa	24	22	8	8	16	14	2	0	0	0	0	0	0	0
America	21,120	22,649	31,315	27,487	27,067	25,727	37,301	71,851	45,224	35,402	33,511	33,691	33,938	35,744
Asia	1,756,796	1,990,400	2,392,241	2,258,741	2,703,671	2,990,853	3,303,494	3,528,123	3,555,462	3,693,707	4,097,693	4,291,896	4,376,465	4,805,653
Europe	54,245	62,630	64,516	67,063	67,377	49,161	31,648	34,679	77,149	69,293	70,847	39,389	41,493	43,780
Oceania	2	7	1,421	1,431	1,419	7	6	8	6	10	18	3	2	2
Total aquaculture	1,832,187	2,075,708	2,489,501	2,354,730	2,799,550	3,065,762	3,372,451	3,634,661	3,677,841	3,798,412	4,202,069	4,364,979	4,451,898	4,885,179
Captures														
Africa	152	215	221	902	660	1,174	757	657	791	573	886	923	1,055	1,105
America	450,595	416,310	429,232	439,910	465,100	469,679	477,087	480,219	416,169	432,926	455,983	438,019	429,281	415,085
Asia	269,869	266,051	271,458	248,002	267,239	256,155	299,845	279,751	220,264	254,649	262,117	244,725	229,141	196,815
Europe	89,518	149,780	134,671	102,854	86,636	79,660	120,285	91,632	62,449	65,413	73,640	76,703	52,824	54,141
Oceania	4,225	5,887	6,116	6,428	6,793	5,098	3,473	3,780	3,769	4,037	2,915	2,261	2,163	2,023
Total captures	814,359	838,243	841,698	798,096	826,428	811,766	901,447	856,039	703,442	757,598	795,541	762,631	714,464	669,169
Total production														
Africa	176	237	229	910	676	1,188	759	657	791	573	886	923	1,055	1,105
America	471,715	438,959	460,547	467,397	492,167	495,406	514,388	552,070	461,393	468,328	489,494	471,710	463,219	450,829
Asia	2,026,665	2,256,451	2,663,699	2,506,743	2,970,910	3,247,008	3,603,339	3,807,874	3,775,726	3,948,356	4,359,810	4,536,621	4,605,606	5,002,468
Europe	143,763	212,410	199,187	169,917	154,013	128,821	151,933	126,311	139,598	134,706	144,487	116,092	94,317	97,921
Oceania	4,227	5,894	7,537	7,859	8,212	5,105	3,479	3,788	3,775	4,047	2,933	2,264	2,165	2,025
Total world production	2,646,546	2,913,951	3,331,199	3,152,826	3,625,978	3,877,528	4,273,898	4,490,700	4,381,283	4,556,010	4,997,610	5,127,610	5,166,362	5,554,348

Source: FAO, FAO Fisheries & Aquaculture—Global Statistics Collection, 2012.

philippinarum) is the most important species, although most of the production is composed of undetermined species. Captures in Indonesia reached maximum values in early 2000s with more than 80,000 tonnes, but in 2010 they decreased to 47,000 tonnes. The blood cockle *Anadara granosa* and hard clams (*Meretrix* spp.) are the most exploited species. Captures in South Korea also peaked in early 2000s, with 72,000 tonnes, to decrease halfway in 2010 with 33,600 tonnes. *R. philippinarum* is the most abundant species, but most of capture reports correspond to undetermined species. Thailand captures have dramatically decreased from late 1990s, where 70,000 tonnes were reported, to 2010, with 15,000 tonnes. Short-neck clams (*Paphia* spp.) account for nearly all Thai captures. On the contrary, capture of clams and similar bivalves has strongly increased in Turkey from 1997 onward, although in recent years a decrease has been observed. The striped venus *Chamelea gallina* is practically the only species captured.[2]

American production of these bivalves relies on wild captures, which have remained relatively stable in values between 415,000 and 450,000 tonnes in recent years. The United States remains as the main bivalve producer, although captures decreased from 322,000 to 251,000 tonnes from 1997 to 2010. The ocean quahog (*Arctica islandica*) and the Atlantic surf clam (*Spisula solidissima*) are the most important species. Venezuela is the second country in volume of captures of wild clams with 69,000 tonnes in 2010, most of them ark clams from the genus *Arca*. Chile captured 51,000 tonnes of clams, cockles, or ark shells, being the taca clam (*Protothaca thaca*) the most abundant species, and Canada produced 28,000 tonnes, with the Stimpson's surf clam (*Spisula polynyma*) as the most abundant species.

European captures have strongly decreased from 150,000 tonnes in 1998 to 54,000 in 2010, whereas aquaculture has also decreased from highest outputs in mid-2000s, with more than 70,000 tonnes/year, to productions around 40,000 tonnes in recent years. Italy, Spain, France, the Netherlands, Portugal, and the United Kingdom are the European countries that report highest captures of wild clams, cockles, and ark shells, with more than 50,000 tonnes altogether. The range of captured species is very diverse, comprising cockles, different genera of clams, razor clams, and hard clams.

Aquaculture in America has also stabilized in values around 35,000 tonnes/year. The United States accounts for almost all this production, being the hard clam *Mercenaria mercenaria* the most cultured species, whose production increased from 18,000 tonnes in 1997 to 29,000 in 2010. Canada produced 2000 tonnes in 2010, 1500 of them were Japanese carpet shell, and the rest the butter clam *Saxidomus giganteus*.[2] In Europe, Italy dominates aquaculture production with 35,000 tonnes of Japanese carpet shell and 1,000 tonnes of grooved carpet shell (*Ruditapes decussatus*) in 2010. France is the second aquaculture producer, with 4500 tonnes distributed among common edible cockle (*Cerastoderma edule*), *R. decussatus*, *R. philippinarum*, and undetermined species. Spain production reached 2100 tonnes in 2010, half of which corresponded to *R. philippinarum*, and the rest were distributed among *C. edule*, *R. decussatus*, and the pullet carpet shell *Venerupis pullastra*. Portugal aquaculture production underwent a dramatic decrease in 2010, with 254 tonnes in 2010 compared to 2500 tonnes in 2009, *C. edule* and *R. decussatus* being the most cultured species.[2]

Aquaculture in Oceania has virtually disappeared in the decade of 2000s, whereas captures have also decreased to one-third from highest records of late 1990s and early 2000s, with figures of 2000 tonnes in recent years. New Zealand accounts for 1200 tonnes, mainly Stutchbury's venus (*Chione stutchburyi*), short-neck clams (*Paphia* spp.), and other undetermined bivalves. Captures in Australia consist of pipi wedge clams (*Paphies australis*), whereas Fiji reports captures of *Anadara* spp. and undetermined species. African production relies exclusively in captures, with an average of 1000 tonnes in recent years. Only data from Tunisia, Senegal, Mozambique, and South Africa are available, being *C. edule* and *R. decussatus* the most common species.[2]

8.1.2 Oysters

Oysters (Fam. Ostreidae) are the second most important group of bivalves in terms of production and trade (Table 8.2). Almost all oyster production worldwide (>95%) comes from aquaculture, and on the other hand, Asia accounts for more than 90% of oyster aquaculture production.[2] Although captures underwent a strong increase in 2000 with regard to previous years, reaching 250,000 tonnes, in following years a continuous reduction has been observed, with 103,000 tonnes captured in 2010. America is the first producer of wild oysters.[2] These data correspond to oysters intended for consumption; pearl oysters (Order Pterioida) are not included.

TABLE 8.2

World Production of Oysters from Aquaculture and Wild Captures (Tonnes)

	1997	1998	1999	2000	2001	2002	2003	2004	2005	2006	2007	2008	2009	2010
Aquaculture														
Africa	732	713	651	567	473	651	622	525	642	750	876	898	979	1,132
America	100,372	102,264	106,335	96,733	119,267	113,993	131,893	170,815	121,042	152,508	142,232	137,442	144,088	156,234
Asia	2,654,904	2,997,576	3,106,084	3,351,374	3,529,596	3,626,351	3,741,456	3,821,686	3,883,566	3,961,610	4,110,120	3,869,879	4,027,759	4,202,229
Europe	160,223	152,383	155,835	149,008	124,446	131,382	129,971	134,932	135,923	130,312	132,232	122,426	121,542	111,643
Oceania	17,788	22,233	25,738	13,185	13,110	11,306	12,447	14,782	14,727	14,939	17,454	16,866	16,849	17,307
Total aquaculture	2,934,019	3,275,169	3,394,643	3,610,867	3,786,892	3,883,683	4,016,389	4,142,740	4,155,900	4,260,119	4,402,914	4,147,511	4,311,217	4,488,545
Captures														
Africa	125	98	133	104	153	165	138	120	226	83	145	190	171	297
America	159,533	142,036	138,898	227,870	183,257	164,332	171,103	120,763	131,390	104,953	119,202	97,404	102,623	71,885
Asia	20,535	13,073	14,569	18,449	11,360	8,304	20,652	26,092	28,360	31,700	30,044	29,589	24,801	23,109
Europe	2,220	1,788	1,674	855	1,048	1,461	2,361	2,797	1,817	2,310	3,154	4,379	5,049	7,714
Oceania	2,174	1,000	1,057	766	832	816	852	465	546	518	512	434	107	980
Total captures	184,587	157,995	156,331	248,044	196,650	175,078	195,106	150,237	162,339	139,564	153,057	131,996	132,751	103,985
Total production														
Africa	857	811	784	671	626	816	760	645	868	833	1,021	1,088	1,150	1,429
America	259,905	244,300	245,233	324,603	302,524	278,325	302,996	291,578	252,432	257,461	261,434	234,846	246,711	228,119
Asia	2,675,439	3,010,649	3,120,653	3,369,823	3,540,956	3,634,655	3,762,108	3,847,778	3,911,926	3,993,310	4,140,164	3,899,468	4,052,560	4,225,338
Europe	162,443	154,171	157,509	149,863	125,494	132,843	132,332	137,729	137,740	132,622	135,386	126,805	126,591	119,357
Oceania	19,962	23,233	26,795	13,951	13,942	12,122	13,299	15,247	15,273	15,457	17,966	17,300	16,956	18,287
Total world production	3,118,606	3,433,164	3,550,974	3,858,911	3,983,542	4,058,761	4,211,495	4,292,977	4,318,239	4,399,683	4,555,971	4,279,507	4,443,968	4,592,530

Source: FAO, FAO Fisheries & Aquaculture—Global Statistics Collection, 2012.

Captures of oysters have increased in Europe from 2200 to 7700 tonnes between 1997 and 2010. This increase is due to cupped oysters (*Crassostrea* spp.), which after being introduced to France in 1960 have overcome the native European flat oyster *Ostrea edulis*, whose captures ranged between 1400 and 3000 tonnes. Denmark is the first producer of *O. edulis* with ca. 1000 tonnes in 2010, followed by France, Ireland, and the United Kingdom with captures between 170 and 200 tonnes. Ireland is the most important producer of cupped oysters with 5800 tonnes; France, Portugal, Spain, and the United Kingdom capturing minor quantities.[2]

In America, captures of oysters have decreased halfway from 160,000 to 71,000 tonnes between 1997 and 2010. Mexico reports stable captures (40,000–50,000 tonnes) of American cupped oysters (*Crassostrea virginica*) and other *Crassostrea* oysters. On the contrary, captures of *C. virginica* in the United States underwent a 10-fold decrease from 104,000 to 11,000 tonnes, whereas Pacific cupped oyster (*Crassostrea gigas*) captures recovered in 2010 with 7,500 tonnes after years of lower records. In Asia, practically all oyster captures correspond to South Korea, with 20,000–30,000 tonnes of *C. gigas* depending on years. Oyster captures in Oceania correspond to New Zealand, which reported ca. 1000 tonnes of *Ostrea lutaria* (New Zealand dredge oyster) in 2010; captures seem to recover after a strong decrease in 2000s. In Africa, majority of captures correspond to Senegal, with 242 tonnes of cupped oysters in 2010.[2]

European aquaculture of oysters is dominated by the culture of *C. gigas* in France, with more than 95,000 tonnes in 2010, although French production has decreased from 150,000 tonnes in late 1990s. Ireland and the Netherlands are also important producers of aquaculture oysters, with 7000 and ca. 4000 tonnes in 2010, respectively. The Channel Islands produced 3500 tonnes of *C. gigas* in 2010. The United Kingdom, Germany, Spain, and Portugal produce lower quantities of *C. gigas*. Spain is the main European producer of aquaculture flat oyster, with 5500 tonnes, followed by Ireland, the Netherlands, and Croatia.[2]

Aquaculture of oysters in America is dominated by North American countries and particularly by the United States, which registered an increase from 88,000 tonnes in 1997 to 137,000 in 2010. This increase corresponds to *C. virginica*, whereas the aquaculture of *C. gigas* has decreased in last decade from 54,000 to 29,000 tonnes. Oyster production in Canada has also doubled between 1997 and 2010, up to 11,000 tonnes, of which two-thirds correspond to *C. gigas* and one-third to *C. virginica*. Aquaculture of oysters in Mexico has also increased in recent years and in 2010 produced ca. 4000 tonnes of *C. gigas* and Cortez oyster (*C. corteziensis*). In recent years, Brazil produced approximately 2000 tonnes of *Crassostrea* spp. As for Asia, China is the absolute leader of oyster aquaculture worldwide; its production increased from 2.1 million tonnes in 1997 to 3.6 million tonnes in 2010 of *Crassostrea* spp. South Korea and Japan are the second and third producers in Asia, with 270,000 and 200,000 tonnes of *C. gigas*, respectively, in 2010. Taiwan, Thailand, and Philippines also produce between 22,000 and 36,000 tonnes of *Crassostrea* spp. In Oceania, the bulk of oyster aquaculture corresponds to Australia, with 10,000 tonnes of *C. gigas* and 5,000 of the Sydney cupped oyster (*Saccostrea commercialis*) in 2010. New Zealand produced 2400 tonnes of *C. gigas* in the same period.[2] Oyster aquaculture in Africa is still very low. Namibia, Morocco, and South Africa produce 250, 280, and 500 tonnes of *C. gigas*, respectively; Namibia also produces 250 tonnes of *O. edulis*.

8.1.3 Scallops

Scallops (Fam. Pectinidae) are highly priced bivalves. Global production of scallops has constantly increased in recent years, from 1.8 to 2.5 million tonnes between 1997 and 2010 (Table 8.3). Aquaculture accounts for 62%–65% of total scallop production, depending on years, and increased from 875,000 tonnes in 1998 to 1.7 million in 2010. Captures have also increased, from 522,000 tonnes in 1997 to 841,000 in 2010.

America is the territory that accounts for almost half of scallop captures in the world. Here, captures have increased from 150,000 tonnes in 1997 to more than 400,000 in 2010. The United States accounts for the greatest scallop captures, from 48,000 to 215,000 tonnes of American sea scallop (*Placopecten magellanicus*). Canada captures range between 60,000 and 94,000 tonnes depending on the year of *P. magellanicus* and the Iceland scallop (*Chlamys islandica*). Peru accounts for an increase in captures of Peruvian calico scallop up to 63,000 tonnes in 2010. Mexico captures of *Argopecten ventricosus* (Pacific calico scallop) have also strongly increased from 2,300 to 16,000 tonnes between 1997 and 2010.

Asia is the second continent in scallop captures, which have slightly increased from 262,000 tonnes in 1997 to 330,000 in 2010. Japan accounts for practically all the scallop captures in Asia, which

TABLE 8.3

World Production of Scallops from Aquaculture and Wild Captures (Tonnes)

	1997	1998	1999	2000	2001	2002	2003	2004	2005	2006	2007	2008	2009	2010
Aquaculture														
Africa	28	2	1	4	0	0	0	0	0	0	0	0	0	0
America	12,008	18,435	23,365	23,006	22,704	20,936	21,929	35,152	28,623	28,472	38,776	36,378	33,313	67,648
Asia	1,256,199	855,867	928,724	1,132,665	1,195,973	1,207,582	1,196,501	1,131,291	1,248,602	1,232,621	1,425,208	1,374,322	1,549,382	1,658,524
Europe	1,061	862	422	434	450	173	481	648	616	600	188	199	919	933
Oceania	0	0	0	0	0	0	0	0	0	0	0	0	0	0
Total aquaculture	1,269,296	875,166	952,512	1,156,109	1,219,127	1,228,691	1,218,911	1,167,091	1,277,841	1,261,693	1,464,172	1,410,899	1,583,614	1,727,105
Captures														
Africa	0	0	0	0	0	0	0	0	0	0	0	0	0	0
America	154,835	171,137	211,116	264,278	310,704	354,878	377,808	396,277	346,162	405,029	381,532	367,383	408,077	408,880
Asia	262,511	290,070	301,266	305,850	291,889	308,288	346,755	316,346	288,698	274,026	260,859	312,187	321,830	329,192
Europe	77,242	79,567	79,182	80,515	83,601	77,146	67,634	67,084	70,124	70,463	78,214	71,471	77,620	95,119
Oceania	27,638	14,557	17,854	14,926	16,188	10,133	12,152	11,246	18,128	11,029	12,494	11,957	8,977	7,685
Total captures	522,226	555,331	609,418	665,569	702,382	750,445	804,349	790,953	723,112	760,547	733,099	762,998	816,504	840,876
Total production														
Africa	28	2	1	4	0	0	0	0	0	0	0	0	0	0
America	166,843	189,572	234,481	287,284	333,408	375,814	399,737	431,429	374,785	433,501	420,308	403,761	441,390	476,528
Asia	1,518,710	1,145,937	1,229,990	1,438,515	1,487,862	1,515,870	1,543,256	1,447,637	1,537,300	1,506,647	1,686,067	1,686,509	1,871,212	1,987,716
Europe	78,303	80,429	79,604	80,949	84,051	77,319	68,115	67,732	70,740	71,063	78,402	71,670	78,539	96,052
Oceania	27,638	14,557	17,854	14,926	16,188	10,133	12,152	11,246	18,128	11,029	12,494	11,957	8,977	7,685
Total world production	1,791,522	1,430,497	1,561,930	1,821,678	1,921,509	1,979,136	2,023,260	1,958,044	2,000,953	2,022,240	2,197,271	2,173,897	2,400,118	2,567,981

Source: FAO, FAO Fisheries & Aquaculture—Global Statistics Collection, 2012.

correspond to yesso scallop. Scallop captures in Europe have ranged between 67,000 and 87,000 in recent years, peaking in 2010 with 95,000 tonnes. France and the United Kingdom have doubled their captures between 1997 and 2010, from 15,000 to 31,000 and from 24,000 to 44,000 tonnes, respectively, of *Pecten maximus* and *Aequipecten opercularis*. Faroe Islands, Isle of Man, and Ireland are also producers of these species, with captures ranging from ca. 2000 tonnes (Ireland) to more than 4000. In contrast, captures of wild scallops (*Patinopecten yessoensis* and undetermined species) in Russia have decreased from 19,000 to 5,300 tonnes between 1997 and 2010. Scallop captures in Oceania have sharply decreased in the same period, from 27,000 to 7,600 tonnes. This is due to the fall of captures of New Zealand scallop (*Pecten novaezelandiae*), from 19,000 tonnes in 1997 to 122 in 2010. Scallop captures in Australia fluctuate between 5,000 and 15,000 tonnes depending on the year. African scallop captures are incidental.

Asia is the most important territory regarding scallop aquaculture, and its production doubled from 850,000 tonnes in 1998 to 1.6 million tonnes in 2010. Most of this production comes from China, where 1.4 million tonnes of undetermined scallop species were cultured in 2010. Japan is the second producer, with 220,000 tonnes of the yesso scallop (*P. yessoensis*). In America, scallop aquaculture underwent a constant increase from 12,000 to 33,000 tonnes between 1997 and 2009, to double production in 2010 with 67,000 tonnes. Peru is the first producer, with 58,000 tonnes of Peruvian calico scallop (*Argopecten purpuratus*) in 2010. Chile is the second producer, with 8800 tonnes of the same species in 2010. Canada cultured 700 tonnes of undetermined scallop species in 2010.

Scallop aquaculture is incidental in Europe, with fluctuations from year to year. Highest records correspond to 2009 and 2010 with 919 and 933 tonnes, respectively. Russia is the most important producer, with 850 tonnes of *P. yessoensis* in 2010. Ireland produced 58 tonnes of the great Atlantic scallop, *P. maximus*, in 2010. Norway accounts for 10 tonnes of the same species. Scallop aquaculture in the United Kingdom has undergone a sharp decrease. Aquaculture of queen scallop (*A. opercularis*) has nearly disappeared in recent years after fluctuations between ca. 50 and more than 140 tonnes in late 1990s and early 2000s. UK production of *P. maximus* has also dropped from 40 tonnes records in late 1990s to less than 15 tonnes in recent years. Spain and France, also traditionally producing countries, did not report aquaculture production of scallops from 2002, despite maximum productions of 200 and 150 tonnes of *P. maximus* a few years before. The occurrence of amnesic shellfish poisoning (ASP) episodes may be associated to this halt in the scallop aquaculture in European countries. Detoxification of domoic acid poses particular difficulties in scallops, since *Pecten* spp. may retain this toxin for months or even years,[5] as observed in Galicia (NW Spain) and Scotland, United Kingdom, resulting in considerable financial hardship for scallop fishermen.[6] No scallop aquaculture has been reported in Africa or Oceania.

8.1.4 Mussels

Global production of mussels (Fam. Mytilidae) has slightly increased in the period between 1997 and 2010, from 1.3 to 1.9 million tonnes produced worldwide. That increase is due to the strong growth of aquaculture, which currently represents 95% of the world mussel production, in comparison to 83% in 1997. In parallel, captures have decreased from 230,000 tonnes in 1997 to 89,000 in 2010 (Table 8.4), even though this drop has not been equally distributed among territories. Captures of wild mussels have sharply declined in Europe, with nearly 80% from 1997 to 2010, and in Asia, with a decrease of 50% within the same period. Nevertheless, captures have remained stable in America. In Africa, where mussel production is incidental, captures are nonexistent most years, whereas in some cases yearly productions around 150 or 200 tonnes have been recorded. Oceanian highest mussel captures were recorded in 1999 and early 2000s but strongly decreased afterward, with recent yearly captures around 150 tonnes.

The United States accounts for the largest mussel captures in America, with 15,000 tonnes of blue mussel (*Mytilus edulis*) in 2010. Peru captured 9000 tonnes of cholga mussel (*Aulacomya atra*), and Chile reported captures of 4500 tonnes of mussel, being the choro mussel (*Choromytilus chorus*) the most important species. In Europe, Denmark is the first producer of wild blue mussel, but captures dramatically decreased from 122,000 tonnes produced in 2001 to 28,000 tonnes in 2010. Likewise, the production of Mediterranean mussel (*Mytilus galloprovincialis*) in Greece peaked in 1997 with 24,000 tonnes to become negligible in recent years. In Italy, captures of Mediterranean mussel reached

TABLE 8.4

World Production of Mussels from Aquaculture and Wild Captures (Tonnes)

	1997	1998	1999	2000	2001	2002	2003	2004	2005	2006	2007	2008	2009	2010
Aquaculture														
Africa	2,585	2,768	2,329	633	671	602	782	764	602	745	999	873	879	882
America	28,617	36,607	45,477	59,416	69,592	76,972	90,287	113,872	127,515	166,764	193,299	225,357	206,598	264,850
Asia	498,159	568,629	652,609	604,115	685,233	907,640	904,238	939,884	1,026,705	1,007,790	810,033	801,841	937,386	971,352
Europe	494,213	602,360	605,892	565,062	553,075	486,251	547,264	527,696	465,791	495,987	491,026	456,557	489,563	476,656
Oceania	66,622	76,482	72,928	78,017	66,509	80,789	80,727	87,628	97,900	100,189	102,708	103,359	93,212	98,630
Total aquaculture	1,090,196	1,286,846	1,379,235	1,307,243	1,375,080	1,552,254	1,623,298	1,669,844	1,718,513	1,771,475	1,598,065	1,587,987	1,727,638	1,812,370
Captures														
Africa	6	7	14	0	0	0	0	0	0	0	217	117	142	0
America	33,379	40,456	31,347	33,697	40,186	34,542	30,726	30,335	28,481	23,912	35,836	33,781	36,856	37,217
Asia	31,776	29,259	16,539	49,395	6,820	9,740	11,414	8,828	16,605	17,374	11,532	8,322	17,098	14,961
Europe	165,809	156,810	156,592	173,614	190,787	178,726	142,305	148,824	90,919	72,574	66,957	48,376	45,121	36,612
Oceania	1	665	2,978	4,468	2,273	1,727	2,148	1,353	486	403	200	182	152	153
Total captures	230,971	227,197	207,470	261,174	240,066	224,735	186,593	189,340	136,491	114,263	114,742	90,778	99,369	88,943
Total production														
Africa	2,591	2,775	2,343	633	671	602	782	764	602	745	1,216	990	1,021	882
America	61,996	77,063	76,824	93,113	109,778	111,514	121,013	144,207	155,996	190,676	229,135	259,138	243,454	302,067
Asia	529,935	597,888	669,148	653,510	692,053	917,380	915,652	948,712	1,043,310	1,025,164	821,565	810,163	954,484	986,313
Europe	660,022	759,170	762,484	738,676	743,862	664,977	689,569	676,520	556,710	568,561	557,983	504,933	534,684	513,268
Oceania	66,623	77,147	75,906	82,485	68,782	82,516	82,875	88,981	98,386	100,592	102,908	103,541	93,364	98,783
Total world production	1,321,167	1,514,043	1,586,705	1,568,417	1,615,146	1,776,989	1,809,891	1,859,184	1,855,004	1,885,738	1,712,807	1,678,765	1,827,007	1,901,313

Source: FAO, FAO Fisheries & Aquaculture—Global Statistics Collection, 2012.

maximum values in early 2000s, with 46,000 tonnes, but captures have stopped in recent years, or no records are available. In Asia, Korea is the main producer of wild mussels, with 13,000 tonnes of undetermined species. In Oceania, virtually all mussel captures (153 tonnes) correspond to New Zealand.

In contrast to captures, mussel aquaculture is expanding mainly in America and Asia. In Europe, where aquaculture of the blue mussel dates back as early as the thirteenth century, the production of this species and that of the Mediterranean mussel reached maximum values in late 1990s with 600,000 tonnes and gradually decreased to 470,000 tonnes in 2010. Spain, and particularly the northwest region of Galicia, continues to be the most important producer of aquaculture mussel in Europe, with more than 189,000 tonnes in 2010 (although other sources point up to 300,000 tonnes)[7] and followed by France with 76,800, Italy with 64,200, and the Netherlands with 56,000 tonnes.

The transfer of the culturing techniques carried out in Europe to third countries has allowed the rapid expansion of mussel aquaculture in Chile or China; in this latter country, the Mediterranean mussel *M. galloprovincialis* has also been introduced. Nowadays China is the first mussel producer with more than 700,000 tonnes in 2010; although the species cultured in China appear in FAO databases as "sea mussels nei," it is thought that most of its production corresponds to *M. galloprovincialis*,[8] with small amounts of *M. coruscus*, *Musculus senhouse*, and *Perna viridis*. Floating rafts are the most common mussel culture system in China.[9] South Korea is another important producer in Asia, with 54,000 tonnes in 2010. Green mussel (*P. viridis*) aquaculture in India has dramatically expanded in recent years, from 27 tonnes in 1997 to 55,000 in 2010.

In America, mussel aquaculture has rocketed in Chile, where production increased from 8,600 tonnes in 1997 to 220,000 tonnes in 2010. The Chilean mussel *Mytilus chilensis* is the most produced species, which is cultured in long lines. Canada is the second aquaculture mussel producer in America, with 24,000 tonnes of blue mussel produced in 2010. As for Oceania, New Zealand is one of the most important mussel-producing countries in the world. The dominant species is the New Zealand mussel or green mussel *Perna canaliculus*, of which 90,000 tonnes were produced in long lines in 2010. In Africa, South Africa is the main producer, with 700 tonnes of *M. galloprovincialis*, followed by Tunisia, with 157 tonnes of the same species produced in 2010.

8.2 Shellfish Poisoning Outbreaks in Galicia

Along the last years, there has been an increase of harmful algae blooms (HABs) worldwide in frequency and duration,[10] leading to the situation that "virtually, every coastal region of the world is affected by HABs."[11] If this situation applies also to the Galician coast or if it is a phenomenon that has reached a somehow stable situation is a matter of concern.[12] Galicia has been suffering HAB episodes since the mid-1970s and this situation is considered one of the main environmental factors affecting Galician bivalve aquaculture. Diarrheic shellfish poisoning (DSP) toxins are the most frequent cause of closure of mussel production areas, although during particular years, the occurrence of paralytic shellfish poisoning (PSP) or ASP toxins has been registered in autumn, either alone or simultaneously to DSP toxins. The increase of number of harvesting areas closure along the years has been proposed to be related to an increase in the renewal time of the embayments, at least in the case of Rías Baixas (Muros–Noia, Arousa, Pontevedra, Aldán, and Vigo), and that this situation will follow an increasing tendency associated to global warming.[13] Mussel farming in Galicia is organized in floating rafts geographically grouped in harvesting areas. There are more than 3300 rafts exploited by family-based producers who owned 1–2 rafts. Water stream, dominant wind, and other factors are taken into account to determine the extent and the number of rafts belonging to these harvesting areas, in order to manage closure and disclosure during algal blooms. Monitoring and control of harvesting areas, not only regarding marine biotoxins but also microbiology, water quality, and other contaminants, lies on the public body INTECMAR (Technological Institute for the Control of Marine Environment in Galicia, www.intecmar.org), which offers online information of the state of the harvesting areas in its website. Table 8.5 shows the number of days that each of these harvesting areas was closed along years 2000–2011. The areas are listed from North to South, grouped by their location in the Galician Rias, which are shown in Figure 8.2.

Since the distribution of the harvesting areas is subjected to revision, some years new harvesting areas are created. This situation is depicted in Table 8.5 as NA (not available) in the years where the harvesting

TABLE 8.5

Number of Days of Closure of the Different Mussel Harvesting Areas in Galicia in the Period 2000–2011

	2000	2001	2002	2003	2004	2005	2006	2007	2008	2009	2010	2011
1. *Ría de Betanzos*												
Sada A	130	100	125	84	88	209	139	90	83	102	82	116
Sada B	96	55	101	64	46	155	115	67	49	79	18	113
2. *Ría de Corme*												
Corme B	NA	NA	130	126	188	238	149	95	117	137	116	131
3. *Ría de Muros–Noia*												
Muros B	192	134	157	143	169	244	157	57	50	135	135	225
Muros A	164	85	120	144	77	214	125	51	29	126	117	186
Noia A	120	53	118	109	59	182	125	51	0	70	96	142
Muros C	NA	NA	NA	NA	NA	NA	NA	NA	NA	NA	NA	44
4. *Ría de Arousa*												
Ribeira B	47	50	67	79	71	162	62	49	16	17	64	85
Ribeira C	44	53	71	83	78	166	58	55	16	80	67	72
Puebla H	34	27	46	69	47	141	56	50	0	38	24	42
Puebla G	18	3	39	21	0	82	11	17	0	0	0	24
Puebla A	17	3	27	23	0	51	0	23	0	0	0	32
Puebla B	23	3	26	41	0	128	16	21	0	3	22	29
Puebla C	23	3	39	49	0	117	11	26	0	8	26	26
Puebla D	27	7	54	65	27	145	13	27	0	47	38	24
Puebla E	19	7	46	70	18	100	19	6	0	31	25	35
Villagarcía A	8	3	45	45	11	98	11	0	0	0	13	0
Villagarcía B	39	4	59	57	2	126	13	3	0	18	34	22
Cambados A2, E	0	3	43	7	0	70	5	0	0	8	0	0
Cambados A1	51	12	61	68	40	155	17	26	0	66	47	32
Cambados B	37	23	62	85	55	165	46	37	23	69	76	36
Cambados C (Norte)	53	39	89	97	73	173	68	55	35	109	101	69
Cambados C (Sur)	46	48	83	109	79	186	65	50	31	92	77	61
Cambados D	13	4	51	45	0	139	0	44	7	0	51	37
Grove A	17	15	78	50	12	148	19	48	0	0	63	32
Grove C1	52	50	127	109	123	180	120	60	43	129	113	153
Grove C2	136	108	157	137	173	257	164	71	49	140	137	162
Grove C3	53	46	117	97	117	185	112	64	45	125	120	144
Grove C4	145	104	141	140	174	203	145	66	52	145	130	152
5. *Ría de Aldán*												
Cangas A	178	117	168	208	287	271	174	77	93	195	128	230
Cangas B	249	138	175	222	276	286	188	87	117	197	155	241
6. *Ría de Pontevedra*												
Bueu B	228	124	160	266	304	260	168	78	120	181	141	229
Bueu A2	250	130	170	256	293	262	174	88	124	187	147	241
Bueu A1	278	150	169	266	291	274	169	92	129	198	147	241
Portonovo A	106	90	142	213	148	200	99	62	40	143	116	153
Portonovo B	153	91	152	223	209	220	124	77	69	164	127	183
Portonovo C	154	89	142	218	226	238	127	73	75	166	131	191
7. *Ría de Vigo*												
Cangas F	193	144	170	209	274	280	186	88	87	154	131	231
Cangas G	131	121	178	205	278	267	170	86	81	133	134	215

(continued)

TABLE 8.5 (continued)

Number of Days of Closure of the Different Mussel Harvesting Areas in Galicia in the Period 2000–2011

	2000	2001	2002	2003	2004	2005	2006	2007	2008	2009	2010	2011
Cangas H	142	112	171	202	265	263	177	90	47	133	131	155
Cangas C	65	67	78	112	130	200	78	41	19	108	119	56
Cangas D	53	83	84	113	161	190	74	51	22	123	114	58
Cangas E	43	47	60	90	80	130	32	22	18	85	66	38
Redondela A	28	36	61	83	38	67	18	5	0	71	50	10
Redondela B, G	28	15	58	39	5	33	0	0	0	9	34	10
Redondela C, F	25	15	49	38	0	40	3	0	0	0	32	9
Redondela D	26	20	60	47	13	41	4	0	0	24	25	9
Redondela E	27	29	56	83	34	81	17	0	0	51	64	11
Vigo A	91	45	58	136	114	140	40	17	23	105	115	60
Baiona A	187	104	170	213	255	184	147	73	75	108	116	191
Total Galicia	4239	2809	4810	5658	5408	8346	4010	2316	1784	4309	4015	4988

Source: Data obtained from INTECMAR.

Note: Numbers correspond with geographical location in Figure 8.2. NA, not available.

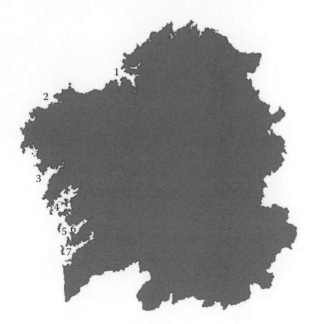

FIGURE 8.2 Localization of the different Galician Rías: 1, Betanzos; 2, Corme; 3, Muros–Noia; 4, Arousa; 5, Aldán; 6, Pontevedra; 7, Vigo. (Map obtained from INTECMAR.)

area had not already been established. The creation of a new harvesting area generates a bias when a number of closure days are directly compared in time series, and it has been proposed that incidence is a better indicator. Incidence is calculated as follows:

$$\text{Incidence} = \sum \left(\frac{N}{M} \right) \times 100$$

where

N is the number of days in which each of the harvesting areas remained closed throughout the year
M is the number of maximum possible closure days, which is calculated by weighting the closure days of each year by the number of existing polygons

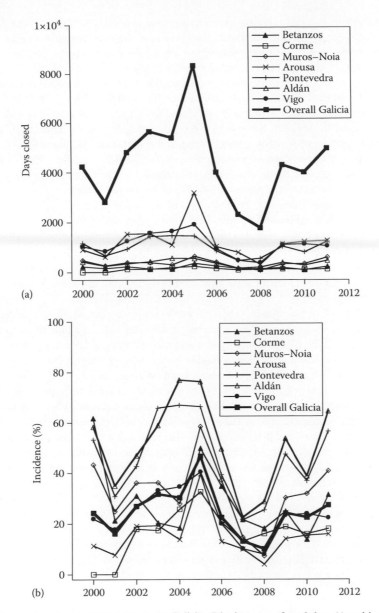

FIGURE 8.3 Closure days during 2000–2011 in the Galician Rías in terms of total days (a) and incidence (b). (Data obtained from INTECMAR.)

The maximum incidence would occur if all of the polygons remained closed for the whole year, which would be equivalent to all of the mussel rafts being closed all year.[12] Figure 8.3a represents the number of days that harvesting areas were closed in each ría and an overall incidence in Galicia during 2000–2011, while Figure 8.3b represents the same data in terms of incidence.

It should be noted that as the number of harvesting areas in each ría is quite different (2 harvesting areas in Betanzos, 1 in Corme, 4 in Muros–Noia, 22 in Arousa, 2 in Aldán, 6 in Pontevedra, 13 in Vigo), the weight of each one on the overall data differs from one to other figure, and hence, some lines should be evaluated carefully when different harvesting areas show different behavior along the year. For instance, Aldán Ría contains only two harvesting areas, Cangas A and Cangas B, which show similar behavior and reached a peak of near 80% of incidence in 2004 and 2005; on the other hand, Bueu B, in Pontevedra Ría or Cangas F, in Vigo Ría, despite showing similar profiles of closing days, when the other harvesting areas in their respective rías are analyzed together, there is a flattening effect due to the better results of the other harvesting areas. The same effect occurs in the overall analysis of the whole number of harvesting areas, which can hide some catastrophic situations at local level.

Another question that must be taken into account in order to evaluate the economic impact of a bloom is the month of the year. This is because mussel consumption is not regular along the year, but it maintains seasonal evolution that is related to the biology of the mollusk. Briefly, from February to June, there is a loss in flesh due to spawn, which is associated to fall in demand, as the product is not in its best quality. From July, there is an increase in the flesh, and it begins the campaign, mainly for the industry. Domestic consumption of live mussels reaches the maximum in September–December, with a peak in Christmas. Although domestic consumption of live mussels represent 40% of the production against 60%, which is addressed to the transformation industry, it has a higher price, so closures during September–December have a more important economic effect on producers.[7]

As seen in Figure 8.3 and Table 8.5, 2005 was one of the worst years in the history of mussel production in Galicia, with several harvesting areas closed for more than 75% of the year and production decreased between 30% and 50% compared to 2004 production.[12,14] Indeed, almost 86% of the harvesting areas were closed in November and December, affecting one of the more important campaigns in the year, the Christmas season.

In 2010 the costs of HABs in Galicia were estimated in 40,000,000 € (research project purgademar) http://www.purgademar.com

In 2011, the major problem was that closure days were very concentrated. In fact, in September, 85% of the harvesting areas were closed, and the remaining open areas were not able to cover market needs. Indeed, the distribution of the bloom was very fast and the situation of harvesting areas changed from 10% closed to 85% in less than a week. This situation became a problem not only for the producers but also for several companies downstream in the transformation chain. Several depuration facilities closed temporarily due to the lack of product, and in the same way, those companies devoted to boil and take the shell out for the canning industry. The mussel campaign in the cannery industry concentrates in this part of the year, and the working schedule had to be readjusted, delaying hiring of seasonal workers. Not only mussels but cockles, clams, and razor clams were also affected in the Christmas season. In 1/3 of the harvesting areas, the closure lasted until Christmas, and with the first storms, part of the mussels came off from their ropes and around 40% of the production got lost. In part of the harvesting areas, mainly in the South, the situation was as bad as in 2005. Although mollusks in the legal circuit were controlled and safe for consumption, health authorities took special measures to make doctors at primary health care aware about PSP and DSP symptomatology by means of a circular letter stressing symptomatology and the need of communication of clinical cases to the epidemiological service, in case of intoxication due to recreational shellfish harvesting. This situation was published by several newspapers and other media,[15,16] and it is hard to determine if it could exert a negative effect on commercially distributed mollusk consumption.

8.3 Economic Losses for Producers

Toxic episodes have detrimental economic impacts not only on shellfish harvesters and the aquaculture industry but also on coastal economies and on human health. Many efforts have been made to estimate the economic impact of HABs, although these studies did not take into account all necessary factors. Mostly, direct costs to the aquaculture industry were calculated, but these represent a low estimate of the true cost of HABs, which should include impacts on demand for uncontaminated shellfish and on recreational shellfish harvesting. In addition, the coastal economy and the health costs associated with toxic outbreaks should be quantified. An integrated assessment approach would examine the economic impact of HABs on consumers and the shellfish industry and both coastal and regional economies. Also, it should include evaluation of the costs and benefits of reducing coastal pollution and other human-related activities that may exacerbate the HABs problem and weigh the costs and benefits of increased monitoring and surveillance that could potentially reduce the number of shellfish harvesting closures.[17]

A conservative estimate of the average annual economic impact resulting from HABS in the United States is approximately US$75 million over the period 1987–2000.[10,18]

The 1997 PSP blooms in Washington State severely impacted the oyster harvesting. The small farms in closed areas suffered great financial losses since the blooms occurred in November and December. Some clams and oysters areas closed for 8 weeks, missing Thanksgiving, Christmas, and New Year's sales, and estimated losses were $5000/week. A PSP bloom in Willapa Bay and Grays Harbor occurred just before Thanksgiving Day, which is the oyster industry's busiest time of the year, accounting for 40% of the business. Sales during the Christmas season were also lost, although the coastal bays were reopened by mid-December, due to that out-of-state competitors had moved into the market. About 34 coastal shellfish farms lost approximately 50% of their sales, reducing average sales by approximately $8 million. Over 100 workers were laid off and many more had hours reduced.

Alaska, of all states in the Pacific region, has the largest and most productive fishery in the United States, contributing 54% of the nation's total landings. The cost of PSP to the commercial fishery, recreational harvesters, and the aquaculture industry is believed to exceed $10 million annually. The Quileute Tribe in La Push, Washington, also suffered high losses during the 1998 domoic acid episode. Toxin levels in Dungeness crab were above the regulatory limit. Crabbers had a choice of eviscerating the crabs or closing down the fishery entirely. They chose to eviscerate, which greatly decreased the market value of the crabs to 50% of the money typically earned.[17]

Washington possesses large populations of the Pacific razor clam, *Siliqua patula*, one of the West Coast's most popular shellfish for recreational harvest. During a routine test for PSP, domoic acid was discovered in razor clams. An emergency closure of the Long Beach Peninsula in the fall of 1991 affected thousands of diggers and coastal businesses. Domoic acid levels continued to increase and spread to other beaches, resulting in the closure of all five major clamming beaches. The closures lasted into the following spring, causing an estimated revenue loss of $5–$8 million, based on estimates of $25 per day per digger.[17]

In Japan, fish mortalities due to red tides in the Seto Inland Sea cost fishermen tens of millions of dollars per year, especially during the early 1970s. After an intensive effort to reduce pollution bloom, incidence has decreased, but blooms of raphidophytes and dinoflagellates still kill cultured finfish and shellfish. In China, a widespread red tide in 1989 along the coast of Hebei Province affected 15,000 ha of shrimp ponds, resulting in a loss valued at US$ 40 million.[10,18]

In Europe, Using FAO shellfish aquaculture data, the estimation of the economic impact of HABs on farmed shellfish was $754 million from 2000 to 2009, which was an annual value of $75.4 million. This yearly average represents 7% of the total value of the shellfish sector. Indeed, annual losses per country for the mussel industry during the period 2000–2009 have been studied and are summarized in Table 8.6.[19]

Regarding economic effects of HABs in tourism, data related to effects at business level are scarce; in this sense Morgan et al. evaluated the effect of *Karenia brevis* blooms on Florida restaurant sales, by comparing daily sales of three restaurants and environmental conditions in a 7-year series, concluding that there was a daily reduction in sales in the range of $868–3734 (13.7%–15.3%).[20] Nevertheless, this data cannot be extrapolated to other toxins, since *K. brevis* blooms evoke respiratory symptoms, which appeared to move from the upper to the lower respiratory track with increasing exposure levels of the aerosolized brevetoxins,[21] and hence losses are due to reduced customers attendance, not to a reduction in mollusk consumption. An overall estimation of *Karenia* red tides costs of respiratory illnesses in Sarasota County (Florida) alone to range from $0.5 to $4 million/bloom, depending upon bloom severity.[22]

8.4 Mollusks Processing

In Spain, mussels are mainly produced in Galicia in the "rías" as it was mentioned previously. These special producing areas are very rich due to topography, water, and nutrients flux and depth.[23] Galicia can be considered as worldwide leader in mussel production intended to human consumption.[24] Mussel aquaculture is developed in more than 3300 floating rafts and, downstream in the production chain, depuration facilities, boiling facilities, and canning industries. The mussel sector generates about 11,500 direct jobs (of which 8,500 are fixed) and 7,000 indirect with an annual turnover of between 120 and

TABLE 8.6

European Annual Losses per Country for the Mussel
Industry during the Period 2000–2009

Country	Average Loss ($)
France	9,216,234
Spain	6,069,746
Netherlands	5,285,977
Italy	4,313,943
United Kingdom	2,700,281
Ireland	2,272,724
Germany	908,131
Greece	819,030
Norway	132,440
Croatia	104,454
Sweden	66,086
Denmark	56,989
Albania	47,639
Bulgaria	28,806
Montenegro	14,413
Portugal	12,930
Channel Islands	12,396
Slovenia	11,375
Russian Federation	9,216
Ukraine	6,961
Bosnia and Herzegovina	3,694
Iceland	1,988
Serbia and Montenegro	130
Total	32,065,171

Source: Maguire, J., EU project ASIMUTH applied simulations and integrated modelling for the understanding
of toxic and harmful algal blooms deliverable 5.1,
Initial user requirements consolidation report, 2011.

150 million euros in the first sale (The Regulatory Council of the Galician Mussel, http://www.mexil-londegalicia.org) and a global turnover of 450 million euros.

In relation to the final destination, 65% of mussel from Galicia goes to processing industries, whereas 35% is consumed fresh. A phenomenon that is necessary to take into account is the fact that processing of mollusk influences the content and type of toxins in the final product. In this context, European Food Safety Authority (EFSA) published a review in relation to the influence of processing on the levels of lipophilic marine biotoxins in bivalve mollusks.[25] Seafood-processing establishments as canning or ready-to-eat producing industries have to face the challenge of buying fresh mollusk with the sanitary control and to find, after processing, that the final product contains toxins above the legal limit. These occasions correspond to fresh mollusks with lipophilic toxins below the legal limit that concentrate and get higher levels after heating and losing water. The literature concerning the effect of mollusk process-ing, mainly heating, on the levels of biotoxins is very scarce. In general terms, it is known that there is conversion or redistribution among toxins analogues when mollusks are differently heat-treated.

The EFSA opinion referred to Hess and Jorgensen (2007) reporting that loss of fluid during cook-ing could result in a 25%–80% increase in the concentration of the lipophilic toxins in cooked shell-fish compared to uncooked.[25] The EFSA Panel on Contaminants in the Food Chain (CONTAM Panel) established the following toxic equivalence factors (TEFs): OA = 1, DTX1 = 1, DTX2 = 0.6. For DTX3 the TEF values are equal to those of the corresponding unesterified toxins (OA, DTX1, and DTX2).[26]

McCarron et al. investigated the influence of conventional steaming (over boiling water for 10 min) and autoclaving (121°C for 15 min) on the level of OA and DTX2 in mussels.[27] The authors studied the effect of processing on whole flesh, the digestive glands and the remainder tissues (remaining after careful dissection of the digestive glands).

Steaming of mussels caused a 30%–70% increase in the concentration of OA-group toxins in the whole flesh. After autoclaving, this increase was between 70% and 84%. Water loss was identified as the cause of these increases in concentration. In addition, there was some evidence that the redistribution of OA-group toxins from the digestive gland to the remaining tissues might occur during processing. Measurements of the moisture content indicated that these increases were caused by water loss during processing. Although not consistent for both samples, the results of the study suggested that redistribution from the digestive gland to the remainder tissues might occur during processing. The authors concluded that analysis of whole shellfish flesh, as opposed to the digestive gland, was more appropriate for regulatory purposes, particularly when processed shellfish is analyzed.

Azaspiracids (AZAs) are a group of shellfish toxins causing AZA poisoning. Approximately 20 different analogues have been identified, of which AZA1, AZA2, and AZA3 are the most important based on occurrence and toxicity. In the EFSA opinion on the AZAs adopted in June 2008, the CONTAM Panel adopted the following TEFs applied in some countries for AZAs: AZA1 = 1, AZA2 = 1.8, and AZA3 = 1.4. The current European Union (EU) regulatory limit is of 160 μg AZA1 equivalents/kg shellfish meat. The CONTAM Panel concluded that in order for a 60 kg adult not to exceed the ARfD of 0.2 μg AZA1 equivalents/kg bw, a 400 g portion of shellfish should not contain more than 12 μg toxin or 30 μg AZA1 equivalent/kg shellfish meat.[28]

AZAs in shellfish are not decomposed at temperatures relevant for cooking. Also, information from Hess et al. indicated that steaming of raw fresh mussels resulted in a twofold higher level of AZAs (AZA1, AZA2, and AZA3 expressed as AZA equivalents/kg) in both whole flesh and digestive gland tissue compared to the uncooked flesh.[29] This effect was attributed to the loss of water from the mussels into the cooking fluid. In a recent study, McCarron et al. investigated the effect of heating on AZAs in the absence of water loss.[30] For that purpose, aliquots of mussel tissue homogenates were put into capped centrifuge tubes, which were heated for 10 min at 90°C. No differences in the concentration of AZA1 and AZA2 were observed, but the concentration of AZA3 increased threefold. It was shown by the authors that a carboxylated AZA analogue, AZA17, was converted under these conditions into AZA3.

There is no information on the effects of processing (e.g., cooking, steaming, autoclaving) on the levels of yessotoxins (YTXs) or pectenotoxins (PTXs) in shellfish. However, it can be assumed that, as for other lipophilic marine biotoxins, OA-group toxins and AZAs, cooking may lead to an increase in concentration of YTXs and PTXs in shellfish flesh due to water loss during processing. The CONTAM noted that there is no information available on other forms of processing such as frying or grilling.[25]

EFSA indicates that the analysis of whole shellfish flesh, as opposed to the digestive gland, might be more appropriate for regulatory purposes, particularly when processed shellfish is analyzed.[25] However, there is no information regarding the transformation of 160 μg OA equivalents/kg after processing although we should take into account that final levels of different toxins in processed shellfish will be always higher than in fresh mollusks. Regulation 1881/2006 setting maximum levels for certain contaminants in food stuffs establishes that to allow maximum levels to be applied to dried, diluted, processed, and compound foodstuffs, where no specific community maximum levels have been established, food business operators should provide the specific concentration and dilution factors accompanied by the appropriate experimental data justifying the factor proposed.[31] Nevertheless, in the case of marine biotoxins, this legislation cannot be applied, although the principle is similar to other contaminants. Thus, increasing the legal limit for processed mollusks could be an economically feasible alternative as was published for other contaminants if a transformation factor is provided.[31]

These economic losses of processing industries were not evaluated yet, but sometimes it happened that the business operators have to destroy the final product after processing and this is a very expensive process.

8.5 Consumption Dose and Legal Limit Decreasing

The current EU regulatory limits for marine biotoxins are stated in Regulation (EC) No. 853/2004.[32] For instance, regulatory limit for okadaic acid is 160 µg OA equivalents/kg shellfish meat. This limit was initially estimated by the EFSA CONTAM Panel, with a 100 g portion of shellfish meat. However, more recently, a new figure of 400 g of shellfish meat was identified as the high portion size to be used in the acute risk assessment of marine biotoxins.

The process of obtaining data for assessing the exposure is difficult and complex, even more if the population is big and heterogeneous as occurs in the EU. Statistical estimations and models are used in order to obtain a unique figure, which is, depending on the case, more or less representative. This is the case of the polemic dose of 400 g of shellfish meat used by EFSA for assessing the risk of the diverse marine biotoxins. Previously, this figure, 400 g dose, was obtained out of the consumption data from five countries (France, Italy, Germany, the United Kingdom, and the Netherlands) and used for the risk assessments for the whole EU population (27 member states nowadays).

Recently, a Concise Database, with information from 20 countries and with different food categories, including aquatic mollusks, was published by EFSA scientific panels and member states for screening purposes.[33] The amount of consumed product is calculated from surveys or similar querying methods in which the population is asked about their feeding habits. Normally, the amount of consumed product is more difficult to obtain because generally methodological differences between the collaborating member states make the outcome data unsuitable for EU-wide analyses and country-to-country comparisons. In studies in which more than one country is involved, normally estimations have to be used, so that uncertainty increases. This database estimates the distribution of portion size per eating occasions, which is needed in order to assess acute exposure, and it estimates the portion size per eating day.[33]

Concerning water mollusk, if we consider the mean of portion size (g) per day, we observe that the consumption is very heterogeneous depending on the country. In general, the mean consumption of mollusks in the EU falls below 100 g/day although there are some exceptions. The biggest ingestion refers to Slovenia with a mean consumption in grams per day of 217.7; however, these data derive from two consuming days that corresponds to 0.5% of consuming days. In addition, the number of observations is lower than 60, then the 95th and higher percentiles (consumption of 250 g/day) may not be statistically robust. Other countries with a high ingestion per day are Austria, Cyprus, Denmark, Germany, Greece, and Italy, in all cases lower than 140.1 g/day. Taking into account that all countries, except Germany, also present low number of observations, 95th and higher percentiles may not be statistically robust. In contrast, Germany has a mean of consumption in grams per day of 103 with a standard deviation of 138, and P95th and P97.5th of 375 and 650, respectively, however a median of 60 consumption in grams per day. It is the only country with such a very high statistical significant percentiles. Once these data are completely analyzed by authorities, legal limits of marine biotoxins might be decreased,[34,35] as summarized in Table 8.7; then shellfish aquaculture will be a major concern, and producers and related industries will suffer serious economical losses, even some will have to quit the business.

As stated earlier, regulatory limit for okadaic acid is 160 µg OA equivalents/kg shellfish meat based on a 100 g portion, but the statement of a 400 g portion brings a reduction on regulatory limits. For instance, EFSA CONTAM Panel concluded that in order for a 60 kg adult not to exceed the acute reference dose (ARfD) of 0.3 µg OA equivalents/kg body weight, a 400 g portion of shellfish should not contain more than 18 µg toxin, corresponding to 45 µg OA equivalent/kg shellfish meat.[26,36] Similar reasoning leads to a decrease of regulatory limits as stated in Table 8.7, except for the case of yessotoxins, where an increase of regulatory limit has been proposed, based on its minor toxicity. Sensitivity of mouse bioassay official methods[37] seemed to be a threshold in order to establish new regulatory limits. Nevertheless, the relatively new developed methodology for PSP toxins and lipophilic toxins recognized as official[38,39] may be an open gate in order to reduce current levels.

Regarding PSP, the current official method, mouse bioassay, has a detection limit of approximately 370 mg/kg,[34] which would not be enough for the new situation created by a reduction in the regulatory limit. The implementation of the precolumn or the postcolumn oxidation HPLC method, which are

TABLE 8.7

Maximum Concentration of Marine Biotoxins Based on 400 g Portion and Risk Assessment

Toxin	Current EU Limits	Exposure by Eating 400 g Portion at the EU Limit	ARfD	Maximum Concentration Based on 400 g Portion
OA	160 µg OA equivalents/kg SM	64 µg OA equivalents/person (1 µg OA equivalents/kg bw)	0.3 µg OA equivalents/kg bw	45 µg OA equivalents/kg SM
AZA	160 µg AZA equivalents/kg SM	64 µg AZA1 equivalents/person (1 µg AZA1 equivalents/kg bw)	0.2 µg AZA1 equivalents/kg bw	30 µg AZA1 equivalents/kg SM
PTX	160 µg OA equivalents/kg SM	64 µg PTX2/person (1 µg PTX2 equivalents/kg bw)	0.8 µg PTX2 equivalents/kg bw	120 µg PTX2 equivalents/kg SM
YTX	1 mg YTX equivalents/kg SM	400 µg YTX equivalents/person (6.7 µg YTX equivalents/kg bw)	25 µg YTX equivalents/kg bw	3.75 mg YTX equivalents/kg SM
STX	800 µg PSP/kg SM	320 µg STX equivalents/person (5.3 µg STX equivalents/kg bw)	0.5 µg STX equivalents/kg bw	75 µg STX equivalents/kg SM
DA	20 mg DA/kg SM	8 mg DA/person (130 µg DA/kg bw)	30 µg DA/kg bw	4.5 mg DA/kg SM

Source: Adapted from EFSA, *EFSA J.*, 1306, 1, 2009.

slower than mouse bioassay, would trigger a delay in getting results and hence would modify the current pattern of monitoring/analysis/harvesting permission. Indeed, the need of HPLCs and highly qualified staff would have a negative economic impact on the costs of monitoring programs as well as on the self-control of producers when these analyses must be carried out in other laboratories. On the other hand, the reduction of the regulatory limit as it has been suggested by EFSA would lead to an enhancement of the number of closure days. In the case of Galicia, where PSP blooms are less frequent, after studying recorded data from previous blooms, it has been evaluated that the length of the closures would double in the case of *Gymnodinium catenatum* blooms, and the scenario would become even worse in the case of *Alexandrium catenatum* blooms.[7]

In the case of lipophilic toxins, the change of regulatory limit would make the mouse bioassay useless, since its detection limit is around the current regulatory limit.[26] Again, the implementation of chromatographic methods (LC-MS/MS) would enhance duration and costs of analysis. Eventually, there would be an enhancement of the length of the closures ranging between 26% and 138%, depending on the toxic profile, the duration of the toxic episode, and the month of the year when the bloom occurs.[7]

ACKNOWLEDGMENTS

This study was financed through research grants AGL2009-13581-C02-02 and AGL2012-40185-C02-02 from the Ministerio de Ciencia e Innovación (Ministry of Science and Innovation, Spanish Government) and through the European research project grants CiguaTools-Development of a Rapid Test Kit and supporting Reference Standards Capable of Detecting the Emerging Fish toxin Ciguatoxin in European and Global Waters (FP7-SME-2012-1-315285), Pharmatlantic-Knowledge Transfer Network for Prevention of Mental Diseases and Cancer in the Atlantic Area (2009-1/117) financed by ERDF funds within the Atlantic Area Operational Programme and Beads-Bio-engineered micro encapsulation of active agents delivered to shellfish (FP7-SME-2010-1-262649).

REFERENCES

1. FAO, 2012. *The State of World Fisheries and Aquaculture*. FAO Fisheries & Aquaculture Department, Rome, Italy.
2. FAO, 2012. FAO Fisheries & Aquaculture—Global Aquaculture Production 1950–2011. Available online at http://www.fao.org/fishery/statistics/global-aquaculture-production/query/en

3. FAO, 2012. FAO Fisheries & Aquaculture—Global Aquaculture Production. Available online at http://www.fao.org/fishery/statistics/global-aquaculture-production/en

4. Crespi, V. and Coche, A., 2008. *Glossary of Aquaculture*. FAO Fisheries & Aquaculture Department, Rome, Italy.

5. Blanco, J., Acosta, C. P., Bermúdez de la Puente, M., and Salgado, C., 2002. Depuration and anatomical distribution of the amnesic shellfish poisoning (ASP) toxin domoic acid in the king scallop *Pecten maximus*. *Aquatic Toxicology*, 60, 111–121.

6. Smith, E. A., Papapanagiotou, E. P., Brown, N. A., Stobo, L. A., Gallacher, S., and Shanks, A. M., 2006. Effect of storage on amnesic shellfish poisoning (ASP) toxins in king scallops (*Pecten maximus*). *Harmful Algae*, 5, 9–19.

7. Blanco, J. (Coord.), (2011). Informe final proyecto JACUMAR "Cultivo de mitílidos: expansión y sostenibilidad (CULMITES)". Subproyecto C.A. Galicia. Available online at http://proyectosmapa.tragsatec.es/app/jacumar/planes_nacionales/Documentos/97_IF_CULMITES_Anexo_GALICIA.PDF

8. FAO, 2012. Cultured aquatic species information programme—*Mytilus galloprovincialis*. Available online at http://www.fao.org/fishery/culturedspecies/Mytilus_galloprovincialis/en

9. Zhang, F., 1984. Mussel culture in China. *Aquaculture*, 39, 1–10.

10. Anderson, D. M., 2009. Approaches to monitoring, control and management of harmful algal blooms (HABs). *Ocean and Coastal Management*, 52, 342–347.

11. Anderson, D. M., Cembella, A. D., and Hallegraeff, G. M., 2012. Progress in understanding harmful algal blooms: Paradigm shifts and new technologies for research, monitoring, and management. *Annual Review of Marine Science*, 4, 143–176.

12. Rodríguez-Rodríguez, G., Villasante, S., and García-Negro, M. C., 2011. Are red tides affecting economically the commercialization of the Galician (NW Spain) mussel farming? *Marine Policy*, 35, 252–257.

13. Álvarez-Salgado, X. A., Labarta, U., Fernández-Reiriz, M. J. et al., 2008. Renewal time and the impact of harmful algal blooms on the extensive mussel raft culture of the Iberian coastal upwelling system (SW Europe). *Harmful Algae*, 7, 849–855.

14. Vieites, J. M. and Cabado, A. G., 2008. Incidence of marine toxins on industrial activity, In *Seafood and Freshwater Toxins. Pharmacology, Physiology and Detection*. Botana, L. M., Ed. CRC Press, Taylor & Francis Group, Boca Raton, FL, pp. 899–917.

15. Paniagua, A. and Blanco, M., El Sergas da la alerta de una marea roja muy grave en las rías del sur in *La Voz de Galicia*. A Coruña, 2011.

16. Paniagua, A. and Blanco, M., Sanidade aconseja extremar precauciones ante una marea roja especialmente virulenta, in *La Voz de Galicia*. A Coruña, 2011.

17. The cost of harmful algal blooms on the West Coast (2000). In *Red Tides, West Coast Newsletter on Marine Biotoxins and Harmful Algal Blooms*, Northwest Fisheries Science Center and Washington Sea Grant Program, pp. 1–8. Available online at http://www.nwfsc.noaa.gov/hab/outreach/pdf_files/RedTides2000.pdf

18. Anderson, D. M., 2007. The ecology and oceanography of harmful algal blooms multidisciplinary approaches to research and management. *IOC Technical Series,* 74. UNESCO, Paris, France.

19. Maguire, J., 2011. EU project ASIMUTH applied simulations and integrated modelling for the understanding of toxic and harmful algal blooms deliverable 5.1. Initial user requirements consolidation report. Available online at http://www.asimuth.eu/Deliverables%20and%20Publications/Documents/D5-1_Initial-user-requirements-consolidation-report.pdf

20. Morgan, K. L., Larkin, S. L., and Adams, C. M., 2009. Firm-level economic effects of HABS: A tool for business loss assessment. *Harmful Algae*, 8, 212–218.

21. Fleming, L. E., Kirkpatrick, B., Backer, L. C. et al., 2011. Review of Florida red tide and human health effects. *Harmful Algae*, 10, 224–233.

22. Hoagland, P., Jin, D., Polansky, L. Y. et al., 2009. The costs of respiratory illnesses arising from Florida Gulf coast Karenia brevis blooms. *Environmental Health Perspectives*, 117, 1239–1243.

23. Pitcher, G., Figueiras, F., Hickey, B., and Moita, M., 2010. The physical oceanography of upwelling systems and the development of harmful algal blooms. *Progress in Oceanography*, 85, 5–32.

24. Leis, M., 2006. Mussel culture in Galicia: A successful career with perspectives. *Revista Galega de Economía*, 15, 251–256.

25. EFSA, 2009. Scientific opinion: Influence of processing on the levels of lipophilic marine biotoxins in bivalve molluscs. Statement of the panel on contaminants in the food chain. *The EFSA Journal*, 1016, 1–10.

26. EFSA, 2008. Opinion of the scientific panel on contaminants in the food chain on a request from the European Commission on marine biotoxins in shellfish-okadaic acid and analogues. *The EFSA Journal*, 589, 1–62.

27. McCarron, P., Kilcoyne, J., and Hess, P., 2008. Effects of cooking and heat treatment on concentration and tissue distribution of okadaic acid and dinophysistoxin-2 in mussels (*Mytilus edulis*). *Toxicon*, 51, 1081–1089.

28. EFSA, 2008. Opinion of the scientific panel on contaminants in the food chain on a request from the European Commission on marine biotoxins in shellfish—Azaspiracids. *The EFSA Journal*, 723, 1–52.

29. Hess, P., Nguyen, L., Aasen, J. et al., 2005. Tissue distribution, effects of cooking and parameters affecting the extraction of azaspiracids from mussels, *Mytilus edulis*, prior to analysis by liquid chromatography coupled to mass spectrometry. *Toxicon*, 46, 62–71.

30. McCarron, P., Kilcoyne, J., Miles, C. O., and Hess, P., 2009. Formation of azaspiracids-3,-4,-6, and-9 via decarboxylation of carboxyazaspiracid metabolites from shellfish. *Journal of Agricultural and Food Chemistry*, 57, 160–169.

31. (EC), Commission Regulation, 2006. COMMISSION REGULATION (EC) No. 1881/2006 of 19 December 2006 setting maximum levels for certain contaminants in foodstuffs. *Official Journal of the European Union*, L 364, 5–24.

32. European Parliament, 2004. Regulation (EC) No. 853/2004 of the European Parliament and of the Council of April 29, 2004 laying down specific hygiene rules for food of animal origin. *Official Journal of the European Union*, 139, 55–205.

33. EFSA, 2011. The EFSA comprehensive European food consumption database. Available online at http://www.efsa.europa.eu/en/datexfoodcdb/datexfooddb.htm

34. EFSA, 2009. Scientific opinion of the panel on contaminants in the food chain on a request from the European Commission on marine biotoxins in shellfish—Summary on regulated marine biotoxins. *EFSA Journal*, 1306, 1–23.

35. Paredes, I., Rietjens, I. M. C. M., Vieites, J. M., and Cabado, A. G., 2011. Update of risk assessments of main marine biotoxins in the European Union. *Toxicon*, 58, 336–354.

36. EFSA, 2010. Statement on further elaboration of the consumption figure of 400 g shellfish meat on the basis of new consumption data. *EFSA Journal*, 1706, 1–20.

37. European Commission, 2005. COMMISSION REGULATION (EC) No. 2074/2005 of December 5, 2005 laying down implementing measures for certain products under Regulation (EC) No. 853/2004 of the European Parliament and of the Council and for the organisation of official controls under Regulation (EC) No. 854/2004 of the European Parliament and of the Council and Regulation (EC) No. 882/2004 of the European Parliament and of the Council, derogating from Regulation (EC) No. 852/2004 of the European Parliament and of the Council and amending Regulations (EC) No. 853/2004 and (EC) No. 854/2004. *Official Journal of the European Union*, L 338, 27–59.

38. European Commission, 2006. COMMISSION REGULATION (EC) No. 1664/2006 of November 6, 2006 amending Regulation (EC) No. 2074/2005 as regards implementing measures for certain products of animal origin intended for human consumption and repealing certain implementing measures. *Official Journal of the European Union*, L 320, 13–45.

39. European Commission, 2011. COMMISSION REGULATION (EU) No. 15/2011 of January 10, 2011 amending Regulation (EC) No. 2074/2005 as regards recognised testing methods for detecting marine biotoxins in live bivalve molluscs. *Official Journal of the European Union*, L 6, 3–6.

9

Designing a Preharvest Monitoring and Management Plan for Marine Shellfish Toxins

Joe Silke

CONTENTS

Because of the absence of practical cost-effective means to remove marine toxins from shellfish, the primary tool employed to prevent human intoxications is the monitoring of toxin levels at preharvesting stage. Based on the concentration of toxins detected, restrictions can be placed on the harvesting of shellfish if levels of toxin are too high. A range of monitoring approaches has been adopted in many parts of the world to manage shellfish toxicity and to comply with local legislative requirements. The incidence of harmful algal blooms (HABs) has been increasing in terms of both frequency and geographic distribution in recent decades. This coupled with increased popularity of shellfish as a consumer food item has resulted in greater emphasis on high-quality food safety practices to be enshrined in the production cycle of bivalve molluscs.

The problem stems from the group of toxin-producing HAB species that produce toxic compounds that are poisonous to other species, including humans. The pathway to human illness from these HABs is usually indirect and involves ingestion of fish or shellfish that have in turn acquired toxins through feeding on the toxic microalgae. Non-shellfish vectors include a small number of highly potent toxins that transfer via finfish including ciguatera fish poisoning (CFP) common only in tropical waters. The number of cases of CFP is suspected to be considerably underreported, but estimates of at least 50,000 per annum have been made. The condition is endemic in tropical and subtropical regions of the Pacific Basin, Indian Ocean, and Caribbean (Ting and Brown, 2001). An example of direct human health impact from HABs occurs when algal toxins becomes airborne in sea spray, causing respiratory irritation and asthma-like symptoms in beachgoers and coastal residents (Flemming et al., 2004). Recent incidents of illness from people after consuming toxic fish or developing respiratory symptoms have increased. These may be explained by increased awareness, shifts in climatic conditions, developments in the scientific methods of detection, coastal eutrophication stemming from changes in coastal demographics, and increased runoff due to deforestation (Hallegraeff, 2003; Sellner et al., 2003).

A more prevalent vector of potential HAB illnesses results from several varieties of microalgal toxins passed to human consumers via various shellfish species (FAO, 2004). These illnesses can range from mild gastrointestinal discomfort to life-threatening neurological toxins and have been grouped into five main categories, distinguished by the human syndrome that they may cause, namely,

- Paralytic shellfish poisoning (PSP) caused by the saxitoxin group
- Diarrheic shellfish poisoning (DSP) caused by the okadaic acid group
- Amnesic shellfish poisoning (ASP) caused by the domoic acid group
- Neurotoxic shellfish poisoning (NSP) caused by the brevetoxin group
- Azaspiracid shellfish poisoning (AZP) caused by the azaspiracid group

At present, there are no practical solutions to removing these toxins from shellfish other than allowing them to naturally depurate by metabolic processes within the shellfish growing area. This can take from several weeks to several months depending on the level of toxin and environmental parameters.

The worldwide production of cultured bivalve shellfish has increased from about 1 million tonnes per annum in 1970 to an estimation of almost 14 million tonnes today as shown in Figure 9.1. According to the Food and Agriculture Organization of the United Nations, the vast majority of this increase has taken place in Asia, with over 12 million tonnes annual production of mainly clams, oysters, and scallops in this region. There is also significant production in Europe, New Zealand, the United States, and South America (FAO, 2012). This increase in production and the prevalence of shellfish toxins have resulted in many of the key producing countries developing and implementing toxin monitoring and management strategies to minimize the risk of unsafe product being placed on the market.

The design and operation of monitoring systems are based on the legal requirements and the system in place between the authorities and industry in various shellfish-producing countries. Interpretation of the legislation by the country has led to a variety of government-controlled or in some cases industry-led programs to allow commercial development to progress while adhering to legal requirements.

In Europe, EC Regulation 854/2004 prescribes the legal controls that are placed on the production and marketing of live bivalve shellfish to ensure that contaminated shellfish are not placed on the market.

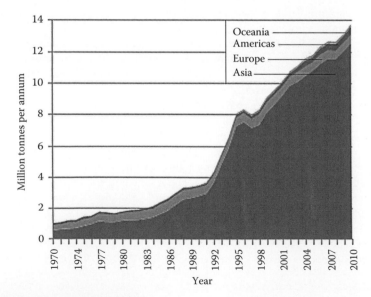

FIGURE 9.1 Total molluscan bivalve shellfish production 1970–2010. (From FAO, [online], Rome, Italy, 2010–2012. Updated [Cited September 12, 2012]. http://www.fao.org/fishery/statistics/global-aquaculture-production/en)

In January 2011, Commission Regulation Number 15/2011 amended this regulation so that a liquid chromatography–mass spectrometric (LC–MS/MS) method would replace the live animal assay and become the reference method for the measurement of marine lipophilic toxins in shellfish from July 1, 2011. The new regulation will allow time to the member states to adapt their methods to LC–MS/MS and allow the mouse bioassay to be used until December 31, 2014.

Legislation in other parts of the world has maintained the use of mouse bioassays as their principal means of detection of toxins, in some cases supported by phytoplankton detection programs. However, there is now greater availability of most of the harmful toxins in the form of highly purified and certified reference standards for laboratory calibration, and this has resulted in a concerted move to more accurate and quantifiable instrumental methods of detection in most countries.

9.1 Management Plans

The design of an appropriate national program must primarily address consumer safety, using the principals of risk assessment and management. In addition, this program should manage the local shellfish toxicity profile in a transparent, efficient, and functional manner. A HAB monitoring program and management plan is composed of a number of design elements. These are incorporated to reflect (1) the monitoring program objectives, (2) the available resources and facilities, (3) the end-user requirements and demands of the data, and (4) the legislation and regulations imposed by the national or regional authorities (Anderson et al., 2003). The establishment of such a program should ideally provide consumer protection while not unnecessarily obstructing the growth of the shellfish industry. The management plan is an important part of the monitoring program and should clearly define the following:

- Samples and the identification and quantification of toxins in shellfish samples
- Assigned responsibilities for sampling, analysis, management decisions, and enforcement
- Agreed procedures for opening/closing production areas
- Efficient and timely procedures for reporting of results
- Traceability procedures to ensure that shellfish placed on the market have robust product recall in place

Due to the variety of toxins that can potentially occur in shellfish, attention must be paid to developing efficient initiatives to detect, monitor, and share information on marine biotoxins, in order to limit health risks associated with the consumption of contaminated shellfish. The management plan is necessary to define a code of practice and identify roles and responsibilities at each of the various control points of shellfish production. These critical areas must be considered in planning the implementation of the shellfish monitoring programs with reference to overall control and implementation of food safety strategies. The drivers are primarily governed by relevant legislative requirements, which are in place to protect consumer safety, promote marketing, and safeguard the industry reputation. These requirements are enacted in the development and implementation of a management plan in order to detect harmful algal species and the toxins they produce (Figure 9.2). This plan is therefore fundamental and represents the most critical component of HAB management.

Regulatory requirements have significant impacts on the monitoring program design and ultimately in ensuring consumer confidence in the produce of the shellfish industry. The legislative requirements along with scientifically robust food safety principles must be coupled to form the framework of an effective shellfish safety program. The management plan will inform the monitoring strategy by setting the appropriate sampling and analysis necessary at critical points along the stages of production. When analytical results indicate a potential risk to human health, for example, detection of toxins above permitted levels, the required actions can be swiftly implemented and be used unambiguously to inform the industry and regulatory authorities on the further requirements for testing. Risk management principles

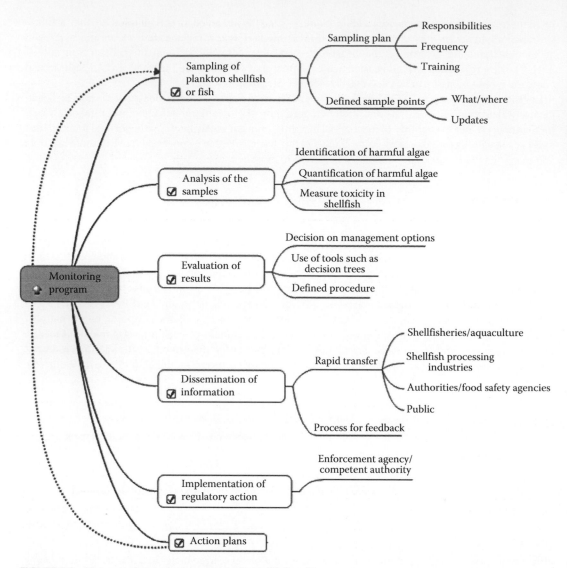

FIGURE 9.2   Elements of a monitoring program for shellfish toxins.

can then be incorporated including collective decision by regulators based on the known analytical status and other appropriate information to assess the risk in adjacent areas and recommend action. In utilizing the best available data and assigning appropriate enforcement based on this risk management, the legislative objectives are fulfilled, an appropriate level of protection is provided to the customer, and the reputation of the industry is safeguarded.

An essential component of ensuring successful implementation is the provision of pertinent advice to consumers and producers. This requires a timely provision of analytical results, and real-time decision processes must be in place to publish advice to the regulators and enforcement agencies at an appropriate timescale. Again the roles and responsibilities concerning decision making, communications, and enforcement should be documented in the management plan to facilitate these aspects of official control.

At present, most shellfish-producing countries have programs in place to monitor for the presence, in the product, of shellfish toxins prior to harvesting. There is, however, a considerable variety in the sophistication and implementation of these programs. There is a growing awareness of the need to adopt internationally harmonized consumer food safety standards for shellfish products whether for export or

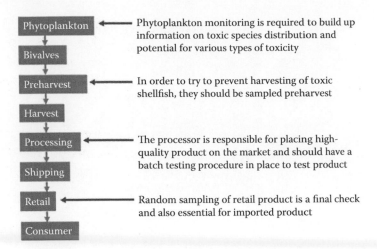

Phytoplankton monitoring is required to build up information on toxic species distribution and potential for various types of toxicity

In order to try to prevent harvesting of toxic shellfish, they should be sampled preharvest

The processor is responsible for placing high-quality product on the market and should have a batch testing procedure in place to test product

Random sampling of retail product is a final check and also essential for imported product

FIGURE 9.3 Chain of production with assigned control points and procedures along the pathway.

for domestic consumption. In minimizing this variability, it is useful to follow the chain of production and assign controls and procedures along the pathway (Figure 9.3). Drafting this process into a management plan is a constructive means to demonstrate that the plan is effective and conforms to national or international requirements as appropriate.

9.2 Sampling

Effective monitoring starts with appropriate sampling of shellfish and phytoplankton. The management plan should detail and document how, who, where, and when shellfish and phytoplankton samples are to be collected, handled, transported, and delivered to the laboratories. An appropriate number of samples should be taken to identify potential toxin occurrences, which will be used for official controls, and also to advise on more intense sampling as appropriate. It is necessary to document in the management plan how representative samples are to be collected, the frequency of sampling, the sample size, and how it is handled after collection and before it is analyzed. This is critical to obtain quality results. Subsamples may be required, and specification should be given on how these should be taken to keep the sample as representative, homogeneous, and unbiased as possible.

In determining an appropriate level of sampling, the approach taken by Anderson et al. (2003) is a useful operational model that responds dynamically in differing HAB situations (Figure 9.4). The different monitoring modes define differing monitoring requirements in response to various trigger levels. These trigger levels, or alerts, which may differ from region to region depending on the toxin profile in each area, should be defined and incorporated into the management plan. Regardless of location, the concept is the same however and is described as follows:

1. *Low-risk level*: (to operate when toxins are not detected)

   Trigger 1: Algal toxins above a given level or a particular detection of a HAB species increase results in going to routine level.

2. *Routine level*: (to operate when toxins are not present above threshold)

   Trigger 2: For instance, changes in water temperature, detection of increasing algal toxins, or presence of HAB species above a concentration level of concern results in going to high alert level.

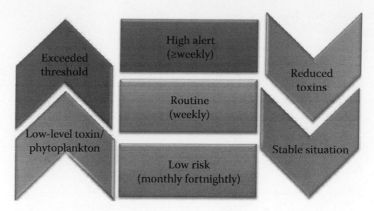

FIGURE 9.4 Operational model action plan, with three monitoring modes and example triggering or alert scenarios that result in a change of monitoring mode. (Developed from Harmful algal monitoring programme and action plan design, in: Hallegraeff, G.M., Anderson, D.M., and Cembella, A.D. (eds.) *Manual on Harmful Marine Microalgae*, 2nd edn., IOC-UNESCO, Paris, France, pp. 627–647, 2003.)

3. *High alert level*: (to operate when HABs are present in critical concentrations or when toxins are detected at regulatory levels or levels close to regulatory levels)

Trigger 3: HABs decrease and algal toxins below regulatory level reduce monitoring back to routine level.

Trigger 4: HABs and toxins not detected reduce back to low-risk level (Figure 9.4).

Each of these monitoring levels needs to be adapted to the local conditions and described in detail in the management plan to indicate the location and frequency of sampling. As the trigger level increases, so does the intensity of sampling; however, when an area is closed for protracted periods, the intensity of monitoring may decrease as the area is no longer open for harvesting, increasing again when decreasing toxicity may result in a requirement to harvest.

9.3 Analysis of the Samples

The management plan should define aspects of good laboratory practice and appropriate methods of analysis. A target turnaround time for sample analysis should be set in order to ensure the timely availability of results, which is essential to allow appropriate management actions aimed at preventing toxic product being placed on the market.

The sampling plan should incorporate certain key details to define the analytical requirements for phytoplankton analysis and shellfish toxin analysis. Phytoplankton analysis generally relies on microscopic identification or more recently on molecular methods of detection, while the toxin analysis relies on biological assays, for example, mouse bioassay, or biochemical and chemical analysis of tissues, for example, LC–MS and ELISA for toxin detection and quantification. The most appropriate methods differ from region to region depending on the species and toxins present.

In all cases, however, there are some key requirements that should be borne in mind when developing or reviewing the management plan:

1. The qualifications, training, and experience of the staff
2. Availability of laboratory instrumentation and infrastructure—properly calibrated and maintained
3. Adequate quality assurance procedures
4. Proper subsampling practices

5. Appropriate testing procedures
6. Validated test methods
7. Traceability of measurements to international standards
8. Accurate recording and reporting procedures
9. Suitable testing facilities

A critical review of these elements and checking that appropriate requirements are in place when designing the analytical elements will facilitate the implementation of a robust biotoxin management plan. It is worth mentioning that certification of laboratory quality accreditation with independent auditing of facilities should be in place, to ensure that all methods are carried out to a standard that can be fully traceable and assured. The benefits of this include increased confidence in data that are used to inform key management decisions. There are also reduced uncertainties associated with decisions that affect the protection of human health that leads to increases in public confidence, because accreditation is a recognizable mark of approval. In addition, the reduction in false positives and false negatives can directly improve compliance with regulations and ultimately reduced incidence of toxic shellfish reaching the market.

Analytical labs should be flexible and open to introducing new methods when necessary. As new analytical procedures and test methods are developed, it is important, where appropriate, that these be incorporated in the routine monitoring programs. There are many examples of this in the field of shellfish testing including improved and more sensitive chemical methods that have become more common in shellfish testing labs (HPLC, LC–MS, etc.), biochemical methods including ELISA, and immunochromatographic assays (Sellner et al., 2003). New means of phytoplankton analysis have also been recently developed and are becoming more routine in analytical labs in recent years. This has resulted in the more accurate identification of toxic species than was previously possible. Microscopic identification of phytoplankton species is time consuming and requires a high level of expertise; however, the incorporation of novel methods such as nucleic acid diagnostic methods may be beneficial (Penna et al., 2007). An example of this is the case of *Pseudo-nitzschia* species that cannot be easily indentified to species level using conventional light microscopy. Intensive electron microscopic investigation is required for species identification, and this technique cannot be easily integrated into a routine monitoring program. Molecular techniques utilizing unique sequence signatures within genomes have been developed for identification and discrimination between closely related species. Molecular identification can be performed on a variety of platforms and therefore provides a rapid alternative to laborious morphological investigation. Nucleic acid-based diagnostic assays have been developed and are now applied to the identification and quantification of toxic phytoplankton species as part of routine analysis (Scholin et al., 1997; Saito et al., 2002; Galluzzi et al., 2004). One such platform using nucleic acid diagnostic assays is real-time PCR-based assays that have been developed to detect and/or quantify species including *Pseudo-nitzschia, Dinophysis, Alexandrium, Pfiesteria, Heterosigma, Lingulodinium, Chattonella, and Azadinium* (Bowers et al., 2000; Maher et al., 2007; Kavanagh et al., 2008; Toebe et al., 2012). The availability of these new tests and new platforms and the capacity to identify with a high level of accuracy to species level add significant value to the monitoring of HABs. They provide a rapid alternative to electron microscopy that requires considerable skill in the area of taxonomy and thereby facilitate the identification of certain species in routine laboratory situations.

9.4 Evaluation of Results

The triggers identified in the earlier example are based on the results obtained from the monitoring program. Along with an appropriate level of sampling and quality-assured analysis, the resource manager has sufficient evidence to make a decision on what the correct status of a production area should be, that is, opened/closed, and for how long that status should remain. In many cases, the biggest problem is the latter, as it is difficult to make a judgment call on the length of time the status should remain unchanged because the environmental conditions may change very quickly; a HAB may get established undetected and shellfish become toxic in between tests. This problem can only be tackled by making very careful and precautionary decisions in shoulder periods, for instance, during nontoxic but high-risk periods (such as early summer when dinoflagellates typically are beginning to increase). In times such as these, it is critical to consider all available information including phytoplankton counts, subthreshold toxicity trends, and the trends in adjacent production areas. Further information including historical patterns of toxicity, oceanographic conditions, water temperature, and wind patterns may be important in making a decision in a high-risk period.

Unfortunately in many areas, the hydrographic mechanisms underlying the HAB problem are poorly understood. There have been few sustained field programs combining physical oceanography and HABs, and therefore, bloom dynamics and physical forcings remain significant and important unknowns. Retrospective studies of meteorological data, shellfish toxicity records, and remote-sensing images of sea surface temperature can often indicate patterns associated with HAB outbreaks, for example, instances when winds shift in the late summer and cause upwelling to relax on the west coast of the United States (Horner et al., 1997). Marine HABs are natural multifactorial events that occur in a turbulent and chaotic environment. Establishing robust forecasting is a complex and difficult task, but many groups worldwide are working towards the coupling of physical oceanographic models with biological processes in an attempt to improve the advice given by resource managers.

Currently, regulators use the best information from the last available suite of testing and historical trends in making management decisions, and it is not possible to give complete assurance that all product harvested will be free of toxins and safe for human consumption. It is important therefore that where shellfish are going for further processing, end-product testing is carried out to give further product assurance. In the case of fresh product, it is prudent to take an even more cautious approach and await the next test results before harvesting and carry out additional testing to reduce the possibility of harvesting toxic shellfish.

The regulator with responsibility for decision making may use tools such as decision trees, to make consistent decisions on production area status. In designing these trees, many different factors may be incorporated including the results from phytoplankton, chemical, and biochemical testing and in vivo test results. It is important that the decision tree is consistent with the regulatory requirements in the region where the product is to be marketed. In the case of exporting countries, this may mean different criteria based on the requirements of the importing country.

In defining the options regarding restrictions in the event of the detection of toxins above permitted levels, it is beneficial to have advance agreement between the stakeholders on the restrictions that may be put in place. This advance consultative process often can prevent later disagreements. Nonroutine situations can also be decided upon in advance such as what to do in the event of conflicting results between different test methods, for example, mouse bioassay and chemical test result.

9.5 Dissemination of Information

The primary objective of effective monitoring should be to protect consumer health while keeping shellfisheries open as much as possible. An appropriate level of protection must be in place to meet both requirements, and this can be facilitated by incorporating a rapid transfer of accurate information. It is essential to alert those in the production chain of the current levels of toxic phytoplankton species and shellfish toxicity in their waters and the current regulatory status of production areas. It is especially important that all involved are aware when the status changes. The important stakeholders to notify include the shellfisheries/aquaculture industry, shellfish processing industries, regulatory authorities/ food safety agencies, and the general public. The dissemination of information should be carried out with great care. The information provided should seek to ensure that all potential food safety issues are covered, while at the same time preventing a so-called halo effect or overreaction in the market. It is also important that a process for feedback is in place to answer queries or deal with complaints in a professional manner. In response to a relaxation in restrictions, it is equally important that this information is conveyed to all parties so that the industry can resume production in a timely manner. In facilitating effective communications, the stakeholders would be wise to consider a Shellfish Safety Committee made up of representatives of the stakeholders to discuss the program at regular meetings and form workgroups to tackle diverse and pertinent issues. Annual research workshops, websites, conferences, and publications may also be used to convey important aspects of the management plan.

Examples of activities that benefit by stakeholder involvement include the following:

- Mapping of sites
- Improved communications (SMS, fax, website)
- Refined methodologies
- Formalized sample management
- Improved coordination between stakeholders
- Improved phytoplankton sampling
- Codes of practice
- Improved risk management procedures

9.6 Discussion

There are many programs in place worldwide that incorporate elements of a coordinated and integrated system of shellfish monitoring, from phytoplankton monitoring through to end-product testing. In most cases, these are nationally coordinated and locally relevant to meet the regulations prevalent in their respective legal jurisdictions. In designing an effective monitoring program, it is important that regional organization of all stakeholders is included in the process and that agreement on a coordinated program is established from the outset. This bottom-up approach development through regional consultation of stakeholders with top-down coordination by regulatory agencies is the basis for a successful program. This is an effective means to establish appropriate risk management structures to safeguard consumer health from shellfish toxins. In taking the process further, larger-scale programs that adopt regional or global perspectives may be necessary in developing understanding of intoxication processes and the mitigation of these events. In the first instance, however, it is important that a local plan is developed to regulate the molluscan fishery and prevent consumer toxicity events.

Although definitive scientific evidence is lacking, there appears to be increasing molluscan shellfish toxicity in number, extent, and severity. The coastal zone has become a more popular area, with people working, living, and using it for recreational activities; these new demographics coupled with changes in dietary habits may be responsible for increases in toxic HAB events being detected more frequently. It is essential that a robust program be maintained to advise on the early detection of potentially harmful toxic events. More advanced developments using physical circulation models coupled with ecological variables may yield useful forecasting of these events in the future allowing mitigative strategies be put in place. In the meantime, rapid communications regarding toxic HAB events to the stakeholders is a key essential component of an effective monitoring program.

REFERENCES

Andersen, P., Enevoldsen, H., and Anderson, D. (2003). Harmful algal monitoring programme and action plan design. In: Hallegraeff, G. M., Anderson, D. M., and Cembella, A. D. (eds.) *Manual on Harmful Marine Microalgae*, 2nd edn. IOC-UNESCO, Paris, France, pp. 627–647.

Bowers, H. A., Tengs, T., Glasgow, Jr., H. B., Burkholder, J. A. M., Rublee, P. A., and Oldach, D. W. (2000). Development of real-time PCR assays for rapid detection of *Pfiesteria piscicida* and related dinoflagellates. *Applied and Environmental Microbiology*, 66: 4641–4648.

FAO. (2004). Food and Nutrition Paper 80, Marine biotoxins, Food and Agriculture Organization of the United Nations, Viale delle Terme di Caracalla, 00100 Rome, Italy, p. 294.

FAO. (2010–2012). FAO Fisheries and Aquaculture Department, Rome, Italy. Updated. [Cited September 12, 2012]. http://www.fao.org/fishery/statistics/global-aquaculture-production/en

Fleming, L. E., Backer, L. C., Kirkpatrick, B., Clark, R., Dalpra, D., Johnson, D. R., Bean, J. A. et al. (2004). An epidemiologic approach to the study of aerosolized Florida Red Tides. In: Steidinger, K. A., Landsberg, J. H., Tomas, C. R., and Vargo, G. A. (eds.) *Harmful Algae 2002*. Florida Fish and Wildlife Conservation Commission, Florida Institute of Oceanography, and Intergovernmental Oceanographic Commission of UNESCO, St. Petersburg, FL, pp. 508–510.

Galluzzi, L., Penna, A., Bertozzini, E., Vila, M., Garcés, E., and Magnani, M. (2004). Development of a real-time PCR assay for rapid detection and quantification of *Alexandrium minutum* (a Dinoflagellate). *Applied and Environmental Microbiology*, 70: 1199–1206.

Hallegraeff, G. M. (2003). Harmful algal blooms: A global overview. In: Hallegraeff, G. M., Anderson, D.M., and Cembella, A. D. (eds.) *Manual on Harmful Marine Microalgae*, Vol. 2. IOC-UNESCO, Paris, France, pp. 25–49.

Horner, R. A., Garrison, D. L., and Plumley, F. G. (1997). Harmful algal blooms and red tide problems on the U.S. west coast. *Limnology and Oceanography,* 42(5) part (2): 1076–1088.

Kavanagh, S., Brennan, C., Lyons, J., Chamberlain, T., Salas, R., Moran, S., Silke, J., and Maher, M. (2008). Development and implementation of the phytotest project. In: McMahon, T., Deegan, B., Silke, J., and O'Cinneide, M. (eds.) *Proceedings of the 8th Irish Shellfish Safety Workshop*, Marine Environment and Health Series, Marine Institute, Galway, Ireland, Vol. 33, pp. 70–78.

Maher, M., Kavanagh, S., Brennan, C., Moran, S., Salas, R., Lyons, J., and Silke, J. (2007). Nucleic acid tests for toxic phytoplankton in Irish waters-Phytotest. In: *Proceedings of the 7th Irish Shellfish Safety Workshop*, Marine Environment and Health Series, Marine Institute, Galway, Ireland, Vol. 27, pp. 70–78.

Penna, A., Bertozzini, E., Battocchi, C., Galluzzi, L., Giacobbe, M. G., Vila, M., Garces, E., Lugliè, A., and Magnani, M. (2007). Monitoring of HAB species in the Mediterranean Sea through molecular methods. *Journal of Plankton Research*, 29(1): 19–38.

Saito, K., Drgon, T., Robledo, J. A. F., Krupatkina, D. N., and Vasta, G. R. (2002). Characterization of the rRNA locus of Pfiesteria piscicida and the development of standard and quantitative PCR-based detection assays targeted to the nontranscribed spacer. *Applied and Environmental Microbiology*, 68: 5393–5407.

Scholin C., Miller P., Buck K., and Chavez F. (1997) Detection and quantification on *Pseudo-nitzschia australis* in cultured and natural populations using LSU rRNA-targeted probes. *Limnol. Oceanogr.* 42 (5, part 2): 1265–1272.

Sellner, K. G., Doucette, G. J., and Kirkpatrick, G. J. (2003). Harmful algal blooms: Causes, impacts and detection. *Journal of Industrial Microbiology and Biotechnology,* 30(7): 383–406.

Ting, J. and Brown, A. (2001). Ciguatera poisoning: A global issue with common management problems. *European Journal of Emergency Medicine*: *Official Journal of the European Society for Emergency Medicine,* 8(4): 295–300.

Toebe, K., Joshi, A. R., Messtorff, P., Tillmann, U., Cembella, A., and John, U. (2012). Molecular discrimination of taxa within the dinoflagellate genus azadinium, the source of azaspiracid toxins. *Journal of Plankton Research*. *Journal of Plankton Research*, 35(1): 225–230. doi: 10.1093/plankt/fbs077.

10

Marine Toxin Monitoring in Asia

Supanoi Subsinserm

CONTENTS

10.1 Background Information and Competent Authority Role in Shellfish Controls by the Department of Fisheries, Thailand

Mollusks are the most successfully cultured and commercially important types of shellfish. A large variety of different mollusk species are cultured throughout the world. Some, such as oysters and abalones, have a very high market value. Mollusks are generally cultivated in inshore coastal areas using bottom and hanging systems. The main species cultured in Thailand are baby clams, mussels, and oysters. Shellfish are marine species consumed widely in the country. The major species exported to the European Union from Thailand are baby clams (*Paphia undulata*) and green mussels (*Perna viridis*). Cockles (*Anadara granosa*), hard clam (*Meretrix* sp.), and scallops (*Amusium pleuronectes*) are also exported, but in very low quantities.

The green mussel (*P. viridis*) is the most important mollusk species in Thailand. It has been cultured in Thailand for more than 60 years [1]. The culture method was developed from a type of stationary fishing gear called "bamboo stake trap." The bamboo poles or palms are driven into the muddy bottom of shallow water areas (about 4–8 m in depth), specifically as collectors of mussel spat. Another adaptation is to extend the wings of fish traps to collect mussel spat. Green mussel culture in Thailand has a good potential for development from both biological and economical points of view. Spat collection techniques using ropes or other materials should be introduced. New culture methods such as the hanging method that has proven to be the most efficient in Europe should be investigated for their biological and economic feasibility.

The production of baby clam or short-necked clam (*P. undulata*) has gradually increased every year. All the baby clams are derived from capture fisheries. The world market demand for this clam species is showing an increasing trend. To control the stock depletion problem, the Department of Fisheries (DOF) is trying to develop an appropriate management scheme. A regulation on boat size and type of gear used has been issued.

The "bivalve production and sanitation program" started operating in 1997. Thailand has 22 marine coastal provinces out of the total 77 provinces. The units under DOF that are responsible for Bivalve

Monitoring Program are the Fish Inspection and Quality Control Division (FIQD), Coastal Aquaculture Division, and Marine Fisheries Division. FIQD of the DOF is responsible for inspection and control of fishery products and bivalve mollusks. The DOF has established a monitoring program for bivalve mollusk production with the objectives to ensure that the mollusks from approved harvesting areas do not contain microorganisms and toxic substances in quantities that are considered harmful to human health and to prevent the environmental pollution and maintain water quality of the production areas.

In order to minimize the potential health risks associated with consuming bivalves, it is necessary that water quality and bivalves flesh in the growing areas be surveyed. Nonapproved areas that are not in compliance with the following criteria are prohibited for bivalve harvesting. The bivalve harvesters or farmers and processing plants shall be notified of updated information on approved and nonapproved areas by publication and posting notices.

According to the Notification on Classification of Bivalve Harvesting Areas under the authority of Fisheries Act B. E. 2490 (1947), the growing areas of Thailand are classified into three zones, similar to the EU Legislation. The zoning of harvesting areas of baby clams is separated to two provinces: Trat province and Suratthani province, and the zoning of harvesting areas of green mussels is the Chumporn province [2].

The Trat province is located in the eastern part of Thailand and has borders with Chanthaburi province to the northwest, Cambodia to the east, and the Gulf of Thailand to the south. The Marine Fisheries Division performs physical, heavy metal, and marine plankton test in sea water and microbiological, heavy metal, and marine biotoxins in the flesh performed by FIQD. This area is classified as zone A.

Suratthani province is located in the southern part of Thailand. Suratthani province borders the Gulf of Thailand to the north and east, Chumporn province to the north, Nakhon Sri thammarat and Krabi provinces to the south, Phang-Nga and Ranong provinces to the west, and Nakhon Srithammarat province to the east. The Coastal Aquaculture Division performs physical, heavy metal, and marine plankton test in sea water and microbiological, heavy metal, and marine biotoxins in the flesh performed by FIQD. This area is classified as zone A.

Chumporn province is located in the southern part of Thailand. Neighboring provinces are (from north clockwise) Prachuap Khirikhan, Suratthani, and Ranong province. To the west it also borders Myanmar. The Coastal Aquaculture Division performs physical, heavy metal, and marine plankton test in sea water and microbiological, heavy metal, and marine biotoxins in the flesh performed by FIQD. This area is classified as zone C.

The red tide monitoring program is coordinated by the Marine Fishery Division. The objectives are to monitor and inform the event continuously to the concerned parties when red tides occur. If potentially harmful species occur, the concerned authorities shall be informed immediately in order to initiate the urgent countermeasures to prevent any unwanted impacts to aquaculture. In case of shellfish poisoning, all information received should first be confirmed before warning the public and banning of harvesting in the affected areas.

Monitoring of biotoxins in bivalve mollusks that are done by DOF was established in accordance with the requirements of the EU. The DOF is a competent authority of the EU. Bivalve mollusks imported into the EU from a third country must have been produced under conditions that are at least equivalent to those stipulated by the Regulations. Third-world countries such as Thailand may apply for equivalence under which they can trade with the EU on the same basis as a member state. The duty of DOF is to control and monitor fish and fishery products before exporting to each importing countries. Thus, all products' export must meet the requirement of the importing countries.

DOF has established rules to control the export of bivalves to the EU according to these criteria: (1) raw materials must come from the approved harvest zone of bivalves with attached Bivalve Mollusk Movement document; (2) bivalve mollusks must be heated until the core temperature is not less than 90° for 90 s; (3) analysis for biotoxins; and (4) in case of imported bivalves as a raw material, they must come from countries that the EU has recognized and should have the certification of the approved zone with a health certificate from the CA of that country. The importation of bivalve mollusks, echinoderms, tunicates, and marine gastropods is furthermore subject to EU Decision 97/275, which indicates the approved treatments to inhibit the development of pathogenic microbes in bivalve mollusks and marine gastropods.

In case of export bivalve mollusks to importing countries, DOF is following the requirement of importing countries. In New Zealand, DOF has sent information about the monitoring system to the New Zealand Food Safety Authority (FSA). At present, FSA has approved on the basis of agreed assurance (preclearance arrangement). The mollusks are allowed to export both fresh water and marine over cooked and consumed, canned or dried. The products must be origin of Thailand and derived from establishments listed to the EU. The products must meet the hygiene and sanitary requirements for export to the EU.

DOF and Peru have not yet signed the Mutual Recognition Agreement (MRA). The Peruvian Institute of Fishery Technology (ITP) has issued a Communication No.041-2010-IPT/SANIPE, which is the regulation concerning the fishery products that are effective from November 1, 2010. Mollusks exported to Peru will be specified in the certificate of health that comes from holding a certificate from the CA of the exporting country and bivalve movement document. Also, DOF and the Canadian Food Inspection Agency (CFIA) have made the MRA regarding the certification of fish products during the period from April 9, 1997. All fishery products including bivalve mollusks can be imported to Canada. It must be cooked and consumed, canned or dried, and CFIA will random at 5% of the total imported sample.

10.2 Monitoring Results of the Approved Bivalve Mollusks Harvesting Areas in Thailand

Regarding the monitoring program for the approved bivalve mollusks harvesting areas as shown next [3].

10.2.1 Monitoring Results of Heavy Metals in Sea Water Collected from the Harvesting Areas in 2010

1. Trat province: the minimum to maximum level of heavy metals such as cadmium, copper, mercury, lead, and zinc was detected in the range 0.014–0.124 ppb, 0.001–6.025 ppb; not detected–0.005 ppb, 0.128–0.589 ppb; and <0.01–6.153 ppb, respectively.

2. Suratthani province: the minimum to maximum level of heavy metals such as cadmium, copper, mercury, lead, and zinc was detected in the range 0.022–0.345 ppb, 0.151–1.386 ppb, <0.01–0.069 ppb, 0.104–1.788 ppb, and 0.542–3.539 ppb, respectively.

3. Chumporn province: the minimum to maximum level of heavy metals such as cadmium, copper, mercury, lead, and zinc was detected in the range 0.027–0.177 ppb, 0.435–5.788 ppb, <0.01–0.010 ppb, 0.226–1.109 ppb, and 0.825–3.916 ppb, respectively.

4. Monitoring Results of Heavy Metals in Flesh Collected from the Harvesting Areas in 2010.

5. Trat province: the minimum to maximum level of heavy metals such as mercury, lead, and cadmium was detected in the range, not detected—0.05 ppm, not detected—0.18 ppm, and <0.05–0.35 ppm, respectively.

6. Suratthani province: the minimum to maximum level of heavy metals such as mercury, lead, and cadmium was detected in the range, not detected—<0.02 ppm, not detected—0.08 ppm, and 0.06–0.20 ppm, respectively.

7. Chumporn province: the minimum to maximum level of heavy metals such as mercury, lead, and cadmium was detected in the range, not detected—<0.02 ppm, not detected—0.08 ppm, and 0.06–0.20 ppm, respectively.

8. Monitoring Results of Biotoxins in Flesh Collected from the Harvesting Areas in 2010.

9. Trat province: the biotoxins such as amnesic shellfish poison (ASP), paralytic shellfish poison (PSP), diarrhetic shellfish poison (DSP), pectenotoxins (PTX), yessotoxin (YTX), and azaspiracid (AZA) were not detected for all samples in the whole year.

10. Suratthani province: the biotoxins such as amnesic shellfish poison (ASP), paralytic shellfish poison (PSP), diarrhetic shellfish poison (DSP), pectenotoxins (PTX), yessotoxin (YTX), and azaspiracid (AZA) were not detected for all samples in the whole year.

11. Chumporn province: the biotoxins such as amnesic shellfish poison (ASP), paralytic shellfish poison (PSP), diarrhetic shellfish poison (DSP), pectenotoxins (PTX), yessotoxin (YTX), and azaspiracid (AZA) were not detected for all samples in the whole year.

12. Monitoring Results of *E. coli* (MPN/100 g) in Flesh Collected from the Harvesting Areas in 2010.

13. Trat province: the mean level of *E. coli* was detected approximately <100 MPN/100 g.

14. Suratthani province: the mean level of *E. coli* was detected approximately <10 MPN/100 g.

15. Chumporn province: the mean level of *E. coli* was detected approximately <10 MPN/100 g.

16. Monitoring Results of Phytoplanktons Collected from the Harvesting Areas in 2010.

17. Trat province: the average level of phytoplanktons such as cyanophyceae (blue-green algae), bacillariophyceae (diatom), dinophyceae (dinoflagellate), and dictyochophyceae (silicoflagellate) was detected in the average <1000, <1500, <1000, and <100 cell/L, respectively. In addition, alexandrium, amphidinium, and lingulodinium were not detected for the whole year.

18. Suratthani province: the average level of phytoplanktons such as cyanophyceae (blue-green algae), bacillariophyceae (diatom), dinophyceae (dinoflagellate), and dictyochophyceae (silicoflagellate) was detected in the average <1000, <2000, <500, and <100 cell/L, respectively. In addition, amphidinium was not detected for the whole year and detection of alexandrium <100 cell/L only in January and September 2010.

19. Chumporn province: the average level of phytoplanktons such as cyanophyceae (blue-green algae), bacillariophyceae (diatom), dinophyceae (dinoflagellate), and dictyochophyceae (silicoflagellate) was detected in the average <100, <1000, <300, and <100 cell/L, respectively. In addition, amphidinium, goniodoma, and lingulodinium were not detected for the whole year and detection of alexandrium <100 cell/L only in January and June 2010.

According to these results, all monitoring criteria such as heavy metals, marine biotoxins, microbiological, and phytoplankton analysis are detected lower than the EU decision limit.

10.3 Occurrences of Red Tide in Thailand and Asian Countries

Red tide is a common name for a phenomenon also known as an algalbloom, an event in which estuarine, marine, or fresh water algae accumulate rapidly in the water column and result in discoloration of the surface water. It is usually found in coastal areas. These algae, known as phytoplankton, are single-celled protists, plant-like organisms that can form dense, visible patches near the water's surface. Red tide is a colloquial term used to refer to one of a variety of natural phenomena known as a harmful algalblooms or HABs. The term red tide specifically refers to blooms of a species of dinoflagellate known as *Kareniabrevis*.

The high abundance blooms of toxic phytoplankton species are named HABs. Phytoplankton can accumulate in various marine species such as fish, crab, and bivalve mollusks. In shellfish, toxin mainly accumulates in the digestive glands without causing adverse effects on the shellfish itself.

Thailand has two coasts. One curves around the scooped-out of the Gulf of Thailand and has a length of 1870 km. The other lines along the shore of the Andaman Sea and has a length of 800 km. The Gulf of Thailand is roughly triangular and divided into two sections: inner gulf and outer gulf. The inner gulf is roughly square-shaped and has an average depth of 20 m and slope of about 0.2 m/km. The surface area is about 10,360 km. Along its shores, aquaculture farms and fisheries abound [4].

Red tides were frequently observed in the inner Gulf of Thailand, especially around the river mouth areas such as Chao-phraya river, Tha-Chin river, Mae klong river, and Bangpakong river. Generally, red tides could be observed all year. It was highlighted that red tide phenomena in Thailand were reported since 1958 as natural phenomena and there was no serious impact of red tide on marine environment or organisms. *Noctiluca scintillans* and *Ceratium furca* were the main causative red tide organisms in the inner gulf of Thailand. Besides *N. scintillans* and *C. furca*, the bloom of other red tide organisms such as *Trichodesmium*, *Chaetoceros*, *Cosinodiscuss*, and *Skeletonema* was also sometimes observed [5].

N. scintillans usually changed the apparent color of water into dark green. This kind of plankton is not toxic for fish and shellfish, but the dense bloom can result in the anoxic condition. The anoxic condition of algal bloom could cause a massive fish killed. In August 1991, there was a mass fish killed in the coastal area of Chonburi. This was caused by *N. scintillans*.

Only one case of PSP was reported in 1983 at the Pranburi river mouth in Prachuabkirikan province, but the causative organism has not been clarified. Since 1985–1995, intensive monitoring programs and research on red tide were carried out. The outbreak of *N. scintillans* was often observed during the period from December to February in the western part of the inner gulf of Thailand, whereas in the eastern part of the inner gulf the blooms were often observed during the period of March to August. Recently, *C. furca* occurred more often at both areas of the inner gulf of Thailand [5].

The other red tide monitoring program in Thailand is coordinated by the Marine Fishery Division. The objectives are to monitor and inform the event continuously to the concerned parties when red tides occur. If potentially harmful species occur, the concerned authorities shall be informed immediately in order to initiate the urgent countermeasures to prevent any unwanted impacts to aquaculture. In case of shellfish poisoning, all information received should first be confirmed before warning the public and banning of harvesting in the affected areas.

Red tide in Malaysia occurs in 300 km of the western coastal of Sabah. The first PSP case was reported in year the 1976. After that alga bloom occurs frequently almost every year and for the first time alga bloom detected occurs in the east coast. The causative organism is *Pyrodimium bahamense*. Monitoring of HABs in Malaysia is carried out by the Department of Fisheries in Sabah with some assistance from the Department of Medical Service, University of Kebangsaan, and cooperation with the Brunei Department of Fisheries. However, no recurrent episodes of toxin production by *P. bahamense* species have been reported since 2002.

In Manila Bay (in Philippines), during the 1992 *P. bahamense* outbreak, around 38,500 fisher folks were displaced from their livelihood due to the red tide scare. Anyway, from 1983 to 2001, a total of 42 toxic outbreaks have resulted in a total of 2107 paralytic shellfish poisoning cases with 117 deaths. The Department of Health (DOH) created the National Red Tide Task Force (NRTTF) composed of different government agencies and academic institutions chaired by the Bureau of Fisheries and Aquatic Resources, Department of Agriculture. The NRTTF is mandated to monitor toxic red tides in Philippines. This is to protect the public from the illness and death caused by the red tide toxin and also to mitigate its negative impact on the shellfish industry. A regular issuance of the red tide update is also undertaken [6].

Indonesia began to study red tide since 1991. In Jakarta bay, *Skeletonema costatum* is the first phytoplankton bloom. This type of situation is common for estuarine waters in Indonesia. Also, the bloom of the dinoflagellate, *N. scintillans* after a skeletonema bloom instead of the usual diatom species. Other red tide occurrences in Jakarta bay were caused by *Prorocentrum minimum* in September 1993.

The program on a monitoring system was carried out since 1996, named SEAWATCH INDONESIA. Component three deals with monitoring of environmental condition such as pollution, red tide, sediment transport, primary productivity, and impact of pollutants on marine life. The study areas are Makassar Strait, Sulawesi Sea, and North Moluccas.

In *the People's Republic of China*, red tide occurred in the coastal water of the northern part of Zhejiang Province in 1933 and next to Bohai Sea in 1952. The researches and monitoring activities related to red tide are carried out by a number of institutes, monitoring centers, universities, and government agencies [7].

In 2003, the national sea waters witnessed altogether 119 cases of red tides up area about $14.55 \times 10^3 \text{ km}^2$. Compared to that of 2002, either events affected areas are increased. According to the monitoring data from 2000 to 2004, the higher number of HABs was recorded from Zhejiang, Fujian, and Guangdong Provinces, which were located in East and South China Seas. The most common causative species in the area are diatoms and dinoflagelltes. *N. scintillans*, *S. costatum*, and *Mesodinium rubrum* are the principal causative species in the region.

The Republic of Korea cited that outbreak of red tides and algal blooms in Korean Coastal Waters have increased gradually and caused severe damages to cultured shellfish as well as natural marine living resources. Red tide problems have serious economic impact on marine culture industry as red tide occurred in areas where intensive shellfish and finfish farms are located.

In Vietnam, in Cat Ba, the red tide is caused by an algae species named sea sparkle or *N. scintillans*. This kind of algae has bloomed massively since late March 2012. *N. scintillans* itself do not appear to be toxic, but as they feed voraciously on phytoplankton high levels of ammonia accumulate in these organisms, which is then excreted into the surrounding area, adding to the neurotoxic chemicals being produced by other dinoflagellates, such as *Alexandrium* spp. or *Gonyaulax* spp. that do result in the death of other aquatic life in the area. Thus, red tide only appears on a narrow area so it does not affect catching and aqua-cultural activities.

10.4 Global Bivalve Mollusk Production

Bivalve mollusks represented almost 10% of the total world fishery production, but 26% in volume and 14% in value of the total world aquaculture production. World bivalve mollusks production (capture and aquaculture) has increased substantially in the last 50 years, going from nearly 1 million tons in 1950 to about 14.6 million tons in 2010. China is by far the leading producer of bivalve mollusks with 10.35 million tons in 2010, representing 70.8% of the global molluscan shellfish production and 80% of the global bivalve mollusk aquaculture production. All of the Chinese bivalve production is cultured. Anyway, in 2010, Japan reported bivalve mollusks producers in 819,131 tons, the United States 676,755 tons, the Republic of Korea 418,608 tons, Thailand 285, 625 tons, France 216,811 tons, and Spain 206,003 tons. By species, the bivalve mollusk production by aquaculture in 2010 consisted of 38.0% clams, cockles, and ark shells, 35.0% oysters, 14.0% mussels, and 13.0% scallops and pectens [8].

In addition, scallops and pectens are a major group produced by capture, followed by clams, cockles, and ark shells. The increase of bivalve mollusk production was driven by international demand since the early 1990s. Total bivalve trade has expanded continuously during the past three decades to reach US$ 2.1 billion in 2009. In terms of quantity, scallops accounted for 24% of export, while mussels contributed to 48%. But in terms of value, scallops are the most important species with 46% value, followed closely by mussels with 26%.

According to the Thai fishery, product exports to the EU amounted to approximately 263,000 tonnes in 2010. From the total exported to the EU, tuna contributed with 111,350 tonnes (mainly canned products) while bivalve mollusks (baby clams (*P. undulata*), white clams (*Meretrix* spp.), mussels (*Perna* sp. and *Mytilus chilensis*), and scallops (*Amusium pleuronectus* and *Placopecten magellanicus*) contributed with 2,700 tonnes. According to Thailand Foreign Agricultural Trade Statistic in 2011, the quantities of bivalve mollusks exports to all countries amounted to 11,736 metric tons [9].

10.5 Status in ASEAN Countries Concerning the Monitoring of Biotoxins and the Methodology for the Detection of Biotoxins

Biotoxins are poisonous substances naturally present in fish and fishery products or accumulated by the animals feeding on toxin-producing algae or in water containing toxins produced by such organisms. In addition, biotoxins could also cause mass killings of fish and shellfish, and death of marine mammals and birds after consuming food that contains biotoxins. Considering the possible impacts of biotoxins in fish and fishery products to human health, Marine Fisheries Research and Development (MFRD) in cooperation with the Japanese Trust Fund II project has implemented the program focused on "Biotoxins Monitoring in Fish and Fish Products in Southeast Asia" since 2009–2012. The ASEAN member countries consisting of Cambodia, Indonesia, Lao P.D.R, Malaysia, Myanmar, Philippines, Singapore, Thailand, and Vietnam participated in this program except Brunei Darussalam.

The activities undertaken by MFRD therefore aimed to develop the methodologies for biotoxins analyses, enhance the capacity of ASEAN Member Countries in the analysis through training, and obtain better understanding of the levels of occurrence and incidence of biotoxins in fish and fishery products in the region. It is envisaged that these activities would enhance the attention of responsible authorities in expanding and improving initiatives to monitor, detect, and share information on marine biotoxins in order to reduce the public health risks associated with the consumption of contaminated shellfish and fish in the future.

Under this project, which focused on PSP monitoring in green mussels (*P. viridis*), except for Vietnam and Indonesia, who would use baby clams (*Meritrix* spp). Myanmar and Singapore had also expanded the scope of their surveys to include monitoring of ASP and DSP in green mussels. Although most of the countries conducted their own analysis by using mouse bioassay as the screening method and HPLC as the confirmation method for PSP, the results of the PSP analysis in the species surveyed have been negative in all the participating countries [10].

The methodology for the determination of biotoxins in ASEAN countries is as described (except Cambodia and Lao P.D.R lack of resources and facilities to perform biotoxins analysis):

1. Indonesia has been analyzed for PSP, DSP, and ASP. The PSP and DSP methods used mouse bioassay while the ASP method used high-performance liquid chromatography (HPLC).

2. Malaysia has been analyzed for PSP and tetradotoxin (TTX). PSP method used mouse bioassay and TTX method used GC/MS.

3. Myanmar has been analyzed for PSP, DSP, NSP, and ASP. Those methods used test kit, HPLC, and LC/MS/MS.

4. Philippines have been analyzed for PSP, DSP, Ciguatera toxin (CFP), TTX, Polycavernoside, and ASP. PSP, DSP, Polycavernoside, and TTX methods used mouse bioassay while ASP method used HPLC and CFP method used test kit.

5. Singapore has been analyzed for PSP, DSP, and ASP. PSP methods used both mouse bioassay and test kit while ASP method used HPLC and DSP method used LC/MS/MS.

6. Thailand has been analyzed for PSP, DSP, PTX, YTX, AZA, TTX, and ASP. PSP methods used both mouse bioassay and HPLC, DSP, PTX, YTX, and AZA used both mouse bioassay and LC/MS/MS, while ASP and TTX methods used HPLC.

7. Vietnam has been analyzed for PSP, DSP, and ASP. PSP methods used both mouse bioassay and HPLC, DSP method used both mouse bioassay and LC/MS/MS or HPLC, and ASP method used HPLC or LC/MS/MS.

Although the MFRD has implemented the program mentioned earlier, each countries also have implemented their own biotoxins monitoring system in their countries. Cambodia is currently setting up plan for biotoxins monitoring, Myanmar would embark on the proposed plan, and Lao P.D.R is currently having no biotoxins analysis facilities. The problem for ASEAN countries to implement the biotoxins monitoring program is in terms of methodology for the detection of biotoxins. In addition, lack of analytical experience for developing countries to perform the alternative test, complicated derivatization, and purification steps for PSP method, the availability of pure reference standard compounds for all list of biotoxins is a major prerequisite and rare of proficiency testing scheme for biotoxins available commercially.

Nowadays, the technique for HPLC and LC/MS/MS is less expensive but still costly and sophisticated, requiring specialized staff. The main advantages of this technique consist in the fact that individual analogues can be distinguished and quantified. The toxic potency of each analogue must be known in order to calculate the total toxicity associated with a sample of shellfish. Other alternative methods are available for some toxin groups, including methods based on antibody technology, such as enzyme-linked immunosorbent assays (ELISAs). However, these tests can only give a single response per toxin group, which lacks information on individual analogues and also on total toxicity present.

Most ASEAN countries have a monitoring program to determine the quality and safety of finished products in terms of chemical, microbiological, and physical quality. Laboratory capacities in these

ASEAN countries are more or less adequate to monitor and guarantee the quality and safety of fishery products using the analytical methods for which they are equipped. It is increasingly apparent that constraints are being faced throughout the region with the increasing stringency of import control programs that are being introduced by importing countries. The effect of this is that there is a continuous trend to increase the sensitivity of analytical methods in importing countries. The effect of this continual move to greater sensitivity is that ASEAN countries must increase investment to acquire the knowledge of techniques and replace or upgrade equipment to keep up with this advancing technology of the importing countries. It is important that there is adequate and timely access to information regarding analytical methods and transparency in the conduct of research and risk analysis on health hazards of toxins and their functional groups. If the precautionary principle is to be utilized as the basis of consumer protection, scientific justification based on risk assessment should be conducted within reasonable timeframes and the results of this communicated in an expeditious manner. This approach is essential to ensure that the continuing trend of increasing sensitivity and stringency of standards does not in effect become a nontariff barrier to trade.

The identification of the toxin alone is only the first step of full hazard identification. In the case of shellfish toxins, it is important to identify the biological source organism of the toxin, mostly unicellular algae (diatoms and dinoflagellates). Once these producing organisms are known, the surveillance system can observe the frequency of their occurrence and the conditions leading to toxin production, such that the full extent of the occurrence of the toxin can be understood.

REFERENCES

1. Juntarashote, K., Bahrometanarat S., and H. Grizel. 1987. *Shellfish Culture in Southeast Asia*. Southeast Asian Fisheries Development Centre. Special Publication, p. 72.
2. FIQD. 2010. Bivalve production and sanitation program, Department of Fisheries, Thailand.
3. FIQD. 2010. Summary of monitoring results of harvest areas in 2010, Department of Fisheries, Thailand.
4. Menasveta, P. 1978. Distribution of heavy metals in the Chao Phraya River Estuary. *Proceedings of the International Conference on Water Pollution Control in Developing Countries*. Asian Institute of Technology, Bangkok, Thailand, pp. 129–145.
5. Lertvidhayaprasit, T. 2003. *Red Tide in the Inner Gulf of Thailand*, Workshop on Red Tide Monitor in Asian Coastal waters, pp. 53–56.
6. Water Environment Partnership in Asia. Occurrence of red tide in Philippine Bay. http://www.wepa-db.net/policies/measures/background/philippines/redtide.htm (accessed March 2012).
7. Zhou, M., Li, J., Lucas, B., Yu, R., and Yan, T. 1999. A recent shellfish toxin investigation in China. *Marine Pollution Bulletin*, 39(1): 331–334.
8. FAO Fisheries and Aquaculture Information and Statistics Service. 2011. Aquaculture production 1950–2009. http://www.fao.org/fishery/statistics/software/fishstat/en (accessed December 2012).
9. Thailand Foreign Agricultural Trade Statistics. 2012. Publication No. 405. Centre for Agricultural Information Office of Agricultural Economics, p. 135.
10. Marine Fisheries Research Department. 2009. Report of Regional Technical Consultation on Japanese Trust Fund II Chemical and Drug Residues in Fish and Fish Products in Southeast Asia (Biotoxins Monitoring in ASEAN), August 26–28, 2009, Singapore.

Part III

Technology

11

Functional and Receptor-Based Assays for Marine Toxins

Natalia Vilariño, María Fraga, and Laura Pérez Rodríguez

CONTENTS

11.1 Introduction

Marine toxin detection methods can be grouped into two main categories, analytical methods, which are based on the physicochemical properties of the compounds of interest, and biological methods, which include a biological component in the detection system (Figure 11.1). Regarding biological methods, two different classes should be discriminated due to their toxin detection characteristics, biochemical methods (immunological, aptamer-based, etc.), and functional/receptor-based methods. A distinction between functional and receptor-based methods should also be made. Functional methods are based on in vitro or in vivo measurement of a biological function that is modified by the presence of toxins in a sample. Receptor/target-based assays use the interaction of a receptor or biological target with a toxin or group of toxins to sense their occurrence.

In this chapter, general characteristics of functional and target/receptor-based assays that determine the main advantages and disadvantages of these methods will be reviewed. Functional and receptor-based methods that have been published for different toxin groups will be discussed as well.

11.2 General Characteristics of Functional and Target-Based Assays

The strategy used for marine toxin detection in functional and target-based methods endows them with certain characteristics that confer advantages and disadvantages versus other detection methods.

One of the main characteristics of functional and receptor-based methods is that all the toxins with the same functional effect or same target are undistinguishable. Since most analogs of a toxin group usually have the same mechanism of action, these methods cannot identify different members within a group. Therefore, functional and receptor-based assays will provide information about the toxicity

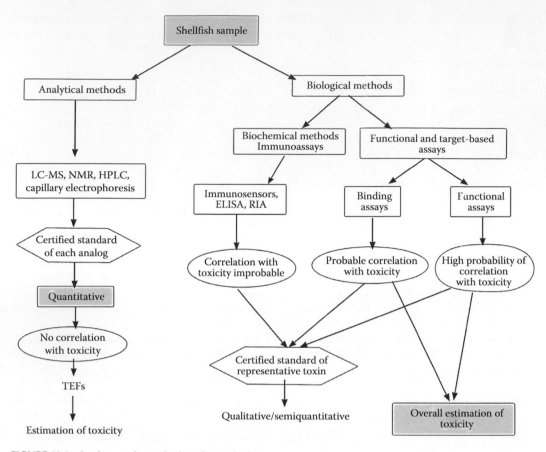

FIGURE 11.1 In vitro marine toxin detection methods.

related to a certain toxin group, but will not indicate the identity of the molecules responsible and their amount. Currently, the unequivocal identification and accurate quantification of the different analogs of a toxin group present in a sample can only be achieved using analytical methods. Immunological methods do not provide the analog profile of a sample. However, when using functional and target-based assays, the capability of detection of each analog is related to its ability to interact with a target or receptor or modify a biological function. Because the function, receptor, or targets selected to develop detection methods are considered to participate in the mechanism of action responsible for toxicity, the ability to detect different analogs with functional methods should have a good correlation with toxic potency, or at least the probability of obtaining a good toxicity-detection correlation should be high. Commonly, immunological methods also lack selectivity among toxin analogs, but in this case, the ability of an antibody to interact with a toxin and its analogs is not related to toxicity, and the probability of obtaining an immunoassay that cross-reactivity profile among toxin analogs has a good correlation with toxicity is low. Actually, for marine toxins, this good correlation has been achieved only for diar-rhetic shellfish poisoning (DSP) toxins.[1,2] In general, as a consequence of the absence of specificity, biological methods will only provide an overall estimation of toxin content related to a toxin group. For functional and receptor/target-based assays, there is a better chance that the result provides a good estimation of sample toxicity.

In any case, the correlation between analog detection efficiency and toxicity should be demon-strated even for functional and receptor-based assays, since there are many factors that contribute to determine the potency of a toxic compound besides interaction with its biological target. For example, receptor/target-based assays, which quantify the interaction with a macromolecule, disregard intrinsic efficiency. Bioavailability of a toxic molecule can also affect enormously its toxic potency and may cause a divergence between detection efficiency by functional in vitro assays and toxic potency. Obviously, the best estimation of toxicity would be provided by in vivo bioassays, and even in this case, the route of administration and the animal species might deviate toxicity estimation from actual toxic potency in human food poisoning.[3]

Although this lack of selectivity of receptor-based and functional assays may be regarded as a disadvantage versus analytical methods, in some circumstances, it results in additional detection capabilities. Routine monitoring with analytical methods will not identify toxic molecules that have not been characterized previously.[3,4] However, functional/receptor-based assays will detect the presence of any molecule with a certain biological activity, even if it has not been identified before.[5–7] In this line of thought, some functional methods, usually in vivo bioassays and cell-based assays, lack also specificity among groups, being able to detect toxins of different groups. Considering the growing number of analogs and groups described for marine toxins,[8] detection of active molecules with potential toxicity is extremely important to protect human health. In spite of many disadvantages, such as high false-positive rates and ethical concerns, animal bioassays have been acting as "universal" detectors and protecting human health for decades. A recent approach to toxin detection is the development of cell-based biosensors also as "universal" toxin detectors.[9] Certainly, cell-based multitoxin detectors agree with the current trend in the marine toxin field to develop screening assays focused on multidetection,[10–12] providing in vitro viable alternatives to bioassays.

Biological methods are considered qualitative or semiquantitative methods, unlike analytical methods, which are designed to provide accurate identification and quantification of a molecule. Due to this feature, biological assays are usually aimed at screening purposes. The objective is to determine the presence or absence of toxins of a certain group in a high number of samples, avoiding the need of processing many samples with more expensive and time-consuming analytical methods. Those samples that require precise quantification should be subsequently analyzed by quantitative techniques. In the case of paralytic shellfish poisoning (PSP) toxins, the reduction of the samples to be processed by the official reference method in many countries, the mouse bioassay,[13,14] would decrease the number of animals sacrificed for this purpose every year. We should keep in mind that while analytical methods are excellent tools for unequivocal identification and quantification of toxins, unknown toxic analogs will be missed by these techniques. Additionally, the evaluation of sample toxicity with analytical methods relies entirely on the availability of toxic equivalency factors (TEFs) for all the analogs detected in a sample, and in many groups of toxins, an accurate estimation of TEF for a high number of analogs is currently impossible due to the lack of experimental data.[3] Therefore, important disagreements between the results provided by functional/receptor methods and analytical methods should be explored further or reexamined. Functional and receptor-based assays should be regarded as complementary to analytical methods.

In functional and target-based methods, toxicity is evaluated using a representative toxin of the group; therefore, only a certified standard material of one toxin is necessary for routine testing with these assays. This is a common feature with immunoassays, but not with analytical methods, that require certified standards of all the analogs of a toxin group for routine sample testing. An important current limitation of analytical methods is the worldwide shortage of toxin-certified standards and the unavailability of standards for many analogs. Although not necessary for routine sample screening, certified standards of all the analogs are indispensable in functional methods to determine the analog cross-reactivity profile of the assay.

An important caveat of functional and target-based methods is the short life of the reagents required to perform the assays. In many cases, the components of the assay cannot be stored for long periods, and the situation gets complicated if cell cultures are involved, since shipping of cells is not a trivial issue and many routine testing laboratories do not have the resources to maintain cell cultures. In other cases, the biological components are not easily available. For a functional/receptor-based assay to be viable as a routine screening tool, it is necessary to warrant the availability and stability of the reagents. This is true for any detection method, but it is particularly challenging for functional/receptor-based assays, mainly if membrane proteins are involved,[15] since functionality and structure has to be maintained after production and storage.

Another problem for the implementation of functional assays in routine sample testing is the lack of validated methods.[5,14] Only a few functional assays have been validated or prevalidated to assess performance, among them is phosphatase inhibition assay for DSP toxins,[7,16–18] although in most cases, no full validation following official guidelines has followed yet.[19,20] Many functional methods have not even been tested for matrix interferences. Obviously, if a functional/receptor-based method is to be considered as a viable screening alternative, a complete evaluation of assay performance will be required. Due to the scarcity of pure material available worldwide for many toxins and the relatively high amounts required for full validation or at least single-laboratory validation, validation is usually only pursued when the scientific and/or regulatory communities have manifested interest in the method. Nevertheless, interest will not be raised if there is not enough information to support adequate performance.

11.3 Functional Methods for Marine Toxin Detection

11.3.1 In Vivo Bioassays

Animal bioassays consist of the administration of a sample extract to an animal and observation of the appearance of toxicity signs. At least three bioassays have been commonly used for the detection of marine toxins in seafood to prevent human intoxication: the PSP mouse bioassay (PSP-MBA), the lipophilic toxin mouse bioassay (LT-MBA), and the lipophilic toxin rat bioassay.

The PSP-MBA has been used for decades to protect humans from this deadly group of toxic compounds. Initially developed by Sommer and Meyer,[21] currently it consists of the intraperitoneal injection to three mice of a shellfish extract obtained in heat/acidic conditions and observation of death occurrence.[13] The PSP-MBA has been standardized for its use as the official detection method worldwide.[13] Although it has been protecting human consumers from PSP outbreaks for more than 50 years, this method presents serious disadvantages. Ethical concerns about animal research have influenced current legal regulations to demand a reduction of the use of experimental animals by seeking alternative techniques.[22] Additionally, PSP-MBA is a semiquantitative method with important technical limitations, including low sensitivity, high false-positive rates, and high variability.[23–25] Moreover, validation of the MBA is probably impossible to achieve due to the number of variables that should be controlled and reproduced in different laboratories. Therefore, a huge international effort has been made to substitute the PSP-MBA in routine detection. In spite of a recent change in the regulations of many countries, with high performance liquid chromatography (HPLC) coupled to fluorescence detection (FLD) becoming an official method for the detection of PSP toxins, the PSP-MBA remains the official reference method for this group of toxins.[26,27] The replacement of the PSP-MBA by other detection methods has turned difficult because the same level of consumer protection is legally required and it must be demonstrated by an international validation study.[14,26]

Two bioassays have been used for years to detect the presence of lipophilic toxins. The LT-MBA was initially developed by Yasumoto et al.[28,29] and later harmonized by European Reference Laboratories for marine toxins (CRLMB and NRLs).[30] An organic extract obtained by acetone extraction, subsequent water/ diethyl ether partition, and finally, diethyl ether evaporation and reconstitution in 1% Tween 60 is administered by intraperitoneal injection to mice followed by observation of death occurrence for 24 h. The oral rat bioassay[31] has fewer false positives and does not require the sacrifice of the animals; however, the method implies a new source of variability: operator subjectivity in the evaluation of feces consistency. Bioassays for the detection of lipophilic toxins present more performance problems than the PSP-MBA, and they are being replaced in several countries as official detection methods for lipophilic toxins by liquid chromatography coupled to mass spectrometry, which has become the official reference method in Europe.[32]

11.3.2 In Vitro Functional Assays

In this section, in vitro assays that use the modification of a biological function as a reporter of the presence of marine toxins are classified depending on the nature of the biological component used as detector. Target-based methods measure a signal triggered by activation of an enzyme or receptor. Cell-based methods use a reporter of cellular activity in live cells. Finally, tissue-based assays quantify functionality in biological tissues.

11.3.2.1 Target-Based Functional Methods

Target-based functional methods provide information about the modification of the activity of a biological target by the presence of the toxin of interest. The specificity of the method depends mainly on the target chosen as bioactivity reporter. The sensitivity will be affected not only by the target, but also by the design of the detection assay. Target-based functional assays have been optimized for the detection of DSP toxins and yessotoxin, all of them based on enzymatic activity.

The efficient inhibition of protein phosphatase 2A (PP2A), a Ser/Thr protein phosphatase expressed in most eukaryotic cells, by okadaic acid and its analogs has been selected in multiple occasions to produce fast, economic, and sensitive assays. These techniques quantify the inhibition of PP2A activity by DSP toxins using a fluorescent or colorimetric substrate of the enzyme.[33–36] Dephosphorylation of the substrate by the enzyme induces a change in its color or fluorescent properties that can be easily monitored by colorimeters or spectrofluorometers. The assay protocols are easy to perform, most of them have been optimized for a 96-well format, and their sensitivity is around the low ng/mL range for the reference toxin of the group, okadaic acid. The ability of the different analogs of the group to inhibit PP2A activity has a good correlation with relative toxicity.[37] Additionally, PP2A-based assays perform well with shellfish samples and provide results consistent with other DSP detection methods such as mouse bioassay or HPLC-FLD.[38] Recently, single-laboratory validation of a commercial PP2A inhibition assay has been published.[16] In spite of the adequate performance of phosphatase inhibition assays demonstrated by interlaboratory validation,[17] more than a decade has passed before the appearance of a commercial kit. PP2A inhibition has been also the starting point for the design of three biosensors aimed at DSP toxin detection. One of the biosensors is based on the electrochemical detection of catechyl monophosphate, a substrate of PP2A that is cleaved by the enzyme immobilized on screen-printed electrodes.[39] The other two biosensors use an off-line incubation with PP2A and subsequent flow injection analysis (FIA) with an enzymatic amplification system of one (pyruvate oxidase)[40] or two (alkaline phosphatase and glucose oxidase)[41] enzymes to increase sensitivity. The PP2A-immobilized biosensor provides a detection limit of 6.4 ng/mL OA,[39] while the pyruvate oxidase- and the alkaline phosphatase/glucose oxidase-immobilized systems yielded detection limits of 0.1 and 30 pg/mL, respectively.[40,41] Although the future of these biosensors is promising, the performance with shellfish samples has not been tested yet.

The target-based functional assay for yessotoxins consists of quantification of phosphodiesterase activation by this group of compounds using a fluorescent cAMP derivative.[42] The sensitivity of this assay is in the low µg/mL range, it can detect different analogs, and it is compatible with shellfish matrixes. The specificity of the method should be evaluated carefully due to later reports of phosphodiesterase interaction with other polyether toxins[43] that might as well modify phosphodiesterase activity.

11.3.2.2 Cell-Based Methods

A variety of cell-based assays have been developed for the detection of marine toxins. One of the main characteristics of these assays is the lack of specificity among toxin groups. The absence of specificity is due mainly to the cell function selected to test for the presence of toxin. Most of the methods are based on the measurement of cell viability or membrane potential. Cell death is a consequence of the modification of a cellular process by the toxin, but malfunction of many different cellular activities can lead to cell death. Therefore, assays based on the detection of toxin-induced cell death are not specific of a certain group. In order to achieve specificity, the assay should measure an event upstream in the signaling cascade triggered by the toxin. Regarding membrane potential, it will be affected by several groups of toxins that target ion channels.

Functional methods based on the evaluation of toxin-induced cytotoxicity have been developed for several toxin groups, including DSP toxins, pectenotoxins, PSP toxins, tetrodotoxin (TTX), palytoxins, ciguatoxins, and brevetoxins.[44–50] The cytotoxicity/viability markers used to evaluate toxin-induced cell death are very varied, from vital dyes or morphology (microscopy) to metabolic activity markers, actin cytoskeleton labeling, or nuclear stains (fluorescence microscopy). Most of these methods are direct assays that quantify cell viability after exposure to the toxins, except for an indirect assay based on the inhibition of veratridine-/ouabain-induced hemolysis or cell death by TTX and saxitoxin (STX).[50–52] As mentioned previously, these assays are not specific, although in the case of palytoxin, the inhibition of toxin-induced cytotoxicity by anti-palytoxin antibodies or ouabain has been used as a strategy to provide specificity.[48,49] Another approach is the presentation of multitoxin detection assays.[7,46,47] Many of these assays can be easily performed, the instrumentation required is often available in most laboratories, and some of them have even been tested with shellfish matrixes. The sensitivity varies greatly depending on the assay and the toxin tested between the low pg/mL range for ciguatoxins, low ng/mL for palytoxin and okadaic acid, and the low µg/mL range for STX and TTX.[48–53] However, they require the maintenance of cell cultures or a reliable source of fresh cells. Additionally, those assays that involve diagnosis by microscopy are not very practical.

Interestingly, two functional methods based on cytotoxicity evaluation have been prevalidated recently to overcome current limitations of marine toxin analytical methods. One of these two assays is aimed at the detection of ciguatoxin-like toxicity in order to avoid toxicity underestimation by immunological or analytical methods.[18,53] Antibody cross-reactivity limitations, the lack of certified standards of all toxic analogs, and the scarcity of experimental data for TEF estimation would be the main factors implicated in the appearance of false negatives with immunological and analytical techniques. The second prevalidated cell-based assay has been developed as a "universal" detector, analyzing cytotoxicity in three different cell lines. It is aimed at the detection of overall toxicity, being capable of sensing both known and unknown toxins, and also at aiding in the process of toxin isolation and identification.[6,7]

The cell-based methods that use modifications of membrane potential or ion fluxes as toxicity marker are designed for the detection of neurotoxins. The specific detection of PSP toxins can be achieved by patch clamp techniques that display a high sensitivity (23 pg/mL STX).[54,55] Although the technique has been optimized to test shellfish samples,[54] most routine testing laboratories do not have the instrumentation or expertise essential to execute electrophysiology experiments. An easy-to-perform alternative has been optimized using a membrane potential fluorescent marker in 96-well plates.[56] This experimental approach has been used to detect PSP toxins, brevetoxins, and ciguatoxin.[56–58] These assays do not require highly trained personnel or sophisticated instruments; just a spectrofluorometer will suffice to obtain the results. Although sensitivity is low compared to patch clamp methods (low ng/mL range), it is enough for consumer protection. A disadvantage is that the maintenance of cell cultures is still necessary. Also suitable for spectrofluorimetry detection is one method for the detection of PSP toxins and domoic acid based on intracellular free calcium measurement with a fluorescent marker.[59] A new development in cell-based functional assays is the detection of extracellular potentials of spinal cord neuronal cells with microelectrodes, which has been adapted to detect neurotoxins. This experimental design was used to produce a cell-based biosensor that allowed the detection of TTX.[60] Similar experiments have also shown high sensitivities for brevetoxin PbTx-3 (296 pg/mL) and STX (12 pg/mL).[61] These neuronal network biosensors constitute an interesting innovation in the marine toxin field, being able to perform adequately with seawater samples, although they have not been tested with shellfish samples. The advances in the development of cell-based biosensors have achieved portability and high sensitivities. In spite of a promising future, some limitations should still be overcome for neuronal network biosensors, such as sample preparation and distribution of the cells.

Finally, a yessotoxin detection method consisting of the evaluation of the appearance of the E-cadherin fragment $ECRA_{100}$ by protein blot has also been published.[62,63] The $ECRA_{100}$ fragment is probably generated as a product of E-cadherin degradation due to apoptotic processes; therefore, this technique might be related to cell death, which is supported by a similar effect obtained with azaspiracids.[64] The assay is not specific, and the practicality of use is poor due to a too long duration to be considered for routine testing, in spite of being suitable for shellfish samples.

11.3.2.3 Tissue-Based Methods

There is only one method for marine toxin detection that has been reported as a tissue biosensor. This assay was optimized for the detection of TTX[65] and consists of the measurement of the transport of Na[+] through frog bladder membranes using a Na[+]-specific electrode. This tissue preparation has a high concentration of Na[+] channels sensitive to TTX. Subsequently, the detection of STX, gonyautoxin 1 (GTX1), GTX2, GTX3, GTX4, decarbamoyl saxitoxin (dcSTX), and decarbamoyl neosaxitoxin (dcNEO)[65,66] was also demonstrated. This assay is highly sensitive (2 pg/mL TTX and 0.1 pg/mL STX); it shows a nice correlation between the efficiency of analog detection and relative analog toxicity, and its performance with shellfish and finfish samples is adequate to assay incurred material.[66,67] However, the assay practicality is limited, the bladder membrane is not so easy to obtain, it is stable only for a few months, and the instrumentation required is not commonly available in routine testing laboratories.

11.4 Receptor Binding-Based Methods for Marine Toxin Detection

In this section, detection methods based on the interaction of the toxin with its biological target will be discussed. Although these assays do not provide information about the effect of the toxin on the activity of the target, the affinity of the members of a toxin group for their target has a higher probability of being related to their toxic potency than the affinity for any antibody.

In the marine toxin field, the first receptor-based assays were developed for the detection of STX and brevetoxins.[68–71] The experiments consisted of inhibition assays based on the competition of the toxin present in a sample with radioactive-labeled toxin for binding to the voltage-dependent sodium channel. Although these assays have been recently validated for the detection of PSP toxins,[72,73] the use of radioactive material is not a well-accepted practice for routine testing laboratories.

Receptor-based methods that do not require radioactive materials have been published for the detection of yessotoxin and macrocyclic imines. Several receptor-based assays for the detection of the macrocyclic imines spirolides, gymnodimine, and pinnatoxins have been optimized for shellfish sample screening.[74–78] Most of these experiments use the competition of macrocyclic imines and the snake toxin α-bungarotoxin for binding to the nicotinic acetylcholine receptor (nAChR) to increase selectivity and reduce matrix interference. In these assays, binding of α-bungarotoxin to *Torpedo marmorata* nAChR-rich membranes is monitored by different techniques: fluorescence polarization, chemiluminescence, colorimetry, or fluorescence (Figure 11.2 shows a summary of assay designs).[74–77] As expected, these assays can sense the presence of several macrocyclic imines in a sample, such as 13-desmethyl spirolide C, 13,19-didesmethyl spirolide C, 20-methyl spirolide G, gymnodimine-A, pinnatoxin-A, and pinnatoxin-G.[76,77,79,80] The sensitivities depend on the experimental design reaching the low ng/mL range with recent developments.[76,77] Due to the absence of specificity among analogs of nAChR-based methods, a microplate assay has been coupled to posterior identification of toxic compounds by mass spectrometry (MALDI-TOF).[76] An nAChR-based assay has been also optimized for the xMap Luminex system with sensitivity in the low ng/mL range and a simple sample extraction method.[77] The xMap Luminex technology allows multidetection by multiple solid-phase assays performed with functionalized microspheres combined with flow cytometry-like separation of analyte-specific microspheres. Therefore, nAChR-based detection of macrocyclic imines can be incorporated in the future to a multitoxin detection panel.

Regarding yessotoxin, its interaction with phosphodiesterases has been used to develop detection methods based on different technologies. Direct assays that measure yessotoxin binding to phosphodiesterases have been adapted to three technologies aimed at detecting the interaction between two molecules: fluorescence polarization, a resonant mirror biosensor, and an surface plasmon resonance (SPR)-based biosensor.[81–84] An indirect assay was subsequently developed for the detection of ladder-shaped polyether compounds, including yessotoxin and brevetoxin-2, with SPR-based biosensors. The assay consists of the competition of free polyether toxins with immobilized desulfo-yessotoxin for binding to phosphodiesterases in solution.[43] This work demonstrated that phosphodiesterase-based assays are not selective for yessotoxins, being also capable of detecting brevetoxins, and in theory even ciguatoxins. However, the sensitivity of these experiments is not enough to comply with the low detection limits required for highly toxic compounds, such a ciguatoxins.

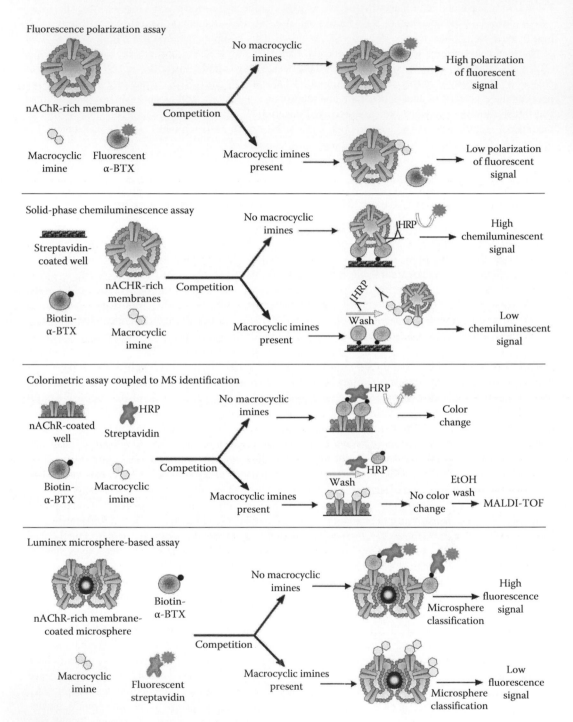

FIGURE 11.2 Receptor-based inhibition assays for the detection of macrocyclic imines. *Abbreviations:* nAChR, nicotinic acetylcholine receptor; α-BTX, α-bungarotoxin; HRP, horseradish peroxidase.

11.5 Concluding Remarks

Recent changes in legal regulations and the escalating number of samples to be tested for the presence of marine toxins have increased the need for validated, rapid, screening assays capable of high-throughput toxin detection in laboratories with heavy workloads. Functional methods can be excellent screening tools due to their lack of specificity among the analogs of a certain toxin group and in some cases the lack of selectivity among toxin groups. In vitro functional methods should be considered a necessary complement to analytical methods for adequate detection in marine toxin monitoring programs. Therefore, not only development but also validation of functional methods is absolutely required.

REFERENCES

1. Stewart, L. D.; Elliott, C. T.; Walker, A. D.; Curran, R. M.; Connolly, L. 2009. Development of a monoclonal antibody binding okadaic acid and dinophysistoxins-1, -2 in proportion to their toxicity equivalence factors. *Toxicon*, 54, 491–498.
2. Stewart, L. D.; Hess, P.; Connolly, L.; Elliott, C. T. 2009. Development and single-laboratory validation of a pseudofunctional biosensor immunoassay for the detection of the okadaic acid group of toxins. *Anal Chem*, 81, 10208–10214.
3. Botana, L. M.; Vilarino, N.; Alfonso, A. et al. 2010. The problem of toxicity equivalent factors in developing alternative methods to animal bioassays for marine-toxin detection. *Trends Analyt Chem*, 29, 1316–1325.
4. Campbell, K.; Vilarino, N.; Botana, L. M.; Elliott, C. 2011. A European perspective on progress in moving away from the mouse bioassay for marine-toxin analysis. *Trends Analyt Chem*, 30, 239–253.
5. Botana, L. M.; Louzao, M. C.; Alfonso, A. et al. 2011. Measurement of algal toxins in the environment. In Meyers, R. A. (ed.) *Encyclopedia of Analytical Chemistry*. Chichester, U.K.: John Wiley & Sons, Ltd.
6. Ledreux, A.; Serandour, A. L.; Morin, B. et al. 2012. Collaborative study for the detection of toxic compounds in shellfish extracts using cell-based assays. Part II: Application to shellfish extracts spiked with lipophilic marine toxins. *Anal Bioanal Chem*, 403, 1995–2007.
7. Serandour, A. L.; Ledreux, A.; Morin, B. et al. 2012. Collaborative study for the detection of toxic compounds in shellfish extracts using cell-based assays. Part I: Screening strategy and pre-validation study with lipophilic marine toxins. *Anal Bioanal Chem*, 403, 1983–1993.
8. James, K. J.; Carey, B.; O'Halloran, J.; van Pelt, F. N.; Skrabakova, Z. 2010. Shellfish toxicity: Human health implications of marine algal toxins. *Epidemiol Infect*, 138, 927–940.
9. Pancrazio, J. J.; Kulagina, N. V.; Shaffer, K. M.; Gray, S. A.; O'Shaughnessy, T. J. 2004. Sensitivity of the neuronal network biosensor to environmental threats. *J Toxicol Environ Health A*, 67, 809–818.
10. Campbell, K.; McGrath, T.; Sjolander, S. et al. 2011. Use of a novel micro-fluidic device to create arrays for multiplex analysis of large and small molecular weight compounds by surface plasmon resonance. *Biosens Bioelectron*, 26, 3029–3036.
11. Zhang, B.; Hou, L.; Tang, D.; Liu, B.; Li, J.; Chen, G. 2012. Simultaneous multiplexed stripping voltammetric monitoring of marine toxins in seafood based on distinguishable metal nanocluster-labeled molecular tags. *J Agric Food Chem*, 60, 8974–8982.
12. McNabb, P.; Selwood, A. I.; Holland, P. T. et al. 2005. Multiresidue method for determination of algal toxins in shellfish: Single-laboratory validation and interlaboratory study. *J AOAC Int*, 88, 761–772.
13. AOAC. 2005. Official method 959.08. Paralytic shellfish poison. Biological method. In International, A. (ed.) *AOAC Official Methods of Analysis*, 18th edn. Gaithersburg, MD: AOAC International.
14. EC. 2005. Commission Regulation (EC) No. 2074/2005 of December 5, 2005 laying down implementing measures for certain products under Regulation (EC) No. 853/2004 of the European Parliament and of the Council and for the organisation of official controls under Regulation (EC) No. 854/2204 of the European Parliament and of the Council and Regulation (EC) No. 882/2204 of the European Parliament and of the Council, derogating from Regulation (EC) No. 852/2004 of the European Parliament and of the Council and amending Regulations (EC) No. 853/2004 and (EC) No. 854/2004. *Off J Eur Communities*, L338, 27.
15. Steller, L.; Kreir, M.; Salzer, R. 2012. Natural and artificial ion channels for biosensing platforms. *Anal Bioanal Chem*, 402, 209–230.

16. Smienk, H. G.; Calvo, D.; Razquin, P.; Dominguez, E.; Mata, L. 2012. Single laboratory validation of a ready-to-use phosphatase inhibition assay for detection of okadaic acid toxins. *Toxins (Basel)*, 4, 339–352.
17. González, J. C.; Leira, F.; Fontal, O. I. et al. 2002. Inter-laboratory validation of the fluorescent protein phosphatase inhibition assay to determine diarrhetic shellfish toxins: Intercomparison with liquid chromatography and mouse bioassay. *Anal Chim Acta*, 466, 233–246.
18. Caillaud, A.; Eixarch, H.; de la Iglesia, P. et al. 2012. Towards the standardisation of the neuroblastoma (neuro-2a) cell-based assay for ciguatoxin-like toxicity detection in fish: Application to fish caught in the Canary Islands. *Food Addit Contam Part A Chem Anal Control Expo Risk Assess*, 29, 1000–1010.
19. EC. 2002. 2002/657/EC: Commission Decision of 12 August 2002 implementing Council Directive 96/23/EC concerning the performance of analytical methods and the interpretation of results. *Off J Eur Communities*, L221, 8.
20. OECD. 2010. Guidance Document No. 129. Cytotoxicity tests to estimate starting doses for acute oral systemic toxicity tests. OECD Environment, Health and Safety Publications (Series on Testing and assessment).
21. Sommer, H.; Meyer, K. F. 1937. Paralytic shellfish poison. *Arch Pathol*, 24, 560–598.
22. EC. 1986. Council Directive 86/609/EEC of November 24, 1986 on the approximation of laws, regulation and administrative provisions of the Member States regarding the protection of animals used for experimental and other scientific purposes. *Off J Eur Communities*, L358, 1.
23. Parks, D. L.; Adams, W. N.; Graham, S.; Jackson, R. C. 1986. Variability of the mouse bioassay for determination of paralytic shellfish poisoning toxins. *J Assoc Off Anal Chem*, 69, 547–550.
24. LeDoux, M.; Hall, S. 2000. Proficiency testing of eight French laboratories in using the AOAC mouse bioassay for paralytic shellfish poisoning: Interlaboratory collaborative study. *J AOAC Int*, 83, 305–310.
25. Botana, L. M.; Alfonso, A.; Botana, A. M. et al. 2009. Functional assays for marine toxins as an alternative, high-throughput-screening solution to animal tests. *Trends Analyt Chem*, 28, 603–611.
26. EC. 2004. Regulation (EC) No. 853/2004 of the European Parliament and of the Council of April 29, 2004 laying down specific hygiene rules for food of animal origin. *Off J Eur Communities*, L139, 55.
27. EC. 2007. Commission Regulation (EC) No. 1244/2007 of 24 October 2007 amending Regulation (EC) No. 2074/2005 as regards implementing measures for certain products of animal origin intended for human consumption and laying down specific rules on official controls for the inspection of meat. *Off J Eur Communities*, L281/12–18.
28. Yasumoto, T.; Oshima, Y.; Yamaguchi, M. 1978. Occurrence of a new type of shellfish poisoning in the Tohoku district. *Bull Jap Soc Sci Fish*, 44, 1249–1255.
29. Yasumoto, T.; Oshima, Y.; Yamaguchi, M. 1979. Occurrence of a new type of shellfish poisoning in Japan and chemical properties of the toxin. In Taylor, D., Seliger, H. H. (eds.) *Toxic Dinoflagellate Blooms*. Amsterdam, the Netherlands: Elsevier.
30. Community Reference Laboratory for Marine Biotoxins (CRLMB). 2009. EU harmonised standard operating procedure for detection of lipophilic toxins by mouse bioassay. http://www.aesan.msssi.gob.es/en/CRLMB/web/procedimientos_crlmb/crlmb_standard_operating_procedures.shtml (accessed in February 2013).
31. Kat, M. 1983. Diarrhetic mussel poisoning in the Netherlands related to the dinoflagellate *Dinophysis acuminata*. *Antonie Van Leeuwenhoek*, 49, 417–427.
32. EC. 2011. Commission Regulation (EU) No. 15/2011 of 10 January 2011 amending Regulation (EC) No. 2074/2005 as regards recognised testing methods for detecting marine biotoxins in live bivalve molluscs. *Off J Eur Communities*, L6/3–6.
33. Della Loggia, R.; Sosa, S.; Tubaro, A. 1999. Methodological improvement of the protein phosphatase inhibition assay for the detection of okadaic acid in mussels. *Nat Toxins*, 7, 387–391.
34. Mountfort, D. O.; Suzuki, T.; Truman, P. 2001. Protein phosphatase inhibition assay adapted for determination of total DSP in contaminated mussels. *Toxicon*, 39, 383–390.
35. Tubaro, A.; Florio, C.; Luxich, E.; Sosa, S.; Della Loggia, R.; Yasumoto, T. 1996. A protein phosphatase 2A inhibition assay for a fast and sensitive assessment of okadaic acid contamination in mussels. *Toxicon*, 34, 743–752.
36. Vieytes, M. R.; Fontal, O. I.; Leira, F.; Baptista de Sousa, J. M.; Botana, L. M. 1997. A fluorescent microplate assay for diarrheic shellfish toxins. *Anal Biochem*, 248, 258–264.
37. Albano, C.; Ronzitti, G.; Rossini, A. M.; Callegari, F.; Rossini, G. P. 2009. The total activity of a mixture of okadaic acid-group compounds can be calculated by those of individual analogues in a phosphoprotein phosphatase 2A assay. *Toxicon*, 53, 631–637.

38. Prassopoulou, E.; Katikou, P.; Georgantelis, D.; Kyritsakis, A. 2009. Detection of okadaic acid and related esters in mussels during diarrhetic shellfish poisoning (DSP) episodes in Greece using the mouse bioassay, the PP2A inhibition assay and HPLC with fluorimetric detection. *Toxicon*, 53, 214–227.

39. Campas, M.; Marty, J. L. 2007. Enzyme sensor for the electrochemical detection of the marine toxin okadaic acid. *Anal Chim Acta*, 605, 87–93.

40. Hamada-Sato, N.; Minamitani, N.; Inaba, Y. et al. 2004. Development of Amperometric sensor system for measurement of diarrheic shellfish poisoning (DSP) toxin, okadaic acid (OA), *Sensor Mater*, 16, 99–107.

41. Volpe, G.; Cotroneo, E.; Moscone, D. et al. 2009. A bienzyme electrochemical probe for flow injection analysis of okadaic acid based on protein phosphatase-2A inhibition: An optimization study. *Anal Biochem*, 385, 50–56.

42. Alfonso, A.; Vieytes, M. R.; Yasumoto, T.; Botana, L. M. 2004. A rapid microplate fluorescence method to detect yessotoxins based on their capacity to activate phosphodiesterases. *Anal Biochem*, 326, 93–99.

43. Mouri, R.; Oishi, T.; Torikai, K. et al. 2009. Surface plasmon resonance-based detection of ladder-shaped polyethers by inhibition detection method. *Bioorg Med Chem Lett*, 19, 2824–2828.

44. Tubaro, A.; Florio, C.; Luxich, E.; Vertua, R.; Della Loggia, R.; Yasumoto, T. 1996. Suitability of the MTT-based cytotoxicity assay to detect okadaic acid contamination of mussels. *Toxicon*, 34, 965–974.

45. Leira, F.; Alvarez, C.; Cabado, A. G.; Vieites, J. M.; Vieytes, M. R.; Botana, L. M. 2003. Development of a F actin-based live-cell fluorimetric microplate assay for diarrhetic shellfish toxins. *Anal Biochem*, 317, 129–135.

46. Cañete, E.; Diogène, J. 2008. Comparative study of the use of neuroblastoma cells (Neuro-2a) and neuroblastomaxglioma hybrid cells (NG108–15) for the toxic effect quantification of marine toxins. *Toxicon*, 52, 541–550.

47. Fladmark, K. E.; Serres, M. H.; Larsen, N. L.; Yasumoto, T.; Aune, T.; Doskeland, S. O. 1998. Sensitive detection of apoptogenic toxins in suspension cultures of rat and salmon hepatocytes. *Toxicon*, 36, 1101–1114.

48. Bignami, G. S. 1993. A rapid and sensitive hemolysis neutralization assay for palytoxin. *Toxicon*, 31, 817–820.

49. Espina, B.; Cagide, E.; Louzao, M. C. et al. 2009. Specific and dynamic detection of palytoxins by in vitro microplate assay with human neuroblastoma cells. *Biosci Rep*, 29, 13–23.

50. Manger, R. L.; Leja, L. S.; Lee, S. Y.; Hungerford, J. M.; Wekell, M. M. 1993. Tetrazolium-based cell bioassay for neurotoxins active on voltage-sensitive sodium channels: Semiautomated assay for saxitoxins, brevetoxins, and ciguatoxins. *Anal Biochem*, 214, 190–194.

51. Gallacher, S.; Birkbeck, T. H. 1992. A tissue culture assay for direct detection of sodium channel blocking toxins in bacterial culture supernates. *FEMS Microbiol Lett*, 71, 101–107.

52. Shimojo, R. Y.; Iwaoka, W. T. 2000. A rapid hemolysis assay for the detection of sodium channel-specific marine toxins. *Toxicology*, 154, 1–7.

53. Caillaud, A.; de la Iglesia, P.; Darius, H. T. et al. 2012. Update on methodologies available for ciguatoxin determination: Perspectives to confront the onset of ciguatera fish poisoning in Europe. *Mar Drugs*, 8, 1838–1907.

54. Velez, P.; Sierralta, J.; Alcayaga, C. et al. 2001. A functional assay for paralytic shellfish toxins that uses recombinant sodium channels. *Toxicon*, 39, 929–935.

55. Vélez, P.; Suárez-Isla, B. A.; Sierralta, J. et al. 1999. Electrophysiological assay to quantify saxitoxins in contaminated shellfish. *Biophys J*, 76, A82.

56. Louzao, M. C.; Vieytes, M. R.; Baptista de Sousa, J. M.; Leira, F.; Botana, L. M. 2001. A fluorimetric method based on changes in membrane potential for screening paralytic shellfish toxins in mussels. *Anal Biochem*, 289, 246–250.

57. Louzao, M. C.; Rodriguez Vieytes, M.; Garcia Cabado, A.; Vieites Baptista De Sousa, J. M.; Botana, L. M. 2003. A fluorimetric microplate assay for detection and quantitation of toxins causing paralytic shellfish poisoning. *Chem Res Toxicol*, 16, 433–438.

58. Louzao, M. C.; Vieytes, M. R.; Yasumoto, T.; Botana, L. M. 2004. Detection of sodium channel activators by a rapid fluorimetric microplate assay. *Chem Res Toxicol*, 17, 572–578.

59. Beani, L.; Bianchi, C.; Guerrini, F. et al. 2000. High sensitivity bioassay of paralytic (PSP) and amnesic (ASP) algal toxins based on the fluorimetric detection of [Ca(2+)](i) in rat cortical primary cultures. *Toxicon*, 38, 1283–1297.

60. Pancrazio, J. J.; Gray, S. A.; Shubin, Y. S. et al. 2003. A portable microelectrode array recording system incorporating cultured neuronal networks for neurotoxin detection. *Biosens Bioelectron*, 18, 1339–1347.

61. Kulagina, N. V.; Mikulski, C. M.; Gray, S. et al. 2006. Detection of marine toxins, brevetoxin-3 and saxitoxin, in seawater using neuronal networks. *Environ Sci Technol*, 40, 578–583.

62. Pierotti, S.; Albano, C.; Milandri, A.; Callegari, F.; Poletti, R.; Rossini, G. P. 2007. A slot blot procedure for the measurement of yessotoxins by a functional assay. *Toxicon*, 49, 36–45.

63. Pierotti, S.; Malaguti, C.; Milandri, A.; Poletti, R.; Paolo Rossini, G. 2003. Functional assay to measure yessotoxins in contaminated mussel samples. *Anal Biochem*, 312, 208–216.

64. Ronzitti, G.; Hess, P.; Rehmann, N.; Rossini, G. P. 2007. Azaspiracid-1 alters the E-cadherin pool in epithelial cells. *Toxicol Sci*, 95, 427–435.

65. Cheun, B.; Endo, H.; Hayashi, T.; Nagashima, Y.; Watanabe, E. 1996. Development of an ultra high sensitive tissue biosensor for determination of swellfish poisoning, tetrodotoxin. *Biosens Bioelectron*, 11, 1185–1191.

66. Cheun, B. S.; Loughran, M.; Hayashi, T.; Nagashima, Y.; Watanabe, E. 1998. Use of a channel biosensor for the assay of paralytic shellfish toxins. *Toxicon*, 36, 1371–1381.

67. Cheun, B. S.; Takagi, S.; Hayashi, T.; Nagashima, Y.; Watanabe, E. 1998. Determination of Na channel blockers in paralytic shellfish toxins and pufferfish toxins with a tissue biosensor. *J Nat Toxins*, 7, 109–120.

68. Vieytes, M. R.; Cabado, A. G.; Alfonso, A.; Louzao, M. C.; Botana, A. M.; Botana, L. M. 1993. Solid-phase radioreceptor assay for paralytic shellfish toxins. *Anal Biochem*, 211, 87–93.

69. Doucette, G. J.; Logan, M. M.; Ramsdell, J. S.; Van Dolah, F. M. 1997. Development and preliminary validation of a microtiter plate-based receptor binding assay for paralytic shellfish poisoning toxins. *Toxicon*, 35, 625–636.

70. Ruberu, S. R.; Liu, Y. G.; Wong, C. T. et al. 2003. Receptor binding assay for paralytic shellfish poisoning toxins: Optimization and interlaboratory comparison. *J AOAC Int*, 86, 737–745.

71. Twiner, M. J.; Bottein Dechraoui, M. Y.; Wang, Z. et al. 2007. Extraction and analysis of lipophilic brevetoxins from the red tide dinoflagellate *Karenia brevis*. *Anal Biochem*, 369, 128–135.

72. Van Dolah, F. M.; Leighfield, T. A.; Doucette, G. J.; Bean, L.; Niedzwiadek, B.; Rawn, D. F. 2009. Single-laboratory validation of the microplate receptor binding assay for paralytic shellfish toxins in shellfish. *J AOAC Int*, 92, 1705–1713.

73. Van Dolah, F. M.; Fire, S. E.; Leighfield, T. A.; Mikulski, C. M.; Doucette, G. J. 2012. Determination of paralytic shellfish toxins in shellfish by receptor binding assay: Collaborative study. *J AOAC Int*, 95, 795–812.

74. Vilariño, N.; Fonfria, E. S.; Molgo, J.; Araoz, R.; Botana, L. M. 2009. Detection of gymnodimine-A and 13-desmethyl C spirolide phycotoxins by fluorescence polarization. *Anal Chem*, 81, 2708–2714.

75. Rodriguez, L. P.; Vilarino, N.; Molgo, J. et al. 2011. Solid-phase receptor-based assay for the detection of cyclic imines by chemiluminescence, fluorescence, or colorimetry. *Anal Chem*, 83, 5857–5863.

76. Araoz, R.; Ramos, S.; Pelissier, F. et al. 2012. Coupling the Torpedo microplate-receptor binding assay with mass spectrometry to detect cyclic imine neurotoxins. *Anal Chem*, 84, 10445–10453.

77. Rodriguez, L. P.; Vilarino, N.; Molgo, J. et al. 2013. Development of a solid-phase receptor-based assay for the detection of cyclic imines using a microsphere-flow cytometry system. *Anal Chem*, 85(4), 2340–2347.

78. Otero, P.; Alfonso, A.; Alfonso, C. et al. 2011. First direct fluorescence polarization assay for the detection and quantification of spirolides in mussel samples. *Anal Chim Acta*, 701, 200–208.

79. Fonfría, E. S.; Vilariño, N.; Espiña, B. et al. 2009. Feasibility of gymnodimine and 13-desmethyl C spirolide detection by fluorescence polarization using a receptor-based assay in shellfish matrixes. *Anal Chim Acta*, 657, 75–82.

80. Fonfría, E. S.; Vilarino, N.; Molgo, J. et al. 2010. Detection of 13,19-didesmethyl C spirolide by fluorescence polarization using Torpedo electrocyte membranes. *Anal Biochem*, 403, 102–107.

81. Alfonso, C.; Alfonso, A.; Vieytes, M. R.; Yasumoto, T.; Botana, L. M. 2005. Quantification of yesso-toxin using the fluorescence polarization technique and study of the adequate extraction procedure. *Anal Biochem*, 344, 266–274.

82. Fonfria, E. S.; Vilarino, N.; Vieytes, M. R.; Yasumoto, T.; Botana, L. M. 2008. Feasibility of using a surface plasmon resonance-based biosensor to detect and quantify yessotoxin. *Anal Chim Acta*, 617, 167–170.

83. Pazos, M. J.; Alfonso, A.; Vieytes, M. R.; Yasumoto, T.; Botana, L. M. 2005. Kinetic analysis of the interaction between yessotoxin and analogues and immobilized phosphodiesterases using a resonant mirror optical biosensor. *Chem Res Toxicol*, 18, 1155–1160.

84. Pazos, M. J.; Alfonso, A.; Vieytes, M. R.; Yasumoto, T.; Vieites, J. M.; Botana, L. M. 2004. Resonant mirror biosensor detection method based on yessotoxin-phosphodiesterase interactions. *Anal Biochem*, 335, 112–118.

12

Surface Plasmon Resonance Biosensor Technology for Marine Toxin Analysis

Katrina Campbell

CONTENTS

12.1 Introduction

Marine biotoxins are diverse chemical compounds that are classified according to the acute symptoms that they present to humans and other mammals upon their ingestion within contaminated seafood. Traditionally, these toxins were detected in seafood using the biological reference methods, more commonly referred to as AOAC (Association of Analytical Communities) mouse bioassays, for both hydrophilic (AOAC, 2005a) and lipophilic toxins (Yasumoto et al., 1978). The release in 1986 of the European Union Directive 86/609 for animal protection to ensure progress away from animal experimentation to scientifically acceptable non-animal procedures that are fully validated to an international standard started the scientific exploration for alternative methods of testing to these animal bioassays. The legislation deemed that the 3Rs of reduction, replacement, and refinement should be implemented and where possible animal assays should be replaced. The difficulties and problems associated with implementing this directive and 3Rs approach to marine biotoxin testing were addressed at the European Centre for the Validation of Alternative Methods (ECVAM) fifty-fifth workshop (Hess et al., 2006). At this time the aquaculture industry was developing globally, and with the implementation of enhanced monitoring regimes to meet production demands, it was established that there were increased trends in frequency of the occurrence of toxin outbreaks and that wider and new geographical areas were being affected with known toxins in new locations and with new toxins such as azaspiracid in known problematic areas for other toxins. In the drive to prevent severe public health and economic impacts to the growing industry from toxin outbreaks, it was deemed that the mouse bioassay at this time was an antiquated method that was unethical and unsustainable to cope with all the toxins for the level of testing required (Hess, 2010).

The difficulties in devising alternative analytical procedures was and remains the lack of certified toxin standards for all marine toxins and their analogues and correlating the different toxic potencies of the parent toxins and analogues relative to the toxicity determined by time of death in the mouse bioassay. Scientists steered three classifiable approaches to finding alternative methods through physicochemical methods such as high-performance liquid chromatography (HPLC) and mass spectrometry (MS), functional cellular and receptor-based assays, and biochemical approaches through immunological methods (Campbell et al., 2011c). For both functional and biochemical approaches, biosensor technologies were proposed as alternative solutions in an attempt to overcome issues with toxin standard supply and varying toxicities of toxin analogues within a group of toxins.

Biosensor technologies are analytical tools for the recognition and measurement of a target through its association with a biological component and physiochemical detector. Therefore, a biosensor typically consists of a bio-recognition element, transducer, and an electronic system composed of a signal amplifier, processor, and display (Figure 12.1). A measurable signal comparative to the extent of the specific molecular interaction of the bio-recognition element with the target of interest is recorded by the transducer, which operates by physicochemical means. Biosensors are classified according to either their bio-recognition component or their transducer. The bio-recognition elements vary from human and animal cells, microorganisms, cell receptors, enzymes, antibodies, peptides, nucleic acids, or biometric materials. Transducers are either based on different forms of electrochemical detection (potentiometric, amperometric, conductometric), mass/acoustic detection (piezoelectric, cantilever), thermal detection, or optical detection (absorbance, reflectance, luminescence, surface plasmon resonance [SPR]).

Different functional assays and biochemical- and biosensor-based technologies employing various bio-recognition elements have shown some potential as alternative screening methods for marine biotoxins, but SPR optical biosensor technology has shown considerable promise in this field in a relatively short period of time. The first SPR immunoassay was proposed 30 years ago by Liedberg and co-workers, and unlike many other traditional enzyme immunoassays (EIAs), it is label-free in that a labeled molecule is not required for the detection of the analyte. Over the last three decades, it has been utilized in a variety of diverse applications in the disciplines of life science, pharmaceutical drug discovery, electrochemistry, chemical vapor detection, defense, food quality and safety, and environmental analysis. Although there are several SPR-based systems,

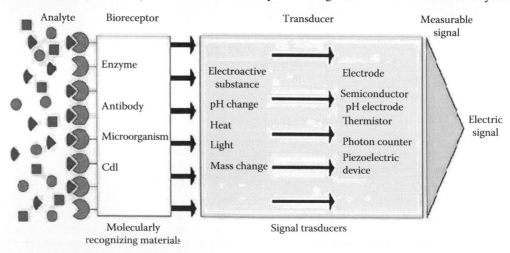

FIGURE 12.1 Diagram illustrating the key components of biosensor technologies.

the most extensively utilized is the Biacore, produced by Biacore AB, which developed into a range of instruments now owned by GE Healthcare. The advantages these biosensors offered over traditional immunoassays such as radio, enzyme-linked, fluorescence, and luminescence immunoassays for food, feed, and environmental diagnostics was not only that that they were label-free but demonstrated improved reproducibility, repeatability, and increased speed of analysis in real time due to automated microfluidic systems. In addition, they required minimal sample preparation and could utilize smaller volumes of sample reducing extraction times and costs of reagents. It is likely that it would be even more widely used were it not for its high cost and limited support for food safety diagnostic applications for the industry and regulatory laboratories. Other manufacturers such as ICx Technologies, Bio-Rad, Ibis, Horiba, Texas Instruments, and Seattle Sensors have commercialized SPR-based measuring systems capable of a very wide range of applications.

12.2 SPR

Since its first discovery by Wood in 1902, the physical phenomenon of SPR as later defined by Kretschmann and Raether (1968), has established its way into practical applications in sensitive detectors. The term biosensor was introduced around 1975, relating to the exploitation of transducer principles for the direct detection of biomolecules at a surface and in 1983 Lunstrom demonstrated the first application of SPR-based sensor technology for biomolecular interaction monitoring with protein–protein interactions. SPR is by no means a simple physical phenomenon, but for most biological analysts due to the simplicity of commercial instrumentation, it is considered a black box technique. Nonetheless, it is a phenomenon that occurs when polarized light, under conditions of total internal reflection, strikes an electrically conducting layer such as gold at the interface between media of different refractive indices. For biosensors this typically occurs on the gold layer of a sensor surface positioned between a glass layer of high refractive index and a buffer with low refractive index via the Kretschmann configuration (Figure 12.2). When the polarized light strikes the glass, an electric field intensity, known as an evanescent wave, is generated that interacts with, and is absorbed by, free electron clouds in the gold layer, generating electron charge density oscillations called surface plasmons. At a certain resonance angle, the plasmons are set to resonate with light, resulting in absorption of light at that angle creating a dark line in the reflected beam (Figure 12.2a and b denoted I and II). This resonance angle can therefore be obtained by observing a dip in SPR reflection intensity (Figure 12.2c). A shift in the reflectivity curve, a change in resonance angle between I and II, represents a molecular-binding event taking place on or near the metal film, or a conformational change in the molecules bound to the film.

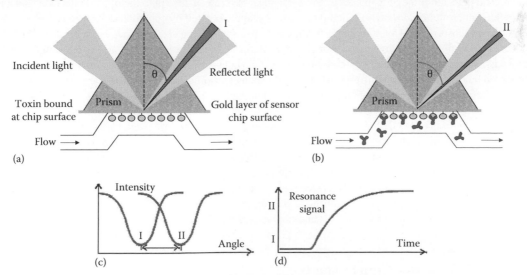

FIGURE 12.2 Schematic of an SPR sensor based on the Kretschmann geometry of the attenuated total reflection method when there is (a) no binding event and (b) during a binding event. (c) Reflection intensity as a function of resonance angle for two different refractive indices at the chip surface. (d) A typical sensorgram, which is a recording of resonant signal shift versus time, showing association due to binding to the target on the surface.

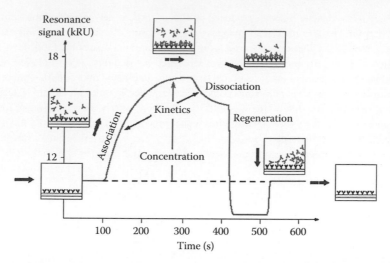

FIGURE 12.3 An SPR optical biosensor sensorgram of the molecular interaction between a specific binder and immobilized ligand. (From Abery, J., *Mod. Drug Discov.*, 4, 34, 2001; Courtesy of Biacore International AB, Uppsala, Sweden.)

By monitoring this shift against time (Figure 12.2d), molecular-binding events and binding kinetics can be studied without the addition of labels, and the reverse process, molecular dissociation, can also be studied.

SPR is a powerful optical biosensing technique to detect biomolecular interactions in real time in a label-free environment by measuring these alterations in refractive index. These changes in the refractive index correspond to changes in the resonance angle by which polarized light is reflected from this gold surface, which is in turn correlated to a change in mass on that surface due to binding interactions (Subrahmanyam et al., 2002). For the majority of biomolecules, the change in response is proportional to the mass of the material that has bound to the surface of the sensor chip. These biomolecular interactions can be used to identify the binding of two or more components to each other, to establish the affinity of the interactions, to calculate the actual association and dissociation rates of the interaction, and, for the purpose where marine toxin detection can be exploited, to measure the concentration of toxin present in a sample (Karlsson, 1994). Commercial SPR biosensors such as Biacore systems consist of three key components: the optical detector at the SPR interface, an interchangeable chip surface onto the optical interface, and an integrated microfluidic system with liquid handling systems operated by computer-driven software.

A typical sensorgram, a measure of the binding response against time, is illustrated in Figure 12.3 (Abery, 2001). The running buffer flowing over the surface established the baseline value, and as the sample solution passed over the sensor surface, the profile of the molecular interaction appeared. During injection the observed binding rate was the difference between the molecules binding to the surface and molecules leaving the surface. Consequently, binding appears fastest at the beginning of the injection as the binding partners readily interact with each other due to the readily available sites on the sensor surface. As the injection continues, the observed rate of binding decreased as fewer binding sites are available on the surface. After the injection was complete, the binding partners dissociated and the non-immobilized partner was washed away by the continuous flow of buffer. The sensor surface was regenerated back to the baseline value for the analysis of the next sample. The sensorgram provides essentially two kinds of information that are relevant to different types of applications: (1) the rate of interaction (association, dissociation, or both), which provides information on kinetic rate constants and target concentration, and (2) the binding level, which provides information on affinity constants and can be used for qualitative or semiquantitative applications.

12.3 SPR Biosensor Chip Surfaces

Although SPR can be generated in thin films made from conducting metals, most SPR sensor chips consist of a glass surface coated with a thin, uniform gold layer. Gold has a number of advantages in that it results in a well-defined reflectance minimum when a visible light source is used to provide the

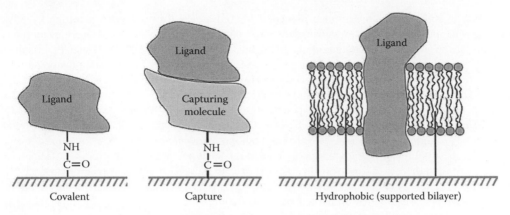

FIGURE 12.4 Approaches for attaching biomolecules to the carboxymethylated chip surface.

physical conditions to generate the SPR signal, it is mostly inert gold in physiological buffer conditions, and it is amenable to the covalent attachment of surface matrix layers. The latter forms the basis for a range of specialized surfaces to be designed to optimize the binding of a variety of molecules. In the most widely used sensor chip, the gold surface is modified with a carboxymethylated dextran layer, but other self-assembled monolayers (SAM) such as alkanethiols are also used. These layers then act as a substrate to which molecules can be attached and provide a hydrophilic environment for the interaction. Biomolecules may be attached to the surface of the sensor chip using three different approaches (Figure 12.4): covalent immobilization, where the molecule is attached to the surface through a covalent chemical link; high affinity capture, where the molecule of interest is attached by non-covalent interaction with another molecule (which in turn is usually attached using covalent immobilization); and hydrophobic adsorption, which exploits more or less specific hydrophobic interactions to attach either the molecule of interest or a hydrophobic carrier such as a lipid monolayer or bilayer to the sensor chip surface. For carboxymethylated dextran substrates, covalent immobilization using amine-, thiol-, or aldehyde-coupling procedures is the normal immobilization performed as it provides better chip stability. The choice of chemical procedure is highly dependent on the molecular properties of the molecule to be immobilized.

12.4 Bio-Recognition Elements for SPR

A number of different types of binders have been exploited in the development of various methodologies for the detection of marine biotoxins. These include receptors such as the sodium channel receptor (SCR) (Campbell et al., 2007), saxiphilin receptor for paralytic shellfish toxins (Lewis et al., 2008; Humpage et al., 2010), and enzymes for the diarrhetic shellfish toxins okadaic acid and yessotoxins (YTXs) (Fonfría et al., 2008), polyclonal and monoclonal antibodies raised against various toxin analogues (Le Berre and Kane, 2006; Traynor et al., 2006; Campbell et al., 2007; Ilamas et al., 2007; Stewart et al., 2009a; Yakes et al., 2011, 2012), chemical molecular imprinted polymers (Lotierzo et al., 2004), and aptamers (Handy et al., 2013). The general advantages and disadvantages of binders that have been previously investigated in the development of assays for SPR analysis for paralytic shellfish poisoning (PSP) toxins have been reported (Campbell et al., 2011b).

12.4.1 Receptors

Receptors can be either cell membrane bound or cytoplasmic proteins that may be exploited for their ligand binding capabilities for screening methodologies based on their functional response. Such a functional assay can be defined as a detection method that, with the purpose of quantification, uses the mechanism of action of the toxin group. Functional-based assays for marine toxin testing have been reviewed as an alternative high-throughput screening solution as most receptors or enzymes for the target toxins have been identified (Botana et al., 2009), but there are still certain toxins such as azaspiracid for which their mode of action still remains elusive. SCR from crude rat brain membrane preparations have been used in radioligand binding assays, which have now been validated and recommended for use (Van Dolah et al., 2009, 2012), and the fact that all saxitoxin (STX) analogues bind to SCRs with affinities that vary according to their toxic potency (Doucette et al., 1997) indicates that receptor-based competitive binding assays provide a measure of a sample's toxicity, irrespective of which PSP toxin(s) are present. A saxiphilin receptor, investigated as a binding molecule for PSP toxins, was used to study the behavior of mixtures of PSP toxins and found that the most potent toxins control the toxicity of the mixture more than the less active toxins that are required to be several orders of magnitude greater for the mixture to reflect their potency (Llewellyn, 2006). As receptor binders for PSP toxins applied in other systems reflect toxicity in a similar manner to the mouse bioassay, it was envisaged that they could be an ideal candidate for the development of an SPR assay to replace the mouse bioassay.

Receptor ligand binding assays using SPR technology had previously been investigated (Gestwicki et al., 2001; De Jong et al., 2005) in other areas of research. However, for concentration analysis, receptor-based assays in general tend to display poorer sensitivity compared to antibody-based tests. Natural receptors are the ideal capture tool, but these binders in automated regeneration systems tend to be unstable. Research is ongoing in the synthesis of cloned receptors, which would prove beneficial in both functional assays and as more stable alternative binders to antibodies for sensor technologies.

12.4.2 Antibodies

Antibody-based immunoassay procedures offer the opportunity of rapid screening methods and allow for the possibility of adaptation for on-site detection of toxins in shellfish extracts and water samples. Antibodies unlike receptors are biochemical binders and bind selectively to chemical features on the structure of the toxin to which they are produced. These binders do not show a similar relationship between the toxicity of a toxin and binding affinity in the same way as receptors for toxins. The difficulty in trying to detect such small molecular weight compounds using antibodies is that there are limited functional components for protein conjugation to use as an immunogen in antibody production based on site specificity, and therefore, few chemical reactions can be utilized for immunogen synthesis. Restricted and limited availability of toxins makes the synthesis of alternative derivatives impractical unless sufficient yield can be achieved for immunogen production. The formation of the toxin protein conjugate must also reduce the toxicity of the toxin or when immunized the animal may be affected with toxin symptoms. The first antibodies produced against marine toxins were reported in 1964 by Johnston et al. (1964) for PSP toxins in rabbits, but it was decades later when immunological methods were actually utilized to monitor toxins in shellfish. Compared to other fields of research, few researchers have produced high-quality antibodies either polyclonal or monoclonal to marine toxins. Polyclonal antibodies offer a finite supply of binder whereas monoclonals offer an infinite supply through their production from immortal cell lines. This area of research tends to be dominated by those researchers who have access to the toxins or analogues either through purification of naturally contaminated materials or by synthetic chemistry.

In the last decade, immunochemical approaches have become increasingly established in their use for food and environmental analysis and toxicology screening due to their ability to function rapid and effectively in complex biological matrices without major purification. Immunochemical assays utilizing antibodies are available for some marine biotoxins, but the majority of these assays display specificity mainly to chemical structure, but not proportionately to toxicity, and this limits an accurate measure of the total toxicity in a sample as required by regulatory authorities. So in many cases, the decisive usefulness of an antibody will lie in its specificity and cross-reactivity profile. For such diverse potency within relatively large toxin groups, whose small molecular weight structures are highly similar, it is extremely difficult to match the cross-reactivity profile of an antibody to the potency of each toxin for similar comparability as a receptor assay to the mouse bioassay. This still remains as the greatest challenge for marine toxin immunodiagnostics to replace the mouse bioassay. Therefore, to measure total toxicity for the full spectra of toxins to an equivalent extent, antibodies produced to different analogues or cocktail mixtures are being investigated. Nonetheless, for SPR the greatest success in the detection of the toxins has been through the development and utilization of monoclonal and polyclonal antibodies.

12.4.3 Synthetic Binders

12.4.3.1 *Molecularly Imprinted Polymers*

MIPs have received controversial exposure over the past 10 years from researchers and industries in their potential role for environmental and food analysis of chemical contaminants and toxins (Lotierzo et al., 2004; Henry, 2005; Baggiani et al., 2008). They are artificially created ligand-binding sites that are able to selectively recognize a target molecule. The synthesis involves the polymerization of functional and cross-linking monomers around the target of interest or a structural mimic template through non-covalent interactions or reversible covalent bonds or both with the functional groups of the template. These 3D polymer-based systems can be optimized to yield recognition sites highly specific and selective to the target of interest in the same manner as either a polyclonal or monoclonal antibody. However, due to their rigidity, they are extensively promoted in sample preparation and cleanup devices.

12.4.3.2 *Aptamers*

Aptamers are produced in vitro from libraries of nucleic acids (RNA and DNA) or peptide sequences and, although first described by Tuerk and Gold (1990), are generating new interest as alternative binders to antibodies due to patent expiry and progress in aptamer-screening methods (Wang and Jia, 2009) and their potential in the field of aptasensors (Wilner and Zayats, 2007). Nucleic acid aptamers are small synthetic oligonucleotides of up to 100 base pairs that can bind specifically to a variety of targets, such as whole cells, proteins, drugs, toxins, and low molecular weight compounds, with affinities in the nanomolar and subnanomolar ranges. They are able to bind with a high affinity and specificity to a target molecule through complementary shape interactions as a result of their 3D shape and can provide high molecular discrimination in being able to distinguish differences of a methyl group between two compounds (Jenison et al., 1994). As such they offer an opportunity of finding a single binder for the detection of the whole PSP toxin family or individual binders for each of the varying toxic groups within this family.

12.5 Key Features in SPR Assay Development

The key features that need to be considered in SPR assay development, some of which are similar to all other analytical methods, are the following:

1. Properties of the target compound including molecular structure, solubility, and stability for surface chemistry design for immobilization onto the biosensor surface, sample extraction, and storage.
2. Properties of the bio-recognition molecule such as stability and longevity.
3. Legislation to determine if the target is banned or has maximum residue level (MRL) or action level for a decision to be taken. If the substance is banned, the as low as reasonably achievable (ALARA) principle applies in the development of the method, whereas if the substance has an action level or MRL, the test may not need to be as sensitive but should be designed to be fit for purpose for this target concentration.
4. Sensitivity that the assay can achieve by optimizing the parameters such as concentration of bio-recognition element, flow rate of the biosensor over the surface, and contact time of the interaction on the surface.
5. Dynamic range of the calibration curve to determine the dilution factor that can be applied to the sample preparation to either achieve the ALARA or MRL detection.
6. Specificity (cross-reactivity) of the bio-recognition element not only to detect targets of interest to be fit for purpose but also to ensure that there are no interfering compounds with the assay, which may provide false results.

7. Composition of the sample to design extraction procedures to eliminate the interfering compounds but to retain the target.

8. Known issues with sample preparation such as the instrumental tolerance for certain solvents and effects of buffering pHs on the bio-recognition element.

9. Length of time for the analysis relative to turnaround times to develop a rapid test.

10. Effects of the biosensor flow rate on the sensitivity and longevity of the chip.

11. Effects of injection or contact time of the surface interaction on the sensitivity of the assay, longevity, and stability of the surface.

12. Effects of the regeneration solution on dissociating the binding event for repeatable analysis.

12.6 SPR Assay Formats for Marine Toxin Analysis

The SPR biosensor assay can be established using different assay formats. The simplest format is a direct capture assay where the bio-recognition element is immobilized onto a gold surface and the target captured from the solution. As SPR measures a change in mass on the surface for relatively low molecular weight marine biotoxins, the change in mass produced by a capture assay is difficult to measure with many SPR sensors. For this reason direct and indirect competitive inhibition assays tend to be applied. In this case, the capture biorecognition assay is immobilized on the surface and unlabeled toxin in a sample competes with protein-labeled toxin for the binding sites (Figure 12.4a). Different research studies have reported employing high molecular weight labels for the enhancement of the sensitivity of SPR immunosensors based on indirect competitive assays (Mitchell, 2010). Avidin molecules can be used as high molecular weight labels that bind with previously bound biotinylated toxin in an additional step, enabling toxin detection, otherwise hampered by the low molecular weight of the toxin biotin conjugate. Though avidin is easily nonspecifically adsorbed onto the chip surface, additional blocking steps are required (Figure 12.4b).

However, for marine biotoxin analysis and to preserve limited supplies of toxin, the most commonly used competitive inhibition assay is when the target is immobilized on the surface and the bio-recognition element competes with the target bound on the surface with target in the sample solution (Figure 12.5).

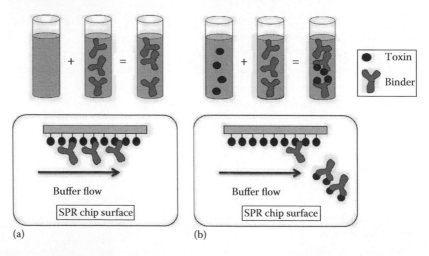

FIGURE 12.5 The competitive inhibition assay format designed for SPR-based devices to measure the concentrations of low molecular weight analytical targets. (a) When no toxin is present, the bio-recognition element binds to the toxin on the surface and a high response is detected. (b) When toxin is present in the sample, the bio-recognition element binds to toxin in the sample and a lower response is detected.

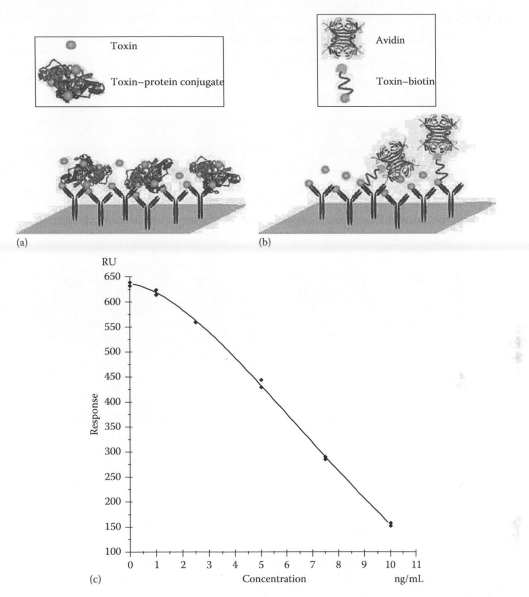

FIGURE 12.6 Antibody-immobilized SPR formats for small molecular weight toxin analysis. (a) Competitive inhibition with toxin protein conjugate. (b) Competitive inhibition with toxin biotin enhanced with avidin for increased sensitivity. (c) A typical inhibition assay calibration curve obtained for the measurement and quantification of toxins in complex biological samples.

Using these three assay formats, the level of binding to the surface is inversely proportional to the concentration of toxin present in the sample, and a typical calibration curve is illustrated in Figure 12.6.

12.7 SPR Analysis of Regulated Toxins

To date, a number of marine toxin SPR assays have now been successfully developed (Table 12.1) either as model systems or for seafood analysis by various researchers, but limitations in bio-recognition specificity, instrumental costs, and availability of toxin material to develop and validate methods to

TABLE 12.1

Summary of the SPR Methods for Marine Biotoxins

Toxin	Biosensor	Bio-Recognition Element	Chip Surface	References
Domoic acid	Biacore 3000	MIP Monoclonal	MIP Monoclonal	Lotierzo et al. (2004)
	SPR Prague	Monoclonal	OEG SAM-coupled domoic acid	Yu et al. (2005)
	Biacore Q	Polyclonal (rabbit)	Biacore CM5-coupled domoic acid	Traynor et al. (2006)
	Biacore	Polyclonal (sheep) Monoclonal Single-chain fragments (sheep and chicken)	Biacore CM5-coupled domoic acid	Le Berre et al. (2006)
	Prototype SPR	Polyclonal (rabbit)	Spreeta 2000 Texas Instruments	Stevens et al. (2007)
Okadaic acid	Biacore Q	Polyclonal Monoclonal	Biacore CM5-coupled okadaic acid	Llamas et al. (2007) Stewart et al. (2009a) Stewart et al. (2009b)
	Biacore 3000	Monoclonal	CM5 monoclonal	Prieto et al. (2010)
YTX	Biacore X	Phosphodiesterase enzymes	Phosphodiesterase enzymes	Fonfria et al. (2008)
	Biacore X	Phosphodiesterase enzymes	CM5 chip-coupled streptavidin biotinylated dsYTX	Mouri et al. (2009)
STX	Biacore Q	Monoclonal Polyclonal SCR	CM5-coupled STX	Campbell et al. (2007)
		Monoclonal		Fonfria et al. (2007)
		Polyclonal		Campbell et al. (2009, 2010) van den Top et al. (2011)
		Monoclonal Polyclonal		Haughey et al. (2011); Rawn et al. (2009)
		Monoclonal Polyclonal	CM5-coupled STX CM5-coupled neoSTX	Campbell et al. (2011b)
	Biacore T100	Monoclonal Polyclonal	CM5-coupled STX	Yakes et al. (2012)
	Biacore T200	Aptamer	CM5-coupled STX	Handy et al. (2013)
TTX	SPR Prague	Monoclonal	TTX	Taylor et al. (2008) Yakes et al. (2010) Vaisocherova et al. (2011)
	Biacore Q	Monoclonal	TTX	Campbell et al. (2013)
Palytoxin	Biacore T100	Monoclonal	Anti-species antibody	Yakes et al. (2012)
Multitoxin	Biacore prototype	Monoclonal Polyclonal	Series S CM5 chip coupled with STX, domoic acid, okadaic acid, and neoSTX	Campbell et al. (2011a) McNamee et al. (2013)

TABLE 12.2

Key Regulated Toxins in Europe and Their Regulatory Limits

Toxin Group	Parent Toxin	Regulatory Limit (μg of Toxin/kg of Seafood)
Amnesic shellfish poisons (ASP)	Domoic acid	20,000
Diarrhetic (lipophilic) shellfish poisons (DSP)	Okadaic acid Dinophysistoxins Pectenotoxin	160 okadaic acid equivalents
	YTX	3,750 YTX equivalents
	Azaspiracid	160 azaspiracid equivalents
Paralytic shellfish poisons (PSP)	STX	800 STX equivalents

European or AOAC standards have restricted their implementation. In Europe, action limits for regulatory purposes have been established for some marine toxins in bivalve molluscs and seafood as stipulated in Regulation (EC) No 853/2004. The key regulated toxins in Europe and their regulatory limits are outlined in Table 12.2. Therefore, the biosensor assays developed for toxin analysis in seafood were designed to detect these toxins optimally at these regulatory limits to be fit for purpose rather than optimizing for the lowest possible sensitivity achievable.

12.7.1 Amnesic Shellfish Poisoning Toxins

Domoic acid is an amnesic shellfish toxin and the most common marine biotoxin for which biosensor assays have been developed due mainly to cost and availability of this toxin. Similarly, as domoic acid is the only standard for this group, the monitoring and detection are for a single analyte. Therefore, most biosensing researchers have used this toxin as their model system to demonstrate their technology or technique to this field of application. The first published SPR assay for domoic acid (Lotierzo et al., 2004) on a Biacore 3000 compared the use of monoclonal antibodies and a molecularly imprinted polymer (MIP) film as capture bio-recognition element for domoic acid. Competitive binding assays were performed with free domoic acid and its conjugate with horseradish peroxidase, which was used as a refractive label. The monoclonal antibodies were deemed to be more sensitive at 9.2 ng/mL compared to 50 ng/mL for domoic acid detection, but the MIP was more robust for continuous regeneration on the surface.

The first SPR inhibition assay for domoic acid as a low molecular weight analyte utilized a novel method in surface chemistry to covalently immobilize domoic acid molecules onto a gold-coated SPR chip functionalized with mixed oligo(ethylene glycol) (OEG) SAMs. The long-chain thiol served as a functional site to react with carboxyl groups on domoic acid (Yu et al., 2005). The SPR sensor was a dual-channel instrument developed at the Institute of Radio Engineering and Electronics, Academy of Sciences in Prague, and the sensitivity achieved in this assay was 0.1 ng/mL.

The first reported detection of domoic acid in seafood was presented using a Biacore Q SPR with immobilized domoic acid on the chip surface (Traynor et al., 2006). The assay was designed as a screening test for bivalve molluscs and compared with liquid chromatography and validated to regulatory requirements. The initial assay in buffer relative to the regulatory limit of 20 mg/kg was too sensitive, which allowed a large dilution factor as part of the sample preparation, which reduced any interfering matrix effects from other components in the sample. The comparison of the method and validation parameters such as reproducibility and repeatability was exceptional for an immunological method, and for toxin testing in food analysis, SPR was believed to be the way forward.

At a similar time, another research group (Le Berre and Kane, 2006) investigated panels of antibodies from different species for domoic acid detection including a mouse monoclonal, sheep polyclonal antiserum, and single-chain variable region fragments from sheep and chicken, using a Biacore instrument.

The sheep polyclonal demonstrated the best sensitivity on this occasion, but so many factors play a key part in antibody sensitivity from immunogen design, immunogen dose including species administered to ascertain if this would always be the pattern. Generally, polyclonal antibodies tend to display better sensitivity due to multiple epitope binding.

The next step for domoic acid detection came with the first portable SPR assay. This assay was performed on a six-channel instrument displaying a limit of detection of 3 µg/kg in clams, following a methanol extraction and solid-phase extraction sample cleanup (Stevens et al., 2007). They utilized an antibody-based assay in both competition and displacement formats. Portability for seafood analysis is a key desire because it allows detection at the shellfish bed, thus allowing samples to be tested before going to the expense of harvesting and returning to shore for analysis. It thereby offers the opportunity for timely analysis based on tidal changes. Unfortunately, the sample preparation used included a solid-phase extraction, which is difficult to implement easily in field analysis particularly for nonscientists.

12.7.2 Diarrhetic Shellfish Poisoning Toxins

Okadaic acid and dinophysistoxins belong to the group of diarrhetic shellfish poisoning (DSP) toxins. An interesting evolution can be observed in the development of these Biacore Q SPR biosensor methods for these toxins starting where an optical (SPR) antibody-based competitive method for okadaic acid detection in mussel (LOD 126 ng/g) was reported following homogenization, methanol extraction, evaporation, and reconstitution in buffer (Llamas et al., 2007). The continuation of this work with considered selection of a monoclonal antibody, the test was developed to show multiplexed cross-reactivity for three compounds within the group (okadaic acid, dinophysistoxins 1 and 2) that mirrored the toxic profiles (Stewart et al., 2009a) before fully validating the method in a matrix showing a working range of 31–174 µg/kg and a limit of detection of 31 µg/kg (Stewart et al., 2009b). Having compared the method with liquid chromatography–mass spectrometry (LC–MS) and in the belief that any replacement for the mouse bioassay for DSP toxins should be able to account for relative toxicities in the group, they postulated that their method could be used as a screening tool for okadaic acid toxins with only suspect samples being forwarded for confirmation. The misrepresentation of this comparison is that the mouse bioassay and LC–MS method detect all the lipophilic toxins and not just the okadaic acid group. Therefore, to be truly effective as a replacement for lipophilic toxins, sensor assays to the other toxins in this classification would be required.

Prieto et al. (2010) used a Biacore 3000 SPR for the detection of okadaic acid using monoclonal antibodies immobilized on the sensor surface and a direct competitive assay with okadaic ovalbumin protein conjugate and an indirect competitive assay with an okadaic acid–biotin–avidin system to enhance sensitivity, but improved sensitivity was not achieved, and using this format, the sensitivity was comparable to that described previously (Stewart et al., 2009b). SPR has also been used to investigate the interactions of okadaic–biotin conjugates with protein phosphatase 2A (PP2A) to determine the toxin's effect on cell signaling pathways (Konoki et al., 2000)

Yessotoxin and analogues are disulfated polyether toxins produced by marine dinoflagellates. Although there is no clear evidence that YTX is toxic to humans, it is a major cause of false positives in diarrhetic shellfish toxin detection by mouse bioassay. An SPR method was developed as a new detection and quantification method for YTX due to its interaction with immobilized phosphodiesterase enzymes on a Biacore X SPR-based biosensor (Fonfria et al., 2008). The assay allowed the quantification of the toxin at concentrations of 1 mg/kg of the European regulatory limit.

This method was altered by immobilizing sulfated YTX to the streptavidin surface and employed phosphodiesterase PDEII in an inhibition detection mode for the detection of ladder-shaped polyethers, YTX and brevetoxin, and potentially ciguatoxin (Mouri et al., 2009).

To date, no SPR methods have been developed for the remaining toxins/analogues in the diarrhetic class of shellfish toxins such as *pectenotoxin*, *gymnodimine*, or *azaspiracid* mainly due to the lack of toxin.

12.7.3 Paralytic Shellfish Poisoning Toxins

STX and its numerous analogues due to their lethal potency and diversity in structure and toxicity are a difficult group of toxins to detect relative to their total potency as performed by the mouse bioassay.

The availability of this toxin and its analogues is approximately 100-fold less compared to okadaic acid at a costly price, and this in itself provided a scientific challenge to researchers designing alternative methods. Biologically, each analogue displays a different binding affinity to the SCRs, which results in different toxicities relative to STX (Genenah and Shimizu, 1981) resulting in the regulatory limit being expressed as μg STX equivalents per kg of shellfish meat (EFSA, 2009). This measure of total toxin contamination is therefore a simple concept for the biological methods whereby toxin levels correlate to toxicity. However, as the number of analogues rises in a toxin group, this causes severe complications for both biochemical and analytical methodologies whereby conversion factors are required especially when certain toxin standards are limited or unavailable for all detectable PSP toxins in a contaminated sample. To increase the challenge for cross-reactivity of binders relative to toxicity, toxicity equivalence factors (TEFs) used worldwide for the conversion of the individual toxin amounts to STXdiHCl equivalents (TEFs) initially determined by Oshima (1995) have been modified and implemented only in European legislation in 2010 with the major difference being that the TEF for dcSTX doubled in value.

Initially, Campbell et al. (2007) examined crude extracts of SCR from rat brains using Biacore Q SPR analysis, but technical difficulties were encountered with the receptor assay in that this preparation appeared to be stable for only a short time at 4°C, which in effect was detrimental to reliability and reproducibility. For receptor-based assays, another issue with developing SPR assays for small molecular weight toxins is that when the toxin is immobilized onto the surface, the toxin may then be orientated in such a manner that it no longer locks into the binding site of the receptor pocket making the toxin unrecognizable with minimal to no binding occurring. The limited availability of the saxiphilin receptor to only a few research groups has inhibited the characterization of this binder in the role of PSP toxin detection by SPR.

To date, although antibodies may have specificity issues relating to the analysis of such a large toxin group, they are the most successful binder in terms of sensitivity for the detection of PSP toxins. For this reason, antibodies were chosen as the model binder to demonstrate the feasibility of SPR optical biosensor technology for PSP toxin analysis. The first SPR assays for PSP toxins performed on a Biacore Q instrument were also designed as an inhibition assay with STX covalently immobilized on the surface. This provided a robust technique that can be regenerated over 1000 times per flow cell for reuse conserving toxin supplies and reducing cost. The potential of both a monoclonal antibody (GT-13A) raised to gonyautoxin 2/3 and a polyclonal antibody (R895) raised to STX illustrated the varying cross-reactivity profiles to the toxin analogues (Campbell et al., 2007). For regulatory purposes, underestimation could have severe health implications to the consumer whereby contaminated material is declared safe for consumption, whereas overestimation could cause detrimental economic losses to the industry through the unnecessary closure of harvesting beds. Using the monoclonal antibody, with poor cross-reactivity to hydroxylated toxins, a follow-up study investigated various extraction procedures previously used for PSP toxin analysis to determine the technology's suitability to different extraction solvents and procedures (Fonfria et al., 2007). The sample preparation techniques were compatible with the system, but the Garthwaite method (Garthwaite et al., 2001) was recommended for further evaluation based on analysis time, but only 50% recovery of STX was achieved using this extraction procedure. As a proof of concept, this monoclonal antibody was also employed to demonstrate that SPR biosensor-based biochemical analysis could be combined with state-of-the-art MS chemical analysis for joint screening and confirmatory determination of PSP toxins (Marchesini et al., 2009).

The polyclonal antibody showed a much more diverse but narrower pattern in cross-reactivity profile with improved sensitivities to all toxins, but the hydroxylated toxins dcNEO and GTX1/4 still remained as outliers in cross-reactivity. Rawn et al. (2009) performed an evaluation of both binders by SPR using the Garthwaite extraction procedure for analyzing 88 natural samples and compared the results to the AOAC HPLC method (AOAC, 2005b). In general the polyclonal antibody correlated better with HPLC than the monoclonal antibody due to the differences in cross-reactivity profiles. Although, it was recommended that improved antibody response to the hydroxylated toxins would be necessary if SPR was to be a replacement to the mouse bioassay for regulatory testing. As a screening tool it was suggested that this SPR method using either antibody could eliminate greater than 80% of samples from the mouse bioassay at the current regulatory limit. In relation to the three Rs of replace, reduce, and refine at this stage, the SPR assay may not be a replacement tool but a reduction tool to the number of animal assays performed for regulatory purposes.

Further work was then performed on the extraction procedure in order to calibrate the SPR assay using a buffer curve to eliminate the requirement of sourcing uncontaminated material and using relatively excessive quantities of toxin in the preparation of a calibration curve (Campbell et al., 2009). This was achieved in a comparative study using a second polyclonal binder raised to STX (BC67) for SPR analysis compared to EIA, HPLC, and mouse bioassay (Campbell et al., 2009). This study demonstrated that the key for immunological assay development was the binder and highlighted that the advantages with using SPR over all the other methods were simplicity, ease of use, and speed of analysis. This new extraction procedure using pH 5 sodium acetate buffer followed by centrifugation, dilution, and analysis was then applied to the STX antibody, and single-laboratory validation of this SPR method performed highly satisfactorily (Campbell et al., 2010). An interlaboratory study between seven international laboratories was performed (van den Top et al., 2011). All seven participating laboratories completed the study and HorRat values obtained were <1 demonstrating that the method performance was acceptable. Mean recoveries expressed as STXdiHCl equivalents/kg were 94.6% ± 16.8% for the low-level PSP toxin mix and 98.6% ± 5.6% for the high level of STX. Relative standard deviations for within-laboratory variations (RSD_R: repeatability) and between-laboratory variations (RSD_R: reproducibility) ranged from 1.8% to 9.6% and 2.9% to 18.3%, respectively. Threshold values for the assay have been discussed for regulatory purposes, but this level could vary depending on geographical location and the risk management strategies that have to be considered whether by industrial or regulatory monitoring laboratories. To date, there have been no reports of PSP toxins occurring in isolation, but if GTX1/4 was to do, this method could then become invalid even as a screening tool due to the lack of sensitivity of this binder to this toxin. Therefore, alternative binders are still being sought with improved sensitivity towards the hydroxylated toxins. Different heterologous assay formats have been investigated whereby different toxins have been immobilized on the surface, and cocktails of antibodies raised to different analogues have been assessed that could improve the overall toxicity determination of PSP toxins in a sample (Campbell et al., 2011b). Further research has been performed in the transferability of the assay to different SPR systems (Haughey et al., 2011), and additional assessment of commercial antibodies on these alternate SPR systems has been assessed with the conclusion that superior antibodies or alternative binders are still required for enhanced specificity to all toxin groups (Yakes et al., 2012). A synthetic binder in the form of an aptamer for STX has been produced and characterized by SPR (Handy et al., 2013), but as yet assay development for PSP toxins using this binder has not been achieved.

12.8 SPR Analysis of Emerging Toxins

12.8.1 Tetrodotoxin

Tetrodotoxin (TTX) poisoning is most commonly associated with consumption of puffer fish, but in recent years in Europe, the first confirmed toxic episode arose from the consumption of gastropods (Rodriguez et al., 2008; Fernández et al., 2010). Similar to PSP toxins, the standard method accepted worldwide for monitoring TTX toxicity in food matrices is the mouse bioassay and is really only detected in Europe as a consequence for testing for paralytic toxins. Ethical concerns from live animal testing, low sample throughput, and analytical inaccuracies have led to the need for an alternative method and move away from the mouse bioassay to HPLC methods for PSP toxins, which do not detect TTX. Taylor et al. (2008) reported the quantitative antibody-based detection of a low molecular weight molecule TTX by inhibition assay with an SPR sensor. A novel anti-TTX antibody sensing surface was developed by chemically immobilizing TTX on a gold film with a mixed SAM consisting of amine-terminated OEG alkanethiol and a hydroxyl-terminated OEG alkanethiol. The detection limit achieved for TTX was defined as IC_{20} (20% inhibitory concentration), at 0.3 ng/mL. As a follow-up to this development, they extended the assay for the detection of TTX in both clinical- and food-relevant matrices such as puffer fish liver extract, puffer fish muscle extract, and human urine (Yakes et al., 2011a). In succession a prevalidation study was conducted to demonstrate the assay performance for the detection of TTX in puffer fish, such as selectivity, limit of detection, limit of quantification, repeatability, reproducibility, and accuracy (Vaisocherova et al., 2011). Three participating laboratories reported standard curves in buffer and puffer fish matrix. The developed method was demonstrated to be capable of detecting TTX in puffer fish matrix standard samples in a broad concentration range (2–9000 ng/mL) with a limit of detection of 1.5 ng/mL. Between-laboratory recovery values were in the range of 51%–190% with a mean of 107% and 64%–180% with a mean of 103% for TTX-spiked samples in buffer and puffer fish matrix, respectively. Between-laboratory recoveries were in the satisfactory range of 101%–119% for naturally contaminated samples. This robust, rapid, and noninvasive method may serve as an attractive alternative to established methods for detection of TTX in puffer fish extracts.

As part of an EU project ATLANTOX examining advanced tests in the Atlantic area, a Biacore Q SPR method was developed and validated for the detection of TTX in gastropods and puffer fish. As no current regulatory limits are set for TTX in Europe, single-laboratory validation was undertaken using those for PSP toxins at 800 µg/kg. The decision limit (CCα) was 100 µg/kg, with the decision limit (CCβ) found to be ≤200 µg/kg. The repeatability and reproducibility were assessed at three levels of toxin fortification, 200, 400, and 800 µg/kg and analyzed in triplicate. The relative standard deviations for repeatability were 8.3%, 3.8%, and 5.4% and for reproducibility were 7.8%, 8.3%, and 3.7%, respectively at the three levels. Similarly, the recovery of the assay at the same three levels was 112%, 98%, and 99%.

12.8.2 Palytoxin

Palytoxin is a polyether marine toxin originally isolated from the zoanthid *Palythoa toxica* and is one of the most toxic nonprotein substances known. Fatal poisonings have been linked to ingestion of contaminated seafood, and effects in humans have been associated with dermal and inhalational exposure to palytoxin-containing organisms and waters. Its co-occurrence with other well-characterized seafood toxins (e.g., ciguatoxins, STXs, TTX) has hindered its direct associations to seafood-borne illnesses. For palytoxin there are currently no validated methods. A new Biacore T100 SPR assay for palytoxin using an anti-mouse substrate to characterize the kinetic values for a previously developed monoclonal antibody raised to palytoxin was developed (Yakes et al., 2012). The characterized antibody was then incorporated into a sensitive, rapid, and selective assay capable of measuring low- to sub-ng/mL palytoxin levels in buffer and two seafood matrices (grouper and clam). Preliminary results indicate that this SPR biosensor assay allows for (1) rapid characterization of antibodies and (2) rapid, sensitive palytoxin concentration determination in seafood matrices.

12.9 SPR Multitoxin Analysis

As eluded to previously, the mouse bioassay, and more recently LC–MS methods, had the ability to detect multiple toxins based on their solubility in the extraction procedure. As such there is an increasing demand to develop biosensor-monitoring devices capable of detecting multiple contaminants or toxins in food produce to be competitive with the current confirmatory techniques. This is particularly pertinent in seafood whereby the replacement of the mouse bioassay should preferably be capable of detecting all the marine toxins in a single test. A microfluidic immobilization device allowing the covalent attachment of up to 16 binding partners in a linear array on a single surface was developed and assessed for compatibility with a Biacore prototype multiplex SPR analyzer using marine toxin concentration analysis as a model system (Campbell et al., 2011a). The parent compound of four toxin groups were immobilized within a single-chip format, and calibration curves were achieved for each of the regulated toxins—domoic acid, okadaic acid, and STX—at low ng/mL levels. The chip design and SPR technology allowed the compartmentalization of the binding interactions for each toxin group offering the added benefit of being able to distinguish between toxin families and perform concentration analysis. This model is particularly contemporary with the current drive to replace biological methods for phycotoxin screening. As part of an EU project Conffidence for detecting contaminants in feed and food through inexpensive detection for control measures, this instrumentation is being assessed for the detection of these three toxin groups in shellfish samples, and to date, suitable sensitivity has been achieved for all three groups.

A modification of this method was then used as part of an EU project Microarrays for the Detection of Toxic Algae (MIDTAL) to test 256 seawater samples from around Europe for each of the toxins (McNamee et al., 2013). A simple sample preparation procedure was developed, which involved lysing and releasing the toxins from the algal cells with glass beads followed by centrifugation and filtering the extract before testing for marine biotoxins by both multi-SPR and ELISA (enzyme linked immunosorbent assay). Method detection limits based on IC_{20} values for PSP, okadaic acid, and domoic acid toxins were 0.82, 0.36, and 1.66 ng/mL, respectively. For seawater samples, the sensitivity can be improved by collecting and filtering a larger volume of water or through enhancement methods in SPR detection.

12.10 Conclusion

Research in analytical methodology over the last decade has demonstrated that there was a clear desire for scientists and regulatory laboratories to move away from the mouse bioassay for the monitoring of shellfish toxins in seafood. The efforts on the development of SPR biosensor assays, which could be validated for regulatory purposes using criteria outlined in the EU directive 2002/657 and the robust transferability and simplicity during interlaboratory comparison trials, showed that this technique could contribute to the removal of the mouse bioassay as a rapid screening test. It is a highly promising bio-tool as it produces real-time, rapid, and reliable results with minimal sample preparation and use of toxin, which is important when toxin availability is low. The development of SPR biosensor methods has been dominated highly by Biacore systems through the support of five European research-funded projects—BioCop, Detectox, Conffidence, MIDTAL, and ATLANTOX—and work conducted by the Center for Food Safety and Applied Nutrition at the Food and Drug Administration in the United States. For the SPR biosensor assay to be a feasible replacement for the MBA, other factors also have to be considered multiple such as the cost per analysis incorporating the equipment and assay components. The reusability of the sensor chip surface is essential to the cost per analysis calculations particularly when toxin is immobilized. The Biacore SPR equipment used by most researchers in this review has been described as prohibitive for industrial and regulatory users due mainly to instrumentation costs. Several new SPR platforms, with a much lower cost basis, are now becoming commercially available, and it will be interesting to determine if they can generate equally as reliable data as the Biacore equipment. Competitive SPR instruments showing excellent promise particularly in the area of portability (Stevens et al., 2007) and multiplexing for future use (Chinowsky et al., 2007) and if supported with innovative sample preparation techniques may be more attractive to the industrial and regulatory stakeholders compared to expensive laboratory-based equipment.

The production of high-quality bio-recognition elements of intrinsic design is of fundamental importance to the development of these SPR assays in their ability to recognize the toxins relative to their toxicity to be fit for purpose. SPR is one detection principle, and these high-quality bio-recognition tools can be applied to the increasing emergence of biosensors utilizing different detection principles such as flow cytometry with fluorescent detection, electrochemistry, biolayer interferometry, planar wave guide, and surface acoustic waves that are showing versatility into the area of analytical detection. It will be even more interesting to determine their feasibility, validity, and transferability to other laboratories for marine toxin testing in shellfish. These new sensor-technology platforms should be evaluated to determine if they can generate reliability and reproducibility equivalent to SPR systems at reduced costs for improved sustainability and as a true competitive screening tool prior to high-maintenance confirmatory analysis such as liquid chromatography mass spectrometry.

REFERENCES

Abery, J. 2001. Detecting the molecular ties that bind, *Mod. Drug Discov.*, 4, 34–36.

AOAC (Association of Official Analytical Chemists). 2005a. AOAC official method 959.08. Paralytic shellfish poison, biological method. Chapter 49, Natural toxins. *AOAC Official Methods of Analysis*, 18th edn., Trucksess M.W. (ed.), Association of Official Analytical Chemists, Gaithersburg, MD, pp. 79–80.

AOAC Official Method. 2005b. 2005.06. Paralytic shellfish poisoning toxins in shellfish. *Official Methods of Analysis of AOAC International*, 18th edn., AOAC, Gaithersburg, MD, Section 49.10.03.

Baggiani, C., Anfossi, L., Giovannoli, C. 2008. Molecular imprinted polymers as synthetic receptors for the analysis of myco- and phyco-toxins. *Analyst*, 133, 719–730.

Botana, L.M., Alfonso, A., Botana, A., Vieytes, M.R., Vale, C., Vilarino, N., Louzao, C. 2009. Functional assays for marine toxins as an alternative, high-throughput screening solution to animal tests. *Trends Anal. Chem.*, 28(5), 603–611.

Campbell, K., Barnes, P., Haughey, S.A., Higgins, C., Kawatsu, K., Vasconcelos, V., and Elliott, C.T. 2013. Development and single laboratory validation of an optical biosensor assay for tetrodotoxin detection as a tool to combat emerging risks in European seafood. *Anal. Bioanal. Chem.*, 405(24), 7753–7763.

Campbell, K., Haughey, S.A., van den Top, H., van Egmond, H., Vilariño, N., Botana, L.M., Elliott, C.T. 2010. Single laboratory validation of a surface plasmon resonance biosensor screening method for paralytic shellfish poisoning toxins. *Anal. Chem.*, 82, 2977–2988.

Campbell, K., Huet, A.C., Charlier, C., Higgins, C., Delahaut, P., Elliott, C.T. 2009. Comparison of ELISA and SPR biosensor technology for the detection of paralytic shellfish poisoning toxins. *J. Chromatogr. B*, 877(32), 4079–4089.

Campbell, K., Mcgrath, T., Sjölander, S., Hanson, T., Tidare, M., Jansson, O., Moberg, A., Mooney, M., Elliott, C., Buijs, J. 2011a. Use of a novel micro-fluidic device to create arrays for multiplex analysis of large and small molecular weight compounds by surface plasmon resonance. *Biosens. Bioelectron.*, 26, 3029–3036.

Campbell, K., Rawn, D.F.K., Niedzwiadek, B., Elliott, C.T. 2011b. Paralytic shellfish poisoning (PSP) toxin binders for SPR analysis: Problems & possibilities for the future, a review. *Food Addit. Contam. Part A*, 28(6), 711–725.

Campbell, K., Stewart, L.D., Fodey, T.L., Haughey, S.A., Doucette, G.J., Kawatsu, K., Elliott, C.T. 2007. An assessment of specific binding proteins suitable for the detection of paralytic shellfish poisons (PSP) using optical biosensor technology. *Anal. Chem.*, 79(15), 5906–5914.

Campbell, K., Vilariño, N., Botana, L.M., Elliott, C.A. 2011c. European perspective on progress in moving away from the mouse bioassay for marine toxin analysis. *Trends Analyt. Chem.*, 30(2), 239–253

Chinowsky, T.M., Soelberg, S.D., Baker, P., Swanson, N.R., Kauffman, P., Mactutis, A., Grow, M.S., Atmar, R., Yee, S.S., Furlong, C.E. 2007. Portable 24-analyte surface plasmon resonance instruments for rapid, versatile biodetection. *Biosens. Bioelectron.*, 22, 2268–2275.

Council Directive. December 18, 1986. 86/609/EEC of 24 November 1986 on the approximation of laws, regulations and administrative provisions of the member states regarding the protection of animals used for experimental and other scientific purposes. *OJL*, 358, 1–28.

De Jong, L.A.A., Uges, D.R.A., Franke, J.P., Bischoff, R. 2005. Receptor ligand binding assays: Technologies and applications. *J. Chromatogr. B.*, 829, 1–25.

Doucette, G.J., Logan, M.L., Ramsdell, J.S., Van Dolah, F.M. 1997. Development and preliminary validation of a microtiter plate-based receptor binding assay for paralytic shellfish poisoning toxins. *Toxicon*, 35, 625–636.

European Commission Decision. 2002. (EC) no 2002/657/EC implementing council directive 96/23/EC concerning the performance of analytical methods and the interpretation of results. *Off. J. Eur. Communities*, L221, 8–34.

European Commission Regulation. 2004. (EC) no 853/2004 of the European parliament and of the council of 29 April 2004 laying down specific hygiene rules for food of animal origin. *Off. J. Eur. Communities*, L139, 55–205.

European Food Safety Authority. 2009. Scientific opinion of the panel on contaminants in the food chain on a request from the European Commission on marine biotoxins in shellfish-saxitoxin group. *EFSA J.*, 1019, 1–76.

Fernández-Ortega, J.F., Morales-de los Santos, J.M., Herrera-Gutiérrez, M.E., Fernández-Sánchez, V., Rodríguez Loureo, P., Alfonso Rancaño, A., Téllez-Andrade, A. 2010. Seafood intoxication by TTX: First case in Europe. *J. Emerg. Med.*, 39, 612–617.

Fonfria, E.S., Vilarino, N., Campbell, K., Elliott, C., Haughey, S.A., Ben-gigirey, B., Vieites, J.M., Kawatsu, K., Botana, L.M. 2007. Paralytic shellfish poisoning detection by surface plasmon resonance-based biosensors in shellfish matrices. *Anal. Chem.*, 79, 6303–6311.

Fonfría, E.S., Vilariño, N., Vieytes, M.R., Yasumoto, T., Botana, L.M. 2008. Feasibility of using a surface plasmon resonance-based biosensor to detect and quantify yessotoxin. *Anal. Chim. Acta*, 617(1–2), 167–170.

Garthwaite, I., Ross, K.M., Miles, C.O., Briggs, L.R., Towers, N.R., Borrell, T., Busby, P. 2001. Integrated enzyme-linked immunosorbent assay screening system for amnesic, neurotoxic, diarrhetic, and paralytic shellfish poisoning toxins found in New Zealand. *J. AOAC Int.*, 84(5), 1643–1648.

Genenah, A.A., Shimizu, Y. 1981. Specific toxicity of paralytic shellfish poisons. *J. Agric. Food Chem.*, 29, 1289–1291.

Gestwicki, J.E., Hsieh, H.V., Pitner, J.B. 2001. Using receptor conformational change to detect low molecular weight analytes by surface plasmon resonance. *Anal. Chem.*, 73, 5732–5737.

Handy, S.M., Yakes, B.J., Degrasse, J.A., Degrasse, S.L., Campbell, K., Elliott, C.T., Kanyuck, K.M. 2013. First report of the use of a saxitoxin protein conjugate to develop a DNA aptamer to a small molecule toxin. *Toxicon*, 61, 30–37.

Haughey, S.A., Campbell, K., Yakes, B.J., Prezioso, S.M., Degrasse, S.L., Kawatsu, K., Elliott, C.T. 2011. Comparison of biosensor platforms for surface plasmon resonance based detection of paralytic shellfish toxins. *Talanta*, 85, 519–526.

Henry, O.Y.F., Cullen, D.C., Piletsky, S.A. 2005. Optical interrogation of molecularly imprinted polymers and development of MIP sensors: A review. *Anal. Bioanal. Chem.*, 382(4), 947–956.

Hess, P. 2010. Requirements for screening and confirmatory methods for the detection and quantification of marine biotoxins in end-product and official control. *Anal. Bioanal. Chem.*, 397(5), 1683–1694.

Hess, P., Grune, B., Anderson, D.B., Aune, T., Botana, L.M., Caricato, P., van Egmond, H.P. et al. 2006. Three Rs approaches in marine biotoxin testing. The report and recommendations of a joint ECVAM/DG SANCO Workshop (ECVAM Workshop 54). *Altern. Lab. Anim.*, 34, 1923–224.

Humpage, A.R., Magalhaes, V.F., Froscio, S.M. 2010. Comparison of analytical tools and biological assays for detection of paralytic shellfish poisoning toxins. *Anal. Bioanal. Chem.*, 397, 1655–1671.

Jenison, R.D., Gill, S.C., Pardi, A., Polisky, B. 1994. High resolution molecular discrimination by RNA. *Science*, 263, 1425–1434.

Johnston, H.M., Frey, P.A., Angelotti, R., Campbell, J.E., Lewis, K.H. 1964. Haptenic properties of paralytic shellfish poison conjugated to proteins by formaldehyde treatment. *Proc. Soc. Exp. Biol. Med.*, 117, 425–430.

Karlsson, R. 1994. Real-time competitive kinetic analysis of interactions between low molecular weight ligands in solution and surface immobilised receptors. *Anal. Biochem.*, 221, 142–151.

Konoki, K., Sugiyama, N., Murata, M., Tachibana, K., Hatanaka, Y. 2000. Development of biotin-avidin technology to investigate okadaic acid-promoted cell signaling pathway. *Tetrahedron*, 56, 9003–9014.

Kretschmann, E., Reather, H. 1968. Radiative decay of nonradiative surface plasmons excited by light. *Z. Naturforsch., Teil A.*, 23, 2135–2136.

Le Berre, M., Kane, M. 2006. Biosensor-based assay for domoic acid: Comparison of performance using polyclonal, monoclonal, and recombinant antibodies. *Anal. Lett.*, 39, 1587–1598.

Lewis, P., Fritsch, I., Gawley, R.E., Henry, R., Kight, A., Lay, J.O., Liyanage, R., Mclachin, J. 2008. Dynamics of saxitoxin binding to saxiphilin c-lobe reveals conformational change. *Toxicon*, 51, 208–217.

Liedberg, B., Nylander, C., Lunstrom, I. 1983. Surface plasmon resonance for gas detection and biosensing. *Sens. Actuat.*, 4, 299–304.

Llamas, N.M., Stewart, L., Fodey, T.L., Elliott, C.T. 2007. Development of a novel immunobiosensor method for the rapid detection of okadaic acid contamination in shellfish extracts. *Anal. Bioanal. Chem.*, 389, 581–587.

Llewellyn, L.E. 2006. The behaviour of mixtures of paralytic shellfish toxins in competitive binding assays. *Chem. Res. Toxicol.*, 19, 661–667.

Lotierzo, M., Henry, O.Y.F., Piletsky, S., Tothill, I., Cullen, D., Kania, M., Hock, B., Turner, A.P.F. 2004. Surface plasmon resonance sensor for domoic acid based on grafted imprinted polymer. *Biosens. Bioelectron.*, 20(2), 145–152.

Marchesini, G.R., Hooijerink, H., Haasnoot, W., Nielen, M.W.F., Buijs, J., Campbell, K., Elliott, C.T., Nielen, M.W.F. 2009. Towards surface plasmon resonance biosensing combined with bioaffinity-assisted nano hilic liquid chromatography/time-of-flight mass spectrometry identification of paralytic shellfish poisons. *Trends Anal. Chem.*, 28(6), 792–803.

Mcnamee, S., Elliott, C.T., Delahaut, P., Campbell, K. 2013. Multiplex biotoxin surface plasmon resonance method for marine biotoxins in algal and seawater samples. *Environ. Sci. Pollut. Res. Int.*, 20(10), 6794–6807.

Mitchell, J. 2010. Small molecule immunosensing using surface plasmon resonance. *Sensors*, 10, 7323–7346.

Mouri, R., Oishi, T., Torikai, K., Ujihara, S., Matsumori, N., Murata, M., Oshima, Y. 2009. Surface plasmon resonance-based detection of ladder-shaped polyethers by inhibition detection method. *Bioorg. Med. Chem. Lett.*, 19, 2824–2828.

Oshima, Y. 1995. Post column derivatization liquid chromatography method for paralytic shellfish toxins. *J. AOAC Int.*, 78, 528–532.

Prieto-Simón, B., Miyachi, H., Karube, I., Saiki, H. 2010, High-sensitive flow-based kinetic exclusion assay for okadaic acid assessment in shellfish samples. *Biosens. Bioelectron.*, 25, 1395–1401.

Rawn, D.F.K., Niedzwiadek, B., Campbell, K., Higgins, H.C., Elliott, C.T. 2009. Evaluation of surface plasmon resonance relative to high pressure liquid chromatography for the determination of paralytic shellfish toxins. *J. Agric. Food Chem.*, 57, 10022–10031.

Rodriguez, P., Alfonso, A., Vale, C., Alfonso, C., Vale, P., Tellez, A., Botana, L.M. 2008. First toxicity report of TTX and 5,6,11-trideoxyTTX in the trumpet shell Charonia lampas lampas in Europe. *Anal. Chem.*, 80, 5622–5629.

Stevens, R.C., Soelberg, S.D., Eberhart, B.L., Spencer, S., Wekell, J.C., Chinowsky, T.M., Trainer, V.L., Furlong, C.L. 2007. Detection of the toxin domoic acid from clam extracts using a portable surface plasmon resonance biosensor. *Harmful Algae*, 6, 166–174.

Stewart, L.D., Elliott, C.T., Walker, A.D., Curran, R.M., Connolly, L. 2009a. Development of a monoclonal antibody binding okadaic acid and dinophysistoxins-1, -2 in proportion to their toxicity equivalence factors. *Toxicon*, 54(4), 491–498.

Stewart, L.D., Hess, P., Connolly, L., Elliott, C.T. 2009b. Development and single-laboratory validation of a pseudofunctional biosensor immunoassay for the detection of the okadaic acid group of toxins. *Anal. Chem.*, 81, 10208–10214.

Subrahmanyam, S., Piletsky, S.A., Turner, A.P. 2002. Application of natural receptors in sensors and assays. *Anal. Chem.*, 74, 3942–3951.

Taylor, A.D., Ladd, J., Etheridge, S., Deeds, J., Hall, S., Jiang, S. 2008. Quantitative detection of TTX (TTX) by a surface plasmon resonance (SPR) sensor. *Sens. Actuat. B*, 130, 120–128.

Traynor, I.M., Plumpton, L., Fodey, T.L., Higgins, C., Elliott, C.T. 2006. Immunobiosensor detection of domoic acid as a screening test in bivalve mollusks: Comparison with LC based analysis. *J. AOAC*, 89, 868–872.

Tuerk, C., Gold, L. 1990. Systematic evolution of ligands by exponential enrichment: RNA ligands to bacteriophage T4 DNA polymerase. *Science*, 249(4968), 505–510.

Vaisocherova, H., Taylor, A.D., Jiang, S., Hegnerova, K., Vala, M., Homola, J., Yakes, B.J., Deeds, J., Degrasse, S. 2011. Surface plasmon resonance biosensor for determination of TTX: Prevalidation study. *J. AOAC Int.*, 94(2), 596–604.

Van Den Top, H., Haughey, S., Vilariño, N., Botana, L., Van Egmond, H., Elliott, C.T., Campbell, K. 2011. Surface plasmon resonance biosensor screening method for paralytic shellfish poisoning toxins: A pilot interlaboratory study. *Anal. Chem.*, 82, 2977–2988.

Van Dolah, F.M., Fire, S.E., Leighfield, T.A., Mikulski, C.M., Doucette, G.J. 2012. Determination of paralytic shellfish toxins in shellfish by receptor binding assay: Collaborative study. *J. AOAC Int.*, 95(3), 795–812.

Van Dolah, F.M., Leighfield, T.A., Doucette, G.J., Bean, L., Niedzwiadek, B., Rawn, D.F. 2009. Single-laboratory validation of the microplate receptor binding assay for paralytic shellfish toxins in shellfish. *J. AOAC Int.*, 92, 1705–1713.

Wang, W, Jia, L.Y. 2009. Progress in aptamer screening methods. *Chin. J. Anal. Chem.*, 37(3), 454–460.

Wilner, I., Zayats, M. 2007. Electronic aptasensors. *Agnew. Chem. Int. Ed*, 46, 6408–6418.

Wood, R.W. 1902. On a remarkable case of uneven distribution of light in a diffraction grating spectrum. *Philos. Mag.*, 4, 396–402.

Yakes, B.J., Deeds, J., White, K., Degrasse, S.L. 2011a. Evaluation of surface plasmon resonance biosensors for detection of TTX in food matrices and comparison to analytical methods. *J. Agric. Food Chem.*, 59(3), 839–846.

Yakes, B.J., Prezioso, S.M., Degrasse, S.L. 2012. Developing improved immunoassays for paralytic shellfish toxins: The need for multiple superior antibodies. *Talanta*, 99, 668–676.

Yakes, B.J., Prezioso, S.M., Degrasse, S.L., Poli, M., Deeds, J.R. 2011b. Antibody characterization and immunoassays for palytoxin using an SPR biosensor. *Anal. Bioanal. Chem.*, 400, 2865–2869.

Yasumoto, T., Oshima, Y., Yamaguchi, M. 1978. Occurrence of a new type of toxic shellfish poisoning in the Tohoku district. *Bull. Jap. Soc. Sci. Fish.*, 44(11), 1249–1255.

Yu, Q., Chen, S., Taylor, A.D., Homola, J., Hock, B., Jiang, S. 2005. Detection of low-molecular-weight domoic acid using surface plasmon resonance sensor. *Sens. Actuat. B*, 107, 193–201.

Zhou, W.H., Guo, X.C., Zhao, H.Q., Wu, S.X., Yang, H.H., Wang, X.R. 2011. Molecularly imprinted polymer for selective extraction of domoic acid from seafood coupled with high-performance liquid chromatographic determination. *Talanta*, 84(3), 777–782.

Validation of HPLC Detection
Methods for Marine Toxins

Andrew Turner

CONTENTS

13.1 Introduction

Marine biotoxins are a diverse range of naturally occurring compounds with various groups of structurally related toxin families exhibiting very different solubilities and mechanisms of toxicity. The presence of toxins in a wide number of marine phytoplankton, which may be accumulated in filter-feeding bivalves and other shellfish, can subsequently impact upon the health of the shellfish consumer. To ensure consumer protection, the monitoring of many of these toxin classes is a statutory requirement. Biological assays, including the rat or mouse bioassay (MBA), have long been used for the determination of sample toxicity for many of the different toxin groups, providing either a quantitative or qualitative monitoring technique for shellfish food safety. While such assays have been relied on for many years as a primary tool for compliance testing, they are not free from complication or controversy. Routine shellfish safety monitoring using biological assays alone involves the killing of large numbers of animals, thereby presenting a clear ethical and political problem. An assay such as the paralytic shellfish poisoning (PSP) MBA [1], while providing generally reproducible quantitative data when carefully controlled, exhibits poor sensitivity relative to regulatory limits and is prone to interferences from metals and other salts that may affect method performance [2–6]. Other assays such as those utilized for diarrhetic shellfish poisoning (DSP) [7] are at best semiquantitative and are subjected to interferences, false positives, false negatives, and a lack of sensitivity [8–11]. All these methods, while providing information on the presence or level of toxicity in shellfish samples, by their very nature exhibit a lack of specificity, being unable to provide additional information, particularly relating to the presence of specific toxin groups and/or profiles.

Given clear concerns with continued use of live animal assays [12,13], there has been a significant move in recent decades to investigate alternative monitoring methodologies. There has been a strong commitment in some countries to move away from animal assays for statutory biotoxin monitoring, most notably with replacement of bioassays in New Zealand, Canada, Portugal, Ireland, France, Norway, and the United Kingdom. Modern analytical techniques using non-animal bioassays, immunoassays, and analytical instrumentation have been extensively investigated in these and many other countries with the aim of replacing the biological assay with accurate and reliable alternative approaches for routine monitoring. Many of these methods are more rapid, more sensitive, and more specific, and some have been demonstrated to provide safe and effective monitoring tools while generating more detailed data on the prevalence and variability of specific toxins.

The importance of potential alternative methods being thoroughly tested and validated cannot be overstated. They must be able to deal with complex matrices and be fully capable of differentiating toxins of interest from nontoxic compounds and from toxins of other groups [14,15]. In addition, there is the important requirement for use of certified toxin standards, without which many of the alternative methods could not be run. Indeed, the increased commercial availability of such standards in recent years has significantly aided the testing and validation of such methods. Certified matrix reference materials are also a valuable tool for method validation and quality control purposes, availability of which has also been expanding in recent years. Official control methods in particular must be validated and quality assured prior to adoption into monitoring programs in order to ensure the method is fit for the intended purpose [16]. Quantitative methods should be characterized by a number of specific criteria including but not restricted to accuracy, applicability (matrix and concentration range), limit of detection (LOD), limit of determination, precision, repeatability, reproducibility, recovery, selectivity or specificity, sensitivity, linearity, and ruggedness [14]. It is vital that the uncertainty of measurement associated with the method is fully and appropriately determined [17], and there is also the requirement where appropriate for comparison of results generated by alternative methods with those provided by the official reference methods, including bioassays. Once method performance criteria are deemed acceptable, they should undergo further validation by interlaboratory collaborative trial, with the proceedings overseen by an appropriate scientific body. As with single-laboratory validation, the trial should incorporate samples to generate data on a wide range of toxin analogues and matrix variability, with results being used to fully describe the recovery, repeatability, and reproducibility of the method. Qualitative methods indicating the presence or absence of the target analyte(s) should also be validated to determine fitness for purpose, including in particular the determination of method sensitivity, specificity, and false-positive and false-negative rates [18,19]. Comparison against reference methods may also be conducted where appropriate.

One alternative instrumental approach involves the use of high-performance or high-pressure liquid chromatography (HPLC). This dynamic chromatographic process involves the separation of components present within a mixture (the sample) and injected into a liquid mobile phase across a solid or liquid stationary phase (the HPLC column). Various modes of liquid chromatographic separation exist, the most common of which is the reversed phase where the stationary phase is nonpolar, typically a bonded C18 chain, and the mobile phase is usually prepared from a mixture of aqueous buffers and organic solvents. Other modes of action applicable to biotoxins include ion-pairing chromatography and ion-exchange chromatography, both of which utilize separation based on charged functional groupings. Hydrophilic interaction liquid chromatography (HILIC) has also been applied for polar toxins, but is not considered further in this chapter given the absence of its application to conventional detection methods. Given appropriate selection of both stationary and mobile phases, competitive interactions between molecules within the injected sample and the phases utilized enable the separation of individual toxins or their derivatives. With the column outlet connected to a suitable continuous flow detector, analytes can be detected, resulting in sensitive and specific analyses. With Chapter 15 covering the use of mass spectrometric (MS) detection methods coupled to HPLC, this chapter focuses solely on other detection methods, specifically those conventional methods incorporating fluorescence and ultraviolet (UV) detection. The choice of detector is dependent upon the chemical properties of the toxin, each now being examined in turn in the succeeding text.

13.2 Paralytic Shellfish Poisoning Toxins

PSP toxins (PSTs) are potent neurotoxins present in specific species of marine algae [20–22], which following ingestion from contaminated food products cause a range of symptoms, including potential fatality [23,24]. The list of PSTs detected in shellfish samples has been steadily growing in recent years, now comprising a group of more than 50 compounds [25] all related to the parent compound saxitoxin (STX) (Figure 13.1). The origin and chemistry of this group of toxins are described in detail within Chapter 36, but noting here that the hydrophilic PSTs most commonly encountered to date can be classified as either carbamoyl, decarbamoyl, or N-sulfocarbamoyl toxins. To ensure the protection of the consumer, the European Union's (EU) reference method for detecting PSTs is the MBA [1,26]. This method gives direct quantitative evidence for the toxicity of samples as calculated from the time of death in replicate mice injected with acidic extracts of shellfish. Alternative methods based upon HPLC exhibit both important similarities and differences in comparison with the MBA. Firstly, both methods require the quantitative extraction of toxins from subsamples of homogenized shellfish flesh. One of the official methods available for this process involves the use of hydrochloric acid (HCl) as the extraction solvent [1], with centrifuged and filtered supernatants being amenable to both MBA and HPLC-based methodologies. With both methods, the final measurement value is expressed in terms of a toxicity, specifically in STX equivalence per kilogram (STX eq./kg) of shellfish flesh. However, while the MBA directly determines sample toxicity, HPLC methods provide qualitative information on individual toxins, following the separation of toxins or toxin oxidation products on suitable chromatographic columns. In addition, assuming the availability of each individual toxin as a certified reference standard for instrument calibration purposes, quantitative molar concentrations of individual PSTs or groups of PSTs including epimeric pairs may be calculated. Sample toxicity can then only be accurately calculated given the availability of appropriate data on toxicity equivalence factors (TEFs) that describe the toxicity of each PST relative to

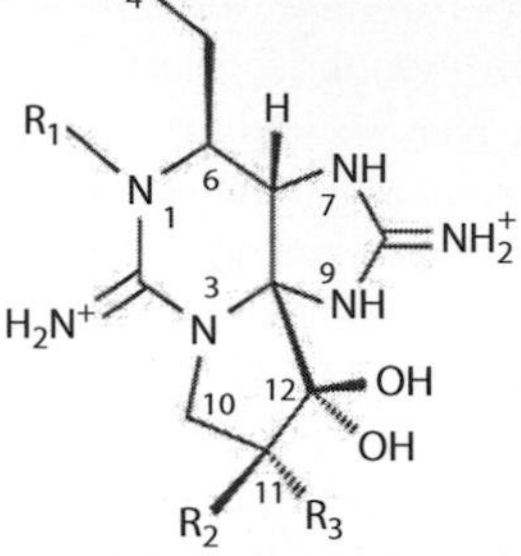

Toxin	R_1	R_2	R_3	R_4
STX	H	H	H	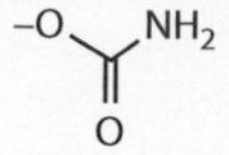
GTX2	H	H	OSO_3^-	
GTX3	H	OSO_3^-	H	
NEO	OH	H	H	
GTX1	OH	H	OSO_3^-	
GTX4	OH	OSO_3^-	H	
M2	H	OH	H	
M4	H	OH	OH	
GTX5	H	H	H	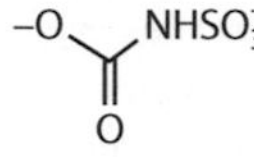
C1	H	H	OSO_3^-	
C2	H	OSO_3^-	H	
C3	OH	H	OSO_3^-	
C4	OH	OSO_3^-	H	
GTX6	OH	H	H	
M1	H	OH	H	
M3	H	OH	OH	
dcSTX	H	H	H	
dcGTX2	H	H	OSO_3^-	
dcGTX3	H	OSO_3^-	H	
dcNEO	OH	H	H	
dcGTX1	OH	H	OSO_3^-	
dcGTX4	OH	OSO_3^-	H	

FIGURE 13.1 Chemical structures of hydrophilic paralytic shellfish toxin analogues.

the toxicity of the most potent analog, the parent STX. To date, a number of studies have been published that quote relative toxicities for PSTs based on MBA toxicity studies (Table 13.1). On the whole, those reported by Oshima [27] have been used in instrumental method validation and comparative studies, although some authors have included the assessment of toxicity data using alternative values supplied by Genenah and Shimizu [28] and Schantz [29]. More recently still, the European Food Standards Agency (EFSA) supplied an opinion on STXs, which included the publication of revised TEFs for the most commonly occurring STX analogues [30]. The accuracy of these TEFs is clearly of concern to those wishing to assure the accuracy of quantitative instrumental analysis [31], given the large differences in total toxicity that can occur when applying different TEFs for toxicity calculation [32], as demonstrated in Table 13.1. The EFSA TEFs, which have recently been recommended for use by the European Union Reference Laboratory for Marine Biotoxins (EURLMB; [33]), are mostly similar to those of Oshima, albeit reported to a more appropriate level of precision. The notable difference is the twofold increase in TEF for decarbamoyl saxitoxin (dcSTX) and the absence of data for C1 and C3 toxins, with the former potentially effecting the accuracy of toxicity determination in shellfish either feeding on decarbamoyl toxin-rich algae or in species known to exhibit enzymatic transformation of carbamate and N-sulfocarbamoyl toxins to their decarbamoyl counterparts [34].

Detection of PSTs following HPLC separation is undertaken using fluorescence detection (FLD). As the STX analogues do not contain a chromophore (Figure 13.1), the toxins have to be oxidized before detection. HPLC–FLD methods, which began to be developed as far back as the 1970s [35], subsequently employ an oxidative derivatization step to form fluorescent products suitable for FLD. This derivatization can take place either pre- or post-column, with very different instrumental, sample processing, and chromatographic requirements resulting between the two approaches. However, both approaches require the availability and use of certified reference materials as instrumental standards for both qualitative and quantitative determination of PSTs in samples, with just 13 PSTs currently available commercially from

TABLE 13.1

Summary of the Most Commonly Used TEFs of PSTs

Toxin	Oshima [27]	Genenah and Shimizu [28]	Schantz [29]	EFSA [30]
STX	1.0000	1.0000	1.0000	1.0
NEO	0.9238	0.5076	0.9376	1.0
GTX1	0.9940	0.8010		1.0
GTX2	0.3592	0.3878		0.4
GTX3	0.6380	1.0924		0.6
GTX4	0.7260	0.3291		0.7
GTX5 (B1)	0.0644	0.1731		0.1
GTX6 (B2)	—	—		0.1
C1	0.0060	—	0.0168	—
C2	0.0963	—	0.1712	0.1
C3	0.0133	—	—	—
C4	0.0576	—		0.1
dcSTX	0.5131	—	0.5081	1.0
dcNEO	—	—		0.4
dcGTX2	0.1538	—		0.2
dcGTX3	0.3766	—		0.4
11-Hydroxy-STX	—	—	0.5657	0.3

the National Research Council of Canada (NRCC). Ongoing developments are therefore still required for refining methods to assess the presence of those toxins currently unavailable as pure standards.

13.2.1 Pre-Column LC–FLD

13.2.1.1 Method Overview

HPLC with pre-column oxidation (Pre-COX) involves the derivatization of shellfish extracts with chemical oxidants prior to chromatographic analysis. Acetic acid is used as the duplicate extraction solvent (first extraction in boiling water) given the chemical conversion of N-sulfocarbamoyl toxins to carbamoyl counterparts in the presence of HCl when using AOAC 959.08. Lawrence et al. and Lawrence and Menard first proposed an approach in 1991 for the alkaline conversion of PSTs to purines using both hydrogen peroxide and periodate reagents [36,37]. These highly fluorescent polar oxidation products, subsequently well characterized [38], were shown to be amenable to reverse-phase HPLC using aqueous mobile phases with ammonium formate buffer utilizing gradient elution with low proportions of organic solvent. Of particular note was the formation of single oxidation products following oxidation of GTX2 and GTX3, STX, GTX5, and C1 and C2, but with multiple oxidation products formed for other toxins. With oxidative ring cleavage and subsequent aromatization occurring during the derivatization, epimeric toxins (GTX2 and GTX3, GTX1 and GTX4, C1 and C2, C3 and C4, dcGTX2 and dcGTX3) yielded identical oxidation products. Peroxide oxidation was found to result in more sensitive analysis, but is not suitable for the N1-hydroxylated toxins GTX1 and GTX4, NEO, dcNEO, and C3 and C4. Furthermore, secondary oxidation products from the N1-hydroxylated toxins were found to be either identical to or similar in chromatographic retention to the primary oxidation products formed following peroxide oxidation of the non-N1-hydroxylated PSTs. Lawrence et al. [39–41] published a number of refinements to the method to improve the chromatography and sensitivity, as well as the inclusion of a solid-phase extraction (SPE) cleanup step for crude shellfish extracts using C18-bonded cartridges, required to remove high levels of chromatographic interferences from naturally fluorescent matrix co-extractives. A second SPE cleanup using weak ion exchange was also incorporated to separate C18-cleaned extracts into discrete fractions (fractionation). This was done given the requirement to separate NEO from GTX6 and C3 and C4 from GTX1 and GTX4 prior to oxidation, as each forms oxidation products that cannot be separated. The complexity of the method is well described [42] as well as other issues such as pH, which, if not appropriately controlled, may affect method performance [43]. In addition, the method stipulates the analysis of unoxidized sample extracts to account for the presence of naturally fluorescent matrix components plus the use of an oyster-extract matrix modifier during the periodate oxidation of standards and samples. However, the method is very useful as a rapid screening tool in high-throughput monitoring environments [6,40] and, if properly validated and standardized protocol carefully applied, can be fit for the purpose for the quantitative analysis of contaminated shellfish samples [6].

13.2.1.2 Pre-COX Method Validation

Lawrence et al. subjected various versions of the Pre-COX HPLC method to within-laboratory validation schemes [37,41], in particular examining LODs, toxin recovery from spiked extracts, repeatability, and the comparability of final toxicity results with those of the MBA and a post-column oxidation (PCOX) HPLC method. This was conducted using HCl extracts obtained from a range of mussels, oysters, and clams [41] as well as scallops [37]. With acceptable levels of recovery, sensitivity, and repeatability, validation was extended to a full interlaboratory study involving the analysis of 21 samples in 18 laboratories worldwide [44,45]. Test samples comprised primarily with mussels with Pacific oysters, clams, and scallops also included (exact species not detailed), with a range of both naturally contaminated and spiked shellfish homogenates. Duplicate acetic acid extraction was employed, and with the sample set containing blanks and blind duplicates, validation data were generated following analysis of both C18 and ion-exchange cleaned extracts. Important method performance characteristics were reported, most notably species-dependent toxin recovery, repeatability, and interlaboratory reproducibility. With acceptable performance data generated for a range of toxins including STX, NEO, GTX1–5, dcSTX, and C1–4, and a good correlation evidenced with the reference MBA, the method became an official AOAC method (2005.06) [46] and was accepted as an alternative method for PSP detection in shellfish for official control purposes in the EU [26].

13.2.1.3 Refinements and Method Extensions

While only a few laboratories adopted the method for shellfish monitoring [4], it was clear that with the commercial availability of new certified toxin standards and with some method performance issues affecting the practicalities of method implementation, further refinement and validation of the method would be required. In the United Kingdom, refinements were conducted to standardize the extraction procedure, improve the stability of oxidation products through temperature control of the HPLC autosampler, refine the ion-exchange cleanup step, and semiautomate both SPE procedures [32]. The result was the production of a refined version of the Pre-COX method, which was shown to be more repeatable, rugged, less labor-intensive, and more applicable to a high-throughput, fast-turnaround monitoring environment [32]. The method was also extended to include the additional toxins dcGTX2 and dcGTX3 and dcNEO and subsequently formally validated within the laboratory. Full method performance characteristics of the refined and extended method were generated following IUPAC (International Union of Pure and Applied Chemistry) guidance [14] for the major species of interest to the UK shellfish industry: common mussels [32], plus common cockles, Pacific and native oysters, razor clams, and hard clams [47]. Given the absence of certified matrix reference materials for PSTs, validation was conducted using naturally contaminated and spiked tissues. The single-laboratory validation data generated showed generally acceptable performance criteria for the majority of toxins in most species including recovery, selectivity, sensitivity, repeatability, and within-laboratory reproducibility. Evidence from low levels of naturally fluorescent matrix components confirmed the need to run unoxidized samples to improve the accuracy of the toxin quantitation. Comparability with the MBA was also demonstrated for most species of interest. Furthermore, ruggedness of the method was confirmed, and validation data are used to generate values for measurement uncertainty (MU) for each toxin in each validated species. Subsequent implementation of the method into the official control monitoring program for the United Kingdom in 2008 incorporated MU calculations into the compliance decisions taken on final toxicity results.

Validation conducted on two species of scallops confirmed acceptable method performance for the analysis of non-N1-hydroxylated PSTs following peroxide oxidation. However, strong evidence was generated for poor performance following periodate oxidation [48], specifically low toxin recovery and poor LODs for GTX1 and GTX4, NEO, and dcNEO. These effects were consistent in a range of scallop tissues with different temporal and spatial sources. A small interlaboratory study conducted using spiked scallop samples also confirmed these data [49]. Developments were conducted that demonstrated improved method recovery through the use of a scallop-based modifier for oxidation of instrumental calibrants in preference to the normal oyster matrix modifier. The method sensitivity was also improved through the use of an optimized periodate reagent and higher volumes for C18 cleanup and HPLC injection [49]. Single-laboratory validation subsequently demonstrated acceptable performance characteristics of the method including ruggedness of the new experimental parameters [49], and the refined scallops method was implemented into the UK monitoring programs in 2011.

More recently, other studies have been published that further describe the interlaboratory performance of the method. Performance characteristics including intra- and interlaboratory precision, recovery, and instrument limits of quantitation were generated from an EURLMB-led interlaboratory study and extended the validation to dcGTX2 and dcGTX3 in mussels and clams. Results confirmed the levels of reproducibility described in the original collaborative trial [45] but provided some evidence for poor reproducibility for some toxins including dcNEO [50]. Recoveries for dcGTX2 and dcGTX3 were generally low, and there were occurrences of high intralaboratory repeatability for some participants that indicated a potential lack of familiarity with the method. In addition, the study included an interlaboratory assessment of a proposed method based on [51] to quantify GTX6 for which no certified reference standards were available. This involved the acid hydrolysis of GTX6 collected following ion-exchange cleanup to form NEO, before quantifying against NEO calibrants. While the hydrolysis protocol was successful and results at one laboratory compared well with those calculated from calibrations prepared from noncertified GTX6 standards (unpublished data), high interlaboratory relative standard deviations (RSDs) indicated issues with the method at some laboratories.

13.2.1.4 Method Efficiencies and Practicalities

The method is particularly suitable as a high-throughput screening method for official control monitoring. Only samples showing the potential presence of PSTs following LC–FLD analysis of periodate-oxidized sample extracts need to be subsequently submitted to full quantitation. To date, this approach is utilized routinely by laboratories in the United Kingdom, Ireland, Portugal, and New Zealand. Given the complex and labor-intensive nature of some steps within the quantitative method, there has been some focus on automation and efficiency improvement. The automated SPE processes mentioned earlier are easily achieved using standard liquid cleanup instrumentation, yet enable high-throughput screening of more than 40 samples per day and ion-exchange fractionation of the same number of samples with relative ease and minimal manual effort [52]. Other researchers have investigated the potential for automated periodate oxidation using standard analytical [53] and temperature-controlled preparative HPLC autosamplers [54]. In the latter study, oxidations were performed at low temperatures resulting in low reaction yields and lower numbers of oxidation products. The automation of both periodate and peroxide oxidation has also been reported as applied to standards, algae, and shellfish [4] with oxidation products similar to those reported in the original method [36,37]. Thus, the potential for automated oxidation in routine official control has been demonstrated. Other potential developments including modifications to extraction protocols and the pH adjustment automation have been discussed, although they remain unpublished. In high-throughput monitoring environments, given high sample numbers, fast results turnaround, and the potential requirement to run multiple HPLC analyses for each quantitative sample, improvements to the speed and of individual chromatographic analyses are another important development. The advent of ultraperformance liquid chromatography (UPLC) may provide one solution to significantly improve the number of analyses that can be conducted per day. Harwood et al. [55] recently reported the refinement of the method using UPLC, with mobile phase incorporating methanol rather than acetonitrile. However, UPLC hardware is considerably more expensive than traditional HPLCs and may preclude many monitoring laboratories from taking this approach. One alternative is the use of newer chromatographic columns packed with solid core or superficially porous particles. With lower particle sizes, shorter column lengths, and lower back pressures, similar chromatographic selectivity and separation efficiency may be realized with substantially reduced run times. Published work has already demonstrated the potential for reducing the run times for Pre-COX HPLC analysis by up to three times with the use of such columns [56,57] and represents a potentially more cost-effective way forward for those laboratories with high sample throughput demands. In addition, such an approach provides similar or improved peak resolution, with significant increases to method sensitivity and linearity, plus an acceptable correlation with results generated using a traditional HPLC method [57]. Nevertheless, potential issues with column lifetime still need to be addressed. Overall, while AOAC 2005.06 is complex and requires a high level of training and quality control, routine use in a number of official control laboratories has demonstrated fitness for purpose of the method. Further work is required however to assess the performance and applicability of the method in relation to other PSTs currently unavailable commercially as reference standards.

13.2.2 Post-Column LC–FLD

13.2.2.1 Method Overview and Development

HPLC with post-column oxidation (PCOX) involves the chromatographic analysis of non-derivatized toxins, with the separated toxins oxidized online through a continuous flow reaction system. PSTs that elute from the end of the HPLC column are mixed with an oxidant such as periodate before passing through a reaction coil where the derivatization takes place. On eluting from the end of the reaction coil, the reaction mixture is quenched with a strong acid generating the formation of stable oxidation products of each PST that subsequently passes through the FLD. A number of early PCOX methods have been well described in previous reviews [58], but the breakthrough came in 1987 with researchers describing a three-stage approach to analyzing the full range of PST analogues [24,31]. Three different isocratic mobile phases and three separate analyses were required for the analysis of all the PSTs investigated, specifically for (1) C toxin group, (2) GTX toxins, and (3) NEO, STX, and dcSTX toxins. Tetrabutylammonium phosphate was used for C toxin separation, with ion-pair separation (using heptanesulfonic acid) being used for the separation of the other groups, with all separations being conducted on a silica-based reverse-phase (C8) HPLC column. Further refinements were made, including the use of C18 columns with a variety of different modified mobile phases, including the use of step-gradient chromatography to separate GTX and STX/NEO/dcSTX toxins in one analytical run [59–61]. These methods were applied to the analysis of standards, cultures, and contaminated shellfish, although some issues with GTX toxin resolution were noted. In 1995, Oshima described further modifications to his original method using a longer C8 reverse-phase HPLC column, modified reaction coil dimensions, and three separate analytical runs per sample, with major modifications also including optimized pH and mobile phase concentrations, changed oxidant composition, and the use of a C18-SPE cleanup to prevent the occurrence of false-positive analyses [27]. While the majority of toxins could be adequately separated, Oshima reported that dcNEO could not be separated from NEO. While other workers subsequently conducted further investigations into the use of sample cleanup prior to PCOX HPLC [62,63], this approach has subsided in more recent years. The Oshima method has been used extensively in research worldwide and a version implemented into routine official control monitoring in Norway for some time [64]. Yu et al. reported in 1998 a modified version of the method reported in [59] resulting in improved chromatographic resolution for GTX toxins and an application to the analysis of algae and shellfish samples [65]. Other workers published investigations into the use and optimization of different PCOX technologies, specifically the use of electrochemical and manganese dioxide solid-phase reactors. Lawrence and Wong assessed both reactor types concluding there was good agreement with results generated using chemical oxidation and potential for application to regulatory testing [66,67]. Boyer and Goddard extended the work on electrochemical oxidation reporting detailed procedures for daily use and maintenance, plus the application to algae and shellfish samples [68]. Jaime et al. reported a different approach utilizing high-performance ion-exchange chromatography with electrochemical oxidation [69] prior to FLD and MS. In comparison with the two or three analyses required for other PCOX methods, this approach enabled separation of toxins with one analysis performed on two ion-exchange columns arranged in series and using an ammonium acetate mobile phase at pH 6.9. The toxin elution order was as expected, with C toxins eluting first, followed by GTXs then STX/dcSTX/NEO [69]. Another variant of the method includes the determination of PSTs in dietary supplements [70].

However, since this time, the use of the original ion-pair/phosphate buffer reverse-phase HPLC with chemical oxidation method has continued in popularity and use throughout the world, most notably through the development and validation undertaken on the method in Canada. Thomas et al. [71] described a further refined version of the Oshima and Thielert methods as applied to HCl extracts obtained according to the MBA method [1]. The number of injections was reduced to two, using a 60 min analysis time to facilitate separation of GTX and STX/NEO/dcSTX toxins. Rourke et al. [72] subsequently refined the chromatography to a binary step gradient, enabling separation in less than 25 min, although resolution issues with GTX5 remained unsolved. In addition to modified reagents, a different cleanup procedure was employed in preference to C18-SPE utilizing trichloroacetic acid for shellfish extract deproteination prior to filtration [72].

13.2.2.2 PCOX Method Validation

The original Oshima method was subjected to a degree of validation, with the determination of analytical selectivity and toxin LODs. Recoveries were determined for toxins spiked into nontoxic extracts, although no full method recovery was determined using spiked tissues [27]. The modified method from Yu et al. reported values for analytical limits of detection, although no further method performance characteristics were given. PCOX with electrochemical oxidation was shown to result in good instrumental limits of detection and instrumental linearity, although sensitivity was relatively poor for the N1-hydroxylated PSTs [68]. Method performance characteristics reported for the high-performance ion exchange with electrochemical oxidation method included evidence for good linearity and sensitivity [69]. The refined rapid version of the Oshima method developed in Canada was initially subjected to a series of method performance tests by Rourke et al. [72] based on the analysis of HCl extracts of shellfish. Results indicated excellent linearity for all toxins investigated over a wide linear range, with detection limits and toxin recoveries shown to be acceptable. The method was also compared with results generated by the Pre-COX HPLC method, and PCOX retention time variability was shown to be low in terms of both retention time and peak area response [72]. This work was followed up by a full single-laboratory validation for the PCOX HPLC method, focusing on the method performance characteristics in blue mussels, soft-shell clams, American oysters, and sea scallops [73]. Linearity, recovery, repeatability, instrumental LOD and limit of quantification (LOQ), intermediate precision, and ruggedness were all assessed and reported as acceptable in each of the four species investigated. In the absence of certified matrix reference materials and rather than using expensive spiked standards, the recovery and precision work was conducted using blank tissues fortified with extracts of naturally contaminated shellfish [73]. Given the success of the single-laboratory validation, the method was subjected to a full AOAC collaborative study eventually completed by 15 laboratories worldwide [74]. Method performance was determined for STX, GTX1–5, NEO, dcSTX, dcGTX2 and dcGTX3, and C1 and C2. Within-laboratory repeatability and between-laboratory reproducibility were shown to be generally excellent for the majority of toxins in each of the four species assessed. However, availability of materials containing suitable concentrations of C1 and C2 toxins resulted in poor levels of repeatability and reproducibility for those toxins, and the number of materials containing GTX5, dcSTX, and dcGTX2 and dcGTX3 was relatively limited [74]. Overall, the results demonstrated the suitability of the method for official control testing and was accepted by the AOAC in 2011 as an alternative method (Official Method 2011.02; [75]) for the testing of blue mussels, soft-shell clams, American oysters, and sea scallops for the PSTs included in the interlaboratory validation study. The PCOX method is approved as a limited use method in the US by the Interstate Shellfish Sanitation Conference (ISSC) and National Shellfish Sanitation Program (NSSP) [76].

13.2.2.3 Method Practicalities

The complications of the PCOX HPLC method reported with the original Oshima method were associated in the main with the need to run three separate analyses per sample, each using different mobile phases. This situation was improved through the modifications detailed previously, although two separate analyses are still to be run if C toxins are to be analyzed. There is potential for automating the analysis using quaternary HPLC pumps and column-switching valves, although in high-throughput, fast-turnaround environments, it may be more practical to run two HPLC systems in parallel. Rourke et al. [72] reported the inability to separate NEO from dcNEO, although an additional 75 min analysis could resolve this issue if required [70]. This would be important for laboratories that regularly see these toxins in naturally contaminated samples. There is also the requirement to establish the performance of the method for GTX6, for which chromatographic elution has been reported as occurring either prior to [72] or co-eluting with GTX4 [74]. During the Canadian validation exercises, working standards were prepared in shellfish extracts, so as to enable chromatography to be optimized, with specific recommendations made to adjust column temperatures in order to resolve toxins from fluorescent matrix co-extractives. There is the requirement to check chromatographic resolution on a regular basis, especially following implementation of a new analytical column [72]. Given successful chromatography, sample processing is relatively straightforward, assuming toxins are correctly identified and resolved from matrix peaks in each of the shellfish species under analysis.

13.2.3 Comparison of HPLC Methods

A number of authors have published work comparing the performance and practicalities of the Pre-COX and PCOX HPLC methods [72,77,52]. There are clear advantages and disadvantages with both methods, so comparisons are more appropriately taken in the context of the monitoring environment in which they are to be used. The PCOX method theoretically provides more accurate results in terms of determining profile and quantifying toxicity, given the overestimation of toxicity provided by the Pre-COX analysis resulting from its inability to separate epimeric pairs. It is also less labor-intensive in relation to both sample processing and data interpretation. However, the Pre-COX method requires simple and less-expensive instrument setup, and the chromatography is robust with excellent column lifetimes. In terms of expense, while the Pre-COX method requires the use of C18-SPE cartridges, the lifetime of PCOX HPLC columns is recognized as being limited. Both methods provide superior sensitivity in relation to the MBA, and both provide valuable profile assessment previously unavailable through use of MBA alone. The application of the fully quantitative Pre-COX method to a large number of positive samples is both complex and time-consuming, especially without any of the automation instrumentation described previously, but the method is simple and quick for the high-throughput screening of large numbers of samples. Ultimately, the choice between HPLC methods should be made in the context of the aim of the work, available instrumentation, and analyst availability and skill, ideally with some prior knowledge of the performance of both methods on the full range of samples and toxins to be encountered. Whichever method is chosen, the importance of fully testing the method(s) on local samples from a variety of temporal and spatial sources is important, given the potential for matrix-related selectivity and toxin recovery issues. Proper training is also required in both methods, and strict quality control and quality assurance procedures applied at all times, including active participation in proficiency tests. Methods should also be validated or at least performance is verified for each of the specific species of interest. For example, with the PCOX method validated in Pacific oysters and sea scallops, further method validation would be required prior to the implementation of the method in other oyster and scallop species. With the growing availability of certified matrix reference materials [78], testing and validation studies should become easier and less reliant on reference material standards for toxin spiking studies.

13.2.4 Comparison with the MBA

Analytical methods have been often compared against the MBA since it is the EU reference method for PSP analysis and used as the gold standard method in most other countries. Some studies have indicated overestimation by Pre-COX HPLC in mussels and scallops as compared to MBA [79], while others have reported higher values by MBA [80]. However, the majority of published comparisons have shown a good correlation between the HPLC and the MBA, with comparisons conducted in a range of species including a range of different mussel, oyster, clam, and scallop species [32,44,81,82]. Differences between the results provided by the HPLC and MBA are thought to relate to a number of factors including the effects of chromatographic interferences or underestimation of the MBA [27,39], differences between extraction methods, or the effects of different toxin profiles [82]. Analysis of PSP-contaminated mussels, cockles, clams, and oysters demonstrated good agreement between HPLC and MBA methods for all species, except for two species of oysters where the HPLC returned toxicity results two to three times higher than the MBA [83]. The apparent positive bias in the HPLC for oysters was further investigated through comparative analysis with other methods including PCOX HPLC, LC–MS/MS, and electrophysiological assay. Results indicated that the MBA was underestimating toxicity with results from all other methods being at least two to three times higher in comparison with a good agreement in methods for mussels and cockles (Figure 13.2) [83]. Investigations into the cause of the apparent MBA suppression showed

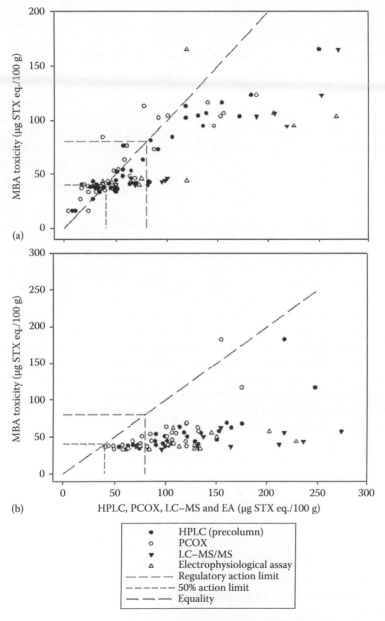

FIGURE 13.2 Total STX equivalents in (a) cockles and mussels and (b) Pacific and native oysters quantified by pre-column HPLC–FLD, post-column HPLC–FLD, HPLC–MS/MS, and electrophysiological assay as compared with the MBA PSP toxicity reference method.

no evidence for the effects of nutritional components, salinity, or the effects of extraction solvent but showed that the naturally occurring high concentrations of zinc were suppressing the MBA. Removal of metals from PSP-positive oyster extracts and spiking of zinc into PSP-positive mussels and cockles demonstrated this effect and subsequently warned against the use of MBA for the determination of PSP in oysters [84].

Similar comparisons have been conducted between the MBA and PCOX HPLC. Following serious PSP outbreaks in the United Kingdom in the late 1980s, samples of molluscs and crustacean were analyzed by both post-column HPLC and MBA. Results indicated HPLC results to be markedly higher than those returned by MBA, with authors proposing this may result from nontoxic fluorescent matrix compounds affecting the HPLC [85]. Oshima [27] reported a fairly good correlation between his PCOX HPLC method and results determined by MBA but again with HPLC results generally higher of the two. This discrepancy was explained by underestimation in the MBA due to low recovery of the assay [27]. Boyer and Goddard reported good correlations between their electrochemical PCOX method and the MBA at levels less than or equal to the regulatory action limit, with deviations above this limit attributed to incomplete oxidation of toxins in the reactor [67]. A study examining the results of the Oshima PCOX method in comparison with the MBA for a large number of Norwegian mussels was published in 2004 and described a highly significant correlation between the methods [64]. Van de Riet et al. [73] compared the PCOX and MBA performance in a range of samples obtained from Norway, New Zealand, and the United Kingdom, with the overall correlation appearing good. The Canadian PCOX interlaboratory study also enabled a comparison between the HPLC method and the MBA, with a good correlation reported [74].

13.2.5 Future Work

While both HPLC methods are being utilized nowadays for official control testing in high-throughput monitoring environments, there is scope for further development and efficiency gain in both methods. New columns providing greater column lifetime and improved separation efficiency would be advantageous for use with the PCOX method, while further automation would improve efficiency for routine high-throughput Pre-COX analysis. Faster chromatographic LC methods would be especially welcomed for both methodologies in relation to improving turnaround and increasing throughput. One clear requirement, relating to the availability of suitable certified standards, is the extension of both methods to encompass new toxins. While proposals have been made for the analysis of GTX6 by Pre-COX and GTX6 and dcNEO by PCOX, these need to be refined and validated. In addition, there is increasing evidence for the potential presence of other PSP analogues in the marine environment [86]. These include a number of benzoate-type analogues known to be produced by *Gymnodinium catenatum* [87,88] that have, in some cases, been found to comprise high proportions of total PSP concentrations [89]. These more hydrophobic PSTs are known to retain on C18-SPE sorbents, so they may be missed in subsequent analysis. While most of the benzoate PSTs have been reported as converting to their decarbamoyl counterparts during shellfish metabolism [90], there may still be the need for methodologies to be extended to include these toxins where appropriate. In addition, other metabolites have been identified, designated M1–M5, which exhibit poor fluorescence, and can only be adequately detected using analytical methods that employ MS detection [91,92]. Even with such developments in place, there is still the need for accurate toxicity information for these analogues, which for most toxins is still unknown.

13.3 Amnesic Shellfish Poisoning Toxins

Amnesic shellfish poisoning (ASP) is caused following consumption of shellfish that have accumulated high-enough concentrations of domoic acid, epidomoic acid (Figure 13.3), and other associated isomers [93]. The principal toxin is domoic acid itself, a secondary amino acid produced by a number of different marine organisms such as *Pseudo-nitzschia* spp. [94]. The toxin isomers are generally low in proportion to the parent compound and not always present in contaminated shellfish [95]. The chemistry of domoic acid and related isomers is described fully in Chapter 32. Given the wide global distribution of

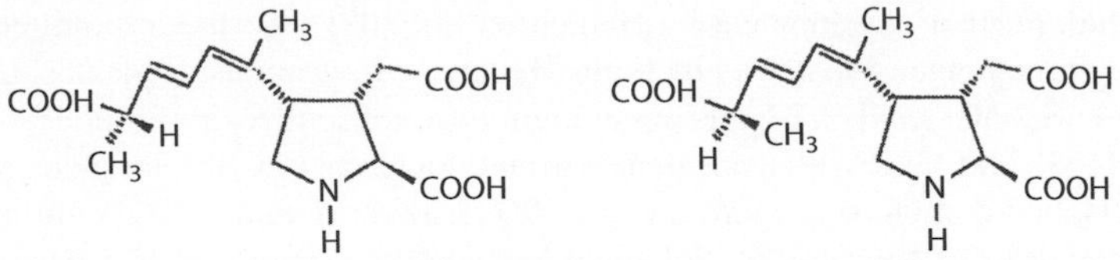

FIGURE 13.3 Chemical structures of the amnesic shellfish toxins domoic and epidomoic acid.

the causative organisms and their accumulation in a large number of shellfish species, there is a strong need for effective monitoring programs to be in place. Following on from a serious outbreak of ASP in Canada in 1987, method development and validation was necessary to establish suitable methodologies to enable future consumer protection [96]. Procedures for quantifying domoic acid using both an MBA similar to the PSP MBA and a rat bioassay [97] were available, although the sensitivity of the method, lack of accurate quantitation, and instability of domoic acid in acidic extracts [98] made it insufficient for use in regulatory monitoring [99]. Consequently, HPLC methods were developed that quickly became established as the reference method for ASP determination. Given the hydrophilic nature of domoic acid, extraction methods reported include a variety of water, acidic, and methanolic solvent mixtures. While the AOAC MBA extraction method has been used for ASP extraction [100–102], a methanol/water (1:1 v/v) mixture used for extraction of mussels during the 1987 outbreak [96] is most commonly used given the production of cleaner extracts and good toxin recoveries, although variants and other options exist [98,103,104].

13.3.1 HPLC–UV Methods

For many years, HPLC has been the preferred method for the analysis of shellfish extracts for ASP. Following separation by either isocratic or gradient elution on reverse-phase chromatography, quantitation is conducted using most commonly UV detection, given the strong absorption of domoic acid at 242 nm [105]. In 1989, Quilliam et al. published studies detailing the use of reverse-phase HPLC with UV diode-array detection (DAD), based on the analysis of boiled distilled-water extracts of shellfish tissues. Extracts were subjected to C18-SPE cleanup prior to analysis with aqueous acetonitrile and 0.1% (v/v) trifluoroacetic acid (TFA) mobile phase. The study reported excellent sensitivity and rapid analysis, suitable for establishing a high-throughput analysis method for official controls [98]. Development and validation of an HPLC–UV method conducted on AOAC acidic extracts by Lawrence et al. focused on a detailed examination of method parameters to determine the ruggedness of the methodology [100]. This included in particular an assessment of different stationary and mobile phases and the ruggedness of the extraction step in relation to boiling and cooling times. The optimized method was subjected to a collaborative study, involving 10 separate laboratories. Following a 5 min extraction in 0.1 M HCl, centrifugation, and filtration, isocratic HPLC was employed on a 150 × 4.6 mm C18 column, with mobile phase conditions (water/acetonitrile adjusted to pH 2.5) optimized in each laboratory to result in the elution of domoic acid around 8 min [101]. Results demonstrated acceptable recovery (mean 75%) from spiked shellfish samples, plus low levels of within-laboratory repeatability and acceptable between-laboratory reproducibility. With the method detection limit (1 µg domoic acid per gram shellfish flesh) significantly below the EU regulatory limit of 20 µg/g, the method was recommended and adopted by the AOAC as an official method (991.26; [102]). Following a need to develop a method for the detection of domoic acid in clinical samples, additional cleanup steps were incorporated using SPE, which enabled the sensitive analysis of urine without chromatographic interferences affecting toxin quantitation [106]. The same work also reported the use of two chemical derivatization protocols for the SPE-cleaned extracts to confirm domoic acid-positive samples, specifically with the use of phenyl isothiocyanate and isopropanol. Quilliam et al. [107] reported a rapid aqueous methanol extraction and cleanup procedure for shellfish samples using strong anion-exchange (SAX) cleanup prior to analysis resulting in high pre-concentration and good subsequent analytical sensitivity. Domoic acid stability issues in SAX eluants following elution with acids were improved with the use of a 0.5 M citrate buffer (pH 4.5). This method was shown to be applicable to a range of sample matrices including bivalves, anchovies, and partly digested food. Further development by Hatfield et al. [108] reported a modified cleanup protocol applicable to a large range of matrices including bivalves, gastropods, tunicates, and crustaceans. This utilized a 0.1 M NaCl in 10% MeCN wash step with subsequent toxin elution in 0.5 M NaCl with 10% MeCN [108]. HPLC–UV analysis demonstrated lower matrix interferences, good stability of cleaned up extracts, and domoic acid recovery of >90%. Lawrence et al. [109] continued their investigations with the analysis of a variety of biological and shellfish sample matrices using both UV and MS methods. Domoic acid recoveries from shellfish were >90% using methanol–water extraction, with similar recoveries (>84%) recorded in biological samples. Two SPE sample cleanup procedures were also compared, further highlighting the effectiveness of SAX for shellfish samples, in comparison with a more effective cleanup following strong cation-exchange (SCS) for biological matrices. LODs for the method were shown to be acceptable in all matrices and HPLC–UV results compared well with those generated using MS detection [107]. Quilliam et al. in 1995 published a full report describing the work conducted on the quantitation of domoic acid with an optimized extraction and cleanup procedure [110]. The work described investigations into a range of extraction methods, including the use of variable proportions of acetonitrile and methanol in water, with a 50% methanol exhaustive extraction providing the best results (domoic acid recovery >95%). Following a comprehensive evaluation of SAX cleanup methods, the optimum conditions were achieved through the use of a 1:9 (v/v) MeCN/water wash step followed by elution of toxins with a pH 3.2 citrate buffer. Subsequent analysis demonstrated cleaner chromatograms and improved sensitivities, with a wide range of linearity and excellent levels of precision and applicability to a range of sample matrices [110]. The method has subsequently been validated in other laboratories [111] providing further evidence for acceptable performance characteristics including selectivity, linearity, SPE column loading, toxin recovery, and comparison with an alternative LC–MS method. It has since formed the basis of standard methods, including those described by the European Committee for Standardization (CEN), where a single-step 50% methanol extraction is used with isocratic HPLC–UV with or without SAX cleanup [112]. The EURLMB-harmonized standard operating procedure (SOP) for the determination of domoic acid in shellfish and finfish by HPLC–UV is also based on this method [113], which includes performance characteristics based upon collaborative study in clams, mussels, scallops, and anchovies. Data showed acceptable levels of repeatability and reproducibility of analysis among the 12 participating laboratories. Hess et al. [114] reported interlaboratory performance characteristics from four laboratories all employing SAX cleanup and 0.1% TFA mobile phases with the majority of results falling within acceptable limits and showing equivalence with an LC–MS alternative method.

Overall, in comparison to other chromatographic biotoxin methods, the ASP method is relatively simple and applied in many laboratories worldwide for the determination of domoic acid in shellfish for official control monitoring purposes [115–118]. The availability of suitable certified reference materials [118] to enable both accurate quantitation and recovery assessment is of high importance to these laboratories. In addition, regular interlaboratory proficiency testing is essential, with testing schemes provided by the EURLMB for EU National Reference Laboratories and Quasimeme all aiding quality assurance of HPLC methods for each participating organization. Although the method is well implemented, there is still potential for refinements including the use of faster chromatographic methods to enable high throughput and potentially faster turnaround times.

13.3.2 Other ASP HPLC Methods

While HPLC–UV analysis of domoic acid is fit for purpose for the regulatory testing of shellfish, other authors have reported success with other HPLC methods involving FLD. This originated from the need to achieve lower LODs necessary to determine domoic acid in seawater and phytoplankton samples. Fluorometric methods require derivatization of domoic acid, which has the benefit of both increasing analytical sensitivity and removing potential interferences from matrix co-extractives [120].

Pocklington et al. [121] published a method involving derivatization with 9-fluorenylmethylchloroformate to form fluorescent products of domoic acid with an LOD in seawater and algal cultures of 15 pg/mL. Furthermore, they utilized an internal standard (dihydrokainic acid) for improved quantitation, given its nonexistence in marine samples and chromatographic separation from domoic acid [122].

The method was shown to have good linearity and good within-batch precision. However, the use of an additional extraction step (ethyl acetate) to remove excess interfering reagent was found to compromise between-operator repeatability [121]. Interlaboratory validation showed acceptable levels of reproducibility (9%) and recoveries >90% were demonstrated in spiked samples. A comparison between the UV detection and FLD methods showed a good correlation (correlation coefficient = 0.9986).

Other derivatization reagents have also been applied for the analysis of domoic acid in plankton and shellfish samples, including the use of 4-fluoro-7-nitro-2,1,3-benzoxadiazole (NBD-F) prior to reverse-phase HPLC–FLD [120]. Validation results showed acceptable method performance in terms of toxin recovery, accuracy, linearity, and reproducibility, with sensitivity appropriate for direct analysis of plankton samples and shellfish. This approach has also been used for the development and validation of a seawater analysis method conducted in tandem with a pre-concentration step using solgel amorphous titania (TiO$_2$) as a solid-phase sorbent [122]. Validation results reported showed high sensitivity (120 pg-DA/mL water) and acceptable domoic acid recovery (89%) and repeatability (6.2%).

A post-column derivatization method using the related 4-chloro-7-nitrobenzo-2-oxa-1,3-diazole (NBD-Cl) was utilized for the fully automated analysis of domoic acid by HPLC–FLD with good sensitivity (<1 µg/g) and selectivity in shellfish samples [123].

Sun and Wong [124] also reported use of 6-aminoquinolyl-N-hydroxysuccinimidyl carbamate (AQC) for the derivatization of domoic acid prior to HPLC–FLD. AQC–domoic acid products were found to be stable and produce sensitive and selective chromatography.

To date, none of the HPLC–FLD methods have been subjected to full interlaboratory validation studies, noting in particular the growing trend to incorporate domoic acid into MS detection methods for other marine biotoxins (Chapter 15).

13.4 DSP/Lipophilic Toxins

Lipophilic marine biotoxins, encompassing the DSP toxins, are a diverse range of naturally occurring constituents of marine phytoplankton and related shellfish metabolic products. The chemistry, action, and occurrences of these toxins are covered in detail in other chapters of this book.

DSP is caused by the lipid-soluble polyether okadaic acid (OA) and more than ten related analogues, including the dinophysis toxins (DTXs) that accumulate in the fatty tissues of shellfish (Figure 13.4). These toxins have been known to trigger poisonings since the 1970s. OA itself was originally identified by Yasumoto et al. [7] following periods of consumer intoxication, with evidence subsequently reported for the toxic effects of both DTX1 [125] and DTX2 [126]. While these toxins are produced by dinoflagellates, the other commonly occurring OA-group toxins, collectively termed DTX3, are a mixture of OA/DTX1 and DTX2 fatty acid esters formed during shellfish metabolism [127]. Proportions of DTX3 toxins can be high, in some instances accounting for 100% of the total OA-group toxins [128]. A range of other diol-ester derivatives of OA/DTX have also been reported, including those termed DTX4 and DTX5 [126,129,130]. Following shellfish consumption contaminated with OA esters, intoxication can occur following hydrolysis to the parent forms.

Two other groups of polyether DSP toxins have also been extensively described, although the health threats of these have not been proved [131]. The pectenotoxins (PTXs) are macrolactones comprising a group of more than 14 analogues, with PTX2 being the precursor compound present in dinoflagellate source species giving rise to other analogues through biotransformation reactions [132]. Commonly detected PTX-group toxins detected in European shellfish comprise the parent PTX together with the metabolites 7-*epi* PTX2 seco acid and PTX2 seco acid [133]. Yessotoxin (YTX) and related analogues are ladder-shaped polycyclic ethers, initially isolated in 1987 from a scallop species, *Patinopecten yessoensis* [134]. Structurally, these are similar to the brevetoxins (PbTxs) and ciguatoxins (CTXs) (Section 13.5). To date, more than 90 analogues have been identified, with the most important determined as being the parent YTX, together with 1a-homo-YTX, 45-OH-YTX, and 45-OH 1a-homo-YTX [135]. Occurrences of YTX-contaminated shellfish are widespread in both the Northern and Southern hemisphere.

Azaspiracid poisoning (AZP) is a shellfish intoxication syndrome discovered more recently in 1995 following intoxication in consumers of mussels from Ireland [136] when symptoms similar to

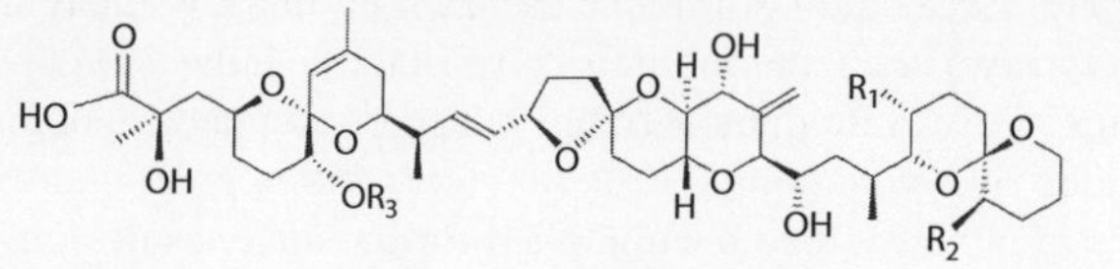

R₁	R₂	R₃	
CH₃	H	H	Okadaic acid (OA)
CH₃	CH₃	H	Dinophysistoxin-1 (DTX1)
H	CH₃	H	Dinophysistoxin-2 (DTX2)
H	CH₃	Acyl	Dinophysistoxin-3 (DTX3)

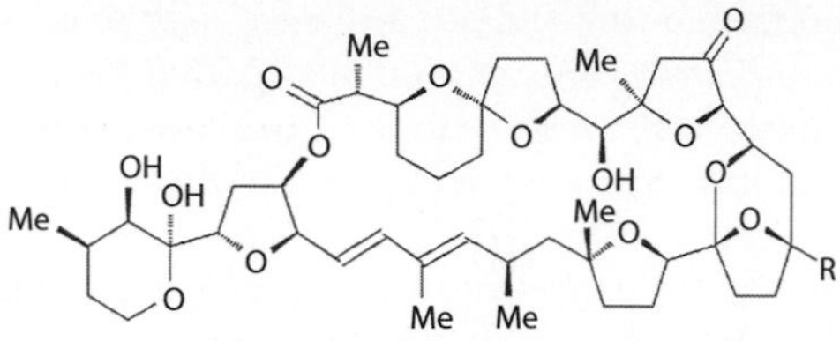

R	
CH₃	Pectenotoxin-2 (PTX2)
CH₂OH	Pectenotoxin-1 (PTX1)
CHO	Pectenotoxin-3 (PTX3)
COOH	Pectenotoxin-6 (PTX6)

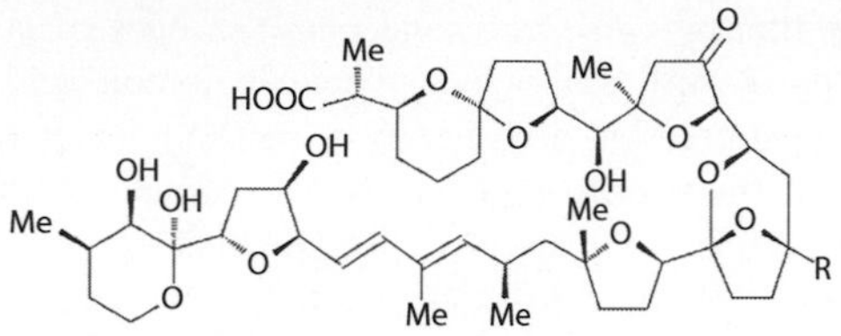

PTX2 seco acid (PTX-2-SA)

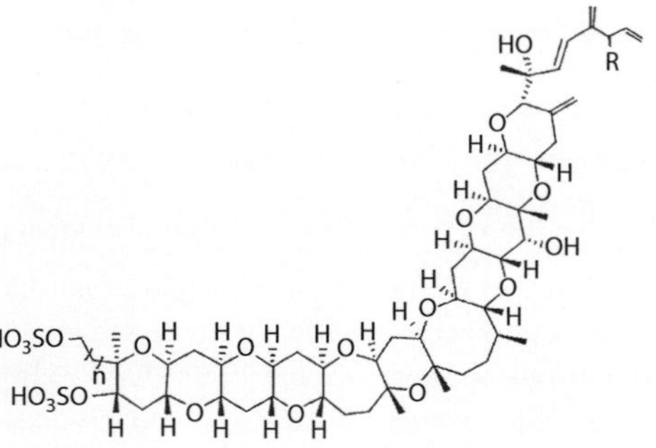

R	n	
H	1	Yessotoxin (YTX)
OH	1	45-Hydroxy-YTX (45-OH-YTX)
H	2	1a-homo-Yessotoxin (homo-YTX)
OH	2	45-Hydroxy-homo-YTX (45-OH-homo-YTX)

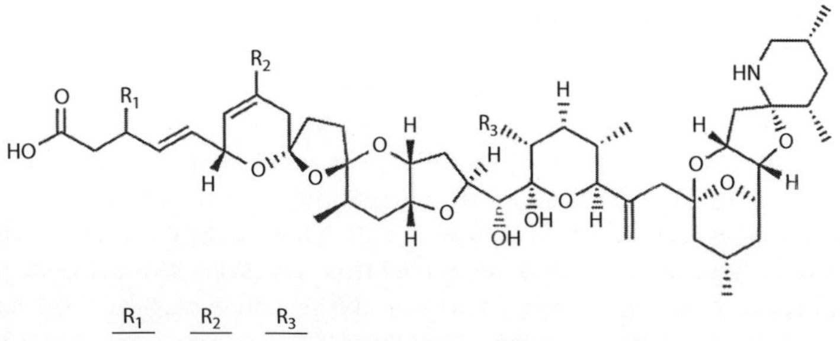

R₁	R₂	R₃	
H	H	CH₃	Azaspiracid-1 (AZA1)
H	CH₃	CH₃	Azaspiracid-2 (AZA2)
H	H	H	Azaspiracid-3 (AZA3)

FIGURE 13.4 Chemical structures of the lipophilic toxins including OA and DTXs, PTXs, YTXs, and AZAs.

those produced by OA-group toxins were reported. Azaspiracid (AZA) toxins are nitrogen-containing polyethers, with AZA1, AZA2, and AZA3 being the most commonly encountered in shellfish tissues [137]. While >20 analogues have been identified in shellfish to date, these three analogues are considered of highest importance by EFSA [138], and since monitoring methods have been implemented, these and related analogues have been detected globally.

In the EU, a number of qualitative MBAs and a rat bioassay were listed until 2011 as the EU reference methods for the determination of lipophilic toxins in shellfish flesh. The range of toxins detected by biological assay depended on the method used and the tissue on which the method was implemented (whole body or hepatopancreas) [139]. However, the most commonly used MBA method based on Yasumoto et al. [7] provides no information regarding the identity of toxins, is subject to false positives from other toxins and shellfish matrix components [10,8,140], and has clear ethical implications. European regulation EC 2075/2005 states that other methods such as LC–MS/MS and in vitro and biochemical methods can also be used given that they provide an equivalent level of public health and can detect all the regulated toxins and the method performance can be defined following validation performed to internationally agreed protocols [139]. Recent changes to European legislation in 2010, specifically a draft amended of regulation 2074/2005, resulted in the adoption of new methods utilizing LC–MS/MS as the reference method for lipophilic toxin detection. This method and related approaches to coordinated validation are described in detail in Chapter 15. However, with the option for shellfish to be tested with other methods, given the caveats described by EC 2075/2005, other methods are available, enabling the detection of regulated lipophilic toxins. While none of these methods are currently able to analyze all regulated toxins, there is the potential for non-MS methods to be utilized, an approach which may be of particular interest to those laboratories for whom modern LC–MS/MS instrumentation is unaffordable yet are faced with removal of the current MBA reference method by the end of 2014. Methods are subsequently described here concerning those alternatives using HPLC separation and optical detection methods.

13.4.1 HPLC Methods for OA-Group Toxins

Many different HPLC methods exist that are capable of the analysis of OA-group toxins in shellfish and plankton. As with other biotoxin HPLC methods, these confirm the presence and quantify the concentrations of individual toxins, or groups of toxins, against the concentrations present in certified reference standard calibrants. Due to the lack of chromophores in the toxins, all the published methods employ pre-column derivatization, with LC separation and FLD of toxin derivatives. The range of fluorescent derivatization reagents is wide, many of which have been described extensively (e.g., [11]).

13.4.1.1 9-Anthryldiazomethane

In 1987, Lee et al. described the first method for HPLC–FLD of OA-group toxins [141]. Digestive glands of contaminated shellfish were subjected to a single-step 80% MeOH extraction prior to an ether wash and chloroform extraction step. After dilution to volume chloroform, extracts were dried and esterified (~1 h) to form fluorescent 9-anthrylmethyl ester products using the 9-anthryldiazomethane (ADAM) reagent prior to further cleanup by silica or carbon-based SPE and reverse-phase HPLC–FLD. The authors reported a linear analytical range of between 1 and 80 ng on-column, with ester recoveries at ≥95% and low associated within-batch variability (2%–3%). However, while the method was shown to be very sensitive and applicable for monitoring shellfish contaminated with OA and DTX1, there was evidence for instability of the reagent, with Marr et al. [142] reporting ADAM to provide the greatest selectivity and sensitivity of all derivatization reagents but noting practical limitations relating to instability and cost. Other limitations are related to the inability of the method to detect OA/DTX esters and diol-esters, although these can be determined following hydrolysis to parent toxins, and the method has been used for the analysis of esters in Portuguese [143] and Spanish [144] bivalves. Consequently, a large amount of work has been conducted to improve overall method performance, with numerous different extractions, reaction conditions, and SPE methods proposed [142,145–151]. In terms of method performance, reproducibility was improved [144], and the work of Quilliam [148] reported increased method sensitivity with modified extraction, cleanup, and FLD conditions (10 pg ADAM-OA on-column) plus a higher level of ruggedness through modifications to the ADAM concentrations used. The accuracy and precision of the method were also improved through the use of internal standards, in particular 7-O-acetylokadaic (AcOA; 149), with the analysis of an NRCC-certified reference material and subsequent comparison with LC–MS analysis results proving an invaluable validation tool [148]. Consequently, the HPLC–FLD method using ADAM was subjected to single-laboratory validation by Van de Riet et al. [152]. LODs were low (0.03 μg/g digestive glands), linearity and recoveries acceptable (99% and 114% for OA and DTX1, respectively), and replicate analyses showed acceptable repeatability (<10%, with absolute values dependent on toxin concentrations) [152]. In addition, protocols were developed to check the reactivity of ADAM reagent prior to use. While selectivity was generally acceptable, the authors noted the need for confirmation by LC–MS, given the complexity associated with HPLC–FLD chromatograms [152]. Quilliam et al. [153] reported an improved approach using the "in situ" generation of ADAM based on the work of Yoshida et al. [154] in order to overcome the problem of reagent degradation. After identifying the source of post-reaction artifact peaks, an improved reagent step using THF was described to eliminate this problem [153]. Additionally, approaches have been taken to automate using column-switching instrumentation resulting in more rapid analysis and retaining good analytical sensitivity and recovery of OA and DTX1 derivatives (>90%; [155]). This approach has been extended and validated in more recent years by Suzuki et al. [156]. The method incorporates the hydrolysis of methanolic extracts prior to ADAM derivatization and HPLC–FLD using an automated column-switching cleanup step. Validation demonstrated good recovery (90%–113%) and precision for OA-group toxins in scallops, mussels, and oysters and a good correlation between results obtained by LC–MS/MS [156].

In the past decade, interest in the method has continued with the use of this method. Ramstad et al. [157] described the use of ADAM for the duplicate analysis of OA-group toxins in mussels from Norway. Results showed good repeatability of the method for the 86 samples examined. ADAM HPLC has also been used for the determination of DTX2 in samples from the Adriatic Sea [158], for OA/DTXs in phytoplankton net hauls from NW Spain [159], and for OA/DTX and related esters in bivalves from various regions within Chile [160,161] and Argentina [162]. A modified version of the original method [163] was validated showing good calibration linearity, reproducibility, and excellent sensitivity (0.7 μg OA/g hepatopancreas tissue). Spiked recoveries ranged from ~100% to 110% [164]. Results in OA-contaminated mussels from Greece also showed good comparability with those reported using an Enzyme-linked immunosorbent assay (ELISA) technique [164]. The chromatography of the Quilliam "in situ" ADAM method has also been modified and compared with other derivatization procedures for the determination of OA-group toxins in harvested phytoplankton [165]. Good sensitivity was reported (~0.7 ng injected) and results compared well with the method using pre-made ADAM reagent. One version of the ADAM LC method was collaboratively validated (conducted by the German Federal Laboratory for fish and fish products) for the determination of OA and DTX1 in mussel. Three separate interlaboratory studies were conducted using contaminated materials involving nine participating laboratories, with results showing good toxin recoveries (97%–102%) and reproducibility (<12.5%) [166]. The method was progressed to achieve status as a CEN method (14524), although this has subsequently been withdrawn due to the low applicability of the method. More recently in 2010, the ADAM HPLC method was compared with the MBA and an LC–MS/MS method to quantify and/or determine the presence of OA-group toxins and related esters in Greek mussels [167]. The method showed good levels of linearity and repeatability of chromatographic performance, and method accuracy for OA was determined using a certified reference material (NRCC CRM-DSP-Mus-b) and reported as 97%, similar to those reported by other authors.

13.4.1.2 1-Bromoacetylpyrine

In 1993, an alternative derivatization method was reported involving the use of the more stable 1-bromoacetylpyrine (BAP) reagent following extraction and SPE cleanup prior to reverse-phase HPLC [168]. A modified derivatization was applied to the detection of OA/DTXs in shellfish extracts and found to provide greater method selectivity, with a lower presence of artifact peaks, although the sensitivity was four times lower than that achieved with ADAM [169]. Validation work to demonstrate a method recovery of 86% was conducted using repeat analysis (n = 25) of a CRM with an instrumental LOD of 0.4 ng on-column. A similar approach taken by other authors but allowing simultaneous separation of both BAP and ADAM derivatives demonstrated acceptable linearity following analysis of OA standards (0.52–2.6 μg OA/mL) and confirmed a BAP LOD of 0.4 ng on-column and the fourfold decrease in sensitivity in comparison with ADAM [152]. Further development of the method by Gonzalez et al. [170] reported improvements for OA using a modified extraction and cleanup protocol with ethyl acetate without the use of chloroform. Validation conducted by the same authors reported acceptable selectivity, linearity, precision, recovery (91%–105% in clams and mussels), and LOD (0.3 μg OA/g hepatopancreas) of the method. In terms of selectivity, the resolution of the derivatized OA peak from matrix co-extractives was sufficient in a range of shellfish, mussels, clams, and scallops with a variety of temporal and spatial sources. Mak et al. [171] reported modifications to the extraction with the addition of a proteolytic digestion step (through the addition of proteinase K) in order to improve the OA recovery of the method in mussel hepatopancreas. OA recovery was found to vary between ~50% and 73% depending on the spiked concentrations, and the authors reported OA concentrations on average more than 2.5 times higher using the modified procedure. More recently in 2009, the method was used for the detection of OA and OA esters in Greek mussels and compared with the MBA and a functional assay [172]. An isocratic reverse-phase column was used and applied to both hydrolyzed and unhydrolyzed extracts. Validation by the authors demonstrated excellent linearity for OA in both solvent and shellfish extracts, with an LOD of 5.86 μg/kg flesh. Accuracy was shown to be 94% and 103% for OA and DTX1, respectively, and there was generally an excellent agreement between the three methods.

13.4.1.3 Coumarin Derivatives

A number of coumarin derivatives have been investigated, including 4-bromomethyl-7-methoxycoumarin (BrMmC), 4-bromomethyl-7,8-benzcoumarin (BrBMC), 4-bromomethyl-7-acetoxycoumarin (BrMAC), and bromomethyl-6,7-dimethoxycoumarin (BrDMC). With the BrMmC derivatization being conducted on SPE-cleaned shellfish extracts, there was potentially less product degradation prior to analysis [173], although HPLC run times were longer and selectivity issues were noted. Ramstad et al. [157] also compared the results from the analysis of BrMmC derivatives with those obtained following ADAM HPLC. For the majority of the 13 positive samples analyzed, there was good agreement between duplicate analyses, evidencing good repeatability with the method. An investigation into the performance of each of the coumarin reagents by Marr et al. [142] showed different chromatographic behaviors between derivatives and a strong influence of mobile phase composition on derivative fluorescence. For BrMmC analysis, optimum HPLC conditions were obtained using gradient chromatography and were applicable to the analysis of algal cultures and DSP-positive mussel tissues. The performance of the alternative coumarin derivatives was variable with lower fluorescence yield for BrBMC, but with BrDMC showing greater reagent stability and improved analytical selectivity due to higher purity.

13.4.1.4 2-(Anthracene-2,3-Dicarboximdo)Ethyl-Trifluoromethanesulfonate

Fluorimetric determination of OA and DTX-1 has been conducted using room-temperature derivatization with 2-(anthracene-2,3-dicarboximdo)ethyl-trifluoromethanesulfonate (AE-Otf), prior to column cleanup and reverse-phase HPLC [174]. Recovery tests for OA and DTX1 derivatives showed variation between ~70% and 89% depending on the toxin and the cleanup washing solvents used. The selectivity of the method was considerably improved through the use of a column-switching valve to analyze fractions from which matrix-related interfering compounds had been removed. Good analytical linearity was reported between 2.5 and 500 pg on-column, as well as excellent levels of sensitivity (0.8 and 1.3 pg LOD), precision (1%–4%), and recovery (91%–116% in mussels and scallops). The same authors also reported the direct determination of DTX3 toxins in mussels and scallops, with recoveries of ~120% in scallop extract, good linearity, and an LOD of 0.6 pg on-column [175].

13.4.1.5 Luminarin-3

Luminarin-3 (LN-3) is a fluorescent hydrazine reagent that has been applied to the derivatization of OA, DTX1, and DTX2 toxins in shellfish samples [176]. Subsequent work investigating the analysis of phytoplankton extracts reported LN3 derivatives to be separated well by 250 mm reverse-phase chromatography with sensitivity equivalent to the analysis using ADAM (2.5–5.5 ng on-column) with good selectivity and linearity over a range of 20–140 ng/mL for OA [177]. One noted advantage of the method was the quality of the chromatography without any SPE cleanup applied prior to analysis, thereby simplifying the detection of OA-group toxins by HPLC–FLD.

13.4.1.6 1-Pyrenyldiazomethane

1-Pyrenyldiazomethane (PDAM) is a more stable reagent than ADAM and has been applied successfully to the analysis of cultured algal cells [178]. However, with high temperatures required during derivatization, losses of OA-group toxins are expected with recoveries for OA shown to be poor [142]. Garcia et al. [179] described a comparison between PDAM and ADAM derivatization and concluded that the methods compared well with the improved stability of PDAM resulting in a method that was fully applicable to the determination of OA and DTX1 in shellfish samples.

13.4.1.7 9-Chloromethylanthracene

Zonta et al. [180] reported the determination of OA in Italian mussels after derivatization with 9-chloromethylanthracene (CA) prior to C8 reverse-phase HPLC–FLD. While the sensitivity of the method was below the European regulatory limit, there were concerns that the lower sensitivity would affect the applicability of the method to routine monitoring in some countries. Lawrence et al. [181] reported a modified version of the method using optimized sample preparation, including a two-step SPE cleanup prior to C18 HPLC. This resulted in a method with equivalent sensitivity to ADAM but using more stable and less-expensive reagents. Other authors have reported analysis of OA-group toxins to be successful in shellfish samples with good chromatography resolution, selectivity, and sensitivity (5.28 ng LOQ on-column) but with no reaction reported in phytoplankton samples [165]. Rawn et al. [182] also described a rapid method of analysis based on CA derivatization and C8 HPLC–FLD. This was subsequently used to study the effect of UV radiation on derivatized standards and samples [182] and proposed as a confirmatory tool for DSP in mussel samples.

13.4.1.8 3-Bromomethyl-6,7-Dimethoxy-1-Methyl-2(1H)-Quinoxalinone

This reagent has been applied to the derivatization and LC–FLD of carboxylic acids but was modified for the application to DSP toxins. Nogueiras et al. [165] compared the performance of 3-bromomethyl-6,7-dimethoxy-1-methyl-2(1H)-quinoxalinone (BrDMEQ) with ADAM and CA reagents, reporting good analytical selectivity and sensitivity (1.0 ng on-column LOQ), similar to that obtained following ADAM derivatization. However, the authors noted that the separation was not effective for the separation of DTX-2B, an isomer formed from bioconversion of DTX2 in shellfish.

13.4.2 HPLC Methods for PTXs

As with OA-group toxins, PTXs lack a strong chromophore, so they are not generally amenable to UV detection or FLD without some form of pre-analysis derivatization. Given the applicability of MS detection to the analysis of PTXs, there are not a wide range of HPLC–FLD methods available. There is no published account of method validation for HPLC analysis of these toxins in shellfish, with PTX toxin recovery data reported following LC–MS/MS analysis only (Chapter 15). However, a number of fluorimetric approaches have been described including Lee et al. [183] who reported the use of 1-anthroyl nitrile (AN) for the derivatization of PTXs with a primary hydroxyl group (PTX1 and PTX4), forming fluorescent esters. The derivatization was conducted for 30 min at 60°C in the presence of MeCN and triethylamine, prior to isocratic reverse-phase C18 HPLC using a MeCN/H$_2$O mobile phase. The applicability of the method for determination of PTXs in Japanese scallops was also demonstrated.

Two of the reagents used for the pre-analysis derivatization of OA-group toxins have also been utilized for the derivatization of PTXs. Lee et al. [183] and Yasumoto et al. [184] also reported the use of

ADAM reagent for application to the derivatization of PTXs with a carboxyl group such as PTX6, PTX 7, and PTX2 *seco* acids (PTX2SAs) [129,182,184,185]. The 60 min room-temperature reaction produced fluorescent esters that following column cleanup were analyzed by C18 HPLC with a MeCN/MeOH/H$_2$O (8:1:1) mobile phase. As extracts may also contain OA-group toxins as well as a large number of other matrix-related interferences, the selectivity of the analysis may be compromised unless the extraction and cleanup procedures are very carefully controlled. Other reagents used for OA-group derivatization such as BAP have also been used for PTX toxins applicable to esterification [186]. For the PTX-2SAs, both the ADAM and BAP have been used as reagents prior to SPE cleanup [129,185]. Separation from OA-group toxins was achieved following isocratic reverse-phase HPLC with PTX ADAM derivatives eluting prior to both OA and DTX1 products. When applied to analysis of toxic phytoplankton from marine waters in tandem with MS studies, the method aided the elucidation of the PTX2 analogues, PTX-2SA and 7-*epi*-PTX-2SA. The same approach has also been used for the identification of 7-*epi*-PTX-2SA in DSP-positive mussels from the Adriatic Sea [158]. HPLC–FLD analysis of PTX2sa and OA/DTX ADAM derivatives was also conducted on clams from Portugal, with the authors noting the destruction of PTX2sa during the alkaline hydrolysis step [187]. PTX6 has also been determined using a slightly modified ADAM reaction in plankton and scallops, with higher relative proportions of PTX6 in scallops suggesting rapid transformation of PTX2 to PTX6 during shellfish metabolism [188]. The same authors also demonstrated quantitative recovery of PTX2 and PTX6 standards from seawater spikes, therefore providing some performance data for the method in water samples.

Other PTXs without any of the functional groups allowing the fluorescent labeling methods described such as PTX2 and PTX3 have been analyzed using an isocratic reverse-phase HPLC–UV method [184]. It has also been used for the quantitation of PTX2 in seawater and scallops [187]. Although the method gives low sensitivity of detection and is not normally selective enough for analysis of natural products, other approaches are preferable. However, preparative reverse-phase HPLC–UV has been a valuable tool for purification of PTX toxins from raw extracts (e.g., [189]).

Conjugated dienes present in PTXs have also been derivatized with the use of the dienophile reagent 4-[2-(6,7-dimethoxy-4-methyl-3-*oxo*-3,4-dihydroquinoxalinyl)ethyl]-1,2,4-triazoline-3,5-dione (DMEQ-TAD) [190]. This has been applied to the analysis of PTXs in algal samples [191] and confirmed the presence of PTX2 in net haul phytoplankton samples from the seas of Japan and Italy [192].

13.4.3 HPLC Methods for YTXs

The majority of YTXs contain conjugated dienes, weak chromophores that provide potential for low sensitivity UV detection. HPLC–UV of YTX and the analogue 45-OH-YTX was reported by Lee et al. [183]. Reverse-phase chromatography was used with a pH 5.7 methanol/sodium phosphate (9:1 v/v) buffer prior to detection at 230 nm. The method was used to confirm the presence of YTX in mussels from Norway and Japan [182].

As with the PTX analysis, detection sensitivity can be improved with dienophile derivatization prior to HPLC–FLD. Consequently, the DMEQ-TAD reagent applied to PTXs has been shown to be effective for the determination of YTX in shellfish [193]. A MeOH/H$_2$O (8:2 v/v) extraction was employed, prior to a C18-SPE cleanup and derivatization with 0.1% DMEQ-TAD in dichloromethane (DCM). A second C18-SPE cleanup was applied to the fluorescent adducts prior to HPLC–FLD analysis. Two derivatives were evidenced as expected from epimeric formation. HPLC conditions were C18 reverse-phase chromatography, with a 40 mM phosphate buffer in MeOH, which at 35°C facilitated the separation of YTX and 45-OH-YTX in less than 20 min, although homoyessotoxin (homo-YTX) products were not found to separate from YTX under these conditions [194]. With the use of modified mobile phase conditions, separation was also achieved between YTX and 45,36,37-trinor-YTX (norYTX). The method was found to be highly sensitive with authors reporting the ability to measure 1 ng of YTX on-column [192]. Good linearity was reported between 0 and 120 ng YTX, and the method selectivity is acceptable in relation to the analysis of YTX in scallops and mussels given the absence of naturally fluorescent matrix components. YTX recoveries averaged 94% for spiked experiments conducted on variable amounts of YTX (0.2–20 μg/g of scallops' digestive gland tissue). Subsequently, the method was applied to the determination of YTX in plankton [193] plus YTX and 45-OH-YTX in mussels from Chile and New Zealand, with additional confirmation provided by LC–MS/MS [192]. Further performance characteristics were determined by Ramstad et al. [195] who reported the repeatability of HPLC–FLD results for concentrations of YTX in the duplicate analysis of 28 mussel samples from Norway. The method was applied to a total of 75 mussel samples and recommended as a repeatable and reliable method for analysis of mussels for YTX. Satake et al. [196,197] reported the use of the HPLC–FLD method to aid the identification of YTX production and norYTX by cultures of *Protoceratium reticulatum*. Daiguji et al. [198] continued the use of the method for the determination of a new YTX analogue (1-desulfoyessotoxin; 1-dsYTX) in Norwegian mussel samples, with chromatograms showing good resolution between the fluorescent products of YTX and 1-dsYTX. The method has also been applied more recently in 2008 to samples of filtered seawater from the Californian coast of the United States [199]. Overall, given the relatively recent discovery of many of the YTX analogues and the introduction of YTX-certified reference standards to enable method performance characteristics to be generated, there is a relatively low amount of data available for the performance of HPLC methods for YTXs. Certainly to date, there have been no interlaboratory validation studies conducted for HPLC–FLD analysis of YTXs.

13.4.4 HPLC Methods for AZAs

AZAs also do not possess a chromophore suitable for analytical-scale HPLC–UV, so derivatization to fluorescent adducts is one possibility given the presence of amine and carboxyl groups in the AZA molecules. Until recently, given the low availability of standards and the incorporation of AZA detection into the LC–MS/MS methodology, there have been no developments in this direction. However, in 2011, McCarron et al. reported their investigations into the derivatization of AZAs prior to HPLC–FLD analysis [200]. The authors described the potential use of both carboxyl derivatization using the in situ ADAM method described previously by Quilliam et al. [153] and an amine derivatization using three different reagents. Certified reference standards for AZA1 were used for assessing the suitability of reactions. For amine derivatization, the reactions utilized were reductive amination with sodium cyanoborohydride, using dansyl chloride and 4-fluoro-7-nitrobenzo-2-oxa-1,3-diazole (NBD-F). Results indicated very low yields of AZA derivatives, possibly due to local steric hindrance of the amine group, so this route of investigation was not continued [199]. ADAM derivatization proved more successful, with LC–MS analysis confirming formation of the AZA1-ADAM derivative and evidence for $\geq 98\%$ conversion efficiency. Method ruggedness was demonstrated showing the minimal effects on reaction yields resulting from varying reaction condition parameters. SPE cleanup methods used for OA/DTX ADAM reactions were modified given the stronger apparent retention of AZA derivatives on silica columns. With the use of larger wash volumes to minimize matrix interferences and higher proportions of MeOH in the elution solvent (30%), >98% recovery was achieved [199]. A variety of HPLC columns and separation conditions were investigated and an optimized method employing an additional cleanup procedure was shown to be applicable to the analysis of shellfish extracts. Method performance validation highlighted excellent linearity for AZA1–3 between 2 and 160 ng/mL and good sensitivity with an LOQ ~40 µg/kg. Method accuracy determined following the analysis of certified matrix standards (NRCC CRM-AZA-Mus) returned values within the assigned uncertainties of the CRM. The authors did note, however, the potential for selectivity issues given the large variability in matrix interferences that can occur between samples and the time-consuming nature of the method. However, it was shown to be accurate, linear, sensitive, rugged, and applicable to the analysis of AZA toxins in shellfish. To date, no further validation including interlaboratory assessment has been conducted.

13.5 New and Emerging Toxins

The detection and quantitation of the marine biotoxins loosely termed "new and emerging toxins" is a major challenge to monitoring and research communities, given the diversity of toxin groups and a large number of analogues identified to date. Method development and validation is complicated further by the large number of different matrices involved plus the need for suitable TEFs and purified toxin standards. While the major analytical chemistry developments have focused on the use of MS detection, there are reports of conventional HPLC methods being used for some applications as summarized in the following text. However, none of these have been formally validated to date (Figure 13.5) [201].

13.5.1 Palytoxin-Group Toxins

Palytoxins (PLTXs) are one of the most potent marine toxins originally extracted from coral, although associated with seafood poisonings following consumption of a range of fish species [202–205] and crabs [206,207]. Production of the toxins has been associated with dinoflagellates of the genus *Ostreopsis*, and a large number of PLTX-group compounds exist with varying molecular weight depending on their

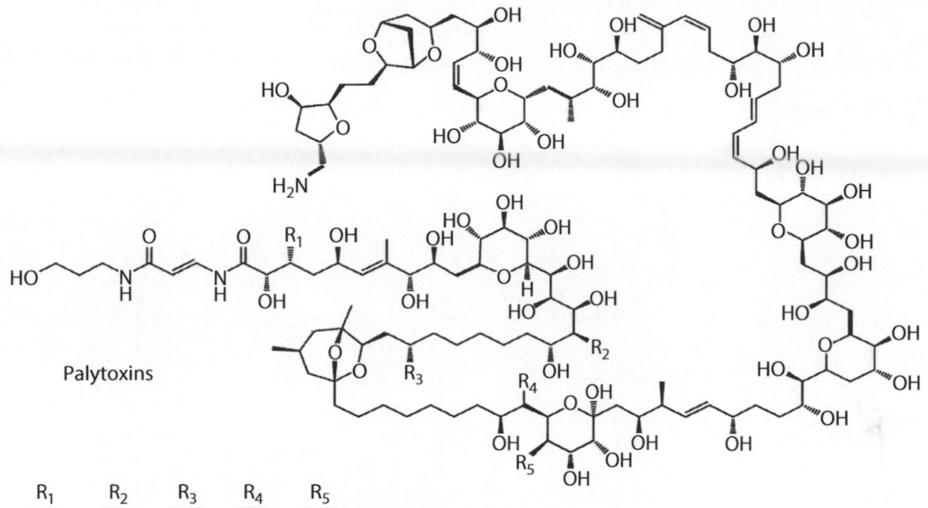

R_1	R_2	R_3	R_4	R_5	
CH$_3$	OH	CH$_3$	H	OH	Palytoxin (PLTX)
H	H	H	OH	H	Ostreocin-D
CH$_3$	OH	CH$_3$	H	OH	42-Hydroxy-palytoxin (42-OH-PLTX)

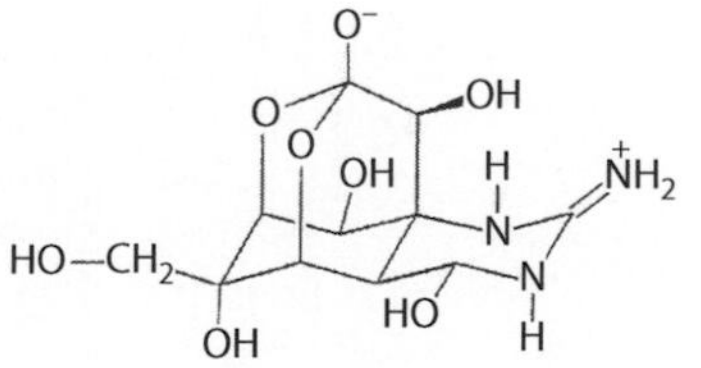

Tetrodotoxin

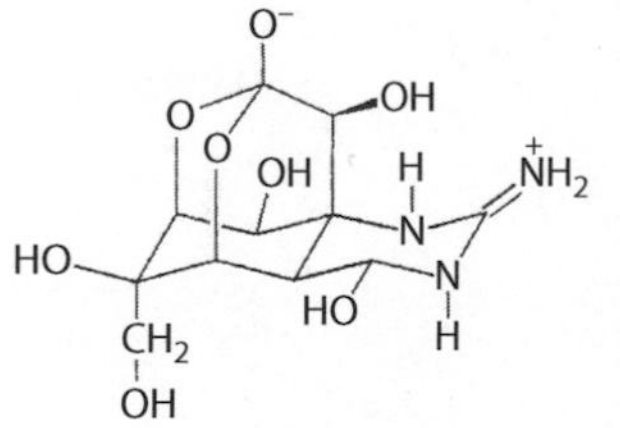

6-*epi*-Tetrodotoxin

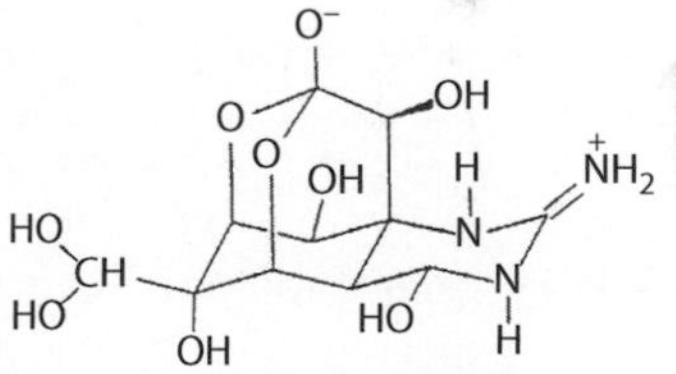

11-*oxo*-Tetrodotoxin

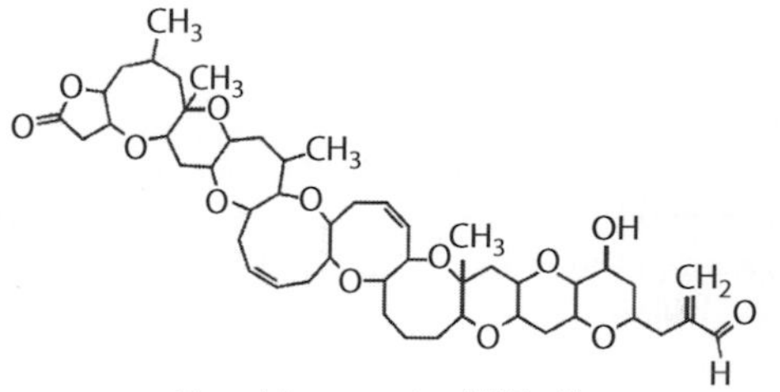

Type A brevetoxins (PbTx-1)

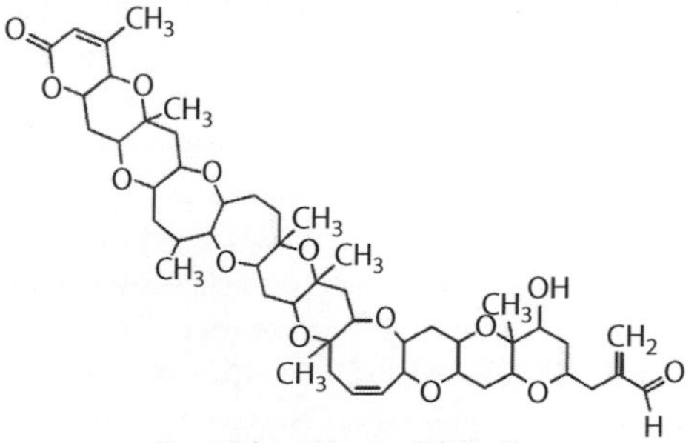

Type B brevetoxins (PbTx-2)

FIGURE 13.5 Chemical structures of the new and emerging toxins, including PLTXs, TTXs, PbTxs, CTXs, and MTXs.

(continued)

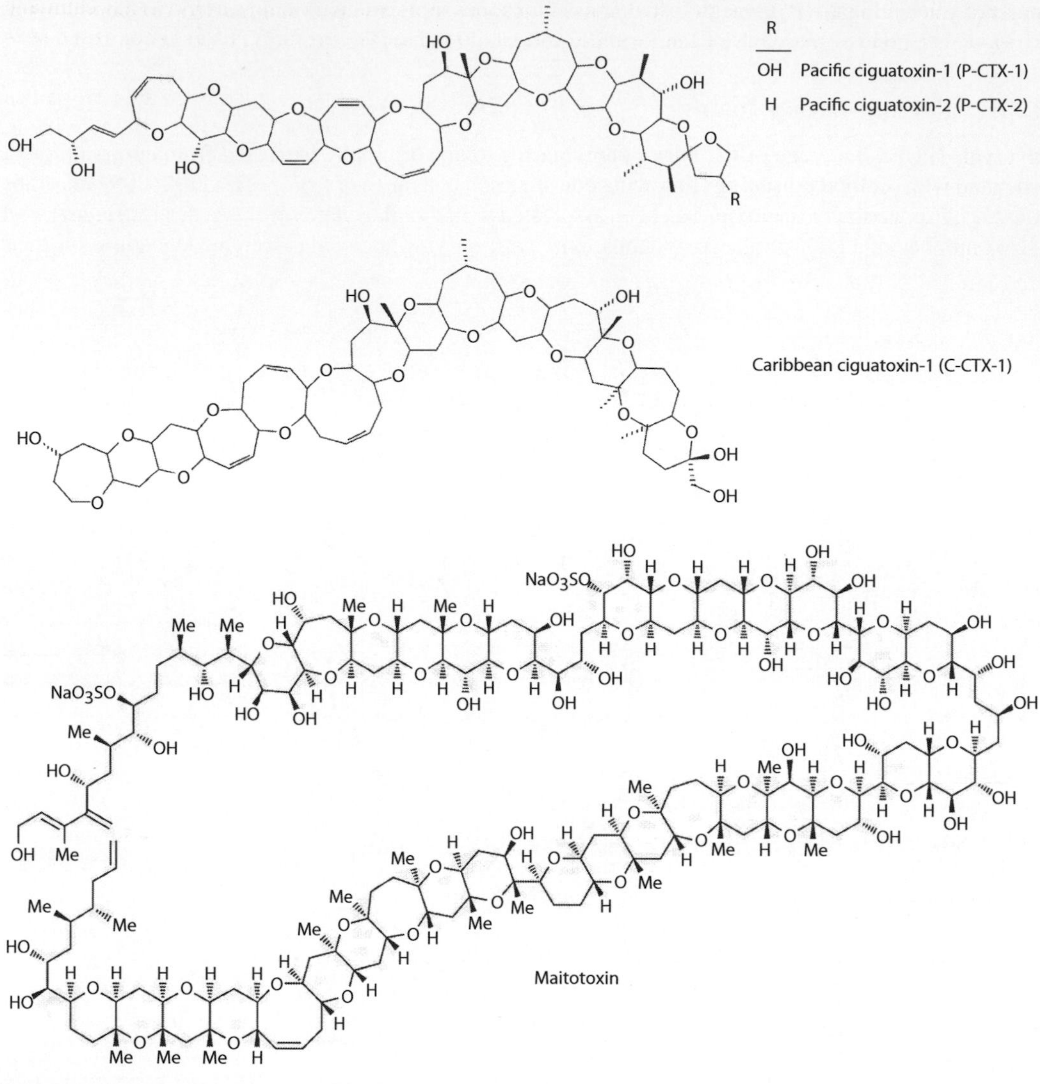

FIGURE 13.5 (continued)

specific source [208]. The toxins are water-soluble, long-chain complex molecules with high molecular weight (>2600), containing both hydrophilic and lipophilic regions of the molecule and >40 hydroxyl and 2 amide groups [209]. PLTXs have a large number of chiral centers and two chromophores giving rise to a large number of analogues and specific and characteristic UV absorption peaks at 233 and 263 nm [210]. PLTXs are associated with a large range of dinoflagellates and with health problems potentially resulting from a number of modes of entry including seafood consumption [207], from exposure to algal aerosols in bathing waters [211], and even from skin contact with aquarium corals [212]. The full detail of the origin, occurrence, and chemistry of PLTX-group toxins is given in Chapter 25. While there are no regulations on PLTX-group toxins in shellfish, a proposed guide of 250 μg/kg shellfish was put forward by the EURLMB [213] with EFSA subsequently proposing a 30 μg/kg limit [214].

13.5.1.1 HPLC–UV Methods

While currently no official method of analysis exists for PLTX-group toxins, analysis has been reported using a number of techniques including the MBA, hemolysis assays, cytotoxicity tests, matrix-assisted laser desorption ionization time of flight (MALDI-TOF) MS, thin-layer chromatography (TLC), capillary electrophoresis, HPLC, and LC–MS/MS with a combination of techniques often used to confirm detection [215]. However, given the strong UV absorbance of the toxins at characteristic wavelengths, HPLC analysis was used early on in combination with an MBA to identify PLTX in crabs from the Philippines [206]. Methanolic crab extracts were cleaned up by liquid–liquid extraction and column cleanup [210], prior to reverse-phase HPLC purification and subsequent HPLC–UV analysis on two column chemistries, showing equivalent chromatographic properties in comparison with a PLTX reference standard [206]. The same purification scheme and HPLC analysis was also used to confirm a PLTX-like toxin as causing human fatality in the Philippines following crab consumption [216] and the occurrence of PLTX in trigger fish [217] and parrot fish species [218]. Lau et al. [219] reported the use of reverse-phase gradient chromatography for the detection of a novel fluorescent toxin from crab and later described the separation of a number of PLTX-group toxins using mixed-mode HPLC with UV DAD [220]. HPLC–UV analysis conducted by Mereish et al. [221] using reverse-phase LC with isocratic mobile phase (MeCN/H_2O (52:48 v/v) + 0.1% TFA) reported an LOD for PLTX of 125 ng. HPLC–UV analysis has also been applied to enable the detection of PLTX in purified fractions of coral reef specimens, including fish, using reverse-phase (C8) analysis with 80 and MeCN + 0.1% TFA mobile phase and detection at 230 nm [222]. The authors compared chromatographic retention with a PLTX standard obtained from *Palythoa caribaeorum* and also reported the superior extraction of PLTX using distilled water in comparison with alcohol extraction [223]. Lenoir et al. [224] described the use of HPLC–UV on a 250 × 4.6 mm C18 column using H_2O + TFA (pH 2.5) and MeCN and a 45 min linear gradient. The analysis of cleaned-up methanolic extracts of a benthic bloom of *Ostreopsis mascarenensis* resulted in the identification of two components, mascarenotoxin-A and mascarenotoxin-B, with the same UV spectrum and retention characteristics as a Pacific palytoxin (P-PLTX) reference standard [224]. Riobbo and Franco [225] also reported the use of HPLC–UV for the analysis of *Ostreopsis* extracts but noted sensitivity issues due to effects of matrix components, reporting a 1–2 μg limit. With a wide range of matrices containing PLTX-group toxins ranging from relatively simple cultures to the more complex components present in molluscs and crustaceans, extraction and cleanup methodologies need to be carefully optimized prior to analysis. To date, only qualitative HPLC–UV methods have been reported for the determination of PLTX toxins in shellfish, given the strong matrix effects known to exist and the subsequent low overall method sensitivity [217,224], particularly in relation to the limits recommended by EFSA. However, the technique has been used for the quantitation of PLTX in home aquarium zoanthids, prior to confirmation of PLTX type by high-resolution LC–MS [211].

13.5.1.2 HPLC–FLD Methods

Given the presence of a suitable amino group in the PLTX molecule, the potential for derivatization of PLTX has been exploited. One specific fluorescent derivatization reagent, 6-aminoquinolyl-N-hydroxysuccinimidyl carbamate (AQC), was investigated for use prior to HPLC–FLD analysis [214]. Filtered and washed samples of 14 samples of *Ostreopsis* cultures were subjected to mixed-mode SPE cleanup for fractionation to separate PLTX from free amino acids. Derivatization of standards and samples with ~10 mM AQC was conducted at pH 8.8 and at 50°C for 10 min. HPLC separation was achieved using Waters XTerra 5 μm C18 columns, with FLD excitation and emission wavelengths set to 250 and 395 nm, respectively. The column was held at 35°C and MeOH/ammonium acetate (pH 5.8) mobile phases were used with gradient elution [214]. All derivatized algal samples showed chromatographic peaks with the same retention time as derivatized PLTX standard, and analysis of derivatized samples spiked with PLTX confirmed the retention characteristics. Some selectivity issues were confirmed through the identification of a partially resolved interference, but these were not found to affect quantitation. The stability of the fluorescent derivatives was excellent up to 12 days, and validation of method recovery showed PLTX recoveries of ~95%. Sensitivity and linearity were also acceptable with a reported LOD and LOQ for PLTX of 0.75 and 2 ng, respectively [214]. The quantitative results from the HPLC–FLD method of the algal cultures compared well with data generated using a hemolytic assay, with confirmation of PLTX undertaken using LC–MS. Overall, the authors reported the method to be simple and quick to use with good method performance characteristics and sensitivity and accuracy superior to the LC–MS method used for confirmation purposes [214], also proposing its application to the analysis of shellfish samples.

To date, no formal single-laboratory or interlaboratory validation studies have been conducted for the HPLC–FLD analysis of PLTXs in shellfish, and there is a strong requirement for the availability of suitable reference materials to enable method optimization, validation, and quality control.

13.5.2 Tetrodotoxins

Tetrodotoxin (TTX) poisoning is the most commonly occurring lethal marine poisoning [226], with the toxin being found in the organs of fish from the Tetraodontidae family, including the pufferfish. TTX and associated analogues are heat-stable, water-soluble, and relatively low molecular weight heterocyclic compounds produced by a range of bacteria [227] that subsequently accumulate in the fish as well as in amphibians and octopus [225]. Given the high potency of the toxins, high mortality rates, and ease of accidental intake of toxic parts, careful monitoring is of high importance [183].

13.5.2.1 HPLC–FLD

The TTX MBA has been used for the determination of toxicity for which 1 mouse unit (MU) is equivalent to 220 ng TTX [228]. A more specific and sensitive approach using chromatography and post-column fluorescence derivatization was developed by Yasumoto et al. [229,230] and further reported by Yotsu et al. [231]. Extraction of TTX was performed using 0.02 M acetic acid in boiling water (10 min) prior to cooling, centrifugation, and filtration. Reverse-phase C18 chromatography (250 × 4.6 mm column), with an ion-pairing reagent (heptafluorobutyric acid) in the pH 5.0 ammonium acetate buffer mobile phase, enabled separation of TTX and the congeners 4-*epi*-TTX and 4,9-anhydro-TTX [183]. FLD was monitored using excitation and emission at 365 and 510 nm, respectively, following post-column treatment with hot 4 M sodium hydroxide (NaOH), yielding highly fluorescent amino-quinazoline derivatives. Analytical sensitivity was good (5 ng per injection on-column), with good reproducibility ($\leq 5\%$) and a good correlation observed between the HPLC method and the MBA [183]. The method has also been used following ethanolic extractions of toads in combination with pre-column cleanup (activated charcoal or cation-exchange gels) where the same three TTX analogues were detected [232]. A modified procedure involving three extractions with 1% acetic acid in methanol was developed, incorporating additional cleanup with chloroform and ultrafiltration for the detection of TTX in gastropods and pufferfish [233]. Method recovery was shown to be 91% ± 5%, with an LOD (S/N = 2) of 10 ng (<0.2 µg TTX/g) and a good method linearity evidenced between 10 ng and 2 µg TTX injected. The method allowed separation of the three TTX analogues all found to coexist in the toxic samples analyzed, and an excellent correlation with the MBA was observed [232]. The same method has also been applied to the analysis of TTX and other TTX analogues in newts, with results compared against isolated standards [234–236]. Modified chromatographic conditions involving the use of sodium 1-heptane sulfonate and post-column reaction conditions (3 M NaOH) together with a C18-SPE cleanup of extracts were also employed to quantify the TTX present in gastropods implicated in a food poisoning event [237,238]. The method provided a rapid quantitative determination of TTX, 4-*epi*-TTX, and anhydro-TTX, with a 1 µg/mL LOD, TTX recovery of 90%, and a linear range of 1–500 µg/mL for TTX. Confirmation of the presence of TTX in patient's blood was conducted using LC–MS/MS [237]. There have been few reports on the use of post-column derivatization HPLC–FLD for the detection of TTX in the urine and serum from patients suspected of TTX ingestion, given the importance of effective diagnosis. Kawatsu et al. [239] described the use of immunoaffinity chromatography following the production of a monoclonal antibody specific to TTX to enable separation of TTX from interfering matrix components. They employed the chromatography as a cleanup step prior to ion-pair HPLC–FLD with post-column derivatization. TTX recovery rates for the entire method were 50%–60% and were sensitive enough and applicable for the selective detection of TTX in urine samples collected from patients. Another approach incorporated the use of SPE as an alternative cleanup, although recoveries were limited and LOQs were 5 and 20 ng/mL for serum and urine, respectively [240]. However, precision was acceptable (13%–15%) and the linear ranges were 20–300 ng/mL and 5–20 ng/mL for urine and serum analysis, respectively.

13.5.2.2 HPLC–UV

Yu et al. [241] have reported the use of a simple HPLC–UV method for the detection of TTX in the urine and plasma of humans intoxicated with pufferfish poisoning. A C18-SPE cleanup was applied to samples followed by weak ion-exchange cleanup. Chromatography was conducted on a 5 μm 250 × 4.6 mm analytical column and the authors reported an LOD of 10 ng/mL [241].Validation demonstrated average TTX method recovery to be >87% in both matrices.

13.5.3 Brevetoxins

The PbTxs are a large family of stable lipid-soluble cyclic polyether compounds primarily produced by the dinoflagellate *Karenia brevis* and are responsible for toxicity in fish, marine mammals, birds, and humans. Humans may be affected from PbTx exposure through consumption of contaminated shell- fish, termed neurotoxic shellfish poisoning (NSP), or from exposure to aerosols. Two distinct structural types (PbTx-1 and PbTx-2) are thought to be the parent algal toxins from which a multiple of other naturally occurring analogues and metabolic products have been identified [242]. The MBA has been used in affected regions for the assessment of shellfish toxicity, but alternative methods have been exten- sively investigated in light of the inefficiencies, poor performance, and ethical issues recognized with the bioassay performance [243,244]. With the relatively recent development of a wide range of detec- tion methods applicable to a variety of sample types including a cytotoxicity assay, receptor binding assay, and immunoassays, the major focus for the development of analytical instrumentation methods has been on the use of LC–MS methodologies (Chapter 15) given the high degree of specificity they provide [242]. Conventional chromatographic methods relying on spectroscopic detection or following functional derivatization are therefore not commonly reported, with HPLC and UV DAD mostly under- taken for fractionation of toxic extracts prior to confirmation by LC–MS [245]. Methods were developed for the HPLC–UV detection of PbTxs on sorbent filters used to concentrate toxins present in aerosols and seawater [246]. Following filter extraction in DCM and evaporation and reconstitution in MeOH, isocratic analysis was conducted using a C18 HPLC column (MeOH/H_2O, 85:15 v/v) with UV detec- tion at 215 nm. Quantitation was performed against commercially available toxin standards. Method verification demonstrated toxin recoveries ~100% for PbTx-2 and PbTx-3 in water [247]. Dickey et al. [248] reported the use of diethylaminocoumarin carbamate for the derivatization of PbTxs to facilitate HPLC–FLD. Analysis of diethylaminocoumarin carbamate PbTx-3 showed two peaks corresponding to the two expected hydroxyl substitutions, with identities confirmed by mass spectral analysis [248].

There are no reports of more recent validation or developments of conventional HPLC methods.

13.5.4 Ciguatera Fish Poisoning Toxins

CTXs, together with gambiertoxins (GTXs, not to be confused with the hydrophilic gonyautoxins), are potent lipophilic polyethers that are known to accumulate in fish from microalgae of certain strains of the dinoflagellates species *Gambierdiscus toxicus* causing ciguatera fish poisoning (CFP) in human con- sumers [249]. A number of structurally distinct groups have been identified from different geographical sources including the Pacific, Caribbean, and Indian Oceans [250]. The MBA as refined by Yasumoto et al. [251] is still widely used for CTX detection, with specific clinical signs denoting qualitative iden- tification and time of death enabling the calculation of total toxicity levels. Other methodologies have been extensively developed to provide in vitro and chemical alternatives to CFP detection (Chapter 34). In particular, given the success of MS detection methods for a large number of CTX and GTX analogues, the majority of published methods focus on this technique (Chapter 15). However, some conventional HPLC methods have been reported. CTXs do not possess strong chromophores to enable selective deter- mination of toxins in fish extracts, but even so, HPLC–UV has been utilized for the detection of purified CTX standards [252] and for chromatographic purification of toxic fractions (e.g., [253] and reviewed by [249]).The presence of a primary hydroxyl group in many of the CTX congeners has been exploited to demonstrate the potential for derivatization of CTXs to form fluorescent esters prior to HPLC–FLD. One HPLC–FLD method using post-column derivatization of separated CTXs was developed using alkaline oxidation with peroxide and ammonium hydroxide [254]. While sensitivity was demonstrated, the authors reported poor precision and accuracy of the method. Yasumoto subsequently investigated the use of the reagent 1-anthroylnitrile, which enabled the characterization of 10 CFP toxins with good detection linearity over the 1–100 ng range [255]. Analysis of CTXs in fish was subsequently conducted using 250 × 4.6 mm reverse-phase HPLC at 30°C, with different isocratic mobile phases (85% and 95% MeCN) used for the separation of the primary fluorescent esters [183]. Yasumoto et al. also noted that efficient cleanup protocols would be required to improve the selectivity and sensitivity of methods, especially important given the complexity of fluorescent matrix components and the low concentrations of CTX causing illness [183]. Dickey et al. [248] used diethylaminocoumarin carbamate for the derivatization of P-CTX-1 prior to HPLC–FLD as also reported for PbTxs, with a detection limit of 0.5–1.0 ng. The low yield of the labeling reaction highlighted the need for optimized reaction conditions or more appropriate fluorescent reagents to be used. Additionally, analysis of CTX analogues without the primary hydroxyl groups would not be suitable.

Maitotoxins (MTXs) are potent water-soluble, high molecular weight polycyclic neurotoxins also originating from *G. toxicus*. They are found to accumulate in fish and another toxin involved in ciguatera poisoning. Preparative-scale HPLC–UV has been used for isolating two analogues of MTX with 15 µm C18 columns (5–28 cm), a MeOH mobile phase, and detection at 210 nm [256].

Carchatoxins are toxins that have been linked to CTX episodes but that exhibit different toxicological properties to the CTXs and have resulted in high mortality rates. Following a mass poisoning from shark meat in 1993, reverse-phase HPLC was used to isolate two toxins termed carchatoxin-A and carchatoxin-B, although structural elucidation was not possible [257]. Analytical-scale HPLC with a 75% MeOH mobile phase and UV detection at 210 nm showed different (less polar) chromatographic properties to CTX-1 [258].

13.5.5 Macrocyclic Imines

Cyclic imines are a relatively recently discovered group of toxins uncovered through their fast-acting toxicity in mice following DSP MBA (Figure 13.6). Toxin groups include the prorocentrolides, spirolides (SPXs), gymnodimines (GYMs), pinnatoxins (PnTXs), and pterotoxins (PtTXs), with the commonality coming from a combination of the imino structural feature and high intraperitoneal (IP) toxicity. As these compounds have not been shown to be toxic in humans following shellfish consumption, the presence of these compounds remains unregulated [259]. Full details regarding the chemistry, origin, and detection methods in general are described in Chapter 35.

As with many of the other new and emerging toxins, given their more recent discovery, lack of evidence for toxicity in humans, and the availability of highly specific and sensitive MS detection methods,

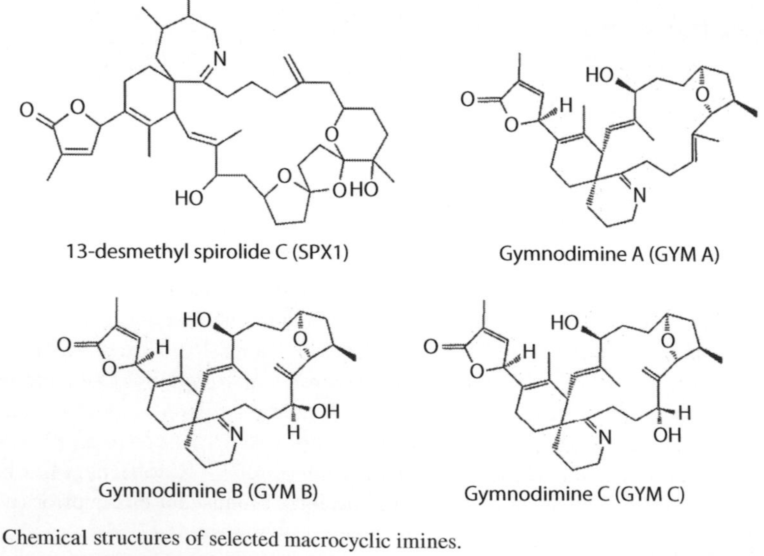

13-desmethyl spirolide C (SPX1)

Gymnodimine A (GYM A)

Gymnodimine B (GYM B)

Gymnodimine C (GYM C)

FIGURE 13.6 Chemical structures of selected macrocyclic imines.

there has been little development in the use of conventional HPLC detection methods for the cyclic imines. In addition, the cyclic imines lack any notable chromophores, further hindering the use of sensitive and selective spectroscopic detection. However, Torigoe et al. used reverse-phase HPLC for the purification of the cyclic polyether prorocentrolide prior to structural elucidation [260]. Tunisian clam samples containing two GYMs (GYM A and GYM B), the smallest of the cyclic imine family, have been analyzed by reverse-phase HPLC–UV [261]. Extraction of digestive glands was conducted in acetone, prior to cleanup by liquid–liquid extraction prior to analysis. Chromatography was performed using C18 HPLC with a MeCN/H_2O mobile phase with 0.1% TFA and gradient elution. Method validation demonstrated toxin recoveries of >96%, with LOD and LOQ 5 and 8 ng/g digestive gland, respectively, and acceptable method repeatability, with the authors proposing the method as a suitable detection method [260]. While a range of other preparative HPLC methods have been used to aid the detection and identification of SPXs, PnTXs, and PtTXs in plankton and shellfish, no other conventional HPLC methods have been published specifically targeting these toxin groups.

13.6 Final Considerations

Given the steady move away from sole reliance on live animal assays for marine biotoxin testing, there is a clear need for robust alternative methods. While there are clear advantages for the use of the more selective MS detection methods, the scope of available conventional HPLC methods with either UV detection or FLD is wide for an increasing number of toxin groups. The two HPLC–FLD methods available for PSP testing along with the ASP HPLC–UV method are well developed, validated, and implemented into official control monitoring programs worldwide as well as providing useful research tools. Methods for many of the lipophilic toxin groups have been available for many years, but with the more recent report of an HPLC–FLD method for AZAs, there is the potential for all EU-regulated lipophilic toxins to be tested using conventional detection methods. This could provide an alternative approach for laboratories where the use of the LC–MS/MS method remains impractical or for work where additional confirmatory methods are required. This appears especially important for developing countries for whom the routine use of LC–MS/MS is too expensive, both in terms of instrumentation and maintenance costs. Indeed some of these methods, such as the ADAM HPLC–FLD for OA-group toxins, are currently enjoying a resurgence in use, with development and validation studies ongoing. However, once such alternatives are developed, they must be fully assessed through both single-laboratory and interlaboratory validation. For the majority of the HPLC testing methods for lipophilic toxins and the new and emerging toxins, this work has yet to be conducted. Comparison of performance using different methods can only be carried out once full validation data are published. Even then, care must be taken to ensure the comparison is made appropriately given the different approaches taken in validation studies by different workers. Recovery data should ideally reflect the recovery of the whole method, using the analysis of spiked tissues rather than spiked extracts. Comparison of method sensitivities in terms of LOD/LOQ also needs to be carefully considered given the large differences in background noise that are found between detectors provided by different manufacturers.

Overall, continued coordinated efforts are required to enable further growth in the use of conventional HPLC methods, along with the ongoing development in the production of suitable certified reference standards essential for running such tests and for maintaining quality assurance and quality control.

REFERENCES

1. Anon. 2005. AOAC Official Method 959.08. Paralytic shellfish poison. Biological method. Final action. Chapter 49: Natural toxins. In: M.W. Truckses (ed.), *AOAC Official Methods for Analysis*, 18th edn. AOAC International, Gaithersburg, MD, pp. 79–80.
2. Aune, T., Ramstad, H., Heinenreich, B., Landsverk, T., Waaler, T., Eggas, E., and Julshamn, K. 1998. Zinc accumulation in oysters giving mouse deaths in paralytic shellfish poisoning bioassay. *J. Shell. Res.* 17(4): 1243–1246.

3. McCulloch, A.W., Boyd, R.K., de Freitas, A.S.W., Foxall, R.A., Jamieson, W.D., Laycock, M.V., Quilliam, M.A., Wright, J.L.C., Boyko, V.J., McLaren, J.W., and Miedema, M.R. 1989. Zinc from oyster tissue as causative factor in mouse deaths in official bioassay for paralytic shellfish poison. *J. Assoc. Off. Anal. Chem.* 72(2): 384–386.

4. Vale, P. and de Sampayo, M.A. 2001. Determination of paralytic shellfish toxins in Portuguese shellfish by automated pre-column oxidation. *Toxicon* 39: 561–571.

5. Wiberg, G.S. and Stephenson, N.R. 1961. The effect of metal ions on the toxicity of paralytic shellfish poison. *Toxicol. Appl. Pharmacol.* 3: 707–712.

6. Turner, A.D., Dhanji-Rapkova, M., Algoet, M., Suarez-Isla, B.A., Cordova, M., Caceres, C., Murphy, C., Casey, M., and Lees, D.N. 2012. Investigations into matrix components affecting the performance of the official bioassay reference method for quantitation of paralytic shellfish poisoning toxins in oysters. *Toxicon* 59: 215–230.

7. Yasumoto, T., Oshima, Y., and Yamaguchi, M. 1978. Occurrence of a new type of shellfish poisoning in the Tohoku district. *Bull. Jpn. Soc. Sci. Fish.* 44(11): 1249–1255.

8. Fernandez, M.L., Richard, D.J.A., and Cembella, A.D. 2003. In vivo assays for phycotoxins. In: G.M. Hallegraeff, D.M. Anderson, and A.D. Cembella (eds.), *Manual on Harmful Marine Microalgae.* UNESCO Publishing, Paris, France, pp. 347–380.

9. Takagi, T., Hayashi, K., and Itabashi, Y. 1984. Toxic effect of free unsaturated fatty acids in the mouse bioassay of diarrhetic shellfish toxin by intraperitoneal injection. *Bull. Jpn. Soc. Sci. Fish.* 50(8): 1413–1418.

10. Suzuki, T., Yoshizawa, R., Kawamura, T., and Yamasaki, M. 1996. Interference of free fatty acids from the hepatopancreas of mussels with the mouse bioassay for shellfish toxins. *Lipids* 31(6): 641–645.

11. James, J.J., Bishop, A.G., Carmody, E.P., and Kelly, S.S. 2000. Detection methods for Okadaic acid and analogues. In: L.M. Botana (ed.), *Seafood and Freshwater Toxins: Pharmacology, Physiology and Detection.* CRC Press, Boca Raton, FL.

12. Dennison, N. and Anderson, D.B. 2007. The 3 "R"s approach to marine biotoxin testing in the UK. AATEX14, pp. 757–761. *Proceedings of the 6th World Congress on Alternatives and Animal Use in the Life Sciences*, August 21–25, 2007, Tokyo, Japan. Japanese Society for Alternatives to Animal Experiments, Bunkyo-Ku, Tokyo.

13. Hess, P., Grune, B., Anderson, D. B., Aune, T., Botana, L. M., Caricato, P., Van Egmond, H. P. et al. 2006. Three Rs approaches in marine biotoxin testing. *Altern. Lab. Anim.* 34: 193–224.

14. Thompson, M., Ellison, S.L.R., and Wood, R. 2002. Harmonized guidelines for single laboratory validation of methods of analysis (IUPAC technical report). *Pure Appl. Chem.* 74(5): 835–855.

15. Anon. 2006. Committee on Toxicity of chemicals in food, consumer products and the environment. Statement on risk assessment and monitoring of Paralytic Shellfish Poisoning (PSP) toxins in support of human health. COT statement 2006/08. July 2006. http://www.food.gov.uk/science/ouradvisors/toxicity/statements/cotstatements2006/cotstatementpsp200608 (accessed August 2012).

16. Anon. 2004. Commission Regulation (EC) No 882/2004 of the European parliament and of the Council of 29th April 2004 on official controls performed to ensure verification of compliance with feed and food law, animal health and animal welfare rules. *Off. J. Eur. Union* L191: 1–52.

17. Anon. 2000. Quantifying uncertainty in analytical measurement. In: S.L.R. Ellison, M. Rosslein, and A. Williams (eds.), *Eurachem/Citac Guide*, 2nd edn. Eurachem: London, U.K.

18. Trullols, E., Ruisanchez, I., and Xavier Rius, F. 2004. Validation of qualitative analytical methods. *Trends Analyt. Chem.* 23(2): 137–145.

19. Eurachem. 1998. The fitness for purpose of analytical methods. A laboratory guide to method validation and related topics. EURACHEM Secretariat. Teddington, U.K.

20. Llewellyn, L.E. 2006. Saxitoxin, a toxic marine natural product that targets a multitude of receptors. *Nat. Prod. Rep.* 23: 200–233.

21. Wright, J.L.C. 1995. Dealing with seafood toxins: Present approaches and future options. *Food Res. Int.* 28: 347–358.

22. Kodama, M. 2000. Ecobiology, classification and origin. In: L.M. Botana (ed.), *Seafood and Freshwater Toxins: Pharmacology, Physiology and Detection.* Marcel Dekker, Inc., New York, pp. 125–149.

23. Etheridge, S.M. 2010. Paralytic shellfish poisoning: Seafood safety and human health perspectives. *Toxicon* 56: 108–122.

24. Luckas, B., Hummert, C., and Oshima, Y. 2004. Analytical methods for PSP. In: G.M. Hallegraeff, D.M. Anderson, and A.D. Cembella (eds.), *Manual on Harmful Marine Microalgae*. UNESCO Publishing, Paris, France, p. 191.

25. Wiese, M., D'Agnostino, P.M., Mihali, T.K., Moffitt, M.C., and Neilan, B.A. 2010. Neurotoxic alkaloids: Saxitoxin and its analogs. *Mar. Drugs*. 8: 2185–2211.

26. Anon. 2006. Commission Regulation (EC) No 1664/2006 of 6th Nov. 2006 amending Regulation (EC) No 2074/2005 as regards implementing measures for certain products of animal origin intended for human consumption and repealing certain implementing measures. *Off. J. Eur. Union* L320: 13–45.

27. Oshima, Y. 1995. Post-column derivatisation liquid chromatography method for paralytic shellfish toxins. *J. AOAC Int*. 78: 528–532.

28. Genenah, A.A. and Shimizu, Y. 1981. Specific toxicity of paralytic shellfish poisons. *J. Agric. Food Chem*. 29: 1289–1291.

29. Schantz, E.J. 1986. Chemistry and biology of saxitoxin and related toxins. *Ann. N. Y. Acad. Sci*. 479: 15–23.

30. EFSA. 2009. Scientific opinion. Marine biotoxins in shellfish—Saxitoxin group. Scientific opinion of the panel on contaminants in the food chain. *EFSA J*. 1019: 1–76.

31. Humpage, A.R., Magalhaes, V.F., and Froscio, S.M. 2010. Comparison of analytical tools and biological assays for detection of paralytic shellfish poisoning toxins. *Anal. Bioanal. Chem*. 397: 1655–1671.

32. Turner, A.D., Norton, D.M., Hatfield, R.G., Morris, S., Reese, A.R., Algoet, M., and Lees, D.N. 2009. Single laboratory validation of the AOAC LC method (2005.06) for mussels: Refinement and extension of the method to additional toxins. *J. AOAC Int*. 92(1): 190–207

33. EURLMB. 2009. Minutes of the 3rd EURLMB Working Group on the determination of PSP toxins by AOAC OMA 2005.06 (HPLC method.) Brussels, Belgium, November 6, 2009.

34. Artigas, M.L., Vale, P.J.V., Gomes, S.S., Botelho, M.I., Rodrigues, S.M., and Amorim, A. 2007. Profiles of paralytic shellfish poisoning toxins in shellfish from Portugal explained by carbamoylase activity. *J. Chromatogr. A*. 1160: 99–105.

35. Bates, H.A. and Rapoport, H. 1975. A chemical assay for saxitoxin, the paralytic shellfish poison. *J. Agric. Food Chem*. 23: 237–239.

36. Lawrence, J.F., Menard, C., Charbonneau, C., and Hall, S. 1991. A study of ten toxins associated with paralytic shellfish poison using prechromatographic oxidation and liquid chromatography with fluorescence detection. *J. AOAC Int*. 74: 404–409.

37. Lawrence, J.F. and Menard, C. 1991. Liquid chromatographic determination of paralytic shellfish poisons in shellfish after prechromatographic oxidation. *J. AOAC Int*. 74(6): 1006–1012.

38. Quilliam, M.A., Janecek, M., and Lawrence, J.J. 1993. Characterisation of the oxidation products of paralytic shellfish poisoning toxins by liquid chromatography/mass spectrometry. *Rapid Commun. Mass Spectrom*. 7: 482–487.

39. Lawrence, J.F., Menard, C., and Cleroux, C. 1995. Evaluation of prechromatographic oxidation for liquid chromatographic determination of paralytic shellfish poisons in shellfish. *J. AOAC Int*. 78(2): 514–520.

40. Lawrence, J.F., Wong, B., and Menard, C. 1996. Determination of decarbamoyl saxitoxin and its analogues in shellfish by prechromatographic oxidation and liquid chromatography with fluorescence detection. *J. AOAC Int*. 79: 1111–1115.

41. Lawrence, J.F. and Niedzwiadek, B. 2001. Quantitative determination of paralytic shellfish poisoning toxins in shellfish using prechromatographic oxidation and liquid chromatography with fluorescence detection. *J. AOAC Int*. 84(4): 1099–1108.

42. Ben-Gigirey, B., Rodriguez-Velasco, A., Villar-Gonzalez, A., and Botana, L.M. 2007. Influence of the sample toxic profile on the suitability of a high performance liquid chromatography method for official paralytic shellfish toxins control. *J. Chromatogr. A*. 1140: 78–87.

43. Gago-Martinez, A., Moscoso, S.A., Leao Martins, J.M., Rodriguez Vazquez, J-A., Niedzwiadek, B., and Lawrence, J.F. 2001. Effect of pH on the oxidation of paralytic shellfish poisoning toxins for analysis by liquid chromatography. *J. Chromatogr. A*. 905: 351–357.

44. Lawrence, J.F., Niedzwiadek, B., and Menard, C. 2004. Quantitative determination of paralytic shellfish poisoning toxins in shellfish using prechromatographic oxidation and liquid chromatography with fluorescence detection: Interlaboratory study. *J. AOAC Int*. 87(1): 83–100.

45. Lawrence, J.F., Niedzwiadek, B., and Menard, C. 2005. Quantitative determination of paralytic shellfish poisoning toxins in shellfish using prechromatographic oxidation and liquid chromatography with fluorescence detection: Collaborative study. *J. AOAC Int.* 88(6): 1714–1732.

46. Anon. 2005. AOAC Official Method 2005.06. *Quantitative Determination of Paralytic Shellfish Poisoning Toxins in Shellfish Using Pre-Chromatographic Oxidation and Liquid Chromatography with Fluorescence Detection.* AOAC International, Gaithersburg, MD.

47. Turner, A.D., Norton, D.M., Hatfield, R.G., Rapkova-Dhanji, M., Algoet, M., and Lees, D.N. 2010. Single laboratory validation of a refined AOAC LC method for oysters, cockles and clams in UK shellfish. *J. AOAC Int.* 93(5): 1482–1493.

48. Cefas contract report. 2010. Refinement and in-house validation of the AOAC HPLC method (2005.06): The determination of paralytic shellfish poisoning toxins in king scallops and queen scallops by liquid chromatography and fluorescence detection. Final project report. http://www.cefas.defra.gov.uk/media/557600/psp%20method%20validation%20scallops.pdf (accessed August 2012).

49. Turner, A.D. and Hatfield, R.G. 2012. Refinement of AOAC 2005.06 liquid chromatography-fluorescence detection method to improve performance characteristics for the determination of paralytic shellfish toxins king and queen scallops. *J. AOAC Int.* 95(1): 129–142.

50. Ben-Gigirey, B., Rodriguez-Velasco, M.M., and Gago-Martinez, A. 2012. Interlaboratory study for the extension of the validation of 2005.06 AOAC Official Method for dc-GTX2,3. *J. AOAC Int.* 95(1): 1–13.

51. Boyer, G.L., Sullivan, J.J., Andersen, R.J., Taylor, F.J.R., Harrison, P.J., and Cembella, A.D. 1986. Use of high-performance liquid chromatography to investigate the production of paralytic shellfish toxins by *Protogonyaulax* spp. in culture. *Mar. Biol.* 93(3): 361–369.

52. DeGrasse, S.L., van de Riet, J., Hatfield, R., and Turner, A.D. 2011. Pre- versus post-column oxidation liquid chromatography fluorescence detection of paralytic shellfish toxins. *Toxicon* 57: 619–624.

53. Janecek, M., Quilliam, M.A., and Lawrence, J.F. 1993. Analysis of paralytic shellfish poisoning toxins by automated pre-column oxidation and microcolumn liquid chromatography with fluorescence detection. *J. Chromatogr. A.* 644: 321–331.

54. Flynn, K. and Flynn, K.J. 1996. An automated HPLC method for the rapid analysis of paralytic shellfish toxins from dinoflagellates and bacteria using precolumn oxidation at low temperature. *J. Expt. Mar. Biol. Ecol.* 197: 145–157.

55. Harwood, D.T., Boundy, M., Selwood, S.I., van Ginkel, R., MacKenzie, L. and McNabb, P.S. 2013. Refinement and implementation of the Lawrence method (AOAC 2005.06) in a commercial laboratory: Assay performance during an *Alexandrium catenella* bloom event. *Harmful Algae* 24: 20–31.

56. DeGrasse, S.L., DeGrasse, J.A., and Reuter, K. 2010. Solid core column technology applied to HPLC-FD of paralytic shellfish toxins. *Toxicon* 57(1): 179–182.

57. Hatfield, R.G. and Turner, A.D. 2012. Rapid liquid chromatography for paralytic shellfish toxin analysis using superficially porous chromatography with AOAC Method 2005.06. *J. AOAC Int.* 95(4): 1–8.

58. Oshima, Y., Hasegawa, M., Yasumoto, T., Hallegraeff, G., and Blackburn, S.I. 1987. Dinoflagellate *Gymnodinium Catenatum* as the source of paralytic shellfish toxins in Tasmanian shellfish. *Toxicon* 25: 1105–1111.

59. Thielert, G., Kaiser, I., and Luckas, B. 1991. HPLC determination of PSP toxins. In: J.M. Fremy (ed.), *Proceedings of Symposium on Marine Biotoxins*, Paris, 30–31 January 1991. Centre National d'Etudes Veterinaires et Alimentaires, Maisons-Alfort, France, pp. 121–125.

60. Hummert, C., Ritscher, M., Reinhardt, K., and Luckas, B. 1998. A new method for the determination of paralytic shellfish poisoning (PSP). *Proceedings of the 22nd International Symposium on Chromatography (ISC)*, Rome, Italy, September 13–18.

61. Franco, J.M. and Fernandez-Vila, P. 1993. Separation of paralytic shellfish toxins by reversed phase high performance liquid chromatography, with postcolumn reaction and fluorimetric detection. *Chromatographia* 35: 613–620.

62. Leao, J.M., Gago, A., Rodriguez-Vazquez, J.A., Aguete, E.C., Omil, M.M., and Comesana, M. 1998. Solid-phase extraction and high performance liquid chromatography procedures for the analysis of paralytic shellfish toxins. *J. Chromatogr.* 798: 131–136.

63. Bire, R., Krys, S., Fremy, J.M., and Dragacci, S. 2003. Improved solid-phase extraction procedure in the analysis of paralytic shellfish poisoning toxins by liquid chromatography with fluorescence detection. *J. Agric. Food Chem.* 51: 6386–6390.

64. Asp, T.N., Larsen, S., and Aune, T. 2004. Analysis of PSP toxins in Norwegian mussels by a post-column derivatisation HPLC method. *Toxicon* 43: 319–327.

65. Yu, R.C., Hummert, C., Luckas, B., Qian, P.Y., Li, J., and Zhou, M.J. 1998. A modified HPLC method for analysis of PSP toxins in algae and shellfish from China. *Chromatographia* 48(9/10): 671–676.

66. Lawrence, J.F. and Wong, B. 1995. Evaluation of a postcolumn electrochemical reactor for oxidation of paralytic shellfish poison toxins. *J. AOAC Int.* 78(3): 698–704.

67. Lawrence, J.F. and Wong, B. 1996. Development of a manganese dioxide solid-phase reactor for oxidation of toxins associated with paralytic shellfish poison. *J. Chromatogr. A.* 755: 227–233.

68. Boyer, G.L. and Goddard, G.D. 1999. High performance liquid chromatography coupled with post-column electrochemical oxidation for the detection of PSP toxins. *Nat. Toxins* 7: 353–359.

69. Jaime, E., Hummert, C., Hess, P., and Luckas, B. 2001. Determination of paralytic shellfish poisoning toxins by high-performance ion-exchange chromatography. *J. Chromatogr. A.* 929: 43–49.

70. Diener, M., Erler, K., Hiller, S., Christian, B., and Luckas, B. 2006. Determination of paralytic shellfish poisoning (PSP) toxins in dietary supplements by application of a new HPLC/FLD method. *Eur. Food Res. Technol.* 224: 147–151.

71. Thomas, K., Chung, S., Ku, J., Reeves, K., and Quilliam, M.A. 2006. In: K. Henshilwood, B. Deega, T. McMahon, C. Cusack, S. Keaveney, J. Silke, M. O'Cinneide, D. Lyons, and P. Hess (eds.), *Molluscan Shellfish Safety*. The Marine Institute, Galway, Ireland, pp. 132–138.

72. Rourke, W.A., Murphy, C.J., Pitcher, G., van de Riet, J.M., Burns, G.B., Thomas, K.M., and Quilliam, M.A. 2008. Rapid postcolumn methodology for determination of paralytic shellfish toxins in shellfish tissue. *J. AOAC Int.* 91(3): 589–597.

73. Van de Riet, J.M., Gibbs, R.S., Chou, F.W., Muggah, P.M., Rourke, W.A., Burns, G., Thomas, K., and Quilliam, M.A. 2009. Liquid chromatographic post-column oxidation method for analysis of paralytic shellfish toxins in mussels, clams, scallops and oysters: Single-laboratory validation. *J. AOAC Int.* 92(6): 1690–1704.

74. Van de Riet, J.M., Gibbs, R.S., Muggah, P.M., Rourke, W.A., MacNeil, J.D., and Quilliam, M.A. 2011. Liquid chromatography post-column oxidation (PCOX) method for the determination of paralytic shellfish toxins in mussels, clams, oysters and scallops: Collaborative study. *J. AOAC Int.* 94(4): 1154–1176.

75. Anon. 2011. AOAC Official Method 2011.02. *Determination of Paralytic Shellfish Poisoning Toxins in Mussels, Clams, Oysters and Scallops. Post-Column Oxidation Method (PCOX)*. First Action 2011. AOAC International, Gaithersburg, MD.

76. NSSP. 2011. http://www.fda.gov/downloads/Food/GuidanceRegulation/FederalStateFoodPrograms/UCM350344.pdf (accessed August 2012).

77. Rodriguez, P., Alfonso, A., Botana, A.M., Vieytes, M.R., and Botana, L.M. 2010. Comparative analysis of pre- and post-column oxidation methods for detection of paralytic shellfish toxins. *Toxicon* 56: 448–457.

78. EURLMB. 2012. Standards and reference materials. http://www.aesan.msps.es/en/CRLMB/web/estandares_materiales_referencia/materiales_referencia.shtml

79. Turrell, E.A., Lacaze, J.P., and Stobo, L. 2007. Determination of paralytic shellfish poisoning (PSP) toxins in UK shellfish. *Harmful Algae* 6: 438–448.

80. Ujevic, I., Roje, R., Nincevic-Gladan, Z., and Marasovic, I. 2012. First report of paralytic shellfish poisoning (PSP) in mussels (*Mytilus galloprovincialis*) from eastern Adriatic Sea (Croatia). *Food Control* 25: 285–291.

81. Costa, P.R., Baugh, K.A., Wright, B., RaLonde, R., Nance, S.L., Tatarenkova, N., Etheridge, S.M., and Lefebvre, K.A. 2009. Comparative determination of paralytic shellfish toxins (PSTs) using five different toxin detection methods in shellfish species collected in the Aleutian Islands, Alaska. *Toxicon* 54: 313–320.

82. Ben-Gigirey, B., Rodriguez-Velasco, M.L., Otero, A., Vieites, J.M., and Cabado, A.G. 2012. A comparative study for PSP toxins quantification by using MBA and HPLC official methods in shellfish. *Toxicon* 60: 864–873.

83. Turner, A.D., Hatfield, R.G., Rapkova, M., Higman, W., Algoet, M., Suarez-Isla, B.A., Cordova, M. et al. 2011. Comparison of AOAC 2005.06 LC official method with other methodologies for the quantitation of paralytic shellfish poisoning toxins in UK shellfish species. *Anal. Bioanal. Chem.* 399: 1257–1270.

84. Turner, A.D., Dhanji-Rapkova, M., Higman, W., Algoet, M., Suarez-Isla, B.A., Cordova, M., Caceres, C., Murphy, C.J., Case, M., and Lees, D.N. 2012. Investigations into matrix components affecting the performance of the official bioassay reference method for quantitation of paralytic shellfish poisoning toxins in oysters. *Toxicon* 59: 215–230.

85. Waldock, M.J., Evans, K.M., Law, R.J., and Fileman, T.W. 1991. An assessment of the suitability of HPLC techniques for monitoring PSP and DSP on the east coast of England. In: J.M. Fremy (ed.), *Proceedings of Symposium on Marine Biotoxins*. Paris, France, pp. 30–31, January, 1991.

86. Vale, P. 2010. New saxitoxin analogues in the marine environment: Developments in toxin chemistry, detection and biotransformation during the 2000s. *Phytochem. Rev.* 9: 525–535.

87. Negri, A., Stirling, D., Quilliam, M.A., Blackburn, S., Bolch, C., Burton, I., Eaglesham, G., Thomas, K., Walter, J., and Willis, R. 2003. Three novel hydroxybenzoate saxitoxin analogues isolated from the dinoflagellates *Gymnodinium catenatum*. *Chem. Res. Toxicol.* 16(8): 1029–1033.

88. Bustillos-Guzman, J., Vale, P., and Band-Schmidt, C. 2011. Presence of benzoate type toxins in *Gymnodinium catenatum* isolated from the Mexican Pacific. *Toxicon* 57: 922–926.

89. Negri, A.P., Bolch, C.J.S., Geier, S., Green, D.H., Park, T.G., and Blackburn, S.I. 2007. Widespread presence of hydrophobic paralytic shellfish toxins in *Gymnodinium catenatum*. *Harmful Algae* 6(6): 774–780.

90. Vale, P. 2008. Fate of benzoate paralytic shellfish poisoning toxins from *Gymnodinium catenatum* in shellfish and fish detected by pre-column oxidation and liquid chromatography with fluorescence detection. *J. Chromtogr. A* 1190(1–2): 191–197.

91. Dell'Aversano, C., Hess, P., and Quilliam, M.A. 2005. Hydrophilic interaction liquid chromatography mass spectrometry for the analysis of paralytic shellfish poisoning (PSP) toxins. *J. Chromatogr. A* 1081: 190–201.

92. Dell'Aversano, C., Walter, J.A., Burton, L.W., Stirling, D.J., Fattol'Uso, E., and Quilliam, M.A. 2008. Isolation and structure elucidation of new and unusual saxitoxin analogues from mussels. *J. Nat. Prod.* 71: 1518–1523.

93. Nikkar, M.S. and Nijjar, S.S. 2000. Ecobiology, clinical symptoms and mode of action of domoic acid, an amnesic shellfish toxin. Chapter 15. In: L.M. Botana (ed.), *Seafood and Freshwater Toxins: Pharmacology, Physiology and Detection*. CRC Press, Boca Raton, FL, pp. 325–358.

94. Perl, T.M., Bedard, L., Kosatsky, T., Hockin, J.C., Todd, E.C., and Remis, R.S. 1990. An outbreak of toxic encephalopathy caused by eating mussels contaminated with domoic acid. *N. Engl. J. Med.* 322: 1775–1780.

95. Zhao, J., Thibault, P., and Quilliam, M.A. 1997. Analysis of domoic acid and isomers in seafood by capillary electrophoresis. *Electrophoresis* 18: 268–276.

96. Wright, J.L.C., Boyd, R.K., de Freitas, A.S.W., Falk, M., Foxall, R.A., Jamieson, W.D., Laycock, M.W. et al. 1989. Identification of domoic acid, a neuroexcitatory amino acid, in toxic mussels from Eastern Prince Edward Island. *Can. J. Chem.* 67: 481–490.

97. Lawrence, J.J. 1989. The toxicology of domoic acid administration systemically to rodents and primates. *Proceedings of the Symposium on Domoic Acid Toxicology*, Canada Diseases Weekly Report, Ottawa, April 10–11, 1989, Vol 16, pp. 27–31.

98. Quilliam, M.A., Sim, P.G., McCulloch, A.W., and McInnes, A.G. 1989. High performance liquid chromatography of domoic acid, a marine neurotoxin, with application to shellfish and plankton. *Int. J. Environ. Anal. Chem.* 36: 139–154.

99. Fernandez, M.L. and Cembella, A.D. 1995. Mammalian bioassays. In: G.M. Hallegraeff, D.M. Anderson, and A.D. Cembella (eds.), *Manual on Harmful Marine Microalgae*. IOC Manuals and Guides No. 33, UNESCO, Paris, France, pp. 213–224.

100. Lawrence, J.F., Charbonneau, C.F., Menard, C., Quilliam, M.A., and Sim, P.G. 1989. Liquid chromatographic determination of domoic acid in shellfish products using the AOAC paralytic shellfish poison extraction procedure. *J. Chromatogr.* 462: 349–356.

101. Lawrence, J.F., Charbonneau, C.F., and Menard, C. 1991. Liquid chromatographic determination of domoic acid in mussels using the AOAC paralytic shellfish poison extraction procedure: Collaborative study. *J. Assoc. Off. Anal. Chem.* 74: 68–72.

102. AOAC. 1991. Official method 991.26: Domoic acid in mussels, liquid chromatographic method, first action 1991. Official methods of analysis. Association of Official Analytical Chemists.

103. Grimmelt, B., Nijjar, M.S., Brown, J., MacNair, N., Wagner, S., Johnson, G.R., and Amend, J.J. 1990. Relationship between domoic acid levels in blue mussels (*Mytilus edulis*) and toxicity in mice. *Toxicon* 28: 501–508.

104. Vale, P. and Sampayo, M.A. 2002. Evaluation of extraction methods for analysis of domoic acid in naturally contaminated shellfish from Portugal. *Harmful Algae* 1: 127–135.

105. Novelli, A., Fernandez-Sanchez, M.T., Doucette, T.A., and Tasker, R.A.R. 2000. Chemical and biological detection methods. Chapter 18. In: L.M. Botana (ed.), *Seafood and Freshwater Toxins: Pharmacology, Physiology and Detection*. CRC Press, Boca Raton, FL, pp. 383–400.

106. Lawrence, J.F., Charbonneau, C.F., Page, B.D., and Lacroix, G.M.A. 1989. Confirmation of domoic acid in molluscan shellfish by chemical derivatization and reversed-phase liquid chromatography. *J. Chromatogr.* 462: 419–425.

107. Quilliam, M.A., Xie, M., and Hardstaff, W.R. 1991. A rapid extraction and clean-up procedure for the determination of domoic acid in tissue samples. National Research Council Canada Technical Report #64 (NRCC No. 33001).

108. Hatfield, C.L., Wekell, J.C., Gauglitz, E.J., and Barnett, H.J. 1994. Salt clean-up procedure for the determination of domoic acid by HPLC. *Nat. Toxins* 2: 206–211.

109. Lawrence, J.F., Lau, B.P., Cleroux, C., and Lewis, D. 1994. Comparison of UV absorption and electrospray mass spectrometry for high-performance liquid chromatographic detection of domoic acid in shellfish and biological samples. *J. Chromatogr. A* 659: 119–126.

110. Quilliam, M.A., Xie, M., and Hardstaff, W.R. 1995. Rapid extraction and cleanup for liquid chromatographic determination of domoic acid in unsalted seafood. *J. AOAC Int.* 78(2): 543–554.

111. Hess, P., Gallacher, S., Bates, L.A., Brown, N., and Quilliam, M.A. 2001. Determination and confirmation of the amnesic shellfish poisoning toxin, domoic acid, in shellfish from Scotland by liquid chromatography and mass spectrometry. *J. AOAC Int.* 84(5): 1657–1667.

112. CEN/TC 275. 2008. Foodstuffs—Determination of domoic acid in shellfish and finfish by RP-HPLC using UV detection. CEN/TC 275 WI 00275xxx:2008 (E).

113. EURLMB. 2008. EU-Harmonised Standard Operating Procedure for determination of domoic acid in shellfish and finfish by RP-HPLC using UV detection. Version 1, 2008. http://www.aesan.msps.es/CRLMB/docs/docs/procedimientos/EU-Harmonised-SOP-ASP-HPLC-UV_Version1.pdf

114. Hess, P., Morris, S., Stobo, L.A., Brown, N.A., McEvoy, J.D.G., Kennedy, G., Young, P.B., Slattery, D., McGovern, E., McMahon, T., and Gallacher, S. 2005. LC-UV and LC-MS methods for the determination of domoic acid. *Trends Anal. Chem.* 24(4): 358–367.

115. Vale, P. and Sampayo, M.A.M. 2001. Domoic acid in Portuguese shellfish and fish. *Toxicon* 39: 893–904.

116. Busse, L.B., Venrick, E.L., Antrobus, R., Miller, P.E., Vigilan, V., Silver, M.W., Mengelt, C., Mydlarz, L., and Prezelin, B.B. 2006. Domoic acid in phytoplankton and fish in San Diego, Ca, USA. *Harmful Algae* 5: 91–101.

117. Bogan, Y.W., Bender, K., Hervas, A., Kennedy, D.J., Slater, J.W., and Hess, P. 2007. Spatial variability of domoic acid concentrations in king scallops *Pecten maximus* off the southeast coast of Ireland. *Harmful Algae* 6: 1–14.

118. Stobo, L.A., Lacaze, J.-P.C.L., Scott, A.C., Petrie, J., and Turrell, E.A. 2008. Surveillance of algal toxins in shellfish from Scottish waters. *Toxicon* 51: 635–648.

119. NRCC. 2012. National Research Council of Canada, Biotoxin CRMs. http://www.nrc-cnrc.gc.ca/eng/solutions/advisory/crm/biotoxin_index.html (accessed August 2012).

120. James, K.J., Gillman, M., Lehane, M., and Gago-Martinez, A. 2000. New fluorometrix method of liquid chromatography for the determination of the neurotoxin domoic acid in phytoplankton. *J. Chromatogr. A.* 871: 1–6.

121. Pocklington, R., Milley, J.E., Bates, S.S., Bird, C.J., De Freitas, S.W., and Quilliam, M.A. 1990. Trace determination of domoic acid in seawater and phytoplankton by high-performance liquid chromatography of the fluorenylmethoxycarbonyl (FMOC) derivative. *Int. J. Environ. Anal. Chem.* 38: 351–368.

122. Chan, I.O.M., Tsang, V.W.H., Chu, K.K., Leung, S.K., Lam., M.H.W., Lau, T.C., Lam, P.K.S., and Wu, R.S.S. 2007. Solid-phase extraction-fluorimetric high performance liquid chromatographic determination of domoic acid in natural seawater mediated by an amorphous titania sorbent. *Anal. Chim. Acta* 583: 111–117.

123. Maroulis, M., Monemvasiois, I., Vardaka, E., and Rigas, P. 2008. Determination of domoic acid in mussels by HPC with post-column derivatisation using 4-chloro-7-nitrobenzo-2-oxa-1,3-diazole (NBD-Cl) and fluorescence detection. *J. Chromatogr. B* 876: 245–251.

124. Sun, T. and Wong, W.H. 1999. Determination of domoic acid in phytoplankton by high-performance liquid chromatography of the 6-aminoquinolyl-N-hydroxysuccinimidyl carbamate derivative. *J. Agric. Food Chem.* 47(11): 4678–4681.

125. Kumagai, M., Yanagi, T., Murata, M., Yasumoto, T., Kat, M., Lassus, P., and Rodriguez-Vazquez, J.A. 1986. Okadaic acid as the causative toxin of diarrhetic shellfish poisoning in Europe. *Agric. Biol. Chem.* 50: 2853–2857.

126. Hu, T., Doyle, J., Jackson, D., Marr, J., Nixon, E., Pleasance, S., Quilliam, M.A., Walter, J.A., and Wright, J.L.C. 1992. Isolation of a new diarrhetic shellfish poison from Irish mussel. *J. Chem. Soc. Chem. Commun.* Issue 1. 39–41.

127. Quilliam, M.A. 2003. Chemical methods for lipophilic shellfish. In: G.M. Hallegraeff, D.M. Anderson, and A.D. Cembella (eds.), *Manual on Harmful Marine Microalgae.* UNESCO, Saint-Berthevin, France, pp. 211–265.

128. Villar-González, A., Rodríguez-Velasco, M.L., Ben-Gigirey, B., Yasumoto, T., and Botana, L.M. 2008. Assessment of the hydrolysis process for the determination of okadaic acid-group toxin ester: Presence of okadaic acid 7-O-acyl-ester derivatives in Spanish shellfish. *Toxicon* 51: 765–773.

129. Yasumoto, T., Murata, M., Lee, J.S., and Torigoe, K. 1989. Polyether toxins produced by dinoflagellates. In: S. Natori, K. Hashimoto, and Y. Ueno (eds.), *Mycotoxins and Phycotoxins '88*. Elsevier, Amsterdam, the Netherlands, pp. 375–382.

130. Hu, T., Curtis, J.M., Oshima, Y., and Quilliam, M.A. 1995. Spirolide-B and spirolides-D, 2 novel macrocycles isolated from the digestive glands of shellfish. *J. Chem. Soc. Chem. Commun.* Issue 20. 2159–2161.

131. Ogino, J., Kumagai, M., and Yasumoto, T. 1997. Toxicologic evaluation of yessotoxins. *Nat. Toxins* 5: 255–259.

132. Draisci, R., Lucentini, L., and Mascioni, A. 2000. Pectenotoxins and yessotoxins: Chemistry, toxicology, pharmacology and analysis. In: L.M. Botana (ed.), *Seafood and Freshwater Toxins: Pharmacology, Physiology and Detection*. Marcel Dekker, New York, pp. 289–324.

133. Vale, P., Gomes, S.S., Lameiras, J., Rodrigues, S.M., Botelho, M.J., and Laycock, M.V. 2009. Assessment of a new lateral flow immunochromatographic (LFIC) assay for the okadaic acid group of toxins using naturally contaminated bivalve shellfish from the Portuguese coast. *Food Addit. Contam. A.* 26: 214.

134. Murata, M., Kumagai, M., Lee, J.S., and Yasumoto, T. 1987. Isolation and structure of yessotoxins, a novel polyether compound implicated in diarrhetic shellfish poisoning. *Tetrahedron Lett.* 28: 5869–5872.

135. European Food Safety Authority. 2008. Opinion of the Scientific Panel on Contaminants in the Food chain on a request from the European Commission on Marine biotoxins in shellfish—Yessotoxin group. *EFSA J.* 907: 1–62.

136. McMahon, T. and Silke, J. 1996. Winter toxicity of unknown aetiology in mussels. *Harmful Algae News* 14: 2.

137. Rehmann, N., Hess, P., and Quilliam, M.A. 2008. Discovery of new analogs of the marine biotoxin azaspiracid in blue mussels (*Mytilus edulis*) by ultra-performance liquid chromatography/tandem mass spectrometry. *Rapid Commun. Mass Spectrom.* 22: 549.

138. European Food Safety Authority. 2008. Opinion of the Scientific Panel on Contaminants in the Food chain on a request from the European Commission on Marine biotoxins in shellfish—Azaspiracid group. *EFSA J.* 723: 1–52.

139. Anon. 2005. Commission regulation (EC) No 2074/2005 of 5 December 2005. *Off. J. Eur. Communities.* L338: 27–59.

140. Suzuki, T., Jin, T., Shirota, Y., Mitsuya, T., Okumura, Y., and Kamiyama, T. 2005. Quantification of lipophilic toxins associated with diarrhetic shellfish poisoning in Japanese bivalves by liquid chromatography-mass spectrometry and comparison with mouse bioassay. *Fish. Sci.* 71: 1370–1378.

141. Lee, J.S., Yanagi, T., Kenma, R., and Yasumoto, T. 1987. Fluorometric determination of diarrhetic shellfish toxins by high-performance liquid chromatography. *Agric. Biol. Chem.* 51: 877–881.

142. Marr, J.C., McDowell, L.M., and Quilliam, M.A. 1994. Investigation of derivatisation reagents for the analysis of diarrhetic shellfish poisoning toxins by liquid chromatography with fluorescence detection. *Nat. Toxins* 2: 302–311.

143. Vale, P. and Sampayo, M.A. 1999. Esters of okadaic acid and dinophysistoxin-2 in Portuguese bivalves related to human poisonings. *Toxicon* 37: 1109–1121.

144. Fernandez, M.L., Miguez, A., Cacho, E., and Martinez, A. 1996. Detection of Okadaic acid esters in the hexane extracts of Spanish mussels. *Toxicon* 34(3): 381–387.

145. Draisci, R., Lucentini, L., Giannetti, L., and Stacchini, A. 1993. Diarrhetic shellfish toxins in mussels: Optimisation of HPLC method for okadaic acid determination. *Riv. Soc. Ital. Sci. Alim.* 4: 443–454.

146. Stockemer, J. and Geurke, M. 1993. Optimierung einer HPLC-methode zur bestimmung von DSP toxinen. *Arch. Lebensmittelhyg.* 44: 146–147.

147. Pereira, A., Klein, D., Sohet, K., Houvenaghel, G., and Braekman, J.C. 1995. Improvement to the HPLC-fluorescence analysis method for the determination of acid DSP toxins. In: P. Lassus, G. Arzul, E. Erard, P. Gentien, and C. Marcaillou-LeBaut (eds.), *Harmful Marine Algal Blooms*. Lavosier, Paris, France, pp. 333–338

148. Quilliam, M.A. 1995. Analysis of diarrhetic shellfish poisoning toxins in shellfish tissue by liquid chromatography with fluorometric and mass spectrometric detection. *J. AOAC Int.* 78: 555–570.

149. Aase, B. and Rogstad, E. 1997. Optimisation of sample clean-up procedure for the determination of diarrhetic shellfish poisoning toxins by use of experimental design. *J. Chromatogr.* 764: 223–231.

150. Shyre, M. and Unger, E. 1996. An alternative for the clean-up of ADAM derivatives of DSP toxins without halogenated solvents. In: T. Yasumoto, Y. Oshima, and Y. Fukuyo (eds.), *Harmful and Toxic Algal Blooms*. International Oceanographic Commission of UNESCO, Paris, France, pp. 535–538.

151. James, K.J., Bishop, A.G., Gillmann, M., Kelly, S.S., Roden, C., Draisci, R., Lucentini, L., Giannetti, L., and Boria, P. 1997. Liquid chromatography with fluorometric, mass spectrometric and tandem mass spectrometric detection to investigate the seafood toxin producing phytoplankton, *Dinophysis acuta*. *J. Chromatogr.* 777: 213–221.

152. Van de Riet, J.M., Burns, B.G., and Gilgan, M.W. 1995. A routine HPLC-Fluorescence method for the determination of the diarrhetic shellfish toxins Okadaic acid and DTX1–1 in shellfish. *Can. Tech. Fish. Aquat. Sci.* 1–26.

153. Quilliam, M.A., Gago-Martinez, A., and Vazquez, J.A. 1998. Improved method for preparation and use of 9-anthryldiazomethane for derivatisation of hydroxycarboxylic acids. Application to diarrhetic shellfish poisoning toxins. *J. Chromatogr. A.* 807: 229–239.

154. Yoshida, T., Uetake, A., Yamaguchi, H., Nimura, N., and Kinoshita, T. 1988. New preparation method for 9-anthryldiazomethane (ADAM) as a fluorescent labelling reagent for fatty acids and derivatives. *Anal. Biochem.* 173(1): 774.

155. Hummert, C., Shen, J.L., and Luckas, N. 1996. Automatic high-performance liquid chromatographic method for the determination of diarrhetic shellfish poison. *J. Chromatogr. A.* 729: 387–392.

156. Suzuki, T., Uchida, H., Watanabe, R., and Nagai, H. 2011. A convenient HPLC method of okadaic acid analogues as 9-Anthrulmethyl esters with an automatic column switching cleanup method. Marine and freshwater toxins analysis. *Second Joint Symposium and AOAC Task Force Meeting*, Baiona, Spain, May 1–5, 2011.

157. Ramstad, H., Larsen, S., and Aune, T. 2001. The repeatability of two HPLC methods and the PP2A assay in the quantification of diarrhetic toxins in blue mussels (*Mytilus edulis*). *Toxicon* 39: 515–522.

158. Pavela-Vrancic, M., Mestrovic, V., Marasovic, I., Gillman, M., Furey, A., and James, K.J. 2002. DSP toxin profile in the coastal waters of the central Adriatic Sea. *Toxicon* 40: 1601–1607.

159. Fernandez, M.I., Reguera, B., Ramilo, I., and Martinez, A. 2001. Toxin content of *Dinophysis acumiata*, *D. acuta* and *D. caudate* from the Galician Rias Bajas. In: G.M. Hallegraeff, S.I. Blackburn, C.J. Bolch, and R.J. Lewis (eds.), *Harmful Algal Blooms*. Intergovernment Oceanographic Commission of UNESCO, Paris, France, pp. 360–363.

160. Garcia, C., Gonzalez, V., Cornejo, C., Palma-Fleming, H., and Lagos, N. 2004. First evidence of dinophysistoxin-1 ester and carcinogenic polycyclic aromatic hydrocarbons in smoked bivalves collected in the Patagonia fjords. *Toxicon* 43: 121–131.

161. Garcia, C., Pruzzo, M., Rodriguez-Unda, N., Contreras, C., and Lagos, N. 2010. First evidence of Okadaic acid acyl-derivatives and dinophysistoxin-3 in mussel samples collected in Chiloe Island, Southern Chile. *J. Toxicol. Sci.* 35(3): 335–344.

162. Sar, E.A., Sunesen, I., Goya, A.B., Lavigne, A.S., Tapia, E., Garcia, C., and Lagos, N. 2012. First report of diarrheic shellfish toxins in molluscs from Buenos Aires Province (Argentina) associated with dinophysis spp.: Evidence of Okadaic acid, dinophysistoxin-1 and their acyl derivatives. *Bol. Soc. Argent.* 47(1–2): 5–14.

163. Mouratidou, T., Kaniou-Grigoriadou, I., Samara, C., and Kouimtzis, T. 2004. Determination of Okadaic acid and related toxins in Greek mussels by HPLC with fluorimetric detection. *J. Liq. Chromatogr. Relat. Technol.* 27(14): 1–14.

164. Mouratidou, T., Kaniou-Grigoriadou, I., Samara, C., and Kouimtzis, T. 2006. Detection of the marine toxin Okadaic acid in mussels during a diarrhetic shellfish poisoning (DSP) episode in Thermaikos Gulf, Greece, using biological, chemical and immunological methods. *Sci. Total. Environ.* 366: 894–904.

165. Nogueiras, M.J., Gago-Martinez, A., Paniello, A.I., Twohig, M., James, K.J., and Lawrence, J.F. 2003. Comparison of different fluorimetric HPLC methods for analysis of acidic polyether toxins in marine phytoplankton. *Anal. Bioanal. Chem.* 377: 1202–1206.

166. CEN. 2004. EN 14524: 2004 (E) Foodstuffs—Determination of Okadaic acid and dinophysis toxin in mussels—HPLC method with solid phase extraction clean-up after derivatisation and fluorimetric detection. CEN/TC 275 Secretariat

167. Louppis, A.P., Badeka, A.V., Katikou, P., Paleologos, E.K., and Kontominas, M.G. 2010. Determination of Okadaic acid, dinophysistoxin-1 and related esters in Greek mussels using HPLC with fluorometric detection, LC-MS/MS and mouse bioassay. *Toxicon* 55: 724–733.

168. Dickey, R.W., Granade, H.R., and Bencasth, F.A. 1993. Improved analytical methodology for the derivatisation and HPLC-fluorometrix determination of Okadaic acid in phytoplankton and shellfish. In: T.J. Smayda and Y. Simizu (eds.), *Toxic Phytoplankton Blooms in the Sea*, Elsevier, Amsterdam, the Netherlands, pp. 495–499.

169. Kelly, S.S., Bishop, A.G., Carmody, E.P., and James, K.J. 1996. Isolation of dinophysistoxin-2 and the high-performance liquid chromatographic analysis of diarrhetic shellfish toxins using derivatisation with 1-bromoacetylpyrene. *J. Chromatogr. A*. 749: 33–40.

170. Gonzalez, J.C., Leira, F., Vieytes, M.R., Vieites, J.M., Botana, A.M., and Botana, L.M. 2000. Development and validation of a high-performance liquid chromatographic method using fluorimetric detection for the determination of the diarrhetic shellfish poisoning toxin Okadaic acid without chlorinated solvents. *J. Chromatogr. A*. 876: 117–125.

171. Mak, K.C.Y., Yu, H., Choi, M.C., Shen, X., Lam, M.H.W., Martin, M., Wu, R.S.S., Wong, P.S., Richardson, B.J., and Lam, P.K.S. 2005. Okadaic acid, a causative toxin of diarrhetic shellfish poisoning, in green-lipped mussels *Perna viridis* from Hong Kong fish culture zones: Method development and monitoring. *Mar. Pollut. Bull.* 51: 1010–1017.

172. Prassopoulou, E., Katikou, P., Georgantelis, D., and Kyritsakis, A. 2009. Detection of okadaic acid and related esters in mussels during diarrhetic shellfish poisoning (DSP) episodes in Greece using the mouse bioassay, the PP2A inhibition assay and HPLC with fluorimetric detection. *Toxicon* 53: 214–227.

173. Hummert, C., Luckas, B., and Kirschbaum, J. 1995. HPLC/MS determination of diarrhetic shellfish poisoning (DSP) toxins as 4-bromo-7-methoxycoumarin derivatives. In: P. Lassus, G. Arzul, E. Erard, P. Gentien, and C. Marcaillou-Le Baut (eds.), *Harmful Marine Algal Blooms*. Lavoiser, Paris, France, pp. 297–302.

174. Akasak, K., Ohrui, H., Meguro, H., and Yasumoto, T. 1996. Fluorimetric determination of diarrhetic shellfish toxins in scallops and mussels by high-performance liquid chromatography. *J. Chromatogr. A* 729: 381–386.

175. Akasak, K., Ohrui, H., Meguro, H., and Yasumoto, T. 1996. Determination of dinophysis toxin-3 by the LC-LC method with fluorometric detection. *Anal. Sci.* 12: 557–560.

176. James, K.J., Furey, A., Healy, B., Kelly, S.S., and Twohig, M. 1998. A new fluorimetric reagent for the HPLC analysis of diarrhetic shellfish poisoning toxins. In: B. Reguera, J. Blanco, M.L. Fernandez, and T. Wyatt (eds.), *Harmful Algae*. Santiago de Compestella: Xunta de Galicia & Intergovernmental Oceanographic Commission of UNESCO, Vigo, Spain, pp. 519–520.

177. James, K.J., Bishop, A.R., Healy, B.M., Roden, C., Sherlock, I.R., Twohig, M., Draisci, R., Giannetti, C., and Lucentini, L. 1999. Efficient isolation of the rare diarrhetic shellfish toxin, dinophysistoxin-2, from marine phytoplankton. *Toxicon* 37: 343–357.

178. Morton, S.L. and Tindall, D.R. 1996. Determination of Okadaic acid content of dinoflagellates cells: A comparison of the HPLC-fluorescence method and two monoclonal antibody Alisa test kits. *Toxicon* 34(8): 947–954.

179. Garcia, C., Pereira, P., Valle, L., and Lagos, N. 2003. Quantitation of diarrhetic shellfish poisoning toxins in Chilean mussel using pyrenyldiazomethane as fluorescent labelling reagent. *Biol. Res.* 36(2): 171–183.

180. Zonta, F., Stancher, B., Bogoni, P., and Masoti, P. 1992. High-performance liquid chromatography of Okadaic acid and free fatty acids in mussels. *J. Chromatogr.* 594: 137–144.

181. Lawrence, J.F., Roussel, S., and Menard, C. 1996. Liquid chromatographic determination of Okadaic acid and dinophysistoxin-1 in shellfish after derivatisation with 9-chloromethylanthracene. *J. Chromatogr. A* 732: 359–364.

182. Rawn, D.F.K., Menard, C., Niedzwiadek, B., Lewis, D., Lau, B.P., Delauney-Beroncini, N., Hennion, M.C., and Lawrence, J.F. 2005. Confirmation of Okadaic acid, dinophysistoxin-1 and dinophysistoxin-2 in shellfish as their anthrylmethyl derivatives using UV radiation. *J. Chromatogr. A* 1080: 148–156.

183. Lee, J.S., Murata, M., and Yasumoto, T. 1989. Analytical methods for determination of diarrhetic shellfish toxins. In: S. Natori, K. Hashimoto, and Y. Ueno (eds.), *Bioactive Molecules: Mycotoxins and Phycotoxins '88*. Elsevier, Amsterdam, the Netherlands, pp. 327–334.

184. Yasumoto, T., Fukui, M., Sasaki, K., and Sugiyama, K. 1995. Determinations of marine toxins in foods. *J. AOAC Int.* 78(2): 574–582.

185. Daiguji, M., Satake, M., James, K.J., Bishop, A., Mackenzie, L., Naoki, H., and Yasumoto, T. 1998. Structures of new pectenotoxin analogs, pectenotoxin-2 seco acid and 7-epi-pectenotoxin-2 seco acid, isolated from dinoflagellates and greenshell mussels. *Chem. Lett.* 7: 653–654.

186. James, K.J., Bishop, A.G., Draisci, R., Palleschi, L., Marchiafava, C., Ferretti, E., Satake, M., and Yasumoto, T. 1999. Liquid chromatographic methods for the isolation and identification of new pectenotoxin-2 analogues from marine phytoplankton and shellfish. *J. Chromatogr. A* 844: 53–65.

187. Vale, P. and Sampayo, M.A. 2002. Pectenotoxin-2 seco acid, 7-epi-pectenotoxin-2 seco acid and pectenotoxin-2 in shellfish and plankton from Portugal. *Toxicon* 40: 979–987.

188. Suzuki, T., Mitsuya, T., Matsubara, H., and Yamasaki, M. 1998. Determination of pectenotoxin-2 after solid-phase extraction from seawater and from the dinoflagellates *Dinophysis fortii* by liquid chromatography with electrospray mass spectrometry and ultraviolet detection. Evidence of oxidation of pectenotoxin-2 to pectenotoxin-6 in scallops. *J. Chromatogr. A* 815(1): 155–160.

189. Miles, C.O., Wilkins, A.L., Munday, R., Dines, M.H., Hawkes, A.D., Briggs, L.R., Sandvik, M. et al. 2004. Isolation of pectenotoxin-2 from *Dinophysis acuta* and its conversion to pectenotoxin-2 seco acid and preliminary assessment of their acute toxicities. *Toxicon* 43: 1–9.

190. Yasumoto, T. and Satake, M. 1997. New toxins and their toxicological evaluations. *Proceedings of the 8th International Conference of Harmful Algae*, Vigo, Spain, pp. 461–464.

191. Sasaki, K., Wright, J.L.C., and Yasumoto, Y. 1998. The identification and characterisation of pectenotoxin PTX4 and PTX7 as spiroketal stereoisomers of two previously reported Pectenotoxins. *J. Org. Chem.* 63: 2475–2480.

192. Sasaki, K., Takizawa, A., Tubaro, A., Sidari, L., Loggia, R.D., and Yasumoto, Y. 1999. Fluorometric analysis of pectenotoxin-2 in microalgal samples by high performance liquid chromatography. *Nat. Toxins* 7(6): 241–246.

193. Yasumoto, T. and Takizawa, A. 1997. Fluorometric measurement of yessotoxins in shellfish by high-pressure liquid chromatography. *Biosci. Biotechnol. Biochem.* 61: 1775–1777.

194. Tubaro, A., Sidari, L., Della Loggia, R., and Yasumoto, T. 1997. Occurrence of Yessotoxin-like toxins in phytoplankton and mussels from northern Adriatic Sea. *Proceedings of the 8th International Conference of Harmful Algae*, Vigo, Spain, pp. 470–472.

195. Ramstad, H., Larsen, S., and Aune, T. 2001. Repeatability and validity of a fluorimetric HPLC method in the quantification of yessotoxins in blue mussels (*Mytilus edulis*) related to the mouse bioassay. *Toxicon* 39: 1393–1397.

196. Satake, M., MacKenzie, L., and Yasumoto, T. 1997. Identification of *Protoceratium reticulatum* as the biogenetic origin of yessotoxins. *Nat. Toxins* 5: 164–167.

197. Satake, M., Ichimura, T., Sekiguchi, K., Yoshimatsu, S., and Oshima, Y. 1999. Confirmation of yessotoxins and 45,46,47-trinoryessotoxin production by *Protoceratium reticulatum* collected in Japan. *Nat. Toxins* 7: 147–150.

198. Daiguji, M., Satake, M., Ramstad, H., Aune, T., Naoki, H., and Yasumoto, T. 1998. Structure and fluorometric HPLC determination of 1-desulfoyessotoxin, a new yessotoxins analog isolated from mussels from Norway. *Nat. Toxins* 6: 235–239.

199. Howard, M.D.A., Silver, M., and Kudela, R.M. 2008. Yessotoxin detected in mussel (*Mytilus californianus*) and phytoplankton samples from the U.S west coast. *Harmful Algae* 7: 646–652.

200. McCarron, P., Giddings, S.D., Miles, C.O., and Quilliam, M.A. 2011. Derivatisation of azaspiracid biotoxins for analysis by liquid chromatography with fluorescence detection. *J. Chromatogr. A* 1218: 8089–8096.

201. Parsons, M.L., Aligizaki, K., Dechraoui Bottein, M.-Y., Fraga, S., Morton, S.L., Penna, A., and Rhodes, L. 2012. *Gambierdiscus* and *Ostreopsis*: Reassessment of the state of knowledge of their taxonomy, geography, ecophysiology and toxicology. *Harmful Algae* 14: 107–129.

202. Hashimoto, Y., Fusetani, N., and Kimura, S. 1969. Aluterin: A toxin of filefish, *Alutera scripta*, probably originating from a zoantharia, *Palythoa tuberculosa*. *Bull. Jpn. Soc. Sci. Fish.* 35: 1086–1093.

203. Kukui, M., Murata, M., Inoue, A., Gawel, M., and Yasumoto, T. 1987. Occurrence of palytoxin in the trigger fish *Melichthys vidua*. *Toxicon* 25: 1121–1124.

204. Fusetani, N., Sato, S., and Hashimoto, K. 1985. Occurrence of water soluble toxin in a parrotfish *Ypsiscarus oviforns* which is probably responsible for parrotfish liver poisoning. *Toxicon* 23: 105–112.

205. Kodama, A.M., Hokama, Y., Yasumoto, T., Fukui, M., Manea, S.J., and Sutherland, N. 1989. Clinical and laboratory findings implicating palytoxin as cause of ciguatera poisoning due to *Decapterus macrosoma* (mackerel). *Toxicon* 9: 1051–1053.

206. Gozales, R.B. and Alcala, A.C. 1977. Fatalities from crab poisoning on Negros Island, Philippines. *Toxicon* 15: 169–170.

207. Yasumoto, T., Yasumura, D., Ohizumi, Y., Takahashi, M., Alcala, A.C., and Alcala, L.C. 1986. Palytoxin in two species of xanthis crab from the Philippines. *Agric. Biol. Chem.* 50: 1373–1377.

208. Aligizaki, K., Katikou, P., Milandri, A., and Diogene, J. 2011. Occurrence of palytoxin-group toxins in seafood and future strategies to complement the present state of the art. *Toxicon* 57: 390–399.

209. Moore, R.E. and Bartolini, G. 1981. Structure of palytoxin. *J. Am. Chem. Soc.* 103: 2491–2494.

210. Hirata, Y., Uemura, D., Ueda, K., and Takano, S. 1979. Several compounds from *Palythoa tuberculosa* (coelenterate). *Pure Appl. Chem.* 51: 1875–1883.

211. Ciminiello, P., Dell'Aversano, C., Fattorusso, E., Forino, M., and James, C.F. 2009. Recent developments in Mediterranean Harmful Algal Events. *Advances in Molecular Toxicology*. Vol 3., Elsevier, pp. 1–41.

212. Deeds, J.R., Handy, S.M., Whilte, K.D., and Reimer, J.D. 2011. Palytoxin found in *Palythoa sp. I zoanthids* (Anthozoa, Hexacorallia) solid in the home aquarium trade. *PLoS One* 6(4): e18235.

213. CRLMB (Community Reference Laboratory for Marine Biotoxins). 2005. *Minutes of the 1st Meeting of Working Group on Toxicology of the National Reference Laboratories (NRLs) for Marine Biotoxins*. Cesenatico, Italy, October 2005, pp. 24–25. http://www.aesan.msps.es (accessed August 2012).

214. EFSA. 2009. Scientific opinion on marine biotoxins in shellfish—Palytoxin group. EFSA Panel on Contaminants in the Food Chain (CONTAM). *EFSA J.* 7(12): 1393: 1–38.

215. Riobo, P., Paz, B., and Franco, J.M. 2006. Analysis of palytoxin-like in *ostreopsis* cultures by liquid chromatography with precolumn derivatisation and fluorescence detection. *Anal. Chim. Acta* 566: 217–233.

216. Alcala, A.C., Alcala, L.C., Garth, J.S., Yasumura, D.Y., and Yasumoto, T. 1988. Human fatality due to ingestion of the crab *Demania reynaudii* that contained a palytoxin-like toxin. *Toxicon* 26(1): 1050107.

217. Fukui, M., Murata, M., Inoue, A., Gawel, M., and Yasumoto, T. 1987. Occurrence of palytoxin in the trigger fish *Melichthys vidua*. *Toxicon* 25(10): 1121–1124.

218. Noguchi, T., Deng-Fwu Hwang, O., Arakawa, H., Sugita, H., Deguchi, Y., Narita, H., Shimidu, U., Kungsuwan, A., Miyazawa, K., and Hashimoto, K. 1988. Palytoxin as the causative agent in parrotfish poisoning. *Toxicon* 26: 34.

219. Lau, C.O., Khoo, H.E., Yuen, R., Wan, M., and Tan, C.H. 1993. Isolation of a novel fluorescent toxin from the coral reef crab, *Lophozozymus pictor*. *Toxicon* 31: 1341–1345.

220. Lau, C.O., Tan, C.H., Khoo, H.E., Yuen, R., Lewis, R.J., Corpuz, G.P., and Bignami, G.S. 1995. *Lophozozymus pictor* toxin: A fluorescent structural isomer of palytoxin. *Toxicon* 33(10): 1373–1377.

221. Mereish, K.A., Morris, S., McCullers, G., Taylor, T.J., and Bunner, D.L. 1991. Analysis of palytoxin by liquid chromatography and capillary electrophoresis. *J. Liq. Chromatogr.* 14: 1025–1031.

222. Gleibs, S., Mebs, D., and Werding, S. 1995. Studies on the origin and distributions of palytoxin in a Caribbean coral reef. *Toxicon* 33(11): 1531–1537.

223. Gleibs, S. and Mebs, D. 1999. Distribution and sequestration of palytoxin in coral reef animals. *Toxicon* 37: 1521–1527.

224. Lenoir, S., Ten-Hage, L., Turguet, J., Quod, J.-P., Bernard, C., and Hennion, M.-C. 2004. First evidence of palytoxin analogues from an *Ostreopsis mascarenensis* (Dinophyceae) bloom in southwestern Indian Ocean. *J. Phycol.* 40: 1042–1051.

225. Riobo, P. and Franco, J.M. 2011. Palytoxins: Biological and chemical determination. *Toxicon* 57: 368–375.

226. Isbister, G.K. and Kiernan, M.C. 2005. Neurotoxic marine poisoning. *Lancet Neurol.* 4: 218–228.

227. Wu, Z., Xie, L., Xia, G., Zhang, J., Nie, Y., Hu, J., Wang, S., and Zhang, R. 2005. A new tetrodotoxin-producing actinomycete, *Nocardiopsis dassonvillei*, isolated from the ovaries of puffer fish *Fugu rubripes*. *Toxicon* 45: 851–859.

228. Kawabata, T. 1978. *Food Hygiene Examination Manual Vol. 2*. Environmental Health Bureau, Ministry of Health and Welfare of Japan, Food Hygiene Association, Tokyo, Japan, pp. 232–240.

229. Yasumoto, T., Nakamura, M., Oshima, Y., and Takahata, J. 1982. Construction of a continuous tetrodotoxins analyser. *Bull. Jpn. Soc. Sci. Fish.* 48(10): 1481–1483.

230. Yasumoto, T. and Michishita, T. 1985. Fluorometric determination of tetrodotoxin by high performance liquid chromatography. *Agric. Biol. Chem.* 49:3077–3080.

231. Yotsu, M., Endo, A., and Yasumoto, T. 1989. An improved Tetrodotoxin analyser. *Agric. Biol. Chem.* 53: 893.
232. Mebs, D., Yotsu-Yamashita, M., Yasumoto, T., Lotters, S., and Schluter, A. 1995. Further report of the occurrence of tetrodotoxin in *Atelopus* species (Family: Bufonidae). *Toxicon* 33(2): 246–249.
233. Chen, C.-Y. and Chou, H.-N. 1998. Detection of Tetrodotoxin by high performance liquid chromatography in Lined-Moon Shell and Puffer Fish. *Acta Zoologica Taiwanica* 9(1): 41–48.
234. Hanifin, C.T., Yotsu-Yamashita, M., Yasumoto, T., Brodie, E.D., and Brodie, E.D. 1999. Toxicity of dangerous prey: Variation of tetrodotoxin levels within and among populations of the newt *Taricha granulosa. J. Chem. Ecol.* 25(9): 2161–2173.
235. Yotsu-Yamashita, M. and Mebs, D. 2003. Occurrence of 11-oxotetrodotoxin in the red-spotted newt, *Notophthalmus viridescens*, and further studies on the levels of tetrodotoxin and its analogues in the newt's efts. *Toxicon* 41: 893–897.
236. Yotsu-Yamashita, M., Gilhen, J., Russell, R.W., Krysko, K.L., Melaun, C., Kurz, A., Kauferstein, S., Kordis, D., and Mebs, D. 2012. Variability of tetrodotoxin and of its analogues in the red-spotted newt, *Notophthalmus viridescens* (Amphibia: Urodela: Salamandridae). *Toxicon* 59: 257–264.
237. Jen, H.-C., Lin, S.-J., Lin, S.-Y., Huang, I.Y.W., Liao, I.C., Arakawa, O., and Hwang, D.F. 2007. Occurrence of tetrodotoxin and paralytic shellfish poisons in a gastropod implicated in food poisoning in southern Taiwan. *Food Addit. Contam.* 24(8): 902–909.
238. Jen, H.-C., Lin, S.-J., Tsai, Y.-H., Chen, C.-H., Lin, Z.-C., and Hwang, D.F. 2008. Tetrodotoxin poisoning evidenced by solid-phase extraction combining with liquid chromatography-tandem-mass spectrometry. *J. Chromatogr. A* 871: 95–100.
239. Kawatsu, K., Shibata, T., and Hamano, Y. 1999. Application of immunoaffinity chromatography for detection of tetrodotoxin from urine samples of poisoned patients. *Toxicon* 37: 325–333.
240. O'Leary, M.A., Schneider, J.J., and Isbister, G.K. 2004. Use of high performance liquid chromatography to measure tetrodotoxin in serum and urine of poisoned patients. *Toxicon* 44: 549–553.
241. Yu, C.H., Yu, C.F., Tam, S., and Yu, P.H.F. 2010. Rapid screening of tetrodotoxin in urine and plasma of patients with pufferfish poisoning by HPLC with creatinine correction. *Food Addit. Contamin.* 27: 89–96.
242. Baden, D.G., Bourdelais, A.J., Jacocks, H., Michelliza, S., and Naar, J. 2005. Natural and derivative brevetoxins: Historical background, multiplicity and effects. *Environ. Health. Perspect.* 113: 621–625.
243. Dickey, R., Jester, E., Granade, R., Mowdy, D., Moncreiff, C., Rebarchik, D., Robl, M., Musser, S., and Poli, M. 1999. Monitoring brevetoxins during a *Gymnodinium breve* red tide: Comparison of sodium channel specific cytotoxicity assay and mouse bioassay for determination of neurotoxic shellfish toxins in shellfish extracts. *Nat. Toxins.* 7: 157–165.
244. Plakas, S.M. and Dickey, R.W. 2010. Advances in monitoring and toxicity assessment of brevetoxins in molluscan shellfish. *Toxicon* 56: 137–149.
245. Poli, M.A., Musser, S.M., Dickey, R., Eilers, P., and Hall, S. 2000. Neurotoxic shellfish poisoning and brevetoxin metabolites: A case study from Florida. *Toxicon* 38: 981–983.
246. Pierce, R.H., Henry, M.S., Proffitt, L.S., and deRosset, A.J. 1992. Evaluation of solid sorbents for the recovery of polyether toxins (brevetoxins) in seawater. *Bull. Environ. Contam. Toxicol.* 49: 479–484.
247. Pierce, R.H., Henry, M.S., Blum, P.C., Lyons, J., Cheng, Y.S., Yassie, D., and Zhou, Y. 2003. Brevetoxin concentrations in marine aerosol: Human exposure levels during a *Karenia brevis* harmful algal bloom. *Bull. Environ. Contam. Toxicol.* 70(1): 161–165.
248. Dickey, R.W., Bencasth, F.A., Granade, H.R., and Lewis, R.J. 1992. Liquid chromatographic mass spectrometric methods for the determination of marine polyether toxins. *Bull. Soc. Pathol. Exot.* 85: 514–515.
249. Dickey, R.W. and Plakas, S.M. 2009. Ciguatera: A public health perspective. *Toxicon* 56(2): 123–136.
250. Caillaud, A., de la Iglesia, P., Darius, H.T., Pauillac, S., Aligizaki, K., Fraga, S., Chinain, M., and Diogene, J. 2010. Update on methodologies available for ciguatoxin determination: Perspectives to confront the onset of ciguatera fish poisoning in Europe. *Mar. Drugs.* 8: 1838–1907.
251. Yasumoto, T., Raj, U., and Bagnis, R. 1984. *Seafood Poisoning in Tropical Regions*. Laboratory of Food Hygiene, Faculty of Agriculture, Tohoku University, Sendai-shi, Japan.
252. Guzman-Perez, S.E. and Park, D.L. 2000. Ciguatera toxins: Chemistry and detection. In: L.M. Botana (ed.), *Seafood and Freshwater Toxins: Pharmacology, Physiology and Detection*. CRC Press, Boca Raton, FL.
253. Vernoux, J.-P. and Lewis, R.J. 1997. Isolation and characterisation of Caribbean ciguatoxins from the horse-eye jack (*Caranx latus*). *Toxicon* 35(6): 889–900.

254. Sick, L., Hansenm, D., Babinchak, J., and Higerd, D. 1986. An HPLC-Fluorescence method for identifying a toxic fraction extracted from the marine dinoflagellates *Gambierdiscus toxicus*. *Mar. Fish. Rev.* 48: 29–34.

255. Yasumoto, T., Satake, M., Fukui, M., Nagai, H., Murata, M., and Legrand, A.D. 1993. A turning point in ciguatera study. In: T.J. Smayda and Y. Shimizu (eds.), *Toxin Phytoplankton Blooms in the Sea*. Elsevier, New York, pp. 455–461.

256. Miller, D.M., Tindall, D.R., and Jacyno, M. 1989. Preparative HPLC separation of maitotoxin from crude extracts of *Gambierdiscus toxicus*. *Toxicon* 27(1): 64–65.

257. Boisier, P., Ranaivoson, G., Rasolofonirina, N., Andriamahefazafy, B., Roux, J., Chanteau, S., Satake, M., and Yasumoto, T. 1995. Fatal mass poisoning in Madagascar following ingestion of a shark (*Carcharhinus leucas*): Clinical and epidemiological aspects and isolation of toxins. *Toxicon* 33: 1359–1364.

258. Yasumoto, T. 1998. Fish poisoning due to toxins of microalgal origins in the Pacific. *Toxicon* 36(11): 1515–1518.

259. Otero, A., Chapela, M.J., Atanassova, M., Vieites, J.M., and Cabado, A.G. 2011. Cyclic imines: Chemistry and mechanism of action: A review. *Chem. Res. Toxicol.* 24(11): 1817–1829.

260. Torigoe, K., Murata, M., Yasumoto, T., and Iwashita, T. 1988. Prorocentrolide, a toxic nitrogenous macrocycle from a marine dinoflagellates, *Prorocentrum lima*. *J. Am. Chem. Soc.* 110: 7876–7877.

261. Marrouchi, R., Dziri, F., Belayouni, N., Hamza, A., Benoit, E., Molgo, J., and Kharrat, R. 2010. Quantitative determination of Gymnodimine-A by high performance liquid chromatography in contaminated clams from Tunisia Coastline. *Mar. Biotechnol. (NY)* 387: 2475–2486.

14

Analysis of Marine Biotoxins by Liquid Chromatography Mass Spectrometric Detection

Arjen Gerssen

CONTENTS

14.1 Introduction

In recent years, there is a definite increase in the use of liquid chromatography coupled to mass spectrometry for the analysis of marine biotoxins. When performing a search in the Scopus database on the search terms mass spectrometry and marine biotoxins, it becomes clear that over the last 20 years a total of 492 publications are present in the database. The majority of these references (85%; $n = 418$) were published in the last 10 years, and in the last 5 years more than 50% ($n = 268$) were published. This increase in popularity of mass spectrometric detection is present in all analytical research fields.

For the liquid chromatographic mass spectrometric detection of marine biotoxins, we can distinguish between various types of methods. First, we have methods that are intended to be used for research purposes such as the detection and structure elucidation of new toxins or toxin metabolites. Secondly, LC-MS methods intended for use in routine applications or surveys of known toxins in various commodities. Within this chapter, both types of application fields will be discussed. Also, the recent developments in the field of liquid chromatography mass spectrometric detection will be discussed, which are the use of high-resolution chromatography (ultra performance or very high pressure LC) and high-mass accuracy, high-resolution mass spectrometric detection such as time-of-flight or Orbitrap MS. The overview given in this chapter will focus on the two groups of marine biotoxins. Based on their chemical properties, marine biotoxins can be divided into two different classes: hydrophilic and lipophilic marine biotoxins. Toxins associated with the syndromes amnesic shellfish poisoning (ASP) and paralytic shellfish poisoning (PSP) are more or less hydrophilic and have a molecular weight below 500 Da. Toxins responsible for diarrhetic shellfish poisoning (DSP), azaspiracid shellfish poisoning (AZP), neurologic shellfish poisoning (NSP), ciguatera fish poisoning (CFP), and other toxins such as pectenotoxins (PTXs), yessotoxins (YTXs), cyclic imines, and palytoxins all have as common denominator a molecular weight above 500 Da (up to 3000 Da). These toxins have certain lipophilic properties and therefore will be discussed in this chapter as lipophilic marine biotoxins.

14.2 Hydrophilic Marine Biotoxins

14.2.1 Domoic Acid

In this section, the various LC-MS methods for hydrophilic marine biotoxins are discussed. The toxin responsible for ASP is domoic acid (DA). After the discovery of this toxin responsible for ASP intoxication, several LC-MS methods were developed.[1] The first LC-MS papers published on this topic focused on the detection of DA and several isomers (A–G). Electrospray ionization (ESI) was and is still used as the preferred ionization technique not only for DA but in general for all marine biotoxins. Pineiro et al. optimized as one of the first a LC-MS method for DA and various analogs. Using isocratic HPLC under reversed phase conditions followed by single ion monitoring (SIM) DA could be detected as well as other compounds present in the shellfish extract. DA with a molecular ion of m/z of 312 [M+H]$^+$ and possible masses that could be related to hydroxylated DA (m/z 327) were also detected.[2] Also, fragmentation studies were performed for DA by using techniques such as ion trap MS. With ion trap MS, it is possible to perform multiple fragmentation steps and after each fragmentation step isolating the produced fragment for the next fragmentation step; this is also called MS^n experiments. This type of fragmentation is called fragmentation in time as each step occurs at a different time. Furey et al. studied and elucidated the fragmentation pathway of DA using these LC-MS^n experiments.[3] With five fragmentation steps (MS^5) they were able to propose a fragmentation pathway. The other applied MS technique is tandem mass spectrometry using a triple quadrupole MS, which is currently by far the most applied MS technique for marine biotoxins. Fragmentation within a triple quadrupole is done by first selecting the ion of interest in the first quadrupole, often the protonated molecular ion (i.e., m/z 312 for [M+H]$^+$). In the second quadrupole, an inert gas and energy is applied to induce fragmentation of the ion, so-called collision-induced dissociation (CID). In the third quadrupole, the produced fragment ion can be filtered and subsequently measured by the detector (i.e., m/z 266 [M+H–HCOOH]$^+$) (Figure 14.1). These techniques are so-called tandem in space techniques where the ion selection and fragmentation occur in different parts of the instruments.

Being a single compound, DA is often incorporated in multitoxin methods like including the toxin within the LC-MS/MS analysis of DSP or PSP toxins. Both in reversed phase conditions (used for DSP) and hydrophilic interaction chromatography (HILIC) conditions (used for PSP), it is possible to incorporate DA.[4,5] In 2003, an in-house validated method was published using reversed phase conditions and ESI-MS/MS. This method showed a low measurement uncertainty at levels between 5 and 50 mg/kg (RSD$_r$ ~ 8%), and the estimated limit of detection was 0.15 mg DA/kg. The method was developed using conventional LC with a total analysis time of 10 min.[6] In 2011, an LC-MS/MS method using the latest generation equipment was developed and validated according to EU criteria (657/2002/EC).[7] By

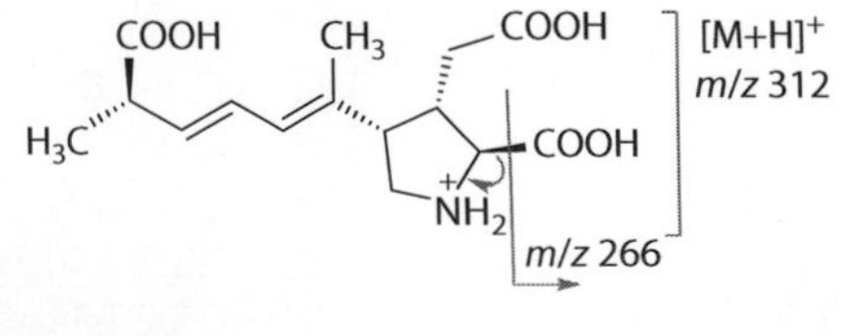

FIGURE 14.1 Fragmentation pathway domoic acid.

applying ultra-performance chromatography, de la Iglesia et al. were able to separate DA and epi-DA within less than 3 min. Also, the limits of detection reported in this study were far below the regulatory limit of 20 mg DA/kg edible shellfish between 0.05 and 0.09 mg DA/kg. In literature, till today one inter-laboratory validation study has been performed that included DA. Unfortunately the study performed by McNabb et al. was partly using shellfish extracts instead of shellfish homogenates.[5] Hence, till now no formal inter-laboratory study has been organized for DA in shellfish products. Therefore, the (EU) legislation is still referring to reference methods such as LC-UV while LC-MS/MS has proven to be more selective, specific, and sensitive.

14.2.2 Paralytic Shellfish Poisoning Toxins

For PSP toxins, more than 50 different analogs are described in literature.[8] For each of these analogs, the toxicity differs and worldwide different toxicity factors have been applied.[9,10] These variations complicate the analysis of PSP toxins in shellfish. Also, the applied chemical detection methods such as the HPLC-FLD methods have pros and cons in the separation and detection of certain analogs.[11–14] Till today, these HPLC-FLD methods are the only chemical methods for PSP toxins that were successfully validated through inter-laboratory validation studies.[11,12] The complexity of the PSPs is mainly due to the polarity of the toxins as well as their structural similarities. Mass spectrometric analysis methods for PSP toxins and the application in shellfish monitoring programs are still in their infancy. In literature, a few different LC-MS/MS methods or derivatives of these methods have been described.[15–17] As mentioned earlier, the PSP toxins are polar and therefore a different retention mechanism is required compared to other marine biotoxins applications. Furthermore, also important, the mobile phase composition should be compatible with the mass spectrometer. Therefore, the HPLC-FLD methods that are using reversed phase conditions are not compatible with mass spectrometric detection. The so-called HPLC-FLD Lawrence method[11] is using precolumn oxidation, which results in the same but multiple reaction products for some isomeric analogues, for example, gonyautoxin-1 and -4 (GTX1, 4). For mass spectrometric detection, this is not desirable as multiple oxidation reaction products should then be analyzed making data analysis more complex. The post-column oxidation HPLC-FLD method described by van de Riet et al.[12] has the advantage that the toxins are separated before the oxidation occurs; therefore, analogs that differ in toxicity factors are separated and data analysis is more simple. Unfortunately, the mobile phase conditions used in this method, a low percentage of organic solvent and ion-pair reagents, are not preferred within LC-MS analysis. Therefore, the use of the reversed phase conditions for PSP toxins, which generally consists of a low-percentage organic solvent and nonvolatile salts, is not suitable for LC-MS. One of the first mass spectrometric applications for the detection of PSPs was using capillary electrophoresis (CE) as a separation tool.[18,19] Although this approach seemed promising, the use of CE-MS was never applied on a large scale. This was due to the effect of salts that originate from the sample extract, and the multiple injections that were needed to analyze the different toxins having different charge states. Applications developed more recently used ion-exchange chromatography (IEC) mass spectrometry.[17] A problem with both CE and IEC is the use of relatively MS unfavorable salts that are nonvolatile or causing major signal suppression. IEC, for example, can be applied using heptanesulfonic acid that will cause problems with ionization efficiencies. Therefore, the most promising approach is the use of HILIC chromatography. This type of chromatography is using comparable mobile phase compositions as the MS applications using reversed phase chromatography. In general, HILIC can be applied for the separation of polar and charged compounds. The first HILIC-MS/MS method for a wide variety of PSP toxins was developed by Quilliam et al., and studied in depth by Dell' Aversano et al.[15,20] The developed method uses a TSK-gel Amide-80 column and LC conditions containing MS favorable mobile phase compositions such as a high-percentage acetonitrile (>60%), ammonium formate, and formic acid. From this paper, it also becomes clear that although the tandem mass spectrometry is a powerful and promising tool for PSP toxins analysis and can be more selective than the HPLC-FLD methods, there are also some drawbacks. These drawbacks are described by the authors and are in general applicable for all PSP toxin analyses with LC-MS/MS. The first drawback is the in-source fragmentation resulting in the loss of SO_3 for the PSP toxins with a sulfonic acid in the α-orientation on the C-11 group (Figure 14.2). This can be a problem for identification as, for example, gonyautoxin-2

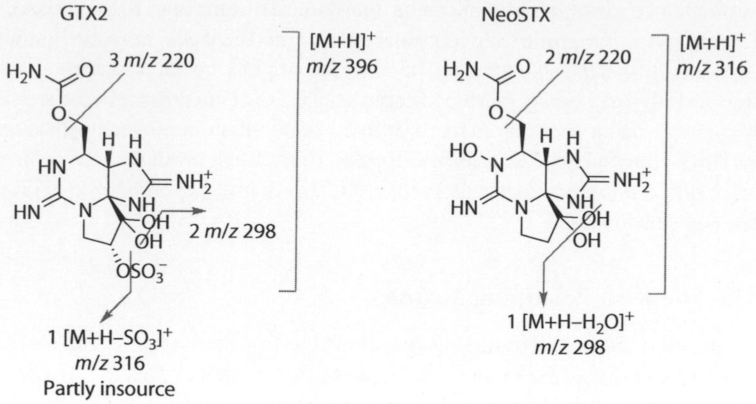

FIGURE 14.2 Fragmentation of GTX2 and neo-saxitoxin under ESI⁺.

(GTX2) gives in ESI predominantly a precursor ion of m/z 316 [M+H–SO₃]⁺, which is the same m/z as the [M+H]⁺ for neo-saxitoxin. As the various structures show large similarities, the product ions also are similar; this results in, for example, multiple peaks (up to 4) in the MRM transition m/z 316 → 298. So it can be concluded that for PSP toxins chromatographic separation is of key importance as separation by selecting different precursors and product ions will not give the selectivity needed. The second general problem the authors recognized, is that HILIC is very sensitive to the presence of salts in the extract. Due to the relatively high amount of salts present in the shellfish, retention times tend to shift under HILIC conditions up to minutes. Furthermore, quite a high number of interfering peaks appear in the chromatogram when analyzing shellfish extracts with LC-MS/MS. This suggests that there is a need for extensive sample clean-up in order to remove salts (avoid retention time shifts) and interfering peaks. A second HILIC approach, studied in detail by Diener et al., uses a zwitter-ionic HILIC stationary phase.[16] With this method the separation of the various PSP toxin analogues (e.g., GTX1 and GTX4) is superior to the method published by Dell'Aversano et al. Furthermore, this method also produced stable retention times for the toxins in various matrices such as mussels and algae (*Alexandrium catenella*). Although the authors suggest that it is feasible to apply this method on a routine basis, still a 40-min run is required for the analysis of these toxins. This will hamper the implementation into routine monitoring programs that require results within a short time frame.

According to Turrell et al. with both methods mentioned earlier, the sensitivity for some of the PSP toxins is poor and matrix effects occur that have an effect on sensitivity and retention time stability. These issues hampered the implementation of these applications into official control programs.[21] Therefore, Turrell et al. and Sayfritz et al. improved the application by investigating different types of clean-up such as solid phase extraction.[22] These improvements in the methodologies will contribute to make these applications at the end fit-for-purpose for routine monitoring programs. Till today no full inter-laboratory studies for LC-MS/MS methods for PSP toxins have been performed. Therefore, till now within the field of PSP toxins, the LC-MS/MS techniques are mainly used for research applications.[23–25]

14.3 Regulated Lipophilic Marine Biotoxins

In what follows, various toxin classes will be discussed. First, the traditional lipophilic marine biotoxins will be discussed, such as diarrheic shellfish poisoning (DSP) toxins, AZP toxins, PTXs, and YTXs. All these toxins show a similar retentive behavior in LC systems, and therefore these toxins are often analyzed in a single multitoxin analysis. The multitoxin methods are often only focusing on the regulated lipophilic marine biotoxins.[5,26,27] Thirteen different lipophilic marine biotoxins are currently stated in EU legislation. The EU is more stringent than other international bodies such as the US Food and Drug Administration (FDA) and CODEX. These bodies do not mention the PTXs and YTXs; therefore, there is continuous discussion on the compliance of shellfish with legislation. PTXs and YTXs are included in EU legislation due to their intraperitoneal (i.p.) toxicity in the mouse bioassay (MBA), which was the official reference method for lipophilic marine biotoxins. Within the EU legislation, a multitoxin method for lipophilic marine biotoxins is now established and is applicable for monitoring programs.[28] From a research perspective, it is interesting to have dedicated methods for certain toxin classes, for example, to investigate the formation of metabolites within shellfish, production of certain toxins by algae or effects of treatments such as heat or radiation.[29,30] The validation of multitoxin methods used for official control is discussed later; first, the individual toxin groups will be discussed and specific dedicated LC-MS methodologies.

14.3.1 Okadaic Acid and Dinophysistoxins

For the diarrheic shellfish poisoning toxins (okadaic acid [OA] and dinophysistoxins [DTXs]), several studies have been conducted on the fragmentation of OA by using various types of ionization such as fast atom bombardment (FAB), thermospray, ion spray, and electrospray,[31,32] where the latter is nowadays used most frequently. OA and DTXs contain a carboxylic acid functionality and therefore both negative electrospray ionization and positive electrospray ionization can be used. For both types of ionization, fragmentation pathways have been proposed.[33,34] In positive ionization, the obtained main fragments are not specific and consist of multiple losses of water ($[M+H-nH_2O]^+$ where $n = 1$–4). In the negative ionization mode, the fragments obtained are more from skeletal fragmentation (Figure 14.3). Also, sensitivity is somewhat better in the negative ionization mode because of the lower number of background ions present. In negative ionization mode, OA and DTXs tend to produce the same fragments such as m/z 255, 563, and 151. OA and DTX2 have the same elemental composition and molecular weight (mw 805); therefore, the MS is not able to distinguish between these toxins.

Recently, Carey et al. showed that in positive ionization the fragmentation of the sodium adduct ($[M+Na]^+$ m/z 827) of both OA and DTX2 resulted in different product ions, respectively, m/z 595, 443, and 151 for OA and m/z 581, 429, and 165 for DTX2.[35] By using the different transitions of m/z 827 → 595 and m/z 827 → 581 for, respectively, OA and DTX2, a clear separation in both chromatography and mass spectrometry could be obtained. With the fragmentation pathways more or less fully elucidated, methods for detecting different types of OA and DTXs in algae and shellfish have been described. The main the methods investigating OA and DTXs are focusing on the esters, which in general are named dinophysistoxin-3 (DTX3). The majority of these esters are produced in shellfish (acyl esters) and a small number in algae, the diol esters. The diol esters are, for example, produced by *Prorocentrum lima* and *Dinophysis acuta* and can only be found in algae as it is known that certain esterases present in shellfish can hydrolyze these diol esters toward the unconjugated toxin again. Torgersen et al. studied various esters in detail using ion trap and tandem mass spectrometric techniques.[36,37] The diol esters were studied in positive electrospray ionization mode. For the OA diol esters, a common fragment could be obtained that corresponds to the loss of the diol group ($[M-diol+Na]^+$ m/z 827). Furthermore, the authors also found hybrid esters within shellfish. These are toxins containing a diol ester and a fatty acid ester; the most abundant observed was the OA 16:0 C-8-diol. Besides the diol and fatty acid esters, also some sulfated esters of OA were isolated from algae. These sulfonic acid–containing esters are DTX4, DTX5a, DTXb, and DTX5c.[38,39] These toxins were investigated by high-resolution mass spectrometry to obtain an elemental composition of the protonated molecule as well as fragmentation information with a high mass accuracy.

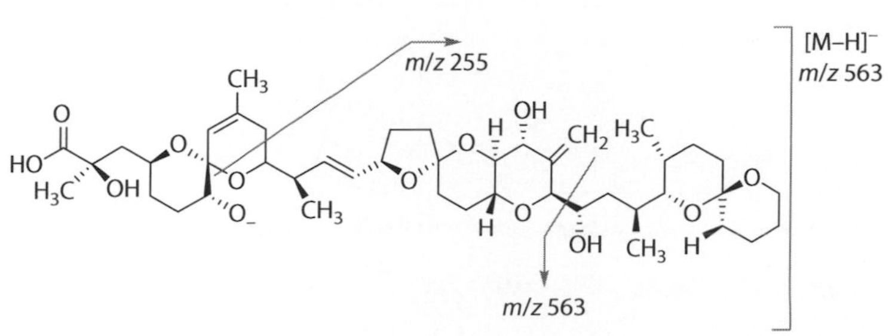

FIGURE 14.3 Proposed fragmentation pathway okadaic acid in ESI⁻.

With mass spectrometry, structures can be proposed only; both authors (Hu et al. and Cruz et al.) used NMR to confirm the structure. Suarez-Gomez et al. detected DTX6 as well as several unknown okadaic acid–related compounds in algae.[40,41] From a mass spectrometric point of view, an interesting study was done by Paz et al. on DTX5c as well as on 7-hydroxymethyl-2-methylene-octa-4,7-dienyl okadate.[42] In this research, interesting molecular ions were found such as [M+Na+NH$_4$–H]$^+$, [M+2NH$_4$–H]$^+$, and [M+3Na–2H]$^+$; which were attributed to the presence of the sulfate group. In general, in routine applications, shellfish extracts are analyzed first without hydrolysis followed by analysis after hydrolysis. The difference between the concentrations found for OA, DTX1, and DTX2 is the amount of esters (DTX3) present in the sample. Legislation (EU, FDA, and CODEX) is based on the sum of the total amount of OA equivalents per kilogram of edible shellfish, which is the sum of OA, DTX1, and DTX2 after hydrolysis and taking into account their toxicity factors. Therefore, in routine applications, there is no need to distinguish between the various esters that can be present in shellfish samples.

14.3.2 Pectenotoxins

In literature, over 15 different PTXs have been described.[43,44] The first PTXs were described in 1985 by Yasumoto et al.[45] Intoxication had occurred in Japan in 1976 and 1977 after the consumption of contaminated scallops. From these scallops, besides OA and DTX1, PTX1 and PTX2 were isolated. It seems that PTX1 is only occurring in Japanese scallops and within Europe the most predominant PTX in algae is PTX2. In shellfish, PTX2 is rapidly metabolized by esterases to PTX2 seco acid.[46] As the PTX molecule is neutral, it can be ionized in both positive and negative ionization although the majority of the published research on PTXs is preferring positive ionization.[47] In positive ionization, the formation of [M+H]$^+$, [M+NH$_4$]$^+$, and [M+Na]$^+$ can occur under different circumstances.[48] Under acid conditions using ammonium formate, the [M+NH$_4$]$^+$ is the most predominant and sensitive ion observed. Fragmentation of ammonium adducts is comparable with the fragmentation of the protonated molecule. When applying relatively high temperatures, the formation of sodium adducts seems to increase. In general, sodium adducts are more difficult to fragment and also give a different fragmentation pathway compared to the protonated molecule. Therefore, most often sodium adducts are not the preferred precursor ions to select for PTXs. When performing collision-induced dissociation of the PTX molecule, in general multiple losses of water can be observed ($n = 1$–5). Also, the closed ring structure is opened and results in a specific PTX fragment of m/z 213 and a fragment that differs depending on the structure at the C-18 position of the molecule (Figure 14.4). PTX 1, -4, and -8 contain a hydroxymethyl residual group at the C-18 position that gives a specific fragment of m/z 567. PTX2, -2sa, -11, -12, -13, and -14 contain a methyl group at C-18 that gives the fragment m/z 551 and PTX3 contains an aldehyde at this position resulting in a fragment of m/z 565. The last type of residual group that can be present on the C-18 position is a carboxylic acid, which results in a fragment of m/z 581 (specific for PTX6, -7, and -9).

The general fragment of m/z 213 can be used for detection of new PTX toxins by performing a precursor scan for this mass. This approach was used to detect PTXs, which can be present as esters within shellfish. Torgersen et al. showed the presence of certain esters in shellfish.[49] Gerssen et al. showed that with sophisticated in-house prepared tools for data analysis it is also possible to search for specific PTX fragments to find certain analogs.[50] Generally, within routine monitoring programs in Europe, the research on PTXs is limited to PTX1 and PTX2. These two PTXs are mentioned only

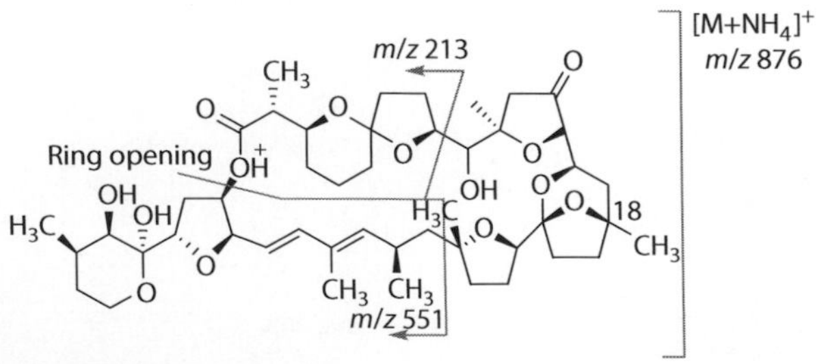

FIGURE 14.4 Proposed fragmentation of pectenotoxin-2 in ESI$^+$.

in EU legislation. This is because at the time of establishing the EU legislation, these were the only described PTXs that showed toxicity in mice when injected i.p. Currently discussions are ongoing on increasing the regulatory limits or deregulating PTXs from EU legislation as the research shows that the oral toxicity is very low and the compound is not regulated by other international bodies such as CODEX.[51]

14.3.3 Yessotoxins

For the mass spectrometric analysis of YTXs, methods have been described using capillary electro-phoresis, nano LC, conventional LC, and ultra-performance high-resolution chromatography.[52–54] The first LC-MS application was actually with nano LC and was developed by Draisci et al.[55] The YTX molecule consists of a ladder-shaped polyether structure containing two sulfonic acid groups and was first discovered by Murate et al.[56] Sulfonic acid groups are strong acids with a low pKa value which remain negatively charged even under acidic mobile phase conditions. For this reason, it is preferred to produce negatively charged ions in the MS. As the compound contains two sulfonic acids under certain chromatographic conditions, the single-charged or double-charged ion will be observed.[27] Under acidic and neutral chromatographic conditions, it is mainly the single-charged ion (for YTX m/z 1141 [M-H]$^-$) while under alkaline chromatographic conditions it is mainly the double-charged ion ([M-2H]$^{2-}$ m/z 570). MS fragments observed are mainly by the loss of a sulfonic acid group ([M-H-SO$_3$]$^-$, m/z 1061) and some low in abundance backbone fragments of the polyether-ladder shape[57] (Figure 14.5). In research over 100 different YTXs have been described, most of them present in low abundance within shellfish and/or algae.[58] By applying different types of MS acquisition modes, new YTXs can be discovered. As mentioned before, the YTXs are producing fragments by the loss of a sulfonic acid (−80 Da), which is a neutral loss. By performing a neutral loss scan of 80 Da, all the corresponding m/z values of the pre-cursor ions will be recorded and shown in the chromatogram. By using the additional criterion that the precursor ions should be in the mass range of m/z 900–m/z 1500, the detected masses will then probably have a YTX-like structure.[58]

YTXs were of interest as these toxins show i.p. toxicity in mice and this method was the reference method for a long time for controlling compliance of shellfish. Currently these compounds are under debate, because of the low oral toxicity of these toxins. Therefore, currently efforts are undertaken to deregulate or increase the regulatory level within Europe.[59] Fortunately for routine control programs, not all analogs that have been found, are mentioned in the legislation, only YTX and 45OH YTX and their

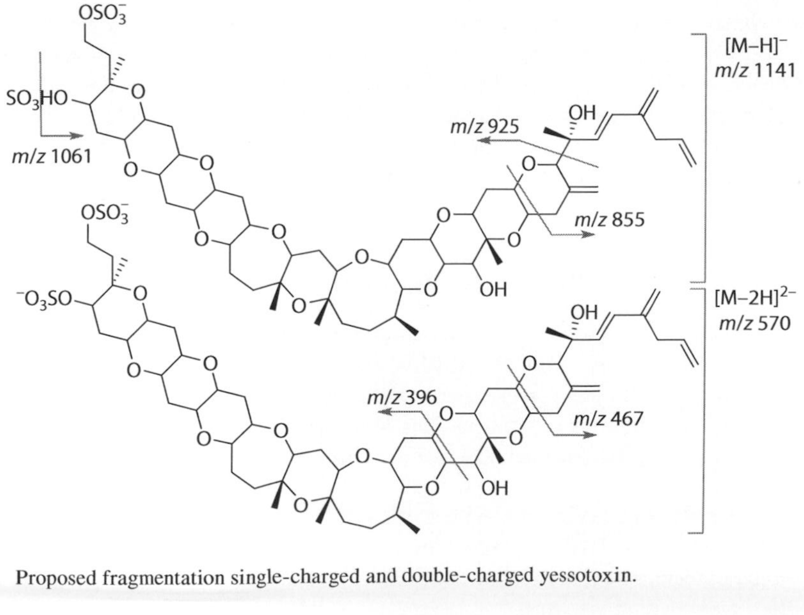

FIGURE 14.5 Proposed fragmentation single-charged and double-charged yessotoxin.

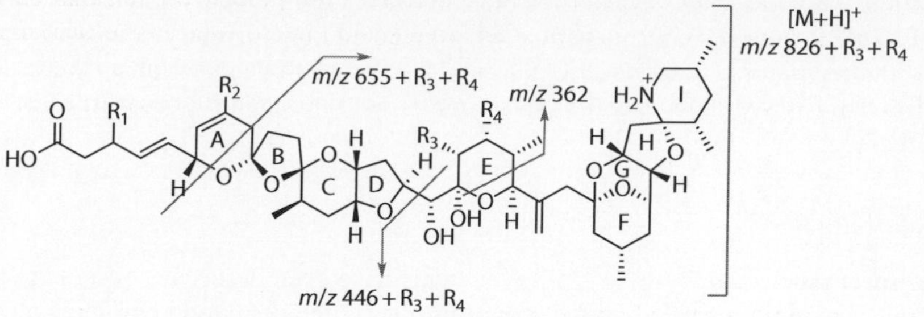

FIGURE 14.6 Proposed fragmentation of azaspiracids using ESI+, AZA1 R_3 = CH_3, R_4 = H; AZA2 R_3 = CH_3, R_4 = H; and AZA3 R_3 and R_4 are H.

corresponding homologues that contain an additional methanediyl group $-CH_2-$ should be monitored. The homologues were discovered by Satake et al. in mussels from the Adriatic Sea in the late 1990s.[60] It should be mentioned that outside Europe these toxins are not regulated.

14.3.4 Azaspiracids

The last group of regulated marine lipophilic toxins to be discussed is the azaspriacids (AZAs) group that currently comprises over 30 analogs. The first discovery of the presence of azaspiracids (AZA1) in shellfish was after an intoxication incident in the Netherlands where people turned ill after the consumption of Irish shellfish.[61] The first MS method was developed by Ofuji et al. after a second intoxication incident with Irish shellfish and showed the presence of other azaspiracids, AZA2 and AZA3.[62] Iontrap MS experiments were used to elucidate and propose structures for various azaspiracids (AZA1 to -6).[63] By now MS revealed many analogs with typical AZA MS fragmentation existing of multiple losses of water (n = 1–6) and different ring cleavages.[64] The cleavage of the A ring in the AZA molecule gives after the losses of water the most abundant fragment of 656 Da plus the mass of the residual groups at positions R_3 and R_4 (Figure 14.6). For AZA1 and AZA2, the residual group R_3 is a methyl group while for AZA3 this is a hydrogen. The R_4 for AZA1–3 is a hydrogen group. After the discovery of these AZAs, many others have been discovered or suggested. These AZAs appear in shellfish after carboxylation, hydroxylation, and other metabolic processes.[65,66] In AZA research also, different MS scanning techniques are used to reveal structures. For the discovery of new AZAs often precursor scanning of the E ring fragment m/z 362 was used. For the AZAs conversion and metabolism, studies were performed using mass spectrometry, which resulted, for example, in the discovery of the decarboxylation of AZA17 and AZA19 to AZA3 and AZA6, respectively.[67] Also recently other types of AZA-like molecules were discovered in different strains of the *Azadinium* species.[68,69] These AZA-like molecules have similar fragmentation characteristics; the only difference is that these compounds are lacking a methyl group on the I ring and therefore these new azaspiracids have a common fragment of m/z 348 [m/z 362–14 Da (CH_2)]. In regulation, EU and CODEX, AZA1, -2, and -3 are the only three analogs mentioned.

14.4 Nonregulated Lipophilic Marine Biotoxins: Cyclic Imines

Nonregulated lipophilic marine biotoxins are the "emerging toxins" cyclic imines (CIs) comprising spirolides (SPXs), gymnodimines (GYMs), pinnatoxins (PnTXs), and pteriatoxins (PtTXs). These toxins are fast-acting toxins and will cause mouse death within minutes after i.p. injection. As oral toxicity studies for most of the compounds are still lacking and there is not enough evidence if these toxins are a real concern for human health, they can also be classified as interfering compounds toward the MBA. Therefore, we should be cautious to designate a compound that is causing i.p. lethality in a mouse as a new toxin without having the evidence that this compound are a real concern for human health. Fortunately, nowadays decision-makers are reserved to establish legislation when there is not enough toxicology, epidemiology, and occurrence data. CIs are under the attention of researchers and decision-makers, but more data should be gathered to make appropriate decisions on establishing legislation for the various CIs. One of the aspects that should be covered is the occurrence data, so analytical methods such as LC-MS need to be established for these compounds groups. Due to their lipophilic character, these compounds can be easily incorporated in the existing methods of extraction and they show comparable retention behavior as the regulated lipophilic marine biotoxins. CIs are macrocyclic compounds with an imine functionality and a spiro-linked ether group. The presence of the imine functionality makes the molecule readily ionizable in ESI[+].

14.4.1 Spirolides

The first CI group discussed are the spirolides (SPXs), which were investigated by Hu et al. using LC-MS.[70] In this paper, the authors described the presence of SPX B-D in scallops with LC ionspray MS. From the fragmentation data, it is clear that the main fragment produced (*m/z* 164) in MS/MS is the ring containing the imine functionality. This fragment is very specific for most of the SPXs found in algae and shellfish (Figure 14.7).

The causative organism *Alexandrium ostenfeldii* was identified by using LC-MS/MS as a tool to prove the presence of SPXs, which was mainly 13-desmethyl SPX C.[71] In 2005, Aasen et al. published on the discovery of 20-methyl spirolide G. These authors used the precursor scanning functionality of the MS to discover possible new SPX analogs within shellfish and algae samples. By scanning the precursor ions that produce fragment ion *m/z* 164, the authors discovered a compound with a precursor ion *m/z* 706 and with comparable MS/MS spectra as the other SPX compounds. NMR confirmed the structure of 20-methyl SPX G.[72] Also, the presence of fatty acid esters of SPX in shellfish was discovered using the same precursor scanning technique.[73] Esters with different chain length (C-12–C-22) and different saturations were discovered (up to 6). The fatty acid ester profiles of the SPXs in shellfish are comparable with the ester profiles of the okadaic acid group toxins. When performing the analysis of various SPXs in shellfish, the most abundant spirolide is 13-desmethyl SPX C and the other compounds are present in minor amounts.

14.4.2 Gymnodimines

Gymnodimines (GYMs) have comparable properties as the SPXs although for the GYMs not that many analogs have been discovered. There are three major compounds—GYM A, B, and C—of which GYM A was the first one isolated from oysters and a tentative elemental composition ($C_{32}H_{45}NO_4$) was determined with FABMS.[74] In 2000, Miles et al. discovered new analogs, GYM B and 18-deoxy GYM B for which electron impact MS was used to accurately determine the mass and NMR was used to confirm the structure.[75] In 2003 the same research group discovered GYM C, the isomer of GYM B, in *Karenia selliformis*.[76] Again, electron impact MS was used for the determination of the accurate mass; the difference in structure between GYM A and GYM B/C is the position (endo/exo) of the methylene group at the C-17 position and an additional hydroxyl group is present at C-18. In 2011, in North Carolina (the United States), *Alexandrium peruvianum* was found to produce a novel GYM compound. By applying

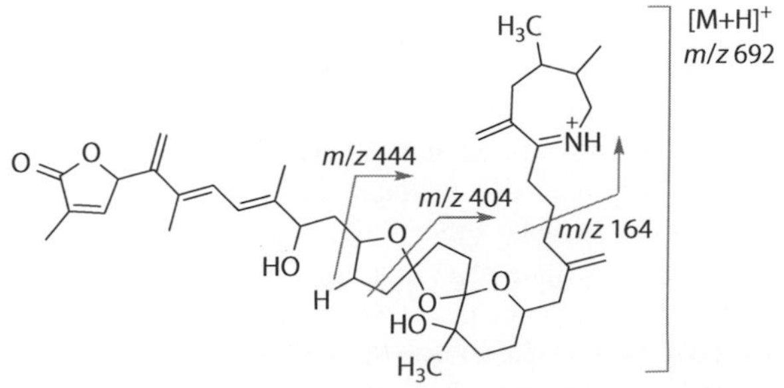

FIGURE 14.7 Fragmentation of 13-desmethyl SPX C after retro-Diels–Alder ring opening.

NMR and ESI in combination with high-resolution MS and MS/MS, the structure of 12-methylgymnodimine A was identified.[77] As no legislation is established on GYMs, these compounds are not incorporated in routine monitoring programs. Most methodologies developed for the routine detection of lipophilic marine biotoxins can easily incorporate the CIs and therefore also the GYMs. Just as with the SPXs it is assumed that GYMs can also be metabolized to fatty acid esters when accumulating in shellfish. de la Iglesia et al. recently discovered in shellfish originating from North Africa (Tunisia), where harmful algae blooms of *K. selliformis* are present continuously, various GYMs containing fatty acid esters. By using a linear iontrap MS and orbitrap MS, the fragmentation pathway of GYM A was proposed. Furthermore by performing a precursor scan of the fragment m/z 490, various fatty acid esters were discovered with chain lengths of C14 till C22. Accurate mass measurements using the orbitrap MS confirmed the findings by showing small mass deviations of below 3 ppm between the predicted and the measured masses.[78]

14.4.3 Pinnatoxins

The last group of CIs discussed are the pinnatoxins (PnTXs) and their metabolites the pteriatoxins (PtTXs). For the PnTXs, various structures have been discovered. The elucidation of PnTX A was done by Uemura et al. who extracted PnTX A from *Pinna muricata*.[79] The application of both NMR and high-resolution FAB MS resulted in the elucidation of the toxin with an elemental composition of $C_{41}H_{61}NO_9$. Later Chou et al. found PnTX D and Takada et al. PnTX B and C.[80,81] Takada et al. used ESI-MS/MS to propose fragmentation pathways. The most abundant ion for the PnTXs are the protonated molecules (i.e., PnTX B [M+H]$^+$ m/z 741), which is followed by a characteristic fragment m/z 164 that is the same fragment obtained as for the SPXs. More recently, Selwood et al. found PnTX E, F, and G in pacific oysters (*Pinna bicolor*) using tandem mass spectrometry. Selwood et al. showed the oxidation of PnTX G and further metabolism to PnTX A–C and the formation of cysteine conjugates PtTX A–C. Similarly, PnTX F is hydrolyzed and metabolized (oxidized) toward PnTX E and D.[82] For the detection of PnTX A, -E, -F and -G, a dedicated rapid LC-MS/MS method using start-of-the-art LC column material with sub-2-μm particles has been developed, which has a run-to-run time of less than 5 min. Furthermore, fatty acids of PnTXs have been discovered in shellfish; this was done by performing a precursor scan of the fragment m/z 164.[83] Additionally, the identity of PnTXs, which have comparable fragmentation and structures as SPXs, was identified by performing an alkaline hydrolysis. During the hydrolysis, PnTXs remain stable while SPXs are degrading.[84] PnTXs are not routinely monitored within monitoring programs, although more data should be gathered to get an idea on occurrence and exposure.[85]

14.5 Nonregulated Lipophilic Marine Biotoxins: Ciguatoxins

Ciguatera (CTX) fish poisoning is the most frequently occurring marine biotoxin intoxication and mainly in tropical regions. It is very difficult or even impossible to set up monitoring programs to test the presence of CTX in fish. This is due to the high variability of the toxin concentration among different fish species and to a large inter-species variation. Therefore, currently the best method to reduce the number of intoxications is probably by creating awareness of which fish species are more vulnerable to CTX and should not be consumed. Most of the work done with LC-MS on CTXs is related to the identification of different toxins in fish.[86–88] The LC-MS method development of these toxins is mainly hampered by the lack of standards, which are not commercially available. Furthermore, the complexity of the molecules makes it difficult to analyze them by LC-MS. First of all there is a wide variety of CTXs many of which are produced by algae (i.e., *Gambierdiscus* spp.) and are metabolized within fish to various different metabolites. The structurally different types of CTX are specific for the region they originate from. Currently we have Pacific CTX (P-CTX), Caribbean CTX (C-CTX), and Indian CTX (I-CTX). The first MS methods on ciguatera (pacific CTX) and maitotoxin were described in the early 1990s by Lewis et al. and Yasumoto et al.[89,90]

Much later Yogi et al. described the use of more modern LC-MS/MS equipment for the discovery of a wide variety of P-CTXs including fish metabolites.[87] Yogi et al. reported, when using water and methanol in the mobile phase, that in positive ionization mode the most abundant precursor ion observed is [M+Na]+ while when using acetonitrile mainly protonated molecular ions [M+H]+ are observed. The latter ion produced mainly losses of water when applying CID. The sodium adduct under water/methanol conditions is by far the most abundant ion. Even when a relatively high collision energy is applied, the sodium is very stable and almost no fragmentation occurs. Therefore, for the monitoring of the presence of P-CTXs and C-CTXs in fish the protonated molecule as precursor ion in combination with the multiple dehydrations ($n = 1$–3) of the molecule as product ions have been used.[91] Alternatively, the sodium adduct can be used as both precursor ion and product ion, while applying a high collision energy. Both approaches do not produce very specific fragments. And as most laboratories do not have access to (certified) standards of CTXs, researchers should be more alert on possible false positives when using these types of fragment ions. Due to the absence of standards, analytical methods are difficult to develop. Therefore, for determining the presence of CTXs in fish after an intoxication incident a combination of (in vitro) bioassays and mass spectrometry can be used.[92]

14.6 Validated and Regulated Methodologies

In order to test compliance of shellfish with various types of legislation, most often still animal-based testing or traditional analytical techniques such as LC-UV or LC-FLD are used. The disadvantage of the animal-based testing is that certain compounds can be very toxic to the test animal but less or even nontoxic to humans. For example, the MBA for lipophilic marine biotoxins is performed by injecting a certain amount of extract intraperitoneal. Clearly, this administration route is different from oral administration. YTXs and PTXs show i.p. a relatively high toxicity while in oral studies with rats or mice, almost no toxicity is observed.[93,94] It seems that the MBA method using i.p. injection is a worst-case scenario testing, which can cause quite a large number of false positives and a negative impact for the industry. Of course, there are also pros of this animal-based testing. The advantage of animal-based tests compared to chemical methods is that they are toxicity driven, although the administration route is completely different from oral exposure. So comparing chemical methods with animal-based methods is impossible as chemical methods are based on the chemical properties of compounds and animal-based testing on the toxicology. The authors' opinion is that more toxic effect-based in vitro assays should become available because these assays are based on the same principles as the animal tests and show the direct effect of toxic compounds. Of course, after screening with these assays the suspect samples should be confirmed using more specific techniques such as LC-MS/MS.

Chemical testing with LC-UV and LC-FLD has been widely accepted and is for some of the toxin groups like ASP and PSP also the official methodology for routine monitoring.[95] Although these methods have many pros over the MBA, there are also some cons toward the LC-MS/MS methodologies. In contrast to MS, with these techniques (LC-FLD being more specific than LC-UV) the identity of the toxin cannot be completely confirmed. This is greatly improved when using tandem mass spectrometric tools, because it is possible to confirm the identity of a compound based on the measurement of at least two transitions per toxin. The relation between the intensity of the two transitions, the so-called ion ratio, is an additional confirmatory criterion that can be used. These identity confirmation criteria, such as ion ratio and retention time, are used to compare a toxin in a standard solution and the possible toxin in a shellfish sample.[96,97] If all the criteria are fulfilled and the concentration is above the regulatory level including the measurement uncertainty, the sample can be regarded as noncompliant. The major drawbacks of this approach are that for all the toxins measured a standard is needed and that only those toxins will analyzed that are defined in the MRM (or SRM) method before the analysis. With a bioassay (in vivo or in vitro), a broader scope of toxins, based on their mode of action, can be analyzed although less specific.

With respect to the legislation applied by different countries for certain toxins, there is some discrepancy, like for YTXs and PTXs which are regulated in the EU, but not outside the EU, while brevetoxins are included in FDA and CODEX and are not mentioned in the EU legislation.[98,99] Of course, this has an impact on global trade. Therefore, it is desirable that worldwide the same toxins and allowed maximum levels are established in legislation as shellfish are distributed all over the world.

14.6.1 Validated LC-MS/MS Methodologies

Here, the different in-house or inter-laboratory validated MS methodologies will be discussed. For DA, there seems to be a tendency to not have full collaborative studies. Probably this is due to the fact that DA is just a single toxin and most laboratories are either using LC-UV or already in-house validated LC-MS methodologies. DA could also be included in LC-MS/MS methods dedicated to lipophilic marine biotoxins.[54,100] With respect to LC-MS/MS analysis, most validation studies have been conducted for the lipophilic marine biotoxins (both in-house and inter-laboratory). The two first LC-MS/MS method validations were done by Stobo et al. and McNabb et al.[100,101] Both these methods showed good performance characteristics and are since then applied in more advanced laboratories. The research group of McNabb et al. already in 2005 implemented the LC-MS/MS methodology in their routine monitoring program. The major drawback of the validation studies from that time was the lack of certified standards. In 2005, only for OA and PTX2 commercial certified standards were available at the National Research Council (NRC) in Halifax, Canada. Therefore, formally only the certified biotoxins included in this method were validated. From 2005 till now, the NRC in Canada has put a lot of effort in the development of certified reference standards and nowadays over a dozen standards for lipophilic marine biotoxins are available from the NRC. Recently, CIFGA, an European producer, also started certifying marine biotoxin standards. The limited availability of the standards and the poor performance of the MBA for lipophilic marine biotoxins resulted in multiple efforts to develop and validate LC-MS/MS methodologies that can be used for official control programs. At this moment three full collaborative studies have been held for lipophilic marine biotoxins, including OA, DTX1, -2, AZA1, -2, -3 PTX2, and YTX. The first study was organized by BfR in Berlin, Germany.[102] The method validated consisted of a fixed extraction procedure using 80% v/v MeOH. With respect to the LC-MS/MS measurements, chromatographic conditions used by the participants were free of choice. So either acidic and/or alkaline chromatographic conditions were used. The study was conducted with good results, which were obtained for different lipophilic biotoxins in extracts and in shellfish materials. The second study was organized by RIKILT, Wageningen, the Netherlands. Compared to the BfR study, there were minor changes in the extraction and the method of constructing calibration curves. In this study, matrix matched standards were used, which was done to compensate for matrix effects in LC-MS/MS. Furthermore, a slight change in extraction (100% methanol) and fixed alkaline chromatographic conditions were used.[103] Also, this study obtained good results with exceptional low RSDs. The last collaborative trial was organized by the European Reference Laboratory, Vigo, Spain, which study had a fixed extraction procedure but chromatographic conditions were open (acidic or alkaline). Also, this study showed good results and this method was proposed as the official reference method. The outcomes of these studies convinced the EU and their member states that these MS methods are a good replacement for the MBA. Therefore, on July 1, 2011, the official method for the detection of lipophilic marine biotoxins in Europe was mass spectrometry based.[28] After New Zealand, the EU is now using LC-MS/MS as the official monitoring method.

14.6.2 Future Perspectives

Within the LC-MS method development for marine biotoxins, it is expected that trends that are already present in other research areas such as the mycotoxins, veterinary drugs, and pesticides will also enter this field. A major difference with these other fields is the way by which methods are allowed for official control. In marine biotoxins analysis, predescribed methods should be used as reference methods where in the other fields the method performance criteria are predescribed and laboratories are allowed to use their own developed methods for official control. Of course, these methods should perform satisfactorily within proficiency testing schemes and preferably standardized but this is not always feasible.

The problem within the marine biotoxin field is that by the time a method is incorporated in legislation a better method has likely become available available. For example, for the lipophilic marine biotoxins in legislation, the LC-MS method is mentioned. This method is using conventional LC while nowadays many laboratories have access to UHPLC equipment and are able to perform a more rapid analysis with comparable or better performance characteristics.[104] Currently, the chosen approach for establishing reference methods is hampering the implementation of the latest techniques in official control programs.

Currently, within CODEX discussions are ongoing on the establishment of performance criteria for screening methods. Screening can, for example, also be done using high-resolution mass spectrometry like ToF or Orbitrap MS. These techniques were already incorporated within the studies on a wide variety of marine biotoxins or in metabolite research.[50,105,106] But for screening in official monitoring, these techniques are not yet established. Preferably a single rapid screening method should be developed for a wide variety of marine biotoxins. If the sample is compliant, the work is done. If a sample is suspected to be noncompliant, a dedicated LC-MS/MS method only for the specific toxin group can be applied. This approach is already used in areas of veterinary drugs, doping analysis, and currently also pesticide analysis.[107–109] A beneficial aspect of this approach is that with a high-resolution mass spectrometry data can also be investigated retrospectively. This means when international bodies such as the European Food Safety Authority want to collect data on the occurrence of a certain new emerging toxin, for instance, pinnatoxins, only data analyses have to be performed in order to see if these toxins are present. The data analysis of high-resolution mass spectrometry still has drawbacks. Each data file can be very large (>100 Mb), which can result in laborious data handling. Thankfully, vendors of MS equipment realize this drawback and are working on the development of these data analysis tools. Currently the data analysis hampers the implementation of these techniques in routine control programs.

The last developments that are foreseen are regarding new types of MS technologies. Within the marine biotoxins field, to the best of my knowledge no ambient ionization techniques have been applied. So, for example, the use of Desorption ElectroSpray Ionization (DESI) or Direct Analysis in Real Time (DART) is promising.[110,111] With these techniques, it is possible to perform a direct analysis from a surface of a sample that can be shellfish meat or algae supplements or whatever. No chromatographic separation is involved with these techniques. These techniques can be of interest for rapid screening of samples. The latest development in mass spectrometry is the use of so-called ion mobility mass spectrometry.[112,113] With this technique it is possible to separate isomeric compounds in the gas phase. Especially with natural compounds such as marine biotoxins, it is expected that many isomeric compounds can be present. Some of these isomeric compounds will not be resolved with the applied LC separation. The ion mobility MS has the power to separate these different isomeric ions based on the cross section of the molecule. Of course, more complex data sets are generated as there is an additional dimension (drift time) added. The application of these techniques in marine biotoxins research is still in its infancy, but it is expected that in the next years the number of applications and publications will increase.

REFERENCES

1. Quilliam, M. A. and Wright, J. L. C., 1989. The amnesic shellfish poisoning mystery. *Analytical Chemistry*, 61, 1053A–1060A.
2. Pineiro, N., Vaquero, E., Leao, J. M., Gago-Martinez, A., and Vazquez, J. A. R., 2001. Optimization of conditions for the liquid chromatographic-electrospray ionization-mass spectrometric analysis of amnesic shellfish poisoning toxins. *Chromatographia*, 53, S231–S235.
3. Furey, A., Lehane, M., Gillman, M., Fernandez-Puente, P., and James, K. J., 2001. Determination of domoic acid in shellfish by liquid chromatography with electrospray ionization and multiple tandem mass spectrometry. *Journal of Chromatography A*, 938, 167–174.
4. Ciminiello, P., Dell'Aversano, C., Fattorusso, E. et al., 2005. Hydrophilic interaction liquid chromatography/mass spectrometry for determination of domoic acid in Adriatic shellfish. *Rapid Communications in Mass Spectrometry*, 19, 2030–2038.
5. McNabb, P., Selwood, A. I., Holland, P. T. et al., 2005. Multiresidue method for determination of algal toxins in shellfish: Single-laboratory validation and interlaboratory study. *Journal of AOAC International*, 88, 761–772.

6. Holland, P. T., McNabb, P., Selwood, A. I., and Neil, T., 2003. Amnesic shellfish poisoning toxins in shellfish: Estimation of uncertainty of measurement for a liquid chromatography/tandem mass spectrometry method. *Journal of AOAC International*, 86, 1095–1100.

7. de la Iglesia, P., Barber, E., Gimenez, G., Rodriguez-Velasco, M. L., Villar-Gonzalez, A., and Diogene, J., 2011. High-throughput analysis of amnesic shellfish poisoning toxins in shellfish by ultra-performance rapid resolution LC-MS/MS. *Journal of AOAC International*, 94, 555–564.

8. Wiese, M., D'Agostino, P. M., Mihali, T. K., Moffitt, M. C., and Neilan, B. A., 2010. Neurotoxic alkaloids: Saxitoxin and its analogs. *Marine Drugs*, 8, 2185–2211.

9. Alexander, J., Benford, D., Cockburn, A. et al., 2009. Marine biotoxins in shellfish—Saxitoxin group. *The European Food Safety Authority Journal*, 1019, 1–76.

10. Oshima, Y., 1995. Postcolumn derivatization liquid-chromatographic method for paralytic shellfish toxins. *Journal of AOAC International*, 78, 528–532.

11. Lawrence, J. F., Niedzwiadek, B., and Menard, C., 2005. Quantitative determination of paralytic shellfish poisoning toxins in shellfish using prechromatographic oxidation and liquid chromatography with fluorescence detection: Collaborative study. *Journal of AOAC International*, 88, 1714–1732.

12. van de Riet, J., Gibbs, R. S., Muggah, P. M., Rourke, W. A., MacNeil, J. D., and Quilliam, M. A., 2011. Liquid chromatography post-column oxidation (PCOX) method for the determination of paralytic shellfish toxins in mussels, clams, oysters, and scallops: Collaborative study. *Journal of AOAC International*, 94, 1154–1176.

13. DeGrasse, S. L., van de Riet, J., Hatfield, R., and Turner, A., 2011. Pre- versus post-column oxidation liquid chromatography fluorescence detection of paralytic shellfish toxins. *Toxicon*, 57, 619–624.

14. Turner, A. D., Hatfield, R. G., Rapkova, M. et al., 2011. Comparison of AOAC 2005.06 LC official method with other methodologies for the quantitation of paralytic shellfish poisoning toxins in UK shellfish species. *Analytical and Bioanalytical Chemistry*, 399, 1257–1270.

15. Dell'Aversano, C., Hess, P., and Quilliam, M. A., 2005. Hydrophilic interaction liquid chromatography–mass spectrometry for the analysis of paralytic shellfish poisoning (PSP) toxins. *Journal of Chromatographic A*, 1081, 190–201.

16. Diener, M., Erler, K., Christian, B., and Luckas, B., 2007. Application of a new zwitterionic hydrophilic interaction chromatography column for determination of paralytic shellfish poisoning toxins. *Journal of Separation Science*, 30, 1821–1826.

17. Jaime, E., Hummert, C., Hess, P., and Luckas, B., 2001. Determination of paralytic shellfish poisoning toxins by high-performance ion-exchange chromatography. *Journal of Chromatography A*, 929, 43–49.

18. Buzy, A., Thibault, P., and Laycock, M. V., 1994. Development of a capillary electrophoresis method for the characterization of enzymatic products arising from the carbamoylase digestion of aralytic shellfish poisoning toxins. *Journal of Chromatography A*, 688, 301–316.

19. Locke, S. J. and Thibault, P., 1994. Improvement in detection limits for the determination of paralytic shellfish poisoning toxins in shellfish tissues using capillary electrophoresis electrospray mass-spectrometry and discontinuous buffer systems. *Analytical Chemistry*, 66, 3436–3446.

20. Quilliam, M. A., Hess, P., and Dell' Aversano, C., Recent developments in the analysis of phycotoxins by liquid chromatography-mass spectrometry, In *Mycotoxins and Phycotoxins in Perspective at the Turn of the Century*, de Koe, W. J., Samson, R. A., van Egmond, H. P., Gilbert, J., and Sabino, M., Eds. Wageningen, Ponsen and Looijen, the Netherlands, 2001, pp. 383–391.

21. Turrell, E., Stobo, L., Lacaze, J. P., Piletsky, S., and Piletska, E., 2008. Optimization of hydrophilic interaction liquid chromatography/mass spectrometry and development of solid-phase extraction for the determination of paralytic shellfish poisoning toxins. *Journal of AOAC International*, 91, 1372–1386.

22. Sayfritz, S. J., Aasen, J. A., and Aune, T., 2008. Determination of paralytic shellfish poisoning toxins in Norwegian shellfish by liquid chromatography with fluorescence and tandem mass spectrometry detection. *Toxicon*, 52, 330–340.

23. Blay, P., Hui, J. P., Chang, J., and Melanson, J. E., 2011. Screening for multiple classes of marine biotoxins by liquid chromatography-high-resolution mass spectrometry. *Analytical and Bioanalytical Chemistry*, 400, 577–585.

24. Lajeunesse, A., Segura, P. A., Gelinas, M. et al., 2012. Detection and confirmation of saxitoxin analogues in freshwater benthic Lyngbya wollei algae collected in the St. Lawrence River (Canada) by liquid chromatography-tandem mass spectrometry. *Journal of Chromatography A*, 1219, 93–103.

25. Vale, P., 2010. New saxitoxin analogues in the marine environment: Developments in toxin chemistry, detection and biotransformation during the 2000s. *Phytochemistry Reviews*, 9, 525–535.

26. Stobo, L. A., Lacaze, J. P., Scott, A. C., Gallacher, S., Smith, E. A., and Quilliam, M. A., 2005. Liquid chromatography with mass spectrometry—Detection of lipophilic shellfish toxins. *Journal of AOAC International*, 88, 1371–1382.

27. Gerssen, A., Mulder, P. P., McElhinney, M. A., and de Boer, J., 2009. Liquid chromatography-tandem mass spectrometry method for the detection of marine lipophilic toxins under alkaline conditions. *Journal of Chromatography A*, 1216, 1421–1430.

28. Anon, Commission Regulation (EU) No 15/2011 of 10 January 2011 amending Regulation (EC) No 2074/2005 as regards recognised testing methods for detecting marine biotoxins in live bivalve molluscs 15/2011, C. R. E. N. *Official Journal of European Communications*, 2011, pp. 3–6.

29. McCarron, P., Kotterman, M., de Boer, J., Rehmann, N., and Hess, P., 2007. Feasibility of gamma irradiation as a stabilisation technique in the preparation of tissue reference materials for a range of shellfish toxins. *Analytical and Bioanalytical Chemistry*, 387, 2487–2493.

30. McCarron, P., Kilcoyne, J., Miles, C. O., and Hess, P., 2009. Formation of Azaspiracids-3, -4, -6, and -9 via decarboxylation of carboxyazaspiracid metabolites from shellfish. *Journal of Agricultural and Food Chemistry*, 57, 160–169.

31. Bencsath, F. A. and Dickey, R. W., 1991. Mass spectral characteristics of okadaic acid and simple derivatives. *Rapid Communications in Mass Spectrometry*, 5, 283–290.

32. Pleasance, S., Quilliam, M. A., and Marr, J. C., 1992. Ionspray mass spectrometry of marine toxins. IV. Determination of diarrhetic shellfish poisoning toxins in mussel tissue by liquid chromatography/mass spectrometry. *Rapid Communications in Mass Spectrometry*, 6, 121–127.

33. Quilliam, M. A., 1995. Analysis of diarrhetic shellfish poisoning toxins in shellfish tissue by liquid-chromatography with fluorometric and mass-spectrometric detection. *Journal of AOAC International*, 78, 555–570.

34. Gerssen, A., Mulder, P., van Rhijn, H., and de Boer, J., 2008. Mass spectrometric analysis of the marine lipophilic biotoxins pectenotoxin-2 and okadaic acid by four different types of mass spectrometers. *Journal of Mass Spectrometry*, 43, 1140–1147.

35. Carey, B., Fidalgo Saez, M. J., Hamilton, B., O'Halloran, J., van Pelt, F. N., and James, K. J., 2012. Elucidation of the mass fragmentation pathways of the polyether marine toxins, dinophysistoxins, and identification of isomer discrimination processes. *Rapid Communications in Mass Spectrometry*, 26, 1793–1802.

36. Torgersen, T., Miles, C. O., Rundberget, T., and Wilkins, A. L., 2008. New esters of okadaic acid in seawater and blue mussels (Mytilus edulis). *Journal of Agricultural and Food Chemistry*, 56, 9628–9635.

37. Torgersen, T., Wilkins, A. L., Rundberget, T., and Miles, C. O., 2008. Characterization of fatty acid esters of okadaic acid and related toxins in blue mussels (*Mytilus edulis*) from Norway. *Rapid Communications in Mass Spectrometry*, 22, 1127–1136.

38. Hu, T. M., Curtis, J. M., Walter, J. A., McLachlan, J. L., and Wright, J. L. C., 1995. Two new water-soluble DSP toxin derivatives from the dinoflagellate *Prorocentrum maculosum*: Possible storage and excretion products. *Tetrahedron Letters*, 36, 9273–9276.

39. Cruz, P. G., Daranas, A. H., Fernandez, J. J., Souto, M. L., and Norte, M., 2006. DTX5c, a new OA sulphate ester derivative from cultures of *Prorocentrum belizeanum*. *Toxicon*, 47, 920–924.

40. Suarez-Gomez, B., Souto, M. L., Cruz, P. G., Fernandez, J. J., and Norte, M., 2005. New targets in diarrhetic shellfish poisoning control. *Journal of Natural Products*, 68, 596–599.

41. Suarez-Gomez, B., Souto, M. L., Norte, M., and Fernandez, J. J., 2001. Isolation and structural determination of DTX-6, a new okadaic acid derivative. *Journal of Natural Products*, 64, 1363–1364.

42. Paz, B., Daranas, A. H., Cruz, P. G. et al., 2007. Identification and characterization of DTX-5c and 7-hydroxymethyl-2-methylene-octa-4,7-dienyl okadaate from *Prorocentrum belizeanum* cultures by LC-MS. *Toxicon*, 50, 470–478.

43. Miles, C. O., Wilkins, A. L., Hawkes, A. D. et al., 2006. Isolation and identification of pectenotoxins-13 and -14 from *Dinophysis acuta* in New Zealand. *Toxicon*, 48, 152–159.

44. Miles, C. O., Wilkins, A. L., Samdal, I. A. et al., 2004. A novel pectenotoxin, PTX-12, in *Dinophysis spp.* and shellfish from Norway. *Chemical Research in Toxicology*, 17, 1423–1433.

45. Yasumoto, T., Murata, M., Oshima, Y., Sano, M., Matsumoto, G. K., and Clardy, J., 1985. Diarrhetic shellfish toxins. *Tetrahedron*, 41, 1019–1025.

46. Suzuki, T., Mackenzie, L., Stirling, D., and Adamson, J., 2001. Pectenotoxin-2 seco acid: A toxin converted from pectenotoxin-2 by the New Zealand Greenshell mussel, *Perna canaliculus*. *Toxicon*, 39, 507–514.

47. Goto, H., Igarashi, T., Yamamoto, M. et al., 2001. Quantitative determination of marine toxins associated with diarrhetic shellfish poisoning by liquid chromatography coupled with mass spectrometry. *Journal of Chromatography A*, 907, 181–189.

48. Suzuki, T., Mitsuya, T., Matsubara, H., and Yamasaki, M., 1998. Determination of pectenotoxin-2 after solid-phase extraction from seawater and from the dinoflagellate *Dinophysis fortii* by liquid chromatography with electrospray mass spectrometry and ultraviolet detection—Evidence of oxidation of pectenotoxin-2 to pectenotoxin-6 in scallops. *Journal of Chromatography A*, 815, 155–160.

49. Torgersen, T., Sandvik, M., Lundve, B., and Lindegarth, S., 2008. Profiles and levels of fatty acid esters of okadaic acid group toxins and pectenotoxins during toxin depuration. Part II: Blue mussels (*Mytilus edulis*) and flat oyster (*Ostrea edulis*). *Toxicon*, 52, 418–427.

50. Gerssen, A., Mulder, P. P., and de Boer, J., 2011. Screening of lipophilic marine toxins in shellfish and algae: Development of a library using liquid chromatography coupled to orbitrap mass spectrometry. *Analytica Chimica Acta*, 685, 176–185.

51. Alexander, J., Benford, D., Cockburn, A. et al., 2009. Marine biotoxins in shellfish—Pectenotoxin group. *The European Food Safety Authority Journal*, 1109, 1–47.

52. de la Iglesia, P., Gago-Martinez, A., and Yasumoto, T., 2007. Advanced studies for the application of high-performance capillary electrophoresis for the analysis of yessotoxin and 45-hydroxyyessotoxin. *Journal of Chromatography A*, 1156, 160–166.

53. Draisci, R., Giannetti, L., Lucentini, L., Ferretti, E., Palleschi, L., and Marchiafava, C., 1998. Direct identification of yessotoxin in shellfish by liquid chromatography coupled with mass spectrometry and tandem mass spectrometry. *Rapid Communications in Mass Spectrometry*, 12, 1291–1296.

54. Fux, E., McMillan, D., Bire, R., and Hess, P., 2007. Development of an ultra-performance liquid chromatography-mass spectrometry method for the detection of lipophilic marine toxins. *Journal of Chromatography A*, 1157, 273–280.

55. Draisci, R., Giannetti, L., Lucentini, L., Ferretti, E., Palleschi, L., and Marchiafava, C., 1998. Direct identification of yessotoxin in shellfish by liquid chromatography coupled with mass spectrometry and tandem mass spectrometry. *Rapid Communications in Mass Spectrometry*, 12, 1291–1296.

56. Murata, M., Kumagai, M., Lee, J. S., and Yasumoto, T., 1987. Isolation and structure of yessotoxin, a novel polyether compound implicated in diarrhetic shellfish poisoning. *Tetrahedron Letters*, 28, 5869–5872.

57. Amandi, M. F., Furey, A., Lehane, M., Ramstad, H., and James, K. J., 2002. Liquid chromatography with electrospray ion-trap mass spectrometry for the determination of yessotoxins in shellfish. *Journal of Chromatography A*, 976, 329–334.

58. Miles, C. O., Samdal, I. A., Aasen, J. A. B. et al., 2005. Evidence for numerous analogs of yessotoxin in *Protoceratium reticulatum*. *Harmful Algae*, 4, 1075–1091.

59. Alexander, J., Benford, D., Cockburn, A. et al., 2008. Marine biotoxins in shellfish—Yessotoxin group. *The European Food Safety Authority Journal*, 907, 1–62.

60. Satake, M., Tubaro, A., Lee, J. S., and Yasumoto, T., 1997. Two new analogs of yessotoxin, homoyessotoxin and 45-hydroxyhomoyessotoxin, isolated from mussels of the Adriatic Sea. *Natural Toxins*, 5, 107–110.

61. Satake, M., Ofuji, K., Naoki, H. et al., 1998. Azaspiracid, a new marine toxin having unique spiro ring assemblies, isolated from Irish mussels, *Mytilus edulis*. *Journal of the American Chemical Society*, 120, 9967–9968.

62. Ofuji, K., Satake, M., McMahon, T. et al., 1999. Two analogs of azaspiracid isolated from mussels, *Mytilus edulis*, involved in human intoxication in Ireland. *Natural Toxins*, 7, 99–102.

63. Lehane, M., Brana-Magdalena, A., Moroney, C., Furey, A., and James, K. J., 2002. Liquid chromatography with electrospray ion trap mass spectrometry for the determination of five azaspiracids in shellfish. *Journal of Chromatography A*, 950, 139–147.

64. Brombacher, S., Edmonds, S., and Volmer, D. A., 2002. Studies on azaspiracid biotoxins. II. Mass spectral behavior and structural elucidation of azaspiracids analogs. *Rapid Communications in Mass Spectrometry*, 16, 2306–2316.

65. James, K. J., Sierra, M. D., Lehane, M., Brana-Magdalena, A., and Furey, A., 2003. Detection of five new hydroxyl analogues of azaspiracids in shellfish using multiple tandem mass spectrometry. *Toxicon*, 41, 227–283.

66. Rehmann, N., Hess, P., and Quilliam, M. A., 2008. Discovery of new analogs of the marine biotoxin azaspiracid in blue mussels (*Mytilus edulis*) by ultra-performance liquid chromatography/tandem mass spectrometry. *Rapid Communications in Mass Spectrometry*, 22, 549–558.

67. McCarron, P., Kilcoyne, J., Miles, C. O., and Hess, P., 2009. Formation of azaspiracids-3, -4, -6, and -9 via decarboxylation of carboxyazaspiracid metabolites from shellfish. *Journal of Agricultural and Food Chemistry*, 57, 160–169.

68. Gu, H. F., Luo, Z. H., Krock, B., Witt, M., and Tillmann, U., 2013. Morphology, phylogeny and azaspiracid profile of Azadinium poporum (Dinophyceae) from the China Sea. *Harmful Algae*, 21–22, 64–75.

69. Krock, B., Tillmann, U., Voss, D. et al., 2012. New azaspiracids in Amphidomataceae (Dinophyceae). *Toxicon*, 60, 830–839.

70. Hu, T. M., Curtis, J. M., Oshima, Y. et al., 1995. Spirolide-B and spirolide-D, 2 novel macrocycles isolated from the digestive glands of shellfish. *Journal of the Chemical Society-Chemical Communications*, 2159–2161.

71. Cembella, A. D., Lewis, N. I., and Quilliam, M. A., 2000. The marine dinoflagellate *Alexandrium ostenfeldii* (Dinophyceae) as the causative organism of spirolide shellfish toxins. *Phycologia*, 39, 67–74.

72. Aasen, J. A. B., MacKinnon, S. L., LeBlanc, P. et al., 2005. Detection and identification of spirolides in Norwegian shellfish and plankton. *Chemical Research in Toxicology*, 18, 509–515.

73. Aasen, J. A. B., Hardstaff, W., Aune, T., and Quilliam, M. A., 2006. Discovery of fatty acid ester metabolites of spirolide toxins in mussels from Norway using liquid chromatography/tandem mass spectrometry. *Rapid Communications in Mass Spectrometry*, 20, 1531–1537.

74. Seki, T., Satake, M., Mackenzie, L., Kaspar, H. F., and Yasumoto, T., 1995. Gymnodimine, a new marine toxin of unprecedented structure isolated from New-Zealand oysters and the dinoflagellate, *Gymnodinium* sp. *Tetrahedron Letters*, 36, 7093–7096.

75. Miles, C. O., Wilkins, A. L., Stirling, D. J., and MacKenzie, A. L., 2000. New analogue of gymnodimine from a *Gymnodinium* species. *Journal of Agricultural and Food Chemistry*, 48, 1373–1376.

76. Miles, C. O., Wilkins, A. L., Stirling, D. J., and MacKenzie, A. L., 2003. Gymnodimine C, an isomer of gymnodimine B, from *Karenia selliformis*. *Journal of Agricultural and Food Chemistry*, 51, 4838–4840.

77. Van Wagoner, R. M., Misner, I., Tomas, C. R., and Wright, J. L. C., 2011. Occurrence of 12-methylgymnodimine in a spirolide-producing dinoflagellate *Alexandrium peruvianum* and the biogenetic implications. *Tetrahedron Letters*, 52, 4243–4246.

78. de la Iglesia, P., McCarron, P., Diogene, J., and Quilliam, M. A., 2013. Discovery of gymnodimine fatty acid ester metabolites in shellfish using liquid chromatography/mass spectrometry. *Rapid Communications in Mass Spectrometry*, 27, 643–653.

79. Uemura, D., Chou, T., Haino, T. et al., 1995. Pinnatoxin-a—A toxic amphoteric macrocycle from the okinawan bivalve Pinna-muricata. *Journal of the American Chemical Society*, 117, 1155–1156.

80. Takada, N., Umemura, N., Suenaga, K. et al., 2001. Pinnatoxins B and C, the most toxic components in the pinnatoxin series from the Okinawan bivalve Pinna muricata. *Tetrahedron Letters*, 42, 3491–3494.

81. Chou, T., Haino, T., Kuramoto, M., and Uemura, D., 1996. Isolation and structure of pinnatoxin D, a new shellfish poison from the Okinawan bivalve Pinna muricata. *Tetrahedron Letters*, 37, 4027–4030.

82. Selwood, A. I., Miles, C. O., Wilkins, A. L. et al., 2010. Isolation, structural determination and acute toxicity of pinnatoxins E, F and G. *Journal of Agricultural and Food Chemistry*, 58, 6532–6542.

83. McCarron, P., Rourke, W. A., Hardstaff, W., Pooley, B., and Quilliam, M. A., 2012. Identification of pinnatoxins and discovery of their fatty acid ester metabolites in mussels (*Mytilus edulis*) from eastern Canada. *Journal of Agricultural and Food Chemistry*, 60, 1437–1446.

84. Rundberget, T., Aasen, J. A. B., Selwood, A. I., and Miles, C. O., 2011. Pinnatoxins and spirolides in Norwegian blue mussels and seawater. *Toxicon*, 58, 700–711.

85. Alexander, J., Benford, D., Cockburn, A. et al., 2010. Scientific Opinion on marine biotoxins in shellfish—Cyclic imines (spirolides, gymnodimines, pinnatoxins and pteriatoxins). *The European Food Safety Authority Journal*, 1628, 1–39.

86. Pottier, I., Vernoux, J. P., Jones, A., and Lewis, R. J., 2002. Characterisation of multiple Caribbean ciguatoxins and congeners in individual specimens of horse-eye jack (*Caranx latus*) by high-performance liquid chromatography/mass spectrometry. *Toxicon*, 40, 929–939.

87. Yogi, K., Oshiro, N., Inafuku, Y., Hirama, M., and Yasumoto, T., 2011. Detailed LC-MS/MS analysis of ciguatoxins revealing distinct regional and species characteristics in fish and causative alga from the Pacific. *Analytical Chemistry*, 83, 8886–8891.

88. Hamilton, B., Hurbungs, M., Jones, A., and Lewis, R. J., 2002. Multiple ciguatoxins present in Indian Ocean reef fish. *Toxicon*, 40, 1347–1353.

89. Lewis, R. J., Holmes, M. J., Alewood, P. F., and Jones, A., 1994. Ionspray mass spectrometry of ciguatoxin-1, maitotoxin-2 and -3, and related marine polyether toxins. *Natural Toxins*, 2, 56–63.

90. Murata, M., Naoki, H., Matsunaga, S., Satake, M., and Yasumoto, T., 1994. Structure and partial stereo-chemical assignments for maitotoxin, the most toxic and largest natural non-biopolymer. *Journal of the American Chemical Society*, 116, 7098–7107.

91. Lewis, R. J., Jones, A., and Vernoux, J. P., 1999. HPLC/tandem electrospray mass spectrometry for the determination of sub-ppb levels of Pacific and Caribbean ciguatoxins in crude extracts of fish. *Analytical Chemistry*, 71, 247–250.

92. Abraham, A., Jester, E. L. E., Granade, H. R., Plakas, S. M., and Dickey, R. W., 2012. Caribbean cigua-toxin profile in raw and cooked fish implicated in ciguatera. *Food Chemistry*, 131, 192–198.

93. Tubaro, A., Dell'Ovo, V., Sosa, S., and Florio, C., 2010. Yessotoxins: A toxicological overview. *Toxicon*, 56, 163–172.

94. Miles, C. O., Wilkins, A. L., Munday, R. et al., 2004. Isolation of pectenotoxin-2 from *Dinophysis acuta* and its conversion to pectenotoxin-2 seco acid, and preliminary assessment of their acute toxicities. *Toxicon*, 43, 1–9.

95. Anon, Commission Regulation (EC) No 2074/2005 of 5 December 2005 laying down implementing measures for certain products under Regulation (EC) No 853/2004 of the European Parliament and of the Council and for the organisation of official controls under Regulation (EC) No 854/2004 of the European Parliament and of the Council and Regulation (EC) No 882/2004 of the European Parliament and of the Council, derogating from Regulation (EC) No 852/2004 of the European Parliament and of the Council and amending Regulations (EC) No 853/2004 and (EC) No 854/2004 (Text with EEA relevance), 2074/2005, C. R. E. N. *Official Journal of European Communications*, 2005, L338, pp. 27–59.

96. Anon, Commission Decision of 12 August 2002 implementing Council Directive 96/23/EC concerning the performance of analytical methods and the interpretation of results (2002/657/EC). *Official Journal of the European Communities*, 2002, L221, pp. 8–36.

97. Anon, Method validation and quality control procedures for pesticide residues analysis in food and feed, SANCO/12495/2011, D. N. http://ec.europa.eu/food/plant/plant_protection_products/guidance_documents/docs/qualcontrol_en.pdf, 2011, last accessed February 10, 2013.

98. Anon, Commission directive 2004/853/EC specific hygiene rules for food of animal origin, 2004/853/EC, C. d. *Official Journal of European Communications*, 2004, L226, pp. 22–82.

99. Anon, Standard for live and raw bivalve molluscs, 292-2008, C. S.2008.

100. McNabb, P., Selwood, A. I., and Holland, P. T., 2005. Multiresidue method for determination of algal toxins in shellfish: Single-laboratory validation and interlaboratory study. *Journal of AOAC International*, 88, 761–772.

101. Stobo, L. A., Lacaze, J. P. C. L., Scott, A. C., Gallacher, S., Smith, E. A., and Quilliam, M. A., 2005. Liquid chromatography with mass spectrometry—Detection of lipophilic shellfish toxins. *Journal of AOAC International*, 88, 1371–1382.

102. These, A., Klemm, C., Nausch, I., and Uhlig, S., 2011. Results of a European interlaboratory method validation study for the quantitative determination of lipophilic marine biotoxins in raw and cooked shellfish based on high-performance liquid chromatography-tandem mass spectrometry. Part I: Collaborative study. *Analytical and Bioanalytical Chemistry*, 399, 1245–1256.

103. van den Top, H. J., Gerssen, A., McCarron, P., and van Egmond, H. P., 2011. Quantitative determination of marine lipophilic toxins in mussels, oysters and cockles using liquid chromatography-mass spectrometry: Inter-laboratory validation study. *Food Additives and Contaminants Part A*, 28, 1745–1757.

104. Gerssen, A., Klijnstra, M., Cubbon, S., and Gledhill, A., UPLC-MS/MS method for the routine quanti-fication of regulated and non-regulated lipophilic marine biotoxins in shellfish, http://www.waters.com/webassets/cms/library/docs/720004601en.pdf, 2013, last accessed February 10, 2013.

105. Blay, P., Hui, J. P., Chang, J., and Melanson, J. E., 2011. Screening for multiple classes of marine bio-toxins by liquid chromatography-high-resolution mass spectrometry. *Analytical and Bioanalytical Chemistry*, 400, 577–585.

106. Kittler, K., Preiss-Weigert, A., and These, A., 2010. Identification strategy using combined mass spec-trometric techniques for elucidation of phase I and phase II in vitro metabolites of lipophilic marine biotoxins. *Analytical Chemistry*, 82, 9329–9335.

107. Peters, R. J., Oosterink, J. E., Stolker, A. A., Georgakopoulos, C., and Nielen, M. W., 2010. Generic sam-ple preparation combined with high-resolution liquid chromatography-time-of-flight mass spectrometry for unification of urine screening in doping-control laboratories. *Analytical and Bioanalytical Chemistry*, 396, 2583–2598.

108. Stolker, A. A., Rutgers, P., Oosterink, E. et al., 2008. Comprehensive screening and quantification of veterinary drugs in milk using UPLC-ToF-MS. *Analytical and Bioanalytical Chemistry*, 391, 2309–2322.
109. Vonaparti, A., Lyris, E., Angelis, Y. S. et al., 2010. Preventive doping control screening analysis of prohibited substances in human urine using rapid-resolution liquid chromatography/high-resolution time-of-flight mass spectrometry. *Rapid Communications in Mass Spectrometry*, 24, 1595–1609.
110. Martinez-Villalba, A., Vaclavik, L., Moyano, E., Galceran, M. T., and Hajslova, J., 2013. Direct analysis in real time high-resolution mass spectrometry for high-throughput analysis of antiparasitic veterinary drugs in feed and food. *Rapid Communications in Mass Spectrometry*, 27, 467–475.
111. Monge, M. E., Harris, G. A., Dwivedi, P., and Fernandez, F. M., 2013. Mass spectrometry: Recent advances in direct open air surface sampling/ionization. *Chemical Reviews*, 113, 2269–2308.
112. Lapthorn, C., Pullen, F., and Chowdhry, B. Z., 2013. Ion mobility spectrometry-mass spectrometry (IMS-MS) of small molecules: Separating and assigning structures to ions. *Mass Spectrometry Reviews*, 32, 43–71.
113. Armenta, S., Alcala, M., and Blanco, M., 2011. A review of recent, unconventional applications of ion mobility spectrometry (IMS). *Analytica Chimica Acta*, 703, 114–123.

15

Standards for Marine and Freshwater Toxins

Álvaro Antelo, Carmen Alfonso, and Mercedes Álvarez

CONTENTS

15.1 Introduction

The use of reference materials (RMs) is part of good quality assurance (QA) practices, which include evaluation of instrument performance independent of the methodology used. Highest quality RMs are certified for estimating concentration values of a toxin or toxins of interest, reflecting high confidence in accuracy and thorough investigation of all known or suspected sources of bias. Nevertheless, the availability of RMs or standards may not ensure the highest level of accuracy and precision in an analytical laboratory; a user must inspect whether the certified RM (CRM) fulfils the requirements for its quality control (QC) program. The intended use of CRMs becomes an important factor for properly using the certified values and providing reliable analytical data.[1]

Marine toxin and freshwater CRMs play a decisive role in the standardization of the testing methods, thus minimizing variability through a reference measurement system. The use of appropriate RMs is an important aspect of accreditation to ISO/IEC 17025.[2] The essential components of this reference marine toxin measurement system are the definition of the toxin to be measured, measurement procedures (including reference measurement procedures and value transfer protocols), and materials (including RMs and calibrators).

15.2 CRMs Are Required

The term harmful algal bloom (HAB) is used to describe the blooms of toxin-producing algae that kill fish, make shellfish poisonous, and cause numerous problems in marine coastal waters. These algae are consumed by bivalve mollusks as part of their natural diet. The consumption of shellfish contaminated with toxins can cause severe intoxications in humans. The toxin release mechanism is also poorly understood, and it seems to be a defense mechanism against other organisms or harmful environmental conditions. Therefore, toxins in products for human consumption are currently a major threat of global interest because of the involvement of public health and economic issues. The occurrence of cyanobacterial mass populations can pose a significant water quality problem. Consumers have to be protected via a system of control involving analytical measurements, which require accuracy and reliability. For these reasons, search for new, rapid, and effective methods to detect marine toxins is a priority for many food safety control laboratories.[3,4]

The chemical nature of marine and freshwater biotoxins and their physical properties allow the classification of these marine natural products into several families of lipophilic and hydrophilic toxins. The marine lipophilic toxin (MLT) group includes yessotoxins (YTXs), azaspiracids (AZAs), pectenotoxins (PTXs), gymnodimines (GYM), spirolides (SPXs), ciguatoxins (CTXs), diarrhetic shellfish poisoning (DSP) toxins, brevetoxins (PbTX), maitoxins, and palytoxins. In addition to the lipophilic toxins mentioned above, hydrophilic toxins, paralytic shellfish poisoning (PSP) toxins, amnesic shellfish poisoning (ASP) toxins, and tetrodotoxins may also be present in shellfish.[5] Conversely, cylindrospermopsins, nodularins, microcystins, and anatoxins are identified mostly as cyanobacterial freshwater toxins. The saxitoxin group of toxins is also produced by cyanobacterial blooms.[6]

Marine biotoxins detected worldwide, but particularly in European waters, were originally classified based on their acute symptomatic effects in humans following intoxication. The three main toxin groups monitored in the European Union (EU) are PSP toxins, DSP toxins, and ASP toxins. However, as alternative detection methods are considered, classification is beginning to focus more on the chemical structures and properties of the toxins.[7] In Europe, the number of toxins to be monitored exceeds the figure of 40.

Nowadays, analytical methods for detecting marine toxins comprise in vivo assays (mouse and rat bioassays), in vitro assays (cell, receptor, enzyme inhibition assays, and immunoassays), and chemical assays, which include analysis by high-performance liquid chromatography (HPLC), with detection by ultraviolet (UV) and diode arrays, fluorescence, mass spectrometry (MS), or capillary electrophoresis (CE).[8]

The EU has established legislation for three major shellfish biotoxin groups that can be detected in shellfish, whereas GYM, SPXs, and CTXs are not yet under legislation. The toxins under legislation are PSP toxins, lipophilic toxins, including those responsible for DSP, and ASP toxins. Shellfish and fishery products placed on the market must not contain marine toxins above the current maximum European limits set in shellfish meat (sm): PSP toxins, 800 μg/kg sm; ASP toxins, 20 mg/kg sm; okadaic acid (OA), dinophysistoxins, PTXs together, 160 μg (OA eq.)/kg sm; YTXs, 1 mg (YTX eq.)/kg sm; and AZAs, 160 μg (AZA eq.)/kg sm.[9,10]

Up until now, the reference method for lipophilic toxins was mouse bioassay (MBA). For many years, this assay has traditionally been used to monitor toxin levels in shellfish for human consumption. In this assay, a sample extract is injected into the peritoneal cavity of a mouse, followed by an observation period to determine symptoms and time to death, which usually correlates with the amount of toxin present.[11] However, the European Food Safety Agency (EFSA) has recently published several scientific opinions on marine toxins, with proposals to reduce some toxin limits and use detection methods that could replace the MBA.[10] In this sense, biological tests are not completely satisfactory due to low sensitivity and absence of specificity. Moreover, there is a growing resistance against the use of animals in experiments.[12] For these reasons, the EU has proposed a series of methods for the detection of marine toxins as an alternative to animal testing methods, pending the validation that their implementation will provide an equivalent level of public health protection. These methods are in vitro assays and chemical analyses. The methods are highly sensitive, being modified to high-throughput formats, and provide total toxicity response.[13] Regarding chemical assays, new analytical methods have also been developed for the determination of toxins in shellfish, especially LC-MS/MS methods.[3,14] These methods need certified standards that are not available for many of the toxins. Despite this, several studies support this approach as an essential research tool in the marine toxin field, which has led LC-MS/MS to become the leading and most demanded technology for improved screening methods.[11,15–17]

In January 2011, Commission Regulation Number 15/2011 stated that LC-MS/MS-based methods are the technology to be recognized as the reference standard for detection of MLTs in shellfish, thus replacing the live animal assay.[18] The new regulation will be applicable from July 1, 2011, and allow the member states to adapt their methods to LC-MS/MS; the MBA may still be used until December 31, 2014. After 3 years of coexistence with the MBA, the LC-MS/MS method shall become the reference method. Therefore, this technique has been evaluated in an interlaboratory validation exercise that was considered to be successful and should now be applied as the reference method following indications agreed to by the National Reference Laboratories Network.[19] MBA has been the most important international method for detecting marine toxins, and all analytical methods designed as official methods shall be evaluated against bioassays using internationally accepted protocols. Some references are working in this way to facilitate the interpretation of the MBA during this transition period, for example, the evaluation of the specificity and selectivity of MBA in comparison with an LC-MS/MS method in detecting lipophilic marine toxins in mussels of the middle Adriatic Sea.[20] The data show a high percentage of false-positive results on MBA due to interference by YTXs. It was also possible to evaluate the toxicity profile of the samples analyzed.

Some interlaboratory studies involving several groups have been performed to check the accuracy, precision, and recovery of LC-MS/MS.[15,19,21] The EU official method has been established according to an interlaboratory validation study where different parameters in either LC or MS tandem detection had been studied but not fixed.[19] However, even in the circumstance of an approved method that has been validated internationally, several parameters are open to the criteria of the technician in-charge of the analysis, such as the commercial source of the mobile phase, whereas others are already approved as being openly usable, such as the conversion factor on MS/MS when using one standard per group or the toxic equivalent factor, which is another source of uncertainty when providing the final result of the analysis.[22] Overall, the final result in a validated method is still affected by several uncontrolled aspects, which could produce considerable errors in the final outcome of an analysis, considering that marine toxins are rather toxic compounds.[10]

In addition to these variables, the new legislation allows each toxin to be quantified regardless of the presence of other toxins, whereas the MBA detects all toxins together; hence, the legal toxic value is potentially increased severalfold using the chemical approach when several toxin groups are present in a sample.

The EU relies on MS/MS as a reference method for monitoring marine toxins for food safety protection since the rate of false positives or false negatives might be unpredictably high for values close to the legal limits, being of special concern false negatives where toxic samples might be identified as negatives by using a given combination of parameters that are not covered by current validation protocols.

In summary, analytical methods are useful tools to show toxin profile, characterize new toxins, or search for analogs, but in order to protect public health and food safety, more stringent conditions, in order to increase methodology reliability, are needed.[23] From a technical perspective, the HPLC-MS/MS method is convenient, practical, and fit for purpose. Marine toxins and freshwater CRMs play a decisive role in the validation of testing methods that are applied within the framework of QA in routine analytical measurements through a reference measurement system, and therefore, the highest level of accuracy and precision is ensured. The use of appropriate RMs is an important aspect of accreditation to ISO/IEC 17025.[2] The essential components of this reference marine toxin measurement system are the definition of the toxin to be measured, measurement procedures (including reference measurement procedures and value transfer protocols), and materials (including RMs and calibrators).

The advantages of LC-MS/MS are high sensitivity, precision, automation, quantitation, and confirmation of toxin identity. Most MLTs are well suited to LC separation due to their lability, polarity, and nonvolatility.[3] Where LC-MS/MS carries a high operating cost, in vitro functional assays or biochemical assays are ideal for "screening out" negative samples.[5] These assays are low cost, provide rapid sample throughput, and allow detection of new bioactive compounds. However, in the presence of co-extracted shellfish matrix interferences, false-positive and false-negative results can occur. Specific and accurate quantitation cannot be achieved with immunoassays where shellfish samples contain groups of toxins and where variable levels of individual toxins exist. In most instances, such techniques require a level of confirmation by more quantitative approaches and comprehensive validation exercises to describe method performance characteristics.

Cefas recommends it to be implemented in the UK statutory lipophilic toxin-monitoring programs and applied to the measurement and reporting of MLTs in official control samples of shellfish species targeted for method validation.[24] Following implementation, they recommended the need for, and effectiveness of, the use of matrix-matched standards (arising from findings from interlaboratory studies), incorporation of new lipophilic toxin reference standards (e.g., AZA2, AZA3) into methodologies as they become commercially available, and validation performance checks and verifications for minor species to allow the method to be extended to all national official control shellfish samples.

In order to quantify toxins in the absence of available standards, it is sometimes assumed that analogs from the same toxin group can provide an equimolar response by MS/MS tandem detection. Thus, the calibration curve constructed for one toxin is used for the quantification of other toxins from the same group. However, there are studies showing that a toxin's concentration reported with a calibration curve that is not its own can be completely different depending on different parameters.[23]

There are currently no federal regulations or guidelines in the United States for protecting human health and ecosystem viability from cyanobacterial HABs (cyanoHABs) that occur in fresh, estuary, and marine water environments.

A number of countries have developed regulations or guidelines for detecting cyanotoxins and cyanobacteria in drinking water and, in some cases, in water used for recreational activity and agriculture. The main focus internationally has been on microcystin toxins, produced predominantly by *Microcystis aeruginosa*. This is because microcystins are widely regarded as the most significant potential source of human injury by cyanobacteria on a worldwide scale. Many international guidelines have taken their lead from the World Health Organization's (WHO) provisional guideline value of 1 μg/L for microcystin-LR in drinking water, which was released in 1998 (WHO 2004). The WHO guideline value is stated as being "provisional" because it covers only microcystin-LR for the reasons that the toxicology is limited and new data for toxicity of cyanobacterial toxins are being generated. The derivation of this guideline is based on data that there is reported human injury related to consumption of drinking water containing cyanobacteria or from limited work with experimental animals.[25]

Although guidelines for estimating cyanotoxins and cyanobacterial cell numbers in recreational water are in place in a number of countries, it is believed that there is currently insufficient information to derive sound guidelines for the use of water contaminated by cyanobacteria or toxins for agricultural production, fisheries, and ecosystem protection. In relation to the need for specific regulations for toxins in the United States, surveys that have been carried out to date would indicate that the priority compounds for regulations, based on their incidence and distribution, are microcystins, cylindrospermopsins, and anatoxin-a. Additional research is required to support guideline development, including whole-of-life animal studies with each of the known cyanotoxins. In view of the animal studies that indicate that microcystins may act as tumor promoters, and also some evidence of genotoxicity and carcinogenicity of cylindrospermopsins, it may be appropriate to carry out whole-of-life animal studies using both toxicity and carcinogenicity as endpoints. In relation to microcystins, it is known that there are a large number of congeners, and the toxico-dynamics and kinetics of these variants are not well understood.

Further research is needed to consider the approach to take in formulating health advisories or regulations for toxin mixtures, that is, multiple microcystins, or mixtures of toxin types. An important requirement for regulations is the availability of robust monitoring and analytical protocols for toxins. Currently, rapid and economical screening or quantitative analytical methods are not available to the water industry or natural resource managers, and this is a priority before the release of guidelines and regulations. There is insufficient information available on a range of categories usually required to satisfy comprehensive risk assessment processes for the major toxins to currently adopt any of the international guidelines as regulations in the United States. The major limitations that need to be overcome include the capacity to deal with multiple toxin congeners, the absence of robust analytical methods for compliance monitoring, and the absence of certified toxin standards to support analyses.

15.3 Types of RMs and Standards

RMs are defined as materials whose identity and/or properties have been established. They are classified into different types based on their properties, state, or content and are used for specific applications, such as calibration of equipment, assessing measurement methods or chemical analysis. There are pure substances, standard solutions, matrix RMs, physicochemical RMs, and reference objects.[26] Pure substances are characterized by their chemical purity or trace impurities and are often used to prepare gravimetrically standard solutions and gas mixtures, which are used for calibration purposes. Matrix RMs are prepared from natural matrices containing analytes of interest or from synthetic mixtures. Physicochemical RMs are used for their storage or transfer properties such as melting point and viscosity, whereas reference objects are characterized by properties such as taste, odor, hardness, and microscopy characteristics.

In the field of analytical chemistry, the definition of RMs must be clearly stated, without ambiguities that could be misunderstood and led to mistakes when the material is applied for specific purposes, such as the validation of an analytical method or QC. From this point of view, the internationally accepted definition of RM is "material, sufficiently homogeneous and stable with respect to one or more specified properties, which has been established to be fit for its intended use in a measurement process."[27] RMs can take a variety of forms such as pure substances, solutions, mixtures, and matrix materials.

This is a new definition approved by the Committee on Reference Materials of the International Organization for Standardization (ISO REMCO) that has been attempted to clarify the previous definitions, due to the accumulated experience in this field over the past years. In this sense, it explains that RM is a term that includes certified and non-CRMs, homogeneity and stability being two properties that must be guaranteed for all RMs. The specified properties are not only quantitative, but qualitative ones are also of interest in many methods. One example is the identity of compounds, which is determined by methods that must be validated in the same way as quantitative methods, for example, the ones to calculate the amount of a compound. In both cases, RMs can be used to validate and verify proper functioning of the methods. Different uses can be defined for each RM, for example, calibration of equipment, verification of measurement methods, or QC. The most important limitation in the use of an RM is that a single RM cannot be used for calibration and validation at the same time in the same measurement.[28] Production and characterization of RMs are very important to maintain and improve a worldwide coherent system of measurements.[29]

CRMs are one subgroup of RMs, defined as follows:

> Reference materials characterized by a metrologically valid procedure for one or more specified properties, accompanied by a certificate that provides the value of the specified property, its associated uncertainty, and a statement of metrological traceability.[27]

The metrologically valid procedure must fulfill the requirements of ISO Guides 34[30] and 35,[29] whereas the certificate accompanying the materials must content the items listed in ISO Guide 31.[31] These requirements can appear in other guides, which can be used for production and certification if the final product matches the previous definition. Moreover, the value of the specified property can be qualitative, with an associated uncertainty expressed as probability and estimated using the best available knowledge. The term traceability means "property of a measurement result whereby the result can be related to a reference through a documented unbroken chain of calibrations, each contributing to the measurement uncertainty."[32] In this sense, the metrological traceability guarantees the consistency and usefulness of the measurement results obtained. There are CRMs produced before the establishment of the previous definition that have no stated traceability.

CRMs must be produced and characterized following technically valid procedures. Users need to know the details of the procedures used for production, characterization, determination of stability and homogeneity, and estimation of the uncertainties associated with each of these steps. These characteristics can be used to select an appropriate RM manufacturer.[33] CRMs are useful to implement the concept of traceability of measurement results in chemistry, biology, physics, and other sciences dealing with materials and/or samples.[29]

Matrix RMs are another subgroup of RMs characterized by their composition and their similarity to laboratory samples. These type of materials can be gaseous, solid, liquid, alloys, biological matrices, etc., and their more common uses are method validation and QA/QC processes. Usually these materials are not used for calibration, due to the lack of traceability of the property values of most of them. This problem can be associated with the laboratory comparisons usually made to obtain those values.[34] Nevertheless, there are also certified matrix RMs whose properties are traceable to international or national references.

All types of RMs must be clearly labeled so that the appropriate certificates and/or analytical information could be correctly identified. This information must include their shelf life, storage conditions, applicability, and restrictions of use.[33]

Other two types of materials can be referred to as primary and secondary standards. A primary standard is a "standard that is designated or widely acknowledged as having the highest metrological qualities and whose value is accepted without reference to other standards of the same quantity, within a specified context,"[35] whereas a secondary standard is a "standard whose value is assigned by comparison with a primary standard of the same quantity." A lot of CRMs are classified as secondary standards due to the use of a procedure traceable to primary standards to obtain property values during the certification process. The suitability of a particular standard for quantification of a material's property depends not only on the type of the standard but also on its physical behavior and its similarities to the material to be quantified.

Other terminologies, as well as different hierarchies[36,37] and classifications, of RMs and standards can be found according to their intended use.[38]

The term measurement standard is defined as a "realization of the definition of a given quantity, with stated quantity value and associated measurement uncertainty, used as reference."[32] This kind of material is used for calibration of equipment, measurements, or processes and for identification purposes and can be also named calibrants. These substances can be solutions of pure substances or matrices in which a specific parameter or property has been characterized.[39] One use of measurement standards is the establishment of traceability through the calibration of measuring instruments, standards, or systems. The standard measurement uncertainty must be small[34] because it will be a component of the combined uncertainty of each measurement performed using the standard.

The term working standard is used to refer to standards "used routinely to calibrate or verify measuring instruments or measuring systems."[32]

A control material is one that has been completely characterized and analyzed using the same treatment and methods as unknown samples. The value of concentration of an appropriate analyte must have had been assigned and it must be representative of the test samples, that is, it must have the same matrix and a similar physical form. Moreover, it must be stable over the required time period (usually a long one), be possible to be divided into identical portions for routine analysis, and be available in large quantities.[40]

CRMs with a suitable composition can be used as control materials, thereby imparting traceability to the measurements performed as well. There are limitations to this use that must be considered. In a lot of analyses, there is not a CRM that matches the needs in spite of the increasing availability. Moreover, the high cost and quantity of CRMs can be a problem for laboratories performing a wide range of analyses and requiring a wide range of CRMs.[40]

Internal QC materials (sometimes named house RMs) can also be used. These materials are prepared by laboratories if appropriate RMs are not available (with the correct matrix and measurand), are very expensive to be used for QC in a large number of experiments, or are not stable over longer time periods. If possible, RMs must be used to assign a value to internal QC materials (QCMs). With this approach, RMs would be used to validate the methods and ensure that the data produced are traceable to a fundamental standard, and internal QCMs would continuously monitor the correct performance of those methods. So, the two types of materials can be used by the same laboratory to achieve different results.[34]

If there is not a suitable RM, laboratories can use a validated method for the chemical characterization of the internal QCM, performing a parallel analysis by a second method, which is independent in theory and practice from the first one.[34]

In the field of marine and freshwater toxins, the amount of available RMs and standards is low, which implies negative impacts on research, method validation, and sample quantification. Usually research is done using different materials, which can be classified as CRMs, purified materials, and in-house developed materials depending on cost and availability.

Available CRMs for this kind of toxins are solutions of a certain concentration in suitable solvents. Suppliers of this kind of materials must identify the method used to quantify the material, guarantee its suitability for this purpose, and assure traceability of the measurement data obtained. Moreover, homogeneity and stability of the materials must be guaranteed, and the overall uncertainty must take into account all factors involved in the certification process. There are also certain tissue CRMs that can be used during the validation of quantification methods and to compare different extraction or cleanup procedures.

Purified materials (with different names depending on the manufacturer) can be defined as materials whose identity, quantity, and purity have been completely established by appropriate methods such as chromatography using different types of detectors (mass spectrometers, fluorescence, UV, etc.) or by nuclear magnetic resonance (NMR). These materials are not certified and their traceability can sometimes be poorly established, but they are used in the absence of CRMs, especially when toxins are available in such less quantity that it does not allow a complete certification process.

In-house-developed materials for marine and freshwater toxins can be defined as materials containing one or more toxins, without an accurate quantification. They can be naturally contaminated samples or extracts in different stages of purification, and their uses can be in QC, identification of rare compounds, recovery studies, etc. Each laboratory can develop and store these kind of materials so that they can use them in applications for which they are appropriate, thus making an economical saving.

Although the global availability of this group of compounds is low, it depends on the specific toxin. Usually only an analog of each of the most important groups of toxins is commercially available, but this is not always true. For example, in the group of diarrhetic toxins, there are reference standards for OA, dinophysistoxin-2 and 1, and also for contaminated mussel RMs. In other groups, for example, in the YTX, PTX, or AZA groups, there are a number of non-available analogs. For some emerging toxins, such as CTXs and palytoxins, there are no CRMs or calibrants.

Current suppliers of this kind of toxins can be companies that distribute different organic and inorganic compounds or specialized manufacturing organizations. Members of this last group are scarce and try to increase the number of commercially available analogs around the world. This is an expensive task, which requires deep technical knowledge and experience, defining laborious production, purification, characterization, and certification processes. The National Research Council of Canada and the Japan Food Research Laboratory developed this function many years ago. At present, there is another company in Spain named Laboratorio CIFGA that provides certified and non-certified solutions for a number of marine toxins and contaminated and non-contaminated shellfish and algae materials.

15.4 Uses of Reference Materials and Standards

RMs and standards are used to guarantee the quality of analytical results obtained in laboratories, which is influenced by several variables. Equipment and methods must be calibrated, performed by competent and trained staff, and fully validated. Traceability and measurement uncertainty must be completely defined so that compatibility could be demonstrated between results achieved by laboratories in different locations. This is essential when the consequence of a measurement is related to human health or has an economic impact and when results from different countries are compared, for example, for exportation purposes. The demonstration of the accuracy of a laboratory is also essential to obtain and maintain laboratory accreditations, according to international requirements (ISO, GLP, etc.) and verified using external organisms. Finally, reliable measurements need complete implementation of QC/QA procedures performed using some kind of standard materials.

RMs can be used for method characterization, validation, and verification. Once a measurement process is completely defined, ideally in a written procedure with all the necessary specifications, it must be characterized, by one laboratory or by an interlaboratory program, through the calculation of its precision and its trueness, which is expressed as the standard deviation and the bias of the measurement. A specific method can be used if the calculated values of these two parameters are within the appropriate limits mandated by regulations, imposed by commercial concerns, or fixed according to previous experience. To guarantee these conditions, the method must be applied to a CRM selected after considering all relevant properties: identity of the measurand, concentration, matrix match and interferences, physical state and form, quantity, homogeneity and stability, measurement uncertainty and characterization, and certification procedures used. Some of these properties are influenced by the duration of the characterization process of characterization, for example, the available quantity must be enough to complete the entire experimental program and to store a stock and the material must remain stable during the entire process or with properties defined at specific times. A user must be sure about the suitability of the selected CRMs with respect to the conditions of the measurement process and about the homogeneity of the CRMs used in each laboratory in an interlaboratory program. To eliminate this variation, the same initial sample can be divided for use between laboratories.[41]

When characterization is performed by one laboratory, precision involves comparison of within-laboratory standard deviation under defined conditions, for example, repeatability conditions, and the required standard deviation, whereas trueness involves comparison of the mean of measurement results and the certified value of the CRMs, considering the between-laboratory component of precision of the measurement process.

If an interlaboratory program is used to characterize the method, the precision is estimated using within-laboratory and between-laboratory standard deviation. Trueness is determined by comparing the overall mean of the interlaboratory measurement program and the certified value of the CRMs.[42]

In both cases, the trueness of the method will be estimated within the limits of the uncertainty of the certified value of the RM and the uncertainty of the measurement method. It is desirable that the uncertainty of the RM contributes to the uncertainty of the global measurement by less than one-third.

Bias differences between two or more methods can also be estimated with RMs without traceable certified values, although this approach is less rigorous. In this case, the RMs must agree with routine samples in terms of matrix type, concentration, etc., and cover the full range of the tested method. The uncertainty associated with the method can be estimated by performing replicate measurements of the RM covering all possible situations in the method.[41]

Method validation can be defined as the process used to define an analytical requirement and confirm that a specific method has performance capabilities consistent with what the application requires.[39] Several performance parameters can be determined, such as selectivity, recovery, accuracy, trueness, limit of detection (LOD) or limit of quantification (LOQ), and working range. Also, the limitations of the method must be characterized and the effects on those parameters must be identified.

Selectivity defines the availability of a method to determine one or more analytes in a complex mixture without interference from other components of the mixture. This property must be studied using different types of samples, from pure measurement standards to mixtures with complex matrices, quantifying in each condition the recovery of the analyte and investigating the interferences. With these data, the applicability of the method can be determined.

To calculate the initial quantity of an analyte in a sample, the recovery of that analyte must be determined. This is usually done by spiking sample portions with the analyte at various levels of concentration, extracting these spiked samples using the same procedures as for test samples, and measuring the analyte concentration. The analyte used to spike must be dissolved in a suitable amount of a solvent enough to completely wet the surface of the solid. The rate of evaporation of this solvent must be carefully considered: if too high, the spike may come out from the pores and cluster, and it will not be sufficiently well bonded to the surface, which can affect the stability of the material. On the other hand, if it is too low, other components of the matrix may migrate or even be lost.[29] The spiking process has a major drawback: differences may appear in the binding of the naturally incurred and spiking analytes, affecting characteristics such as extraction behavior. Hence, this method can provide over- or underestimated recovery values. To solve this problem, recovery studies can be performed using appropriate RMs, which are usually obtained by characterization of natural materials and similar to real test samples.[39] If this is not possible, the equivalence of the spiked and naturally contaminated material must be checked, and this relation must be used to guarantee the reliability of the obtained results.[29]

Matrix effects produce under- or overestimation of analyte concentration when it is quantified in a biological sample. They can be defined as the difference in method response for the same quantity of analyte determined in a tissue extract or in a pure solution. Causes of matrix effects depend on the method of analysis and are not usually completely known. For example, for electrospray ionization in MS, authors suggest that substances that extract together with the compound of interest from a sample interfere with the ionization process, producing a suppression or enhancement in its signal.[43] The existence of matrix interferences in the signal measured by a method can be detected during its validation. In this case, a matched matrix RM must be used to perform the validation,[33] with a composition as close as possible to the samples. If this material is not available, a sample spiked with an RM can be used for performing the necessary studies to guarantee its stability.

If a new or rarely used method is applied, RMs are used to confirm all the characteristics that influence the obtained results, for example, personal characteristics such as capabilities of the staff or material characteristics such as equipment and standards. This application is useful when an internationally validated method is applied. In this case, the method must be verified by each laboratory, assuring it will be performed correctly. The best option in this context is the use of appropriate CRMs, but if this kind of material is not available, another measurement standard can be used. RMs can also be used for troubleshooting if the results obtained with a completely defined method are incorrect.[41] If a laboratory can achieve correct results using CRMs, it is supposed that it will achieve correct results for the same parameters in the same matrix.

Traceability of measurements performed by a laboratory must be established to guarantee the reliability of its results. This can be achieved by method validation, calibration, and use of standards for physical quantities such as mass or volume.

Calibration is the principal activity to guarantee the traceability of a system or instrument. It can be defined as the process to establish a relation between the indications shown by a measuring instrument or system and the values yielded by measurement standards, with the final objective of obtaining a measurement result from an indication.[32] The quality of a calibration depends on the uncertainty of the reference used and the appropriateness of this reference taking into account either the analytical method used or the samples tested. The calculated uncertainty of a calibration (obtained from these parameters) must be compared with the required uncertainty of the measurement, which depend on applicable regulations, needs of the customer, etc. Calibration in analytical chemistry must use standards that accomplish the needs of the equipment being calibrated, traceable to international references and with small uncertainty; both properties must appear in their certificates of calibration. Identity and purity of standards are important issues too because their associated uncertainty will influence the global uncertainty of the measurement.[33]

Stability of the instruments used is essential to guarantee the validity of calibration; this is achieved with appropriate QC and correct recalibration intervals. The calibration schedule must guarantee that all measurements with a significant effect on results are traceable to a measurement standard. National and international measurement standards are the best option, CRMs being the most appropriate standards. If this kind of materials is not available, a stable material with appropriate properties can be prepared by the laboratory using chemicals supplied by reputable manufacturers with known purity and composition. To assure these properties, additional analysis may be needed, which can be done by the laboratory or a network of laboratories, in both cases using one or more validated methods. This is especially important for trace analysis because very low quantities of impurities can produce interferences in the results.

There are two kinds of calibrations in an analytical process: calibration of a measurement stage or instrument and calibration of the complete process.[41]

The first type of calibration is usually done using pure substance RMs. In this case, the uncertainty associated with the RM's purity must be considered when the total uncertainty of the measurement is calculated. To confirm the identity of a material, either certified pure materials can be used or comparisons with reference data can be done. If their availabilities and costs are adequate, the use of CRMs for calibration is the best option to guarantee the traceability of the measurement.[41]

The calibration of a complete analytical procedure depends on its type, which is associated with a basic principle or a number of basic prerequisites.

There are analytical methods that do not need to use CRMs, for example, titrations or weights because traceability is guaranteed using balances and volumetric instruments calibrated conveniently.

There are procedures that use measurements taken during analysis to obtain results by performing a calculation based on the physical and chemical laws applicable in each case. The basic calibration procedure is the identification of each quantity whose measurement is necessary to establish the analytical result by calculation.[44]

Other methods use the response of a detection system to a set of calibration samples of known content and interpolate the sample signal in the response curve obtained. In this case, it is assumed that differences in composition, form, or any other characteristic between the calibration samples and measured samples have no effect on the response. To satisfy this condition, the analytical procedure can be modified, reducing its sensitivity to differences, by either applying a procedure to give a similar form to the calibration set and the samples or by limiting the scope. The working standards in this case generally consist of a determined quantity of analyte diluted in a larger quantity of diluent. Traceability is guaranteed by the calibration of the mass measurements and the system (which can include variables like temperature and humidity) and by knowledge of the purity of the materials used. This type of calibration is usually performed using commercial standard solutions with calculated uncertainties.

Finally, there are methods whose detection system is sensitive to different types of matrices. If this parameter is ignored, a systematic error will be generated.[44] These methods must be calibrated using matrix RMs that will follow the same procedures as the test samples (intermediate operations such as extractions, derivatizations, and evaporation) to guarantee that both share the same characteristics. The matrix must be similar in the selected materials and the tested samples, and measured analyte must be the same, with concentrations at the same levels. This kind of RM also provides an estimation of the recovery of an analyte at the end of the measurement process, taking into account processing losses, contamination, and interferences. The recovery can be defined as the amount of analyte in the original sample relative to that in the processed sample after procedures like extractions, digestions, and derivatizations. Spiked samples can also be used for this purpose, but their recovery does not necessarily simulate the extraction of the native analyte from the samples since the spiked analyte in solid samples can be freely available on the surface of the sample particles, whereas the native analyte can be strongly adsorbed within the particles and, therefore, less extracted.

Methods and instruments can be calibrated using other materials without evidence of traceability and uncertainty information. In such a case, each laboratory must demonstrate their suitability for their intended purpose.[45]

QA procedures include all measures used in a laboratory to ensure the quality of obtained results. The principles of QA have been listed in different standards, which can be divided in three groups, ISO/IEC 17025, ISO/IEC 9001, and GLP (OECD Principles of Good Laboratory Practice). The first standard is related to the technical competence of laboratories to carry out specific experiments, the second standard includes quality management for facilities producing or supplying services, and the third standard is related to organizational processes and conditions under which laboratory measurements are realized. Nevertheless, a laboratory can design its own QA procedures, which might include the implementation of a quality system, controlled by qualified staff, with requirements for reagents, RMs, and environment and procedures for QC, staff training, calibration, method validation, establishment of traceability, calculation of measurement uncertainty, internal audit and review, proficiency test, and management of preventive and corrective actions and complaints. Quality control (QC) is a group of activities realized to fulfill the requirements for quality and is applied to specific samples or batches of samples. Examples of QC procedures are analysis of blind samples, blanks, spiked samples, RMs, and QC samples.[33] QC is necessary to proof the performance of a laboratory, together with permanent QA, with continuous monitoring during routine activity of the laboratory, with normal samples and usual methods.

QC must be done with a material of stated homogeneity and stability so that there is no need to use an RM for this purpose. The same requirements are needed when a proficiency test is done in various laboratories. In this case, comparison is done by using the consensus mean values of the studied properties instead of certified properties values.[41]

A part of the QC process usually is measurement of reference or perfectly described samples in every batch of test samples. If these control samples are placed at regular intervals in an analytical batch, it is possible to check whether the response of the system or instrument is stable.[39]

The frequency of analysis of the control sample (whatever it is) varies depending on the certainty of the method and the importance of the work, two parameters that must be known to establish a required level of QC. For routine analysis, an acceptable QC level is 5%, so 1 in every 20 samples in each batch must be a QC sample. If the used method is routine, a lower level of QC can be accepted. On the other hand, if the procedures performed are complex or unusual, 20% or 50% levels may be required. If the method is used rarely, a complete validation should be made each time. In this case, an RM with certified concentration should be used, and then the samples and spiked samples must be analyzed several times.

The best option to perform QC in a chemical testing is through the use of a CRM for initial validation of the method and a secondary standard (e.g., a QCM) for routine control of the measurements obtained.[33]

CRMs can also be used to store and transfer information on measured property values. For this application, the material must be stable under normal conditions of storage, transport, and use and be homogeneous so that the property value measured in one portion of a batch can be applied to other portions of the same batch (within the limits of uncertainty). Moreover, the associated uncertainty must be adequate for the end use of the CRM and it must be accompanied by a certificate with all measuring information. All measurements must be traceable to national measurements standards such that the CRMs can be used to compare national measurement standards.[42]

In this sense, CRMs with accepted property values can be used to obtain both SI (International System of Units) base units and derived units. In some cases, the reproduction of an SI unit according to its definition is difficult and expensive, so a better option is to carry out the measurements on a practical scale based on values assigned to the RMs. This kind of scale is defined by two items: a CRM and a document containing the specifications of the measurement method.[42]

Although there are many applications of RMs, their suitability for a specific purpose must be considered before use. There are characteristics that influence this suitability, one of them being the uncertainty of the certified value, but there are others that are not usually considered and can be more important for a specific purpose, such as concentration, matrix match, homogeneity, cost, and availability. Moreover, there are factors concerning the certifying body, such as validity of the measurement and certification processes used, compliance with the requirements listed in ISO Guide 34 (or equivalent standards), and availability of a certificate or a report that must be considered as well. Ideally, compliance with the requirements listed in ISO Guide 34 must be accredited by an external accreditation body; other aspects, such as the use of the RM in interlaboratory trials and its use by different laboratories over a period of years in different measurement methods can, however, be considered.

To assess the suitability of an RM for a determined use, the first stage is defining the analytical requirement with all available details such as the analyte to be measured, its concentration range, the measurement uncertainty of the method, and the matrix of the tested samples. Using these data, an RM among different commercial options can be selected, and all available information can be obtained from the supplier. If the characteristics of the RM are appropriate for the analytical requirements described and the data concerning the quality of the supplier are satisfactory, then the RM is considered suitable for this use. If one of these conditions does not match, an alternative RM must be found or the analytical requirements must be changed.[41]

There are procedures performed using CRMs that can be done with other kinds of standards such as pure compounds, solutions of pure elements, and homogeneous materials. These applications include all measurements that do not consider the certified value and its uncertainty or that compare relative values without external references (e.g., values obtained with the same instrument in two separate instances). For example, CRMs with a suitable composition can be used as QCMs, providing traceability to the measurements performed. However, this use presents several constraints such as the lack of an appropriate CRM that matches the needs of each measurement process or high cost, a problem for laboratories performing a wide range of analysis and needing a wide range of CRMs in high quantity.[40] In these situations, the use of control materials developed by each laboratory or commercially available is recommended because they are adequate for QC purposes and less expensive.

On the other hand, there are activities that should only be performed using CRMs, such as method validation.[41] The use of CRMs is essential for the assessment of trueness, but optional for the assessment of precision.

If cost and availability of CRMs do not pose a problem, they can be used to obtain more confident results. Nevertheless, it should be taken into account that the same CRM cannot be used in the same measurement process for calibration purpose and as a "blind" check sample. Moreover, it must be considered that the certified value of a CRM and its uncertainty had been calculated using one or more methods with determined repeatability. This is important if the user wants to assess a method with different repeatability. Certification parameters of CRMs can only be applied to a user's method if the precision and trueness obtained by the two methods are comparable.[42]

Characteristics listed on CRM certificates, such as conditions for handling and storage, period of validity, minimum test portion, and intended use, must be considered to achieve reliable measurements. If a CRM is utilized for a new application, the user must assess its suitability.[42]

Although marine and freshwater standards and RMs are used for the above applications, they are also needed for biological studies. More information on the toxicology and mechanism of action of these toxins is needed to determine the safe limits of exposition and to discover new applications for this kind of compounds. Data on dose–response are often confounded[46–48] due to the lack of reliable RMs and standards. In this sense, several studies can be cited[49,50] to support the need of well-defined standards, with stated traceability, to achieve reliable data on toxicology. There is also a need of matrix RMs for these toxins to develop all applications for these kinds of compounds such as rigorous recovery studies and complete method validations. Obtaining contaminated natural tissue can be difficult, and spiking of natural tissue can yield matrix materials with different properties than natural ones because the analyte added to the natural tissue will probably not be bound as strongly as that, which is naturally present in the tissue, as we have shown previously. Due to these reasons, other approaches are being designed, such as feeding shellfish in laboratories with dinoflagellates that produce toxins, which are being sought.[51] The most important drawback of this approach is the need for maintaining these microorganisms in culture, which is not always possible. Moreover, all matrix RMs must be tested to assure homogeneity and stability of the toxin in the selected matrix. So first, the certified calibrant must be available and the appropriate measurement methods must be designed. Once this has been done, the matrix material can then be characterized, analyzed, and certified.[38]

15.5 Development of Marine and Freshwater Toxins Standards

The preceding chapters detail the need for RMs in toxin analyses. This chapter, therefore, begins by outlining the regulatory requirements and development stages that apply to CRMs in toxin production.

Development and production of marine and freshwater toxin RMs must be carried out according to internationally accepted ISO Guides 34[30] and 35,[29] which involve a significant number of analytical stages and statistical operations. ISO Guide 34 specifies the general requirements with which an RM manufacturer has to show compliance. A number of ISO Guide 34 key points that have to be taken into account are listed in Figure 15.1.

ISO Guide 34 covers the production of certified and non-CRMs also known as QCMs.[52] The main attributes of the latter materials are their homogeneity and stability, which guarantee their proper use. Compared with CRMs, their accuracy is not as important because their application aims at a different purpose such as a complementary instrument in QA and QC laboratory programs.

Conversely, ISO Guide 35[29] provides guidance to achieve a value assignment and explains the concepts for processes such as assessment of homogeneity, stability, and value assignment for the certification of RMs.

ISO Guide 33[42] makes a reference about information regarding selection and proper use of RMs for QA/QC purposes. As a result, CRM manufacturers should offer supporting materials with detailed instructions on how to make the best use of CRMs.

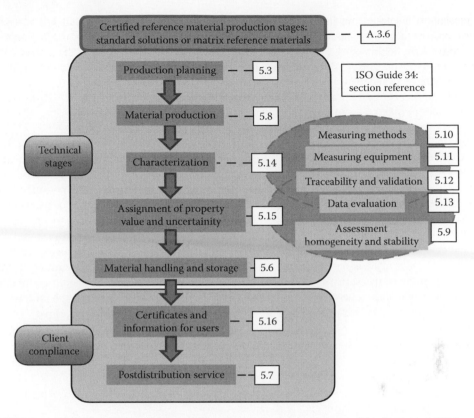

FIGURE 15.1 An ISO Guide 34 flow diagram of the major steps in the entire process of development of CRMs.

A CRM production project begins with the definition of the materials to be produced. The target properties in a marine and freshwater toxin CRM project are the concentration value of one to many toxins and the associated total uncertainty.

The next stage usually is to obtain toxin or shellfish tissue materials enough to cover a batch of CRM production: (1) batch size, (2) feasibility studies, if required, (3) amount required for characterization, (4) number of units for homogeneity test, and (5) number of units for stability test.

There are different sources of marine and freshwater toxins:

- Cultures of proper dinoflagellates
- Toxic materials from toxin-contaminated shellfish
- Toxic materials from algal blooms
- Synthetic methodology
- Toxins, which can be purchased from commercial sources and in subsequent purification steps

Currently, for the purpose of analytical determination of marine and freshwater toxins, CRMs for these are available as follows:

1. Toxin solution CRMs, which are often prepared gravimetrically from a stock solution of a target marine toxin and quantified by ^{1}H-qNMR. This type of CRM indicates high-purity toxin content in a specific solvent.
2. Matrix toxin CRMs, which are characterized for the composition of specified different toxin levels and families. Such materials may be prepared from matrices of shellfish tissue or phytoplankton cell. Blank matrices (free of toxins of interest) or matrices with a low background level are also available.

Once a sample is acquired, a manufacturer begins to prepare the material in the state it will be used. If a CRM standard or calibrant solution is required, treatment including purification steps must be performed to get a high-purity toxin solution. Further purification steps are not necessary if the matrix CRM is planned, as long as the correct shellfish tissue is selected. Sometimes an external source of toxins is required to achieve an adequate concentration level.[53]

According to ISO Guide 34,[30] a number of requirements exist for the certification of CRMs. Certified reference values may be assigned using the following strategies:

> *Certification using one primary method*: The definition of a primary method according to the BIPM's CCQM Group is "a measuring method with the highest metrological quality whose operation can be completely described and understood, for which a complete uncertainty statement can be written down in terms of traceability to the International System of Units (SI)."[54] All potentially significant sources of error should have been evaluated explicitly for the application of the method. The primary direct method measures the value of an unknown without reference to a pattern of the same magnitude that is being measured,[55] whereas the primary ratio method measures the ratio of an unknown to a standard of the same quantity; its operation must be described completely by a measurement equation. The method must be shown to have negligible systematic errors and provide sufficient measurement accuracy.[56] They are, therefore, procedures that do not require calibration of the instruments. Absolute measurement methods allow a traceability chain between the result obtained and the magnitude of the SI value assigned to what is being measured.
>
> *Certification using several (at least two) independent measuring methods*: Apart from certification using a suitable primary method, several evaluated independent measurement methods could be used to produce the true value of an analyte. It is important that the methods used be independent in order to compensate for method biases, since each analytical method has its own sources of error and variability. Each method must show a complete uncertainty budget and keep track of full metrological traceability.
>
> *Certification through interlaboratory comparison with external partners*: When a primary method or second independent are not available, the certified value can be obtained by coordinating the details of results from select external laboratories whose capability has been demonstrated, since all participants must work strictly according to the standard procedure concerned.

Often combinations of the aforementioned methods are used to certify RMs. For example, the two independent method approach is often coupled with the interlaboratory testing procedure, after which data are combined to yield the proposed best value.

15.5.1 qNMR as the Primary Method to Develop Marine and Freshwater Toxin Solution CRMs

While NMR has been widely used in chemical analysis, a review of the literature of the last decade shows continuous update of the concerned literature overview on the quantitative ^{1}H-qNMR methodology and its application in the analysis of natural products.[57–61]

A well-known major advantage of the quantitative NMR (qNMR) method is the higher information content of the data set recorded. The NMR workflow allows simultaneous determination of concentration (quantitative parameter) and identity (qualitative parameter) information for one to many target analytes without the need for identical calibration standards. The basic pillar of qNMR lies on the fact that the area of the signal from an analyte can be measured with respect to another signal originating from a standard by means of internal addition or external calibration.

Provided accurate relative intensities of peak areas have been obtained, one of the well-known characteristics of NMR is the proportionality of the area of peaks to the number of resonating atoms, which does not rely on the nature of the molecule. Therefore, it is an attractive, valuable, and unbiased analytical quantitative tool for organic materials and validation of other analytical techniques and to produce CRMs.[62] qNMR as the primary ratio method of quantification has to lead to an accurate measurement.[63–65]

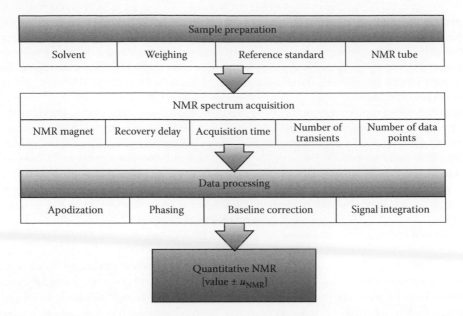

FIGURE 15.2 Major influences on the general qNMR analytical process. The figure has not been attempted to be exhaustive.

The typical quantitative inaccuracy of concentration estimation by qNMR has been reported to be better than 2%, which is an acceptable limit for precise, accurate quantification. But it is not straightforward to estimate uncertainties associated with sample preparations and qNMR experiments.

Unlike other techniques, qNMR spectroscopy has certain acquisition and processing parameters and referencing techniques that need careful consideration in order to achieve a high degree of accuracy and precision. There are three main stages in qNMR analysis, which are shown in Figure 15.2.

15.5.1.1 NMR Sample Preparation: Solvent and Solution

Most proton qNMR experiments consider the fact that spectra are typically recorded in solutions prepared with deuterated solvents. It is very important to first select an NMR (deuterated or non-deuterated) solvent that fully dissolves the toxin of interest. Methanol and water with/without toxin stabilizers or/and pH modifiers are the quasi-unique solvents selected for lipophilic and hydrophilic toxins, respectively.

The rationale is, of course, that this enables observation of the protons of interest without interference from solvent protons. Although deuterated solvents play an important role in the lock, shim, and reference purposes in NMR, they could not be fitted with some intended uses of the final RMs.

A deuterated solvent must be used with caution because of possible H–D exchanges. Deuterium does not normally get exchanged with ^{1}H–C, at least usually not as quickly as some PSP molecules, unless it is a chemically active center. This could be a problem for later intended use in MS. Conversely, labile proton groups such as amide groups, amines, alcohols, or carboxylic acids undergo rapid H–D exchange and, therefore, present limited problem in HPLC-MS/MS.

Because of its lower nuclear transition energy, NMR presents a relative insensitivity comparable to other analytical techniques, and so detection levels are limited to components present in at least micromolar concentrations. This implies that the solution concentration used in quantitative analysis is high, usually in the range 1–25 mM, and enough to quantify with an accuracy error less than 2%. So, the NMR technique allows the quantification of a standard toxin stock solution, which is then subjected to the gravimetric dilution process (with non-deuterated solvents) to yield a batch of well-defined toxin concentration. This high dilution should be more than enough to reach a value of deuterium close to the natural deuterium abundance of 0.0115%.[66]

As a practical example, 1000 times the dilution of the NMR quantification solution yields a deuterium content of approximately 0.05% in a CRM solution, and its subsequent use in chromatographic flow yields an appropriate lower concentration of below 0.02%, a value similar to the deuterium natural abundance, and which, anyway, is clearly lower than the isotopic content of ^{13}C (1.1%), which determines the mass spectrum profile. Nonetheless, the uncertainty associated with the deuterated solvent ratio must be indicated in the certificate.

Although deuterated solvents play an important role in the lock, shim, and reference purposes in NMR, collecting NMR spectra in non-deuterated solvents (No-D NMR) avoids proton–deuterium exchange. The saxitoxin group shows a known hydrogen–deuterium slow exchange of diol vicinal $H_{(11)}$–C through enolization. This exchange could occur at different rates, from 1 h for neosaxitoxin to 2 weeks for saxitoxin.[67] The suppression of water resonance has been of fundamental importance for the quantification of this type of toxins by NMR.[68]

There are several methods that can be used to shim the proton probe to a non-deuterium solvent. These include (1) initial use of a reference tube of same volume as the deuterated solvent, which is locked and shimmed as usual and then replaced with the No-D sample; (2) recalling/reentering a set of previously used shim settings known to be optimal for the solvent in use; (3) use of a capillary insert containing a deuterated sample of the same solvent, which can be locked and shimmed; (4) gradient shimming; (5) shimming the No-D sample using the free induction decay (FID); and (6) shimming the No-D sample using the spectrum.[69]

The key criteria for an effective solvent suppression method are (1) high efficiency to suppress the water peak, which is about 10^5–10^6 times as intense as the resonances of the molecules of interest with no other signal loss and the solvent suppression method must not affect the solute or standard signals; (2) a narrow suppression band across the water region to avoid suppression of the resonances close to the water; and (3) a short duration to minimize magnetization transfer to the exchangeable protons. Requirement (1) may be the most important of the three. A large signal loss results in decreased sensitivity and may lead to significant errors in quantitative analysis especially when metabolites are suppressed to unequal degrees, and incomplete water suppression can also produce baseline roll and phase distortions that can hinder quantitative measurement.

Solvent suppression techniques require some modifications in the pulse sequence. The most common solvent suppression schemes are (1) PRESAT, (2) PRESAT-NOESY1D, (3) WET (water suppression through enhanced T_1 effects), (4) PURGE, (5) excitation sculpting, and (6) Watergate and their optimizations or even more sophisticated techniques.[70]

Each laboratory for analysis must weigh the advantages and disadvantages of each suppression technique, the instruments available, and the parameters while choosing the most convenient method for quantitative analysis. Eliminating water without perturbing other resonances is ideal but not realistic, and it is here that the validation scheme of the qNMR technique plays a basic role. A brief summary of some solvent suppression techniques is given in the following.

The simplest method of solvent suppression is pre-saturation of the solvent frequency before the 90° hard pulse. A disadvantage of pre-saturation is that it can result in the transfer of saturation to exchangeable proton groups, such as amides, making their quantification impossible.

Commonly used solvent pre-saturation techniques are not recommended for quantitative studies as they can lead to magnetization transfer between analyte protons having a nuclear Overhauser effect (NOE) enhancement and a proton under the water signal (intramolecular NOEs) or which is exposed to a hydration shell (intermolecular NOEs). This effect must be evaluated since it could produce increased signal intensity relative to other protons in the same molecule, rendering quantification of such signals by the pre-saturation method inapplicable.[68] Additionally, pre-saturation can cause baseline distortions around the suppressed region, negatively impacting quantitation of analyte signals.

Metabolite signals that are close to the solvent signal should be considered first to observe the effect of solvent suppression techniques. It is important to weigh irradiation bandwidth and pre-saturation time in order to get effective solvent suppression and reduce the collateral effect of pre-saturation.

Generally, if adequate solvent suppression is achieved with low values of pre-saturation power and delay, higher power should not be applied in order to avoid attenuation of integral values nearby resonances, which may adversely affect the potential for quantitative analysis. It is obvious that quantification can only be done if the pre-saturation strength is calibrated.

In a calibration example test to check qNMR solvent suppression, signal reduction could be checked by means of sucrose or D-glucose integral ratio analysis. As sucrose H1 (δ = 5.4 ppm) and H2 (δ = 4.2 ppm) signals are closer to water, they are affected much more than that of H3 (δ = 4.0 ppm). The same could be observed using D-glucose and comparing an α-anomeric (δ = 5.2 ppm) proton with a β-anomeric (δ = 4.6 ppm) proton; the latter would be closer to the water signal.[71] Moreover, these signals can also be quantified using other qNMR standards (e.g., maleic acid, dimethylsulfone) whose signals are clearly far away from water chemical shift. NOE enhancement could be evaluated using caffeine by comparing the signal of the de-shielded hydrogen of the imidazole ring (δ = 7.9 ppm) with the signal of the CH3 singlet at δ = 3.5 ppm. The H-imidazole signal is prone to develop NOE enhancement; instead, the singlet at 3.5 ppm is used for the quantification of caffeine.

The 1D version of the 2D NOE spectroscopy (NOESY) is used in a modified form for 1D acquisition.[72] It is a NOESY pulse train with pre-saturation during the recycle delay and mixing time. Owing to the use of gradients, the mixing time can be kept short and signal loss due to T_2 relaxation can be minimized. It is also assured that the residual water is always in phase with the rest of the spectrum. It must be noted that the mixing time will falsify the absolute amplitudes of the NMR signals detected due to differential T_1, NOE, and chemical effects.[73]

WET uses a shorter pulse than pre-saturation, so it is less likely to attenuate exchangeable protons and NOEs.[74] This is because the overall duration of the sequence is more than one order of magnitude shorter compared with that of pre-saturation pulses (typically 2 s). Besides, the absence of mixing time allows accurate quantification.

As a consequence of different calibration parameters to obtain suitable solvent suppression and reliable quantification, data obtained through different suppression techniques cannot be analyzed statistically in a combined data set but must be treated separately.

In summary, these three solvent suppression techniques provide a simple, highly reproducible, and robust method for acquisition of high-quality qNMR spectra in aqueous solutions. It has to be kept in mind, however, that absolute quantification is possible only with limited accuracy.

15.5.1.2 Weighing

The standard solutions are prepared by diluting the high-purity materials with a solvent, and the resulting standard solutions are subdivided. Since the weighing result is directly proportional to the determined quantification value, the sample and the reference must be weighed out with as high a degree of accuracy as possible. It is generally agreed that a five-figure calibrated balance (weighing to 0.01 mg) with a sensible weighing capacity is needed for this purpose.

15.5.1.3 Reference Standard

An important aspect of this is the general fact that the integrated intensity (or the area under the NMR signal) is proportional to the number of nuclei giving rise to that NMR signal. Therefore, quantitative analysis by NMR requires a reference compound for calculating the concentration of an analyte. RMs are important tools for transfer of measurement accuracy as their proper values should have to be metrologically traceable to the SI and they can be used where a traceable source is a different material.

A universal standard for assay purposes (i.e., validation of quantitative conditions) would be one that is readily available in a highly pure form, inexpensive, stable and chemically inert (if used as an internal standard), nonvolatile (tetramethylsilane [TMS] is highly volatile, so it is unsuitable for quantitative analysis) and non-hygroscopic, and soluble in all (or most) NMR solvents that are used routinely. Its ^{1}H-NMR spectrum should contain minimum interfering signals to the signal associated with the spectrum of the target analyte and preferably singlets. The relaxation time of the reference compound should also be in the range of the analyte's relaxation time so as to avoid unnecessary increases in experimental time; that is, a disadvantage of using dimethyl sulfone or maleic acid for quantitative analysis by NMR is the relative long delays between acquisitions due to the T_1 relaxation times of the protons in these compounds.

All these conditions make the finding of a unique qNMR reference standard a nonrealistic task. Depending on the particular application, a reference substance could be suggested. Proton-containing

CRMs allow both validation of ^{1}H-qNMR experimental conditions and quantitative calibration; that is, sucrose, benzoic acid by National Institute of Standards and Technology (NIST), and compounds such as sodium 3-(trimethylsilyl)propionate-2,2,3,3-d$_4$ (TSP) can be successfully employed for subsequent secondary/external calibration.

Based on their use, reference compounds can be classified as internal and external standards. Internal standard method presents an important disadvantage for preparing CRMs of marine and freshwater toxins. This method implies that a known concentration or weighed amount of a reference compound is dissolved in a known volume of an analyte solution for quantitative estimation, which would introduce contamination of a valued and purified toxin, which can be avoided by using the calibration curve method or a coaxial stem insert (see Figure 15.3). However, it is possible to use the residual solvent resonance as an internal standard to get an accurate measurement.[75] Watanabe et al.[76] developed the quantitative analysis of PSPs by NMR using *tert*-butanol as an internal standard. This method showed good precision (<3%).

Calibration curve method: In this method, a calibration curve is developed using least-square linear regression and the NMR integral area is obtained from serial dilutions of a stock solution of the reference compound.[68] Analyte test samples are then recorded using the same experimental parameters and the integral area is compared with the calibration curve to calculate the concentration.

External calibration: A coaxial insert is generally filled by a reference compound dissolved in a suitable deuterated solvent and inserted into NMR tubes containing an analyte solution.[77] Concentrations of the analyte and reference compounds should be comparable in range. During manual integration, a slight variation in the area of the highest signal will also cause a significant quantitative error in the smaller ones.

Here, the concentration of the reference compound solution filled in the capillary cannot be directly used for quantitation. The effective concentration of the reference should be calibrated by placing the sealed capillary in the NMR tube containing a solution of the primary standard (a known solution of a CRM compound) and a qNMR spectrum is recorded (stage 1 of external calibration in Figure 15.3). After the standardization of the external standard solution,

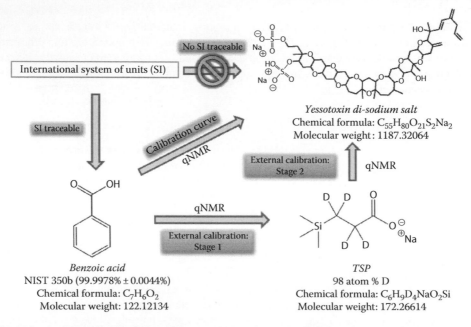

FIGURE 15.3 An illustrative description of the traceability scheme of qNMR for marine and freshwater toxins for the production of CRMs. External calibration requires generating a calibration curve for accurate quantification. Besides, traceability to the SI can be achieved by a mole-to-mole comparison between the reference compound and the analyte in one NMR measurement; this can make a new traceability scheme for the production of SI-traceable RMs for marine and freshwater toxins available.

the capillary is removed, rinsed, dried, and placed in an NMR tube containing the analyte solution, and a reverse calculation is performed to quantify the analyte (stage 2 of external calibration in Figure 15.3). The most important disadvantage of this method is that the sensitivity is reduced due to the small unit volume of the analyte in the radiofrequency coil region.

Electronic reference (ERETIC) method: A simulated electronic signal can also be used for normalization of the area, namely, the ERETIC method.[78] As an external calibration method, the ERETIC signal must be calibrated using a solution of known concentration so it can also be used for quantitative analysis of test samples.[79] During amplification, the ERETIC signal is treated as a real NMR signal so as to have no discrepancies in comparing the quantitative results.

15.5.1.4 NMR Tube

When a large set of samples has to be analyzed for comparison, variations in the cross-sectional area of NMR tubes also contribute to errors during qNMR analysis; hence NMR tubes with very precise diameters should be used. It has to be remembered that the observed absolute intensities will be proportional to the amount of material in the effective volume of transmitter/receiver coil, and variations in the tubes' inner diameter (ID) will constitute a source of errors for samples at the same concentration. Before purchasing NMR tubes, a user should check the manufacturers' specifications, for example, Wilmad NMR precision tubes have an ID variation of 0.15%.

This variation affects quantification methods, calibration curves, and external referencing also using an ERETIC signal. In order to ensure high reproducibility of the results, this source of error can be corrected by (1) using the same tube in all batch experiments, which is easier to implement when coaxial inserts are used for external reference filling, and (2) calculating the effective volume of each tube.[80]

15.5.1.5 NMR Spectrum Acquisition Parameters

The purpose of qNMR is to obtain a high degree of accurate integrals. Certain acquisition and processing parameters have to be chosen for acquiring a spectrum that guarantees accuracy of the integrals. A precise and accurate quantification demands an accuracy of less than 2.0%.

Validation processes (e.g., precision, accuracy, linearity, reproducibility, robustness, selectivity, and specificity) had proved that NMR spectroscopy is a good analytical technique for quantitative estimation.[63] In order to get the best accurate quantification, the validation protocol needs to include factors that affect integrations.[81] The settings of NMR acquisition parameters have been extensively depicted in several studies.[82–84]

A brief summary of these parameters is depicted and summarized in Table 15.1.

1. *Magnet adjustment*: Before the acquisition itself, there are a few steps that must be taken into account. Achieving a good line shape is a basic requirement for accurate quantitation and, therefore, shimming to get a highly homogeneous magnetic field plays a crucial role in this.

   Shimming is adjusting the resolution of the signal by optimizing the homogeneity of the magnetic field. When the field is shimmed properly, a known line shape and the best signal-to-noise ratio (SNR) are obtained.

   Tuning is adjusting the impedance of the probe. A poorly tuned probe reflects a large amount of the power of the pulses. Probe tuning does not affect resolution; however, the SNR will be worse and, thus, also accuracy uncertainty.

   Optimal probe tuning may vary from one sample to the next. But, simply, recording the reference immediately before or after the samples of interest, without adjusting the tuning between them, results in well-controlled reference and sample conditions, enabling accurate comparisons. Besides, once a particular sample in a particular magnet and probe is shimmed, most of the shims do not need adjustment between samples. Shimming can be done manually or automatically, and nowadays, gradient shimming tools yield the best time consumption-versus-spectrum quality ratio.

TABLE 15.1

Summary of Acquisition and Processing Parameters to Be Evaluated in Order to Achieve
Reliable, Precise, and Accurate Results

Parameter	Value	Notes
Sample preparation		
NMR tube	ID variation $\leq 0.2\%$	Volume correction factor or the same tube could be used for all experiments
Acquisition parameters		
Pulse sequence	Instrument-specific	Solvent suppression techniques could be used
Pulse angle	90°	Calculated for each sample
		Ernst angle calculated with regard to relaxation delay and T_1
Pulse strength	Instrument-specific	dB
Pulse length	Instrument-specific	μs
Relaxation delay	42 s ($7 \times T_1 = 6$ s)	T_1 must be calculated ($\geq 7 \times$ longest T_1)
Acquisition time	2–4 s	Varies with sample/spectral window
Spin rotation	No	Optional
^{13}C decoupling	Method-specific	Short acquisition times must be used
Number of scans	64	Depends on sample concentration
		Increase to reach S/N, precision, and accuracy
Steady-states scans	4–16	
Receiver gain	Highest possible	Automatic setting
Spectral window	12 ppm	±2 ppm on each side
Number of data points	32k	
Measurement temperature	303 K	Method-specific
Signal-to-noise ratio	≥ 250	Increase to reach accuracy
Processing parameters		
Phasing	Manual setting	
Line broadening	0.3 Hz (exponential multiplication)	0.1–0.5 Hz (other functions may be used)
Linear prediction	One level can be performed	
Zero filling	One level can be performed	Factor of 2
Baseline correction	Manual setting	Polynomial nth order preferable, but other functions may be implemented
Integration region	Decreased to reach precision and accuracy	Satellite signal integration must be defined

Note: Some of the factors are dependent on individual spectrometer configurations.

Sample *spinning* is a common way to improve the resolution of an NMR spectrum. However, spinning the sample produces small unwanted signals to the spectrum, which are known as spinning sidebands that are proportional to the spinning rate of the sample. The most convenient way to avoid spinning sidebands on modern high-quality NMR equipment is to acquire data in a non-spinning mode.

The *temperature* of the sample in the probe must be regulated for the best-quality spectra. Samples require time for temperature to equilibrate before performing successive NMR experiments.

Broadband isotopic ^{13}C decoupling: All C–H signals have ^{13}C satellites located $\pm J_{\text{C–H}}/2$ ($J_{\text{C–H}}$ coupling is typically 115–200 Hz) from the center of the peak. One-bond coupling between the proton and the attached ^{13}C accounts for 1.1% of the area of the central peak (0.55% each). Quantization of the part of the ^{1}H signal that is away from satellites is desirable, but larger errors are introduced if satellites from a nearby very intense peak fall under the signal being integrated, and this situation must be accounted for if integration at the >99% level of accuracy is desired. Compressing the ^{13}C satellites into the central peak simplifies the spectrum. Some spectrometers can make this experiment quite easy to perform. But one must be aware that broadband ^{13}C decoupling itself may raise the temperature in the probe quite significantly, which would affect the line shape and, therefore, be undesirable for quantization uncertainty. One can decrease the acquisition time to minimize this effect, but either peaks with less points or a truncated FID are acquired. But, there is a bright side to ^{13}C satellites: they can be used as internal standards for the quantitation of very small amounts of isomers or contaminants since their size relative to the central peak is accurately known.[85,86]

Receiver gain: Receiver gain should be set such that the NMR signal is as strong as possible avoiding the top of the FID is clipped off. NMR receiver gain is a parameter that is often chosen to maximize the SNR; therefore, too small receiver gain is undesirable as well. Note that auto-gain routine protocols supplied by NMR spectrometers work well in setting receiver gain.

2. *Pulse sequence*: The typical acquisition scheme for qNMR experiments follows the repetitive sequence of relaxation–excitation–acquisition. In order for a spectrum to be quantitative, each of the NMR signals must be sufficiently relaxed to equilibrium before applying a new pulse. Not allowing enough time for relaxation between pulses can cause varied attenuation of the signals and inaccurate integration. *Relaxation delay* (recycle time) should be at least five times (seven is preferable) the spin–lattice relaxation time (T_1) instead of subsequent T_1 correction. At this point, magnetization would have been recovered by 99.33% ($\geq 99.82\%$ for $\geq 7 \times T_1$).

The application of a short radiofrequency pulse at appropriate frequency rotates the magnetization by a specific angle. *Pulse width* is generally described by this angle of rotation. The amount of rotation is dependent on the power and width of the pulse in microseconds. Maximum signal and SNR are obtained with a 90° pulse. Ninety degree pulse width must be set for each instrument (probe) and each sample (i.e., solvent, etc.) for proton NMR experiments. Conversely, maximum signal results from a 90° pulse when used with a smaller flip angle when performing a quantitative experiment, which is often more efficient as it reduces the recovery time for magnetization. The optimum pulse flip angle can be calculated using Ernst angle equation.[87] As stated earlier, one should always beware while comparing samples recorded with different pulse sequences.

3. *The spectral window, acquisition time, and number of points* are closely related. Spectral window defines the size of the observed frequency window. Acquisition time is the time after the pulse for which the FID is detected. It must be long enough to collect the time domain FID signal until it has decayed to the point where only noise is being digitized. Shorter acquisition times lead to truncation and baseline artifacts. Typical acquisition times in ^{1}H-qNMR experiments are 2–4 s.

The signal received from the NMR sample is first amplified by the receiver and then digitized by the analog-to-digital converter into a series of points along the FID curve. This is the number of points. In general, the more points used to define the FID, the higher the resolution. If the number of data points in the spectrum is too low, there will not be enough points to accurately define each resonance, resulting in inaccurate integrals. The spectral window should not be too narrow to ensure that no peaks are close to the ends of the spectrum. This is because spectrometers use filters to filter out frequencies outside the spectral window and, unfortunately, the filters tend to decrease the intensities of the peaks near the ends of the spectrum (e.g., TSP signal at 0 ppm). To avoid this distortion, an additional 2 ppm region is recommended on both ends of the spectral window. This will also lead to a flatter baseline.

SNR: A high SNR is a prerequisite for accurate quantitative measurement. The higher the SNR, the better is the quantitative accuracy that can be achieved. The number of scans and sample concentration affects the SNR. Once concentration has been settled, then the only way with the instrument at hand is to increase the number of scans to get the desired SNR. SNR is proportional to the square root of the number of scans; in other words, to double the SNR, it is necessary to acquire four times as many scans. A target SNR of at least 250:1 is recommended for any peak that will be integrated for qNMR purposes, with accuracy better than 2%, although qNMR quantization at SNR = 10 (typical definition of analytical method LOQ) is possible but at the expense of the accuracy efficiency.

Increasing the number of scans makes the experiment time longer; this can be viewed through the next example: a 90° hard pulse with an interpulse delay of 40 s and an acquisition time of 2 s takes 45, 90, or 180 min when 64, 128, or 256 number of transients are selected, respectively.

Steady-state scans must be added in order to reach an equilibrium condition prior to collecting FID information. This permits to improve reproducibility and to reduce variability of the data being collected. This number of scans will be variable.

15.5.1.6 Data Processing

The greatest source of error in qNMR is the integration stage, which includes software operations that are performed to improve spectral quality such as improving SNR and spectroscopic resolution. But correct results are reported only if attention is paid to spectrum acquisition conditions. Some basic aspects of data processing must be taken into account in order to determine accurate integration. These functions should be used with some caution, however, and validation carried out to ensure that the quantitative information is accurate.

15.5.1.6.1 Apodization

The objective is to increase SNR and ensure that all signals decay to quasi-zero at the end of the FID. For qNMR experiments, the most common apodization function is an exponential decay that matches the decay of the FID (a matched filter) and forces the data to zero intensity at the end of the FID. Typically, for proton qNMR spectra, line-broadening factors in the range 0.15–0.40 Hz are applied.

15.5.1.6.2 Linear Prediction and Zero Filling

The digital resolution of the spectrum can be improved by zero filling, which involves the addition of zeros to the end of the acquired FID. Forward linear prediction increases the digital resolution by means of an FID data point extrapolation algorithm, namely, by predicting the values of missing data points. General forward linear prediction can provide a better approximation of the data than zero filling. The use of linear prediction can also decrease the degree of apodization required by reducing FID truncation errors.

If adequate acquisition times are employed, linear prediction should not be used since the application of weighting functions can increase the SNR but at the cost of spectral resolution. Both aspects must be evaluated through a validation methodology.

15.5.1.6.3 Baseline Correction

Poor phasing and wrong baseline correction produce a negative influence on the integral values. Therefore, a flat baseline is desired. Automatic and manual phasing and baseline correction methods are available and must be applied prior to the integration process. Sometimes, the phase values saved by the spectrometer need to be revised; phasing ensures that the integrals representing the various signals in the transformed spectrum will have minimal distortion and will, therefore, contribute to quantitative reproducibility. Performing a manual phase correction is almost always necessary.

Fitting a polynomial function to a free signal spectrum region is the most common, simplest, and most robust solution to baseline correction. Note that there are more sophisticated baseline correction routines available and even careful manual baseline correction often entails a slightly better baseline shape. This yields accurate results with regard to precision and accuracy. Accuracy and precision must be evaluated using various baseline correction protocols.

15.5.1.6.4 Integrated Regions

Quantification is performed after the most convenient signals or multiplets are selected and the integral has been calculated, which can then be mapped to the corresponding concentration units by using a scaling factor that had been previously calculated using some internal or external references. NMR integrals are calculated by summation of the intensities of the data points within the defined integration region. The number of discrete points that defines a peak is a very important factor in minimizing the integration error.

After a careful manual phase and baseline correction, integration of signals relies on the correct choice of an integration range.[88] The best result is obtained when each signal is manually integrated into each individual spectrum and when the integral ratios between the standard and analyte signals are calculated using identical criteria to select the integral region.

Since NMR signals have Lorentzian shapes, it is crucial to define how far should each side of the line integral extend to properly represent the area of the peak. Griffiths[89] showed that integration of 24 times the peak width in each direction makes the region allocated on each side of the peak to encompass more than 99% of the peak area. Long-tail peaks are problematic when the samples present a complex resonance profile, such as marine toxin NMR spectra where closely spaced or overlapping signals are presented, where wide integrals cannot be used when peaks are not so well separated. Moreover, in the non-spinning mode, possibly ^{13}C satellites are presented, which must always be either included in the integral or excluded to make comparisons meaningful. In cases where resonances are highly overlapping, a more accurate quantitative analysis can often be achieved by peak fitting rather than integration.

At this point, specificity and selectivity must be kept in mind as key prerequisites for qNMR measurements and must be checked for each sample. Quantification of algal toxins in seawater or shellfish tissue is dependent on prior identification and structure determination of the target toxin and subsequent availability of high-purity RM, that is, precise measurements require in-depth knowledge of the structural assignments of chemical shifts, as the number of protons assigned to each group of the resonances in the spectra must be known.[90]

Marine and freshwater toxins often have different isomeric forms or analogs whose signal cannot be resolved. In these cases, the target-certified concentration is the sum of the different analogs. Generally, these analogs are chromatographically resolved; therefore, HPLC and NMR act as complementary techniques. HPLC coupled to different detectors (MS, UV, fluorescence detection [FLD]) can provide the individual concentration as long as the relative response factors are known. Therefore, besides the total analog concentration certified by qNMR, individual analog concentrations can appear as certified or non-certified values. In the former case, at least two independent techniques must be employed, and for the latter, a single technique could be enough while homogeneity and stability are assured. Since calibration standard CRMs may not be available for all toxin forms in a group, the establishment and evaluation of relative response factors must be documented.

Despite further cycles of cleanup and purification, detectable levels of analogs presenting as impurities are often encountered. But after using these processes, impurity level presents low values, usually ≤1%. These low impurity values could be translated into the principal component concentration uncertainty provided the impurity present is pointed out since the intended use may as a result get affected.

15.5.1.7 Traceability of CRMs of Marine and Freshwater Toxins by qNMR

To obtain the absolute concentration of a compound in an NMR sample, the area of the signals must be determined and compared to the area of a reference that has a known concentration. If spectra are acquired in a quantitative manner, the sensitivity factor (spectrometer constant) of the NMR spectrometer is cancelled for the sample and reference ratio.[62,91]

After an optimal acquisition and processing methodology, which would have yielded the most accurate peak integral, analyte concentration can be determined by comparing the resonance integral of the analyte to that of a standard compound of a known concentration according to the well-known equation that follows:

$$C_{tx} = \frac{A_{tx}}{A_r} \cdot \frac{N_r}{N_{tx}} \cdot C_r \cdot P_r \cdot \left(\frac{V_r}{V_{tx}} \right)$$

where

subscripts tx and r relate to the test toxin and reference compound, respectively
C_{tx} is the toxin concentration
C_r is the quantitation reference concentration
A_{tx} and A_r are the resonance areas of the toxin and the reference, respectively
P_r is the reference purity
N is the number of ^{1}H nuclei giving rise to each resonance

The function in parentheses is optional and refers to correction for the different volumes of the reference and test substances measured by the procedure; it must, however, be used when different NMR tubes have been calibrated.

Toxin concentration result is complete only when accompanied by a quantitative statement of its uncertainty. This uncertainty is required in order to decide whether the result is adequate for its intended purpose.

The uncertainty in the result of a measurement generally consists of several components, which may be grouped into two categories according to the manner in which their numerical value is estimated. The gray terms must be known whereas the black-highlighted terms could be derived from NMR statistical data; the latter is, therefore, type-A error whereas the former are type-B errors. Once all contributors to an uncertainty budget have been converted to a standard uncertainty, the standard uncertainties must then be converted to a unified unit of measure. Following the law of the uncertainty propagation protocol, a measurement uncertainty when there is no correlation between the standard uncertainties, the combined uncertainty for determination of toxin concentration is given by

$$\frac{u_{C_{tx}}}{C_{tx}} = 2 \sqrt{\left(\frac{u_{(A_{tx}/A_r)}}{(A_{tx}/A_r)} \right)^2 \cdot \left(\frac{u_{C_r}}{C_r} \right)^2 \cdot \left(\frac{u_{P_r}}{P_r} \right)^2 \cdot \left(\frac{u_{(V_r/V_{tx})}}{(V_r/V_{tx})} \right)^2}$$

The uncertainty of a volumetric correction factor could be assumed as being manufacturer-specified and experimentally calculated or could not be necessary if the same NMR tube is used.

Although the combined standard uncertainty $u_{C_{tx}}$ is used to express the uncertainty of many measurement results, the property's certified value should be reported together with the expanded uncertainty by multiplying the resulting uncertainty value by a factor of 2 ($k = 2$), approximating a 95% confidence level. This expanded uncertainty is shown in the uncertainty statement of a scope of accreditation.

In summary, it has been shown that ^{1}H-qNMR fulfils all requirements to be used as a validated method for quantitative determination of the concentration of dissolved sample components. A validation protocol for quantitative ^{1}H-qNMR measurements has to be developed, which takes into account all relevant parameters for data acquisition and data processing, with subsequent evaluation. Therefore, an operator would have the most influence on accuracy and precision, and hence a qNMR user needs to be highly trained.

15.5.2 Matrix Toxin CRMs

Once a high-purity solution standard of a marine or freshwater toxin has been created, it is possible to quantify this toxin in a contaminated matrix. A wide variety of analytical methods for the determination of marine and freshwater toxins in contaminated matrix are currently available.[92] These methods mainly employ HPLC with mass detection (HPLC-MS), FLD (HPLC-FLD), UV detection (HPLC-UV), evaporative light-scattering detection (HPLC-ELSD), chemiluminescent nitrogen detection (HPLC-CLND), CE using mass or UV detection, thin-layer chromatography, gas chromatography with MS (GC-MS), or biochemical methods[93] (e.g., enzyme-linked immunosorbent assays [ELISA]) subsequent to liquid–liquid extraction or solid-phase extraction (SPE).

In the EU, LC-MS has recently replaced the MBA as the reference method for most classes of lipophilic shellfish toxins. CRMs are essential for the validation of alternative methods to the MBA.[38]

Official guidelines for the analytical determination of lipophilic and hydrophilic toxins, which include the extraction method, are a good starting point for any laboratory manufacturer of matrix CRMs of marine toxins.[94] Marine toxins (lipophilic and hydrophilic) will tend to accumulate in shellfish, such as mussels, clams, oysters, clams, or scallops, so it is interesting to have a stock of CRMs of the toxins in these matrices.

Public health concern in relation to cyanoHABs focuses on the ability of these species and/or strains to produce toxins called cyanotoxins that lead to waterborne diseases when ingested.[95] A number of countries have developed regulations or guidelines for cyanotoxins and cyanobacteria in drinking water and in some cases, in water used for recreational activity and agriculture. Therefore, water acts as the matrix for these toxins while preparing high-purity CRM solutions suitable for matrix-matched cyanotoxins. Although there are no national guidelines for cyanotoxins in fish or shellfish, they are prone to bioaccumulation in river fish and freshwater mussel tissues.[96] Therefore, for aquaculture and fish harvesting, one must be aware of cyanoHABs and their potential business risks. Even with the objective of analyzing HABs or cyanoHABs, dinoflagellate and cyanobacterial cell extract matrixes could be useful for accuracy control in the determination of toxins in environmental waters.

The preparation of an RM requires substantial planning prior to undertaking a specific project (see Figure 15.1). The process begins with the definition of the material to be produced, for example, preparation of a cockle tissue RM containing PSP toxins at concentration levels appropriate for regulatory analysis and certified for these constituents.

Despite the development of a wide variety of sensitive methods and instrumental procedures, it is possible to accurately determine toxins at extremely low levels in contaminated tissues. Analytical techniques used for determination of marine and freshwater toxins generally involve many analytical steps such as extraction, derivatization, separation, and detection, which should always be performed. Therefore, sources of errors possibly occurring at different steps should be controlled, which include poor extraction recovery, inhibition of derivatization reaction, incomplete separation, and interferences in detection.

The control of the quality of measurements ensures the availability of suitable calibrants as well as RMs certified in a suitable manner. Therefore, the first step to get matrix CRMs is a feasibility study, which mainly involves the next exercises:

- Chromatography and detection method optimization
- Extraction procedure optimization
- Tests for stability

To undertake a single-laboratory validation,[97] a validated method must be employed to carry out matrix toxin determination and establish the performance characteristics of the selected extraction and analytical methods, for which the following performance characteristics must be evaluated and described: selectivity, instrument calibration, linearity and working linear range, method limits of detection and quantitation, within-laboratory method repeatability and reproducibility, influence of co-extracted shellfish matrix on toxin measurement, method ruggedness, measurement uncertainty, and, finally, extraction recovery efficiencies. In the validation of LC-MS/MS, it is appropriate to perform the recovery experiments together with ion suppression enhancement experiments.[98]

The essential component of the development process for matrix CRMs is the process of estimating toxin concentration with an uncertainty that is fit for purpose. The matrix extraction method relies on transferring the toxins from the complex matrix to a much simpler solution that is used for instrumental determination. However, the transfer procedure results in loss of analyte. It is important that all concerned with the production and interpretation of analytical results are aware of the problems and the basis on which the result is being reported. There is no generally applicable procedure for estimating recovery (R) that is free from shortcomings, and therefore, an uncertainty is associated with this step.[99]

The recovery, R, for a particular sample is considered as comprising three elements R_m, R_s, and R_{rep}.[100] These relate to the recovery of the method, the effect of the sample matrix, and/or the analyte concentration on recovery, and the behavior of the spiked samples represents that of the test samples. The uncertainty associated with R, u_R, will have contributions from u_{R_m}, u_{R_s}, and $u_{R_{rep}}$. The evaluation of these components depends on the method scope and availability, or otherwise, of representative CRMs:

1. R_m is an estimate of the recovery obtained from, for example, the analysis of a CRM (traceability and uncertainty) or a spiked sample (method repeatability). R_m may be considered as a "reference" recovery or more generally a "method recovery" since it would normally be expected to apply to all determinations using the method, at least in a particular laboratory.
2. R_s is a correction factor used to take account of differences in recovery for a particular sample compared with the recovery observed for the material used to estimate R_m.
3. R_{rep} is a correction factor used to take account of the fact that a spiked sample may behave differently than a real sample toward the incurred analyte.

These three elements are combined multiplicatively to give an estimate of the recovery for a particular sample, R, and its uncertainty, u_R[101]:

$$R = R_m \cdot R_s \cdot R_{rep}$$

$$u_R = R \cdot \sqrt{\left(\frac{u_{R_m}}{R_m}\right)^2 \cdot \left(\frac{u_{R_S}}{R_S}\right)^2 \cdot \left(\frac{u_{R_{rep}}}{R_{rep}}\right)^2}.$$

Official extraction methods for lipophilic and hydrophilic marine toxins are valuable tools for method verification and validation and besides constitute a well-defined starting point to perform an evaluation of the recovery efficiency of the matrix extraction method, although each laboratory could perform method modifications.

Reported concentrations presented by the double extraction procedure as described by the EU-RL standard operating procedure assume that recovery is likely to be reasonably close to unity, and the assumption that $R = 1$ is then made, in a way because recovery had been acceptable and efficient to quantitatively isolate the maximum levels of toxins.[24] As the method scope covers only a single matrix type and toxin concentration, the estimate of R_m and its uncertainty can be based on the analysis of a sample, which is truly representative of real samples. There is, therefore, no need to include a correction factor to take account of differences in recovery for a particular sample compared with the sample used in the estimation of R_m (i.e., R_s is assumed to equal 1 with negligible uncertainty). In the same way, it can be assumed that this will behave in a similar manner toward the incurred toxin in a real sample. A correction factor to take account of the fact that the toxin recovery from shellfish tissue used to estimate R_m may not be representative of the recovery from a real sample is, therefore, unnecessary. The main uncertainties associated with recovery arise from this assumption, and neither recovery uncertainties were mentioned.

Anyway, each matrix toxin CRM manufacturer must evaluate recovery efficiency and precision as crucial parameters to certify property values as matrix influences on toxin determinations exist, in the same way that qNMR parameters must be evaluated in order to quantify a high-purity toxin solution. Moreover, to quantify the uncertainty, it is necessary to consider the degree to which a particular sample matrix under test is represented by the RM employed and, where relevant, the extent to which spiking provides a representation of the native toxin behavior.

Recovery value (R) could be estimated indirectly by experiments on related RMs with a certified concentration by comparison with an alternative definitive method or by observing the amount of an added spike recovered from a sample matrix. Each of them has different uncertainty contributions to the recovery equation and uncertainty recovery equation.

There are several kinds of CRMs of marine toxins (lipophilic and hydrophilic), which are embedded in different matrixes, which can be used to obtain a new RM, CRM or not (QCM). Although the use of same shellfish species matrix CRMs is the easiest way to estimate recovery in a new material, there is a certain degree of non-composition matrix similarity. Differences in matrix or toxin levels between CRMs and the test matrix add unknown and possibly large uncertainties to the results of CRM studies. Such variability will potentially add an additional contribution to the overall measurement of toxin concentration (R_s). The uncertainty, u_{R_s}, is, therefore, the standard deviation of the mean recoveries for each sample type. In this case, R_s is implicitly assumed to be equal to 1, with negligible uncertainty if only one type of matrix CRM is employed. R_{rep} is generally assumed to equal 1, indicating that the recovery from a matrix CRM perfectly represents the recovery observed for the target toxin.[102] This type of methodology is feasible to transfer in-house laboratory matrix CRM producers in order to achieve subsequent batches of the same matrix CRM, but the same problem arises since these new materials had been prepared from samples acquired at different times and/or from different shellfish-producing areas.

Matrix mismatch can be avoided in principle by a surrogate experiment for each separate test material analyzed. Even though such an approach will often be considered impracticable on an economical basis with the purpose of generating a new CRM, a representative test material in each analytical run must be used to determine recovery and minimize uncertainties.

A surrogate method to evaluate the impact of matrix effects on the overall analytical performance and the potential usability of the data can be devised using different methodologies:

1. When an *internal standard* is used in recovery experiments, the alternative analyte is an entity chemically distinct from the target toxins, and, therefore, will not have identical chemical properties. However, it will normally be selected so as to be chemically closely related to the toxins and not expected to be found in the tissues. In order to obtain CRMs of toxins in shellfish tissue, the internal standard would be used, for example, in recovery estimation where numerous toxin analogs are to be determined in the same matrix and marginal recovery experiments would be impracticable for each of them individually; therefore, the most important toxin of a specific toxin family is used as the internal standard besides the spiked standard.

   Moreover, internal standard calibration involves the comparison of instrument responses from the target compounds in the sample to the responses of the reference standards added to the sample or sample extract before injection. Therefore, the relative response factor (RRF) must be known so that the target compound response could be calculated relative to that of the internal standard.

2. The best type of surrogate is an isotopically modified version of the toxin, which is used in an *isotope dilution* approach.[103] But the application of the isotope dilution approach is limited by the availability and cost of isotopically enriched analytes. Nowadays, isotopically stable and high-purity solutions of isotopic toxin CRMs are not available. It must be noted that isotopically labeled toxin molecules could be obtained by two possible ways: feeding toxin-producing microalgae, which would carry synthesis using ^{13}C, ^{15}N, or ^{2}H precursors, or by a synthetic route. Both of them are labour-intensive to implement and highly expensive. But this is the ideal surrogate such that the recovery of the surrogate would be the same as that of the analyte and can be estimated separately by MS. Isotope dilution method with MS is identified as the primary ratio method by the CCQM (Consultative Committee for Amount of Substance—Metrology in Chemistry), which represents a high level of metrology.[104]

3. *Spiking*: This less costly method, and one very commonly applied in order to evaluate the analytical bias for an actual matrix, focuses on the certification process and is used to estimate in a separate experiment the recovery of the target toxin added as a spike *prior* to being taken through the entire analytical process. Duplicate or replicate matrix spikes are also used to evaluate overall precision.[99]

There are two spiking approaches: spiking a single concentration, similar to the native toxin, and using the standard addition method. The sample with the spike will show a larger analytical response than the original sample due to the additional amount of toxin added to it. The difference in analytical response between the spiked and unspiked samples is due to the amount of toxin in the spike. This provides a calibration point to determine the toxin concentration in the original sample.

At this point, a matrix blank or no matrix blank can be spiked. The former focuses on confirming that the matrix effectively contains none of the toxins (below LOQ or LOD), and the latter needs to assure a toxin concentration.

There are a number of issues that should be considered when measuring recovery for quantitative analysis. Furthermore, each CRM laboratory manufacturer has to develop a system for adequate toxin determination where the analytical method has been validated previously. The spiking method focusing on the certification of a toxin concentration in a matrix must ensure that the measurand is the concentration of the "toxin" that can be measured in the test material by the specific procedure applied and the result is traceable to the method. Therefore, the concentration measured is necessarily close to the true value. In that case, the measurand is the concentration of the "extractable" toxin. When a "spike" is used for recovery estimation, the recovery of the toxin from the sample may differ from the recovery of the spike, introducing an uncertainty, which needs to be evaluated.

As a minimum, when carrying out the spiking/recovery experiments, the spiking procedure must be precise and accurate, the spike should be added prior to any sample extraction procedures, the method of fortification must be described, and qualitative data should be obtained to demonstrate that only the toxin of interest is being measured.

It is usually necessary to perform recovery experiments with care to obtain accurate and precise quantitative results. This discussion presumes that the reader already has an understanding of the basic theory of recovery experiments. We present here a cookbook approach to toxin quantification by spiking recovery, providing general guidelines for the choice of spiking parameters.

Therefore, in the same way that qNMR methodology, there are certain experimental factors that need to be considered and which require optimization (see Figure 15.4): these are the traceability of the spiked toxin concentration, the nature of the spiked toxin, the spiking concentration level, the number of spiking levels, the number of replicates at each spiking level (not necessarily equal), the time for the spiking to reach equilibrium, and inclusion of method blanks.[99]

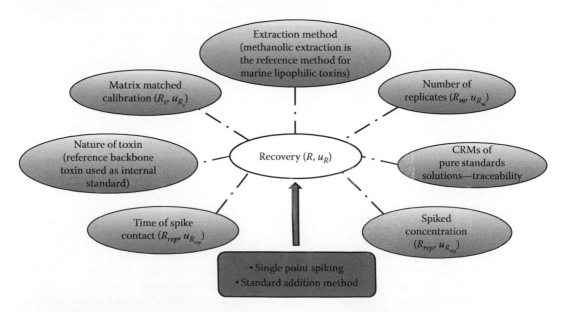

FIGURE 15.4 Factors influencing recovery and uncertainty by the matrix spiking methodology.

15.5.2.1 Traceability of Spiked Toxin Concentrations

For matrix CRM production by the spiking method, the concentration is potentially traceable, through calibrated balances and volumetric glassware, to the pure standards used for spiking. And, consequently, these pure standards are well characterized and the traceability chain extends to the SI. However, this traceability chain can be broken if the method used for spiking is not validated or not well understood and controlled.

15.5.2.2 Nature of the Spiked Toxin

In general, each spiked toxin can be clearly linked to each of the unspiked target toxins. If one of the spiked toxins clearly represents the nature and form of a subset of the target toxins in the natural material being analyzed, then the target toxins of the subset can only be qualified on the basis of the matrix recovery factor.

In order for this procedure to be valid, the representative toxin subset must behave quantitatively in the same way as the rest of the subset toxins that are native to the matrix, especially with regard to its partition between the various phases. Recovery of the toxin need not be 100%, but the extent of recovery of a toxin and the representative toxin used as the internal standard should be consistent, precise, and reproducible. Moreover, the RRF response detector must be evaluated, although an equimolar response is a general assumption when a marine toxin family group is being checked, for example, a representative DSP toxin, OA, could be used to evaluate the DTX2 and DTX1 recovery factor and YTX to estimate the recovery factor of hYTX or 45-OH-YTX or saxitoxin for all PSP toxins.

In practice, this equivalence is often difficult to demonstrate, and therefore certain assumptions have to be made. Thus, in principle, recovery estimated in this manner is not strictly accurate and should be regarded solely as an estimate. The use of each target toxin as a spiked toxin is technically not much complicated but is financially more expensive. Sometimes, due to the lack of some high-purity CRM toxins, reliance on spiking with toxin(s) of interest is the sole alternative for recovery determination.

15.5.2.3 Spiking Concentration Level

In order to avoid incurring a relatively large uncertainty recovery factor, the selected spike level should be approximately the same, within an order of magnitude. Therefore, assessment of the amount of toxin (native level) already present in the sample prior to conduction of recovery tests is absolutely vital as the proper definition of spike recovery refers to the recovery of the added quantity.

If the native concentration of a target toxin is high relative to the spiking concentration, this may contribute a significant uncertainty to the recovery calculations; the recovery factor may not be representative of the actual method performance for the matrix.

An appropriate range of toxin concentrations should be investigated because the recovery of the toxin may be concentration-dependent (R_{rep} and $u_{R_{rep}}$ must be calculated). At very low levels, the analyte may be largely chemisorbed at a limited number of sites on the matrix or be irreversibly adsorbed onto the surfaces of the analytical vessels. Recovery at this concentration level might be close to zero. At a somewhat higher level, where analyte is in excess of that adsorbed, recovery will be partial. At considerably higher concentrations, where the adsorbed analyte is only a small fraction of the total analyte, recovery may be effectively complete.

The analytical chemist may need to have information on recovery over all these concentration ranges. In default of complete coverage or absence of official validated guidance, it may be suitable to estimate matrix recovery when the spiking concentration is at least two times greater than the native toxin concentration or at some critical level of the toxin concentration, for example, at a regulatory limit. Values at other levels would have to be estimated by experience, again with an additional uncertainty. The extent of deviation from this again depends on the CRM manufacturer-specific method quality requirements; however, the greater the ratio, the greater the certainty of recovery factor measurement.

If the concentration of the toxin is close to the detection limit, the spike level can be a certain multiple of the LOQ or the regulatory limit, although relative uncertainty, ux/x, will be high.

If the standard addition method is applied, the spiked toxin concentration scale should include the native concentration to permit adherence to identical conditions of dilution, calibration, etc. If spiking is applied to a matrix blank (matrix-matched calibration [MMC] method), the whole range of concentrations can be considered conveniently.

15.5.2.4 Number of Replicates

It may be deemed important to carry out a sufficient number of repeat measurements at each concentration level in order to get a good estimate of the uncertainty, a parameter we believe to be essential in estimating recovery. Depending on the variability of the background toxin signal and the spike level, it may be necessary to prepare many replicates to get a good estimate of the average toxin recovery and the uncertainty of this value. Repeats are especially necessary when ratios of spike to native or total level are small or unfavorable due to existing native levels; this leads to high uncertainty in the recovery factors.

15.5.2.5 Spike Time Contact

An appropriate range of time should be investigated after the addition of toxin as the recovery of the toxin may be time-dependent. An assumption inherent in spiking or surrogate methods is that of homogeneous distribution of the labeled spike with the native toxin. Although this is a fundamental prerequisite for the validity of any surrogate method results, it is a rather neglected aspect. Therefore, the time of equilibration between the analyte and spike is essentially a homogenization and equilibration issue. This aspect has been aptly emphasized almost a decade ago: "in the presence of complete equilibration with the labeled analyte after spiking, less than complete recovery of the analyte does not affect the measured concentrations, unless there is a significant isotope effect, since it is the ratio of unlabeled to labeled analyte that is measured."[105] However, if none of them is complete, it is likely that the results would be biased. Hence, the two paradigms to ensure accuracy are either attainment of 100% extraction recovery or complete spiking equilibration. Unfortunately, the latter is harder to verify experimentally and often is only assumed to be complete. This requirement is critical in the case of solid samples.

Plotting the toxin concentration measured versus increasing spike time contact, spiked concentration, or extraction time allows the assessment of spike equilibration; these data allow us to obtain R_{rep} and $u_{R_{rep}}$ to correct the recovery factor. Without data from previous experience, spiking an analyte to a matrix at several different time intervals is the methodology that a matrix CRM manufacturer must apply.

In a very short-time contact, the spiked toxin may not be so firmly bound to the matrix as the native toxin; as a result, the spiked concentration level will tend to be high in relation to that of the native toxin. This would lead to a negative bias in a corrected analytical result.

The extraction procedures investigated, depending on the nature of the toxin, normally reveal that spike toxin equilibrate with natural toxin in the order of a few minutes. This fact indicates a labile binding of conjugation of toxins in most tissues under study and makes that the added toxin is so firmly bound to the matrix tissue as the native toxin and the non presence of interfering matrix compounds which hinder the accessibility of toxin, free and conjugated. Therefore, no bias and high recovery values and, therefore, low uncertainty values are obtained.

15.5.2.6 Inclusion of Method Blanks

It is also called MMC. Matrix CRMs of free toxin tissues are spiked with pure toxin CRMs after inclusion of method blanks.[21] Recovery is then calculated as the percentage of the measured spike of the matrix sample relative to that of the blank control or the amount of spike added to the sample.

As the method scope covers different matrix types, there is, the need to include a correction factor to take account of differences in recovery for a particular sample. R_s will be determined from the recovery for a range of representative sample matrices spiked at representative concentrations and u_{R_S} would be calculated from the spread of the recovery estimates.

An indication of trueness can also be obtained by comparing the method with a second, well-characterized reference method under the condition that the precision of the established reference method is known, although for the toxin extraction reference method, R_s is assumed to be equal to 1, with negligible uncertainty.

If R_s indicates that the matrix effect is sample-dependent, it becomes necessary to spike a single point or perform standard addition calibration on the real sample. Although, results from the two methods, matrix CRM producer extraction and standardized protocols, performed on the same sample or set of samples can indicate a trueness result.

15.5.3 Homogeneity and Stability Testing

Systematic studies of a candidate CRM must include the required overview of the contributions of analytical characterization, homogeneity, and stability to the total uncertainty of the certified property value of the material.[106]

15.5.3.1 *Homogeneity Study*

Assessment of the homogeneity of every new candidate CRM, packaged in its final form, is of particular importance and is always performed prior to every other operation. In fact, there is no need to proceed to stability study or certification exercise for a material that has not shown acceptable homogeneity. In addition, the homogeneity study would determine in a quantitative way the "residual" inhomogeneity, which, in principle, will contribute to the final uncertainty of the material.

Homogeneity uncertainty (u_{bb}) or known heterogeneity takes into account several design questions, such as efficacy of the mixing process during bulk assay and micro-heterogeneity in matrices.

There are two types of homogeneity, within-bottle and between-bottle. The former dictates the variability of measurement, whereas the latter deals with between-unit variation. The key requirement for any RM is equivalence between the various units. In this respect, it is not relevant whether the variation between the units is significant compared with the analytical variation, but whether this variation is significant to the certified uncertainty. The between-bottle variability is determined by analysis of variance (ANOVA) (ISO Guide 35) or a combination of fitness for purpose and statistical criteria. ANOVA separates the between-bottle variation (s_{bb}) from within-bottle variation (s_{wb}).[107] The analytical variability should not be smaller than the variability among replicates, which can be decreased by increasing the replicates on an individual unit. As s_{bb} and s_{wb} are estimates, between-bottle variation could be hidden by method repeatability, and in this case, u_{bb} could be calculated as described by Linsinger et al.[108] to be comparable to the LOD of an analytical method, yielding the maximum inhomogeneity (amount of substance) that might be undetected by the given analytical test.

> Even when a material is expected to be homogeneous, as in the case of solutions, an assessment of the between-bottle inhomogeneity is required. When dealing with solid-state reference materials, including slurries and sludges, a within-bottle homogeneity study should be foreseen to determine the minimum sample intake…The minimum number of bottles selected at random [could be] between 10 and 30, but should generally not be smaller than 10.[29]

The typical homogeneity study involves sampling of the material at the production line. Samples, that is, units of the material already packed and labeled according to the filling sequence, are taken usually following the "random stratified" sampling scheme (division of the total batch into sub-batches according to the filling order and selection of one sample randomly from each sub-batch). Moreover, the homogeneity of the proposed candidate material as a CRM to be used in more than one trial will be assessed by all tests that are considered relevant for the purpose.

Due to the intrinsic heterogeneity, individual aliquots of a material will not contain the same amount of toxin. This is one of the most pertinent issues of matrix CRMs where homogeneity is not intrinsically resolved as in solutions of pure toxins. The minimum sample intake defines the minimum amount of sample that is representative of the whole unit.

Within-unit heterogeneity does not influence the uncertainty of the certified value when the minimum sample intake is maintained, but determines the minimum size of an aliquot that is representative of the whole unit. Quantification of within-unit heterogeneity is, therefore, necessary to determine the minimum sample intake. A sample intake must give acceptable repeatability, demonstrating that within-unit heterogeneity no longer contributes to analytical variations at this sample intake. The assumption is that at these small intakes, analytical variation becomes negligible compared with variations due to micro-heterogeneity. The observed standard deviation can, therefore, be used to estimate a minimum sample amount necessary for a given measurement repeatability as described by Pauwels and Vandecasteele.[109] Sometimes a minimum sample intake is depicted for convenience of handling.

Sample sizes equal to or above the minimum sample intake guarantee a certified value within its stated uncertainty. For a between-bottle homogeneity test, the used sample intake should be larger than the minimum sample intake to minimize analytical variation. Grubbs test could be performed to detect potentially outlying individual results as well as outlying bottle averages.

15.5.3.2 Stability Study

Since one of the main goals of RM production is to provide a stable RM, tests for stability begin early in the production process. Uncertainty of stability refers to two distinctly different uncertainty components: possible degradation during long-term storage (the expected lifetime of the RM prior to its distribution, u_{lts}) and possible degradation during short-term storage (transport to the user, u_{sts}). Even in the absence of visible degradation, these uncertainties are not null because of the uncertainties associated with measurement reproducibility.

Although stability is generally associated with thermal stability, a CRM manufacturer must pay attention to other parameters such as solvent, additives, pH, type of packaging, and the presence or absence of an inert atmosphere.

The purposes of stability study are as follows:

1. To obtain sufficient evidence for the stability of the material
2. To determine the optimum conditions for storage and shipment
3. To calculate the contribution of stability in the final uncertainty of the material

The stability study usually includes storage of small batches of samples at different temperatures and their analysis after several time intervals. One temperature (usually the lowest) is considered to be a "reference" temperature, that is, the temperature at which the material is supposed to be stable.[110] The study can last for 1–2 years for "long-term stability" and for a few weeks for "short-term stability" but at more extreme temperatures to simulate transport.

Although the approach summarized below focuses on the estimation of u_{lts}, it is also applicable for u_{sts}. There are mainly two assumptions: (1) absence of significance degradation due to the material to be used as a CRM and (2) any small degradation can be approximated by a linear function. The slope of the straight line is the degradation rate and the intercept is an estimate for the concentration at time zero. u_{lts} is obtained by multiplication of the standard uncertainty of the slope by the chosen shelf life.[29,111]

At this point, it should be noted that the uncertainty of stability may not necessarily be related to any real degradation of the material, but can simply be a lack of proof that the material is stable. Instability would be detected if the slope of the regression line deviates from zero. This means that the most important conclusion that can be drawn from the results is the presence/absence of a significant trend in the data, which would hint toward any degradation. So the next question that arises is what is the uncertainty associated with the assumption of zero degradation?[112]

The longer the stated shelf life, the larger the u_{lts} and the certified uncertainty. Shelf life must be sufficiently long, but should not result in uncertainties too large to make the material useless. While an assessment of long-term instability is required, short-term stability is relevant as an uncertainty component only when the stability of a CRM is affected by the specified transport conditions in excess of the storage conditions. Even if the CRM is seemingly stable, u_{lts} must present a contribution to the final CRM uncertainty; zero contribution shows a lack of understanding of the stability performance critical factors.

Stability studies of CRMs will depend on the intended use of the candidate. Therefore, the choice of a measurement methodology is a critical step. The estimates for u_{bb} and u_{lts} are frequently limited by the quality of the analytical data on which they are based. In only a few cases, they are caused by a significant between-bottle inhomogeneity or lack of long-term stability. Since these measurements are usually carried out by a single laboratory, the laboratory's method repeatability is quite decisive for the combined uncertainty of the property value. High values of u_{lts} show that measurements have been performed by a method with poor reproducibility than real instability. For materials with small instability, method precision is undoubtedly the crucial issue for detecting small changes in property value. To compensate for possible drift of the method of analysis during the duration of the study, two alternatives have been offered:

- At every time point, using the ratio of the property value obtained on samples stored at temperature T to the property value obtained at the same time interval on samples stored at the reference temperature. This procedure cancels out variations in analytical response as a function of time. However, to be able to prove that samples are also stable at this reference temperature, it is necessary to know this stability either from previous experience or well-documented bibliographic data, and can also be derived from the study itself where it is mandatory that samples stored under at least one higher temperature be stable as well.

- Application of the "isochronous" scheme:[113,114] At the end of each isochronous sample storage scheme, the samples could be measured together under repeatability conditions. Two designs of isochronous studies are possible: (1) samples are first exposed to various storage conditions before being placed back under reference conditions until the moment of analysis and (2) for each of the storage temperatures, the studied samples are moved from the reference conditions to the test temperature at different time points. At the defined end time, the samples are immediately analyzed or put back (for a short time) at reference temperature before analysis. This is the most economic methodology and leads to better estimations of u_{lts}. A practical problem of an isochronous study can be that results are only available at the end of the study.

Subsequently, the material is analyzed for the analytes of interest for certification purposes after which a certificate of analysis can be prepared. It is also imperative that a CRM or RM be continually monitored for stability throughout its useable lifetime. This process should also include periodic reassessment of the certified concentrations.

It will, thus, be necessary to establish a timetable for the preparation of further batches of the material to ensure that supplies are always available. These subsequent batches (particularly if they are matrix-based) will need to be treated almost like new material, that is, they should be tested for stability, and a completely new certification will be needed for each replacement batch. This involves substantial work each time it is done; hence it is desirable to make as large a batch as practical, consistent with the probable shelf life and expected usage.

In accordance with regulatory requirements, CRM manufacturers following ISO Guide 34 must conduct long-term stability testing programs, which include the determination of stability (the time period over which the product is expected to remain within specifications upon reevaluation) and expiration dates (the date after which the product should not be used by a consumer). However, ISO Guide 31 only refers to an explicit obligation to mention an expiry date "for all CRMs where instability has been demonstrated or is considered possible."[31] Expiration dates are assigned to established products and are determined through real-time stability studies. The expiration date defines the total shelf life of the product.[115]

If shelf life is stated as only a year, it is expected that the product will meet the specifications over the last day of the year. Shelf life can be extended upon reevaluation if the product still meets the release specifications. Generally, the indicated expiration and shelf life dates apply to unopened products that have been stored under indicated conditions.

Sometimes special considerations must be taken into account, such as inclusion of incidences of freeze–thaw cycles; in appropriate cases, stability studies of lyophilized CRMs should include the time that must elapse after reconstitution and the protocol to check the stability of blank matrix CRMs.

Blank matrix CRMs should sufficiently match the analytical behavior of the real test samples, but should not contain the toxin of interest to a detectable extent. A blank RM can and will give a true indication as to how a specific method may perform as the spiked nutrient levels approach zero. Then, besides the recovery parameter, the qualitative parameters of LOD and LOQ must be determined. Different criteria are used for evaluating these parameters, for example, visual evaluation, SNR, or standard deviation–slope ratio.

However, for a CRM, not only must the toxin be stable within the specified storage conditions, but also de-matrix. Well-defined matrix blank materials (e.g., those obtained from shellfish tissue, dinoflagellate cells) would most probably not be marketed as CRMs, as their absence (i.e., toxin mass fraction < LOD of the methods) could not have been analytically confirmed for all possible toxins and uncertainty statements may not have been established for any stages in the CRM production; "the certified value should be an accurate estimate of the true value, with a reliable estimate of the uncertainty compatible with the end-use requirements."[29]

While homogeneity and stability testing of toxin matrix CRMs focus on the characterization of principal constituents, for blank matrix CRMs, these studies are conducted to detect the presence of any potential degradation or transformation of matrix-relevant parameters, such as water content, particle size (lyophilized material), and additive content (i.e., antibiotics, antioxidants) as well as to confirm that no impurities are generated, which can impact the specific toxin by a specific method or the intended use of the material.

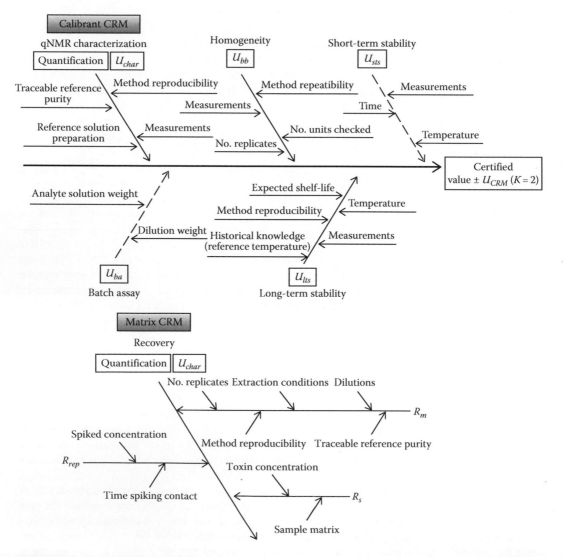

FIGURE 15.5 Uncertainty budget of detected major influences on the uncertainty of a certified value of a CRM: high-standard purity CRM solutions[123] and matrix CRMs. (From Barwick, V.J. et al., *Accredit. Qual. Assur.*, 5, 104, 2000.) The dashed lines indicate uncertainty pathways, which may not be included depending on the value (u_{sts}) or characterization protocol (u_{ba}). The upper figure is related to the production of a high-purity calibrant toxin solution, whereas for a matrix CRM, the qNMR pathway must be replaced by the pathway shown below. The figure has not been attempted to be exhaustive.

15.5.4 Certification and Calculation of Uncertainty of RMs

The uncertainty of the value assigned to the toxin concentration of calibrant CRMs or matrix CRMs must be calculated according to the recommendations in ISO Guide 35. The combined uncertainty of the certified value includes contributions from between-bottle homogeneity, long-term stability, and characterization study. In the case of using qNMR to characterize CRMs, a posterior dilution of the characterized material, on the basis of a direct gravimetric method, is carried out and, therefore, a contribution of the batch assay must be aggregated. This contribution is generally negligible compared with other uncertainties, but although it could not be included in the calculation of combined uncertainty, it is preferable to count in order to get a reliable estimate of uncertainty. This is the same case when the homogeneity and/or characterization uncertainties are deemed significant respect u_{lts}, their values have to be included.

The relative combined uncertainty is calculated as the square root of the sum of the squares of the relative uncertainties of the individual contributions,[116] according to the following equation:

$$U_{CRM} = k \cdot \sqrt{u_{bb}^2 + u_{lts}^2 + u_{char}^2},$$

where

U_{CRM} denotes the expanded uncertainty of the CRM
k is the coverage factor
u_{char} is the uncertainty of the certified toxin concentration
u_{bb} is the uncertainty of the between-bottle inhomogeneity
u_{lts} is the uncertainty of the instability

Figure 15.5 summarizes the factors that have to be taken into account while estimating the certification values of the mass fractions of toxins and their associated certified uncertainty values.

15.6 Marine and Freshwater Toxin Fit-for-Purpose for Food Analysis

To ensure a high level of protection for human health and the environment, the EU has adopted a set of integrated policies, which addresses the safety of shellfish associated with algal toxins produced by naturally occurring phytoplankton (algal biotoxin contamination).

Shellfish and fishery products form a complicated matrix and the number of toxins of interest is high. A chain of EFSA studies showed that these bioassays had shortcomings and were not considered an appropriate tool for control purposes because of the high variability in results, insufficient detection capability, limited specificity, and lack of validation. Hence, classical methods relying on traditional MBAs are becoming increasingly superseded by hyphenated systems such as LC-MS/MS, which have opened up new dimensions to determine several analytes simultaneously within one run. Moreover, the drastic increase in international trade has produced an urgent need for global comparability of analytical results.

Worldwide interest in the traceability and, thus, in the comparability of chemical measurements and the role that matrix RMs play in the process has been on the rise.[1] A CRM is prepared and used for three main purposes: (1) to help develop methods of analysis under ISO 17025 with a high degree of precision and accuracy; (2) to calibrate measurement systems used to facilitate the exchange of comparable data, institute QC, determine performance characteristics, or measure a property at a state-of-the-art limit; and (3) to ensure long-term adequacy and integrity of measurement QA programs. These points have become a nonissue since there are three types of marine toxins and freshwater CRMs now available, namely, calibrant CRM solutions, matrix CRMs, and blank matrix CRMs. And recently, manufacturers of toxin CRMs for QA in food analysis have started supplying "toolboxes" containing, for example, a calibration solution, a blank matrix material, and a naturally incurred matrix material all of which carry certified values for the same toxins.

Sometimes it is easy to find the different LD50 values for a specific toxin; for example, LD50 (intraperitoneal) for domoic acid ranges from 2.4[117] and 3.6 mg/kg[118] to 6.0 mg/kg in mice.[119] This difference in LD50 values may be due to the use of commercial products. These products are usually sold in dried form, which requires a perfectly calibrated balance, even though the toxin state (acid or salt form, anhydrous form) and stability are normally not indicated and a relation with impurity content, which may affect analytical data, is not present. This issue has a crucial relevance as LD50 is a starting point to establish a regulatory limit. It is, therefore, concluded that having appropriate CRMs is important for not only regulated toxins but also some non-regulated toxins, which have been shown to be harmful and/or occur in the EU, such as tetrodotoxins, palytoxins, brevetoxins, CTXs, and some cyclic imines.[120]

CRMs available for the purpose of analytical determination of marine and freshwater toxins are shown in Table 15.2. Marine toxin CRMs are present in two types: high-standard purity solutions (calibrant) and toxins embedded in shellfish tissue (matrix), whereas freshwater toxin CRMs are mostly sold as calibrant solutions to ensure safe drinking water. The list of marine toxin RMs supplied by Laboratorio CIFGA S.A. and National Research Council Canada has increased substantially.

As already outlined, CRMs are generally characterized by their high level of homogeneity and stability of both the analyte and matrix. Generally, it has been found easier to fulfill these criteria by using matrix CRMs in the form of dried samples. As a result, most of the food CRMs are available as a dried (oven-, spray-, or freeze-dried) and finely ground powder (ball or jet milling, or cryo-grinding). However, many CRM users require the material to reflect the natural state of the samples, which are routinely analyzed to provide a realistic picture regarding the validity of the applied analytical method.[38]

Physical disruption of tissues during milling and the dehydration effects during freeze-drying can also contribute to an altered sorption/extraction behavior in comparison with wet or less rigorously processed samples. Also, particle size has a pronounced influence on the extractability of analytes from the matrix; finely ground, dry CRMs usually have a particle size distribution, which differs from a real sample under investigation.

Alternatives to conventional powder CRMs do exist, for example, frozen homogenates. Such materials will undoubtedly satisfy users requiring a matrix of the CRMs similar to the state of the samples, which are analyzed routinely. But the logistics of delivering such CRMs, which need cooling at least at dry-ice temperatures, is complicated, and the corresponding handling costs are relatively high. Distribution problems could be avoided for heat-stable analytes/matrices as they could be processed by canning and autoclaving or γ-irradiation stabilization.

TABLE 15.2

Types of Marine and Freshwater Toxin CRMs Available

Toxin Class	Family	Toxin (Abbreviated Noun)	Type of CRM
Lipophilic marine toxin	DSP	OA, DTX2, DTX1	Calibrant solution Matrix (mussel)
	YTX	YTX, 1a-homoYTX	Calibrant solution
	AZA	AZA1, AZA2, AZA3	Calibrant solution Matrix (mussel)
	Cyclic imine	Gymnodimines, 20-MeSPX G, 13-desmeSPX C	Calibrant solution
	Pectenotoxin	PTX2	Calibrant solution
Hydrophilic marine toxin	ASP	Domoic acid	Calibrant solution Matrix (mussel)
	PSP	STX, Neo, dcNeo, dcSTX, GTX1 and 4, GTX2 and 3, C1 and 2, GTX5, dcGTX2 and 3	Calibrant solution Matrix (mussel, oyster)
Cyanobacterial toxin	Microcystin	Total mycrocystins	Matrix (cyanobacterial cells)
	Cylindrospermopsin	CYN	Calibrant solution
	Anatoxin	ATXa	Calibrant solution
Other toxins	Tetrodotoxin	TTX, 4,9-anhTTX	Calibrant solution
	None	None	Blank matrix (mussel)

Note: Laboratorio CIFGA S.A., NRC, CEFAS, NIES, and NIST are organizations that support these CRMs.

15.7 Cost of Producing Marine and Freshwater Toxin CRMs

As mentioned earlier, the production and certification of CRMs follows several stages, which include requirements of traceability and rigorous certification criteria. As a result, the production cost of a CRM is higher than a simple reference.[121]

The cost of a CRM is influenced by the cost of its preparation, distribution, storage, stability assessment, and the required annual or semiannual reassessment, in conclusion, by an intensive certification procedure.[121] Although CRMs are expensive products, users normally do not pay the real cost of feasibility studies lead to obtaining the first batch of a material, for example, due to the length of time it may take to establish a CRM and the effort involved in this process, CRMs for shellfish toxins are considered very precious.[38] The production of pure compounds is also difficult, so many purification steps need to be executed, and sometimes, despite the best efforts of purification, detectable levels of impurity components are found, which implies that the samples would need to be subjected to further cycles of cleanup and purification. Samples become more expensive when they have to be stored in cold conditions, especially when they have to be stored in freezers, or when they have to be stored following special safety measures. Price easily rises when they have to be shipped in a cooled container or as dangerous goods.

In proficiency testing, the use of RMs is necessary for fulfilling two basic requirements of ISO 17025 in order to obtain results traceable to the SI:

1. The traceability of the results of an analytical method is verified by comparison with a reference.
2. The measurement procedure must be validated according to a clearly defined standard methodology in order to minimize variability that may result from differences in laboratory.

Although from a practical point of view, CRMs of marine toxins are the best possible reference materials to ensure traceability of analytical results, nevertheless, not everything is advantageous: marine and freshwater toxin CRMs are not available for all known toxins for the current analysis being performed (taking into account the enormous range of matrices, analytes, and existing concentrations). Although desirable, another drawback is that the price of certifying the property values of proficiency testing samples often prohibits this from being done, and consensus mean values are often used instead. The great pressure of the costs in routine analysis leads laboratories to invest in highly sophisticated, automated analytical equipment and reduce running costs (personnel, consumables). Marine toxin CRMs are demanding and costly to produce, and if materials are available from other sources, it is not normally cost effective for laboratories to make their own.

As part of running costs, the costs of CRMs are obviously considered excessive, reflecting a poor understanding of the economic importance of these materials and the way they are prepared. Its high cost should not limit its application since the indirect impact resulting from inappropriate conclusions based on incorrect measurements cannot be estimated precisely by using substandard or unsafe goods, but rather by using the highest quality RMs, which are certified for the concentration values of the constituents of interest. Such a situation could yield unsafe analysis results in food safety controls.[122]

REFERENCES

1. Emons, H., Held, A., and Ulberth, F., 2006. Reference materials as crucial tools for quality assurance and control in food analysis. *Pure and Applied Chemistry*, 78, 135–143.
2. ISO/IEC 17025, 2002. General requirements for the competence of testing and calibration laboratories.
3. Fux, E., McMillan, D., Bire, R., and Hess, P., 2007. Development of an ultra-performance liquid chromatography–mass spectrometry method for the detection of lipophilic marine toxins. *Journal of Chromatography A*, 1157, 273–280.
4. European Centre for the Validation of Alternative Methods, European Commission. Directorate-General for Health Consumer Protection, 2006. Three Rs Approaches in Marine Biotoxin Testing. FRAME, Nottingham, U.K.
5. Campas, M., Prieto-Simon, B., and Marty, J.-L., 2007. Biosensors to detect marine toxins: Assessing seafood safety. *Talanta*, 72, 884–895.

6. Chorus, I. and Bartram, J., 1999. *Toxic Cyanobacteria in Water: A Guide to Their Public Health Consequences, Monitoring and Management.* Published on behalf of UNESCO, WHO and UNEP by E & FN Spon.
7. Campbell, K., Vilariño, N., Botana, L. M., and Elliott, C. T., 2011. A European perspective on progress in moving away from the mouse bioassay for marine-toxin analysis. *TrAC Trends in Analytical Chemistry*, 30, 239–253.
8. Botana, L. M., Louzao, M. C., Alfonso, A. et al., 2006. Measurement of algal toxins in the environment, in *Encyclopedia of Analytical Chemistry.* Meyers, R. A., ed. John Wiley & Sons, Ltd., Chichester, U.K.
9. Regulation (EC) No. 853/2004 of the European Parliament and of the Council of 29 April 2004 laying down specific hygiene rules for food of animal origin, 2004. *Official Journal of the European Union L*, 226, 22–82.
10. Scientific Opinion of the Panel on Contaminants in the Food Chain, 2009. *The EFSA Journal*, 1306, 1–23.
11. Quilliam, M. A., 2003. The role of chromatography in the hunt for red tide toxins. *Journal of Chromatography A*, 1000, 527–548.
12. Botana, L. M., 2008. *Seafood and Freshwater Toxins, Pharmacology, Physiology, and Detection*, 2nd edn. CRC Press, Boca Raton, FL.
13. Dolah, F. M. v. and Ramsdell, J. S., 2001. Review and assessment of *in vitro* detection methods for algal toxins. *Journal of AOAC International*, 84, 1617–1625.
14. Ciminiello, P., Dell'Aversano, C., Fattorusso, E. et al., 2006. The Genoa 2005 outbreak. Determination of putative palytoxin in Mediterranean *Ostreopsis ovata* by a new liquid chromatography tandem mass spectrometry method. *Analytical Chemistry*, 78, 6153–6159.
15. McNabb, P., Selwood, A. I., and Holland, P. T., 2005. Multiresidue method for determination of algal toxins in shellfish: Single-laboratory validation and interlaboratory study. *Journal of AOAC International*, 88, 761–772.
16. Villar-González, A., Rodríguez-Velasco, M. L., Ben-Gigirey, B., and Botana, L. M., 2007. Lipophilic toxin profile in Galicia (Spain): 2005 Toxic episode. *Toxicon*, 49, 1129–1134.
17. Blay, P., Hui, J. P. M., Chang, J., and Melanson, J. E., 2011. Screening for multiple classes of marine biotoxins by liquid chromatography-high-resolution mass spectrometry. *Analytical and Bioanalytical Chemistry*, 400, 577–585.
18. Commission Regulation (EU) No. 15/2011, 2011, Official Journal of the European Union. pp. 3–6.
19. These, A., Klemm, C., Nausch, I., and Uhlig, S., 2011. Results of a European Interlaboratory Method Validation Study for the quantitative determination of lipophilic marine biotoxins in raw and cooked shellfish based on high-performance liquid chromatography–tandem mass spectrometry. Part I: Collaborative study. *Analytical and Bioanalytical Chemistry*, 399, 1245–1256.
20. Velieri, F., Bacchiocchi, S., Graziosi, T., Latini, M., Orletti, R., and Bacci, C. 2012. Valutation of official mouse bioassay for the detection of lipophilic marine toxins. *Italian Journal of Food Safety*, 1, 5.
21. Gerssen, A., van Olst, E. H. W., Mulder, P. P. J., and de Boer, J., 2010. In-house validation of a liquid chromatography tandem mass spectrometry method for the analysis of lipophilic marine toxins in shellfish using matrix-matched calibration. *Analytical and Bioanalytical Chemistry*, 397, 3079–3088.
22. Botana, L. M., Vilariño, N., Alfonso, A. et al., 2010. The problem of toxicity equivalent factors in developing alternative methods to animal bioassays for marine-toxin detection. *TrAC Trends in Analytical Chemistry*, 29, 1316–1325.
23. Otero, P., Alfonso, A., Alfonso, C., Rodríguez, P., Vieytes, M. R., and Botana, L. M., 2011. Effect of uncontrolled factors in a validated liquid chromatography–tandem mass spectrometry method question its use as a reference method for marine toxins: Major causes for concern. *Analytical Chemistry*, 83, 5903–5911.
24. CEFAS, 2011. In-house validation of an LC-MS/MS method for the determination of lipophilic toxins in shellfish species typically tested in the United Kingdom. CEFAS contract report C3011.
25. Burch, M., 2008. Effective doses, guidelines & regulations, in *Cyanobacterial Harmful Algal Blooms: State of the Science and Research Needs.* Hudnell, H. K., ed. Springer, New York, pp. 831–853.
26. Eurachem Guide, EEE-RM Working Group. The selection and use of reference materials, 2002.
27. ISO Guide 30, 2008. Terms and definitions used in connection with reference materials. Amendment 1 Revision of definitions for reference material and certified reference material, 2nd edn.
28. Emons, H., Fajgelj, A., van der Veen, A. M. H., and Watters, R., 2006. New definitions on reference materials. *Accreditation and Quality Assurance*, 10, 576–578.
29. ISO Guide 35, 2006. Reference materials—General and statistical principles for certification, 3rd edn.

30. ISO Guide 34, 2009. General requirements for the competence of reference material producers, 3rd edn.
31. ISO Guide 31, 2000. Reference materials—Contents of certificates and labels, 2nd edn.
32. *International Vocabulary of Metrology—Basic and General Concepts and Associated Terms (VIM)*, JCGM Guidance Documents, Paris, France, 2012.
33. CITAC and Eurachem Guide. Guide to quality in analytical chemistry: An aid to accreditation, 2002.
34. IAEA-TECDOC-1350. *Development and Use of Reference Materials and Quality Control Materials*, IAEA, 2003.
35. ISO Guide 30, 1992. Terms and definitions used in connection with reference materials, 2nd edn.
36. De Bièvre, P., Kaarls, R., Peiser, H. S., Rasberry, S. D., and Reed, W. P., 1996. Measurement principles for traceability in chemical analysis. *Accreditation and Quality Assurance*, 1, 3–13.
37. Pan, X., 1997. Hierarchy of reference materials certified for chemical composition. *Metrologia*, 34, 35.
38. Hess, P., McCarron, P., and Quilliam, M. A., 2007. Fit-for-purpose shellfish reference materials for internal and external quality control in the analysis of phycotoxins. *Analytical and Bioanalytical Chemistry*, 387, 2463–2474.
39. Eurachem Guide, The *Fitness for Purpose of Analytical Methods. A Laboratory Guide to Method Validation and Related Topics*, 1998.
40. Thompson, M. and Wood, R., 1995. Harmonized guidelines for internal quality control in analytical chemistry laboratories (Technical report). Resulting from the *Symposium on Harmonization of Internal Quality Assurance Systems for Analytical Laboratories*, Washington, DC, July 22–23, 1993; *Pure and Applied Chemistry*, 67, 649–666.
41. International Laboratory Accreditation Cooperation (ILAC) guidance. ILAC-G9 Guidelines for the selection and use of reference materials, 2005.
42. ISO Guide 33, 2000. Uses of certified reference materials, 2nd edn.
43. King, R., Bonfiglio, R., Fernandez-Metzler, C., Miller-Stein, C., and Olah, T., 2000. Mechanistic investigation of ionization suppression in electrospray ionization. *Journal of the American Society for the Mass Spectrometry*, 11, 942–950.
44. ISO Guide 32, 1997. Calibration in analytical chemistry and use of certified reference materials, 1st edn.
45. EURACHEM/CITAC Guide: Traceability in Chemical Measurement. A Guide to Achieving Comparable Results in Chemical Measurement, 2003.
46. Botana, L. M., 2012. A perspective on the toxicology of marine toxins. *Chemical Research in Toxicology*, 25, 1800–1804.
47. Donohue, J., Orme-Zavaleta, J., Burch, M. et al., 2008. Risk assessment workgroup report. *Advances in Experimental Medicine and Biology*, 619, 759–829.
48. Sivonen, K., 2008. Emerging high throughput analyses of cyanobacterial toxins and toxic cyanobacteria. *Advances in Experimental Medicine and Biology*, 619, 539–557.
49. Munday, R., Quilliam, M. A., LeBlanc, P. et al., 2012. Investigations into the toxicology of spirolides, a group of marine phycotoxins. *Toxins (Basel)*, 4, 1–14.
50. Otero, P., Alfonso, A., Rodriguez, P. et al., 2012. Pharmacokinetic and toxicological data of spirolides after oral and intraperitoneal administration. *Food and Chemical Toxicology*, 50, 232–237.
51. Higman, W. A. and Turner, A., 2010. A feasibility study into the provision of Paralytic Shellfish Toxins laboratory reference materials by mass culture of *Alexandrium* and shellfish feeding experiments. *Toxicon*, 56, 497–501.
52. Emons, H., 2006. The RM family—Identification of all of its members. *Accreditation and Quality Assurance*, 10, 690–691.
53. McCarron, P., Emteborg, H., Nulty, C. et al., 2011. A mussel tissue certified reference material for multiple phycotoxins. Part 1: Design and preparation. *Analytical and Bioanalytical Chemistry*, 400, 821–833.
54. BIPM, 1998. *Proceedings of the 4th Meeting of CCQM*, Bureau International des Poids et Mesures (BIPM), Paris, France.
55. BIPM, 1995. *Proceedings of the 1st Meeting of the CCQM*, Bureau International des Poids et Mesures (BIPM), Paris, France.
56. Taylor, P., Kipphardt, H., and De Bièvre, P., 2001. The definition of primary method of measurement (PMM) of the 'highest metrological quality': A challenge in understanding and communication. *Accreditation and Quality Assurance*, 6, 103–106.
57. Holzgrabe, U., 2008. qNMR spectroscopy in drug analysis—a general view, in *NMR Spectroscopy in Pharmaceutical Analysis*. Holzgrabe, U., Diehl, B., and Wawer, I., eds. Elsevier Ltd., Oxford, U.K., pp. 131–137.

58. Pauli, G. F., Jaki, B. U., Lankin, D. C., Walter, J. A., and Burton, I. W., 2008. Quantitative NMR of bioactive natural products, in *Bioactive Natural Products: Detection, Isolation, and Structural Determination*, 2nd edn. Colegate, S. M. and Molyneux, R. J., eds. CRC Press, Boca Raton, FL, pp. 113–141.

59. Pauli, G. F., Gödecke, T., Jaki, B. U., and Lankin, D. C., 2012. Quantitative 1H NMR: Development and potential of an analytical method: An update. *Journal of Natural Products*, 75, 834–851.

60. Bharti, S. K. and Roy, R., 2012. Quantitative 1H NMR spectroscopy. *TrAC Trends in Analytical Chemistry*, 35, 5–26.

61. Saito, T., Ihara, T., Miura, T., Yamada, Y., and Chiba, K., 2011. Efficient production of reference materials of hazardous organics using smart calibration by nuclear magnetic resonance. *Accreditation and Quality Assurance*, 16, 421–428.

62. Saito, T., Ihara, T., Koike, M. et al., 2009. A new traceability scheme for the development of international system-traceable persistent organic pollutant reference materials by quantitative nuclear magnetic resonance. *Accreditation and Quality Assurance*, 14, 79–86.

63. Malz, F. and Jancke, H., 2005. Validation of quantitative NMR. *Journal of Pharmaceutical and Biomedical Analysis*, 38, 813–823.

64. Holzgrabe, U., Deubner, R., Schollmayer, C., and Waibel, B., 2005. Quantitative NMR spectroscopy—Applications in drug analysis. *Journal of Pharmaceutical and Biomedical Analysis*, 38, 806–812.

65. Wells, R. J., Cheung, J., and Hook, J. M., 2004. Dimethylsulfone as a universal standard for analysis of organics by QNMR. *Accreditation and Quality Assurance*, 9, 450–456.

66. Rosman, K. J. R. and Taylor, P. D. P., 1998. Isotopic compositions of the elements, 1997. *Pure and Applied Chemistry*, 70, 217–235.

67. Shimizu, Y., Hsu, C.-P., Fallon, W. E., Oshima, Y., Miura, I., and Nakanishi, K., 1978. Structure of neosaxitoxin. *Journal of the American Chemical Society*, 100, 6791–6793.

68. Burton, I. W., Quilliam, M. A., and Walter, J. A., 2005. Quantitative 1H NMR with external standards: Use in preparation of calibration solutions for algal toxins and other natural products. *Analytical Chemistry*, 77, 3123–3131.

69. Hoye, T. R., Eklov, B. M., Ryba, T. D., Voloshin, M., and Yao, L. J., 2004. No-D NMR (no-deuterium proton NMR) spectroscopy: A simple yet powerful method for analyzing reaction and reagent solutions. *Organic Letters*, 6, 953–956.

70. McKay, R. T., 2009. Recent advances in solvent suppression for solution NMR: A practical reference, Chapter 2, in *Annual Reports on NMR Spectroscopy*. Graham, A. W., ed. Academic Press, London, U.K., pp. 33–76.

71. Liu, M., Tang, H., Nicholson, J. K., and Lindon, J. C., 2001. Recovery of underwater resonances by magnetization transferred NMR spectroscopy (RECUR-NMR). *Journal of Magnetic Resonance*, 153, 133–137.

72. Claridge, T., 2009. *High-Resolution NMR Techniques in Organic Chemistry*. Elsevier Science Ltd., Oxford, U.K.

73. Holmes, E., Nicholson, J. K., and Lindon, J. C., 2007. *The Handbook of Metabonomics and Metabolomics*. Elsevier, Amsterdam, the Netherlands.

74. Smallcombe, S. H., Patt, S. L., and Keifer, P. A., 1995. WET solvent suppression and its applications to LC NMR and high-resolution NMR spectroscopy. *Journal of Magnetic Resonance, Series A*, 117, 295–303.

75. Pierens, G. K., Carroll, A. R., Davis, R. A., Palframan, M. E., and Quinn, R. J., 2008. Determination of analyte concentration using the residual solvent resonance in 1H NMR spectroscopy. *Journal of Natural Products*, 71, 810–813.

76. Watanabe, R., Suzuki, T., and Oshima, Y., 2010. Development of quantitative NMR method with internal standard for the standard solutions of paralytic shellfish toxins and characterisation of gonyautoxin-5 and gonyautoxin-6. *Toxicon*, 56, 589–595.

77. Henderson, T. J., 2001. Quantitative NMR spectroscopy using coaxial inserts containing a reference standard: Purity determinations for military nerve agents. *Analytical Chemistry*, 74, 191–198.

78. Akoka, S., Barantin, L., and Trierweiler, M., 1999. Concentration measurement by proton NMR using the ERETIC method. *Analytical Chemistry*, 71, 2554–2557.

79. Remaud, G. S., Silvestre, V., and Akoka, S., 2005. Traceability in quantitative NMR using an electronic signal as working standard. *Accreditation and Quality Assurance*, 10, 415–420.

80. Schievano, E., Guardini, K., and Mammi, S., 2009. Fast determination of histamine in cheese by nuclear magnetic resonance (NMR). *Journal of Agricultural and Food Chemistry*, 57, 2647–2652.
81. Pauli, G. F., Jaki, B. U., and Lankin, D. C., 2007. A routine experimental protocol for qHNMR illustrated with taxol. *Journal of Natural Products*, 70, 589–595.
82. Grove, D. M., 1988. *Modern NMR Techniques for Chemistry Research*, Vol. 6 (Organic Chemistry Series, Derome, A. E., ed., Pergamon Press, Oxford, U.K., 280pp., ISBN 0-08-0325149 HC, 0-08-0325130 FC. *Recueil des Travaux Chimiques des Pays-Bas*, 107, 25.
83. Colegate, S. M. and Molyneux, R. J., 2008. *Bioactive Natural Products: Detection, Isolation, and Structural Determination*. CRC Press, Boca Raton, FL.
84. Pauli, G. F., Jaki, B. U., and Lankin, D. C., 2004. Quantitative 1H NMR: Development and potential of a method for natural products analysis. *Journal of Natural Products*, 68, 133–149.
85. Claridge, T. D. W., Davies, S. G., Polywka, M. E. C. et al., 2008. Pure by NMR? *Organic Letters*, 10, 5433–5436.
86. Dalisay, D. S. and Molinski, T. F., 2009. NMR quantitation of natural products at the nanomole scale. *Journal of Natural Products*, 72, 739–744.
87. Ernst, R. R. and Anderson, W. A., 1966. Application of Fourier transform spectroscopy to magnetic resonance. *Review of Scientific Instruments*, 37, 93–102.
88. Bauer, M., Bertario, A., Boccardi, G., Fontaine, X., Rao, R., and Verrier, D., 1998. Reproducibility of 1H-NMR integrals: A collaborative study. *Journal of Pharmaceutical and Biomedical Analysis*, 17, 419–425.
89. Griffiths, L., 1998. Assay by nuclear magnetic resonance spectroscopy: Quantification limits. *Analyst*, 123, 1061–1068.
90. Perez, R. A., Rehmann, N., Crain, S. et al., 2010. The preparation of certified calibration solutions for azaspiracid-1, -2, and -3, potent marine biotoxins found in shellfish. *Analytical and Bioanalytical Chemistry*, 398, 2243–2252.
91. Jancke, H., Malz, F., and Haesselbarth, W., 2005. Structure analytical methods for quantitative reference applications. *Accreditation and Quality Assurance*, 10, 421–429.
92. Franco, J. M., López, E., and Riobó, P., 2011. Chemical methods for detecting phycotoxins: LC and LC/MS/MS, in *New Trends in Marine and Freshwater Toxins: Food and Safety Concerns*. Cabado, A. G. and Vieites, J. M., eds. Nova Publishers, New York.
93. Vilarino, N., Louzao, M. C., Vieytes, M. R., and Botana, L. M., 2010. Biological methods for marine toxin detection. *Analytical and Bioanalytical Chemistry*, 397, 1673–1681.
94. EURLMB Standard Operating Procedures, EU-Harmonised Standard Operating Procedure for determination of lipophilic marine biotoxins in molluscs by LC-MS/MS, version 4, 2011.
95. Antoniou, M. G., de la Cruz, A. A., and Dionysiou, D. D., 2005. Cyanotoxins: New generation of water contaminants. *Journal of Environmental Engineering (Reston, VA, United States)*, 131, 1239–1243.
96. Ibelings, B. W. and Chorus, I., 2007. Accumulation of cyanobacterial toxins in freshwater "seafood" and its consequences for public health: A review. *Environmental Pollution*, 150, 177–192.
97. Thompson, M., Ellison, S. L. R., and Wood, R., 2002. Harmonized guidelines for single-laboratory validation of methods of analysis (IUPAC technical report). *Pure and Applied Chemistry*, 74, 835–855.
98. Peters, F. T., Drummer, O. H., and Musshoff, F., 2007. Validation of new methods. *Forensic Science International*, 165, 216–224.
99. Thompson, M., Ellison, S. L. R., Fajgelj, A., Willetts, P., and Wood, R., 1999. Harmonized guidelines for the use of recovery information in analytical measurement. *Pure and Applied Chemistry*, 71, 337–348.
100. Barwick, V. J., Ellison, S. L. R., Rafferty, M. J. Q., and Gill, R. S., 2000. The evaluation of measurement uncertainty from method validation studies. Part 2: The practical application of a laboratory protocol. *Accreditation and Quality Assurance*, 5, 104–113.
101. Barwick, V. J. and Ellison, S. L. R., 1999. Measurement uncertainty: Approaches to the evaluation of uncertainties associated with recovery. *Analyst (Cambridge, United Kingdom)*, 124, 981–990.
102. Ellison, S. L. R. and Williams, A. (eds). 2012. *Eurachem/CITAC guide: Quantifying Uncertainty in Analytical Measurement*, 3rd edn. Available from www.eurachem.org.
103. Meija, J. and Mester, Z., 2008. Paradigms in isotope dilution mass spectrometry for elemental speciation analysis. *Analytica Chimica Acta*, 607, 115–125.
104. Milton, M. J. T. and Quinn, T. J., 2001. Primary methods for the measurement of amount of substance. *Metrologia*, 38, 289–296.

105. Ellerbe, P., Phinney, C. S., Sniegoski, L. T., and Welch, M. J., 1999. Validation of new instrumentation for isotope dilution mass spectrometric determination of organic serum analytes. *Journal of Research of the National Institute of Standards and Technology*, 104, 141–145.

106. Linsinger, T. P. J., Pauwels, J., Schimmel, H. et al., 2000. Estimation of the uncertainty of CRMs in accordance with GUM: Application to the certification of four enzyme CRMs. *Fresenius' Journal of Analytical Chemistry*, 368, 589–594.

107. van der Veen, A. M. H., Linsinger, T., and Pauwels, J., 2001. Uncertainty calculations in the certification of reference materials. 2. Homogeneity study. *Accreditation and Quality Assurance*, 6, 26–30.

108. Linsinger, T. P. J., Pauwels, J., van der Veen, A. M. H., Schimmel, H., and Lamberty, A., 2001. Homogeneity and stability of reference materials. *Accreditation and Quality Assurance*, 6, 20–25.

109. Pauwels, J. and Vandecasteele, C., 1993. Determination of the minimum sample mass of a solid CRM to be used in chemical analysis. *Fresenius' Journal of Analytical Chemistry*, 345, 121–123.

110. Bremser, W., Becker, R., Kipphardt, H., Lehnik-Habrink, P., Panne, U., and Toepfer, A., 2006. Stability testing in an integrated scheme. *Accreditation and Quality Assurance*, 11, 489–495.

111. van der Veen, A. M. H., Linsinger, T. P. J., Lamberty, A., and Pauwels, J., 2001. Uncertainty calculations in the certification of reference materials. 3. Stability study. *Accreditation and Quality Assurance*, 6, 257–263.

112. Linsinger, T. P. J., Pauwels, J., Lamberty, A., Schimmel, H. G., van der Veen, A. M. H., and Siekmann, L., 2001. Estimating the uncertainty of stability for matrix CRMs. *Fresenius' Journal of Analytical Chemistry*, 370, 183–188.

113. Linsinger, T. P. J., van der Veen, A. M. H., Gawlik, B. M., Pauwels, J., and Lamberty, A., 2004. Planning and combining of isochronous stability studies of CRMs. *Accreditation and Quality Assurance*, 9, 464–472.

114. Lamberty, A., Schimmel, H., and Pauwels, J., 1998. The study of the stability of reference materials by isochronous measurements. *Fresenius' Journal of Analytical Chemistry*, 360, 359–361.

115. Pauwels, J., Lamberty, A., and Schimmel, H., 1998. Quantification of the expected shelf-life of certified reference materials. *Fresenius' Journal of Analytical Chemistry*, 361, 395–399.

116. van der Veen, A. M. H., Linsinger, T. P. J., Schimmel, H., Lamberty, A., and Pauwels, J., 2001. Uncertainty calculations in the certification of reference materials 4. Characterisation and certification. *Accreditation and Quality Assurance*, 6, 290–294.

117. Iverson, F., Truelove, J., Nera, E., Tryphonas, L., Campbell, J., and Lok, E., 1989. Domoic acid poisoning and mussel-associated intoxication: Preliminary investigations into the response of mice and rats to toxic mussel extract. *Food and Chemical Toxicology*, 27, 377–384.

118. Grimmelt, B., Nijjar, M. S., Brown, J. et al., 1990. Relationship between domoic acid levels in the blue mussel (*Mytilus edulis*) and toxicity in mice. *Toxicon*, 28, 501–508.

119. Munday, R., Holland, P. T., McNabb, P., Selwood, A. I., and Rhodes, L. L., 2008. Comparative toxicity to mice of domoic acid and isodomoic acids A, B and C. *Toxicon*, 52, 954–956.

120. Paredes, I., Rietjens, I. M. C. M., Vieites, J. M., and Cabado, A. G., 2011. Update of risk assessments of main marine biotoxins in the European Union. *Toxicon*, 58, 336–354.

121. Venelinov, T. and Quevauviller, P., 2003. Are certified reference materials really expensive? *TrAC Trends in Analytical Chemistry*, 22, 15–18.

122. Emons, H., Linsinger, T. P. J., and Gawlik, B. M., 2004. Reference materials: Terminology and use. Can't one see the forest for the trees? *TrAC Trends in Analytical Chemistry*, 23, 442–449.

123. Al-Deen, T. S., Hibbert, D. B., Hook, J. M., and Wells, R. J., 2004. An uncertainty budget for the determination of the purity of glyphosate by quantitative nuclear magnetic resonance (QNMR) spectroscopy. *Accreditation and Quality Assurance*, 9, 55–63.

16

Strategies on the Use of Antibodies as Binders for Marine Toxins

Edwina Stack and Richard O'Kennedy

CONTENTS

16.1 Chapter Summary

In this chapter, we review sensor-based methods of marine toxin analysis with particular emphasis on immunosensing approaches and their applications.

16.2 Introduction

Episodes of marine toxin contamination, produced by phytoplankton, occur worldwide causing both animal and human fatalities. In many countries, legislation has been implemented governing maximum permitted levels of marine toxins in seafood and water. The mouse bioassay is the reference method in current legislation for the majority of marine toxins. However, this method has raised ethical concerns due to the use of laboratory animals. Also, animal bioassays are known for their lack of sensitivity and specificity. This new regulatory landscape has stimulated the development of tools for the monitoring of seafood and water contamination by individual toxin classes.

Chromatographic techniques have been widely employed for the sensitive detection of toxins produced by marine microalgae. Chromatography allows for separation, highly selective identification, and sensitive quantification of the various toxin mixtures present in a sample. Moreover, limits of detection are generally one order of magnitude lower than those obtained with the mouse bioassay. However, toxin chromatographic techniques require expensive equipment and trained personnel. Furthermore, these methods are laborious and time-consuming. The lack of standards is also a key concern, since noncertified or unknown toxins cannot be evaluated. Other reported issues include peak spreading, poor resolution, and the need for continuous calibration.

Antibody techniques for marine toxins cover a vast area of ongoing research efforts, including immunoassays, enzyme-inhibition assays, biosensors, immunosensors, and enzyme-inhibition-based biosensors. In the current climate, immunological assays with the accuracy and reliability of traditional analytical methods and the sensitivity and specificity of biological interactions are sought. The versatility of immunosensor-based analytical platforms for pharmacological, environmental, and food safety detection has been extensively reviewed (Ivnitski et al. 1999; Baeumner 2003; Amine et al. 2006; Rodriguez-Mozaz et al. 2006; Byrne et al. 2009; Van Dorst et al. 2010). Biosensors provide a cost-effective alternative for marine toxin detection, as well as group specificity, sensitivity, portability, repeatability, and robustness. However, immunoassays have been vilified by some because of their inability to analyze different analogs of a toxin group present in a sample. Like the mouse bioassay, they generate an overall estimate of the toxin content of a sample. For the purpose of this chapter, attention will be focused on antibody development to the cyanobacterial toxin, microcystin (MC), and immunosensor development to a wider range of toxins, including paralytic shellfish poisoning (PSP), amnesic shellfish poisoning (ASP), and diarrheic shellfish poisoning (DSP) toxins. An introduction to antibody technology will be given, with a particular emphasis on immune response generation to small hapten targets, including marine biotoxins.

16.3 Antibody Structure and Function

Antibodies are produced by the host's immune system in response to a foreign material or antigen. The antibody-producing cells are known as B lymphocytes or B cells, and they play a major role in generating the humoral response of the immune system (LeBien and Tedder 2008). Each B cell is programmed to make a single type of antibody for a particular target, known as an antigen. When a B cell encounters an antigen, it differentiates into a plasma cell, which produces antibodies with specificity and affinity for the antigen. Antibodies (also referred to as immunoglobulins or IgGs) are natural biological scaffolds with structurally variable antigen-binding domains (Table 16.1). More than 10^8 different antibodies can be in circulation at any one time. A process known as gene rearrangement is responsible for the production of a primary repertoire of antibodies. This is followed by a secondary process known as somatic hypermutation, in which IgGs with highly evolved molecular recognition properties are generated.

Antibodies are large glycoprotein structures with a characteristic "Y" shape (Figure 16.1). There are five main antibody classes, designated according to their heavy-chain structure (IgG, IgA, IgM, IgD, and IgE). IgG_1 is the predominant isoform, resulting from its longer lifetime in the plasma (approximately 21 days). An IgG antibody consists of two heavy chains and two light chains, which are covalently linked by disulfide bonds. In addition to an interchain disulfide bond, an IgG has two intra-chain disulfide bonds. Each light chain has an *N*-terminal variable domain (V_L) and a constant domain (C_L). Each heavy chain is composed of an *N*-terminal variable domain (V_H), three constant domains (C_H1-C_H3), and a hinge region. There are five classes of heavy chains, α, γ, μ, δ, and ε, and two classes of light chains, κ and λ. The heavy chains confer different biological functions to a specific isotype and they differ in their size and carbohydrate content. Most species produce both types of light chains, but the ratio of κ to λ varies with the species (Scott and Potter 1983).

Each antibody has only one light-chain and heavy-chain type, which determine the subclass. The V_H and V_L chains form the antigen-binding site of the molecule. The sequence and structural variation in the

TABLE 16.1

Structure and Function of IgG Components and Recombinant Fragments

Structure	Function
scFv molecule	Smallest recombinant fragment of ~26–27 kDa. Consists of a complete binding site of the individual heavy- and light-chain V domains. Connected with a short linker peptide of 10–25 amino acids.
Fab molecule	Recombinant fragment of ~50 kDa with a shortened heavy chain. This heavy-chain fragment is referred to as a Fd fragment. Two domains, V_L–V_H and C_L–C_H1, interact to form the two-chain structure of the Fab molecule, which is further stabilized by a disulfide bridge between C_L and C_H1.
Fab fragment	Region on an antibody that binds to antigens. It is composed of one constant and one variable domain of each of the heavy and the light chain.
Fragment-crystallizable region (Fc region)	Tail region of an antibody that interacts with cell surface receptors called Fc receptors and some proteins of the complement system. This property allows antibodies to activate the immune system.
Disulfide bridges	Important for structural determination and conformation. Stabilize the interaction between heavy and light chains.
Carbohydrate	Fc regions of IgGs have a highly conserved *N*-glycosylation site. Glycosylation of the Fc fragment is essential for Fc receptor-mediated activity. The *N*-glycans attached to this site are predominantly core-fucosylated diantennary structures.

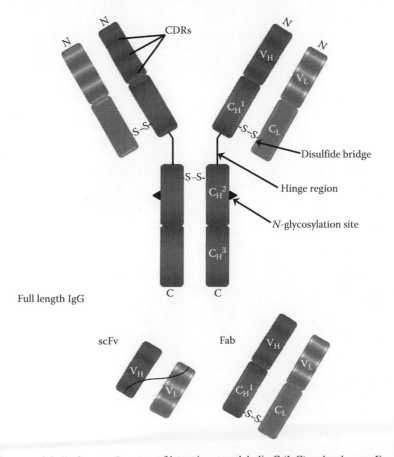

FIGURE 16.1 Immunoglobulin formats. Structure of intact immunoglobulin G (IgG) molecule, an scFv molecule, and a Fab molecule. Heavy-chain domains are represented in dark gray and light-chain domains in light gray. S–S represents a disulfide bridge. N and C represent the N and C terminus, respectively.

variable domains is generally restricted to three short hypervariable loops, known as complementarity determining regions (CDRs). The variable domain also consists of a framework region, which is highly conserved. The combination of amino acid residues in the CDRs determines the ability of the antibodies to recognize a specific antigenic determinant. A number of specific amino acid residues account for the predominant interaction of the antibody with the antigen. These locations are referred to as "hot spots" (Murphy et al. 2006).

There are three main approaches for generating antibodies for any target, including marine toxins. These include polyclonal, monoclonal, and recombinant techniques (Figure 16.2).

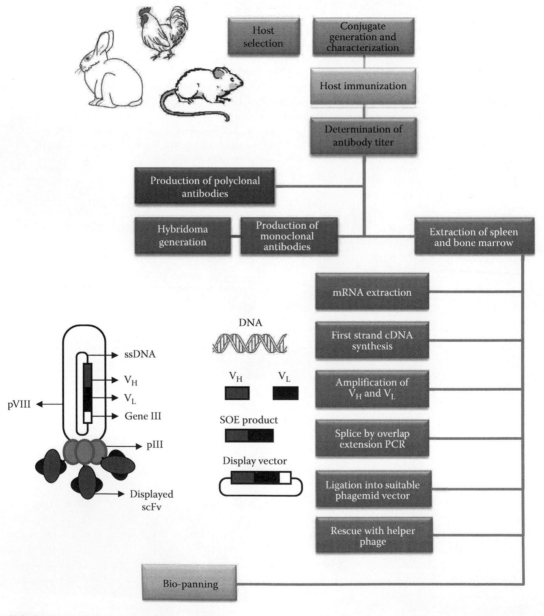

FIGURE 16.2 Overview of antibody generation strategies. Polyclonal antibodies can be isolated from immune serum and monoclonal antibodies can be generated using hybridoma technology. In recombinant antibody generation, the genetic material is harvested from the host's lymphoid organs (spleen and bone marrow). The introduction of this construct into a phagemid system and rescue with helper phage allows the encoded antibody to be presented on the exterior of a bacteriophage particle as fusion partner of a coat protein, pIII (Inset).

A number of key issues need to be considered in relation to the generation and use of antibodies for the detection of marine toxins. These include the following:

- Availability of toxin in sufficient quantities in a pure form for immunization, screening, and analysis.
- Toxicity of toxin and toxin conjugate used for immunization.
- Availability of alternative toxin structural mimics that can be substituted for the toxin where availability, stability, or structural limitations exist.
- Low molecular weight toxins may have only a single epitope available to which specific antibodies can be generated.
- Limitations in capacity of conjugating toxin to carrier for immunization and screening due to lack of suitable chemical groups on the toxin molecule; toxin modification and derivatization may help to overcome this issue.
- Many toxins exist in multiple forms (congeners), which may compromise antibody recognition in toxin mixtures. The challenge in detecting related compounds is to retain the ability to distinguish structurally related molecules of the target while not cross-reacting with unrelated compounds in the complex matrices to be tested.
- The inherent diversity of polyclonal antibody (pAb) preparations may provide the required sensitivity and capacity to recognize multiple forms of a toxin.
- Monoclonal antibodies offer defined specificity; cocktails of multiple monoclonal antibodies may be necessary to achieve desired cross-reactivity profiles (Campbell et al. 2007).
- Implementation of recombinant antibodies may have the capacity to provide significant information on antibody–antigen interactions; this can be exploited to aid in the engineering of antibodies with highly tailored antibody specificity or affinity characteristics.
- Antibody preparations may be utilized in various formats, for example, immobilized on solid supports such as nanoparticles and magnetic beads (Fraga et al. 2012; Zhang et al. 2012), to isolate/concentrate toxins from complex matrices with many potentially interfering components.
- Recombinant antibodies may be generated from immunized hosts, from hybridomas secreting highly specific monoclonal antibodies, as well as from immunized, naive, and synthetic antibody libraries. Application of molecular biological techniques may be applied to optimize antibody performance (broad or narrow specificity depending on the precise application), stability, antibody format (full-length Ig, fragment antigen binding [Fab], single-chain variable fragment [scFv], single-chain antibody fragment [scAb], etc.), and addition of fusion labels (enzymes or fluorescent proteins for signal generation or His/myc/peptides to facilitate conjugation or to optimize orientation).

16.3.1 Polyclonal Antibodies

PAb production usually involves the immunization of a host animal in order to generate an immune response toward a particular antigen. Following immunization, blood samples are collected from the animal, and the specific antibodies are purified from the serum employing affinity purification techniques, such as protein A or G chromatography. A pAb mixture usually consists of a number of different serotypes with varying affinities and specificities toward the target antigen. Many different species can be used for pAb development, including guinea pigs, rats, goats, chickens, sheep, and donkeys (Leenaars and Hendriksen 2005).

In general, the analytical capacity of any enzyme-linked immunosorbent assay (ELISA) in routine sample screening is dependent on the antibodies' ability to recognize all antigenic variants. For example, polyclonal antibodies to the cyanobacterial target, MC, have the advantage of being composed of a mixed pool of antibodies, which bind to different sites on the MC molecule, including those that are common to all toxin variants (Table 16.2). However, pAb responses are highly variable

TABLE 16.2

Strategies for PAb Development to MC

Toxin	Conjugation Strategy	Carrier	IC$_{50}$ (µg/L)	Format	Cross-Reactivity	References
MC-LR and NOD	Aminoethylation of the N-methyldehydroalanine residue and one-step glutaraldehyde coupling	KLH	2.50	Indirect competitive	MC-LA, MC-LR, MC-LF, MC-LW, MC-D-Asp3-RR, MC-LY, NOD, MC-Asp (Z)-Dhb7-HtyR	Metcalf et al. (2000)
MC-LR	Carbodiimide EDPC (1-(3 dimethylaminopropyl)-3-ethylcarbodiimide)	BSA Poly-L-lysine	1.75	RIA,[a] direct and indirect competitive	MC-RR, MC-LR, and -YR, NOD	Chu et al. (1989)
MC-LR	Aminoethylation of the N-methyldehydroalanine residue and glutaraldehyde coupling	BSA	0.63	Direct competitive	MC-LR, MC-RR, MC-YR, MC-LF, MC-LW, NOD	Sheng et al. (2006)
MC-LR/RR NOD	Carbodiimide	Poly-L-lysine	10–50	Competitive inhibition	MC-LR, MC-RR, NOD	Baier et al. (2000)
Adda	Synthetic N-acetyl D-alanyl Adda	cBSA OVA	0.61	Indirect competitive	MC-LR, MC-RR, MC-YR, MC-LW, MC-LF, 3-dm-MC-LR, 3-dm-MC-RR, NOD	Fischer et al. (2001)
MC-LR	Carbodiimide method using activated EDC, via carboxylic acid group (mixed anhydride)	BSA OVA HRP	0.50	Indirect and direct competitive	Abs with similar cross-reactivity pooled	Mhadhbi et al. (2006)
MC-RR	Aminoethylation of the N-methyldehydroalanine residue and glutaraldehyde coupling	KLH	3.03	CIPPIA[b]	MC-LR, MC-RR, NOD	Young et al. (2006)

Note: Antibodies were compared, according to their immunogen preparation (conjugation strategy and carrier molecule), IC$_{50}$, immunoassay format, and cross-reactivity, to MC variants.

[a] RIA: radioimmunoassay.

[b] CIPPIA: colorimetric immuno–protein phosphatase inhibition assay.

and non-reproducible, especially when different batches of sera are used. A sheep pAb was raised to the (2S,3S,8S,9S)-3-amino-9-methoxy-2,6,8-trimethyl-10-phenyldeca-4,6-dienoic (Adda) moiety, which is found in 80% of all MC and nodularin variants (Fischer et al. 2001). Immunization with a common structural feature, such as Adda, restricts the number of sites available for binding, giving greater reproducibility. The sheep pAb cross-reacted with MC-LR, MC-RR, MC-YR, MC-LW, MC-LF, 3-desmethyl-MC-LR, 3-desmethyl-MC-RR, and nodularin. ELISA formats have also been developed for MC using monoclonal and recombinant antibodies (Tables 16.3 and 16.4). Monoclonal antibodies from hybridoma cell lines are more reliable and reproducible than polyclonal antibodies, as they can be generated in uniform batches with comparable specificities and can bind to a single epitope on the target antigen.

16.3.2 Monoclonal Antibodies

Hybridoma technology is a second approach to antibody production that can be used to generate monoclonal antibodies (Hudson and Souriau 2003). Monoclonal antibodies are produced by immunizing a host (generally murine) with the target of interest. When a sufficient antibody serum titer is reached in the mouse serum, the spleen, bone marrow, or primary lymphoid organs (lymph nodes) are removed from the host and the antibody-producing B cells are harvested. These B cells are immediately fused to immortal myeloma cells, either by pulsing them with an electrical current or using polyethylene glycol (PEG). The "hybrid" population is selected and cloned out to ensure monoclonality. The resulting hybridoma will secrete antibodies to the desired target.

A number of successful ELISA screening tools have been created using monoclonal antibodies to MC (Table 16.3). In general, the sensitivity and specificity of MC-binding monoclonal antibodies is dependent on immunogen preparation, including choice of MC variant for immunization and conjugation chemistry. Monoclonal antibody (mAb) development for MC began almost three decades ago, when Kfir et al. (1986) produced an MC-LA immunogen using carbodiimide chemistry. A highly cross-reactive mAb was isolated by Nagata et al. (1995). In this study, carbodiimide chemistry was utilized to catalyze the formation of stable amide bonds between the carboxylic acid group of MC at the MeAsp (erythro-b-methylaspartic acid) site and amine groups of the carrier protein. Successful exposure of the Adda moiety to the immune system of the host animal resulted in the isolation of antibodies capable of binding multiple congeners. The most sensitive mAb (M8H5) had a limit of detection of MC-LR of 0.025 µg/L and cross-reacted with five variants and nodularin in the nanomolar range. The M8H5 antibody has subsequently been incorporated into an immunoaffinity column for sample cleanup and to concentrate trace amounts of toxin from water samples for HLPC analysis (Tsutsumi et al. 2000; Kondo et al. 2002).

Other monoclonal MC-LR and nodularin-specific antibodies have used conjugation methods directed through the methyldehydroalanine moiety (Mikhailov et al. 2001). This approach has produced clones directed against other epitopes of MC and nodularin, which is not possible using carbodiimide chemistry. Zeck et al. (2001) developed a highly sensitive and specific monoclonal anti-MC antibody using mice immunized with a MC-LR conjugated to ovalbumin (OVA) through the methyldehydroalanine residue. The best performing clone (MC10E7) has a limit of detection of 8 ng/L. Binding of this antibody is dependent on the arginine residue at position 4 of MC (Figure 16.3). Therefore, the cross-reactivity profile shows binding to other variants that contain arginine at position 4, including MC-RR, MC-WR, and MC-YR, in the picomolar range. However, MC10E7 is unable to detect MCs that lack the arginine residue and it does not recognize Adda.

Monoclonal antibodies to MC are generally incorporated into competitive assay formats due to their small molecular weight. However, noncompetitive assay formats are generally considered to be more sensitive. Additionally, it is not possible to establish a sandwich immunoassay with small molecules, as they usually posses only one epitope or overlapping epitopes. Therefore, Nagata et al. (1999) generated a secondary antibody that bound the immune complex formed by MC and a primary antibody. Monoclonal antibodies have also been developed to the Adda moiety using synthetic immunogens (Fischer et al. 2001) and modified versions of Adda (Zeck et al. 2001).

TABLE 16.3

Strategies for mAb Development to MC

Toxin	Conjugation Strategy	Carrier	IC_{50} (µg/L)	Format	Cross-Reactivity	References
MC-LA	—	Poly-L-lysine Muramyl dipeptide	—	—	6 variants	Kfir et al. (1986)
MC-LR	Carbodiimide EDPC	BSA OVA KLH	0.13	Indirect competitive	—	Nagata et al. (1995)
MC-LR	Aminoethylation of N-methyldehydroalanine residue and glutaraldehyde coupling	BSA	1.00	Direct competitive	MC-RR, dm-MC-LR, dm-MC-RR, H_2N-etMC-LR, MC-YR, NOD	Mikhailov et al. (2001)
Adda	Amide (activated ester) between carboxylic acid of Adda and primary amino groups	KLH BSA HRP	0.33	Direct competitive	All congeners	Zeck et al. (2001)
MC-LR	Carboxylic acid group via carbodiimide	HRP	0.22	Direct competitive	All congeners	Weller et al. (2001)
MC-LR	EDC/NHS linkage via carboxylic acid groups	Biotin	0.05	Indirect inhibition	—	Lindner et al. (2004)
MC-LR	Aminoethylation of the N-methyldehydroalanine residue and glutaraldehyde coupling	BSA	1.8	Indirect competitive	Very low level	Sheng et al. (2007)
MC-LR NOD	Aminoethylation on N-methyldehydroalanine	BSA	0.01	EIA[a]	MC-LR, -YR, -LA, NOD	Khreich et al. (2009)

Note: Antibodies were compared, according to their immunogen preparation (conjugation strategy and carrier molecule), IC_{50}, immunoassay format, and cross-reactivity, to MC variants.

[a] EIA: enzyme immunoassay.

TABLE 16.4

Strategies for Recombinant Antibody Development to MC-LR

Conjugation Strategy	Carrier	Antibody Format	IC$_{50}$ (µg/L)	Format	Cross-Reactivity	References
Aminoethylation of the N-methyldehydroalanine residue and one-step glutaraldehyde coupling	KLH BSA	scAb from Tomlinson I library	4–9	Direct competitive	MC-RR MC-LW MC-LF	McElhiney et al. (2000)
Aminoethylation of the N-methyldehydroalanine residue and one-step glutaraldehyde coupling	KLH BSA	scAb from Griffin I library	0.0045	Direct competitive	MC-RR MC-LW MC-LF	McElhiney et al. (2002)
Aminoethylation of the N-methyldehydroalanine residue and one-step glutaraldehyde coupling	KLH BSA	scAb from Tomlinson I scAb from Griffin I	0.013 4	Direct competitive	—	Strachen et al. (2002)

Note: Antibodies were compared, according to their immunogen preparation (conjugation strategy and carrier molecule), IC$_{50}$, antibody format, immunoassay format, and cross-reactivity, to MC variants.

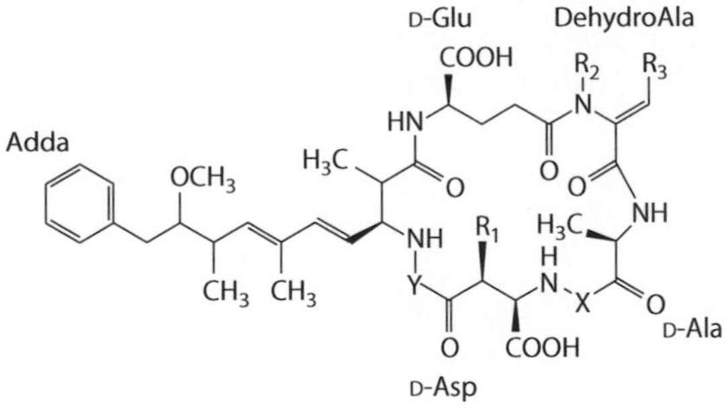

MC Variant	X	Y	R1	R2	R3
MC-LR	Leu	Arg	CH$_3$	CH$_3$	H
MC-LW	Leu	Trp	CH$_3$	CH$_3$	H
MC-LF	Leu	Phe	CH$_3$	CH$_3$	H
MC-LA	Leu	Ala	CH$_3$	CH$_3$	H
MC-RR	Arg	Arg	CH$_3$	CH$_3$	H
MC-YR	Try	Arg	CH$_3$	CH$_3$	H

FIGURE 16.3 MC structure and derivatives: MC XY—X and Y represent the one-letter abbreviations of the variable amino acids 2 (X) and 4 (Y). R1–R3 represent variations in the methyl group position. At least 80 MC variants have been identified and MC-LR, MC-LW, MC-LF, MC-LA, MC-RR, and MC-YR represent the most abundant. MCs also consist of a d-alanine (Ala); d-erythro β-methylaspartic acid (MeAsp); Adda; iso-linked d-glutamic acid (Glu) and N-methyldehydroalanine (Mdha).

16.3.3 Recombinant Antibodies

Production of polyclonal or monoclonal antibodies requires continuous maintenance of animals or cultures of hybridomas, respectively. For both approaches, the life-span of the animal and subsequent maintenance through a course of immunizations and bleedings is costly and time-consuming. A highly effective alternative to both polyclonal and mAb development is the recombinant approach. Recombinant antibodies can be expressed easily in bacterial systems, including *Escherichia coli (E. coli)*, as well as in fungal and mammalian cells. In 2003, 30% of the antibodies used in clinical trials in the biopharmaceutical industry were recombinant (Hudson and Souriau 2003). Molecular biological techniques have been developed to increase antibody affinity for specific antigenic targets. The amino acid sequence of a CDR region may be altered to enhance the binding characteristics of an antibody by site-directed mutagenesis. This has permitted the use of a wide range of high-affinity antibodies in antibody-based platforms, particularly for marine targets (Campàs et al. 2007; Vilariño et al. 2010). Recombinant antibodies, generated through phage display and bio-panning against a target of interest (Bradbury and Marks 2004; Hoogenboom 2005), have been utilized for the detection of a range of structurally diverse antigens, including haptens (Byrne et al. 2009), cell surface markers (Marty et al. 2006), and proteins (Tully et al. 2008).

Antibody fragments isolated from immune libraries typically have high specificity and affinity due to the process of affinity maturation. In the process of recombinant antibody generation, the RNA is first converted into complementary DNA (cDNA), which in turn serves as a template for the amplification of variable heavy (V_H) and variable light (V_L) gene sequences. These are fused through an overlapping-extension splicing PCR reaction and subsequently cloned into a suitable phage or phagemid vector. The introduction of this construct into suppressor strains of *E. coli* by electroporation, in conjunction with the packaging of phage particles via the addition of helper phage (a process referred to as rescuing), allows the encoded antibody structure to be "presented" on the exterior of a bacteriophage particle. In the phage display technique, the scFv fragments encoded by the antibody library are expressed as fusion partners of a coat protein, pIII, on the surface of the phage (Figure 16.4).

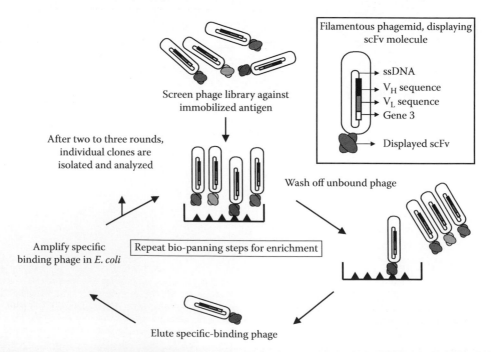

FIGURE 16.4 Recombinant antibody phage display. The illustration demonstrates how the filamentous phage particle, displaying the scFv molecule (inset), can be exploited in the process of "bio-panning". Repeated cycles of incubation, washing and re-amplification result in phage enrichment over a number of rounds.

E. coli is often chosen as the host because of its ease of use in transformation and manipulation. A number of alternative host options are also available, including mammalian, yeast, and insect (Verma et al. 1998).

A variety of recombinant antibodies were generated to MC (McElhiney et al. 2000, 2002; Strachan et al. 2002), and a summary of these antibodies is listed in Table 16.4. Anti-MC recombinant antibodies were also generated from nonimmune sources including a naïve human semisynthetic phage display library, Griffin I, and the synthetic naïve library, Tomlinson I. A major advantage of using immune libraries, over conventional naïve antibody libraries, is that the host animal immune system can refine and enhance antigen affinity and specificity. This increases the possibility of selecting higher-affinity antibodies from a recombinant antibody fragment library, due to in vivo affinity maturation (Schmitz et al. 2000; Hoogenboom 2005). Although naïve libraries are becoming increasingly popular for recombinant antibody selection, they may not have the same diversity as that of the immune system, which uses somatic hypermutation and gene rearrangement to generate large panels of diverse antibodies. Moreover, the affinity of antibodies generated from nonimmune sources is frequently low, often requiring the use of antibody engineering for improved affinity (Gram et al. 1992).

The isolation of scAbs to MC-LR, from a synthetic Tomlinson human phage library, was reported by McElhiney et al. (2000). The most sensitive antibody clone selected from the library detected MC-LR with an IC_{50} of 4 μM. The suitability of two naïve antibody libraries, the synthetic Tomlinson and the semisynthetic Griffin phage libraries for recombinant antibody generation to MC-LR, was compared by Strachan et al. (2002). The Griffin library consists of human V_H and V_L chain gene fragments, with CDR3 diversity generated using synthetic oligonucleotides. The Tomlinson library is based on a single human framework with side chain diversity incorporated at 18 amino acid positions in the antigen-binding site. Strachen et al. (2002) demonstrated that a highly sensitive recombinant scAb antibody to MC could be selected from the Griffin I library, with sensitivities that ranged from 13 to 2000 nM. It was reported that the most sensitive scAb isolated was capable of detecting MC-LR at levels below the World Health Organization limit in drinking water (1 μg/L). In addition, the antibody fragment cross-reacted with three purified MC variants (MC-RR, MC-LW, and MC-LF) and a related cyanotoxin, nodularin. The quantification of MCs in toxic samples assayed by ELISA showed good correlation with analysis by high-performance liquid chromatography (HPLC) (McElhiney et al. 2002).

16.3.4 Antibody Formats

The scFv is the most widely used recombinant antibody fragment (Table 16.1). The variable regions (V_H and V_L) of the antibody are linked by a flexible amino acid linker. The most frequently used linkers are based on glycine–serine repeat structures and can be of different lengths. With the inclusion of an *N*-terminal signal sequence, the antibody fragment can be exported to the bacterial periplasm (Tudyka and Skerra 1997). In the periplasmic space, the antibody fragment can fold correctly, remain soluble, and form intra-domain disulfide bonds, which is only possible in the oxidative environment of the periplasm. Proteins with no signal sequence are expressed in the cytoplasm and are known to form aggregates of insoluble protein or inclusion bodies, which produces a low expression yield.

Fab antibodies are heterodimer structures containing an antibody light chain and the V_H and the C_H1 domains of the heavy chain. In general, Fabs are difficult to assemble, have lower yields as soluble fragments, and are more likely to be unstable in phage, due to the fact that Fabs have two protein chains (Barbas et al. 2001). However, Fabs have a number of advantages; they do not undergo dimerization and can be converted into a full-length IgG (Guo et al. 1997). The constant regions of the Fab structure aid in the stabilization of the variable domain (Röthlisberger et al. 2005). It was shown that the Fab format is applicable to small-molecule competition immunoassays due to its reproducibility and high sensitivity. The strict monovalency of this format led to significant improvements in assay sensitivity in both ELISA and SPR assay formats (Townsend et al. 2006).

16.3.5 Immunoassay Formats

Most immunological detection platforms for low molecular weight marine toxin targets are based on a competition assay format (Marquette and Blum 2006). Competitive immunoassays usually occur in two different formats, one in which immobilized antibodies react with free antigen in competition with labeled antigen in solution or when immobilized antigens compete with free antigens for labeled antibodies in solution. In order to facilitate immobilization and antibody–antigen interactions, small molecular weight targets, including toxins, are conjugated to large molecular weight proteins, for example, bovine serum albumin (BSA), OVA, and keyhole limpet hemocyanin (KLH). Both these formats are defined as direct competitive immunoassays. In the second or "indirect" format, a second anti-species enzyme-labeled-IgG (secondary antibody) is used as a label to bind to the Fc portion of the primary antibody. This format leads to signal amplification and circumvents problems associated with antibody immobilization, including loss of affinity and incorrect antibody orientation. This technique is generally referred to as an indirect competitive immunoassay.

16.4 Immune Response Generation

16.4.1 Immunogen Preparation for Immunization

The ability of the antigen to generate an immune response depends on its immunogenicity. An antigen capable of generating a humoral or a cell-mediated immune response by itself is known as an immunogen. The immunogenicity of an antigen is conferred by distinctive molecular structural features, recognized as foreign by the host's immune system. These features act as targets for the immune response to produce large numbers of antibodies with varying specificity, whose purpose is to bind the immunogen, rendering it ineffective. However, not all antigens are immunogens. Small molecules or "haptens" are unable to stimulate an immune response unless they are coupled to a larger reactive molecule, known as a carrier (Singh et al. 2004). When an immune response is generated against a hapten–carrier molecule, the B cells will produce antibodies that are specific for both the hapten and the carrier and possibly also to chemical linkers or any combination of the three.

The first step in the successful production of an antibody to a hapten target involves the careful consideration of a number of key issues, including conjugation strategy and point of attachment, functionalization of the hapten, choice of carrier molecule, hapten–carrier ratio, and purification and characterization of the conjugate.

16.4.2 Conjugate Carriers

The most commonly used carriers are large molecules, which give haptens immunogenicity when they are coupled covalently to them. Examples of carriers include proteins, liposomes, polymers (such as dextran, agarose, and poly-L-lysine), or synthetic organic molecules (dendrimers). A good carrier molecule will have suitable immunogenicity, functional groups for conjugation, and reasonable solubility, even after derivatization (Hermanson 2008). The most common protein carriers are KLH, BSA, cationized BSA (cBSA), thyroglobulin, OVA, and toxoid protein, such as tetanus toxoid (Table 16.5). cBSA is prepared by modification of BSA's carboxylate groups with ethylene diamine. This leads to the masking of BSA's native negatively charged carboxylates, and positively charged amines are created in their place. This highly positive charge dramatically increases BSA's immunogenicity by increasing the binding to antigen-presenting cells (APCs) in vivo. cBSA conjugates get incorporated by APCs faster and generate quicker immune responses with a greater concentration of specific antibody (Muckerheide et al. 1987). Thyroglobulin and OVA are widely used as conjugate carriers for antibody characterization and screening. Table 16.5 outlines some of the most commonly used carrier proteins, along with details of their molecular weight, structural and stability properties, and some requirements for conjugation.

TABLE 16.5

Properties of Carrier Proteins

Carrier Protein	KLH	BSA and cBSA	Thyroglobulin	OVA
Molecular weight (Da)	4.5×10^5–1.3×10^7	67,000	660,000	43,000
Structure	Large, multi-subunit At physiological pH, exists in multi-subunit aggregate states	Presence of numerous carboxylate groups confers BSA with a negative charge	Large multi-subunit protein composed of several polypeptide chains	Phosphoprotein containing 1 *N*-glycosylation site and 386 amino acids
Stability	Increased immunogenicity and solubility, when dissociated into subunits Highly stable and soluble in 0.9 M NaCl Should not be frozen or freeze-thawed	Cationization significantly increases pI of protein DMSO may be added to solubilize hapten molecules Highly soluble	Acidic pI (4.7) due to presence of multiple carboxylate groups	Sensitive to temperature (above 56°C), electric fields, and vigorous shaking Extremely soluble in DMSO (70%)
Conjugation requirements	High salt concentrations required for multi-subunit KLH to preserve solubility	DMSO may be added to solubilize hapten molecules	Limited solubility DMSO may be added to solubilize hapten molecules	Care should be taken in handling to prevent denaturation and precipitation
Functional group availability (per mole)	2000 amines (lysine residues) 700 sulfhydryls (cysteine groups) 1900 tyrosines 300–600 maleimide groups (after SMCC[a] activation)	59 Lysine ε-amine groups (35 available) 1 Free cysteine sulfhydryl (17 disulfides buried in structure) 19 Tyrosine phenolate residues 17 Histidine imidazole groups	Large number of tyrosine residues Glycosylated; contains 8–10 carbohydrates	20 Lysine residues, 14 aspartic acids, 33 glutamic acid groups, 20 ε-amine groups, *N*-terminal amine, 47 side chain carboxylates, C–terminal carboxylate, 4 sulfhydryls, 10 tyrosine, 7 histidine

[a] Succinimidyl-4-(*N*-maleimidomethyl) cyclohexane-1-carboxylate.

16.4.3 Coupling Chemistry

The coupling chemistry used to prepare the immunogen is extremely important for the successful production of an antibody with the desired specificity. The conjugation process is dependent on the functional groups present primarily on the hapten and also on the carrier molecule. The most commonly used linkage involves the formation of an amide bond between a carboxylic acid moiety on the hapten and a primary amino group on the carrier. Usually, the correct functional group is not present on the hapten and needs to be introduced using a derivatization step, or alternatively, a structural analogue of the hapten can be used. As well as introducing a functional group for attachment, this step may also introduce a bridge or spacer arm between the hapten and the carrier. A spacer arm may have the advantage of reducing steric hindrance of the protein molecule on the hapten, allowing the hapten to be easily recognized by circulating lymphocytes. A disadvantage of a coupling molecule or spacer arm is the possibility of generating an antibody response to the coupling entity.

A number of coupling strategies have been employed including carbodiimide-mediated synthesis, *N*-hydroxysuccinimide (NHS) ester-mediated synthesis, and glutaraldehyde-mediated synthesis. Carbodiimides are short cross-linking agents that react with carboxylate groups for coupling with amine-containing proteins. This results in the formation of an amide or a phosphoramidate linkage between a carboxylate and an amine or a phosphate and an amine, respectively. Hapten–carrier conjugation can also be carried out using homobifunctional reagents, containing NHS ester groups at both ends. The active esters are highly reactive to amines on proteins and form stable amide linkages. Cross-linking agents of various lengths can be used in this method, including sulfo-NHS ester analogs, which are more water soluble. Glutaraldehyde is a homobifunctional cross-linking agent that can be used in a one- or two-step conjugation reaction. This reagent can react with primary amine groups to form Schiff bases or double-bond (Michael-type) addition products. Schiff bases can form resonance-stabilized products with α,β-unsaturated aldehydes of the glutaraldehyde polymers, which predominate at basic pH. The reduction of the Schiff base can yield stable secondary amine linkages (Hermanson 2008).

Another important consideration in conjugate design is that the hapten is orientated in the correct manner for proper presentation to the immune system. Landsteiner's principle determines the most suitable point of attachment to link the hapten and carrier molecules (Landsteiner 1945). This law states that antibody specificity is directly related to the portion of the hapten molecule furthest away from the point of attachment or functional group that is used to link it to the carrier. The part of the hapten closest to the point of attachment is sterically hindered by the carrier protein. Landsteiner's principle also states that the carrier protein should be attached at a site remote from the point of chemical or metabolic activity. Therefore, in carrying out hapten–carrier conjugation, consideration must be given to the reaction group chosen as the point of attachment, in addition to the number of reaction groups that are present on the hapten. This should result in the exposure of the portion of the hapten most desirable for antibody development. Pedersen et al. (2006) investigated the influence of different conjugation ratios and orientations on antibody affinity and titer to haptens. This report showed that differing types of molecular orientation influenced the antibody titer to the immunized molecule. It also appeared that a lower conjugation ratio of peptide to carrier increased the antibody affinity.

16.4.4 Purification and Characterization of Conjugates

Purification of the crude immunogen is essential for a number of reasons. Firstly, it is necessary to remove excess reagents and unreacted starting material, which may cause toxicity when injected into an animal, and carrier, which may result in an excessive carrier-only response. Purification ensures specificity of the immune response to the targeted epitope or antigenic determinant on the antigen. Secondly, it is essential for any subsequent conjugate characterization, including the determination of the carrier–hapten ratio. The most commonly used methods for purification involve initial dialysis and gel filtration chromatography, such as Sephadex® G25, which is efficient at removing noncovalently linked material based on size. If the hapten has a characteristic UV or visible absorbance spectrum that distinguishes it from the carrier protein, this property can be used to determine the degree of incorporation to the conjugate. Indirect methods can also be used if the reaction involves lysine ε-amino residues, as the extent of incorporation can be calculated by the degree of free amino groups remaining on the conjugate (Hermanson 2008). Two of the main and most widely used methods for conjugate characterization include nuclear magnetic resonance (NMR) and matrix-assisted laser desorption time-of-flight mass spectrometry (MALDI-TOF-MS) (Singh et al. 2004). These advanced techniques are capable of unequivocally demonstrating effective conjugation. MALDI-TOF-MS has the advantage of also providing quantitative information on conjugation ratios. NMR has the advantage of discriminating between covalently and noncovalently bound hapten.

16.5 Display Techniques

The development of advanced display techniques has allowed the screening of large antibody libraries, leading to the selection of antibodies with desirable traits, such as high affinity and specificity. Display techniques include bacterial (Daugherty 2007), yeast (Feldhaus and Siegel 2004; Gai and Wittrup 2007), mRNA (Gold 2001; Fukuda et al. 2006), phage (Smith 1985; McCafferty et al. 1990), and ribosomal display (Mattheakis et al. 1994). The choice of selection technology for a given antibody depends on a number of different parameters, including the diversity of the library, the properties of antigen, and the intended use. It is desirable to have combinational libraries with the maximum functional diversity to increase the possibility of finding molecules with the desired function (Benhar 2007). All major display techniques have two traits in common; they can be applied to a wide variety of cognate antigens and the selection pressure can be tailored for the application requirements.

Phage display, described by Smith (1985), was the first molecular diversity selection platform and the forerunner of all subsequent molecular diversity techniques (Figure 16.2). McCafferty et al. (1990) were the first to use phage display to isolate antibodies from a large naïve library. Phage selection involves repeated rounds of growth, bio-panning, and infection, which selects for binding of antibody fragments that are expressed on phage. Phage display is accomplished by fusing the antibody library to the *N*-terminus of either the minor coat protein (pIII) or the major coat protein (pVIII) of fila-mentous bacteriophages. Expression of these fusion proteins in bacteria results in the incorporation of the antibody fragment into the mature phage coat, which is then displayed on the phage surface. Importantly, the genetic material that relates to the antibody fragment is still contained within the phage genome. This link between antibody genotype and phenotype allows for isolation of antigen-specific phage antibodies using immobilized antigen in the selection process. Bound phage are eluted, re-infected into bacteria, and regrown for the next round of selection, resulting in enrichment of the phage pool.

Bio-panning (Figure 16.4) is used for the selection of binders from an antibody library that may contain between 10^7 and 10^{10} different antibody-encoding gene sequences. In bio-panning, the antigen is immobilized onto a solid phase (e.g., on a column or immunotube) or bead-conjugated (in solution phase), and the antibody pool is subjected to recurrent rounds of selection against the antigen with increasing levels of stringency in terms of binding ability. Selected binders are retained and subjected to additional screening to increase their specificity for the target (affinity maturation), which can be moni-tored by ELISA-based analysis.

16.6 Immunosensors for Toxins from Marine Microalgae

Biosensors have the potential to fulfill increasing demands for certification and traceability of seafood products. A biosensor is an analytical device incorporating a bio-recognition element that is associated with or integrated within a transducer that converts a biological response into an elec-trical signal. A large number of detection techniques can be incorporated into a biosensor format. The biological response can include enzymatic activity, antibody binding, receptor binding, or cell responses. Biosensor technologies include transduction platforms based on electrochemical (potentio-metric, amperometric, impedance), piezoelectric, thermal, or optical methods (reflectometric interfer-ence spectroscopy, interferometry, optical waveguide lightmode spectroscopy, total internal reflection fluorescence, surface plasmon resonance [SPR]). The sensitivity and the portability of a biosensor will depend on the signal transducer used. Recently, micro-fabrication tools have made it possible to manu-facture micro-biosensors and nano-biosensors (Pumera et al. 2007; Jaffrezic-Renault and Dzyadevych 2008). An immunosensor is a biosensor, incorporating an antibody as its biological detection element. Immunosensors can also be applied to the detection of small molecular weight toxins produced by toxic marine microalgae. A summary of electrochemical immunosensors for phycotoxin detection is presented in Table 16.6.

16.6.1 Electrochemical Immunosensors

An electrochemical biosensor was developed for the detection of a number of marine toxins with disposable screen-printed electrodes (SPEs), using a mAb to okadaic acid and polyclonal antibodies to domoic acid and saxitoxin (STX), as recognition elements (Kreuzer et al. 2002). The assay was based on the detection of *p*-aminophenol and alkaline phosphatase-labeled antibodies. *p*-Nitrophenol can be detected electrochemically at a low working potential of +300 mV, versus Ag/AgCl. The sensors all

TABLE 16.6

Electrochemical Immunosensors for the Detection of Marine Toxins

Toxin	Antibodies	LOD	References
Okadaic acid	Anti-OA monoclonal-AP; anti-BTX-AP;	1.5 µg/L	Kreuzer et al. (2002)
Brevetoxin	anti-DA sheep polyclonal; anti-sheep	1 µg/L	
Domoic acid	IgG-AP labeled	2 µg/L	
Tetrodotoxin		0.016 µg/L	
Brevetoxin	Goat polyclonal anti-PTX-glucose	15 µg/L	Carter et al. (1993)
STX	oxidase; donkey polyclonal anti-STX-glucose oxidase; rabbit anti-STX		
Okadaic acid	Monoclonal (on quartz crystal microbalance)	3.6 µg/L	Tang et al. (2002)
Okadaic acid	Monoclonal (on super paramagnetic nanobeads)	0.38 µg/L	Hayat et al. (2011)
Domoic acid	Polyclonal anti-DA; anti-goat IgG-AP labeled	5 µg/L	Micheli et al. (2004)
Domoic acid	Rabbit polyclonal; goat anti-rabbit IgG-biotin; strep-HRP conjugate	0.6 µg/L	Kania et al. (2003)
MC	Monoclonal (on silver nanoparticles)	7.0×10^{-6} µg/L	Loyprasert et al. (2008)
MC	Rabbit polyclonal (on magnetic nanoparticles)	0.6 ng/g	Ma et al. (2009)
MC	Rabbit polyclonal (SWNHs)	0.03 µg/L	Zhang et al. (2010)
MC	Monoclonal (MC10E7) and polyclonal (undisclosed source)	0.10 µg/L (mAb)/ 1.73 µg/L (pAb)	Campàs and Marty (2007)
Okadaic acid	Monoclonal: AP-labeled OA	2 µg/L	Tang et al. (2003)
Okadaic acid	Monoclonal; goat anti-mouse-HRP or AP	0.03 µg/L	Campàs et al. (2008)

achieved detection limits in the µg/L range, well within the limits of detection for each target. Micheli et al. (2004) also developed a disposable immunosensor for domoic acid, with a 5 µg/L detection limit. The assay was based on an electrochemical immunosensor, using SPEs coated with a domoic acid–BSA conjugate, as a transducer for differential pulse voltammetry (DPV). The assay format had a good percentage recovery making it suitable for accurate determination of domoic acid in real shellfish samples.

A novel electrochemical immunosensor was developed for the detection of MC, employing functionalized single-walled carbon nanohorns (SWNHs) and HRP-labeled polyclonal antibodies (Zhang et al. 2010). The numerous carboxylic acid groups on the cone-shaped tips of the SWNHs enhanced the immobilization capacity of MC-LR, resulting in an accurate, precise, and reproducible assay. The same antibodies were employed to develop a technique for the determination of MC residues in water, based on the magnetic relaxation of superparamagnetic nanoparticles, using NMR technology (Ma et al. 2009). Hayat et al. (2011) developed a competitive immunosensor, based on superparamagnetic nanobeads, for the detection of okadaic acid. Electrochemical sensing was carried out using DPV and a limit of detection of 0.38 µg/L was achieved.

Carter et al. (1993) described one of the first amperometric immunosensors for the detection of STX and brevetoxin. The biosensor utilized solid support membranes for the immobilization of toxin conjugates. The detection was based on a glucose oxidase-labeled antibody in a competitive format with immobilized and free toxin. The glucose oxidase label caused the conversion of a β-D-glucose substrate to its product with the release of H_2O_2, which was detected using a platinum electrode. The limit of detection for this assay format was 15 µg/L. Campàs and Marty (2007) utilized both anti-MC monoclonal and polyclonal antibodies to develop a competitive ELISA (cELISA) on screen-printed graphite electrodes. Tang et al. (2003) also produced a disposable immunosensor based on SPEs for okadaic acid with a commercial mAb, with a 2 ng/mL detection limit.

16.6.2 Optical Immunosensors

Optics-based immunosensors for toxin detection, particularly those that incorporate SPR, are widely used (Table 16.7). Kreuzer et al. (1999) developed a highly sensitive, optical immunosensor for okadaic acid using commercial murine monoclonal antibodies. They discovered that changing from a competitive to a displacement ELISA format affected the selectivity of the assay for okadaic acid and dinophysis-1. This work highlighted the importance of assay format on overall specificity. A semi-automated membrane-based chemiluminescent biosensor was also developed for the detection of okadaic acid in mussels by Marquette et al. (1999). An okadaic acid–BSA conjugate was immobilized onto a pre-activated membrane connected to a fiber-optic-based chemiluminescent flow injection configuration. The membranes minimized nonspecific protein adsorption and showed good regeneration potential. Anti-okadaic acid monoclonal antibodies were mixed with spiked samples and antibody binding onto the membrane was monitored. The combination of the membranes and sensitive chemiluminescent detection resulted in a high sensitivity of 0.1 ng/mL in spiked mussel extracts.

SPR has become a widely used technique, because "real-time" and "label-free" assays can be performed in complex matrices without the need for sample cleanup. SPR has been successfully employed to detect small molecules and haptens in a multitude of food and environmental samples (Dostálek and Homola 2006; Shankaran et al. 2007). A number of SPR immunosensors have recently been described for MC in drinking water (Herranz et al. 2010). In one such method, a competitive inhibition format was used, in which MC-LR was immobilized onto an SPR chip functionalized with a self-assembled monolayer (SAM). In this format, the assay gave an IC_{50} of 0.67 μM and cross-reacted with MC-RR and MC-YR. A SPR inhibition immunoassay was also developed using a mAb to MC with a Biacore™ 3000 biosensor (Hu et al. 2009). In this assay, an MC-BSA conjugate was immobilized onto a CM5 chip surface and inhibition occurred with MC-LR in solution. The assay was sensitive in the 1–100 μM range. Additionally, a rapid SPR immunobiosensor assay was developed for the detection of MC in blue-green algae food supplements (Vinogradova et al. 2011). The biosensor results were in good agreement with an established LC-MS/MS assay. The assay was advantageous because it employed a simple cleanup procedure and compared favorably to chemical assays in terms of sensitivity and specificity. Alternative biosensor techniques developed for MC detection include molecular-imprinted polymer (MIP) sensors (Chianella et al. 2002), electrochemical immunosensors (Campàs et al. 2005; Campàs and Marty 2007; Loyprasert et al. 2008), and evanescent wave immunosensors (Long et al. 2008, 2009).

A number of SPR-based methods for PSP toxins were developed. The aim of this research was to develop methods that could detect STX below the regulatory limit. Additionally, it aimed to assess if these SPR-based methods were comparable to the mouse bioassay and current HPLC techniques for PSP detection. Cross-reactivity to PST congeners was also evaluated (Campbell et al. 2007; Fonfria et al.

TABLE 16.7

Optical Immunosensors for the Detection of Marine Toxins

Toxin	Competition Format	Antibodies	LOD (μg/L)	References
Okadaic acid	Direct	Monoclonal-AP; OA-AP	5×10^{-4}–4	Kreuzer et al. (1999)
Okadaic acid	Direct	Monoclonal-HRP	0.1	Marquette et al. (1999)
Domoic acid	Indirect	Monoclonal	1.8	Lotierzo et al. (2004)
Domoic acid	Indirect	Monoclonal	0.1	Yu et al. (2005)
Domoic acid	Indirect	Rabbit polyclonal	3.0	Stevens et al. (2007)
MC	Direct	Monoclonal; Cy5-labeled	0.03	Long et al. (2009)
STX	Direct	Donkey polyclonal	0.5	Yakes et al. (2011)

2007). In these SPR studies, an anti-GTX2/3 mAb detected STX and its congeners below the required regulatory limit. In addition, Campbell et al. (2007) also employed a rabbit pAb raised to STX, along with an STX-binding sodium channel receptor. Haughey et al. (2011) also compared the same polyclonal and monoclonal antibodies using two SPR instruments: a Biacore Q biosensor and a Biacore T100. A novel approach was used for the detection of STX by Chen et al. (2007). This group employed SAMs of a calix[4]arene derivative to sensitively detect STX, using SPR. STX, a bis-guanidinium structure, binds calix[4]arene based on its guanidinium ion selectivity. In addition, Yakes et al. (2011) developed an improved SPR immunoassay for STX detection, by optimization of a sensor chip surface chemistry, antibody–analyte mixing ratios, and incubation times.

SPR was also applied to the detection of domoic acid by Yu et al. (2005). In this biosensor format, the toxin was linked covalently to a mixed SAM-modified chip. The assay used a competition format between free domoic acid in solution and anti-domoic acid monoclonal antibodies. They achieved a detection limit of 0.1 ng/mL, which was superior to that of a conventional colorimetric ELISA. This improvement was due to the lack of nonspecific antibody adsorption on the SAM and the high sensitivity of the SPR instrument. Le Berre and Kane (2006) developed SPR assays for the detection of domoic acid, using polyclonal, monoclonal, and recombinant antibodies. Interestingly, they demonstrated that a pAb demonstrated the best sensitivity for domoic acid analysis. A sensitive toxin inhibition SPR assay was also developed, using a mAb, which detected MC-LR below the regulatory limit of 1 μg/L (Hu et al. 2009). In addition, monoclonal antibodies were also employed to detect MC-LR in Spirulina and *Aphanizomenon flos-aquae* blue-green algae food supplements, using SPR (Vinogradova et al. 2011).

16.6.3 Commercial Kits

MC antibodies have been incorporated into an immuno-protein phosphatase inhibition assay (Metcalf et al. 2001), immunoaffinity chromatography (McElhiney et al. 2002; Aranda-Rodriguez et al. 2003), and a lateral flow "dipstick"-style assay (Kim et al. 2003). A number of commercial kits for marine toxin analysis have also become available in an ELISA format. Two commercially available ELISA kits for MC detection using polyclonal antibodies were produced by Abraxis LLC (United Kingdom) and Envirologix (United Kingdom). Both the Abraxis and Envirologix QualiTube demonstrated good sensitivity and cross-reactivity to MC congeners. The Abraxis immunoassay is based on the Adda-specific antibodies of Fischer et al. (2001). The Adda moiety is common to most MCs and nodularins. Therefore, this assay can be described as congener independent. Additionally, a mAb generated against 4-R-MCs is also commercially available (Alexis Biochemicals, United Kingdom).

Such kits have proven useful for screening water and cyanobacterial samples, but they have poor cross-reactivity to toxin variants (Rapala et al. 2002). The issue of cross-reactivity to all STX congeners has posed a problem for most PSP immunoassay kits. The RIDASCREEN STX assay (R-BioPharm, Germany) is designed for testing in a shellfish matrix. The assay displays a good sensitivity profile, with an LOD of 0.02 μg/L. In a comparative study with HPLC methods for the determination of STX in mussels, the RIDASCREEN overestimated STX concentration but underestimated total PSP content compared with the mouse bioassay (Usleber et al. 1997).

A widely used rapid detection system for PSP immuno-detection is the Jellett MIST Alert lateral flow immunochromatographic strips (Jellett, Canada). The test is based on competition for binding to labeled anti-STX antibodies between PSP toxins in the sample and the test line in the device. The assay has been compared to alternative methods of PSP detection including the mouse bioassay, HPLC, and a receptor binding assay by a number of research groups (Costa et al. 2009; Laycock et al. 2010). An anti-domoic acid pAb was incorporated into a sensitive cELISA method (Osada et al. 1995) and commercialized as a high-throughput method for analyzing shellfish samples (Biosense, Norway). Kleivdal et al. (2007) compared this cELISA method to the liquid chromatography reference method for domoic acid determination. Despite some overestimation of toxin content, the study showed that the ELISA method was suitable for routine determination of domoic acid toxins in shellfish.

Several diagnostics kits for MC detection are now currently available (Abraxis, United States; Wako Chemicals, Japan; EnviroLogix, United States). The kits have proven to be successful in screening water samples, as well as cyanobacterial samples. Due to the high structural variability of MC, their cross-reactivity profiles are frequently lacking, and they do not correlate well with toxicity (Rivasseau et al. 1999; Rapala et al. 2002). However, good assay sensitivity has ensured that no time-consuming sample preparation steps are necessary. Therefore, the success of an ELISA technique for cyanobacterial toxins, such as MC, in routine screening will depend on the antibodies' ability to recognize all toxin variants that are present.

16.7 Conclusions

Increased awareness has led to the development of a diverse range of sensor techniques for phycotoxin and hepatotoxin monitoring. Immunosensors have many advantages including low cost, ease of use, speed, less requirement for highly trained personnel, capacity for automation, reproducibility, robustness, sensitivity, and portability. Unfortunately, very few antibody-based sensors for phycotoxins have been approved as regulatory methods. This is due in part to the scarcity of sufficient quantities of pure toxin for the development of antitoxin antibodies and assay validation (Hirama 2005). Also, a poor supply of reference materials and cross-reactivities with non-target molecules pose significant problems. To reduce the risk to human health of exposure to marine biotoxins, there is a requirement for more sensitive and reliable detection methods.

An important aspect for immuno-detection of marine algal toxins is the structural similarity between toxin congeners; therefore, care must be taken to characterize the toxin antibody for cross-reactivity to structurally similar molecules of the same phycotoxin grouping. If a mixture of toxin congeners is analyzed in an immunosensor format, the underestimation or overestimation of toxicity may occur, due to the inability of the antibody to recognize one or multiple isomers of the toxin molecule. Ideally, biosensors for marine toxins should also be capable of detecting mixtures of toxins in complex matrices, such as shellfish meat. The described biosensor formats for marine toxins were all created in an attempt to replace the current regulated methods of detection, including the mouse bioassay, and physiochemical analysis, including HPLC-MS. However, it remains to be seen whether they will be incorporated into legislation or routine monitoring programs in the future.

The enormous advancements in the immune-sensing field have been paralleled by the ever-increasing complexity of toxin panels found in environmental samples. Ideally, analytical measurements that would allow accurate estimates of the overall toxicity of multiple classes of toxins in a single sample would provide a high standard of consumer protection. This approach would considerably strengthen the arsenal of tools available for monitoring the risks posed by marine toxin contamination events.

ACKNOWLEDGMENTS

This material is based upon works supported by the Beaufort Research Initiative, the PharmAtlantic EU consortium, and the Science Foundation Ireland under Grant No. 10/CE/B1821.

ABBREVIATIONS

Adda	((2S,3S,8S,9S)-3-Amino-9-methoxy-2,6,8-trimethyl-10-phenyldeca-4,6-dienoic)
APC	Antigen-presenting cell
BSA	Bovine serum albumin
cDNA	Complementary DNA
CDRs	Complementary determining regions
$C_H^1 - C_H^3$	Constant heavy region of antibody chain 1–3

CL	Constant light region of antibody chain
DVP	Differential voltage probe
E. coli	*Escherichia coli*
ELISA	Enzyme-linked immunosorbent assay
Fab	Fragment antigen-binding region of antibody
Fc	Fragment-crystallizable region of antibody
Ff	Filamentous
HPLC	High-performance liquid chromatography
IC_{50}	Half maximal inhibitory concentration
Ig	Immunoglobulin
IgG	Immunoglobulin G
KLH	Keyhole limpet hemocyanin
LC-MS	Liquid chromatography–mass spectrometry
mAb	Monoclonal antibody
MALDI-TOF	Matrix-assisted laser desorption time-of-flight mass spectrometry
MC	Microcystin
MHC	Major histocompatibility complex
MIP	Molecularly imprinted polymer
NHS	*N*-Hydroxysuccinimide
NMR	Nuclear magnetic resonance
OVA	Ovalbumin
pAb	Polyclonal antibody
PCR	Polymerase chain reaction
PEG	Polyethylene glycol
PPIA	Protein phosphatase inhibition assay
RNA	Ribonucleic acid
SAM	Self-assembled monolayer
scAb	Single-chain antibody fragment
scFv	Single-chain variable fragment of antibody
SPE	Solid-phase extraction
SPR	Surface plasmon resonance
STX	Saxitoxin
TH	Helper T cells
UV	Ultraviolet
VH	Variable heavy
VL	Variable light
κ	Kappa
λ	Lambda

REFERENCES

Amine, A., Mohammadi, H., Bourais, I., and Palleschi, G. 2006. Enzyme inhibition-based biosensors for food safety and environmental monitoring. *Biosens. Bioelectron.* 8: 1405–1423.

Aranda-Rodriguez, R., Kubwabo, C., and Benoit, F.M. 2003. Extraction of 15 microcystins and nodularin using immunoaffinity columns. *Toxicon* 6: 587–599.

Baeumner, A.J. 2003. Biosensors for environmental pollutants and food contaminants. *Anal. Bioanal. Chem.* 3: 434–445.

Baier, W., Loleit, M., Fischer, B. et al. 2000. Generation of antibodies directed against the low-immunogenic peptide-toxins microcystin-LR/RR and nodularin. *Int. J. Immunopharmacol.* 5: 339–353.

Barbas, C.F. 3rd., Burton, D.R., Scott, J.K., and Silverman, G.J. 2001. *Phage Display: A Laboratory Manual*, 1st edn., Cold Spring Harbor Laboratory Press, New York.

Benhar, I. 2007. Design of synthetic antibody libraries. *Exp. Opin. Biol. Ther.* 5: 763–779.

Bradbury, A.R. and Marks, J.D. 2004. Antibodies from phage antibody libraries. *J. Immunol. Methods* 290(1–2): 29–49.

Byrne, B., Stack, E., Gilmartin, N., and O'Kennedy, R. 2009. Antibody-based sensors: Principles, problems and potential for detection of pathogens and associated toxins. *Sensors* 6: 4407–4445.

Campàs, M., de la Iglesia, P., Le Berre, M. et al. 2008. Enzymatic recycling-based amperometric immunosensor for the ultrasensitive detection of okadaic acid in shellfish. *Biosens. Bioelectron.* 24: 716–722.

Campàs, M. and Marty, J. 2007. Highly sensitive amperometric immunosensors for microcystin detection in algae. *Biosens. Bioelectron.* 22(6): 1034–1040.

Campàs, M., Prieto-Simón, B., and Marty, J.L. 2007. Biosensors to detect marine toxins: Assessing seafood safety. *Talanta* 72: 884–895.

Campàs, M., Szydlowska, D., Trojanowicz, M., and Marty, J. 2005. Towards the protein phosphatase-based biosensor for microcystin detection. *Biosens. Bioelectron.* 8: 1520–1530.

Campbell, K., Stewart, L.D., Fodey, T.L. et al. 2007. Assessment of specific binding proteins suitable for the detection of paralytic shellfish poisons using optical biosensor technology. *Anal. Chem.* 79: 5906–5914.

Carter, R.M., Poli, M.A., Pesavento, M. et al. 1993. Immunoelectrochemical biosensors for detection of saxitoxin and brevetoxin. *Immunomethods* 2: 128–133.

Chen, H., Kim, Y.S., Keum, S. et al. 2007. Surface plasmon spectroscopic detection of saxitoxin. *Sensors* 7: 1216–1223.

Chianella, I., Lotierzo, M., Piletsky, S.A. et al. 2002. Rational design of a polymer specific for microcystin-LR using a computational approach. *Anal. Chem.* 6: 1288–1293.

Chu, F.S., Huang, X., Wei, R.D., and Carmichael, W.W. 1989. Production and characterization of antibodies against microcystins. *Appl. Environ. Microbiol.* 8: 1928–1933.

Costa, P.R., Baugh, K.A., Wright, B. et al. 2009. Comparative determination of paralytic shellfish toxins (PSTs) using five different toxin detection methods in shellfish species collected in the Aleutian Islands, Alaska. *Toxicon* 54: 313–320.

Daugherty, P.S. 2007. Protein engineering with bacterial display. *Curr. Opin. Struct. Biol.* 4: 474–480.

Dostálek, J. and Homola, J. 2006. SPR biosensors for environmental monitoring. In *Surface Plasmon Resonance Based Sensors*, 1st edn., ed., Homola, J., Springer-Verlag, Berlin, Germany, p. 251.

Feldhaus, M.J. and Siegel, R.W. 2004. Yeast display of antibody fragments: A discovery and characterization platform. *J. Immunol. Methods* 1–2: 69–80.

Fischer, W.J., Garthwaite, I., Miles, C.O. et al. 2001. Congener-independent immunoassay for microcystins and nodularins. *Environ. Sci. Technol.* 24: 4849–4856.

Fonfria, E.S., Vilariño, N., Campbell, K. et al. 2007. Paralytic shellfish poisoning detection by surface plasmon resonance-based biosensors in shellfish matrixes. *Anal. Chem.* 16: 6303–6311.

Fraga, M., Vilariño, N.M., Louzao, C. et al. 2012. Detection of paralytic shellfish toxins by a solid-phase inhibition immunoassay using a microsphere-flow cytometry system. *Anal. Chem.* 84: 4350–4356.

Fukuda, I., Kojoh, K., Tabata, N. et al. 2006. In vitro evolution of single-chain antibodies using mRNA display. *Nucleic Acids Res.* 19: 127.

Gai, S.A. and Wittrup, K.D. 2007. Yeast surface display for protein engineering and characterization. *Curr. Opin. Struct. Biol.* 4: 467–473.

Gold, L. 2001. mRNA display: Diversity matters during in vitro selection. *Proc. Natl. Acad. Sci. U.S.A.* 9: 4825–4826.

Gram, H., Marconi, L.A., Barbas, C.F. 3rd. et al. 1992. In vitro selection and affinity maturation of antibodies from a naive combinatorial immunoglobulin library. *Proc. Natl. Acad. Sci. U.S.A.* 89: 3576–3580.

Guo, J., Jaume, J.C., Rapoport, B., and McLachlan, S.M. 1997. Recombinant thyroid peroxidase-specific Fab converted to immunoglobulin G (IgG) molecules: Evidence for thyroid cell damage by IgG1, but not IgG4, autoantibodies. *J. Clin. Endocrinol. Metab.* 3: 925–931.

Haughey, S.A., Campbell, K., Yakes, B.J. et al. 2011. Comparison of biosensor platforms for surface plasmon resonance based detection of paralytic shellfish toxins. *Talanta* 85: 519–526.

Hayat, A., Barthelmebs, L., and Marty, J.L. 2011. Enzyme-linked immunosensor based on super paramagnetic nanobeads for easy and rapid detection of okadaic acid. *Anal. Chim. Acta* 2: 248–252.

Hermanson, G.T. 2008. Preparation of hapten–carrier immunogen conjugates. *In Bioconjugate Techniques*, 2nd edn., ed., Hermanson, G.T., Academic Press, New York, pp. 743–782.

Herranz, S., Bocková, M., Marazuela, M. et al. 2010. An SPR biosensor for the detection of microcystins in drinking water. *Anal. Bioanal. Chem.* 398: 2652–2634.

Hirama, M. 2005. Total synthesis of ciguatoxin CTX3C: A venture into the problems of ciguatera seafood poisoning. *Chem. Rec.* 5: 240–250.

Hoogenboom, H.R. 2005. Selecting and screening recombinant antibody libraries. *Nat. Biotechnol.* 9: 1105–1116.

Hu, C., Gan, N., Chen, Y. et al. 2009. Detection of microcystins in environmental samples using surface plasmon resonance biosensor. *Talanta* 1: 407–410.

Hudson, P.J. and Souriau, C. 2003. Engineered antibodies. *Nat. Med.* 9: 129–134.

Ivnitski, D., Abdel-Hamid, I., Atanasov, P., and Wilkins, E. 1999. Biosensors for detection of pathogenic bacteria. *Biosens. Bioelectron.* 7: 599–624.

Jaffrezic-Renault, N. and Dzyadevych, S.V. 2008. Conductometric microbiosensors for environmental monitoring. *Sensors* 4: 2569–2588.

Kania, M., Kreuzer, M., Moore, E. et al. 2003. Development of polyclonal antibodies against domoic acid for their use in electrochemical biosensors. *Anal. Lett.* 36: 1851–1863.

Kfir, R., Johannsen, E., and Botes, D.P. 1986. Monoclonal antibody specific for cyanoginosin-LA: Preparation and characterization. *Toxicon* 6: 543–552.

Khreich, N., Lamourette, P., Renard, P. et al. 2009. A highly sensitive competitive enzyme immunoassay of broad specificity quantifying microcystins and nodularins in water samples. *Toxicon* 5: 551–559.

Kim, Y.M., Oh, S.W., Jeong, S.Y. et al. 2003. Development of an ultrarapid one-step fluorescence immunochromatographic assay system for the quantification of microcystins. *Environ. Sci. Technol.* 9: 1899–1904.

Kleivdal, H., Kristiansen, S.I., Nilsen, M.V. et al. 2007. Determination of domoic acid toxins in shellfish by biosense ASP ELISA—A direct competitive enzyme-linked immunosorbent assay: Collaborative study. *J AOAC Int.* 90: 1011–1027.

Kondo, F., Ito, Y., Oka, H. et al. 2002. Determination of microcystins in lake water using reusable immunoaffinity column. *Toxicon* 40: 893–899.

Kreuzer, M.P., O'Sullivan, C.K., and Guilbault, G.G. 1999. Development of an ultrasensitive immunoassay for rapid measurement of okadaic acid and its isomers. *Anal. Chem.* 19: 4198–4202.

Kreuzer, M.P., Pravda, M., O'Sullivan, C.K., and Guilbault, G.G. 2002. Novel electrochemical immunosensors for seafood toxin analysis. *Toxicon* 40: 1267–1274.

Landsteiner, K. 1945. *The Specificity of Serological Reactions*, 1st edn., Harvard University Press, Cambridge, MA, p. 156.

Laycock, M.V., Donovan, M.A., and Easy, D.J. 2010. Sensitivity of lateral flow tests to mixtures of saxitoxins and applications to shellfish and phytoplankton monitoring. *Toxicon* 55: 597–605.

Le Berre, M. and Kane, M. 2006. Biosensor-based assay for domoic acid: Comparison of performance using polyclonal, monoclonal, and recombinant antibodies. *Anal. Lett.* 8: 1587–1598.

LeBien, T.W. and Tedder, T.F. 2008. B lymphocytes: How they develop and function. *Blood* 112: 1570–1580.

Leenaars, M. and Hendriksen, C.F. 2005. Critical steps in the production of polyclonal and monoclonal antibodies: Evaluation and recommendations. *ILAR J.* 46: 269–279.

Lindner, P., Molz, R., Yacoub-George, E. et al. 2004. Development of a highly sensitive inhibition immunoassay for microcystin-LR. *Anal. Chim. Acta* 1: 37–44.

Long, F., He, M., Shi, H.C., and Zhu, A.N. 2008. Development of evanescent wave all-fiber immunosensor for environmental water analysis. *Biosens. Bioelectron.* 7: 952–958.

Long, F., He, M., Zhu, A.N., and Shi, H.C. 2009. Portable optical immunosensor for highly sensitive detection of microcystin-LR in water samples. *Biosens. Bioelectron.* 8: 2346–2351.

Lotierzo, M., Henry, O.Y., Piletsky, S. et al. 2004. Surface plasmon resonance sensor for domoic acid based on grafted imprinted polymer. *Biosens. Bioelectron.* 20: 145–152.

Loyprasert, S., Thavarungkul, P., Asawatreratanakul, P. et al. 2008. Label-free capacitive immunosensor for microcystin-LR using self-assembled thiourea monolayer incorporated with Ag nanoparticles on gold electrode. *Biosens. Bioelectron.* 24(1): 78–86.

Ma, W., Chen, W., Qiao, R. et al. 2009. Rapid and sensitive detection of microcystin by immunosensor based on nuclear magnetic resonance. *Biosens. Bioelectron.* 1: 240–243.

Marquette, C.A. and Blum, L.J. 2006. State of the art and recent advances in immunoanalytical systems. *Biosens. Bioelectron.* 21: 1424–1433.

Marquette, C.A., Coulet, P.R., and Blum, L.J. 1999. Semi-automated membrane based chemiluminescent immunosensor for flow injection analysis of okadaic acid in mussels. *Anal. Chim. Acta* 398: 173–182.

Marty, C., Langer-Machova, Z., Sigrist, S. et al. 2006. Isolation and characterization of a scFv antibody specific for tumor endothelial marker 1 (TEM1), a new reagent for targeted tumor therapy. *Cancer Lett.* 2: 298–308.

Mattheakis, L.C., Bhatt, R.R., and Dower, W.J. 1994. An in vitro polysome display system for identifying ligands from very large peptide libraries. *Proc. Natl. Acad. Sci. USA* 91: 9022–9026.

McCafferty, J., Griffiths, A.D., Winter, G., and Chiswell, D.J. 1990. Phage antibodies: Filamentous phage displaying antibody variable domains. *Nature (London)* 6301: 552–554.

McElhiney, J., Drever, M., Lawton, L.A., and Porter, A.J. 2002. Rapid isolation of a single-chain antibody against the cyanobacterial toxin microcystin-LR by phage display and its use in the immunoaffinity concentration of microcystins from water. *Appl. Environ. Microbiol.* 11: 5288–5295.

McElhiney, J., Lawton, L.A., and Porter, A.J. 2000. Detection and quantification of microcystins (cyanobacterial hepatotoxins) with recombinant antibody fragments isolated from a naïve human phage display library. *FEMS Microbiol. Lett.* 1: 83–88.

Metcalf, J.S., Bell, S.G., and Codd, G.A. 2000. Production of novel polyclonal antibodies against the cyanobacterial toxin microcystin-LR and their application for the detection and quantification of microcystins and nodularin. *Water Res.* 10: 2761–2769.

Metcalf, J.S., Bell, S.G., and Codd, G.A. 2001. Colorimetric immuno-protein phosphatase inhibition assay for specific detection of microcystins and nodularins of cyanobacteria. *Appl. Environ. Microbiol.* 2: 904–909.

Mhadhbi, H., Ben-Rejeb, S., Cléroux, C. et al. 2006. Generation and characterization of polyclonal antibodies against microcystins-application to immunoassays and immunoaffinity sample preparation prior to analysis by liquid chromatography and UV detection. *Talanta* 2: 225–235.

Micheli, L., Radoi, A., Guarrina, R. et al. 2004. Disposable immunosensor for the determination of domoic acid in shellfish. *Biosens. Bioelectron.* 20: 190–196.

Mikhailov, A., Härmälä-Braskén, A., Meriluoto, J. et al. 2001. Production and specificity of mono and polyclonal antibodies against microcystins conjugated through *N*-methyldehydroalanine. *Toxicon* 4: 477–483.

Muckerheide, A., Apple, R.J., Pesce, A.J., and Michael, J.G. 1987. Cationization of protein antigens. I. Alteration of immunogenic properties. *J. Immunol.* 3: 833–837.

Murphy, M., Jason-Moller, L., and Bruno, J. 2006. Using Biacore to measure the binding kinetics of an antibody–antigen interaction. *Curr. Protoc. Protein Sci.* 19: 14.

Nagata, S., Soutome, H., Tsutsumi, T. et al. 1995. Novel monoclonal antibodies against microcystin and their protective activity for hepatotoxicity. *Nat. Toxins* 2: 78–86.

Nagata, S., Tsutsumi, T., Yoshida, F., and Ueno, Y. 1999. A new type sandwich immunoassay for microcystin: Production of monoclonal antibodies specific to the immune complex formed by microcystin and an anti-microcystin monoclonal antibody. *Nat. Toxins* 2: 49–55.

Osada, M., Marks, L.J., and Stewart, J.E. 1995. Determination of domoic acid by two different versions of a competitive enzyme-linked immunosorbent assay (ELISA). *Bull. Environ. Contam. Toxicol.* 54: 797–804.

Pedersen, M.K., Sorensen, N.S., Heegaard, P.M.H. et al. 2006. Effect of different hapten–carrier conjugation ratios and molecular orientations on antibody affinity against a peptide antigen. *J. Immunol. Methods* 1–2: 198–206.

Pumera, M., Sánchez, S., Ichinose, I., and Tang, J. 2007. Electrochemical nanobiosensors. *Sens. Actuators B: Chem.* 2: 1195–1205.

Rapala, J., Erkomaa, K., Kukkonen, J. et al. 2002. Detection of microcystins with protein phosphatase inhibition assay, high-performance liquid chromatography–UV detection and enzyme-linked immunosorbent assay: Comparison of methods. *Anal. Chim. Acta* 466: 213–231.

Rivasseau, C., Racaud, P., Deguin, A., and Hennion M. 1999. Evaluation of an ELISA kit for the monitoring of microcystins (cyanobacterial toxins) in water and algae environmental samples. *Environ. Sci. Technol.* 33: 1520–1527.

Rodriguez-Mozaz, S., Lopez de Alda, M.J., and Barceló, D. 2006. Biosensors as useful tools for environmental analysis and monitoring. *Anal. Bioanal. Chem.* 4: 1025–1041.

Röthlisberger, D., Honegger, A., and Plückthun, A. 2005. Domain interactions in the Fab fragment: A comparative evaluation of the single-chain Fv and Fab format engineered with variable domains of different stability. *J. Mol. Biol.* 347: 773–789.

Schmitz, U., Versmold, A., Kaufmann, P., and Frank, H. 2000. Phage display: A molecular tool for the generation of antibodies—A review. *Placenta* 1: S106–S112.

Scott, C. and Potter, M. 1983. Diversity of immunoglobulin structural gene loci. *Immunol. Res.* 2: 43–51.

Shankaran, D.R., Gobi, K.V., and Miura, N. 2007. Recent advancements in surface plasmon resonance immunosensors for detection of small molecules of biomedical, food and environmental interest. *Sens. Actuators B: Chem.* 1: 158–177.

Sheng, J., He, M., and Shi, H.C. 2007. A highly specific immunoassay for microcystin-LR detection based on a monoclonal antibody. *Anal. Chim. Acta* 1: 111–118.

Sheng, J.W., He, M., Shi, H.C., and Qian, Y. 2006. A comprehensive immunoassay for the detection of microcystins in waters based on polyclonal antibodies. *Anal. Chim. Acta* 2: 309–315.

Singh, K.V., Kaur, J., Varshney, G.C. et al. 2004. Synthesis and characterization of hapten-protein conjugates for antibody production against small molecules. *Bioconjug. Chem.* 1: 168–173.

Smith, G.P. 1985. Filamentous fusior phage: Novel expression vectors that display cloned antigens on the virion surface. *Science* 228: 1315–1317.

Stevens, R.C., Soelberg, S.D., Eberhart, B.L. et al. 2007. Detection of the toxin domoic acid from clam extracts using a portable surface plasmon resonance biosensor. *Harmful Algae* 6: 166–174.

Strachan, G., McElhiney, J., Drever, M.R. et al. 2002. Rapid selection of anti-hapten antibodies isolated from synthetic and semi-synthetic antibody phage display libraries expressed in *Escherichia coli*. *FEMS Microbiol. Lett.* 2: 257–261.

Tang, A.X.J., Kreuzer, M., Lehane, M. et al. 2003. Semi-automated membrane based chemiluminescent immunosensor for flow injection analysis of okadaic acid in mussels. *Int. J. Environ. Anal. Chem.* 83: 663–670.

Tang, A.X.J., Pravda, M., Guilbault, G.G. et al. 2002. Immunosensor for okadaic acid using quartz crystal microbalance. *Anal. Chim. Acta* 471: 33–40.

Townsend, S., Finlay, W.J., Hearty, S., and O'Kennedy, R. 2006. Optimizing recombinant antibody function in SPR immunosensing. The influence of antibody structural format and chip surface chemistry on assay sensitivity. *Biosens. Bioelectron.* 22: 268–274.

Tsutsumi, T., Nagata, S., Hasegawa, A., and Ueno, Y. 2000. Immunoaffinity column as clean-up tool for determination of trace amounts of microcystins in tap water. *Food Chem. Toxicol.* 38: 593–597.

Tudyka, T. and Skerra, A. 1997. Glutathione S-transferase can be used as a C-terminal, enzymatically active dimerization module for a recombinant protease inhibitor, and functionally secreted into the periplasm of *Escherichia coli*. *Protein Sci.* 10: 2180–2187.

Tully, E., Higson, S.P., and O'Kennedy, R. 2008. The development of a 'labeless' immunosensor for the detection of *Listeria monocytogenes* cell surface protein, Internalin B. *Biosens. Bioelectron.* 6: 906–912.

Usleber, E., Donald, M., Straka, M., and Märtlbauer, E. 1997. Comparison of enzyme immunoassay and mouse bioassay for determining paralytic shellfish poisoning toxins in shellfish. *Food Addit. Contam.* 14: 193–198.

Van Dorst, B., Mehta, J., Bekaert, K. et al. 2010. Recent advances in recognition elements of food and environmental biosensors: A review. *Biosens. Bioelectron.* 4: 1178–1194.

Verma, R., Boleti, E., and George, A.J.T. 1998. Antibody engineering: Comparison of bacterial, yeast, insect and mammalian expression systems. *J. Immunol. Methods* 216(1–2): 165–181.

Vilariño, N., Louzao, M.C., Vieytes, M.R., and Botana, L.M. 2010. Biological methods for marine toxin detection. *Anal. Bioanal. Chem.* 397: 1673–1681.

Vinogradova, T., Danaher, M., Baxter, A. et al. 2011. Rapid surface plasmon resonance immunobiosensor assay for microcystin toxins in blue-green algae food supplements. *Talanta* 3: 638–643.

Weller, M.G., Zeck, A., Eikenberg, A. et al. 2001. Development of a direct competitive microcystin immunoassay of broad specificity. *Anal. Sci.* 12: 1445–1448.

Yakes, B.J., Prezioso, S., Haughey, S.A. et al. 2011. An improved immunoassay for detection of saxitoxin by surface plasmon resonance biosensors. *Sens. Actuators B: Chem.* 2: 805–811.

Young, F.M., Metcalf, J.S., Meriluoto, J.A.O. et al. 2006. Production of antibodies against microcystin-RR for the assessment of purified microcystins and cyanobacterial environmental samples. *Toxicon* 3: 295–306.

Yu, Q., Chen, S., Taylor, A.D. et al. 2005. Detection of low-molecular-weight domoic acid using surface plasmon resonance sensor. *Sens. Actuators B: Chem.* 1: 193–201.

Zeck, A., Weller, M.G., Bursill, D., and Niessner, R. 2001. Generic microcystin immunoassay based on mono-clonal antibodies against Adda. *Analyst* 11: 2002–2007.

Zhang, B., Hou, L., Tang, D. et al. 2012. Simultaneous multiplexed stripping voltammetric monitoring of marine toxins in seafood based on distinguishable metal nanocluster-labeled molecular tags. *J. Agric. Food Chem.* 60: 8974–8982.

Zhang, J., Lei, J., Xu, C. et al. 2010. Carbon nanohorn sensitized electrochemical immunosensor for rapid detection of microcystin-LR. *Anal. Chem.* 3: 1117–1122.

17

Toxic Phytoplankton Detection

Alberto Otero, María-José Chapela, Paula Fajardo, Alejandro Garrido, and Ana G. Cabado

CONTENTS

17.1 Introduction

Phytoplankton, in the marine ecosystems, is composed of major primary producers, but also harmful algae that can negatively influence marine environment. There are around 5000 referenced microscopic algae, including marine and freshwater photosynthetic unicellular organisms, but only 2% (about 100 species) are able to produce toxins that can kill marine mammals, birds, and humans.[1] Toxins are secondary metabolites but their metabolic or ecological role is not well defined yet. A significant increase in the toxic phytoplankton is usually referred to as harmful algae blooms (HABs) that induce a negative impact on the ecosystem. High biomass HABs are caused by exotoxin-producing planktonic microalgae that excrete compounds that, above a threshold concentration, kill fish and benthic organisms. In contrast, there are toxigenic HAB species that, even at low-cell densities, produce endotoxins that are transferred through the food web, mainly through filter-feeding bivalves, to human beings. This kind of HABs or toxic episodes constitutes a major threat to public health and shellfish aquaculture.[2]

Many of the management actions taken to respond to HABs can be termed mitigation, prevention, and control. Mitigation, that is, dealing with an existing or ongoing bloom, and taking whatever steps are necessary or possible to reduce negative impacts. Obvious examples are the routine monitoring programs for toxins in shellfish, as currently conducted in more than 50 countries. The detection of dangerous levels of HAB toxins in shellfish will lead to harvesting restrictions to keep the contaminated product off the market. Another common mitigation strategy is the towing of fish net pens away from the sites of intense HABs. Prevention refers to actions taken to keep HABs from happening or from directly impacting a particular resource. Bloom control is the most challenging and controversial aspect of HAB management. The concept refers to actions taken to suppress or destroy HABs. This is one area where HAB science is rudimentary and slow moving. One form of mechanical control is the removal of HAB cells from the water by dispersing clay over the water surface. The clay particles aggregate with each other and with toxic phytoplankton, removing those cells through sedimentation. In countries such as Korea, where a fish-farming industry worth hundreds of millions of dollars is threatened by HABs, this control strategy makes sense, economically and socially, and so work has progressed.[3]

To protect consumer health from toxin-contaminated shellfish and decrease economic losses, food safety regulations were published in order to create national phycotoxins monitoring programs (in EU, for instance).[4] This legislation states a series of guidelines for sampling and plankton monitoring that should carry out the competent authority: Sampling plans must be drawn up taking into account the geographical distribution of the sampling points and the frequency, ensuring that the results of the analysis are as representative as possible for the area considered. Periodic toxicity tests should be performed using those mollusks from the affected area most susceptible to contamination. Phytoplanktonic samples have to be representative of the water column and provide information on the presence of toxic species as well as on population trends. Sampling frequency of mollusks has to be increased if toxin accumulation is detected, or precautionary closures of the areas have to be established until outcome of toxin analysis is obtained. When the results of sampling show that the health standards for mollusks are exceeded, or that it might be a risk to human health, the competent authority must close the production area concerned, preventing the harvesting of live bivalve mollusks. The competent authority may re-open a closed production area if the health standards for mollusks once again comply with Community legislation, for instance in EU.[5,6]

Identification and counting of microalgae from the water column is performed to provide information related to the presence of toxins producing cells. Thus, ecological exploration of phytoplankton is essential to increase our knowledge on these toxic events. An accurate and early detection of toxic episodes is necessary to develop adequate preventive mechanisms in shellfish aquaculture. Furthermore, mitigation of some of these HABs can be achieved by early detection and tracking providing an early warning of the presence of phycotoxins in shellfish-harvesting areas.[7] We should take into account that some species of harmful algae may become successful due to global climate change; then, human society should be prepared for significant expansions of toxic dinoflagellates.[7]

17.2 Phytoplankton Monitoring Programs

Many programs have been developed to monitor toxic phytoplanktonic microalgae in coastal waters. Monitoring of these microorganisms was based on conventional methods, mainly involving the microscopic examination of morphological characteristic and counting of cells. Traditionally, water samples were collected from the water column for phytoplankton observation, fixed immediately with neutralized formalin, and concentrated by sedimentation. Then, phytoplankton species were counted using a microscope at magnifications of 100× to 600×. Although very efficient, these methods are time-consuming and require considerable training and taxonomic experience based on the knowledge of morphological characteristics.[8]

Furthermore, this is not a simple scenario and some aspects should be mentioned; it is known that blooms of the same species can have chronic devastating effects in some parts of the world and can be practically harmless elsewhere. In addition, blooms of particular species in the same location exhibit large interannual variability in their toxigenic capability. These differences are mainly due to distinct toxin composition or toxin profiles and cellular toxin content, or toxin per cell of the causative agents. Complex mechanisms can induce the expression of toxin synthesis by microalgae. The production and accumulation of toxins in microalgae will be affected by the responses of different strains to external or environmental conditions, such as physical, chemical, and biological factors, but also by intrinsic or genetically determined factors.[2]

The toxin profile or fingerprint of a given species or strain is genetically determined and inherited. In fact, the identification of genes controlling toxin production is, at present, an interesting topic under research. Changes within certain ranges of this profile should be expected in response to environmental conditions. Moreover, each species may exhibit considerable genetic variability and each strain being able to develop subpopulations distributed in geographic locations that may extend from restricted areas to larger distributions. Therefore, within the same genus, important interspecific differences in toxin profile and maximum toxin content may be found. Furthermore, intraspecific variability, that is, different strains of the same species, can be at least as large as interspecific differences.[2]

In an effort to further detect and discriminate among different microalgae, several studies were focused on the development of alternative techniques that could provide a rapid and easy identification of harmful species. It should be also mentioned that HABs are complex oceanographic phenomena that require multidisciplinary study, ranging from molecular and cell biology to large-scale field surveys, numerical modeling, and remote sensing from space.[3] At the smallest scale, "molecular probes" have been developed for many HAB species that allow them to be detected and counted more easily and faster than has been possible with traditional microscopy. These probes are often either antibodies or short segments of DNA that are specific for the HAB species of interest.[3,7]

This chapter is mainly focused on the molecular probes, including immunodetection and genetic tools, although other developed strategies are briefly introduced.

17.3 Immunological Techniques

The main advantage of the immunological techniques is the wide variety of immunoglobulins for the specific detection of different targets characterizing by sensitivity, specificity, and fast performing. Also, in immunodetection it is possible to work with the entire microalgae and the automation is easy. Then, an unequivocal identification can be obtained by using a species-specific antibody against the target organism. Specific polyclonal antibodies were produced to differentiate among phytoplankton species including diatoms and other toxic microalgae. However, polyclonal antibodies have several drawbacks: differences among batches, mixture of immunoglobulins (Ig) specificities, and polyreactivity. Also, polyclonal antibodies production is dependent on the short life of animals used for immunization and they require new animals for the immunization and testing the specificity.[9]

These disadvantages can be overcome by the generation of monoclonal antibodies that can be obtained by the fusion of immunized B cells with tumoral cells (myelomas) resulting in a hybridoma or hybrid cell. These antibodies are reactive to only one epitope and therefore more specific. Hybridoma presents two characteristics, secretion of the desirable antibody and immortality. After fusion and growth in specific media, hybridoma is selected by careful screening of clones against the target of interest.

Combination of flow cytometry and immunology as a tool to identify, count, and examine marine phytoplankton was previously reviewed.[10] Use of antibodies with fluorescent markers or fluorochromes has made possible to apply different technologies, such as microscopy, flow cytometry, or flow cam to phytoplankton samples, where the antigens can be identified using either direct or indirect labeling. The light emitted by a labeled antibody can be detected by a fluorescent microscope, equipped with a UV light source, a flow cytometer, a confocal microscope, or a flow cam allowing the detection and enumeration of phytoplankton species.[9] This technique allowed examining the thecal plate morphology of *Alexandrium* cells using phase contrast and UV epifluorescence microscopy after calcofluor staining. The thecal plate tabulation and the shapes of plates and apical pore complex could prove the *Alexandrium* species. Nevertheless, these features can be very similar among different species and can even vary in relation to the environmental conditions and growth phases.[8] Several monoclonal antibodies were obtained against different species of *Alexandrium* allowing the unequivocal identification of the dinoflagellate *A. minutum*.[11] Then, using immunofluorescence could help to identify different species in natural samples during coastal monitoring.

To discriminate and count small cells or a large number of samples, the flow cytometry can be used. Designed to automate the rapid analysis and identification of cells, flow cytometry is a reliable method for the routine monitoring of the abundance of phytoplankton species, leading to an early detection of HABs. This is an optimal instrument for analyzing cells ranging from 0.5 to 20 μm in diameter that exists at concentrations between 10^6 and 10^9 cells per liter.[9]

In this context, a modified flow cytometer, known as FlowCam, has been developed to handle larger cells. It is an integrated system combining the capabilities of flow cytometry, microscopy, imaging, and fluorescence that counts, takes images, and analyzes the particles or cells that range in size from 20 to 200 μm in a discrete sample (fewer than 10^4 cells per liter) or a continuous flow. In addition to monitor harmful species of microalgae, other potential applications of immunodetection include studies of plankton community structure and ocean optics.[9]

Other authors used Imaging FlowCytobot that combines video and flow cytometric technology to capture images of nano- and microplankton and to measure the chlorophyll fluorescence associated with each image. The images are of sufficient resolution to identify many organisms to genus or even species level.[12]

17.4 Genetic Tools

Nowadays, the increasing number of microbial sequences in the GeneBank and other public databases and the development of new tools in the last 15 years enable the study of molecular methods for detection and quantification of harmful phytoplankton species and their toxins. Nevertheless, population genetic studies, taxonomic identification, and environmental monitoring are hampered by two major constraints: the necessity to establish monoclonal cultures from environmental samples and the sensitivity of available molecular tools.

Molecular techniques used for phytoplankton have been reviewed over the last decade[13–17] and specifically for harmful algae.[18,19] Available methods and new high-throughput technologies for their practical use in molecular detection, quantification, and diversity assessment of microalgae have been recently revised.[15] Advantages and drawbacks of the different methods and certain examples of applications are described in the following sections.

17.4.1 Fluorescent In Situ Hybridization

The introduction of fluorescent in situ hybridization (FISH) almost 30 years ago marked the beginning of a new era for the study of chromosome structure and function. As a combined molecular and cytological approach, the major advantage of this visually appealing technique resides in its unique ability to provide an intermediate degree of resolution between DNA analysis and chromosomal investigations, while also retaining information at the single-cell level. FISH-based diagnostic assays have been developed within different fields of investigation, including clinical genetics, neuroscience, reproductive medicine, toxicology, microbial ecology, evolutionary biology, comparative genomics, cellular genomics, and chromosome biology. The diversification of the original FISH protocol is due to the improvements in sensitivity, specificity, and resolution of the technique; together with the advances in the fields of fluorescence microscopy and digital imaging, and the growing availability of genomic and bioinformatic resources, has led to almost 40 different variations, like CO-FISH (chromosome orientation), CARD-FISH (catalyzed reporter deposition), and LNA-FISH (locked nucleic acid), among others; for additional details, see Volpi and Bridger.[20]

The demonstration that fixed whole cells are permeable to short-oligonucleotide probes extended these studies to single-cell identification. The first demonstration of this approach used radioactively labeled probes in combination with autoradiography. Fluorescent-dye-conjugated probes would extend this technique to the direct observation and identification of single cells by fluorescence microscopy.[21] Fluorescently labeled probes designed to recognize a specific sequence of a particular organism is hybridized inside intact cells, and cells containing a complex of the probe and the specific sequence are detected using epifluorescence microscopy.[22,23] It is well established that genomic resolution of DNA-fluorescence in situ hybridization (FISH) is limited by spatial resolution of the microscope and determined by chromatin condensation state.[24]

Comparative sequencing and molecular systematic are rapidly changing the character of studies in determinative and environmental microbiology. The most encompassing of molecular descriptions of microbial diversity has been provided by the comparative sequencing of rRNAs. Sequence divergence among the different species has served to define the primary lines of evolutionary descent and provided the framework for a natural classification of microorganism. For historical and technical reasons, the largest available data sets of complete sequences are for the 5S and 16S-like rRNAs. Although both have proved valuable for determinative, phylogenetic, and environmental studies, the greater information content of the larger rRNA species makes them the preferred reference sequence.[21] Comparative sequencing of the rRNAs, principally the 16S-like rRNAs, has yielded the most complete understanding of microbial phylogeny. Differences in nucleotide sequences among these ubiquitous biopolymers serve not only to relate microorganisms but also to identify them in environmental studies.[25] The use of rRNA-targeted probes has been used as a method for easy identification of microalgal cells. Oligonucleotide probe methods were later modified for application in sandwich hybridization assays and biosensors (e.g., DNA biosensor and sensor chip), in a cell-free format where many probes could be used simultaneously.[15]

Ribosomes located in the cytoplasm and comprised largely of rRNA represent easily accessible generally abundant targets for the oligonucleotide probes used to bind these molecules. Phytoplankton rRNA levels can vary as a function of algal physiological status, just like cell surface antigens. It is thus also imperative that labeling intensities of target species can be compared under a range of both favorable and unfavorable conditions in the laboratory prior to the development of field applications.[26]

Even though probes designed are supposed to be specific for one or more algal taxa based on the available sequence data, its binding must be empirically verified as the target region may be inaccessible due to folding of the rRNA molecule upon itself. In whole cell hybridization application (WCH), the probe penetrates into chemically fixed, intact cells, hybridizes or binds to its target sequence on the rRNA molecules, and is then visualized via a fluorescent reporter either attached directly to the probe or applied during a secondary labeling step. Algal cells labeled using FISH protocols can be examined directly by epifluorescence microscopy or analyzed using automated methods such as flow cytometry. It must be kept in mind that the abundance or ribosomes within the cell, and thus labeling intensity, generally varies in proportion to growth rate. The extent to which fluctuations in ribosome levels under different growth conditions affect the labeling of target cells must therefore be investigated experimentally to aid the interpretation of data from natural populations.[26]

The WCH approach has been developed and applied extensively for the detection of many harmful algae, including dinoflagellates, diatoms, and raphidophytes.[26] A general and simplified protocol consists of these three steps: (1) fixation, dehydration, and decoloration for 10 min; (2) hybridization of probes for 5 min; and (3) washing excess and misannealed probes for another 5 min.[23] As it can be observed, the general protocol is fast and simple. Previous studies have reported that the application of 4% paraformaldehyde in PBS for 5 min at room temperature was the best fixation method for subsequent FISH analysis. Also, even some authors have hypothesized that the use of cetyltrimethylammonium bromide (CTAB) solution was considered to facilitate entry of probes into cells[27] although others have detected certain detrimental effects on this characteristic.[28] The combination of a 40°C hybridization temperature and 50°C wash temperature showed higher probe reactivity with no specificity; washing twice for 5 min has proven to be fast and effective at removal of nonspecific signals.[28]

17.4.1.1 Advantages and Drawbacks of FISH

Whole cell FISH combines the advantages of both phenotypic and genetic analyses by allowing monitoring of multiple species and the reliable discrimination of toxic and nontoxic taxa that may be morphologically identical but generically distinct.[29] FISH does not require cell homogenization or lysis, and intact cells can be analyzed roughly by their morphological characteristics with a light microscope. Therefore, cells with a nonspecific signal can be discerned from those labeled specifically more easily than by methods requiring cell homogenization. Other molecular identification methods such as the sandwich hybridization assay and the PCR assay can detect targeted cells with high efficiency; however, some authors state that a major disadvantage associated with these techniques is that it is not possible with them to verify that the signal is derived only from the targeted organisms because the cells are completely homogenized or lysed during the assay. Furthermore, an additional advantage of this technique is that it does not require expensive equipment such as PCR equipment or the use of radioisotope-labeled compounds, or even a high degree of skill or experience.[28]

Application of this technique has proven a high specificity and rapidity for identification of the targeted species.[22] Some studies have used probes that hybridize with nuclear-encoded DNA, thus signals were only observed from the nuclei and the intensity of the fluorescence signal was too weak for practical use. To improve the intensity of the fluorescent signal, a new FISH methodology was established designing probes against other rRNA targets.[28] When the rRNA-targeted probes correctly hybridize to rRNA in ribosomes distributed throughout the cell, the whole cell fluoresces.[28]

The major drawbacks of this methodology is that it does not allow high throughput,[30] and the existence of autofluorescence due to chlorophyll.[22,31] Regarding the second issue, different solutions have been proposed, like the application of acetone, methanol, ethanol, or even dimethylformamide as fixing agents. It has been observed that fixation with acetone extracts 90% of the chlorophyll in only 10 min, meanwhile ethanol, methanol, or dimethylformamide extractions take about 1 h to achieve similar results.[22] It is worth to mention that if cells of targeted organisms do not have a hard cell wall, like *Alexandrium* spp., they may be broken due to chemical reagents or centrifugation,[28] even though these problems may be overcome by using filtration instead of centrifugation for concentration purposes and by the application of increasing acetone concentrations, from 20% to 80%, to decrease cells disruption.[22]

17.4.1.2 Applications in Marine Biotoxins

The value of a probe-based identification system is not decreased by the fact that the level of toxicity changes with varying nutrient status of the cell, because the probes identify ribotypes that, for *A. tamarense*, are always either nontoxic of potentially toxic.[31] This is one of the reasons why in recent years several methods have been developed, optimized, and applied in different parts of the world as Ireland and Japan for the identification and quantification of these dinoflagellates.[22,23,28,29] Methods for the detection and enumeration of other *Alexandrium* species based on FISH have been developed, like two DNA probes for *A. tamiyavanichii*.[32] Recent studies have gone one step further adapting and combining previously developed FISH and sandwich hybridization assay probes into a microarray format, the so-called ALEX-CHIP. This chip can simultaneously detect five different targets, including three clades of *A. tamarense*, *A. ostenfeldii*, and *A. minutum*, which would improve detection of member of this group.[33]

Application of FISH for the detection of dinoflagellates that produce okadaic acid, dinophysistoxins, AZAs, PTXs, and YTXs are scarce.[34,35]

The large subunit of ribosomal RNA gene sequences have been compared from cultured isolates of *P. australis* (Frenguelli), *P. pungens* (Grunow) Hasle, *P. multiseries* (Hasle) Hasle, *P. fraudulenta* (P. T. Cleve) Heiden, *P. heimii* Manguin, *P. delicatissima* (P. T. Cleve) Heiden, and *N. Americana* (Hasle) Fryxell. These sequences revealed unique nucleotide "signatures" for each species examined.[36] Probes targeting rRNA can be applied using both whole cell or sandwich hybridization techniques.[37]

Studies describing the application of rRNA probes in WCH for detection and enumeration of *Pseudo nitzschia* have been published. Optimized simple fixation protocol that permeabilizes cell membranes and reduces autofluorescence while at the same time preserves cell structure and shape has been extensively tested.[36,37] These types of methods have been applied to monitor potentially toxic blooms of *Pseudo nitzschia* in Monterey Bay, California; in surveillance programs operating in New Zealand, even preliminary tests were done in Ireland and Scotland.[37,38]

A reduction in the ethanol concentration and keeping the salinity constant prevents precipitate formation without diminishing the effectiveness of the preservative and remains precipitate-free for several months at room temperature. This fixation protocol has proven superior to other using Carnoy's solution or formalin solutions with ethanol or methanol. Cultured and natural samples, fixed with the modified ethanol protocol, are stable 4–6 weeks. The fact that samples remain reactive for long time after fixation makes the method very convenient when sample examination is not possible right after hybridization.[37]

17.4.2 Detection of Potentially Toxic Species by Polymerase Chain Reaction and Quantitative PCR

Most detection tools used for phytoplankton rely on detecting DNA because of the instability of other molecules such as RNA and proteins. Advantages of DNA-based methods are based on the DNA isolation from frozen, fresh, or preserved samples and also on the large number of DNA sequences available in public databases (mainly in the GenBank and in the EMBL). PCR methods include single-cell PCR, traditional PCR with sequencing, qPCR, and other PCR-based methods not very commonly used that focus on DNA bands analysis, for instance, random amplified polymorphic DNA (RAPD), single-strand conformation polymorphism (SSCP), and denaturing gradient gel electrophoresis (DGGE) among others.[39] PCR-based methods can amplify minute amounts of template DNA and multiply even a single copy of a given DNA sequence; its high specificity makes this tool highly effective for species and strain identification over a wide range of organisms. The relatively low cost of the equipment and reagents makes PCR accessible to small laboratories. In phytoplankton studies, PCR-based assays have largely been used for the identification and characterization of toxic species with the use of species-specific PCR primers and genetic markers. One of the most studied genus is *Alexandrium*, which was one of the first phytoplankton genus that have been identified in culture samples using PCR and which continues to be an organism of great interest for research purposes.[34,40–44]

17.4.2.1 Conventional PCR Methods

17.4.2.1.1 Single-Cell PCR

Conventional PCR methods have been used to detect specific single cells by single-cell PCR. Single-cell PCR makes it possible to amplify DNA fragments by PCR from one or a few cells of an organism. It has enabled the detection and determination of DNA sequences from noncultivable microalgae.[45–47] But it is also applicable to frozen samples or samples preserved in solvents, such as formalin.[34,48–50] Although single-cell PCR assay is very useful for the determination of DNA sequences from uncultured microalgae collected from the environment, it is still labor-intensive to isolate these target cells from natural phytoplankton samples. In addition, pico-size cells cannot be isolated by capillary methods prior to cell extraction and subsequent PCR amplification. For this reason, initially it is a very useful tool to isolate and detect comparatively large cells, such as armored dinoflagellates, because they are easy to isolate by capillary tubes using the inverted light microscope. However, pico-size eukaryotic cells in environmental samples have recently been isolated by flow cytometry.[51,52] This technique allows that single-cell PCR detection to be applied for various size phytoplankton making easy the isolation of cells previous to PCR.

17.4.2.1.2 Species-Specific PCR

Conventional PCR detection with species-specific primers may only detect a single species rather than the multiple phytoplankton species present in a given body of water. The use of species-specific PCR followed by sequencing could therefore be impractical for the routine analysis of field samples that may contain many different species, but multiple phytoplankton species detections are essential for monitoring harmful algal species in coastal waters.

Monitoring of coastal waters could be achieved by multiplex traditional PCR with a mixture of species-specific primers that detect several species simultaneously. This technique has been tested for the detection of harmful phytoplankton by some different authors.[53,54] In conventional PCR, multiple primer sets within a single PCR mixture produce amplicons of varying sizes specific to different DNA sequences. Annealing temperatures for each of the specific primer sets must be optimized to work properly within a single reaction, and amplicon sizes should be sufficiently different to form distinct bands when visualized by gel electrophoresis. However, this method has several limitations that have been solved with multiplex qPCR also called real-time PCR.

17.4.2.2 Quantitative or Real-Time PCR

Real-time PCR, also called qPCR, is known as the second generation of PCR because it could be used to amplify and simultaneously quantify several target DNA molecules. The procedure follows the same principle as standard PCR technique, but the key distinction is that the amplified DNA is detected as the reaction progresses in real time; therefore, it is more advantageous than conventional PCR because of its linearity, sensitivity, specificity, and the speed at which a large number of samples can be processed.

Two different types of chemistries can be used in qPCR applications: (1) sequence-specific oligonucleotide probes that are labeled with a fluorescent reporter, such as TaqMan, and (2) nonspecific fluorescent dyes (e.g., SYBR green) that intercalate with any double-stranded DNA. Data are collected over the entire series of PCR cycles by using fluorescent markers that are incorporated into the amplicon product during amplification and directly in the exponential phase where PCR is precise and linear. In order to quantify cells, the qPCR parameters are optimized using different standard curves (plasmid dilution or pure algal cultures). qPCR generates a standard curve of cycle thresholds (Ct) with known concentrations, and thus cell density can be compared and calculated from the Ct value. SYBR green-based qPCR is commonly considered a relatively easier and cost-effective method. However, double strand DNA (dsDNA) dyes, such as SYBR green, will bind to all dsDNA PCR products, including nonspecific PCR products like primer dimers. This can potentially prevent accurate quantification of the intended target sequence. On the other hand, probe-based qPCR is considered more accurate than intercalating dye methods. Both types of qPCR have been tested for the quantification of harmful microalgae. Also, some authors has shown that multiplexing (using several species-specific sets of primers and probes) was more efficient than multiprobing (using the same set of primers with species-specific probes) for simultaneous detection of several species.[17,55] Concerning the target genes selected to identify phytoplankton species they were usually within the rRNA operon. But some authors used other genes, for instance, the mitochondrial cytochrome b upstream region.[56,57]

qPCR was successfully used to detect and quantify certain toxic species in either the water column, sediments, or in mollusk tissues and it was also used to perform, in less than 4 h, and semi-quantification or quantification of cells, in addition to identify them. qPCR methods developed to date for species detection and quantification include genus *Alexandrium*,[34,40,44] *Cochlodinium*,[58] *Cyanobacterium*,[59] *Dinophysis*,[40,60] *Gambierdiscus*,[57,61] *Karenia*,[40,62] *Pfiesteria*,[63] *Prymnesium*,[64] *Prorocentrum*,[65] and *Pseudonitzia*[66,67] (Table 17.1). As it was stated before, molecular quantification of different phytoplankton species in an aquatic environment is a relevant parameter for the monitoring of possible algal bloom episodes. Among current technologies, qPCR may be considered the best method for the molecular quantification of some targeting phytoplankton species. Most qPCR methods have focused on the detection and discrimination of microalgae but are not commonly used in the field. In this sense, the use of qPCR-based methods in field applications and for quantification purposes is slowly developing.

Recently, the potential of species-specific qPCR as a practical adjunct tool for monitoring programs, allowing high-throughput analysis of phytoplankton samples when morphology is an imprecise character and/or is not practical for taxonomic identification has been demonstrated. The application of qPCR for monitoring purposes is relatively inexpensive, rapid, and provides same-day results for species identification.[67] The application of this method in monitoring programs will allow the accumulation of data that, correlated to other physical parameters, may help in the development of models for prediction of blooms of certain species.

17.4.3 Detection of Potentially Toxic Species by Microarray-Based Methods

FISH and real-time PCR are powerful and highly quantitative tools for the identification of microbial organisms, but they are limited to the analysis of only one or a few targets at a time. However, DNA

TABLE 17.1

qPCR Methods Developed for Species Detection
and Quantification

Phytoplankton Genus	References
Alexandrium	Penna et al.[34]
	Guillou et al.[40]
	Zhang et al.[44]
Cochlodinium	Howard et al.[58]
Cyanobacterium	Churro et al.[59]
Dinophysis	Guillou et al.[40]
	Kavanagh et al.[60]
Gambierdiscus	Otero et al.[57]
	Vandersea et al.[61]
Karenia	Guillou et al.[40]
	Yuan et al.[62]
Pfiesteria	Bowers et al.[63]
Prymnesium	Zamor et al.[64]
Prorocentrum	Yuan et al.[65]
Pseudonitzia	Andree et al.[66]
	Fitzpatrick et al.[67]

microarrays provide an option to avoid the limitations of these single probe approaches since they allow the parallel analysis of almost infinite numbers of probes at a time in just one experiment. Consequently, there are a growing number of publications about the use of microarrays for identification, for example, marine bacteria,[68] picoplankton,[69] diatoms,[70] dinoflagellates,[71] fish pathogens,[72–74] coral microbial ecology,[75] or sulfate reducing prokaryotes.[76]

DNA microarrays use many species-specific oligonucleotide probes, in most cases immobilized on a solid surface in the defined positions,[77–79] allowing the simultaneous detection of a number of DNA sequences in a sample. However, a large variety of detection chemistries and target preparation methods have been used in microarray studies,[80] and also variations of the classical planar surface arrays have been described.[81,82]

The DNA array technology was originally designed for gene expression or single-nucleotide polymorphism profiling,[15,83–85] primarily of pure cultures of individual organisms, but major recent advances have allowed to apply them to environmental samples.[86] In general, DNA arrays can be divided into at least three categories based on the genes targeted by the array[86]: functional gene arrays designed for the detection of key functional genes in a given environment, phylogenetic arrays, the most common DNA arrays, which are based on a diagnostic marker, such as the 16S or 18S rRNA genes, and are used for microbial identification and metagenomic arrays that unlike the other arrays contain DNA fragments produced directly from environmental DNA and can be applied with no prior sequence knowledge.

17.4.3.1 Functional Gene Arrays Designed for the Detection of Key Functional Genes in a Given Environment

Despite the serious impact of HABs on public health, the toxicological responses to toxins have received little attention due to the limited availability of purified toxin to carry out such studies. Functional gene arrays are a useful tool to study the toxigenomic effects of aquatic toxins. This technique has been used to study the toxic effects of brevetoxins in liver and brain of mice,[87] the liver response to ciguatoxin,[88] or the role of immune functions in chronic phase ciguatera poisoning.[89] Microarrays have been also used to profile gene expression in mouse brain following domoic acid (DA) exposure[90] to understand DA-induced excitotoxicity, and in human T lymphocyte cells following azaspiracid toxin exposure.[91]

17.4.3.2 Phylogenetic Arrays

With regard to phylogenetic arrays, this strategy has proven to be successful for microbial identification, even when species can only be discriminated by a single-nucleotide polymorphism.[92] Numerous studies demonstrate that the microarray technique also constitutes an effective method for the simultaneous large-scale detection of microalgae.[69,93] Furthermore, this method is recommended as one of the high-throughput molecular quantification techniques. For quantification, the arrays can be hybridized using different concentrations of target cells, and the cells are subsequently enumerated from the signals generated.[81,82,93,94]

17.4.3.3 Metagenomic Arrays

Use of DNA arrays for the field detection of cyanobacterial species has also been investigated. Rudi et al. have tested 10 specific 16S rDNA oligonucleotide probes on water samples from 8 lakes, obtaining good results for qualitative estimation of the presence or absence of the various cyanobacterial genera.[95] However, this array did not enable quantification. After this first method, a universal microarray was developed in the framework of the European project MIDI-CHIP.[96] The aim of this project was to design and test DNA microarrays to monitor microbial diversity with adequate biodiversity indexes using cyanobacteria in freshwater as a model system. Comparison of the microarray data with those obtained by microscopic examination of the same samples revealed consistent results, demonstrating the potential of this approach for monitoring cyanobacteria.

The applicability of microarrays for the detection and monitoring of harmful algae has been demonstrated in various publications.[77,79] In addition, different array technologies have been used for the simultaneous identification and quantification of many taxa in phytoplankton communities.[97]

A phytoplankton DNA chip for all microalgal classes, including many toxic species, was developed in the framework of the European "Fish and Chips" project.[98] The specificity, sensitivity, and reliability of this chip were evaluated later[77] to the detect and classify *Alexandrium* species (ALEX-CHIP), obtaining a sensitive monitoring tool of toxic and nontoxic species of this dinoflagellate.

Most of the molecular detection methods use DNA as target[15,99] because of instability of RNA and protein. DNA microarrays allowed the researchers to rapidly screen for the presence or absence and for the levels of gene expression.[100] Pomati et al. have utilized a DNA-microarray approach to explore gene expression patterns associated with the production of PSP toxins within phylogenetically closely related strains of toxic and nontoxic *Anabaena circinalis*.[101] The DNA microarray analysis allowed the identification of genes potentially implicated in the development of STX-producing *A. circinalis* blooms. This DNA-microarray could also be applied for the validation of molecular probes that have been designed for the environmental screening and analysis of toxic cyanobacterial blooms.

However, DNA-based methods can reveal only the presence of genes involved in toxin production. In environmental samples, DNA can originate from dead or can be mutated, preventing or diminishing their transcription and subsequent toxin production.[102] Although microcystin biosynthesis genes (*mcy* genes) were used to distinguish between microcystin-producing and nonproducing strains of the genera *Anabaena*, *Microcystis*, and *Planktothrix*,[103] several investigations showed that certain strains possess *mcy* genes but lack detectable toxicity.[104] Then, the interpretation of toxicity exclusively based on the presence of genes might produce erroneous results and should be further verified using targeted physiological and biochemical tests.[105]

Use of RNA allows detection of potential toxin-producing microorganisms that are alive and actively transcribing the toxicity genes. Consequently, observation of actual toxin producers is more reliable.[106] Production of nodularin toxin by *Nodularia spumigena* was detected by real-time PCR in Baltic Sea samples.[107] Rantala et al.[108] developed a new tool to detect and identify hepatotoxin-producing cyanobacteria of the genera *Anabaena*, *Microcystis*, *Planktothrix*, *Nostoc*, and *Nodularia*. Genus-specific probe pairs were designed for the detection of the microcystin (*mcyE*) and nodularinsynthetase genes (*ndaF*) of these five genera to be used with a DNA-chip. Later, Yang et al.[109] used a microarray approach to compare the transcriptomes of toxic and nontoxic *Alexandrium minutum* clones and thus identified differences in gene expression potentially linked to toxin synthesis and/or regulation.

In vitro bioassays offer the possibility to screen for the presence of whole classes of contaminants and toxins based on their biological effects. As a result, such bioassays are able to detect both known and yet unknown compounds. A tailored microarray platform was designed[110] for the detection of marine toxins based on the differential expression of a set of genes. The new dedicated low-density tube microarray for marine toxins requires further improvement. However, the current microarray data enable future developments of other fast in vitro bioassays. Recently, a high-resolution microarray assay was developed to evaluate species and strain diversity in *Pseudo nitzschia* populations of the northeast Pacific coastal ocean with a total assay time under 7 h.[111]

17.4.3.3.1 Advantages and Utilities of Microarrays

Microarrays have the capacity to overcome some limitations associated with the restricted resolution of many fingerprinting methods, the requirement of large simple methods, and associated costs for sequencing clones.[112] Moreover, they provide the possibility for high throughput analysis of molecular probe–based species identification without a cultivation step and do not require a broad taxonomic knowledge to identify cells.[113] It is the most suitable technique for the identification of an, a priori, unlimited amount of DNA sequences in a single assay,[114] because the target is labeled, not the probes, and many probes can be used simultaneously.[69] This fact provides the unlimited expanding capacity to detect new microorganisms or genes of interest.[112]

This technique may also provide quantitative information since hybridization signals are proportional to the quantity of target DNA[115,116] and could be suited to serve as a valuable tool to ensure the quality of a culture collection.[69]

Summarizing, this technique is accurate, it has inexpensive maintenance, and good sensitivity and specificity. It is characterized by low detection limit, shorter analysis time, and minimal false-positive signals. Besides, it is user-friendly and has a simple configuration of assay platform. Taking all these reasons into account, microarrays have great potential to quantify microalgal cells and alter the standard procedures used for microalgae monitoring programs.[15]

17.4.3.3.2 Disadvantages or Weakness of Microarrays

When in situ hybridization results for probes are not always consistent with their in silico predictions, then probes can display strong variation if they are hybridized to different target organisms.[69] Furthermore, it is not always possible to have perfect specificity for all detector oligonucleotides since they all need to hybridize under the same conditions, so cross-hybridizations are almost impossible to avoid in a microarray hybridization format under stringent conditions.[117] Therefore, the development of a functional chip is an elaborate task because the set of probes on the microarray has to be developed such that all constituents work specifically under the same hybridization conditions.[118]

Its most important drawback is that there is a need for specification of the target organisms or genes. As a result, the most demanding challenge for the applicability of microarrays for species identification is the high number of unknown environmental species that may result in unspecific signals. Then, the importance of an organism, which may be dominant and critical to the ecosystem under study, can be completely overlooked if the organism does not have a corresponding probe on the array.[86] Nevertheless, this problem can be addressed by spotting multiple oligonucleotides for the same target.[112] Arrays containing probes generated from random genomic fragments have been used in situations where the genome sequences of the target organisms were unknown.[119,120]

Similar to many other techniques, microarrays currently detect only the dominant populations in many environmental samples.[121,122] Some environments contain low levels of biomass, making it difficult to obtain enough material for use in microarray analysis without first amplifying the nucleic acids. Such techniques may introduce biases into the analyses.[123]

Furthermore, it is often a challenge to analyze microarray results from environmental samples due to the massive amounts of data generated and a lack of standardized controls and data analysis procedures.[86]

High set-up costs for the machines and requirement of quite bulky pieces of equipment, make it unsuitable on-board ship or for field applications.[15] This is of particular interest for the monitoring programs for toxic algae, where samples are taken regularly at places that are not in close proximity of laboratories that host the previously described equipment.[113] Moreover, the need of validation for routine use and the cost of these methods still hamper their use in monitoring programs.[17]

17.4.4 Molecular Detection of Specific Genotype Producers of Biotoxins

HABs are frequently presented as almost monospecific events, and the identification of the causative organism has been proved to be crucial in the decisions to adopt in order to prevent or mitigate the effects of the toxic bloom. Resolution of the species concept for unicellular algae has become an important issue, whether morphological versus genetic identification can diverse.[7] With the basis of the combination of both genetic and morphological information in addition to other characteristics like lipid, pigment and toxic biochemistry, traditional taxonomy based on several species and on morphotypes genus have been recently revised.

It is well established that there is not a direct linkage between morphology and genetics, and the fact of looking similar does not mean to have the same genetic information. For instance, this is the case of *Alexandrium tamarense*, known to exist as toxic and nontoxic strains, morphologically indistinguishable. This reveals the existence of various genotypes, some of which are consistently toxic and others that are mostly nontoxic.[124] The specific identification of these toxic genotypes rather than the species should be taken into account for selecting the molecular probes for the investigation of HABs.

17.4.4.1 Detection of Toxic Genotypes in Marine Ecosystems

Detection of strains containing genes responsible for the production of marine biotoxins remains very difficult. One of the main reasons for this difficulty is the extremely large size of the nuclear genomes of eukaryotic phytoplankton. This is especially remarkable in the case of dinoflagellates, here in some species the genome can be more than 40 times the size of the human genome. Further difficulties are the permanent condensation of chromatin, general lack of histones, the frequent base–pair substitutions, and the high G–C base–pair ratio.[7]

Paralytic shellfish poisoning (PSP) is the group of toxins where the investigations on toxic-production-related genes and toxic genotypes had achieved more valuable results. The main reason for this is the recent availability of the cyanobacterial saxitoxin synthesis gene cluster structure. Cyanobacteria are the most frequent organism causative of toxigenic HABs in freshwater ecosystems, and their relative small genomes facilitate the application of conventional genomics to elucidate the structure of the toxic-production gene clusters.[125] The investigation of homologous structures to those obtained from cyanobacteria in species with a much larger genome could allow the identification and differentiation of toxic and nontoxic strains. The first attempt for the identification of the cyanobacterial PSP toxin genes in the genome of a dinoflagelate was performed by Yang et al. They constructed and analyzed an expressed sequence tag (EST) library of *A. minutum* and this was used to construct an oligonucleotide microarray. While no presence of cyanobacterial genes was detected in *A. minutum* genoma, 192 genes were differentially expressed between toxic and nontoxic strains.[109] Hackett et al. assembled comprehensive transcriptome data sets for several STX-producing dinoflagellates and a related nontoxic species. This allowed them to identify 265 putative homologues of 13 cyanobacterial STX synthesis genes, including all the genes directly involved in toxin synthesis. Putative homologues of four proteins group closely in phylogenies with cyanobacteria and are likely to their functional homologues of sxtA, sxtG, and sxtB in dinoflagellates. However, the phylogenies do not support the transfer of these genes directly between toxic cyanobacteria and dinoflagellates. Their findings suggest that the STX synthesis pathway was likely assembled independently in the distantly related cyanobacteria and dinoflagellates, although using some evolutionarily related proteins. The biological role of STX is not well understood in either cyanobacteria or dinoflagellates. However, STX production in these two ecologically distinct groups of organisms suggests that this toxin confers a benefit to producers that we do not yet fully understand.[126]

In the case of those dinoflagellate phycotoxins whose structures are linear or ladder-frame polyethers derived via polyketide biosynthesis, the genomic search for polyketide synthase (PKS) genes involved in these pathways could lead to the identification of toxic genotypes producing this kind of toxins. Polyketide synthase enzymes are large multi-domain complexes that structurally and functionally resemble the fatty acid synthases involved in lipid metabolism. Polyketide biosynthesis of secondary metabolites and hence functional PKS genes are widespread among bacteria, fungi, and streptophytes.[31] Jaeckisch et al. focused their research on the identification and characterization of genes involved in spirolide biosynthesis, specifically PKS genes. The dinoflagellate *Alexandrium ostenfeldii* is the only known producer of toxic spirolides. Spirolides are macrocyclic imines that are derived via polyketide biosynthetic pathways production is therefore almost certainly mediated by PKS genes. Genomic characterization of *A. ostenfeldii* was conducted by generating two expressed sequence tag (EST) data banks, based on normalized cDNA libraries of two strains of *A. ostenfeldii* (AOSH1 and AOSH2) from Nova Scotia, Canada, which produce distinctive spirolide profiles. About 5,300 and 12,287 ESTs were sequenced, which yielded 2,634 and 9,833 unique sequences, respectively. The ESTs were annotated and compared between the two strains. Several genes putatively related to toxin synthesis were detected, including genes encoding PKS. A Fosmid library was also generated to detect and further analyze toxin-related genes. The identification of polyketide biosynthetic genes from dinoflagellates provided the first steps for further research on this pharmacologically interesting enzyme group.[127] Brevetoxins are a group of polyketide toxins thought to be synthesized by a PKS complex. Nevertheless, the gene cluster for this PKS has not been identified. Moroe et al. identified eight PKS transcripts in *Karenia brevis*, a known organism producer of brevetoxins, by high throughput cDNA library screening. Full length sequences were obtained through 3′ and 5′ RACE Transcript lengths ranged from 1875 to 3397 nucleotides, based on sequence analysis, and were confirmed by northern blotting. Their results identified an unprecedented PKS structure in a toxic dinoflagellate.[128] However, the role of the PKS genes in the production of the corresponding toxins remains uncovered.

17.4.4.2 Application of Molecular Tools in the Detection of Toxic Genotypes in Freshwater Ecosystems: Cyanobacteria

In freshwater ecosystems, the main phytoplanktonic organisms causative of HABs are cyanobacteria. Several cyanobacteria genera are able to produce a wide range of different kinds of toxins that can be classified into hepatotoxins (e.g., microcystins, nodularins, and cylindrospermopsin) and neurotoxins (anatoxins, jamaicamids, and saxitoxins). Studies of toxic cyanobacteria populations have reported the presence of both toxin-producing and nontoxin–producing genotypes into the same species. Investigation on the causative species of a specific bloom could lead to an invalid result if the toxicity is evaluated in function of the species that are present in the bloom.

The detection and monitoring of hepatotoxic cyanobacterial genotypes have been improved in the last years due to the characterization of the gene clusters involved in the production of such kind of toxins. On the contrary, the detection of toxic genotypes producing neurotoxins remains elusive due to the scarce information on the biosynthetic pathways and the coding gene clusters, which have begun to be uncovered recently.[129]

The *mcy* gene cluster responsible for the production of microcistins has been described for several genera of cyanobacteria. This has made possible the implementation of PCR procedures to detect single or multiple (multiplex PCR) genes of the cluster. The gene cluster involved in the production of nodularins has a high sequence homology with the *mcy* cluster. This has allowed the implementation made by Jungblut et al. of a PCR test to detect all potential microcystin and nodularin-producing cyanobacteria from laboratory cultures as well as from HABs. They chose the aminotransferase (AMT) domain, which is located on the modules *mcyE* and *ndaF* of the microcystin and nodularin synthetase enzyme complexes, respectively, as the target sequence because of its essential function in the synthesis of all microcystins as well as nodularins. Using the described PCR, it was possible to amplify a 472 bp PCR product from the AMT domains of all tested hepatotoxic species and bloom samples.[130] A disadvantage of PCR procedures is that the data obtained indicate the presence/absence of potentially toxic genotypes, but not their abundance on a given bloom. In order to overcome this problem, several q-PCR assays have been proposed to estimate the cyanobacterial population and the proportion of potentially toxic genotypes. Moreover, mutations, insertions, or deletions in the gene clusters, which both can inactivate these genes preventing toxin synthesis or their detection by PCR methods, could lead to an incorrect toxicity evaluation,[131,132] so a careful selection of the target genes for the PCR procedure should be made. Al-Tebrineh et al. have recently developed a quantitative PCR (qPCR) assay based on SYBR-green chemistry for the detection of potentially hepatotoxic cyanobacteria spanning all known microcystin and nodularin–producing taxa using primers specifically targeting *mcyE* and *ndaF*.[133]

Mihali et al. characterized the gene cluster for the biosynthesis of the cyanobacterial toxin cylindrospermopsin in *Cylindrospermopsis raciborskii*. The *cyr* gene cluster spans 43 kb and is comprised of 15 open-reading frames containing genes required for the biosynthesis, regulation, and export of the toxin. These findings enable the design of specific probes that could be applied for the detection of toxic strains of cyanobacteria.[134] Simultaneously, Rasmussen et al. developed a duplex real-time PCR assay that targeted a cylindrospermopsin-specific and *Cylindrospermopsis raciborskii*–specific DNA sequence. In toxic strains, sequences of each of these three genes were always present, while in nontoxic strains the distribution of these sequences was patchy, resulting in what are likely to be natural deletion mutants.[135]

Saxitoxins are known to be produced by several species of freshwater filamentous cyanobacteria, including *Anabaena circinalis*, *Aphanizomenon* spp., *Lyngbyawollei*, and *Cylindrospermopsis raciborskii*. The recent description of a unique polyketide synthase sequence (*sxtA*), which is an integral part of the cyanobacterial STX biosynthesis gene cluster (*sxt*),[134,136] has allowed the development of PCR methods to detect genotypes containing this cluster. Al-Tebrineh et al. developed a specific quantitative PCR (qPCR) method based on SYBR green chemistry to quantify saxitoxin-producing *Anabaena circinalis* cyanobacteria. The aim of this study was to infer the potential toxigenicity of samples by determining the copy number of a unique and unusual polyketide synthase sequence (*sxtA*) in the STX biosynthesis gene cluster identified in cyanobacteria. They applied a qPCR approach to water samples collected from different Australian lakes, dams, and rivers. The STX concentration and cyanobacterial cell density of these blooms were also determined by high-pressure liquid chromatography and microscopic cell counting, respectively. STX concentrations correlated positively with STX gene copy numbers, indicating that the latter can be used as a measure of potential toxigenicity in *Anabaena circinalis* and possibly other cyanobacterial blooms. The qPCR method targeting STX genes can also be employed for both monitoring and ecophysiological studies of toxic *Anabaena circinalis* blooms and potentially several other STX-producing cyanobacteria.[137]

The biosynthesis of anatoxins and the genes involved in their production were recently described for *Oscillatoria* sp. strain PCC 6506.[138] Rantala et al. identified the anatoxin synthetase gene cluster (*anaA* to *anaG* and *orf1*; 29 kb) in *Anabaena* sp. strain 37. The gene (81.6%–89.2%) and amino acid (78.8%–86.9%) sequences were highly similar to those of *Oscillatoria* sp. strain PCC 6506, while the organization of the genes differed. Molecular detection methods for potential anatoxin-a and homoanatoxin-a producers of the genera *Anabaena*, *Aphanizomenon*, and *Oscillatoria* were developed by designing primers to recognize the *anaC* gene. *Anabaena* and *Oscillatoria anaC* genes were specifically identified in several cyanobacterial strains by PCR. Restriction fragment length polymorphism (RFLP) analysis of the *anaC* amplicons enabled simultaneous identification of three producer genera: *Anabaena*, *Oscillatoria*, and *Aphanizomenon*.[139]

Recently, Al-Tebrineh et al. described the development and validation of a quadruplex quantitative-PCR (qPCR) assay capable of detecting and quantifying simultaneously the toxin genes from the microcystin, nodularin, cylindrospermopsin, and saxitoxin biosynthesis pathways. The primers and probes were designed from conserved regions within toxin biosynthesis genes from most of the representative cyanobacterial genera. The qPCR assay was optimized to reliably determine the copy number of cyanotoxin biosynthesis genes, as well as an internal cyanobacteria 16S rDNA control, in a single reaction. Amplification efficiency and reproducibility were similar among the cyanotoxin genes, while the sensitivity of the reaction for the toxin genes ranged from 10^2 to 10^6 gene copies per reaction. The authors verified that this multiplex qPCR assay can be applied as a powerful tool for detecting and quantifying potentially toxic cyanobacteria in laboratory and field samples.[140]

17.5 Satellite Approaches

Compared with traditional in situ point observations, satellite remote sensing is considered a promising technique for studying HABs due to its advantages of large-scale, real-time, and long-term monitoring.[141] Satellite remote sensing is now used operationally to detect HABs with simple transport models; forecasts are now issued of impending landfall or exposure. That capability is not easily transferred to other HABs, as the blooms being detected are very dense and mono-specific, and thus have a chlorophyll signature that reveals their presence. For other HABs, remote sensing applications rely on detecting the water masses in which the cells reside using sea surface temperature, for example.[3]

An in situ optical classification algorithm was developed and validated for a variety of ocean environments for the rapid identification of *Karenia brevis* blooms that can be applied to various ocean-observing platforms. This identification was based on two criteria: chlorophyll *a* concentration and chlorophyll-specific particulate backscattering.[142]

Combining multiple accessible satellite approaches as visual interpretation, spectra analysis, parameters retrieval, and spatial temporal pattern led to a systematic and comprehensive monitoring of HABs. For instance, monitoring of C-phycocyanin and chlorophyll-a concentrations and other pigments retrieved for satellite, changes in water quality, or levels of inorganic nutrients are other alternatives to detect toxic episodes.

17.6 Solid-Phase Adsorption Toxin Tracking TS

Although it is not a phytoplankton monitoring method, this technique can have the potential to be used to forecast HABs. It was reported that passive adsorption of dissolved toxins from seawater, coupled to sensitive analytical technologies such as LC–MS and ELISA assays, provided a simple means of biotoxins monitoring. The technique was given the acronym SPATT (solid-phase adsorption toxin tracking) and the idea was deduced by the observation that significant amounts of algal biotoxins were dissolved in the seawater when toxic species were present.[143] These authors suggest that the SPATT method could be used as a regulatory food safety monitoring tool applicable to all algal-toxin groups, after being standardized and validated. More recent studies suggest that SPATT can be established as a supplementary technique with other phytoplankton-monitoring methods. Then, the utilization of SPATT highlights the potential of this technique to provide a useful tool for the screening and early warning of shellfish contamination by lipophilic toxins.[143,144]

17.7 Biosensors

DNA biosensors are known from various areas of interest that take advantage of the hybridization principle, for example, a biosensor was developed for the specific identification of letters containing *Bacillus anthracis* in the fall of 2001.[145] DNA biosensors have specific probes that target only DNA sequences present in the organism of interest and can be used onsite and therefore circumvent the need to return samples into the laboratory. A DNA biosensor was adapted by Metfies et al.[118] to the electrochemical detection of the toxic dinoflagellate *A. ostenfeldii*. The technical background of this device is explained in detail in the German patent application DE 10032 042 A1 (Elektrochemischer Einwegbiosensorfür die quantitative Bestimmung von Analytkonzentrationen in Flüssigkeiten). The device could facilitate the work that must be done in the course of monitoring toxic algae by eliminating the need to count algae and reduce the need for mouse bioassay.

17.8 Other Methods

Karenia brevis forms HABs in the Gulf of Mexico, producing toxins that kill fish, contaminate bivalves, and also release toxic aerosols. An observatory system for the monitoring of this dinoflagellate based on the optical phytoplankton discriminator (OPD) uses an algorithm to select *K. brevis* from mixed samples. A variety of platforms have been adapted for the OPD and the data are transferred in a variety of methods including direct cable, wireless network, VHF radio, cell phone, and satellite phones. It was expanded from detection of only *K. brevis* to a community structure library that includes taxonomy. This observatory instrument fulfills the need for near real-time ocean-observing tools to detect and track different classes of toxic phytoplankton. In the EU FP6-project ALGADEC, a portable semi-automated biosensor system was developed in order to facilitate the detection of toxic algae in water samples. This prototype enables the electrochemical detection of microalgae in less than 2 h without the need of expensive equipment. This device serves as a cornerstone of a new molecular-based strategy for the monitoring HABs.[146]

A new algorithm termed the surface algal bloom index (SABI) has been proposed to delineate the spatial distributions of floating micro-algal species like cyanobacteria or exposed inter-tidal vegetation like sea grass. This algorithm was specifically modeled to adapt to the marine habitat through its inclusion of ocean-color-sensitive bands in a four-band ratio-based relationship. The algorithm has demonstrated high stability against various environmental conditions like aerosol and sun glint.[147]

The OPD placed on a variety of ocean platforms, and the beach conditions reporting system (BCRS) constitutes an HAB observing system.[148]

Complementary methods could be necessary in order to achieve an almost real-time HAB monitoring or tracking. For instance, in the monitoring of the toxic *Ostreopsis* blooms, PCR-based methods proved to be effective tools complementary to microscopy for rapid and specific detection of *Ostreopsis* and other toxic dinoflagellates in marine coastal environments.[34]

In summary, in order to evaluate changes in marine ecosystems and to monitor and manage HABs in coastal waters, strategies should be adopted by countries worldwide. Different and complementary approaches will be necessary to have useful information related to phytoplankton forecasting and occurrence of HABs episodes.

ACKNOWLEDGMENTS

This study was financed through research grants AGL2009-13581-C02-02 and AGL2012-40185-C02-02 from the Ministerio de Ciencia e Innovación (Ministry of Science and Innovation, Spanish Government) and through the European research project grants CiguaTools-Development of a Rapid Test Kit and supporting Reference Standards Capable of Detecting the Emerging Fish Toxin Ciguatoxin in European and Global Waters (315285-FP7-SME-2012) and Pharmatlantic-Knowledge Transfer Network for Prevention of Mental Diseases and Cancer in the Atlantic Area (2009-1/117) financed by ERDF funds within the Atlantic Area Operational Programme.

REFERENCES

1. Hallegraeff, G., Anderson, D., and Cembella, A., 2003. *Harmful Algal Blooms: A Global Overview*. UNESCO, Paris, France.
2. Reguera, B., Rodriguez, F., and Blanco, J., 2012. Harmful algae blooms and food safety: Physiological and environmental factors affecting toxin production and their accumulation in shellfish, in *New Trends in Marine and Freshwater Toxins*. Cabado, A. G. and Vieites, J. M., eds., Nova Science Publishers, Inc., New York. pp. 53–89.
3. Anderson, D. M., 2009. Approaches to monitoring, control and management of harmful algal blooms. *Ocean & Coastal Management*, 52, 342–347.
4. European Parliament and the Council of the European Union, 2004. Regulation (EC) No 854/2004 of the European Parliament and of the Council of 29 April 2004 laying down specific rules for the organisation of official controls on products of animal origin intended for human consumption, *Official Journal of the European Union*, 47, L139, 30.4.2004, pp. 206–320.
5. European Commission, 2004. COMMISSION REGULATION (EC) No 2074/2005 of 5 December 2005 laying down implementing measures for certain products under regulation (EC) No 853/2004 of the European Parliament and of the Council and for the organisation of official controls under Regulation (EC) No 854/2004 of the European Parliament and of the Council and Regulation (EC) No 882/2004

of the European Parliament and of the Council, derogating from Regulation (EC) No 852/2004 of the European Parliament and of the Council and amending Regulations (EC) No 853/2004 and (EC) No 854/2004, *Official Journal of the European Union*, 48, L338, 22.12.2005, pp. 27–59.

6. European Commission, 2011. COMMISSION REGULATION (EU) No 15/2011 of 10 January 2011 amending Regulation (EC) No 2074/2005 as regards recognised testing methods for detecting marine biotoxins in live bivalve mollusks. *Official Journal of the European Union*, L6m, 11.1.2011, pp. 3–6.

7. Anderson, D. M., Cembella, A. D., and Hallegraeff, G. M., 2012. Progress in understanding harmful algal blooms: Paradigm shifts and new technologies for research, monitoring, and management. *Annual Review of Marine Science*, 4, 143–176.

8. Fritz, L. and Triemer, R. E., 1985. A rapid simple technique using calcofluor White M2R for the study of dinoflagellate thecal plates. *Journal of Phycology*, 21, 662–664.

9. González-Fernández, A., Garet, E., Kleivdal, H., Elliot, C., and Campbell, K., 2012. Immunological methods for detection of toxic algae and phycotoxins: Immunofluorescence, ELISAS and other innovative techniques, in *New Trends in Marine and Freshwater Toxins*. Cabado, A. G. and Vieites, J. M., eds. NovaScience Publishers, Inc., New York. pp. 267–303.

10. Perpezak, L., Vrieling, E. G., Sandee, B., and Rutten, T., 2000. Immuno flow cytometry in marine phytoplankton research. *Scientia Marina*, 64, 165–181.

11. Carrera, M., Garet, E., Barreiro, A. et al., 2010. Generation of monoclonal antibodies for the specific immunodetection of the toxic dinoflagellate *Alexandrium minutum* Halim from Spanish waters. *Harmful Algae*, 9, 272–280.

12. Campbell, L., Olson, R. J., Sosik, H. M. et al., 2010. First harmful *Dinophysis* (Dinophyceae, Dinophysiales) bloom in the US is revealed by automated imaging flow cytometry. *Journal of Phycology*, 46, 66–75.

13. Medlin, L. K., Lange, M., and Nothig, E. M., 2000. Genetic diversity in the marine phytoplankton: A review and a consideration of Antarctic phytoplankton. *Antarctic Science*, 12, 325–333.

14. Medlin, L. K., Metfies, K., Mehl, H., Wiltshire, K., and Valentin, K., 2006. Picoeukaryotic plankton diversity at the Helgoland time series site as assessed by three molecular methods. *Microbial Ecology*, 52, 53–71.

15. Ebenezer, V., Medlin, L. K., and Ki, J.-S., 2012. Molecular detection, quantification, and diversity evaluation of microalgae. *Marine Biotechnology*, 14, 129–142.

16. De Bruin, A., Ibelings, B. W., and Van Donk, E., 2003. Molecular techniques in phytoplankton research: From allozyme electrophoresis to genomics. *Hydrobiologia*, 491, 47–63.

17. Humbert, J. F., Quiblier, C., and Gugger, M., 2010. Molecular approaches for monitoring potentially toxic marine and freshwater phytoplankton species. *Analytical and Bioanalytical Chemistry*, 397, 1723–1732.

18. Bott, N. J., Ophel-Keller, K. M., Sierp, M. T. et al., 2010. Toward routine, DNA-based detection methods for marine pests. *Biotechnology Advances*, 28, 706–714.

19. Kudela, R. M., Howard, M. D. A., Jenkins, B. D., Miller, P. E., and Smith, G. J., 2010. Using the molecular toolbox to compare harmful algal blooms in upwelling systems. *Progress in Oceanography*, 85, 108–121.

20. Volpi, E. V. and Bridger, J. M., 2008. FISH glossary: An overview of the fluorescence in situ hybridization technique. *Biotechniques*, 45, 385.

21. Amann, R. I., Krumholz, L., and Stahl, D. A., 1990. Fluorescent-oligonucleotide probing of whole cells for determinative, phylogenetic, and environmental-studies in microbiology. *Journal of Bacteriology*, 172, 762–770.

22. Hosoi-Tanabe, S. and Sako, Y., 2005. Rapid detection of natural cells of *Alexandrium tamarense* and *A. catenella* (*Dinophyceae*) by fluorescence in situ hybridization. *Harmful Algae*, 4, 319–328.

23. Hosoi-Tanabe, S. and Sako, Y., 2006. Development and application of fluorescence in situ hybridization (FISH) method for simple and rapid identification of the toxic dinoflagellates *Alexandrium tamarense* and *Alexandrium catenella* in cultured and natural seawater. *Fisheries Science*, 72, 77–82.

24. Raap, A. K., 1998. Advances in fluorescence in situ hybridization. *Mutation Research—Fundamental and Molecular Mechanisms of Mutagenesis*, 400, 287–298.

25. Stahl, D. A., Flesher, B., Mansfield, H. R., and Montgomery, L., 1988. Use of phylogenetically based hybridization probes for studies of ruminal microbial ecology. *Applied and Environmental Microbiology*, 54, 1079–1084.

26. Sellner, K. G., Doucette, G. J., and Kirkpatrick, G. J., 2003. Harmful algal blooms: Causes, impacts and detection. *Journal of Industrial Microbiology & Biotechnology*, 30, 383–406.

27. Adachi, M., Sako, Y., and Ishida, Y., 1996. Identification of the toxic dinoflagellates *Alexandrium catenella* and *A. tamarense* (*Dinophyceae*) using DNA probes and whole-cell hybridization. *Journal of Phycology*, 32, 1049–1052.

28. Sako, Y., Hosoi-Tanabe, S., and Uchida, A., 2004. Fluorescence in situ hybridization using rRNA-targeted probes for simple and rapid identification of the toxic dinoflagellates *Alexandrium tamarense* and *Alexandrium catenella*. *Journal of Phycology*, 40, 598–605.

29. Touzet, N., Keady, E., Raine, R., and Maher, M., 2009. Evaluation of taxa-specific real-time PCR, whole-cell FISH and morphotaxonomy analyses for the detection and quantification of the toxic microalgae *Alexandrium minutum* (Dinophyceae), Global Clade ribotype. *FEMS Microbiology Ecology*, 67, 329–341.

30. Touzet, N., Davidson, K., Pete, R. et al., 2010. Co-occurrence of the West European (Gr.III) and North American (Gr.I) Ribotypes of *Alexandrium tamarense* (Dinophyceae) in Shetland, Scotland. *Protist*, 161, 370–384.

31. John, U., Medlin, L. K., and Groben, R., 2005. Development of specific rRNA probes to distinguish between geographic clades of the *Alexandrium tamarense* species complex. *Journal of Plankton Research*, 27, 199–204.

32. Kim, C. J. and Sako, Y., 2005. Molecular identification of toxic *Alexandrium tamiyavanichii* (Dinophyceae) using two DNA probes. *Harmful Algae*, 4, 984–991.

33. Gescher, C., Metfies, K., and Medlin, L. K., 2008. The ALEX CHIP—Development of a DNA chip for identification and monitoring of *Alexandrium*. *Harmful Algae*, 7, 485–494.

34. Penna, A., Bertozzini, E., Battocchi, C. et al., 2007. Monitoring of HAB species in the Mediterranean Sea through molecular methods. *Journal of Plankton Research*, 29, 19–38.

35. Takahashi, Y., Takishita, K., Koike, K. et al., 2005. Development of molecular probes for *Dinophysis* (Dinophyceae) plastid: A tool to predict blooming and explore plastid origin. *Marine Biotechnology*, 7, 95–103.

36. Miller, P. E. and Scholin, C. A., 1998. Identification and enumeration of cultured and wild *Pseudo-nitzschia* (Bacillariophyceae) using species-specific LSU rRNA-targeted fluorescent probes and filter-based whole cell hybridization. *Journal of Phycology*, 34, 371–382.

37. Miller, P. E. and Scholin, C. A., 2000. On detection of *Pseudo-nitzschia* (Bacillariophyceae) species using whole cell hybridization: Sample fixation and stability. *Journal of Phycology*, 36, 238–250.

38. Turrell, E., Bresnan, E., Collins, C., Brown, L., Graham, J., and Grieve, A., 2008. Detection of *Pseudo-nitzschia* (Bacillariophyceae) species and amnesic shellfish toxins in Scottish coastal waters using oligonucleotide probes and the Jellet Rapid Test (TM). *Harmful Algae*, 7, 443–458.

39. Ebenezer, V., Medlin, L. K., and Ki, J. S., 2012. Molecular detection, quantification, and diversity evaluation of microalgae. *Marine Biotechnology*, 14, 129–142.

40. Guillou, L., Nezan, E., Cueff, V. et al., 2002. Genetic diversity and molecular detection of three toxic dinoflagellate genera (*Alexandrium, Dinophysis,* and *Karenia*) from French coasts. *Protist*, 153, 223–238.

41. Godhe, A., Asplund, M. E., Harnstrom, K., Saravanan, V., Tyagi, A., and Karunasagar, I., 2008. Quantification of diatom and dinoflagellate biomasses in coastal marine seawater samples by real-time PCR. *Applied and Environmental Microbiology*, 74, 7174–7182.

42. Wang, L., Li, L., Alam, M. J. et al., 2008. Loop-mediated isothermal amplification method for rapid detection of the toxic dinoflagellate *Alexandrium*, which causes algal blooms and poisoning of shellfish. *FEMS Microbiology Letters*, 282, 15–21.

43. Nagai, S., 2011. Development of a multiplex PCR assay for simultaneous detection of six *Alexandrium* species (Dinophyceae). *Journal of Phycology*, 47, 703–708.

44. Zhang, F., Shi, Y., Jiang, K., Xu, Z., and Ma, L., 2012. Sensitive and rapid detection of two toxic microalgae *Alexandrium* by loop-mediated isothermal amplification. *Acta Oceanologica Sinica*, 31, 139–146.

45. Edvardsen, B., Shalchian-Tabrizi, K., Jakobsen, K. S. et al., 2003. Genetic variability and molecular phylogeny of *Dinophysis* species (Dinophyceae) from Norwegian waters inferred from single cell analyses of rDNA. *Journal of Phycology*, 39, 395–408.

46. Ki, J. S., Jang, G. Y., and Han, M. S., 2004. Integrated method for single-cell DNA extraction, PCR amplification, and sequencing of ribosomal DNA from harmful dinoflagellates *Cochlodinium polykrikoides* and *Alexandrium catenella*. *Marine Biotechnology*, 6, 587–593.

47. Takano, Y. and Horiguchi, T., 2006. Acquiring scanning electron microscopical, light microscopical and multiple gene sequence data from a single dinoflagellate cell. *Journal of Phycology*, 42, 251–256.

48. Richlen, M. L. and Barber, P. H., 2005. A technique for the rapid extraction of microalgal DNA from single live and preserved cells. *Molecular Ecology Notes*, 5, 688–691.
49. Masseret, E., Enquebecq, M., Laabir, M., Genovesi, B., Vaquer, A., and Avarre, J.-C., 2010. A simple and innovative method for species identification of phytoplankton cells on minute quantities of DNA. *Environmental Microbiology Reports*, 2, 715–719.
50. Lang, I. and Kaczmarska, I., 2011. A protocol for a single-cell PCR of diatoms from fixed samples: Method validation using *Ditylum brightwellii* (T. West) Grunow. *Diatom Research*, 26, 43–49.
51. Man-Aharonovich, D., Philosof, A., Kirkup, B. C. et al., 2010. Diversity of active marine picoeukaryotes in the Eastern Mediterranean Sea unveiled using photosystem-II psbA transcripts. *ISME Journal*, 4, 1044–1052.
52. Shi, X., Lin, L.-I., Chen, S.-y., Chao, S.-h., Zhang, W., and Meldrum, D. R., 2011. Real-time PCR of single bacterial cells on an array of adhering droplets. *Lab on a Chip*, 11, 2276–2281.
53. Oldach, D. W., Delwiche, C. F., Jakobsen, K. S. et al., 2000. Heteroduplex mobility assay-guided sequence discovery: Elucidation of the small subunit (18S) rDNA sequences of *Pfiesteria piscicida* and related dinoflagellates from complex algal culture and environmental sample DNA pools. *Proceedings of the National Academy of Sciences of the United States of America*, 97, 4303–4308.
54. Rublee, P. A., Kempton, J. W., Schaefer, E. F. et al., 2001. Use of molecular probes to assess geographic distribution of *Pfiesteria* species. *Environmental Health Perspectives*, 109, 765–767.
55. Handy, S. M., Hutchins, D. A., Cary, S. C., and Coyne, K. J., 2006. Simultaneous enumeration of multiple raphidophyte species by quantitative real-time PCR: Capabilities and limitations. *Limnology and Oceanography-Methods*, 4, 193–204.
56. Lin, S. J., Zhang, H., and Jiao, N. Z., 2006. Potential utility of mitochondrial cytochrome b and its mRNA editing in resolving closely related dinoflagellates: A case study of *Prorocentrum* (Dinophyceae). *Journal of Phycology*, 42, 646–654.
57. Otero, A., Chapela, M. J., Lago, J. et al., 2011. Genetic Variability of *Gambierdiscus* spp. strains using RAPD analysis and cytochrome b sequencing, in *Marine and Freshwater Toxins Analysis. Second Joint Symposium and AOAC Task Force Meeting*, AOAC International, Bayona, Spain.
58. Howard, M. D. A., Jones, A. C., Schnetzer, A. et al., 2012. Quantitative real-time Polymerase Chain Reaction for *Cochlodinium fulvescens* (Dinophyceae), a harmful dinoflagellate from California coastal waters. *Journal of Phycology*, 48, 384–393.
59. Churro, C., Pereira, P., Vasconcelos, V., and Valerio, E., 2012. Species-specific real-time PCR cell number quantification of the bloom-forming cyanobacterium *Planktothrix agardhii*. *Archives of Microbiology*, 194, 749–757.
60. Kavanagh, S., Brennan, C., O'Connor, L. et al., 2010. Real-time PCR detection of *Dinophysis* species in Irish coastal waters. *Marine Biotechnology*, 12, 534–542.
61. Vandersea, M. W., Kibler, S. R., Holland, W. C. et al., 2012. Development of semi-quantitative PCR assays for the detection and enumeration of *Gambierdiscus* species (Gonyaulacales, Dinophyceae). *Journal of Phycology*, 48, 902–915.
62. Yuan, J., Mi, T., Zhen, Y., and Yu, Z., 2012. Development of a rapid detection and quantification method of *Karenia mikimotoi* by real-time quantitative PCR. *Harmful Algae*, 17, 83–91.
63. Bowers, H. A., Tengs, T., Glasgow, H. B., Burkholder, J. M., Rublee, P. A., and Oldach, D. W., 2000. Development of real-time PCR assays for rapid detection of *Pfiesteria piscicida* and related dinoflagellates. *Applied and Environmental Microbiology*, 66, 4641–4648.
64. Zamor, R. M., Glenn, K. L., and Hambright, K. D., 2012. Incorporating molecular tools into routine HAB monitoring programs: Using qPCR to track invasive *Prymnesium*. *Harmful Algae*, 15, 1–7.
65. Yuan, J., Mi, T., Zhen, Y., and Yu, Z., 2012. Development of a real-time PCR method (Taqman) for rapid identification and quantification of *Prorocentrum donghaiense*. *Journal of Ocean University of China*, 11, 366–374.
66. Fitzpatrick, E., Caron, D. A., and Schnetzer, A., 2010. Development and environmental application of a genus-specific quantitative PCR approach for *Pseudo-nitzschia* species. *Marine Biology*, 157, 1161–1169.
67. Andree, K. B., Fernandez-Tejedor, M., Elandaloussi, L. M. et al., 2011. Quantitative PCR coupled with melt curve analysis for detection of selected *Pseudo-nitzschia* spp. (Bacillariophyceae) from the Northwestern Mediterranean Sea. *Applied and Environmental Microbiology*, 77, 1651–1659.
68. Rehnstam, A. S., Backman, S., Smith, D. C., Azam, F., and Hagstrom, A., 1993. Blooms of sequence-specific culturable bacteria in the sea. *FEMS Microbiology Ecology*, 102, 161–166.

69. Gescher, C., Metfies, K., Frickenhaus, S., Knefelkamp, B., Wiltshire, K. H., and Medlin, L. K., 2008. Feasibility of assessing the community composition of prasinophytes at the Helgoland roads sampling site with a DNA microarray. *Applied and Environmental Microbiology*, 74, 5305–5316.

70. Berzano, M., Marcheggiani, S., Rombini, S., and Spurio, R., 2012. The application of oligonucleotide probes and microarrays for the identification of freshwater diatoms. *Hydrobiologia*, 695, 57–72.

71. Galluzzi, L., Cegna, A., Casabianca, S., Penna, A., Saunders, N., and Magnani, M., 2011. Development of an oligonucleotide microarray for the detection and monitoring of marine dinoflagellates. *Journal of Microbiological Methods*, 84, 234–242.

72. Chang, C. I., Hung, P. H., Wu, C. C. et al., 2012. Simultaneous detection of multiple fish pathogens using a naked-eye readable DNA microarray. *Sensors*, 12, 2710–2728.

73. Lievens, B., Frans, I., Heusdens, C. et al., 2011. Rapid detection and identification of viral and bacterial fish pathogens using a DNA array-based multiplex assay. *Journal of Fish Diseases*, 34, 861–875.

74. Warsen, A. E., Krug, M. J., LaFrentz, S., Stanek, D. R., Loge, F. J., and Call, D. R., 2004. Simultaneous discrimination between 15 fish pathogens by using 16S ribosomal DNA PCR and DNA microarrays. *Applied and Environmental Microbiology*, 70, 4216–4221.

75. Kellogg, C. A., Piceno, Y. M., Tom, L. M., DeSantis, T. Z., Zawada, D. G., and Andersen, G. L., 2012. PhyloChip™ microarray comparison of sampling methods used for coral microbial ecology. *Journal of Microbiological Methods*, 88, 103–109.

76. Miletto, M., Loy, A., Antheunisse, A. M., Loeb, R., Bodelier, P. L. E., and Laanbroek, H. J., 2008. Biogeography of sulfate-reducing prokaryotes in river floodplains. *FEMS Microbiology Ecology*, 64, 395–406.

77. Gescher, C., Metfies, K., and Medlin, L. K., 2008. The ALEX CHIP-Development of a DNA chip for identification and monitoring of *Alexandrium*. *Harmful Algae*, 7, 485–494.

78. Metfies, K. and Medlin, L. K., 2008. Feasibility of transferring fluorescent in situ hybridization probes to an 18S rRNA gene phylochip and mapping of signal intensities. *Applied and Environmental Microbiology*, 74, 2814–2821.

79. Ki, J. S. and Han, M. S., 2006. A low-density oligonucleotide array study for parallel detection of harmful algal species using hybridization of consensus PCR products of LSU rDNA D2 domain. *Biosensors and Bioelectronics*, 21, 1812–1821.

80. Zhou, J., 2003. Microarrays for bacterial detection and microbial community analysis. *Current Opinion in Microbiology*, 6, 288–294.

81. Scorzetti, G., Brand, L. E., Hitchcock, G. L., Rein, K. S., Sinigalliano, C. D., and Fell, J. W., 2009. Multiple simultaneous detection of Harmful Algal Blooms (HABs) through a high throughput bead array technology, with potential use in phytoplankton community analysis. *Harmful Algae*, 8, 196–211.

82. Ahn, S., Kulis, D. M., Erdner, D. L., Anderson, D. M., and Walt, D. R., 2006. Fiber-optic microarray for simultaneous detection of multiple harmful algal bloom species. *Applied and Environmental Microbiology*, 72, 5742–5749.

83. Saiki, R. K., Walsh, P. S., Levenson, C. H., and Erlich, H. A., 1989. Genetic analysis of amplified DNA with immobilized sequence-specific oligonucleotide probes. *Proceedings of the National Academy of Sciences of the United States of America*, 86, 6230–6234.

84. Guo, Z., Guilfoyle, R. A., Thiel, A. J., Wang, R., and Smith, L. M., 1994. Direct fluorescence analysis of genetic polymorphisms by hybridization with oligonucleotide arrays on glass supports. *Nucleic Acids Research*, 22, 5456–5465.

85. Yershov, G., Barsky, V., Belgovskiy, A. et al., 1996. DNA analysis and diagnostics on oligonucleotide microchips. *Proceedings of the National Academy of Sciences of the United States of America*, 93, 4913–4918.

86. Gentry, T. J., Wickham, G. S., Schadt, C. W., He, Z., and Zhou, J., 2006. Microarray applications in microbial ecology research. *Microbial Ecology*, 52, 159–175.

87. Walsh, P. J., Bookman, R. J., Zaias, J. et al., 2003. Toxicogenomic effects of marine brevetoxins in liver and brain of mouse. *Comparative Biochemistry and Physiology—B Biochemistry and Molecular Biology*, 136, 173–182.

88. Morey, J. S., Ryan, J. C., Dechraoui, M. Y. B. et al., 2008. Liver genomic responses to ciguatoxin: Evidence for activation of phase I and phase II detoxification pathways following an acute hypothermic response in mice. *Toxicological Sciences*, 103, 298–310.

89. Ryan, J. C., Bottein Dechraoui, M. Y., Morey, J. S. et al., 2007. Transcriptional profiling of whole blood and serum protein analysis of mice exposed to the neurotoxin Pacific Ciguatoxin-1. *NeuroToxicology*, 28, 1099–1109.

90. Ryan, J. C., Morey, J. S., Ramsdell, J. S., and Van Dolah, F. M., 2005. Acute phase gene expression in mice exposed to the marine neurotoxin domoic acid. *Neuroscience*, 136, 1121–1132.
91. Twiner, M. J., Ryan, J. C., Morey, J. S. et al., 2008. Transcriptional profiling and inhibition of cholesterol biosynthesis in human T lymphocyte cells by the marine toxin azaspiracid. *Genomics*, 91, 289–300.
92. Lievens, B., Claes, L., Vanachter, A. C. R. C., Cammue, B. P. A., and Thomma, B. P. H. J., 2006. Detecting single nucleotide polymorphisms using DNA arrays for plant pathogen diagnosis. *FEMS Microbiology Letters*, 255, 129–139.
93. Anderson, D. M., Kulis, D., Erdner, D., Ahn, S., and Walt, D., 2006. Fibre optic microarrays for the detection and enumeration of harmful algal bloom species. *African Journal of Marine Science*, 28, 231–235.
94. Diaz, M. R., Jacobson, J. W., Goodwin, K. D., Dunbar, S. A., and Fell, J. W., 2010. Molecular detection of harmful algal blooms (HABs) using locked nucleic acids and bead array technology. *Limnology and Oceanography: Methods*, 8, 269–284.
95. Rudi, K., Skulberg, O. M., Skulberg, R., and Jakobsen, K. S., 2000. Application of sequence-specific labeled 16S rRNA gene oligonucleotide probes for genetic profiling of cyanobacterial abundance and diversity by array hybridization. *Applied and Environmental Microbiology*, 66, 4004–4011.
96. MIDI-CHIP. Microbial Diversity Chip, http://www.cip.ulg.ac.be/midichip/2000 (accessed July 31, 2003).
97. Ellison, C. K. and Burton, R. S., 2005. Application of bead array technology to community dynamics of marine phytoplankton. *Marine Ecology Progress Series*, 288, 75–85.
98. Fish and Chips. Towards DNA chip technology as a standard analytical tool for the identification of the marine organisms in biodiversity and ecosystem science, 2004, www.fish-and-chhips.uni-bremen.de.
99. Pearson, L. A. and Neilan, B. A., 2008. The molecular genetics of cyanobacterial toxicity as a basis for monitoring water quality and public health risk. *Current Opinion in Biotechnology*, 19, 281–288.
100. Stoughton, R. B., 2005. Applications of DNA microarrays in biology. *Annual Review of Biochemistry*, 74, 53–82.
101. Pomati, F., Kellmann, R., Cavalieri, R., Burns, B. P., and Neilan, B. A., 2006. Comparative gene expression of PSP-toxin producing and non-toxic *Anabaena circinalis* strains. *Environment International*, 32, 743–748.
102. Mikalsen, B., Boison, G., Skulberg, O. M. et al., 2003. Natural variation in the microcystin synthetase operon mcyABC and impact on microcystin production in *Microcystis* strains. *Journal of Bacteriology*, 185, 2774–2785.
103. Hisbergues, M., Christiansen, G., Rouhiainen, L., Sivonen, K., and Börner, T., 2003. PCR-based identification of microcystin-producing genotypes of different cyanobacterial genera. *Archives of Microbiology*, 180, 402–410.
104. Tillett, D., Parker, D. L., and Neilan, B. A., 2001. Detection of toxigenicity by a probe for the Microcystin Synthetase a Gene (mcyA) of the Cyanobacterial Genus Microcystis: Comparison of toxicities with 16S rRNa and Phycocyanin Operon (Phycocyanin Intergenic Spacer) Phylogenies. *Applied and Environmental Microbiology*, 67, 2810–2818.
105. Golubic, S., Abed, R. M. M., Palińska, K., Pauillac, S., Chinain, M., and Laurent, D., 2010. Marine toxic cyanobacteria: Diversity, environmental responses and hazards. *Toxicon*, 56, 836–841.
106. Sipari, H., Rantala-Ylinen, A., Jokela, J., Oksanen, I., and Sivonen, K., 2010. Development of a chip assay and quantitative PCR for detecting microcystin synthetase E gene expressions. *Applied and Environmental Microbiology*, 76, 3797–3805.
107. Jonasson, S., Vintila, S., Sivonen, K., and El-Shehawy, R., 2008. Expression of the nodularin synthetase genes in the Baltic Sea bloom-former cyanobacterium *Nodularia spumigena* strain AV1. *FEMS Microbiology Ecology*, 65, 31–39.
108. Rantala, A., Rizzi, E., Castiglioni, B., De Bellis, G., and Sivonen, K., 2008. Identification of hepatotoxin-producing cyanobacteria by DNA-chip. *Environmental Microbiology*, 10, 653–664.
109. Yang, I., John, U., Beszteri, S. et al., 2010. Comparative gene expression in toxic versus non-toxic strains of the marine dinoflagellate *Alexandrium minutum. BMC Genomics,* 1, 248.
110. Bovee, T. F. H., Hendriksen, P. J. M., Portier, L. et al., 2011. Tailored microarray platform for the detection of marine toxins. *Environmental Science and Technology*, 45, 8965–8973.
111. Smith, M. W., Maier, M. A., Suciu, D. et al., 2012. High resolution microarray assay for rapid taxonomic assessment of *Pseudo-nitzschia* spp. (Bacillariophyceae) in the field. *Harmful Algae*, 19, 169–180.

112. Justé, A., Thomma, B. P. H. J., and Lievens, B., 2008. Recent advances in molecular techniques to study microbial communities in food-associated matrices and processes. *Food Microbiology*, 25, 745–761.
113. Medlin, L. K. and Kooistra, W. H. C. F., 2010. Methods to estimate the diversity in the marine photosynthetic protist community with illustrations from case studies: A review. *Diversity*, 2, 973–1014.
114. Lievens, B., Grauwet, T. J. M. A., Cammue, B. P. A., and Thomma, B. P. H. J., 2005. Recent developments in diagnostics of plant pathogens: A review. In: *Recent Research Developments in Microbiology*. Pandalai, S.G., ed. Vol. 9, Part I, 2005, pp. 57–59.
115. Cho, J. C. and Tiedje, J. M., 2002. Quantitative detection of microbial genes by using DNA microarrays. *Applied and Environmental Microbiology*, 68, 1425–1430.
116. Lievens, B., Brouwer, M., Vanachter, A. C. R. C., Lévesque, C. A., Cammue, B. P. A., and Thomma, B. P. H. J., 2005. Quantitative assessment of phytopathogenic fungi in various substrates using a DNA macroarray. *Environmental Microbiology*, 7, 1698–1710.
117. Loy, A., Schulz, C., Lücker, S. et al., 2005. 16S rRNA gene-based oligonucleotide microarray for environmental monitoring of the betaproteobacterial order "Rhodocyclales". *Applied and Environmental Microbiology*, 71, 1373–1386.
118. Metfies, K., Huljic, S., Lange, M., and Medlin, L. K., 2005. Electrochemical detection of the toxic dinoflagellate *Alexandrium ostenfeldii* with a DNA-biosensor. *Biosensors and Bioelectronics*, 20, 1349–1357.
119. Cho, J. C. and Tiedje, J. M., 2001. Bacterial species determination from DNA–DNA hybridization by using genome fragments and DNA microarrays. *Applied and Environmental Microbiology*, 67, 3677–3682.
120. Byoung, C. K., Ji, H. P., and Man, B. G., 2004. Development of a DNA microarray chip for the identification of sludge bacteria using an unsequenced random genomic DNA hybridization method. *Environmental Science and Technology*, 38, 6767–6774.
121. Denef, V. J., Park, J., Rodrigues, J. L. M., Tsoi, T. V., Hashsham, S. A., and Tiedje, J. M., 2003. Validation of a more sensitive method for using spotted oligonucleotide DNA microarrays for functional genomics studies on bacterial communities. *Environmental Microbiology*, 5, 933–943.
122. Rhee, S. K., Liu, X., Wu, L., Chong, S. C., Wan, X., and Zhou, J., 2004. Detection of genes involved in biodegradation and biotransformation in microbial communities by using 50-mer oligonucleotide microarrays. *Applied and Environmental Microbiology*, 70, 4303–4317.
123. Reysenbach, A. L., Giver, L. J., Wickham, G. S., and Pace, N. R., 1992. Differential amplification of rRNA genes by polymerase chain reaction. *Applied and Environmental Microbiology*, 58, 3417–3418.
124. Lilly, E. L., Halanych, K. M., and Anderson, D. M., 2007. Species boundaries and global biogeography of the *Alexandrium tamarense* complex (Dinophyceae)1. *Journal of Phycology*, 43, 1329–1338.
125. Stucken, K., John, U., Cembella, A. et al., 2010. The smallest known genomes of multicellular and toxic cyanobacteria: Comparison, minimal gene sets for linked traits and the evolutionary implications. *PLoS One*, 5, e9235.
126. Hackett, J. D., Wisecaver, J. H., Brosnahan, M. L. et al., 2013. Evolution of saxitoxin synthesis in cyanobacteria and dinoflagellates. *Molecular Biology and Evolution*, 30, 70–78.
127. Jaeckisch, N., Glöckner, G., Vogel, H., Cembella, A., and John, U., Genomic characterization of the spirolide-producing dinoflagellate *Alexandrium ostenfeldii* with special emphasis on PKS genes, in *Proceedings of the 12th International Conference on Harmful Algae*, Moestrup, O. et al., eds. ISSHA and IOC-UNESCO, Copenhagen, Denmark, 2006.
128. Monroe, E. A. and Van Dolah, F. M., 2008. The toxic dinoflagellate *Karenia brevis* encodes novel type I-like polyketide synthases containing discrete catalytic domains. *Protist*, 159, 471–482.
129. Humbert, J., Quiblier, C., and Gugger, M., 2010. Molecular approaches for monitoring potentially toxic marine and freshwater phytoplankton species. *Analytical and Bioanalytical Chemistry*, 397, 1723–1732.
130. Jungblut, A.-D. and Neilan, B., 2006. Molecular identification and evolution of the cyclic peptide hepatotoxins, microcystin and nodularin, synthetase genes in three orders of cyanobacteria. *Archives of Microbiology*, 185, 107–114.
131. Christiansen, G., Kurmayer, R., Liu, Q., and Barner, T., 2006. Transposons inactivate biosynthesis of the nonribosomal meptide microcystin in naturally occurring *Planktothrix* spp. *Applied and Environmental Microbiology*, 72, 117–123.
132. Mbedi, S., Welker, M., Fastner, J., and Wiedner, C., 2005. Variability of the microcystin synthetase gene cluster in the genus *Planktothrix* (*Oscillatoriales*, Cyanobacteria). *FEMS Microbiology Letters*, 245, 299–306.

133. Al-Tebrineh, J., Gehringer, M. M., Akcaalan, R., and Neilan, B. A., 2011. A new quantitative PCR assay for the detection of hepatotoxigenic cyanobacteria. *Toxicon*, 57, 546–554.

134. Wiese, M., D'Agostino, P. M., Mihali, T. K., Moffitt, M. C., and Neilan, B. A., 2010. Neurotoxic alkaloids: Saxitoxin and its analogs. *Marine Drugs*, 8, 2185–2211.

135. Rasmussen, J. P., Giglio, S., Monis, P. T., Campbell, R. J., and Saint, C. P., 2008. Development and field testing of a real-time PCR assay for cylindrospermopsin-producing cyanobacteria. *Journal of Applied Microbiology*, 104, 1503–1515.

136. Kellmann, R., Mihali, T. K., Jeon, Y. J., Pickford, R., Pomati, F., and Neilan, B. A., 2008. Biosynthetic intermediate analysis and functional homology reveal a saxitoxin gene cluster in cyanobacteria. *Applied and Environmental Microbiology*, 74, 4044–4053.

137. Al-Tebrineh, J., Mihali, T. K., Pomati, F., and Neilan, B. A., 2010. Detection of saxitoxin-producing cyanobacteria and *Anabaena circinalis* in environmental water blooms by quantitative PCR. *Applied and Environmental Microbiology*, 76, 7836–7842.

138. Méjean, A., Mann, S., Maldiney, T., Vassiliadis, G., Lequin, O., and Ploux, O., 2009. Evidence that biosynthesis of the neurotoxic alkaloids anatoxin-a and homoanatoxin-a in the *Cyanobacterium Oscillatoria* PCC 6506 occurs on a modular polyketide synthase initiated by l-proline. *Journal of the American Chemical Society*, 131, 7512–7513.

139. Sipari, H., Rantala-Ylinen, A., Jokela, J., Oksanen, I., and Sivonen, K., 2010. Development of a chip assay and quantitative PCR for detecting microcystin synthetase E gene expression. *Applied and Environmental Microbiology*, 76, 3797–3805.

140. Al-Tebrineh, J., Pearson, L. A., Yasar, S. A., and Neilan, B. A., 2012. A multiplex qPCR targeting hepato- and neurotoxigenic cyanobacteria of global significance. *Harmful Algae*, 15, 19–25.

141. Shen, L., Xu, H., and Guo, X., 2012. Satellite remote sensing of Harmful Algal Blooms (HABs) and a potential synthesized framework. *Sensors*, 12, 7778–7803.

142. Cannizzaro, J. P., Hu, C., English, D. C., Carder, K. C., Heil, C. A., and Muller-Karger, F. E., 2009. Detection of *Karenia brevis* blooms on the west Florida shelf using in situ backscattering and fluorescence data. *Harmful Algae*, 8, 898–909.

143. McKenzie, A. L., 2010. In situ passive solid phase adsorption of micro-algal biotoxins as a monitoring tool. *Current Opinion in Biotechnology*, 21, 326–331.

144. Rodríguez, P., Alfonso, A., Otero, P. et al., In press. Utilisation of solid-phase adsorption toxin tracking (SPATT) as a tool to monitor the presence of lipophilic shellfish toxins in the coastal waters of Western Europe. *Environmental Science & Technology*.

145. Hartley, H. A. and Baeumner, A. J., 2003. Biosensor for the specific detection of a single viable *B. anthracis* spore. *Analytical and Bioanalytical Chemistry*, 376, 319–327.

146. Hails, A., Boyes, C., Boyes, A. et al., 2009. The optical phytoplankton discriminator, in *OCEANS 2009, MTS/IEEE Biloxi—Marine Technology for Our Future: Global and Local Challenges*, Biloxi, MS. pp. 1–4.

147. Alawadi, F., 2010. Detection of surface algal blooms using the newly developed algorithm surface algal bloom index (SABI): *Remote Sensing of the Ocean, Sea Ice, and Large Water Regions*. Bostate, C.R.Jr. et al., eds. *Proc. of SPIE*, 7825, 782506.

148. Currier, R. D., Boyes, C., Hails, A., Nierenberg, K., Kirkpatrick, B., and Kirkpatrick, G., 2009. An ocean observing system for harmful algal bloom detection and tracking. *Oceans, MTS/IEEE Biloxi-Marine Technology for our Future: Global and Local Challenges,* pp.1–4.

18

Nanotechnology Applications in Aquatic Toxins

**Begoña Espiña, Verónica C. Martins, Manuel Bañobre-López,
Paulo P. Freitas, and José Rivas**

CONTENTS

18.1 Introduction

Nanosciences and nanotechnologies (N&N) are new approaches to research and development that concern the study of phenomena and manipulation of materials at atomic, molecular, and macromolecular scales, where properties differ significantly from those at a larger scale.

A good definition for nanotechnology comes from the National Nanotechnology Initiative (NNI), an American institution usually associated to the nanotechnology takeoff: "Nanotechnology is the understanding and control of matter at dimensions between approximately 1 and 100 nm, where unique

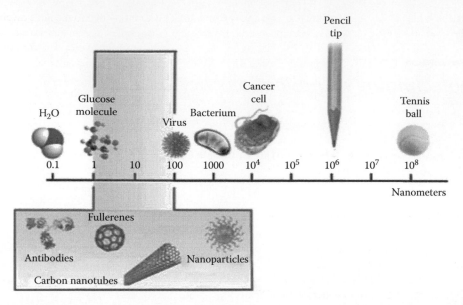

FIGURE 18.1 Nanoscale. At nanoscale we deal with antibodies and other biomolecules such as DNA. Additionally, fullerenes, carbon nanotubes, and other types of nanoparticles can be synthesized at this range. (From http://inl.int/what-is-nanotechnology-2)

phenomena enable novel applications (Figure 18.1). Encompassing nanoscale science, engineering, and technology, nanotechnology involves imaging, measuring, modeling, and manipulating matter at this length scale."

At the nanoscale, materials exhibit unusual and attractive chemical and physical properties. Besides, their extremely small feature size allows direct interaction with enzymes, proteins, DNA, and other biomolecules, opening great possibilities in several fields. For example, the biomedical field takes advantage of novel systems for drug delivery, gene therapy, and medical diagnostics; the food industry has seen improvements in the taste of food, food safety, and the health benefits from new food carriers; and at the environmental field nanotechnology can create materials and products that will advance our ability to monitor, detect, and clean up environmental contaminants.

Waterborne toxins are an example of such environmental contaminants, and in the last years nanotechnology has been commonly applied to this problem, mainly devoted to the development of new detection systems for monitoring. However, nanotechnology could also help to a better comprehension of the pharmacokinetic and biodistribution of toxins in the human body when they are consumed. Furthermore, new nano-based applications can be used to detoxify water, mollusks, or blood. In this chapter, we will discuss the current role of nanotechnology in the fields of both seawater and freshwater toxins and the future perspectives that this emerging approach can contribute to the risk management and toxicological knowledge about biotoxins.

18.2 Nanotech-Based Biosensors for Detection and Quantification of Aquatic Toxins

Safe drinking water and food is an issue of growing concern at a global scale. As a result, great efforts are being made to explore the potential impact of nanotechnology in water management at different fronts, namely, prevention of pollution, treatment and remediation, and sensing and detection.

Concerning the sensing and detection field, the main challenges consist in the development of novel sensing devices and enhanced detection strategies to promptly detect biological and chemical contaminants at very low concentration levels.

In particular, the detection of aquatic toxins is a very demanding task mainly due to the huge diversity of this group of analytes. Toxins of different biochemical natures and pathological effects require customized processes of sample extraction, purification, and detection. Therefore, a wide range of sensing principles have been established and many others still are under development to aid in the challenge of toxin detection, identification, and quantification. At this point, nanotechnology emerges as a valuable tool, where micro-/ nanofabrication processes and nanoscale materials and biomolecules are combined to give rise to a novel class of devices seeking for enhanced detection and quantification efficiencies.[1,2] Toxin analysis is benefiting from the advances of applying nanomaterials (e.g., thin-film materials, gold and magnetic nanoparticles, and carbon nanotubes [CNTs]) to biosensors development.[3] Compared to traditional detection methods, nano-materials-based biosensors may have higher selectivity, sensitivity, and stability, and are faster and cost less.[4]

In fact, actual monitoring programs for marine toxins suffer from lack of uniformity in the adopted analytical methods, as well as in their inter-laboratorial outcomes. Thus, in order to move away from mouse bioassay, an inexpensive but fast method still is needed, and biosensors show up as a promising choice.

Biosensors are devices in the interface of biology with microsystems technology, which combine a biological element with a physical transducer.[5] There are several types of transducing principles, including electrochemical, gravimetrical, optical, and magnetic sensors, among others. In general, when the biological recognition element interacts with an environmental toxin, it creates a biological signal that can be converted into data by the integrated transducer and then be interpreted.

Biomolecules such as nucleic acids, enzymes, antibodies, cell receptors, or even whole cells or tissues are common examples of recognition elements in biosensors. When they react with the targeted toxin, such molecules are expected to change their structure or activity, or simply exhibit a secondary reporter feature. The transducer can then convert this change into an electrical signal and determine/quantify which toxin is present (Figure 18.2).

Biosensors have several potential advantages over other methods of analysis, including high sensitivity in the range of nanogram (ng) down to picogram (pg) of target analyte per milliliter of sample, potentially associated to a fast or real-time detection, portability, and multiple detection.

In addition to these advantages, biosensors possess another relevant characteristic that would support their use either in a central laboratory or as portable systems in the field, and simultaneously facilitate their

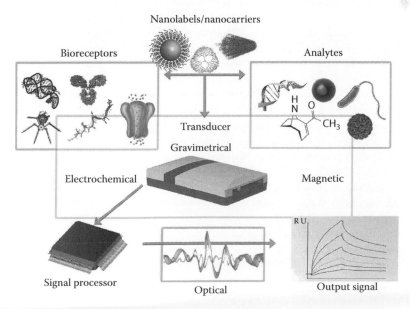

FIGURE 18.2 Biosensors. What all these devices have in common is the use of specific bioreceptors to recognize the target molecule. In general, biosensors are classified taking into account the signal transducer; electrochemical, gravi-metrical, magnetic, or optical mainly. Nanoparticles are in increasing use in biosensors as nanolabels, nanocarriers, or even to enhance the signal obtained.

commercialization, the miniaturization. Usually the small size of the detection system enables in situ real-time analysis, avoids sample transportation and degradation, and provides almost immediate interactive information about the tested samples thus, allowing a prompt decision and adoption of most adequate preventive and corrective measures before dissemination of the contaminated products and the occurrence of toxin outbreaks.

In particular for the field of aquatic toxin analysis, biosensor technologies can offer cost-effective solutions with suitable characteristics of group specificity, sensitivity, repeatability, and robustness.[6] However, the identification of different analogs from a same group of toxins remains an unattained challenge even for the actual biosensing methods.[1] Also important to note is that despite the wide range of biosensors developed so far or under development with potential for application in toxicity screening, relatively few of these have evolved into commercial devices.[7,8]

To overcome this challenge, nanotechnology will play an important role. Nanotech-based analytical biosensors, making use of different nanoparticles, CNTs, dendrimers, microstructured surfaces, and/or micro/nanosensors, are described here highlighting the resulting enhancement as well as exemplifying their applicability to the detection and quantification of biotoxins.

Representative examples, widely reported along this chapter, are gold and magnetic nanoparticles, CNTs, and dendrimers.

In most of the examples, nanoparticle-based biosensing systems present excellent performance and are advantageous as alternatives to existing conventional strategies/assays and the corresponding equipment.

Gold nanoparticles are one of the most widely investigated nanoparticles (NP) and are normally synthesized by the reduction of metal salts in citrate solution. Gold nanoparticles typically have dimensions ranging from 1 to 100 nm, directly comparable with the scale of many biological structures, including DNA, cell surface receptors, and viruses. The huge interest in this nanostructured material from a technological standpoint is mainly the anticipated application in different areas based on optical properties explained with plasmon resonance. Besides the optical properties, their electrical characteristics are also very interesting. Additionally, they present a large surface area and superior geometric and physical properties that make them well-suited for enhancing interactions with biological molecules in assays.[9]

Similarly, magnetic nanoparticles and their broad range of properties enable scientists to develop increasingly sensitive, rapid, and cost-effective biological sensors.[10,11] Biosensing strategies based on magnetic nanoparticles have received considerable attention because they offer unique advantages over other nanomaterials.[10] Magnetic nanoparticles are inexpensive to produce, physically and chemically stable, biocompatible, and environmentally safe. In addition, biological samples exhibit virtually no magnetic background, and thus highly sensitive measurements can be performed.

Conversely, CNTs exhibit excellent mechanical, electrical, and electrochemical properties combined with a large specific surface area and low absorption in the visible range, which is stimulating increasing interest in its application as components in biosensors.[12]

Dendrimers are monodispersed, three-dimensional, hyperbranched, nanoscale polymeric architectures. These molecules have a definite molecular weight, shape, and size, which make them excellent molecules for several applications.[13] In particular, the very high density of surface functional groups, internal porosity, hydrophilicity, and high mechanical and chemical stability properties make them an ideal matrix for the immobilization of biomolecules.[14] Dendrimers are being extensively used in biosensors because such polymers have proven to enhance their target-capturing ability, sensitivity, specificity, stability, and reusability. Dendrimeric bioplatforms have been used successfully for the detection of proteins, DNA, pathogens, chemicals, etc., using different sensor mechanisms, for example, electrochemical, fluorescence, and SPR.

This section summarizes the examples of application of the these nanomaterials and the derived developments in the area of biosensors for toxin analysis. Particular attention is given to the progress on different micro/nanoarray transducers and their impact on the performance of novel devices.

18.2.1 Optical Biosensors

Typical optical schemes are based on simple absorption spectroscopy (from UV to deep infrared), Raman and conventional fluorescence spectroscopy and imaging, but also on more sophisticated methods such as surface plasmon resonance (SPR), evanescent wave, or fiber optic spectroscopy.

Like other sensing principles, optical biosensors are taking advantage of the rapid ongoing advances in nanotechnology and instrumentation.

Current studies focusing on optically based transduction methods aim to achieve a more robust, easy to use, portable, and inexpensive analytical system.

18.2.1.1 Surface Plasmon Resonance

One of the methods that gather most of the required biosensing capabilities is SPR. This technology became popular in the 1990s upon biosensors commercialization by the Swedish enterprise Biacore®. The phenomena of SPR allow the study of molecular interactions in real time and without the need of molecular labeling.

In basic terms, SPR detects changes in the refractive index at the surface of a sensor. The sensor comprises a glass substrate and a thin metal layer, often a gold coating. Light passes through the substrate and is reflected off of the gold coating. At certain angles of incidence, a fraction of the light energy couples through the gold layer and creates a surface plasmon wave at the sample and gold surface interface. The angle of incident light required to sustain the surface plasmon wave is very sensitive to changes in refractive index at the surface, promoted by mass changes. In biosensors, these changes are used to monitor the recognition of target molecules. As mass accumulates at the sensor surface during a binding interaction, the refractive index increases and an increased signal is recorded.

More recently, the association of SPR technology with nanostructured materials is even pushing forward its capabilities. The conjugation of the analyte with nanoparticles and/or the modification of the SPR gold layer with multifunctional nanomaterials is being used to enhance the refractive index changes. For example, the use of magnetic nanoparticles results in a signal amplification effect and higher sensitivity.[15] Also, gold nanoparticles functionalized with different polymers, such as dendrimers and borin acid, have proved to amplify the SPR response and lower the detection limits.[16]

SPR-based biosensors are presently being investigated as food and environmental analytical tools,[17] in particular applied to the complex problem of marine toxins.[18,19]

Researchers at the Queen's University in Northern Ireland had pioneered the use of SPR biosensors to detect marine biotoxins. The first research was performed developing a biosensor assay for domoic acid (a member of the Amnesic shellfish poisons)[20] and later for more complex toxins, such as Diarrhetic Shellfish Poisons (DSP)[21] and Paralytic Shellfish Poisons (PSP).[22,23] In general, these assays use antibodies as bioreceptors (immunoassays) to perform inhibition strategies. That is, the binding of the antibody to the standard toxin on the sensor surface is inhibited by the presence of target toxin in the sample solution and the signal inversely proportional to the sample concentration. Domoic acid was detected in the range of ng/g of the analyzed sample, while okadaic acid had an assay action limit of 126 ng/g. Conversely, PSP toxins were quantified at concentrations from 2 to 50 ng/mL.

But dendrimers can also improve the performance of SPR-based biosensors. When used as an intermediate layer, dendrimers overcome the mass transport-limiting effects in the ligand immobilization increasing its efficiency. Furthermore, dendrimer-based affinity sensor matrices were found to exhibit greater stability and regeneration of bioreceptor layers.[16,24,25]

18.2.1.2 Lateral Flow Immunoassays

Lateral flow immunoassay (LFIA) is one of the simplest optical devices intended to detect the presence of a target analyte in a sample, often by visual inspection of the results, without the need for dedicated reading equipment.

LFIA combines the sensitivity and selectivity of immunoassays, such as enzyme-linked immunosorbent assay (ELISA), with simplicity and portability.

Briefly, the technology is based on porous material, such as a nitrocellulose membrane or synthetic polymer (test strip), which has the capacity to transport a fluid by capillarity. When wetted with an analyte-containing sample, the porous material provides a motive force for the movement of bulk liquid from wet to dry areas of the strip. In the strip, there are one or more areas (often called test lines) where a bioligand (frequently an antibody) specific to the analyte has been immobilized. Once the sample reaches the test lines, the analyte is captured by the ligand, accumulates, and due to the presence of a colored reporter system the test-line area changes color.

Here, as well as reported in SPR technology, the combination of the detection system with nanoengineered particles makes it to benefit from their unique optical properties and highly improve the assay sensitive. The conjugation of the target analyte with a labeling particle is used to overcome the limitations of traditional LFIA; nanoparticles-based systems have achieved notable progress in signal amplification strategy and improved sensing performance. In the past decades, many different nanoparticles have been used as labels to increase the sensitivity of immunoassays, including quantum dots (QD),[26,27] colloidal gold,[28] enzyme-gold nanoparticles,[29] silica nanoparticles,[30] superparamagnetic nanoparticles,[31] carbon nanotubes[32] polystyrene microparticles,[33] and fluorescent europium(III) nanoparticles.[34]

In particular for cyanobacterial toxins detection, a standard fluorescence-based LFIA system has been compared with gold colloidal enhanced LFIA system.[28]

These two assays are easy to perform, rapid, and their quantitative range is within detectable microcystin (MC) concentrations in water samples. The limit of detection (LOD) was investigated to be 0.2 ng/mL for the fluorescent strip and 1 ng/mL for the colloidal gold strip. However, the colloidal gold-based system has the strong advantage of direct detection of MCs at the test site without the need to pack and transport the samples back to the laboratory for test analysis.

Another example of membrane-based LFIA was developed for the fast screening of aflatoxin B(2) as a model compound.[35] The label entity consisted of magnetic nanogold microspheres with nano-iron oxide particles as core and gold nanoparticles as shell, and bio-functionalized with monoclonal antibodies. As the major advantage, experimental results indicated that the visual detection limit (cutoff value) could be improved threefolds when compared to a conventional LFIA test using simple gold nanoparticles as a reporter system.

For the particular case of aquatic toxins, researchers at the University of Michigan led the development of a new lateral flow test for the quick and cheap monitorization of MC-LR in water.[36] In their study, a porous paper strip was impregnated with single-walled carbon nanotubes (SWNTs) and antibodies, and measured using electrochemical current–time (i–t) transients. The system benefits from the strong dependence of electrical conductivity through nanotubes percolation network on the width of nanotube–nanotube tunneling gap. This dispersion of antibodies in the membrane was used to dip-coat the paper rendering it conductive. Upon the presence of the target analyte occurs a proportional change in the conductivity.

This way the SWCNT-paper sensor was able to detect MC-LR in water samples with a LOD of 0.6 ng/mL and a linear detection range up to 10 ng/mL both comparable to those of ELISA. Conversely, the time of analysis was at least 28 times shorter, which makes it suitable for everyday environmental monitoring.

18.2.1.3 Fluorescence-Based Methods

Nanomaterials are starting to replace traditional organic fluorescent dyes as reporter labels because they offer superior optical properties, such as brighter fluorescence, wider ranges of excitation and emission wavelengths, higher photostability, etc.[37]

Many reported optical biosensing systems for the detection of toxins rely on fluorescence-based transducing principles associated to immunoassay-type methods involving antibodies microarrays. Among them, the array biosensor designed by the Naval Research Laboratory (NRL) is one of the most well-known in the field.[38] The detection strategy of the NRL biosensor is an ELISA-like immunoassay conducted on glass slides where the fluorescence-labeled analytes are then interrogated using evanescent wave technology. In simple terms, a diode laser that gives rise to an evanescent wave excites the fluorescence-labeled analyte, and a charge-coupled device (CCD) camera collects the emission light.[39] The array biosensor is capable of detecting multiple targets fast and simultaneously on the surface of a single waveguide. Sandwich and competitive fluoroimmunoassays have been developed to detect high and low molecular weight toxins, respectively, in complex samples. Recognition molecules (usually antibodies) are first immobilized in specific locations on the waveguide, and the resultant patterned array can interrogate up to 12 different samples for the presence of multiple different analytes. Upon binding of a fluorescent analyte or fluorescent immunocomplex, the pattern of fluorescent spots is detected using a CCD camera and an automated image analysis determines the mean fluorescence value for each assay spot. The location of the spot and its mean fluorescence value were used to determine the toxin identity and concentration.

This array biosensor has been used to detect pure and complex samples of a variety of pathogens and toxins. As model application, the simultaneous detection of staphylococcal enterotoxin B and botulinum toxoid A in buffer presented limits of detection of 0.1 and 20 ng/mL, respectively.[40]

More recently, a group from the Universidad Complutense de Madrid has developed an automated array biosensor based on the same technology of evanescent-wave excitation targeting the detection of MCs in freshwater samples. The sensing surface consisted of microcystin-leucine-arginine (MCLR) covalently immobilized onto a microscope slide working as planar waveguide. The used detection strategy is a competitive immunoassay labeled by the fluorophore Cy5 that can assay up to six different samples in parallel, with a total analysis time of about 60 min. The optimized biosensor assay presents a detection limit of 16 pg/mL and a dynamic range from 0.06 to 1.5 ng/mL of MCLR, improving the performance of previously reported devices. The immunosensor has been successfully applied to the direct analysis of MCs in surface water samples and the results were in close agreement with those provided by LC-MS/MS.[41]

Improved versions of such fluorescence-based microarray assays were achieved using superior fluorescent nanoparticles of high-intensity and stable fluorescent light. Lian et al. were able to detect various toxins, as exemplified by ricin, cholera toxin, and staphylococcal enterotoxin B (SEB), in both pure and spiked samples, with superior specificity and sensitivity down to 10 pg/mL in the case of SEB. High specificities were also demonstrated in the detection of mixed toxin samples with similar sensitivities.[42]

A latest contribution describes a new versatile instrument for array-based simultaneous detection of various (up to five) toxins. The bioanalytical platform incorporates a microstructured polymer slide serving both as support of printed arrays and as an incubation chamber, where fluorescence image analysis and signal quantitation allow the determination of the toxin's identity and concentration. The system's performance has been investigated by immunological detection of botulinum neurotoxin type A, SEB, and the plant toxin ricin. Toxins were detectable at levels as low as 0.5–1 ng/mL in buffer or in raw milk.[43]

Additionally, dendrimers have proven to decrease detection limits in fluorescence-based biosensors mainly due to their high loading efficiency, greater accessibility, and uniform distribution of the bioreceptor on them but also because dendrimeric layers decrease the fluorescence quenching by increasing the distance between the fluorophore and the sensor substrate. Due to these advantages, dendrimers have been utilized in surface functionalization of micro and nanostructures meant for protein or DNA/RNA microarrays.[44,45]

18.2.1.4 Chemiluminescence-Based Methods

A simple and rapid chemiluminescence enzyme immunoassay (CLEIA) was developed for the determination of MC-LR in water samples. Under optimum conditions, the calibration curve obtained for MC-LR had detection limits of 0.032 ng/mL and the quantitative detection range was 0.062–0.65 ng/mL. The LOD attained from the calibration curves and the results obtained for the real samples demonstrate the potential use of CLEIA as a screening tool for the analysis of MC-LR in environmental samples.[46]

In parallel, a portable chemiluminescence multichannel immunosensor (CL-MADAG) was developed. The sensor device is based on a capillary ELISA technique in combination with a miniaturized fluidics system. Minimum concentrations of at least 0.2 ng/mL of MC-LR could be unambiguously measured in a spiked buffer system as well as in spiked real water samples. A single sample analysis for detection of MC-LR could be accomplished in just 13 min on the CL-MADAG. Besides providing a highly reproducible, fast and easy to perform test format, one major advantage of the newly established capillary immunoassay is represented by the feasibility of an internal retrospective quality control mechanism. Finally, simultaneous CL-MADAG measurements employing an immunoassay and a sandwich ELISA could be successfully demonstrated.[47]

Enhanced chemiluminescence (ECL)[48] detection can significantly enhance the sensitivity of immunoassays but often requires expensive and complex detectors. The need for these detectors limits broader use of ECL in immunoassay applications. To make ECL more suitable for immunoassays, the usage of cooled CCD detectors associated to the incorporation of nanomaterials, such as gold nanoparticles and CNTs, has been implemented.

Despite their interesting properties, mainly large specific surface area and low absorption in the visible range, there has been little use of CNTs to enhance ELISA and other optically based assays.

Nevertheless, a group from the University of Maryland Baltimore County has developed a biosensor for toxin detection integrating CNTs.[49] The system integrates a cooled CCD detector combined to CNTs and antibodies to develop a simple and portable point-of-care immunosensor. This combination of ECL, CNT, and CCD detector technologies was used to improve the detection of Staphylococcal enterotoxin B (SEB) in food. Anti-SEB primary antibodies were immobilized onto the CNT surface, and the antibody–nanotube complex was attached onto a polycarbonate surface. SEB was then detected by an ELISA assay on the CNT-polycarbonate surface with a secondary antibody. The ECL assay presented a LOD of 0.01 ng/mL, a level similar to that obtained with a fluorometric detector when using the CNTs. Later the reported system was combined with a lab-on-a-chip immunoassay method used to reduce the exposure of users to toxins and other biohazards when working outside the lab.[50]

The same group, using an identical biosensing system for the same application, but replacing the CNTs by gold nanoparticles, achieved the same detection limit of ~0.01 ng/ML, which is ~10 times more sensitive than traditional ELISA.[51]

18.2.2 Magneto-Optic Biosensors

Researchers at the Argonne National Laboratory have developed a magneto-optic biosensor that takes advantage of bio-functionalized magnetic nanoparticles. The use of an external magnetic field for magnetic nanoparticles excitation enables manipulation and sensitive detection of those particles for improved biosensors. The process involves applying a time-varying external magnetic field and a linearly polarized incident laser light to a suspension of magnetic nanoparticles. The resulting transmitted or reflected light and its polarization is recorded with a suitable photodetector. This allows for the determination of the Brownian relaxation time, which may indicate hydrodynamic radius changes upon chemical binding of the target to the magnetic nanoparticles.[52]

More recently, other new microarray-based analytical techniques relying on the use of magnetic beads for the simultaneous detection of multibacterial toxins were disclosed. The assay involves three major steps: electrophoretic collection of toxins on an antibody microarray, labeling of captured antigens with secondary biotinylated antibodies, and detection of biotin labels by scanning the microarray surface with streptavidin-coated magnetic beads in a shear flow. All the stages are performed in a single flow cell allowing application of electric and magnetic fields as well as optical detection of microarray-bound beads. Replacement of diffusion with a forced transport at all the recognition steps allows the significant decrease of both LOD and assay time. It was demonstrated that application of this "active" assay technique to the detection of toxins in water samples from natural sources and in food samples (milk and meat extracts) allowed the conclusion of the assay in less than 10 min and to decrease the LOD to 0.1–1 pg/mL for water and to 1 pg/mL for food samples.[53]

18.2.3 Electrochemical Biosensors

Electrochemical biosensors are currently among the most popular of the various types of biosensors. Electrochemical sensors are devices that extract information about the sample from the measurement of some electrical parameters. It is easy to categorize them according to the measured electrical parameter: difference of two potentials—potentiometric sensors, current—amperometric sensors, and resistance or conductance—chemiresistors or conductometric sensors.

An up-to-date review describing in depth the electrochemical biosensors for the analysis of toxins, in particular mycotoxins, marine toxins, and cyanobacterial toxins, that incorporate nanobiotechnological concepts can be found in Campas et al.[54]

Amperometric detection of toxins involves the measurement of the current generated through electrooxidation/reduction catalyzed by an associated enzyme or by their involvement in a bioaffinity reaction at the surface of the working electrode.[55]

A potentiometric biosensor consists of a perm-selective outer layer and a bioactive material, usually an enzyme. The enzyme-catalyzed reaction generates or consumes a species, which is detected by an ion selective electrode.[56]

Most common nanotech-based improvements of these systems are associated to the use of carbon nanomaterials, which have been used as components in electrochemical biosensors for over a decade mostly due to their electronic properties.

An example is presented by Zhang et al., which has proposed a sensitive electrochemical immunosensor by functionalizing single-walled carbon nanohorns (SWNHs) with analyte for MC-LR detection. Compared with single-walled CNTs, SWNHs as immobilization matrixes showed a better sensitizing effect. Using enzyme-labeled MC-LR antibody for the competitive immunoassay, under optimal conditions, the immunosensor exhibited a wide linear response to MC-LR ranging from 0.05 to 20 ng/mL with a detection limit of 0.03 ng/mL at a signal-to-noise of 3. This method showed good accuracy, acceptable precision, and reproducibility. The assay results of MC-LR in polluted water were in a good agreement with the reference values. The proposed strategy provided a biocompatible immobilization and sensitized recognition platform for analytes as small antigens and possessed promising application in food and environmental monitoring.[57]

Another work conducted by a group from the Fuzhou University in China presented a label-free amperometric immunosensor for rapid determination of MC-LR in a water sample enhanced by gold nanoparticles. The sensor was prepared by immobilizing antibody on a gold electrode coated with L-cysteine-modified gold nanoparticles where a solution of hydroquinone was used as the electron mediator. The immunosensor was incubated with MC-LR and the differential pulse voltammetric current was observed to change linearly over the concentration range from 0.05 to 15 ng/L, with a detection limit of 20 pg/L. The developed biosensor was used to determine MC-LR in spiked crude algae samples. The method has proved to be cost-effective and efficient, making it potentially suitable for field analysis of MC-LR in crude algae and water samples.[58]

Dendrimers are reported to be not good enough as conductors to be used in electrochemical sensors. Nevertheless, their coupling with metallic compounds or colloids has shown to improve this property to the point that this is one of the most extended applications of dendrimers in biosensing. As an example, in 2009, Wei and Ho developed a streptavidin–dendrimer electrochemical sensor for the detection of botulinum toxin based on aptamer-specific recognition.[59] Regarding marine toxins, a sensitive electrochemical immunosensor for the fast screening of brevetoxin B (BTX-2) in food samples was developed by means of immobilizing BTX-2-bovine serum albumin conjugate (BTX-2-BSA) on the gold nanoparticles-decorated amine-terminated poly(amidoamine) dendrimers (AuNP-PAADs). The presence of gold nanoparticles greatly improved the conductivity of the PAADs, and three-dimensional PAADs increased the surface coverage of the biomolecules on the electrode.[60]

Other kinds of sensors that have also shown an improved response with the use of dendrimers as intermediate layers were the electrochemical impedance spectroscopy–based sensors.[61]

18.2.4 Mass Biosensors

18.2.4.1 Quartz Crystal Microbalance

Quartz crystal microbalance (QCM) is a label-free piezoelectric mass sensing technique. In simple terms, it gives a response that characterizes the binding event between the analyte to be detected and a sensing layer, which is immobilized on the surface of the QCM transducer. The resonant QCM frequency depends on the mass attached to the quartz crystal surface.

Standard QCM is ideal for detecting analytes of high molecular weights[62]; however, upon nanoparticle enhancement, it has also proved to work for smaller analytes, such as cyanobacterial toxins. Thus, various amplification methods were developed, in particular gold nanoparticles (AuNPs) have attracted attention due to their unique physical and chemical properties, including easily controllable size distribution and long-term stability and biocompatibility with immunospecies.[63]

A good example is the highly sensitive, portable method developed for detecting MC-LR using gold nanoparticles. The method includes an inexpensive sensor, composed of a QCM along with gold nanoparticles, and a sandwich immunoassay for rapid and in situ detection of MC-LR. By using this method a detection sensitivity of 0.1 pg/mL of MC-LR can be reached that meets the standard of World Health Organization (WHO) requirements for drinking water (1 ng/mL of MC-LR) and compatible with those of conventional techniques, such as high-performance liquid chromatography (HPLC) and ELISA. The size of the gold nanoparticles clearly influenced the amplification efficiency of the MC-LR signal and it has been found that 30 nm in diameter is the optimal particle size.[64]

18.2.4.2 Cantilever Biosensors

Cantilever sensors have attracted considerable interest over the last decade because of their potential as a highly sensitive sensor platform for high throughput and multiplexed detection.

A particular type of cantilever sensors are the piezoelectric-excited millimeter-sized cantilevers (PEMC), which are macrocantilevers composed of two layers: a PZT (lead zirconate titanate) and a nonpiezoelectric layer (glass) of a few millimeters in length. The PZT layer is attached to the cantilever's base and acts both as an actuating and as a sensing element, while the nonpiezoelectric layer provides a surface for bioreceptor immobilization. PEMC sensor is used in resonance mode. When the target analyte binds to bioreceptor immobilized on the cantilever sensor, the effective mass of the cantilever increases and alters the sensor resonant frequency. Therefore, measuring the resonance frequency provides information not only about the presence of the antigen but also its concentration. Reports have been published on the detection of both larger toxins such as staphylococcal enterotoxin B[65] and smaller toxins, the MC-LR detected in the dynamic range from 1 pg/mL to 100 ng/mL.[66]

However, micromachined cantilever platform integrates nanoscale science and microfabrication technology for the label-free detection of biological molecules, besides allowing miniaturization promise further advantages. Mass-produced, miniature silicon and silicon nitride microcantilever arrays offer a clear path to the development of miniature sensors with unprecedented sensitivity for biodetection applications, such as toxin detection, and selective detection of pathogens through immunological techniques.[67]

18.2.5 Magnetic-Based Biosensors

18.2.5.1 Nuclear Magnetic Resonance

A stable and sensitive toxin residues immunosensor based on the relaxation of magnetic nanoparticles was developed. The method was performed in one reaction and offered sensitive, fast detection of target toxin residues in water. The target analyte, MC-LR competed with the antigens on the surface of the magnetic nanoparticles and then influenced the formation of particle aggregates. Accordingly, the magnetic relaxation time of the magnetic nanoparticles was changed under the effect of the target analyte. The calibration curve was deduced at different concentrations of the target analyte. The LOD of MC-LR was 0.6 ng/g and the detection range was 1–18 ng/g. Another important feature of the developed method was the easy operation: only two steps were needed to mix the magnetic nanoparticle solution with the sample solution and read the results through the instrument. Therefore, the developed method may be a useful tool for toxin residues sensing and may find widespread applications.[68]

18.2.5.2 Magnetoresistive Biosensors

This type of biosensors makes use of highly sensitive micro- or nanostructured magnetoresistive (MR) sensors associated to superparamagnetic nanoparticles as reporter systems.[69–72] MR sensors are made of nanometric multilayers stack, intercalating magnetic with nonmagnetic thin-film materials.

The electrical resistance of an MR sensor varies with an applied external magnetic field due to the scattering of "spin up" and "spin down" electrons at the interfaces of the multilayer sensor stack. This variation is linear in a relatively short magnetic field range (i.e., 50 Oe range), conferring quantitative sensing capacity.[69]

Spin valves (SV) are now the most frequently used type of MR sensors applied to the detection of biological events. SV are a particular type of MR sensors composed of two ferromagnetic layers, one with a fixed magnetization and the other free to rotate with an external magnetic field, separated by a nonmagnetic metal spacer. The angle between the magnetization directions dictates the resistance of the sensor. When they are in a parallel configuration, the resistance is minimal while in antiparallel configuration they produce a maximal resistance.

In a standard MR biochip-based bioassay, a recognition bioligand immobilized over the sensor is used to interrogate an unknown sample potentially containing a target molecule of interest (e.g., toxin), labeled with a magnetic nanoparticle. Whenever there is recognition between the target and its bioligand, a biomolecular event occurs. After washing, the recognized targets stay over the sensor while the unbound molecules are washed out. Applying an external magnetic field, the magnetic labels attached to the bound molecules will create a fringe field further detected by the MR sensor.[73]

In addition to fast response times, this technology is extremely sensitive, down to the level of single molecule detection. The magnetic nanolabels are discretely identified by the MR sensors, thus avoiding the "yes or no" qualitative type of answer. Another important asset is the multiplexability, detecting the presence of several analytes in the same sample.

In the literature, magnetoresistive biochips have been used mostly as immuno-chips or DNA-chips more recently. At NRL, the detection of a toxin (Ricin A) was demonstrated.[74] The toxin was spiked in a complex matrix (bovine serum) instead of using a clean buffer as was performed in the previous application.

The detection of proteins in spiked complex matrices was further proven by other groups for different applications.[75] A group from Stanford University used their technology to detect smaller proteins, namely, the mycotoxins Aflatoxin B1, Zearalenone, and HT-2.[76]

Nevertheless, fully integrated and compact devices still are missing to reach the market and being implemented as standard methods. INESC-MN group[69] in collaboration with the recently created International Iberian Nanotechnology Laboratory-INL (www.inl.int) is addressing the development of an MR-based nanotechnological platform for the detection of multiple cyanotoxins (Figure 18.3).

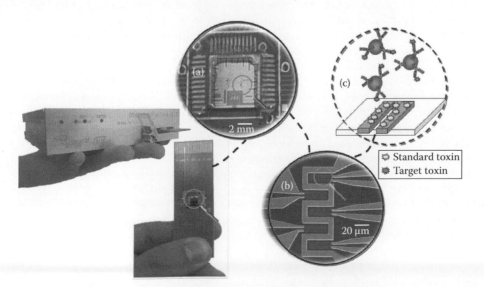

FIGURE 18.3 Magnetoresistive-biochip and measurement electronic platform. (a) Close-up of the chip encapsulated in a PCB chip-carrier. (b) Optical microscopy picture (500× magnification) of a group of spin-valve U-shaped sensors. (c) Schematic representation of the sensor and magnetic nanoparticles functionalization with standard toxin and target toxin.

18.3 Detoxification Techniques Using Nanotechnology Approaches

The development of new detection systems to monitor the presence of hazardous toxins in seafood and water is of vital importance to avoid toxic episodes to humans and other animals as discussed earlier. However, a lot of money is spent every year on the monitoring programs for seafood toxins mainly, above all in countries with a well-developed industry in seafood production and commercialization. Furthermore, toxic outbreaks imply great loses to the seafood industry as the mollusks cannot be commercialized for, frequently, long periods of time.

Taking all this into consideration, detoxification processes for seafood are really promising technologies that are in their first steps of development. But seafood is not the only target for detoxification techniques. Removal of toxins from water resources would also help to avoid the accumulation of those compounds in the seafood and toxic episodes in freshwater due to human consumption or recreational activities. Finally, detoxification processes applied for the removal of toxins already circulating in blood would be a helpful tool to reduce the noxious effects of those compounds to the human body meaning a medical treatment itself.

Nanotechnology approaches are being extensively studied to promote and improve the detoxification processes in seafood, water, and blood with very promising results using diverse kinds of nanoparticles with very specific activities and properties. Here we describe some of the most representative examples.

18.3.1 Photocatalysis

The shellfish aquaculture industry cannot prevent outbreaks of harmful algal blooms that produce biotoxins and must therefore find approaches to manage the issue. A great challenge is to develop new inexpensive and ecologically sustainable technologies that would assist with this. Nanotechnology can help with this by applying nano-based detoxification technologies. Nanocrystalline titanium dioxide (TiO_2) films with 200–670 nm thickness have been described as very efficient photocatalysts in the degradation of domoic acid mediated by UV irradiation. Under UV irradiation of photon energy greater than or equal to the TiO_2 band-gap energy, electron–hole pairs are formed, which once dissociated generate free photoelectrons and holes that are able to interact with organic matter present at a TiO_2 particle surface. The O_2 molecule scavenges an electron from the conduction band of TiO_2 to form a superoxide radical (O_2), because the energy of the conduction band edge is close to the reduction potential of oxygen. This superoxide reacts with a proton, and a hydroperoxyl radical (HO_2) is formed. These O_2 and HO_2 species interact with organic pollutants and degrade them to CO_2, a harmless product.[77] Thus, through a complex multi-step heterogeneous photocatalytic process, an oxidative decomposition of domoic acid can be induced.

Domoic acid can enter the marine food chain via uptake by molluscan shellfish such as mussels that filter their food out of the water. This water can contain both diatoms themselves and the toxin, which is released to the water column. The toxin accumulates in the digestive gland and certain tissues of shellfish, and it appears to have no effect on the animals. Domoic acid may be metabolized by bacteria (e.g., of the genera *Alteromonas* and *Pseudomonas*) present in the tissue of blue mussels (*Mytilus edulis*). Scallops are reported not to contain these elimination bacteria.[78,79]

Taking this into account, one possible approach to get the depuration of shellfish from domoic acid would be to allow the shellfish to depurate the toxin in seawater that is free of both domoic acid-containing *Pseudo nitzschia* cells and dissolved domoic acid and this would be granted by depurating the outflow and inflow of water with this system of photocatalytic degradation.[80]

Recently, US Department of Energy's (DOE) Argonne National Laboratory has created visible-light catalysis using silver chloride nanowires decorated with gold nanoparticles that may decompose organic molecules in polluted water. Traditional silver chloride photocatalytic properties are restricted to ultraviolet and blue light wavelengths, but with the addition of the gold nanoparticles, they become photocatalytic in visible light. The visible light excites the electrons in the gold nanoparticles and initiates reactions that culminate in charge separation on the silver chloride nanowires. Tests have already shown that gold-decorated nanowires can decompose organic molecules such as methylene blue.[81] As organic compounds, toxins dissolved in water could be decomposed as well, meaning this a promising technology for waters detoxification.

18.3.2 Adsorption

In recent years, nanotechnology has introduced different types of nanomaterials to the water industry that can have promising outcomes. Nanosorbents such as CNTs, polymeric materials (e.g., dendrimers), or zeolites have exceptional adsorption properties and are applied for the removal of heavy metals, organics, and biological impurities.[82] CNTs, in particular, received special attention for their exceptional water treatment capabilities and proved to work effective against both chemical and biological contaminants. CNT's fibrous shape with high aspect ratio, large accessible external surface area, and well-developed mesopores contribute to their efficiency.[83]

CNTs form aggregated pores due to the entanglement of multiple individual tubes that are adhered to each other as a result of van der Waals forces of attraction.[84–86] These aggregated pores have the dimensions of a mesopore or higher[87–94] and are able to provide large external surface areas that can immobilize large biological contaminants including bacteria and viruses. In CNTs, adsorption can occur at four regions in CNTs, at hollow interiors of nanotubes they are open ended, at interstitial pore spaces between the tube bundles, at groves present at the boundary of nanotube bundles or at the external surface of the outermost CNTs.[84,95]

The removal of MC-LR and microcystin-RR (MC-RR) via adsorption technique using CNTs was studied recently. The kinetics of MCs and other similar toxins on CNTs is very fast as the equilibrium is reached in less than 10 min, where the time taken to reach equilibrium concentration by the toxin in activated carbon is more than an hour.[96–98]

CNTs with small outside diameters and within the range of 2–10 nm have shown higher adsorption of MC-LR molecules. The longest dimension of MC-LR molecule (1.9 nm) is able to just fit into the pore sizes of the earlier-mentioned dimensions and, as a result, a close bond is formed between MC molecules and adsorption groups on the intrasurface of CNTs. On the other hand, desorption of MC molecules from smaller diameter tubes is less as compared to the tubes with larger outside diameters.[96]

Even direct adsorption is being studied as a very feasible method to capture other toxins from drinking water. A very recent work evaluated the adsorption capacity of the natural materials chitin and oyster shell powder (OSP) in the removal of saxitoxin (STX) from water. Simplified reactors of adsorption containing 200 mg of adsorbents and known concentrations of STX in solutions were proven to be able to remove up to 50% of STX from water in 18 h. However, the adsorption rate dramatically decreased with time probably due to the saturation of the adsorption sites.[99] The utilization of nanomaterials could improve the deficiency due to their high surface:volume ratio allowing the disposition of much more binding sites. However, this kind of application has not been tested in the real world.

18.3.3 Assisted Biodegradation

Adsorbent materials can be used also to grow active biofilms that help in the biodegradation of biotoxins. The fact that the natural organic matter dissolved in water is competing with the toxins in the absorbent media means an advantage in this kind of applications. The organic matter can be utilized as a primary substrate for the biofilm growing as it is present in high concentrations.[100]

The absorbent-assisted biodegradation was already proven to be effective in the biodegradation of MCs by using CNTs. Although CNTs normally display cytotoxic effects that would avoid the biofilm formation, biocompatible CNTs can be produced and successfully used to bioremediate MCs. *Raistonia solanacearum*, a plant pathogenic gram-negative bacteria, grown on biocompatible CNTs, has yielded higher efficiencies in MCs removal than any of both systems by separate (plant and CNTs) and up to 20% higher than *R. solanacearum* alone.[97]

Assisted biodegradation could be used to detoxify water supplies where disinfection processes such as chlorination or cavitation are implemented as most part of the toxin is released to the water as a consequence of the cyanobacterial cells rupture.

18.3.4 Nanocarriers-Mediated Detoxification

Nanotechnology can also play an important role in the detoxification of blood from humans intoxicated with waterborne toxins. The direct removal of disease-causing factors from blood would be highly attractive in a number of clinical situations avoiding the use of hemodialysis, filtration, or adsorption.

One possible strategy would involve injecting nanocarriers (<1 μm) to reduce the free drug concentration in the body. Those nanocarriers would be either in the circulatory system or have diffused in the peripheral organs that extract the toxin from the tissues and then exit the body via the kidneys or liver. Nanosized carriers can take the form of liposomes, nanoemulsions, nanoparticles, and macromolecules. Their high specific surface area and adjustable composition/surface properties confer them special properties to be used as detoxifiers. The affinity of the toxic agent to the carrier should be very high to ensure rapid and efficient removal of toxins from the peripheral tissues.[101]

Liposomes are spherical vesicles that possess one or more concentric phospholipid bilayer membranes that delimit aqueous compartments. Liposomes were first proposed as a means of treating plutonium poisoning more than 35 years ago[102] and since then they have proven to be effective antidotes for amphiphilic compounds that can be inactivated by encapsulated enzymes or actively trapped within their aqueous compartments.

For highly hydrophobic and poorly or nonionizable molecules, colloidal systems such as nanoemulsions would be more appropriate. For instance, intralipid was evaluated as a detoxifier for hydrophobic drugs such as bupivacaine, a local anaesthetic associated with occasional but severe and potentially lethal cardiotoxicity and increased survival was found after its infusion in animals injected with the drug.[103,104]

Biofunctionalized nanomagnets of 30 nm of diameter were successfully used to remove specific toxic compounds from whole blood such as metal ions or steroids as digoxin without causing any significant damage to the blood cells or without releasing iron to the blood system.[105] In the same way, magnetic nanoparticles could be functionalized with specific bioligands for waterborne toxins such as antibodies or cell receptors and used to remove those compounds from blood before reaching their target organ and display their toxicity.

Finally, nonimmune macromolecules such as cyclodextrins (cyclic oligosaccharides) can also reverse the pharmacological effect of drugs. For example, Sugammadex is a novel γ-cyclodextrin-based molecule that forms an exceptionally stable 1:1 complex with the neuromuscular blocking agent, rocuronium. The intravenous injection of Sugammadex was shown to deplete the free rocuronium in plasma and enhance its urinary excretion.[106]

Unfortunately, intoxications with waterborne toxins are commonly detected only after observing their symptoms and many of those toxins induce their effects very quickly making it difficult to be able to release the toxin from the blood stream in time.

18.4 Nanoparticles-Based Biomedical Applications for Aquatic Toxins

The development of nanotechnology has allowed nanobiomedicine to emerge with novel approaches and applications in research fields like bioimaging, drug delivery, or biosensing. Some of these techniques could be, in principle, extended for implementation in toxins-related fields. The discovery of new nanostructures and the possibility to modulate their physicochemical properties led to a more effective design of functional platforms capable of addressing insurmountable challenges in these fields, as well as consider new and more ambitious ones. Nowadays, NP-based technologies in biomedicine bet for an integration of multiple functionalities that combine diagnosis and therapy therapeutics in one single platform. From that revolutionary idea, the so frequently used concept in biomedical research, "theranostic nanoparticles," arises. This is a try to provide one single platform with multiple functionalities that allow it to be applied in both diagnostic and therapeutic tasks. Moreover, this approach would allow providing a more personalized medical treatment to the patients following their own needs. Overcoming this challenge involves the design of more complex nanostructures in which, in addition to the intrinsic physical and chemical properties of the support nanomaterials, new functionalities are added by proper particle surface modification with organic and inorganic molecules or compounds. Surface functionalization is

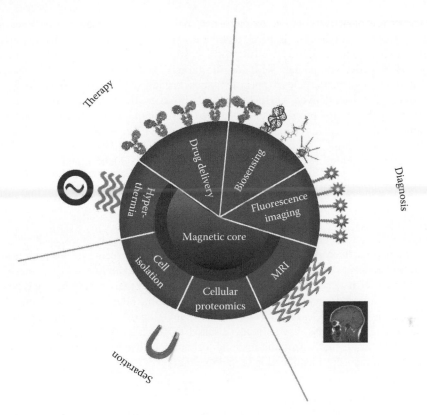

FIGURE 18.4 Nanoparticles-based applications. Nanoparticles present a great applicability in medicine, biological research, and biosensing fields for diagnosis, separation, and therapy among others. Magnetic nanoparticles are one of the most promising and used ones.

a very required technology to provide the nanoparticles with a major specificity to reach targeted tissues and so also the possibility to offer a more efficient and localized treatment on the injured tissues, avoiding the damage to surrounding healthy cells and reducing harmful side effects (Figure 18.4).

The main biomedical applications of these nanoparticles and nanoplatforms are mostly developed in fields such as bioimaging, drug delivery, and biosensing. Nanoparticles offer significant improvements in performance compared with existing conventional technologies. They show interesting properties that make them suitable for biomedical applications, that is, their size in the same range of dimension like biomolecules such as antibodies, membrane receptors, nucleic acids and proteins, high surface area, facile surface modification, and the possibility of modulating their magnetic or optical properties by controlling different experimental parameters during their synthesis. Like biosensing has been a topic extensively described previously, here we will mainly focus on the use of nanotechnology (nanoparticles) in *bioimaging* and *drug delivery*. Although more examples of nanotechnology applied to aquatic toxins are missing in the literature, some of them can be extrapolated from other already successfully achieved examples in related fields.

18.4.1 Bioimaging

Most of the efforts of nanobiomedicine are driven to the improvement of clinical imaging methods with higher specificity and sensitivity. They will allow a more efficient and early diagnosis and a more rapid therapeutic evaluation, as well as an in vivo tracking of the molecular processes involved as a therapeutic treatment is performed or administered. Also, emerging tools in molecular nanotechnology will be useful to monitor and quantify pathogen levels and toxin production inter- and intra-cellularly. Many of these nanoparticles contain both pharmaceutics and imaging agent(s) within an individual nanoparticle for simultaneous disease diagnosis and therapy (Figure 18.5).

Aquatic toxins are bioactive compounds that exert their toxicity by inducing changes usually in specific cells, tissues, or organs. The imaging techniques are very useful to evaluate the pharmacokinetic and the biodistribution of these harmful substances in order to describe and fight their toxicity. Furthermore, as bioactive compounds with specific targets, aquatic toxins could behave as useful labels capable of driving nanoparticles to specific tissues, organs, or cells, allowing their visualization or acting as intelligent drug delivery carriers to targeted tissues. For example, lanthanide ion-doped oxide nanoparticles, YVO4:Eu, properly functionalized with guanidinium groups mimic the blocking effect of guanidine toxins such as tetrodotoxin and saxitoxin (STX) and specifically target Na^+ channels in live cardiac myocites.[107] This functionalization can be easily adaptable to targeting other biological species and constitutes a powerful tool to use in targeting and labeling Na^+ channels, opening new possibilities of studying long-term single-molecule diffusion dynamics of molecules, destination of receptors, and pathological agents in cells and tissues. In vivo tracking of the toxins' distribution, bioaccumulation, and clearance in animal models such as mice or rats is a promising tool only in the first steps of study.

Conventional techniques of bioimaging were based on optical imaging methods, such as fluorescence biolabeling using organic fluorophores. However, many of these luminescent systems present some limitations related to their poor fluorescence intensity, photostability, or inability to be optimized in multicolor assays. The use of nanoparticles has contributed to overcome these restrictions and also improve the specificity and contrast observed in the targeted tissues. On the other hand, very good examples lie in the use of magnetic nanoparticles in magnetic resonance imaging (MRI), in which superparamagnetic iron oxide nanoparticles (SPIONs) have already resulted to be effective in increasing the contrast.[108] Also, the use of QD has revolutionized the imaging technologies due to their powerful quantum yield and possibility of simultaneous identification of multiple markers.

18.4.1.1 Magnetic Resonance Imaging

Magnetic resonance imaging (MRI) is widely used in bioapplications. In particular, in medicine, not only for a 3D examination of internal structures (tissues, organs) but also to monitorize biological processes with high special resolution and without the use of ionizing radiation of radiotracers. It has become an irreplaceable diagnosis technique in medical clinics and now it constitutes one of the most researched topics in biomedicine, since some limitations such as its low imaging sensitivity still need to be overcome. For these reasons, intensive research efforts aim to develop new MRI contrast agents to enhance the imaging.

The basis for MRI signal is the precession of water hydrogen nuclei under an applied magnetic field. After application of radiofrequency pulses, the relaxation process through which the nuclei return to the original aligned state can be exploited to produce an image. In order to improve imaging sensitivity, adding contrast agents accelerates the relaxation rate of water molecules, T1 (longitudinal relaxation) and T2 (transverse relaxation), therefore greatly increasing the contrast between specific issues or organs of interest.[109]

Currently, the commonest contrast agents used in MRI are paramagnetic Gd(III) chelates (typically Gd-DTPA); however, they show problems mainly related to their toxicity at high doses administration and rapid excretion due to short-term accumulation in the body, which hinders high-resolution imaging due to the long scan time required. Inorganic nanoparticles have been intensively developed in recent years for several reasons. In comparison to the paramagnetic complexes, they show tunable magnetic properties with size, shape, composition, and assembly (and so modification of T1 and T2), spend a longer circulating time in the plasma, and have a large surface area that can be easily functionalized with proper molecules for specific target recognition and multimodal conjugation.[110]

Engineered nanostructures for enhanced imaging have included dendrimers, vesicles, micelles, core-shell structures, and CNTs. These nanoplatforms have many anchoring sites available capable to be functionalized with targeting moieties, therapeutic compounds and contrast agents.[111–114] This development of nanoparticulate-based contrast agents offers the platform for engineering specificity and sensitivity required for in vivo molecular imaging. For example, Bae et al. and Yang et al.

synthesized T1/T2 dual contrast agents through modifying Gd-DTPA molecules on the surface of magnetic iron oxide nanoparticles,[115,116] and Choi et al. designed a core–shell structure $MnFe_2O_4@SiO_2@Gd_2O(CO_3)_2$ in which the T1 and T2 relaxivities were maximized by adjusting the thickness of the silica shell.[117] Recently, inorganic nanoparticles with a great potential for molecular imaging were developed. The first ones included Gd and Mn in their composition. Gd_2O_3 have been one of the most studied materials as good T1 contrast agent. Gd_2O_3 nanoparticles were further investigated as a function of composition,[118,119] particle size,[120] morphology, and surface modification.[121–123] For example, ultra small paramagnetic Gd_2O_3 NPs between 1 and 2.5 nm,[124] and $Gd_2O_3@PEG$, exhibited enhanced proton relaxivities and so high contrast imaging.[123]

However, Gd- and Mn-based inorganic nanoparticle contrast agents show some limitations related to their accumulative toxicity. Although their imaging contrast is comparable to that from conventional Gd-based complexes, ultrasmall iron oxide NPs (Fe_3O_4/Fe_2O_3) were found to be potential candidates for T1 contrast agents due to their ability to enhance MRI contrast and also their surface functionality, biocompatibility, and stability in aqueous solutions.[125,126] These NPs are especially interesting because of their high resistance to protein adsorption and surface modification, which allow them to overcome some physiological barriers.[127] Also some ferrite MFe_2O_4 (M = Fe, Zn, Ni) have shown good MRI properties to be potentially used as a contrast agent. More recently, FeCo NPs[128,129] showed better MRI contrast than iron oxide NPs, although still some toxicity-related issues remain unsolved.[130]

Aquatic toxins are bioactive compounds that exert their toxicity by inducing changes usually in specific cells, tissues, or organs. The study of the toxin pharmacokinetic is of vital importance to describe and fight its toxicity. As mentioned in this section, the nanoparticle surface modification is of fundamental importance to achieve specific targeting of the imaging contrast agents in the tissues of interest. Furthermore, NPs should be well designed and properly functionalized in order to improve biocompatibility and stability in physiological mediums, besides showing enhanced MRI contrasts. The fulfillment of these requirements will lead to an increase of the specificity and sensitivity and will allow to label and visualize internal structures with molecular imaging in vivo. This concept could be extrapolated to the specific case of aquatic toxins; specific attachment to the particle surface (i.e., specific antigen–antibody recognition and target moiety receptors) would allow us to study their pharmacokinetic and biodistribution inside the human body and would give us a deeper insight into their toxicity mechanism, needed to evaluate a proper therapeutic treatment. In addition, as bioactive compounds with specific targets, aquatic toxins could be used as labels to drive nanoparticles to specific tissues, organs, or cells to be visualized or to be reached as the target of drug delivery systems.

18.4.1.2 Quantum Dots

Optical imaging has gained a renewed interest after borrowing the amazing optical properties of QD, which overcome the low sensitivity and limited spatial resolution of the technique as using the conventional organic fluorescence dyes.

QD are colloidal fluorescence semiconductor nanocrystals. They possess unique optical and electrical properties that make them suitable for applications such as biolabels, biosensors, and image contrast agents. QD show several advantages in comparison to conventional organic fluorophores: they are brighter, show higher quantum yield, large molar extinction coefficients, size- and composition-tuneable narrow emission spectra, large surface-to-volume ratio, and resist photobleaching. All these properties make QD excellent contrast agents for imaging[131] and ideal for simultaneous detection of multiple fluorophores by excitation of a single light source[132] and also to observe biomolecular dynamics in live cells by single molecule labeling by allowing the visualization of fluorescence through tissues or other interfering compounds.[133] Their applications in biomedicine cover from diagnosis and drug delivery to gene therapies.[134] In this sense, QD have been applied to cancer research in animals, specifically for in vivo molecular imaging of tumors.[135,136] A deeper review about optical imaging in the oncology field is given by Weissleder and Pittet.[137] Also a complex consisting of QD-aptamer-dexorubicin conjugate has been used to sense a therapeutic drug release by a change in the fluorescence imaging.[138]

The first generation of QD was made of CdSe, CdTe, and PbS, which excitation spectra covered most of the visible spectra. However, the tissue penetration distance was not deep enough for in vivo applications. To overcome this limitation, other QD formulations were synthesized showing emission spectra shifted to near-infrared region (i.e., CdTe/CdSe, Cd_3P_2, and InAs/ZnSe), where the transmission of light through tissues and blood is maximum. The most commonly studied QD formulation in biological applications (molecular sensing and tissue imaging) is the core–shell structure CdSe–ZnS.[139] In order to avoid possible toxicity issues, the aqueous solution and also the circulation time of the nanostructures were increased, and many different coatings, such as hydrophilic polymer and PEGylated phospholipid, have been used to coat QD.[140] Furthermore, this allows QD to be further surface functionalized with targeting ligands or loaded with therapeutics that will drive to targeted tissues, organs, or cells, making possible to monitor their biodistribution.[141–143] These biomolecular surface functionalization strategies are based on physical/chemical attachment of chemical functional groups found in polymers, carbohydrates, antibodies, or RNA/DNA acid nucleics among others, in such a way they can interact specifically with certain proteins or recognize molecule receptors localized in the cell membrane of the tissue of interest. In this sense, multifunctional QD have become a powerful platform to detect the presence of a pathogenic bacteria or toxin. It is important to remark that the choice of the biomolecule to attach to the QD nanoparticles is critical and can be dependent upon sample and target bacteria or toxin. Many representative examples can be found in the report from Burris and Stewart[144] related to the ability of QD for sensing and monitor pathogens and toxins in foods and crops (i.e., neurotoxins, cholera, ricin, Shiga-like, and staphylococcal enterotoxin B).[145,146] More specifically, recent examples of using semiconductor QD as biological imaging can be found in the literature.[147,148] In this sense, Alivisatos[149] designed a green-emitting CdSe/ZnS QD functionalized with trimethoxysilylpropyl urea and acetate groups that showed high affinity to the cell nucleous and Chen and Nie used immunomolecules-labeled CdSe to recognize specific antibodies or antigens.[150] Related to cancer imaging, several properly functionalized QD were used to label cancer markers on the surface of fixed and live cancer cells with the aim to identify tumors that respond to antitumoral drugs[136] or to study the efficiency of targeting mechanisms in them.[135,151] Also, kinetic studies have been carried out on the mobility of human mammary epithelial tumors.[152] Also, QD emitting in the NIR region were successfully used in lymph mapping of a large pig.[153]

It is worth mentioning here one example of simultaneous cancer imaging, therapy, and therapy monitoring that takes place in donor/acceptor QD-based conjugates that show fluorescence resonance energy transfer (FRET) properties, which is essentially a photoluminescence quenching happening when a reversible attachment is formed between the QD and the substance that will be responsible for the effect that we intend to monitor. Following this principle, Bagalkot et al. monitored the intercellular release of Dox using QD-Apt(Dox)-FRET nanosystems.[138]

Besides QD, different kind of nanoparticles can also be used as platforms for biological imaging applications. This is the case of Au NPs, which are excellent labels for imaging applications since they can be detected by numerous techniques, such as optic absorption and fluorescence.[154] Au NPs have a very well-developed thiol-chemistry at the surface that can provide the nanoparticles with a wide variety of functional ligands. A lot of examples of imaging applications have been reported by using Au NPs linked to fluorophores, either QD or organic ones, achieve with high contrast, high special resolution, and efficient targeting.[148,155] Also, other nanostructures based on CNTs have been proven suitable for potential biological applications related to bioimaging or drug delivery. Oxidation processes at the graphite-like surface create defects that become anchoring sites for functional ligands or drug loadings. Taking advantage that CNTs can be internalized by cells, efforts to investigate their potential role in biological processes and mechanisms are being developed.[155]

18.4.2 Drug Delivery

Sometimes, the difference between the most harmful poison and the healthiest therapeutic substance lies, exclusively, in the doses. This is the case of many toxins, which are mainly known by their powerful mechanism of action and their noxious effects on the human body. However, the same compounds, when prepared appropriately in the right doses, can behave as therapeutic substances.[156–158] The design of intelligent drug delivery nanosystems capable of carrying and selectively delivering therapeutic drugs in targeted diseased tissues has been an intensive area of research for the last decades. Nanoparticle-based drug delivery systems can improve significantly the pharmacological and therapeutic drug administration.[159] Their intrinsic physicochemical properties, together with their ability to be functionalized with both organic and inorganic ligands, provide them with unique properties, capable of overcoming the most ambitious challenges for applications as drug delivery systems. The use of toxins as therapeutic agents in combination with an NP-based transport system could provide a novel and original solution for the treatment of several diseases. However, the success of an effective drug administration must fulfill several chemical and biological requirements that derive essentially from their ability to improve the water solubility of drugs and biocompatibility, avoid the actuation of the immunologic system, modify pharmacokinetics, increase the specificity toward target tissues, and control more precisely the drug release. In this sense, toxins appear as excellent candidates to improve the efficiency of drug delivery systems due to their high specificity and virulence factor, since they are able to avoid the response of the immune system on the required time or even slip past. Although it is difficult to find the use of toxins as components of more complex multifunctional drug delivery systems, two of the main roles that toxins could play in an integrated nanoparticle-based drug delivery system due to their powerful activity mechanism are (1) they act as a therapeutic drug by releasing the right amount in localized areas of the human body where the toxin develops more efficiently its therapeutic effect and (2) they act as drug delivery carriers by taking advantage of their high specificity to targeted tissues and their well-known pharmacokinetics in the human body. The activity mechanisms are well known for the main toxins affecting humans, so that allows us to design more effective drug delivery systems capable of achieving specific targets or deliver therapeutic substances of interest in particular areas of the body. Recent research in drug delivery nanostructures involves the use of magnetic nanoparticles as drug delivery carriers, because in addition to their easy surface decoration with recognition molecules (i.e., antibodies, proteins, and polysaccharides) that would allow a straight targeting, they also offer the possibility of a magnetic guiding. One representative example in vivo that help to understand the concept of integration of functionalities (in other words, called "theranostic NPs") is the work from Yang et al., in which multifunctional magnetic–polymeric nanohybrids (MRI contrast agent) are combined with therapeutic antibodies (for specific recognition of target breast cancer cells) and loaded with doxorubicin drug (for delivery) in such a way that they demonstrated ultrasensitive targeted detection by MRI and excellent therapeutic effect by inhibiting the tumor.[160] The specific recognition of a target tissue, organ, or cell is crucial to avoid as possible harmful side effects in healthy body areas. As mentioned elsewhere, many aquatic toxins show specific recognition of cells in which they will perform their toxic effect. In principle, this ability of toxins could be exploited to be used as a driving force to guide magnetic functional nanoplatforms toward target cells for both therapeutic delivery and MRI treatment control. However, more recently, different approaches have been developed in which nanoparticles can take advantage of specific physiological and anatomic features of the diseased tissues (passive targeting). For example, Holme et al.[161] developed shear-stress-induced drug delivery lenticular vesicles activated by the mechanical changes that take place naturally in blood vessel areas suffering from atherosclerosis.

It is well known that some toxins are able to cross the cell membrane and even reach the nucleus, where they perform their harmful purpose (i.e., okadaic acid, cylindrospermopsin, or pectenotoxin). On the other hand, Au NPs have been extensively investigated for biomedical applications due to their easy surface functionalization (i.e., thiol-chemistry and PEG) and their ability to be intracellular internalized and penetrate the nucleus while carrying drugs or other cargos.[162] Combining both toxins and Au NPs properties, the resultant hybrid multifunctional nanoplatforms could improve the significant potential that Au NPs already have to be used as gene delivery vehicles, drug carriers, and carriers for other biomolecules.

Finally, many aquatic toxins have been found to display therapeutic effects that could be used in medicine to treat diseases such as cancer, Alzheimer's disease, or diabetes. Multifunctional nanoparticle-based applications in drug delivery could allow driving specifically the therapeutics to a damaged tissue, avoiding some of the noxious effects that toxins show in unspecific tissues as a consequence of a nonefficient targeted release and, in turn, increase the yield of delivery in the damaged area of interest.

18.5 Future Perspectives

In this chapter, we already revised the role that nanotechnology has been playing until now in the seafood and freshwater toxins fields. However, nanotechnologies are only in their starting point and huge advances are expected in the next years.

Biosensors could extensively benefit from the great advantages of using nanomaterials such as magnetic and gold nanoparticles, dendrimers, and CNTs in their structures. In general, biosensors for environmental analysis, despite their advanced state of development and promising features, still present one or more limitations among many possible: sensitivity, accuracy, reliability, response time, lifetime, portability, cost, etc.; this should be improved in order to bring biosensor to the confidence of potential users and achieve standardization as commercial devices. The areas of development that are expected to have a greater impact in biosensor technology are immobilization techniques, nanotechnology, miniaturization, and multisensor array determinations. In this sense, it is clear that the future of biosensors for toxins analysis greatly depends on the emergent micro- and nanotechnologies. However, as the world becomes more concerned about the impact that environmental contamination may cause on public health and the ecosystem, the demand for rapid detecting biosensors allied to new strategies of decontamination will increase.

"Smart" detoxification of water, mollusks, and human blood based on nanotechnological applications in combination with bioremediation agents (i.e., bacteria) constitute a really promising subject that for sure will be explored more in depth. Also, bioimaging techniques improved by the use of nanoparticles could help to better understand the biotoxins bioavailability, pharmacokinetics, and pharmacodynamics.

Furthermore, biotoxins could be used as tools to improve nanotechnologies mainly applied to the field of nanomedicine. For instance, bioimaging techniques can be highly improved by using biotoxins to functionalize nanoparticles, allowing a site direct imaging. Moreover, the use of biotoxins as therapeutic drugs could greatly benefit from nano-based drug delivery systems.

But nanoscale is not the end of the road. The way from bulk-to-nanosize materials and the subsequent increase of the surface-to-volume ratio was a breakthrough in the area of materials science. As a consequence, novel physico-chemical properties and applications have been emerging since then. However, below nanometer scale there is still plenty of room with multiple potential applications. In the last years, the synthesis of sub-nanometric metal clusters (Au, Ag, and Cu) has been greatly investigated due to their amazing chemical, optical, and catalytic properties.[163–169]

Metal atomic clusters consist of groups of atoms with very well-defined composition and one or few stable geometric structures.[170] They represent the most elemental building block in nature (after atoms) and are characterized by a size comparable to the Fermi wavelength of an electron (~0.52 nm for Au and Ag). At this particle size scale, their physico-chemical behavior is dominated by quantum effects, which are responsible for a drastic change of their chemical, optical, and electrical properties, for example, magnetism, photoluminescence, or catalytic activity. All these unique properties make sub-nanometric species very promising for biomedical applications. For example, their fluorescence properties and catalytic activity could make them of potential interest to be used as imaging label in diagnosis and detoxification, respectively.

Another biomedical application that promotes the multifunctional character of magnetic nanoparticles and that is being intensively developed is the magnetic hyperthermia.[171] The most used magnetic nanoparticles in hyperthermia applications are magnetite nanoparticles due to mainly their size-dependent magnetic properties and biocompatibility. Below the single-to-multi domain limit (superparamagnetic region) and under an external oscillating magnetic field, they are capable of transforming the applied electromagnetic energy into heat. This is due to magnetic relaxation processes resulting in an efficient temperature increase that can kill specifically damaged cells (more sensitive to temperature increases than the healthy ones, ~42°C). However, although most of the applications researched so far have been related to cancer treatment,[172,173] novel applications are emerging in other fields.[174] Again, a specific attachment of these heat nano-generators to the tissue of interest is essential. In this sense, the specificity shown by many toxins could be a very suitable driving force for targeting these multifunctional nanosystems (Figure 18.5).

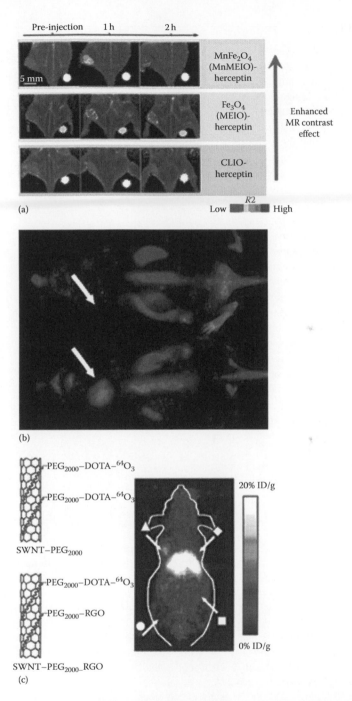

FIGURE 18.5 Several examples of nanoparticle contrast agents and TNPs. (a) Color-mapped MR images of the mouse at different times following injection. (From[175] Jun, Y.-W., Lee, J.-H., and Cheon, J.: Chemical design of nanoparticle probes for highperformance magnetic resonance imaging. *Angewandte Chemie International Edition*. 2008. 47. 5122–5135. Copyright Wiley-VCH Verlag GmbH & Co. KGaA. Reproduced with permission.) (b) In vivo NIRF imaging of U87MG tumor-bearing mice injected with 200 pmol of QD705—RGD or QD705. Arrows indicate tumors. (Reprinted with permission from[176] Cai, W., Shin, D. W., Chen, K. et al., Peptide-labeled near-infrared quantum dots for imaging tumor vasculature in living subjects. *Nano Letters*, 6, 669–676. Copyright 2006 American Chemical Society.) (c) A two-dimensional projection of the microPET image of a U87MG tumor-bearing mouse 8 h post injection of a high dose of SWNT–PEG$_{5400}$–RGD solution. The arrows point to the tumor and several organs. (Reprinted by permission from Macmillan Publishers Ltd. *Nature Nanotechnology*,[177] Liu, Z., Cai, W., He, L. et al., 2006. In vivo biodistribution and highly efficient tumour targeting of carbon nanotubes in mice, 2, 47–52, copyright 2006.)

ABBREVIATIONS

AuNP-PAADs	Gold nanoparticle-decorated amine-terminated poly(amidoamine) dendrimers
BTX	Brevetoxin
CLEIA	Chemiluminescence enzyme immunoassay
CNT	Carbon nanotube
DNA	Deoxyribonucleic acid
DSP	Diarrheic shellfish poisoning
ECL	Enhanced chemiluminescence
ELISA	Enzyme-linked immunosorbent assay
FRET	Fluorescence resonance energy transfer
HPLC	High-performance liquid chromatography
LFIA	Lateral flow immunoassay
MC	Microcystin
MC-LR	Microcystin-leucin arginine
MC-RR	Microcystin-arginine arginine
MR	Magnetoresistive
MRI	Magnetic resonance imaging
NP	NanoParticle
OSP	Oyster shell powder
PSP	Paralytic shellfish poisoning
PEG	Polyethylene glycol
PEMC	Piezoelectric-excited millimeter-sized cantilevers
PZT	Lead zirconate titanate
QCM	Quartz crystal microbalance
QD	Quantum dots
SPIONs	Superparamagnetic iron oxide nanoparticles
SPR	Surface plasmon resonance
STX	Saxitoxin
SWCNTs	Single wall carbon nanotubes
WHO	World Health Organization

REFERENCES

1. Botana, L., Vilariño, N., Alfonso, A. et al., 2012. Use of biosensors as alternatives to current regulatory methods for marine biotoxins, in *Molecular Biological Technologies for Ocean Sensing*. Tiquia-Arashiro, S. M., ed. Humana Press, New York, pp. 219–242.
2. Campas, M., Prieto-Simon, B., and Marty, J. L., 2007. Biosensors to detect marine toxins: Assessing seafood safety. *Talanta*, 72, 884–895.
3. Tothill, I. E., 2011. Biosensors and nanomaterials and their application for mycotoxin determination. *World Mycotoxin Journal*, 4, 361–374.
4. Wang, L. B., Ma, W., Xu, L. G. et al., 2010. Nanoparticle-based environmental sensors. *Materials Science and Engineering R-Reports*, 70, 265–274.
5. Vo-Dinh, T. and Cullum, B., 2000. Biosensors and biochips: Advances in biological and medical diagnostics. *Fresenius' Journal of Analytical Chemistry*, 366, 540–551.
6. Singh, S., Srivastava, A., Oh, H. M., Ahn, C. Y., Choi, G. G., and Asthana, R. K., 2012. Recent trends in development of biosensors for detection of microcystin. *Toxicon*, 60, 878–894.
7. Taitt, C. R., Shriver-Lake, L. C., Ngundi, M. M., and Ligler, F. S., 2008. Array biosensor for toxin detection: Continued advances. *Sensors*, 8, 8361–8377.
8. Leonard, P., Hearty, S., Brennan, J. et al., 2005. Advances in biosensors for detection of pathogens in food and water. *Enzyme and Microbial Technology*, 32, 3–13.
9. Saha, K., Agasti, S. S., Kim, C., Li, X., and Rotello, V. M., 2012. Gold nanoparticles in chemical and biological sensing. *Chemical Reviews*, 112, 2739–2779.

10. Haun, J. B., Yoon, T. J., Lee, H., and Weissleder, R., 2010. Magnetic nanoparticle biosensors. *Wiley Interdisciplinary Reviews—Nanomedicine and Nanobiotechnology*, 2, 291–304.
11. Hsing, I. M., Xu, Y., and Zhao, W. T., 2007. Micro- and nano-magnetic particles for applications in biosensing. *Electroanalysis*, 19, 755–768.
12. Balasubramanian, K. and Burghard, M., 2006. Biosensors based on carbon nanotubes. *Analytical and Bioanalytical Chemistry*, 385, 452–468.
13. Tomalia, D. A., Baker, H., Dewald, J. et al., 1985. A new class of polymers—Starburst-dendritic macromolecules. *Polymer Journal*, 17, 117–132.
14. Satija, J., Sai, V. V. R., and Mukherji, S., 2011. Dendrimers in biosensors: Concept and applications. *Journal of Materials Chemistry*, 21, 14367–14386.
15. Wang, J. L., Munir, A., Zhu, Z. Z., and Zhou, H. S., 2010. Magnetic nanoparticle enhanced surface plasmon resonance sensing and its application for the ultrasensitive detection of magnetic nanoparticle-enriched small molecules. *Analytical Chemistry*, 82, 6782–6789.
16. Frasconi, M., Tel-Vered, R., Riskin, M., and Willner, I., 2010. Surface plasmon resonance analysis of antibiotics using imprinted boronic acid-functionalized Au nanoparticle composites. *Analytical Chemistry*, 82, 2512–2519.
17. Haughey, S. A., Campbell, K., Yakes, B. J. et al., 2011. Comparison of biosensor platforms for surface plasmon resonance based detection of paralytic shellfish toxins. *Talanta*, 85, 519–526.
18. Hodnik, V. and Anderluh, G., 2009. Toxin detection by surface plasmon resonance. *Sensors*, 9, 1339–1354.
19. Campbell, K., Rawn, D. F. K., Niedzwiadek, B., and Elliott, C. T., 2011. Paralytic shellfish poisoning (PSP) toxin binders for optical biosensor technology: Problems and possibilities for the future: A review. *Food Additives and Contaminants: Part A*, 28, 711–725.
20. Traynor, I. M., Plumpton, L., Fodey, T. L., Higgins, C., and Elliott, C. T., 2006. Immunobiosensor detection of domoic acid as a screening test in bivalve molluscs: Comparison with liquid chromatography-based analysis. *Journal of AOAC International*, 89, 868–872.
21. Llamas, N., Stewart, L., Fodey, T. et al., 2007. Development of a novel immunobiosensor method for the rapid detection of okadaic acid contamination in shellfish extracts. *Analytical and Bioanalytical Chemistry*, 389, 581–587.
22. Campbell, K., Stewart, L. D., Doucette, G. J. et al., 2007. Assessment of specific binding proteins suitable for the detection of paralytic shellfish poisons using optical biosensor technology. *Analytical Chemistry*, 79, 5906–5914.
23. Fonfría, E. S., Vilariño, N., Campbell, K. et al., 2007. Paralytic shellfish poisoning detection by surface plasmon resonance-based biosensors in shellfish matrixes. *Analytical Chemistry*, 79, 6303–6311.
24. Mark, S. S., Sandhyarani, N., Zhu, C. C., Campagnolo, C., and Batt, C. A., 2004. Dendrimer-functionalized self-assembled monolayers as a surface plasmon resonance sensor surface. *Langmuir*, 20, 6808–6817.
25. Singh, P., Onodera, T., Mizuta, Y., Matsumoto, K., Miura, N., and Toko, K., 2009. Dendrimer modified biochip for detection of 2,4,6 trinitrotoluene on SPR immunosensor: Fabrication and advantages. *Sensors and Actuators B-Chemical*, 137, 403–409.
26. Chen, Y. P., Ning, B. A., Liu, N. et al., 2010. A rapid and sensitive fluoroimmunoassay based on quantum dot for the detection of chlorpyrifos residue in drinking water. *Journal of Environmental Science and Health Part B-Pesticides Food Contaminants and Agricultural Wastes*, 45, 508–515.
27. Chen, J. X., Xu, F., Jiang, H. Y. et al., 2009. A novel quantum dot-based fluoroimmunoassay method for detection of enrofloxacin residue in chicken muscle tissue. *Food Chemistry*, 113, 1197–1201.
28. Pyo, D., 2007. Comparison of fluorescence immunochromatographic assay strip and gold colloidal immunochromatographic assay strip for detection of microcystin. *Analytical Letters*, 40, 907–919.
29. He, Y. Q., Zhang, S. Q., Zhang, X. B. et al., 2011. Ultrasensitive nucleic acid biosensor based on enzyme-gold nanoparticle dual label and lateral flow strip biosensor. *Biosensors & Bioelectronics*, 26, 2018–2024.
30. Wu, Y. F., Chen, C. L., and Liu, S. Q., 2009. Enzyme-functionalized silica nanoparticles as sensitive labels in biosensing. *Analytical Chemistry*, 81, 1600–1607.
31. Wang, Y. Y., Xu, H., Wei, M., Gu, H. C., Xu, Q. F., and Zhu, W., 2009. Study of superparamagnetic nanoparticles as labels in the quantitative lateral flow immunoassay. *Materials Science & Engineering C-Biomimetic and Supramolecular Systems*, 29, 714–718.
32. Lai, G., Wu, J., Ju, H., and Yan, F., 2011. Streptavidin-functionalized silver-nanoparticle-enriched carbon nanotube tag for ultrasensitive multiplexed detection of tumor markers. *Advanced Functional Materials*, 21, 2938–2943.

33. Yan, J. L., Estevez, M. C., Smith, J. E. et al., 2007. Dye-doped nanoparticles for bioanalysis. *Nano Today*, 2, 44–50.
34. Juntunen, E., Myyrylainen, T., Salminen, T., Soukka, T., and Pettersson, K., 2012. Performance of fluorescent europium(III) nanoparticles and colloidal gold reporters in lateral flow bioaffinity assay. *Analytical Biochemistry*, 428, 31–38.
35. Tang, D., Sauceda, J. C., Lin, Z. et al., 2009. Magnetic nanogold microspheres-based lateral-flow immunodipstick for rapid detection of aflatoxin B2 in food. *Biosensors and Bioelectronics*, 25, 514–518.
36. Wang, L., Chen, W., Xu, D. et al., 2009. Simple, rapid, sensitive, and versatile SWNT–paper sensor for environmental toxin detection competitive with ELISA. *Nano Letters*, 9, 4147–4152.
37. Zhong, W., 2009. Nanomaterials in fluorescence-based biosensing. *Analytical and Bioanalytical Chemistry*, 394, 47–59.
38. Ligler, F. S., Taitt, C. R., Shriver-Lake, L. C., Sapsford, K. E., Shubin, Y., and Golden, J. P., 2003. Array biosensor for detection of toxins. *Analytical and Bioanalytical Chemistry*, 377, 469–477.
39. Taitt, C. R., Anderson, G. P., and Ligler, F. S., 2005. Evanescent wave fluorescence biosensors. *Biosensors and Bioelectronics*, 20, 2470–2487.
40. Sapsford, K. E., Taitt, C. R., Loo, N., and Ligler, F. S., 2005. Biosensor detection of botulinum toxoid A and staphylococcal enterotoxin B in food. *Applied and Environmental Microbiology*, 71, 5590–5592.
41. Herranz, S., Marazuela, M. D., and Moreno-Bondi, M. C., 2012. Automated portable array biosensor for multisample microcystin analysis in freshwater samples. *Biosensors and Bioelectronics*, 33, 50–55.
42. Lian, W., Wu, D. H., Lim, D. V., and Jin, S. G., 2010. Sensitive detection of multiplex toxins using antibody microarray. *Analytical Biochemistry*, 401, 271–279.
43. Weingart, O. G., Gao, H., Crevoisier, F., Heitger, F., Avondet, M. A., and Sigrist, H., 2012. A bioanalytical platform for simultaneous detection and quantification of biological toxins. *Sensors*, 12, 2324–2339.
44. Bhatnagar, P., Mark, S. S., Kim, I. et al., 2006. Dendrimer-scaffold-based electron-beam patterning of biomolecules. *Advanced Materials*, 18, 315–319.
45. Rozkiewicz, D. I., Brugman, W., Kerkhoven, R. M., Ravoo, B. J., and Reinhoudt, D. N., 2007. Dendrimermediated transfer printing of DNA and RNA microarrays. *Journal of the American Chemical Society*, 129, 11593–11599.
46. Long, F., Shi, H. C., He, M., Sheng, J. W., and Wang, J. F., 2009. Sensitive and rapid chemiluminescence enzyme immunoassay for microcystin-LR in water samples. *Analytica Chimica Acta*, 649, 123–127.
47. Lindner, P., Molz, R., Yacoub-George, E., and Wolf, H., 2009. Rapid chemiluminescence biosensing of microcystin-LR. *Analytica Chimica Acta*, 636, 218–223.
48. Kricka, L. J., Thorpe, G. H. G., and Stott, R. A. W., 1987. Enhanced chemiluminescence enzyme-immunoassay. *Pure and Applied Chemistry*, 59, 651–654.
49. Yang, M. H., Kostov, Y., Bruck, H. A., and Rasooly, A., 2008. Carbon nanotubes with enhanced chemiluminescence immunoassay for CCD-based detection of staphylococcal enterotoxin B in food. *Analytical Chemistry*, 80, 8532–8537.
50. Yang, M. H., Sun, S., Kostov, Y., and Rasooly, A., 2010. Lab-on-a-chip for carbon nanotubes based immunoassay detection of Staphylococcal Enterotoxin B (SEB). *Lab on a Chip*, 10, 1011–1017.
51. Yang, M., Kostov, Y., Bruck, H. A., and Rasooly, A., 2009. Gold nanoparticle-based enhanced chemiluminescence immunosensor for detection of Staphylococcal Enterotoxin B (SEB) in food. *International Journal of Food Microbiology*, 133, 265–271.
52. Chung, S.-H., Grimsditch, M., Hoffmann, A. et al., 2008. Magneto-optic measurement of Brownian relaxation of magnetic nanoparticles. *Journal of Magnetism and Magnetic Materials*, 320, 91–95.
53. Shlyapnikov, Y. M., Shlyapnikova, E. A., Simonova, M. A. et al., 2012. Rapid simultaneous ultrasensitive immunodetection of five bacterial toxins. *Analytical Chemistry*, 84, 5596–5603.
54. Campas, M., Garibo, D., and Prieto-Simon, B., 2012. Novel nanobiotechnological concepts in electrochemical biosensors for the analysis of toxins. *Analyst*, 137, 1055–1067.
55. Campas, M. and Marty, J. L., 2007. Highly sensitive amperometric immunosensors for microcystin detection in algae. *Biosensors and Bioelectronics*, 22, 1034–1040.
56. Queiros, R. B., Noronha, J. P., Marques, P. V. S., Fernandes, J. S., and Sales, M. G. F., 2012. Determination of microcystin-LR in waters in the subnanomolar range by sol-gel imprinted polymers on solid contact electrodes. *Analyst*, 137, 2437–2444.
57. Zhang, J., Lei, J. P., Xu, C. L., Ding, L., and Ju, H. X., 2010. Carbon nanohorn sensitized electrochemical immunosensor for rapid detection of microcystin-LR. *Analytical Chemistry*, 82, 1117–1122.

58. Tong, P., Tang, S. R., He, Y., Shao, Y. H., Zhang, L., and Chen, G. N., 2011. Label-free immunosensing of microcystin-LR using a gold electrode modified with gold nanoparticles. *Microchimica Acta*, 173, 299–305.
59. Wei, F. and Ho, C.-M., 2009. Aptamer-based electrochemical biosensor for Botulinum neurotoxin. *Analytical and Bioanalytical Chemistry*, 393, 1943–1948.
60. Tang, D., Tang, J., Su, B., and Chen, G., 2011. Gold nanoparticles-decorated amine-terminated poly(amidoamine) dendrimer for sensitive electrochemical immunoassay of brevetoxins in food samples. *Biosensors and Bioelectronics*, 26, 2090–2096.
61. Zucolotto, V., Pinto, A. P. A., Tumolo, T. et al., 2006. Catechol biosensing using a nanostructured layer-by-layer film containing Cl-catechol 1,2-dioxygenase. *Biosensors and Bioelectronics*, 21, 1320–1326.
62. Salmain, M., Ghasemi, M., Boujday, S. et al., 2011. Piezoelectric immunosensor for direct and rapid detection of staphylococcal enterotoxin A (SEA) at the ng level. *Biosensors and Bioelectronics*, 29, 140–144.
63. Tang, D. Q., Zhang, D. J., Tang, D. Y., and Ai, H., 2006. Amplification of the antigen–antibody interaction from quartz crystal microbalance immunosensors via back-filling immobilization of nanogold on biorecognition surface. *Journal of Immunological Methods*, 316, 144–152.
64. Han, J. H., Zhang, J. P., Xia, Y. T., and Jiang, L., 2011. Highly sensitive detection of the hepatotoxin microcystin-LR by surface modification and bio-nanotechnology. *Colloids and Surfaces a-Physicochemical and Engineering Aspects*, 391, 184–189.
65. Maraldo, D. and Mutharasan, R., 2007. Detection and confirmation of staphylococcal enterotoxin B in apple juice and milk using piezoelectric-excited millimeter-sized cantilever sensors at 2.5 fg/mL. *Analytical Chemistry*, 79, 7636–7643.
66. Ding, Y. and Mutharasan, R., 2011. Highly sensitive and rapid detection of microcystin-LR in source and finished water samples using cantilever sensors. *Environmental Science and Technology*, 45, 1490–1496.
67. Datar, R., Kim, S., Jeon, S. et al., 2009. Cantilever sensors: Nanomechanical tools for diagnostics. *MRS Bulletin*, 34, 449–454.
68. Ma, W., Chen, W., Qiao, R. R. et al., 2009. Rapid and sensitive detection of microcystin by immunosensor based on nuclear magnetic resonance. *Biosensors & Bioelectronics*, 25, 240–243.
69. Freitas, P. P., Cardoso, F. A., Martins, V. C. et al., 2012. Spintronic platforms for biomedical applications. *Lab on a Chip*, 12, 546–557.
70. Graham, D. L., Ferreira, H. A., and Freitas, P. P., 2004. Magnetoresistive-based biosensors and biochips. *Trends in Biotechnology*, 22, 455–462.
71. Martins, V. C., Cardoso, F. A., Germano, J. et al., 2009. Femtomolar limit of detection with a magnetoresistive biochip. *Biosensors and Bioelectronics*, 24, 2690–2695.
72. Megens, M. and Prins, M., 2005. Magnetic biochips: A new option for sensitive diagnostics. *Journal of Magnetism and Magnetic Materials*, 293, 702–708.
73. Cardoso, F. A., Germano, J., Ferreira, R. et al., 2008. Detection of 130 nm magnetic particles by a portable electronic platform using spin valve and magnetic tunnel junction sensors. *Journal of Applied Physics*, 103, 07A310-1–07A310-3.
74. Mulvaney, S. P., Cole, C. L., Kniller, M. D. et al., 2007. Rapid, femtomolar bioassays in complex matrices combining microfluidics and magnetoelectronics. *Biosensors and Bioelectronics*, 23, 191–200.
75. Osterfeld, S. J., Yu, H., Gaster, R. S. et al., 2008. Multiplex protein assays based on real-time magnetic nanotag sensing. *Proceedings of the National Academy of Sciences of the United States of America*, 105, 20637–20640.
76. Mak, A. C., Osterfeld, S. J., Yu, H. et al., 2010. Sensitive giant magnetoresistive-based immunoassay for multiplex mycotoxin detection. *Biosensors and Bioelectronics*, 25, 1635–1639.
77. Hoffmann, M. R., Martin, S. T., Choi, W. Y., and Bahnemann, D. W., 1995. Environmental applications of semiconductor photocatalysis. *Chemical Reviews*, 95, 69–96.
78. Mos, L., 2001. Domoic acid: A fascinating marine toxin. *Environmental Toxicology and Pharmacology*, 9, 79–85.
79. Stewart, J. E., Marks, L. J., Gilgan, M. W., Pfeiffer, E., and Zwicker, B. M., 1998. Microbial utilization of the neurotoxin domoic acid: Blue mussels (*Mytilus edulis*) and soft shell clams (*Mya arenaria*) as sources of the microorganisms. *Canadian Journal of Microbiology*, 44, 456–464.
80. Djaoued, Y., Robichaud, J., Thibodeau, M., Balaji, S., Tchoukanova, N., and Bates, S. S., 2009. Photocatalytic properties of nanocrystalline titanium dioxide films in the degradation of domoic acid in aqueous solution: Potential for use in molluscan shellfish biotoxin depuration facilities. *Food Additives and Contaminants Part A—Chemistry Analysis Control Exposure and Risk Assessment*, 26, 248–257.

81. Sun, Y., 2010. Conversion of Ag nanowires to AgCl nanowires decorated with Au nanoparticles and their photocatalytic activity. *Journal of Physical Chemistry C*, 114, 2127–2133.

82. Savage, N. and Diallo, M. S., 2005. Nanomaterials and water purification: Opportunities and challenges. *Journal of Nanoparticle Research*, 7, 331–342.

83. Upadhyayula, V. K. K., Deng, S., Mitchell, M. C., and Smith, G. B., 2009. Application of carbon nanotube technology for removal of contaminants in drinking water: A review. *Science of the Total Environment*, 408, 1–13.

84. Agnihotri, S., Mota, J. P. B., Rostam-Abadi, M., and Rood, M. J., 2005. Structural characterization of single-walled carbon nanotube bundles by experiment and molecular simulation. *Langmuir*, 21, 896–904.

85. Donaldson, K., Aitken, R., Tran, L. et al., 2006. Carbon nanotubes: A review of their properties in relation to pulmonary toxicology and workplace safety. *Toxicological Sciences*, 92, 5–22.

86. Yan, X. M., Shi, B. Y., Lu, J. J., Feng, C. H., Wang, D. S., and Tang, H. X., 2008. Adsorption and desorption of atrazine on carbon nanotubes. *Journal of Colloid and Interface Science*, 321, 30–38.

87. Benny, T., Bandosz, T., and Wong, S., 2008. Effect of ozonolysis on the pore structure, surface chemistry, and bundling of single walled carbon nanotubes. *Journal of Colloid Interface and Science*, 317, 375–382.

88. Lee, S. M., Lee, S. C., Jung, J. H., and Kim, H. J., 2005. Pore characterization of multi-walled carbon nanotubes modified by KOH. *Chemical Physics Letters*, 416, 251–255.

89. Li, Y. H., Wang, S. G., Zhang, X. F. et al., 2003. Adsorption of fluoride from water by aligned carbon nanotubes. *Materials Research Bulletin*, 38, 469–476.

90. Liao, Q., Sun, J., and Gao, L., 2008. Adsorption of chlorophenols by multi-walled carbon nanotubes treated with HNO_3 and NH_3. *Carbon*, 46, 553–555.

91. Liu, Y., Shen, Z., and Yokogawa, K., 2006. Investigation of preparation and structures of activated carbon nanotubes. *Materials Research Bulletin*, 41, 1503–1512.

92. Mauter, M. S. and Elimelech, M., 2008. Environmental applications of carbon-based nanomaterials. *Environmental Science and Technology*, 42, 5843–5859.

93. Niu, J. J., Wang, J. N., Jiang, Y., Su, L. F., and Ma, J., 2007. An approach to carbon nanotubes with high surface area and large pore volume. *Microporous and Mesoporous Materials*, 100, 1–5.

94. Yang, K., Zhu, L. Z., and Xing, B. S., 2006. Adsorption of polycyclic aromatic hydrocarbons by carbon nanomaterials. *Environmental Science and Technology*, 40, 1855–1861.

95. Kang, S., Herzberg, M., Rodrigues, D. F., and Elimelech, M., 2008. Antibacterial effects of carbon nanotubes: Size does matter. *Langmuir*, 24, 6409–6413.

96. Yan, H., Gong, A. J., He, H. S., Zhou, J., Wei, Y. X., and Lv, L., 2006. Adsorption of microcystins by carbon nanotubes. *Chemosphere*, 62, 142–148.

97. Yan, H., Pan, G., Zou, H., Li, X. L., and Chen, H., 2004. Effective removal of microcystins using carbon nanotubes embedded with bacteria. *Chinese Science Bulletin*, 49, 1694–1698.

98. Ye, C., Gong, Q.-M., Lu, F.-P., and Liang, J., 2007. Adsorption of middle molecular weight toxins on carbon nanotubes. *Acta Physico-Chimica Sinica*, 23, 1321–1324.

99. Melegari, S. and Matias, W., 2012. Preliminary assessment of the performance of oyster shells and chitin materials as adsorbents in the removal of saxitoxin in aqueous solutions. *Chemistry Central Journal*, 6, 86.

100. Wang, H., Ho, L., Lewis, D. M., Brookes, J. D., and Newcombe, G., 2007. Discriminating and assessing adsorption and biodegradation removal mechanisms during granular activated carbon filtration of microcystin toxins. *Water Research*, 41, 4262–4270.

101. Leroux, J.-C., 2007. Injectable nanocarriers for biodetoxification. *Nature Nanotechnology*, 2, 679–684.

102. Rahman, Y. E., Rosentha, M. W., and Cerny, E. A., 1973. Intracellular plutonium—Removal by liposome-encapsulated chelating agent. *Science*, 180, 300–302.

103. Weinberg, G., Ripper, R., Feinstein, D. L., and Hoffman, W., 2003. Lipid emulsion infusion rescues dogs from bupivacaine-induced cardiac toxicity. *Regional Anesthesia and Pain Medicine*, 28, 198–202.

104. Weinberg, G. L., VadeBoncouer, T., Ramaraju, G. A., Garcia-Amaro, M. F., and Cwik, M. J., 1998. Pretreatment or resuscitation with a lipid infusion shifts the dose-response to bupivacaine-induced asystole in rats. *Anesthesiology*, 88, 1071–1075.

105. Herrmann, I. K., Urner, M., Koehler, F. M. et al., 2010. Blood purification using functionalized core/shell nanomagnets. *Small*, 6, 1388–1392.

106. Sorgenfrei, I. F., Norrild, K., Larsen, P. B. et al., 2006. Reversal of rocuronium-induced neuromuscular block by the selective relaxant binding agent sugammadex—A dose-finding and safety study. *Anesthesiology*, 104, 667–674.

107. Beaurepaire, E., Buissette, V., Sauviat, M. P. et al., 2004. Functionalized fluorescent oxide nanoparticles: Artificial toxins for sodium channel targeting and imaging at the single-molecule level. *Nano Letters*, 4, 2079–2084.

108. McAteer, M. A., Sibson, N. R., von zur Muhlen, C. et al., 2007. In vivo magnetic resonance imaging of acute brain inflammation using microparticles of iron oxide. *Nature Medicine*, 13, 1253–1258.

109. Hu, F. and Zhao, Y. S., 2012. Inorganic nanoparticle-based T-1 and T-1/T-2 magnetic resonance contrast probes. *Nanoscale*, 4, 6235–6243.

110. Park, K., Lee, S., Kang, E., Kim, K., Choi, K., and Kwon, I. C., 2009. New generation of multifunctional nanoparticles for cancer imaging and therapy. *Advanced Functional Materials*, 19, 1553–1566.

111. Richard, C., Doan, B.-T., Beloeil, J.-C., Bessodes, M., Toth, E., and Scherman, D., 2008. Noncovalent functionalization of carbon nanotubes with amphiphilic Gd3+ chelates: Toward powerful T-1 and T-2 MRI contrast agents. *Nano Letters*, 8, 232–236.

112. Rieter, W. J., Kim, J. S., Taylor, K. M. L. et al., 2007. Hybrid silica nanoparticles for multimodal imaging. *Angewandte Chemie-International Edition*, 46, 3680–3682.

113. Rieter, W. J., Taylor, K. M. L., An, H., Lin, W., and Lin, W., 2006. Nanoscale metal-organic frameworks as potential multimodal contrast enhancing agents. *Journal of the American Chemical Society*, 128, 9024–9025.

114. Sitharaman, B., Kissell, K. R., Hartman, K. B. et al., 2005. Superparamagnetic gadonanotubes are high-performance MRI contrast agents. *Chemical Communications*, 2005, 31, 3915–3917.

115. Bae, K. H., Lee, K., Kim, C., and Park, T. G., 2010. Surface functionalized hollow manganese oxide nanoparticles for cancer targeted siRNA delivery and magnetic resonance imaging. *Biomaterials*, 32, 176–184.

116. Yang, H., Zhuang, Y., Sun, Y. et al., 2011. Targeted dual-contrast T1- and T2-weighted magnetic resonance imaging of tumors using multifunctional gadolinium-labeled superparamagnetic iron oxide nanoparticles. *Biomaterials*, 32, 4584–4593.

117. Choi, J.-S., Lee, J.-H., Shin, T.-H., Song, H.-T., Kim, E. Y., and Cheon, J., 2010. Self-confirming "AND" logic nanoparticles for fault-free MRI. *Journal of the American Chemical Society*, 132, 11015–11017.

118. Li, I. F., Su, C.-H., Sheu, H.-S. et al., 2008. $Gd_2O(CO_3)_2$ center dot H_2O particles and the corresponding Gd_2O_3: Synthesis and applications of magnetic resonance contrast agents and template particles for hollow spheres and hybrid composites. *Advanced Functional Materials*, 18, 766–776.

119. Yoon, Y.-S., Lee, B.-I., Lee, K. S. et al., 2010. Fabrication of a silica sphere with fluorescent and MR contrasting GdPO4 nanoparticles from layered gadolinium hydroxide. *Chemical Communications*, 46, 3654–3656.

120. Park, J. Y., Kattel, K., Xu, W. et al., 2011. Longitudinal water proton relaxivities of Gd(OH)(3) nanorods, Gd(OH)(3) nanoparticles, and Gd_2O_3 nanoparticles: Dependence on particle diameter, composition, and morphology. *Journal of the Korean Physical Society*, 59, 2376–2380.

121. Bridot, J.-L., Faure, A.-C., Laurent, S. et al., 2007. Hybrid gadolinium oxide nanoparticles: Multimodal contrast agents for in vivo imaging. *Journal of the American Chemical Society*, 129, 5076–5084.

122. Choi, E. S., Park, J. Y., Baek, M. J. et al., 2010. Water-soluble ultra-small manganese oxide surface doped gadolinium oxide (Gd_2O_3@MnO) nanoparticles for MRI contrast agent. *European Journal of Inorganic Chemistry*, 2010, 4555–4560.

123. Fortin, M.-A., Petoral, R. M., Jr., Soederlind, F. et al., 2007. Polyethylene glycol-covered ultra-small Gd_2O_3 nanoparticles for positive contrast at 1.5 T magnetic resonance clinical scanning. *Nanotechnology*, 18, 395501-1–395501-9.

124. Park, J. Y., Baek, M. J., Choi, E. S. et al., 2009. Paramagnetic ultrasmall gadolinium oxide nanoparticles as advanced T-1 MR1 contrast agent: Account for large longitudinal relaxivity, optimal particle diameter, and in vivo T-1 MR images. ACS *Nano*, 3, 3663–3669.

125. Chambon, C., Clement, O., Leblanche, A., Schoumanclaeys, E., and Frija, G., 1993. Superparamagnetic iron-oxides as positive mr contrast agents—In vitro and in vivo evidence. *Magnetic Resonance Imaging*, 11, 509–519.

126. Taboada, E., Rodriguez, E., Roig, A., Oro, J., Roch, A., and Muller, R. N., 2007. Relaxometric and magnetic characterization of ultrasmall iron oxide nanoparticles with high magnetization. Evaluation as potential T-1 magnetic resonance imaging contrast agents for molecular imaging. *Langmuir*, 23, 4583–4588.

127. Gref, R., Minamitake, Y., Peracchia, M. T., Trubetskoy, V., Torchilin, V., and Langer, R., 1994. Biodegradable long-circulating polymeric nanospheres. *Science*, 263, 1600–1603.

128. Ahmad, T., Rhee, I., Hong, S., Chang, Y., and Lee, J., 2011. $Ni\text{-}Fe_2O_4$ nanoparticles as contrast agents for magnetic resonance imaging. *Journal of Nanoscience and Nanotechnology*, 11, 5645–5650.

129. Zeng, L., Ren, W., Zheng, J., Cui, P., and Wu, A., 2012. Ultrasmall water-soluble metal-iron oxide nanoparticles as T-1-weighted contrast agents for magnetic resonance imaging. *Physical Chemistry Chemical Physics*, 14, 5645–5650.

130. Seo, W. S., Lee, J. H., Sun, X. et al., 2006. FeCo/graphitic-shell nanocrystals as advanced magnetic-resonance-imaging and near-infrared agents. *Nature Materials*, 5, 971–976.

131. Medintz, I. L., Uyeda, H. T., Goldman, E. R., and Mattoussi, H., 2005. Quantum dot bioconjugates for imaging, labelling and sensing. *Nature Materials*, 4, 435–446.

132. Tang, Z. Y., Kotov, N. A., and Giersig, M., 2002. Spontaneous organization of single CdTe nanoparticles into luminescent nanowires. *Science*, 297, 237–240.

133. Chang, Y.-P., Pinaud, F., Antelman, J., and Weiss, S., 2008. Tracking bio-molecules in live cells using quantum dots. *Journal of Biophotonics*, 1, 287–298.

134. Azzay, H. M., Mansour, M. M., and Kazmierczak, S. C., 2007. From diagnostics to therapy: Prospects of quantum dots. *Clinical Biochemistry*, 40, 917–927.

135. Gao, X. H., Cui, Y. Y., Levenson, R. M., Chung, L. W. K., and Nie, S. M., 2004. In vivo cancer targeting and imaging with semiconductor quantum dots. *Nature Biotechnology*, 22, 969–976.

136. Wu, X. Y., Liu, H. J., Liu, J. Q. et al., 2003. Immunofluorescent labeling of cancer marker Her2 and other cellular targets with semiconductor quantum dots. *Nature Biotechnology*, 21, 41–46.

137. Weissleder, R. and Pittet, M. J., 2008. Imaging in the era of molecular oncology. *Nature*, 452, 580–589.

138. Bagalkot, V., Zhang, L., Levy-Nissenbaum, E. et al., 2007. Quantum dot—Aptamer conjugates for synchronous cancer imaging, therapy, and sensing of drug delivery based on Bi-fluorescence resonance energy transfer. *Nano Letters*, 7, 3065–3070.

139. Ghasemi, Y., Peymani, P., and Afifi, S., 2009. Quantum dot: Magic nanoparticle for imaging, detection and targeting. *Acta Bio-Medica: Atenei Parmensis*, 80, 156–165.

140. Park, J.-H., von Maltzahn, G., Ruoslahti, E., Bhatia, S. N., and Sailor, M. J., 2008. Micellar hybrid nanoparticles for simultaneous magnetofluorescent imaging and drug delivery. *Angewandte Chemie-International Edition*, 47, 7284–7288.

141. Pan, J., Liu, Y., and Feng, S.-S., 2010. Multifunctional nanoparticles of biodegradable copolymer blend for cancer diagnosis and treatment. *Nanomedicine*, 5, 347–360.

142. Yildiz, I., Deniz, E., McCaughan, B., Cruickshank, S. F., Callan, J. F., and Raymo, F. M., 2010. Hydrophilic CdSe-ZnS core-shell quantum dots with reactive functional groups on their surface. *Langmuir*, 26, 11503–11511.

143. Yildiz, I., McCaughan, B., Cruickshank, S. F., Callan, J. F., and Raymo, F. M., 2009. Biocompatible CdSe-ZnS core-shell quantum dots coated with hydrophilic polythiols. *Langmuir*, 25, 7090–7096.

144. Burris, K. P. and Stewart Jr, C. N., 2012. Fluorescent nanoparticles: Sensing pathogens and toxins in foods and crops. *Trends in Food Science and Technology*, 28, 143–152.

145. Goldman, E. R., Anderson, G. P., Tran, P. T., Mattoussi, H., Charles, P. T., and Mauro, J. M., 2002. Conjugation of luminescent quantum dots with antibodies using an engineered adaptor protein to provide new reagents for fluoroimmunoassays. *Analytical Chemistry*, 74, 841–847.

146. Warner, M. G., Grate, J. W., Tyler, A. et al., 2009. Quantum dot immunoassays in renewable surface column and 96-well plate formats for the fluorescence detection of botulinum neurotoxin using high-affinity antibodies. *Biosensors and Bioelectronics*, 25, 179–184.

147. Medintz, I. L., Mattoussi, H., and Clapp, A. R., 2008. Potential clinical applications of quantum dots. *International Journal of Nanomedicine*, 3, 151–167.

148. Wang, Y., Tang, Z., and Kotov, N. A., 2005. Bioapplication of nanosemiconductors. *Nanotoday*, 8, 20–31.

149. Alivisatos, P., 2004. The use of nanocrystals in biological detection. *Nature Biotechnology*, 22, 47–52.

150. Chan, W. C. W. and Nie, S. M., 1998. Quantum dot bioconjugates for ultrasensitive nonisotopic detection. *Science*, 281, 2016–2018.

151. Ballou, B., Lagerholm, B. C., Ernst, L. A., Bruchez, M. P., and Waggoner, A. S., 2004. Noninvasive imaging of quantum dots in mice. *Bioconjugate Chemistry*, 15, 79–86.

152. Parak, W. J., Boudreau, R., Le Gros, M. et al., 2002. Cell motility and metastatic potential studies based on quantum dot imaging of phagokinetic tracks. *Advanced Materials*, 14, 882–885.

153. Kim, S., Lim, Y. T., Soltesz, E. G. et al., 2004. Near-infrared fluorescent type II quantum dots for sentinel lymph node mapping. *Nature Biotechnology*, 22, 93–97.

154. Huang, X., Jain, P. K., El-Sayed, I. H., and El-Sayed, M. A., 2007. Gold nanoparticles: Interesting optical properties and recent applications in cancer diagnostic and therapy. *Nanomedicine*, 2, 681–693.

155. Xie, J., Lee, S., and Chen, X., 2010. Nanoparticle-based theranostic agents. *Advanced Drug Delivery Reviews*, 62, 1064–1079.

156. Alonso, E., Vale, C., Vieytes, M. R., Laferla, F. M., Gimenez-Llort, L., and Botana, L. M., 2011. 13-Desmethyl spirolide-C is neuroprotective and reduces intracellular A beta and hyperphosphorylated tau in vitro. *Neurochemistry International*, 59, 1056–1065.

157. Kim, G.-Y., Kim, W.-J., and Choi, Y. H., 2011. Pectenotoxin-2 from marine sponges: A potential anti-cancer agent—A review. *Marine Drugs*, 9, 2176–2187.

158. Watters, M. R., 2008. Marine neurotoxins as a starting point to drugs, in *Seafood and Freshwater Toxins: Pharmacology, Physiology and Detection*, 2nd edn. Botana, L. M., ed. CRC Press, Boca Raton, FL. pp. 889–896.

159. Allen, T. M. and Cullis, P. R., 2004. Drug delivery systems: Entering the mainstream. *Science*, 303, 1818–1822.

160. Yang, J., Lee, C.-H., Ko, H.-J. et al., 2007. Multifunctional magneto-polymeric nanohybrids for targeted detection and synergistic therapeutic effects on breast cancer. *Angewandte Chemie-International Edition*, 46, 8836–8839.

161. Holme, M. N., Fedotenko, I. A., Abegg, D. et al., 2012. Shear-stress sensitive lenticular vesicles for targeted drug delivery. *Nature Nanotechnology*, 7, 536–543.

162. Tiwari, P. M., Vig, K., Dennis, V. A., and Singh, S. R., 2011. Functionalized gold nanoparticles and their biomedical applications. *Nanomaterials*, 1, 31–63.

163. Ledo, A., Martinez, F., Lopez-Quintela, M. A., and Rivas, J., 2007. Synthesis of Ag clusters in microemulsions: A time-resolved UV-vis and fluorescence spectroscopy study. *Physica B-Condensed Matter*, 398, 273–277.

164. Ledo-Suarez, A., Rivas, J., Rodriguez-Abreu, C. F. et al., 2007. Facile synthesis of stable subnanosized silver clusters in microemulsions. *Angewandte Chemie-International Edition*, 46, 8823–8827.

165. Rodríguez Cobo, E., Rivas Rey, J., Blanco Varela, M. C., Mouriño Mosquera, A., Torneiro Abuín, M., and López-Quintela, M. A., 2006. Functionalization of atomic cobalt clusters obtained by electrochemical methods. *Physica Status Solidi*, 203, 1223–1228.

166. Rodríguez-Vázquez, M. J., Vázquez-Vázquez, C., Rivas, J., and López-Quintela, M. A., 2009. Synthesis and characterization of gold atomic clusters by the two-phase method. *The European Physical Journal D*, 52, 23–26.

167. Vazquez-Vazquez, C., Banobre-Lopez, M., Mitra, A., Arturo Lopez-Quintela, M., and Rivas, J., 2009. Synthesis of small atomic copper clusters in microemulsions. *Langmuir*, 25, 8208–8216.

168. Vilar-Vidal, N., Blanco, M. C., Lopez-Quintela, M. A., Rivas, J., and Serra, C., 2010. Electrochemical synthesis of very stable photoluminescent copper clusters. *Journal of Physical Chemistry C*, 114, 15924–15930.

169. Vilar-Vidal, N., Rivas, J., and Arturo Lopez-Quintela, M., 2012. Size dependent catalytic activity of reusable subnanometer copper(0) clusters. ACS *Catalysis*, 2, 1693–1697.

170. Calvo-Fuentes, J., Rivas, J., and López-Quintela, M. A., 2012. Synthesis of subnanometric metal nanoparticles, in *Encyclopedia of Nanotechnology*. Bhushan, B., ed. Springer Verlag, pp. 2639–2648.

171. Pineiro-Redondo, Y., Banobre-Lopez, M., Pardinas-Blanco, I., Goya, G., Arturo Lopez-Quintela, M., and Rivas, J., 2011. The influence of colloidal parameters on the specific power absorption of PAA-coated magnetite nanoparticles. *Nanoscale Research Letters*, 6, 383-1–383-7.

172. Banobre-Lopez, M., Pineiro-Redondo, Y., De Santis, R. et al., 2011. Poly(caprolactone) based magnetic scaffolds for bone tissue engineering. *Journal of Applied Physics*, 109.

173. Rivas, J., Banobre-Lopez, M., Pineiro-Redondo, Y., Rivas, B., and Lopez-Quintela, M. A., 2012. Magnetic nanoparticles for application in cancer therapy. *Journal of Magnetism and Magnetic Materials*, 324, 3499–3502.

174. Tampieri, A., D'Alessandro, T., Sandri, M. et al., 2012. Intrinsic magnetism and hyperthermia in bioactive Fe-doped hydroxyapatite. *Acta Biomaterialia*, 8, 843–853.

175. Jun, Y.-W., Lee, J.-H., and Cheon, J., 2008. Chemical design of nanoparticle probes for highperformance magnetic resonance imaging. *Angewandte Chemie-International Edition*, 47, 5122–5135.

176. Cai, W., Shin, D. W., Chen, K. et al., 2006. Peptide-labeled near-infrared quantum dots for imaging tumor vasculature in living subjects. *Nano Letters*, 6, 669–676.

177. Liu, Z., Cai, W., He, L. et al., 2006. In vivo biodistribution and highly efficient tumour targeting of carbon nanotubes in mice. *Nature Nanotechnology*, 2, 47–52.

19

Culture of Microalgal Dinoflagellates

F. García-Camacho, A. Sánchez-Mirón, J. Gallardo-Rodríguez,
L. López-Rosales, Y. Chisti, and E. Molina-Grima

CONTENTS

19.1 Introduction

Production of metabolites from microalgal dinoflagellates requires them to be grown in a controlled environment, usually as relatively large-volume pure cultures, in some form of a bioreactor. This chapter is focused on bioreactor culture of dinoflagellates. Only about half of the dinoflagellate species photosynthesize and the rest of the species are symbiotic and parasitic or rely on some form of heterotrophy (Taylor 1987; Taylor et al. 2003; Sherr and Sherr 2007; Gallardo-Rodríguez et al. 2012a). Most of the toxic dinoflagellates are capable of mixotrophic growth (Stoecker 1999; Sherr and Sherr 2007; Burkholder et al. 2008). That is, they can simultaneously photosynthesize and use organic carbon sources for growth. In the absence of light, mixotrophic species grow exclusively by heterotrophy, although in some cases the productivity may be lower than in phototrophic growth (Gallardo-Rodríguez et al. 2012a). A photoautotrophic culture growing on sunlight as the energy source and carbon dioxide as an almost exclusive source of carbon may nevertheless require trace amounts of organic carbon in the form of essential vitamins.

Heterotrophic growth is feasible in conventional bioreactors, or fermenters, as light is not necessary. Photoautotrophic growth requires light and the use of some form of a photobioreactor. Production of a metabolite and its productivity may be influenced by whether the mode of growth is photosynthetic or heterotrophic. Any metabolite production process must be inexpensive and consistently achieve a satisfactory level of productivity under well-defined conditions. The design of the culture system, that is, the bioreactor or photobioreactor, influences production as do the culture media and the growth environment.

Although several microalgae are grown commercially in large quantities, this is not so for dinoflagellates. Only a few dinoflagellate species are grown, mostly photoautotrophically at a scale of <50 L, to produce reference standards of some dinoflagellate-derived toxins (Quilliam 2003; Gallardo-Rodríguez et al. 2012a). Products such as docosahexaenoic acid (DHA) have been produced via heterotrophic culture of nontoxic dinoflagellates in conventional fermenters (Mendes et al. 2009).

Compared to the other commercially used microalgae, dinoflagellates grow slowly (Tang 1996). This may be surprising considering their ability to cyclically provoke blooms with thousands of cells per milliliter in only a few days in natural waters (Hallegraeff 2003). However, the dynamics of bloom development in coastal waters appear to be related more to oceanic flow patterns and winds that concentrate biomass in areas of low turbulence and less to any sudden increase in the growth rate of the cells (Gallardo-Rodríguez et al. 2012a).

In production of bioactive metabolites (Garcia Camacho et al. 2007a) from dinoflagellates, the titer of the target product is often low. For example, the production of 150 g of a dinoflagellate toxin is estimated to require a culture broth volume of 10^3–10^5 m^3 (Shimizu 2000). This is far larger than the volume of the fermentation broth needed to produce the same quantity of a typical antibiotic (Gallardo-Rodríguez et al. 2012a), for example. The handling of such a large volume of broth of a highly toxic material could be a major problem (Gallardo-Rodríguez et al. 2012a). The broth handling task can be greatly simplified by raising the concentration of the bioactive in the broth so that the volume that needs to be handled is reduced. An elevated concentration of the bioactive in the broth will also reduce its cost of production (Chisti 2007). As a result of low productivity, most of the commercially available dinoflagellate bioactives are extremely expensive. For example, prices of the commercially available dinoflagellate toxins are in the range of € 276–30,980 mg^{-1} (Garcia Camacho et al. 2007a). Enhancements in concentration of a target compound may be made also by improving the producer strain through selection and genetic modification.

19.2 Growth of Dinoflagellates

Dinoflagellates are generally associated with harmful algal blooms, and the dynamics of development of such blooms have received much attention (Gallardo-Rodríguez et al. 2012a). In contrast, far less effort has been devoted to controlled culture of dinoflagellates in bioreactors. Production of large quantities of nondinoflagellate microalgae in photobioreactors has been quite successful (Molina Grima et al. 2003; Acién Fernández et al. 2005; Fernández Sevilla et al. 2010), but this has not been generally the case for dinoflagellate microalgae (Gallardo-Rodríguez et al. 2012a). Nonetheless, the production of gram quantities of dinoflagellate bioactives for various purposes has mostly relied on culturing them in low-productivity systems. The maximum biomass concentration attainable in a typical photosynthetic culture of a dinoflagellate is low (Hu et al. 2006; Mountfort et al. 2006; Gallardo Rodríguez et al. 2010), for example, well below 1 g·L^{-1}. Also, toxin production per cell is of the order of picograms (Shimizu 2000); therefore, a photobioreactor culture typically has a low toxin productivity (Gallardo-Rodríguez et al. 2012a).

Dinoflagellates generally grow slower than the other microalgae, but the reasons for this are not clearly known (Tang 1996). The low photoautotrophic growth rates of dinoflagellates are unlikely to be related to any differences in the photosynthetic capacity relative to the other microalgae. For example, the chlorophyll *a* contents per unit mass of dinoflagellates are comparable to those of the diatoms. In nutrient-sufficient conditions, nonphotosynthesizing dinoflagellates, for example, the heterotrophs, can grow more rapidly than the ones that rely exclusively on photosynthesis (Mendes et al. 2009; Skelton 2009).

To improve productivity of the desired bioactive in a bioreactor culture, several aspects of the producer species need to be first characterized. For example, the nutritional requirements of the producer species and its life cycle need to be known (Gallardo-Rodríguez et al. 2012a). The particular nutrients provided in the culture medium may influence the cell-specific production of the bioactive.

In nature, complex circadian systems control the behavior of dinoflagellates (Roenneberg and Merrow 2002). For example, daylight and changes in the levels of nutrients in the water column are known to affect vertical migrations (Doblin et al. 2006). In photosynthetic dinoflagellates, cells generally divide at the end of the dark period (Homma 1989) and grow during the light phase. The latter corresponds to the G1 phase of the cell cycle (Gallardo-Rodríguez et al. 2012a). Production of many toxins has been found to coincide with the G1 phase (Taroncher-Oldenburg 1998; Wong and Kwok 2005). Dinoflagellates are able to couple the progression of the cell cycle to cell growth, allowing them to make the best use of available resources and possibly preparing them for a symbiotic existence (Wong and Kwok 2005).

In a photobioreactor where the levels of the nutrients are typically uniform and illumination is often continuous, the natural rhythms may cease and the metabolic behavior may be quite different to the behavior in nature (Gallardo-Rodríguez et al. 2012a).

The development of a capability to mass culture dinoflagellates for producing bioactives requires attention to the following aspects: (1) media formulations for enhancing cell growth and production of the metabolite, (2) optimization of the culture conditions to attain a high concentration of the desired compound in a short period, (3) understanding of the possible triggers for the synthesis of the bioactive, and (4) better engineered bioreactors and photobioreactors (Gallardo-Rodríguez et al. 2012a). Some of these aspects have been discussed in the literature in relation to specific cases. For example, temperature has been shown to affect the saxitoxin content of *Alexandrium catenella* cells (Navarro et al. 2006) and the yessotoxin content of *Protoceratium reticulatum* cells (Paz et al. 2006). Environmental factors including osmotic pressure have been found to affect the growth of *Karenia brevis* (Magaña and Villareal 2006; Errera and Campbell 2011).

The toxin profile of *Alexandrium ostenfeldii* has been determined to be sensitive to the culture conditions (Otero et al. 2010). Nutritional supplementation of the culture medium has been shown to influence the toxin productivity of several dinoflagellates (Wang and Hsieh 2002; Gallardo Rodríguez et al. 2009a). A two-step culture methodology has been determined to improve toxin production by *Alexandrium tamarense* (Hu et al. 2006). The first step used 4 days of static operation to favor growth. Subsequently, the culture was aerated in an airlift bioreactor (Hu et al. 2006). Similar approaches have been used in a stirred-tank photobioreactor for producing toxins of *P. reticulatum* (Gallardo Rodríguez et al. 2007).

Production of several dinoflagellate toxins in laboratory cultures has been discussed in the literature (Beuzenberg et al. 2012; Gallardo-Rodríguez et al. 2012a; Lee et al. 2012; Yamaguchi et al. 2012; Paz et al. 2013). Production of yessotoxins has been described (Paz et al. 2004, 2013; Gallardo Rodríguez et al. 2007). The production of paralytic shellfish toxins has been reviewed by Hsieh et al. (2001). Other notable studies include the production of C2 toxin by *A. tamarense* (Wang and Hsieh 2002; Wang et al. 2002), gymnodimine production by *Karenia selliformis* (Mountfort et al. 2006), saxitoxin production by *Alexandrium minutum* (Parker 2002; Lim et al. 2010), palytoxin production by *Ostreopsis ovata* (Pistocchi et al. 2011), and ciguatoxin production by *Gambierdiscus polynesiensis* (Chinain 2009).

19.3 Production Media

Studies of metabolite production in dinoflagellate cultures have not generally used media optimized specifically for maximal productivity (Gallardo-Rodríguez et al. 2012a). For example, the media compositions that are almost exclusively used in culturing toxic dinoflagellates are the *f*/2 medium (Guillard 1975), the L1 (Guillard and Hargraves 1993), and the K medium (Keller and Guillard 1986). These similar formulations were originally developed for nondinoflagellate species. For example, the L1 formulation was originally intended as a standard medium for culturing marine diatoms (Guillard and Hargraves 1993). The commonly used formulations are therefore not necessarily optimal for producing dinoflagellates and their toxins. Media formulations for heterotrophic growth have received barely any attention (Gallardo-Rodríguez et al. 2012a).

The medium formulation can greatly impact the productivity of a metabolite. Media for culturing dinoflagellates typically contain many different components. Optimizing such media by the conventional statistical experimental design is an unwieldy task. A superior approach is to use optimization methods based on genetic algorithms (Weuster-Botz 2000). A genetic algorithm-based stochastic search strategy has been used to successfully optimize the culture medium for producing yessotoxins from *P. reticulatum* (García-Camacho et al. 2011a). The composition of this optimized medium is shown in Table 19.1. The use of the optimized medium allowed a 60% enhancement in the final cell concentration relative to the control operation based on the L1 medium (García-Camacho et al. 2011a). The optimized medium enhanced the productivity of yessotoxins by 40% relative to control and improved the stability of the cultures in the stationary phase (García-Camacho et al. 2011a).

TABLE 19.1

Optimal Medium Composition for Producing Yessotoxins from *P. reticulatum*

Component	Concentration (μM)
$NaNO_3$	8500.00
Urea	10.00
$C_3H_7Na_2O_6P \cdot 5H_2O$	110.00
$Na_2HPO_4 \cdot 2H_2O$	20.00
$NaSiO_3 \cdot 9H_2O$	110.00
Na_2CO_3	40.00
$Na_2EDTA \cdot 2H_2O$	145.84
$FeCl_3 \cdot 6H_2O$	9.36
$Fe-Na-EDTA \cdot 3H_2O$	9.36
$MnCl_2 \cdot H_2O$	20.00
$ZnSO_4 \cdot 7H_2O$	636.67×10^{-3}
$CoCl_2 \cdot 6H_2O$	14.02×10^{-3}
$NiSO_4 \cdot 6H_2O$	8.00×10^{-3}
H_3BO_3	400.00
$Na_2MoO_4 \cdot 2H_2O$	1341.65×10^{-3}
$(NH_4)_6Mo_7O_{24} \cdot 4H_2O$	14.56×10^{-3}
H_2SeO_3	5.00×10^{-3}
Na_3VO_4	2.00×10^{-2}
K_2CrO_4	1.00×10^{-2}
Thiamine $\cdot$ HCl	4941.65×10^{-3}
Biotin	2.97×10^{-3}
Vitamin B_{12}	25.00×10^{-5}
Citric acid $\cdot H_2O$	65.00

Source: Reprinted from *Harmful Algae*, 10, García-Camacho, F., Gallardo-Rodríguez, J.J., Sánchez-Mirón, A., Chisti, Y., and Molina-Grima, E., Genetic algorithm-based medium optimization for a toxic dinoflagellate microalga, 697–701, Copyright 2011a, with permission from Elsevier.

19.4 Bioreactor Culture

Culture of dinoflagellates at any significant scale inevitably requires the use of bioreactors and photobioreactors, depending on the nature of the production operation. Heterotrophic culture is generally feasible only in monoseptically operated closed bioreactors as any accidental microbial contaminant will inevitably outgrow a dinoflagellate in a medium that is rich in organic carbon. Open pond culture systems commonly used for commercial photoautotrophic production of nondinoflagellate microalgae (Ostwald 1988; Sompech et al. 2012) may not be suitable for producing dinoflagellate toxins because of safety considerations, unless a product is relatively benign. Depending on the scale of production operation, different configurations of photobioreactors have been used for growing various nondinoflagellate microalgae. Figure 19.1 shows a set of closed photobioreactors developed by the author's group for growing various microalgae at different scales. The hydrodynamic environment in bioreactors and photobioreactors is necessarily turbulent to ensure a homogeneous distribution of nutrients and cells. Turbulence is needed also to achieve mass transfer of carbon dioxide from the gas phase to the liquid phase at a sufficiently rapid rate in photoautotrophic growth. Gas–liquid mass transfer is important also in a heterotrophic culture that must be supplied with oxygen, usually by absorption from air (Gallardo-Rodríguez et al. 2012a). The carbon dioxide generated by respiration in a heterotrophic culture must be removed, typically by desorption into the exhaust gas. All these gas–liquid mass

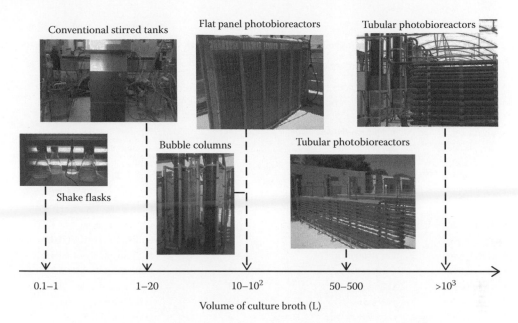

FIGURE 19.1 Photobioreactors typically used for culturing nondinoflagellate microalgae at different scales of operation.

transfer processes need mixing of the culture broth. Dinoflagellates, unfortunately, are often sensitive to flow and withstand only a limited level of turbulence as discussed next.

19.4.1 Turbulence Sensitivity of Dinoflagellates

Dinoflagellates are often sensitive to turbulence in the culture broth. Inhibition of growth by agitation, shaking, stirring, and aeration has been commonly reported in laboratory growth operations (e.g., White 1976; Pollingher and Zemel 1981; Berdalet 1992). The growth rate and morphology are known to be affected by small-scale turbulence (Berdalet and Estrada 1993; Sullivan et al. 2003; Sullivan and Swift 2003; Berdalet et al. 2007). In nature, the small-scale turbulence induced by winds and waves has been found to adversely affect growth (Pollingher and Zemel 1981; Berman and Shteinman 1998; Stoecker et al. 2006). Consequently, a successful culture in a bioreactor requires careful control of the turbulence intensity through engineering of the bioreactor, a sensible choice of its operational regime, and possible use of protective additives in the culture medium (Gallardo Rodríguez et al. 2007, 2011, 2012a; García Camacho et al. 2007b). The intensity of turbulence, or its scale, is characterized in terms of the specific energy dissipation rate in the culture fluid. The length scale of energy-dissipating terminal eddies is smaller in an intensely agitated fluid compared to the case of a less turbulent one.

Growth inhibition thresholds of the specific energy dissipation rates for various dinoflagellates are summarized in Table 19.2 (Gallardo-Rodríguez et al. 2012a). The data in Table 19.2 span several dino-flagellate orders and cells ranging in diameter from 12 to 500 μm (Berdalet et al. 2007). No definite link has been found between the flow sensitivity and the size, shape, and taxonomy of dinoflagellate species (Sullivan and Swift 2003; Berdalet et al. 2007; Gallardo-Rodríguez et al. 2012a).

The reasons for the shear sensitivity of dinoflagellates have been speculated on, but not definitively established (Gallardo-Rodríguez et al. 2012a). Dinoflagellates commonly consist of large cells. In some species, the cells may be as large as 2 mm. For photosynthetic species associated with the formation of harmful blooms, the size ranges approximately from 10 to 60 μm (Gallardo-Rodríguez et al. 2012a). In thecate dinoflagellates, that is, the ones with cell walls made of cellulosic plates, or thecae (Lee 2008), a cell-protective function has been suggested for the thecae (e.g., Thomas et al. 1995), but not supported by evidence. The thecate dinoflagellates can be as sensitive to turbulence as the athecate or naked species. For example, *P. reticulatum* having thecae is highly shear-sensitive, whereas the nontoxic dinoflagellate

TABLE 19.2

Energy Dissipation Rate (ε) Damage Threshold for Dinoflagellates

Dinoflagellate Order	Microorganism	Inhibitory ε (cm^2·s^{-3})	Reference
Gonyaulacales	*Lingulodinium polyedrum*	0.045	Thomas et al. (1995)
Gonyaulacales	*Alexandrium fundyense*	0.1	Juhl et al. (2001)
Gonyaulacales	*Ceratocorys horrid*	0.1	Zirbel et al. (2000)
Gonyaulacales	*Crypthecodinium cohnii*	0.1	Yeung and Wong (2003)
Gonyaulacales	*L. polyedrum*	0.15	Thomas and Gibson (1990)
Gonyaulacales	*L. polyedrum*	0.18	Juhl et al. (2000)
Gonyaulacales	*L. polyedrum*	0.2	Juhl and Latz (2002)
Gonyaulacales	*L. polyedrum*	0.2	Thomas and Gibson (1990)
Gonyaulacales	*L. polyedrum*	0.73	Gibson and Thomas (1995)
Gonyaulacales	*Protoceratium reticulatum*	0.8	García Camacho et al. (2007b)
Gonyaulacales	*A. fundyense*	1	Sullivan and Swift (2003)
Gonyaulacales	*Ceratium fusus*	1	Sullivan and Swift (2003)
Gonyaulacales	*Ceratium tripos*	1	Sullivan and Swift (2003)
Gonyaulacales	*C. tripos*	1	Sullivan and Swift (2003)
Gonyaulacales	*C. tripos*	1	Havskum et al. (2005)
Gonyaulacales	*Oxyrrhis marina*	1	Havskum (2003)
Gonyaulacales	*Pyrocystis noctiluca*	1	Sullivan and Swift (2003)
Gonyaulacales	*L. polyedrum*	3.5	Juhl and Latz (2002)
Gonyaulacales	*L. polyedrum*	10	Sullivan et al. (2003)
Gymnodiniales	*Akashiwo sanguinea*	0.011	Thomas and Gibson (1992)
Gymnodiniales	*A. sanguinea*	1	Berdalet (1992)
Gymnodiniales	*A. sanguinea*	2	Berdalet (1992)
Gymnodiniales	*A. sanguinea*	4.6	Tynan (1993)
Peridiniales	*Heterocapsa triquetra*	0.1	Dempsey (1982)
Peridiniales	*H. triquetra*	0.1	Yeung and Wong (2003)
Peridiniales	*Scrippsiella trochoidea*	2	Berdalet and Estrada (1993)
Prorocentrales	*Prorocentrum micans*	2	Berdalet and Estrada (1993)
Prorocentrales	*Prorocentrum triestinum*	2	Berdalet and Estrada (1993)

Source: Reprinted from *Biotechnology Advances*, 30, Gallardo-Rodríguez, J., Sánchez-Mirón, A., García-Camacho, F., López-Rosales, L., Chisti, Y., and Molina-Grima, E., Bioactives from microalgal dinoflagellates, 1673–1684, Copyright 2012a, with permission from Elsevier.

Crypthecodinium cohnii, having a similar cell wall structure, is more robust. *P. reticulatum* is damaged by energy dissipation rate values exceeding 0.8 cm^2·s^{-3} (García Camacho et al. 2007b), but *C. cohnii* can be grown at an energy dissipation rate of 5.8×10^5 cm^2·s^{-3} without obvious damage (Hu et al. 2007).

Tests performed on thecal plates isolated from the dinoflagellates *A. catenella* and *Lingulodinium polyedrum* have shown them to have mechanical properties comparable to those of softwood cell walls (Lau et al. 2007). Many plant cells with cellulosic walls are of course known to be highly sensitive to hydrodynamic shear forces (Namdev and Dunlop 1995; Joshi et al. 1996; Chisti 2010), and plant cells also tend to be comparatively large (Gallardo-Rodríguez et al. 2012a).

Animal cells freely suspended in culture media in bioreactors are used in many commercial biotechnology processes and are among the most shear-sensitive types of cells (Joshi et al. 1996; Chisti 1999, 2000, 2001, 2010; Juhl et al. 2000). Compared to such cells, dinoflagellates tend to be far more sensitive to turbulence. In general, the shear stress levels that dinoflagellates can tolerate are one or two orders of magnitude lower (Gallardo-Rodríguez et al. 2012a). Specific energy dissipation rate (ε) values in the range of $0.011 \leq \varepsilon \leq 10$ cm^2·s^{-3} have generally inhibited dinoflagellate growth (Table 19.2). In studies that did not find an adverse impact of turbulence on dinoflagellate cells, the specific energy dissipation rate was always <1 cm^2·s^{-3} (Berdalet et al. 2007) and, therefore, not relevant to bioreactor culture (Gallardo-Rodríguez et al. 2012a).

Flow sensitivity of dinoflagellates may be related to their unusual genomes (Gallardo-Rodríguez et al. 2012a). Dinoflagellates possess massive genomes packed in relatively small volumes. Their genomes are in the range of 3–245 Gb, compared to 10–100 Mb for most of the other eukaryotic algae (Veldhuis et al. 1997). A large genome is believed to increase the possibility of entanglement of the DNA strands during replication (Wong and Kwok 2005). The DNA in a dinoflagellate exists mostly in a liquid crystal state and may be susceptible to external mechanical forces transmitted to the nuclear envelope via the cytoskeleton. The nucleus is generally large, occupying nearly half of the cell volume, and this may ease the transmission of the external mechanical stimuli to the nucleus (Gallardo-Rodríguez et al. 2012a). The chromosomes in the nucleus are not scattered, but are attached to the nuclear membrane. This may further enhance their susceptibility to mechanical forces. Such forces may induce changes in the phase state of the DNA, leading to mutagenesis (Gallardo-Rodríguez et al. 2012a). This appears to concur with the observed increase in the cell's susceptibility to shear forces at certain stages of the cell cycle (García Camacho et al. 2007b). At certain levels, turbulence appears to be able to reversibly arrest the progression of the cell cycle without killing the cell (Yeung and Wong 2003). At lower levels, turbulence may merely slow the progression of the cell cycle rather than arrest it (Yeung and Wong 2003).

Adverse responses to flow can be wide ranging: growth inhibition, disturbance of the cell cycle (Berdalet 1992; Yeung and Wong 2003), calcium mobilization (Yeung 2006), production of peroxide radicals (Juhl and Latz 2002; Gallardo Rodríguez et al. 2009b), changes in the fluidity of the cell membrane (Mallipattu 2002; Gallardo-Rodríguez et al. 2012b), and others. The intensity of the response depends on the magnitude of turbulence, its duration, and the frequency of exposure (Gallardo-Rodríguez et al. 2012a). The light–dark cycle also influences how a cell responds to turbulence. Many types of cells are known to adapt to better tolerate shear stresses, but this does not appear to be the case for dinoflagellates such as *P. reticulatum* (García Camacho et al. 2007b). The intensity of shear stress appears to affect the production of toxins in at least some dinoflagellates (Juhl et al. 2001; Gallardo Rodríguez et al. 2011).

Some of the previously noted effects of turbulence are interrelated. The precise mechanisms involved in the mechanochemical transduction of an external shear stress into the cell are mostly unclear. The cytoskeleton may participate in mechanochemical transduction of external forces, but does not seem to be the primary sensor of flow. In animal cells, lipid bilayers of cell membranes are said to possess flow-sensing receptors (Gudi et al. 1996) and a similar mechanism may exist in the outer plasma membrane of dinoflagellates (Gallardo-Rodríguez et al. 2012a). In animal cells, changes in the fluid shear stress level are known to alter the membrane viscosity or fluidity. A similar phenomena may operate in dinoflagellates. For example, supplementation of the culture medium with additives that reduce the fluidity of the cell membrane has been shown to protect animal cells against shear stresses (Chisti 2010). Similar additives have the potential to broaden the shear tolerance range of dinoflagellates, to improve their cultivability (Gallardo-Rodríguez et al. 2012b).

Either most studies of shear sensitivity generally failed to satisfactorily quantify the turbulence intensity or measurement systems were not particularly meaningful in the context of culture in a bioreactor. For example, studies have been reported mostly in Couette flow devices, shakers, and oscillating rod mixers. The uniform and better-defined shear field in a Couette flow facilitates data analysis, but does not subject the cells to the full range of stresses found in a typical bioreactor. Furthermore, a bioreactor typically needs to be sparged with a gas, that is, carbon dioxide or air, and bubbling a gas through the culture fluid affects the hydrodynamic forces experienced by the cells (Chisti 2000).

In a Couette flow device, the growth of the heterotrophic nontoxic dinoflagellate *C. cohnii* was inhibited at relatively low energy dissipation rate values of 0.1–1.0 $cm^2 \cdot s^{-3}$ (Yeung and Wong 2003), but this species is known to be exceptional among dinoflagellates in tolerating fairly turbulent conditions in bioreactors (Gallardo-Rodríguez et al. 2012a). For example, *C. cohnii* has been found to withstand energy dissipation rates of up to 5.8×10^5 $cm^2 \cdot s^{-3}$ without lysis (Hu et al. 2007). Indeed, *C. cohnii* grown heterotrophically in bioreactors is used in industrial production of DHA (Mendes et al. 2009).

Unlike Couette flow devices, shaken flasks expose the cells to a hydrodynamic environment that is closer to that of a bioreactor. Shake flasks have proven useful for rapid screening of microbial strains and identifying the suitable growth conditions (Suresh et al. 2009). Methods have been developed for estimating the hydrodynamic forces experienced by cells suspended in a shake flask (Peter et al. 2006). Thus, experiments in shake flasks and laboratory bioreactors can be used to quantify the shear sensitivity of dinoflagellates of interest. This information can then be used in designing scaled-up bioreactors in such a way that the size of the fluid microeddies is mostly kept greater than the damaging threshold identified at the small scale.

19.4.1.1 Quantification of Turbulence in Shake Flasks

In shake flasks, the specific energy dissipation rate (ε) is relatively uniform, and the average shear stress τ_a experienced by a cell of diameter d_p is readily calculated (García Camacho et al. 2007b) as follows:

$$\tau_a = 0.0676 \left(\frac{d_p}{\lambda} \right)^2 \left(\rho_L \mu_L \varepsilon \right)^{0.5} \tag{19.1}$$

where
  λ is the length scale of energy-dissipating microeddies
  ρ_L is the density of the culture medium
  μ_L is the viscosity of the medium

The length scale (λ) of turbulence is estimated as the Kolmogorov microscale of energy-dissipating terminal eddies; thus,

$$\lambda = \left(\frac{\mu_L}{\rho_L} \right)^{0.75} \varepsilon^{-0.25} \tag{19.2}$$

where the mass specific energy dissipation rate (ε) is calculated as follows:

$$\varepsilon = \frac{1.94 n^3 d_s^4}{V_L^{2/3} Re^{0.2}} \tag{19.3}$$

where
  n is the rotational speed of the shake flask
  d_s is the flask diameter
  V_L is the volume of the liquid in the flask
  Re is the Reynolds number

Equation 19.3 is valid for the liquid volume fraction in the range of 0.04–0.20 of the total flask volume (Büchs et al. 2000). The Reynolds number in Equation 19.3 is estimated as follows:

$$Re = \frac{n \rho_L d_s^2}{\mu_L} \tag{19.4}$$

Once the average shear stress τ_a is known, the average shear rate γ is easily calculated as follows:

$$\gamma = \frac{\tau_a}{\mu_L} \tag{19.5}$$

The previous procedure for estimating the average shear stress and the average shear rate is applicable to turbulent flow. If a water-like fluid is being shaken, the flow is considered turbulent for Reynolds number values exceeding about 10,000 (García Camacho et al. 2007b).

  In some cases, a shake flask culture may be mixed intermittently. For example, multiple shaking cycles may be used with each cycle consisting of a shaken phase of duration t_t and a static phase of duration t_s. The total duration (t_c) of a single cycle is then $t_t + t_s$. The cycle frequency ν can be defined as $1/t_c$

(García Camacho et al. 2007b). For a mixing regime consisting of a single cycle, the fraction ϕ of the total time that the cells are subjected to turbulence may be calculated as follows (García Camacho et al. 2007b):

$$\phi = \frac{t_t}{t_c} \tag{19.6}$$

For such an intermittent agitation regime, the average shear stress and the average shear rate may be calculated as follows (García Camacho et al. 2007b):

$$\tau_{ai} = \phi\tau_a \tag{19.7}$$

$$\gamma_{ai} = \phi\gamma_a \tag{19.8}$$

where
τ_{ai} is the average shear stress for intermittent agitation
γ_{ai} is the average shear rate for intermittent agitation

19.4.2 Bioreactor Scale-Up Considerations

In heterotrophic growth in a conventional bioreactor, the supply of light is not an issue, and therefore, the scale-up of the bioreactor is essentially identical to the scale-up of any other bioprocess involving relatively fragile live cells (Chisti 2010). In any culture system, the damaging threshold of the specific energy dissipation rate should not be generally exceeded for prolonged periods, or the cells will be inhibited. The average value of the specific energy dissipation rate (ε) in a typical bioreactor used for suspension culture of relatively fragile animal cells is about 10^2 cm$^2 \cdot$s^{-3} (Varley and Birch 1999). In conventional stirred tanks and bubble column bioreactors used for growing relatively robust microorganisms, the average specific energy dissipation rate value is generally $\geq 10^3$ cm$^2 \cdot$s^{-3} (Gallardo-Rodríguez et al. 2012a). Growth of many dinoflagellates is inhibited at energy dissipation rate threshold value in the range of 10^{-2}–10 cm$^2 \cdot$s^{-3} (Table 19.2).

Bulk average specific energy dissipation rates (ε_{ave}) in bubble columns and industrial-scale stirred tanks are commonly in the range of $1,000 \leq \varepsilon_{ave} \leq 40,000$ cm$^2 \cdot$s^{-3} (Chisti 1999, 2000). These values of ε_{ave} far exceed the damage thresholds for toxic dinoflagellates (Table 19.2). Furthermore, the local value of ε in a bioreactor can greatly exceed the average rate of energy dissipation. For example, the local specific energy dissipation rate behind a rupturing bubble and in the vicinity of an impeller can be much greater than the average specific energy dissipation rate for the bioreactor as a whole. Therefore, the conventional regimes of operation of bubble columns and stirred-tank bioreactors are not suitable for culturing most dinoflagellates, but exceptions exist. For example, *P. reticulatum* has been found to be sensitive to turbulence in bioreactors (García Camacho et al. 2007b), but this does not seem to be the case for *A. minutum* (Parker 2002).

Culture of shear-sensitive cells in a stirred tank is often possible so long as the bioreactor has a suitable geometry and the regime of operation has been carefully selected (Chisti 2000, 2010). Characterization of turbulence intensity in terms of shear rate and shear stress in various types of bioreactors has been discussed in the literature (Chisti 1999, 2001, 2010; Sánchez Pérez et al. 2006; Merchuk and Garcia-Camacho 2010). In aerated cultures, gas bubbles have the potential to damage sensitive cells, but methods have been developed to minimize the damage (Chisti 2000; Gallardo Rodríguez et al. 2011). Exposure to a high pressure has been found to affect the thecal plate pattern and the microtubule assembly of the dinoflagellate *Scrippsiella hexapraecingula* (Sekida et al. 2012).

Although the methods for design and scale-up of photobioreactors are well established for microalgae that are relatively physically robust (Molina et al. 2001), these methods cannot be extrapolated to photobioreactors for culturing the fragile dinoflagellates (Gallardo-Rodríguez et al. 2012a). Supply of light is an enormously important factor in determining the productivity of a photoautotrophic culture. Consequently, the diameter of the bioreactor vessels can be increased only to a limited extent, or the availability of light will be reduced to unacceptably low levels (Gallardo-Rodríguez et al. 2012a). In addition, the ability to mix the culture is severely limited by the shear damage threshold considerations. Thus, a low-shear impeller must be used in a vessel that is relatively narrow and tall to accommodate the required volume (Gallardo-Rodríguez et al. 2012a). The diameter of such a culture vessel would generally not exceed 0.2 m, or the volume of the photosynthetically unproductive dark zone would be large.

A further complicating factor is mass transfer: the photosynthetically generated oxygen must be removed, or it will build up to inhibitory levels. Unfortunately, the conventional method of removing the oxygen by bubbling the algal broth with air is not always applicable as the gas bubbles rupturing at the surface of the broth are extremely damaging to fragile cells (Chisti 2000). For example, mixing and oxygen removal by bubbling the broth with air have been found to be impossible with *P. reticulatum* (García Camacho et al. 2007b). Either the oxygen must be removed via desorption from the surface of the broth in the bioreactor vessel or the cells must be excluded from a certain volume of the broth, for example, by means of a spinfilter (Chisti 2000; García Camacho et al. 2011b) so that the cell-free volume of the broth can be sparged with air to remove the oxygen. Oxygen removal from the surface becomes increasingly difficult as the volume of the broth is increased in a vessel of a relatively narrow diameter (Gallardo-Rodríguez et al. 2012a).

Design and operation of a bioreactor for a dinoflagellate require an initial characterization of its susceptibility to turbulence (Gallardo-Rodríguez et al. 2012a). Studies in shake flasks can be quite useful for this. For example, shake flasks were used to identify an average energy dissipation rate (ε_{ave}) value of 0.8 cm$^2 \cdot$s^{-3} as the damage threshold for the dinoflagellate *P. reticulatum* (García Camacho et al. 2007b). As *P. reticulatum* does not withstand gas bubbles (Gallardo-Rodríguez et al. 2012a), the use of the gas-sparged bioreactors was ruled out. This steered the choice to a surface-aerated 2 L stirred-tank bioreactor equipped with a low-shear axial flow impeller and a central spinfilter (Gallardo Rodriguez et al. 2007, 2010). The local value of the maximum specific energy dissipation rate (ε_{max}) in the bioreactor was 1.49 cm$^2 \cdot$s^{-3} (García Camacho et al. 2011b), or higher than the damage threshold, but this did not pose a problem because the cells were exposed to the damaging turbulence only for a brief period during circulation in the bioreactor (Gallardo-Rodríguez et al. 2012a). The average value of the specific energy dissipation rate in the bioreactor was only 0.3 cm$^2 \cdot$s^{-3} (García Camacho et al. 2011a), or much lower than the earlier noted damage threshold. The data obtained were used to further scale-up the production to a 15 L stirred bioreactor (García Camacho et al. 2011b).

In the larger reactor, the vessel diameter could not be much greater than in the 2 L bioreactor, or light supply would have become limiting (Gallardo-Rodríguez et al. 2012a). Thus, the 15 L stirred photobioreactor for suspension culture of *P. reticulatum* was designed to be tall and thin with an aspect ratio of 4.5 (García Camacho et al. 2011b). Two scaling-up criteria were considered in designing this photobioreactor (García Camacho et al. 2011b). The first criterion related with the frequency of passage of the cells through the high-shear zone of the impeller, or the inverse of the liquid circulation time in the photobioreactor (Gallardo-Rodríguez et al. 2012a). The second scaling-up criterion consisted of keeping the tip speed of the impeller at the 15 L scale at the same value as was successfully used at the 2 L scale (Gallardo-Rodríguez et al. 2012a). The tip speed is related to the maximum specific energy dissipation rate (ε_{max}) in a stirred tank (Gallardo-Rodríguez et al. 2012a). In the taller bioreactor, the impeller-to-tank diameter ratio was kept at nearly the same value as in the smaller bioreactor. This led to an impeller diameter of 8.14 cm in the larger vessel. An impeller of this size rotating at 50 rpm would have an acceptable tip speed of 0.2 m$\cdot$s^{-1} ($\varepsilon_{ave} \approx 0.007$ cm$^2 \cdot$s^{-3}; $\varepsilon_{max} = 4.77$ cm$^2 \cdot$s^{-3}), but the circulation time would be eight times as high as in the small reactor (Gallardo-Rodríguez et al. 2012a). A lowering of the circulation time by increasing the rotation speed would result in an excessively high value of ε_{max} (García Camacho et al. 2011b). The scaled-up photobioreactor is shown in Figure 19.2.

Of course, a high circulation time reduces the frequency of passage of the cells through the high-shear zone of the impeller, but raises other issues (Gallardo-Rodríguez et al. 2012a). For example, the gas–liquid mass transfer becomes poorer with increasing values of the circulation time (Gallardo-Rodríguez et al. 2012a). This leads to an increased oxygen accumulation in the culture broth and an increased formation of the reactive oxygen species. Oxygen accumulation at a lower impeller speed could be reduced by increasing the aeration rate within the cell-free zone of the spinfilter (Gallardo-Rodríguez et al. 2012a). In addition, the culture medium was supplemented with ascorbic acid to protect the cells against damage by the reactive oxygen species (Gallardo-Rodríguez et al. 2012a).

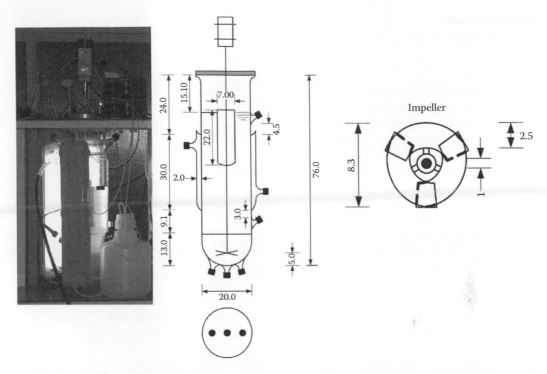

FIGURE 19.2 A 15 L stirred-tank photobioreactor with a central spinfilter for producing yessotoxins from the red tide dinoflagellate *P. reticulatum*. Dimensions in cm. (Reprinted from *Process Biochemistry*, 46, García Camacho, F., Gallardo Rodríguez, J.J., Sánchez Mirón, A., Belarbi, E.H., Chisti, Y., and Molina Grima, E., Photobioreactor scale-up for a shear-sensitive dinoflagellate microalga, 936–944, Copyright 2011b, with permission from Elsevier.)

Although the scale-up to 15 L proved successful, further scale-up to larger bioreactors does not seem possible for *P. reticulatum* unless the culture medium is formulated with effective shear-protective additives (Gallardo-Rodríguez et al. 2012a). As a general rule, the scaling-up of a phototrophic culture of a dinoflagellate is more difficult compared to the scale-up of some of the other types of microbial and cell cultures (Figure 19.3).

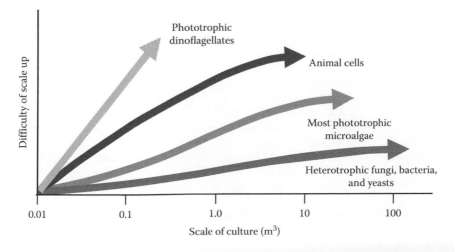

FIGURE 19.3 Difficulty of scaling-up of a bioreactor increases with increasing scale of operation. Scale-up is relatively easy for heterotrophic bacteria, fungi, and yeasts, and the upper limit of operation is generally higher than, for example, for animal cell cultures. Scale-up is more difficult for dinoflagellates than for animal cells and the upper limit on the bioreactor volume is relatively low.

19.5 Concluding Remarks

Depending on the species, dinoflagellate microalgae may be grown in bioreactors either photoautotrophically or heterotrophically. Optimization of the medium composition and the culture conditions can greatly enhance the metabolite productivity. Irrespective of the form of growth, the generally extreme sensitivity of dinoflagellates to turbulence in the culture fluid imposes severe limits on the design and operation of a bioreactor for growing them. These limitations may be further compounded in photoautotrophic culture in which the need for light further constrains bioreactor design. Not all dinoflagellates are equally sensitive to turbulence, and therefore, if a product can be sourced from multiple species, the selection of a more robust species for use in large-scale production may have important advantages.

ACKNOWLEDGMENTS

This work was supported by the Spanish Ministry of Science and Innovation (SAF2011-28883-C03-02); the General Secretariat of Economy, Innovation and Science of Junta de Andalucía (Spain) (TEP-5375); and the European Regional Development Fund Program.

REFERENCES

Acién Fernández, F. G., Fernández Sevilla, J. M., Egorova-Zachernyuk, T. A., and Molina Grima, E. 2005. Cost-effective production of 13C, 15N stable isotope-labeled biomass from phototrophic microalgae for various biotechnological applications. *Biomolecular Engineering* 22: 193–200.

Berdalet, E. 1992. Effects of turbulence on the marine dinoflagellate *Gymnodinium nelsonii*. *Journal of Phycology* 28: 267–272.

Berdalet, E. and Estrada, M. 1993. Effects of turbulence on several dinoflagellate species. In *Toxic Phytoplankton Blooms in the Sea*, eds. T. J. Smayda and Y. Shimizu, pp. 737–740. New York: Elsevier.

Berdalet, E., Peters, F., Koumandou, V. L., Roldan, C., Guadayol, O., and Estrada, M. 2007. Species-specific physiological response of dinoflagellates to quantified small-scale turbulence. *Journal of Phycology* 43: 965–977.

Berman, T. and Shteinman, B. 1998. Phytoplankton development and turbulent mixing in Lake Kinneret (1992–1996). *Journal of Plankton Research* 20: 709–726.

Beuzenberg, V., Mountfort, D., Holland, P., Shi, F., and MacKenzie, L. 2012. Optimization of growth and production of toxins by three dinoflagellates in photobioreactor cultures. *Journal of Applied Phycology* 24: 1023–1033.

Büchs, J., Maier, U., Milbradt, C., and Zoels, B. 2000. Power consumption in shaking flasks on rotary shaking machines. II. Nondimensional description of specific power consumption and flow regimes in unbaffled flasks at elevated liquid viscosity. *Biotechnology and Bioengineering* 68: 594–601.

Burkholder, J. M., Glibert, P. M., and Skelton, H. M. 2008. Mixotrophy, a major mode of nutrition for harmful algal species in eutrophic waters. *Harmful Algae* 8:77–93.

Chinain, M. 2009. Growth and toxin production in the ciguatera-causing dinoflagellate *Gambierdiscus polynesiensis* (Dinophyceae) in culture. *Toxicon* 56: 739–750.

Chisti, Y. 1999. Shear sensitivity. *Encyclopedia of Bioprocess Technology: Fermentation, Biocatalysis, and Bioseparation* 5: 2379–2406.

Chisti, Y. 2000. Animal-cell damage in sparged bioreactors. *Trends in Biotechnology* 18: 420–432.

Chisti, Y. 2001. Hydrodynamic damage to animal cells. *Critical Reviews in Biotechnology* 21: 67–110.

Chisti, Y. 2007. Strategies in downstream processing. In *Bioseparation and Bioprocessing: A Handbook*, 2nd edn, Vol. 1, ed. G. Subramanian, pp. 29–62. New York: Wiley-VCH.

Chisti, Y. 2010. Shear sensitivity. *Encyclopedia of Industrial Biotechnology, Bioprocess, Bioseparation, and Cell Technology* 7: 4360–4398.

Dempsey, H. P. 1982. The effects of turbulence on three algae. *Skeletonema costatum, Gonyaulax tamarensis, Heterocapsa triquetra*. SB Thesis, Massachusetts Institute of Technology, Cambridge, MA.

Doblin, M. A., Thompson, P. A., Revill, A. T., Butler, E. C. V., Blackburn, S. I., and Hallegraeff, G. M. 2006. Vertical migration of the toxic dinoflagellate *Gymnodinium catenatum* under different concentrations of nutrients and humic substances in culture. *Harmful Algae* 5: 665–677.

Errera, R. M. and Campbell, L. 2011. Osmotic stress triggers toxin production by the dinoflagellate *Karenia brevis. Proceedings of the National Academy of Sciences of the United States of America* 108: 10597–10601.

Fernández Sevilla, J. M., Acién Fernández, F. G., and Molina Grima, E. 2010. Biotechnological production of lutein and its applications. *Applied Microbiology and Biotechnology* 86: 27–40.

Gallardo Rodríguez, J. J., Cerón García, M.-C., García Camacho, F., Sánchez Mirón, A., Belarbi, E. H., and Molina Grima, E. 2007. New culture approaches for yessotoxin production from the dinoflagellate *Protoceratium reticulatum. Biotechnology Progress* 23: 339–350.

Gallardo-Rodríguez, J. J., García-Camacho, F., Sánchez-Mirón, A., López-Rosales, L., Chisti, Y., and Molina-Grima, E. 2012b. Shear-induced changes in membrane fluidity during culture of a fragile dinoflagellate microalga. *Biotechnology Progress* 28: 467–473.

Gallardo Rodríguez, J. J., Sánchez Mirón, A., Cerón García, M.-C., Belarbi, E. H., García Camacho, F., Chisti, Y., and Molina Grima, E. 2009a. Macronutrients requirements of the dinoflagellate *Protoceratium reticulatum. Harmful Algae* 8: 239–246.

Gallardo Rodríguez, J. J., Sánchez Mirón, A., Cerón García, M.-C., Belarbi, E. H., García Camacho, F., Chisti, Y., and Molina Grima, E. 2009b. Causes of shear sensitivity of the toxic dinoflagellate *Protoceratium reticulatum. Biotechnology Progress* 25: 792–800.

Gallardo Rodríguez, J. J., Sánchez Mirón, A., García Camacho, F., Cerón García, M. C., Belarbi, E. H., Chisti, Y., and Molina Grima, E. 2011. Carboxymethyl cellulose and Pluronic F68 protect the dinoflagellate *Protoceratium reticulatum* against shear-associated damage. *Bioprocess and Biosystems Engineering* 34: 3–12.

Gallardo Rodríguez, J. J., Sánchez Mirón, A., García Camacho, F., Cerón García, M. C., Belarbi, E. H., and Molina Grima, E. 2010. Culture of dinoflagellates in a fed-batch and continuous stirred-tank photobioreactors: Growth, oxidative stress and toxin production. *Process Biochemistry* 45: 660–666.

Gallardo-Rodríguez, J., Sánchez-Mirón, A., García-Camacho, F., López-Rosales, L., Chisti, Y., and Molina-Grima, E. 2012a. Bioactives from microalgal dinoflagellates. *Biotechnology Advances* 30: 1673–1684.

García Camacho, F., Gallardo Rodríguez, J. J., Sánchez Mirón, A., Belarbi, E. H., Chisti, Y., and Molina Grima, E. 2011b. Photobioreactor scale-up for a shear-sensitive dinoflagellate microalga. *Process Biochemistry* 46: 936–944.

García Camacho, F., Gallardo Rodríguez, J. J., Sánchez Mirón, A., Cerón García, M. C., and Molina Grima, E. 2007b. Determination of shear stress thresholds in toxic dinoflagellates cultured in shaken flasks. Implications in bioprocess engineering. *Process Biochemistry* 42: 1506–1515.

Garcia Camacho, F., Gallardo Rodríguez, J. J., Sánchez Mirón, A., Cerón García, M. C., Belarbi, E. H., Chisti, Y., and Molina Grima, E. 2007a. Biotechnological significance of toxic marine dinoflagellates. *Biotechnology Advances* 25: 176–194.

García-Camacho, F., Gallardo-Rodríguez, J. J., Sánchez-Mirón, A., Chisti, Y., and Molina-Grima, E. 2011a. Genetic algorithm-based medium optimization for a toxic dinoflagellate microalga. *Harmful Algae* 10: 697–701.

Gibson, C. H. and Thomas, W. H. 1995. Effects of turbulence intermittency on growth inhibition of a red tide dinoflagellate, *Gonyaulax polyedra* Stein. *Journal of Geophysical Research—Oceans* 100(C12): 24841–24846.

Gudi, S. R. P., Clark, C. B., and Frangos, J. A. 1996. Fluid flow rapidly activates G proteins in human endothelial cells: Involvement of G proteins in mechanochemical signal transduction. *Circulation Research* 79: 834–839.

Guillard, R. R. L. 1975. Culture of phytoplankton for feeding marine invertebrates. In *Culture of Marine Invertebrate Animals*, eds. W. L. Smith and M. H. Chanley, pp. 26–60. New York: Plenum Press.

Guillard, R. R. L. and Hargraves, P. E. 1993. Stichochrysis immobilis is a diatom, not a chrysophyte. *Phycologia* 32: 234–236.

Hallegraeff, G. M. 2003. Harmful algal blooms: A global overview. In *Manual on Harmful Marine Microalgae*, eds. G. M. Hallegraeff, D. M. Anderson, and A. D. Cembella, pp. 25–49. Paris, France: UNESCO Publishing.

Havskum, H. 2003. Effects of small-scale turbulence on interactions between the heterotrophic dinoflagellate *Oxyrrhis marina* and its prey, *Isochrysis* sp. *Ophelia* 57(3): 125–135.

Havskum, H., Hansen, P. J., and Berdalet, E. 2005. Effect of turbulence on sedimentation and net population growth of the dinoflagellate *Ceratium tripos* and interactions with its predator, *Fragilidium subglobosum. Limnology and Oceanography* 50: 1543–1551.

Homma, K. 1989. The S phase is discrete and is controlled by the circadian clock in the marine dinoflagellate *Gonyaulax polyedra*. *Experimental Cell Research* 182: 635–644.

Hsieh, D. P. H., Wang, D., and Chang G. H. 2001. Laboratory bioproduction of paralytic shellfish toxins in dinoflagellates. *Advanced Applied Microbiology* 49: 85–110.

Hu, H., Shi, Y., and Cong, W. 2006. Improvement in growth and toxin production of *Alexandrium tamarense* by two-step culture method. *Journal of Applied Phycology* 18: 119–126.

Hu, W., Gladue, R., Hansen, J., Wojnar, C., and Chalmers, J. J. 2007. The sensitivity of the dinoflagellate *Crypthecodinium cohnii* to transient hydrodynamic forces and cell-bubble interactions. *Biotechnology Progress* 23: 1355–1362.

Joshi, J. B., Elias, C. B., and Patole, M. S. 1996. Role of hydrodynamic shear in the cultivation of animal, plant and microbial cells. *Chemical Engineering Journal and the Biochemical Engineering Journal* 62: 121–141.

Juhl, A. R. and Latz, M. I. 2002. Mechanisms of fluid shear-induced inhibition of population growth in a red-tide dinoflagellate. *Journal of Phycology* 38: 683–694.

Juhl, A. R., Trainer, V. L., and Latz, M. I. 2001. Effect of fluid shear and irradiance on population growth and cellular toxin content of the dinoflagellate *Alexandrium fundyense*. *Limnology and Oceanography* 46: 758–764.

Juhl, A. R., Velazquez, V., and Latz, M. I. 2000. Effect of growth conditions on flow-induced inhibition of population growth of a red-tide dinoflagellate. *Limnology and Oceanography* 45: 905–915.

Keller, M. D. and Guillard, R. R. L. 1986. Factors significant to marine dinoflagellate culture. In *Toxic Dinoflagellates*, eds. D. M. Anderson, A. W. White, and D. G. Baden, pp. 113–116. New York: Elsevier.

Lau, R. K. L., Kwok, A. C. M., Chan, W. K., Zhang, T. Y., and Wong, J. T. Y. 2007. Mechanical characterization of cellulosic thecal plates in dinoflagellates by nanoindentation. *Journal of Nanoscience and Nanotechnology* 7: 452–457.

Lee, R. E. 2008. *Phycology*. Cambridge, U.K.: Cambridge University Press.

Lee, T. C.-H., Kwok, O.-T., Ho, K.-C., and Lee, F. W.-F. 2012. Effects of different nitrate and phosphate concentrations on the growth and toxin production of an *Alexandrium tamarense* strain collected from Drake Passage. *Marine Environmental Research* 81: 62–69.

Lim, P.-T., Leaw, C.-P., Kobiyama, A., and Ogata, T. 2010. Growth and toxin production of tropical *Alexandrium minutum* Halim (Dinophyceae) under various nitrogen to phosphorus ratios. *Journal of Applied Phycology* 22: 203–210.

Magaña, H. A. and Villareal, T. A. 2006. The effect of environmental factors on the growth rate of *Karenia brevis* (Davis) G. Hansen and Moestrup. *Harmful Algae* 5: 192–198.

Mallipattu, S. K. 2002. Evidence for shear-induced increase in membrane fluidity in the dinoflagellate *Lingulodinium polyedrum*. *Journal of Comparative Physiology A: Neuroethology, Sensory, Neural, and Behavioral Physiology* 188: 409–416.

Mendes, A., Reis, A., Vasconcelos, R., Guerra, P., and Lopes Da Silva, T. 2009. *Crypthecodinium cohnii* with emphasis on DHA production: A review. *Journal of Applied Phycology* 21: 199–214.

Merchuk, J. C. and García-Camacho, F. 2010. Bioreactors, airlift reactors. *Encyclopedia of Industrial Biotechnology: Bioprocess, Bioseparation, and Cell Technology* 2: 851–912.

Molina, E., Fernández, J., Acién, F. G., and Chisti, Y. 2001. Tubular photobioreactor design for algal cultures. *Journal of Biotechnology* 92: 113–131.

Molina Grima, E., Belarbi, E. H., Acién Fernández, F. G., Robles Medina, A., and Chisti, Y. 2003. Recovery of microalgal biomass and metabolites: Process options and economics. *Biotechnology Advances* 20: 491–515.

Mountfort, D., Beuzenberg, V., MacKenzie, L., and Rhodes, L. 2006. Enhancement of growth and gymnodimine production by the marine dinoflagellate, *Karenia selliformis*. *Harmful Algae* 5: 658–664.

Namdev, P. K. and Dunlop, E. H. 1995. Shear sensitivity of plant cells in suspensions—Present and future. *Applied Biochemistry and Biotechnology* 54: 109–131.

Navarro, J. M., Muñoz, M. G., and Contreras, A. M. 2006. Temperature as a factor regulating growth and toxin content in the dinoflagellate *Alexandrium catenella*. *Harmful Algae* 5: 762–769.

Ostwald, W. J. 1988. Large scale algal culture systems. In *Microalgal Biotechnology*, eds. M. A. Borowitzka and L. J. Borowitzka, pp. 357–394. Cambridge, U.K.: Cambridge University Press.

Otero, P., Alfonso, A., Vieytes, M. R., Cabado, A. G., Vieites, J. M., and Botana, L. M. 2010. Effects of environmental regimens on the toxin profile of *Alexandrium ostenfeldii*. *Environmental Toxicology and Chemistry* 29: 301–310.

Parker, N. S. 2002. Growth of the toxic dinoflagellate *Alexandrium minutum* (Dinophyceae) using high biomass culture systems. *Journal of Applied Phycology* 14: 313–324.

Paz, B., Blanco, J., and Franco, J. M. 2013. Yessotoxins production during the culture of *Protoceratium reticulatum* strains isolated from Galician Rias Baixas (NW Spain). *Harmful Algae* 21–22: 13–19.

Paz, B., Riobó, P., Luisa Fernández, M., Fraga, S., and Franco, J. M. 2004. Production and release of yessotoxins by the dinoflagellates *Protoceratium reticulatum* and *Lingulodinium polyedrum* in culture. *Toxicon* 44: 251–258.

Paz, B., Vázquez, J. A., Riobó, P., and Franco, J. M. 2006. Study of the effect of temperature, irradiance and salinity on growth and yessotoxin production by the dinoflagellate *Protoceratium reticulatum* in culture by using a kinetic and factorial approach. *Marine Environmental Research* 62: 286–300.

Peter, C. P., Suzuki, Y., and Büchs, J. 2006. Hydromechanical stress in shake flasks: Correlation for the maximum local energy dissipation rate. *Biotechnology and Bioengineering* 93: 1164–1176.

Pistocchi, R., Pezzolesi, L., Guerrini, F., Vanucci, S., Dell'Aversano, C., and Fattorusso, E. 2011. A review on the effects of environmental conditions on growth and toxin production of *Ostreopsis ovata*. *Toxicon* 57: 421–428.

Pollingher, U. and Zemel, E. 1981. In situ and experimental evidence of the influence of turbulence on cell division processes of *Peridinium cinctum* forma westii (Lemm.) Lefevre. *British Phycological Journal* 16: 281–287.

Quilliam, M. A. 2003. Chemical methods for lipophilic shellfish toxins. In *Manual on Harmful Marine Microalgae*, eds. G. M. Hallegraeff, D. M. Anderson, and A. D. Cembella, pp. 211–245. Paris, France: UNESCO Publishing.

Roenneberg, T. and Merrow, M. 2002. "What watch?… such much!" Complexity and evolution of circadian clocks. *Cell and Tissue Research* 309: 3–9.

Sánchez Pérez, J. A., Rodríguez Porcel, E. M., Casas López, J. L., Fernández Sevilla, J. M., and Chisti, Y. 2006. Shear rate in stirred tank and bubble column bioreactors. *Chemical Engineering Journal* 124: 1–5.

Sekida, S., Takahira, M., Horiguchi, T., and Okuda, K. 2012. Effects of high pressure in the armored dinoflagellate *Scrippsiella hexapraecingula* (Peridiniales, Dinophyceae): Changes in thecal plate pattern and microtubule assembly. *Journal of Phycology* 48: 163–173.

Sherr, E. B. and Sherr, B. F. 2007. Heterotrophic dinoflagellates: A significant component of microzooplankton biomass and major grazers of diatoms in the sea. *Marine Ecology Progress Series* 352: 187–197.

Shimizu, Y. 2000. Microalgae as a drug source. In *Drugs from the Sea*, ed. N. Fusetani, pp. 30–45. Basel, Switzerland: Karger.

Skelton, H. M. 2009. Axenic culture of the heterotrophic dinoflagellate *Pfiesteria shumwayae* in a semi-defined medium. *Journal of Eukaryotic Microbiology* 56: 73–82.

Sompech, K., Chisti, Y., and Srinophakun, T. 2012. Design of raceway ponds for producing microalgae. *Biofuels* 3: 387–397.

Stoecker, D. K. 1999. Mixotrophy among dinoflagellates. *Journal of Eukaryotic Microbiology* 46: 397–401.

Stoecker, D. K., Long, A., Suttles, S. E., and Sanford, L. P. 2006. Effect of small-scale shear on grazing and growth of the dinoflagellate *Pfiesteria piscicida*. *Harmful Algae* 5: 407–418.

Sullivan, J. M. and Swift, E. 2003. Effects of small-scale turbulence on net growth rate and size of ten species of marine dinoflagellates. *Journal of Phycology* 39: 83–94.

Sullivan, J. M., Swift, E., Donaghay, P. L., and Rines, J. E. B. 2003. Small-scale turbulence affects the division rate and morphology of two red-tide dinoflagellates. *Harmful Algae* 2: 183–199.

Suresh, S., Srivastava, V. C., and Mishra, I. M. 2009. Critical analysis of engineering aspects of shaken flask bioreactors. *Critical Reviews in Biotechnology* 29: 255–278.

Tang, E. P. Y. 1996. Why do dinoflagellates have lower growth rates? *Journal of Phycology* 32: 80–84.

Taroncher-Oldenburg, G. 1998. Toxin availability during the cell cycle of the dinoflagellate *Alexandrium fundyense*. *Limnology and Oceanography* 42: 1178–1188.

Taylor, F. J. R. 1987. General group characteristics; special features of interest; short history of dinoflagellate study. In *The Biology of Dinoflagellates*, ed. F. J. R. Taylor, pp. 1–23. New York: Wiley.

Taylor, F. J. R., Fukuyo, Y., Larsen, J., and Hallegraeff, G. M. 2003. Taxonomy of harmful dinoflagellates. In *Manual on Harmful Marine Microalgae*, eds. G. M. Hallegraeff, D. M. Anderson, and A. D. Cembella, pp. 389–432. Paris, France: UNESCO Publishing.

Thomas, W. H. and Gibson, C. H. 1990. Quantified small-scale turbulence inhibits a red tide dinoflagellate, *Gonyaulax polyedra* Stein. *Deep Sea Research Part A, Oceanographic Research Papers* 37: 1583–1593.

Thomas, W. H. and Gibson, C. H. 1992. Effects of quantified small-scale turbulence on the dinoflagellate, *Gymnodium sanguineum* (Splendens): Contrasts with *Gonyaulax* (*Lingulodinium*) *polyedra*, and the fishery implication. *Deep Sea Research Part A, Oceanographic Research Papers* 39: 1429–1437.

Thomas, W. H., Vernet, M., and Gibson, C. H. 1995. Effects of small-scale turbulence on photosynthesis, pigmentation, cell division, and cell size in the marine dinoflagellate *Gonyaulax polyedra* (Dinophyceae). *Journal of Phycology* 31: 50–59.

Tynan, C. T. 1993. The effects of small scale turbulence on dinoflagellates. PhD dissertation, University of California at San Diego, Scripps Institution of Oceanography, San Diego, CA.

Varley, J. and Birch, J. 1999. Reactor design for large scale suspension animal cell culture. *Cytotechnology* 29: 177–205.

Veldhuis, M. J. W., Cucci, T. L., and Sieracki, M. E. 1997. Cellular DNA content of marine phytoplankton using two new fluorochromes: Taxonomic and ecological implications. *Journal of Phycology* 33: 527–541.

Wang, C. and Hsieh, D. D. P. 2002. Nutritional supplementation to increase growth and paralytic shellfish toxin productivity by the marine dinoflagellate *Alexandrium tamarense*. *Biochemical Engineering Journal* 11: 131–135.

Wang, D. Z., Ho, A. Y. T., and Hsieh, D. P. H. 2002. Production of C2 toxin by *Alexandrium tamarense* CI01 using different culture methods. *Journal of Applied Phycology* 14: 461–468.

Weuster-Botz, D. 2000. Experimental design for fermentation media development: Statistical design or global random search? *Journal of Bioscience and Bioengineering* 90: 473–483.

White, A. W. 1976. Growth inhibition caused by turbulence in the toxic marine dinoflagellate *Gonyaulax excavata*. *Journal of the Fisheries Research Board of Canada* 33: 2598–2602.

Wong, J. T. Y. and Kwok, A. C. M. 2005. Proliferation of dinoflagellates: Blooming or bleaching. *BioEssays* 27: 730–740.

Yamaguchi, H., Yoshimatsu, T., Tanimoto, Y., Sato, S., Nishimura, T., Uehara, K., and Adachi, M. 2012. Effects of temperature, salinity and their interaction on growth of the benthic dinoflagellate *Ostreopsis* cf. *ovata* (Dinophyceae) from Japanese coastal waters. *Phycological Research* 60: 297–304.

Yeung, P. K. K. 2006. Involvement of calcium mobilization from caffeine-sensitive stores in mechanically induced cell cycle arrest in the dinoflagellate *Crypthecodinium cohnii*. *Cell Calcium* 39: 259–274.

Yeung, P. K. K. and Wong, J. T. Y. 2003. Inhibition of cell proliferation by mechanical agitation involves transient cell cycle arrest at G(1) phase in dinoflagellates. *Protoplasma* 220: 173–178.

Zirbel, M. J., Veron, F., and Latz, M. I. 2000. The reversible effect of flow on the morphology of *Ceratocorys horrida* (Peridiniales, Dinophyta). *Journal of Phycology* 36: 46–58.

Part IV

Nonneurotoxic Lipophilic Toxins

20

Ecobiology and Geographical Distribution of Potentially Toxic Marine Dinoflagellates

Aristidis Vlamis and Panagiota Katikou

CONTENTS

20.1 Introduction

Dinoflagellates are the second-most abundant phytoplankton group following the diatoms. The term "dinos" comes from the Greek word meaning "whirling," as this type of movement is characteristic in these organisms. Dinoflagellates are unique organisms as they possess two flagella or whip-like appendages that help them to move up or down in the water column. They are a diverse group, comprising approximately 115–130 genera, 2000 living species, and 2000 fossil species.[1–3]

Dinoflagellates are mostly unicellular and range from 2 to 2000 µm in diameter[4] and are commonly estuarine and marine, with only 250–300 of the approximately 2000 known species inhabiting freshwaters.[5,6] Dinoflagellates are very abundant throughout the world, occurring in all latitudes from the Arctic and Antarctic Seas to the tropics. In warm waters, dinoflagellates are usually large and found in various forms; in fact, they are considered as more important in the warmer waters than in colder polar waters.[7] Many dinoflagellates also occur in marginal habitats, whereas some are confined to near-shore or neritic waters due to the richness of nutrient and lower salinity compared to the open sea.[8]

Dinoflagellates are a highly diverse group of flagellates, comprising both photosynthetic and nonphotosynthetic taxa in equal proportions.[9] According to their feeding mechanisms, they are categorized as (1) autotrophic photosynthetically growing species, (2) mixotrophic species that obtain their nutrition through a combination of photosynthesis and uptake of dissolved organic substances (osmotrophy) and/or particulate organic matter (phagotrophy), and (3) heterotrophic dinoflagellates whose feeding is phagotrophic.[10–12] Roughly half of the species in this group are photosynthetic.[10,13]

The greatest diversity and abundance of harmful dinoflagellates occurs in estuaries and coastal marine waters, coinciding with higher nutrient supplies from land sources and/or upwelling.[5,14] Most harmful dinoflagellates are planktonic, free-living benthic species and are important ciguatoxin producers, whereas various parasitic taxa that also have a benthic habit, grow attached to or inside prey.[15]

Many dinoflagellate species are potentially toxic and can cause human illness through shellfish or fish poisoning; dinoflagellates are the ultimate cause of diseases like diarrheic shellfish poisoning (DSP), neurotoxic shellfish poisoning (NSP), paralytic shellfish poisoning (PSP), and ciguatera. Some toxic dinoflagellates can also cause fish kills and mortality of other marine fauna.[16] Apart from marine toxins production, dinoflagellates can affect the full spectrum of living systems from the biochemical to the ecosystem level.[17] For example, at the ecosystem level, high concentrations of cells may interfere with light penetration and influence subsurface communities such as submerged aquatic vegetation. At the biochemical level, secondary metabolites produced by microalgae may interfere with particular cellular processes in the organism, but may not adversely affect the organism as a whole.[18]

Dinoflagellate morphology can be as miscellaneous and complex as of any unicellular eukaryote. A simple definition for dinoflagellates states that they are "eukaryotic, primarily single-celled organisms in which the motile cell possesses two dissimilar flagella: a ribbon-like flagellum with multiple waves which beats to the cell's left, and a more conventional flagellum with one or a few waves which beats posteriorly."[19] Taxonomic approach for this group has traditionally been based on cytological characters.[20]

The existence of large numbers of undescribed dinoflagellate species has been shown by use of molecular analyses in environments like marine picoplankton[21,22] or as symbionts ("zooxanthellae") in many types of protists and invertebrates like corals.[23]

20.2 Taxonomy

Molecular phylogenetic analyses place dinoflagellates in the Alveolata kingdom,[24] together with the ciliates and apicomplexans.[25] The Alveolata constitute a diverse group of single-celled eukaryotes present in both marine and terrestrial ecosystems, the principal shared morphological feature of which is the presence of flattened vesicles (cortical alveoli) packed into a continuous layer supporting the cell membrane.[26] These structures have been associated by immunolocalization to a family of proteins, named alveolins, common to all alveolates.[27,28]

Alveolates exhibit extremely diverse trophic strategies, including predation, photo-autotrophy, and intracellular parasitism. Most alveolates fall into one of three main subgroups (or phyla): ciliates, dinoflagellates, and Apicomplexa, all sharing a common ancestor.[29] Apicomplexans are obligate parasites of animal cells, including humans (e.g., *Plasmodinium*, which causes malaria). Ciliates are mainly aquatic predators that possess essential roles as consumers in microbial food webs; however, some taxa can be parasitic or may contain sequestered plastids, such as *Myrionecta rubra*. Dinoflagellates can be either photoautotrophs, free-living predators (heterotrophs) or both, either simultaneously or alternatively (mixotrophs), while some also live as parasites or symbionts.[30]

The most acceptable taxonomic classification of dinoflagellates has been presented by Taylor[31] and Adl et al.[32] Taxonomy of thecate (armored) dinoflagellates has been historically based upon their plate tabulations, most often following the system proposed by Kofoid[33] (reviewed in Fensome et al.[19] and Carty[6]), coupled with molecular sequence data where available.[34] In contrast, taxonomy of athecate (syn. unarmored or naked) dinoflagellates has been problematic for more than a century because of difficulties in identifying reliable morphological characters with light microscopy. The ongoing revolution in dinoflagellate taxonomy, classification, and phylogeny has resulted from a combination of molecular studies and high-resolution electron microscopy, including reconstruction of the cell ultrastructure based on serial sectioning.

Dinoflagellate research has a 225 year-old history, beginning with O.F. Müller in Copenhagen in the late 1700s. The first modern dinoflagellates were described by Baker in 1753 as "Animalcules which cause the Sparkling Light in Sea Water,"[35] while the first species were formally named by Müller later in 1773.[36] A major boost was provided by Ehrenberg's[37] work in Berlin in 1838, notably by his book *Infusionsthierchen als vollkommende Organismen*, in which the family "Peridinaea" was introduced, marking the beginning of dinoflagellate classification. During the latter half of the 1800s and the early part of the 1900s, many people worked on dinoflagellates, prominent early names being Claparède and Lachmann in Switzerland and Germany, respectively, and von Stein in Prague. These were followed by Kofoid and Swezy in North America, and a long line of people in Central Europe (Lemmermann, Lindemann, Wotoszynská, etc.). In the 1900s, Kofoid produced a standardized description of dinoflagellate tabulation, which is still in use today. The taxonomic work of this era was assembled by Johs Schiller in the famous *Kryptogamen flora von Deutschland, Österreich und der Schweiz*.[38] Although printed in the 1930s, this book still constitutes an important reference work for the identification of dinoflagellates. In 1933, Wetzel established the genus *Hystrichosphaera* for the spiny spherical forms Ehrenberg had seen, giving rise to the general term hystrichosphere. In 1961, Evitt recognized that the openings on the walls of cysts correspond to the plates on the theca of dinoflagellates (while the cysts themselves do not have separate plates), and termed these openings as archeopyles. Evitt also realized that the spines or processes seen on many cysts reflect the tabulation pattern of the original dinoflagellate from which the cyst emerged. In 1964, Evitt and Davidson attempted to associate dinoflagellates with their cysts, while in 1968 Wall and Dale documented the excystment of the living dinoflagellate *Gonyaulax* from a Spiniferites-type cyst.[39] Termination of the premolecular age is marked by the appearance of another major book, by Fensome et al., *A Classification of Living and Fossil Dinoflagellates*.[19]

At the generic level, the genera of "naked" species have been recently examined in detail and the main genera have been redefined,[40,41] followed by studies on the "thin-walled" species, the woloszynski-oids ("*Glenodinium*").[42] With regard to thecate orders (Gonyaulacales, Peridiniales, Dinophysiales, and Prorocentrales), the theca is contained in a relatively few alveoli with a pattern that can be determined relatively easily (thecal plate tabulation). Athecate taxa, however, notably the order Gymnodiniales, but also Syndiniales, Noctilucales, etc., often contain hundreds of alveoli, making it difficult to determine homologies and locational relationships. As a consequence, thecate taxa are much easier to classify than athecate ones.[20]

Nine major orders (Gonyaulacales, Peridiniales, Gymnodiniales, Suessiales, Prorocentrales, Dinophysiales, Blastodiniales, Phytodiniales, and Noctilucales) are recognized within the dinoflagellates, while another order, namely, Thoracosphaerales, is suspected to belong to the Peridiniales.[20] Dinoflagellate orders can be distinguished on the basis of major morphological characters and lifecycle features of their members. The Gonyaulacales and Peridiniales, which were separated by Taylor,[43] are both characterized by the presence of cellulose-like thecal plates within the cortical alveoli. The thecae of both groups are constituted of five latitudinal series of plates (apical, anterior intercalary, precingular, postcingular, and antapical) plus the cingular and sulcal series. Members of the Blastodiniales order have a parasitic lifestyle and a temporary dinokaryon, which fostered the hypothesis that Blastodiniales diverged early from the dynokaryotic dinoflagellate lineage.[20] The Prorocentrales and Dinophysiales share a major synapomorphic feature, unique within dinoflagellates: the division of theca into lateral halves joined by a sagittal suture. Both orders have two pores, the flagella emerging from the larger one. In addition, the Prorocentrales lack the sulcus and the cingulum and have tiny periflagellar platelets. The order Phytodiniales includes species characterized by a shift from a noncalcareous coccoid cell or continuous-walled colonial stage to a vegetative stage. Similar life shifts have, however, also been observed in genera of other orders (e.g., Suessiales [*Symbiodinium*] and Gonyaulacales [*Pyrocystis*]). The Phytodiniales presently include poorly understood genera for which little molecular data are available. The Noctilucales is an early diverging order containing aberrant dinoflagellates characterized by a highly mobile ventral tentacle, which is missing in typical dinoflagellates and other alveolates. They lack, at least in some life stages, typical dinoflagellate characters such as the ribbon-like transverse flagellum or the condensed chromosomes of the dinokaryon. The tentacle does not play a role in keeping the cell in suspension, but seems rather related to food capture. The Noctilucales have the ability to incorporate, replace, or lose chloroplasts, a phenomenon rare in other alveolate groups. Whether these chloroplasts are kleptoplastids or derive from ancient endosymbiosis, as in other dinoflagellate families, remains to be demonstrated.[44] Finally, the Gymnodiniales are a polyphyletic order and together with the Peridiniales are the most evolutionary complex groups of dinoflagellates.[28]

20.3 Ecology of Dinoflagellates

Marine dinoflagellates have three major trophic modes, that is, autotrophy, mixotrophy, and heterotrophy.[45–49] Phototrophic dinoflagellates (autotrophic or mixotrophic dinoflagellates) have been thought to be one of the most important phytoplankton groups for a long time, and a number of studies concerning the ecology and physiology of the phototrophic dinoflagellates have assumed them to be exclusively autotrophic.[50] Phototrophic dinoflagellates have often formed huge red tides causing large-scale mortalities of finfish and shellfish and thus have been implicated in great losses to the aquaculture and tourism industries of many countries.[51,52] Mechanisms of the outbreak, persistence, and decline of red tides dominated by phototrophic dinoflagellates have also been studied based on the exclusively autotrophic character assumption. However, many of the initially considered phototrophic dinoflagellates have recently been revealed to be mixotrophic and thus the study on phagotrophy of phototrophic dinoflagellates is rapidly increasing.[11,53–57] In addition, some newly described phototrophic dinoflagellate species, such as *Paragymnodinium shiwhaense*, have been recently revealed to be mixotrophic dinoflagellates.[58,59] Thus, the possibility of mixotrophy by the causative phototrophic dinoflagellate species should be considered when the mechanisms of outbreak, persistence, and decline of red tides are investigated.

20.3.1 Mechanisms of Food Intake

20.3.1.1 Photosynthetic Dinoflagellates

Photosynthetic dinoflagellates are common and abundant in pelagic and benthic habitats of both marine and freshwater ecosystems. Typically, they reach their highest abundances in estuaries and coastal marine waters, in concomitance with high nutrient supply from land sources and/or deep water upwelling. Blooms of noxious species (HABs) are more common under these conditions. Using their two perpendicular flagella, dinoflagellates exhibit directed movement in response to chemical stimuli, physical variations, gravity, and light. Due to this motility, dinoflagellates are able to find optimal conditions for growth and survival under high physical disturbance (turbulence and shear forces), intense light stress, and nutrient limitation. Due to their various habitat preferences, multiple life strategies, and nutritional versatility, compared to other protist groups, dinoflagellates are very competitive for resource acquisition. Although they can sometimes be important in terms of biomass, both micro- and nano-dinoflagellates are rarely reported to dominate in terms of abundance within the phototrophic fraction of plankton communities.[60] This could be partly attributed to the fragmentary quantitative information for dinoflagellates because of inadequate identification methodologies, especially for athecate species. In coastal waters, bloom initiation can be due to germination of vegetative cells from hypnozygotes. The biological and physical factors that trigger bloom initiation are poorly known for most dinoflagellates, including harmful species.[15] During bloom development, many dinoflagellate species are capable of rapid growth, attaining abundances up to 10^9 cells/L (up to 400–500 mg Chl-a/L).[14] Dinoflagellates can grow at rates of up to 3.5 divisions/day, but only 15% of the larger free-living harmful species show growth rates greater than 1.0 division/day.[50] Photosynthetic dinoflagellates are primarily limited by phosphorous and nitrogen, although they can store these nutrients in a species-specific way that in some cases allows one species to outcompete others.[5,61] As for other phytoplankton taxa, micro-nutrients, including forms of selenium and iron, have been shown to influence blooms of some harmful phototrophic dinoflagellates.[62,63] Apart from nutrient limitation, bloom termination can be caused by water dispersion and dilution, zooplankton grazing and biological endogenous cycles, as well as parasite[64] and viral[65] infections. Field observations indicate that bloom-forming dinoflagellate species have neither strict habitat preferences nor uniform responses. Smayda and Reynolds[66] recognized nine different pelagic habitats where dinoflagellates bloom, arranged along an onshore–offshore gradient of decreasing nutrients, reduced mixing and deepening of the photic water layer (Figure 20.1). Each of the nine types of habitat is characterized by a specific dinoflagellate life form, which suggests that dinoflagellates have evolved multiple adaptive strategies, rather than a common ecological strategy. Subsequently, these authors introduced five rules of assembly for marine dinoflagellate communities, which state that specific habitat conditions correspond to specific life forms that are mainly selected on the basis of abiotic factors (turbulence and nutrient availability). Within the species pool of a given habitat, seasonal succession is stochastic and characterized by a high degree of unpredictability.[68] Conversely, for cyst-forming dinoflagellates, the existence of endogenous or exogenous factors determining the presence and succession of species has been hypothesized, suggesting that the apparent random succession of species within a pool of species is understandable and predictable.[69] The ecological role of dinoflagellates in the functioning of marine ecosystems and in the marine food web can be significant. Many, if not most, photosynthetic dinoflagellates are considered mixotrophic.[70] The larger size and lower cell surface-to-volume ratios of dinoflagellates has been suggested to generally result in lower affinities for dissolved nutrients than smaller protists, therefore positively selecting for mixotrophy among photosynthetic species.[50]

20.3.1.2 Heterotrophic Dinoflagellates

Heterotrophic dinoflagellates have been known to have various feeding mechanisms and feed on diverse prey.[71] About one-half of extant dinoflagellates lack a plastid or pigments to carry out photosynthesis.[10] These heterotrophic species have both naked and armored cell walls and occur in every type of aquatic environment. Most naked heterotrophic dinoflagellates have flexible cell walls that allow them to engulf living cells and particles (termed phagotrophy), which can then be seen inside the colorless dinoflagellate. Some naked species deploy a thin, tube-like extension called a peduncle to penetrate prey and withdraw the contents. The feeding behavior of the armored or thecate heterotrophic dinoflagellates was completely unknown until recently. Some of these species have developed a remarkable pseudopod-like structure, which is extruded from the cell and flows around the prey, enveloping it so the contents can then be digested. Termed a "feeding veil" or "pallium,"[54] the retractile organelle easily spreads over long spines on diatoms and sometimes envelops as many as 70 diatoms in a chain.[25] Recently, their feeding mechanisms and prey items have been newly discovered and it was found that small heterotrophic dinoflagellates actually fed on a single bacterium cell using feeding mechanisms (filter/interception feeding) different from those used for large algal prey.[12,72]

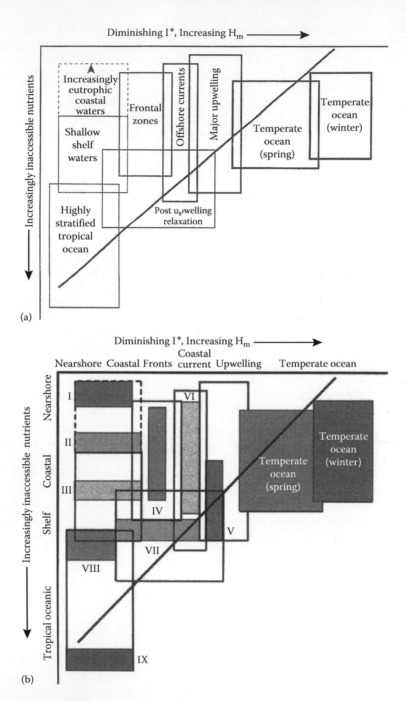

FIGURE 20.1 (a) Schematic matrix of pelagic marine habitats along an onshore–offshore gradient separating deep-mixed and well-stratified, but nutrient-deficient systems. I* refers to irradiance level received by cells within water column; H_m represents depth of mixed layer. Overlap of types within the habitat template schema does not always imply their contiguity. The diagonal approximates the main successional sequence depicted in Margalef et al.[67] (b) Predominant dinoflagellate life-form types (see Figure 20.3) associated with the turbulence-nutrient matrix (a) along an onshore–offshore continuum characterizing pelagic habitats. Type I, gymnodinioids; Type II, peridinioids and prorocentroids; Type III, ceratians; Type IV, frontal zone species; Type V, upwelling relaxation taxa; Type VI, coastal current entrained taxa; Type VII, dinophyso-ids; Type VIII, tropical oceanic flora; Type IX, tropical shade flora. (From Smayda, T.J. and Reynolds, C.S., Community assembly in marine phytoplankton: Application of recent models to harmful dinoflagellate blooms, *J. Plankton Res.*, 23(5), 447–461, 2001 by permission of Oxford University Press.)

20.3.1.3 Mixotrophic Dinoflagellates

Mixotrophs are reported among all the major extant orders of dinoflagellates (Figure 20.2), although evidence for mixotrophy is stronger in some taxa than in others. Mixotrophy is often difficult to detect in dinoflagellates for several reasons. Chloroplasts may mask food vacuoles and it can be difficult to distinguish food vacuoles from other types of inclusions.[10,71,74,75] Experimentally, it is often difficult to induce feeding in mixotrophic dinoflagellates because some species only feed under certain conditions or have low-feeding rates[74,76,77] or are specialized predators on particular types of live prey.[78–82] Conversely, reports of ingestion of bacterial-size prey by dinoflagellates, including photosynthetic species, are questionable because dinoflagellates prey on relatively large-size particles and absorption of prey on surfaces or uptake of dissolved label may have confounded the results.[71,75] However, mixotrophy is often difficult to assess clearly because of low-feeding rates, intermittent feeding dependent on conditions poorly simulated in cultures, specificity of prey or the fact that organelles can obscure food vacuoles.[28,77]

20.3.2 Motility

Dinoflagellates as motile cells are capable of directed swimming behavior in response to a variety of parameters. These include chemotaxis, phototaxis, and geotaxis, for which movement is controlled by chemical stimuli, light, or gravity, respectively.[25]

The eukaryote motility organelle is the cilium, or "eukaryotic flagellum," which consists of a cell membrane-bound extension supported by a microtubular-based axoneme and a basal body or kinetosome with associated cytoskeletal elements serving as anchors.[32]

Most dinoflagellates have a characteristic flagellar arrangement: a transversal flagellum that encircles the cell and, perpendicular to it, a trailing flagellum. Both flagella are inserted on what has been defined as the ventral side of the cell. The transversal flagellum is usually situated within an equatorial or slightly descending groove (the girdle or cingulum) and runs to the left, usually encircling the cell completely. The proximal part of the longitudinal flagellum lies freely in another groove referred to as the sulcus.[83] The mechanisms by which this arrangement causes the cells to swim and the adaptive arrangement of the flagella have been debated for almost a century, but this has not so far provided a convincing model of dinoflagellate swimming and some contradictory observations and ideas have prevailed in the literature. There is a general agreement of most authors that flagellates swim in a helical path in which the ventral side is directed toward the axis of the helix and that cells rotate around their longitudinal axis.[84,85] However, there has been no consensus as to whether it is a right or left helix or in which direction cells rotate, and it has even been suggested that cells can alternate between these rotational directions. In practice it is difficult to determine rotational directions microscopically because different focal planes may leave the impression that directions change. Following Lindemann[86] (cited in Levandowsky and Kaneta[84]) who claimed that propulsion is unaffected by loss of the trailing flagellum in *Hemidinium* cells, it has generally been assumed that the transversal flagellum is at least in part responsible for translational motion, whereas the trailing flagellum serves mainly for "orientation." Hand and Schmidt[87] also observed residual translational motion in *Gyrodinium dorsum* cells deprived of the longitudinal flagellum, while Jahn et al.[88] reported that flow-lines in the form of a torus encircling the girdle could explain a thrust in a posterior direction. On the other hand, the transversal flagellum is assumed to have a helical beat pattern.[89] Under all circumstances, however, it appears difficult to see how the transversal flagellum can contribute to the translation of the cell through the water by generating a thrust in the posterior direction, if the girdle has an equatorial position. In principle, the transversal flagellum may only generate a net torque in a direction perpendicular to the longitudinal axis of the cell. The transversal flagellum has been shown to cause the cell to rotate around its own longitudinal axis while it was further found that the rotation is in the direction of the metachronal waves that run distally along the flagellum from its point of insertion.[90] This is explained by the presence of flagellar hairs that protrude distally from the ribbon-shaped transversal flagellum (a mechanism similar to that of chrysomonad flagellates with a hirsute, anteriorly directed flagellum). Dinoflagellates thus rotate clockwise when observing their posterior end. If the girdle has a somewhat descending course (as is the case in several species), then, in case that only

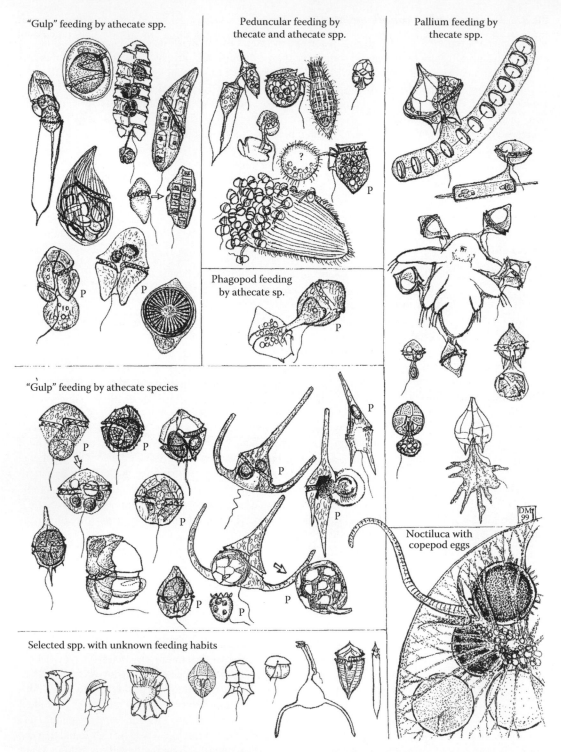

"Gulp" feeding by athecate spp.

Peduncular feeding by thecate and athecate spp.

Pallium feeding by thecate spp.

Phagopod feeding by athecate sp.

"Gulp" feeding by athecate species

Noctiluca with copepod eggs

Selected spp. with unknown feeding habits

FIGURE 20.2 Selected examples of dinoflagellate feeding techniques, drawn roughly to scale. Species are listed for each panel starting with top left cell and proceeding clockwise. P = photosynthetic; all others are nonphotosynthetic. "Gulp" feeding by athecate spp.: *Gyrodinium* sp. With unknown food; *Polykrikos kofoidii* with *Scrippsiella* sp., note slender capture filament; *Gyrodinium* sp. with *Melosira*; *Gyrodinium helveticum*; *Gymnodinium* sp. with diatom; *Gymnodinium scmgunium* with ciliates; *Gyrodinium* with *Strombidium* sp.; *Gyrodinium instriurum* with *Helicostomella* sp.; *Gyrodinium spirale* (center) with *Thalassiosira* sp.

the transversal flagellum is active, this would result in a slight backward motion. The observation that the beat pattern of the transversal flagellum is not a perfectly regular circular helix[91] cannot on its own provide an explanation, making it also difficult to explain the rotational direction without assuming a hydrodynamic effect of the flagellar hairs.[83]

Flagellates in situ will swim either through or to pycnoclines in response to photo-induced motility,[92] with frequent attraction to pycnocline microhabitats often characterized by elevated nutrient levels and low irradiance.[93] Collectively, these responses reveal the persistent need and ability of HAB dinoflagellates to respond and adapt to low levels of irradiance. This requirement seems paradoxical, given the tendency of dinoflagellates and flagellates generally to predominate seasonally and regionally under conditions of high irradiance, long daylength, and reduced water-column turbidity. Flagellates, through their motility and nutrient-retrieval migrations, can potentially access nutrients throughout the water column, whereas diatoms are less efficient in this regard.[50] The motility-dependent behaviorisms of flagellates that may facilitate this greater internal control are phototaxis, vertical migration, pattern swimming, and aggregation. Phototaxis as a general mechanism provides directed behavior, such as depth-keeping, environmental surveillance (=habitat information gathering) leading to microhabitat relocation, and environmental coupling between irradiance and nutrients (i.e., the two fundamental energy sources of phytoplankton growth). Although motility per se is not an effective nutrient uptake mechanism, swimming behavior also allows expression of the other behaviorisms dependent upon motility and thus implementation of the nutrient retrieval strategy.[94]

In the same context, HAB flagellates exhibit flexible, controlled behavior as a result of motility, with their exact behavioral expression at a given time or spatial domain being a complex balance between physiological optimization and environmental stress.[95] The behavior of the chain-forming dinoflagellate *Gymnodinium catenatum* in Spanish upwelling rias[96] provides an elegant example of the ecophysiological benefits to population dynamics of auto-regulated cellular behavior. The formation of longer chains by this toxic species, which can reach 64 cells/chain and 2 mm in length,[97] increases swimming speed. Fraga et al.[96] indicated that such strong motility can allow *G. catenatum* to be retained during downwelling periods, when it then blooms. Diel migrations into the underlying nutrient reservoir accompany this behavior.[98] During nutrient deficiency, the serpentine swimming motion with synchronized propulsion and torsion of the chains is abandoned and a reduction in chain size occurs and the stationary phase cells then hang vertically within the water column.[50,97]

Harmful dinoflagellates exhibit directed motion in response to chemical stimuli, gravity, and light, with the latter being observed in photosynthetic species, which are generally attracted to low light and repelled by high light.[6,99] Vertical migration, which involves geotaxis, a circadian rhythm, and chemosensory behavior, is exhibited by some photosynthetic species that move to shallower depths during the day and to deeper waters at night for nutrient acquisition and predator avoidance. This complex behavior depends on the species and environmental conditions. Remarkable distances (relative to the cell size) of up to 16 m/day can be traversed with swimming velocities up to 1–2 m/h or more (280–560 μm/s[100,101]). Certain heterotrophic species have shown the opposite directional behavior, moving to deeper waters

---

FIGURE 20.2 (continued)   Peduncular feeding by thecate and athecate spp.: *Oxyphysis oxyfoxoides* on tintinnid; *Dinophysis (Phalacroma) rotundata* with *Tiarina* sp.; *Pfiesteria piscicida* with large amoeboid stage, fish gill, and epithelial tissue not shown; *Dinophysis norvegica* on undetermined ciliate; *Gymnodinium fungiforme* swarm on large ciliates; *G. fungiforme* on *Amphidinium* sp. Pallium feeding by thecate spp.: *Protoperidinium depressum* with *Thalassiosira* sp.; *Diplopsalis lenticula* with *Ditylum brightweillii*; *Peridinium divergens* with copepod nauplius; *Protoperidinium steinii* with *Alexandrium* sp.; *Podolampus*, no known prey; *Blepharocysta* sp. with mass of cyanobacteria; *Oblea rotunda* with *Pyramimonas* sp. *Noctiluca* with copepod eggs: *Noctiluca miliaris* with ingested *Acartia tonsu* eggs. Selected spp. with unknown feeding habits: *Amphidiniopsis* and an unnamed psamophilic heterotroph, *Ornithocercus* sp., *Lissodinium* spp., *Heterodinium* sp., *Triposolenia* sp., *Oxytoxum* spp. "Gulp" feeding by thecate species: *Alexandrium pseudogonyaulax* ingesting *Mesodinium rubrum*; *Gonyaulax grindleyi* with unknown prey; *Gonyaulax alaskensis*, a coprophage; *Ceratium longipes* with ciliates; *Ceratium* sp. ingesting ciliate; *Ceratium furca* with ciliate; *Fragilidium subglobosum* with *Ceratium* sp.; *Prorocentrum minimum* with cryptophytes; *Scrippsiella* sp. with ciliate; *Peridinium garguntua* with *Alexandrium* sp.; *Amylax* sp. with ciliate; *Fragilidium mexicanum* (center) with *Protoperidinium divergens*. Phagopod feeding by athecate sp.: *Amphidinium cryophilum* with *Peridinium* sp. (Jacobson, D.M.: A brief history of dinoflagellate feeding research. *J. Eukaryot. Microbiol.* 1999. 46(4). 376–381. Copyright Wiley-VCH Verlag GmbH & Co. KGaA. Reproduced with permission.)

during light periods for predator avoidance and to shallow waters at night for prey acquisition, while they have also demonstrated strong chemosensory responses to prey.[10,102]

20.3.3 Diversity

Dinoflagellates in their majority (perhaps 80%) are free-living marine planktonic or benthic flagellates, the remainder inhabiting equivalent freshwater habitats.[30] Dinoflagellates are dominated by planktonic species, while benthic forms represent 8% of the species. After sexual recombination, dinoflagellates produce resistant diploid benthic stages (hypnozygotes, also termed resting cysts) to escape predation and adverse environmental conditions as well as to colonize ecosystems. Their adaptation to a wide range of environments is reflected by tremendous morphological and trophic diversity.[31]

About half of the estimated 2000 extant species of dinoflagellates are considered photosynthetic.[28] In fact, from the total number of species, 49% are heterotrophic (devoid of plastids), while 51% of the species have been reported with plastids, which however does not strictly imply autotrophy. All the basal dinoflagellates (ellobiopsids, Duboscquodinida, and Syndiniales) are heterotrophic, with the exception of a few Noctilucales (*Spatulodinium*). The continental waters are highly dominated by plastid-containing species (88%), while in marine environments there is a slight dominance of heterotrophic species (58%). Most of the dinoflagellates are free-living forms; only 7% of the total species are parasites. The dinokaryotic parasites appear in separate clades, and about 40% of them contain plastids. The beneficial or mutualistic symbionts (21 species, 1%) are photosynthetic species dispersed into at least three clades[103] (Table 20.1).

Where autotrophic dinoflagellates are concerned, it has been shown that the marine species *Amphidinium carterae* and *Heterocapsa oceanica* do not possess an external carbonic anhydrase, and thus their photosynthesis is dependent on free CO_2 alone.[104] Consequently, the growth of these two species is suggested to be CO_2-limited,[104,105] and their growth could potentially be stimulated by increasing CO_2 concentrations in the future ocean. In contrast, the growth rates of three other marine dinoflagellates (*Prorocentrum minimum*, *Heterocapsa triquetra*, and *Ceratium lineatum*) are most likely not limited by dissolved inorganic carbon, since they preferentially take up HCO_3^- instead of CO_2 to support photosynthesis.[106] This observation is supported by the finding that increasing CO_2 did not significantly affect the growth rate of another isolate of *P. minimum*.[107]

Photosynthesis is not only the essential process in primary metabolism but is also required for toxin production.[108] For example, the yield of saxitoxin per cell in the dinoflagellate *Alexandrium catenella* has been shown to be proportional to hours of daylight.[109] Also, *A. minutum* is not capable of producing saxitoxin after a 22 day incubation period in the dark, while parallel light-grown cultures produced 1.17 μg/10,000 algal cells.[110]

Cellular toxicity can also be sensitive to rising temperature. For instance, cultures and field samples of *Karlodinium veneficum* exhibit increased cellular toxicity at temperatures >25°C.[111,112] Annual variability in PSP-contaminated shellfish could result from either changing seasonal incidence of toxic *Alexandrium* blooms, variations in toxicity by resident dinoflagellates, or a combination of both.[113] Arguably each of these scenarios could be temperature-related. Correlations between cooler temperature and enhanced *Alexandrium* toxicity have been reported by numerous culture and field investigations.[114–117] In contrast, enhanced toxicity at median or increased temperature is less common, but has also been documented.[113,118,119]

In the same context, the increased abundance, geographical range expansion, and growing severity of ciguatera fish poisoning occurrences are likely indicators that several members of the benthic/epiphytic dinoflagellate genus *Gambierdiscus* are responding to warming sea surface temperatures and habitat transformation by concurrent spreading of the marine macroalgae with which they are associated.[120–123] The range of *Gambierdiscus* is rapidly expanding along with another toxic dinoflagellate genus, *Ostreopsis*, which is not closely related to *Gambierdiscus* and produces quite different toxins, but also shares a benthic/epiphytic lifestyle.[123–125]

P. micans and *P. minimum* have been reported to double their growth rates in simulated warm stratified conditions.[126] The brevetoxin-producing dinoflagellate *Karenia brevis*, which has been implicated in mass mortality of marine life in the Gulf of Mexico, has been observed in the field between 7°C and

TABLE 20.1

Number and Percent of Dinoflagellates Species according to the Lifestyle, Habitat, and Trophic Diversity

	Total	CHL	HET	FRE	PAR	SYM	MAR	CON	PLK	BEN
Total	2377	1198 (50.3%)	1179 (49.6%)	2192 (92.1%)	164 (6.8%)	21 (0.8%)	1957 (82.3%)	420 (17.6%)	2177 (91.6%)	200 (8.4%)
CHL	1198	—	0	1143 (95.4%)	34 (2.6%)	21 (1.6%)	826 (68.9%)	372 (31.0%)	1065 (88.8%)	133 (11.1%)
HET	1179	0	—	1049 (88.9%)	130 (11.0%)	0	1131 (95.9%)	48 (4.0%)	1112 (94.3%)	67 (5.6%)
FRE	2192	1143 (52.1%)	1049 (47.8%)	—	0	0	1799 (82.0%)	393 (17.9%)	2045 (93.2%)	147 (6.7%)
PAR	164	34 (20.7%)	130 (79.2%)	0	—	0	137 (83.5%)	27 (16.4%)	127 (77.4%)	37 (22.5%)
SYM	21	21 (100%)	0	0	0	—	21 (100%)	0	5 (23.8%)	16 (76.2%)
MAR	1957	826 (42.2%)	1131 (57.8%)	1799 (91.9%)	137 (7.0%)	21 (10.7%)	—	0	1787 (91.3%)	170 (8.7%)
CON	420	372 (88.5%)	48 (11.4%)	393 (93.5%)	27 (6.4%)	0	0	—	390 (92.8%)	30 (7.1%)
PLK	2177	1065 (48.9%)	1112 (51.03)	2045 (93.9%)	127 (5.8%)	5 (0.2%)	1787 (82.0%)	390 (18.0%)	—	0
BEN	200	133 (66.5%)	67 (35.0%)	147 (73.5%)	37 (18.5%)	16 (8%)	170 (85.0%)	30 (15.0%)	0	—

Source: Reprinted from Gómez, F., *Syst. Biodivers.*, 10(3), 267, Copyright (2012), with permission from Taylor & Francis Group.

CHL, plastid-containing species; HET, heterotrophic; FRE, free-living; PAR, parasites; SYM, mutualistic symbionts; MAR, marine; CON, species living in continental waters; PLK, planktonic, living in the water column; BEN, benthic, living in the benthos.

33°C.[127] Toxin production in *K. brevis*, however, demonstrates a trend of slightly higher toxicity at low temperatures that impair growth,[128] suggesting the possibility of reduced brevetoxin impacts in a future warming ocean.[129]

Distribution assessment of the many species of *Dinophysis* is prevented to a large extent by the lack of adequate molecular data. On the other hand, more data are available on the genus *Alexandrium*,[130,131] particularly on the so-called *tamarense* complex,[132] as well as on certain species of *Gymnodinium*.[133] As regards taxonomy of the *tamarense* complex, comprising the morphotypes *A. catenella*, *A. tamarense*, and *A. fundyense*, there is still considerable uncertainty. Molecular studies so far have not supported separation into three different species. In a study on the D1–D2 LSU rDNA from 110 *Alexandrium* spp. isolates, these were reported to fall into 5 groups.[131,134] Two of the groups were restricted to a single locality (Tasmania and Italy, respectively) and both belonged to the *tamarense* morphotype. The third group also comprised *tamarense* morphotypes only, whereas the strains were mostly restricted to Europe (i.e., Sweden and Ireland in the north; Spain in the south). A single strain of this group occurred in Japan, suggesting human-induced spreading. Remarkably, all examined strains of these three groups were found to be nontoxic. Both of the remaining two groups comprised *tamarense*, *fundyense*, and *catenella* morphotypes and all examined strains were toxic. In other words, toxicity was confined to these two groups, the "American" and the "East Asian," which are widely distributed. The American group is the only genetic group in the Americas, extending into the North Atlantic as far east as Scotland and to the North Pacific as far west as Japan and Korea. It is distributed from the Arctic to warm water, although strains from truly tropical waters have not been reported to date. This American clade also occurs in South Africa, indicating spreading by the circumpolar current. The second group/clade comprising all three morphotypes, namely, the "East Asian," is mainly confined to East Asia, from Thailand to Korea. This genotype has been also sporadically found elsewhere, in Port Phillip Bay, Australia, on the North Island of New Zealand, and in the French Mediterranean and it appears to be temperate tropical. These two toxic genotypes overlap in distribution in Korea and Japan.[131]

Where the genus *Gymnodinium* is concerned, it includes a group characterized by microreticulate cysts. One of the species, *G. catenatum*, is a serious PSP toxin-producer, while *G. nolleri* and *G. microreticulatum* appear to be nontoxic. These three species are closely related and have been repeatedly confused, resulting in erroneous conclusions about their geographic distribution. Identifications based solely on cyst diameter measurements are not entirely reliable, as the cyst diameter overlaps and considerable variation has been detected. The three species show a somewhat erratic geographic distribution, which may reflect that cysts have been introduced into new areas. Thus, the presence of *G. catenatum* in Australia is believed to be due to spreading with ships' ballast water to Tasmania, and from there to the southeastern mainland of Australia and the North Island of New Zealand. Cysts are generally absent from sediments in Tasmania except near Hobart, where ballast water is usually discharged.[135]

All three species are confined to temperate and tropical waters. However, *G. catenatum* is very widely distributed, particularly in warmer waters, with Tasmania being its coldest area of occurrence. In Europe, *G. catenatum* has not been reported to occur north of the Iberian Peninsula, but it is considered as a serious cause of PSP in western North Africa, in agreement to the remark that it generally occurs at subtropical areas and may bloom at sea-surface temperatures up to 26°C.[136]

In the Mediterranean Sea, *G. catenatum* is considered an invasive species with its presence attributed to a geographical expansion from the Atlantic across the Strait of Gibraltar.[137] The first record was in the Alboran Sea in 1986,[137,138] later spreading along the southern basin of the Mediterranean Sea[139] into Algeria[137] and Tunisia.[140,141]

20.4 Cell and Molecular Biology

The eukaryotic cell cycle, divided into M (mitosis), G1 (Gap 1), S (DNA synthesis), and G2 (Gap 2) phases, is universal for all microalgae, including the dinoflagellates,[142,143] which present a unique mitosis. Reduction in growth rate is correlated to changes in the duration of the cell cycle and is attributable to expansion of a single cell-cycle phase (G1).[144]

Circadian rhythms among the phototrophic microalgae, for example, in cell division, nutrient assimilation, bioluminescence, toxin production, onset of sexual reproduction, and vertical migration, are linked to both nutrients and light regime. The cell-division cycles are therefore phased or synchronized to photocycles. Mitotic division in the dark is typical,[145] but there are exceptions, for example, shade-adapted dinoflagellate species such as *Prorocentrum lima*, *Prorocentrum cordatum/minimum*,[143,146] and *Amphidinium operculatum*[147] may divide in the light. In the last species, it is the time from dark-to-light transition that dictates occurrence of M-phase, not whether it is in the dark or light period.[147]

20.4.1 Sexual Reproduction

The first phase of a planktonic phytoplankton bloom development is the initiation and requires an inoculum of cells to seed a bloom, as without the inocula there would be no increased population. The inoculum can derive from several sources and may involve different life stages.[148–150] Smayda and Reynolds[68] summarized sources of blooms by presenting three categories: holoplanktonic, meroplanktonic, and advected sources. Holoplanktonic infers that the source population exists all year long at low concentrations and has a wide temperature tolerance; it does not however mean that there is not a sexual cycle or that the maintenance life stage is a vegetative cell. Meroplanktonic infers an alternation between planktonic and benthic forms. This alternation could be between dimorphic haploid planktonic stages and diploid benthic resting stages for dinoflagellates, or benthic temporary resting cells such as in some diatoms.[151,152] Meroplanktonic coupling of stages that involves asexual and sexual processes is common in many neritic and estuarine microalgae. The timing of other events such as dormancy and maturation can have an effect on timing of blooms as modulated by abiotic factors such as light and temperature.[149,153] Dormancy itself can last from days (e.g., 12 days for *Gymnodinium catenatum*[154]) to months or years and depends on both species as well as on abiotic factors, such as temperature. The third category, advected populations, may actually be a later rather than an initial stage of a bloom. It may be a higher-than-normal abundance of a species that has been passively concentrated at a boundary layer or discontinuity and advected to another area, such as an embayment. Zingone et al.[153] suggested three possible scenarios for cysts, that is, they can germinate continually, sporadically, or seasonally. At the beginning of cyst formation, there can be many cysts with little viability or there can be few with high viability. Although dormant cells can remain in a resting state for years, viability of any cyst population can vary, as can also hatchability.[155]

In the literature of the dinoflagellate life cycle, some terms like "temporary," "pellicle," and "ecdysal" cyst have also been arbitrarily employed to describe a nonmotile and single-layered wall stage, with no mandatory dormancy period, of asexual or sexual origin. When sexual resting cyst formation occurs within a clone of a given dinoflagellate species, this species is called homothallic. When two different mating types are required, the species is called heterothallic.[156] It has been argued that the use of the term "temporary" to define thin-walled cysts should be definitively rejected.[157] Bravo et al.[157] further recommended that the term "ecdysal" should be also abandoned for the definition of the thin-walled cysts, as it could not be exclusively applied to these types of cysts, since thick-walled zygotic cysts (resting) can also be formed through ecdysis. The same authors concluded that the term "pellicle cyst" should be better used to describe a cyst stage in which the cyst has a single-layered wall and either no dormancy period at all or a dormancy period significantly shorter than that described for resting cysts of the same species.[157]

In the study of photosynthetic *Lingulodinium polyedrum* cultures, it was found that this heterothallic dinoflagellate could produce two types of resting cysts: one is an ecdysal sexual diploid ($2n$) stage and the other a spiny resting cyst or hypnozygote ($2n$).[158] If the medium was phosphate depleted, spiny cysts resulted from syngamy; however, if nutrients were repleted, ecdysal cysts were produced. The ecdysal product took up to 72 h to germinate, and 24–48 h later, the germling produced two cells, presumably by mitotic division. Hypnozygotes were dormant for 2–4 months and excystment depended on exogenous factors, as well as on endogenous factors. It was concluded that the ecdysal process took a sexual $2n$ product rapidly to a haploid ($1n$) product.[158] This represents Type V in the terminology of Smayda and Reynolds[66] (Figure 20.3). In other studies, not all planozygotes in culture undergo transition into hypnozygotes; some die, and some divide. Most species are either homothallic or heterothallic, for example, an advantage for homothallism relates to increased gamete encounters and reduced energy expenditure.

Occasionally, a species has been documented to be both homothallic and heterothallic. Homothallism and heterothallism both involve sexual reproduction and could provide DNA repair. Probert[159] thought that harmful algal species could select for homothallism for maintenance of populations if the habitat did not promote environmental concentrations of cells for sustaining blooms. In a study on heterothallic *Gymnodinium nolleri*, an alternation of life stages proceeded from vegetative to gamete to planozygote, and from there the next product depended on the nutritional status of the external medium.[160] If nutrients were high, the $2n$ planozygote divided producing presumably two $1n$ cells; an hypnozygote resulted, however, if nutrients were low. The nutritional status of culture experiments has been reported to have an influence on the path a species will follow. *Karenia mikimotoi* is known to aggregate at pycnoclines in thin layers and constitutes a year-round population off the Bay of Biscay and at the perimeter of the Celtic Sea.[161] As small cells of *K. mikimotoi* have higher growth rates (1.0 division/day vs. 0.6 divisions/day[162]), it is believed that they contribute to blooms. This represents Type IV of Smayda and Reynolds[66] (Figure 20.3). Dinoflagellate "small cells" can represent gametes or asexual disproportionate daughter cells. In some cases, the small cells act as anisogametes and fuse with larger cells, or they can grow and mitotically divide, as in the case of *Dinophysis*.[163] *Dinophysis* small cells were previously identified as other species, but are now known to be part of the life cycle.[164] This represents Type VII of Smayda and Reynolds[66] (Figure 20.3).

Temporary cysts of dinoflagellates are considered nonmotile stages, formed by exposure of motile, vegetative cells to unfavorable conditions such as mechanical shock or sudden changes in temperature.

- **Type I** (= *Gymnodinioids*)
  Gymnodinium spp., Gyrodinium instriatum, Katodinium rotundatum
  \
  - **Type II** (= *Peridinians/Prorocentroids*)
    Heterocapsa triquetra, Scrippsiella trochoidea, Prorocentrum micans, Prorocentrum minimum
    \
    - **Type III** (= *Ceratians*)
      Ceratium tripos, Ceratium fusus, Ceratium lineatum
      \
      - **Type IV** (= *Frontal zone taxa*)
        Gymnodinium mikimotoi, Alexandrium tamarense
        \
        - **Type V** (= *Upwelling relaxation taxa*)
          Gymnodinium catenatum, Lingulodinium (Gonyaulax) polyedra
          \
          - **Type VI** (= *Coastal current entrained taxa*)
            Gymnodinium breve, Ceratium spp., *Pyrodinium bahamense* var. *compressum*
            \
            - **Type VII** (= *Dinophysoids*)
              Dinophysis acuta, Dinophysis acuminata
              \
              - **Type VIII** (= *Tropical oceanic flora*)
                Amphisolenia, Histioneis, Ornithocercus, Ceratium spp.
                \
                - **Type IX** (= *Tropical shade flora*)
                  Pyrocystis noctiluca, Pyrocystis pyriformis

FIGURE 20.3 Dinoflagellate bloom and vegetation life-form types and representative species, found along an onshore–offshore gradient of decreasing nutrients, reduced mixing and deepened euphotic zone. (From Smayda, T.J. and Reynolds, C.S., Community assembly in marine phytoplankton: Application of recent models to harmful dinoflagellate blooms, *J. Plankton Res.*, 23(5), 447–461, 2001 by permission of Oxford University Press.)

Studies on ecdysal cysts of *Pfiesteria piscicida,*[165] *Pseudopfiesteria shumwayae,*[166] and *Alexandrium taylori*[150] have considered this stage as part of the asexual reproduction. However, there are other studies on *Pfiesteria*, cryptoperidiniopsoids, and *Lingulodinium polyedrum* that show temporary cysts as a product of the sexual cycle.[158,167] In the case of *A. taylori*, it exhibited a daily shift from a motile stage at the water surface to a nonmotile stage, the ecdysal cyst, in the sediments. Production of ecdysal cysts could be advantageous as it allows a stock of the population to be stored in sediments.[150,168] Moreover, it has been suggested that temporary cysts in the *Alexandrium* genus could be a means to avoid predation or attack by viruses, bacteria, and parasites.[168] Furthermore, survival of temporary pellicle cysts of dinoflagellates in mussel and oyster feces has been proposed as indicative that such processes may serve as a means of potential dispersion of the species.[169]

Different life stages and life-cycle adaptations allow a species to extend its tolerance of environmental conditions, its distribution, and its survival. Dispersal can be of key importance to survival, but maintenance of populations within an area, realm, or strata may help ensure survival for sexually reproducing populations. The integrity of a water mass, such as a gyre, a discontinuity layer, or waters downstream of upwelling event for certain periods of time may be crucial to success. When integrity is disrupted, dissipation and dilution of populations and their favorable environmental conditions can result. Interspecies interactions in a water mass can create conditions favorable for one species or one group of microalgae over another, based on physiological efficiencies and tolerances.[170,171] In certain cases, bloom termination resulted from zooplankton grazing, prompting a transition from vegetative to resting stages, while in others it was attributed to exudates from zooplankton inhibiting dinoflagellate excystment.[172] Transition from planktonic to benthic stages can be regulated by endogenous or exogenous mechanisms. For instance, cyst formation in *A. minutum* started in a period with high-vegetative cell densities in the water column. Once production was initiated, encystment fluxes remained constant for 2 weeks, over the periods of maintenance and decline of the bloom.[173,174]

20.4.2 Morphology and Ecological Aspects of Recognized Potentially Toxic Dinoflagellates

As previously indicated, dinoflagellates are single-celled organisms possessing two distinctive flagella during the least part of their life cycle and a special type of nucleus known as dinokaryon. Cells are divided by a transverse girdle groove into two parts, an upper (epitheca) and a lower (hypotheca) region, whereas within the groove lies the flattened, ribbon-like, transverse flagellum that encircles the cell. This may be situated centrally, apically, or posteriorly. The smooth longitudinal flagellum extends to the base of the cell within a longitudinal furrow (sulcus). The transverse flagellum causes the rotational motion of the cell, while the longitudinal flagellum propels the cell forward. Dinoflagellates are described as armored or unarmored, according to the type of cell covering (theca or amphiesma), which always consists of several layers of membranes. The thecate or armored group has a number of cellulosic plates that are thecal plates, or simply theca as a whole. Many thecal plates tightly assemble to form a firm, strong peripheral skeleton. The number, shape, and arrangement of these plates form a distinctive geometry or topology known as "plate tabulation," which is the main means for classification and constitute an important taxonomic criterion.[43] The number, arrangement, and thickness of the thecal plates can considerably vary. They may also be ornamented with pores, depressions, spines, ridges, and reticulations.[175] Scanning electron microscopy has revealed that ornamentation of the thecal plates and fine structure of the apical pore, present on the top of many cells, are also useful diagnostic characters.[4] The other, athecate, unarmored, or naked group lacks of the plates. Athecate species are identified principally by the size and shape of their cells, that is, cell outline, position of girdle and sulcus groove, and girdle displacement. In the thecate group, genera are classified according to plate pattern, which is decided by the arrangement of thecal plates, whereas species in each genus are identified by cell size and shape, similar to the taxonomy of athecate forms. Therefore, for critical taxonomy of thecate forms, additionally to observation of cell shape, staining or dissociation of thecal plates is necessary in order to recognize their tabulation.[3]

20.4.2.1 Dinophysiales

The Dinophysiales order includes two genera that have been implicated in toxic episodes, *Dinophysis* spp. and *Phalacroma* spp. The genus *Dinophysis* is characterized by a polarized cell morphology, with the hypocone being the major part of the cell and the epicone accounting for less than one-tenth of the whole cell. The theca is composed of a few large plates accompanied by a series of small platelets. Due to the anterior position of the cingulum, the two large hypothecal plates occupy the largest part of the theca. Cells are strongly compressed laterally and therefore usually seen in lateral view. The taxonomic identification of *Dinophysis* spp. is therefore principally based on the size, shape, and ornamentation of their large hypothecal plates, which provide the cell contour, the shape of the left sulcal lists, and the three ribs supporting them.[176] Nevertheless, in different biogeographic regions, each *Dinophysis* species may exhibit a continuum of shapes between the large vegetative specimens and small gamete-like cells—with different sizes and shapes—resulting from their polymorphic life cycles, feeding behavior, and cell-cycle phases.[163,177,178]

Morphology within *Dinophysis* is highly variable and delineation between species is based on cell shape and size. Many of the so-far-described species need to be confirmed using molecular methods. Morphological variability causes uncertainty in identification, particularly when two close *Dinophysis* species co-occur, such as the pairs *D. acuminata/D. sacculus*[179] and *D. caudata/D. tripos*.[180] The term "*D. acuminata* complex" employed by several authors[181–183] is therefore a good example of how to label a group of co-occurring species, difficult to discriminate with conventional microscopy. A large array of morphologically distinct morphotypes of *Dinophysis* have been labeled as *D. acuminata*, *D.* cf *acuminata*, *D. ovum*, *D.* cf *ovum* on the basis that their large hypothecal plates were dorsally convex and cells had a more or less oval/suboval shape in lateral view. The relationship between *Dinophysis* and *Phalacroma* Stein—the latter for long considered a synonym of *Dinophysis*[184,185]—has been a matter of controversy. The genus *Phalacroma* was assigned to heterotrophic species with an elevated epitheca visible in lateral view and narrow horizontally projected cingular lists.[186,187] Recent molecular analyses of the LSU rDNA in a large group of Dinophysiales supports the view that *Phalacroma* is a separate genus.[178,188]

Diarrhetic shellfish toxins (DST) and pectenotoxins (PTXs) have to date been unambiguously found in 12 species of *Dinophysis* Ehrenberg. Of these, seven species (*D. acuminata*, *D. acuta*, *D. caudata*, *D. fortii*, *D. miles*, *D. ovum*, and *D. sacculus*) have been associated with DSP events. There are doubts about the toxigenic nature of the heterotroph *Dinophysis rotundata* (= *Phalacroma rotundatum*) that may act as a vector of toxins taken up from ciliate preys previously fed on co-occurring toxic *Dinophysis* spp.[189] Dinophysistoxin 1 (DTX1) was found in just one sample of picked cells of *Phalacroma mitra*, *D. rotundata*, and *D. tripos* analyzed by liquid chromatography with fluorescence detection (LC-FLD),[190] but there are no DSP outbreak reports associated with either *D. rotundata* or *D. tripos* when these were the only potentially toxic *Dinophysis* spp. present in the microplankton community.[191,192] False positives may also result from the old LC-FLD method.[193] Furthermore, although *D. norvegica* has been associated with DSP events in eastern Canada, it is not considered an important contributor to DSP events in its bloom areas in Scandinavia and Japan where it co-occurs with other toxic *Dinophysis* spp.[194] whereas *D. infundibulus* toxigenicity has been only shown in laboratory cultures.[178,193,195]

20.4.2.2 Gonyaulacales

The potentially toxic species of the order Gonyaulacales belong mainly in the genera *Alexandrium*, *Coolia*, *Gambierdiscus*, *Ostreopsis*, and *Pyrodinium*. It should be noted, however, that also the common and widespread species *Gonyaulax spinifera* (Claparède et Lachmann) Diesing 1866, *Lingulodinium polyedrum* (Stein) Dodge 1989, and *Protoceratium reticulatum* (Claparède et Lachmann) Bütschli 1885 may produce toxins.

20.4.2.2.1 Genus Alexandrium

The genus *Alexandrium* is certainly one of the most important in terms of the severity, diversity, and distribution of bloom impacts. Of the more than 30 morphologically defined species in this genus, at least half are known to be toxic or have otherwise harmful effects. One unique feature of this genus is that three different families of known toxins are produced among species within it, that is, saxitoxins, spirolides, and goniodomins. This toxigenic diversity is not found in any other HAB genus. The most significant of these toxins in terms of impacts are the saxitoxins, responsible for outbreaks of paralytic shellfish poisoning (PSP), the most widespread of the HAB-related shellfish poisoning syndromes. The macrocyclic imine spirolides, thus far known only from *Alexandrium ostenfeldii*[196] and possibly *A. peruvianum*, are potent fast-acting neurotoxins when administered intraperitoneally into laboratory rodents. Goniodomins, on the other hand, produced by *A. monilatum* and *A. hiranoi* (formerly *Goniodoma pseudogonyaulax*[197]) cause paralysis and mortality in finfish.[198]

From a morphological point of view, the species now included in the genus *Alexandrium* share a Kofoidean plate pattern of apical pore complex (APC), 4′, 6″, 5‴, 2⁗, 6C, 9–10S.[198,199] Cells are relatively featureless when observed by light microscopy, but minor morphological characters become visible after staining and dissection of thecal plates and/or after examination by scanning electron microscopy. The morphological characters for species identification are cell size, shape, chain formation, ornamentation of the theca, cingular and sulcal excavation, sulcal lists, shape of APC, 1′, 6″, and some sulcal plates, such as S.p., S.a., and S.s.a. A detailed illustration, description, and discussion of the various species are presented in the monograph by Balech.[199]

The genus *Alexandrium* comprises species with a conspicuous girdle and sulcus and many small thecal plates; species of *Alexandrium* are primarily defined on the basis of the morphology of certain thecal plates. Three of the *Alexandrium* species that are commonly reported in HAB events, *A. catenella*, *A. fundyense*, and *A. tamarense*, form what is known as the "*A. tamarense* species complex."[200,201] These three toxic species were found to be more closely related to each other than to three other nontoxic species (*A. affine*, *A. insuetum*, and *A. pseudogonyaulax*) based on their rDNA-ITS and 5.8S rDNA sequences.[202] In that study, *A. catenella* and the majority of *A. tamarense* sequences formed discrete clusters, with *A. fundyense* included within the *A. tamarense* cluster, and with some strains of *A. tamarense* outside of this cluster. The same study, together with results from 28S rDNA sequencing, revealed a geographical correlation between strains within the species complex, rather than a correlation with morphology.[203,204] In the genus *Alexandrium*, as for many other taxa, the advent of molecular techniques challenged the classification of species based on morphological characters by showing that (1) a high level of genetic diversity is present within the same morphospecies, and (2) some characters for separation of closely related morphospecies show a broad range of variability and do not match molecular genetic clustering.[198]

No correlation has also been found between the type of toxin produced and genetic affiliation, but rather the toxin profile varies with growth conditions.[205] Cellular toxin content has been reported to be a less stable phenotypic character of a clonal isolate of *Alexandrium* than its toxin profile.[206] Average cellular toxin content of toxigenic *Alexandrium* isolates varies considerably (up to an order of magnitude) among different growth phases and environmental regimes in batch cultures, with maxima usually found in exponential phase and under phosphorus limitation. Furthermore, within *Alexandrium* species, clone-specific toxin content can vary from undetectable to >100 fmol/cell, even among clones isolated from the same geographical population. This practically implies that cell PSP toxin content is not reliable as a species-, ribotype-, or population-characteristic and must be interpreted cautiously.[117,207]

20.4.2.2.2 Genera Ostreopsis and Coolia

Ostreopsis and *Coolia* are the only two genera comprising the family Ostreopsidaceae Lindeman. *Coolia monotis* has the same fundamental epithecal plate arrangement as *O. siamensis* Schmidt, although differences are apparent in the hypothecal plate arrangement. Both genera include toxic species and their presence in aquaculture and fishing areas should therefore be of concern to shellfish harvesters, biotoxin regulators, and public health authorities. Australian strains of *C. monotis* produce the lipid soluble compound cooliatoxin, considered a monosulphated analog of yessotoxin (YTX),[208] whereas *O. siamensis* also produces lipid soluble polyether compounds.[209,210]

The benthic dinoflagellates *Ostreopsis* spp. are reported worldwide in many tropical and lately in temperate regions.[210–215] In the Mediterranean Sea, blooms of *O.* cf. *ovata* and *O. siamensis* have been reported since the late 1970s[216,217] but, in the last decade, they have become increasingly frequent and resulted in relevant benthic biocenosis sufferings and human health problems. *Ostreopsis* species, typically, proliferate in shallow and sheltered waters with low hydrodynamism; they form a rusty-brown colored mucilaginous film, which covers reefs, rocks,[218] soft sediments,[212] as well as seaweeds,[212,213,218,219] marine angiosperms, and invertebrates.[220,221] The whole of the evidence suggests that the presence of *Ostreopsis* spp. in coastal waters may pose a real threat to coastal food web and fishery.[222] The exact effects on marine organisms and ecosystem dynamics, however, still remain unknown, although mortality of several marine organisms, in particular sea urchins that lost their spines during blooms of *O.* cf. *ovata* or *O. siamensis*, has been reported.[223–225]

The genus *Ostreopsis* was described in 1901 with the type species *O. siamensis* Schmidt.[226] This genus did not receive major attention until the taxonomical study of Fukuyo,[227] who redescribed the type species together with the description of two new species, *O. ovata* and *O. lenticularis*. Since then, six other new species of *Ostreopsis* have been added: *O. heptagona*,[228] *O. mascarenensis*,[229] *O. labens*,[230] *O. marinus*,[231] *O. belizeanus*,[231] and *O. caribbeanus*.[231] Taxonomy of *Ostreopsis* spp. is based on the morphological characters, such as thecal plate pattern, shape, and size. Since, however, the plate pattern is quite similar in most of the *Ostreopsis* species, almost any *Ostreopsis* species could easily fit the original description of *O. siamensis*, with the exception of *O. heptagona*. The latter is the only species in which plates 10 and 500 touch. But even in this case, the connection is usually limited to only just a point instead of a suture. In the *O. siamensis* original description of Schmidt,[226] one figure shows *O. siamensis* in anteroposterior (AP) view as rounded, whereas another figure presents it as elongated. The rounded or elongated shape is one of the main differences between *O. lenticularis* and *O. siamensis*,[227] the former being a species that Norris et al.[228] do not consider as an independent taxon. Thus, taxonomy of the genus *Ostreopsis* is unclear.[210,212] When used together with other characters, molecular approaches may help to resolve taxonomical problems.[40,201]

Toxins produced by *O.* cf. *ovata* strains have been initially identified as a putative palytoxin (pPLTX) in small amounts and ovatoxin-a (OVTX-a) as the major toxin[215,232]; recently, the presence of putative PLTX and OVTX-a was confirmed and the occurrence in the algal extract of four new palytoxin-like compounds, OVTX-b, -c, -d, and -e, was highlighted[233] (see also Chapter 26). After the 2005 excessive blooms in Italy, studies on *Ostreopsis* spp. have greatly increased and more careful monitoring of benthic biocenosis has been conducted, providing evidence of widespread *Ostreopsis* spp. proliferations in the Mediterranean areas, including several Italian regions.[219,234,235] It is difficult to establish if *O.* cf. *ovata* is really a species of recent introduction in the Mediterranean area; however, its massive cell proliferations constitute a new phenomenon, since the brownish mucilaginous film covering all benthic substrates and the associated presence of high cell numbers in the overlying water column, both typical of *O.* cf. *ovata* blooms,[213] have been reported to occur only recently in the Mediterranean basin.

A morphological and genetic study of 82 *Ostreopsis* strains collected from 26 localities around the globe, involving phylogenetic analyses of LSU, 5.8S, and ITS as both single and concatenated sequences, indicated that strains identified as *O. lenticularis* and *O. labens* by different authors clustered together in a single clade. Designations of these species, therefore, should likely be revised. On the other hand, the *O.* cf. *siamensis* isolates from the Mediterranean Sea clustered together, but as no *O. siamensis* isolates from the Indo-Pacific region were included in the analysis, it was unclear whether these isolates were truly *O. siamensis* (hence the *O.* cf. *siamensis* designation). *O.* cf. *ovata* all grouped together, but as four distinct clades: Mediterranean/Atlantic, Malacca Strait, South China Sea, and Celebus Sea. A clear distinction existed between the Atlantic/Mediterranean and Indo-Pacific clades suggesting genetic isolation, but divergences were not as great as between genetic species (morphospecies), suggesting *O.* cf. *ovata* is still a single species hosting high variability within the taxon.[123,236]

20.4.2.2.3 Genus Gambierdiscus

Dinoflagellates in the genus *Gambierdiscus* Adachi and Fukuyo were originally described using live and preserved materials collected from the Gambier Islands, French Polynesia by T. Yasumoto.[237] Physiological data on *Gambierdiscus* species are limited to studies on relatively few clones, most which have not been identified to species level.[120,238–240] The reason for the lack of definitive identifications was that most prior studies were conducted when the taxonomy of *Gambierdiscus* was poorly resolved and the cells were reported as either *Gambierdiscus toxicus* (Adachi and Fukuyo) or *Gambierdiscus* spp. Variability in cell size (e.g., a dorsoventral diameter range of 45–150 μm) and shape (some cells were more rounded) were noted by the authors in these field collections, the range of which later led to the conclusion that the original species description likely included multiple species present in the examined field samples.[241]

Gambierdiscus spp. is a marine benthic dinoflagellate of considerable interest as its members produce ciguatoxins, the lipophilic toxins responsible for ciguatera fish poisoning (CFP). These toxins readily accumulate in tropical, marine food webs and reach their highest concentrations in fish.[242,243] The same genus may also produce other toxins, that is, maitotoxins (MTXs), gambierol, and gambieric acid. MTXs have been found in the viscera of herbivorous fish but are unlikely to produce human illness due to their low capacity for bioaccumulation in fish tissue and low oral potency.[244,245]

The effects of temperature, salinity, and irradiance on the growth of eight *Gambierdiscus* species— *G. australes, G. belizeanus, G. caribaeus, G. carolinianus, G. carpenteri, G. pacificus,* and *G. ruetzleri*— and one putative new species, *Gambierdiscus* ribotype 2, were studied by Kibler et al.[246] Depending on species, temperatures where maximum growth occurred varied between 26.5°C and 31.1°C. The upper and lower thermal limits for all species were between 31°C–34°C and 15°C–21°C, respectively. Salinities where maximum growth occurred varied between 24.7 and 35, while the lowest salinities supporting growth ranged from <14 to 20.9.

20.4.2.2.4 Genus Pyrodinium

Pyrodinium is classified into a recognizable taxon under the subfamily Pyrodinioideae by Fensome et al.[19] based on the fossilizable dinosporin cysts. Species of genus whose importance as a paralytic shellfish poisoning toxin (PSTs) producer has increased in several regions of the world, especially in the Indowest Pacific, is *Pyrodinium bahamense*. The classification of *P. bahamense* is generally phenetic,[132,247] but in some cases a phylogenetic hypothesis is implied.[19,248]

Populations of *P. bahamense* are thought to be generally segregated, with the var. *compressum* exclusive to the Pacific and var. *bahamense* exclusive to the Atlantic. It is now known however that there are at least two locations where the two varieties co-occur, namely, in the Arabian Gulf[249] and the Pacific coast of Mexico.[250] Locations at which motile cells of *P. bahamense* have been reported are grouped into three regions, the Caribbean Sea and Central America, Persian Gulf and the Red Sea, and the western Pacific. The var. *compressun* is well known to cause PSP in Southeast Asia coastal waters and the Pacific coast of central America. Until 2002, the var. *bahamense* in the Atlantic was assumed to be nontoxic; then it was confirmed that *P. bahamense* occurring in the Indian River Lagoon, Florida, USA, can produce saxitoxin, although it has never been known to cause any PSP incident.[251,252] Indeed, from 2002 to 2004 there were at least 28 recorded cases of saxitoxic puffer fish poisoning due to toxins of *P. bahamense* origin.[253] The presence of PSTs was reported in mussels from Trinidad, but the source of the toxins was not identified.[254] It remains a mystery as to why so far no PSP cases have been recorded from areas where *P. bahamense* var. *bahamense* is found.[255]

20.4.2.2.5 Genus Lingulodinium

Lingulodinium polyedrum (F. Stein) Dodge is a planktonic, single-celled, photoheterotrophic dinoflagellate species. Cells are polyhedral-shaped and range in size from 40 to 54 μm in length and 37 to 53 μm in width. It is made up of thick plates, well defined, with a delicate reticulation and with numerous large trichocyst pores surrounded by circular sculpturing.[256] The girdle is deeply excavated, descending, and without intercrossings. It is bioluminescent[257] and its life cycle involves vegetative reproduction, temporary cyst formation, and sexual reproduction. The cysts are spherical (31–54 μm in diameter) with a double cell wall and a granular surface covered with spines. Living cysts present a prominent red body.[158] It requires high levels of nutrients to develop; it is cosmopolitan and can be found mainly in temperate and subtropical coastal zones.[256] Toxicity of *L. polyedrum* has long been argued but recent results confirmed that *L. polyedrum* is capable of producing yessotoxin.[258,259] Other reports have also identified both nontoxic and toxic isolates of *L. polyedrum* from Spain, the United Kingdom, and California.[259–263] In addition, several YTX-positive isolates of *L. polyedrum* have been identified in Italy[264,265] and Ireland, yet only nontoxic isolates have been observed in Norwegian waters.[266] Its occurrence has also been reported in the Moroccan Atlantic coast without confirmed toxicity.[267] The *L. polyedrum* species shows very low intraspecific diversity, and at this level of genetic assessment it appears that there are no geographically distinct populations but rather a global distribution of ribotypes within this species. Consequently, rRNA operons provide no indirect genetic markers for YTX production, and lack of diversity at this level hints that variation in toxicity may be due to environmental conditions or genomic variability.[268]

20.4.2.2.6 Genus Protoceratium

It is thought that *Protoceratium reticulatum* is synonymous with *Gonyaulax grindleyi*, however there is no consensus on its taxonomy. Paz et al.[269] hypothesized that *P. reticulatum* could be a group comprising several species, but deeper taxonomic studies are necessary to confirm this. Very little biological knowledge of this species exists aside from the fact that it is a photosynthetic and thecate planktonic dinoflagellate belonging to the family Gonyaulacaceae. Its size oscillates between 28 and 43 µm in length and 25–35 µm in width[270]; it is shaped like a polyhedron with a strong theca made up of several plates; the theca has a prominent reticulation with pores in the center of each reticulation. Since it has been found in very different locations, it is reasonable to believe that *P. reticulatum* is able to grow within a wide range of temperature conditions, salinities, light, pH, and nutrient conditions.[271] Environmental conditions are considered important for the production of toxins by dinoflagellates. However, only few studies are published with regard to environmental factors that might affect YTX formation by *P. reticulatum*. Recently, Röder et al.[272] reported that *P. reticulatum* growth was favored at salinities between 20 and 30, with water temperature and nutrient limitation strongly influencing YTXs formation. Generally, nitrogen-limited cultures displayed the lowest and phosphorous-limited cultures the highest YTX cell quota. Lower salinities caused a higher volume of the cell accompanied by an increase of YTX concentration.

20.4.2.2.7 Genus Gonyaulax

The most important potentially toxic representative of the genus is the species *Gonyaulax spinifera*. Certain variability in morphology among individuals belonging to this species was observed by Dodge,[273] who stated that *Gonyaulax spinifera* could likely be a species complex, and by Tomas,[274] who hypothesized that this taxon could represent several species or sibling species.

   G. spinifera has been reported as a YTX producer as two out of eight strains from New Zealand analyzed by ELISA[275] showed very high concentrations of YTXs. However, previous LC/MS analyses of this organisms only gave a weak signal of YTX in one sample.[263] More recently, *G. spinifera* was found, together with *L. polyedrum*, in plankton net samples during a YTX toxic episode in mussels in Russia.[276] Morphology of *G. spinifera* is very similar to that of *P. reticulatum*, so it could well be a YTX producer.[270] Some authors have also suggested that the real producers of YTXs are bacteria associated with these dinoflagellates; however, there is no solid evidence for this.[277]

20.4.2.3 Peridiniales

The most frequently occurring potentially toxic genera in this order are *Protoperidinium*, *Pfiesteria*, and the recently described genera *Azadinium* and *Vulcanodinium*.

20.4.2.3.1 Genus Protoperidinium

The genus *Protoperidinium* is typically characterized by having the following plate formula: Po, X, 4′, 2 or 3a, 7″, (3 + t) c, 6 s, 5‴, and 2‴″[187], although there are several exceptions.[278] The genus appears to be polyphyletic, based on the sequence of the 28S rDNA, forming sister groups with gymnodinoid and prorocentroid dinoflagellates.[40] The only documented toxic species of *Protoperidinium* is *P. crassipes*. The heterotroph *Protoperidinium crassipes* had been associated with AZAs; however, recent studies including a statistical review of Irish monitoring data[279] could not corroborate this hypothesis.

   Limited studies on two isolates of this toxic species have shown that it is a sister group to *P. divergens* and that it encompasses very little divergence at the level of its 18S rDNA.[278]

20.4.2.3.2 Genus Pfiesteria

The genus *Pfiesteria* includes two toxigenic species, *Pfiesteria piscicida* and *P. shumwayae*, which are thinly thecate dinoflagellates with apparently cosmopolitan distribution, especially in shallow, poorly flushed, eutrophic estuaries.[102,280] They are heterotrophic prey generalists that typically feed via phagotrophy and prefer live fish or their fresh tissues as food. They can also engage in limited mixotrophy through temporary retention of kleptochloroplasts from algal prey.[281–283] A hydrophilic *Pfiesteria* toxin (PfTx), isolated in 1997 and consisting of a metallated organic complex, has been shown to affect fish and mammals. *Pfiesteria* toxins were found to be susceptible to decomposition in the presence of white light, pH variations, and prolonged heat. It is likely that sunlight and metal exposure are the two primary environmental factors that combine to initiate *P. piscicida* toxicity during toxic algal blooms. Light exposure could initiate redox cycling of the metal ion(s) resulting in radical formation and release of the toxin species. It is this photochemistry that appears to be responsible for both generation of the radical toxic species and the eventual toxin disappearance.[284]

Toxigenic strains are generalist predators that have shown strong preference for live fish prey; when such prey are not available, they consume cryptophytes and an array of other organisms. These dinoflagellates mainly thrive in quiet, shallow, eutrophic estuaries where microbial prey and fish prey, especially planktivorous fish (juvenile menhaden), are abundant. Their stimulation by nutrient over-enrichment seems mainly to be an indirect effect, mediated by prey abundance, but they can also be directly stimulated by dissolved organic nutrients, and by inorganic nutrient forms when they have retained kleptochloroplasts. In the habitat described earlier, and following three decades of hurricane-free years, they were linked as causative agents of major estuarine fish kills. All available evidence[49,285–294] except for the unrooted tree of Litaker et al.[295] suggests that *P. piscicida* and *P. shumwayae* are "sister" species, apparently forming a monophyletic group.

20.4.2.3.3 Genus Azadinium

Members of the marine dinoflagellate genus *Azadinium* have recently been recognized as causative organisms of azaspiracid (AZA) shellfish poisoning, a serious seafood toxicity syndrome associated with consumption of contaminated shellfish.[296]

Azadinium spinosum Elbrächter & Tillmann is so far the only documented toxin-producing species of the genus. *A. spinosum* is a new species in a newly erected genus, clearly belonging to the subclass Peridiniphycidae.[297] Potentially toxic species of *Azadinium* genus are small (*A. spinosum* 12–16 μm length and 7–11 μm width and *A. obesum* 13–18 μm length; 10–14 μm width) photosynthetic dinoflagellates.[297,298]

A. spinosum consistently produce AZA with a reported toxin profile consisting of AZA-1 and AZA-2, indicating that the production and profile of known AZAs is a stable characteristic of the species. Other species of *Azadinium* have initially been reported as nontoxigenic in terms of known AZAs, such as *A. caudatum*.[299,300] *A. obesum* cannot produce AZA-1 and/or AZA-2 in significant amounts, nor any toxin of the AZA-3 to AZA-12 group. However, Rehman et al.[301] have shown that there are many more structural AZA variants, such that to date the number of described analogues has increased to 32.[298] In support to this, Krock et al.[302] recently reported the presence of new AZA analogues in *A. poporum*, which was until then considered as a nontoxic species.

DNA sequence and phylogenetic analyses elucidated and supported the separation (but close affinity) of *A. obesum* and *A. spinosum*, as well as description of the former as a distinct species. Phylogenetic interpretation of the four genes analyzed—internal transcribed spacer, 18S rDNA, 28S rDNA (D1/D2), and cytochrome oxidase I—further validated the recently erected genus *Azadinium* Elbrächer et Tillmann but did not clarify the position of the genus with respect to higher taxonomic levels within the subclass Peridiniphycidae.[298]

From an ecological point of view, it is important to point out that the nontoxic species *A. obesum* co-occurs with both *A. spinosum* and *A. poporum*.[298,303] The increasing diversity of the genus and the coexistence of toxic and nontoxic species in the same water mass complicate all attempts to identify/quantify the source organism of AZAs by routine monitoring programmes using light microscopy.[303]

20.4.2.3.4 Genus Vulcanodinium

Recently it was confirmed that pinnatoxins, known previously only from shellfish, originate from toxic dinoflagellates. The recent association of a benthic peridinoid dinoflagellate from New Zealand, *Vulcanodinium rugosum*, with production of pinnatoxins E and F has now confirmed this link.[304,305] The thecal plate formula is Po, X, 4′, 3a, 7″, 6c, 6s, 5‴, 2‴″. The apical pore plate Po is very large and a mucous matrix is extruded from its center. The plate X is rather long and just below is the narrow and short first apical plate 1′. The intercalary anterior plates are contiguous. The first cingular cl plate is narrow. The number, the shape of plates, and the presence of lists characterize the sulcus. The thecal surface is covered by longitudinal striae with often cross reticulations and is perforated by large pores. A phylogenetic study, based on LSU rDNA sequence data, confirms that this taxon is new and that it belongs to the order Peridiniales.[305]

20.4.2.4 Prorocentrales

The conventional taxonomy of *Prorocentrum* species is complex and relies on differences between taxa that can only be resolved by electron microscopy. In one study of nine species of *Prorocentrum* and their respective 18S rDNA sequences,[306] strains were divided between two distinct groups, the first comprising benthic species (*P. lima*, *P. arenarium*, *P. maculosum*, and *P. concavum*) and the second group comprising planktonic and bentho-planktonic species (*P. micans*, *P. cordatum/minimum*, *P. mexicanum*, and *P. panamensis*). There was an argument raised, however, that *P. mexicanum* as described in most literature records is, in reality, a misnomer for *P. rhathymum*.[307] The two names belong to separate species that are distinguished by a slightly different structure of the apical spine, details of poroid and trichocyst number and placement, and habitat (*P. rhathymum* = benthic; *P. mexicanum* = planktonic). Other investigators list *P. rhathymum* as a synonym of *P. mexicanum*.[187,308] Nevertheless, the primary compilation of algal names, AlgaeBase currently considers both to be taxonomically accepted names.

A number of authors consider *P. minimum* to be a synonym of *P. cordatum* (Ostenfeld) Dodge. The latter name is based on *Exuviaella cordata*, which was originally described as lacking an apical spine. Subsequent SEM examination demonstrated that all specimens studied did, in fact, have a tiny apical spine.[309] These authors describe the many comparisons and misidentifications that have taken place involving this species, and conclude that the correct name is *P. cordatum*, since Ostenfeld's name preceded Pavillard's name by 15 years. Only recently has the name *P. cordatum* become evident in the literature.[310,311] Other authors continue to use *P. minimum*.[308,312,313] As the latter name is so frequent in the literature, it is maintained in this chapter, though priority indicates that *P. cordatum* is the correct name. Some sources consider both *P. minimum* and *P. cordatum* as currently accepted names.

The new planktonic species *Prorocentrum texanum* was very recently described from the Gulf of Mexico. *P. texanum* is a round to oval bivalvate dinoflagellate, with a prominent anterior, serrated solid flange on periflagellar a platelet and an opposing short, flat flange on the h platelet. *P. texanum* has two varieties that exhibit distinct morphotypes, one round to oval (var. *texanum*) and the other pointed (var. *cuspidatum*). *P. texanum* var. *cuspidatum* is morphologically similar to *P. micans* in surface markings, but is smaller, and has a serrated periflagellar flange, and is genetically distinct from *P. micans*. No genetic difference was found between the two varieties in the five genes examined. Phylogenetic analysis of the SSU, LSU, and ITS ribosomal regions place *P. texanum* sp. as a sister group to *P. micans*. One isolate of *P. texanum* var. *texanum* is reported as an okadaic acid producer.[314]

A new benthic species, *Prorocentrum bimaculatum*, was reported from Kuwait's marine sediments. Cells are large, oblong oval in shape, 49.9–55.3 μm long and 38.4–43.2 μm wide. The molecular phylogenetic position of this new taxon was inferred from SSU and LSU rDNA genes. In both phylogenetic analyses, *P. bimaculatum* branched with high support with *P. consutum* and formed a clade sister to the one including *P. lima* and related species such as *P. arenarium*, *P. belizeanum*, *P. hoffmannianum*, and *P. maculosum*. Since most species related to *P. bimaculatum* are known for their toxic effects and production of okadaic acid, this species could also be considered as a potential toxin producer, but this has yet to be analyzed.[315]

In comparison to planktonic *Prorocentrum* species, the ecology, physiology, and food web impacts of benthic harmful *Prorocentrum* species are poorly known for two reasons: benthic microalgae typically are more logistically difficult to study than plankters both in natural habitats and in culture[316] and also the focus of research has been on their taxonomy and on the toxins produced by these species, which potentially can adversely affect shellfish and humans. Benthic harmful species tend to be larger than harmful plankters and generally grow slowly even at their optimal, warm temperature range of 23°C–28°C, with maximum growth rates often <0.20 divisions/day and extending to as little as

0.1 divisions/day at colder temperatures. Based on available information for two of the nine known harmful benthic taxa, these species show a strong preference for NH_4^+ over NO_3^-, which may be advantageous in their generally NH_4^+-rich habitats. As with many harmful algal species, toxin production increases when growth occurs above Redfieldian proportions.

20.4.2.5 Gymnodiniales

Potential toxic genera of Gymnodiniales include *Karlodinium*, *Takayama*, and *Karenia*. These three genera have so far been well supported by their clear morphological differentiation. The family as a whole contains fucoxanthin and its derivatives as their main carotenoid pigments.[40,317–319]

Karenia species are characterized by their linear apical groove, lack of a ventral pore, and their generally dorsoventrally flattened appearance (except for *K. digitata*,[320] *K. longicanalis*,[321] and *K. umbella*[322]). The genus *Takayama* is distinguished by its characteristic sigmoid apical groove,[319] and the genus *Karlodinium* by its generally short, linear apical groove and the presence of a ventral pore.[323]

20.4.2.5.1 Genus Karenia

Karenia brevis is the producing species of brevetoxins, responsible for causing neurotoxic shellfish poisoning (NSP) and can generate an aerosol that causes respiratory distress in humans. *Karenia* species are found throughout the world. Most have been described as a result of investigations into extensive animal mortalities or human health problems. *Karenia mikimotoi* was the focus of the earliest studies on species now included in the *Karenia* genus. It was initially described as *Gymnodinium mikimotoi*, which caused fish kills and oyster mortalities in Japan.[324] Once *Gymnodinium breve* (now *K. brevis*) was discovered to be the cause of the Florida red tide that causes widespread animal mortality and affects human health,[325–327] it became one of the most studied species of harmful algae with extensive investigations into its toxicity, physiology, and bloom formation. For half a century, animal mass mortality, NSP, and respiratory distress caused by frequent blooms of *K. brevis* in the Gulf of Mexico, and animal mass mortality by *K. mikimotoi* in many parts of the world were thought to be the primary problems caused by *Karenia*. In the past few decades, however, blooms of newly discovered species of *Karenia* have developed in many parts of the world, also causing animal mass mortalities, NSP, and respiratory distress. Although brevetoxin is the most intensively studied toxin produced by some *Karenia* species, gymnodimine, gymnocins, and a variety of toxic sterols, polyunsaturated fatty acids (PUFAs), and other compounds are produced by various *Karenia* species.[328]

The genus *Karenia* G. Hansen & Moestrup 2000 was created as a result of a molecular and morphological study of athecate dinoflagellates previously contained within the *Gymnodinium* genus.[40] *Karenia* initially contained three species: *K. brevis*[325] G. Hansen & Moestrup, *K. mikimotoi* (*G. mikimotoi* Miyake & Kominami ex Oda[324]), and *Karenia brevisulcata*.[329] A major characteristic that differentiates the Kareniaceae from other dinoflagellates is that, instead of peridinin (which most dinoflagellates have), they have the accessory pigments fucoxanthin, 190-butanoyloxyfucoxanthin, 190-hexanoyloxyfucoxanthin, and 19-hexanoyloxyparacentrone 3-acetate (gyroxanthin-diester).[330,331] *Karenia* are unarmored dinoflagellates with no distinct cell wall plates, so are quite pleiomorphic. As a result, cells can be relatively difficult to identify to species level using standard light microscopy, particularly using standard fixatives such as Lugol's iodine.

Over the past two decades, blooms of other *Karenia* species have been discovered in many parts of the world. In 1999, *K. brevisulcata* (first named *Gymnodinium brevisulcatum*) was observed in New Zealand in a bloom that produced fish kills and human respiratory distress symptoms very similar to those produced by *K. brevis* blooms.[329] In the Atlantic, Botes et al.[332] described the new species *K. cristata* and *K. bicuneiformis* from blooms in South Africa. *K. cristata* blooms caused animal deaths and respiratory problems in humans. Haywood et al.[333] described three new species, from New Zealand, *Karenia selliformis* and *Karenia papilionacea*. Although initially isolated from New Zealand,[333] *K. selliformis* has also been found in association with fish kills in Kuwait.[249,334] *K. papilionacea* was first described from New Zealand waters and the Gulf of Mexico.[333] An additional new species from New Zealand, *Karenia concordia*, was described by Chang and Ryan,[335] which co-occurred with *K. mikimotoi* and *K. brevisulcata* in a 2002 New Zealand bloom. De Salas et al.[336] described the new species *Karenia umbella* from blooms in Tasmania that caused fish kills.[328]

20.4.2.5.2 Genus Karlodinium

While phylogenetic analyses clearly separate *Karenia* and *Karlodinium* into distinct monophyletic clades, they are morphologically so close that the main distinction remaining between them is the presence (*Karlodinium*) or absence (*Karenia*) of a ventral pore. When first described by J. Larsen,[40] the genus *Karlodinium* contained only three species, *Karl. micrum*, *Karl. veneficum*, and *Karl. vitiligo*. *Karl. micrum* is now known to be synonymous with the earlier named *Gymnodinium veneficum*,[337] and as a result, the type species in the genus *Karlodinium* is now *Karl. veneficum*.[323] The existence of *Karl. vitiligo* as a separate species from *Karl. veneficum* is doubtful for the following reasons: (1) Ballantine[337] herself states that the differences between *Karl. veneficum* and *Karl. vitiligo* are mainly physiological (*Karl. veneficum* is described as being toxic, and *Karl. vitiligo* as nontoxic); (2) the description of *Karl. vitiligo* is almost identical to that of *Karl. veneficum*; and (3) it is now recognized that there are both toxic and nontoxic forms of *Karl. veneficum*.[338] It was not until recently that a further species in this genus was characterized, *Karl. australe*[339] from shallow lagoon and estuary habitats of southeastern Australia. Its close relative, *Karl. armiger*, was described from similar habitats in the Mediterranean coast of Spain.[323]

High densities of the dinoflagellate *Karl. veneficum* have been associated with aquatic faunal mortalities worldwide. This small (<8–12 mm) athecate phytoplankton, common in coastal aquatic ecosystems, has a mixed nutritional mode, relying on both photosynthesis and phagotrophy for growth (mixotrophy). It is frequently present in relatively low cell abundance (10^2–10^3 cells/mL), but is capable of forming intense blooms of 10^4–10^5 cells/mL that are often associated with fish kills. A suite of toxic compounds (karlotoxins) have been characterized, both in the laboratory and in the field, with hemolytic, ichthyotoxic, and cytotoxic properties. These toxins have been shown to generate pores in membranes with desmethyl sterols and increase the ionic permeability, resulting in membrane depolarization, disruption of motor functions, osmotic cell swelling, and lysis.[340]

20.4.2.5.3 Genus Takayama

The potentially ichthyotoxic dinoflagellate genus *Takayama* includes two species isolated from Tasmanian (Australia) and South African coastal waters that possess a sigmoid apical groove and contain fucoxanthin and its derivatives as the main accessory pigments. They are distinct from *Akashiwo* (spiroid apical groove), *Gymnodinium* (horseshoe-shaped apical groove), *Karenia*, and *Karlodinium*. One species, *T. tasmanica*, is characterized by an S-shaped apical groove and a central pyrenoid surrounded by starch, while the other species, *T. helix*, has a shallow sigmoid apical groove and plastids with individual pyrenoids.[319] *T. tasmanica* is similar to the previously described species *Gymnodinium pulchellum*. A species identified as *G. pulchellum* was responsible for a massive bloom (up to 7.3×10^6 cells/L) and was probably the same species illustrated from Carrada et al.[341]

Following the erection of the genus *Takayama*, the species previously classified as *G. pulchellum* was assigned to two distinct species *T. cladochroma* (Larsen) de Salas, Bolch et Hallegraeff, and *T. pulchella* (Larsen) de Salas, Bolch et Hallegraeff,[319] which differ by the number of chloroplasts, the size of the nucleus and the ratio of length to width.[342] The genus *Takayama* has close affinities to the genera *Karenia* and *Karlodinium*.[319]

20.4.2.5.4 Genus Cochlodinium

Dinoflagellates of the genus *Cochlodinium* were first identified in 1895 by Schütt and have been forming harmful algal blooms in the coastal waters of Southeast Asia and North America for many decades. *Cochlodinium* blooms have since then expanded in their geographic distribution across Asia, Europe, and North America, with fisheries losses associated with blooms in South Korea alone exceeding $100M annually.[343] More than 40 species of *Cochlodinium* have been described, although the two primary HAB-forming species are *C. polykrikoides* and *C. fulvescens*. Both of these species are large (~40 μm) athecate dinoflagellates that commonly form chains of 2–16 cells. *Cochlodinium* blooms are generally characterized by spatially large (10s–100s of kilometers) and dense (>1000 cells/mL) cell aggregates that are heterogeneous in their vertical and horizontal distributions. These blooms are strongly ichthyotoxic and can also kill many other marine organisms, although the compound(s) responsible for these impacts have yet to be identified and bloom-associated toxins are not known to affect human health.

Partly due to the expansion of *Cochlodinium* blooms and the general difficulty in culturing this species, there is far less known about the autecology and toxicity of *Cochlodinium* compared to other HAB species, particularly for *C. fulvescens*.[344]

The genus *Cochlodinium* was established more than a century ago with the identification of *C. strangulatum* (Schütt). The majority of reported organisms within this genus (~50 species, with 40 accepted[345]) are rare heterotrophic organisms, and not well studied or described. Within this large group, only four species are known to produce chloroplasts and form chains: *C. polykrikoides* (synonymous with *C. catenatum* Okamura[346] and *C. heterolobactum* Silva[347]), *C. fulvescens*, *C. geminatum*, and *C. convolutum*.[348,349] Of those species, only two, *C. polykrikoides* and *C. fulvescens*, are confirmed ichthyotoxic organisms.[344]

20.4.2.5.5 Genus Amphidinium

The genus *Amphidinium* comprises naked benthic species. *Amphidinium* species with minute left-deflected epicones are reported to be monophyletic, including the type species *A. operculatum*.[41] Polyketides produced by *Amphidinium* species are extremely diverse in structure, and fall broadly into three categories: macrolides, short linear polyketides, and long-chain polyketides. Macrolides isolated from *Amphidinium* include amphidinolides, caribenolide I, amphidinolactone, and iriomoteolides. Amphidinolides are the most abundant type of bioactive metabolite found in *Amphidinium*, with 34 different compounds (designated A–H, J–S, T1, U–Y, G2, G3, H2–H5, T2–T5) having been isolated.[350–352]

20.5 Ecological Consequences of Harmful Dinoflagellates

Planktonic organisms can form mass occurrences in the water column. When their cell densities reach values considerably higher than their usual distribution, they are then termed as blooms.[50] Blooms can be either monospecific or formed by a combination of species.[353,354] Numerous prominent blooms can be traced back to high nutrient loads,[355–357] but can actually occur whenever a species is able to outgrow its competitors while partially reducing grazer pressure.[358] Dinoflagellates sometimes bloom in unexpected places, such as below the Baltic winter ice cover, while others are rather benthic than planktonic, like the palytoxin-producing *Ostreopsis ovata*.[234,359] Being the base of marine food chains, many phytoplankton blooms are beneficial for ocean productivity and consequently for the fishing and shellfish industries.[355] Dinoflagellate blooms, however, can very often significantly disrupt ecosystems,[360] harm commercially important species,[361] or produce substances that are toxic to humans.[362] Coastal eutrophication may in some cases lead to an increase in such harmful bloom events.

Under nitrate or phosphate limited conditions, many diatoms can outcompete dinoflagellates due to their generally faster nutrient uptake capabilities and subsequently higher growth rates. When concentrations of these macronutrients are increased, diatom growth is likely to be limited by silicate, increasing the likelihood of dinoflagellate dominance.[50,363] The apparent global increase of harmful algal blooms (HABs) might be partly due to increased scientific awareness; increased commercial activities in coastal areas, eutrophication, climatic effects, and the introduction of new harmful species by ship ballast water or import of shellfish stocks for aquaculture, however, are possible causes that alter the current patterns of bloom occurrence.[203,355,364,365] The increased economic impact of HABs is probably linked with the increased consumption of seafood and growth in coastal populations.[310]

A recent 50 year time series study in the northeast Atlantic and North Sea indicated that phytoplankton community structure has shifted away from dinoflagellates, including harmful species, such as some *Prorocentrum* spp. and nonharmful taxa such as *Ceratixum fuca*, and toward diatoms such as the potentially toxic *Pseudo-nitzschia* spp. and non-HABs such as *Thalassiosira* spp.[366] Combined effects of increasing sea surface temperature and increasingly windy conditions in summer have been proposed as the main reasons for this observation. However, Hinder et al.'s[366] results do not necessarily apply to many HAB species, since their survey focused on an open ocean phytoplankton community, while most HABs occur in estuaries or coastal waters. Local physical dynamics in such regions can be completely different. Nutrients in general are much more enriched in estuaries than in the open ocean, whereas estuaries and bays are usually less influenced by wind-driven physics. Certain harmful taxa, and in particular many dinoflagellates, are warm-water species and hence a slightly increasing temperature may favor their growth. Calm winds and warmer temperatures stratify the water column and suppress mixing long enough for motile dinoflagellates to grow and accumulate in surface waters, hence allowing them to bloom.[129]

20.5.1 Dinoflagellate Toxicity

The list of microalgal species potentially involved in HABs comprises about 300 noxious and toxic species out of an approximate total of 4000–5000 marine planktonic microalgae.[310,367] Of these, only around 80 (mainly dinoflagellates) have the potential to produce toxins.[68,368] This list has remarkably increased in recent years due to new cases of harmful events, development of scientific research in the field, and enhanced human interactions with the coastal zone; however, several thousand phytoplankton species are still undescribed.[310]

HAB toxins can affect humans, other mammals, seabirds, fish, as well as many other animals and organisms. One major category of impact occurs when toxic species are filtered from the water as food by shellfish, which then accumulate the algal toxins to levels that can be detrimental to humans or other consumers.[369] The main poisoning syndromes linked to dinoflagellates have been given the names paralytic (PSP), diarrhetic (DSP), neurotoxic (NSP), and azaspiracid shellfish poisoning (AZP). A fifth syndrome, namely, ciguatera fish poisoning (CFP), is caused by ciguatoxins produced by dinoflagellates that attach to surfaces in many coral reef communities.[25,370]

Dinoflagellates produce an array of highly toxic metabolites, many of which are involved in human intoxications from ingestion of seafood and can cause mortality of marine animals.[371–374] Toxins are considered to be secondary metabolites, with their metabolic and ecological roles, as well as the identification of genes controlling their production being topics under intense research.[178]

A brief summary of dinoflagellate toxic/potentially toxic genera and species accompanied by the toxins produced is presented in Table 20.2. A detailed description of these toxins is beyond the scope of this chapter, since the reader can refer to the individual specific chapters of this book.

20.5.2 Effect of Temperature, Light, and Salinity to Toxicity

Temperature is probably the most widely recognized component of climate change and also plays a crucial role in determining potential algal growth rates. Consequently, temperature can be of significant influence to community dynamics of harmful bloom species relatively to their competitors and grazers. In diatoms, for instance, nitrate uptake and reduction rapidly decline at elevated temperatures,[477] thus potentially favoring competing algae. The benthic/epiphytic dinoflagellate genus *Gambierdiscus* spp. respond to warming sea surface temperatures and habitat transformation by concurrent spreading of the marine macroalgae with which they are associated.[120–123] Where *Ostreopsis* spp. is concerned, the majority of laboratory experiments examining temperature suggest that *Ostreopsis* grow more efficiently at high temperatures, but are more toxic at lower temperatures.[125,225,478]

Temperature also has an effect on toxicity of some diarrhetic shellfish poisoning (DSP)-producing *Prorocentrum* spp.[444] and *Dinophysis* spp.[479,480]; this effect is dependent on the optimum growth temperature range for each species. Where *Prorocentrum* spp. is concerned, okadaic acid production, for instance in *P. hoffmannianum*, appears to be a response to physiological stress. The content of okadaic acid increases with both low temperatures and low light intensities, where growth is limited (22°C and 2000 lx). Also, the cellular content of okadaic acid increased with high temperature and high-light intensity where growth was limited (32°C and 4000 lx). This is also the case with salinity, where cellular okadaic acid content increased with salinity stress, both high and low salinities.[444] Similarly, increasing temperature generally stimulated toxin production in *D. acuminata* populations due to an increase in cell density, but cellular content and production rates of OA and PTX2 in response to temperature differed and were influenced by growth phase.[479]

Similarly, studies on yessotoxin and analogues produced by *Protoceratium reticulatum* suggest that toxicity increases with temperature,[269,481] but recently Röder et al.[272] reported that cell quotas of YTXs cultured at 20°C were lower compared to 15°C. The brevetoxin-producing dinoflagellate *Karenia brevis*,

TABLE 20.2

Toxin Production of Harmful Marine Dinoflagellates

Species	Toxins Produced	Reference
Gonyaulacales		
Alexandrium acatenella	PSP toxins	[375]
A. andersonii	Saxitoxin (STX), Neosaxitoxin (neo-STX), and Gonyautoxin-2 (GTX2)	[376,377]
A. catenella	Ichthyotoxins, C-toxins: C1–C4 toxins, GTX, STX	[378–381]
A. minutum	GTX1–4, C-toxins: C1, C2, and C4, neo-STX and STX	[382,383]
A. monilatum	Ichthyotoxins, GTX1, STX	[384–387]
A. ostenfeldii	Spirolides (SPX)	[116,206,388]
A. peruvianum	SPX	[389]
A. pseudogonyaulax	Goniodomin A	[390]
A. tamarense	GTX1–5, STX, neoSTX	[391–393]
A. tamiyavanichi	GTX, STX, neoSTX, dcGTX2, and dcGTX3	[394–396]
Coolia monotis	Cooliatoxin	[208,397]
Gambierdiscus toxicus	Ciguatoxins (CTX) and maitotoxin (MTX)	[398–402]
Gambierdiscus excentricus	CTX, MTX	[245]
Gonyaulax spinifera	Yessotoxin (YTX)	[275]
Lingulodinium polyedrum	YTX	[258,264,403]
Ostreopsis lenticularis	Ostreotoxin, unnamed toxin	[404,405]
O. mascarenensis	Mascarenotoxins	[406]
O. ovata	Palytoxin, ovatoxins A–F	[227,233,407]
O. siamensis	Ostreocin D	[397,408]
Protoceratium reticulatum	YTX	[258,409–411]
Pyrodinium bahamense	dc-STX, STX, neo-STX, B1 and B2	[252,412–415]
Dinophysiales		
D. acuminata	Okadaic acid (OA), Dinophysistoxins (DTXs), Pectenotoxins (PTXs)	[190,416–418]
D. acuta	OA, DTX1, DTX2, PTX2, PTX11, PTX12	[190,418–423]
D. caudata	OA, DTX1, PTX2	[424–427]
D. fortii	OA, DTX1, PTX2	[190,193,419]
D. infundibula	PTX2	[193]
D. miles	OA, DTX-1	[425]
D. norvegica	DTX1, OA, PTX2, PTX12	[190,193,416,418,419]
D.ovum	OA	[428,429]
D. rotundata	DTX1	[190]
D. sacculus	OA	[430–432]
D. tripos	DTX1, PTX2	[190,433]
Peridiniales		
Azadinium spinosum	Azaspiracids (AZA)	[297]
Pfiesteria piscicida	Pfiesteria toxins (PfTxs)	[434]
Pseudopfiesteria shumwayae	PfTxs	[434]
Protoperidinium crassipes	AZAs?	[435]
Vulcanodinium rugosum	Pinnatoxins	[305]
Prorocentrales		
Prorocentrum belizeanum	DTX1, OA	[436]

(continued)

TABLE 20.2 (continued)

Toxin Production of Harmful Marine Dinoflagellates

Species	Toxins Produced	Reference
P. concavum	OA, fast-acting toxin (FAT), unnamed toxin	[437–440]
P. faustiae	DTX1, OA	[441]
P. hoffmannianum	OA, FAT	[442–444]
P. lima	OA, DTX1, 2, 4,	[190,371,445–448]
P. maculosum	OA, Prorocentrolide B	[439,449]
P. mexicanum/P. rhathymum	OA, FAT	[397,437,450–452]
P. cordatum/P. minimum	Venerupin shellfish toxin (VST)?	[453–458]
Gymdoiniales		
Amphidinium carterae	Ciguatera fish poisoning (CFP) toxins	[355,459]
A. gibbosum	Unknown—Cytotoxic	[460–462]
A. klebsii	Unknown—ichthyotoxicity	[209,400]
A. operculatum	Unknown—ichthyotoxicity	[209]
Gymnodinium catenatum	GTX, neo-STX, and STX	[463]
Kareniabi cuneiformis	Brevetoxin (BTX)	[333]
K. brevis	BTX, Brevisamide, Brevisin, Brevenal, Hemolysins O,O-dipropyl(E)-2-(1-methyl-2-oxopropylidene) phosphorohydrazidothioate-(E)oxime	[325,464–470]
K. brevisulcata	Allelochemicals, compounds that affect sodium channels	[471]
K. concordia	Allelochemicals, hemolysins cytotoxic compounds	[471]
K. mikimotoi	Gymnocin-A, gymnocin-B, hemolysin, polyunsaturated fatty acids (PUFA)	[468–470,472–474]
K. papilionacea	BTX	[333]
K. selliformis	Gymnodimine (GYM), BTX	[475,476]
K. umbella	PUFA	[470]
Karlodinium veneficum	Karlotoxins (hemolytic, ichthyotoxic and cytotoxic properties)	[340]

responsible for mass mortality of marine life in the Gulf of Mexico, has been observed in the field between 7°C and 34°C,[328] while its toxin production demonstrated a trend of slightly higher toxicity at low temperatures that impair growth.[128]

Light is essential for the production of many algal toxins, including PSPs, domoic acid, and DSP toxins.[108,109,480,482,483] Parkhill and Cembella[484] and Etheridge and Roesler[118] reported that the highest cellular toxin levels in *Alexandrium tamarense* and *A. fundyense* coincided with light intensities between 100 and 150 μmol photons/m²/s. Effect of light on PSPs production in all *Alexandrium* species is not always the same between strains, and generally the effect of light variation on toxicity is less remarkable compared to other factors such as temperature, salinity, and nutrients.[115,119]

Alterations in rainfall and climate patterns can cause a significant increase with regard to salinity variability in coastal areas, especially in estuaries.[313,485] Salinity fluctuations may subsequently favor halotolerant and euryhaline organisms, as is the case with many HAB dinoflagellates. For instance, many species of *Prorocentrum* spp. are euryhaline both in culture and in nature.[486] In a clonal culture of *P. lima*, growth rate and toxicity were inversely correlated with salinity.[444] In the dinoflagellate *Karl. veneficum*, low salinity significantly results in reduced growth rates, which enhance cellular toxin quotas.[112,129]

Relationships between toxicity and salinity range from inverse[487,488] to no difference[117] and to positive.[488,489] A clone of *A. minutum* was reported to grow most favorably at salinities ranging from 20 to 37, but toxicity was highest at salinity 15.[487] A range of growth and toxicity responses to changing salinity has also been reported in other dinoflagellates. *Pyrodinium bahamense* was shown to possess a high tolerance to salinity changes, but natural blooms are usually encountered only at salinities of 20 or more.[255] Guerrini et al.[481] reported that *Protoceratium reticulatum* grew over a salinity range of 22–42, while highest yessotoxin concentrations were obtained at salinity 32. Paz et al.[269] also reported that yessotoxin production decreased with increasing salinity in this species.[129]

Where *Gambierdiscus* spp. is concerned, both growth and toxicity respond to salinity changes. In general, members of this genus grow optimally at or near full-strength seawater and can tolerate mild fluctuations,[123] while toxicity is partially determined by salinity.[490,491] On the other hand, effects of salinity on the ecologically similar genus *Ostreopsis* are quite variable, ranging from negative to positive correlations with growth and toxicity.[492] A Mediterranean *O. ovata* isolate displayed optimal growth rates at high salinities (36–40), but toxicity was highest at salinity 32.[129,493]

20.6 Geographical Distribution of Dinoflagellates

Dinoflagellate distribution has been termed as "modified latitudinal cosmopolitanism,"[494,495] meaning that the same morphospecies occur within similar climatic zones in both northern and southern hemispheres. It is little appreciated that the entire microplankton community of northern and southern temperate ocean waters are virtually identical,[495,496] despite their separation by the circumtropical community, at least since the Miocene (20 Ma). Clear differences also exist between neritic (coastal) versus oceanic plankton. Many neritic dinoflagellate and diatom species include a benthic resting stage (resting cysts or resting spores, respectively) in their life cycle and are therefore confined to the shallower waters of the continental shelf. Neriticism in some species may also be related to a requirement for land-derived nutrients or other products, such as humic acids.[30]

20.6.1 Arctic

The Eurasian Arctic seas are characterized by two peaks of phytoplankton abundance in spring and autumn, with the spring peak being much more pronounced in terms of biomass and cell numbers. Dinoflagellate blooms are rare and have so far been recorded only in Norwegian coastal waters.[457,497–500] Information about dinoflagellate blooms from the Russian Arctic, seasonally covered by fast or drifting ice, is lacking, Russian literature on the phytoplankton of the Arctic seas deals primarily with diatom blooms, with few reports on ice algae, the development of which occurs long before the spring bloom. In this case, ice coloration is usually caused by colony-forming pinnate diatoms,[501–503] which, with increasing solar radiation, are released into the water column initiating or contributing to the water column bloom. The role of dinoflagellates in the Arctic seas had until recently been underestimated. Data on the abundance and biomass of dinoflagellates in the Arctic seas in certain seasons suggest that dinoflagellates are important in the diet of herbivorous animals in the Arctic.[504,505]

In certain regions of the European Arctic, toxic dinoflagellates reach high abundance.[457,499] By the early 1990s, about 20 harmful planktonic algal species had been reported from the Norwegian Sea. Until 1968, harmful bloom events in the coastal Norwegian waters were recorded to the south of 63°N. By the early 1990s, they distributed up to 71°N.[500] It is expectable that with increasing climate warming in the Northern Hemisphere and developing shipping, toxic algal species and especially dinoflagellates, could unintentionally be transported with ships' ballast waters and sediment to the Russian Arctic from southern areas. Intensive development of some species, which at present do not reach high numbers, cannot also be excluded.

Harmful algal blooms can disperse into the Arctic from both the Atlantic and Pacific Oceans. Human deaths caused by toxic dinoflagellates have been reported in eastern Kamchatka in the Russian Republic.[506] Since the mid-1980s, red tides in the far-eastern seas of Russia have become more intensive and regular, some of them being caused by nonindigenous species,[507] and with an increase in number of toxic and harmful algal species. In the western Bering Sea, toxic red tides have been reported from Koryakskoye Nagorye to the Bay of Anadyr.[506,508]

Despite the fact that some toxic dinoflagellate species occurring in the Arctic seem to be indigenous to the Arctic, none of them is endemic to this region. Only a few dinoflagellate species are distributed in both the Arctic Ocean and the temperate regions of the Atlantic and the Pacific, and can be considered endemic in the Arctic-boreal biogeographic zone. Out of about 250 dinoflagellate species recorded from the Arctic, only 5 species are Arctic-boreal: *Alexandrium ostenfeldii, Amylax triacantha, Ceratium arcticum, Dinophysis norvegica,* and *Peridiniella catenata.*[509,510] Some species were conventionally called Arctic-boreal, as they have been also recorded from Hudson and Baffin Bays, the Davis Strait, the area near the NE coast of the United States, the North Atlantic down to Gibraltar and the Mediterranean, including the Black Sea.[511]

20.6.2 Southern Ocean

The Southern Ocean is generally considered to extend from the Antarctic continent to the Subtropical Front and makes up nearly 20% of the world ocean.[512,513] There are two distinct hydrographical zones: (1) the Antarctic zone lying between Antarctica and the Polar Front and (2) the Subantarctic zone lying between the Polar Front and the Subtropical Front. The most common harmful heterotrophic species found in surface waters of these areas were representatives of *Gyrodinium, Gymnodinium,* and *Protoperidinium,* confirmed more or less by the research of Umani et al.,[514,515] who reported *Protoperidinium* spp., *Gyrodinium,* and *Amphidinium* sp. as the major heterotrophic species present in surface waters of the Ross Sea shelf.[516]

Karenia cf. *mikimotoi, K.* cf. *papilionaceae,* and *Karlodinium* cf. *antarcticum* were recorded across the open Antarctic and Subantarctic waters (<200 cells/L), south of New Zealand. Previously, several species of *Karlodinium* spp. were reported in the south of Tasmania, Australia.[517] Some of the *Karenia* species had been associated with marine life mortalities in coastal waters of New Zealand.[333,471,518,519] So far none of these species has been implicated in any marine life kills either in the New Zealand sector or in any other areas of the Southern Ocean, but a build-up of these species in the region could possibly pose a threat to marine life. As Southern Ocean is far from landmass, build-up of any of these species might not be easy to observe.

20.6.3 Atlantic

The phytoplankton spring bloom is one of the most important biological events in the North Atlantic Ocean.[520,521] The bloom starts at a latitude of ~35°N, just north of the North Atlantic Subtropical Gyre (NASG), in December–January. The bloom subsequently develops across the North Atlantic throughout spring and summer, propagating northwards to Arctic waters in June.[520,522] Concurrently, the stratified nutrient-depleted waters of the NASG also extend northwards, reaching the latitudes of the Azores in late spring to early summer.[523] Among the numerous phytoplankton species recorded in this bloom, the most frequently occurring potentially toxic genera are *Dinophysis, Alexandrium, Ostreopsis, Gambierdiscus, Karenia, Gymnodinium,* and *Pfiesteria.*

Dinophysis spp. is highly distributed in coastal and oceanic waters of the Atlantic. For instance, *D. acuminata, D. acuta,* and *D. norvegica* were isolated from Rhode Island, North America,[524] whereas *D. acuminata, D. norvegica,* and *Dinophysis* sp. were also recorded in the other side of the ocean, that is, the Baltic Sea, the North Sea, the Greenland Sea, and the Norwegian fjord Masfjorden.[525] In a study of the free-living dinoflagellates in the southern Gulf of Mexico, the toxic species recognized were *Amphidinium carterae, D. acuta, D. caudata, D. fortii, D. mitra, D. rotundata, D. tripos, Prorocentrum mexicanum,* and *P. minimum.*[526]

Ostreopsis spp. has been reported from the Atlantic islands northwest of mainland Africa, the Canary and Madeira Islands.[527] A bloom of *O. ovata* was reported along a 400 km stretch of the Atlantic coast of Brazil and since then there have been reports of *O. ovata* blooms from the northeast to the southern coast. An *Ostreopsis* isolate from the Florida Keys was described as a new species, *O. heptagona,*[228] whereas *O. lenticularis* and *O. ovata* were isolated from the Virgin Islands.[404] *O. lenticularis* was also found along the northwestern coast of Cuba[528] and has been known for more than a quarter of a century in southwest Puerto Rico,[405,529] where toxic strains have been identified.[530]

Other studies report the presence of *Gymnodinium catenatum* in the northeastern Atlantic,[531,532] and *Alexandrium ostenfeldii* in northwest Atlantic.[196,388,533] *Alexandrium tamarense* complex cells were reported as the cause of PSP in Argentina and Uruguay[534,535] in Brazil[536] and in the Atlantic coast of North America.[200] *Pfiesteria* spp., well known as a fish killer in the Atlantic coast of America, was also isolated from sediment samples taken in the Oslofjord region of Norway.[287]

The toxic alga *Karenia brevis* has been reported to occur along Florida's west coast on a near-annual basis, causing massive fish kills within Sarasota Bay and the adjacent Gulf of Mexico.[537] *Karenia mikimotoi* has been reported in southern Norwegian waters back in 1966[538]; however, anecdotal observations suggest that it could have bloomed off the southwest of Ireland in 1865.[539]

The ciguatera-causing dinoflagellate *Gambierdiscus toxicus* was also isolated from the French West Indies.[540] *Gambierdiscus excentricus* has been reported from the Canary Islands coasts together with *Gambierdiscus* cf. *polynesiensis*.[245]

Specifically where the Mediterranean sea is concerned, apart from the commonly occurring genera *Dinophysis* and *Prorocentrum*, potentially toxic dinoflagellate reports include, among others, *Ostreopsis ovata* and *Coolia monotis*[541] as well as *Gymnodinium catenatum*[137–139] and *Alexandrium minutum*.[542,543] *A. catenella* was found in the Balearic Islands and Catalonia already in 1983,[544] and then appears to have spread in the Western Mediterranean region along the French, Spanish, Italian, Greek, and Maghrebian coasts.[212,545–548] *Ostreopsis* spp. has been increasingly recorded in the Mediterranean Sea during the past decade, with *O. ovata* being a major toxic bloom former in the Mediterranean Sea, causing respiratory illnesses and resulting in the uptake of palytoxin-like compounds by shellfish throughout the Mediterranean coastline of Europe.[215,222,234]

20.6.4 Pacific

The most frequently occurring potential toxic dinoflagellate genera/species in the Pacific Ocean are those commonly described as cosmopolitan species. One of these, *Gymnodinium catenatum*, affected at least 200 km of the mainland coast of Mexico at the entrance of the Gulf of California in April, 1979.[549] Further to the west of Mexico, at the southern end of the Gulf of California in the Pacific Ocean, where the volcanic Isla Isabel is located, *O. siamensis* was collected by net tows, suggesting that the species was tychoplanktonic at that specific site.[550] Additionally, *Gymnodinium catenatum* cells were isolated from three locations in the Gulf of California.[551] In Japan, a paralytic shellfish poisoning (PSP) event caused by *G. catenatum* was first reported from Senzaki Bay, western part of the Sea of Japan in 1986.[552]

Where *Ostreopsis* spp. is concerned, *O. lenticularis* and *O. ovata* were first discovered in French Polynesian and New Caledonian waters.[227] *O. heptagona* was found during a sampling study in 2005 in the Veracruz reef zone of the Gulf of Mexico, although in low concentrations.[125] An intensive sampling survey of an extensive area of coastal Hawaii in 2001 resulted in the detection of *O. ovata* and an unknown species, *Ostreopsis* sp. 1, at most sites, often in high abundance.[553] This supports previous findings of *Ostreopsis* in Hawaiian waters, as *O. siamensis* was first recorded in Hawaii by Taylor.[216] In Australian waters, high concentrations of *Ostreopsis* spp. were reported in most sites, with species present including *O. ovata*, *O. siamensis*, *O. lenticularis*, and *O. heptagona*.[125] *O. lenticularis* is also common in Tahitian waters (e.g., the Papeete Reef and Gambier Islands) in association with *Gambierdiscus toxicus*.[554] The same authors suggested that at some sites *O. lenticularis* may fill the niche left after a *Gambierdiscus* bloom. Toxic strains of both *O. siamensis* and *O. ovata* were recorded in Okinawan waters, Japan, in the late 1970s.[227,397,400]

In the southwestern Pacific region, the dinoflagellate *Pyrodinium bahamense* var. *compressa* was pointed out as the major causative organism of paralytic shellfish poisoning and was reported as continuously spreading around the region.[555] *P. bahamense* var. *bahamense* was observed off San José del Cabo, which is an extension of the range of this variety.[250] Where presence of *Karenia* spp. is concerned, *K. mikimotoi* shows a longtime occurrence in Japanese waters, as it was initially described in 1935 from western Japan (as *Gymnodinium mikimotoi* (Miyake and Kominami ex Oda, 1935).[324]

Studies on dinoflagellates species' composition in epiphytic assemblages on macrophytes in the Peter the Great Bay of the Sea of Japan revealed the presence of the potentially toxic species *Amphidinium carterae*, *A. operculatum*, *Prorocentrum lima*, *Ostreopsis siamensis*, and *O. ovata*.[556] Finally, the presence of the potentially toxic species *Dinophysis dens*, *D. infundibulus*, *D. mitra*, and *D. rapa* was reported from the coasts of Korea.[557]

20.6.5 Indian

A wide range of potentially toxic dinoflagellates has also been recorded in different parts of the Indian ocean. With regard to the genus *Ostreopsis*, the species *O. marinus*, *O. belizeanus*, and *O. caribbeanus* were isolated from islands in the Mascareignes Archipelago, east of Madagascar between 1995 and 1997 being all newly described species at the time.[231] The coral reefs of Reunion Island are also considered as an ideal habitat for typical coral reef dinoflagellate consortia, including *O. mascarenensis*,[229] *O. siamensis*, *O. ovata*, and *O. lenticularis*.[558] In 1996, a bloom of *O. mascarenensis* was reported in the coral reef habitat of Mauritius (Rodrigues Island) and extracts contained new analogues of palytoxin-like compounds.[406,559] Toxic strains of *Ostreopsis* species have been proposed as the causative organisms of illnesses in this region.[560,561] Toward the northwest of Madagascar, in the islands of the Union of Comoros, proliferation of epiphytic dinoflagellates, including *Gambierdiscus* spp. and all the described *Ostreopsis* species except *O. belizeanus*, has been attributed to severe coral bleaching.[562] *Ostreopsis* species, including *O. ovata* and *O. heptagona*, also occur further to the north off the coast of Tanzania, particularly from the waters around Zanzibar.[561,563,564]

The potentially harmful species *Prorocentrum micans* and *P. sigmoides*, suspected to cause red coloration of oysters or oxygen depletion due to massive blooms,[565,566] were detected in Myanmar coasts, mainly in May. On the other hand, latent events of shellfish poisonings have also been reported to be of concern in the same area, as *Alexandrium tamiyavanichii*, a producer of potent toxin causing PSP, has been detected. In 2007, high cell densities of *A. tamiyavanichii* from Myanmar waters (the offshore area of Kadan Island) were reported in February. An outbreak of PSP following consumption of clams harvested from an estuary near the City of Mangalore, southwest India, which caused the death of an infant was also reported, with toxin profiles of the clams corresponding to those of an *A. tamiyavanichii* strain isolated from Thailand.[567] The potentially toxic species *Dinophysis caudata*, *D. miles*, and *Dinophysis* cf. *infundibulus* were also detected, with the presence of *D. caudata* being important in both May and December.[568] Finally, on the west coast of India, off Mangalore, sporadic occurrences of DSP have been attributed to *Dinophysis* sp. and *Prorocentrum* sp. blooms,[569] whereas blooms of *Alexandrium* spp. have been associated with PSP in the west coast of India.[567,570]

20.7 Conclusion

Apart from playing an important general role in the food chain as primary producers, potentially toxic dinoflagellates are of extreme significance due to their ability for toxin production, particularly when they occur in large numbers. Many of these toxins can be very potent, and if not fatal, can still cause a wide range of symptoms to humans, affecting the nervous and gastrointestinal systems. As years progress, it is becoming more evident that blooms of potentially toxic dinoflagellates are of increasing importance, partly due to human inputs of phosphates and warmer global temperatures. It is thus expectable as well as recommended that research should continue to investigate the effects of potentially toxic dinoflagellates upon marine life and human health, as they constitute an important risk with serious impact on the shellfish and fisheries industry.

REFERENCES

1. Sournia, A. 1986. Atlas du phytoplancton marin. In *Introduction, Cyanophycées, Dictyochophycées, Dinophycées et Raphidophycées*, Vol. I. Paris, France: Editions du Centre National de la Recherche Scientifique.
2. Sournia, A., Chretiennot-Dinet, M. J., and Ricard, M. 1991. Marine phytoplankton: How many species in the world ocean? *J Plankton Res*, 13, 1093–1099.
3. Fukuyo, Y. and Taylor, F. J. R. 1989. Morphological characteristics dinoflagellates. In *Biology, Epidemiology and Management of Pyrodinium Red Tides*, eds. G. M. Hallegraef and J. L. Maclean, pp. 201–205. Manilla, Philippines: ICLARM Conference Proceedings.
4. Hallegraeff, G. M. 1988. *Plankton: A Microscopic World*. Bathurst, New South Wales, Australia: CSIRO.
5. Graham, L. E. and Wilcox, L. W. 2000. *Algae*. Upper Saddle River, NJ: Prentice Hall.

6. Carty, S. 2003. Dinoflagellates. In *Freshwater Algae of North America—Ecology and Classification*, eds. J. D. Wehr and R. G. Sheath, pp. 685–714. New York: Academic Press.

7. Lee, J. S., Igarashi, T., Fraga, S. et al. 1989. Determination of diarrhetic toxins in various dinoflagellate species. *J Appl Phycol*, 1, 147–152.

8. Smetacek, V., Bathmann, U., Nothig, E. M. et al. 1991. Coastal eutrophication: Causes and consequences. In *Ocean Margin Process in Global Change*, eds. R. F. C. Mantoura, J. M. Martin, and R. Wollast, pp. 251–279. Chichester, U.K.: John Wiley & Sons.

9. Taylor, R. W. 1987. A checklist of the ants of Australia, New Caledonia and New Zealand (Hymenoptera: Formicidae). First supplement, July 10, 1987. *CSIRO Div Entomol Rep*, 41, 1–5.

10. Gaines, G. and Elbrächter, M. 1987. Heterotrophic nutrition. In *The Biology of Dinoflagellates*, ed. F. J. R. Taylor, pp. 224–268. Oxford, U.K.: Blackwell Scientific Publications.

11. Burkholder, J. M., Gilbert, P. M., and Skelton, H. M. 2008. Mixotrophy, a major mode of nutrition for harmful algal species in eutrophic waters. *Harmful Algae*, 8, 77–93.

12. Jeong, H. J., Yoo, Y. D., Kim, J. S. et al. 2010. Growth, feeding and ecological roles of the mixotrophic and heterotrophic dinofl agellates in marine plankton food webs. *Ocean Sci J*, 45, 65–91.

13. Ignatiades, L. 2012. Mixotrophic and heterotrophic dinoflagellates in eutrophic coastal waters of the Aegean Sea (eastern Mediterranean Sea). *Bot Mar*, 55, 39–48.

14. Taylor, F. J. R. and Pollingher, U. 1987. Ecology of dinoflagellates. In *The Biology of Dinoflagellates*, ed. F. J. R. Taylor, pp. 398–529. London, U.K.: Blackwell Scientific Publications.

15. Burkholder, J. M., Azanza, R. V., and Sako, Y. 2006. The ecology of harmful dinoflagellates. In *Ecology of Harmful Algae*, eds. E. Graneli and J. Turner, pp. 53–66. New York: Springer-Verlag.

16. Steidinger, K. A. 1993. Some taxonomic and biologic aspects of toxic dinoflagellates. In *Algal Toxins in Seafood and Drinking Water*, ed. I. R. Falconer, pp. 1–28. London, U.K.: Academic Press.

17. Yasumoto, T. and Murata, M. 1993. Marine toxins. *Chem Rev*, 93, 1897–1909.

18. Landsberg, J. H. 2002. The effects of harmful algal blooms on aquatic organisms. *Rev Fish Sci*, 10, 113–390.

19. Fensome, R. A., Taylor, F. J. R., Norris, G. et al. 1993. *A Classification of Living and Fossil Dinoflagellates*. Micropaleontology, Special Publication 7. Hanover, PA: Sheridan Press.

20. Saldarriaga, J. F., Taylor, F. J. R., Cavalier-Smith, T. et al. 2004. Molecular data and the evolutionary history of dinoflagellates. *Eur J Protistol*, 40, 85–111.

21. Moreira, D. and López-García, P. 2002. The molecular ecology of microbial eukaryotes unveils a hidden world. *Trends Microbiol*, 10, 31–38.

22. Worden, A. Z. 2006. Picoeukaryote diversity in coastal waters of the Pacific Ocean. *Aquat Microb Ecol*, 43, 165–175.

23. Coffroth, M. A. and Santos, S. R. 2005. Genetic diversity of symbiotic dinoflagellates in the genus *Symbiodinium*. *Protist*, 156, 19–34.

24. Cavalier-Smith, T. 1991. Cell diversification in heterotrophic flagellates. In *The Biology of Free-Living Heterotrophic Flagellates*, eds. D. J. Patterson and J. Larsen, pp. 113–131. Oxford, U.K.: Clarendon Press.

25. Hackett, J. D., Anderson, D. M., Erdner D. L. et al. 2004. Dinoflagellates: A remarkable evolutionary experiment. *Am J Bot*, 91, 1523–1534.

26. Cavalier-Smith, T. and Chao, E. E. 2004. Protalveolate phylogeny and systematics and the origins of Sporozoa and dinoflagellates. *Eur J Protistol*, 40, 185–212.

27. Gould, S. B., Tham, W. H., Cowman, A. F. et al. 2008. Alveolins, a new family of cortical proteins that define the protist infrakingdom Alveolata. *Mol Biol Evol*, 25, 1219–1230.

28. Not, F., Siano, R., Kooistra, W. H. C. F. et al. 2012. Diversity and ecology of eukaryotic marine phytoplankton. *Adv Bot Res*, 64, 1–53.

29. Leander, B. S. and Keeling, P. J. 2003. Morphostasis in alveolate evolution. *Trends Ecol Evol*, 18, 395–402.

30. Taylor, F. J. R., Hoppenrath, M., and Saldarriaga, J. F. 2008. Dinoflagellate diversity and distribution. *Biodivers Conserv*, 17, 407–418.

31. Taylor, F. J. R. 1987. *The Biology of Dinoflagellates*. Oxford, U.K.: Blackwell Scientific Publications.

32. Adl, S. M., Simpson, A. G. B., Farmer, M. A. et al. 2005. The new higher level classification of eukaryotes with emphasis on the taxonomy of protists. *J Eukaryot Microbiol*, 52, 399–451.

33. Kofoid, C. A. 1909. On *Peridinium steini* Jörgensen, with a note on the nomenclature of the skeleton of the Peridinidae. *Arch Protistenk*, 16, 25–47.

34. Fensome, R. A., Saldarriaga, J. F., and Taylor, F. J. R. 1999. Dinoflagellate phylogeny revisited: Reconciling morphological and molecular based phylogenies. *Grana*, 38, 66–80.

35. Baker, M. 1753. *Employment for the Microscope*. London, U.K.: Dodsley.

36. Müller, O. F. 1773. Vermium Terrestrium et Fluviatilium, sue animalium Infusorium, Helminthicorum et Testaceorum, non Marioru. *Succincta Historica*, 1–135.

37. Ehrenberg, C. G. 1838. Die Infusionsthierchen als vollkommene Organismen. Ein Blick in das tiefere organische Leben der Natur. Nebst einem Atlas von vierundsechszig colorirten Kupfertafeln, gezeichnet vom Verfasser. Leopold Voss, Leipzig, Germany.

38. Schiller, J. 1931–1937. Dinoflagellatae (Peridineae) in monographischer Behandlung. *Rabenhorst's Kryptogamenflora*, Band 10, Abt. 3, Teil 1, 1–617. Leipzig, Germany: Akademie Verlag.

39. Moestrup, Ø. and Daugbjerg, N. 2007. On dinoflagellate phylogeny and classification. In *Unravelling the Algae: The Past, Present, and Future of Algal Systematic*, eds. J. Brodie and J. M. Lewis, pp. 215–230. New York: CRC Press.

40. Daugbjerg, N., Hansen, G., Larsen, J. et al. 2000. Phylogeny of some of the major genera of dinoflagellates based on ultrastructure and partial LSU rDNA sequence data, including the erection of three new genera of unarmoured dinoflagellates. *Phycologia*, 39, 302–317.

41. Jørgensen, F. M., Murray, S., and Daugbjerg, N. 2004. Amphidinium revisited. I. Redefinition of *Amphidinium* (Dinophyceae) based on cladistic and molecular phylogenetic analyses. *J Phycol*, 40, 351–365.

42. Lindberg, K., Moestrup, Ø., and Daugbjerg, N. 2005. Studies on woloszynskioid dinoflagellates I: *Woloszynskia coronata* re-examined using light and electron microscopy and partial LSU rDNA sequences, with description of *Tovellia* gen. nov and *Jadwigia* gen. nov. (Tovelliaceae fam. nov.). *Phycologia*, 44, 416–440.

43. Taylor, F. J. R. 1980. On dinoflagellate evolution. *Biosystems*, 13, 65–108.

44. Gomez, F., Moreira, D., and Lopez-Garcia, P. 2010. Molecular phylogeny of noctilucoid dinoflagellates (Noctilucales, Dinophyceae). *Protist*, 161, 466–478.

45. Lessard, E. J. and Swift, E. 1985. Species-specific grazing rates of heterotrophic dinoflagellates in oceanic waters, measured with a dual-label radioisotope technique. *Mar Biol*, 87, 289–296.

46. Burkholder, J. A. M., Noga, E. J., Hobbs, C. W. et al. 1992. New "phantom" dinoflagellate is the causative agent of major estuarine fish kills. *Nature*, 358, 407–410.

47. Steidinger, K. A., Burkholder, J. M., Glasgow, H. B. J. et al. 1996. *Pfiesteria piscicida* gen. et sp. nov. (Pfiesteriaceae fam. nov.), a new toxic dinoflagellate with a complex life cycle and behavior. *J Phycol*, 32, 157–164.

48. Sherr, E. B. and Sherr, B. F. 2002. Significance of predation by protists in aquatic microbial food webs. *Ant van Leeuwenh*, 81, 293–308.

49. Mason, P. L., Litaker, R. W., Jeong, H. J. et al. 2007. Description of a new genus of *Pfiesteria*-like dinoflagellate, *Luciella* gen. nov. (Dinophyceae), including two new species: *Luciella masanensis* sp. nov. and *Luciella atlantis* sp. nov. *J Phycol*, 43, 799–810.

50. Smayda, T. J. 1997. Harmful algal blooms: Their ecophysiology and general relevance to phytoplankton blooms in the sea. *Limnol Oceanogr*, 42, 1137–1153.

51. ECOHAB. 1995. *The Ecology and Oceanography of Harmful Algal Blooms: A National Research Agenda*. Woods Hole, MA: Woods Hole Oceanographic Institute, 66pp.

52. Azanza, R. V., Fukuyo, Y., Yap L. G. et al. 2005. *Prorocentrum minimum* bloom and its possible link to a massive fish kill in Bolinao, Pangasinan, Northern Philippines. *Harmful Algae*, 4, 519–524.

53. Larsen, J. 1988. An ultrastructural study of *Amphidinium poecilochroum* (Dinophyceae), a phagotrophic dinoflagellate feeding on small species of cryptophytes. *Phycologia*, 27, 366–377.

54. Jacobson, D. M. and Anderson, D. M. 1992. Ultrastructure of the feeding apparatus and myonemal system of the heterotrophic dinoflagellate *Protoperidinium spinulosum*. *J Phycol*, 28, 69–82.

55. Granéli, E., Anderson, D. M., Carlsson, P. et al. 1997. Light and dark carbon uptake by *Dinophysis* species in comparison to other photosynthetic and heterotrophic dinoflagellates. *Aquat Microb Ecol*, 13, 177–186.

56. Jeong, H. J., Lee, C. W., Yih, W. H. et al. 1997. *Fragilidium* cf. *mexicanum*, a thecate mixotrophic dinoflagellate which is prey for and a predator on co-occuring thecate heterotrophic dinoflagellate *Protoperidinium* cf. *divergens*. *Mar Ecol Prog Ser*, 151, 299–305.

57. Adolf, J. E., Stoecker, D. K., and Harding, L. W. 2006. The balance of autotrophy and heterotrophy during mixotrophic growth of *Karlodinium micrum* (Dinophyceae). *J Plankton Res*, 28, 737–751.

58. Kang, N. S., Jeong, H. J., Moestrup, Ø. et al. 2010. Description of a new planktonic mixotrophic dino-flagellate *Paragymnodinium shiwhaense* n. gen., n. sp. from the coastal waters off western Korea: Morphology, pigments, and ribosomal DNA gene sequence. *J Eukaryot Microbiol*, 57, 121–144.

59. Yoo, Y. D., Jeong, H. J., Kang, N. S. et al. 2010. Feeding by the newly described mixotrophic dinoflagel-late *Paragymnodinium shiwhaense*: Feeding mechanism, prey species, and effect of prey concentration. *J Eukaryot Microbiol*, 57, 145–158.

60. Siokou-Frangou, I., Christaki, U., Mazzocchi, M. G. et al. 2010. Plankton in the open Mediterranean Sea: A review. *Biogeosciences*, 7, 1543–1586.

61. Labry, C., Denn, E. E. L., Chapelle, A. et al. 2008. Competition for phosphorus between two dinoflagel-lates: A toxic *Alexandrium minutum* and a non-toxic *Heterocapsa triquetra*. *J Exp Mar Biol Ecol*, 358, 124–135.

63. Doblin, M. A., Blackburn, S. I., and Hallegraeff, G. M. 2000. Intraspecific variation in the selenium requirement of different geographic strains of the toxic dinoflagellate *Gymnodinium catenatum*. *J Plankton Res*, 22, 421–432.

64. Chambouvet, A., Morin, P., Marie, D. et al. 2008. Control of toxic marine dinoflagellate blooms by serial parasitic killers. *Science*, 322, 1254–1257.

65. Nagasaki, K., Tomaru, P. Y., Shirai, Y. et al. 2006. Dinoflagellate infecting viruses. *J Mar Biol Assoc UK*, 86, 469–474.

66. Smayda, T. J. and Reynolds, C. S. 2001. Community assembly in marine phytoplankton: Application of recent models to harmful dinoflagellate blooms. *J Plankton Res*, 23, 447–461.

67. Margalef, R., Estrada, M., and Blasco, D. 1979. Functional morphology of organisms involved in red tides, as adapted to decaying turbulence. In *Toxic Dinoflagellate Blooms*, eds. D. Taylor and H. Seliger, pp. 89–94. New York: Elsevier.

68. Smayda, T. J. and Reynolds, C. S. 2003. Strategies of marine dinoflagellate survival and some rules of assembly. *J Sea Res*, 49, 95–106.

69. Anderson, D. M. and Rengefors, K. 2006. Community assembly and seasonal succession of marine dino-flagellates in a temperate estuary: The importance of life cycle events. *Limnol Oceanogr*, 51, 860–873.

70. Smalley, G. W. and Coats, D. W. 2002. Ecology of red-tide dinoflagellate *Ceratium furca*: Distribution, mixotrophy, and grazing impact on ciliate populations of Chesapeake Bay. *J Eukaryot Microbiol*, 49, 63–73.

71. Hansen, P. J. and Calado, A. J. 1999. Phagotrophic mechanisms and prey selection in free-living dinofla-gellates. *J Eukaryot Microbiol*, 46, 382–389.

72. Jeong, H. J., Seong, K. A., Yoo, Y. D. et al. 2008. Feeding and grazing impact by small marine heterotro-phic dinoflagellates on hetertrophic bacteria. *J Eukaryot Microbiol*, 55, 271–288.

73. Jacobson, D. M. 1999. A brief history of dinoflagellate feeding research. *J Eukaryot Microbiol*, 46, 376–381.

74. Li, A., Stoecker, D. K., Coats, D. W. et al. 1996. Ingestion of fluorescently labeled and phycoerythrin-containing prey by mixotrophic dinoflagellates. *Aquat Microb Ecol*, 10, 139–147.

75. Hansen, P. J. 1998. Phagotrophic mechanisms and prey selection in mixotrophic phytoflagellates. In *Physiological Ecology of Harmful Algal Blooms*, eds. D. M. Anderson, A. D. Cembella, and G. M. Hallegraff, pp. 525–537. Berlin, Germany: Springer-Verlag.

76. Stoecker, D. K., Li, A., Coats, D. W. et al. 1997. Mixotrophy in the dinoflagellate, *Prorocentrum mini-mum*. *Mar Ecol Prog Ser*, 152, 1–12.

77. Stoecker, D. K. 1999. Mixotrophy among dinoflagellates. *J Eukaryot Microbiol*, 46, 397–401.

78. Bockstahler, K. R. and Coats, D. W. 1993. Grazing of the mixotrophic dinoflagellate *Gynznodiniuin sanguineurn* on ciliate populations of Chesapeake Bay. *Mar Biol*, 116, 477–487.

79. Bockstahler, K. R. and Coats, D. W. 1993. Spatial and temporal aspects of mixotrophy in Chesapeake Bay dinoflagellates. *J Eukaryot Microbiol*, 40, 49–60.

80. Jacobson, D. M. and Anderson, D. M. 1996. Widespread phagocytosis of ciliates and other protists by marine mixotrophic and heterotrophic thecate dinoflagellates. *J Phycol*, 32, 279–285.

81. Skovgaard, A. 1996. Engulfment of *Ceratium* spp. (Dinophyceae) by the thecate photosynthetic dinofla-gellate *Fragilidium subglobosum*. *Phycologia*, 35, 490–499.

82. Smalley, G. W., Coats, D. W., and Adam, E. J. 1999. A new method for using fluorescent microspheres to determine grazing rates on ciliates by the mixotrophic dinoflagellate *Ceratium furca*. *Aquat Microb Ecol*, 17, 167–179.

83. Fenchel, T. 2001. How dinoflagellates swim. *Protist*, 152, 329–338.

84. Levandowsky, M. and Kaneta, P. J. 1987. Behaviour in dinoflagellates. In *The Biology of Dinoflagellates*, ed. F. J. R. Taylor, pp. 360–397. Oxford, U.K.: Blackwell Scientific Publications.

86. Lindemann, E. 1928. Über die Schwimmbewegung einer experimentell eingeisselig gemachten dinoflagellata. *Arch Protistenkd*, 64, 507–510.

87. Hand, G. H. and Schmidt, J. A. 1975. Phototactic orientation by the marine dinoflagellate *Gyrodinium dorsum* Kofoid. II. Flagellar activity and overall response mechanism. *J Protozool*, 22, 494–498.

88. Jahn, T. L., Harman, U. M., and Landman, M. 1963. Mechanism of locomotion in flagellates I. *Ceratium*. *J Protozool*, 10, 358–363.

89. Dodge, J. D. and Greuet, C. 1987. Dinoflagellate ultrastructure and complex organelles. In *The Biology of Dinoflagellates*, ed. F. J. R.Taylor, pp. 92–142. Oxford, U.K.: Blackwell Scientific Publications.

90. Gaines, G. and Taylor, F. J. R. 1985. Form and function in the dinoflagellate transverse flagellum. *J Protozool*, 32, 290–296.

91. Goldstein, S. F. 1992. Flagellar beat patterns in algae. In *Algal Cell Motility*, ed. M. Melkonian, pp. 99–153. New York: Chapman & Hall.

92. Edler, L. and Olsson, P. 1985. Observations on diel migration of *Ceratium furca* and *Prorocentrum micans* in a stratified bay on the Swedish west coast. In *Toxic Dinoflagellates*, eds. D. M. Anderson, A. W. White, and D. G. Baden, pp. 195–200. New York: Elsevier.

93. Holligan, P. M. 1987. The physical environment of exceptional phytoplankton blooms in the Northeast Atlantic. *Rapp P-v Réun Cons Int Explor Mer*, 187, 9–18.

94. Aksnes, D. L. and Egge, J. K. 1991. A theoretical model for nutrient uptake in phytoplankton. *Mar Ecol Prog Ser*, 70, 65–72.

95. Kamykowski, D. M., Reed, R. E., and Kirkpatic, G. J. 1992. Comparison of sinking velocity, swimming, rotation and path characteristics among six marine dinoflagellate species. *Mar Biol*, 113, 319–328.

96. Fraga, S., Gallagher, S. M., and Anderson, D. M. 1989. Chain-forming dinoflagellates: An adaptation to red tides. In *Red Tides: Biology, Environmental Science and Toxicology*, eds. T. Okaichi, D. M. Anderson, and T. Nemoto, pp. 281–284. New York: Elsevier.

97. Blackburn, S. I., Hallegraeff, G. M., and Bolch, C. J. 1989. Vegetative reproduction and sexual life cycle of the toxic dinoflagellate *Gymnodinium catenatum* from Tasmania, Australia. *J Phycol*, 25, 577–590.

98. Fraga, S. and Bakun, A. 1993. Global climate change and harmful algal blooms: The example of *Gymnodinium catenatum* on the Galician coast. In *Toxic Phytoplankton Blooms in the Sea*, eds. T. J. Smayda and Y. Shimizu, pp. 59–65. Amsterdam, the Netherlands: Elsevier.

99. Cullen, J. J. and MacIntyre, J. G. 1998. Behavior, physiology and the niche of depth-regulating phytoplankton. In *Physiological Ecology of Harmful Algal Blooms*, eds. D. M. Anderson, A. D. Cembella, and G. M. Hallegraeff, pp. 559–580. Heidelberg, Germany: Springer-Verlag.

100. Eppley, R. W., Holm-Hansen, O., and Strickland, J. D. H. 1968. Some observations on the vertical migration of dinoflagellates. *J Phycol*, 4, 333–340.

101. Kamykowski, D., Yamazaki, H., Yamazaki, A. K. et al. 1998. A comparison of how different orientation behaviors influence dinoflagellate trajectories and photoresponses in turbulent water columns. In *Physiological Ecology of Harmful Algal Blooms*, eds. D. M. Anderson, A. D. Cembella, and G. M. Hallegraeff, pp. 581–599. New York: Springer.

102. Burkholder, J. M., Glasgow, H. B., and Deamer-Melia, N. J. 2001. Overview and present status of the toxic *Pfiesteria* complex. *Phycologia*, 40, 186–214.

103. Gómez, F. 2012. A quantitative review of the lifestyle, habitat and trophic diversity of dinoflagellates (Dinoflagellata, Alveolata). *Syst Biodivers*, 10, 267–275.

104. Dason, J. S., Huertas, I. E., and Colman, B. 2004. Source of inorganic carbon for photosynthesis in two marine dinoflagellates. *J Phycol*, 40, 285–292.

105. Colman, B., Huertas, I. E., Bhatti, S. et al. 2002. The diversity of inorganic carbon acquisition mechanisms in eukaryotic microalgae. *Funct Plant Biol*, 29, 261–270.

106. Rost, B., Richter, K., Riebesell, U. et al. 2006. Inorganic carbon acquisition in red tide dinoflagellates. *Plant Cell Environ*, 29, 810–822.

107. Fu, F. X., Zhang, Y., Warner, M. E. et al. 2008. A comparison of future increased CO_2 and temperature effects on sympatric *Heterosigma akashiwo* and *Prorocentrum minimum. Harmful Algae*, 7, 76–90.
108. Pan, Y. L., Rao, D. V. S., and Mann, K. H. 1996. Acclimation to low light intensity in photosynthesis and growth of *Pseudonitzschia multiseries* Hasle, a neurotoxigenic diatom. *J Plankton Res*, 18, 1427–1438.
109. Proctor, N. H., Chan, S. X., and Trevor, A. J. 1975. Production of saxitoxin by cultures of *Gonyaulax catenella. Toxicon*, 13, 1–9.
110. Maas, E. W. and Brooks, H. J. L. 2010. Is photosynthesis a requirement for paralytic shellfish toxin production in the dinoflagellate *Alexandrium minutum* algal–bacterial consortium? *J Appl Phycol*, 22, 293–296.
112. Adolf, J. E., Bachvaroff, T. R., and Place, A. R. 2009. Environmental modulation of karlotoxin levels in strains of the cosmopolitan dinoflagellate *Karlodinium veneficum* (Dinophyceae). *J Phycol*, 45, 176–192.
113. Siu, G., Young, M., and Chan, D. 1997. Environmental and nutritional factors which regulate population dynamics and toxin production in the dinoflagellate *Alexandrium catenella. Hydrobiologia*, 352, 117–140.
114. Hall, S., Reichardt, P. B., Neve, R. A. et al. 1982. Studies on the origin and nature of toxicity in Alaskan bivalves: Toxins from *Protogonyaulax* of the Northeast Pacific. *J Shellfish Res*, 2, 119.
115. Ogata, T., Ishimaru, T., and Kodama, M. 1987. Effect of water temperature and light intensity on growth rate and toxicity change in *Protogonyaulax tamarensis. Mar Biol*, 95, 217–220.
116. Cembella, A. D., Therriault, J., and Beland, P. 1988. Toxicity of cultured isolates and natural populations of *Protogonyaulax tamarensis* from the St. Lawrence estuary. *J Shellfish Res*, 7, 611–621.
117. Anderson, D. M., Kulis, D. M., Sullivan, J. J. et al. 1990. Dynamic of physiology of saxitoxin production by the dinoflagellates *Alexandrium* spp. *Mar Biol*, 104, 511–524.
118. Etheridge, S. M. and Roesler, C. S. 2005. Effects of temperature, irradiance, and salinity on photosynthesis, growth rates, total toxicity, and toxin composition for *Alexandrium fundyense* isolates from the Gulf of Maine and Bay of Fundy. *Deep-Sea Res PT II*, 52, 2491–2500.
119. Lim, P. T., Leaw, C. P., Usup, G. et al. 2006. Effects of light and temperature on growth, nitrate uptake, and toxin production of two tropical dinoflagellates: *Alexandrium tamiyavanichii* and *Alexandrium minutum* (Dinophyceae). *J Phycol*, 42, 786–799.
120. Morton, S. L., Norris, D. R., and Bomber, J. W. 1992. Effect of temperature, salinity and light-intensity on the growth and seasonality of toxic dinoflagellates associated with ciguatera. *J Exp Mar Biol Ecol*, 157, 79–90.
121. Hales, S., Weinstein, P., and Woodward, A. 1999. Ciguatera (fish poisoning), El Niño, and Pacific sea surface temperatures. *Ecosyst Health*, 5, 20–25.
122. Chateau-Degat, M. L., Chinain, M., Cerf, N. et al. 2005. Seawater temperature, *Gambierdiscus* spp. variability and incidence of ciguatera poisoning in French Polynesia. *Harmful Algae*, 4, 1053–1062.
123. Parsons, M. L., Aligizaki, K., Dechraoui Bottein, M. Y. et al. 2012. *Gambierdiscus* and *Ostreopsis*: Reassessment of the state of knowledge of their taxonomy, geography, ecophysiology, and toxicology. *Harmful Algae*, 14, 107–129.
124. Tindall, D. R. and Morton, S. L. 1998. Community dynamics and physiology of epiphytic/benthic dinoflagellates associated with ciguatera. In *Physiological Ecology of Harmful Algal Blooms*, eds. D. A. Anderson, A. D. Cembella, and G. M. Hallegraeff, pp. 293–313. Berlin, Germany: Springer-Verlag.
125. Rhodes, L. 2011. World-wide occurrence of the toxic dinoflagellate genus *Ostreopsis* Schmidt. *Toxicon*, 57, 400–407.
126. Peperzak, L. 2003. Climate change and harmful algal blooms in the North Sea. *Acta Oecol*, 24, 139–144.
127. Vargo, G. A. 2009. A brief summary of the physiology and ecology of *Karenia brevis* Davis (G. Hansen and Moestrup comb. nov.) red tides on the West Florida Shelf and of hypotheses posed for their initiation, growth, maintenance, and termination. *Harmful Algae*, 8, 573–584.
128. Lamberto, J. N., Bourdelais, A., Jacocks, H. M. et al. 2004. Effects of temperature on production of brevetoxin and brevetoxin-like compounds. In *Harmful Algae 2002*, eds. K. A. Steidinger, J. H. Landsberg, C. R. Tomas et al., pp. 155–156. Paris, France: Florida Fish and Wildlife Conservation Commission, Florida Institute of Oceanography, Intergovernmental Oceanographic Commission of UNESCO.
129. Xue, F. F., Avery, O. T., and David, A. H. 2012. Global change and the future of harmful algal blooms in the ocean. *Mar Ecol Prog Ser*, 470, 207–233.

130. Lilly, E. L., Halanych, K. M., and Anderson, D. M. 2005. Phylogeny biogeography and species boundaries within the *Alexandrium minutum* group. *Harmful Algae*, 4, 1004–1020.

131. Lilly, E. L., Halanych, K. M., and Anderson, D. M. 2007. Species boundaries and global biogeography of the *Alexandrium tamarense* complex (Dinophyceae). *J Phycol*, 43, 1329–1338.

132. Balech, E. 1985. The genus *Alexandrium* or *Gonyaulax* of the *tamarensis* group. In *Toxic Dinoflagellates*, eds. D. M. Anderson, A. W. White, and D. G. Baden, pp. 33–38. New York: Elsevier.

133. Heimann, K. 2012. *Gymnodinium* and related dinoflagellates. In *Encyclopedia of Life Sciences*. Chichester, UK: John Wiley & Sons Ltd. http://www.els.net, doi: 10.1002/9780470015902.a0001967.pub2.

134. Lilly, E. L. 2003. Phylogeny and biogeography of the toxic dinoflagellate *Alexandrium*. PhD thesis. Cambridge, MA/Woods Hole/MA: Massachusetts Institute of Technology/Woods Hole Oceanographic Institution, 226pp.

135. McMinn, A., Hallegraeff, G. M., Thomson, P. et al. 1997. Cyst and radionucleotide evidence for the recent introduction of the toxic dinoflagellate *Gymnodinium catenatum* into Tasmanian waters. *Mar Ecol Prog Ser*, 161, 165–172.

136. Band-Schmidt, C. J., Bustillos-Guzmán, J. J., David, J. L. C. et al. 2010. Ecological and physiological studies of *Gymnodinium catenatum* in the Mexican Pacific: A review. *Mar Drugs*, 8, 1935–1961.

137. Illoul, H., Maso, M., Figueroa R. I. et al. 2005. Detection of toxic *Gymnodinium catenatum* (Graham, 1943) in Algerian waters (SW Mediterranean Sea). *Harmful Algae News*, 29, 10–12.

138. Bravo, I., Reguera, B., Martinez, A. et al. 1990. First report of *Gymnodinium catenatum* Graham on the Spanish Mediterranean Coast. In *Toxic Marine Phytoplankton*, eds. E. Granelli, B. Sundtröm, L. Edler et al., pp. 449–452. New York: Elsevier.

139. Gómez, F. 2003. Checklist of mediterranean free-living dinoflagellates. *Bot Mar*, 46, 215–242.

140. Dammak-Zouari, H., Hamza, A., and Bouain, A. 2009. Gymnodiniales in the Gulf of Gabes (Tunisia). *Cah Biol Mar*, 50, 153–170.

141. Ribeiro, S., Amorim, A., and Thorbjørn, J. A. 2012. Reconstructing the history of an invasion: The toxic phytoplankton species *Gymnodinium catenatum* in the Northeast Atlantic. *Biol Invasions*, 14, 969–985.

142. Taroncher-Oldenburg, G., Kulis, D. M., and Anderson, D. M. 1997. Toxin variability during the cell cycle of the dinoflagellate *Alexandrium fundyense*. *Limnol Oceanogr*, 42, 1178–1188.

143. Pan, Y., Bates, S., and Cembella, A. D. 1998. Environmental stress and domoic acid production by *Pseudo-nitzschia*: A physiological perspective. *Nat Toxins*, 6, 127–135.

144. Eschbach, E., John, U., Reckermann, M. et al. 2005. Cell cycle dependent expression of toxicity by the ichthyotoxic prymnesiophyte *Chrysochromulina polylepis*. *Aquat Microb Ecol*, 39, 85–95.

145. Chisholm, S. W. 1981. Temporal patterns of cell division in unicellular algae. In *Physiological Bases of Phytoplankton Ecology*, ed. T. Platt; *Can Bull Fish Aquat Sci*, 20, 150–181.

146. Pan, Y., Cembella, A. D., and Quilliam, M. A. 1999. Cell cycle and toxin production in the benthic dinoflagellate *Prorocentrum lima*. *Mar Biol*, 134, 541–549.

147. Leighfield, T. A. and Van Dolah, F. M. 1999. Cell cycle regulation in a dinoflagellate, *Amphidinium operculatum*: Identification of the diel entraining cue and a possible role of cyclic AMP. *J Exp Mar Biol Ecol*, 262, 177–197.

148. Anderson, D. M. and Morel, D. 1979. The seeding of two red tide blooms by the germination of benthic *Gonyaulax tamarensis* hypnocysts. *Est Coast Shelf Sci*, 8, 279–293.

149. Montresor, M. 1992. Life histories in diatoms and dinoflagellates and their relevance in phytoplankton ecology. *Oebalia*, Suppl 17, 241–257.

150. Garcés, E., Delgado, M., Masó, M. et al. 1998. Life history and in situ growth rates of *Alexandrium taylori* (Dinophyceae, Pyrrophyta). *J Phycol*, 34, 880–887.

151. Sicko-Goad, L., Stoermer, E. F., and Kociolek, J. P. 1989. Diatom resting cell rejuvenation and formation: Time course, species records and distribution. *J Plankton Res*, 11, 375–389.

152. Mann, D. G. 2002. Diatom life cycles. In *LIFEHAB: Life Histories of Microalgal Species Causing Harmful Blooms*, eds. E. Garcés, A. Zingone, M. Montresor et al., pp. 13–17. Luxembourg: Office for the Official Publications of the European Community.

153. Zingone, A., Sarno, D., Licandro, P. et al. 2002. Seasonality and interannual variations in the occurrence of species of the genus *Pseudo-nitzschia* in the Gulf of Naples (Mediterranean Sea). In *Xth International Conference on Harmful Algae*, St. Pete Beach, FL, October 21–25, 2002. ISSHA, Florida. Abstract Book, p. 315.

154. Moita, M. T. and Amorim, A. 2002. The relevance of *Gymnodinium catenatum* (Dinophyceae) over-wintering planktonic population vs. cysts as seedbeds for the local development of toxic blooms off Western Iberia. In *LIFEHAB: Life Histories of Microalgal Species Causing Harmful Blooms*, eds. E. Garcés, A. Zingone, M. Montresor et al., pp. 87–89. Luxembourg: Office for the Official Publications of the European Community.

155. Anderson, D. M. 1998. Physiology and bloom dynamics of toxic *Alexandrium* species, with emphasis on life cycle transitions. In *Physiological Ecology of Harmful Algal Blooms*, eds. D. M. Anderson, A. D. Cembella, and G. M. Hallegraeff, pp. 29–48. New York: Springer.

156. Figueroa, R. I., Bravo, I., Ramilo, I. et al. 2008. New life-cycle stages of *Gymnodinium catenatum* (Dinophyceae): Laboratory and field observations. *Aquat Microb Ecol*, 52, 13–23.

157. Bravo, I., Figueroa, R. I., Garcés, E. et al. 2010. The intricacies of dinoflagellate pellicle cysts: The example of *Alexandrium minutum* cysts from a bloom-recurrent area (Bay of Baiona, NW Spain). *Deep-Sea Res PT II*, 57, 166–174.

158. Figueroa, R. I. and Bravo, I. 2005. Sexual reproduction and two different encystment strategies of *Lingulodinium polyedrum* (Dinophyceae) in culture. *J Phycol*, 41, 370–379.

159. Probert, I. 2002. The induction of sexual reproduction in dinoflagellates: Culture studies and field. In *LIFEHAB: Life Histories of Microalgal Species Causing Harmful Blooms*, eds. E. Garcés, A. Zingone, M. Montresor et al., pp. 57–59. Luxembourg: Office for the Official Publications of the European Community.

160. Figueroa, R. I. and Bravo, I. 2005. A study of sexual reproduction and determination of mating type of *Gymnodinium nolleri* (Dinophyceae) in culture. *J Phycol*, 41, 74–78.

161. Raine, R. 2002. Harmful algal events in Irish waters. The importance of life cycles from an ecologist's perspective. In *LIFEHAB: Life Histories of Microalgal Species Causing Harmful Blooms*, eds. E. Garcés, A. Zingone, M. Montresor et al., pp. 90–91. Luxembourg: Office for the Official Publications of the European Community.

162. Gentien, P. 2002. Models of bloom dynamics: What is needed to incorporate life cycles and life stages? In *LIFEHAB: Life Histories of Microalgal Species Causing Harmful Blooms*, eds. E. Garcés, A. Zingone, M. Montresor et al., pp. 103–108. Luxembourg: Office for the Official Publications of the European Community.

163. Reguera, B. and González-Gil, S. 2001. Small cell and intermediate cell formation in species of *Dinophysis* (Dinophyceae, Dinophysiales). *J Phycol*, 37, 318–333.

164. Reguera, B., González-Gil, S., and Delgado, M. 2004. Formation of *Dinophysis dens* Pavillard and *D. diegensis* Kofoid from laboratory incubations of *Dinophysis acuta* Ehrenberg and *D. caudata* Saville-Kent. In *Harmful Algae 2002*, eds. K. A. Steidinger, J. A. Landsberg, C. R. Tomas et al., pp. 440–442. St. Petersburg, FL: Florida Fish and Wildlife Conservation Commission, Florida Institute of Oceanography, IOC-UNESCO.

165. Litaker, R. W., Vandersea, M. W., Kibler, S. R. et al. 2002. Life cycle of the heterotrophic dinoflagellate *Pfiesteria piscicida. J Phycol*, 38, 442–463.

166. Parrow, M. W. and Burkholder J. M. 2003. Reproduction and sexuality in *Pfiesteria shumwayae* (Dinophyceae). *J Phycol*, 39, 697–711.

167. Parrow, M. W. and Burkholder, J. M. 2004. The sexual life cycles of *Pfiesteria piscicida* and Cryptoperidiniopsoids (Dinophyceae). *J Phycol*, 40, 664–673.

168. Garcés, E., Masó, M., and Camp, J. 2002. Role of temporary cysts in the population dynamics of *Alexandrium taylori* (Dinophyceae). *J Plankton Res*, 24, 681–686.

169. Laabir, M. and Gentien, P. 1999. Survival of toxic dinoflagellates after gut passage in the Pacific oyster *Crassostrea gigas* Thunburg. *J Shellfish Res*, 18, 217–222.

170. Walsh, J. J. and Steidinger, K. A. 2001. Saharan dust and Florida red tides: The cyanophyte connection. *J Geophys Res*, 106, 11597–11612.

171. Mulholland, M. R., Heil, C. A., Bronk, D. A. et al. 2004. Does nitrogen regeneration from the N_2 fixing cyanobacteria *Trichodesmium* spp. fuel *Karenia brevis* blooms in the Gulf of Mexico? In *Harmful Algae 2002*, eds. K. A. Steidinger, J. H. Landsberg, C. R. Tomas et al., pp. 47–49. St. Petersburg, FL: Florida Fish and Wildlife Conservation Commission, Florida Institute of Oceanography, IOC-UNESCO.

172. Rengefors, K., Karlsson, I., and Hansson, L. A. 1998. Algal cyst dormancy: A temporary escape from herbivory. *Proc R Soc B*, 265, 1353–1358.

173. Garcés, E., Bravo, I., Vila, M. et al. 2004. Relationship between vegetative cells and cyst production during *Alexandrium minutum* bloom in Arenys de Mar harbour (NW Mediterranean). *J Plankton Res*, 26, 637–645.

174. Steidinger, K. and Garcés, E. 2006. Life cycles of harmful algae: An overview. In *Ecology of Harmful Algae*, eds. E. Graneli and J. T. Turner, pp. 37–49. Berlin, Germany: Springer Verlag.

175. Vesk, M., Hallegraeff, G. M., and Jeffrey, S. W. 1990. Biology of marine plants. In *Biology of Marine Plants*, eds. M. N. Clayton and R. J. King, pp. 133–148. Melbourne, Victoria, Australia: Longman Cheshire.

176. Larsen, J. and Moestrup, Ø. 1992. Potentially toxic phytoplankton. 2. Genus *Dinophysis* (Dinophyceae). In *ICES Identification Leaflets for Plankton*, ed. J. A. Lindley, p. 12. Copenhagen, Denmark: International Council for the Exploration of the Sea.

177. Reguera, B., Garcés, E., Bravo, I. et al. 2003. In situ division rates of several species of *Dinophysis* estimated by a postmitotic index. *Mar Ecol Prog Ser*, 249, 117–131.

178. Reguera, B., Velo-Suarez, L., Raine, R. et al. 2012. Harmful *Dinophysis* species: A review. *Harmful Algae*, 14, 87–106.

179. Zingone, A., Montresor, M., and Marino, D. 1998. Morphological variability of the potentially toxic dinoflagellate *Dinophysis sacculus* (Dinophyceae) and its taxonomic relationships with *D. pavillardii* and *D. acuminata*. *Eur J Phycol*, 33, 259–273.

180. Reguera, B., González-Gil, S., and Delgado, M. 2007. *Dinophysis diegensis* Kofoid is a life history stage of *Dinophysis caudata* Kent (Dinophyceae, Dinophysiales). *J Phycol*, 43, 1083–1093.

181. Lassus, P. and Bardouil, M. 1991. Le Complexe *Dinophysis acuminata*: Identification des espéces le long des côtes Françaises. *Cryptogamie Algol*, 12, 1–9.

182. Bravo, I., Delgado, M., Fraga, S. et al. 1995. The *Dinophysis* genus: Toxicity and species definition in Europe. In *Harmful Marine Algal Blooms*, eds. P. Lassus, G. Arzul, E. Erard-Le Denn et al., pp. 843–845. Paris, France: Lavoisier.

183. Koukaras, K. and Nikolaidis, G. 2004. *Dinophysis* blooms in Greek coastal waters (Thermaikos Gulf NW Aegean Sea). *J Plankton Res*, 26, 445–457.

184. Abé, T. H. 1967. The armoured Dinoflagellata: II. Prorocentridae and Dinophysidae (B). *Dinophysis* and its allied genera. *Publ Seto Mar Biol Lab*, 15, 37–78.

185. Balech, E. 1976. Some Norwegian *Dinophysis* species (Dinoflagellata). *Sarsia*, 61, 75–94.

186. Hallegraeff, G. M. and Lucas, I. A. N. 1988. The marine dinoflagellate genus *Dinophysis* (Dinophyceae): Photosynthetic, neritic and non-photosynthetic, oceanic species. *Phycologia*, 27, 25–42.

187. Steidinger, K. A. and Tangen, K. 1997. Dinoflagellates. In *Identifying Marine Diatoms and Dinoflagellates*, ed. C. R. Tomas, pp. 387–598. San Diego, CA: Academic Press.

188. Jensen, M. H. and Daugbjerg, N. 2009. Molecular phylogeny of selected species of the order Dinophysiales (Dinophyceae)—Testing the hypothesis of a dinophysoid radiation. *J Phycol*, 45, 1136–1152.

189. González-Gil, S., Pizarro, G., Paz, B. et al. 2011. Considerations on the toxigenic nature and prey sources of *Phalacroma rotundatum*. *Aquat Microb Ecol*, 64, 197–203.

190. Lee, R. W. 1989. *Phycology*, 2nd edn. Cambridge, U.K.: Cambribge University Press.

191. Caroppo, C., Congestri, R., and Bruno, M. 1999. On the presence of *Phalacroma rotundatum* in the Southern Adriatic Sea (Italy). *Aquat Microb Ecol*, 17, 301–310.

192. Pazos, Y., Arévalo, F., Correa, J. et al. 2010. An unusual assemblage of *Gymnodinium catenatum* and *Dinophysis* in the Spanish Galician rías in 2009. In *Book of Abstracts and Programme, 14th International Conference on Harmful Algae*, Hersonissos-Crete, Greece. ISSHA, St. Pete Beach, FL, p. 47.

193. Suzuki, T., Miyazono, A., Baba, K. et al. 2009. LC–MS/MS analysis of okadaic acid analogues and other lipophilic toxins in single-cell isolates of several *Dinophysis* species collected in Hokkaido, Japan. *Harmful Algae*, 8, 233–238.

194. Rao, D. V. S., Pan, Y., Zitko, V. et al. 1993. Diarrhetic shellfish poisoning (DSP) associated with a subsurface bloom of *Dinophysis norvegica* in Bedford Basin, eastern Canada. *Mar Ecol Prog Ser*, 97, 117–126.

195. Johansen, M. 2008. On *Dinophysis* occurrence and toxin content. PhD thesis. Department of Marine Ecology, University of Göteborg, Göteborg, Sweden.

196. Cembella, A. D., Bauder, A. G., Lewis, N. I. et al. 2001. Association of the gonyaulacoid dinoflagellate *Alexandrium ostenfeldii* with spirolide toxins in size-fractionated plankton. *J Plankton Res*, 23, 1413–1419.

197. Hsia, M. H., Morton, S. L., Smith, L. L. et al. 2005. Production of goniodomin A by the planktonic, chain-forming dinoflagellate *Alexandrium monilatum* (Howell) Balech isolated from the Gulf Coast of the United States. *Harmful Algae*, 5, 290–299.

198. Anderson, D. M., Tilman, J. A., Cembella, A. D. et al. 2012. The globally distributed genus *Alexandrium*: Multifaceted roles in marine ecosystems and impacts on human health. *Harmful Algae*, 14, 10–35.

199. Balech, E. 1995. *The Genus Alexandrium Halim (Dinoflagellata)*. Sherkin Island, Co. Cork, Ireland: Sherkin Island Marine Station, 151pp.

200. Anderson, D. M., Kulis, D. M., Doucette, G. J. et al. 1994. Biogeography of toxic dinoflagellates in the genus *Alexandrium* from the northeastern United States and Canada. *Mar Biol*, 120, 467–478.

201. Scholin, C. A. and Anderson, D. M. 1994. Identification of group- and strain-specific genetic markers for globally distributed *Alexandrium* (Dinophyceae). I. RFLP analysis of SSU rDNA genes. *J Phycol*, 30, 744–754.

202. Adachi, M., Sako, Y., and Ishida, Y. 1996. Analysis of *Alexandrium* (Dinophyceae) species using sequences of the 5.8S ribosomal DNA and internal transcribed spacer regions. *J Phycol*, 32, 424–432.

203. Scholin, C. A., Hallegraeff, G. M., and Anderson, D. M. 1995. Molecular evolution of the *Alexandrium tamarense* species complex (Dinophyceae): Dispersal in the North American and West Pacific regions. *Phycologia*, 34, 472–485.

204. Medlin, L. K., Lange, M., Wellbrock, U. et al. 1998. Sequence comparisons link toxic European isolates of *Alexandrium tamarense* from the Orkney Islands to toxic North American stocks. *Eur J Protistol*, 34, 329–335.

205. Hansen, G., Daugbjerg, N., and Franco, J. M. 2003. Morphology, toxin composition and LSU rDNA phylogeny of *Alexandrium minutum* (Dinophyceae) from Denmark, with some morphological observations on other European strains. *Harmful Algae*, 2, 317–335.

206. Cembella, A. D., Sullivan, J. J., Boyer, G. L. et al. 1987. Variation in paralytic shellfish toxin composition within the *Protogonyaulax tamarensis/catenella* species complex: Red tide dinoflagellates. *Biochem Syst Ecol*, 15, 171–186.

207. Boczar, B. A., Beitler, M. K., Liston, J. et al. 1988. Paralytic shellfish toxins in *Protogonyaulax tamarensis* and *Protogonyaulax catenella* in axenic culture. *Plant Physiol*, 88, 1285–1290.

208. Holmes, M. J., Lewis, R. J., Jones, A. et al. 1995. Cooliatoxin, the first toxin from *Coolia monotis* (Dinophyceae). *Nat Toxins*, 3, 355–362.

209. Taylor, F. J. R., Fukuyo, Y., and Larsen, J. 1995. Taxonomy of harmful dinoflagellates. In *Manual on Harmful Marine Microalgae, IOC Manuals and Guides*, eds. G. M. Hallegraeff, D. M. Anderson, and A. D. Cembella, pp. 283–317. Paris, France: UNESCO.

210. Rhodes, L., Adamson, J., Suzuki, T. et al. 2000. Toxic marine epiphytic dinoflagellates, *Ostreopsis siamensis* and *Coolia monotis* (Dinophyceae), in New Zealand. *N Z J Mar Freshwat Res*, 34, 371–383.

211. Faust, M. A., Morton, S., and Quod, J. P. 1996. Further SEM study of marine dinoflagellates: The genus *Ostreopsis* (Dinophyceae). *J Phycol*, 32, 1053–1065.

212. Vila, M., Garcés, E., and Masó, M. 2001. Potentially toxic epiphytic dinoflagellate assemblages on macroalgae in the NW Mediterranean. *Aquat Microb Ecol*, 26, 51–60.

213. Aligizaki, K. and Nikolaidis, G. 2006. The presence of the potentially toxic genera *Ostreopsis* and *Coolia* (Dinophyceae) in the North Aegean Sea, Greece. *Harmful Algae*, 5, 717–730.

214. Chang, F. H., Shimizu, Y., Hay, B. et al. 2000. Three recently recorded *Ostreopsis* spp. (Dinophyceae) in New Zealand: Temporal and regional distribution in the upper North Island from 1995–1997. *N Z J Mar Freshwat Res*, 34, 29–39.

215. Ciminiello, P., Dell'Aversano, C., Fattorusso, E. et al. 2008. Putative palytoxin and its newanalogue, ovatoxin-a, in *Ostreopsis ovata* collected along the Ligurian coasts during the 2006 toxic outbreak. *J Am Soc Mass Spectrom*, 19, 111–120.

216. Taylor, F. J. R. 1979. The description of the benthic dinoflagellate associated with maitotoxin and ciguatoxin, including observations on Hawaiian material. In *Toxic Dinoflagellate Blooms*, eds. D. L. Taylor and H. H. Seliger, pp. 71–77. New York: Elsevier Scientific.

217. Abboud-Abi Saab, M. and El-Bakht, Y. 1998. Dominant and potentially toxic microalgae in Lebanese coastal waters. In *Harmful Algae*, eds. B. Reguera, J. Blanco, M. L. Fernandez et al., p. 92. Paris, France: Xunta de Galicia and Intergovernmental Oceanographic Commission of UNESCO.

218. Bottalico, A., Micella, P., and Feliciti, G. P. 2002. Fioritura di *Ostreopsis* sp. (Dinophyta) nel porto di Otranto. In *Gruppo di Lavoro per l'Algologia—Società Botanica Italiana*, Chioggia, Italy, November 8–9, 2002.

219. Totti, C., Accoroni, S., Cerino, F. et al. 2010. *Ostreopsis ovata* bloom along the Conero Riviera (northern Adriatic Sea): Relationships with environmental conditions and substrata. *Harmful Algae*, 9, 233–239.

220. Bianco, I., Sangiorgi, V., Penna, A. et al. 2007. *Ostreopsis ovata* in benthic aggregates along the Latium Coast (middle Tyrrhenian Sea). Tyrrhenian Sea). In *International Symposium on Algal Toxins*, Trieste, Italy, May 27–29, 2007.

221. Totti, C., Cucchiari, E., Romagnoli, T. et al. 2007. Bloom of *Ostreopsis ovata* on the Conero riviera (NW Adriatic Sea). *Harmful Algae News*, 33, 12–13.

222. Aligizaki, K., Katikou, P., Nikolaidis, G. et al. 2008. First episode of shellfish contamination by palytoxin-like compounds from *Ostreopsis* species (Aegean Sea, Greece). *Toxicon*, 51, 418–427.

223. Granéli, E., Vidyarathna, N. K., and Funari, E. 2008. Climate change and benthic dinoflagellates— The *Ostreopsis ovata* case. In *Proceedings of the 13th International Conference on Harmful Algae*, Hong Kong, China, November 3–7, 2008, p. 42.

224. Sansoni, G., Borghini, B., Camici, G. et al. 2003. Fioriture algali di *Ostreopsis ovata* (Gonyaulacales: Dinophyceae): Un problema emergente. *Biol Amb*, 17, 17–23.

225. Shears, N. T. and Ross, P. M. 2009. Blooms of benthic dinoflagellates of the genus *Ostreopsis*; an increasing and ecologically important phenomenon on temperate reefs in New Zealand and worldwide. *Harmful Algae*, 8, 916–925.

226. Schmidt, J. 1901. Preliminary report of the botanical results of the Danish Expedition to Siam (1899–1900). Pt. IV, Peridiniales. *Bot Pidsslerift*, 24, 212–221.

227. Fukuyo, Y. 1981. Taxonomic study on benthic dinoflagellates collected in coral reefs. *Bull Jpn Soc Sci Fish*, 47, 967–978.

228. Norris, D. R., Bomber, J. W., and Balech, E. 1985. Benthic dinoflagellates associated with ciguatera from the Florida Keys. I. *Ostreopsis heptagona* sp. nov. In *Toxic Dinoflagellates*, eds. D. M. Anderson, A. W. White, and D. G. Baden, pp. 39–44. New York: Elsevier Scientific.

229. Quod, J. P. 1994. *Ostreopsis mascarensis* sp. nov. (Dinophyceae), dinoflagellates toxiques associes a la ciguatera dans l'Ocean Indien. *Rev Cryptog Algol*, 15, 243–251.

230. Faust, M. A. and Morton, S. L. 1995. Morphology and ecology of the marine dinoflagellate *Ostreopsis labens* sp. nov. (Dinophyceae). *J Phycol*, 31, 456–463.

231. Faust, M. A. 1999. Three new *Ostreopsis* species (Dinophyceae): *O. marinus* sp. nov., *O. belizeanus* sp. nov. and *O. caribbbeanus* sp. nov. *Phycologia*, 38, 92–99.

232. Guerrini, F., Pezzolesi, L., and Feller, A. 2010. Comparative growth and toxin profile of cultured *Ostreopsis ovata* from the Tyrrhenian and Adriatic Seas. *Toxicon*, 55, 211–220.

233. Ciminiello, P., Dell'Aversano, C., Dello Iacovo, E. et al. 2010. Complex palytoxin-like profile of *Ostreopsis ovata*. Identification of four new ovatoxins by high-resolution liquid chromatography/mass spectrometry. *Rapid Commun Mass Spectrom*, 24, 2735–2744.

234. Mangialajo, L., Bertolotto, R., Cattaneo-Vietti, R. et al. 2008. The toxic benthic dinoflagellate *Ostreopsis ovata*: Quantification of proliferation along the coastline of Genoa, Italy. *Mar Pollut Bull*, 56, 1209–1214.

235. Monti, M., Minocci, M., Beran, A. et al. 2007. First record of *Ostreopsis* cfr. *ovata* on macroalgae in the Northern Adriatic Sea. *Mar Pollut Bull*, 54, 598–601.

236. Penna, A., Fraga, S., Battocchi, C. et al. 2010. A phylogeographical study of the toxic benthic dinoflagellate genus *Ostreopsis* Schmidt. *J Biogeogr*, 37, 830–841.

237. Adachi, R. and Fukuyo, Y. 1979. The thecal structure of a marine toxic dinoflagellate *Gambierdiscus toxicus* gen. et sp. nov. collected in a ciguatera-endemic area. *Bull Jpn Soc Sci Fish*, 45, 67–71.

238. Bomber, J. W., Rubio, M. R., and Norris, D. R. 1989. Epiphytism of dinoflagellates associated with the disease ciguatera: Substrate specificity and nutrition. *Phycologia*, 28, 360–368.

239. Lartigue, J., Jester, J. E., Dickey, R. W. et al. 2009. Nitrogen source effects on the growth and toxicity of two strains of the ciguatera-causing dinoflagellate *Gambierdiscus toxicus*. *Harmful Algae*, 8, 781–791.

240. Parsons, M. L., Settelmier, C. J., and Bienfang, P. K. 2010. A simple model capable of simulating the population dynamics of *Gambierdiscus*, the benthic dinoflagellate responsible for ciguatera fish poisoning. *Harmful Algae*, 10, 71–80.

241. Litaker, R. W., Vandersea, M. W., Faust, M. A. et al. 2009. Taxonomy of *Gambierdiscus* including four new species, *Gambierdiscus caribaeus*, *Gambierdiscus carolinianus*, *Gambierdiscus carpenter* and *Gambierdiscus ruetzleri* (Gonyaulacales, Dinophyceae). *Phycologia*, 48, 344–390.

242. Lewis, R. J., Holmes, M. J., and Sellin, M. 1994. Invertebrates implicated in the transfer of gambiertoxins to the benthic carnivore *Pomadasys maculatus*. *Mem Qld Mus*, 34, 561–564.

243. Baden, D. G., Fleming, L. E., and Bean, J. A. 1995. Marine toxins. In *Handbook of Clinical Neurology: Intoxications of the Nervous System Part H. Natural Toxins and Drugs*, ed. F. A. Wolff, pp. 141–175. Amsterdam, the Netherlands: Elsevier Press.

244. Alfonso, A., Roman, Y., Vieytes, M. R. et al. 2005. Azaspiracid-4 inhibits Ca^{2+} entry by stored operated channels in human T lymphocytes. *Biochem Pharmacol*, 69, 1543–1680.

245. Fraga, S., Francisco, R., Caillaud, A. et al. 2011. *Gambierdiscus excentricus* sp. nov. (Dinophyceae), a benthic toxic dinoflagellate from the Canary Islands (NE Atlantic Ocean). *Harmful Algae*, 11, 10–22.

246. Kibler, S. R., Litaker, R. W., Holland, W. C. et al. 2012. Growth of eight *Gambierdiscus* (Dinophyceae) species: Effects of temperature, salinity and irradiance. *Harmful Algae*, 19, 1–14.

247. Steidinger, K. A., Tester, L. S., and Taylor, F. J. R. 1980. A redescription of *Pyrodinium bahamense* var. *compressa* (Böhm) stat. nov. from Pacific red tides. *Phycologia*, 19, 329–337.

248. Leaw, C. P., Lim, P. T., Ng, B. K. et al. 2005. Phylogenetic analysis of *Alexandrium* species and *Pyrodinium bahamense* (Dinophyceae) based on theca morphology and nuclear ribosomal gene sequence. *Phycologia*, 44, 550–565.

249. Glibert, P. M., Landsberg, J. H., Evans, J. J. et al. 2002. A fish kill of massive proportion in Kuwait Bay, Arabian Gulf, 2001: The roles of bacterial disease, harmful algae, and eutrophication. *Harmful Algae*, 1, 215–231.

250. Garate-Lizarraga, I. and Gonzalez-Armas, R. 2011. Occurrence of *Pyrodinium bahamense* var. *compressum* along the southern coast of the Baja California Peninsula. *Mar Pollut Bull*, 62, 626–630.

251. Landsberg, J. H., Hall, S., Johannessen, J. et al. 2002. Puffer fish poisoning: Widespread implications of saxitoxin in Florida [Abstract]. In *Xth International Conference on Harmful Algae*, St. Pete Beach, FL, October 21–25, 2002. ISSHA, St. Pete Beach, FL. Abstract Book, p. 160.

252. Landsberg, J. H., Sherwood, H., Johannessen, J. N. et al. 2006. Saxitoxin puffer fish poisoning in the United States, with the first report of *Pyrodinium bahamense* as the putative toxin source. *Environ Health Perspect*, 114, 1502–1507.

253. Walsh, J. J., Tomas, C. R., Steidinger, K. A. et al. 2011. Imprudent fishing harvests and consequent trophic cascades on the West Florida shelf over the last half century: A harbinger of increased human deaths from paralytic shellfish poisoning along the southeastern United States, in response to oligotrophication? *Contl Shelf Res*, 31, 891–911.

254. Ammons, D., Rampersad, J., and Poli, M. A. 2001. Evidence for PSP in mussels in Trinidad. *Toxicon*, 39, 889–892.

255. Usup, G., Ahmada, A., Matsuoka, K. et al. 2012. Biology, ecology and bloom dynamics of the toxic marine dinoflagellate *Pyrodinium bahamense*. *Harmful Algae*, 14, 301–312.

256. Lewis, J. and Hallet, R. 1997. *Lingulodinium polyedrum* (*Gonyaulax polyedra*) a blooming dinoflagellate. *Oceanogr Mar Biol Annu Rev*, 35, 97–161.

257. Latz, M. I. and Rohr, J. 1999. Luminescent response of the red tide dinoflagellates *Lingulodinium polyedrum* to laminar and turbulent flow. *Limnol Oceanogr*, 44, 1423–1435.

258. Paz, B., Riobó, P., Fernández, M. L. et al. 2004. Production and release of yessotoxins by the dinoflagellates *Protoceratium reticulatum* and *Lingulodinium polyedrum* in culture. *Toxicon*, 44, 251–258.

259. Armstrong, M. and Kudela, R. 2006. Evaluation of California isolates of *Lingulodinium polyedrum* for the production of yessotoxin. *Afr J Mar Sci*, 28, 399–401.

260. Howard, M. D. A., Silver, M., and Kudela, R. M. 2008. Yessotoxin detected in mussel (*Mytilus californicus*) and phytoplankton samples from the U.S. west coast. *Harmful Algae*, 7, 646–652.

261. Plumley, F. G. 1997. Marine algal toxins: Biochemistry, genetics, and molecular biology. *Limnol Oceanogr*, 42, 1252–1264.

262. Riobo, P., Paz, B., and Fernandez, M. 2002. Lipophylic toxins of different strains of Ostreopsidaceae and Gonyaulacaceae. In *Xth International Conference on Harmful Algae*, St. Pete Beach, FL, October 21–25, 2002. ISSHA, Florida. Abstract Book, pp. 119–121.

263. Stobo, L. A., Lewis, J., Quilliam, M. A. et al. 2003. Detection of yessotoxin in UK and Canadian isolates of phytoplankton and optimization and validation of LC-MS methods. *Can Tech Rep Fish Aquat Sci*, 2498, 8–14.

264. Draisci, R., Ferretti, E., Palleschi, L. et al. 1999. High levels of yessotoxin in mussels and presence of yessotoxin and homoyessotoxin in dinoflagellates of the Adriatic Sea. *Toxicon*, 37, 1187–1193.

265. Tubaro, A., Sidari, L., Della Loggia, R. et al. 1998. Occurrence of yessotoxin in phytoplankton and mussels from northern Adriatic Sea. In *Harmful Algae*, eds. B. Requera, J. Blanco, M. L. Fernández et al., pp. 470–472. *Proceedings of the VIII International Conference on Harmful Algae*. Vigo, Spain: Xunta de Galicia and Intergovernmental Oceanographic Commission of UNESCO.

266. Ramstad, H., Hovgaard, P., Yasumoto, T. et al. 2001. Monthly variations in diarrhetic toxins and yessotoxin in shellfish from coast to the inner part of the Sognefjord, Norway. *Toxicon*, 39, 1035–1043.

267. Bennouna, A., Berland, B., Attar, J. et al. 2002. *Lingulodinium polyedrum* (Stein) Dodge red tide in shellfish areas along Doukkala coast (Moroccan Atlantic). *Oceanol Acta*, 25, 159–170.

268. Howard, M. D. A., Smith, J. G., and Kudela, R. M. 2009. Phylogenetic relationships of yessotoxin-producing dinoflagellates, based on the large subunit and internal transcribed spacer ribosomal DNA domains. *Appl Environ Microb*, 75, 54–63.

269. Paz, B., Riobo, P., Ramilo, I. et al. 2007. Yessotoxins profile in strains of *Protoceratium reticulatum* from Spain and USA. *Toxicon*, 50, 1–17.

270. Hansen, G., Moestrup, Ø., and Roberts, K. R. 1997. Light and electron microscopical observations on *Protoceratium reticulatum* (Dinophyceae). *Arch Prostistenkd*, 147, 381–391.

271. Rodríguez, J. J. G., Mirón, A. S., Belarbi, E. H. et al. 2007. New culture approaches for yessotoxin production from the dinoflagellate *Protoceratium reticulatum*. *Biotechnol Prog*, 23, 339–350.

272. Röder, K., Hantzsche, F. M., Gebühr, C. et al. 2012. Effects of salinity, temperature and nutrients on growth, cellular characteristics and yessotoxin production of *Protoceratium reticulatum*. *Harmful Algae*, 15, 59–70.

273. Dodge, J. D. 1989. Some revisions of the family Gonyaulacaceae (Dinophyeae) based on a scanning electron microscope study. *Bot Mar*, 32, 275–298.

274. Tomas, C. R. 1997. *Identifying Marine Phytoplankton*. San Diego, CA: Academic Press, p. 858.

275. Rhodes, L., McNabb, P., de Salas, M. et al. 2006. Yessotoxin production by *Gonyaulax spinifera*. *Harmful Algae*, 5, 148–155.

276. Morton, S. L., Vershinin, A., Leighfield, T. et al. 2007. Identification of yessotoxin in mussels from the Caucasian Black Sea Coast of the Russian Federation. *Toxicon*, 50, 581–584.

277. Paz, B., Daranas, A. H., Norte, M. et al. 2008. Yessotoxins, a group of marine polyether toxins: An overview. *Mar Drugs*, 6, 73–102.

278. Yamaguchi, A. and Horiguchi, T. 2005. Molecular phylogenetic study of the heterotrophic dinoflagellate genus *Protoperidinium* (Dinophyceae) inferred from small subunit rRNA gene sequences. *Phycol Res*, 53, 30–42.

279. Moran, S., Silke, J., Cusack, C. et al. 2007. Correlations between known toxic phytoplankton species and toxin levels in shellfish in Irish waters 2002–2006. In *Sixth International Conference on Molluscan Shellfish Safety*, Blenheim, New Zealand, p. 72.

280. Marshall, H. G., Gordon, A. S., Seaborn, D. W. et al. 2000. Comparative culture and toxicity studies between the toxic dinoflagellate *Pfiesteria piscicida* and a morphologically similar cryptoperidiniopsoid dinoflagellate. *J Exp Mar Biol Ecol*, 255, 51–74.

281. Lewitus, A. J., Willis, B. M., Hayes, K. C. et al. 1999. Mixotrophy and nitrogen uptake by *Pfiesteria piscicida* (Dinophyceae). *J Phycol*, 35, 1430–1437.

282. Lewitus, A. J., Wetz, M. S., Willis, B. M. et al. 2006. Grazing activity of *Pfiesteria piscicida* (Dinophyceae) and susceptibility to ciliate predation vary with toxicity status. *Harmful Algae*, 5, 427–434.

283. Glasgow, H. B., Burkholder, J. M., Mallin, M. A. et al. 2001. Field ecology of toxic *Pfiesteria* complex species, and a conservative analysis of their role in estuarine fish kills. *Environ Health Perspect*, 109, 715–730.

284. Møller, E. F., Riemann, L., and Søndergaard, M. 2007. Bacteria associated with copepods: Abundance, activity and community composition. *Aquat Microb Ecol*, 47, 99–106.

285. Litaker, R. W., Tester, P. A., Colorni, A. et al. 1999. The phylogenetic relationship of *Pfiesteria piscicida*, *Cryptoperidiniopsoid* sp., *Amyloodinium ocellatum* and a *Pfiesteria*-like dinoflagellate to other dinoflagellates and apicomplexans. *J Phycol*, 35, 1379–1389.

286. Oldach, D. W., Delwiche, C. F., Jakobsen, K. S. et al. 2000. Heteroduplex mobility assay-guided sequence discovery: Elucidation of the small subunit (18S) rDNA sequences of *Pfiesteria piscicida* and related dinoflagellates from complex algal culture and environmental sample DNA pools. *Proc Natl Acad Sci USA*, 97, 4303–4308.

287. Jakobsen, K. S., Tengs, T., Vatne, A. et al. 2002. Discovery of the toxic dinoflagellate, *Pfiesteria*, from northern European waters. *Proc R Soc Lond B*, 269, 211–214.

288. Jeong, H. J., Seong, J., Park, J. Y. et al. 2005. *Stoeckeria algicida* n. gen., sn. sp. (Dinophyceae) from the coastal waters off southern Korea: Morphology and small subunit ribosomal DNA gene sequence. *J Eukaryot Microbiol*, 52, 382–390.

289. Rublee, P. A., Remington, D. L., Schaefer, E. F. et al. 2005. Detection of the dinozoans *Pfiesteria piscicida* and *P. shumwayae*: A review of detection methods and geographic distribution. *J Eukaryot Microbiol*, 52, 83–89.

290. Zhang, H., Bhattacharya, D., and Lin, S. 2005. Phylogeny of dinoflagellates based on mitochondrial cytochrome b and nuclear small subunit rDNA sequence comparisons. *J Phycol*, 41, 411–420.

291. Seaborn, D. W., Tengs, T., Cerbin, S. et al. 2006. A group of dinoflagellates similar to *Pfiesteria* as defined by morphology and genetic analysis. *Harmful Algae*, 5, 1–8.

292. Steidinger, K. A., Landsberg, J. H., Mason, P. L. et al. 2006. *Cryptoperidiniopsis brodyi* gen. et sp. nov. (Dinophyceae), a small lightly armored dinoflagellate in the Pfiesteriaceae. *J Phycol*, 42, 951–961.

293. Levy, M. G., Litaker, R. W., and Goldstein, R. J. 2007. *Piscinoodinium*, a fish-ectoparasitic dinoflagellate, is a member of the class dinophyceae, subclass Gymnodiniphycidae: Convergent evolution with *Amyloodinium*. *J Parasitol*, 93, 1006–1015.

294. Zhang, C. S., Wang, J. T., Zhu, D. D. et al. 2008. The preliminary analysis of nutrients in harmful algal blooms in the East China Sea in the spring and summer of 2005. *Acta Ecol Sin*, 30, 153–159.

295. Litaker, R. W., Steidinger, K. A., Mason, P. L. et al. 2005. The reclassification of *Pfiesteria shumwayae*: *Pseudopfiesteria*, gen. nov. *J Phycol*, 41, 643–651.

296. Kerstin, T., Joshi, A. R., Messtorff, P. et al. 2012. Molecular discrimination of taxa within the dinoflagellate genus *Azadinium*, the source of azaspiracid toxins. *J Plankton Res*, 35, 225–230.

297. Tillmann, U., Elbrächter, M., Krock, B. et al. 2009. *Azadinium spinosum* gen. et sp. nov. (Dinophyceae) identified as a primary producer of azaspiracid toxins. *Eur J Phycol*, 44, 63–79.

298. Tillmann, U., Elbrächter, M., John, U. et al. 2010. *Azadinium obesum* (Dinophyceae), a new nontoxic species in the genus that can produce azaspiracid toxins. *Phycologia*, 49, 169–182.

299. Nézan, E., Tillmann, U., Bilien, G. et al. 2012. Taxonomic revision of the dinoflagellate *Amphidoma caudata*: Transfer to the genus *Azadinium* (Dinophyceae) and proposal of two varieties, based on morphological and molecular phylogenetic analyses. *J Phycol*, 48, 925–939.

300. Tillmann, U., Salas, R., Gottschling, M. et al. 2012. *Amphidoma languid* sp. nov. (Dinophyceae) reveals a close relationship between *Amphidoma* and *Azadinium*. *Protist*, 163, 701–719.

301. Rehmann, N., Hess, P., and Quilliam, M. A. 2008. Discovery of new analogs of the marine biotoxin azaspiracid in blue mussels *Mytilus edulis* by ultra performance liquid chromatography/tandem mass spectrometry. *Rapid Commun Mass Spectrom*, 22, 549–558.

302. Krock, B., Tillmann, U., Voß, D. et al. 2012. New azaspiracids in Amphidomataceae (Dinophyceae): Proposed structures. *Toxicon*, 60, 830–839.

304. Rhodes, L., Smith, K. F., Munday, R. et al. 2010. Toxic dinoflagellates (Dinophyceae) from Rarotonga, Cook Islands. *Toxicon*, 56, 751–758.

305. Nézan, E. and Chomérat, N. 2011. *Vulcanodinium rugosum* gen. et sp. nov. (Dinophyceae), un nouveau dinoflagellé marin de la côte méditerranéenne française. *Cryptogamie Algol*, 32, 3–18.

306. Grzebyk, D. and Sako, Y. 1998. Phylogenetic analysis of nine species of *Prorocentrum* (Dinophyceae) inferred from 18S ribosomal ADN sequences, morphological comparisons, and description of *Prorocentrum panamensis*, sp. nov. *J Phycol*, 34, 1055–1068.

307. Cortés-Altamirano, R. and Sierra-Beltrán, A. P. 2003. Morphology and taxonomy of *Prorocentrum mexicanum* and reinstatement of *Prorocentrum rhathymum* (Dinophyceae). *J Phycol*, 39, 221–225.

308. Faust, M. A. and Gulledge, R. A. 2002. Identifying harmful marine dinoflagellates. *Contrib US Nat Herb*, 42, 1–144.

309. Velikova, V. and Larsen, J. 1999. The *Prorocentrum cordatum/Prorocentrum minimum* taxonomic problem. *Grana*, 38, 108–112.

310. Hallegraeff, G. M. 2003. Taxonomic principles. In *Manual on Harmful Marine Microalgae*, eds. G. M. Hallegraeff, D. M. Anderson, and A. D. Cembella, pp. 383–432. Paris, France: UNESCO Publishing.

311. Hoppenrath, M., Elbrächter, M., and Drebes, G. 2009. *Marine Phytoplankton*. Kleine Senckenberg-Reihe 49. E. Stuttgart, Germany: Schweizerbart Science Publishers, 264pp.

312. Throndsen, J., Hasle, G. R., and Tangen, K. 2007. *Phytoplankton of Norwegian Coastal Waters*. Oslo, Norway: Almater Forlag AS, 343pp.

313. Hallegraeff, G. M., Bolch, C. J. S., Huisman, J. M. et al. 2010. Planktonic dinoflagellates. In *Algae of Australia: Phytoplankton of Temperate Coastal Waters*, eds. G. M. Hallegraeff, C. J. S. Bolch, D. R. A. Hill et al., pp. 145–212. Melbourne, Victoria, Australia: CSIRO Publishing.

314. Henrichs, D. W., Scott, P. S., Steidinger, K. A. et al. 2013. Morphology and phylogeny of *Prorocentrum texanum* sp. nov. (Dinophyceae): A new toxic dinoflagellate from the Gulf of Mexico coastal waters exhibiting two distinct morphologies. *J Phycol*, 49, 143–155.

315. Chomérat, N., Saburova, M., Bilien, G. et al. 2012. *Prorocentrum bimaculatum* sp. nov. (Dinophyceae, Prorocentrales), a new benthic dinoflagellate species from Kuwait (Arabian Gulf). *J Phycol*, 48, 211–221.

316. Bravo, I., Fernandez, M. L., and Martinez, R. A. 2001. Toxin composition of the toxic dinoflagellate *Prorocentrum lima* isolated from different locations along the Galician coast (NW Spain). *Toxicon*, 39, 1537–1545.

317. Bjornland, T. and Tangen, K. 1979. Pigmentation and morphology of a marine *Gyrodinium* (dinophyceae) with a major carotenoid different from peridinin and fucoxanthin. *J Phycol*, 15, 457–463.

318. Bjørnland, T., Borch, G., and Liaaen-Jensen, S. 1984. Configurational studies on red algal carotenoids. *Phytochemistry*, 23, 1711–1715.

319. de Salas, M. F., Bolch, C. J. S., Botes, L. et al. 2003. *Takayama* (Gymnodiniales, Dinophyceae) gen. nov., a new genus of unarmoured dinoflagellates with sigmoid apical grooves, including the description of two new species. *J Phycol*, 39, 1233–1246.

320. Yang, Z. B., Takayama, H., Matsuoka, K. et al. 2000. *Karenia digitata* sp. nov. (Gymnodiniales, Dinophyceae), a new harmful algal bloom species from the coastal waters of West Japan and Hong Kong. *Phycologia*, 39, 463–470.

321. Yang, Z. B., Hodgkiss, I. J., and Hansen, G. 2001. *Karenia longicanalis* sp. nov. (Dinophyceae): A new bloom-forming species isolated from Hong Kong, May 1998. *Bot Mar*, 44, 67–74.

322. de Salas, M. F., Bolch, C. J. S., and Hallengraeff, G. M. 2004. *Karenia asterichroma* sp. no. (Gymnodiniales, Dinophyceae), a new dinoflagellate species associated with finfish aquaculture mortalities in Tasmania, Australia. *Phycologia*, 43, 624–631.

323. Bergholtz, T., Daugbjerg, N., and Moestrup, Ø. 2005. On the identity of *Karlodinium veneficum* and description of *Karlodinium armiger* sp. nov. (Dinophyceae), based on light and electron microscopy, nuclear-encoded LSU rDNA, and pigment composition. *J Phycol*, 42, 170–193.

324. Oda, M. 1935. *Gymnodinium mikimotoi* Miyake et Kominami n. sp. (MS.) no akashiwo to ryusando no koka. (The red tide of *Gymnodinium mikimotoi* Miyake et Kominami and the influence of copper sulfate on the red tide of November 1972). *Zool Mag*, 47, 35–48.

325. Davis, C. C. 1948. *Gymnodinium brevis* sp. nov., a cause of discolored water and animal mortality in the Gulf of Mexico. *Bot Gaz*, 109, 358–360.

326. Gunter, G., Williams, R. H., Davis, C. C. et al. 1948. Catastrophic mass mortality of marine animals and coincident phytoplankton bloom on the west coast of Florida, November 1946–August 1947. *Ecol Monogr*, 18, 309–324.

327. Woodcock, A. H. 1948. Note concerning human respiratory irritation associated with high concentrations of plankton and mass mortality of marine organisms. *J Mar Res*, 2, 56–62.

328. Brand, L. E., Campbell, L., and Bresnan, E. 2012. *Karenia*: The biology and ecology of a toxic genus. *Harmful Algae*, 14, 156–178.

329. Chang, F. H. 1999. *Gymnodinium brevisulcatum* sp. nov. (Gymnodiniales, Dinophyceae), a new species isolated from the 1998 summer toxic bloom in Wellington Harbour, New Zealand. *Phycologia*, 38, 337–384.

330. Hansen, G., Daugbjerg, N., and Henriksen, P. 2000. Comparative study of *Gymnodinium mikimotoi* and *Gymnodinium aureolum*, comb. nov. (= *Gyrodinium aureolum*) based on morphology, pigment composition, and molecular data. *J Phycol*, 36, 394–410.

331. Steidinger, K. A., Landsberg, J. H., Flewelling, L. J. et al. 2008. Toxic dinoflagellates. In *Oceans and Human Health*, eds. P. J. Walsh, S. L. Smith, L. E. Fleming et al., pp. 239–256. New York: Academic Press.

332. Botes, L., Sym, S. D., and Pitcher, G. C. 2003. *Karenia cristata* sp. nov. and *Karenia bicuneiformis* sp. nov. (Gymnodiniales, Dinophyceae): Two new *Karenia* species of the South African coast. *Phycologia*, 42, 563–571.

333. Haywood, A. J., Steidinger, K. A., and Truby, E. W. 2004. Comparative morphology and molecular phylogenetic analysis of three new species of the genus *Karenia* (Dinophyceae) from New Zealand. *J Phycol*, 40, 165–179.

334. Heil, C. A., Glibert, P. M., Al-Sarawi, M. A. et al. 2001. First record of a fish-killing *Gymnodinium* sp. bloom in Kuwait Bay, Arabian Sea: Chronology and potential causes. *Mar Ecol Prog Ser*, 214, 15–23.

335. Chang, F. H. and Ryan, K. G. 2004. *Karenia concordia* sp. nov. (Gymnodiniales, Dinophyceae), a new nonthecate dinoflagellate isolated from the New Zealand northeast coast during the 2002 harmful algal bloom events. *Phycologia*, 43, 552–562.

336. de Salas, M. F., Bolch, C. J. S., and Hallengraeff, G. M. 2004. *Karenia umbella* sp. nov. (Gymnodiniales, Dinophyceae), a new potentially ichthyotoxic dinoflagellate species from Tasmania, Australia. *Phycologia*, 43, 166–175.

337. Ballantine, D. 1956. Two new marine species of *Gymnodinium* isolated from the Plymouth area. *J Mar Biol Assoc UK*, 35, 467–474.

338. Bachvaroff, T. R., Adolf, J. E., and Place, A. R. 2009. Strain variation in *Karlodinium veneficum* (Dinophyceae): Toxin profiles, pigments, and growth characteristics. *J Phycol*, 45, 137–153.

339. de Salas, M. F., Rhodes, L. L., MacKenzie, L. A. et al. 2005. Gymnodinoid genera *Karenia* and *Takayama* (Dinophyceae) in New Zealand coastal waters. *N Z J Mar Freshwat Res*, 39, 135–139.

340. Place, A. R., Bowers, H. A., Bachvaroff, T. R. et al. 2012. *Karlodinium veneficum*—The little dinoflagellate with a big bite. *Harmful Algae*, 14, 179–195.

341. Carrada, G. C., Ceccherelli, V. V., and Eerrari, L. 1987. Iles lagunes italiennes. *Bull Ecol*, 18, 149–158.

342. Zingone, A., Siano, R., D'Alelio, D. et al. 2006. Potentially toxic and harmful microalgae from coastal waters of the Campania region (Tyrrhenian Sea, Mediterranean Sea). *Harmful Algae*, 5, 321–337.

344. Kudela, R. M. and Gobler, C. J. 2012. Harmful dinoflagellate blooms caused by *Cochlodinium* sp.: Global expansion and ecological strategies facilitating bloom formation. *Harmful Algae*, 14, 71–86.

345. Guiry, M. D. and Guiry, G. M. 2011. AlgaeBase. World-wide Electronic Publication. National University of Ireland, Galway. http://www.algaebase.org.

346. Okamura, K. 1916. Akashio ni Tsuite. (On red-tides). *Suisan Koushu Sikenjo Kenkyu Hokoku*, 12, 26–41.

347. Silva, E. S. 1967. *Cochlodinium heterolobactum* n. sp.: Structure and some cytophysiological aspects. *J Protozool*, 14, 745–754.

348. Iwataki, M., Kawami, H., and Matsuoka, K. 2007. *Cochlodinium fulvescens* sp. nov. (Gymnodiniales, Dinophyceae), a new chain-forming unarmored dinoflagellate from Asian coasts. *Phycol Res*, 55, 231–239.

349. Matsuoka, K., Iwataki, M., and Kawami, H. 2008. Morphology and taxonomy of chainforming species of the genus *Cochlodinium* (Dinophyceae). *Harmful Algae*, 7, 261–270.

350. Kobayashi, J. 2008. Amphidinolides and its related macrolides from marine dinoflagellates. *J Antibiot*, 61, 271–284.

351. Kobayashi, J. and Tsuda, M. 2004. Amphidinolides, bioactive macrolides from symbiotic marine dinoflagellates. *Nat Prod Rep*, 21, 77–93.

352. Murray, S. A., Garby, T., Hoppenrath, M. et al. 2012. Genetic diversity, morphological uniformity and polyketide production in dinoflagellates (*Amphidinium*, Dinoflagellata). *PLoS ONE*, 7, e38253. doi: 10.1371/journal.pone.0038253.

353. Garcés, E., Vila, M., Masó, M. et al. 2005. Taxon-specific analysis of growth and mortality rates of harmful dinoflagellates during bloom conditions. *Mar Ecol Prog Ser*, 301, 67–79.

354. Popovich, C. A., Spetter, C. V., Marcovecchio, J. E. et al. 2008. Dissolved nutrient availability during winter diatom bloom in a turbid and shallow estuary (Bahía Blanca, Argentina). *J Coastal Res*, 24, 95–102.

355. Hallegraeff, G. M. 1993. A review of harmful algal blooms and their apparent global increase. *Phycologia*, 32, 79–99.

356. Hwang, D. F. and Lu, Y. H. 2000. Influence of environmental and nutritional factors on growth, toxicity, and toxin profile of dinoflagellate *Alexandrium minutum*. *Toxicon*, 38, 1491–1503.

357. Yentsch, C. S., Lapointe, B. E., Poulton, N. et al. 2008. Anatomy of a red tide bloom off the southwest coast of Florida. *Harmful Algae*, 7, 817–826.

358. Irigoien, X., Flynn, K. J., and Harris, R. P. 2005. Phytoplankton blooms: A "loophole" in microzooplankton grazing impact? *J Plankton Res*, 27, 313–321.

359. Spilling, K. 2007. Dense sub-ice bloom of dinoflagellates in the Baltic Sea, potentially limited by high pH. *J Plankton Res*, 29, 895–901.

360. Wear, R. G. and Gardner, J. P. A. 2001. Biological effects of the toxic algal bloom of February and March 1998 on the benthos of Wellington Harbour, New Zealand. *Mar Ecol Prog Ser*, 218, 63–76.

361. Tang, Y. Z. and Gobler, C. J. 2009. Characterization of the toxicity of *Cochlodinium polykrikoides* isolates from Northeast US estuaries to finfish and shellfish. *Harmful Algae*, 8, 454–462.

362. Van Dolah, F. M. 2000. Marine algal toxins: Origins, health effects, and their increased occurrence. *Environ Health Perspect*, 108, 133–141.

363. Smayda, T. J. 1990. Novel and nuisance phytoplankton blooms in the sea: Evidence for a global epidemic. In *Toxic Marine Phytoplankton*, eds. E. Granéli, B. Sundström, L. Edler et al., pp. 29–40. New York: Elsevier.

364. Nagai, S., Lian, C., Yamaguchi, S. et al. 2007. Microsatellite markers reveal population genetic structure of the toxic dinoflagellate *Alexandrium tamarense* (Dinophyceae) in Japanese coastal waters. *J Phycol*, 43, 43–54.

365. Leung, K. M. Y. and Dudgeon, D. 2008. Ecological risk assessment and management of exotic organisms associated with aquaculture activities. In *Understanding and Applying Risk Analysis in Aquaculture*, eds. M. G. Bonand-Reantaso, J. R. Arthur, and R. P. Subasinghe, pp. 67–100. Rome, Italy: FAO.

366. Hinder, S. L., Hays, G. C., Edwards, M. et al. 2012. Changes in marine dinoflagellates and diatom abundance under climate change. *Nat Clim Change*, 2, 271–275.

367. Sournia, A. 1995. Red tide and toxic marine phytoplankton of the world ocean: An inquiry into biodiversity. In *Harmful Marine Algal Blooms*, eds. P. Lassus, G. Arzul, E. Erand et al., pp. 103–112. Paris, France: Lavoisier, Intercept Ltd.

368. Zingone, A. and Enevoldsen, H. O. 2000. The diversity of harmful algal blooms: A challenge for science and management. *Ocean Coast Manage*, 43, 725–748.

369. Shumway, S. E. 1989. Toxic algae: A serious threat to shellfish aquaculture. *World Aquacult*, 20, 65–74.

370. Lehane, L. and Lewis, R. J. 2000. Ciguatera: Recent advances but the risk remains. *Int J Food Microbiol*, 61, 91–125.

371. Yasumoto, T., Murata, M., Lee, J. S. et al. 1989. Polyether toxins produced by dinoflagellates. In *Mycotoxins and Phycotoxins '88*, eds. S. Natori, K. Hashimoto, and Y. Ueno, pp. 375–382. Amsterdam, the Netherlands: Elsevier.

372. Daranas, A. H., Norte, M., and Fernández, J. J. 2001. Toxic marine microalgae. *Toxicon*, 39, 1101–1132.

373. Cembella, A. D. 2003. Chemical ecology of eukaryotic microalgae in marine ecosystems. *Phycologia*, 42, 420–447.

374. Fusetani, N. and Kem, W. 2009. Marine toxins: An overview. In *Marine Toxins as Research Tools*, *Progress in Molecular and Subcellular Biology*, *Marine Molecular Biotechnology*, eds. N. Fusetani and W. Kem, Vol. 46, pp. 1–44. Berlin, Germany: Springer-Verlag.

375. Prakash, A. and Taylor, F. J. R. 1966. A "red water" bloom of *Gonyaulax acatenella* in the strait of Geogia and its relation to paralytic shellfish toxicity. *J Fish Res Board Can*, 23, 1265–1270.

376. Ciminiello, P., Fattorusso, E., Fiorino, M. et al. 2000. Saxitoxin and neosaxitoxin as toxic principles of *Alexandrium andersoni* (Dinophyceae) from the Gulf of Naples, Italy. *Toxicon*, 38, 1871–1877.

377. Frangópulos, M., Guisande, C., DeBlas, E. et al. 2004. Toxin production and competitive abilities under phosphorus limitation of *Alexandrium* species. *Harmful Algae*, 3, 131–139.

378. Prakash, A., Medcof, J. C., and Tennant, A. D. 1971. Paralytic shellfish poisoning in eastern Canada. *J Fish Res Board Can*, 177, 1–87.

379. Fukuyo, Y. 1985. Morphology of *Protogonyaulax tamarensis* (Lebour) and *Protogonyaulax catenella* (Whedon and Kofoid) Taylor from Japanese coastal waters. *Bull Mar Sci*, 37, 533–534.

380. Fukuyo, Y., Yoshida, K., and Inoue, H. 1985. *Protogonyaulax* in Japanese coastal waters. In *Toxic Dinoflagellates*, eds. D. M. Anderson, A. W. White, and D. G. Baden, pp. 27–32. Amsterdam, the Netherlands: Elsevier.

381. Ogata, T. and Kodama, M. 1986. Ichthyotoxicity found in cultured media of *Protogonyaulax* spp. *Mar Biol*, 92, 31–34.

382. Oshima, Y., Hirota, M., Yasumoto, T. et al. 1989. Production of paralytic shellfish toxins by the dinoflagellate *Alexandrium minutum* Halim from Australia. *Nippon Suisan Gakk*, 55, 925.

383. Parker, N. S., Negri, A. P., and Frampton, D. M. F. 2002. Growth of the toxic dinoflagellate *Alexandrium minutum* (Dinophyceae) using high biomass culture systems. *J Appl Phycol*, 14, 313–324.

384. Gates, J. A. and Wilson, W. B. 1960. The toxicity of *Gonyaulax monilata* Howell to *Mugil cephalus*. *Limnol Oceanogr*, 5, 171–174.

385. Ray, S. M. and Aldrich, D. V. 1967. Ecological interactions of toxic dinoflagellates and molluscs in the Gulf of Mexico. In *Animal Toxins*, eds. F. E. Russell and P. R. Saunders, pp. 75–83. *First International Symposium on Animal Toxins*. New York: Pergamon Press.

386. Schmidt, R. J. and Loeblich, A. R. 1979. Distribution of paralytic shellfish poison among Pyrrhophyta. *J Mar Biol Assoc UK*, 59, 479–487.

387. Clemons, G. P., Pinion, J. P., Bass, E. et al. 1980. A hemolytic principle associated with the red-tide dinoflagellate *Gonyaulax monilata*. *Toxicon*, 18, 323.

388. Cembella, A. D., Lewis, N. I., and Quilliam, M. A. 2000. The marine dinoflagellate *Alexandrium ostenfeldii* (Dinophyceae) as the causative organism of spirolide shellfish toxins. *Phycologia*, 39, 67–74.

389. Franco, J. M., Paz, B., Riobo, R. et al. 2006. First report of the production of spirolides by *Alexandrium peruvianum* (Dinophyceae) from the Mediterranean Sea. In *12th International Conference on Harmful Algae Programme and Abstracts*, pp. 174–175. Copenhagen, Denmark: ISSHA.

390. Murakami, M., Makabe, K., and Yamaguchi, K. 1988. Goniodomin A, a novel polyether macrolide from the dinoflagellate *Goniodoma pseudogoniaulax*. *Tetrahed Lett*, 29, 1149–1152.

391. Larsen, J. and Moestrup, Ø. 1989. *Guide to Toxic and Potentially Toxic Marine Algae*. Copenhagen, Denmark: The Fish Inspection Service, Ministry of Fisheries, 61pp.

392. Shimizu, Y., Alam, M., Oshima, Y. et al. 1975. Presence of four toxins in red tide infested clams and cultured *Gonyaulax tamarensis* cells. *Biochem Biophys Res Commun*, 66, 731–737.

393. Oshima, Y., Buckley, L. J., Alam, M. et al. 1977. Heterogeneity of paralytic shellfish poisons. Three new toxins from cultured *Gonyaulax tamarensis* cells, *Mya arenaria* and *Saxidomus giganteus*. *Comp Biochem Physiol*, 57, 31–34.

394. Fukuyo, Y., Yoshida, K., Ogata, T. et al. 1989. Suspected causative dinoflagellates of paralytic shellfish poisoning in the Gulf of Thailand. In *Red Tides: Biology, Environmental Science and Toxicology*, eds. T. Okachi, D. M. Anderson, and T. Nemoto, pp. 403–406. New York: Elsevier.

395. Kodama, M., Ogata, T., Fukuyo, Y. et al. 1988. *Protogonyaulax cohorticula*, a toxic dinoflagellate found in the Gulf of Thailand. *Toxicon*, 26, 709–712.

396. Menezes, M., Varela, D., de Oliveira Troença, L. A. et al. 2010. Identification of the toxic algae *Alexandrium tamiyavanichi* (Dinophyceae) from Northeastern Brazil: A combined morphological and rDNA sequence (partial LSU and ITS) approach. *J Phycol*, 46, 1239–1251.

397. Nakajima, I., Ochima, Y., and Yasumoto, T. 1981. Toxicity of dinoflagellates in Okinawa. *Bull Jpn Soc Sci Fish*, 47, 1029–1033.

398. Murata, M., Legrand, A. M., and Ishibashi, Y. 1990. Structures and configurations of ciguatoxin from the moray eel *Gymnothorax javanicus* and its likely precursor from the dinoflagellate *Gambierdiscus toxicus*. *J Am Chem Soc*, 112, 4380–4386.

399. Yasumoto, T., Nakijama, I., and Bagnis, R. 1977. Finding of a dinoflagellate as a likely culprit of ciguatera. *Bull Jpn Soc Sci Fish*, 43, 1021–1026.

400. Yasumoto, T., Seino, N., Murakami, Y. et al. 1987. Toxins produced by benthic dinoflagellates. *Biol Bull*, 172, 128–131.

401. Yasumoto, T., Satake, M., Fukui, M. et al. 1993. A turning point in ciguatera study. In *Toxic Phytoplankton in the Sea Smayda*, eds. T. J. Shimizu and Y. Shimizu, pp. 455–461. Amsterdam, the Netherlands: Elsevier.

402. Yokoyama, A., Murata, M., Oshima, Y. et al. 1988. Some chemical properties of maitotoxin: A putative calcium channel agonist isolated from a marine dinoflagellate. *J Biochem*, 104, 184–187.

403. Bruno, M., Gucci, P. M. B., Pierdominici, E. et al. 1990. Presence of saxitoxin in toxic extracts from *Gonyaulax polyedra*. *Toxicon*, 28, 1113–1116.

404. Tindall, D. R., Miller, D. M., and Tindall, P. M. 1990. Toxicity of *Ostreopsis lenticularis* from the British and United States Virgin Islands. In *Toxic Marine Phytoplankton*, eds. E. Graneli, B. Sundstrom, L. Edler et al., pp. 424–429. New York: Elsevier.

405. Ballantine, D. L., Tosteson, T. R., Durst, H. D. et al. 1988. Population dynamics and toxicity of natural populations of benthic dinoflagellates in southwest Puerto Rico. *J Exp Mar Biol Ecol*, 119, 210–212.

406. Lenoir, S., Ten-Hage, L., Turquet, J. et al. 2004. First evidence of palytoxin analogues from an *Ostreopsis mascarenensis* (Dinophyceae) benthic bloom in Southwestern Indian Ocean. *J Phycol*, 40, 1042–1051.

407. Ciminiello, P., Dell'Aversano, C., Dello Iacovo, E. et al. 2012. Isolation and structure elucidation of ovatoxin-a, the major toxin produced by *Ostreopsis ovata. J Am Chem Soc*, 134, 1869–1875.
408. Usami, M., Satake, M., Ishida, S. et al. 1995. Palytoxin analogs from the dinoflagellate *Ostreopsis siamensis. J Am Chem Soc*, 177, 5389–5390.
409. Satake, M., MacKenzie, L., and Yasumoto, T. 1997. Identification of *Protoceratium reticulatum* as biogenetic origin of yessotoxin. *Nat Toxins*, 5, 164–167.
410. Satake, M., Ichimura, T., Sekiguchi, K. et al. 1999. Confirmation of yessotoxin and 45,46,47-trinoryessotoxin production by *Protoceratium reticulatum* in Japan. *Nat Toxins*, 7, 147–150.
411. Ciminiello, P., Dell'Aversano, C., Fattorusso, E. et al. 2003. Complex yessotoxins profile in *Protoceratium reticulatum* from north-western Adriatic Sea revealed by LC–MS analysis. *Toxicon*, 42, 7–14.
412. Usup, G., Kulis, D. M., and Anderson, D. M. 1994. Growth and toxin production of the toxic dinoflagellate *Pyrodinium bahamense* var. compressum in laboratory cultures. *Nat Toxins*, 2, 254–262.
413. Hummert, C., Ritscher, M., Reinhardt, R. et al. 1997. Analysis of the characteristic PSP profiles of *Pyrodinium bahamense* and several strains of *Alexandrium* by HPLC based on ion-pair chromatographic separation, post-column oxidation, and fluorescence detection. *Chromatographia*, 45, 312–316.
414. Montojo, U. M., Sakamoto, S., Cayme, M. F. et al. 2006. Remarkable difference in toxin accumulation of paralytic shellfish poisoning toxins among bivalve species exposed to *Pyrodinium bahamense* var. *compressum* bloom in Masinloc bay, Philippines. *Toxicon*, 48, 85–92.
415. Gedaria, A. I., Luckas, B., Reinhardtb, K. et al. 2007. Growth response and toxin concentration of cultured *Pyrodinium bahamense* var. *compressum* to varying salinity and temperature conditions. *Toxicon*, 50, 518–529.
416. Cembella, A. D. 1989. Occurrence of okadaic acid, a major diarrheic shellfish toxin, in natural populations of *Dinophysis* spp. from the eastern coast of North America. *J Appl Phycol*, 1, 307–310.
417. Kat, M. 1985. *Dinophysis acuminata* blooms, the distinct cause of Dutch mussel poisoning. In *Toxic Dinoflagellates*, eds. D. M. Anderson, A. W. White, and D. G. Baden, pp. 73–78. New York: Elsevier.
418. Miles, C. O., Wilkins, A. L., and Jensen, D. J. 2004. Isolation of 41a-homoyessotoxin and the identification of 9-methyl-41ahomoyessotoxin and Nor-ring A-yessotoxin from *Protoceratium reticulatum. Chem Res Toxicol*, 17, 1414–1422.
419. Yasumoto, T. 1990. Marine microorganisms toxins—An overview. In *Toxic Marine Phytoplankton*, eds. E. Graneli, B. Sundström, L. Edler et al., pp. 3–8. New York: Elsevier.
420. Fernández Puente, P., Fidalgo Sáez, M. J., and Hamilton, B. 2004. Studies of polyether toxins in the marine phytoplankton, *Dinophysis acuta*, in Ireland using multiple tandem mass spectrometry. *Toxicon*, 44, 919–926.
421. MacKenzie, L., Beuzenberg, V., Holland, P. et al. 2005. Pectenotoxin and okadaic acid-based toxin profiles in *Dinophysis acuta* and *Dinophysis acuminata* from New Zealand. *Harmful Algae*, 4, 75–85.
422. Pizarro, G., Paz, B., González-Gil, S. et al. 2009. Seasonal variability of lipophilic toxins during a *Dinophysis acuta* bloom in Western Iberia: Differences between picked cells and plankton concentrates. *Harmful Algae*, 8, 926–937.
423. Nielsen, L. T., Krock, B., and Hansen, P. J. 2013. Production and excretion of okadaic acid, pectenotoxin-2 and a novel dinophysistoxin from the DSP-causing marine dinoflagellate *Dinophysis acuta*—Effects of light, food availability and growth phase. *Harmful Algae*, 23, 34–45.
424. Okaichi, T. 1967. Red tides found in and around the Seto Inland Sea in 1965. *Tech Bull Fac Agric Kagawa Univ*, 15, 181–185.
425. Marasigan, A. N., Sato, S., Fukuyo, Y. et al. 2001. Accumulation of a high level of diarrhetic shellfish toxins in the green mussel *Perna viridis* during a bloom of *Dinophysis caudata* and *Dinophysis miles* in Saipan Bay, Panay Island, the Philippines. *Fisheries Sci*, 67, 994–996.
426. Fernández, M. L., Reguera, B., Ramilo, I. et al. 2001. Toxin content of *Dinophysis acuminata, D. acuta*, and *D. caudata* from the Galician Rias Bajas. In *Harmful Algal Blooms 2000*, eds. G. M. Hallegraeff, S. I. Blackburn, C. J. Bolch et al., pp. 360–363. Paris, France: Intergovernmental Oceanographic Commission of UNESCO.
427. Fernandez, M. L., Reguera, B., Gonzales-Gil, S. et al. 2006. Pectenotoxin-2 in single-cell isolates of *Dinophysis caudata* and *Dinophysis acuta* from the Galician Rìas (NW Spain). *Toxicon*, 48, 477–490.
428. Papaefthimiou, D., Aligizaki, K., and Nikolaidis, G. 2010. Exploring the identity of the Greek *Dinophysis* cf. *acuminata. Harmful Algae*, 10, 1–8.

429. Fux, E., Smith, J. L., Tong, M. et al. 2011. Toxin profiles of five geographical isolates of *Dinophysis* spp. from North and South America. *Toxicon*, 57, 275–287.

430. Masselin, P., Lassus, P., and Bardouil, M. 1992. High-performance liquid-chromatography analysis of diarrhetic toxins in *Dinophysis* spp. from the French Coast. *J Appl Phycol*, 4, 385–389.

431. Giacobbe, M. G., Oliva, F., and La Ferla, R. 1995. Potentially toxic dinoflagellates in Mediterranean waters (Sicily) and related hydrobiological conditions. *Aquat Microb Ecol*, 9, 63–68.

432. Delgado, M., Garces, E., and Camp, J. 1996. Growth and behavior of *Dinophysis sacculus* from NW Mediterranean. In *Harmful and Toxic Algal Blooms*, eds. T. Yasumoto, Y. Oshima, and Y. Fukuyo, pp. 261–264. Paris, France: IOC UNESCO.

433. Rodríguez, F., Escalera, L., Reguera, B. et al. 2012. Morphological variability, toxinology and genetics of the dinoflagellate *Dinophysis tripos* (Dinophysiaceae, Dinophysiales). *Harmful Algae*, 13, 26–33.

434. Burkholder, J. M. and Marshall, H. G. 2012. Toxigenic *Pfiesteria* species—Updates on biology, ecology, toxins, and impacts. *Harmful Algae*, 14, 196–230.

435. Twiner, M. J., Rehmann, N., Hess, P. et al. 2008. Azaspiracid shellfish poisoning: A review on the chemistry, ecology, and toxicology with emphasis on human health impacts. *Mar Drugs*, 6, 39–72.

436. Morton, S. L., Moeller, P. D. R., Young, K. A. et al. 1998. Okadaic acid production from the marine dinoflagellate *Prorocentrum belizeanum* isolated from the Belizean coral reef ecosystems. *Toxicon*, 36, 201–206.

437. Tindall, D. R., Dickey, R. W., Carlson, R. D. et al. 1984. Ciguatoxigenic dinoflagellates from the Caribbean Sea. In *Seafood Toxins*, ed. E. P. Ragelis. *Am Chem Soc Symp Ser*, 262, 225–240.

438. Tindall, D. R., Miller, D. M., and Bomber, J. W. 1989. Culture and toxicity of dinoflagellates from ciguatera endemic regions of the world. *Toxicon*, 27, 83.

439. Dickey, R. W., Bobzin, S. C., Faulkner, D. J. et al. 1990. Identification of okadaic acid from a Caribbean dinoflagellate, *Prorocentrum concavum*. *Toxicon*, 28, 371–377.

440. Hu, T., deFreitas, A. S. W., Doyle, J. et al. 1993. New DSP toxin derivatives isolated from toxic mussels and the dinoflagellates, *Prorocentrum lima* and *Prorocentrum concavum*. In *Toxic Phytoplankton Blooms in the Sea*, eds. T. J. Smayda and Y. Shimizu, pp. 507–512. Amsterdam, the Netherlands: Elsevier.

441. Morton, S. L. 1998. Morphology and toxicology of *Prorocentrum faustiae* sp. nov., a toxic species of non-planktonic dinoflagellate from Heron Island, Australia. *Bot Mar*, 41, 565–569.

442. Aikman, K. E., Tindall, D. R., and Morton, S. L. 1993. Physiology and potency of the dinoflagellate *Prorocentrum hoffmannianum* during one complete growth cycle. In *Toxic Phytoplankton Blooms in the Sea*, eds. T. Smayda and Y. Shimizu, pp. 463–668. Amsterdam, the Netherlands: Elsevier.

443. Morton, S. L. and Bomber, J. W. 1994. Maximizing okadaic acid content from *Prorocentrum hoffmannianum* Faust. *J Appl Phycol*, 6, 41–44.

444. Morton, S. L., Bomber, J. W., and Tindall, P. M. 1994. Environmental effects on the production of okadaic acid from *Prorocentrum hoffmannianum* Faust. I. Temperature, light, and salinity. *J Exp Mar Biol Ecol*, 178, 67–77.

445. Hu, T., Doyle, J., Jackson, D. et al. 1992. Isolation of a new diarrhetic shellfish poison from Irish mussels. *J Chem Soc Chem Commun*, 21, 39–41.

446. James, K. J., Carmody, E. P., Gillman, M. et al. 1997. Identification of a new diarrhoeic toxin in shellfish using liquid chromatography with fluorimetric and mass spectrometric detection. *Toxicon*, 35, 973–978.

447. Quilliam, M. A. and Ross, N. W. 1996. Analysis of diarrhetic shellfish poisoning toxins and metabolites in plankton and shellfish by liquid chromatography-ionspray mass spectrometry. In *Biochemical and Biotechnological Applications of Electrospray Ionization Mass Spectrometry*, ed. A. P. Snyder, pp. 351–364. Washington, DC: American Chemical Society.

448. Nascimento, S. M., Purdie, D. A., and Morris, S. 2005. Morphology, toxin composition and pigment content of *Prorocentrum lima* strains isolated from a coastal lagoon in southern UK. *Toxicon*, 45, 633–649.

448. Rossi, S. and Fiorillo, A. 2010. Biochemical features of a *Protoceratium reticulatum* red tide in Chipana Bay (northern Chile) in summer conditions. *Sci Mar*, 74, 633–642.

449. Hu, T., de Freitas, A. S. W., Curtis, J. M. et al. 1996. Isolation and structure of prorocentrolide B, a fast-acting toxin from *Prorocentrum maculosum*. *J Nat Prod*, 59, 1010–1014.

450. Steidinger, K. A. 1983. A re-evaluation of toxic dinoflagellate biology and ecology. *Prog Phycol Res*, 2, 147–188.

451. Carlson, R. D. 1984. Distribution, periodicity and culture of benthic/epiphytic dinoflagellates in a ciguatera endemic region of the Caribbean. PhD thesis, Southern Illinois University, Carbondale, IL, 308pp.

452. Carlson, R. D. and Tindall, D. R. 1985. Distribution and periodicity of toxic dinoflagellates in the Virgin Islands. In *Toxic Dinoflagellates*, eds. D. M. Anderson, A. W. White, and D. G. Baden, pp. 171–176. Amsterdam, the Netherlands: Elsevier.

453. Nakazima, M. 1965. Studies on the source of shellfish poison in Lake Hamana. I. Relation of the abundance of a species of dinoflagellate *Prorocentrum* sp. to shellfish toxicity. *Bull Jpn Soc Sci Fish*, 31, 198–203.

454. Nakazima, M. 1968. Studies on the source of shellfish poison in Lake Hamana-IV. Identification and collection of the noxious dinoflagellate. *Bull Jpn Soc Sci Fish*, 34, 130–132.

455. Smith, G. B. 1975. Phytoplankton blooms and reef kills in the mid-eastern Gulf of Mexico. *Florida Mar Res Publ*, 8, 8.

456. Okaichi, T. and Imatomi, Y. 1979. Toxicity of *Prorocentrum minimum* var. mariae-lebouriae assumed to be a causative agent of short-necked clam poisoning. In *Toxic Dinoflagellate Blooms*, eds. D. L. Taylor and H. H. Seliger, pp. 385–388. New York: Elsevier.

457. Tangen, K. 1983. Shellfish poisoning and the occurrence of potentially toxic dinoflagellates in Norwegian waters. *Sarsia*, 68, 1–7.

458. Shimizu, Y. 1987. Dinoflagellate toxins. In *The Biology of Dinoflagellates*, ed. F. J. R. Taylor, pp. 282–315. Boston, MA: Blackwell Scientific Publications.

459. Nayak, B. B., Karunasagar, I., and Karunasagar, I. 1997. Influence of bacteria on growth and hemolysin production by the marine dinoflagellate *Amphidinium carterae*. *Mar Biol*, 130, 35–39.

460. Bauer, I., Maranda, L., Shimizu, Y. et al. 1994. The structures of Amphidinolide B isomers: Strongly cytotoxic macrolides produced by a free-swimming dinoflagellate, *Amphidinium* sp. *J Am Chem Soc*, 116, 2657–2658.

461. Bauer, I., Maranda, L., Young, K. A. et al. 1995. Isolation and structure of Caribenolide I, a highly potent antitumour macrolide from a culture of the free swimming Caribbean dinoflagellate, *Amphidinium* sp. S1-36-5. *J Org Chem*, 60, 1084–1086.

462. Bauer, I., Maranda, L., Young, K. A. et al. 1995. The isolation and structures of unusual 1,4-polyketides from the dinoflagellate, *Amphidinium* sp. *Tetrahedron Lett*, 36, 991–994.

463. Anderson, D. M., Sullivan, J. J., and Reguera, B. 1989. Paralytic shell-fish poisoning in NW Spain: The toxicity of the dinoflagellate *Gymnodinium catenatum*. *Toxicon*, 27, 665–674.

464. Baden, D. G., Mende, T. J., and Block, R. E. 1979. Two similar toxins isolated from *Gymnodinium breve*. In *Toxic Dinoflagellate Blooms*, eds. D. L. Taylor and H. H. Seliger, pp. 327–334. New York: Elsevier.

465. Baden, D. G. 1989. Brevetoxins: Unique polyether dinoflagellate toxins. *FASEB J*, 3, 1807–1817.

466. Van Wagoner, R. M., Satake, M., Bourdelais, A. J. et al. 2010. Absolute configuration of brevisamide and brevisin: Confirmation of a universal biosynthetic process for *Karenia brevis* polyethers. *J Nat Prod*, 73, 1177–1179.

467. Bourdelais, A. J., Jacocks, H. M., Wright, J. L. C. et al. 2005. A new polyether ladder compound produced by the dinoflagellate *Karenia brevis*. *J Nat Prod*, 68, 2–6.

468. Neely, T. and Campbell, L. 2006. A modified assay to determine hemolytic toxin variability among *Karenia* clones isolated from the Gulf of Mexico. *Harmful Algae*, 5, 592–598.

469. Prince, E. K., Poulson, K. L., Myers, T. L. et al. 2010. Characterization of allelopathic compounds from the red tide dinoflagellate *Karenia brevis*. *Harmful Algae*, 10, 39–48.

470. Mooney, B. D., Nichols, P. D., de Salas, M. F. et al. 2007. Lipid, fatty acid and sterol composition of eight species of Kareniaceae (Dinophyta): Chemotaxonomy and putative lipid phycotoxins. *J Phycol*, 43, 101–111.

471. Chang, F. H., Uddstrom, M. J., Pinkerton, M. H. et al. 2008. Characterising the 2002 toxic *Karenia concordia* (Dinophyceae) outbreak and its development using satellite imagery on the north-eastern coast of New Zealand. *Harmful Algae*, 7, 532–544.

472. Satake, M., Shoji, M., Oshima, Y. et al. 2002. Gymnocin-A, a cytotoxic polyether from notorious red tide dinoflagellate, *Gymnodinium mikimotoi*. *Tetrahedron Lett*, 43, 5829–5832.

473. Satake, M., Tanaka, Y., Ishikura, Y. et al. 2005. Gymnocin-B with the largest contiguous polyether rings from the red tide dinoflagellate *Karenia* (formerly *Gymnodinium*) *mikimotoi*. *Tetrahedron Lett*, 46, 3537–3540.

474. Parrish, C. C., Bodennee, G., and Gentien, P. 1994. Time courses of intracellular and extracellular lipid classes in batch cultures of the toxic dinoflagellate *Gymnodinium* cf. *nagasakiense*. *Mar Chem*, 48, 71–82.

475. Miles, C. O., Wilkins, A. L., Stirling, D. J. et al. 2000. New analogue of gymnodimine from a *Gymnodinium* species. *J Agric Food Chem*, 48, 1373–1376.

476. Seki, T., Satake, M., Mackenzie, L. et al. 1995. Gymnodimine, a new marine toxin of unprecedented structure isolated from New Zealand oysters and the dinoflagellate, *Gymnodinium* sp. *Tetrahedron Lett*, 36, 7093–7096.

477. Lomas, M. W. and Glibert, P. M. 1999. Interactions between NH_4^+ and NO_3^- uptake and assimilation: Comparison of diatoms and dinoflagellates at several growth temperatures. *Mar Biol*, 133, 541–551.

478. Granéli, E., Vidyarathna, N. K., Funari, E. et al. 2011. Can increases in temperature stimulate blooms of the toxic benthic dinoflagellate *Ostreopsis ovata*? *Harmful Algae*, 10, 165–172.

479. Kamiyama, T., Nagai, S., and Suzuki, T. 2010. Effect of temperature on production of okadaic acid, dinophysistoxin-1, and pectenotoxin-2 by *Dinophysis acuminata* in culture experiments. *Aquat Microb Ecol*, 60, 193–202.

480. Tong, M., Kulis, D. M., Fux, E. et al. 2011. The effects of growth phase and light intensity on toxin production by *Dinophysis acuminata* from the northeastern United States. *Harmful Algae*, 10, 254–264.

481. Guerrini, F., Ciminiello, P., and Dell'Aversano, C. 2007. Influence of temperature, salinity and nutrient limitation on yessotoxin production and release by the dinoflagellate *Protoceratium reticulatum* in batch-cultures. *Harmful Algae*, 6, 707–717.

482. Bates, S. S., de Freitas, A. S. W., Milley, J. E. et al. 1991. Controls on domoic acid production by the diatom *Nitzschia pungens* f. multiseries in culture: Nutrients and irradiance. *Can J Fish Aquat Sci*, 48, 1136–1144.

483. Carneiro, R. L., dos Santos, M. E. V., Pacheco, A. B. F. et al. 2009. Effects of light intensity and light quality on growth and circadian rhythm of saxitoxins production in *Cylindrospermopsis raciborskii* (Cyanobacteria). *J Plankton Res*, 31, 481–488.

484. Parkhill, J. P. and Cembella, A. D. 1999. Effects of salinity, light and inorganic nitrogen on growth and toxigenicity of the marine dinoflagellate *Alexandrium tamarense* from northeastern Canada. *J Plankton Res*, 21, 939–955.

485. Paerl, H. W. and Scott, J. T. 2010. Throwing fuel on the fire: Synergistic effects of excessive nitrogen inputs and global climate change on harmful algal blooms. *Environ Sci Technol*, 44, 7756–7758.

486. Grzebyk, D. and Berland, B. 1996. Influences of abiotic factors on *Prorocentrum minimum* (Dinophyceae). *J Plankton Res*, 18, 1837–1849.

487. Grzebyk, D., Bechemin, C., and Ward, C. J. 2003. Effects of salinity and two coastal waters on the growth and toxin content of the dinoflagellate *Alexandrium minutum*. *J Plankton Res*, 25, 1185–1199.

488. Lim, P. T. and Ogata, T. 2005. Salinity effect on growth and toxin production of four tropical *Alexandrium* species (Dinophyceae). *Toxicon*, 45, 699–710.

489. White, A. W. 1978. Salinity effects on growth and toxin content of *Gonyaulax excavata*, a marine dinoflagellate causing paralytic shellfish poisoning. *J Phycol*, 14, 475–479.

490. Bomber, J. W., Guillard, R. L., and Nelson, W. G. 1988. Roles of temperature, salinity, and light in seasonality, growth, and toxicity of ciguatera-causing *Gambierdiscus toxicus* Adachi et Fukuyo (Dinophyceae). *J Exp Mar Biol*, 115, 53–65.

491. Roeder, K., Erler, K., Kibler, S. et al. 2010. Characteristic profiles of ciguatera toxins in different strains of *Gambierdiscus* spp. *Toxicon*, 56, 731–738.

492. Pistocchi, R., Pezzolesi, L., Guerrini, F. et al. 2011. A review on the effects of environmental conditions on growth and toxin production of *Ostreopsis ovata*. *Toxicon*, 57, 421–428.

493. Pezzolesi, L., Guerrini, F., Ciminiello, P. et al. 2012. Influence of temperature and salinity on *Ostreopsis* cf. *ovata* growth and evaluation of toxin content through HR LC-MS and biological assays. *Water Res*, 46, 82–92.

494. Taylor, F. J. R. 1987. Dinogagellate ecology: General and marine ecosystems. In *The Biology of Dinogagellates*, ed. F. J. R. Taylor, pp. 399–501. London, U.K.: Blackwell Scientific Publications.

495. Taylor, F. J. R. 2004. Harmful dinogagellate species in space and time and the value of morphospecies. In *Harmful Algae 2002*, eds. K. A. Steidinger, J. H. Landsberg, C. R. Tomas et al., pp. 555–559. St. Petersburg, FL: IOC UNESCO.

496. Taylor, F. J. R. 2001. Conference overview: Harmful algal bloom studies enter the new millenium. In *Harmful Algal Blooms 2000*, eds. G. M. Hallegraef, S. I. Blackburn, C. J. Bolch et al., pp. 3–5. Paris, France: IOC, UNESCO.

497. Sakshaug, E. and Jensen, A. 1971. *Gonyaulax tamarensis* and paralytic mussel toxicity in Trondheimsfjorden, 1963–1969. *K Norske Vidensk Selsk Skr*, 15, 1–15.
498. Sakshaug, E. 1972. Phytoplankton investigations in Trondheimsfjord, 1963–1966. *K Norske Vidensk Selsk Skr*, 1, 1–56.
499. Tangen, K. 1979. Dinoflagellate blooms in Norwegian waters. In *Toxic Dinoflagellate Blooms*, eds. D. L. Taylor and H. H. Seliger, pp. 179–182. New York: Elsevier.
500. Tangen, K. and Dahl, E. 1993. Harmful phytoplankton in Norwegian waters—An overview. In *Abstracts of the Sixth International Conference on Toxic Marine Phytoplankton*, Nantes, France, p. 195.
501. Okolodkov, Y. B. 1987. Vertical distribution of algae and nutrients in the first-year ice from the East Siberian Sea in May. *Bot J Russ Acad Sci*, 81, 34–40.
502. Okolodkov, Y. B. 1992. Ice algae of the Laptev Sea. *Novit Syst Plant Non Vascul*, 28, 29–34.
503. Okolodkov, Y. B. 1992. Cryopelagic flora of the Chukchi, East Siberian and Laptev seas. In *Proceedings of the National Institute of Polar Research Symposium on Polar Biology*, Tokyo, Japan, pp. 28–43.
504. Okolodkov, Y. B. 2000. Dinoflagellates (Dinophyceae) of the Eurasian Arctic seas. DSc thesis. Komarov Botanical Institute, Russian Academy of Sciences, St. Petersburg, FL.
505. Tuschling, K., Von Juterzenka, K., Okolodkov, Y. et al. 2000. Composition and distribution of the pelagic and sympagic algal assemblages in the Laptev Sea during autumnal freeze-up. *J Plankton Res*, 20, 843–864.
506. Konovalova, G. V. 1993. Toxic and potentially toxic dinoflagellates from the Far East coastal waters of Russia. In *Toxic Phytoplankton Blooms in the Sea*, eds. T. Smayda and Y. Shimizu, pp. 275–279. Amsterdam, the Netherlands: Elsevier.
507. Konovalova, G. V. 1998. Dinoflagellates (Dinophyta) of the Far Eastern seas of Russia and adjacent areas of the Pacific Ocean. Vladivostok, Russia: Dalnauka.
508. Konovalova, G. V. 1995. The dominant and potentially dangerous species of phytoflagellates in the coastal waters of East Kamchatka. In *Harmful Marine Algal Blooms*, eds. P. Lassus, G. Arzul, E. Erard et al., pp. 169–174. Paris, France: Lavoisier.
509. Okolodkov, Y. B. 1999. Species range types of recent marine dinoflagellates recorded from the Arctic. *Grana*, 38, 162–169.
510. Okolodkov, Y. B. and Dodge, J. D. 1996. Biodiversity and biogeography of planktonic dinoflagellates in the Arctic Ocean. *J Exp Mar Biol Ecol*, 202, 19–27.
511. Okolodkov, Y. B. 2005. The global distributional patterns of toxic, bloom dinoflagellates recorded from the Eurasian Arctic. *Harmful Algae*, 4, 351–369.
512. Heywood, R. B. and Whitaker, T. M. 1984. The marine flora. In *Antarctic Ecology*, ed. R. M. Laws, pp. 373–419. London, U.K.: Academic Press.
513. El-Sayed, S. Z. 1998. Antarctic marine ecosystem research, where to from here? *Mem Natl Inst Polar Res*, 52, 172–185.
514. Umani, S. F., Monti, M., and Nuccio, C. 1998. Microzooplankton biomass distribution in Terra Nova Bay, Ross Sea (Antarctica). *J Mar Syst*, 17, 289–303.
515. Umani, S. F., Monti, M., Bergamasco, A. et al. 2005. Plankton community structure and dynamics versus physical structure from Terra Nova Bay to Ross Ice Shelf (Antarctica). *J Mar Syst*, 55, 31–46.
516. Chang, F. H., Williams, M. J. M., Schwarz, J. N. et al. 2013. Spatial variation of phytoplankton assemblages and biomass in the New Zealand sector of the Southern Ocean during the late austral summer 2008. *Polar Biol*, 36, 391–408.
517. de Salas, M. F., Laza-Martínez, A., and Hallegraeff, G. M. 2008. Novel unarmored dinoflagellates from the toxigenic family Kareniaceae (Gymnodiniales): Five new species of *Karlodinium* and one new *Takayama* from the Australian sector of the Southern Ocean. *J Phycol*, 44, 241–257.
518. Chang, F. H., Chiswell, S. M., and Uddstrom, M. J. 2001. Occurrence and distribution of *Karenia brevisulcata* (Dinophyceae) during the 1998 summer toxic outbreaks on the central east coast of New Zealand. *Phycologia*, 40, 215–222.
519. Chang, F. H. 2011. Toxic effects of three closely-related dinoflagellates, *Karenia concordia*, *K. brevisulcata* and *K. mikimotoi* (Gymnodiniales, Dinophyceae) on other microalgal species. *Harmful Algae*, 10, 181–187.
520. Siegel, D. A., Doney, S. C., and Yoder, J. A. 2002. The North Atlantic spring phytoplankton bloom and Sverdrup's critical depth hypothesis. *Science*, 296, 730–733.
521. Longhurst, A. R. 2007. *Ecological Geography of the Sea*. London, U.K.: Academic Press.

522. Behrenfeld, M. J. 2010. Abandoning Sverdrup's critical depth hypothesis on phytoplankton blooms. *Ecology*, 91, 977–989.

523. Visser, F., Hartman, K. L., and Pierce, G. J. 2011. Timing of migratory baleen whales at the Azores in relation to the North Atlantic spring bloom. *Mar Ecol Prog Ser*, 440, 267–269.

524. Hackett, J. D., Maranda, L., Yoon, H. S. et al. 2003. Phylogenetic evidence for the cryptophyte origin of the plastid of *Dinophysis* (Dinophysiales, Dinophyceae). *J Phycol*, 39, 440–448.

525. Minnhagen, S. and Janson, S. 2006. Genetic analyses of *Dinophysis* spp. support kleptoplastidy. *FEMS Microbiol Ecol*, 57, 47–54.

526. Licea, S., Zamudio, M. E., Zamudio, R. et al. 2004. Free living dinoflagellates in the Southern Gulf of Mexico: Report of data (1979–2002). *Phycol Res*, 52, 419–428.

527. Riobó, P., Paz, B., and Franco, J. M. 2006. Analysis of palytoxin-like in *Ostreopsis* cultures by liquid chromatography with precolumn derivatization and fluorescence detection. *Anal Chim Acta*, 566, 217–223.

528. Delgado, G., Lechuga-Deveze, C. H., Popowski, G. et al. 2006. Epiphytic dinoflagellates associated with ciguatera in the Northwestern coast of Cuba. *Rev Biol Trop*, 54, 299–310.

529. Ballantine, D. L., Bardales, A. T., Tosteson, T. R. et al. 1985. Seasonal abundance of *Gambierdiscus* and *Ostreopsis* sp. in coastal waters of southwest Puerto Rico. In *Proceedings of the Fifth International Coral Reef Congress*, eds. C. Gabrie and B. Salvat, pp. 417–422. Tahiti, May 27–June 1, 1985. Vol. 4: Symposia and Seminars (B).

530. Mercado, J. A., Viera, M., Tosteson, T. R. et al. 1995. Differences in the toxicity and biological activity of *Ostreopsis lenticularis* observed using different extraction procedures. In *Harmful Marine Algal Blooms*, eds. P. Lassus, G. Arzul, E. Erard et al., pp. 321–326. Paris, France: Lavoisier, Intercept Ltd.

531. Amorim, A. and Dale, B. 2006. Historical cyst record as evidence for the recent introduction of the dino-flagellate *Gymnodinium catenatum* in the north-eastern Atlantic. *Afr J Mar Sci*, 28, 193–197.

532. Bartels-Jónsdóttir, H. B., Voelker, A. H. L., Knudsen, K. L. et al. 2009. Twentieth-century warming and hydrographical changes in the Tagus Prodelta, eastern North Atlantic. *Holocene*, 19, 369–380.

533. Gribble, K. E., Keafer, B. A., Quilliam, M. A. et al. 2005. Distribution and toxicity of *Alexandrium ostenfeldii* (Dinophyceae) in the Gulf of Maine, USA. *Deep-Sea Res Pt II*, 52, 2745–2763.

534. Carreto, J. I., Negri, R. M., Benavides, H. R. et al. 1985. Dinoflagellate blooms in the Argentine Sea. In *Toxic Dinoflagellates*, eds. D. M. Anderson, A. W. White, and D. G. Baden, pp. 147–152. New York: Elsevier.

535. Davison, P. and Yentsch, C. M. 1985. Occurrence of toxic dinoflagellates and shellfish toxin along coastal Uruguay, South America. In *Toxic Dinoflagellates*, eds. D. M. Anderson, A. W. White, and D. G. Baden, pp. 153–158. New York: Elsevier.

536. Odebrecht, C., Mendez, S., and Garcia, V. M. T. 1997. Oceanographic processes and HAB in the subtropical southwestern Atlantic (26–36 degrees S). *Poster presented at the VIII International Conference on Harmful Algae*, Vigo, Spain.

537. Gannon, D. P., Berens McCabe, E. J., Camilleri, S. A. et al. 2009. Effects of *Karenia brevis* harmful algal blooms on nearshore fish communities in southwest Florida. *Mar Ecol Prog Ser*, 478, 171–186.

538. Braarud, T. and Heimdal, B. R. 1970. Brown water on the Norwegian coast in autumn 1966. *Nytt Mag Bot*, 17, 91–97.

539. Al-Kandari, M., Highfield, A. C., Hall, M. J. et al. 2011. Molecular tools separate harmful algal bloom species, *Karenia mikimotoi*, from different geographical regions into different subgroups. *Harmful Algae*, 10, 636–643.

540. Chinain, M., Germain, M., Sako, Y. et al. 1997. Intraspecific variation in the dinoflagellate *Gambierdiscus toxicus* (Dinophyceae). I. Isozyme analysis. *J Phycol*, 33, 36–43.

541. Penna, A., Vila, M., Fraga, S. et al. 2005. Characterization of *Ostreopsis* and *Coolia* (Dinphyceae) isolates in the Western Mediterranean Sea based on morphology, toxicity and internal transcribed spacer 5.8S rDNA sequences. *J Phycol*, 41, 212–225.

542. Giacobbe, M. G., Oliva, F. D., and Maimone, G. 1996. Environmental factors and seasonal occurrence of the dinoflagellate *Alexandrium minutum*, a PSP potential producer, in a mediterranean lagoon. *Estuar Coast Shelf Sci*, 42, 539–549.

543. Casabianca, S., Penna, A., Pecchioli, E. et al. 2011. Population genetic structure and connectivity of the harmful dinoflagellate *Alexandrium minutum* in the Mediterranean Sea. *Proc Biol Sci*, 279, 129–138.

544. Margalef, R. and Estrada, M. 1987. Synoptic distribution of summer microplankton (algae and protozoa) across the principal front in the Western Mediterranean. Invest. *Pesqueria*, 51, 121–140.
545. Abadie, E., Amzil, Z., Belin, C. et al. 1999. Contamination de l'etang de Thau par *Alexandrium tamarense*: Épisode de novembre à décembre 1998. *Bilans et Prospectives*. Plouzané, France: IFREMER, 44pp.
546. Lugliè, A., Giacobbe, M. G., Sannio, A. et al. 2003. First record of the dinoflagellate *Alexandrium catenella* (Whedon & Kofoid) Balech (Dinophyta), a potential producer of paralytic shellfish poisoning, in Italian waters (Sardinia, Tyrrhenian Sea). *Bocconea*, 16, 1045–1052.
547. Frehi, H., Couté, A., Mascarell, G. et al. 2007. Harmful and red-tide dinoflagellates in the Annaba bay (Algeria). *C R Biol*, 330, 615–628.
548. Turki, S., Balti, N., and Ben Janet, H. 2007. First bloom of dinoflagellate *Alexandrium catenella* in Bizerte lagoon (northern Tunisia). *Harmful Algae News*, 35, 7–9.
549. Mee, L. D., Espinosa, M., and Diaz, G. 1986. Paralytic shellfish poisoning with a *Gymnodinium catenatum* red tide on the pacific coast of Mexico. *Mar Environ Res*, 19, 77–92.
550. Cortés, M. C., Cortés Altamirano, R., Sierra Beltrán, A. et al. 2005. *Ostreopsis siamensis* (Dinophyceae) a new tychoplanktonic record from Isabel Island National Park, Pacific Mexico. *Harmful Algae News*, 28, 4–5.
551. Band-Schmidt, C., Bustillos-Guzmán, J., Morquecho, L. et al. 2006. Variations of PSP toxin profiles during different growth phases in *Gymnodinium catenatum* (Dinophyceae) strains isolated from three locations in the Gulf of California, Mexico. *J Phycol*, 42, 757–768.
552. Matsuoka, K., Fujii, R., Hayashi, M. et al. 2006. Recent occurrence of toxic *Gymnodinium catenatum* Graham (Gymnodiniales, Dinophyceae) in coastal sediments of West Japan. *Paleontol Res*, 10, 117–125.
553. Parsons, M. and Preskitt, L. B. 2007. A survey of epiphytic dinoflagellates from the coastal waters of the island of Hawaii. *Harmful Algae*, 6, 658–669.
554. Bagnis, R., Legrand, A. M., and Inoue, A. 1990. Follow-up of a bloom of the toxic dinoflagellate *Gambierdiscus toxicus* on a fringing reef of Tahiti. In *Toxic Marine Phytoplankton*, eds. E. Graneli, B. Sundström, L. Edler et al., pp. 98–103. New York: Elsevier.
555. Maclean, J. L. 1989. An overview of *Pyrodinium* red tides in the western Pacific. In *Biology, Epidemiology and Management of Pyrodinium Red Tides*, eds. G. M. Hallegraeff and J. L. Maclean, pp. 1–7. *ICLARM Conference Proceedings 21*. Manila, Philippines: International Center for Living Aquatic Resources Management.
556. Selina, M. S. and Levchenko, E. V. 2011. Species composition and morphology of dinoflagellates (Dinophyta) of epiphytic assemblages of Peter the Great Bay in the Sea of *Japan. Russ J Mar Biol*, 37, 23–32.
557. Shin, E. Y., Park, J. G., and Yeo, H. G. 2004. A taxonomic study of family Dinophysiaceae Stein (Dinophysiales, Dinophyta) in Korean coastal waters. *Ocean Polar Res*, 26, 655–668.
558. Quod, J. P., Turquet, J., Diogene, G. et al. 1995. Screening of extracts of dinoflagellates from coral reefs (Reunion Island, SW Indian Ocean), and their biological activities. In *Harmful Marine Algal Blooms*, eds. P. Lassus, G. Arzul, and E. Erard-Le Denn, pp. 815–820. Paris, France: Lavoisier, Intercept Ltd.
559. Lenoir, S., Ten-Hage, L., Quod, J. P. et al. 2006. Characterisation of new analogues of palytoxin isolated from an *Ostreopsis mascarenensis* bloom in the south-west Indian Ocean. *Afr J Mar Sci*, 28, 389–391.
560. Onuma, Y., Satake, M., Ukena, T. et al. 1999. Identification of putative palytoxin as the cause of clupeotoxism. *Toxicon*, 37, 55–65.
561. Hansen, G., Turquet, J., Quod, J. P. et al. 2001. Potentially harmful algae of the West Indian Ocean: A guide based on a preliminary survey. In *IOC Manuals and Guides*, Series no. 41. Paris, France: Intergovernmental Oceanographic Commission of UNESCO, 105pp.
562. Turquet, J., Quod, J. P., Ten-Hage, L. et al. 2001. Example of a *Gambierdiscus toxicus* flare-up following the 1998 coral bleaching event in Mayotte Island (Comoros, south-west Indian Ocean). In *Harmful Algal Blooms*, eds. G. M. Hallegraeff, S. I. Blackburn, C. J. Bolch et al., pp. 364–366. Paris, France: Intergovernmental Oceanographic Commission of UNESCO.
563. Wawiye, O. P., Ogongo, B., and Tunje, S. 1999. Workshop on harmful algalm blooms in the Western Indian Ocean. WINDOW. *West Indian Waters*, 10, 1–3.
564. Kyewalyanga, M. and Lugomela, C. 2001. Existence of potentially harmful microalgae in coastal waters around Zanzibar: A need for a monitoring programme? In *Proceedings of the Anniversary Conferences on Advances in Marine Science in Tanzania, 1999*, eds. M. D. Richmond and J. Francis, pp. 319–328. Zanzibar, Tanzania: IMS/WIOMSA.

565. Pastoureaud, A., Dupuy, C., Chrétiennot-Dinet, M. J. et al. 2003. Red coloration of oysters along the French Atlantic coast during the 1998 winter season: Implication of nanoplanktonic cryptophytes. *Aquaculture*, 228, 225–235.

566. Lee, W. J., Simpson, A. G. B., and Patterson, D. J. 2005. Free-living heterotrophic flagellates from freshwater sites in Tasmania (Australia), a field survey. *Acta Protozool*, 44, 321–350.

567. Karunasagar, I., Oshima, Y., Yasumoto, T. et al. 1990. A toxin profile for shellfish involved in an outbreak of paralytic shellfish poisoning in India. *Toxicon*, 28, 868–870.

568. Myat, S., Thaw, M. S. H., Matsuoka, K. et al. 2012. Phytoplankton surveys off the southern Myanmar coast of the Andaman Sea: An emphasis on dinoflagellates including potentially harmful species. *Fish Sci*, 78, 1091–1106.

569. Karunasagar, I., Segar, K., and Karunasagar, I. 1989. Incidence of DSP and DSP in shellfish along the coast of Karnataka state (India). In *Red Tides: Biology, Environmental Science and Toxicology*, eds. T. Okaichi, D. M. Anderson, and T. Nemoto, pp. 61–64. Amsterdam, the Netherlands: Elsevier.

570. Rao, B. 2005. Comprehensive review of the records of the biota of the Indian Seas and introduction of non-indigenous species. *Aquat Conserv: Mar Freshw Ecosyst*, 15, 117–146.

21

Lipophilic Toxins, Pectenotoxins, and Yessotoxins: Chemistry, Metabolism, and Detection

Toshiyuki Suzuki

CONTENTS

21.1 Introduction

The presence of pectenotoxins and yessotoxins in shellfish was discovered due to their high acute toxicity in the traditional mouse bioassay after i.p. injection of lipophilic extracts. Among the natural toxins, pectenotoxins and yessotoxins had been grouped together with diarrhetic shellfish poisoning (DSP) toxins (i.e., okadaic acid and dinophysistoxins) because of their similar polyether structures to okadaic acid analogues (Yasumoto et al. 1985; Murata et al. 1987; Yasumoto and Murata 1993). They generally coexist in shellfish contaminated with DSP toxins. Animal studies indicate that pectenotoxins and yessotoxins are much less toxic via the oral route and that they do not induce diarrhea (Ogino et al. 1997; Aune et al. 2002; Tubaro et al. 2003; Miles et al. 2004a; Ito et al. 2008), except for one report on pectenotoxin-2 (PTX2) (Ishige et al. 1988). Since pectenotoxins and yessotoxins do not fit the clinical case definition of DSP toxins, they are recently considered as separate from the DSP group. Levels of pectenotoxins and yessotoxins have been regulated in shellfish in some countries, including those in the European Union (EU). In the EU, pectenotoxins are regulated together with okadaic acid and dinophysistoxins, and the quarantine level of the sum of both toxin groups in bivalves is 0.16 mg/kg (European Union 2002). The quarantine level of yessotoxins in bivalves in the EU is 1 mg/kg, which is much higher than okadaic acid and pectenotoxin analogues (European Union 2002).

PTX2 has been reported to be present in the toxic dinoflagellates *Dinophysis* spp. (Lee et al. 1989a; Draisci et al. 1996, 1999a; Suzuki et al. 1998, 2003, 2006, 2009; James et al. 1999; Sasaki et al. 1999; Pavela-Vrancic et al. 2001; Fernández et al. 2002; MacKenzie et al. 2002, 2005; Vale and Sampayo 2002; Miles et al. 2004b; Puente et al. 2004a,b; Vale 2004; Krock et al. 2008; Pizarro et al. 2008; Kamiyama and Suzuki 2009; Kamiyama et al. 2010; Fux et al. 2011; Nagai et al. 2011), which is also the causative species of DSP toxins. Several pectenotoxins, pectenotoxin-11 (PTX11) (Suzuki et al. 2003, 2006; Pizarro et al. 2008), pectenotoxin-12 (PTX12) (Miles et al. 2004b), pectenotoxin-13 (PTX13), and pectenotoxin-14 (PTX14) (Miles et al. 2006a), were found in *Dinophysis* spp. by using liquid chromatography–mass spectrometry (LC–MS). It has been shown that many of the other pectenotoxins such as pectenotoxin-6 (PTX6) and pectenotoxin-2 seco acid (PTX2sa) are formed by the metabolism of PTX2 in shellfish tissues (Yasumoto et al. 1989; Suzuki et al. 1998, 2001a,b).

Yessotoxin is produced by the dinoflagellates *Protoceratium reticulatum* (Satake et al. 1997a, 1999; Ciminiello et al. 2003; Paz et al. 2004, 2006, 2007; Samdal et al. 2004; Eiki et al. 2005; Miles et al. 2005a; Suzuki et al. 2007), *Gonyaulax spinifera* (Rhodes et al. 2006; Riccardi et al. 2009), and *Lingulodinium polyedrum* (Draisci et al. 1999b; Paz et al. 2004) and accumulates in filter-feeding bivalves feeding on the toxic dinoflagellates. Several yessotoxin analogues have been identified in bivalves and dinoflagellate (Satake et al. 1996, 1997b, 2006; Ciminiello et al. 1998, 2000a,b, 2001, 2002a, 2007; Daiguji et al. 1998b; Konishi et al. 2004; Miles et al. 2004c,d, 2005a,b, 2006b,c; Finch et al. 2005; Souto et al. 2005; Domínguez et al. 2010). Some yessotoxins such as 45-hydroxyyessotoxin (45-hydroxyYTX) and carboxyyessotoxin (carboxyYTX) are formed by metabolism of yessotoxin in shellfish (Aasen et al. 2005).

Due to the difficulties in distinguishing between DSP toxins and other lipophilic toxins by the traditional mouse bioassay, several chemical analyses have been developed. The most common methods are based on LC with detection by ultraviolet (UV) absorption, fluorescence (FL), and mass spectrometry (MS). In the present chapter, chemistry, metabolism, and chemical detection methods of pectenotoxins and yessotoxins are described.

21.2 Chemistry and Metabolism of Pectenotoxins

21.2.1 Chemistry

The chemical structures of pectenotoxins are shown in Figure 21.1. Pectenotoxins resemble okadaic acid in molecular weight and in having cyclic ethers and a carboxyl group in the molecule. Unlike okadaic acid, the carboxyl moiety in many pectenotoxins is in a form of macrocyclic lactone (macrolide). All pectenotoxins absorb UV light between 235 and 239 nm due to the presence of a 1,3-dienyl moiety at C-28–C-31. The infrared (IR) bands at 3400, 1760, and 1740 cm^{-1} are observed (Yasumoto et al. 1984, 1985; Murata et al. 1986) due to absorption by the hydroxyl, five-membered ring ketone, and ester of lactone ring. Pectenotoxins are susceptible to isomerization due to the presence of a hemiketal (C-36) and several ketal centers (C-7 and C-21), along with a ketone α- to an ether linkage. The ketal at C-7 is especially sensitive to epimerization under acidic conditions (Sasaki et al. 1998; Evans et al. 2002; Suzuki et al. 2003). Pectenotoxins are easily destroyed under strong basic conditions (Vale and Sampayo 2002) such as those used to hydrolyze acyl esters of the okadaic acid groups, while PTX2 is stable for more than 24 h between pH 4.5 and pH 9.1 (Suzuki et al. 2001a).

Pectenotoxin-1 (PTX1) and PTX2 were originally isolated from Japanese scallops, *Patinopecten yessoensis*, and their structures were elucidated by single crystal x-ray diffraction techniques, nuclear magnetic resonance (NMR) spectroscopy, and MS together with UV and IR spectroscopy (Yasumoto et al. 1984, 1985). As part of the same study, three other analogues (PTX3–5) were also isolated and partially identified from UV spectra and MS (Yasumoto et al. 1984, 1985). Additional studies using spectroscopic techniques elucidated the structure of pectenotoxin-3 (PTX3) (Murata et al. 1986). Acidic pectenotoxins, PTX6 and pectenotoxin-7 (PTX7), were later isolated from Japanese scallops and the structure of PTX6 was elucidated by NMR spectroscopy (Yasumoto et al. 1989). The absolute configuration of PTX6 was later determined by NMR spectroscopy using a chiral anisotropic reagent, phenylglycine methyl ester, which was condensed with the carboxylic acid group at C-18 of PTX6 and was identified to be 18*S* (Sasaki et al. 1997); thereby, the stereochemical structures of the natural 7*R*-pectenotoxins were assigned as shown in Figure 21.1.

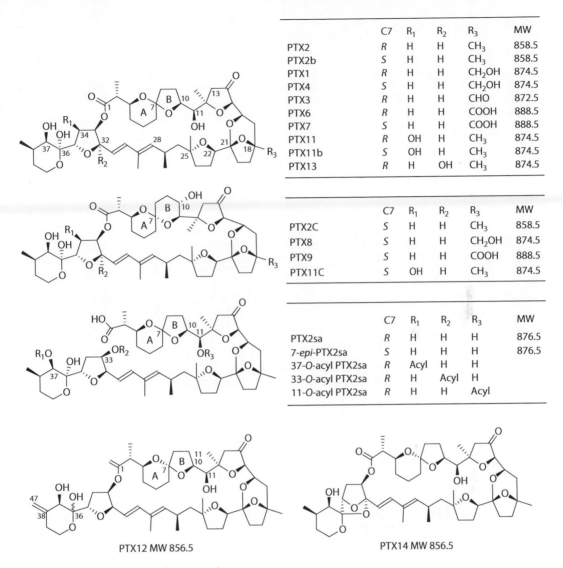

	C7	R_1	R_2	R_3	MW
PTX2	R	H	H	CH_3	858.5
PTX2b	S	H	H	CH_3	858.5
PTX1	R	H	H	CH_2OH	874.5
PTX4	S	H	H	CH_2OH	874.5
PTX3	R	H	H	CHO	872.5
PTX6	R	H	H	COOH	888.5
PTX7	S	H	H	COOH	888.5
PTX11	R	OH	H	CH_3	874.5
PTX11b	S	OH	H	CH_3	874.5
PTX13	R	H	OH	CH_3	874.5

	C7	R_1	R_2	R_3	MW
PTX2C	S	H	H	CH_3	858.5
PTX8	S	H	H	CH_2OH	874.5
PTX9	S	H	H	COOH	888.5
PTX11C	S	OH	H	CH_3	874.5

	C7	R_1	R_2	R_3	MW
PTX2sa	R	H	H	H	876.5
7-*epi*-PTX2sa	S	H	H	H	876.5
37-*O*-acyl PTX2sa	R	Acyl	H	H	
33-*O*-acyl PTX2sa	R	H	Acyl	H	
11-*O*-acyl PTX2sa	R	H	H	Acyl	

PTX12 MW 856.5

PTX14 MW 856.5

FIGURE 21.1 The structures of pectenotoxins.

Treatment of 7R-pectenotoxins under acidic condition such as acetonitrile/water (7:3, v/v) with 0.1% (v/v) trifluoroacetic acid (TFA) leads to an equilibrium mixture of spiroketal stereoisomers, 7R, 7S, and 6-membered B-ring isomers (Sasaki et al. 1998; Evans et al. 2002; Suzuki et al. 2003) as illustrated in Figure 21.2. Identification and characterization of pectenotoxin-4 (PTX4) and PTX7 as the spiroketal isomers of PTX1 and PTX6, respectively, was achieved on the basis of NMR and acid-catalyzed chemical interconversion (Sasaki et al. 1998). Equilibration between PTX6 and PTX7 and between PTX1 and PTX4 resulted in the formation of two additional isomeric products, pectenotoxin-8 (PTX8) and pectenotoxin-9 (PTX9) (Sasaki et al. 1998). It was suggested that PTX4 and PTX7 are naturally occurring toxins rather than artifacts of the extraction process, whereas PTX8 and PTX9 are artifacts obtained by acidic interconversion (Sasaki et al. 1998). Analogous spiroketal isomers of PTX2 were later tentatively identified during acidic interconversion by tandem MS (MS/MS) coupled with chromatographic identification (Suzuki et al. 2003). 7S and 6-Membered B-ring isomers of PTX2 were named as PTX2b and PTX2c, respectively. Figure 21.3 shows the kinetics for the acid-catalyzed interconversion of PTX1, PTX6, and PTX2. Spiroketal isomers of pectenotoxins reached an equilibrium ratio after 48 h in acetonitrile/water (7:3, v/v) with 0.1% TFA (Suzuki et al. 2003). The kinetics for PTX6 interconversion were somewhat different from those of the other pectenotoxins.

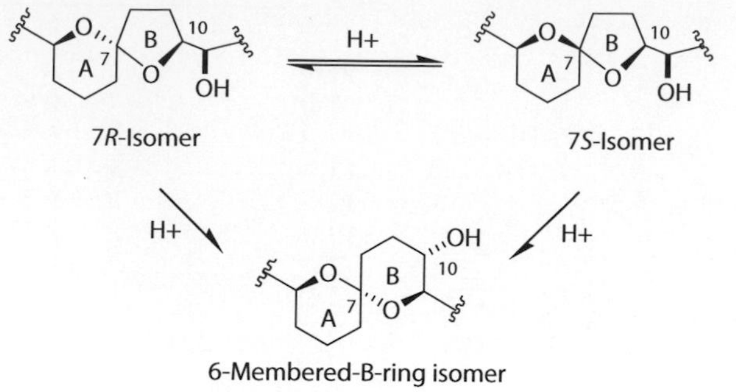

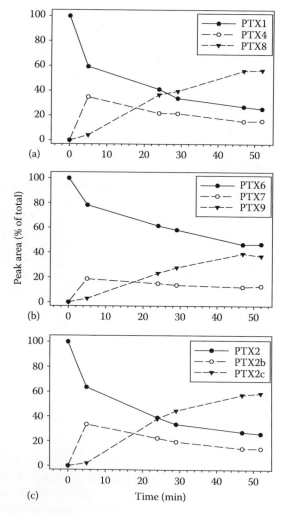

FIGURE 21.2 Acid-catalyzed interconversion of the pectenotoxins.

FIGURE 21.3 Kinetics of acid-catalyzed interconversion of PTX1 (a), PTX6 (b), and PTX2 (c). Peak area of pectenotoxins was obtained by SIM LC–MS. (From Suzuki, T. et al., *J. Chromatogr. A*, 992, 141, 2003. With permission.)

PTX2sa and its epimer 7-*epi*-PTX2sa, analogues of PTX2 in which the lactone ring had been hydrolyzed, were identified in *Dinophysis acuta* from Ireland and mussels, *Perna canaliculus,* from New Zealand (Daiguji et al. 1998a). A compound tentatively characterized as a new pectenotoxin with the same molecular weight as PTX1 was detected by LC–MS analyses of *P. canaliculus* and *D. acuta* from New Zealand and temporarily designated as "PTX-1i" (MacKenzie et al. 2002). After further studies, this compound was named PTX11 along with its spiroketal isomers, PTX11b and PTX11c (Suzuki et al. 2003). PTX11 was isolated from *D. acuta* and identified by NMR and MS/MS (Suzuki et al. 2006). The same sample of *D. acuta* also showed the presence of another compound temporarily designated PTX11x on the basis of LC–MS/MS spectra (Suzuki et al. 2006). This compound was isolated from algal concentrates and identified as PTX13 by NMR and MS/MS (Miles et al. 2006a). A second compound, PTX14, was identified as the cyclized 32,36-dehydration product of PTX13 in the same sample, although this compound was suggested to be an artifact in origin (Miles et al. 2006a). A pair of pectenotoxin isomers with a molecular weight of two less than that of PTX2 were isolated from a bloom of *D. acuta* from Norway and identified as PTX12 as a pair of equilibrating 36-epimers of 38,47-dehydroPTX2 (Miles et al. 2004b). 37-, 33-, and 11-*O*-Acyl esters of PTX2sa have been reported in blue mussels, *Mytilus edulis*, from Ireland (Wilkins et al. 2006). Very recently, a novel pectenotoxin, pectenotxin-15 (PTX15), was isolated from Japanese scallops, *P. yessoensis*. The PTX15 was identified as 38-hydroxypectenotoxin-6 by MS/MS and NMR spectroscopy (Suzuki et al. 2012). The structures of pectenotoxin-5 (PTX5) and pectenotoxin-10 (PTX10) have not been determined yet. The absolute stereochemistry for pectenotoxins was confirmed by total synthesis of PTX4 and its isomerization to PTX8 and PTX1 (Evans et al. 2002).

21.2.2 Metabolism

The origin of pectenotoxins is the toxic dinoflagellate genus *Dinophysis*, which is also the causative species for DSP toxins (okadaic acid and the dinophysistoxins). PTX2 has been reported to be present in the toxic dinoflagellates *D. fortii, D. acuminata, D. norvegica, D. rotundata, D. acuta,* and *D. infundibulus* (Lee et al. 1989a; Draisci et al. 1996, 1999a; Suzuki et al. 1998, 2003, 2006, 2009; James et al. 1999; Sasaki et al. 1999; Pavela-Vrancic et al. 2001; Fernández et al. 2002; MacKenzie et al. 2002, 2005; Vale and Sampayo 2002; Miles et al. 2004b; Puente et al. 2004a,b; Vale 2004; Krock et al. 2008; Pizarro et al. 2008; Kamiyama and Suzuki 2009; Kamiyama et al. 2010; Fux et al. 2011; Nagai et al. 2011). Recently, the production of PTX2, okadaic acid, and dinophysistoxin-1 by *D. fortii* and *D. acuminata* was confirmed for cultured strains collected in Japan by LC–MS/MS (Kamiyama and Suzuki 2009; Kamiyama et al. 2010; Nagai et al. 2011). PTX11, PTX12, and PTX13 were found in *D. acuta* collected in New Zealand and European waters (Suzuki et al. 2003, 2006; Miles et al. 2004b, 2006a; Krock et al. 2008; Pizarro et al. 2008). It has been shown that many of the other pectenotoxins such as PTX1, PTX3, PTX6, and PTX2sa are formed by metabolism of PTX2 in shellfish tissues (Yasumoto et al. 1989; Suzuki et al. 1998, 2001a,b). Recently, PTX1 was found from seawater sample preoccupied by *D. acuminata* from the North Sea along the Scottish east coast (Krock et al. 2008). This is the first finding of the presence of PTX1 in *Dinophysis* sample although the possibility of metabolic transformations of pectenotoxins by organisms that have grazed upon *Dinophysis* has not been ruled out.

PTX2 in bivalves is absorbed from algae and metabolized by two processes as illustrated in Figure 21.4. In the Japanese scallop, *P. yessoensis*, PTX2 undergoes stepwise oxidation of the methyl group attached to C-18 (Yasumoto et al. 1989; Suzuki et al. 1998). Thus, the 18-methyl group in PTX2 is oxidized to an alcohol (PTX1), aldehyde (PTX3), and finally a carboxylic acid (PTX6) group. This biotransformation of PTX2 in Japanese scallops was confirmed by the content of PTX6 in scallops, which was found to be significantly higher than that of PTX2 when *D. fortii* collected in the same location contained only PTX2 (Suzuki et al. 1998). It is reported that PTX6 content in Japanese scallops is significantly higher than that of PTX2 and PTX1 by LC–MS (Suzuki et al. 2005a; Hashimoto et al. 2006), indicating a rapid biotransformation of PTX2 to PTX6 in Japanese scallops. The oxidation of the methyl group attached to C-18 leads to reduced toxicity in the mouse bioassay. PTX6 is half as toxic as PTX2 (Yasumoto et al. 1995; Ito et al. 2008), suggesting a kind of detoxification of PTX2 in the scallops. Although very low levels of PTX7 are often found in Japanese scallops along with PTX6, it appears that PTX7 is formed by nonenzymatic isomerization of PTX6 (Sasaki et al. 1998; Suzuki et al. 2003).

In the New Zealand scallop, *Pecten novaezelandiae*, and mussels *P. canaliculus* and *Mytilus galloprovincialis* from New Zealand and *M. edulis* from Norway, a different process has been demonstrated whereby the lactone moiety of PTX2 undergoes rapid enzymatic hydrolysis to afford PTX2sa. The biotransformation of PTX2 to PTX2sa was confirmed by in vitro experiments by using bivalve extracts and PTX2 (Suzuki et al. 2001a,b; Miles et al. 2004a). Although 7-*epi*-PTX2sa is detected in the extracts,

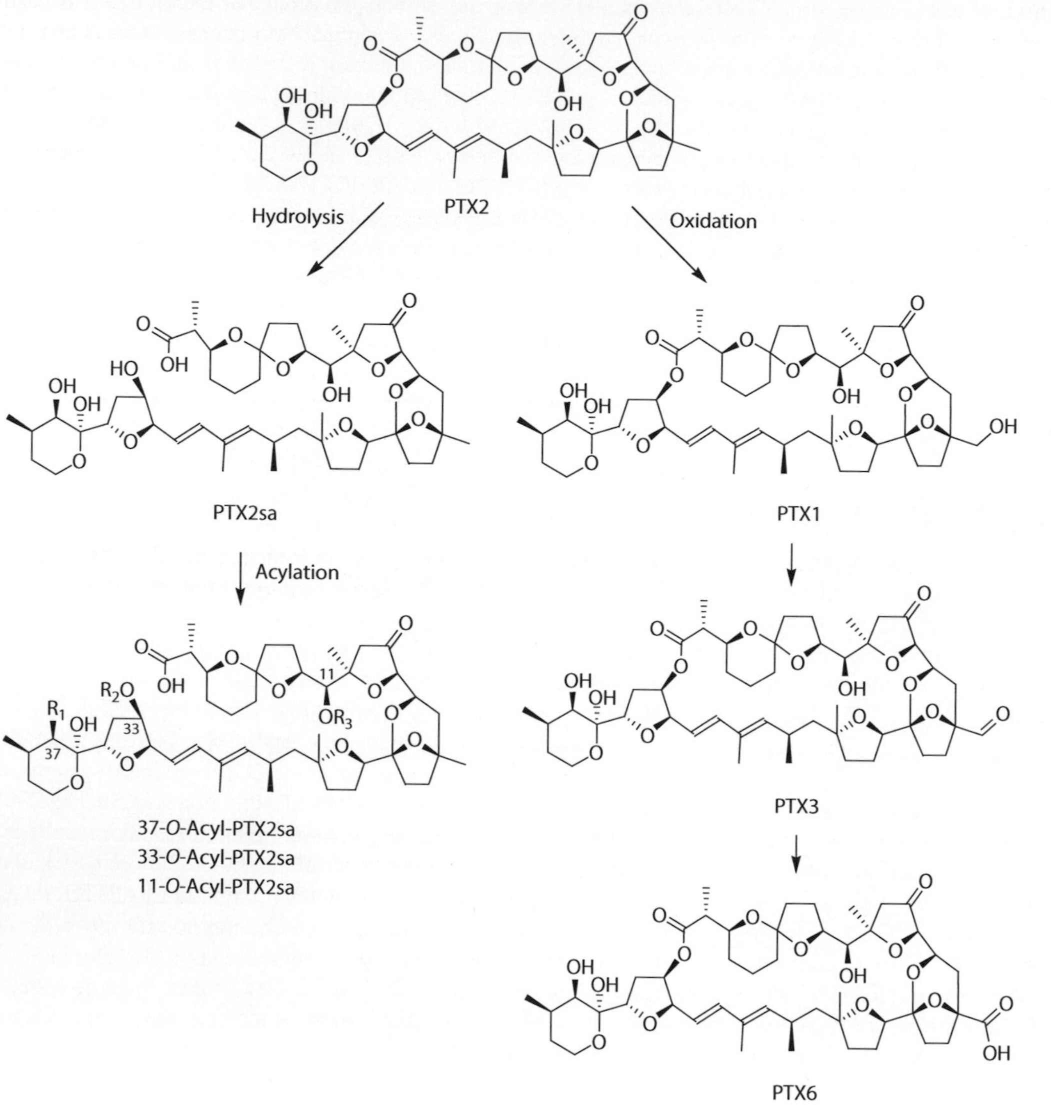

FIGURE 21.4 The metabolism of PTX2 in shellfish.

it appears that this is formed by nonenzymatic isomerization of pectenotoxins (Sasaki et al. 1998; Suzuki et al. 2003). It is interesting that PTX2 is not converted to any other pectenotoxins in Japanese scallop extracts (Suzuki, unpublished data), indicating that activities of some enzymes such as oxidases are not induced in in vitro extracts. The result also suggests lack of the capability to convert PTX2 to PTX2sa in Japanese scallops. Examination of the metabolite profiles reported for shellfish contaminated with pectenotoxins suggests that conversion from PTX2 to PTX2sa is the major metabolic pathway in many shellfish species (MacKenzie et al. 2002; Vale and Sampayo 2002; Miles et al. 2004b; Puente et al. 2004b; Vale 2004). Because PTX2sa was not cytotoxic to KB cells even at 1.8 μg/mL, whereas PTX-2 was cytotoxic at 0.05 μg/mL (Daiguji et al. 1998a), the conversion from PTX2 to PTX2sa in shellfish is a kind of detoxification. Recently, metabolites of PTX2sa, 37-, 33-, and 11-*O*-acyl esters of PTX2sa have been reported in blue mussels, *M. edulis*, from Ireland (Wilkins et al. 2006). The most abundant fatty acid esters in the samples were, in order, the 16:0, 22:6, 14:0, 16:1, 18:4, and 20:5 fatty acids.

PTX11 is more resistant to enzymatic hydrolysis than PTX2. PTX11 was not detectably hydrolyzed in vitro overnight, even though the half-life for PTX-2 hydrolysis in the same preparation was ca 15 min

(Suzuki et al. 2006). This result indicates that PTX11 is at least two orders of magnitude less easily hydrolyzed than PTX2 by the enzymes in the mussel hepatopancreas. This suggests that because of steric hindrance by the 34-hydroxyl group, and possibly hydrogen bonding between the 34-OH and the carbonyl oxygen of PTX11, the latter is not a substrate for the enzyme(s) responsible for hydrolysis of the lactone ring of other pectenotoxins. As a consequence, PTX11 is expected to accumulate to a much greater extent than PTX2 in mussels. This is in accord with the observation that there was a large difference between the ratios of PTX11 and the putative PTX11sa (0.63) and PTX2/PTX2sa (0.04) in naturally contaminated mussels *P. canaliculus* collected in New Zealand (MacKenzie et al. 2002). Analyses of contaminated mussels similarly suggest that PTX12 is more resistant hydrolysis than PTX2 (Miles et al. 2004b). Recently an enzyme capable of hydrolyzing pectenotoxins and okadaic acid esters was isolated from the hepatopancreas of the green shell mussel *P. canaliculus* in New Zealand (MacKenzie et al. 2012). PTX2 and PTX1 were hydrolyzed but the enzyme was inactive against PTX11, PTX6, and acid-isomerized PTX2 and PTX11. PTX11 and PTX2b competitively inhibited PTX2 hydrolysis.

There are only limited data on depuration of pectenotoxins from shellfish. The elimination of PTX2sa from the mussel *P. canaliculus* in New Zealand occurred with half-lives of 26 days (MacKenzie et al. 2002) and of 15 days in Akaroa Harbour (McNabb and Holland 2002). Depuration of PTX2sa and 7-*epi*-PTX2sa from *M. galloprovincialis* in Portugal has also been reported (Vale 2004). When PTX6 was injected into the adductor muscle of scallops *P. yessoensis*, it was rapidly transported to the hepatopancreas (Suzuki et al. 2005b). The residual ration of PTX6 in the hepatopancreas of the scallops was less than 20%. The residual ration of PTX6 was slightly higher than that of the okadaic acid group.

21.3 Chemistry and Metabolism of Yessotoxins

21.3.1 Chemistry

The chemical structures of yessotoxins are shown in Figure 21.5. Yessotoxins resemble brevetoxins and ciguatoxins in having a ladder-shaped polycyclic ether skeleton and an unsaturated side chain. Another characteristic is having one to three sulfate esters in the structure. YTX, 45-hydroxyYTX, and 45,46,47-trinoryessotoxin (45,46,47-trinorYTX) absorb UV light at 230 or 226 nm (Murata et al. 1987; Yasumoto et al. 1989; Satake et al. 1996) due to the presence of a 1,3-dienyl moiety in the eastern side chain. In contrast to pectenotoxins, yessotoxins are relatively stable under strongly basic conditions such as those used to hydrolysis of acyl esters of the okadaic acid groups. There are few reports about the chemical conversion of yessotoxins due to the chemically stable molecular structures. The IR bands at 3400, 1240, 1220, 1070, and 820 cm^{-1} are observed due to absorption by the hydroxyl group and sulfate esters (Murata et al. 1987).

Through the studies on the chemical structures of yessotoxins, almost all of the major yessotoxin analogues were found from bivalves. YTX was first isolated from Japanese scallops, *P. yessoensis* (Murata et al. 1987). The planer structure was elucidated by NMR spectroscopy (Murata et al. 1987). The relative stereochemistry of YTX was later assigned by NMR studies (Satake et al. 1996). The absolute configuration of YTX was determined by NMR using a chiral anisotropic reagent, α-methoxy-α-(2-naphtyl)acetic acid (2NMA), and was identified to be 4*S* (Takahashi et al. 1996); thereby, the stereochemical structures of YTX was assigned as shown in Figure 21.5. In the same paper reporting the relative stereochemistry of YTX, two yessotoxin analogues, 45-hydoroxyyessotoxin (45-hydroxyYTX) and 45,46,47-trinoryessotoxin (45,46,47-trinorYTX), isolated from Japanese scallops were reported as the first yessotoxin analogues (Satake et al. 1996). YTX and 45-hydroxyYTX were also isolated from mussels of the Adriatic Sea and the structure was confirmed by NMR (Ciminiello et al. 1997, 1999). Absolute configuration of C-45 in 45-hydroxyYTX was assigned later (Morohashi et al. 2000). Homoyessotoxin (homoYTX) and 45-hydroxy-homoyessotoxin (45-hydroxyhomoYTX) were found from mussels, *M. galloprovincialis*, collected from Italy in 1997 (Satake et al. 1997b). Successively, a unique yessotoxin analogue adriatoxin (ATX) was found from mussels in the northern Adriatic Sea in 1998 (Ciminiello et al. 1998). The structure of ATX is different from other yessotoxin analogues in the eastern part of the molecule where there is absence of the side chain as well as of an ether ring and presence of a further sulfate group. Later, several other yessotoxin analogues were successively found from Norwegian and Italian mussels. 1-Desulfoyessotoxin

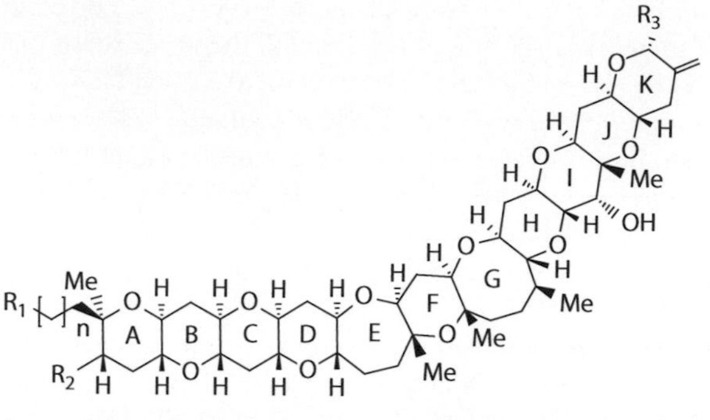

Name	R_1	R_2	R_3	n	Ref.
Yessotoxin (YTX)	OSO_3H	OSO_3H	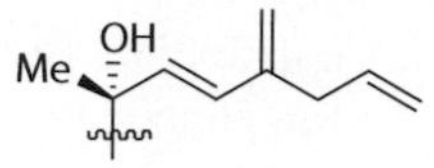	1	Murata et al. (1987) Satake et al. (1996) Takahashi et al. (1996)
45-HydroxyYTX	OSO_3H	OSO_3H	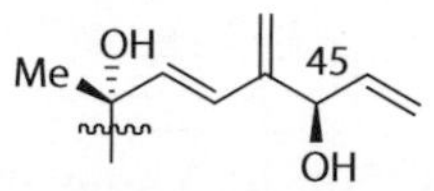	1	Satake et al. (1996) Morohashi et al. (2000)
45,46,47-TrinorYTX	OSO_3H	OSO_3H	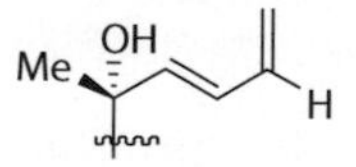	1	Satake et al. (1996)
HomoYTX	OSO_3H	OSO_3H	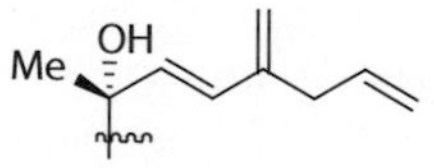	2	Satake et al. (1997b)
45-HydroxyhomoYTX	OSO_3H	OSO_3H	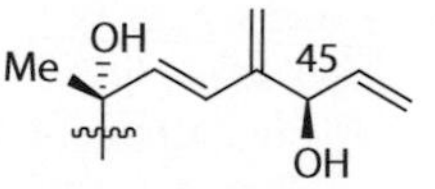	2	Satake et al. (1997b)
1-DesulfoYTX	OH	OSO_3H	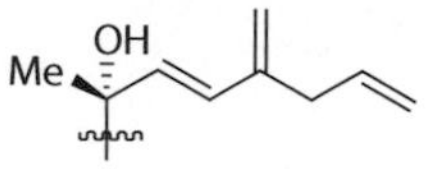	1	Daiguji et al. (1998b)
CarboxyYTX	OSO_3H	OSO_3H	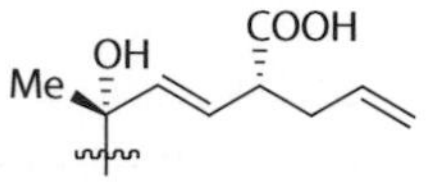	1	Ciminiello et al. (2000a)
CarboxyhomoYTX	OSO_3H	OSO_3H	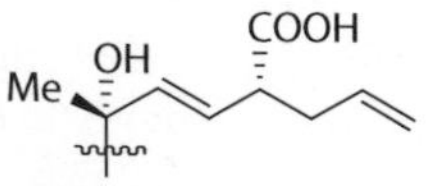	2	Ciminiello et al. (2000b)
NoroxohomoYTX	OSO_3H	OSO_3H	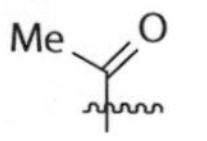	2	Ciminiello et al. (2001)

(a)

FIGURE 21.5   Structures of YTXs.

Name	R_1	R_2	R_3	n	Ref.
1-Desulfocarboxy homoYTX	OH	OSO_3H	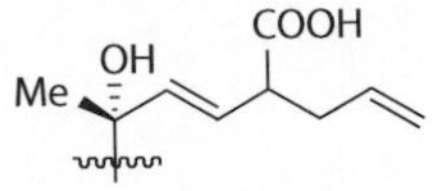	2	Ciminiello et al. (2007)
4-Desulfocarboxy homoYTX	OSO_3H	OH	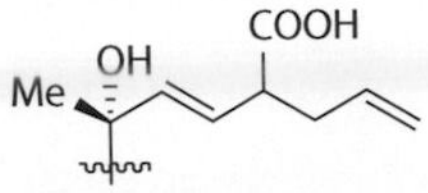	2	Ciminiello et al. (2007)
45-Hydroxycarboxy-YTX	OSO_3H	OSO_3H	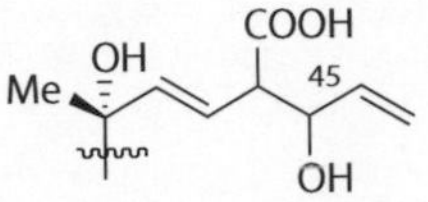	1	Aasen et al. (2005)
NoroxoYTX	OSO_3H	OSO_3H	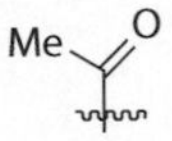	1	Ciminiello et al. (2002)
44,55-DihydroxyYTX	OSO_3H	OSO_3H	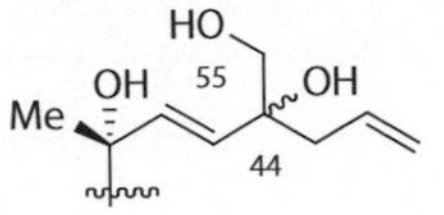	2	Finch et al. (2005)
45,46,47-TrinorhomoYTX	OSO_3H	OSO_3H	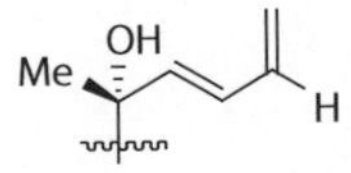	2	Satake et al. (2006)

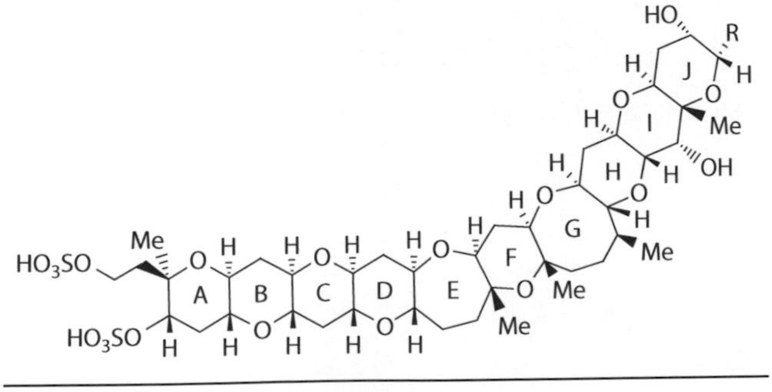

Name	R	Ref.
Adriatoxin (ATX)	OSO_3H	Ciminiello et al. (1998)
ATX-B	CH_3	Dominguez et al. (2010)

(b)

FIGURE 21.5 (continued) Structures of YTXs.

(continued)

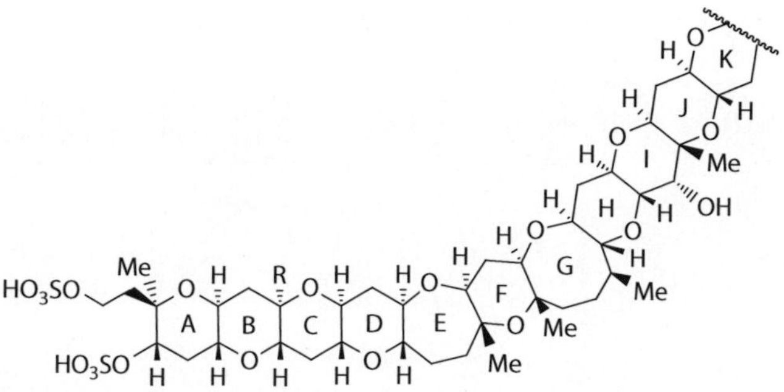

Name	R		Ref.
YTX enone	H	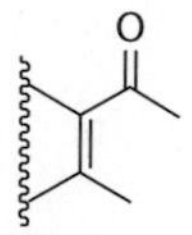	Miles et al. (2004c)
40-*epi*-NoroxoYTX	H	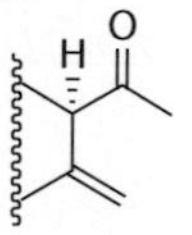	Miles et al. (2004c)
9-Me-YTX enone	CH$_3$	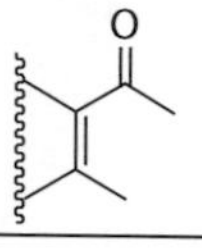	Miles et al. (2006b)

(c)

FIGURE 21.5 (continued)   Structures of YTXs.

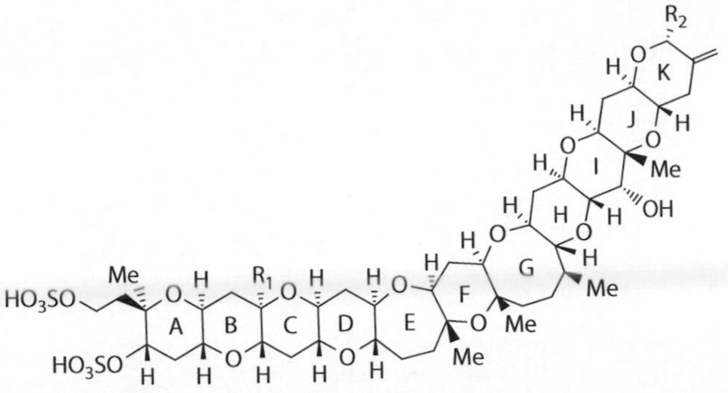

Name	R_1	R_2	Ref.
41a-HomoYTX	H	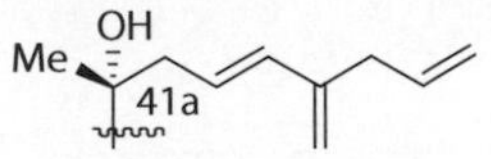	Miles et al. (2004d)
9-Me-41a-HomoYTX	CH_3	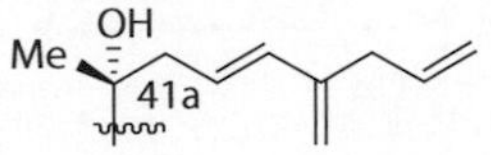	Miles et al. (2004d)
44, 55-Dihydroxy 41a-HomoYTX	H	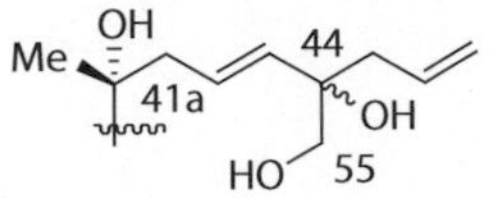	Finch et al. (2005)
44, 55-Dihydroxy 9-Me-41a-HomoYTX	CH_3	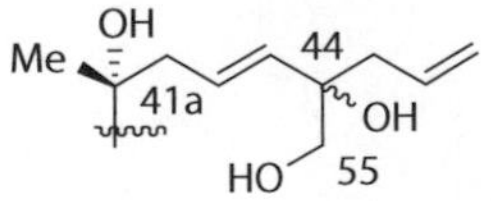	Finch et al. (2005)
Trihydroxyamide of 41a-HomoYTX	H	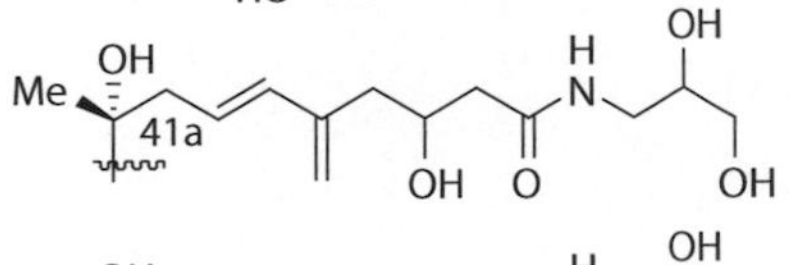	Miles et al. (2005b)
Trihydroxyamide of 9-Me-41a-HomoYTX	CH_3	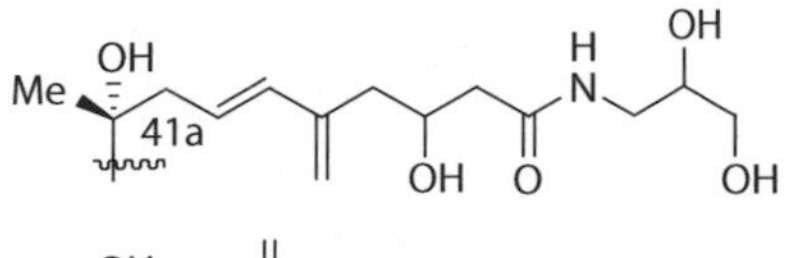	Miles et al. (2005b)
45-Hydroxy-46, 47-dinorYTX	H	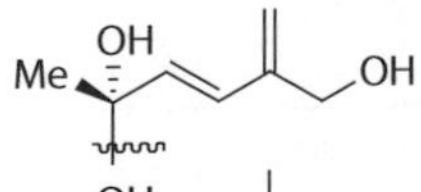	Miles et al. (2006b)
44-Oxo-45, 46, 47-trinorYTX	H	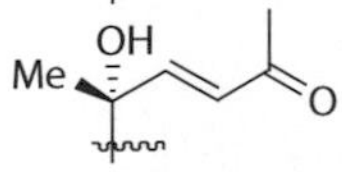	Miles et al.(2006b)

(d)

FIGURE 21.5 (continued) Structures of YTXs.

(continued)

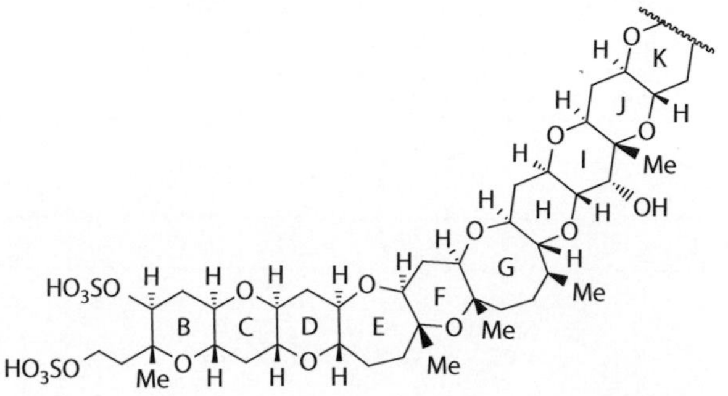

Name		Ref.
Nor-ring-A-YTX	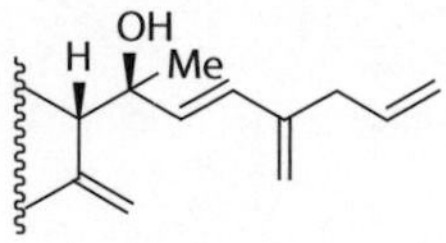	Miles et al. (2004d)
Nor-ring-A-YTX enone	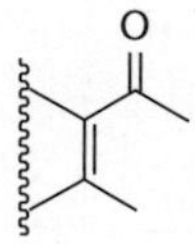	Miles et al. (2004d)
Nor-ring-A-40-*epi*-noroxoYTX	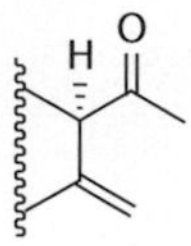	Miles et al. (2004d)
Nor-ring-A-noroxoYTX	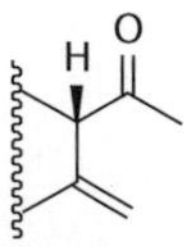	Miles et al. (2004d)

(e)

FIGURE 21.5 (continued) Structures of YTXs.

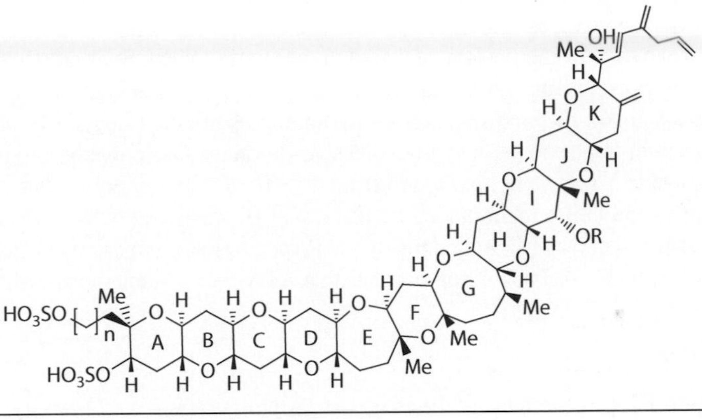

Name	R			n	Refs.
Diarabinoside-homoYTX				2	Konishi et al. (2004)
Monoarabinoside-homoYTX				2	Konishi et al. (2004)
Triarabinoside-homoYTX				2	Konishi et al. (2004)
Monoarabinoside-YTX				1	Soute et al. (2005) Miles et al. (2006c)
Diarabinoside-YTX				1	Miles et al. (2006c)

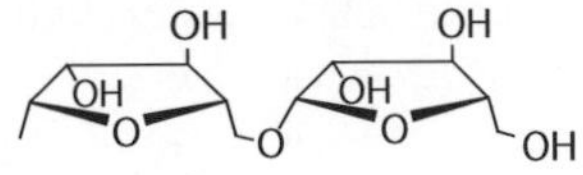

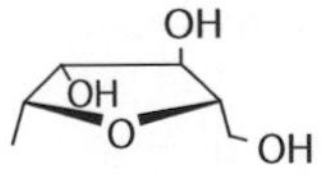

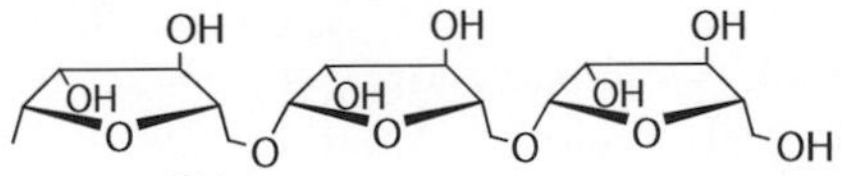

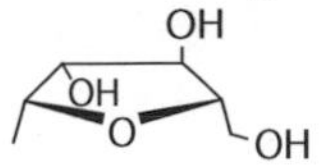

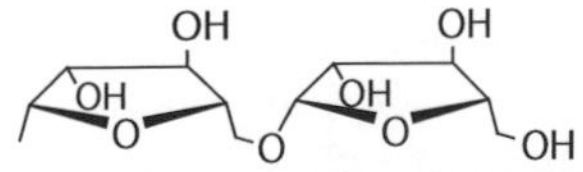

(f)

FIGURE 21.5 (continued)   Structures of YTXs.

(1-ds YTX) (Daiguji et al. 1998b) and 45-hydroxycarboxyyessotoxin (45-hydroxycarboxyYTX) (Aasen et al. 2005) were found from Norwegian mussels. Other yessotoxin analogues carboxyYTX (Ciminiello et al. 2000a), carboxyhomoyessotoxin (carboxyhomoYTX) (Ciminiello et al. 2000b), noroxohomoyes-sotoxin (noroxohomoYTX) (Ciminiello et al. 2001), noroxoyessotoxin (noroxoYTX) (Ciminiello et al. 2002a), 44,55-dihydroxyyessotoxin (44,55-dihydroxyYTX) (Finch et al. 2005), 1-desulfocarboxyho-moyesstoxin (1-desulfocarboxyhomoYTX) (Ciminiello et al. 2007), and 4-desulfodarboxyhomoyesso-toxin (4-desulfodarboxyhomoYTX) (Ciminiello et al. 2007) were found from Italian mussels. Although the structures of 45-hydroxycarboxyYTX and noroxoYTX have tentatively been assigned by LC–MS/MS analysis, the proposed structures have not been confirmed by NMR yet.

Other yessotoxin analogues shown in Figure 21.5 were found from *P. reticulatum* cultures as minor yessotoxins (Miles et al. 2004c,d, 2005b, 2006b; Finch et al. 2005; Satake et al. 2006). Yessotoxin-enone (YTX-enone) and 40-*epi*-noroxoyessotxin (40-*epi*-noroxoYTX) are isomers of noroxoYTX. YTX-enone is isomerized from noroxoYTX in the presence of diluted ammonia (Miles et al. 2004c). The investigation on highly cytotoxic compounds against human tumor cell lines in *P. reticulatum* led to finding of novel homoYTX analogues, mono-, di-, and tri-arabinoside homoyessotoxins (Konishi et al. 2004). They are interesting compounds in terms of the first glycosides of dinoflagellate polyethers. Similar compounds, mono- and di-arabinoside YTX, were also found from *P. reticulatum* cultures (Souto et al. 2005; Miles et al. 2006c). Recently, novel adriatoxin analogue, adriatoxin-B, was isolated from *P. reticulatum* culture and the structure was elucidated by a combination of NMR spectroscopy experiments and a conformational analysis (Domínguez et al. 2010). The finding suggests that ATX found in mussels is originated from algae.

21.3.2 Metabolism

Since the presence of YTX in the marine dinoflagellate was first confirmed in cultured cells of a New Zealand *P. reticulatum* strain in 1997 (Satake et al. 1997a), several studies had reported that YTX was the most dominant toxin with other minor yessotoxin analogues in cultured *P. reticulatum* (Satake et al. 1999; Ciminiello et al. 2003; Eiki et al. 2005; Miles et al. 2005a, Paz et al. 2006, 2007; Suzuki et al. 2007). However, there are some exceptions on the yessotoxin profiles in some *P. reticulatum* strains. Some cultured *P. reticulatum* strains collected in Japan and Spain exclusively produces homoYTX (Konishi et al. 2004; Paz et al. 2007; Suzuki et al. 2007). It is also reported that an acetonic extract of *P. reticulatum* cell contained larger amount of monoarabinoside yessotoxin than YTX (2.90 vs. 0.59 mg) (Souto et al. 2005). However, different extractability of acetone for the monoarabinoside YTX and YTX should be considered in this case. It is also interesting that some *P. reticulatum* strains do not produce any yessotoxins (Suzuki et al. 2007). *G. spinifera* cultured strain isolated in New Zealand was identi-fied as a YTX producer by ELISA in 2006 (Rhodes et al. 2006). *G. spinifera* strains isolated from the Adriatic Sea was confirmed to produce homoYTX and YTX by LC–MS/MS (Riccardi et al. 2009). *L. polyedrum* has also been considered to produce yessotoxins (Draisci et al. 1999; Paz et al. 2004).

Because almost all of the previous studies about toxin profile of *P. reticulatum*, *G. spinifera*, and *L. polyedrum* demonstrate that YTX or homoYTX is the most occurring yessotoxins in the cells, YTX or homoYTX can be absorbed in bivalves from algae with other minor yessotoxins. Profiles of yessotox-ins in bivalves obtained by several previous studies indicate that YTX or homoYTX is always present. They are included in the most or second dominant yessotoxins in bivalves with other minor yessotox-ins (Ciminiello et al. 1998, 2000a,b, 2001, 2002a; Finch et al. 2005; Ciminiello and Fattorusso 2008). Besides YTX and homoYTX, 45-hydroxy-form and carboxy-form are usually detected in bivalves (Finch et al. 2005). An article by Aasen et al. (2005) clarified that Norwegian blue mussels rapidly oxidized YTX to 45-hydroxyYTX and more slowly to carboxyYTX. 45-HydroxyYTX is possibly metabolized to 45-hydroxycarboxyYTX. The same article reports that the depuration rate for carboxyYTX is consider-ably slower than for YTX and 45-hydroxyYTX (Aasen et al. 2005). Therefore, yessotoxin profiles in bivalves in which YTX was initially absorbed tend to change dramatically. Relatively long-term obser-vation of the yessotoxin profiles in blue mussels demonstrates that carboxyYTX is the most dominant yessotoxin analogue in mussels after 1–6 months later from the initial contamination with YTX (Aasen et al. 2005). Another interesting aspect in the metabolism of yessotoxins is that desulfoyessotoxins, which is occasionally reported from bivalves (Daiguji et al. 1998b; Ciminiello et al. 2007), have not been

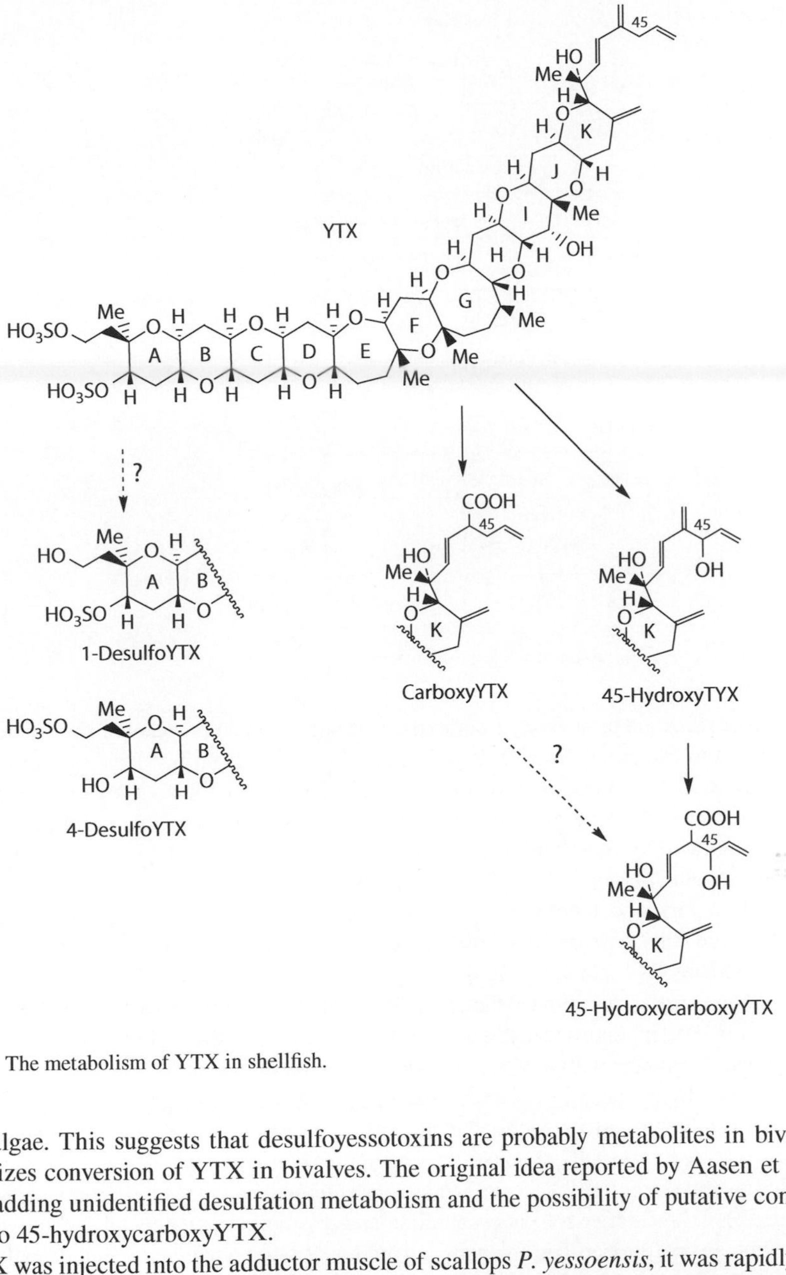

FIGURE 21.6 The metabolism of YTX in shellfish.

found from algae. This suggests that desulfoyessotoxins are probably metabolites in bivalves. Figure 21.6 summarizes conversion of YTX in bivalves. The original idea reported by Aasen et al. is slightly modified by adding unidentified desulfation metabolism and the possibility of putative conversion from carbxyYTX to 45-hydroxycarboxyYTX.

When YTX was injected into the adductor muscle of scallops *P. yessoensis*, it was rapidly transported to the hepatopancreas (Suzuki et al. 2005b). The residual ration of YTX in the hepatopancreas of the scallops was less than 20%. The conversion of YTX to 45-hydroxyYTX is also demonstrated in Japanese scallops (*P. yessoensis*) administered with YTX by syringe injection (Suzuki et al. 2005b).

21.4 Chemical Detection Methods of Pectenotoxins and Yessotoxins

21.4.1 Extraction, Isolation, and Cleanup for Chemical Methods

DSP toxins and other lipophilic toxins including pectenotoxins and yessotoxins are usually isolated from bivalves or algal concentrates harvested from natural blooms by acetone extraction, although aqueous methanol such as 80% or 90% methanol is used. Individual toxins are then isolated through a complex

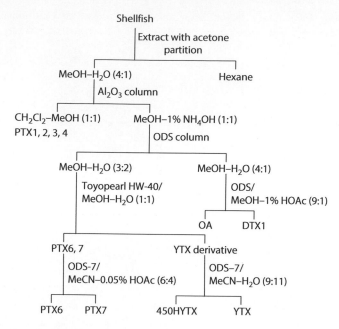

FIGURE 21.7 Purification of DSP toxins and lipophilic toxins.

fractionation and purification procedure of raw extracts based on a combination of chromatographic techniques. Extraction and fractionation of DSP and lipophilic toxins from bivalves reported by Yasumoto are shown in Figure 21.7 (Yasumoto et al. 1989). Acidic PTX6, PTX7, and yessotoxins are separated from neutral pectenotoxins on an alumina column together with okadaic acid and dinophysistoxin-1. Toxin fractions separated by the alumina column are usually chromatographed on a silica gel column with chloroform/methanol (Goto et al. 1998) although this step is not shown in the scheme in Figure 21.7. It is relatively easy to purify pectenotoxins and yessotoxins from algal concentrates harvested from natural blooms or cultured cells (Suzuki et al. 2006; Loader et al. 2007) or by in vitro enzymatic conversion of isolated PTX2 (Miles et al. 2004a, 2006d).

The preparation of extracts for chemical methods for pectenotoxins and yessotoxins is rather simple compared to the isolation. Pectenotoxins and yessotoxins are extracted together with okadaic acid and dinophysistoxins from bivalve samples with 4–9 volumes of 80% or 90% methanol. These solvent systems have been shown to be equally efficient for pectenotoxins and yessotoxins although 90% methanol is more efficient for DSP toxins and their esters (McNabb et al. 2005). In several LC–MS methods, methanol extracts are directly analyzed by LC–MS. Cleanup has been accomplished using liquid/liquid partitioning between methanolic solution and chloroform. Pectenotoxins are partitioned into the chloroform layer and toxins are analyzed directly by LC–MS after solvent evaporation and dissolution in methanol (Suzuki and Yasumoto 2000). Yessotoxins are partitioned into the aqueous methanol layer when using liquid/liquid partitioning between aqueous methanol and dichloromethane according to the extraction protocol for toxic shellfish currently in force in the European Community (European Union 2002; Ciminiello and Fattorusso 2008). In this partitioning procedure, okadaic acid analogues and pectenotoxins are partitioned into dichloromethane; therefore, yessotoxins can be analyzed separately from other lipophilic toxins. However, this approach is not applicable to less hydrophilic yessotoxins such as desulfo derivatives, which are being recovered in the dichloromethane (Ciminiello and Fattorusso 2008). The method of McNabb et al. uses a hexane wash of the crude methanolic extract to remove nonpolar lipids before direct LC–MS analysis of pectenotoxins and yessotoxins in the relatively dilute extract (0.1 g equiv/mL) (McNabb et al. 2005). Solid phase extraction (SPE) cleanup is useful for cleanup of pectenotoxins and yessotoxins in LC–MS (Goto et al. 2001; Gerssen et al. 2009a) in situations where the quantification of the toxins is interfered with by co-extractives from biological matrices (Ito and Tsukada 2002). SPE on C18 cartridge column is also useful to extract pectenotoxins, okadaic acid, and dinophysistoxin-1 from condensed seawater plankton net samples (Suzuki et al. 1998).

This approach is also applicable to yessotoxins with slight modifications. Solid phase adsorption toxin tracking (SPATT) is used as a monitoring tool that simulates the biotoxin contamination of filter-feeding bivalves (MacKenzi et al. 2004).

21.4.2 Liquid Chromatography–Ultraviolet Detection

Because pectenotoxins and some yessotoxins have a conjugated diene in the molecular skeleton, UV detection between 226 and 239 nm is applicable to their detection after LC separation. Pectenotoxins and yessotoxins can be separated by a C18 or C8 reversed-phase column with acetonitrile/water mobile phases. The quantification of PTX2 by isocratic LC–UV detection at 235 nm has been reported (Lee et al. 1989a,b; Yasumoto et al. 1995; Draisci et al. 1996; Suzuki et al. 1998, 2006; James et al. 1999). An example of LC–UV analysis of YTX has also been reported (Yasumoto et al. 1995). The LC–UV detection is not sufficiently sensitive or specific for pectenotoxins and yessotoxins in bivalve extracts due to biological matrices although this approach is useful for algal extracts (Lee et al. 1989a,b; Draisci et al. 1996; Suzuki et al. 1998, 2006; James et al. 1999). LC–diode array detection (DAD) is useful for purity check of pectenotoxins and yessotoxins standard prepared from bivalve and plankton extracts.

21.4.3 Liquid Chromatography–Fluorescence Detection

The carboxyl group in acidic pectenotoxins such as PTX6 and PTX2sa reacts rapidly with 9-anthryl-diazomethane (ADAM) (Lee et al. 1989b; Yasumoto et al. 1995; Daiguji et al. 1998a; Suzuki et al. 1998; James et al. 1999; Pavela-Vrancic et al. 2001; Vale and Sampayo 2002; Nogueiras et al. 2003), 1-bromoacetylpyrene (BAP) (James et al. 1999), 3-bromomethyl-6,7-dimethoxy-1-methyl-2(1H)-quinoxalinone (BrDMEQ) (Nogueiras et al. 2003), and 9-chloromethylanthracene (CA) (Nogueiras et al. 2003). The derivatization of toxins with ADAM has also been used for the confirmation of the presence of a carboxyl group in structural studies (Daiguji et al. 1998a). Separation of fluorescent pectenotoxin derivatives by LC is usually carried out using C18 reversed-phase chromatography with acetonitrile/water mobile phases. Although cleanup of the ADAM derivative of okadaic acid by Sep-Pak silica cartridge (Lee et al. 1987) is useful, in the case of ADAM-PTX6, several peaks that may interfere with the quantification of ADAM-PTX6 were observed. A second chromatographic run on a cyanopropyl column (Capcell Pak CN SG 120 column, Shiseido, Japan) (Zhao et al. 1993) was useful for confirmatory analysis of ADAM-PTX6 (Suzuki et al. 1998). The primary hydroxyl group of PTX1 and PTX4 is derivatized with 1-anthroylnitrile (AN) (Lee et al. 1989b; Yasumoto et al. 1995). Pre-column fluorometric analysis of PTX2 by isocratic LC–FL detection has been reported (Sasaki et al. 1999) after derivatization of a conjugated diene of PTX2 with the fluorescent dienophile DMEQ-TAD, 4-[2-(6,7-dimethoxy-4-methyl-3-oxo-3,4-dihydroquinoxalinyl)ethyl]-1,2,4-triazoline-3,5-dione. Application of this method to bivalve samples has not been reported although it has been used to confirm the occurrence of PTX2 in plankton net samples.

Yessotoxins are also derivatized with DMEQ-TAD for sensitive and selective detection of yessotoxins from bivalves (Yasumoto and Takizawa 1997). The derivatization of yessotoxins with DMEQ-TAD results in the formation of two C-42 epimers that give two peaks on the C18 reversed-phase chromatogram. Simultaneous detection of YTX and 45-hydroxyYTX (Yasumoto and Takizawa 1997) or YTX and arabinoside YTX (Paz et al. 2006) was reported. Because DMEQ-TAD reacts to a conjugated diene in the eastern side chain of yessotoxin molecule, some yessotoxins lacking a conjugated diene such as noroxoYTX, noroxohomoYTX, ATX, carboxyYTX, and carboxyhomoYTX cannot be analyzed by this method. Another weakness in this method is that YTX and homoYTX after derivatization with DMEQ-TAD cannot be chromatographically separated. Therefore, the method cannot distinguish between YTX and homoYTX.

21.4.4 Liquid Chromatography–Mass Spectrometric Detection

The technique of electrospray ionization (ESI) LC–MS has proven to be one of the most powerful tools for the detection, identification, and quantification of marine toxins (Quilliam 2003). This atmospheric pressure ionization technique provides very high sensitivity for a wide range of polar compounds that can carry a charge in aqueous solution. It is generally recognized that ion formation in ESI results from the "ion evaporation" phenomenon, which involves field-assisted desorption of preformed solute ions from microdroplets of solution (Thomson and Iribarne 1979).

The determination of lipophilic toxins including pectenotoxins and yessotoxins by LC–MS is usually carried out using a reversed-phase chromatography on a C8 or C18 silica column and isocratic or gradient elution with acetonitrile/water or methanol/water mobile phases containing volatile modifiers such as acetic acid, formic acid, ammonium formate, or ammonium acetate. It is reported that a change of a mobile phase pH to alkaline conditions results in even better chromatographic separation of yessotoxins by using the new type of cross-linked silica-based C18 column materials that are stable up to pH 12 (Gerssen 2009b). Recently, several LC–MS or LC–MS/MS methods allowing detection of pectenotoxins and yessotoxins together with okadaic acid, dinophysistoxins, and azaspiracids have been reported and in some cases validated (McNabb et al. 2005; Stobo et al. 2005; Gerssen et al. 2010; These et al. 2011; van den Top et al. 2011; Villar-Gonzalez et al. 2011). These methods have also reported on challenges posed by matrix effects (Ito and Tsukada 2002; Fux et al. 2008) on quantification of lipophilic toxins within the method validation process. The consequences of matrix effects are the over- or underestimation of the true concentration of toxins present in the sample. The main cause of ionization suppression in biological extracts is thought to be induced by changes in the properties of the droplets due to the presence of nonvolatile solutes (King et al. 2000). In most cases, the matrix effects in quantification of lipophilic toxins can be corrected by using calibration curve prepared by matrix-matched standards (Ito and Tsukada 2002; Stobe et al. 2005; Gerssen et al. 2010; These et al. 2011; van den Top et al. 2011; Villar-Gonzalez et al. 2011). The potential of SPE cleanup was assessed to reduce matrix effects in the LC–MS/MS analysis of lipophilic toxins (Gerssen et al. 2009a). The paper concluded that SPE of methanolic shellfish extracts can be very useful for reduction of matrix effects. However, the type of LC and MS methods used is also of great importance. Ultra-performance liquid chromatography (UPLC) separation using a C8 or C18 column is also useful to reduced matrix effects compared to the other conditions assessed (Fux et al. 2007, 2008).

21.4.4.1 Pectenotoxins

Several analytical methods for the determination of pectenotoxins by LC–MS or LC–MS/MS are reported (Draisci et al. 1996, 1999a; Suzuki et al. 1998, 2001a,b, 2003, 2005a, 2006; James et al., 1999; Suzuki and Yasumoto 2000; Goto et al. 2001; Pavela-Vrancic et al. 2001; Quilliam et al. 2001; Fernández et al. 2002; Ito and Tsukada 2002; MacKenzie et al. 2002, 2005; McNabb et al. 2002, 2005; Vale and Sampayo 2002; Quilliam 2003; Miles et al. 2004b, 2006a; Puente et al. 2004a,b; Vale 2004; Stobo et al. 2005; Fux et al. 2007; Gerssen et al. 2009b, 2010; These et al. 2011; van den Top et al. 2011; Villar-Gonzalez et al. 2011). Selected ion monitoring (SIM) for $[M-H]^-$, $[M+HCO_2]^-$, $[M+NH_4]^+$, and $[M+Na]^+$ or multiple reaction monitoring (MRM) using loss of water molecules from $[M+NH_4]^+$ is applicable to the quantification. There seems to be no significant difference between the results for single MS (SIM) and MS/MS (MRM) detection. The most popular ion for detection of pectenotoxins is $[M+NH_4]^+$, which gives better sensitivity in comparison with negatively charged ions $[M-H]^-$ or $[M+HCO_2]^-$.

Pectenotoxins are separated by Hypersil BDS C8 column with an isocratic elution (Suzuki et al. 2003). Figure 21.8 shows the LC–MS chromatogram of spiroketal isomers of pectenotoxins detected by SIM for $[M+MH_4]^+$ ions. Spiroketal isomers of pectenotoxins are eluted in the order of 7*R*, 7*S*, and 6-membered B-ring isomers. LC–MS/MS spectra for $[M+NH_4]^+$ of pectenotoxins have been reported for the confirmation of identity and structure elucidation (James et al. 1999; Suzuki et al. 2003, 2006; Miles et al. 2004b, 2006a; Wilkins et al. 2006). Figure 21.9 illustrates the MS/MS product ion spectra obtained for the $[M+NH_4]^+$ ions of PTX1, PTX6, and PTX2 on a triple quadrupole MS (Suzuki et al. 2003). The spectra show a characteristic fragment ion at *m/z* 213, as well as series of ions resulting from the loss of first ammonium and then water molecules from $[M+NH_4]^+$. In addition, PTX1, PTX6, and PTX2 produce characteristic fragment ions at *m/z* 567, 581, and 551, respectively. The characteristic ion at *m/z* 551 produced from PTX2 is also found in the MS/MS spectra of PTX11. These ions are key ions for the identification of each pectenotoxin analogue. The product ion spectra of spiroketal isomers in Figure 21.8 were found to be essentially identical to that of PTX1, PTX6, and PTX2. A proposed assignment of fragment

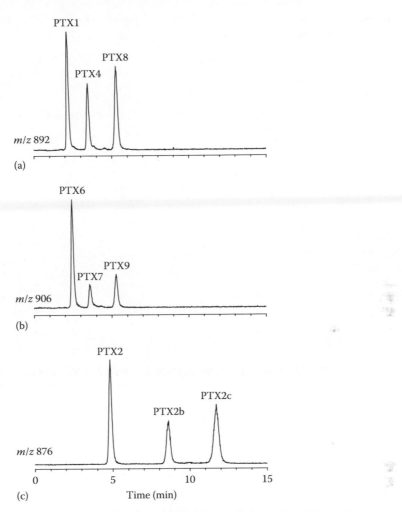

FIGURE 21.8 SIM LC–MS chromatogram of spiroketal isomers of PTX1 (a), PTX6 (b), and PTX2 (c). Column: Hypersil BDS C8 (50 mm × 2.1 mm i.d.). Mobile phase: acetonitrile/water (48:52) with 2 mM ammonium formate and 50 mM formic acid. (From Suzuki, T. et al., *J. Chromatogr. A*, 992, 141, 2003. With permission.)

ions deduced from the structure and through comparison of the spectra of PTX1 and PTX11 is presented in Figure 21.10 (Suzuki et al. 2006). Fragment ions are most easily explained by an initial opening of the macrocyclic ring at the lactone site. The base peak spectrum detected in all pectenotoxin analogues is *m/z* 213. This appears to be due to cleavage of the C-10–C-11 bond adjacent to ring B. Characteristic fragment ions at *m/z* 567 detected in PTX1 can be explained through fragmentation of the C-25–C-26 bond. Corresponding fragment ions at *m/z* 581 from PTX6 and at *m/z* 551 from PTX2 can also be explained by the fragmentation of the C-25–C-26 bond.

21.4.4.2 Yessotoxins

The validity of collision-induced dissociation (CID) by negative-ion fast atom bombardment (FAB) MS/MS analysis for YTX was established in a structural study on YTX (Naoki et al. 1993), and this technique was applied to structural elucidation of a yessotoxin analogue (Daiguji et al. 1998b). Recently, a number of LC–MS or LC–MS/MS methods have been demonstrated as powerful tools for quantification of yessotoxin analogues and structure elucidation of novel toxins in plankton and shellfish (Satake et al. 1997b, 1999; Draisci et al. 1998, 1999b; Ciminiello et al. 2001, 2002a,b, 2003; Goto et al. 2001; Amandi et al. 2002; Canas et al. 2004; Miles et al. 2004c,d, 2005a,b; Paz et al. 2004; Eiki et al. 2005; Finch et al.

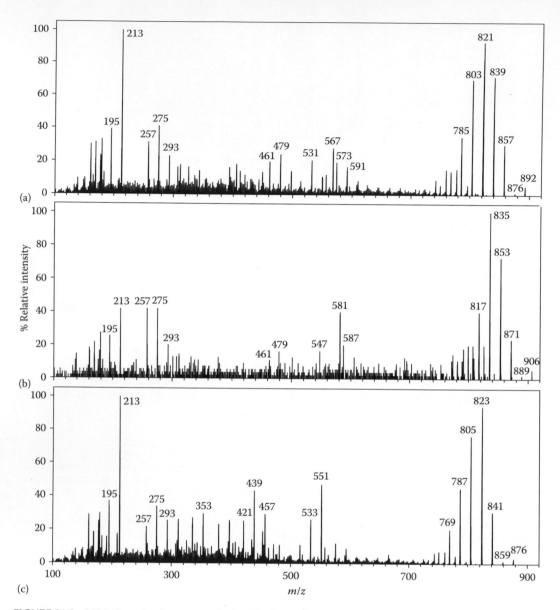

FIGURE 21.9 MS/MS product ion spectra obtained for the [M+NH4]+ ions of PTX1 (a), PTX6 (b), and PTX2 (c). LC conditions as described in Figure 21.8. Collision energy was 45 eV. All *m/z* values have been rounded down. (From Suzuki, T. et al., *J. Chromatogr. A*, 992, 141, 2003. With permission.)

2005; McNabb et al. 2005; Stobo et al. 2005; Suzuki et al. 2005; Rhodes et al. 2006; Fux et al. 2007; Gerssen et al. 2009b, 2010; These et al. 2011; van den Top et al. 2011; Villar-Gonzalez et al. 2011). Most of the studies concerning structural elucidation on yessotoxin analogues by LC–MS have been reported by a 3D ion trap LC–MS^n with an ESI source in the negative mode (Amandi et al. 2002; Ciminiello et al. 2002a,b, 2003; Miles et al. 2004c,d, 2005a,b; Paz et al. 2004). Hybrid quadrupole time-of-flight MS (TOF-MS) was applied to MS/MS analysis of yessotoxins (Canas et al. 2004). It is reported that a hybrid triple quadrupole/linear ion trap MS/MS technique is useful for the characterization of yessotoxin analogues (Suzuki et al. 2007). SIM for [M–H]$^-$or MRM using loss of neutral SO$_3$ moiety from [M–H]$^-$ is applicable to the quantification of yessotoxins. There seems to be no significant difference between the results for SIM and MRM detection. LC–MS detection of yessotoxins on the positive mode has not been reported due to the resulting low sensitivity.

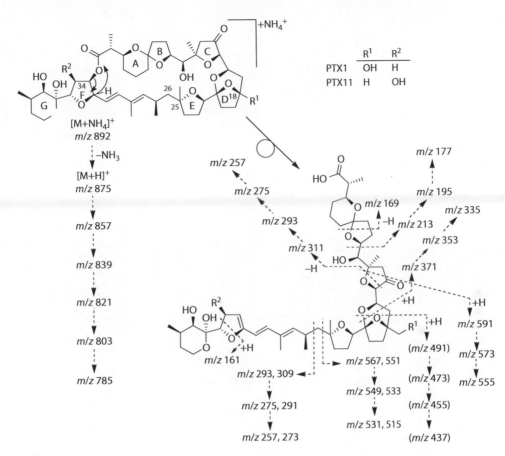

FIGURE 21.10 Proposed fragmentations observed in positive ion MS/MS spectra of PTX1 and PTX11. Ions in bold text arise from PTX11, ions in italic text arise from PTX1, and ions in parentheses are of very low abundance. All transitions shown involved loss of water (18 amu) unless otherwise indicated. (From Suzuki, T. et al., *Chem. Res. Toxicol.*, 19, 310, 2006. With permission.)

One of the most characteristic MS/MS detection, applied to yessotoxins analysis is a neutral loss scan monitoring in the negative mode. The neutral loss scan LC–MS/MS by performing synchronous scanning of Q1 and Q3 with an offset of 80 amu (SO₃ loss) of yessotoxins is useful to survey for known and unknown yessotoxin analogues (Miles et al. 2005a; Suzuki et al. 2007). Figure 21.11 illustrates the neutral loss scan negative-ion LC–MS/MS chromatogram obtained from an extract of a *P. reticulatum* isolate (10628-OK-PR-C) from Japan (Suzuki et al. 2007). The peaks at *m/z* 1047, 1101, 1115, and 1141 correspond to [M–H]⁻ of noroxoYTX, 45,46,47-trinorYTX, 45,46,47-trinorhomoYTX, and YTX, respectively. The negative-ion MRM LC–MS/MS chromatogram obtained from an extract of the same *P. reticulatum* isolate is shown in Figure 21.12 (Suzuki et al. 2007). This MRM LC–MS/MS can detect all known yessotoxin analogues by selecting [M–H]⁻ as the target parent ions to [M–H–SO₃]⁻ as the fragment ions. Although 45,46,47-trinorYTX (peak 2) and 45,46,47-trinorhomoYTX (peak 3) cannot be separated on the C8 column, they can be distinguished by different MRM channels. Due to difficulty in distinguish between yessotoxins and homoyessotoxins by their retention time, LC–MS/MS is probably the only method for quantification of yessotoxins and homoyessotoxins in samples in which both toxins are present.

It is noteworthy that the LC–MS/MS spectrum obtained for YTX with a hybrid triple quadrupole/ linear ion trap MS is identical to that obtained by FAB MS/MS charge remote fragmentation (Suzuki et al. 2007). Similar charge remote fragmentation of yessotoxins was also reported by TOF-MS analysis (Canas et al. 2004). Figure 21.13 shows linear ion trap LC–MS/MS spectra obtained for YTX and 45,46,47-trinorhomoYTX detected in the *P. reticulatum* isolate extract. This showed that product ions were formed as a consequence of charge remote fragmentation processes that included a strong directional

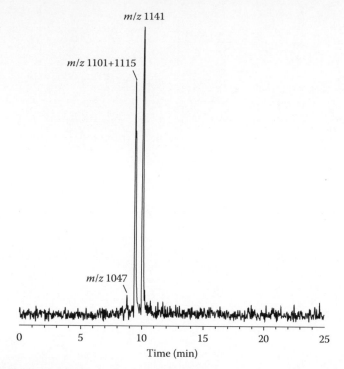

FIGURE 21.11 Neutral loss scan LC–MS/MS chromatogram of YTXs in *P. reticulatum* (020603-MB(20m)-PR-2) from Mutsu Bay. Column: Hypersil BDS C8 (50 mm × 2.1 mm i.d.). Mobile phase: A (water) and B (acetonitrile/water (95:5 v/v)) both containing 2 mM ammonium formate and 50 mM formic acid. Gradient elution from 20% to 100% B over 10 min (step 1) and 100% B for 15 min (step 2) with flow rate at 0.2 mL/min. (From Suzuki, T. et al., *J. Chromatogr. A,* 1142, 172, 2007. With permission.)

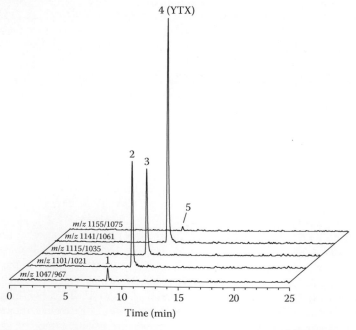

FIGURE 21.12 MRM LC–MS/MS chromatogram of YTXs in *P. reticulatum* (020603-MB(20m)-PR-2) collected from Mutsu Bay. Column: Hypersil BDS C8 (50 mm × 2.1 mm i.d.). Mobile phase: A (water) and B (acetonitrile/water (95:5 v/v)) both containing 2 mM ammonium formate and 50 mM formic acid. Gradient elution from 20% to 100% B over 10 min (step 1) and 100% B for 15 min (step 2) with flow rate at 0.2 mL/min. (From Suzuki, T. et al., *J. Chromatogr. A,* 1142, 172, 2007. With permission.)

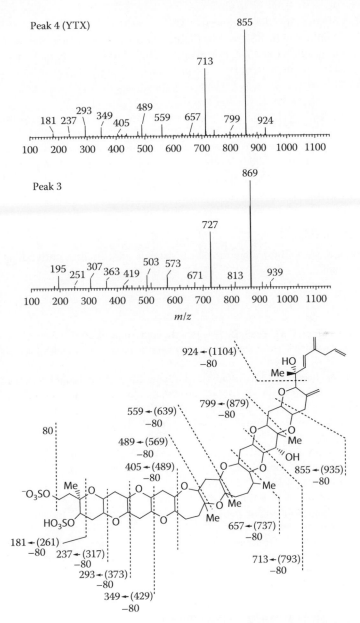

FIGURE 21.13 LC–MS/MS product ion spectra obtained for [M–H]– ions of peak 4 (YTX) and peak 3 (trinor-1-homoYTX) in Figure 21.12. All *m/z* values have been rounded down. Column: Hypersil BDS C8 (50 mm × 2.1 mm i.d.). Mobile phase: A (water) and B (acetonitrile/water (95:5 v/v)) both containing 2 mM ammonium formate and 50 mM formic acid. Gradient elution from 20% to 100% B over 10 min (step 1) and 100% B for 15 min (step 2) with flow rate at 0.2 mL/min. (From Suzuki, T. et al., *J. Chromatogr. A,* 1142, 172, 2007. With permission.)

cleavage of the polyether rings of yessotoxins. The MS/MS spectra of homoYTX analogues including 45,46,47-trinorhomoYTX are 14 mass units higher than those obtained for YTX due to the elongation of the homologous methylene group in the western part of the molecule with negatively charged sulfate esters.

21.4.5 Capillary Electrophoresis

Separation of compounds by capillary electrophoresis (CE) is based on the different mobilities in an electric field depending on the charge and the size of the molecules. Analysis of YTX and

45-hydroxyYTX in bivalves by CE was reported (De la Iglesia et al. 2007). Successively, this approach was developed by coupling with ESI MS for the determination of yessotoxins and pectenotoxins in seafood samples (De la Iglesia and Gago-Martinez 2009). This work demonstrated the potential of CE-ESI-MS to be applied for a sensitive determination of lipophilic toxins in seafood samples as alternative to LC–ESI–MS.

21.4.6 Calibration Standards

Calibration standards of PTX2 and YTX are available from the National Research Institute Canada (Halifax, Canada) (Thomas et al. 2003). There is a standard toxin distribution project organized by the Japanese government for domestic use (Suzuki and Watanabe 2011). PTX1, PTX2, PTX6, and YTX are available in Japan from the National Research Institute of Fisheries Science (Yokohama, Japan).

ACKNOWLEDGMENT

I express my gratitude to Dr. Jim Hungerford for assistance with English corrections and his valuable comments on this chapter.

REFERENCES

Aasen, J., Samdal, I.A., Miles, C.O., Dahl, E., Briggs, L.R., and Aune, T. 2005. Yessotoxins in Norwegian blue mussels (*Mytilus edulis*): Uptake from *Protoceratium reticulatum*, metabolism and depuration. *Toxicon* **45**: 265–272.

Amandi, M.F., Furey, A., Lehane, M., Ramstad, H., and James, K.J. 2002. Liquid chromatography with electrospray ion-trap mass spectrometry for the determination of yessotoxins in shellfish. *J. Chromatogr. A* **976**: 329–334.

Aune, T., Sorby, R., Yasumoto, T., Ramstad, H., and Landsverk, T. 2002. Comparison of oral and intraperitoneal toxicity of yessotoxin towards mice. *Toxicon* **40**: 77–82.

Canas, I.R., Hamilton, B., Amandi, M.F., Furey, A., and James, K.J. 2004. Nano liquid chromatography with hybrid quadrupole time-of-flight mass spectrometry for the determination of yessotoxin in marine phytoplankton. *J. Chromatogr. A* **1056**: 253–256.

Ciminiello, P., Dell'Aversano, C., Fattorusso, E., Forino, M., Grauso, L., Magno, S.G., Poletti, R., and Tartaglione, L. 2007. Desulfoyessotoxins from adriatic mussels: A new problem for seafood safety control. *Chem. Res. Toxicol.* **20**: 95–98.

Ciminiello, P., Dell'Aversano, C., Fattorusso, E., Forino, M., Magno, S., Guerrini, F., Pistocchi, R., and Boni, L. 2003. Complex yessotoxins profile in *Protoceratium reticulatum* from north-western Adriatic sea revealed by LC-MS analysis. *Toxicon* **42**: 7–14.

Ciminiello, P., Dell'Aversano, C., Fattorusso, E., Forino, M., Magno, S., and Poletti, R. 2002a. The detection and identification of 42,43,44,45,46,47,55-heptanor-41-oxoyessotoxin, a new marine toxin from Adriatic shellfish, by liquid chromatography–mass spectrometry. *Chem. Res. Toxicol.* **15**: 979–984.

Ciminiello, P., Dell'Aversano, C., Fattorusso, E., Forino, M., Magno, S., and Poletti, R. 2002b. Direct detection of yessotoxin and its analogues by liquid chromatography coupled with electrospray ion trap mass spectrometry. *J. Chromatogr. A* **968**: 61–69.

Ciminiello, P. and Fattorusso, E. 2008. Chemistry, metabolism, and chemical analysis. In *Seafood and Freshwater Toxins: Pharmacology, Physiology, and Detection*, 2nd edn., ed. L.M. Botana, pp. 287–314. CRC Press, Boca Raton, FL.

Ciminiello, P., Fattorusso, E., Forino, M., Magno, S., Poletti, R., Satake, M., Viviani, R., and Yasumoto, T. 1997. Yessotoxin in mussels of the northern Adriatic Sea. *Toxicon* **35**: 177–183.

Ciminiello, P., Fattorusso, E., Forino, M., Magno, S., Poletti, R., and Viviani, R. 1998. Isolation of adriatoxin, a new analogue of yessotoxin from mussels of the Adriatic Sea. *Tetrahedron Lett.* **39**: 8897–8900.

Ciminiello, P., Fattorusso, E., Forino, M., Magno, S., Poletti, R., Viviani, R., and Yasumoto, T. 1999. Isolation of 45-hydroxyyessotoxin from mussels of the Adriatic Sea. *Toxicon* **37**: 689–693.

Ciminiello, P., Fattorusso, E., Forino, M., and Poletti, R. 2001. 42,43,44,45,46,47,55-Heptanor-41-oxohomoyessotoxin, a new biotoxin from mussels of the northern Adriatic sea. *Chem. Res. Toxicol.* **14**: 596–599.

Ciminiello, P., Fattorusso, E., Forino, M., Poletti, R., and Viviani, R. 2000a. A new analogue of yessotoxin, carboxyyessotoxin, isolated from Adriatic Sea mussels. *Eur. J. Org. Chem.* **2**: 291–295.

Ciminiello, P., Fattorusso, E., Forino, M., Poletti, R., and Viviani, R. 2000b. Structure determination of carboxyhomoyessotoxin, a new yessotoxin analogue isolated from Adriatic mussels. *Chem. Res. Toxicol.* **13**: 770–774.

Daiguji, M., Satake, M., James, K.J., Bishop, A., Mackenzie, L., Naoki, H., and Yasumoto, T. 1998a. Structures of new pectenotoxin analogs, pectenotoxin-2 seco acid and 7-*epi*-pectenotoxin-2 seco acid, isolated from a dinoflagellate and greenshell mussels. *Chem. Lett.* **7**: 653–654.

Daiguji, M., Satake, M., Ramstad, H., Aune, T., Naoki, H., and Yasumoto, T. 1998b. Structure and fluorometric HPLC determination of 1-desulfoyessotoxin, a new yessotoxin analog, isolated from mussels from Norway. *Nat. Toxins* **6**: 235–239.

De la Iglesia, P. and Gago-Marti'nez, A. 2009. Determination of yessotoxins and pectenotoxins in shellfish by capillary electrophoresis-electrospray ionization-mass spectrometry. *Food Addit. Contam. Part A* **226**: 221–228.

De la Iglesia, P., Gago-Martinez, A., and Yasumoto, T. 2007. Advanced studies for the application of high-performance capillary electrophoresis for the analysis of yessotoxin and 45-hydroxyyessotoxin. *J. Chromatogr. A* **1156**: 160–166.

Domínguez, H.J., Souto, M.L., Norte, M., Daranas, A.H., and Fernández, J.J. 2010. Adriatoxin-B, the first C13 terminal truncated YTX analogue obtained from dinoflagellates. *Toxicon* **55**: 1484–1490.

Draisci, R., Ferretti, E., Palleschi, L., Marchiafava, C., Poletti, R., Milandri, A., Ceredi, A., and Pompei, M. 1999b. High levels of yessotoxin in mussels and presence of yessotoxin and homoyessotoxin in dinoflagellates of the Adriatic Sea. *Toxicon* **37**: 1187–1193.

Draisci, R., Giannetti, L., Lucentini, L., Ferretti, E., Palleschi, L., and Marchiafava, C. 1998. Direct identification of yessotoxin in shellfish by liquid chromatography coupled with mass spectrometry and tandem mass spectrometry. *Rapid Commun. Mass Spectrom.* **12**: 1291–1296.

Draisci, R., Lucentin, L., Giannetti, L., Boria, P., and Poletti, R. 1996. First report of pectenotoxin-2 (PTX-2) in algae (*Dinophysis fortii*) related to seafood poisoning in Europe. *Toxicon* **34**: 923–935.

Draisci, R., Palleschi, L., Giannetti, L., Lucentini, L., James, K.J., Bishop, A.G., Satake, M., and Yasumoto, T. 1999a. New approach to the direct detection of known and new diarrhoeic shellfish toxins in mussels and phytoplankton by liquid chromatography-mass spectrometry. *J. Chromatogr. A* **847**: 213–221.

Eiki, K., Satake, M., Koike, K., Ogata, T., Mitsuya, T., and Oshima, Y. 2005. Confirmation of yessotoxin production by the dinoflagellate *Protoceratium reticulatum* in Mutsu Bay. *Fish. Sci.* **71**: 633–638.

European Union. 2002. *Off. J. Eur. Commun.* **L75**: 62.

Evans, D.A., Rajapakse, H.A., Chiu, A., and Stenkamp, D. 2002. Asymmetric syntheses of pectenotoxins-4 and -8, part II: Synthesis of the C20–C30 and C31–C40 subunits and fragment assembly. *Angew. Chem. Int. Ed. Engl.* **41**: 4573–4576.

Fernández, M.L., Míguez, A., Martínez, A., Moroño, Á., Arévalo, F., Pazos, Y., Salgado, C., Correa, J., Blanco, J., González-Gil, S., and Reguera, B. 2002. First report of pectenotoxin-2 in phytoplankton net-hauls and mussels from the Galician Rías Baixas (NW Spain) during proliferations of *Dinophysis acuta* and *Dinophysis caudata*. In *Proceedings of the 4th International Conference on Molluscan Shellfish Safety*, eds. A. Villalba, B. Reguera, J.L. Romalde, and R. Beiras, pp. 75–83. Xunta de Galicia and IOC of UNESCO, Santiago de Compostela, Spain.

Finch, S.C., Wilkins, A.L., Hawkes, A.D., Jensen, D.J., MacKenzie, L., Beuzenberg, V., Quilliam, M.A. et al. 2005. Isolation and identification of (44-R,S)-44,55-dihydroxyyessotoxin from *Protoceratium reticulatum*, and its occurrence in extracts of shellfish from New Zealand, Norway and Canada. *Toxicon* **46**: 160–170.

Fux, E., McMillan, D., Bire, R., and Hess, P. 2007. Development of an ultra-performance liquid chromatography-mass spectrometry method for the detection of lipophilic marine toxins. *J. Chromatogr. A* **1157**: 273–280.

Fux, E., Rode, D., Bire, R., and Hess, P. 2008. Approaches to the evaluation of matrix effects in the liquid chromatography-mass spectrometry (LC-MS) analysis of three regulated lipophilic toxin groups in mussel matrix (*Mytilus edulis*). *Food Addit. Contam.* **25**: 1024–1032.

Fux, E., Smith, J.L., Tong, M., Guzma'n, L., and Anderson, D.M. 2011. Toxin profiles of five geographical isolates of *Dinophysis* spp. from North and South America. *Toxicon* **57**: 275–287.

Gerssen, A., McElhinney, M.A., Mulder, P.P., Bire, R., Hess, P., and de Boer, J. 2009a. Solid phase extraction for removal of matrix effects in lipophilic marine toxin analysis by liquid chromatography-tandem mass spectrometry. *Anal. Bioanal. Chem.* **394**: 1213–1226.

Gerssen, A., Mulder, P.P., McElhinney, M.A., and de Boer, J. 2009b. Liquid chromatography-tandem mass spectrometry method for the detection of marine lipophilic toxins under alkaline conditions. *J. Chromatogr. A* **1216**: 1421–1430.

Gerssen, A., Van Olst, E.H.W., Mulder, P.P.J., and De Bore, J. 2010. In-house validation of a liquid chromatography tandem mass spectrometry method for the analysis of lipophilic marine toxins in shellfish using matrix-matched calibration. *Anal. Bioanal. Chem.* **397**: 3079–3088.

Goto, H., Igarashi, T., Sekiguchi, R., Tanno, K., Satake, M., Oshima, Y., and Yasumoto, T. 1998. A Japanese project for production and distribution of shellfish toxins as calibrants for HPLC analysis. In *Proceedings of the VIII International Conference on Harmful Algae*, eds. B. Reguera, J. Blanco, M.L. Fernández, and T. Wyatt, pp. 216–219. Xunta de Galicia and Intergovernmental Oceanographic Commission of UNESCO, Vigo, Spain.

Goto, H., Igarashi, T., Yamamoto, M., Yasuda, M., Sekiguchi, R., Watai, M., Tanno, K., and Yasumoto, T. 2001. Quantitative determination of marine toxins associated with diarrhetic shellfish poisoning by liquid chromatography coupled with mass spectrometry. *J. Chromatogr. A* **907**: 181–189.

Hashimoto, S., Suzuki, T., Shirota, Y., Honma, M., Itabashi, Y., Chyounan, T., and Kamiyama, T. 2006. Lipophilic toxin profile associated with diarrhetic shellfish poisoning in scallops, *Patinopecten yessoensis*, collected in Hokkaido and comparison of the quantitative results between LC/MS and mouse bioassay. *Shokuhin Eiseigaku Zasshi* **47**: 33–40.

Ishige, M., Satoh, N., and Yasumoto, T. 1988. Pathological studies on the mice administrated with the causative agent of diarrhetic shellfish poisoning (okadaic acid and pectenotoxin-2). *Bull. Hokkaido Inst. Public Health* **38**: 18–19.

Ito, E., Suzuki, T., Oshima, Y., and Yasumoto, T. 2008. Studies of diarrhetic activity on pectenotoxin-6 in the mouse and rat. *Toxicon* **51**: 707–716.

Ito, S. and Tsukada, K. 2002. Matrix effect and correction by standard addition in quantitative liquid chromatographic-mass spectrometric analysis of diarrhetic shellfish poisoning toxins. *J. Chromatogr. A* **943**: 39–46.

James, K.J., Bishop, A.G., Draisci, R., Palleschi, L., Marchiafava, C., Ferretti, E., Satake, M., and Yasumoto, T. 1999. Liquid chromatographic methods for the isolation and identification of new pectenotoxin-2 analogues from marine phytoplankton and shellfish. *J. Chromatogr. A* **844**: 53–65.

Kamiyama, T., Nagai, S., Suzuki, T., and Miyamura, K. 2010. Effect of temperature on production of okadaic acid, dinophysistoxin-1, and pectenotoxin-2 by *Dinophysis acuminata* in culture experiments. *Aquat. Microb. Ecol.* **60**: 193–202.

Kamiyama, T. and Suzuki, T. 2009. Production of dinophysistoxin-1 and pectenotoxin-2 by a culture of *Dinophysis acuminata* (Dinophyceae). *Harmful Algae* **8**: 312–317.

King, R., Bonfiglio, R., Fernandez-Metzler, C., Miller-Stein, C., and Olah, T. 2000. Mechanistic investigation of ionization suppression in electrospray ionization. *J. Am. Soc. Mass Spectrom.* **11**: 942–950.

Konishi, M., Yang, X., Li, B., Fairchild, C.R., and Shimizu, Y. 2004. Highly cytotoxic metabolites from the culture supernatant of the temperate dinoflagellate *Protoceratium cf. reticulatum. J. Nat. Prod.* **67**: 1309–1313.

Krock, B., Tillmann, U., Selwood, A.I., and Cembella, A.D. 2008. Unambiguous identification of pectenotoxin-1 and distribution of pectenotoxins in plankton from the North Sea. *Toxicon* **52**: 927–935.

Lee, J.S., Igarashi, T., Fraga, S., Dahl, E., Hovgaard, P., and Yasumoto, T. 1989a. Determination of diarrhetic shellfish toxins in various dinoflagellate species. *J. Appl. Phycol.* **1**: 147–152.

Lee, J.S., Murata, M., and Yasumoto, T. 1989b. Analytical methods for determination of diarrhetic shellfish toxins. In *Proceedings of the Mycotoxins and Phycotoxins "88*, eds. S. Natori, K. Hashimoto, and Y. Ueno, pp. 327–334. Elsevier, Amsterdam, the Netherlands.

Lee, J.S., Yanagi, T., Kenma, R., and Yasumoto, T. 1987. Fluorometric determination of diarrhetic shellfish toxins by high-performance liquid chromatography. *Agric. Biol. Chem.* **51**: 877–881.

Loader, J.I., Hawkes, A.D., Beuzenberg, V., Jensen, D.J., Cooney, J.M., Wilkins, A.L., Fitzgerald, J.M., Briggs, L.R., and Miles, C.O. 2007. Convenient large-scale purification of yessotoxin from *Protoceratium reticulatum* culture and isolation of a novel furanoyessotoxin. *J. Agric. Food Chem.* **55**: 11093–11100.

MacKenzie, L., Beuzenberg, V., Holland, P., McNabb, P., and Selwood, A. 2004. Solid phase adsorption toxin tracking (SPATT): A new monitoring tool that simulates the biotoxin contamination of filter feeding bivalves. *Toxicon* **44**: 901–918.

MacKenzie, L., Beuzenberg, V., Holland, P., McNabb, P., Suzuki, T., and Selwood, A. 2005. Pectenotoxin and okadaic acid-based toxin profiles in *Dinophysis acuta* and *Dinophysis acuminata* from New Zealand. *Harmful Algae* **4**: 75–85.

MacKenzie, L., Holland, P., McNabb, P., Beuzenberg, V., Selwood, A., and Suzuki, T. 2002. Complex toxin profiles in phytoplankton and Greenshell mussels (*Perna canaliculus*), revealed by LC–MS/MS analysis. *Toxicon* **40**: 1321–1330.

MacKenzie, L.A., Selwood, A.I., and Marshall, C. 2012. Isolation and characterization of an enzyme from the Greenshell™ mussel *Perna canaliculus* that hydrolyses pectenotoxins and esters of okadaic acid. *Toxicon* **60**: 406–419.

McNabb, P. and Holland, P.T. 2002. Using liquid chromatography mass spectrometry to manage shellfish harvesting and protect public health. In *Proceedings of the 4th International Conference on Molluscan Shellfish Safety*, eds. A. Villalba, B. Reguera, J.L. Romalde, and R. Beiras, pp. 179–186, Xunta de Galicia and IOC of UNESCO, Santiago de Compostella, Spain.

McNabb, P., Selwood, A.I., and Holland, P.T. 2005. Multiresidue method for determination of algal toxins in shellfish: Single-laboratory validation and interlaboratory study. *J. AOAC Int.* **88**: 761–772.

Miles, C.O., Samdal, I.A., Aasen, J.A.G., Jensen, D.J., Quilliam, M.A., Petersen, D., Briggs, L.M. et al. 2005a. Evidence for numerous analogs of yessotoxin in *Protoceratium reticulatum*. *Harmful Algae* **4**: 1075–1091.

Miles, C.O., Wilkins, A.L., Hawkes, A.D., Jensen, D.J., Cooney, J.M., Beuzenberg, V., Mackenzie, A.L., Selwood, A.I., and Holland, P.T. 2006a. Isolation and identification of pectenotoxins-13 and -14 from *Dinophysis acuta* in New Zealand. *Toxicon* **48**: 152–159.

Miles, C.O., Wilkins, A.L., Hawkes, A.D., Selwood, A.I., Jensen, D.J., Aasen, J., Munday, R. et al. 2004c. Isolation of a 1,3-enone isomer of heptanor-41-oxoyessotoxin for *Protoceratium reticulatum* cultures. *Toxicon* **44**: 325–336.

Miles, C.O., Wilkins, A.L., Hawkes, A.D., Selwood, A.I., Jensen, D.J., Cooney, J.M., Beuzenberg, V., and MacKenzie, L. 2006b. Identification of 45-hydroxy-46,47-dinoryessotoxin, 44-oxo-45,46,47-trinoryessotoxin, and 9-methyl-42,43,44,45,46,47,55-heptanor-38-ene-41-oxoyessotoxin, and partial characterization of some minor yessotoxins, from *Protoceratium reticulate*. *Toxicon* **47**: 229–240.

Miles, C.O., Wilkins, A.L., Hawkes, A.D., Selwood, A.I., Jensen, D.J., Munday, R., Cooney, J.M., and Beuzenberg, V. 2005b. Polyhydroxylated amide analogs of yessotoxin from *Protoceratium reticulatum*. *Toxicon* **45**: 61–71.

Miles, C.O., Wilkins, A.L., Jensen, D.J., Cooney, J.M., Quilliam, M.A., Aasen, J., and MacKenzie, L. 2004d. Isolation of 41a-homoyessotoxin and the identification of 9-methyl-41a-homoyessotoxin and nor-ring-A-yessotoxin from *Protoceratium reticulatum*. *Chem. Res. Toxicol.* **17**: 1414–1422.

Miles, C.O., Wilkins, A.L., Munday, J.S., Munday, R., Hawkes, A.D., Jensen, D.J., Cooney, J.M., and Beuzenberg, V. 2006d. Production of 7-*epi*-pectenotoxin-2 seco acid and assessment of its acute toxicity to mice. *J. Agric. Food Chem.* **54**: 1530–1534.

Miles, C.O., Wilkins, A.L., Munday, R., Dines, M.H., Hawkes, A.D., Briggs, L.R., Sandvik, M. et al. 2004a. Isolation of pectenotoxin-2 from *Dinophysis acuta* and its conversion to pectenotoxin-2 seco acid, and preliminary assessment of their acute toxicities. *Toxicon* **43**: 1–9.

Miles, C.O., Wilkins, A.L., Samdal, I.A., Sandvik, M., Petersen, D., Quilliam, M.A., Naustvoll, L.J. et al. 2004b. A novel pectenotoxin, PTX-12, in *Dinophysis* spp. and shellfish from Norway. *Chem. Res. Toxicol.* **17**: 1423–1433.

Miles, C.O., Wilkins, A.L., Selwood, A.I., Hawkes, A.D., Jensen, D.J., Cooney, J.M., Beuzenberg, V., and MacKenzie, A.L. 2006c. Isolation of yessotoxin 32-O-[ß-l-arabinofuranosyl-(5' → 1")-ß-l-arabinofuranoside] from *Protoceratium reticulatum*. *Toxicon* **47**: 510–516.

Morohashi, A., Satake, M., Oshima, Y., and Yasumoto, T. 2000. Absolute configuration at C45 in 45-hydroxyyessotoxin, a marine polyether toxin, isolated from shellfish. *Biosci. Biotechnol. Biochem.* **64**: 1761–1763.

Murata, M., Kumagai, M., Lee, J.S., and Yasumoto, T. 1987. Isolation and structure of yessotoxin, a novel polyether compound implicated in diarrhetic shellfish poisoning. *Tetrahedron Lett.* **28**: 5869–5872.

Murata, M., Sano, M., Iwashita, T., Naoki, H., and Yasumoto, T. 1986. The structure of pectenotoxin-3, a new constituent of diarrhetic shellfish toxins. *Agric. Biol. Chem.* **50**: 2693–2695.

Nagai, S., Suzuki, T., Nishikawa, T., and Kamiyama, T. 2011. Differences in the production and excretion kinetics of okadaic acid, dinophysistoxin-1, and pectenotoxins-2 between cultures of *Dinophysis acuminata* and *Dinophysis fortii* isolated from western Japan. *J. Phycol.* **47**: 1326–1337.

Naoki, H., Murata, M., and Yasumoto, T. 1993. Negative-ion fast-atom bombardment tandem mass spectrometry for the structural study of polyether compounds: Structural verification of yessotoxin. *Rapid Commun. Mass Spectrom.* **7**: 179–182.

Nogueiras, M.J., Gago-Martínez, A., Paniello, A.I., Twohig, M., James, K.J., and Lawrence, J.F. 2003. Comparison of different fluorometric HPLC methods for analysis of acidic polyether toxins in marine phytoplankton. *Anal. Bioanal. Chem.* **377**: 1202–1206.

Ogino, H., Kumagai, M., and Yasumoto, T. 1997. Toxicologic evaluation of yessotoxin. *Nat. Toxins* **5**: 255–259.

Pavela-Vrancic, M., Mestrovic, V., Marasovic, I., Gillman, M., Furey, A., and James, K.K. 2001. The occurrence of 7-*epi*-pectenotoxin-2 seco acid in the coastal waters of the central Adriatic (Kastela Bay). *Toxicon* **39**: 771–779.

Paz, B., Riobo, P., Fernandez, M.L., Fraga, S., and Franco, J.M. 2004. Production and release of yessotoxins by the dinoflagellates *Protoceratium reticulatum* and *Lingulodinium polyedrum* in culture. *Toxicon* **44**: 251–258.

Paz, B., Riobó, P., Ramilo, I., and Franco, J.M. 2007. Yessotoxins profile in strains of *Protoceratium reticulatum* from Spain and USA. *Toxicon* **50**: 1–17.

Paz, B., Riobó, P., Souto, M.L., Gil, L.V., Norte, M., Fernández, J.J., and Franco, J.M. 2006. Detection and identification of glycoyessotoxin A in a culture of the dinoflagellate *Protoceratium reticulatum*. *Toxicon* **48**: 611–619.

Pizarro, G., Paz, B., Franco, J.M., Suzuki, T., and Reguera, B. 2008. First detection of pectenotoxin-11 and confirmation of OA-D8 diol-ester in *Dinophysis acuta* from European waters by LC-MS/MS. *Toxicon* **52**: 889–896.

Puente, P.F., Sáez, M.J.F., Hamilton, B., Furey, A., and James, K.J. 2004a. Studies of polyether toxins in the marine phytoplankton, *Dinophysis acuta*, in Ireland using multiple tandem mass spectrometry. *Toxicon* **44**: 919–926.

Puente, P.F., Sáez, M.J.F., Hamilton, B., Lehane, M., Ramstad, H., Furey, A., and James, K.J. 2004b. Rapid determination of polyether marine toxins using liquid chromatography–multiple tandem mass spectrometry. *J. Chromatogr. A* **1056**: 77–82.

Quilliam, M.A. 2003. The role of chromatography in the hunt for red tide toxins. *J. Chromatogr. A* **1000**: 527–548.

Quilliam, M.A., Hess, P., and Dell'Aversano, C. 2001. Recent developments in the analysis of phycotoxins by liquid chromatography-mass spectrometry. In *Proceedings of the Mycotoxins and Phycotoxins in Perspective at the Turn of the Century*, eds. W.J. deKoe, R.A. Samson, H.P. van Egmond, J. Gilbert, and M. Sabino, pp. 383–391. Wageningen, the Netherlands.

Rhodes, L., McNabb, P., de Salas, M., Briggs, L., Beuzenberg, V., and Gladstone, M. 2006. Yessotoxin production by *Gonyaulax spinifera*. *Harmful Algae* **5**: 148–155.

Riccardi, M., Guerrini, F., Roncarati, F., Milandri, A., Cangini, M., Pigozzi, S., Riccardi, E. et al. 2009. *Gonyaulax spinifera* from the Adriatic sea: Toxin production and phylogenetic analysis. *Harmful Algae* **8**: 279–290.

Samdal, I.A., Naustvoll, L.J., Olseng, C.D., Briggs, L.R., and Miles, C.O. 2004. Use of ELISA to identify *Protoceratium reticulatum* as a source of yessotoxin in Norway. *Toxicon* **44**: 75–82.

Sasaki, K., Satake, M., and Yasumoto, T. 1997. Identification of the absolute configuration of pectenotoxin-6, a polyether macrolide compound, by NMR spectroscopic method using a chiral anisotropic reagent, phenylglycine methyl ester. *Biosci. Biotechnol. Biochem.* **61**: 1783–1785.

Sasaki, K., Takizawa, A., Tubaro, A., Sidari, L., Loggia, R.D., and Yasumoto, T. 1999. Fluorometric analysis of pectenotoxin-2 in microalgal samples by high performance liquid chromatography. *Nat. Toxins* **7**: 241–246.

Sasaki, K., Wright, J.L., and Yasumoto T. 1998. Identification and characterization of pectenotoxin (PTX) 4 and PTX7 as spiroketal stereoisomers of two previously reported pectenotoxins. *J. Org. Chem.* **63**: 2475–2480.

Satake, M., Eiki, K., Ichimura, T., Ota, S., Sekiguchi, K., and Oshima, Y. 2006. Structure of 45,46,47-trinorhomoyessotoxin, a new yessotoxin analog, from *Protoceratium reticulatum* which represents the first detection of a homoyessotoxin analog in Japan. *Harmful Algae* **5**: 731–735.

Satake, M., Ichimura, T., Sekiguchi, K., Yoshimatsu, S., and Oshima, Y. 1999. Confirmation of yessotoxin and 45,46,47-trinoryessotoxin production by *Protoceratium reticulatum* collected in Japan. *Nat. Toxins* **7**: 147–150.

Satake, M., MacKenzie, L., and Yasumoto, T. 1997a. Identification of *Protoceratium reticulatum* as the biogenetic origin of yessotoxin. *Nat. Toxins* **5**: 164–167.

Satake, M., Terasawa, K., Kadowaki, Y., and Yasumoto, T. 1996. Relative configuration of yessotoxin and isolation of two new analogs from toxic scallops. *Tetrahedron Lett.* **37**: 5955–5958.

Satake, M., Tubaro, A., Lee, J.S., and Yasumoto, T. 1997b. Two new analogs of yessotoxin, homoyessotoxin and 45-hydroxyhomoyessotoxin, isolated from mussels of the Adriatic Sea. *Nat. Toxins* **5**: 107–110.

Souto, M.L., Ferna'ndez, J.J., Franco, J.M., Paz, B., Gil, L.V., and Norte, M. 2005. Glycoyessotoxin a, a new yessotoxin derivative from cultures of *Protoceratium reticulatum*. *J. Nat. Prod.* **68**: 420–422.

Stobo, A., Lacaze, J.P., Scott, A.C., Gallacher, S., Smith, E.A., and Quilliam, M.A. 2005. Liquid chromatography with mass spectrometry detection of lipophilic shellfish toxins, *J. AOAC Int.* **88**: 1371–1382.

Suzuki, T., Beuzenberg, V., Mackenzie, L., and Quilliam, M.A. 2003. Liquid chromatography-mass spectrometry of spiroketal stereoisomers of pectenotoxins and the analysis of novel pectenotoxin isomers in the toxic dinoflagellate *Dinophysis acuta* from New Zealand. *J. Chromatogr. A* **992**: 141–150.

Suzuki, T., Horie, Y., Koike, K., Satake, M., Oshima, Y., Iwataki, M., and Yoshimatsu, S. 2007. Yessotoxin analogues in several strains of *Protoceratium reticulatum* in Japan determined by liquid chromatography-hybrid triple quadrupole/linear ion trap mass spectrometry. *J. Chromatogr. A* **1142**: 172–177.

Suzuki, T., Igarashi, T., Ichimi, K., Watai, M., Suzuki, M., Ogiso, E., and Yasumoto, T. 2005b. Kinetics of diarrhetic shellfish poisoning toxins, okadaic acid, dinophysistoxin-1, pectenotoxin-6 and yessotoxin in scallops *Patinopecten yessoensis*. *Fish. Sci.* **71**: 948–955.

Suzuki, T., Jin, T., Shirota, Y., Mitsuya, T., Okumura, Y., and Kamiyama, T. 2005a. Quantification of lipophilic toxins associated with diarrhetic shellfish poisoning in Japanese bivalves by liquid chromatography-mass spectrometry and comparison with mouse bioassay. *Fish. Sci.* **71**: 1370–1378.

Suzuki, T., Mackenzie, L., Stirling, D., and Adamson, J. 2001a. Pectenotoxin-2 seco acid: A toxin converted from pectenotoxin-2 by New Zealand Greenshell mussel, *Perna canaliculus. Toxicon* **39**: 507–514.

Suzuki, T., Mackenzie, L., Stirling, D., and Adamson, J. 2001b. Conversion of pectenotoxin-2 to pectenotoxin-2 seco acid in the New Zealand scallop, *Pecten novaezelandiae*. *Fish. Sci.* **67**: 506–510.

Suzuki, T., Mitsuya, T., Matsubara, H., and Yamasaki, M. 1998. Determination of pectenotoxin-2 after solid phase extraction from seawater and from the dinoflagellate *Dinophysis fortii* by liquid chromatography with electrospray mass spectrometry and ultraviolet detection: Evidence of oxidation of pectenotoxin-2 to pectenotoxin-6 in scallops. *J. Chromatogr. A* **815**: 155–160.

Suzuki, T., Miyazono, A., Baba, K., Sugawara, R., and Kamiayam, T. 2009. LC-MS/MS analysis of okadaic acid analogues and other lipophilic toxins in single-cell isolates of several *Dinophysis* species collected in Hokkaido, Japan. *Harmful Algae* **8**: 233–238.

Suzuki, T., Walter, J.A., LeBlanc, P., Mackinnon, S., Miles, C.O., Wilkins, A.L., Munday, R. et al. 2006. Identification of pectenotoxin-11 as 34*S*-hydroxypectenotoxin-2, a new pectenotoxin analogue in the toxic dinoflagellate *Dinophysis acuta* from New Zealand. *Chem. Res. Toxicol.* **19**: 310–318.

Suzuki, T. and Watanabe, R. 2011. Shellfish toxin monitoring system in Japan and some Asian countries. In *New Trends in Marine Freshwater Toxins*, eds. A.G. Cabado and J.M. Vietes, pp. 305–314. Nova Science Publishers, Inc., New York.

Suzuki, T., Wilkins, A.L., Watanabe, R., Miles, C.O., and Rise, F. 2012. Discovery of a novel pectenotoxins identified as 38-hydroxypectenotoxin-6 in Japanese scallops, *Patinopecten yessoensis*. In *The 15th International Conference on Harmful Algae 2012 Korea Abstract Book*, p. 164. Changwon, Korea.

Suzuki, T. and Yasumoto, T. 2000. Liquid chromatography-electrospray ionization mass spectrometry of the diarrhetic shellfish—poisoning toxins okadaic acid, denophysistoxin-1 and pectenotoxin-6 in bivalves. *J. Chromatogr. A* **874**: 199–206.

Takahashi, H., Kusumi, T., Kan, Y., Satake, M., and Yasumoto, T. 1996. Determination of the absolute configuration of yessotoxin, a polyether compound implicated in diarrhetic shellfish poisoning, by NMR spectroscopic method using a chiral anisotropic reagent, methoxy (2-naphthyl) acetic acid. *Tetrahedron Lett.* **37**: 7087–7090.

These, A., Klemm, C., Nausch, I., and Uhlig, S. 2011. Results of a European interlaboratory method validation study for the quantitative determination of lipophilic marine biotoxins in raw and cooked shellfish based on high-performance liquid chromatography-tandem mass spectrometry. Part I: Collaborative study. *Anal. Bioanal. Chem.* **399**: 1245–1256.

Thomas, K., Blay, P., Burton, I.W., Cembella, A.D., Craft, C., Crain S, Hardstaff, W.R. et al. 2003. Certified reference materials for marine toxins. In *Proceedings of the HAB Tech03 Workshop (Cawthron Report No. 906)*, eds. P. Holland, L. Rhodes, and L. Brown, p. 137. Nelson, New Zealand.

Thomson, B.A. and Iribarne, J.V. 1979. Field-induced ion evaporation from liquid surfaces at atmospheric-pressure. *J. Chem. Phys.* **71**: 4451–4463.

van den Top, H.J., Gerssen, A., McCarron, P., and van Egmond, H.P. 2011. Quantitative determination of marine lipophilic toxins in mussels, oysters and cockles using liquid chromatography-mass spectrometry: Inter-laboratory validation study. *Food Addit. Contam. Part A* **28**: 1745–1757.

Tubaro, A., Sosa, S., Carbonatto, M., Altinier, G., Vita, F., Melato, M., Satake, M., and Yasumoto, T. 2003. Oral and intraperitoneal acute toxicity studies of yessotoxin and homoyessotoxins in mice. *Toxicon* **41**: 783–792.

Vale, P. 2004. Differential dynamics of dinophysistoxins and pectenotoxins between blue mussel and common cockle: A phenomenon originating from the complex toxin profile of *Dinophysis acuta. Toxicon* **44**: 123–134.

Vale, P. and Sampayo, M.A. 2002. Pectenotoxin-2 seco acid, 7-epi-pectenotoxin-2 seco acid and pectenotoxin-2 in shellfish and plankton from Portugal. *Toxicon* **40**: 979–987.

Villar-González, A., Rodríguez-Velasco, M.L., and Gago-Martínez, A. 2011. Determination of lipophilic toxins by LC/MS/MS: Single-laboratory validation. *J. AOAC Int.* **94**: 909–922.

Wilkins, A.L., Rehmann, N., Torgersen, T., Rundberget, T., Keogh, M., Petersen, D., Hess, P., Rise, F., and Miles, C.O. 2006. Identification of fatty acid esters of pectenotoxin-2 seco acid in blue mussels (*Mytilus edulis*) from Ireland. *J. Agric. Food Chem.* **54**: 5672–5678.

Yasumoto, T., Fukui, M., Sasaki, K., and Sugiyama, K. 1995. Determinations of marine toxins in foods. *J. AOAC Int.* **78**: 574–582.

Yasumoto, T. and Murata, M. 1993. Marine toxins. *Chem. Rev.* **93**: 1897–1909.

Yasumoto, T., Murata, M., Lee, J.S., and Torigoe, K. 1989. Polyether toxins produced by dinoflagellates, In *Proceedings of the Mycotoxins and Phycotoxins '88*, eds. S. Natori, K. Hashimoto, and Y. Ueno, pp. 375–382. Elsevier, Amsterdam, the Netherlands.

Yasumoto, T., Murata, M., Oshima, Y., Matsumoto, G.K., and Clardy, J. 1984. Diarrhetic shellfish poisoning. In *ACS Symposium Series No. 262, Seafood Toxins*, ed. E.P. Ragelis, pp. 207–214. ACS, Washington, DC.

Yasumoto, T., Murata, M., Oshima, Y., Sano, M., Matsumoto, G.K., and Clardy, J. 1985. Diarrhetic shellfish toxins. *Tetrahedron* **41**: 1019–1025.

Yasumoto, T. and Takizawa, A. 1997. Fluorometric measurement of yessotoxins in shellfish by high-pressure liquid chromatography. *Biosci. Biotechnol. Biochem.* **61**: 1775–1777.

Zhao, J., Lembeye, G., Cenci, G., Wall, B., and Yasumoto, T. 1993. Determination of okadaic acid and dinophysistoxin-1 in mussels from Chile, Italy and Ireland. In *Proceedings of the Toxic Phytoplankton Blooms in the Sea*, eds. T.J. Smayda and Y. Shimuzu, pp. 587–592. Elsevier, Amsterdam, the Netherlands.

22

Yessotoxins and Pectenotoxins

Amparo Alfonso, Araceli Tobío, and M. Carmen Louzao

CONTENTS

22.1 Yessotoxins

22.1.1 Introduction

Yessotoxin (YTX) and its analogs are a group of more than 100 polyether compounds produced by several species of dinoflagellates genera *Gonyaulax*, *Protoceratium*, and *Lingulodinium* and originally isolated from *Patinopecten yessoensis*.[100] So far, no human intoxications have been described, and even though high acute toxicity after mice intraperitoneal (i.p.) injection has been reported, low toxicity after oral administration has been showed.[1,32,77,117] The lack of oral toxicity and the absence of human intoxications have prompted discussions about the role of these compounds as toxins.[80] In addition, several references of YTX effect over cancer cell survival together with the different effect observed in tumoral and nontumoral cells point to this molecule as a useful tool in searching for new drugs.

22.1.2 Mechanism of Action

Several approaches have been done to clear up the cellular activity of the YTX group. The effects reported in the presence of YTX were obtained after incubation with low toxin concentrations (nanomolar range) for several days or with high toxin concentrations (micromolar range) for a few seconds or minutes. This two sort of results pointed to two different receptorial systems depending on the incubation time.[41] However, recent results indicate that probably the same mechanism of action is activated as it was before hypothesized.[3]

22.1.2.1 Early Activation Steps

Cytosolic calcium levels, ion fluxes, cyclic nucleotides levels, and enzymatic activity are early signals in cellular activation. These signals are the molecular target, or are involved in the initial effect, of some marine phycotoxins and through complex cross-talk pathways induce long-term effects.

The increase of cytosolic calcium levels is a basic step in cellular activation. Different effects in calcium levels were reported in different cellular models after YTX incubation. Micromolar YTX concentrations induce a fast but small increase in cytosolic calcium levels (40 nM) in human fresh lymphocytes. This increase is due to the activation of nifedipine and SKF 96365-sensitive calcium channels.[30] However, in the same cellular model, YTX inhibits the influx of calcium after preincubation in a calcium-free medium and also the influx activated by thapsigargin, a tumor-promoting sesquiterpene lactone that inhibits calcium-ATPase from intracellular pools and activates store-operated calcium influx.[30] On the contrary, in the K-562 cell line, YTX does not modify cytosolic calcium levels in a calcium-containing media and induces an increase on calcium pools depletion in a calcium-free media followed by high calcium influx when the calcium is restored to the media. The pools affected by YTX are not thapsigargin dependent.[115] In this cellular line, the calcium pool depletion induced by YTX was abolished by the adenosine 3′–5′cyclic monophosphate (cAMP) analog dibutyryl cAMP, by the phosphodiesterase 4 (PDE4) inhibitor rolipram, by the protein kinase A (PKA) inhibitor H89, and by the oxidative phosphorylation uncoupler, carbonyl cyanide p-trifluoromethoxy (FCCP) treatments. However, the YTX-dependent calcium influx was only abolished by FCCP pretreatment.[115] In addition, in human fresh lymphocytes, the calcium influx induced by maitotoxin, a potent water-soluble marine toxin associated with ciguatera food poisoning, was increased in the presence of YTX through the activation of different calcium channels.[31] A cytosolic calcium increase in the presence of YTX was also observed in HL7702 human liver cells, in Bel7402 human hepatoma cell line, and in primary cultures of rat cerebellar neurons.[82,83,90] However, YTX did not directly modify calcium basal levels in rat primary cardiomyocytes, while the mitochondrial pathway is mediating in cellular survival of these cells.[33] All these results evidence the cross talks between calcium, the cAMP pathway, and the mitochondria in the YTX effect.

The chemical structure of YTX, more than 10 contiguous ether rings,[101] resembles those of brevetoxins and ciguatoxins. The action of these toxins is mediated through voltage-gated sodium channels; however, YTX did not induce any direct effect in sodium channels, besides the toxin did not induce any competitive displacement of brevetoxins from site 5 of sodium channels.[47] Therefore, these results point that the effect of YTX on cytosolic calcium levels is a direct consequence of calcium channel activation and it is not linked to sodium channels as it happens with those toxins. In summary, calcium influx seems to be an important event in the YTX mechanism of action.

The cyclic nucleotides cAMP and guanine 3′–5′ cyclic monophosphate (cGMP) are second messengers related with early activation pathways of cellular signaling. Cells regulate the levels of these second messengers by a balance between adenylyl cyclases (synthesis) and phosphodiesterases (PDEs) (hydrolysis). YTX induces a dose-dependent decrease of cAMP and cGMP levels after 10 min of incubation in human fresh lymphocytes. These effects are calcium dependent and can be modified by specific PDEs inhibitors.[3,6] Surprisingly, YTX effect in K-562 cell line is completely opposite since YTX induces a dose-dependent increase of cAMP levels after 10 min incubation. The effect is reverted in a calcium-free medium.[115] On the other hand, YTX did not directly modify cAMP levels in rat primary cardiomyocytes.[33]

PDEs are a group of isozymes that includes several families with different substrate specificity, affinity, sensitivity to inhibitors, and tissue localization. In human fresh lymphocytes, YTX induces a dose-dependent increase in PDEs activity. In parallel, the toxin decreases cAMP levels while increasing the rate of hydrolysis of this second messenger. All these effects can be mimicked by PDEs activators and modulated by enzyme inhibitors.[4]

All these results pointed to PDEs as an early cellular target for YTX and to the calcium as an important key factor for toxin effects. The interaction between PDEs and YTX has been demonstrated by immobilizing these enzymes in a biosensor surface. When different concentrations of toxin were added over the immobilized YTX, typical association curves indicative of interaction were observed.[3] In these conditions, the value of the kinetic equilibrium dissociation constant K_D for YTX–PDEs association obtained was 3.74×10^{-6} M YTX.[85] When the YTX molecule was modified, the K_D value was increased, indicating a structure–activity relationship. In the same conditions, the K_D for hydroxy-YTX–PDEs interaction obtained was 7.36×10^{-6} M OH-YTX and the K_D value for carboxy-YTX–PDEs interaction was 23×10^{-6} M carboxy-YTX.[87] These results point to a structure–selectivity of YTX–PDEs association and are according to the decrease in the toxic effect observed with some YTX analogs.[120] The PDEs–YTX interaction was also confirmed by measuring changes in fluorescence polarization of an enzyme–dye conjugate in the presence of YTX.[9] By using different enzyme families in a sensor surface and by measuring changes in fluorescence polarization, it was concluded that YTX binds to cyclic nucleotide PDE1, PDE3, and PDE4, and the toxin shows also high affinity by exonuclease PDE I.[8,86]

There are several anchoring proteins related with the PDEs family members, such as receptor for activated C-kinase (RACK1), β-arrestins, and the A-kinase anchoring proteins (AKAPs). AKAPs are structural proteins that interact with a variety of cellular components as PKAs and PDEs and share out these enzymes near to local cAMP pools regulating its levels.[18] AKAP family subtypes are cell- and tissue-specific proteins and can be associated to the mitochondria, to membrane receptors, or to the nuclear matrix.[40] The AKAP149, also called AKAP1, is localized in the outer mitochondrial membrane and in the nuclear envelope. In the mitochondria, AKAP149 anchors the PKA and the type 4A PDE (PDE4A).[15] Therefore, AKAPs are the most important proteins that take part in cAMP/PDE compartmentalization.[79] The complex AKAP–PDEs–PKA is essential for cell survival and participates in crucial pathways such as cell respiration.[25] Since PDEs and mitochondria are related through AKAPs, the levels of this anchoring protein were measured in the presence of YTX. YTX has different and completely opposite effect in fresh human lymphocytes and in the K-562 cell line. In the first one, YTX increases AKAP149 cytosolic levels, while in K-562 cells, this toxin decreases the cytosolic amount of AKAP149 (Figure 22.1). The same effects were observed after 10 min of incubation with high toxin concentration (10 μM) than after 24 and 48 h of incubation in the presence of lower YTX concentration (30 nM). Therefore, the same effects in AKAP149 levels were observed after short- and long-term YTX incubations and this protein is the next link in the molecular pathway activated by the toxin.

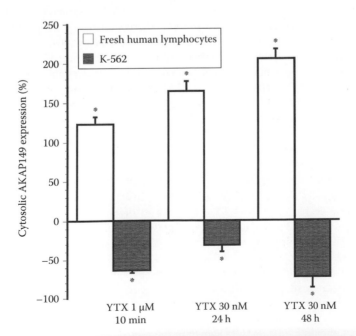

FIGURE 22.1 Cytosolic AKAP149 expression after YTX incubation in human fresh lymphocytes and K-562 cells. X axis represents expression levels of cells without treatment. Mean ± SEM of three experiments. (*) Significant differences with respect to cells without treatment.

Recently, some effect of YTX over protein kinase C (PKC) translocation was reported in primary cortical neurons.[11] PKC is a protein activated in early steps of signal transduction pathways and involved in the activation of PDEs in several cellular models.

22.1.2.2 Long-Term Effects

Several approaches had been done to study long-term effects of YTXs. After 1 h of YTX incubation, no effects over F-actin levels were reported in neuroblastoma BE(2)-M17 cells, as well as after 4 h of incubation of rabbit fresh enterocytes.[14,59] However, cellular detachment from culture dishes was reported after YTX incubation.[78] On the other hand, lysosomal vesicles and a progressive depolymerization of actin microfilaments, either in invertebrate, insect fat body IPLB-LdFB, or vertebrate, mouse fibroblasts NIH3T3, have been described after YTX treatment.[65]

E-cadherin is a large family of proteins responsible for calcium-dependent cell to cell adhesion that mediates in the aggregation-dependent cell survival. A decrease in E-cadherin expression is associated with the tumor expansion in epithelial cells, but in some cases, this protein plays a role in survival and apoptosis suppression of other carcinoma cells.[93] After 20 h of incubation of the human breast cancer cells MCF-7 in the presence of YTX, an accumulation of a 100 kDa fragment of E-cadherin without a parallel loss of the intact protein was described.[91] The collapse of E-cadherin system happened after 2–5 days YTX treatment (sub-nanomolar range) either in MCF-7 cells or in other tumoral epithelial cellular model as Caco-2.[96] This effect was related with toxin structure involving the C9 terminal chain. YTX was the most potent analog to induce accumulation of 100 kDa fragment of E-cadherin, then 45-hydroxyhomoYTX showed some activity and then carboxy-YTX.[41] An increase in the polarity of the C9 chain, rather than an increase in size, is related with the decrease in affinity of YTX by the E-cadherin. Surprisingly, as it was before mentioned, the same structure–selectivity relationship and decrease in potency depending on C9 chain were observed in the association PDEs–YTX and YTX analogs.[87]

It has been shown that YTX did not induce any effect in E-cadherin system in vivo.[24] These results confirm the loss of morphological changes observed in any internal organ after several days of toxin oral treatment. Before these last results and from E-cadherin data, YTX was proposed to facilitate tumor spreading and metastasis formation[96]; therefore, this hypothesis affirmation should be reviewed. In addition, an effect over E-cadherin levels was reported after azaspiracids exposition, suggesting that both toxins share their mechanism of action.[97] However, while human azaspiracids intoxications had been reported, YTX intoxications have never been described, and the data available about azaspiracid effect have shown a very different effect than YTX over cAMP, cytosolic calcium, intracellular pH, and cytoskeleton structure.[5,7,94,95,121,124] In addition, later on, only some interference with the degradation pathway of E-cadherin by slowing down the endocytosis and therefore the inhibition of the complete degradation of E-cadherin was proposed.[23]

As it is shown, in the K-562 cell line, a decrease in the cytosolic levels of AKAP149 is observed after 24 and 48 h of incubation in the presence of 30 nM YTX. This decrease is associated with a decrease in PDE4 and PKA levels in the outer mitochondrial membrane. These two proteins are involved in the cAMP pathway and therefore various studies were designed to clarify the implications and the consequences of these decreases in the YTX effect. Surprisingly, after 24 h of toxin incubation, high levels of AKAP149, PKA, and PDE4 are located in plasma membrane, while after 48 h, the complex AKAP149–PKA–PDE4A is migrating to the nuclear envelope (Figure 22.2a and b). These results point to the complex translocation as the cellular target for YTX effect. In fact, the presence of the complex in the membrane could alter E-cadherin system and therefore connect the effects described.

Apoptosis, or programmed cell death, is a complex process characterized by a variety of morphological and biochemical changes in cells. Different processes such as changes in mitochondrial membrane potential, caspases activation, or changes in total nucleic acids content are associated to apoptosis. Different apoptotic effects were shown in the presence of YTX within several tumoral cellular lines. In the neuroblastoma cell line BE(2)-M17, different apoptotic events were observed after YTX incubation, although with lower potency than okadaic acid (OA). Small changes in mitochondrial membrane potential and nucleic acids content after 48 h of YTX incubation were described. However,

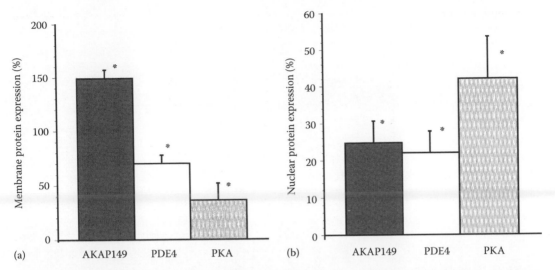

FIGURE 22.2 AKAP149, PDE4, and PKA expression after YTX incubation in K-562 cells. (a) Membrane protein expression after 24 h of YTX incubation. (b) Nuclear protein expression after 48 h of YTX incubation. X axis represents expression levels of cells without treatment. Mean ± SEM of three experiments. (*) Significant differences with respect to cells without treatment.

caspase 3 activity and annexin-V binding were increased in the presence of the toxin.[60] These effects were found at concentrations between 0.1 and 1 µM. The human cervix carcinoma HeLa S_3 cells death was activated after 48–96 h of incubation in the sub-nanomolar range of YTX. This effect was mediated by caspase 3 and caspase 7 activation and caused loss of intact poly (ADP-ribose)-polymerase.[68] Apoptotic effects of YTX were also described in myoblast L6 and DC3H1 cell lines from rat and mouse after 72 h of incubation in the presence of 100 nM YTX; these effects were associated with an activation of caspase 3 and caspase 9, while DNA fragmentation was not detected.[108] In addition, the activation of the apoptotic pathway and the protein families associated, heterogeneous nuclear ribonucleoprotein, lamin, cathepsin, and heat shock protein, was also confirmed by proteomic studies using HepG2 cells, though the connection between all is still unknown.[131] Early changes in mitochondrial membrane potential and swelling of mitochondria, indicating an active role of this structure, were also associated to the apoptotic effect of YTX.[106] In addition, after 72 h of YTX treatment, cellular apoptosis associated to tensin cleavage and cytoskeleton disruption was described in myoblast cell lines.[107] YTX apoptotic effect was also described in other cellular models as the Bel7402 human hepatoma cell line and HL7702 human liver cells.[82,83] However, YTX does not modify cellular viability of human fresh lymphocytes, 30 nM YTX for 48 h of incubation, whereas in K-562 cells and mouse T lymphocytes EL-4, after 48 h of incubation, or in HeLa-229 cells or A2780 cells, after 24 h of incubation, high cytotoxic effects were observed.[3,69,115] When the toxin effect was checked in primary neuronal cultures, after 24 h of treatment, only a small cytotoxic effect was reported at concentrations between 10 and 100 nM (30% cells death). These results agree with other data[90] and point that higher concentrations and probably longer incubation times are necessary to induce a cytotoxic effect in nontumoral cells. In fact, 72 h of toxin incubation is necessary to induce caspase-independent cell death in primary cortical neurons.[11]

The permeability transition pore is a mitochondrial voltage-dependent calcium channel involved in cell death. This channel is present as a high conductance channel in the mitochondria with a controversial role in apoptosis.[54] As it was mentioned, no changes in mitochondrial membrane potential were observed after 12 h of incubation in the presence of different YTX concentrations. Only a small change was induced in the presence of 1 µM YTX after 12 h of treatment. After 48 h, a small effect was observed at lower YTX concentrations.[60] However, an important and immediately activated mitochondrial depolarization has been described in the hepatoma MH1C1 cells line after YTX addition suggesting the mitochondria and the opening of permeability transition pores as the target for YTX.[19] The effect is blocked by cyclosporin A and requires the presence of a permissive level of calcium (10 µM). In addition, when

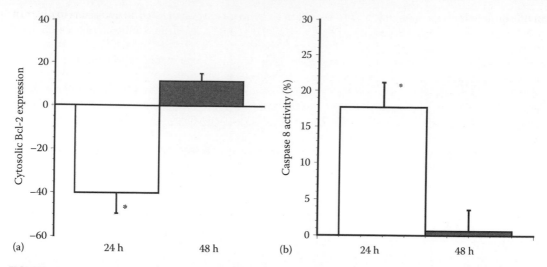

FIGURE 22.3 Effect of YTX incubation over apoptotic mediators in K-562 cells. (a) Cytosolic Bcl-2 expression after 24 and 48 h of YTX incubation. (b) Caspase 8 activity after 24 and 48 h of YTX incubation. X axis represents basal levels of cells without treatment. Mean ± SEM of three experiments. (*) Significant differences with respect to cells without treatment.

the oxidative phosphorylation is uncoupled, either calcium pool depletion or calcium influx induced by YTX is blocked.[115] On the other hand, the permeability transition pores seem to play a role in necrosis more than apoptosis and they are opened as a consequence of apoptosis not to induce it.[54] Therefore, the mitochondrial domain plays an important role in YTX effect.

To clarify the apoptotic role of YTX, the levels of the antiapoptotic Bcl-2 protein and the activity of caspase 8 were measured after YTX treatment in K-562 cells. Interestingly, in the first 24 h of toxin incubation, the antiapoptotic protein Bcl-2 expression decreased a 40% with respect to untreated cells; however, after 48 h of incubation, no variations in Bcl-2 levels were observed (Figure 22.3a). In addition, 20% more activity was found in caspase 8 when cells were treated with the toxin for 24 h, while after 48 h, again no differences were obtained (Figure 22.3b). Hence, after 24 h of YTX incubation, the apoptotic pathway is activated; however, after 48 h of YTX treatment, another cellular death different from apoptosis is activated. Therefore, after 24 h, apoptosis might be related with the translocation of AKAP149–PKA–PDE4A complex from the mitochondria to the cellular membrane, while after 48 h, when another cellular death is activated, this complex is located in the outer nuclear domain.

Mitochondria-mediated apoptosis, death receptor-mediated apoptosis, and paraptosis can be activated after YTX treatment.[56,57] As it was described, the apoptosis associated to the mitochondria can involve PKA and Bcl-2 pathway. The death receptor pathway activates apoptosis through the tumor necrosis factor receptor (TNFR) superfamily, where death ligands bind to the receptor and the apoptotic pathway begins. The best known are the Fas/TNF death receptor, where a ligand binds to death domain that recruits adaptor molecules like Fas-associated death domain (FADD) and TNF receptor-associated protein with a death domain (TRADD). FADD and TRADD recruit procaspases 8 and 10 to make the death-inducing signaling complex (DISC). Procaspases are activated to caspase and the extrinsic apoptotic pathway is carried on.[55] Finally, paraptosis is a nonapoptotic programmed cell death that appears in cells after YTX incubations.[57] This type of programmed cell death is unclear. Caspases are not involved in paraptosis cell death, while the mitogen-activated protein kinases (MAPK), the TAJ/TROY receptor, and the insulin-like growth factor I receptor are involved in this process.[21,57,105]

From the initial E-cadherin results with different toxin analogs and taken into account the different observations about toxin effects in different cellular models, the existence of two separate receptorial systems involved in YTX effect was proposed.[41] One system early activated at micromolar YTX concentrations and the other activated after long incubation times within the nanomolar toxin range and related with E-cadherin. However, E-cadherin role in cellular survival is controversial and a decrease in this protein levels was observed after 3–5 days YTX treatment, when tumoral cells start to die.[96] In addition, E-cadherin is an epithelial protein and therefore the effect of YTX only could be explained in these cells; however, the major effect observed with the toxin was in the heart. The mechanism that renders E-cadherin functional is unknown, and even its function as mediator in adhesion cells can be regulated by several signal transduction and also the protein may regulate other processes such as migration, proliferation, apoptosis, or cytotoxicity.[88] In vitro studies about E-cadherin expression have shown that the levels of this protein depend on cellular line used, epithelioid morphology, high expression, or fibroblast-like morphology, lost expression.[125] Moreover, as it was described, no effects in E-cadherin were reported in vivo even after long YTX treatment periods.[24] On the other hand, the relationship of potency and the C9 chain observed in E-cadherin results but also in PDEs–YTX binding data is probably not a coincidence and pointed to the same mechanism of action. Therefore, PDEs modulation, AKAP149–PKA–PDE4A complex migration, E-cadherin, cytoskeleton effects, and cellular death are related. The effect after PDEs activation in tumoral and nontumoral cells can be different, that is, the same mechanism of action with different implications depending on cellular model and time. In fact, the low toxicity observed in primary cortical neurons and the effect over tau protein expression also point to this hypothesis.

22.1.2.3 Others

YTXs often coexist with diarrhetic shellfish toxins (DSP) but their effects are different. DSP toxins are specific and potent inhibitors of Ser/Thr protein phosphatases PP1 and PP2A. These enzymes play a critical role in phosphorylation/dephosphorylation processes within eukaryotic cells. YTX also inhibits protein phosphatases, but the effect is four orders of magnitude lower than the one induced by DSP, the same as toxicity.[78] Therefore, it has been concluded that YTX mechanism of action was not mediated by these enzymes inhibition.

Since the YTX molecule has a hydrophobic polyether skeleton, some hemolytic activity could be expected. However, the toxin did not induce hemolysis.[78] Even an important hemolytic property was described to desulfated YTX by interacting with alpha-helix membrane peptides.[76]

Phagocytic activity and phagosome maturation of macrophages were inhibited after YTX exposition.[81] After 24 h of incubation in the presence of YTX, an increase in interleukin-2 production in human fresh lymphocytes was observed.[4] This increase can be functionally related with the decrease in cAMP levels, since cellular function can be inhibited by agents that increase the levels of this second messenger in human lymphocytes.[102] In addition, after i.p. YTX injection, the thymus and the immune system are affected and also some inflammatory response is reported.[44] On the other hand, YTX inhibits the activation of mast cells (nonpublished data). In this sense, PDEs modulation is often used to regulate the activity of a number of inflammatory cell types and several drugs used in the asthma therapy interfere within this pathway. In addition, high cytotoxic effects were reported in mouse T lymphocytes after YTX exposures.[69] Also a reversible downregulation of T receptor in T cells was reported after YTX incubation; this effect was partially mediated by PKC.[62] Therefore, all these results on immune cells are very interesting and again point to PDEs as the YTX target.

Few papers have been published about the effect of YTX in marine bivalves. The toxin is mainly localized in immunocytes and in the digestive gland of mussels.[45] On the other hand, lysosomes have been described as one target either in vertebrate or invertebrate cell lines.[66] An increase in mussel phagocytic immunocytes under control conditions after YTX addition was described but no effect under stress conditions was reported.[65] In this shellfish, YTX and analogs suffered extensive metabolism and had a half-life of 20–24 days.[2] YTX induced cell shape changes in mussel immunocytes. The toxin is not able to activate these cells but enhances the activating response of other activators as peptides. This effect is induced through the involvement of both extracellular calcium and cAMP.[67] Therefore, even in nonmammalian cells, the second messengers calcium and cAMP are key steps for YTX effect.

The activation of PKC and its translocation in primary cortical neurons induced the inhibition of glycogen synthase kinase 3 and as consequence the inhibition of the tau protein hyperphosphorylation and intracellular accumulation of amyloid-beta peptide. That is, the YTX incubation improved the hallmarks related with neurodegenerative process as Alzheimer disease.[11]

22.1.3 Toxicology: In Vivo YTX Effects

No reports of human poisoning induced by YTXs have been described. Several studies are available about in vivo toxicity. YTX induced marked cytoplasmic edema in cardiac muscle cells after 3 h i.p. injection. Severe fatty acid degeneration and intracellular necrosis in liver and pancreas but not in the heart were reported after 24 h of desulfated YTX injection. From these results, the heart was postulated as the target organ for the toxin.[113] However, after oral administration, only moderated changes in heart were observed.[17] In addition, no effects in liver, pancreas, lungs, adrenals, kidney, spleen, or thymus have been reported after oral and i.p. YTX administrations.[17,119,120] In addition, morphofunctional changes in neurons, in particular in calcium-binding proteins from the cytoskeleton after 2 h i.p. injection, were reported.[43,44] In the same conditions, some inflammatory responses associated to effects on thymus and the immune system were also described.[42,44] In summary, YTX has been extensively reported as lethal for mice after i.p. injection, although a range from 80 to 700 µg/kg of toxin has been published as median lethal dose (LD_{50}) after i.p. administrations.[117] This wide dose range can be due to different experimental conditions, animals, or toxins purity; in fact, a factor of seven in the variability of LD_{50} was observed in these conditions.[16] Within this range, LD_{50} of some analogs as 444 µg/kg for homoYTX or 301 µg/kg for di-desulfo-YTX is included.[113,120] The discrepancies in LD_{50} of YTXs made difficult to establish the values of the toxic equivalency factor (TEF) for this group of compounds.[20] However, according with the toxicity observed, the following TEFs have been proposed by the Contaminants Panel at the European Food Safety Agency for the YTX group: YTX = 1, 1a-homoYTX = 1, 45-hydroxy-YTX = 1, and 45-hydroxy-1a homoYTX = 0.5.[80]

No lethality or changes in mice behavior were observed after oral administration of doses up to 54 mg/kg,[117] and only some effects in cardiac cells were reported.[17] In addition, after 7 days of daily oral administration, no changes at any level were observed, and only some ultrastructural effect in cardiac cells was reported; these effects were reverted after 90 days.[118] In addition, no effects in E-cadherin were reported after long oral YTX treatment periods.[24] In this sense, after oral administration, most of the toxin is recovered from lower intestine and feces and only trace amount are found in blood, urine and tissues.[77] Besides, not enough information about YTX pharmacokinetic parameters is available, but toxicity data in mice suggest small absorption after oral administration; 24 h after oral administration, the toxin was detectable in the bloodstream.[117]

The EU regulatory level for YTX is 1 mg YTX equivalent/kg shellfish.[28] Based on that and since no lethal effects have been reported but some cardiac effects have been shown, the Contaminants Panel concluded that to avoid exceeding a dose of 1500 µg YTX equivalents, corresponding to the acute reference dose (ARfD) of 25 µg YTX equivalents/kg, a 400 g portion should not contain more than 3.75 mg YTX equivalent/kg shellfish meat. This level is above the current EU limit value of YTXs of 1 mg/kg shellfish flesh.[80]

It is important to bear in mind that some cytotoxic effect after i.p. administration can be due to the combination of different lipophilic toxins. The fact that YTX coexists with DSP, pectenotoxins (PTXs) and azaspiracids, is important since they may show significant unknown pharmacological interactions that each toxin did not shown by separate. In this sense, the toxicity after oral administration of YTX and azaspiracid-1 association was checked. Neither clinical effects nor pathological changes were observed, and very low levels of YTX were detected in internal organs. Therefore, no increase of YTX oral toxicity was observed in combination with other toxins.[1]

In summary, no toxic effects were observed after oral administration, and even though high toxicity after injection was reported, the YTX seems to be a promising molecule for drug development to neurodegenerative diseases as Alzheimer, to the immune system, as well as to induce cellular toxicity in tumoral cells.

22.2 Pectenotoxins

22.2.1 Introduction

PTXs are a group of cyclic polyether macrolide compounds from marine origin[129] that have been found in the digestive glands of scallops together with OA and dinophysistoxins (DTXs) and intoxicate humans.[130] PTXs have been found in a range of shellfish worldwide but the toxins are produced by the planktonic dinoflagellates of the genus *Dinophysis*.[35,123,127] At least 14 PTX analogs have been described. The algae *Dinophysis* produces pectenotoxin-2 (PTX-2),[49] pectenotoxin-11 (PTX-11),[109] pectenotoxin-12 (PTX-12),[73] pectenotoxin-13 (PTX-13), and pectenotoxin-14 (PTX-14).[70] Other PTXs seem to be either product of the shellfish metabolism or artifacts.[34]

Even though initially PTXs were classified as DSP toxins in accordance with their origin (dinoflagellates from the genus *Dinophysis*) and their coexistence in contaminated shellfish, PTXs are nowadays classified as a separate group of phycotoxins based on their different effect and activity.

22.2.2 Biotransformation in Shellfish

The metabolism of toxins that have accumulated in fish and shellfish is considered a detoxification process, as happens with PTXs in the Japanese scallop *P. yessoensis*. PTX-2 is suspected to be the precursor from which many PTXs are derived through biotransformation during metabolism in the gut of bivalves.[10] After consumption of the algae by shellfish, PTX-2 is metabolized to other PTX derivatives by two main routes: (1) oxidation of the C-43 methyl group of PTX-2 yields hydroxymethyl (PTX-1), aldehyde (PTX-3), and carboxylic acid (PTX-6) derivatives[111] and (2) rapid enzymatic hydrolysis of PTX-2 produces pectenotoxin-2 seco acid (PTX-2sa) where the characteristic lactone has been opened giving the free acid form of the toxins.[99,110] Structurally, PTX-2 seco acid (PTX-2sa) is identical to PTX-2 except that the characteristic lactone ring is hydrolyzed in the seco acid form. Also PTX-2sa appears to progressively epimerize to the thermodynamically more stable 7-epi-pectenotoxin-2 seco acid (7-epi-PTX-2sa).[71,110] PTX-11 and PTX-12 are less susceptible to enzymatic hydrolysis, and seco acid forms of these compounds are therefore relatively less abundant in mussels.[72] Also, pectenotoxin-4 (PTX-4) and pectenotoxin-7 (PTX-7) have been isolated from the digestive glands of scallops collected in Japan, and these are stereoisomers of PTX-1 and PTX-6, respectively.[39] After acid treatment of PTX-4 and PTX-7, two isomers, named pectenotoxin-8 (PTX-8) and pectenotoxin-9 (PTX-9), respectively, were formed; however, they are not naturally occurring compounds.[99] Different species of bivalves that accumulate PTXs metabolize PTX-2 SA into fatty acid derivative by conjugating fatty acids through an ester linkage to one or more hydroxyl-group(s). The biochemical reason for this biotransformation is unclear, as metabolism often occurs through transformation to more water-soluble derivatives to facilitate depuration from the organism. One explanation may be that conjugation to fatty acids is a way of detoxicating the compounds and protecting the organism from harmful effects of the toxins.[116] The 37-O-acyl esters of PTX-2-SA were the most abundant form, followed by the corresponding 11-O-acyl esters and low levels of 33-O-acyl esters. All these esters appear to be metabolites produced by the bivalves because they have never been observed in phytoplankton.[126] An enzyme capable of hydrolyzing PTXs within the hepatopancreas of the greenshell mussel *Perna canaliculus* was recently isolated and characterized. PTX-2 and PTX-1 were hydrolyzed but the enzyme was inactive against PTX-11, PTX-6, and acid-isomerized PTX-2 and PTX-11. The ability of the esterase to hydrolyze PTX analogs does not appear to relate to the toxicity of these compounds and suggests that PTX detoxification is not the primary function of the enzyme.[64]

PTXs were sometimes present in plankton in higher proportions than total DTXs. The lower elimination kinetics found for DTXs in relation to PTXs explain why shellfish usually do not present concentrations of PTXs much higher than DTXs. A detoxification experiment showed that mussels are faster detoxifiers than cockles.[122]

22.2.3 Mechanism of Action

About the mechanism of action of PTXs, actin is their principal target. Actin is one of the most abundant and common cytoskeletal proteins involved in many cellular processes such as cell growth, motility, signaling, and maintenance of cell shape. In cells, there is a dynamic equilibrium between polymerized F-actin (filamentous) and monomeric G-actin (globular).[27,98] When the G-actin concentration is above a critical level, it spontaneously polymerizes to F-actin.

PTXs may exert some of their main effects via the actin cytoskeleton disruption through their binding sites with actin.[10,13] In in vitro studies with hepatocytes, the cytoskeletal disruption of PTX-1 was shown.[132]

PTX-2 through its binding to actin can modify the cytoskeleton by promoting actin depolymerization in hepatocytes,[38] intestinal cells,[14] and neuroblastoma cells.[13] It has been proposed that PTX-2 inhibits actin polymerization by sequestering monomeric actin but does not exhibit severing activity. PTX-2 forms a 1:1 complex with G-actin by binding between subdomains 1 and 3 and near the barber end.[104] PTX-2 very efficiently inhibits actin polymerization by capping the fast-growing barbed end,[10] but an actin-sequestering effect is also possible.[39] It was reported that PTX-2 causes a concentration-dependent decrease in both the rate and yield of skeletal muscle actin polymerization with no significant effects on depolymerization. The inhibitory effects of PTX-2 appear to be conserved toward other actin isoforms (i.e., smooth muscle, cardiac muscle, and nonmuscle), whereas no effects of PTX-2sa were observed on actin polymerization.[22] Other analogs such as PTX-6 caused a specific time- and dose-dependent depolymerization of F-actin in neuroblastoma cells.[61] Later studies showed that PTX-6 damaged the F-actin cytoskeleton in enterocytes from rabbit in a way not related to Ca^{2+} flux although they produce no change in cell morphology.[14]

22.2.4 Structure–Activity Relation

Toxicological studies indicated evident differences between PTX potencies that can be related to their structures.[39] Also, in vitro studies have compared the effects of diverse PTXs on cells. Progressive oxidation at C-43 constitutes a detoxification route, because toxicity in a mouse bioassay decreases in order PTX-2 > PTX-1 > PTX-3 > PTX-6.[128,130] However, oxidation at C34 does not change i.p. toxicity, with PTX-11 being as toxic as PTX-2.[112] On the other hand, rupture of the lactone ring inactivated the PTX molecule.[13] It was reported that PTX-2 was cytotoxic to KB cells, whereas PTX-2sa was not toxic.[29] Analogs isomerized so as to contain a six-membered B-ring, PTX-8 and PTX-9, are more than one order of magnitude less toxic than those containing a five-membered B-ring.[39] PTX-3 and PTX-6, the 7R-epimers of PTX-4 and PTX-7, are significantly less toxic than their corresponding 7-S-epimers.[128]

PTX-1, PTX-2, and PTX-11 trigger a remarkable depolymerizing effect on actin cytoskeleton and also modifications in the shape of human neuroblastoma cells, but PTX-2 and PTX-11 were more potent than PTX-1. Therefore, oxidation of the residue at C-18 in the PTX molecule (e.g., PTX-1) led to reduction in toxicity in the mouse bioassay and appears to be responsible for the diminished ability of PTX-1 to disrupt F-actin. In contrast, PTX-2sa did not evidence those effects allowing development of the structure–activity relationship: PTXs activity is related to the presence of an intact lactone ring in their structures.[13] In agreement with these results, the actin cytoskeleton was clearly altered by PTX-1, PTX-2, and PTX-11 in the hepatocyte cell line clone 9 and primary rat hepatocytes. Morphological assessments indicate a higher sensitivity of the cancer-like cell line to these toxins. However, the viability of both cell types was not altered.[38] This supports the idea that lactone ring integrity is essential for the action of PTXs: oxidation on C-43 decreases the toxicity of the molecule and oxidation on C34 does not affect the potency of PTXs.[39]

PTX-1, PTX-6, and PTX-9 induce dose-dependent damage in the actin cytoskeleton and in the viability of primary cultured rat hepatocytes (Figure 22.4). In clone 9 rat hepatocytes, PTX-1 and PTX-9 also affect the morphology of cells, but surprisingly, PTX-6 induced no effect (Figure 22.4). In accordance with this lack of activity, the actin cytoskeleton of CaCo-2 cells, another epithelial cell line, is not affected by PTX-6.

The order of cytotoxicity of the analogs is PTX-2 > PTX-1 > PTX-6 > PTX-9. From a structure–activity perspective, the increase in the level of oxidation of the PTX molecule on C-43 decreases its cytotoxicity. Furthermore, PTX-6 is not able to induce effects on immortal cells while retaining its toxicity against primary cultured cells, whereas PTX-9, a 7-S-isomer, is active in both cellular models. The different cytotoxicities exerted by PTX-6 on cell lines and primary cells could be determined by the presence of a carboxylic acid group on C-43 of the PTX molecule.[37]

22.2.5 Biological Effects

Relatively little is known about the biological effects of PTXs. Nearly all information regarding PTXs toxicology has been obtained from in vitro and in vivo experiments directed either to identify their molecular targets or to assign the possible risk of PTXs on human health by consumption of contaminated shellfish.

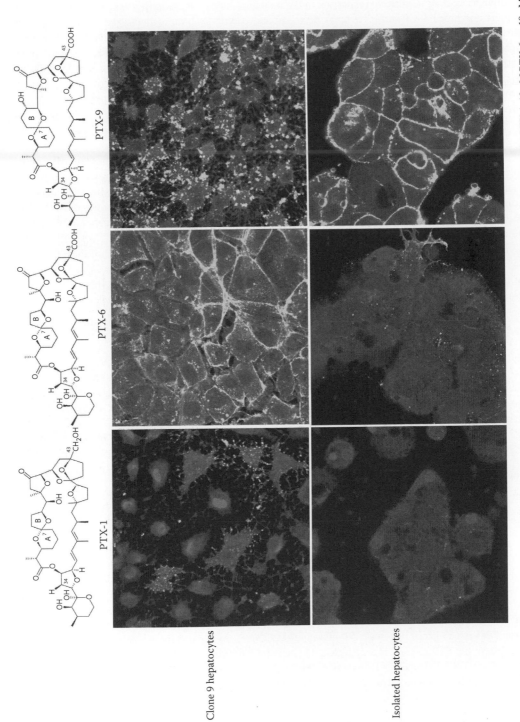

FIGURE 22.4 Confocal imaging of the F- and G-actin double staining of clone nine rat hepatocytes and rat isolated hepatocytes treated with 1 μM PTX-1, 10 μM PTX-6, or 10 μM PTX-9. The images are representative of three independent experiments. (From Espina, B. et al., *Chem. Res. Toxicol.*, 23, 504, 2010.)

The poisoning associated with these toxins was initially described as spreading worldwide posing and a serious threat to public health and to the aquaculture industry.[130] PTXs are highly toxic by i.p. injection in mice,[114] leading to positive responses in the mouse bioassay for lipophilic marine biotoxins. The LD_{50} determined for PTX-1 and PTX-2 has been 250 and 260 µg/kg b.w., respectively,[130] and 500 µg/kg b.w. for PTX-6.[48] Symptomatic animals appeared lethargic, had difficulties in breathing, lacked muscle coordination, and experienced cyanosis. No lethality was observed for PTX-7 and PTX-9 and no toxic effects have been reported for the group of PTX-2sa.[72,99] However, studies undertaken in mice by oral consumption of PTXs do not induce diarrhea. After oral ingestion of PTXs, only high doses induced some toxicity indicating that PTXs are much less toxic via oral than i.p.[72,114] Again no toxic effects were observed in mice receiving PTX-2sa either by oral or by gavage.[72] The PTX-2sa conversion concurs to render PTXs safe for the human consumer.[72] Therefore, acute toxic effects in humans resulting from ingestion of shellfish contaminated with PTX-2sa or 7-epi-PTX-2sa are most unlikely.[71]

PTXs are toxic to the liver when administered i.p. in mice. Histopathological studies on mice have shown that i.p. injection of PTX-1 induces macroscopic liver damage including congestion and finely granulated appearance.[114] Microscopic analysis revealed hepatocytes with large numbers of vacuoles and granules and become necrotic in periportal regions of the hepatic lobules. In the same study, PTX-1 caused no pathological changes in the intestine or other visceral organs; therefore, PTXs are placed in the group of hepatotoxins.[114] PTX-6 does not induce diarrhea, and Ito et al. have shown a large difference in toxicity between the i.p. and oral exposure route in mice. PTX-6 is a potent toxin if administered i.p. to mice with bleeding in the liver and injuries at the gastric organs and kidney. PTX-6 may induce deformation of hepatocytes and blood filled the resulting gaps. However, administered orally, the toxin did not injure mouse organs. When rats were gavaged with PTX-6, no diarrhetic activity was showed, but toxin induced edema was reported in the middle–lower small intestine (jejunum–ileum).[48]

It is not clear whether the PTXs cause disease in vivo in humans. Further studies will be required to definitively evaluate the risk posed by PTXs to shellfish consumers. In any case, the levels of some PTXs have been regulated in shellfish in Europe. The Scientific Panel on Contaminants in the Food Chain (CONTAM Panel) has set a human ARfD of 0.8 µg PTX-2 equivalents/kg b.w. based on animal data including intestinal toxicity studies using PTX-2 in mice following oral administration. The current European regulatory limit is 120 µg PTX-2 equivalents/kg shellfish meat; therefore, a 400 g portion of shellfish should not contain more than 48 µg PTX-2 equivalents.[36]

PTXs can exert a potent cytotoxic effect in several human cell such as lung, colon, and breast cancer cell lines causing apoptosis effects, loss of radial arrangement of microtubules, and disruption of stress fibers.[35,50]

This cytotoxicity has led to the investigation of the effects of PTXs on tumors and cancer cell lines. PTX-2 has anticancer effects that are due to disruption of the actin cytoskeleton through the inhibition of actin polymerization, whereby a complex is formed with G-actin.[74]

In a cell-based screening system based on the use of mammalian ovulated oocytes to identify mitosis inhibitors, PTX-2 was markedly toxic to p53-deficient tumors both in vitro and in vivo.[26] The tumor suppressor p53 gene plays a major role in preventing tumorigenesis, by responding to both cellular stress and DNA damage, and the mutation of p53 is frequently associated with oncogenesis.[46] Also disruption of p53 function reduces the apoptosis induced by anticancer agents.[63] In p53-deficient tumor cells, PTX-2 triggers apoptosis through mitochondrial dysfunction, and this is followed by the release of proapoptotic factors and caspase activation. Therefore, PTX-2 as an actin inhibitor may be a potent chemotherapeutic agent against p53-deficient tumors.[26] PTX-2 markedly inhibits the p53-deficient Hep3B hepatocarcinoma cell growth and induces apoptosis, whereas p53-wild-type HepG2 cells were much more resistant to PTX-2. These results suggest that PTX-2 acts via a cytotoxic mechanism that seems to be p53 independent. The apoptosis induced by PTX-2 in Hep3B cells was associated with activation of caspases and loss of mitochondrial membrane potential. More notably, the nonsteroidal anti-inflammatory drugs (NSAID)-activated gene-1 (NAG-1) pathway had been proven to be one of the molecular targets that mediate the cytotoxic actions of PTX-2.[103] Related with that, PTX-2 concentration dependently inhibited the growth of synovial fibroblasts, arresting them in the G1 phase of their cell cycle. Thus, PTX-2 might help identify new therapeutic agents against rheumatoid arthritis (RA)-mediated hyperplasia of synovial fibroblasts.[84]

PTX-2 is a strong suppressor of leukemia cell proliferation. PTX-2 treatment significantly inhibited the growth of leukemia cells and caused a marked increase in apoptosis in a dose-dependent manner.[74]

It has been recognized that control of the actin cytoskeleton must be coordinated with control of cell cycle events.[92] Cell cycle progression into G1, S, and G2/M phases has been shown to be controlled by actin. PTX-2 induces abnormal cell cycle transition through G2/M arrest, endoreduplication, and apoptosis in a time-dependent manner via promoting actin depolymerization and disruption of the actin cytoskeleton in leukemia cells.[74] Actin dysfunction also accelerates the ERK and the JNK signal pathways and delays entry into mitosis in mammalian cells.[58] Inhibition of ERK and JNK signaling pathways prevented PTX-2-induced abnormal cell cycle transition and apoptosis in leukemia cells.[74] In addition, PTX-2 also displays selective and potent cytotoxicity against human breast cancer. PTX-2-treated cells are arrested in the G2/M phase, at the relatively early time point of 12 h.[75] PTX-2 also suppressed cell viability and telomerase activity in human leukemia cells. The telomerase complex consists of two essential components: hTERT and hTR. Although hTR is ubiquitously expressed in most cells, expression of hTERT is limited in germinal and cancer cells and has received considerable attention for its role in regulating telomerase activity.[89] PTX-2 can be used to effectively inhibit telomerase activity via the transcriptional and posttranslational suppression of hTERT, and this process precedes cellular differentiation of human leukemia cells.[53] The activation of caspase 3 is associated with PTX-2-induced apoptosis.[52] Nuclear factor-kappa B (NF-kB) is a prominent factor in cell proliferation, apoptosis, and cancer development. A number of reports have demonstrated that NF-kB activation can maintain tumor cell viability and inhibiting NF-kB activation alone can be sufficient to induce cell death.[51] NF-kB inhibitors act as potent enhancers of chemotherapy-induced apoptosis.[12] PTX-2 inhibits constitutively expressed NF-kB activation and the expression of antiapoptotic and proliferative genes known to be regulated by NF-kB activity in human leukemia cells.[52] Therefore, PTX-2 may be a good candidate for the development of a potential anti-tumorigenic agent.

REFERENCES

1. Aasen, J. A., Espenes, A., Miles, C. O. et al. 2011. Combined oral toxicity of azaspiracid-1 and yessotoxin in female NMRI mice. *Toxicon,* 57, 909–917.
2. Aasen, J. A., Samdal, I. A., Miles, C. O. et al. 2005. Yessotoxins in Norwegian blue mussels (*Mytilus edulis*): Uptake from *Protoceratium reticulatum*, metabolism and depuration. *Toxicon,* 45, 265–272.
3. Alfonso, A. and Alfonso, C. 2008. Yessotoxin: Pharmacology and mechanism of action. Biological detection. In: Botana, L. M. (ed.) *Seafood and Freshwater Toxins.* 2nd edn. London, U.K.: CRC Press, Taylor & Francis Group, pp. 315–327.
4. Alfonso, A., De La Rosa, L. A., Vieytes, M. R., Yasumoto, T., and Botana, L. M. 2003. Yessotoxin a novel phycotoxin, activates phosphodiesterase activity. Effect of yessotoxin on cAMP levels in human lymphocytes. *Biochemical Pharmacology,* 65, 193–208.
5. Alfonso, A., Roman, Y., Vieytes, M. R. et al. 2005. Azaspiracid-4 inhibits Ca^{2+} entry by stored operated channels in human T lymphocytes. *Biochemical Pharmacology,* 69, 1627–1636.
6. Alfonso, A., Vale, C., Vilariño, N. et al. 2009. Recent developments on the mechanism of action of marine phycotoxins. *Toxins et Signalisation. 17emes Rencontres en Toxinologie,* 1, 51–56.
7. Alfonso, A., Vieytes, M. R., Ofuji, K. et al. 2006. Azaspiracids modulate intracellular pH levels in human lymphocytes. *Biochemical and Biophysical Research Communications,* 346, 1091–1099.
8. Alfonso, C., Alfonso, A., Pazos, M. J. et al. 2007. Extraction and cleaning methods to detect yessotoxins in contaminated mussels. *Analytical Biochemistry,* 363, 228–238.
9. Alfonso, C., Alfonso, A., Vieytes, M. R., Yasumoto, T., and Botana, L. M. 2005. Quantification of yessotoxin using the fluorescence polarization technique, and study of the adequate extraction procedure. *Analytical Biochemistry,* 344, 266–274.
10. Allingham, J. S., Miles, C. O., and Rayment, I. 2007. A structural basis for regulation of actin polymerization by pectenotoxins. *Journal of Molecular Biology,* 371, 959–970.
11. Alonso, E., Vale, C., Vieytes, M. R., and Botana, L. M. 2013. Translocation of PKC by yessotoxin in an in vitro model of Alzheimer's disease with improvement of tau and β-amyloid pathology. *ACS Chemical Neuroscience,* 4, 1062–1070.
12. Amit, S. and Ben-Neriah, Y. 2003. NF-kB activation in cancer: A challenge for ubiquitination- and proteasome-based therapeutic approach. *Seminars in Cancer Biology,* 13, 15–28.

13. Ares, I. R., Louzao, M. C., Espina, B. et al. 2007. Lactone ring of pectenotoxins: A key factor for their activity on cytoskeletal dynamics. *Cellular Physiology and Biochemistry,* 19, 283–292.

14. Ares, I. R., Louzao, M. C., Vieytes, M. R., Yasumoto, T., and Botana, L. M. 2005. Actin cytoskeleton of rabbit intestinal cells is a target for potent marine phycotoxins. *The Journal of Experimental Biology,* 208, 4345–4354.

15. Asirvatham, A. L., Galligan, S. G., Schillace, R. V. et al. 2004. A-kinase anchoring proteins interact with phosphodiesterases in T lymphocyte cell lines. *The Journal of Immunology,* 173, 4806–4814.

16. Aune, T., Aasen, J. A., Miles, C. O., and Larsen, S. 2008. Effect of mouse strain and gender on LD(50) of yessotoxin. *Toxicon,* 52, 535–540.

17. Aune, T., Sorby, R., Yasumoto, T., Ramstad, H., and Landsverk, T. 2002. Comparison of oral and intraperitoneal toxicity of yessotoxin towards mice. *Toxicon,* 40, 77–82.

18. Beavo, J. A., Francis, S. H. & Houslay, M. D. 2007. Role of A-kinase anchoring proteins in the compartmentation in cyclic nucleotide signaling. In: Beavo, J. A., Sharron, H. F., and Miles, D. H. (eds.) *Cyclic Nucleotide Phosphodiesterases in Health and Disease.* Boca Raton, FL: CRC Press, pp. 377–387.

19. Bianchi, C., Fato, R., Angelin, A. et al. 2004. Yessotoxin, a shellfish biotoxin, is a potent inducer of the permeability transition in isolated mitochondria and intact cells. *Biochimica et Biophysica Acta,* 1656, 139–147.

20. Botana, L. M., Vilariño, N., Alfonso, A. et al. 2010. The problem of toxicity equivalent factors in developing alternative methods to animal bioassay for marine-toxin detection. *Trends in Analytical Chemistry,* 29, 1316–1325.

21. Broker, L. E., Kruyt, F. A., and Giaccone, G. 2005. Cell death independent of caspases: A review. *Clinical Cancer Research,* 11, 3155–3162.

22. Butler, S. C., Miles, C. O., Karim, A., and Twiner, M. J. 2012. Inhibitory effects of pectenotoxins from marine algae on the polymerization of various actin isoforms. *Toxicology In Vitro,* 26, 493–499.

23. Callegari, F. and Rossini, G. P. 2008. Yessotoxin inhibits the complete degradation of E-cadherin. *Toxicology,* 244, 133–144.

24. Callegari, F., Sosa, S., Ferrari, S. et al. 2006. Oral administration of yessotoxin stabilizes E-cadherin in mouse colon. *Toxicology,* 227, 145–155.

25. Carlucci, A., Lignitto, L., and Feliciello, A. 2008. Control of mitochondria dynamics and oxidative metabolism by cAMP, AKAPs and the proteasome. *Trends in Cell Biology,* 18, 604–612.

26. Chae, H. D., Choi, T. S., Kim, B. M. et al. 2005. Oocyte-based screening of cytokinesis inhibitors and identification of pectenotoxin-2 that induces Bim/Bax-mediated apoptosis in p53-deficient tumors. *Oncogene,* 24, 4813–4819.

27. Chu, J. W. and Voth, G. A. 2005. Allostery of actin filaments: Molecular dynamics simulations and coarse-grained analysis. *Proceedings of the National Academy of Sciences of the United States of America,* 102, 13111–13116.

28. Commission, E. 2004. Regulation (EC) No 853/2004 of the European Parliament and of the Council of 29 April 2004 laying down specific hygiene rules for food of animal origin. *Official Journal,* L 226, (25/06/2004), 0022–0082.

29. Daiguji, M., Satake, M., James, K. J. et al. 1998. Structures of new pectenotoxin analogs, pectenotoxin-2 seco acid and 7-epi-pectenotoxin-2 seco acid, isolated from a dinoflagellate and greenshell mussels. *Chemistry Letters,* 7, 653–654.

30. De La Rosa, L. A., Alfonso, A., Vilariño, N., Vieytes, M. R., and Botana, L. M. 2001. Modulation of cytosolic calcium levels of human lymphocytes by yessotoxin, a novel marine phycotoxin. *Biochemical Pharmacology,* 61, 827–833.

31. De La Rosa, L. A., Alfonso, A., Vilariño, N. et al. 2001. Maitotoxin-induced calcium entry in human lymphocytes—Modulation by yessotoxin, Ca^{2+} channel blockers and kinases. *Cell Signal,* 13, 711–716.

32. Dell'ovo, V., Bandi, E., Coslovich, T. et al. 2008. Effects of yessotoxin (YTX) on the skeletal muscle: An update. *Toxicological Sciences,* 106, 392–399.

33. Dell'ovo, V., Bandi, E., Coslovich, T. et al. 2008. In vitro effects of yessotoxin on a primary culture of rat cardiomyocytes. *Toxicological Sciences,* 106, 392–399.

34. Dominguez, H. J., Paz, B., Daranas, A. D. et al. 2010. Dinoflagellate polyether within the yessotoxin, pectenotoxin and okadaic acid toxin groups: Characterization, analysis and human health implications. *Toxicon,* 56, 191–217.

35. Draisci, R., Lucentini, L., Giannetti, L., Boria, P., and Poletti, R. 1996. First report of pectenotoxin-2 (PTX-2) in algae (*Dinophysis fortii*) related to seafood poisoning in Europe. *Toxicon,* 34, 923–935.

36. EFSA. 2009. Scientific opinion of the Panel on Contaminants in the Food Chain on a request from the European Commission on marine biotoxins in shellfish—Pectenotoxin group. *The EFSA Journal,* 1109, 1–47.

37. Espina, B., Louzao, M. C., Ares, I. R. et al. 2010. Impact of the pectenotoxin C-43 oxidation degree on its cytotoxic effect on rat hepatocytes. *Chemical Research in Toxicology,* 23, 504–515.

38. Espiña, B., Louzao, M. C., Ares, I. R. et al. 2008. Cytoskeletal toxicity of pectenotoxins in hepatic cells. *British Journal of Pharmacology,* 155, 934–944.

39. Espiña, B. and Rubiolo, J. A. 2008. Marine toxins and the cytoskeleton: Pectenotoxins, unusual macrolides that disrupt actin. *The FEBS Journal,* 275, 6082–6088.

40. Feliciello, A., Gottesman, M. E., and Avvedimento, E. V. 2001. The biological functions of A-kinase anchor proteins. *Journal of Molecular Biology,* 308, 99–114.

41. Ferrari, S., Ciminiello, P., Dell'aversano, C. et al. 2004. Structure–activity relationships of yessotoxins in cultured cells. *Chemical Research in Toxicology,* 17, 1251–1257.

42. Franchini, A., Malagoli, D., and Ottaviani, E. 2010. Targets and effects of yessotoxin, okadaic acid and palytoxin: A differential review. *Marine Drugs,* 8, 658–677.

43. Franchini, A., Marchesini, E., Poletti, R., and Ottaviani, E. 2004. Acute toxic effect of the algal yessotoxin on Purkinje cells from the cerebellum of Swiss CD1 mice. *Toxicon,* 43, 347–352.

44. Franchini, A., Marchesini, E., Poletti, R., and Ottaviani, E. 2004. Lethal and sub-lethal yessotoxin dose-induced morpho-functional alterations in intraperitoneal injected Swiss CD1 mice. *Toxicon,* 44, 83–90.

45. Franchini, A., Milandri, A., Poletti, R., and Ottaviani, E. 2003. Immunolocalization of yessotoxins in the mussel *Mytilus galloprovincialis. Toxicon,* 41, 967–970.

46. Halaby, M. J. and Yang, D. Q. 2007. p53 translational control: A new facet of p53 regulation and its implication for tumorigenesis and cancer therapeutics. *Gene,* 395, 1–7.

47. Inoue, M., Hirama, M., Satake, M., Sugiyama, K., and Yasumoto, T. 2003. Inhibition of brevetoxins binding to the voltage-gated sodium channel by gambierol and gambieric acid-A. *Toxicon,* 41, 469–474.

48. Ito, E., Suzuki, T., Oshima, Y., and Yasumoto, T. 2008. Studies of diarrhetic activity on pectenotoxin-6 in the mouse and rat. *Toxicon,* 51, 707–716.

49. James, K. J., Bishop, A. G., Draisci, R. et al. 1999. Liquid chromatographic methods for the isolation and identification of new pectenotoxin-2 analogues from marine phytoplankton and shellfish. *Journal of Chromatography A,* 844, 53–65.

50. Jung, J. H., Sim, C. J., and Lee, C. O. 1995. Cytotoxic compounds from a two-sponge association. *Journal of Natural Products,* 58, 1722–1726.

51. Keller, S. A., Schattner, E. J., and Cesarman, E. 2000. Inhibition of NF-kB induces apoptosis of KSHV-infected primary effusion lymphoma cells. *Blood,* 96, 2537–2542.

52. Kim, M. O., Moon, D. O., Heo, M. S. et al. 2008. Pectenotoxin-2 abolishes constitutively activated NF-kB, leading to suppression of NF-kB related gene products and potentiation of apoptosis. *Cancer Letters,* 271, 25–33.

53. Kim, M. O., Moon, D. O., Kang, S. H. et al. 2008. Pectenotoxin-2 represses telomerase activity in human leukemia cells through suppression of hTERT gene expression and Akt-dependent hTERT phosphorylation. *FEBS Letters,* 582, 3263–3269.

54. Kinnally, K. W. and Antonsson, B. 2007. A tale of two mitochondrial channels, MAC and PTP, in apoptosis. *Apoptosis,* 12, 857–868.

55. Korsnes, M. S. 2012. Yessotoxin as a tool to study induction of multiple cell death pathways. *Toxins,* 4, 568–579.

56. Korsnes, M. S. and Espenes, A. 2011. Yessotoxin as an apoptotic inducer. *Toxicon,* 57, 947–958.

57. Korsnes, M. S., Espenes, A., Hetland, D. L., and Hermansen, L. C. 2011. Paraptosis-like cell death induced by yessotoxin. *Toxicology In Vitro,* 25, 1764–1770.

58. Lee, K. and Song, K. 2007. Actin dysfunction activates ERK1/2 and delays entry into mitosis in mammalian cells. *Cell Cycle,* 6, 1487–1495.

59. Leira, F., Alvarez, C., Cabado, A. G. et al. 2003. Development of a F actin-based live-cell fluorimetric microplate assay for diarrhetic shellfish toxins. *Analytical Biochemistry,* 317, 129–135.

60. Leira, F., Alvarez, C., Vieites, J. M., Vieytes, M. R., and Botana, L. M. 2002. Characterization of distinct apoptotic changes induced by okadaic acid and yessotoxin in the BE(2)-M17 neuroblastoma cell line. *Toxicology In Vitro,* 16, 23–31.

61. Leira, F., Cabado, A. G., Vieytes, M. R. et al. 2002. Characterization of F-actin depolymerization as a major toxic event induced by pectenotoxin-6 in neuroblastoma cells. *Biochemical Pharmacology,* 63, 1979–1988.

62. López, A. M., Rodríguez, J. J., Mirón, A. S., Camacho, F. G., and Grima, E. M. 2011. Immunoregulatory potential of marine algal toxins yessotoxin and okadaic acid in mouse T lymphocyte cell line EL-4. *Toxicology Letters,* 207, 167–172.

63. Lowe, S. W., Ruley, H. E., Jacks, T., and Housman, D. E. 1993. p53-dependent apoptosis modulates the cytotoxicity of anticancer agents. *Cell,* 74, 957–967.

64. Mackenzie, L. A., Selwood, A. I., and Marshall, C. 2012. Isolation and characterization of an enzyme from the Greenshell mussel *Perna canaliculus* that hydrolyses pectenotoxins and esters of okadaic acid. *Toxicon,* 60, 406–419.

65. Malagoli, D., Casarini, L., Sacchi, S., and Ottaviani, E. 2006. Stress and immune response in the mussel *Mytilus galloprovincialis. Fish and Shellfish Immunology,* 23, 171–177.

66. Malagoli, D., Marchesini, E., and Ottaviani, E. 2006. Lysosomes as the target of yessotoxin in invertebrate and vertebrate cell lines. *Toxicology Letters,* 167, 75–83.

67. Malagoli, D. and Ottaviani, E. 2004. Yessotoxin affects fMLP-induced cell shape changes in *Mytilus galloprovincialis* immunocytes. *Cell Biology International,* 28, 57–61.

68. Malaguti, C., Ciminello, P., Fattorusso, E., and Rossini, G. P. 2002. Caspase activation and death induced by yessotoxin in HeLa cells. *Toxicology In Vitro,* 16, 357–363.

69. Martín-López, A., Gallardo-Rodríguez, J., Sánchez-Mirón, A., García-Camacho, F., and Molina-Grima, E. 2012. Cytotoxicity of yessotoxin and okadaic acid in mouse T lymphocyte cell line EL-4. *Toxicon,* 60, 1049–1056.

70. Miles, C. O., Wilkins, A. L., Hawkes, A. D. et al. 2006. Isolation and identification of pectenotoxins-13 and -14 from *Dinophysis acuta* in New Zealand. *Toxicon,* 48, 152–159.

71. Miles, C. O., Wilkins, A. L., Munday, J. S. et al. 2006. Production of 7-epi-pectenotoxin-2 seco acid and assessment of its acute toxicity to mice. *Journal of Agricultural and Food Chemistry,* 54, 1530–1534.

72. Miles, C. O., Wilkins, A. L., Munday, R. et al. 2004. Isolation of pectenotoxin-2 from *Dinophysis acuta* and its conversion to pectenotoxin-2 seco acid, and preliminary assessment of their acute toxicities. *Toxicon,* 43, 1–9.

73. Miles, C. O., Wilkins, A. L., Samdal, I. A. et al. 2004. A novel pectenotoxin, PTX-12, in *Dinophysis* spp. and shellfish from Norway. *Chemical Research in Toxicology,* 17, 1414–1422.

74. Moon, D. O., Kim, M. O., Kang, S. H. et al. 2008. Induction of G2/M arrest, endoreduplication, and apoptosis by actin depolymerization agent pextenotoxin-2 in human leukemia cells, involving activation of ERK and JNK. *Biochemical Pharmacology,* 76(3), 312–321.

75. Moon, D. O., Kim, M. O., Nam, T. J. et al. 2010. Pectenotoxin-2 induces G2/M phase cell cycle arrest in human breast cancer cells via ATM and Chk1/2-mediated phosphorylation of cdc25C. *Oncology Reports,* 24, 271–276.

76. Mori, M., Oishi, T., Matsuoka, S. et al. 2005. Ladder-shaped polyether compound, desulfated yessotoxin, interacts with membrane-integral alpha-helix peptides. *Bioorganic & Medical Chemistry,* 13, 5099–5103.

77. Munday, R., Aune, T., and Rossini, J. P. 2008. Toxicology of the yessotoxins. In: Botana, L. M. (ed.) *Seafood and Freshwater Toxins.* 2nd edn. London, U.K.: CRC Press, Taylor & Francis Group.

78. Ogino, H., Kumagai, M., and Yasumoto, T. 1997. Toxicological evaluation of yessotoxin. *Natural Toxins,* 5, 255–259.

79. Omori, K. and Kotera, J. 2007. Overview of PDEs and their regulation. *Circulation Research,* 100, 309–327.

80. Opinion, E. 2008. Opinion of the scientific panel on contaminants in the food chain on a request from the European Commission on Marine Biotoxins in Shellfish—Yessotoxin group. *The EFSA Journal,* 907, 1–62.

81. Orsi, C. F., Colombari, B., Callegari, F. et al. 2010. Yessotoxin inhibits phagocytic activity of macrophages. *Toxicon,* 55, 265–273.

82. Pang, M., Qu, P., Gao, C. L., and Wang, Z. L. 2012. Yessotoxin induces apoptosis in HL7702 human liver cells. *Molecular Medicine Reports,* 5, 211–216.

83. Pang, M., Wang, Z. L., Gao, C. L., Qu, P., and Li, H. D. 2011. Characterization of apoptotic changes induced by yessotoxin in the Bel7402 human hepatoma cell line. *Molecular Medicine Reports,* 4, 547–552.

84. Park, C., Kim, G. Y., Jung, J. Y., Kim, W. J., and Choi, Y. H. 2011. Pectenotoxin-2 induces G1 arrest of the cell cycle in synovial fibroblasts of patients with rheumatoid arthritis. *International Journal of Molecular Medicine,* 27, 783–787.

85. Pazos, M., Alfonso, A., Vieytes, M., Yasumoto, T., and Botana, L. 2004. Resonant mirror biosensor detection method based on yessotoxin–phosphodiesterase interactions. *Analytical Biochemistry,* 335, 112–118.

86. Pazos, M., Alfonso, A., Vieytes, M., Yasumoto, T., and Botana, L. 2006. Study of the interaction between different phosphodiesterases and yessotoxin using a resonant mirror biosensor. *Chemical Research in Toxicology,* 19, 794–800.

87. Pazos, M. J., Alfonso, A., Vieytes, M. R., Yasumoto, T., and Botana, L. M. 2005. Kinetic analysis of the interaction between yessotoxin and analogs and immobilized phosphodiesterases using a resonant mirror optical biosensor. *Chemical Research in Toxicology,* 18, 1155–1160.

88. Pecina-Slaus, N. 2003. Tumor suppressor gene E-cadherin and its role in normal and malignant cells. *Cancer Cell International,* 14, 1–7.

89. Pendino, F., Tarkanyi, I., Dudognon, C. et al. 2006. Telomeres and telomerase: Pharmacological targets for new anticancer strategies? *Current Cancer Drug Targets,* 6, 147–180.

90. Perez-Gomez, A., Ferrero-Gutierrez, A., Novelli, A. et al. 2006. Potent neurotoxic action of the shellfish biotoxin yessotoxin on cultured cerebellar neurons. *Toxicological Sciences,* 90, 168–177.

91. Pierotti, S., Malaguti, C., Milandri, A., Poletti, R., and Paolo Rossini, G. 2003. Functional assay to measure yessotoxins in contaminated mussel samples. *Analytical Biochemistry,* 312, 208–216.

92. Pollard, T. D. and Borisy, G. G. 2003. Cellular motility driven by assembly and disassembly of actin filaments. *Cell,* 112, 453–465.

93. Rios-Doria, J. and Day, M. L. 2005. Truncated E-cadherin potentiates cell death in prostate epithelial cells. *Prostate,* 63, 259–268.

94. Roman, Y., Alfonso, A., Louzao, M. C. et al. 2002. Azaspiracid-1, a potent, nonapoptotic new phycotoxin with several cell targets. *Cell Signaling,* 14, 703–716.

95. Roman, Y., Alfonso, A., Vieytes, M. R. et al. 2004. Effects of Azaspiracids 2 and 3 on intracellular cAMP, $[Ca^{2+}]$, and pH. *Chemical Research in Toxicology,* 17, 1338–1349.

96. Ronzitti, G., Callegari, F., Malaguti, C., and Rossini, G. P. 2004. Selective disruption of the E-cadherin-catenin system by an algal toxin. *British Journal of Cancer,* 90, 1100–1107.

97. Ronzitti, G., Hess, P., Rehmann, N., and Rossini, G. P. 2007. Azaspiracid-1 alters the E-cadherin pool in epithelial cells. *Toxicological Sciences,* 95, 427–435.

98. Rubenstein, P. A. and Wen, K. K. 2005. Lights, camera, action. *IUBMB Life,* 57, 683–687.

99. Sasaki, K., Wright, J. L. C., and Yasumoto, T. 1998. Identification and characterization of pectenotoxin (PTX) 4 and PTX7 as spiroketal stereoisomers of two previously reported pectenotoxins. *Journal of Organic Chemistry,* 63, 2475–2480.

100. Satake, M., Mackenzie, L., and Yasumoto, T. 1997. Identification of *Protoceratium reticulatum* as the biogenetic origin of yessotoxin. *Natural Toxins,* 5, 164–167.

101. Satake, M., Terasawa, K., Kadowaki, Y., and Yasumoto, T. 1996. Relative configuration of yessotoxin and isolation of two new analogs from toxic scallops. *Tetrahedron Letters,* 37, 5955–5958.

102. Sheth, S. B., Chaganti, K., Bastepe, M. et al. 1997. Cyclic AMP phosphodiesterases in human lymphocytes. *British Journal of Haematology,* 99, 784–789.

103. Shin, D. Y., Kim, G. Y., Kim, N. D. et al. 2008. Induction of apoptosis by pectenotoxin-2 is mediated with the induction of DR4/DR5, Egr-1 and NAG-1, activation of caspases and modulation of the Bcl-2 family in p53-deficient Hep3B hepatocellular carcinoma cells. *Oncology Reports,* 19, 517–526.

104. Spector, I., Braet, F., Shochet, N. R., and Bubb, M. R. 1999. New anti-actin drugs in the study of the organization and function of the actin cytoskeleton. *Microscopy Research and Technique,* 47, 18–37.

105. Sperantio, S., Poksay, K., De Belle, I. et al. 2004. Paraptosis: Mediation by MAP kinases and inhibition by AIP-1/Alix. *Cell Death and Differentiation,* 11, 1066–1075.

106. Suarez Korsness, M., Hetland, D. L., Espenes, A., and Aune, T. 2006. Induction of apoptosis by YTX in myoblast cell lines via mitochondrial signalling transduction pathway. *Toxicology In Vitro,* 20, 1419–1426.

107. Suarez Korsness, M., Hetland, D. L., Espenes, A., and Aune, T. 2007. Cleavage of tensin during cytoskeleton disruption in YTX-induced apoptosis. *Toxicology In Vitro,* 21, 9–45.

108. Suarez Korsness, M., Hetland, D. L., Espenes, A., Tranulis, M. A., and Aune, T. 2006. Apoptotic events induced by yessotoxin in myoblast cell lines from rat and mouse. *Toxicology In Vitro,* 20, 1077–1087.

109. Suzuki, T., Beuzenberg, V., Mackenzie, L., and Quilliam, M. A. 2003. Liquid chromatography-mass spectrometry of spiroketal stereoisomers of pectenotoxins and the analysis of novel pectenotoxin isomers in the toxic dinoflagellate *Dinophysis acuta* from New Zealand. *Journal of Chromatography,* 992, 141–150.

110. Suzuki, T., Mackenzie, L., Stirling, D., and Adamson, J. 2001. Pectenotoxin-2 seco acid: A toxin converted from pectenotoxin-2 by the New Zealand Greenshell mussel, *Perna canaliculus. Toxicon,* 39, 507–514.

111. Suzuki, T., Mitsuya, T., Matsubara, H., and Yamasaki, M. 1998. Determination of pectenotoxin-2 after solid-phase extraction from seawater and from the dinoflagellate *Dinophysis fortii* by liquid chromatography with electrospray mass spectrometry and ultraviolet detection—Evidence of oxidation of pectenotoxin-2 to pectenotoxin-6 in scallops. *Journal of Chromatography A,* 815, 155–160.

112. Suzuki, T., Walter, J. A., Leblanc, P. et al. 2006. Identification of pectenotoxin-11 as 34S-hydroxypectenotoxin-2, a new pectenotoxin analogue in the toxic dinoflagellate *Dinophysis acuta* from New Zealand. *Chemical Research in Toxicology,* 19, 310–318.

113. Terao, K., Ito, E., Oarada, M., Murata, M., and Yasumoto, T. 1990. Histopathological studies on experimental marine toxin poisoning—5. The effects in mice of yessotoxin isolated from *Patinopecten yessoensis* and of a desulfated derivative. *Toxicon,* 28, 1095–1104.

114. Terao, K., Ito, E., Yanagi, T., and Yasumoto, T. 1986. Histopathological studies on experimental marine toxin poisoning. I. Ultrastructural changes in the small intestine and liver of suckling mice induced by dinophysistoxin-1 and pectenotoxin-1. *Toxicon,* 24, 1141–1151.

115. Tobío, A., Fernández-Araujo, A., Alfonso, A., and Botana, L. M. 2012. Role of yessotoxin in calcium and cAMP-crosstalks in primary and K-562 human lymphocytes: The effect is mediated by anchor kinase A mitochondrial proteins. *Journal of Cellular Biochemistry,* 113, 3752–3761.

116. Torgersen, T., Sandvik, M., Lundve, B., and Lindegarth, S. 2008. Profiles and levels of fatty acid esters of okadaic acid group toxins and pectenotoxins during toxin depuration. Part II: Blue mussels (*Mytilus edulis*) and flat oyster (*Ostrea edulis*). *Toxicon,* 52, 418–427.

117. Tubaro, A., Dell'ovo, V., Sosa, S., and Florio, C. 2010. Yessotoxins: A toxicological overview. *Toxicon,* 56, 163–172.

118. Tubaro, A., Giangaspero, A., Ardizzone, M. et al. 2008. Ultrastructural damage to heart tissue from repeated oral exposure to yessotoxin resolves in 3 months. *Toxicon,* 51, 1225–1235.

119. Tubaro, A., Sosa, S., Altinier, G. et al. 2004. Short-term oral toxicity of homoyessotoxins, yessotoxin and okadaic acid in mice. *Toxicon,* 43, 439–445.

120. Tubaro, A., Sosa, S., Carbonatto, M. et al. 2003. Oral and intraperitoneal acute toxicity studies of yessotoxin and homoyessotoxins in mice. *Toxicon,* 41, 783–792.

121. Vale, C., Nicolaou, K. C., Frederick, M. O. et al. 2007. Effects of azaspiracid-1, a potent cytotoxic agent, on primary neuronal cultures. A structure–activity relationship study. *Journal of Medicinal Chemistry,* 50, 356–363.

122. Vale, P. 2004. Differential dynamics of dinophysistoxins and pectenotoxins between blue mussel and common cockle: A phenomenon originating from the complex toxin profile of *Dinophysis acuta. Toxicon,* 44, 123–134.

123. Vale, P. and Sampayo, M. A. D. 2002. Pectenotoxin-2 seco acid, 7-epi-pectenotoxin-2 seco acid and pectenotoxin-2 in shellfish and plankton from Portugal. *Toxicon,* 40, 979–987.

124. Vilarino, N., Nicolaou, K. C., Frederick, M. O. et al. 2006. Cell growth inhibition and actin cytoskeleton disorganization induced by azaspiracid-1 structure–activity studies. *Chemical Research in Toxicology,* 19, 1459–1466.

125. Wijnhoven, B. P., Dinjens, W. N., and Pignatelli, M. 2000. E-cadherin-catenin cell–cell adhesion complex and human cancer. *British Journal of Surgery,* 87, 992–1005.

126. Wilkins, A. L., Rehmann, N., Torgersen, T. et al. 2010. Identification of fatty acid esters of pectenotoxin-2 seco acid in Blue mussels (*Mytilus edulis*) from Ireland. *Toxicon,* 56, 191–217.

127. Yasumoto, T. and Murata, M. 1990. Polyether toxin involved in seafood poisoning. In: Hall, S. and Stritchartz, G. (eds.) *Marine Toxins.* Washington, DC: American Chemical Society, pp. 120–132.

128. Yasumoto, T., Murata, M., Lee, J. S., and Torigoe, K. 1989. Polyether toxins produced by dinoflagellates. In: Natori, S. K., Hashimoto, K., and Ueno, Y. (eds.) *Mycotoxins and Phycotoxins'88*. Amsterdam, the Netherlands: Elsevier, pp. 375–382.

129. Yasumoto, T., Murata, M., Oshima, Y., Matsumoto, G. K., and Clardy, J. 1984. Diarrhetic shellfish poisoning. In: Ragelis, E. P. (ed.) *Seafood Toxins*. Washington, DC: American Chemical Society, pp. 207–214.

130. Yasumoto, T., Murata, M., Oshima, Y., and Sano, M. 1985. Diarrhetic shellfish toxins. *Tetrahedron*, 41, 1019–1025.

131. Young, C., Truman, P., Boucher, M. et al. 2009. The algal metabolite yessotoxin affects heterogeneous nuclear ribonucleoproteins in HepG2 cells. *Proteomics*, 9, 2529–2542.

132. Zhou, Z. H., Komiyama, M., Terao, K., and Shimada, Y. 1994. Effects of pectenotoxin-1 on liver cells in vitro. *Toxicology In Vitro*, 26, 493–499.

23

Maitotoxin: An Enigmatic Toxic Molecule with Useful Applications in the Biomedical Sciences

Juan G. Reyes, Claudia Sánchez-Cárdenas, Waldo Acevedo-Castillo,
Patricio Leyton, Ignacio López-González, Ricardo Felix,
María A. Gandini, Marcela B. Treviño, and Claudia L. Treviño

CONTENTS

23.1 Introduction

Many marine invertebrates produce potent toxins, turning themselves poisonous as a defense strategy against predators. In contrast, other organisms can become poisonous by accumulating toxins from their own prey. Dinoflagellates are aquatic photosynthetic microbial eukaryotes, and some species produce highly toxic metabolites. These dinoflagellate toxins bioaccumulate up the food chain in various consumer organisms. Many filter-feeding organisms such as bivalves accumulate such toxins with no apparent adverse effects on them[1] but causing intoxication when ingested by their predators, including fish and marine mammals, and ultimately also when humans consume contaminated seafood.[2]

Four major groups of dinoflagellate toxins have been described, namely, saxitoxins, ladder-shaped polyether compounds, long-chain polyketides, and macrolides.[2] The dinoflagellate species *Gambierdiscus toxicus* produces several potent polyether toxins, some of which were initially identified in connection with a common type of food poisoning called ciguatera, caused by consumption of certain contaminated tropical and subtropical fish. Ciguatera involves a combination of gastrointestinal, neurological, and cardiovascular disorders. The two most common toxin classes associated with ciguatera are ciguatoxin (CTx) and maitotoxin (MTx), and they are among the most lethal natural substances known to man.[2]

Most of the neurological symptoms of ciguatera are caused by CTx, which exert their effects due primarily to the activation of voltage-gated sodium channels, causing cell membrane depolarization.[1] MTx displays diverse pharmacological activities, which seem to be derived from its ability to activate Ca^{2+}-uptake processes in a variety of cell types.[3] MTx is the largest and most toxic known nonbiopolymeric toxin, with a molecular weight of 3422 Da. MTx is a very interesting compound given its extremely potent biological activity, and it has been used as a powerful pharmacological tool for the elucidation of Ca^{2+}-dependent cellular processes.

23.2 History

The discovery of MTx is closely related to the characterization of ciguatera, a food-borne illness caused by the consumption of fish contaminated with certain dinoflagellate toxins. Ciguatera symptoms can vary with the geographic origin of the contaminated fish. Gastrointestinal symptoms—such as diarrhea, vomiting, and abdominal pain—occur first, usually within 24 h of eating implicated fish. Neurological symptoms may occur at the same time or may follow several days later and include thermal sense inversion, characterized by the feeling of receiving an electric shock when touching cold water, pain and weakness in the lower extremities, and circumoral and peripheral paresthesia.

This mode of poisoning was called "ciguatera" after *cigua*, a snail commonly occurring in the Caribbean Sea.[4,5] Ciguatera occurs worldwide in tropical and subtropical regions causing 20,000–50,000 victims per year. The agents causing this condition bioaccumulate in fish as they are transferred up the food chain, to be finally consumed by humans. Ancient references to toxic diseases conditions similar to "ciguatera" are found in Homer's Odyssey (ca. 800 BC), in reports of a pandemic occurring in China (600 BC), and in the chronicles written by Pedro Martir de Anglería in 1555.[6]

MTx was discovered in 1965 by Bagnis, who reported that the human symptoms caused by ingestion of contaminated herbivorous fish were different from those caused by carnivorous fish, primarily involving gastrointestinal discomfort and less neurological disorders. The molecule responsible for these symptoms was discovered upon examination of the toxic constituents in the surgeonfish *Ctenochaetus striatus* and was named after the Tahitian namesake of this species—"maito."[7] MTx is a polyketide-derived polycyclic ether consisting of four extended fused-ring systems termed polyether ladders (molecular formula $C_{164}H_{256}O_{68}S_2Na_2$) (Figure 23.1).

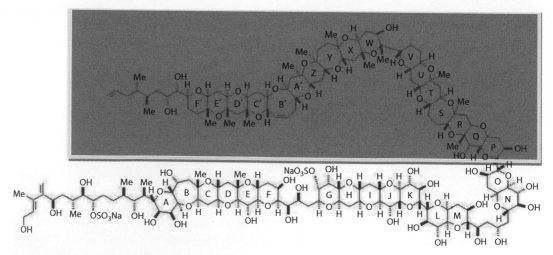

FIGURE 23.1 Structure of MTx. (Taken from Treviño, C.L. et al., Maitotoxin: A unique pharmacological tool for elucidating Ca^{2+}-dependent mechanisms, in: Botana, L.M. (ed.), *Seafood and Freshwater Toxins: Pharmacology, Physiology and Detection*, 2nd edn., CRC Press, Boca Raton, FL, pp. 503–516, 2008.) The grey region was utilized for the theoretical molecular dynamics calculations in the section *MTx interaction with membranes*.

23.3 Natural Origin

The marine dinoflagellate *G. toxicus* is a single-celled phytoplanktonic organism, and it may be found on the surface of algae in tropical waters worldwide. Among other toxins, it produces CTx and MTx, which accumulate through the food chain as carnivorous fish consume contaminated herbivorous reef fish. MTx toxin accumulates primarily in the liver and viscera of fishes, but not in their flesh.[8] Higher concentrations of toxins can be found in large predatory fish such as barracuda, grouper, amberjack, snapper, and shark. Because the fish industry has no borders and marine products are shipped to many countries, ciguatera fish poisoning can occur almost anywhere. People who live in or travel to endemic areas should avoid consumption of barracuda or moray eel, should be cautious with grouper and red snapper, and are advised to enquire about local fish associated with ciguatera. Since there is no reliable way to "decontaminate" or even to distinguish contaminated fish by smell or appearance, it is wise to avoid eating the viscera of any reef fish and to prevent consumption of large predacious reef fish.[9,10].

The temperatures of the northern Caribbean and extreme southeastern Gulf of Mexico have been predicted to increase 2.5°C–3.5°C during the next years.[11] Higher temperatures favor *G. toxicus* growth[12] and are also likely to alter fish migration patterns. Ciguatera outbreaks have been correlated with sea-surface temperature increases in the south Pacific Ocean.[13]

After Yasumoto discovered in 1977 that the dinoflagellate *G. toxicus* was responsible for producing MTx, he cultivated this organism for 10 years in order to have enough material to isolate this toxin and to determine its structure.[14,15] For some years, MTx was commercially available for experimentation and was used to study Ca^{2+} dynamics in diverse cell types (see Section 23.7). Having this tool commercially available again would certainly continue to be useful for research purposes.

23.4 Toxicology

Human ingestion of seafood contaminated with toxins produced by marine phytoplankton[10,16,17] can cause a variety of diseases. These toxins can have a wide range of acute and chronic health effects not just in humans but also in other animal species. Given that these compounds are tasteless, odorless, and heat and acid stable, conventional food testing methods fail to detect and destroy them in contaminated seafood.

Ciguatera can cause mild to severe symptoms lasting from a few days and up to years. Around 400 species of fish are considered to be ciguateric and contain distinct combinations and quantities of toxins. Classical ciguateric symptoms include gastrointestinal and neurological disorders, abdominal cramps, diarrhea, nausea, vomiting, temperature reversal, and itching. The toxins can even be passed on to a fetus or to a newborn child, via placental or breast milk transmission, respectively.[9,10]

Most of the neurological symptoms of ciguatera are due to CTx, while MTx is considered to be less important in the generation of ciguatera symptoms given that it is less concentrated in fishes. However, it should be noted that the observed toxicity differences could also be the result of chemical modifications of the toxins possibly occurring as they pass through the food chain, and it is therefore difficult to establish a direct relationship between the various symptoms and a particular toxin. Diagnosis of ciguatera is based solely on the presence of the general symptoms in correlation to patients with a recent history of fish ingestion.

In contrast to the lipid-soluble CTxs, MTx is water soluble, and it apparently does not accumulate in the flesh of fishes but rather in organs such as the liver.[18] MTx has a very low oral potency as compared to its high lethality when injected intraperitoneally (i.p.), and pure MTx is even more toxic than CTx. For example, in mice, CTx is lethal at 0.45 µg/kg i.p. and MTx at a dose of 0.15 µg/kg i.p. However, the precise lethal dose depends on the mouse strain, the sample source, and even the sample preparation procedure, as MTx binds to glass and plastic and thus its exact concentration may be underestimated. Mice injected i.p. with MTx display reduced body temperature, piloerection, dyspnea, progressive paralysis, slight tremors or convulsions, and long death times. High doses of MTx produce CTx-like symptoms, such as gasping with convulsions and shorter death times.

Three different MTx molecules have been isolated from a variety of strains of *G. toxicus*. Injection of MTx-1 and MTx-2 in mice exerted similar symptoms, except that MTx-2 exhibited shorter death times. MTx-3 induced additional symptoms such as intense gasping that ameliorated near death; however, further purification of MTx-3 by HPLC reduced the gasping symptoms, suggesting that additional bioactive components may be present in the crude preparation.[19] The death times produced by MTx-1 and MTx-3 were very similar. Desulfonation of MTx (solvolysis) reduces the toxicity of all three forms about 200-fold.[19,20]

Efforts to develop a radioimmunoassay (RIA) or enzyme-linked immunosorbent assay (ELISA) to detect CTx have been made over the past few years, such as the Hokama enzyme immunoassay stick test.[21] There is a commercial kit called Cigua-Check® that may be used by fisherman or restaurants to prevent ingestion of contaminated fish. Unfortunately, this kit only detects CTx. Detection can be confirmed by finding CTx and MTx in contaminated fish samples by high-performance liquid chromatography and mass spectrometry, although this process is costly and not widely available in high risk areas, such as small islands.

To date, there is no antidote for ciguatera, but medications such as amitriptyline have been used to diminish some of the symptoms of chronic ciguatera, including fatigue and paresthesias. There are several palliative remedies including medicinal teas used in both the Indo-Pacific and West Indies regions. However, none of these treatments have been properly standardized to provide effective treatment.[9,10] Patients are also advised to avoid alcohol, nuts, and nut oil for at least 6 months after the intoxication in order to avoid reappearance of symptoms.

23.5 Synthesis

23.5.1 Biosynthesis of Ladder-Shaped Polyether Compounds

The structural similarities among dinoflagellate-produced polyether ladder toxins including brevetoxins, CTxs, yessotoxins, and MTxs strongly suggest that their biosynthetic pathways may share similar strategies. In the case of brevetoxins, experimental studies on their biosynthetic pathways are starting to unveil the biochemical reactions involved in the production of such complex polyethers. Based on tracing studies using radiolabeled carbon precursors, it is now clear that polyketides in general are assembled from acetyl-CoA or malonyl-CoA precursors; they also contain carbon units derived from methionine and from some larger carbon unit precursors, such as glycolate.[22] The carbon chain formed from the aforementioned precursors appears to be interrupted by C-1 deletions of acetate-derived carbon atoms. Although a Favorskii-like rearrangement has been suggested to be involved in the ring size reduction observed in polyether ladder toxins, such proposed catalytic mechanism (which in vitro takes place with halogenated compounds and under strong basic conditions) has not yet been unequivocally demonstrated. In this biosynthetic pathway, and similarly to bacterial polyether synthesis, polyketide synthases appear to play an important role. This family of enzymes catalyzes the synthesis of complex natural products from precursors such as acetyl-CoA, propionyl-CoA, and methylmalonyl-CoA through a biosynthetic strategy resembling the one used for fatty acid (FA) biosynthesis.[23] Thus, polyketides are built by a series of successive condensations of simple precursors, decarboxylations, reductions, and rearrangements. However, unlike FA biosynthesis, in which the FA chain is subjected to the whole series of intermediate reactions, the partial chemical processing of intermediaries in polyketide biosynthesis can give rise to a complex pattern of functional groups associated to the polyether chain. Furthermore, different dinoflagellate species can use different combinations of starter CoA-activated precursors and chain-extension substrates during polyketide biosynthesis, which at least in some cases involve the generation of specific chiral centers and cyclization. Despite the proposed existence of similar polyether ladder biosynthetic pathways in different dinoflagellate species, suggested by their products' structural similarities.[22,24] Defining the specific reactions of any such pathway has proven a very difficult task. This challenge stems from the diversity of chemical structures found in this family of compounds, from the diversity of species within this phylum of alveolate eukaryotes, and from the particularly complex genetic organization observed in these organisms, including multigene phylogenies, diverse plastid endosymbiotic relationships, and chromatin configuration.[22,25–28] It has been suggested that for polyether ladder toxins, the participating acetate units can enter the tricarboxylic acid (TCA) cycle, and some TCA intermediate could be the actual precursor involved in the condensation process.[29] In fact, to the best of our knowledge, there are thus far no reports of specific studies on MTx biosynthesis. Furthermore, it is likely that the toxins isolated from the organs of herbivorous fishes represent a chemically modified version of the toxins originally synthesized by the dinoflagellates.[30–32]

The cyclization process in these compounds is probably associated to the formation of an epoxide intermediate presumably catalyzed by epoxidases and epoxide hydrolases.[33,34] The accompanying polyepoxide process proposed for marine polyether ladder toxins has clear precedents in several reports on epoxide and cycle formation during antibiotic polyether biosynthesis.[35] Although the process whereby 10 or more epoxides are formed and then coordinated to a polyepoxide cascade to yield polyether ladder toxins still remains unclear, an oxidase-catalyzed tandem epoxide formation and epoxide protection, followed by a hydrolase-catalyzed epoxide opening and cycle rearrangement, is likely involved.

23.5.2 Chemical Synthesis of Maitotoxin

The chemical structures of marine toxins in general—and MTx in particular—are very interesting and represent a formidable challenge for organic synthesis.[36] The appearance in the literature of the structure of brevetoxin-B (the first marine polycyclic ether to be isolated and characterized[37]) awoke a large interest in synthetic organic chemists. The structure of brevetoxin-B is characterized by several fused polycyclic ethers containing ether rings with 6, 7, and 8 units, in addition to 23 chiral centers, certainly a daring task for chemical synthesis. It contains 32 fused ether rings, 28 hydroxyl groups, 21 methyl groups, 98 chiral centers, and 2 sulfates.[3,38–40]

The efforts of chemical synthesis have been directed toward developing new methods that allow synthesis of only part of these molecules by initially building structural fragments of these ladder-shaped polyether toxins. Great progress in the synthesis of several marine polycyclic ethers has been accomplished since the year 2000.[41,42] They designed a remarkable synthetic strategy involving an efficient iterative method for the stereoselective construction of transfused polycyclic ethers based on induced reductive cyclization of β-alcoxy-acrylate by samarium iodide (SmI_2). In the case of the synthesis of the ring systems of MTx, the stereoselectivity was accomplished by state transition chelation (Figure 23.2).[42–46]

Oxepane ring formation also was stereoselectively synthesized through this reaction generating a single product with an 84% yield (Figure 23.3).

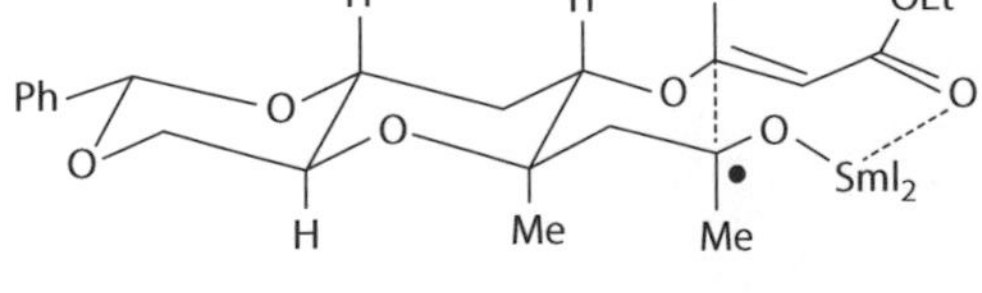

FIGURE 23.2 Transition state of the cyclization induced by SmI_2. (From Sakamoto, Y. et al., *Org. Lett.*, 3, 2749, 2001; Nakata, T., *Chem. Rec.*, 10, 159, 2010.)

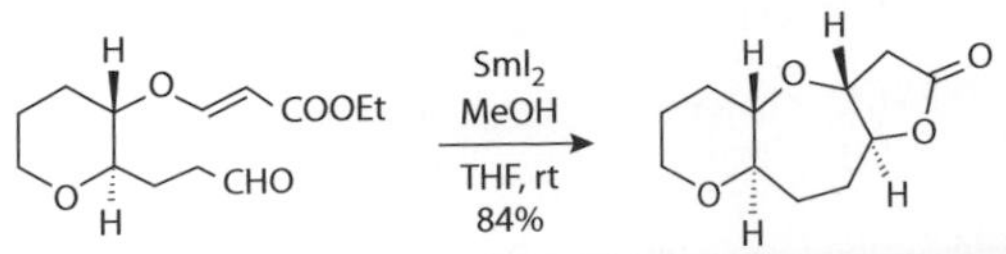

FIGURE 23.3 Synthesis of polycyclic ethers based on cyclization induced by SmI_2. (From Nakata, T., *Chem. Rec.*, 10, 159, 2010.)

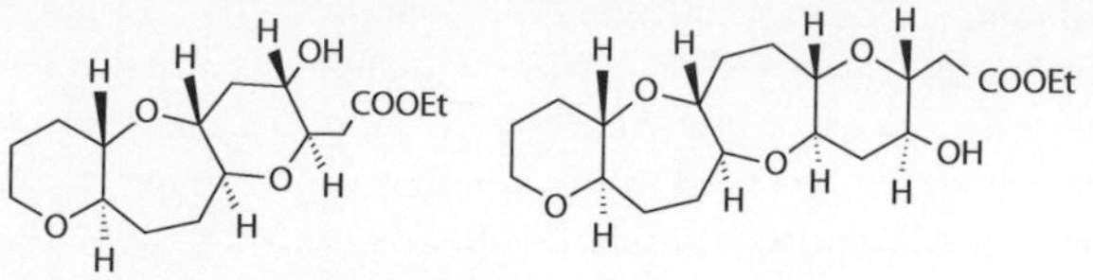

FIGURE 23.4 Examples of ethers synthesized by iterative strategy induced cyclization 6,7,6 and 6,7,7,6 membered polycyclic ethers. (From Nakata, T., *Chem. Rec.*, 10, 159, 2010.)

Moreover, the trans-membered fused polycyclic 6,7,6 and 6,7,7,6 ethers were iteratively synthesized using this cyclization induced by SmI_2 strategy (Figure 23.4).[42]

Additionally, in 1998, Dr. Nicolaou's research group (La Jolla, CA) reported the complete synthesis of brevetoxin-A, another ladder-shaped polyether compound, the first stereoselective synthesis of pyrans involving the opening of epoxides with a hydroxyl group. This synthesis route has the particularity of overcoming the natural preference for cyclization to an unwanted product 5-exo by placing one C—C bond adjacent to the epoxy fragment. Thus, under these conditions, the structure shown in Figure 23.5 exclusively undergoes ring closure to produce a 6-endo by pyran system instead of 5-exo product. The selectivity observed is attributed to the π orbital stabilization generated by a carbon atom next to the electron-deficient transition state provoking an endo attack; this effect would be absent during the exo attack.[47]

Using similar synthetic strategies, this same research group has accomplished the stereoselective synthesis of ladder-shaped portions of a large part of MTx.[40,41,48–50] Altogether, between Dr. Nakata's and Dr. Nicolaou's group, 29 out of the 32 rings of MTx have been chemically synthesized.

Although thus far no complete chemical synthesis has been achieved for MTx, complete synthesis has been successful for some of the other ladder-shaped polycyclic ester toxins. New methods such as biomimetic cascades, cross-coupling reactions catalyzed by palladium, and radical reactions could provide additional tools for approaching the laboratory synthesis of this type of compounds.

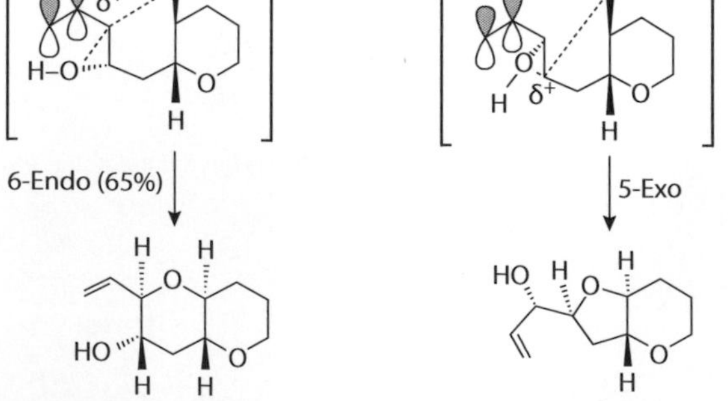

FIGURE 23.5 Reactions involved for the formation of cyclic ethers. (From Nicolaou, K. et al., *J. Am. Chem. Soc.*, 108, 2468, 1986; Nicolaou, K.C. et al., *J. Am. Chem. Soc.*, 130, 7466, 2008.)

23.6 Mechanisms of Action

23.6.1 MTx and Plasma Membrane Channel Activation

After the early work of Dr. Yasumoto's group,[51–53] it became clear that MTx acted on mammalian cells inducing entry of external Ca^{2+}, and based on pharmacological criteria, it was proposed that MTx activated voltage-gated Ca^{2+} (Cav) channels.[54–57] Consistent with this proposal, MTx-induced Ca^{2+} entry was absent in fibroblast that lacked these channels.[55] However, even this early work on the mechanisms of action of MTx pointed out some peculiar aspects of the toxin's effects, such as a delay of about 2 min in the induction of Ca^{2+} entry observed in certain cell types[55] or the reported inhibition of Na^+-K^+-ATPase induced by the toxin.[58] Furthermore, it was soon reported that MTx was able to induce inositol triphosphate (IP_3) release independently of its action on Ca^{2+} channels.[59] These results were corroborated by Gusovsky et al.[60–63] in several cell lines, showing also that MTx activated phosphoinositide (PI) breakdown in a Ca^{2+}-dependent manner but it was not inhibited by Cav channel blockers, suggesting the activation of phospholipase C (PLC) or the activation of other Ca^{2+} channels. The fact that MTx action on PI breakdown was not mimicked by Ca^{2+} ionophores supported the notion that MTx activated PLC directly. However, in the work of Gusovsky et al.[64] using HL60 cells, it became clear that MTx action on PI turnover was associated to a Ca^{2+}-induced activation of PLC, rather than a direct PLC activation by MTx. Furthermore, the work of Pin et al.[65] suggested that the effects of MTx on gamma-aminobutyric acid (GABA) release in striatal neurons were associated to a Ca^{2+}-dependent Na^+ influx, introducing the notion of an additional cellular target for MTx. Similar results of a Ca^{2+}-dependent Na^+ influx was reported by Sladescek et al.[66] The pleiotropic effects and action mechanisms of MTx on different cells was reviewed by Hamilton and Perez.[67]

Although the effects of MTx were pleiotropic, they all seemed to involve an intracellular Ca^{2+} increase. The fact that MTx activated cation channels was clear from direct voltage-clamp current measurements (e.g., [38,68–81]). Some of the proposed channels were Cav and also nonselective cation channels such as store-operated channels (SOCs). Furthermore, in some cells such as skin fibroblasts, MTx seems to activate large conducting channels[82,83] leading to cell lysis. Hence, the action of MTx would be highly dependent on the channel expression profile of each cell type and also on the MTx concentration used (e.g., [84]). Due to scope limitations in this review, we have excluded a discussion of all cellular effects downstream of the MTx interaction with membranes, on which a wealth of data is undoubtedly available in the literature.

The ability of MTx to activate Cav and other cationic channels posed the question as to whether the toxin was activating channels by inserting itself in the membrane and perturbing the phospholipid membrane structure (see MTx interaction with membranes in the following texts) or whether it had specific interactions with the proteins forming the channels. Murata et al.[85] reported that either a removal of the sulfated residues from MTx or a hydrogenation of the molecule decreased (by several orders of magnitude) its ability to induce Ca^{2+} entry or PI breakdown in insulinoma or glioma cells. When these MTx derivatives were used together with intact MTx, they acted as blockers of the MTx effect. The work of Konoki et al.[86] describing inhibition of MTx-induced Ca^{2+} entry in glioma C6 cells by brevetoxin and synthetic fragments of MTx (corresponding to a sulfated portion, rings EF-GH, and rings LM-NO) strongly suggested that MTx acted on specific sites to activate Ca^{2+} entry in these cells. Interestingly, the sulfated fragment of MTx (EF-GH rings, and hence, a portion expected to remain in the aqueous phase or at the lipid–water interphase) was more potent in inhibiting MTx effects on Ca^{2+} uptake than the LM-NO rings. Recent work by Oishi et al.[87] clearly showed that an artificial ladder-shaped heptacyclic polyether was the most potent substance described to date capable of inhibiting MTx-induced Ca^{2+} influx in glioma C6 cells, strongly suggesting the existence of a specific MTx binding site in these cells. However, this work did not give insight into the molecular mechanisms of action of MTx.

23.6.2 MTx Interaction with Membranes

The insertion of MTx in membranes was first suggested by Konoki et al.,[88] with rings RSTUVWXYZA'B'C'D'E'F' inserted in and spanning the phospholipid bilayer and rings ABCDEFGHIJKLMNOPQ—containing the sulfated parts of the molecule—staying in the aqueous

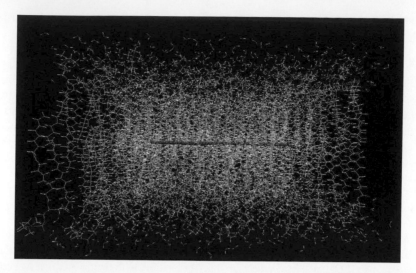

FIGURE 23.6   The initial position of MTx in the 1-palmitoyl-2-oleoyl-*sn*-glycero-3- phosphocholine (POPC) membrane was set with the plane of the molecule parallel to the POPC/water interphase. This position and conformation as well as the environment were then allowed to drift with molecular dynamics calculations toward steady states with minimal energy conformations. Water molecules: oxygen = red, hydrogen = white. Phospholipids: light blue large chains. MTx: darker blue at the center of the bilayer. (http://www.ibt.unam.mx/server/PRG.base?tipo:doc,dir:PRG.curriculum,par:ctrevino)

environment. This work was later cited by Murata et al.,[89] Nicolau et al.,[90] and Nicolau and Aversa[91] to discuss the properties of MTx. This association of MTx with phospholipid membranes was deduced from the structural properties of MTx and by analogy to the properties of other ladder-shaped polyether toxins.[89] However, to the best of our efforts, we were unable to find the specific model or program used to estimate MTx distribution in phospholipid membranes. Thus, in order to theoretically estimate the stability of the relatively hydrophobic portion of MTx in a phosphatidylcholine phospholipid membrane, we performed force field parameterization of rings P–F′ and molecular dynamics as shown in the following texts. The molecular structure of MTx was taken from Nicolau and Frederic[40] (Figure 23.1). Partial parameterization with the CHARMM force field was accomplished taking different sections of the molecule from ring P to F′ using the CCPN web applications (http://www.ccpn.ac.uk/). The 1-palmitoyl-2-oleoyl-sn-glycero-3-phosphocholine (DOPC) bilayer was built with visual molecular dynamics (VMD 1.9).[92] The mentioned fragment of MTx was distributed in the center of the bilayer, and the program not (just) another molecular dynamics (NAMD) allowed to iteratively locate the molecule to acquire a conformation giving steady values of potential energy parameters (http://www.ks.uiuc.edu/Research/vmd/). This modeling clearly shows that rings P–F′ and tail were stable within the lipid bilayer (Figures 23.6 and 23.7), and this conformation is likely restricted and modified by the more hydrophilic portion of MTx (see also Murata et al.[89]). This distribution of the hydrophobic portion of MTx is consistent with the proposed role of this part of MTx (or similar portions of ladder-shaped polyether toxins) in the interaction with integral membrane α-helices.[89,93] However, these results do not exclude that the hydrophilic portion of MTx, anchored in the membrane by the hydrophobic portion, could also interact externally with channels[86] or, as we could cautiously propose, that both mechanisms could be responsible for activation of different types of channels in biological membranes.

23.7 MTx Bioactivity and Applications

Ca^{2+} is an ubiquitous secondary intracellular messenger responsible for mediating a multitude of cellular responses as diverse as proliferation, development, contraction, secretion, and fertilization. Ca^{2+} action is quite simple: cells at rest have an intracellular concentration of ~100 nM but are activated when this level rises to ~1 μM. However, the universality of Ca^{2+} as an intracellular messenger depends on its remarkable capacity to create a wide range of spatial and temporal signals.

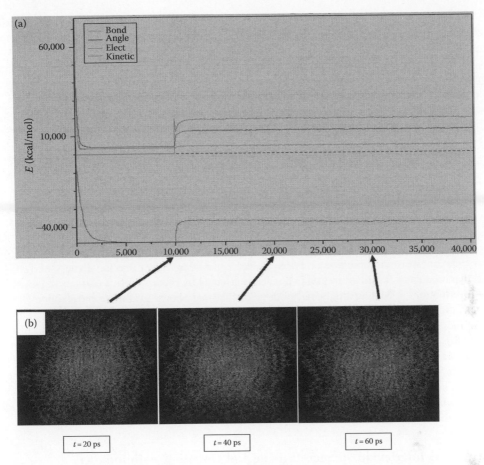

FIGURE 23.7   (a) Plot of energy (kcal/mol) versus the molecular simulation steps (1 ps corresponds to 500 steps). Each curve corresponds to the different components of potential energy: binding energy (blue line), angles (red line), electrostatic energy (green line), and kinetic energy (orange line). (b) Spatial distribution of MTx in the 1,2-dioleoyl-sn-glycero-3-phosphocholine (DOPC) membrane at 20, 40, and 60 ps. From the potential energy curves and the molecular images, it can be seen that this portion of MTx is stably located within the hydrophobic portion of the phospholipid bilayer at 40 ps, with a location and dynamics that certainly would be restricted by the hydrophilic portion that is expected to be located at the water/phospholipid interface. (See also Murata, M. et al., *Bull. Chem. Soc. Jpn.*, 81, 307, 2008.)

MTx has attracted much attention given its powerful bioactivity involving disruption of Ca^{2+} homeostasis. MTx is not only one of the most potent toxins, but it also possesses multiple activities that appear to be linked to elevation of intracellular Ca^{2+} concentration. Thus, the toxin serves as a versatile tool for studies on cellular events associated with intracellular Ca^{2+} changes that are of particular interest, including hormone secretion, programmed cell death activation, and fertilization.

23.7.1 Insulinotropic Actions of MTx

Although some hormones such as insulin-like growth factor and adiponectin have hypoglycemic effects,[94] insulin has long been considered the only hypoglycemic agent in mammals. Insulin is synthesized and secreted by pancreatic β-cells located in specialized structures, the islets of Langerhans. In general, β-cells adjust insulin secretion to the prevailing blood glucose levels by a process called glucose-stimulated insulin secretion (GSIS). Inside pancreatic β-cells, glucose metabolism induces insulin secretion by altering the cellular array of messenger molecules. ATP is particularly important given its role in regulating cation channel activity dependent upon its hydrolysis.

ATP-dependent K$^+$ (K$_{ATP}$) channels play a key role in insulin secretion. Under euglycemic conditions, K$_{ATP}$ channels are maintained in an open state, resulting in K$^+$ efflux and thus clamping the resting membrane potential close to -70 mV. When glucose is elevated, ATP levels increase and displace bound ADP on K$_{ATP}$ channels, which results in channel closure. These events lead to a small membrane depolarization that activates voltage-dependent Ca^{2+} channels, which trigger Ca^{2+} influx and raise the intracellular Ca^{2+} concentration, thus promoting insulin secretion.[95,96]

Several reports have shown that some members of the transient receptor potential (TRP) channel family, which mediate nonselective cationic currents (NSCCs), are expressed, and might contribute to pancreatic β-cell function. Although the role of TRP channels in β-cells remains largely enigmatic, these channels may provide an alternative for the depolarizing background membrane conductance required for the cells to depolarize upon K$_{ATP}$ channel closure.[96] Indeed, it has been reported that thermosensitive TRPM2, TRPM4, and TRPM5 channels control insulin secretion levels by sensing intracellular Ca^{2+} increase, NAD$^+$ metabolites, or hormone receptor activation.[97]

In addition to glucose, insulin secretion may be regulated by diverse chemical messengers such as neurotransmitters and hormones,[96] as well as by exogenous substances such as toxins that act on ion channels. Hence, some peptide toxins present in the venom of marine organisms may affect NSCCs and serve as potential insulinotropic agents. For example, it has been shown that the activity of TRPV1, a channel that modulates insulin secretion in β-cells, is affected by crude cell-free extracts obtained from marine invertebrates.[98,99] Interestingly, one of these extracts has shown insulinotropic activity.[100]

By activating NSCCs, MTx has also shown insulinotropic activity in insulinoma cells. The time course of these currents is very similar to that evoked by incretin hormones such as glucagon-like peptide-1 (GLP-1), which stimulate glucose-dependent insulin secretion by activating cAMP-mediated signaling pathways.[101] Likewise, NSCCs in insulinoma cells can be attenuated by application of a Ca^{2+} SOC blocker SKF 96365, suggesting a contribution of the mammalian TRP-related channels in these currents.[102] The ability to activate NSCCs in insulin-secreting cells stresses the role of MTx as a helpful tool for the analysis of ion channels and insulin secretion.[103] Likewise, the role of MTx as a novel blood glucose-lowering agent remains an interesting topic for future research.

23.7.2 MTx as Interleukin-1β Secretagogue and Oncotic Death Inducer

Most inflammatory reactions are mediated by cytokines, including IL-1, IL-6, TNF-α, and TGF-β. The term interleukin-1 (IL-1) refers to two cytokines, IL-1α and IL-1β, which are the master cytokines of local and systemic inflammation.[104,105] In particular, IL-1β is primarily synthesized in activated macrophages as an immature protein that remains cytosolic until converted through proteolytic cleavage by caspase-1 into its mature active form, which can then be exported outside the cell.

Given its ability to induce cell death secondary to its disruption of Ca^{2+} homeostasis, MTx is likely to trigger innate immune responses and inflammation in vivo. Indeed, it has been suggested that the toxic effect of MTx during shellfish seafood poisoning may involve a component mediated by secretion of proinflammatory cytokine IL-1β. In line with this, Verhoef and coworkers[106] reported that MTx induces a biphasic release of IL-1β from bacterial lipopolysaccharide-primed macrophages. At subnanomolar concentrations, MTx induced mature IL-1β release via a mechanism that can be blocked by high extracellular K$^+$ or nominally zero extracellular Ca^{2+}. MTx may therefore represent an exceptional tool for studying specific components of the innate immune response and/or the physiology of inflammatory effector cells such as monocytes, macrophages, and neutrophils. One representative example of this type of application is the work by Mariathasan and colleagues.[107] These authors found that cryopyrin is responsible for assembly of the so-called inflammasome, a cytosolic complex of proteins that activates caspase-1 to process the proinflammatory cytokine IL-1β. Cryopyrin is essential for inflammasome activation in response to signaling pathways triggered by specific bacterial infections as well as by MTx.

It is worth mentioning here that there are several human diseases caused by different mutations in the cryopyrin gene, including familial cold autoinflammatory syndrome, Muckle–Wells syndrome, as well as chronic infantile neurological cutaneous and articular syndrome.[108] Mutations in the cryopyrin gene are associated with gain of function leading to an enhanced and faster production of IL-1β. In this scenario, MTx could be used as a probe to study possible mechanisms of release and implications of IL-1β overproduction.

Likewise, the second phase of IL-1β release induced by MTx from macrophages occurs at nanomolar concentrations.[106] In this case, MTx produces secretion of unprocessed IL-1β, which is indicative of cell lysis. Interestingly, cell death induced by MTx shares some elements involved in the signaling cascade activated by stimulation of purinergic receptors of the P2Z/P2X$_7$ type.[82,83,109] As discussed earlier, MTx initially activates Ca^{2+}-permeable channels and then induces the formation of large cytolytic/oncotic pores (COPs) that allow molecules <800 Da to enter the cell. These effects are similar to those observed upon activation of P2Z/P2X$_7$ receptors in a variety of cell types, raising the intriguing possibility that MTx and P2Z/P2X$_7$ receptor stimulation activate a common cytolytic pore.

Given the high permeability of the MTx-induced channels for Ca^{2+} transport and the structural similarity of MTx with palytoxin—a marine peptide toxin that converts the plasmalemmal Na$^+$/K$^+$-ATPase (NKA) pump into a channel—it has been proposed that MTx may activate another member of the P-type ATPase family, specifically the plasmalemmal Ca^{2+}-ATPase (PMCA) pump. The results obtained by Sinkins and colleagues[110] are consistent with this idea and suggest that MTx binds to PMCA and converts the pump into a Ca^{2+}-permeable nonselective cation channel. Therefore, MTx could be used as a cell death inducer to unveil some of the molecular mechanisms involved in this process. For instance, whether or not the channel mode of operation of the PMCA plays a role in pathological cell death could be an interesting possibility for future investigations.

23.7.3 MTx and Sperm Physiology

Fertilization is fundamental for the preservation of life by sexual reproduction. The ability of the sperm and the oocyte to recognize, adhere to, and fuse with each other is a crucial aspect of fertilization. All these processes are largely determined by nicely orchestrated ionic fluxes.[111] Hence, it is well known that raises in intracellular Ca^{2+} play crucial roles in sperm functions such as capacitation, motility, and the acrosome reaction.[111]

The acrosome reaction is a secretory process triggered in sperm by components of the outer layer of the egg, and in many species it must occur before the sperm can fertilize the egg. However, the mechanisms responsible for increasing intracellular Ca^{2+} and resulting in the biochemical events that trigger the acrosome reaction are not fully understood. Two different types of Ca^{2+} channels have been proposed to participate in mammalian sperm acrosome reaction: one necessary for a fast transient change in Ca^{2+} levels and another needed to sustain an elevated intracellular Ca^{2+} concentration. The membrane pathway responsible for the first phase of Ca^{2+} entry seems to belong to the Cav channel family, while the sustained Ca^{2+} influx may be carried through a store depletion-operated pathway.[112,113] Interestingly, it has been reported that several TRP channels are expressed in sperm and may be important for the sustained Ca^{2+} entry that drives the acrosome reaction.[113–115]

Evidence obtained in our laboratory indicated that MTx activates a Ca^{2+} influx that induces the mammalian acrosome reaction. The data initially suggested that the actions of MTx were comparable to those of other agents that promote a sustained increase in intracellular Ca^{2+} and drive the mammalian sperm acrosome reaction, including the physiological ligands of the *zona pellucida* (ZP).[116] More recently, however, we found differences in the acrosome reaction induced by MTx and the ZP in human and mouse sperm. Our data indicated that the acrosome reaction induced by the physiological ligands and by MTx occurred through distinct pathways.[117] By using specific PLC antagonists, the participation of a PLC-dependent signaling pathway in the ZP-induced acrosome reaction was confirmed. In contrast, the use of PLC inhibitors blocked the acrosome reaction induced by MTx in mouse but not in human sperm, unveiling species-specific variants of the acrosome reaction induced by the toxin.

Lastly, MTx has also been instrumental in unveiling of some of the mechanisms of the spermatogenic cell regulation exerted by Sertoli cells. We have previously shown that glucose and lactate, two substrates secreted by Sertoli cells toward the adluminal compartment in the seminiferous tubules, can modulate the activity of MTx-sensitive Ca^{2+} channels in enzymatically dissociated rat spermatocytes and spermatids.[118] By inducing changes in intracellular Ca^{2+}, both substrates can activate a Ca^{2+}/calmodulin-dependent protein kinase that results in the phosphorylation of MTx-sensitive channels. We have recently developed in our laboratory a methodology to study Ca^{2+} signaling in spermatogenic

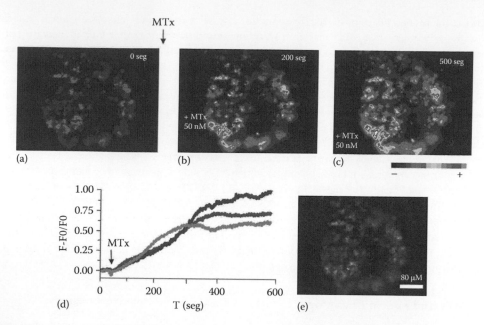

FIGURE 23.8 STSs are obtained as reported. Briefly, the *Tunica albuginea* is removed from mice testis and the seminiferous tubules are mechanically dispersed with tweezers in a Petri dish containing Ringer solution (in mM: 125NaCl, 2.5KCl, 2CaCl$_2$, 1MgCl$_2$, 1.25NaH$_2$PO$_4$, 26NaHCO$_3$, 12 glucose, gassed with 5% CO$_2$, 95% O$_2$, adjusted to pH 7.4). The dispersed tubules are embedded in agar (low melting point, 3%) to form a cube that is mounted on the plate of a vibratome, and 160 μM thick slices are obtained. STSs were loaded with fluo 4-AM (20 μM) immobilized with a nylon mesh, placed on the stage of a microscope, and continuously perfused (2 mL/min) with gassed physiological solution at room temperature. Fluorescence images were acquired (for equipment details, see [119]) every second with an exposure/illumination time of 10 ms for a total of 10 min (600 images). Pseudocolored fluorescence image obtained from the recording of STS before (a) and after addition of 50 nM MTx (b and c). Fluorescence traces obtained from three different cells in the STS shown in (a) and (d). Fluorescence image (black and white) of the same STS after incubation with fluo 4-AM (e). (From Sánchez-Cárdenas, C. et al., *Biol. Reprod.*, 87, 92, 2012.)

cells by preparing slices of seminiferous tubules. This methodology has the advantage of preserving tissue architecture and intercellular connections,[119] and we demonstrated that Ca^{2+} signaling differs in dissociated spermatogenic cells compared to spermatogenic cells inside the tubules. Here, we show that MTx induces a generalized Ca^{2+} increase when applied to this seminiferous tubule slice (STS) preparation, which can be used to further study spermatogenic cell Ca^{2+} dynamics in a physiological environment that preserves cell interactions within the tubule (Figure 23.8). The knowledge generated using this approach could have relevant implications for the understanding of the physiological process of spermatogenic cell regulation by Sertoli cells, as well as the hormonal control that they may exert on spermatogenesis, which is not possible to study in vitro.

23.8 Final Remarks

MTx has inspired vast experimentation by organic and biological researchers due to its structural complexity and intricate mode of action. However, knowledge of both its organic and biochemical synthesis, as well as of its biological target(s), remains incomplete. The current lack of commercially available MTx underscores the importance for achieving its organic synthesis, so that it can become readily available again for studies on Ca^{2+} dynamics in different systems and also to help identify its putative receptor(s). This would lead to a better understanding of the molecular mechanisms involved in MTx action, which in turn may help explain the apparent discrepancies in its functional modalities. Knowledge in this area could also help to find appropriate treatment or an antidote for ciguatera.

ACKNOWLEDGMENTS

The authors would like to thank José Luis de la Vega, Yoloxochitl Sánchez, and Shirley Ainsworth for technical assistance. This work was supported by grants DGAPA-UNAM (IN202212 to CT, IN217210 to ILG) and CONACyT (99333 to CT, 84362 to ILG) and Fondecyt (1110267 to JGR).

REFERENCES

1. Plakas, S.M. and Dickey, R.W. 2010. Advances in monitoring and toxicity assessment of brevetoxins in molluscan shellfish. *Toxicon: Official Journal of the International Society on Toxinology*, 56, 137–149.
2. Fusetani, N. and Kem, W. 2009. Marine toxins: An overview. *Progress in Molecular and Subcellular Biology*, 46, 1–44.
3. Yasumoto, T. 2001. The chemistry and biological function of natural marine toxins. *The Chemical Record*, 1, 228–242.
4. Halstead, B.W. 1988. *Poisonous and Venous Marine Animals of the World*. Darwin Press, Princeton, NJ, p. 1168.
5. Hashimoto, Y. 1979. Marine organisms which cause food poisoning. In *Marine Toxins and Other Bioactive Marine Metabolites*. Japan Scientific Society Press, Tokyo, Japan, pp. 91–105.
6. Rey, J. 2007. Ciguatera. Available at: http://edis.ifas.ufl.edu/ENY-741 (accessed October 2007).
7. Yasumoto, T., Bagnis, R., and Vernoux, J. 1976. Toxicity of the surgeonfishes-II properties of the principal water soluble toxin. *Bulletin of the Japanese Society of Scientific Fisheries*, 42, 359–366.
8. Yasumoto, T. 1971. Toxicity of the surgeonfishes. *Bulletin of the Japanese Society of Scientific Fisheries*, 37, 724–734.
9. Friedman, M.A., Fleming, L.E., Fernandez, M., Bienfang, P., Schrank, K., Dickey, R., Bottein, M.-Y. et al. 2008. Ciguatera fish poisoning: Treatment, prevention and management. *Marine Drugs*, 6, 456–479.
10. Skinner, M.P., Brewer, T.D., Johnstone, R., Fleming, L.E., and Lewis, R.J. 2011. Ciguatera fish poisoning in the Pacific Islands (1998 to 2008). *PLoS Neglected Tropical Diseases*, 5, e1416.
11. Sheppard, C. and Rioja-Nieto, R. 2005. Sea surface temperature 1871–2099 in 38 cells in the Caribbean region. *Marine Environmental Research*, 60, 389–396.
12. Chateau-Degat, M., Chinain, M., Cerf, N., Gingras, S., Hubert, B., and Dewailly, E. 2005. Seawater temperature, *Gambierdiscus* spp. variability and incidence of ciguatera poisoning in French Polynesia. *Harmful Algae*, 4, 1053–1062.
13. Hale, S., Weinstein, P., and Woodward, A. 1999. Ciguatera (fish poisoning), el niño and the pacific sea surface temperatures. *Ecosystem Health*, 5, 20–25.
14. Yokoyama, A., Murata, M., Oshima, Y., Iwashita, T., Yasumoto, T., and Chemistry, F. 1988. Some chemical properties of maitotoxin, a putative calcium channel agonist isolated from a marine dinoflagellate. *Biochemistry Journal*, 187, 184–187.
15. Murata, M. and Yasumoto, T. 2000. The structure elucidation and biological activities of high molecular weight algal toxins: Maitotoxin, prymnesins and zooxanthellatoxins. *Natural Product Reports*, 17, 293–314.
16. Falkoner, I. 1993. *Algal Toxins in Seafood and Drinking Water*. Academic Press, San Diego, CA, p. 224.
17. Baden, D., Fleming, L.E., and Bean, J.A. 1995. Marine toxins. In *Handbook of Clinical Neurology: Intoxications of the Nervous System Part II. Natural Toxins and Drugs*. F.A. de Wolff (Ed). Elsevier Press, Amsterdam, the Netherlands, pp. 141–175.
18. Lewis, R. 2006. Ciguatera: Australian perspectives on a global problem. *Toxicon*, 48, 799–809.
19. Holmes, M. and Lewis, R. 1994. Purification and characterization of large and small maitotoxins from cultured *Gambierdiscus toxicus*. *Natural Toxins*, 2, 64–72.
20. Holmes, M., Lewis, R., and Gillespie, N. 1990. Toxicity of Australian and French Polynesian strains of *Gambierdiscus toxicus* (Dinophyceae) grown in culture: Characterization of a new type of maitotoxin. *Toxicon*, 28, 1159–1172.
21. Hokama, Y. 1985. A rapid, simplified enzyme immunoassay stick test for the detection of ciguatoxin and related polyethers from fish tissues. *Toxicon*, 23, 939–946.
22. Kellmann, R., Stüken, A., Orr, R.J.S., Svendsen, H.M., and Jakobsen, K.S. 2010. Biosynthesis and molecular genetics of polyketides in marine dinoflagellates. *Marine Drugs*, 8, 1011–1048.

23. Khosla, C., Gokhale, R.S., Jacobsen, J.R., and Cane, D.E. 1999. Tolerance and specificity of polyketide synthases. *Annual Review of Biochemistry*, 68, 219–253.

24. Hotta, K., Chen, X., Paton, R.S., Minami, A., Li, H., Swaminathan, K., Mathews, I.I. et al. 2012. Enzymatic catalysis of anti- Baldwin ring closure in polyether biosynthesis. *Nature*, 483, 355–358.

25. Murray, S.A., Garby, T., Hoppenrath, M., and Neilan, B.A. 2012. Genetic diversity, morphological uniformity and polyketide production in dinoflagellates (*Amphidinium, Dinoflagellata*). *PloS One*, 7, e38253.

26. Van Wagoner, R.M., Deeds, J.R., Tatters, A.O., Place, A.R., Tomas, C.R., and Wright, J.L.C. 2010. Structure and relative potency of several karlotoxins from *Karlodinium veneficum*. *Journal of Natural Products*, 73, 1360–1365.

27. Monroe, E.A. and Van Dolah, F.M. 2008. The toxic dinoflagellate *Karenia brevis* encodes novel type I-like polyketide synthases containing discrete catalytic domains. *Protist*, 159, 471–482.

28. Kubota, T., Iinuma, Y., and Kobayashi, J. 2006. Cloning of polyketide synthase genes from amphidinolide-producing dinoflagellate *Amphidinium* sp. *Biological & Pharmaceutical Bulletin*, 29, 1314–1318.

29. Shimizu, Y., Yorimitsu, A., Maruyama, Y., Kubota, T., Aso, T., and Bronson, R.A. 1998. Prostaglandins induce calcium influx in human spermatozoa. *Molecular Human Reproduction*, 4, 555–561.

30. Kwong, R.W.M., Wang, W.-X., Lam, P.K.S., and Yu, P.K.N. 2006. The uptake, distribution and elimination of paralytic shellfish toxins in mussels and fish exposed to toxic dinoflagellates. *Aquatic Toxicology* (Amsterdam, the Netherlands), 80, 82–91.

31. Monteiro, A. and Costa, P.R. 2011. Distribution and selective elimination of paralytic shellfish toxins in different tissues of *Octopus vulgaris*. *Harmful Algae*, 10, 732–737.

32. Costa, P.R., Pereira, P., Guilherme, S., Barata, M., Nicolau, L., Santos, M.A., Pacheco, M., and Pousão-Ferreira, P. 2012. Biotransformation modulation and genotoxicity in white seabream upon exposure to paralytic shellfish toxins produced by *Gymnodinium catenatum*. *Aquatic Toxicology* (Amsterdam, the Netherlands), 106–107, 42–47.

33. Liu, T., Cane, D.E., and Deng, Z. 2009. The enzymology of polyether biosynthesis. *Methods in Enzymology*, 459, 187–214.

34. Minami, A., Migita, A., Inada, D., Hotta, K., Watanabe, K., Oguri, H., and Oikawa, H. 2011. Enzymatic epoxide-opening cascades catalyzed by a pair of epoxide hydrolases in the ionophore polyether biosynthesis. *Organic Letters*, 13, 1638–1641.

35. Minami, A., Shimaya, M., Suzuki, G., Migita, A., Shinde, S.S., Sato, K., Watanabe, K., Tamura, T., Oguri, H., and Oikawa, H. 2012. Sequential enzymatic epoxidation involved in polyether lasalocid biosynthesis. *Journal of the American Chemical Society*, 134, 7246–7249.

36. Yasumoto, T. 2001. The chemistry and biological function of natural marine toxins. *Chemical Record* (New York), 1, 228–242.

37. Nakanishi, K. 1985. The chemistry of brevetoxins: A review. *Toxicon*, 23, 473–479.

38. Murata, M., Sasaki, M., Yokoyama, A., Iwashita, T., Gusovsky, F., Daly, J., and Yasumoto, T. 1992. Partial structures and binding studies of maitotoxin, the most potent marine toxin. *Bulletin de la Societe de Pathologie Exotique*, 85, 470–473.

39. Murata, M. and Yasumoto, T. 2000. The structure elucidation and biological activities of high molecular weight algal toxins: Maitotoxin, prymnesins and zooxanthellatoxins. *Natural Product Reports*, 17, 293–314.

40. Nicolaou, K.C. and Frederick, M.O. 2007. On the structure of maitotoxin. *Angewandte Chemie* (International ed. in English), 46, 5278–5282.

41. Nicolaou, K.C., Frederick, M.O., Burtoloso, A.C., Denton, R.M., Rivas, F., Cole, K.P., Aversa, R.J., Gibe, R., Umezawa, T., and Suzuki, T. 2008. Chemical synthesis of the GHIJKLMNO ring system of Maitotoxin. *Journal of the American Chemical Society*, 130, 7466–7476.

42. Nakata, T. 2010. SmI2-induced cyclizations and their applications in natural product synthesis. *Chemical Record* (New York), 10, 159–172.

43. Sakamoto, Y., Matsuo, G., Matsukura, H., and Nakata, T. 2001. Stereoselective syntheses of the C′D′E′F′-ring system of maitotoxin and the FG-ring system of gambierol. *Organic Letters*, 3, 2749–2752.

44. Morita, M., Haketa, T., Koshino, H., and Nakata, T. 2008. Synthetic studies on maitotoxin. 2. Stereoselective synthesis of the WXYZA′-ring system. *Organic Letters*, 10, 1679–1682.

45. Morita, M., Ishiyama, S., Koshino, H., and Nakata, T. 2008. Synthetic studies on maitotoxin. 1. Stereoselective synthesis of the C′D′E′F′-ring system having a side chain. *Organic Letters*, 10, 1675–1678.

46. Satoh, M., Koshino, H., and Nakata, T. 2008. Synthetic studies on maitotoxin. 3. Stereoselective synthesis of the BCDE-ring system. *Organic Letters*, 10, 1683–1685.

47. Nicolaou, K., Yang, Z., Shi, G., Gunzner, J., Agrios, K., and Gärtner, P. 1998. Total synthesis of brevetoxin A. *Nature*, 392, 264–269.

48. Nicolaou, K.C., Gelin, C.F., Seo, J.H., Huang, Z., and Umezawa, T. 2010. Synthesis of the QRSTU domain of maitotoxin and its 85-epi- and 86-epi-diastereoisomers. *Journal of the American Chemical Society*, 132, 9900–9907.

49. Nicolaou, K.C., Aversa, R.J., Jin, J., and Rivas, F. 2010. Synthesis of the ABCDEFG ring system of Maitotoxin. *Journal of the American Chemical Society*, 132, 6855–6861.

50. Nicolaou, K.C., Seo, J.H., Nakamura, T., and Aversa, R.J. 2011. Synthesis of the c′d′e′f′ domain of maitotoxin. *Journal of the American Chemical Society*, 133, 214–219.

51. Miyahara, J., Akau, C., and Yasumoto, T. 1979. Effects of ciguatoxin and maitotoxin on the isolated guinea pig atria. *Research Communications in Chemical Pathology and Pharmacology*, 25, 177–180.

52. Takahashi, M., Ohizumi, Y., and Yasumoto, T. 1982. Maitotoxin, a Ca^{2+} channel activator candidate. *The Journal of Biological Chemistry*, 257, 7287–7289.

53. Ohizumi, B.Y.Y. and Yasumotot, T. 1983. Contractile response of the rabbit aorta TO maitotoxin, the most potent marine toxin. *Journal of Physiology*, 337, 711–721.

54. Miyamoto, T., Ohizumi, Y., Washio, H., and Yasumoto, Y. 1984. Potent excitatory effect of maitotoxin on Ca channels in the insect skeletal muscle. *Pflugers Arch*, 400, 439–441.

55. Freedman, S.B., Miller, R.J., Miller, D.M., and Tindall, D.R. 1984. Interactions of maitotoxin with voltage-sensitive calcium channels in cultured neuronal cells. *Proceedings of the National Academy of Sciences of the United States of America*, 81, 4582–4585.

56. Schettini, G., Koike, K., Login, I., Judd, A., Cronin, M., Yasumoto, T., and MacLeod, R. 1984. Maitotoxin stimulates hormonal release and calcium flux in rat anterior pituitary cells in vitro. *American Journal of Physiology Endocrinology and Metabolism*, 247, E520–E525.

57. Kobayashi, M., Ohizumi, Y., and Yasumoto, T. 1985. The mechanism of action of maitotoxin in relation to Ca^{2+} movements in guinea-pig and rat cardiac muscles. *British Journal of Pharmacology*, 86, 385–391.

58. Legrand, A. and Bagnis, R. 1984. Effects of highly purified maitotoxin extracted from dinoflagellate *Gambierdiscus toxicus* on action potential of isolated rat heart. *Journal of Molecular and Cellular Cardiology*, 16, 663–666.

59. Berta, P., Sladeczek, F., Derancourt, J., Durand, M., Travo, P., and Haiech, J. 1986. Maitotoxin stimulates the formation of inositol phosphates in rat aortic myocytes. *FEBS Letters*, 197, 349–352.

60. Gusovsky, F., Yasumoto, T., and Daly, J. 1987. Maitotoxin stimulates phosphoinositide breakdown in neuroblastoma hybrid NCB-20 cells. *Cellular and Molecular Neurobiology*, 7, 317–322.

61. Gusovsky, F., Daly, J.W., Yasumoto, T., and Rojas, E. 1988. Differential effects of maitotoxin on ATP secretion and on phosphoinositide breakdown in rat pheochromocytoma cells. *FEBS Letters*, 233, 139–142.

62. Gusovsky, F., Yasumoto, T., and Daly, J.W. 1989. Maitotoxin, a potent, general activator of phosphoinositide breakdown. *FEBS Letters*, 243, 307–312.

63. Gusovsky, F., Yasumoto, T., and Daly, J. 1989. Calcium-dependent effects of maitotoxin on phosphoinositide breakdown and on cyclic AMP accumulation in PCi 2 and NCB-20 cells. *Molecular Pharmacology*, 36, 44–53.

64. Gusovsky, F., Bitran, J.A., Yasumoto, T., and Daly, J.W. 1990. Mechanism of maitotoxin- stimulated phosphoinositide breakdown in HL-60 cells. *The Journal of Pharmacology and Experimental Therapeutics*, 252, 466–473.

65. Pin, J., Yasumoto, T., and Bockaert, J. 1988. Maitotoxin-evoked gamma-aminobutyric acid release is due not only to the opening of calcium channels. *Journal of Neurochemistry*, 50, 1227–1237.

66. Sladeczek, F., Schmidt, B.H., Alonso, R., Vian, L., Tep, A., Yasumoto, T., Cory, R.N., and Bockaert, J. 1988. New insights into maitotoxin action. *European Journal of Biochemistry*, 174, 663–670.

67. Hamilton, S. and Perez, M. 1987. Toxins that affect voltage-dependent calcium channels. *Biochemical Pharmacology*, 36, 3325–3329.

68. Kobayashi, M., Ochi, R., and Ohizumi, Y. 1987. Maitotoxin-activated single calcium channels in guinea-pig cardiac cells. *British Journal of Pharmacology*, 92, 665–671.

69. Yoshii, M., Tsunoo, A., Kuroda, Y., Wu, C.H., and Narahashi, T. 1987. Maitotoxin-induced membrane current in neuroblastoma cells. *Brain Research*, 424, 119–125.

70. Murata, M., Gusovsky, F., Yasumoto, T., and Daly, J. 1992. Selective stimulation of Ca^{2+} flux in cells by maitotoxin. *The European Journal of Pharmacology*, 227, 43–49.

71. Xi, D., Van Dolah, F.M., and Ramsdell, J.S. 1992. Maitotoxin induces a calcium-dependent membrane depolarization in GH4C1 pituitary cells via activation of type L voltage-dependent calcium channels. *The Journal of Biological Chemistry*, 267, 25025–25031.

72. Nishio, M., Kigoshi, S., Muramatsu, I., and Yasumoto, T. 1993. $Ca^{(2+)}$- and $Na^{(+)}$- dependent depolarization induced by maitotoxin in the crayfish giant axon. *General Pharmacology*, 24, 1079–1083.

73. Worley III, J.F., Mcintyre, M.S., Spencer, B., and Dukes, I.D. 1994. Depletion of intracellular Ca^{2+} stores activates a maitotoxin-sensitive nonselective cationic current in beta-cells. *The Journal of Biological Chemistry*, 269, 32055–32058.

74. Musgrave, I.F., Seifert, R., and Schultz, G. 1994. Maitotoxin activates cation channels distinct from the receptor-activated non-selective cation channels of HL-60 cells. *The Biochemical Journal*, 301 (Pt 2), 437–441.

75. Dietl, P. and Volkl, H. 1994. Maitotoxin activates a nonselective cation channel and Ca^{2+} entry in MDCK renal epithelial cells. *Molecular Pharmacology*, 45, 300–305.

76. Young, R., McLaren, M., and Ramsdell, J. 1995. Maitotoxin increases voltage independent chloride and sodium currents in GH4C1 rat pituitary cells. *Natural Toxins*, 3, 419–427.

77. Nishio, M., Muramatsu, I., and Yasumoto, T. 1996. $Na^{(+)}$-permeable channels induced by maitotoxin in guinea-pig single ventricular cells. *European Journal of Pharmacology*, 297, 293–298.

78. Estacion, M., Nguyen, H.B., Gargus, J.J., Estacion, M., and Bryant, H. 1996. Calcium is permeable through a maitotoxin-activated nonselective cation channel in mouse L cells Calcium is permeable through a maitotoxin-activated nonselective cation channel in mouse L cells. *The American Journal of Physiology-Cell Physiology*, 270, 1145–1152.

79. Bielfeld-Ackermann, A., Range, C., and Korbmacher, C. 1998. Maitotoxin (MTX) activates a nonselective cation channel in *Xenopus laevis* oocytes. *Pflügers Archiv: European Journal of Physiology*, 436, 329–337.

80. Cataldi, M., Secondo, A., D'Alessio, A., Taglialatela, M., Hofmann, F., Klugbauer, N., Di Renzo, G., and Annunziato, L. 1999. Studies on maitotoxin-induced intracellular $Ca^{(2+)}$ elevation in Chinese hamster ovary cells stably transfected with cDNAs encoding for L- type $Ca^{(2+)}$ channel subunits. *The Journal of Pharmacology and Experimental Therapeutics*, 290, 725–730.

81. Martínez-françois, J.R., Morales-tlalpan, V., and Vaca, L. 2002. Characterization of the maitotoxin-activated cationic current from human skin fibroblasts. *Journal of Physiology*, 538, 79–86.

82. Schilling, W.P., Sinkins, W.G., and Estacion, M. 1999. Maitotoxin activates a nonselective cation channel and a $P2Z/P2X_7$-like cytolytic pore in human skin fibroblasts Maitotoxin activates a nonselective cation channel and a $P2Z/P2X_7$-like cytolytic pore in human skin fibroblasts. *The American Journal of Physiology*, 277, C755–C765.

83. Schilling, W.P., Wasylyna, T., Dubyak, G.R., Humphreys, B.D., and Sinkins, W.G. 1999. Maitotoxin and $P2Z/P2X_7$ purinergic receptor stimulation activate a common cytolytic pore. *The American Journal of Physiology*, 277, C766–C776.

84. Egido, W., Castrejón, V., Antón, B., and Martínez, M. 2008. Maitotoxin induces two dose-dependent conductances in *Xenopus oocytes*. Comparison with nystatin effects as a pore inductor. *Toxicon: Official Journal of the International Society on Toxicology*, 51, 797–812.

85. Murata, M., Gusovsky, F., Sasaki, M., Yokoyama, A., Yasumoto, T., and Daly, J. 1991. Effect of maitotoxin analogues on calcium influx and phosphoinositide breakdown in cultured cells. *Toxicon*, 29, 1085–1096.

86. Konoki, K., Hashimoto, M., Nonomura, T., Sasaki, M., Murata, M., and Tachibana, K. 1998. Influx in rat glioma inhibition of maitotoxin-induced Ca^{2+} influx in rat glioma C6 cells by brevetoxins and synthetic fragments of maitotoxin. *Journal of Neurochemistry*, 70, 409–416.

87. Oishi, T., Konoki, K., Tamate, R., Torikai, K., Hasegawa, F., Matsumori, N., and Murata, M. 2012. Artificial ladder-shaped polyethers that inhibit maitotoxin-induced Ca^{2+} influx in rat glioma C6 cells. *Bioorganic & Medicinal Chemistry Letters*, 22, 3619–3622.

88. Konoki, K., Hashimoto, M., Murata, M., and Tachibana, K. 1999. Maitotoxin-induced calcium influx in erythrocyte ghosts and rat glioma C6 cells, and blockade by gangliosides and other membrane lipids. *Chemical Research in Toxicology*, 12, 993–1001.

89. Murata, M., Matsumori, N., Konoki, K., and Oishi, T. 2008. Structural features of dinoflagellate toxins underlying biological activity as viewed by NMR. *Bulletin of the Chemical Society of Japan*, 81, 307–319.

90. Nicolaou, K.C., Frederick, M.O., and Aversa, R.J. 2008. The continuing saga of the marine polyether biotoxins. *Angewandte Chemie* (International ed. in English), 47, 7182–7225.

91. Nicolaou, K. and Aversa, R.J. 2011. Maitotoxin: An inspiration for synthesis. *Israel Journal of Chemistry*, 51, 359–377.

92. Humphrey, W., Dalke, A., and Schulten, K. 1996. VMD: Visual molecular dynamics. *Journal of Molecular Graphics*, 14, 33–38, 27–28.

93. Mori, M., Oishi, T., Matsuoka, S., Ujihara, S., Matsumori, N., Murata, M., Satake, M., Oshima, Y., Matsushita, N., and Aimoto, S. 2005. Ladder-shaped polyether compound, desulfated yessotoxin, interacts with membrane-integral alpha-helix peptides. *Bioorganic & Medicinal Chemistry*, 13, 5099–5103.

94. Yamauchi, T., Kamon, J., Waki, H., Terauchi, Y., Kubota, N., Hara, K., Mori, Y. et al. 2001. The fat-derived hormone adiponectin reverses insulin resistance associated with both lipoatrophy and obesity. *Nature Medicine*, 7, 941–946.

95. McTaggart, J.S., Clark, R.H., and Ashcroft, F.M. 2010. The role of the KATP channel in glucose homeostasis in health and disease: More than meets the islet. *The Journal of Physiology*, 588, 3201–3209.

96. Rorsman, P. and Braun, M. 2013. Regulation of insulin secretion in human pancreatic islets. *Annual Review of Physiology*, 75, 1–25.

97. Uchida, K. and Tominaga, M. 2011. The role of thermosensitive TRP (transient receptor potential) channels in insulin secretion. *Endocrine Journal*, 58, 1021–1028.

98. Akiba, Y., Kato, S., Katsube, K., Nakamura, M., Takeuchi, K., Ishii, H., and Hibi, T. 2004. Transient receptor potential vanilloid subfamily 1 expressed in pancreatic islet beta cells modulates insulin secretion in rats. *Biochemical and Biophysical Research Communications*, 321, 219–225.

99. Cuypers, E., Yanagihara, A., Karlsson, E., and Tytgat, J. 2006. Jellyfish and other cnidarian envenomations cause pain by affecting TRPV1 channels. *FEBS Letters*, 580, 5728–5732.

100. Diaz-Garcia, C.M., Fuentes-Silva, D., Sanchez-Soto, C., Domínguez-Pérez, D., García-Delgado, N., Varela, C., Mendoza-Hernández, G., Rodriguez-Romero, A., Castaneda, O., and Hiriart, M. 2012. Toxins from *Physalia physalis* (Cnidaria) raise the intracellular Ca^{2+} of beta-cells and promote insulin secretion. *Current Medicinal Chemistry*, 19, 5414–5423.

101. Leech, C.A. and Habener, J.F. 1997. Insulinotropic glucagon-like peptide-1-mediated activation of non-selective cation currents in insulinoma cells is mimicked by maitotoxin. *The Journal of Biological Chemistry*, 272, 17987–17993.

102. Roe, M.W., Worley, J.F., Qian, F., Tamarina, N., Mittal, A.A., Dralyuk, F., Blair, N.T., Mertz, R.J., Philipson, L.H., and Dukes, I.D. 1998. Characterization of a Ca^{2+} release-activated nonselective cation current regulating membrane potential and $[Ca^{2+}]i$ oscillations in transgenically derived beta-cells. *The Journal of Biological Chemistry*, 273, 10402–10410.

103. Holz, G.G., Leech, C.A. and Habener, J.F. 2000. Insulinotropic toxins as molecular probes for analysis of glucagon-like peptide-1 receptor-mediated signal transduction in pancreatic beta-cells. *Biochimie*. 82(9–10), 915–926.

104. Dinarello, C.A., Simon, A., and Van der Meer, J.W.M. 2012. Treating inflammation by blocking interleukin-1 in a broad spectrum of diseases. *Nature Reviews: Drug Discovery*, 11, 633–652.

105. Gabay, C., Lamacchia, C., and Palmer, G. 2010. IL-1 pathways in inflammation and human diseases. *Nature Reviews Rheumatology*, 6, 232–241.

106. Verhoef, P.A., Kertesy, S.B., Estacion, M., Schilling, W.P., and Dubyak, G.R. 2004. Maitotoxin induces biphasic interleukin-1beta secretion and membrane blebbing in murine macrophages. *Molecular Pharmacology*, 66, 909–920.

107. Mariathasan, S., Weiss, D.S., Newton, K., McBride, J., O'Rourke, K., Roose-Girma, M., Lee, W.P., Weinrauch, Y., Monack, D.M., and Dixit, V.M. 2006. Cryopyrin activates the inflammasome in response to toxins and ATP. *Nature*, 440, 228–232.

108. Federici, S., Caorsi, R., and Gattorno, M. 2012. The autoinflammatory diseases. *Swiss Medical Weekly*, 142, 13602.

109. Verhoef, P.A., Estacion, M., Schilling, W., and Dubyak, G.R. 2003. $P2X_7$ receptor-dependent blebbing and the activation of Rho-effector kinases, caspases, and IL-1 beta release. *Journal of Immunology* (Baltimore, MD: 1950), 170, 5728–5738.

110. Sinkins, W.G., Estacion, M., Prasad, V., Goel, M., Shull, G.E., Kunze, D.L., and Schilling, W.P. 2009. Maitotoxin converts the plasmalemmal $Ca^{(2+)}$ pump into a $Ca^{(2+)}$-permeable nonselective cation channel. *The American Journal of Physiology Cell Physiology*, 297, C1533–C1543.

111. Darszon, A., Nishigaki, T., Beltran, C., and Trevino, C.L. 2011. Calcium channels in the development, maturation, and function of spermatozoa. *Physiological Review*, 91, 1305–1355.

112. O'Toole, C.M., Arnoult, C., Darszon, A., Steinhardt, R.A., and Florman, H.M. 2000. $Ca^{(2+)}$ entry through store-operated channels in mouse sperm is initiated by egg ZP3 and drives the acrosome reaction. *Molecular Biology of the Cell*, 11, 1571–1584.

113. Jungnickel, M.K., Marrero, H., Birnbaumer, L., Lemos, J.R., and Florman, H.M. 2001. Trp2 regulates entry of Ca^{2+} into mouse sperm triggered by egg ZP3. *Natural Cell Biology*, 3, 499–502.

114. Trevino, C.L., Serrano, C.J., Beltran, C., Felix, R., and Darszon, A. 2001. Identification of mouse trp homologs and lipid rafts from spermatogenic cells and sperm. *FEBS Letters*, 509, 119–125.

115. Sutton, K.A., Jungnickel, M.K., Wang, Y., Cullen, K., Lambert, S., and Florman, H.M. 2004. Enkurin is a novel calmodulin and TRPC channel binding protein in sperm. *Devision of Biology*, 274, 426–435.

116. Treviño, C.L., De la Vega-Beltrán, J.L., Nishigaki, T., Felix, R., and Darszon, A. 2006. Maitotoxin potently promotes Ca^{2+} influx in mouse spermatogenic cells and sperm, and induces the acrosome reaction. *Journal of Cellular Physiology*, 206, 449–456.

117. Chávez, J.C., De Blas, G.A., De la Vega-Beltrán, J.L., Nishigaki, T., Chirinos, M., González-González, M.E., Larrea, F., Solís, A., Darszon, A., and Treviño, C.L. 2011. The opening of maitotoxin-sensitive calcium channels induces the acrosome reaction in human spermatozoa: Differences from the zona pellucida. *Asian Journal of Andrology*, 13, 159–165.

118. Reyes, J., Osses, N., Knox, M., Darszon, A., and Trevino, C. 2010. Glucose and lactate regulate maitotoxin-activated Ca^{2+} entry in spermatogenic cells: The role of intracellular $[Ca^{2+}]$. *FEBS Letters*, 584, 3111–3115.

119. Sánchez-Cárdenas, C., Guerrero, A., Treviño, C.L., Hernández-Cruz, A., and Darszon, A. 2012. Acute slices of mice testis seminiferous tubules unveil spontaneous and synchronous Ca^{2+} oscillations in germ cell clusters. *Biology of Reproduction*, 87, 92.

120. Treviño, C.L., Escobar, L., Vaca, L., Morales-Tlalpan, V., Ocampo, A.Y., and Darszon, A. 2008. Maitotoxin: A unique pharmacological tool for elucidating Ca^{2+}-dependent mechanisms. In *Seafood and Freshwater Toxins: Pharmacology, Physiology and Detection*, 2nd edn. L.M. Botana (ed.). CRC Press, Boca Ratón, FL, pp. 503–516.

121. Nicolaou, K., Duggan, M., and Hwang, C. 1986. New synthetic technology for the construction of oxocenes. *Journal of American Chemical Society*, 108, 2468–2469.

24

Palytoxin and Analogs: Ecobiology and Origin, Chemistry, and Chemical Analysis

Panagiota Katikou and Aristidis Vlamis

CONTENTS

24.1 Introduction

Palytoxin (PLTX) was first discovered by Moore and Scheuer[1] in the soft coral *Palythoa toxica*, which had been used for poisoned arrowheads in old Hawaii.[2] PLTX is one of the most potent natural non-protein compounds known to date,[3] exhibiting extreme toxicity in mammals (i.v. mean LD_{50} in 24 h: 25–450 ng/kg).[4] Consequently, an i.v. toxic dose in a human by extrapolation would range between 2.3 and 31.5 μg.[5] Despite the fact that the oral route was reported to be the least sensitive,[4] acute toxicity and deaths have been reported from human outbreaks; however, reliable quantitative data on acute toxicity in humans are unavailable. In view of the acute toxicity reports and the lack of chronic toxicity data for PLTX-group toxins, the EFSA Panel on Contaminants was able to derive an oral acute reference dose (ARfD) of only 0.2 μg/kg b.w. for the sum of PLTX and its analog ostreocin-D. In order for a 60 kg adult to avoid exceeding the ARfD, a 400 g portion of shellfish meat should not contain more than 12 μg of the sum of PLTX and ostreocin-D, corresponding to 30 μg/kg shellfish meat.[6]

Initial NMR studies of PLTX indicated an estimated molecular weight of about 3300 and a chemical formula of $C_{145}H_{264}N_4O_{78}$, with an error assumed not to exceed 10%.[1] The correct chemical structure was defined about 11 years later, in 1981, almost simultaneously by two separate research groups, one in Nagoya University, Japan, led by Prof. Hirata[7] and the other in the University of Hawaii, USA, led by Prof. Moore.[8]

PLTX is a large and very complex molecule with both lipophilic and hydrophilic areas, possessing the longest chain of continuous carbon atoms known to exist in a natural product. Its chemical formula is $C_{129}H_{223}N_3O_{54}$, with 115 of the 129 carbons being in a continuous chain. Another unusual structural feature of PLTX is that it contains 64 stereogenic centers, which means that PLTX can have 2^{64} stereogenic isomers. Moreover, there are eight double bonds able to exhibit cis/trans isomerism, which means that PLTX can have more than 10^{21} (one sextillion) stereoisomers.[9] Despite the complexity arising from the numerous possible isomers, the group of Prof. Kishi from Harvard University in 1989 achieved the monumental task of complete chemical synthesis of the correct isomer of PLTX in its carboxylic acid form.[10]

This chapter is structured in three sections. The first section focuses on the ecobiology and origin of this fascinating molecule, PLTX, and also highlights the most important up-to-date available data regarding its chemistry. The second section deals with current knowledge on the ecobiology, origin, and chemistry of naturally occurring PLTX analogs produced from different species of the dinoflagellate genus *Ostreopsis*. The third and final section provides a detailed summary of the developments regarding chemical analysis methods for this group of compounds, with special reference to their detection and quantification in seafood.

24.2 Palytoxin

24.2.1 Ecobiology and Origin

PLTX presence has been reported worldwide primarily not only in zoanthids belonging to the genus *Palythoa* but also in other species. Moore and Scheuer[1] were the first to isolate PLTX from the Hawaiian zoanthid *P. toxica*, whereas 1 year later, its presence was demonstrated in *P. tuberculosa* collected from tropical Pacific waters of Okinawa, Japan.[11] Following these reports, PLTX and its congeners were detected in other *Palythoa* species: *P. vestitus* from Hawaii,[12] *P. mammilosa*,[13] and *P. carribaeorum*[14] from Jamaica, Puerto Rico, and the Bahamas in the West Indies, in unidentified *Palythoa* spp. from Tahiti[8,15] and Ishigaki Island, Japan,[16] and more recently in *P.* aff. *margaritae* from Nakanoshima Island in Japan.[17] Investigation regarding toxin distribution in the tissues of *P. tuberculosa* from the Pacific[11] revealed that toxicity was essentially defined by the presence of eggs in a polyp. In the female polyps, eggs, including ovulated eggs, showed a very high toxicity, whereas other tissues were also strongly toxic. The toxicity of eggs themselves was high regardless of maturation degree, while other tissues became more toxic as maturation proceeded. On the other hand, none of the male polyps tested showed any sign of toxicity, the hermaphroditic polyps showed low toxicity, reflecting the presence of a few eggs in the gonads, whereas sterile polyps were nontoxic, even when found adjacent to female polyps in a colony. Similarly, Uemura[18] found that *P. tuberculosa* coelenterates produce eggs and have the strongest toxicity between April and June. However, this was not confirmed in *Palythoa* species from the Caribbean Sea, where considerable concentrations of PLTX were measured even in sterile polyps, while some egg-bearing polyps were entirely free from PLTX.[19] Recent investigations of two human intoxication cases—one via the dermal route in Georgia and one via the respiratory route in Virginia—involving *P. heliodiscus* zoanthids in home aquaria revealed that these organisms contain extremely high PLTX/deoxy-PLTX concentrations within the range of 515–3515 µg crude toxin/g wet zoanthid.[20,21] Occurrence of PLTX in marine organisms living close to and/or feeding on the zoanthid colonies, such as sponges, corals, shellfish, polychaetes, crustaceans, and fish, has also been demonstrated.[22,23]

Due to the significant seasonal and regional fluctuations observed in PLTX contents of the *Palythoa* zoanthids, and its wide distribution in various systematic groups of marine organisms, its origin has been an important matter of long-term speculation. A bacterial origin has been hypothesized by researchers in Hawaii, who reported that *Vibrio* sp. strains isolated from *P. toxica* were found to produce a toxic fraction similar to PLTX in UV spectrum.[24] Uemura et al.[16] supported the theory of PLTX biosynthesis by symbiotic microorganisms, after isolation and structural elucidation of at least four minor toxins coexisting with PLTX in *P. tuberculosa*. The structural differences between PLTX, homo-PLTX, and bishomo-PLTX were located in the ω-aminoalcohol moiety, which is often observed in natural products produced by microorganisms. Much later, PLTX hemolytic activity was detected in extracts from *Pseudomonas* sp. associated with the toxic dinoflagellate *O. lenticularis* and with Caribbean *Palythoa* species,[25] whereas the gram-negative bacteria *Aeromonas* sp. and *Vibrio* sp. isolated from toxic samples of *Palythoa* sp. were found to produce compounds antigenically related to PLTX.[26] Furthermore, Seemann et al.,[27] using a newly developed PLTX blood agar assay, screened toxin production and potential PLTX-producing bacteria isolated from two zoanthid corals (*P. caribaeorum*, *Zoanthus pulchellus*) and one sponge (*Neofibularia nolitangere*) in order to investigate a possible microbial origin of PLTX. Seven percent of the bacterial isolates (*n* = 17), all of which were derived from *P. caribaeorum*, showed an ouabain-inhibitable hemolytic phenotype. This PLTX-like hemolysis was stable after several rounds of restreaking and after recovery of the isolates from frozen strain collections. Thus, metabolites of these bacterial strains were suggested to be the true origins of the PLTX-like hemolytic activity. This activity was stable after heating to 100°C, indicating that it was not due to a protein, but most probably due to the production of Na^+/K^+–adenosine triphosphatase (ATPase) toxins by these bacteria. The PLTX-like hemolysis positive strains belonged phylogenetically to the *Bacillus cereus* group (*n* = 11) as well as to the genera *Brevibacterium* (*n* = 4) and *Acinetobacter* (*n* = 2).[27] The first evidence with regard to the production of PLTX and its analog 42-OH-PLTX by the marine cyanobacterium *Trichodesmium* sp. in tropical and subtropical waters has been very recently reported,[28] suggesting a potential role of *Trichodesmium* blooms in clupeotoxicity, via the ingestion of the trichomes of this pelagic cyanobacterium by plankton-eating fish.

Symbiotic algae able to synthesize secondary products similar to PLTX[29] and living in large masses in the mesogloea of the Zoantharia have also been considered as potential PLTX producers. In this context, the detection of PLTX or a closely related compound was reported in the red alga *Chondria crispus*.[30] Nevertheless, the lack of correlation between algal presence (as expressed by chlorophyll a content) and PLTX content appears to contradict their involvement in toxin synthesis.[19]

At present, dinoflagellates of the genus *Ostreopsis* are considered as the most probable biogenetic source of PLTX and its analogs. *Ostreopsis*-related origin of PLTXs was initially reported from Japanese researchers. Potent toxins produced by the species *O. siamensis*, termed ostreocins, and specifically their major constituent, namely, ostreocin-D, were demonstrated as a PLTX analog.[31–33] The implication of *O. siamensis* in a case of clupeotoxism in Madagascar, where the causative agent was found to be PLTX or one of its analogs, provided further support for this theory.[34] Numerous studies in the following years have identified PLTX analogs in *O. mascarenensis* from the Indian Ocean[35] and in *O. ovata* and *O.* cf. *siamensis* from the Mediterranean Sea.[36–42]

PLTX is one of the most potent natural nonprotein compounds, showing an extremely high toxicity in mammals with the i.v. LD_{50} value ranging between 25 and 450 ng/kg.[4] The toxic dose for humans has obviously not been experimentally documented. Nevertheless, extrapolation of animal toxicity data indicates a toxic dose in humans of about 4 µg[43] or between 2.3 and 31.5 µg.[5] Based on the limited available data from human intoxication cases, an oral ARfD of 0.2 µg/kg b.w. has been derived for the sum of PLTX and its analog ostreocin-D.[6] Regardless of its high lethal potency in terrestrial animals, PLTX has been repeatedly detected in marine organisms, such as crabs from the Philippines[44] and Singapore,[45] the fish species *Alutera scripta* filefish from Okinawa, Japan,[46] *Melichthys vidua* triggerfish from Ponape, Micronesia,[47,48] *Decapterus macrosoma* mackerel from Hawaii,[49] the sea anemone *Radianthus macrodactylus* from the Seychelles,[50] as well as sponges, bivalve mollusks, sea urchins, and soft corals[21,40,51–53] without causing any deleterious effects. Resistance of marine animals to PLTX enables its sequestration and accumulation in the food chain, resulting in numerous reported cases of human poisoning and lethality.[54–58] All marine species implicated in human poisoning cases share one common characteristic, which is their bottom feeding nature. The fact that the main sources of PLTX and analogs, that is, *Palythoa* spp. and *Ostreopsis* spp., grow on the sea bottom strongly supports the theory regarding their role in PLTX biogenesis.

24.2.2 Chemistry

24.2.2.1 Physical Properties

Purified PLTX has been described as a white, amorphous, hydroscopic solid, which to date has not been crystallized. It presents insolubility in nonpolar solvents such as chloroform, ether, and acetone; it is sparingly soluble in methanol and ethanol and soluble in pyridine, dimethyl sulfoxide, and water. The partition coefficient for the distribution of PLTX between 1-butanol and water is 0.21 at 25°C, based on the comparison of the absorbance at 263 nm for the two layers. The toxin does not show a definite melting point and is heat resistant but chars at 300°C. It is an optically active compound, having a specific rotation of +26° ± 2° in water. The optical rotatory dispersion curve of PLTX exhibits a positive Cotton effect with $[\alpha]250$ being +700° and $[\alpha]215$ being +600°. In aqueous solution, PLTX behaves like a steroidal saponin, producing a foam on agitation, probably because of its amphipathic nature; however, unlike a steroidal saponin, the toxin cannot be cleaved by acid hydrolysis into lipophilic and hydrophilic moieties.[1,59] Moreover, in aqueous solutions, PLTX forms an associated dimer, which can be unbound by single-site acetylation of a terminal, whereas the acetylated derivative exists as a monomer.[60,61]

24.2.2.2 Structure

PLTX can be considered as one of the most complicated and largest molecules, excluding the naturally occurring polymers. The basic molecule consists of a long, partially unsaturated (with eight double bonds) aliphatic backbone with spaced cyclic ethers, 64 chiral centers, 40–42 hydroxyl, and 2 amide groups.[16,59,62] The third nitrogen present as a primary amino group at the C-115 end of the molecule accounts for the basicity of PLTX.[15] Both molecular weight and molecular formula of PLTXs have been reported to differ depending on the species from which they are obtained, while certain species contain mixtures of different isomers.[8] Initial determination of the gross structures of different PLTXs was based on sodium periodate oxidation and ozonolysis fragmentation, subsequent ordering of the fragments followed by the use of field desorption mass spectrometry (MS), ^{252}Cf plasma MS, and nuclear magnetic resonance (^{1}H NMR).[7,8,63–66] More recent studies aiming to further clarify stereostructure of different PLTXs have employed high-resolution liquid chromatography–MS (HR-LC–MS) analyses along with extensive one- and two-dimensional NMR studies.[67]

Moore and Bartolini[8] reported that PLTX from the Tahitian *Palythoa* had a molecular formula of $C_{129}H_{221}N_3O_{54}$ (Mr 2659). On the other hand, a molecular formula of $C_{129}H_{223}N_3O_{54}$ (Mr 2677) with two possible structures was found for *P. toxica* PLTX, which differed from the Tahitian PLTX in the C-55 hemiketal ring. A mixture of these three PLTXs, the one from Tahitian *Palythoa* and two from *P. toxica*, was indicated for the Hawaiian *P. tuberculosa*.[8] Macfarlane et al.[66] indicated the presence of two PLTX components in Okinawan *P. tuberculosa*, one with an Mr of 2681.1 ± 0.35 µ and another with a mass lower by 16–18 µ, which was speculated to be the related C-54 ketal and hemiketal.[8] On the other hand, Uemura et al.[7] have found four other minor toxins co-occurring with PLTX in *P. tuberculosa*, namely, homo-PLTX, bishomo-PLTX, neo-PLTX, and deoxy-PLTX (Figure 24.1). These were structurally

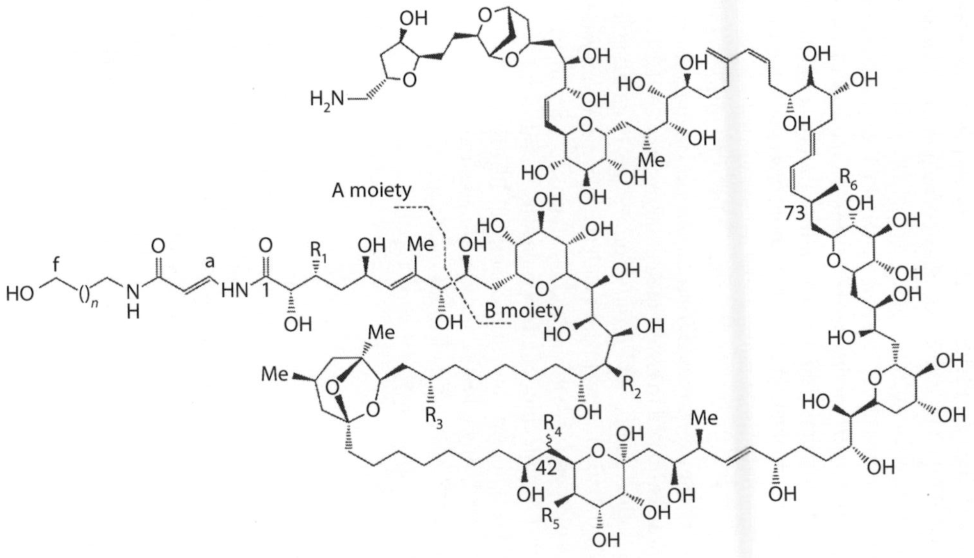

	n	R_1	R_2	R_3	R_4	R_5	R_6
Palytoxin (1)	1	Me	OH	Me	H	OH	OH
Homopalytoxin (2)	2	Me	OH	Me	H	OH	OH
Bishomopalytoxin (3)	3	Me	OH	Me	H	OH	OH
Neopalytoxin (4)	1	–	OH	Me	H	OH	OH
Deoxypalytoxin (5)	1	Me	OH	Me	H	OH	OH
42-Hydroxypalytoxin (6)	1	Me	OH	Me	OH	OH	OH
Ostreocin D (7)	1	H	H	H	OH	H	OH

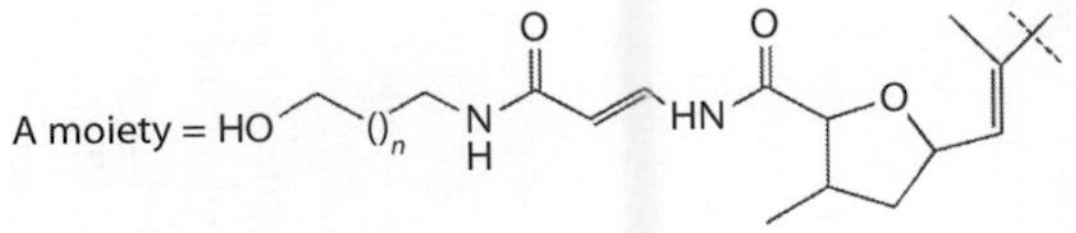

FIGURE 24.1 Stereostructure of palytoxins. MS/MS spectra of palytoxins are dominated by a fragment ion due to cleavage between carbons 8 and 9 with an additional loss of a water molecule. Cleavage between C8 and C9 divides the molecule in two moieties termed A and B moieties, respectively. Stereochemistry at C42, when a hydroxyl group occurs, has not yet been defined. (Reprinted from *Toxicon*, 57(3), Ciminiello, P., Dell'Aversano, C., Dello Iacovo, E., Fattorusso, E., Forino, M., Grauso, L., and Tartaglione, L., A 4-decade-long (and still ongoing) hunt for palytoxins chemical architecture, 362–367, Copyright 2011 with permission from Elsevier.)

characterized as PLTX analogs, having only minor differences from the major PLTX. Specifically, the structural difference among homo-PLTX, bishomo-PLTX, and PLTX are in the proximity of the C-a proton, while molecular weights of homo- and bishomo-PLTXs exceed that of PLTX by 14 and 28 mass units, respectively. The same major and minor toxins have been isolated from another unclassified *Palythoa* species in Ishigaki island, albeit with higher contents of homo-PLTX, bishomo-PLTX, and deoxy-PLTX than those of *P. tuberculosa*.[7] Recent studies on PLTXs of *P. toxica* and *P. tuberculosa* have revealed that the profile of *P. toxica* is dominated (91%) by one major peak corresponding to a new PLTX congener named 42-hydroxy-PLTX, with a molecular formula of $C_{129}H_{223}N_3O_{55}$ and a mass of 2694, whereas *P. tuberculosa* contained almost equal amounts of PLTX and 42-OH-PLTX.[21,67,68] Studies on PLTX profiles of five samples belonging to the species *P. heliodiscus*[21] revealed that four of them contained only PLTX, while the fifth contained primarily deoxy-PLTX with a lesser amount of PLTX. Minor PLTXs could not be quantified due to inadequate chromatographic resolution; however, none were found to contain 42-OH-PLTX, the primary toxin reported from samples collected in the 1990s from the original Hana tide pools from, presumably, *P. toxica*.[67] Finally, the PLTX isolated from *P. caribaoreum* had a molecular mass of 2680, while a PLTX-like substance extracted from *Lophozozymus pictor* crab, possessing a very similar positive ion MS profile, was estimated to have a molecular mass of 2681.0 Da.[45]

The absolute stereochemistry of PLTXs from both *P. toxica* and *P. tuberculosa* has been assigned to all 64 chiral centers[69,70] after a long series of degradation experiments with the use of x-ray crystallography, NMR, and circular dichroic spectroscopy together with organic synthesis.[71–73] Small-angle x-ray scattering has been used to calculate the PLTX molecule length, which was found to be 50 Å, while its molecular weight was determined as 5700. This was due to the fact that PLTX was studied as an aqueous solution where it exists as a dimer.[18,60,61] Using a low-resolution model simulation, it was also found that the dimer of PLTX consists of two "⊃"-shaped molecules overlapping each other to give a figure-eight shape.[18]

24.2.2.3 Mass Spectrometry

MS studies have been widely used for PLTX presence detection, molecular weight determination, as well as elucidation of structural differences between PLTXs from various origins. The loss of numerous water molecules during MS analyses has indicated that PLTXs contain a large number of hydroxyl and/or ether moieties.[35,45] Another important MS characteristic indicative of PLTX-like substances is the presence of a fragment ion at or near $m/z = 327$ in the bivalent and trivalent positive ion MS/MS spectra. This fragment ion, commonly termed as A-moiety, arises from cleavage between carbons 8 and 9 of PLTX (Figure 24.1) and the additional loss of one water molecule.[16,35,74] Presence of this $m/z = 327$ fragment ion has been reported in the majority of PLTXs, for example, from *P. tuberculosa*,[16,37] *P. caribaoreum*,[45] *P. toxica*,[35] and *P. heliodiscus*,[21] as well as in many PLTX analogs. Nevertheless, the absence of this fragment ion does not rule out the PLTX-like character of a compound, as it might be the result of structural differences at the A-moiety part of the molecule, as in the case of *L. pictor* toxin or minor *P. tuberculosa* toxins.[16,45]

24.2.2.4 Ultraviolet Spectrum

Ultraviolet (UV) absorption spectrum of PLTX presents two maxima: one λmax at 233 (ε 47,000) and another at 263 nm (ε 28,000),[75] which have been attributed to the presence of respective chromophores (Figure 24.2). The ratio of UV absorbances between 233 and 263 nm has been reported to be 1.71.[1] This UV spectrum is a common characteristic for PLTXs, regardless of subtle differences present in their proton magnetic resonance (^{1}H-NMR) and carbon magnetic resonance (^{13}C-NMR) spectra. It has been confirmed for the PLTXs isolated in *P. toxica* from Hawaii, *P. mammilosa* from Jamaica, *P. caribaeorum* from Puerto Rico, *Palythoa* sp. from Tahiti, and *P. heliodiscus* from home aquaria[13,14,21,76] and constitutes another indicative feature for the presence of this toxin and/or its analogs.[59]

The λ 233 nm absorption maximum has been attributed to the presence of two chromophores, a conclusion derived from the respective value of the extinction coefficient[63]; studies by ^{1}H NMR indicated

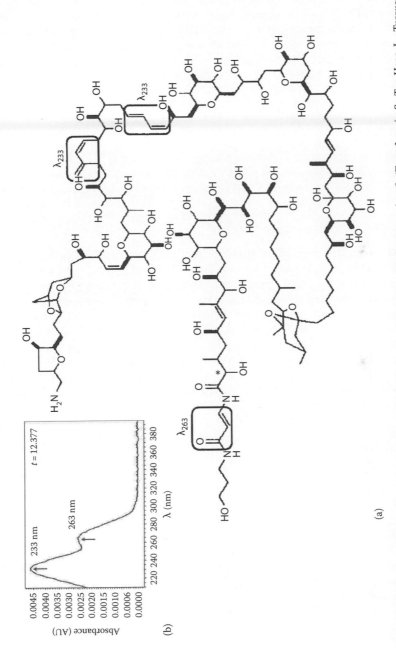

FIGURE 24.2 (a) Planar structure of reference Pacific palytoxin showing the UV chromophores. Asterisk denotes carbon 8. (From Lenoir, S., Ten-Hage, L., Turquet, J., Quod, J.-P., Bernard, C., and Hennion, M.C.: First evidence of palytoxin analogs from an *Ostreopsis mascarenensis* (Dinophyceae) benthic bloom in southwestern Indian Ocean. *J. Phycol.* 2004. 40(6). 1042–1051. Copyright Wiley-VCH Verlag GmbH & Co. KGaA. Reproduced with permission.) (b) Ultraviolet spectrum of reference palytoxin from *Palythoa tuberculosa* at 25 μg/mL in water.

that both of these two chromophores are conjugated dienes.[77] The λ 263 nm chromophore is an *N*-(3'-hydroxypropyl)-trans-3-amidoacrylamide moiety.[76] This moiety is responsible for the positive response of PLTX to the ninhydrin test, while its destruction is accompanied by the loss of toxicity, as well as by a negative ninhydrin test.[63] The 263 nm chromophore is sensitive to methanolic 0.05 M HCl or aqueous 0.05 M NaOH, disappearing with a half-life of 85 and 55 min, respectively. However, neutralization within 2 min regenerated PLTX with no apparent loss in toxicity.[1] PLTX exposure to both visible and UV light produces structural changes in both the 263 and 233 chromophores and a subsequent toxicity reduction by at least 20-fold in only 5 min in UV and 30 min in visible light.[78] This is further confirmed by the toxicity of *N*-acetylpalytoxin, which is 100-fold weaker compared to PLTX; *N*-acetylpalytoxin possesses only a slight structural difference around the N-terminal part of PLTX, where the 263 chromophore is located.[79]

24.2.2.5 Infrared Spectrum

The infrared (IR) spectrum of purified PLTX or its congener shows a band at 1670 cm^{-1} attributed to the presence of an α,β-unsaturated amide carbonyl group.[1] Similar IR data were provided for purified PLTX from *P. caribaeorum*,[14] from the sea anemone *R. macrodactylus*,[50] and from the xanthid crab *L. pictor*.[59]

24.2.2.6 Nuclear Magnetic Resonance Spectra

NMR determinations on various degradation products from periodate oxidation or ozonolysis have provided a large contribution with regard to structural elucidation of PLTX.[8,24,69] Complete chemical shift assignments of ^{1}H and ^{13}C NMR signals of the whole *P. tuberculosa* PLTX molecule and of N-acetylpalytoxin have been reported by Kan and coworkers.[79] Later studies have provided comparative complete NMR chemical shift data (Table 24.1) for *P. tuberculosa* reference PLTX vs. 42-OH-PLTX and the PLTX analog ovatoxin-a (OVTX-a).[67,80] Detailed descriptions of various PLTXs' NMR data and their differences are outside the scope of the present chapter. It is however noteworthy that deuterated methanol (CD$_3$OD or CD$_3$OH) was reported to provide much sharper signals than deuterated water (D$_2$O) in the ^{1}H NMR spectrum, which was attributed to a fast averaged conformation or a monomer.[79] On the other hand, Oku et al.[17] obtained satisfactory ^{1}H NMR spectra of both reference PLTX and *P.* aff. *margaritae* PLTX by use of D$_2$O with 0.2% acetic acid.

24.2.2.7 Chemical Synthesis

Despite the huge number of possible stereoisomers, Prof. Kishi's research group managed to achieve the total chemical synthesis of a fully protected PLTX carboxylic acid in 1989.[10] Subsequently, this was converted to PLTX carboxylic acid and PLTX amide without the use of protecting groups.[81] Comparison of biological activity, chromatographic behavior, and spectroscopic data (MS, 1D, and 2D ^{1}H NMR, and ^{13}C NMR) showed that the synthetic products were identical to the naturally occurring counterparts.[81,82] Conversion of PLTX carboxylic acid to PLTX identical to the natural product from *P. tuberculosa* with a yield of 100% was completed a few years later.[83] Nevertheless, the fact that the whole chemical synthesis procedure for PLTX involves approximately 65 steps indicates a limited potential of practical use.[84]

24.2.3 Metabolism

There is limited information in the literature concerning PLTX metabolism in the animal/human body and subsequently its connection with toxicity. The mode of PLTX toxic action is mainly by disruption of the mammalian cell sodium pump functionality. Targeting the Na$^+$–K$^+$–adenosine triphosphatase (ATPase) pump, PLTX binds to the ATPase and converts the pump into a nonspecific ion channel. This way, PLTX short-circuits the membrane function of cells that rely on Na/K pumps to generate ion gradients and can eventually cause cell lysis.[85]

TABLE 24.1

^{1}H and ^{13}C NMR Chemical Shift Data of Palytoxin (PLTX), Ovatoxin-a (OVTX-a), and 42-Hydroxypalytoxin (42-OH-PLTX)

No.	PLTX ^{13}C	PLTX ^{1}H	OVTX-a ^{13}C	OVTX-a ^{1}H	42-OH-PLTX ^{13}C	42-OH-PLTX ^{1}H	No.	PLTX ^{13}C	PLTX ^{1}H	OVTX-a ^{13}C	OVTX-a ^{1}H	42-OH-PLTX ^{13}C	42-OH-PLTX ^{1}H
1	175.92	—	175.93	—	175.76	—	60	70.18	3.85	68.82	3.82	70.21	3.85
2	75.70	4.09	75.12	4.09	75.68	4.08	61	76.57	3.15	75.70	3.14	76.57	3.15
3	34.73	2.17	34.54	2.14	34.89	2.18	62	73.11	3.74	76.75	3.42	73.15	3.75
3-Me	13.99	0.88	13.94	0.86	14.13	0.88	63	36.77	1.70 1.96	29.55	1.52 2.03	36.89	1.70 1.96
4	41.73	1.40 1.77	41.34	1.39 1.79	41.82	1.40 1.76	64	71.77	3.68	35.20	1.50 1.71	71.88	3.68
5	66.62	4.50	66.40	4.51	66.67	4.50	65	72.20	3.76	73.57	3.86	72.27	3.76
6	131.85	5.49	131.51	5.49	131.82	5.49	66	37.01	1.53 2.04	40.68	1.55 1.93	37.16	1.54 2.04
7	138.28	—	138.31	—	138.6	—	67	77.22	3.44	76.72	3.45	77.16	3.44
7-Me	13.17	1.72	13.22	1.4	13.34	1.72	68	76.04	3.12	75.57	3.10	76.04	3.12
8	80.91	3.92	80.90	3.91	80.97	3.92	69	79.74	3.36	79.31	3.35	79.81	3.36
9	72.34	3.81	70.68	3.92	72.30	3.82	70	75.85	3.09	75.49	3.09	75.95	3.09
10	29.23	2.12	27.95	1.80 2.11	29.36	2.13	71	77.08	3.44	76.70	3.41	77.08	3.43
11	76.19	4.18	77.15	4.11	76.26	4.17	72	41.51	1.43 2.04	41.11	1.42 2.03	41.69	1.40 2.04
12	73.88	3.64	74.26	3.65	73.68	3.65	73	64.99	4.84	64.86	4.82	65.03	4.84
13	75.17	3.54	74.55	3.57	75.18	3.55	74	133.47	5.37	133.10	5.37	133.45	5.37
14	71.68	3.60	71.32	3.58	71.82	3.59	75	130.04	6.00	129.85	5.99	139.99	6.00
15	72.91	3.62	74.55	3.58	72.91	3.62	76	128.87	6.46	128.44	6.43	128.87	6.46
16	71.28	4.03	74.34	4.04	71.35	4.03	77	133.88	5.78	133.58	5.78	133.95	5.78
17	71.68	4.04	45.60	1.33 1.52	71.64	4.04	78	38.64	2.42	38.54	2.40	38.81	2.41
18	73.27	3.54	68.43	3.87	73.29	3.54	79	71.20	3.93	72.60	3.93	71.22	3.93
19	71.35	3.79	69.90	4.05	71.30	3.79	80	76.29	3.27	76.03	3.26	76.34	3.26
20	71.11	3.87	68.10	3.88	71.19	3.88	81	73.04	3.63	72.74	3.69	73.10	3.71
21	27.38	1.39 1.48	29.00	1.32 1.63	27.70	1.37 1.49	82	34.35	2.39 2.75	34.00	2.37 2.75	34.56	2.39 2.76
22	26.93	1.35 1.47	27.11	1.40	27.40	1.35 1.48	83	130.18	5.69	129.91	5.68	130.26	5.69
23	35.03	1.55 1.64	34.82	1.23 1.58	35.16	1.55 1.64	84	132.64	5.95	132.27	5.94	132.67	5.95
24	28.44	1.36	30.43	1.22 1.47	28.70	1.36	85	146.73	—	146.33	—	146.63	—
25	39.72	1.26	40.12	1.14 1.30	39.89	1.26	85′	114.86	4.94 5.07	114.74	4.92 5.05	114.92	4.94 5.07
26	29.70	1.67	30.01	1.61	29.83	1.68	86	34.30	2.25 2.34	34.01	2.23 2.32	34.56	2.25 2.34
26-Me	19.30	0.92	21.41	0.92	19.50	0.92	87	33.13	1.59 1.72	32.77	1.59 1.73	33.17	1.58 1.72
27	40.78	0.91 1.47	39.35	0.78 1.60	40.77	0.90 1.48	88	74.19	3.71	73.92	3.70	74.29	3.71
28	80.17	3.97	79.94	3.97	80.22	3.97	89	74.02	3.50	73.56	3.50	74.02	3.50
29	82.31	—	82.20	—	82.27	—	90	77.82	3.35	77.59	3.35	77.93	3.35
29-Me	21.01	1.18	20.70	1.18	21.15	1.18	91	33.00	1.89	32.71	1.88	33.16	1.89

(continued)

TABLE 24.1 (continued)

^{1}H and ^{13}C NMR Chemical Shift Data of Palytoxin (PLTX), Ovatoxin-a (OVTX-a), and 42-Hydroxypalytoxin (42-OH-PLTX)

No.	PLTX ^{13}C	PLTX ^{1}H	OVTX-a ^{13}C	OVTX-a ^{1}H	42-OH-PLTX ^{13}C	42-OH-PLTX ^{1}H	No.	PLTX ^{13}C	PLTX ^{1}H	OVTX-a ^{13}C	OVTX-a ^{1}H	42-OH-PLTX ^{13}C	42-OH-PLTX ^{1}H
30	45.74	1.14 1.70	45.44	1.14 1.71	45.92	1.15 1.70	91-Me	15.65	0.91	15.38	0.90	15.78	0.91
31	25.55	2.04	25.25	2.06	25.77	2.05	92	27.86	1.30 2.21	27.61	1.28 2.20	27.97	1.30 2.22
31-Me	21.89	0.91	21.61	0.91	22.00	0.92	93	74.83	4.03	74.51	4.03	74.90	4.03
32	43.74	1.09 1.67	44.10	1.08 1.65	43.94	1.09 1.68	94	73.04	3.65	72.58	3.64	73.13	3.64
33	109.23	—	109.00	—	109.24	—	95	74.73	3.61	74.42	3.61	74.74	3.61
34	38.64	1.60	39.32	1.60	38.69	1.60	96	76.01	3.15	75.71	3.16	76.01	3.15
35	23.98	1.41	24.11	1.43	24.23	1.43	97	69.71	4.32	69.35	4.31	69.74	4.32
36	30.98	1.31	30.50	1.27	30.84	1.29	98	132.43	5.55	132.11	5.54	132.41	5.54
37	30.93	1.31	30.50	1.27	30.84	1.29	99	135.28	5.71	135.08	5.70	135.31	5.70
38	30.81	1.31	31.71	1.35	30.84	1.29	100	71.90	4.36	71.65	4.36	71.94	4.37
39	31.29	1.36	28.50	1.27 1.68	31.21	1.35	101	71.77	3.68	71.50	3.67	71.88	3.68
40	39.20	1.48	34.81	1.20 1.87	38.69	1.58	102	40.21	1.58	39.79	1.57	40.33	1.59
41	69.26	3.80	71.95	3.66	71.92	3.65	103	68.39	4.22	68.12	4.21	68.38	4.22
42	39.37	1.44 1.86	77.73	3.05	77.34	3.70	104	40.53	1.38 1.74	40.21	1.37 1.73	40.72	1.38 1.74
43	64.86	4.39	63.11	4.63	66.10	4.32	105	76.14	4.51	75.91	4.51	76.21	4.51
44	73.88	3.65	34.49	1.63 2.01	74.08	3.91	106	36.83	1.78 1.84	36.48	1.76 1.85	36.96	1.79 1.84
45	74.28	3.95	69.81	4.28	74.28	3.91	107	79.62	4.21	79.40	4.21	79.61	4.21
46	68.25	3.67	71.52	3.41	67.75	3.78	108	82.74	4.35	82.51	4.35	82.80	4.36
47	101.24	—	101.16	—	101.59	—	109	26.59	1.67 1.78	26.33	1.64 1.78	26.83	1.66 1.78
48	41.95	1.83	40.34	1.74	41.92	1.77	110	32.30	1.47	32.11	1.48	32.47	1.48
49	72.40	3.94	72.49	3.82	72.45	3.92	111	83.81	3.89	83.64	3.89	83.87	3.89
50	44.07	2.26	43.55	2.29	44.41	2.25	112	73.27	4.27	72.92	4.27	73.31	4.27
50-Me	16.58	1.03	16.82	1.05	16.72	1.03	113	39.78	1.86 2.10	39.46	1.87 2.11	39.89	1.86 2.11
51	134.46	5.62	134.51	5.62	134.59	5.64	114	75.31	4.36	74.46	4.38	75.14	4.37
52	134.74	5.51	134.14	5.47	134.69	5.50	115	45.13	2.87 2.99	44.49	2.91 3.05	45.13	2.90 3.03
53	74.06	4.05	73.92	4.01	74.06	4.06	2'	134.82	7.79	134.81	7.80	134.76	7.80
54	34.93	1.61 1.77	34.82	1.57 1.76	35.09	1.61 1.78	3'	106.82	5.95	106.82	5.94	106.79	5.95
55	27.79	1.46 1.69	27.18	1.43 1.63	27.89	1.46 1.69	4'	169.66	—	169.39	—	169.57	—
56	73.11	3.74	72.75	3.66	73.15	3.75	6'	37.42	3.33	37.53	3.34	37.51	3.33
57	72.81	3.85	71.67	3.87	72.86	3.86	7'	33.28	1.74	33.19	1.73	33.46	1.74
58	74.19	3.87	70.91	3.86	74.11	3.87	8'	60.40	3.60	60.40	3.59	60.60	3.59
59	33.05	1.66 2.27	32.72	1.65 2.27	33.16	1.66 2.26							

Source: Reprinted with permission from Ciminiello, P., Dell'Aversano, C., Dello Iacovo, E., Fattorusso, E., Forino, M., Guerrini, F., Pezzolesi, L., and Pistocchi, R., Isolation and structure elucidation of ovatoxin-a, the major toxin produced by *Ostreopsis ovata*, *J. Am. Chem. Soc.*, 134(3), 1869–1875, Copyright 2012 American Chemical Society.

As until now there are no experimental data to indicate otherwise; it is believed that PLTX has to bind to the ATPase in its intact form in order to remain toxic. This is supported by the fact that even minor structural alterations in the PLTX molecule can result in toxicity loss. In this context, acid hydrolysis of PLTX with refluxing 2 N HCl for 4 h has been reported to result in the destruction of the λ 263 chromophore, an alteration connected to the loss of toxicity.[76] Treatment of PLTX with 0.1 N NaOH at room temperature for 50 min or 0.1 N acetic acid at 80°C for 24 h as well as catalytic hydrogenation can also cause significant loss of toxicity.[75] Additionally, solutions of 1–5N HCl or 0.5–5 N NaOH have been reported to deactivate 5 LD$_{50}$'s of PLTX within a 5-min contact period, whereas acetic acid was totally ineffective.[4] Such effects could partly account for the major toxicity reduction observed upon oral administration of PLTX, compared to the i.v. or intraperitoneal routes,[4] due to the strongly acidic pH in the stomach and strongly alkaline pH in the small intestine. This speculation has been also expressed in the first meeting of the Working Group on Toxicology of Marine Biotoxins held in 2005 in Cesenatico, Italy (Luis Botana, personal communication), but has not been to date confirmed. Finally, PLTX has been shown to stimulate both metabolism of arachidonic acid and prostaglandin production; these properties are considered to be relevant with PLTX's tumor-promoting activity, as PLTX is a known non-TPA type tumor promoter.[86,87]

24.3 Palytoxin Analogs from *Ostreopsis* spp.

Dinoflagellates belonging to the genus *Ostreopsis* (Dinophyceae) have been indicated as the most probable biogenetic originators of PLTX. In 1995, the research group of Yasumoto has established the PLTX-like character of the major compound isolated from *O. siamensis*, termed thereafter as "ostreocin."[31] Since then, numerous research groups have confirmed the presence of PLTX-like compounds in different *Ostreopsis* species.

Ostreopsis spp. are mainly benthic and epiphytic dinoflagellates with a worldwide distribution. They are considered as important components of subtropical and tropical marine coral reef-lagoonal environments and are also thought to be potential pregenitors of toxins associated with ciguatera fish poisoning.[88–90] However, the genus *Ostreopsis* has a much broader geographical distribution than initially thought[91] and is now a global concern since these organisms can affect human health whenever they develop and become prevalent.[20] The presence of *Ostreopsis* spp. in tropical waters is well documented since the 1980s. On the other hand, the number of studies reporting the presence of these benthic dinoflagellates in temperate regions has substantially increased in the last few years.[91] These PLTX-like producing microorganisms occur in the China Sea,[92] Pacific Ocean,[33,92–94] Tasman Sea,[94] Indian Ocean,[35] Atlantic Ocean,[39,95] Gulf of Mexico,[96,97] and the Mediterranean Sea.[37,38,98,99]

Ostreopsis spp. have been regularly recorded during summertime in the past decade in the Mediterranean countries Spain, Italy, Monaco, France, Greece, and Tunisia.[37,98,100–105] In the south of Spain and France as well as in Italy and Greece, their presence has been accompanied by relevant toxicity in shellfish and sea urchins,[40,51–53] as well as by toxic episodes in humans caused by aerosols.[106] The spread of toxin-producing *Ostreopsis* spp. to temperate regions may be partly due to ballast waters of cargo ships but also due to marginal changes in climate conditions, enough to induce bloom formation.[91] These dinoflagellate blooms are characterized by a brownish-colored mucilaginous coverage of marine benthos.[107]

To date, there are nine different *Ostreopsis* species described, five of which, namely, *O. siamensis*, *O. ovata*, *O. mascarenensis*, *O. lenticularis*, and *O. heptagona* are also reported as producers of toxic substances (Table 24.2). No data are available to date concerning the toxin production ability of the four remaining species, *O. labens*, *O. marina*, *O. belizeana*, and *O. caribbeanna*.[96,108]

The present section will provide an updated compilation on the available chemical data concerning only toxic substances produced by *Ostreopsis* sp. shown to possess PLTX characteristics. PLTX-like compounds, also termed as PLTX analogs, will be presented according to producing species, that is, *O. siamensis* (ostreocins), *O. mascarenensis* (mascarenotoxins), and *O. ovata* (ovatoxins). Until today, the neurotoxins ostreotoxin-1 and -3 produced by *O. lenticularis* have not been definitely characterized as PLTX analogs, despite their reported mouse lethality and possible

TABLE 24.2

Toxic *Ostreopsis* Species and Summary of Reported Data on Properties of Respective Toxins Produced

Producing Species	Toxin	Considered a Palytoxin Analog?	Molecular Weight	Chemical Formula	Mouse Lethality (LD$_{50}$ i.p.)	References
O. siamensis	Unnamed					[88]
	Ostreocin-D	Yes	~2635	$C_{127}H_{219}N_3O_{53}$	0.75 µg/kg	[31,32,119]
	Ostreocin-B	Yes	~2651	$C_{127}H_{219}N_3O_{54}$		[117,120]
O. mascarenensis	Unnamed					[90]
	Mascarenotoxin-A and	Yes	~2500–2535	n.d.	0.9 mg/kg	[35,123]
	Mascarenotoxin-B	Yes				
O. ovata	Unnamed	Yes	n.d.	n.d.	n.d.	[37,88]
	Putative palytoxin	Yes	2678	$C_{129}H_{224}N_3O_{54}$		[38,131]
	Ovatoxin-a	Yes	2646	$C_{129}H_{223}N_3O_{52}$	<7.0 µg/kg	[80,131,132]
	Ovatoxin-b	Yes	2690	$C_{131}H_{227}N_3O_{53}$		[133]
	Ovatoxin-c	Yes	2706	$C_{131}H_{227}N_3O_{54}$		[133]
	Ovatoxin-d + -e	Yes	2662	$C_{129}H_{223}N_3O_{53}$		[133]
	Ovatoxin-f	Yes	2674	$C_{131}H_{227}N_3O_{52}$		[135]
	Mascarenotoxin-A and	Yes	2588	$C_{127}H_{221}N_3O_{50}$		[68]
	Mascarenotoxin-C	Yes	2628	$C_{129}H_{221}N_3O_{51}$		[68]
O. lenticularis	Ostreotoxin	Not known	n.d.	n.d.	32.1 mg/kg	[89]
	Ostreotoxin 1					[109]
	Ostreotoxin 3					[110]
O. heptagona	Unnamed	Not known	n.d.	n.d.	n.d.	[111]

n.d., not detected.

connection to ciguatera.[89,109,110] Regarding *O. heptagona*, the only available information is that methanol extracts obtained from clonal cultures of *O. heptagona* isolated from Knight Key, Florida, were weakly toxic to mice.[111]

24.3.1 *Ostreopsis siamensis* Schmidt (1901): Ostreocins

24.3.1.1 *Ecobiology, Origin, Distribution, and Toxin Production*

O. siamensis was first isolated in the Gulf of Siam (Thailand) in 1901 by Schmidt.[112] This dinoflagellate mainly occurs epiphytically and less frequently as planktonic; its presence has been recorded in many tropical and subtropical areas of the world, but also in temperate areas during summertime. Until today, *O. siamensis* has been reported in the coastal waters of Japan,[113] New Zealand,[114,115] Tasmania,[94] Australia, Caribbean, Hawaii, Indian Ocean,[116] Spain, Italy, Portugal, Greece, and Tunisia.[37,98,100,102,117]

O. siamensis was characterized in 1981 as a species producing compounds toxic to mice.[88] Lethality and hemolytic activity of the *O. siamensis* toxins were reported some years later.[113,118] The structure of the major ostreocin produced by *O. siamensis* (strain SOA 1 from Aka Island, Okinawa, Japan) was first elucidated by Usami et al.,[31] who reported on the resemblance of its structural and chemical properties to those of PLTX. This compound that accounted for 70% of the total extract's toxicity was named ostreocin-D. More than 10 other minor ostreocins were present in the *O. siamensis* extracts, but none were found to be identical to PLTX by electrospray ionization-MS (ESI–MS).[32,119] Similarly, *O. siamensis* isolates from New Zealand have also been shown to produce toxins with strong hemolytic activity and mouse lethality.[93,115] Toxins possessing a strong delayed hemolytic activity inhibited by the PLTX antagonist ouabain, thus indicating a PLTX-like character, were reported in *O.* cf. *siamensis* isolates from the NW Mediterranean Sea.[37] In a recent study, however, certain Mediterranean and Atlantic *O.* cf. *siamensis* strains were shown not to produce either ostreocin-D or ostreocin-B, which are produced by Japanese *O. siamensis* strains, or ovatoxins, which are produced by the Mediterranean *O.* cf. *ovata*. Only sub-fg levels of PLTX on a per cell basis were detected in the Mediterranean strain.[117]

Among the known *O. siamensis* toxins, only the chemistry of ostreocin-D has been studied in detail until today, whereas there is some limited information with regard to the structure of ostreocin-B.

24.3.1.2 *Chemistry of Ostreocin-D*

Ostreocin-D is a colorless amorphous solid compound, positive to ninhydrin, possessing an optical activity with a specific rotation of +16.6 in water (c 0.121, $T = 23°C$) and a UV absorption spectrum exhibiting two maxima, at 234 (ε 35,000) and 263 nm (ε 22,000). UV absorption together with NMR spectra indicates that ostreocin-D has conjugated diene and ketone functionality analogous with PLTX.[31]

Structure elucidation of ostreocin-D was achieved by the use of MS and ^{1}H NMR spectra. In the high-mass range of the fast-atom bombardment mass spectrometry (FABMS), ostreocin-D displayed cluster ions having a centroid at m/z 2636.51. The ion distribution pointed to a molecular formula of $C_{127}H_{219}N_3O_{53}$, with the MH$^+$ calculated at 2636.47. This compositional difference of C_2H_4O between PLTX and ostreocin-D was initially attributed to the substitution of two methyls and one hydroxyl of the former with protons in the latter. The substitution of methyls is located at C3 and C26 (Figure 24.1). A comparison of PLTX and ostreocin-D NMR spectra in 0.2% CD_3COOD/D_2O was required to identify partial structures around methyls and double bonds. However, reduction of the molecule size was required for further studies due to severe congestion of the NMR signals. Dissolution of the NMR signals and clarification of the entire structure were achieved by ozonolysis-induced degradation of the molecule in MeOH–H$_2$O–AcOH (70:30:0.1) at −77°C for 20 min followed by reduction with NaBH$_4$. It was finally concluded that in ostreocin-D, two hydroxyls (positions C19 and C44) are substituted by protons while an extra hydroxyl is present at C42, compared to PLTX. Ostreocin-D was thus deduced to be 42-hydroxy-3,26-didemethyl-19,44-dideoxy-PLTX,[31,32] a structure confirmed also by use of negative ion FABMS.[119] It is noteworthy that the small structural differences between ostreocin-D and PLTX have limited effect on the mouse lethality of the former (LD$_{50}$ [i.p.]: 0.75 and 0.50 μg/kg, respectively), but cause significant reduction in cytotoxicity and hemolytic potency.[31,32]

24.3.1.3 Chemistry of Ostreocin-B

Ostreocin-B is one of the other PLTX-like molecules also detected in a Japanese *O. siamensis* culture. These other compounds were present in the algal extract in amounts that were too low for a complete NMR-based structure elucidation. A tentative structure of ostreocin-B was reported by Ukena.[120] Compared to ostreocin-D, ostreocin-B presents an additional hydroxyl at C-44, thus being the 42-hydroxy-3,26-didemethyl-19-deoxy-PLTX. The elemental formula of ostreocin-B is therefore $C_{127}H_{219}N_3O_{54}$ with an $[M+H]^+$ of 2651.44 in its spectrum as defined by LC–HRMS. Fragmentation between C-8 and C-9 of the molecule, which is typical of all PLTX-like compounds so far known, produced an A-moiety of $C_{15}H_{26}N_2O_6$ with a characteristic ion $[A\ moiety + H - H_2O]^+$ at $m/z = 313.1754$ and a B-moiety of $C_{112}H_{193}NO_{48}$.[117]

24.3.2 Ostreopsis mascarenensis Quod (1994): Mascarenotoxins

24.3.2.1 Ecobiology, Origin, Distribution, and Toxin Production

O. mascarenensis has been first identified in shallow (2–5 m) barrier reef environments and coral reefs in the Southwest Indian Ocean and is the largest species of the genus.[90,121] *O. mascarenensis* was detected in low numbers epiphytically on macroalgae (*Turbinaria* sp., *Galaxaura* sp.) and dead corals and sediments at Mayotte and Reunion islands and in high numbers at Rodrigues Island.[122] Crude methanol extracts (CMEs) of this species were toxic to mice.[90,123] In a monospecific bloom of *O. mascarenensis* recorded in 1996 in Rodrigues Island (Mascareignes Archipelago, SW Indian Ocean), CMEs as well as their polar n-butanol soluble fractions (BSFs) showed mouse lethality ($LD_{50} \approx 0.9$ mg/kg) with symptoms similar to those induced by PLTX but without diarrhea. Both CME and BSF also exhibited a typical of PLTX-delayed hemolytic activity; most of the mouse toxicity and hemolytic potency were found in the BSF. Subsequent analyses were carried out to identify the nature of the toxic compounds.[35,123]

24.3.2.2 Chemistry of Mascarenotoxins-A and -B

Further analysis of the BSF from *O. mascarenensis* employed the use of high-performance LC (HPLC)–DAD in comparison to reference PLTX from *P. toxica*.[35] The mobile phase was water acidified to pH 2.5 with trifluoroacetic acid (solvent A) and pure acetonitrile (solvent B), and a linear gradient was applied from 30% to 70% of solvent B over 45 min. HPLC screening of the BSF revealed two distinct peaks eluted at approximately 38% acetonitrile with retention times very near to that of reference PLTX. The two characteristic UV absorption maxima, at 233 and 263 nm, were present in both peaks, while the ratio between their absorbance (233 vs. 263 nm) was identical to that of reference PLTX. Peaks were collected separately, and the purified toxic compounds were named mascarenotoxin-A (McTX-A) and mascarenotoxin-B (McTX-B).[35]

McTX-A and McTX-B were further analyzed by nano-ESI quadrupole time-of-flight (nano-ESI–Q–TOF) and LC-ESI MS/MS in comparison to reference PLTX. Both compounds showed a serial dehydration process in their fragmentation patterns, indicating the presence of numerous hydroxyls. Furthermore, the characteristic fragment ion $m/z = 327.2$ previously detected in reference PLTX and Caribbean PLTX[16,45] was abundantly obtained for both McTX-A and McTX-B by selecting the bi- and tricharged ions.[35]

MS profiles of both McTX-A and McTX-B were very similar to that of reference PLTX, whereas their estimated molecular masses were found to range between 2500 and 2535 Da, being lower compared to reference PLTX (2680 Da) or other PLTXs and ostreocin-D. Despite the mass difference, MS profiles and fragmentation patterns of McTX-A and McTX-B coupled to mouse bioassay (MBA) symptomatology and delayed hemolytic activity were considered enough to account for a PLTX-like character for these compounds. Structural variations between mascarenotoxins and the reference PLTX can explain both the quantitative differences reported for hemolytic action and mouse lethality, as well as the minor deviations in the MS spectra and retention times,[35] as small changes in the structure of PLTX analogs had been previously shown to affect mouse toxicity, hemolytic potency, and cytotoxicity.[31]

O. mascarenensis is largely distributed in the western Indian Ocean, a known clupeotoxism endemic zone.[121] Since *Ostreopsis* sp. have been suspected as the PLTX source in reported clupeotoxism cases,[34,124] this species could play a key role in the development of regional clupeotoxism incidents.

24.3.3 *Ostreopsis ovata* Fukuyo (1981): Ovatoxins

24.3.3.1 *Ecobiology, Origin, Distribution, and Toxin Production*

O. ovata, the smallest species of the genus, presents a worldwide distribution, with records in the Pacific Ocean,[92,113] the Caribbean Sea,[89] the Atlantic Ocean,[95,125,126] and the Mediterranean Sea.[37,98,101,103,105,127]

O. ovata from Okinawa, Japan, was reported as the producer of a butanol-soluble compound exhibiting mouse lethality.[29] Cell extracts of the same organism were later shown to exhibit also a slight hemolytic activity.[113] However, CMEs of *O. ovata* isolated in the Virgin Islands were nontoxic to mice.[89] On the other hand, extracts of *O. ovata* from Brazil and the Mediterranean Sea were shown to contain substances possessing strong delayed hemolytic ouabain-inhibited activity, as well as mouse lethality with a symptomatology typical of PLTX.[36,37,95] Since 2005, summer blooms of *O. ovata* in the Italian coasts have been repeatedly implicated as the cause of respiratory problems in swimmers and sunbathers, most probably through inhalation of toxic aerosols containing a PLTX-like substance.[38,101,128–130] Further analyses of cultured *O. ovata* isolated during a similar event in 2006 showed that extracts contained a putative PLTX (p-PLTX) and a new compound, which was named OVTX-a.[131] Subsequent extensive research of the Ciminiello et al. group has provided an enormous contribution toward elucidation of OVTX-a chemical and structural properties by use of various mass spectral techniques.[80,132] Five more ovatoxins, namely, ovatoxins-b, -c, -d, -e, and very recently OVTX-f, have also been identified, to date, by the same research group.[133–135] Almost simultaneously, four novel similar PLTX analogs have been reported for the Mediterranean *O.* cf. *ovata* by LC-ESI–TOF–MS[68] and later in Japanese *Ostreopsis* spp. strains among which *O.* cf. *ovata*.[136,137]

24.3.3.2 *Chemistry of Ovatoxins*

Initial investigations with regard to the chemistry of *O. ovata* toxins revealed that extracts from all tested strains isolated from Brazil and the Mediterranean Sea (Italy and Spain) exhibited a strong delayed hemolytic activity, neutralized by ouabain.[36,37] When tested by HPLC–UV, the extract obtained from the *O. ovata* strain OS06BR presented a peak at the same retention time as standard PLTX from *P. tuberculosa*, while the UV spectrum of this peak, exhibiting two absorbance maxima at 230 and 263 nm, confirmed the PLTX-like character of the compound. Subsequent MS analyses showed that spectra of the compound in question and PLTX were identical; in both cases, a positive ion spray with bicharged ions at m/z 1346.7 and a fragment at m/z 327, characteristic of thermally fragmented PLTX,[16] was obtained. Similar LC–MS data were reported by Ciminiello et al.[38] for both pellet and butanol extracts of Mediterranean *O. ovata* derived from the Genoa 2005 outbreak, with the presence of a peak at 6.45 min for the transitions m/z 1340 → 327 and 912 → 327, which matched perfectly, in retention time, fragmentation, and ion ratios, those of reference PLTX injected under the same experimental conditions. Due to the complex stereostructure of PLTX, this compound was thereafter referred to as "putative palytoxin" rather than PLTX, as the possibility that the compound was a PLTX isomer that could not be excluded on the basis of the obtained LC–MS results.

24.3.3.2.1 *Ovatoxin-a*

Later research[131] showed the presence, along with p-PLTX, of a much more abundant PLTX-like compound never reported before, which was named ovatoxin-a (OVTX-a) and which was found to be the dominant toxin present during the 2006 summer bloom in the Ligurian coasts in Italy. On the basis of molecular formula, fragmentation pattern, and chromatographic behavior, the structure of OVTX-a appeared to be strictly related to that of PLTX. Further analyses on cultured *O. ovata* strains, which were necessary to unequivocally demonstrate that p-PLTX and OVTX-a were actually produced by *O. ovata* itself, showed that OVTX-a had an estimated molecular weight of 2648.5 Da and a molecular formula of $C_{129}H_{223}N_3O_{52}$, therefore structurally similar to PLTX but containing two fewer oxygen atoms.[131] The spectrum of OVTX-a also contained the characteristic ion peak at m/z 327.1 and presented similar trich-arged and bicharged ion clusters, which basically differed from those of reference PLTX only for m/z absolute values. MS data comparison pointed to the conclusion that the two molecules shared the same part structure A (A-moiety) as indicated by (1) the common loss of a $C_{16}H_{30}N_2O_7$ part structure from the monocharged ions emerging from the experiments performed on ion trap MS and linear ion trap hybrid FTMS instruments and (2) fragment ion at m/z 327.1 contained in MS spectra of both compounds run on the triple quadrupole MS instrument. Thus, structural differences between OVTX-a and PLTX were likely to lie in the part structure B (B-moiety).

At the same time, the relative abundance of OVTX-a and p-PLTX in the plankton samples was also investigated by means of an LC–MS experiment employing a slow gradient elution, which allowed chromatographic separation of the two compounds.[131] MS detection was accomplished in MRM mode on a triple quadrupole MS instrument by monitoring the transitions m/z 1340.7 → 327.1, 1331.7 → 327.1 for p-PLTX and m/z 1324.7 → 327.1, 1315.7 → 327.1 for OVTX-a. Under the chromatographic conditions used, p-PLTX eluted at the same retention time as the PLTX standard (11.08 min), while OVTX-a eluted at 11.48 min. On account of the evident structural similarities between the two compounds, a similar molar mass response was assumed. Comparison between p-PLTX and OVTX-a contents suggested that the latter was by far the predominant PLTX-like compound in the field plankton samples of the 2006 outbreak, by a factor within the range of 5–15. This was also the case with pellet and growth medium extracts of cultured *O. ovata*, which yielded a p-PLTX and OVTX-a content of 0.55 and 3.85 pg/cell, respectively.

Stereostructure of OVTX-a (Figure 24.3) was finally elucidated by use of 1D and 2D NMR experiments (^{1}H NMR, ^{1}H–^{1}H COSY, z-TOCSY, ROESY, HSQC, HMBC, and HSQCTOCSY) combined with analyses by HR-LC–MS.[80,132,134] HR full MS spectrum of OVTX-a, acquired on a hybrid linear ion trap FTMS instrument, generated a monocharged ion [M+H]$^+$ (monoisotopic ion at m/z 2647.4979) corresponding to the molecular formula $C_{129}H_{223}N_3O_{52}$ ($\Delta = -3.918$ ppm). NMR data relative to the part of the structure of OVTX-a stretching out from position 8′ through 7 as well as those of the regions extending from position 29 to 32 and from position 73 up to the terminal position 115 appeared nearly superimposable with the reference NMR data of both PLTX and 42-hydroxy-PLTX (Table 24.1). Hence, it was concluded that OVTX-a shared not only the same planar structure but also the same stereochemistry as PLTX and 42-hydroxy-PLTX in these segments. On the other hand, apart from the part structure comprised between positions 29 and 32, the central region of OVTX-a from positions 8 to 72 showed remarkable differences in comparison to PLTX and 42-hydroxy-PLTX. Like 42-hydroxy-PLTX, OVTX-a featured a hydroxyl group at C42 (δ_H 3.05, δ_C 77.73), but unlike PLTX and 42-hydroxy-PLTX, it presented a methylene (δ_H 1.63, 2.01; δ_C 34.49) at position 44 instead of a hydroxy methine functionality. The last structural divergence between OVTX-a and both PLTX and 42-hydroxy-PLTX emerged at position 64 (δ_H 1.50, 1.71; δ_C 35.20), where the lack of a hydroxyl group was detected.[80] Cumulatively, in comparison with PLTX, OVTX-a lacks three hydroxy groups at 17-, 44-, and 64-positions, but features an extra hydroxy functionality at the 42-position, which demonstrates that OVTX-a is the 42-hydroxy-17,44,64-trideoxy derivative of PLTX. Further NMR-based studies on OVTX-a stereochemistry identified the presence of 7 stereogenic double bonds and 62 asymmetric carbon atoms, located either on pyranose rings or along polyhydroxylated carbon chains; OVTX-a has the same stereochemistry as PLTX at C8 as well as at all of the asymmetric carbon atoms belonging to the A ring, but shows an inversion of the configuration at C9.[132] Subsequently, the fragmentation pattern of OVTX-a was extensively investigated,[134] and it was found to closely parallel that of PLTX: all fragments contained in its HR CID MS^2, MS^3, and MS^4 spectra were due to the same cleavages observed for PLTX, with the exception of only 4 out of the 32 cleavages (cleavage #14, #20, #28, and #6+#12) that were lacking in OVTX-a. This pointed to a close structural similarity among the molecules, suggesting that they share the same backbone. There were, however, some clues in the spectra that indicated the regions and, in some cases, the specific sites where structural differences between the two compounds occur. A complete description of OVTX-a fragmentation pattern is beyond the scope of this chapter; the reader should refer to the excellent work of Ciminiello et al.[134] for detailed information.

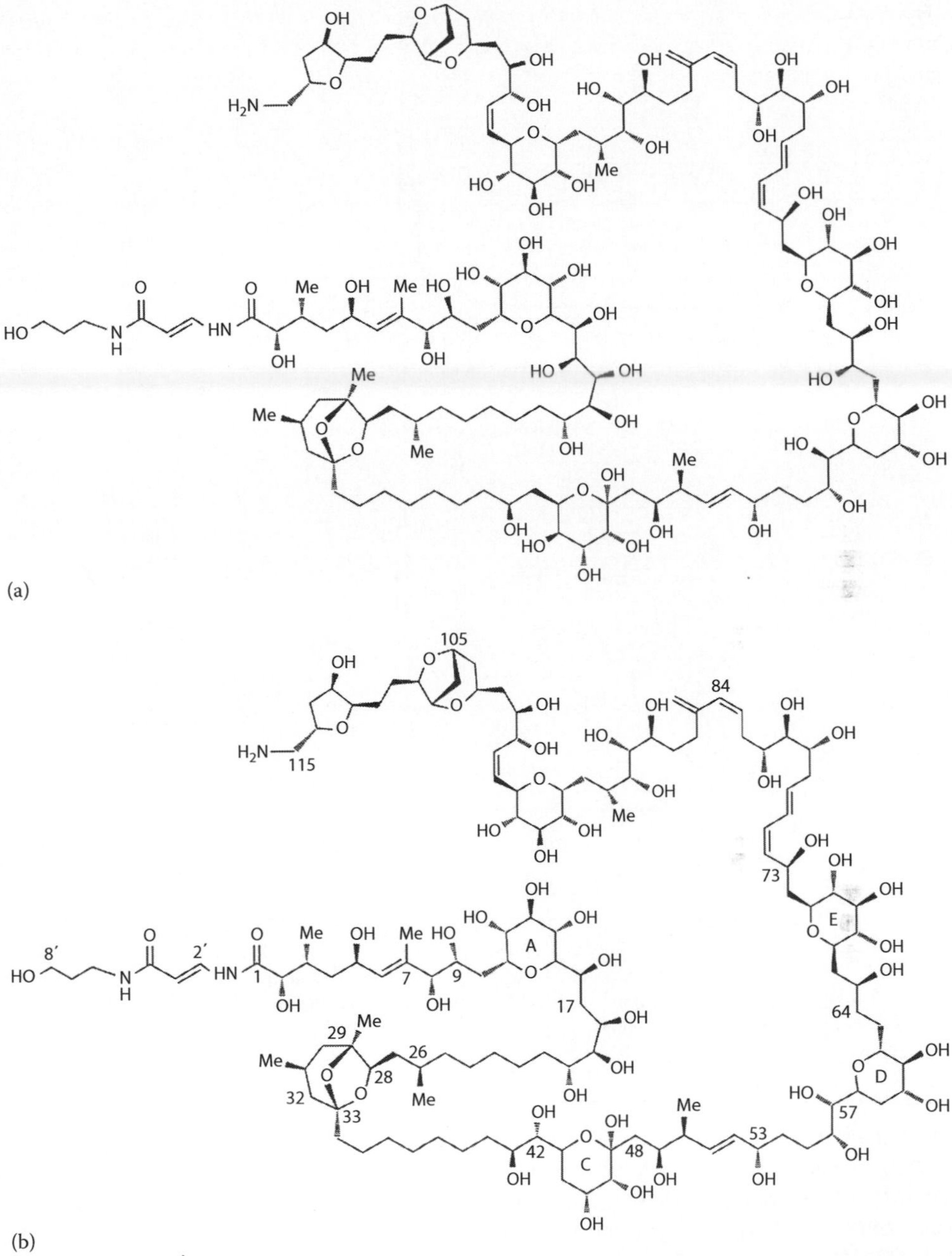

(a)

(b)

FIGURE 24.3 Stereostructures of (a) palytoxin and (b) OVTX-a. Asymmetric carbon atoms showing an inverted configuration in comparison to the corresponding atoms in palytoxin are indicated in bold. C42 is not a stereocenter in palytoxin. (From Ciminiello, P., Dell'Aversano, C., Dello Iacovo, E., Fattorusso, E., Forino, M., Grauso, L., and Tartaglione, L.: Stereochemical studies on ovatoxin-a. *Chem. Eur. J.* 2012. 18(52). 16836–16843. Copyright Wiley-VCH Verlag GmbH & Co. KGaA. Reproduced with permission.)

24.3.3.2.2 Ovatoxins-b, -c, -d, -e, and -f

Further in-depth investigation of a cultured strain (OOAN0601) of *O. ovata* isolated from water samples collected along the Adriatic coasts of Italy (Marche region) were carried out by HR-LC/MS and tandem mass spectrometry (MS²).[133] The presence of p-PLTX and OVTX-a was reconfirmed, but the occurrence in the extract of four new PLTX-like compounds, which were named OVTX-b, -c, -d, and -e,

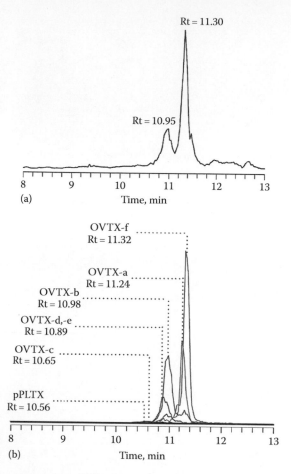

FIGURE 24.4 (a) Total ion chromatogram (TIC) of the cultured *O*. cf. *ovata* CBA2–122 and (b) extracted ion chromatograms (XIC) of the principal components of the toxin profile. (Reprinted with permission from Ciminiello, P., Dell'Aversano, C., Dello Iacovo, E., Fattorusso, E., Forino, M., Tartaglione, L, Battocchi, C., Crinelli, R., Carloni, E., Magnani, M., and Penna, A., Unique toxin profile of a Mediterranean *Ostreopsis* cf. *ovata* strain: HR LC–MS^n characterization of ovatoxin-f, a new palytoxin congener, *Chem. Res. Toxicol.*, 25(6), 1243–1252. Copyright 2012 American Chemical Society.)

was also demonstrated (Figure 24.4). The elemental formulae of the new ovatoxins were also assigned (Table 24.3). A comparison of molecular formulae of ovatoxins with that of PLTX {[M+H]$^+$ at *m/z* 2679.4893 (all *m/z* refer to monoisotopic ion peaks), $C_{129}H_{224}N_3O_{54}$} indicated that (1) OVTX-a ([M+H]$^+$ at *m/z* 2647.4979, $C_{129}H_{224}N_3O_{52}$) presents two O atoms less than PLTX, as previously ascertained; (2) OVTX-b ([M+H]$^+$ at *m/z* 2691.5233, $C_{131}H_{228}N_3O_{53}$) presents two C, four H, and one O atoms more than OVTX-a; (3) OVTX-c ([M+H]$^+$ at *m/z* 2707.5173, $C_{131}H_{228}N_3O_{54}$) presents two C, four H, and two O atoms more than OVTX-a; and (4) OVTX-d and OVTX-e ([M+H]$^+$ at *m/z* 663.4905, $C_{129}H_{224}N_3O_{53}$) present one O atom more than OVTX-a.

Information was also obtained about the structural features of the new ovatoxins by initially analyzing the fragment ions due to [M+H–A moiety–nH$_2$O]$^+$ (n = 0–6) present in the mass range *m/z* 2200–2350 of the HR full MS spectrum of each ovatoxin.[133] Absolute *m/z* values of such ions in the OVTX-b spectrum were practically superimposable with those of OVTX-a, thus suggesting that the two compounds share the same part structure B at least in elemental composition. Regarding OVTX-c, -d, and -e, identification of the monoisotopic ion peak for each ion cluster was hampered by their heavy overlapping, attributed to their incomplete chromatographic separation. Based only on full MS results, therefore, an unambiguous assignment of elemental formula to each fragment ion was not possible.

TABLE 24.3

HRMS Data of Palytoxin (PLTX), Putative PLTX (p-PLTX), and Ovatoxin-a (OVTX-a), OVTX-b, OVTX-c, OVTX-d, and OVTX-e, Obtained from Full MS Spectra Acquired in the Mass Ranges m/z 2000–3000 and m/z 800–1400

	PLTX	p-PLTX[a]	OVTX-a	OVTX-b	OVTX-c	OVTX-d	OVTX-e
Monocharged ions							
$[M+H]^+$	2679.4893	2679.4721	2647.4979	2691.5233	2707.5173	2663.4905	2663.4905
Formula	$C_{129}H_{224}N_3O_{54}$	$C_{129}H_{224}N_3O_{54}$	$C_{129}H_{224}N_3O_{52}$	$C_{131}H_{228}N_3O_{53}$	$C_{131}H_{228}N_3O_{54}$	$C_{129}H_{224}N_3O_{53}$	$C_{129}H_{224}N_3O_{53}$
RDB, Δ ppm	19.5, 0.907	19.5, −5.512	19.5, 0.325	19.5, 0.017	19.5, −0.321	19.5, −0.546	19.5, −0.546
$[M+H–H_2O]^+$	2661.4744		2629.4844	2673.5112	2689.5056	2645.4797	2645.4797
Formula	$C_{129}H_{222}N_3O_{53}$		$C_{129}H_{222}N_3O_{51}$	$C_{131}H_{226}N_3O_{52}$	$C_{131}H_{226}N_3O_{53}$	$C_{129}H_{222}N_3O_{52}$	$C_{129}H_{222}N_3O_{52}$
RDB, Δ ppm	20.5, −0.715		20.5, −0.789	20.5, −0.557	20.5, −0.745	20.5, −0.639	20.5, −0.639
$[M+H–2H_2O]^+$	2643.4629		2611.4721	2655.5029		2627.4702	2627.4702
Formula	$C_{129}H_{220}N_3O_{52}$		$C_{129}H_{220}N_3O_{50}$	$C_{131}H_{224}N_3O_{51}$		$C_{129}H_{220}N_3O_{51}$	$C_{129}H_{220}N_3O_{51}$
RDB, Δ ppm	21.5, −1.074		21.5, −1.459	21.5, 0.292		21.5, −0.238	21.5, −0.238
$[M+H–3H_2O]^+$	2625.4487		2593.4686	2637.4915			
Formula	$C_{129}H_{218}N_3O_{51}$		$C_{129}H_{218}N_3O_{49}$	$C_{131}H_{222}N_3O_{50}$			
RDB, Δ ppm	22.5, −2.466		22.5, 1.255	22.5, −0.023			
$[M+H–A\ moiety]^+$	2335.2944		2303.2983	2303.2947	2319.2917	2319.2954	2303.2988
Formula	$C_{113}H_{196}NO_{48}$		$C_{113}H_{196}NO_{46}$	$C_{113}H_{196}NO_{46}$	$C_{113}H_{196}NO_{47}$	$C_{113}H_{196}NO_{47}$	$C_{113}H_{196}NO_{46}$
RDB, Δ ppm	16.5, 0.971		16.5, −1.738	16.5, −3.301	16.5, −2.379	16.5, −0.784	16.5, −1.521
$[M+H–A\ moiety–H_2O]^+$	2317.2842		2285.2893	2285.2866	2301.2830	2301.2871	2285.2913
Formula	$C_{113}H_{194}NO_{47}$		$C_{113}H_{194}NO_{45}$	$C_{113}H_{194}NO_{45}$	$C_{113}H_{194}NO_{46}$	$C_{113}H_{194}NO_{46}$	$C_{113}H_{194}NO_{45}$
RDB, Δ ppm	17.5, 1.136		17.5, −1.067	17.5, −2.248	17.5, −1.587	17.5, 0.194	17.5, −0.192
$[M+H–A\ moiety–2H_2O]^+$	2299.2734		2267.2793	2267.2759	2283.2710	2283.2776	2267.2808
Formula	$C_{113}H_{192}NO_{46}$		$C_{113}H_{192}NO_{44}$	$C_{113}H_{192}NO_{44}$	$C_{113}H_{192}NO_{45}$	$C_{113}H_{192}NO_{45}$	$C_{113}H_{192}NO_{44}$
RDB, Δ ppm	18.5, 1.043		18.5, −0.826	18.5, −2.326	18.5, −2.229	18.5, 0.662	18.5, −0.165
$[M+H–A\ moiety–3H_2O]^+$	2281.2634		2249.2693	2249.2671	2265.2622	2265.2668	2249.2725
Formula	$C_{113}H_{190}NO_{45}$		$C_{113}H_{190}NO_{43}$	$C_{113}H_{190}NO_{43}$	$C_{113}H_{190}NO_{44}$	$C_{113}H_{190}NO_{44}$	$C_{113}H_{190}NO_{43}$
RDB, Δ ppm	19.5, 1.298		19.5, −0.582	19.5, −1.560	19.5, −1.467	19.5, 0.563	19.5, 0.841

(*continued*)

TABLE 24.3 (continued)

HRMS Data of Palytoxin (PLTX), Putative PLTX (p-PLTX), and Ovatoxin-a (OVTX-a), OVTX-b, OVTX-c, OVTX-d, and OVTX-e, Obtained from Full MS Spectra Acquired in the Mass Ranges *m/z* 2000–3000 and *m/z* 800–1400

	PLTX	p-PLTX[a]	OVTX-a	OVTX-b	OVTX-c	OVTX-d	OVTX-e
Monocharged ions							
$[M+H-A\ moiety-4H_2O]^+$	2263.2522		2231.2578	2231.2556	2247.2502	2247.2551	2231.2620
Formula	$C_{113}H_{188}NO_{44}$		$C_{113}H_{188}NO_{42}$	$C_{113}H_{188}NO_{42}$	$C_{113}H_{188}NO_{43}$	$C_{113}H_{188}NO_{43}$	$C_{113}H_{188}NO_{42}$
RDB, Δ ppm	20.5, 1.028		20.5, −1.006	20.5, −1.992	20.5, −2.118	20.5, 0.063	20.5, 0.876
$[M+H-A\ moiety-5H_2O]^+$	2245.2415		2213.2493	2213.2446	2229.2393	2229.2480	2213.2498
Formula	$C_{113}H_{186}NO_{43}$		$C_{113}H_{186}NO_{41}$	$C_{113}H_{186}NO_{41}$	$C_{113}H_{186}NO_{42}$	$C_{113}H_{186}NO_{42}$	$C_{113}H_{186}NO_{41}$
RDB, Δ ppm	21.5, 0.976		21.5, −0.081	21.5, −2.205	21.5, −2.285	21.5, 1.617	21.5, 0.145
$[M+H-A\ moiety-6H_2O]^+$	2227.2310		2195.2385	2195.2351	2211.2319		
Formula	$C_{113}H_{184}NO_{42}$		$C_{113}H_{184}NO_{40}$	$C_{113}H_{184}NO_{40}$	$C_{113}H_{184}NO_{41}$		
RDB, Δ ppm	22.5, 1.013		22.5, −0.189	22.5, −1.738	22.5, −0.873		
Bicharged ions							
$[M+H+K]^{2+}$	1359.2194		1343.2262	1365.2393	1373.2346	1351.2231	1351.2231
Formula	$C_{129}H_{224}KN_3O_{54}$		$C_{129}H_{224}KN_3O_{52}$	$C_{131}H_{228}KN_3O_{53}$	$C_{131}H_{228}KN_3O_{54}$	$C_{129}H_{224}KN_3O_{53}$	$C_{129}H_{224}KN_3O_{53}$
RDB, Δ ppm	19.0, −4.130		19.0, −2.903	19.0, −2.861	19.0, −4.416	19.0, −3.298	19.0, −3.298
$[M+H+Na]^{2+}$	1351.2377		1335.2435	1357.2540	1365.2510	1343.2411	1343.2411
Formula	$C_{129}H_{224}N_3NaO_{54}$		$C_{129}H_{224}N_3NaO_{52}$	$C_{131}H_{228}N_3NaO_{53}$	$C_{131}H_{228}N_3NaO_{54}$	$C_{129}H_{224}N_3NaO_{53}$	$C_{129}H_{224}N_3NaO_{53}$
RDB, Δ ppm	19.0, −0.255		19.0, 0.277	19.0, −1.649	19.0, −1.974	19.0, 0.381	19.0, 0.381
$[M+2H]^{2+}$	1340.2462	1340.2479	1324.2534	1346.2655	1354.2620	1332.2484	1332.2484
Formula	$C_{129}H_{225}N_3O_{54}$	$C_{129}H_{225}N_3O_{54}$	$C_{129}H_{225}N_3O_{52}$	$C_{131}H_{229}N_3O_{53}$	$C_{131}H_{229}N_3O_{54}$	$C_{129}H_{225}N_3O_{53}$	$C_{129}H_{225}N_3O_{53}$
RDB, Δ ppm	19.0, −0.651	19.0, 0.617	19.0, 0.938	19.0, 0.174	19.0, −0.534	19.0, −0.912	19.0, −0.912
$[M+2H-H_2O]^{2+}$	1331.2417	1331.2417	1315.2480	1337.2595	1345.2566	1323.2439	1323.2439
Formula	$C_{129}H_{223}N_3O_{53}$	$C_{129}H_{223}N_3O_{53}$	$C_{129}H_{223}N_3O_{51}$	$C_{131}H_{227}N_3O_{52}$	$C_{131}H_{227}N_3O_{53}$	$C_{129}H_{223}N_3O_{52}$	$C_{129}H_{223}N_3O_{52}$
RDB, Δ ppm	20.0, −0.068	20.0, −0.068	20.0, 0.855	20.0, −0.361	20.0, −0.625	20.0, −0.327	20.0, −0.327
$[M+2H-2H_2O]^{2+}$	1322.2360		1306.2429	1328.2542	1336.2548	1314.2397	1314.2397

Formula	$C_{129}H_{221}N_3O_{52}$		$C_{129}H_{221}N_3O_{50}$	$C_{131}H_{225}N_3O_{51}$	$C_{131}H_{225}N_3O_{52}$	$C_{129}H_{221}N_3O_{51}$	$C_{129}H_{221}N_3O_{51}$
RDB, Δ ppm	21.0, −0.384		21.0, 1.000	21.0, −0.377	21.0, 1.977	21.0, 0.494	21.0, 0.494
$[M+2H-3H_2O]^{2+}$	1313.2303		1297.2334	1319.2498		1305.2328	1305.2328
Formula	$C_{129}H_{219}N_3O_{51}$		$C_{129}H_{219}N_3O_{49}$	$C_{131}H_{223}O_{50}N_3$		$C_{129}H_{219}N_3O_{50}$	$C_{129}H_{219}N_3O_{50}$
RDB, Δ ppm	22.0, −0.705		22.0, −2.244	22.0, 0.289		22.0, −0.742	22.0, −0.742
Tricharged ions							
$[M+2H+K]^{3+}$	906.4851	906.4861	895.8225	910.4976	915.8286	901.1533	901.1533
Formula	$C_{129}H_{225}KN_3O_{54}$	$C_{129}H_{225}KN_3O_{54}$	$C_{129}H_{225}KN_3O_{52}$	$C_{131}H_{229}KN_3O_{53}$	$C_{131}H_{229}KN_3O_{54}$	$C_{129}H_{225}KN_3O_{53}$	$C_{129}H_{225}KN_3O_{53}$
RDB, Δ ppm	18.5, −0.737	18.5, 0.366	18.5, 0.009	18.5, −0.326	18.5, −1.021	18.5, −0.921	18.5, −0.921
$[M+2H+Na]^{3+}$	901.1592	901.1603	890.4968	905.1717	910.5017	895.8281	895.8281
Formula	$C_{129}H_{225}N_3NaO_{54}$	$C_{129}H_{225}N_3NaO_{54}$	$C_{129}H_{225}N_3NaO_{52}$	$C_{131}H_{229}N_3NaO_{53}$	$C_{131}H_{229}N_3NaO_{54}$	$C_{129}H_{225}N_3NaO_{53}$	$C_{129}H_{225}N_3NaO_{53}$
RDB, Δ ppm	18.5, −2.133	18.5, −0.912	18.5, −1.174	18.5, −1.713	18.5, −3.502	18.5, −1.545	18.5, −1.545
$[M+3H-H_2O]^{3+}$	887.8308	887.8268	877.1687	891.8452	897.1757	882.5019	882.5019
Formula	$C_{129}H_{224}N_3O_{53}$	$C_{129}H_{224}N_3O_{53}$	$C_{129}H_{224}N_3O_{51}$	$C_{131}H_{228}N_3O_{52}$	$C_{131}H_{228}N_3O_{53}$	$C_{129}H_{224}N_3O_{52}$	$C_{129}H_{224}N_3O_{52}$
RDB, Δ ppm	19.5, 0.579	19.5, −3.926	19.5, 1.927	19.5, 3.124	19.5, 1.836	19.5, 3.685	19.5, 3.685
$[M+3H-2H_2O]^{3+}$	881.8273		871.1649	885.8421	891.1729	876.4982	876.4982
Formula	$C_{129}H_{222}N_3O_{52}$		$C_{129}H_{222}N_3O_{50}$	$C_{131}H_{226}N_3O_{51}$	$C_{131}H_{226}N_3O_{52}$	$C_{129}H_{222}N_3O_{51}$	$C_{129}H_{222}N_3O_{51}$
RDB, Δ ppm	20.5, 0.608		20.5, 1.621	20.5, 3.621	20.5, 2.658	20.5, 3.507	20.5, 3.507
$[M+3H-3H_2O]^{3+}$	875.8238		865.1615	879.8395	885.1697	870.4941	870.4941
Formula	$C_{129}H_{220}N_3O_{51}$		$C_{129}H_{220}N_3O_{49}$	$C_{131}H_{224}N_3O_{50}$	$C_{131}H_{224}N_3O_{51}$	$C_{129}H_{220}N_3O_{50}$	$C_{129}H_{220}N_3O_{50}$
RDB, Δ ppm	21.5, 0.636		21.5, 1.773	21.5, 4.693	21.5, 3.040	21.5, 2.867	21.5, 2.867

Source: Ciminiello, P., Dell'Aversano, C., Dello Iacovo, E., Fattorusso, E., Forino, M., Grauso, L., Tartaglione, L., Guerrini, F., and Pistocchi, R.: Complex palytoxin-like profile of *Ostreopsis ovata*. Identification of four new ovatoxins by high-resolution liquid chromatography/mass spectrometry. *Rapid. Commun. Mass Spectrom.* 2010, 24(18). 2735–2744. Copyright Wiley-VCH Verlag GmbH & Co. KGaA. Reproduced with Permission.

Note: Assignment of molecular formulae to the monoisotopic ion peaks of mono-, bi-, and tricharged ions, Relative double bonds (RDB) equivalent, and error (ppm).

[a] The presence of a small amount of putative PLTX in the *O. ovata* extract results in a very poor spectrum in the high mass range where only the [M+H]⁺ ion could be individuated.

This drawback was, however, overcome through interpretation of HRMS^2 spectra of the $[M+2H+K]^{3+}$ ions of ovatoxins, which paralleled that of PLTX in containing (1) abundant tricharged ion peaks due to subsequent losses of water molecules (two to seven) from the relevant precursor ion; (2) a diagnostic monocharged $[M+H–B\ moiety–H_2O]^+$ ion in the region m/z 300–400; and (3) diagnostic bicharged ions due to $[M+H+K–A\ moiety–nH_2O]^{2+}$ ($n = 0$–5); among them, the $[M+H+K–A\ moiety–2H_2O]^{2+}$ ion was the most abundant. From these studies, it was deducted that compared to OVTX-a, the A moiety of OVTX-b contained additional C_2H_4O atoms (ion at m/z 371.2181, $C_{18}H_{31}N_2O_6$ vs. m/z 327.1919, $C_{16}H_{27}N_2O_5$), whereas part structure B was identical (ion at m/z 1153.1189a vs. 1153.1194, $C_{113}H_{192}KNO_{44}$) at least in elemental composition. Based on structural features of PLTX-like compounds isolated by Uemura et al.[16] (homo-, bishomo-, neo-, and deoxy-PLTX), OVTX-b could present the potential addition of a hydroxyl group and two methylene groups in the A moiety, thus being a bishomo-hydroxy derivative of OVTX-a. Compared to OVTX-a, OVTX-c presented additional C_2H_4O atoms (potentially a hydroxyl and two methylene groups) in the A moiety (m/z 371.2179, $C_{18}H_{31}N_2O_6$ vs. 327.1919, $C_{16}H_{27}N_2O_5$) and an extra oxygen atom (potentially a hydroxyl group) in the B moiety (m/z 1161.1173, $C_{113}H_{192}KNO_{45}$, vs. 1153.1194, $C_{113}H_{192}KNO_{44}$). The MS^2 spectrum of the $[M+2H+K]^{3+}$ ion at m/z 901.4 highlighted the presence of two structural isomers, OVTX-d and -e. Comparison of the data obtained with those of OVTX-a indicated that OVTX-d possessed the same A moiety as OVTX-a (327.1919, $C_{16}H_{27}N_2O_5$) and one additional oxygen atom (potentially an additional hydroxyl group) in the B moiety (m/z 1161.1157, $C_{113}H_{192}KNO_{45}$ vs. 1153.1194, $C_{113}H_{192}KNO_{44}$). OVTX-e in comparison with OVTX-a contained one more oxygen atom (potentially an additional hydroxyl group) in the A moiety (m/z 343.1869, $C_{16}H_{27}N_2O_6$ vs. 327.1919, $C_{16}H_{27}N_2O_5$) and the same B-moiety (m/z 1153.1179 vs. 1153.1194, $C_{113}H_{192}KNO_{44}$).[133]

A quantitative study was also conducted to determine the relative abundance of p-PLTX and ovatoxins in the tested *O. ovata* culture extract.[133] Results indicated that the four new ovatoxins (OVTX-b, -c, -d, and -e) represented up to 46% of the total toxin content (Table 24.4). It was thus suggested that their presence should be taken into account in case of LC/MS-based monitoring programs of either plankton or contaminated seafood.

So far, toxin profiles of most field samples and cultured *O.* cf. *ovata* strains were all dominated by OVTX-a, which accounted for up to 89% of the total toxin content, followed by OVTX-b, OVTX-d+e, OVTX-c, and p-PLTX. Only in two cases of *O.* cf. *ovata* strains, some minor components of the toxin profiles were completely lacking, namely, OVTX-b and -c[80] and p-PLTX,[138] respectively, but still OVTX-a was the major component of the toxin profile. A different toxin profile from those previously reported for *O.* cf. *ovata*, both qualitatively and quantitatively, was revealed in a very recent investigation of a North Western Adriatic *O.* cf. *ovata* strain collected at Portonovo (Italy) in 2008 by HR-LC–MS.[135] For the first time, OVTX-a was not the dominant toxin in the profile, whereas a new PLTX congener, named OVTX-f, was detected (Figure 24.4).

Based on the combined analysis of all the singly, doubly, and triply charged ions contained in HR full MS spectra, the elemental formula $C_{131}H_{227}N_3O_{52}$ was assigned to OVTX-f. Therefore, compared to OVTX-a ($C_{129}H_{223}N_3O_{52}$), the OVTX-f elemental formula contains more C_2H_4 than that of OVTX-a. High-resolution collision-induced dissociation (CID) MS^n experiments revealed that structural differences between OVTX-a and -f are restricted to the region between C-95 and C-102, a region that has not previously been described to be modified in other PLTXs.

Interestingly, in the aforementioned analyzed strain (*O.* cf. *ovata* CBA2–122), OVTX-f represented the major component in the toxin profile accounting for 50% of the total toxin content, whereas OVTX-a, the dominant toxin in most of the Mediterranean *O.* cf. *ovata* strains so far analyzed, was the second major component of the toxin profile (23%), followed by OVTX-b (17%), OVTX-c (2.4%), OVTX-d+e (6.7%), and p-PLTX (0.3%). Thus, the presence of OVTX-f was suggested as an additional factor to be taken into account in monitoring programs for PLTX-like compounds in microalgae and/or seawater.[135]

Four new PLTX-like molecules, presenting slight differences from those reported along the last few years by the Ciminiello group, along with OVTX-a and McTX-A, were also reported by Rossi et al.[68] in cultured cells of *O.* cf. *ovata* from the Mediterranean sea, using an HR-LC coupled with ESI/TOF/MS method. Differences among the ovatoxin molecules in this study were located in the A moiety, whereas all four ovatoxins shared the same structure for part B, pointing to the conclusion that the absence of the m/z 327 fragment does not necessarily exclude the presence of a PLTX-like compound.

TABLE 24.4

Percentage (%) and Content on a Per Cell Basis (pg/cell) of Putative Palytoxin (p-PLTX) and Ovatoxins (OVTX-a, -b, -c, -d + -e, and -f) Contained in Field and Cultured *O.* cf. *ovata* Strains Analyzed So Far

Cultured/Field	Sampling Site (Sea, Region, Country), Date (Code)	p-PLTX %	p-PLTX pg/Cell	OVTX-a %	OVTX-a pg/Cell	OVTX-b %	OVTX-b pg/Cell	OVTX-c %	OVTX-c pg/Cell	OVTX-d+e %	OVTX-d+e pg/Cell	OVTX-f %	OVTX-f pg/Cell
Cultured	Portonovo (Adriatic, Marche, Italy), 2008 (CBA2–122)	0.3	0.1	23	8	17	6	2.4	0.8	6.7	2	50	17
Cultured	Numana (Adriatic, Marche, Italy), 2006 (OOAN0601)	0.6	0.2	54	18	27	9	6	2	12	4	n.d.[a]	n.d.
Field	Ancona (Adriatic, Marche, Italy), 2009	n.d.–3	n.d.–2	55–65	8–49	14–20	2–15	n.d.–6	n.d.–4	15–21	3–13	n.d.	n.d.
Field	Trieste (Adriatic, Friuli Venezia Giulia, Italy), 2009	n.d.	n.d.	77–89	45–64	5–14	4–8	n.d.–1	n.d.–0.7	4–9	3–5	n.d.	n.d.
Field	Rovinj (Adriatic, Croatia), 2010 (M. Pfannkuchen, personal commun.)	0.6–0.9	0.2–0.7	58–64	14–46	18–25	5–13	4–5	0.9–2	10–12	2–8	n.d.	n.d.
Cultured	Numana (Adriatic, Marche, Italy), 2008 (OOAN0816)	3	77	n.d.	n.d.	20	n.d.	n.d.					
Cultured	Numana (Adriatic, Marche, Italy), 2007 (OOAN0709), Bari (Adriatic, Puglia, Italy), 2008 (OOAB0801), Latina (Tyrrhenian, Lazio, Italy), 2007 (OOTL0707)	1–4	53–57	24–26	4–5	12–14	n.d.	n.d.					

Source: Reprinted with permission from Ciminiello, P., Dell' Aversano, C., Dello Iacovo, E., Fattorusso, E., Forino, M., Tartaglione, L, Battocchi, C., Crinelli, R., Carloni, E., Magnani, M., and Penna, A., Unique toxin profile of a Mediterranean *Ostreopsis* cf. *ovata* strain: HR LC-MS[n] characterization of ovatoxin-f, a new palytoxin congener, *Chem. Res. Toxicol.*, 25(6), 1243–1252. Copyright 2012 American Chemical Society.

[a] n.d., not detected.

A detailed toxin profile determination with regard to PLTX analogs in several Japanese *Ostreopsis* strains was conducted by LC–MS,[137] using an Italian *Ostreopsis* strain as reference material. The presence of OVTX-a, -b, -c, -d, and -e was reconfirmed. However, the most dominant PLTX analog in Japanese *Ostreopsis* was a novel PLTX analog, which was identified as an isomer of OVTX-a, whereas novel isomers of OVTX-b, -d, and -e were also detected. The isomers of OVTX-a, -b, -d, and -e detected in Japanese *Ostreopsis* were tentatively named OVTX-a AC, -b AC, -d AC, and -e AC, and the LC–MS analysis suggested that OVTX-a AC was a dideoxy-42-hydroxy-44-deoxy-PLTX, with the unidentified deoxy-positions assigned both between C16 and C20 and between C53 and C73.

24.4 Chemical Analysis Methods

24.4.1 Extraction and Purification of Palytoxin and Analogs

PLTX is quite soluble in water or other water-miscible solvents, so ethanol and methanol are the most common solvents used to extract PLTX. Isolation and purification of PLTX from Hawaiian *Palythoa*, as initially reported,[1] were conducted in a series of extraction steps of the polyps for 2–3 h by use of 70% aqueous ethanol, followed by blending and washing of the ground polyps' residue. Ethanol was removed from combined extracts by evaporation under reduced pressure at 50°C, and the concentrate was defatted by a triplicate benzene extraction and duplicate extraction with portions of 1-butanol saturated with water. Butanolic extracts were backwashed thrice with water saturated with 1-butanol. After removal of the dissolved 1-butanol under reduced pressure at 50°C, the combined aqueous portion was desalted and further purified with ion-exchange chromatography. A variety of modified procedures, involving aqueous methanol or ethanol and different methods of LC, thin-layer chromatography, or electrophoresis, were employed for PLTX extraction and purification from zoanthids or other marine species.[11,14,16,17,34,44,50,56,75,139] An isolation protocol, however, with acetone as the initial extraction solvent and subsequent extraction with diethyl ether and 1-butanol followed by column LC and HPLC was also reported.[47]

A completely different approach was adopted to isolate PLTX from *L. pictor* crab, using hot aqueous extraction and acidification followed by column LC.[140] This method was later applied for toxin extraction from the crab species provided earlier, to investigate a documented human poisoning outbreak caused by crab soup.[139,141] Under the boiling conditions employed, the toxin was heat resistant[59]; nevertheless, a subsequent modification with aqueous ethanol as extracting solvent instead of heat resulted in both higher yields and increase in specific activities.[139]

Isolation and purification of cultured *Ostreopsis* spp.-derived PLTX analogs for toxicological studies or chemical analysis are conducted with more or less similar procedures, involving cell harvesting by filtering or centrifugation and subsequent extraction with pure or aqueous methanol[31,33,35,37–39,115] or aqueous ethanol,[36] with or without mild sonication. Cell pellet is removed by centrifugation, followed by supernatant defatting with diethyl ether, hexane dichloromethane, or chloroform and partitioning between water and 1-butanol. Mouse toxicity data and chromatographic separation and identification results are contradictory as PLTX analogs are detected both in the 1-butanol fraction[31,33,35,38] and in the aqueous fraction.[36] Some methods exclude the butanol/water partitioning step and proceed to analysis using the methanolic culture extracts obtained after defatting, with[39] or without[37] cleanup by solid phase extraction (SPE).

24.4.2 Detection and Quantification

Due to their recent expansion of its occurrence in areas with temperate climate where it was not earlier considered as a threat, such as the Mediterranean, PLTX, and analogs are nowadays perceived as one of the most important emerging toxin groups. Currently, there are no regulations on PLTX-group toxins in shellfish, either in the EU or in other regions of the world. During the first meeting of the working group on Toxicology of the national reference laboratories for Marine Biotoxins (Cesenatico, Italy, October 24–25, 2005), a provisional limit of 250 µg/kg shellfish was proposed.[142] Subsequently, on request of the EU Commission, the EFSA Panel on Contaminants in the Food Chain (CONTAM Panel) assessed the risks to human health related to the presence of PLTX-group toxins in shellfish[6] and concluded that analysis methods, other than the MBA, should be further developed and optimized with respect to selectivity and sensitivity for PLTX-group toxins in shellfish tissues, whereas subsequent (interlaboratory) validation studies are also necessary.

In this context, regulatory monitoring for this toxin group as well as purity checks of the toxin extracted in research would require the existence of appropriate methods for detection and quantification. Both analytical and biological methods (see also Chapter 27) can be employed to achieve detection and quantification of PLTX in biological samples, and a combination of methods is often required in order to positively confirm its presence. The MBA constitutes the simplest and most sensitive method to detect PLTX in terms of detection limit; it involves intraperitoneal injection of extracts from contaminated samples to mice and recording of symptomatology and death times. Lethal potency is expressed as mouse units (MUs), where 1 MU is the amount of toxin that kills a 20 g mouse in 24 h. One MU is presumed to be 9 ng of PLTX, based on the reported LD_{50} value of 450 ng/kg.[34] Upon injection with PLTX, mice exhibit a characteristic symptomatology prior to death, which includes sudden jerks and convulsions. Nevertheless, the MBA is only indicative as it is unable to unequivocally prove the implicated causative agent. Numerous alternative assays based on certain functional properties of PLTX and with very favorable detection limits have been reported, among which in vitro cytotoxicity,[41,42,143–145] delayed hemolysis,[146] monoclonal antibody-based enzyme-linked immunoassays,[147] and the fluorescence polarization technique.[148] These assays are all extremely sensitive; however, positive results would require further confirmation by instrumental methods in case of application for regulatory purposes.

Research with regard to the development of chemical analysis methods for the determination of PLTX and analogs, taking advantage of the characteristic chemical properties of this toxin group, is ongoing. Methods developed so far include (1) IR spectrometry, (2) UV spectrometry, (3) MS, (4) high-performance capillary electrophoresis, (5) thin layer chromatography (TLC), and (6) LC, combined with UV or MS detection. The most important currently available quantitative chemical analysis methods and their main features are summarized in Table 24.5.

24.4.2.1 Infrared Spectrometry

The IR spectrum of *P. toxica* PLTX shows a band at 1670 cm^{-1}, assigned to the presence of an α,β-unsaturated amide carbonyl group,[1] while this band has been observed at 1655 cm^{-1} in the case of *P. tuberculosa* PLTX in potassium bromide (KBr).[75] Similar IR spectra have been reported for purified PLTXs from *P. caribaeorum*,[14] from the sea anemone *R. macrodactylus* (1670 cm^{-1}, assigned to amide carbonyl)[50] and from the xanthid crab *L. pictor*.[59]

24.4.2.2 Ultraviolet Spectrometry

As discussed in a previous section, PLTX possesses a characteristic UV spectrum with two absorption peaks at 233 and 263 nm, attributed to the presence of respective chromophores (Figure 24.2). The absorbance ratio of the 233 vs. 263 nm peak with an approximate value of 1.7[1] is considered as characteristic and indicative of PLTX presence. Absorption values at either wavelength have been demonstrated to be linearly related to PLTX concentration in the range of 5–20 μg/mL. A disadvantage of this method that limits its suitability as a regulatory analysis method, however, lies in its detection limit, since a minimum detectable concentration of 5 μg/mL (PLTX standard in water) has been reported, whereas concentrations as low as 0.05–0.1 μg/mL are enough to produce toxicological and physiological effects.[149]

24.4.2.3 Mass Spectrometry

A number of characteristic MS data that were used to determine molecular weights and elucidate structural differences between PLTXs from various origins and PLTX analogs have already been mentioned in a previous section. Ion-spray MS has been commonly implemented for PLTX and analogs' detection,

TABLE 24.5

Comparative Table of Most Important Quantitative Chemical Analysis Methods for Palytoxin and Analogs

Method	Toxin	Matrix	Column Details	Mobile Phase	Flow Rate	Detection Details	Limit of Detection (LOD)	Injection Volume	Retention Time (min)	References
LC–MS										
Reversed-phase LC-ESI-MS/MS3	PLTX, OST	Reference PLTX + Ostreopsis cultures	5 μm Gemini C18 (150 × 2 mm) Temperature: Ambient	A: Water + 30 mM acetic acid B: 95% acetonitrile/water + 30 mM acetic acid	0.2 mL/min, Gradient (20%–100% B over 10 min and hold 4 min)	Positive ion mode, SIM (m/z 1340 and 912) and MRM (m/z 1340 → 327 and 912 → 327), Bicharged and tricharged ions	PLTX standard: SIM: 40 ng/mL MRM: • 25 ng/mL (MeOH/H_2O 1:1) • 39 ng/mL (butanol extract) • 38 ng/mL (pellet extract)	5 μL	PLTX standard: SIM: 6.45 MRM: 6.40 OST (pellet and butanol extract): SIM: 6.45 MRM: 6.45	[38]
LC–FLD–MS	PLTX, OST	Reference PLTX + Ostreopsis ovata and O. cf. siamensis (derivatized and nonderivatized with 6-aminoquinolyl-N-hyroxysuccinimidyl carbamate, Acc-Q)	5 μm Xterra C18 (150 × 2.1 mm) Temperature: 35°C	A: MeOH B: 2 mM aqueous ammonium acetate pH = 5.8	0.3 mL/min Gradient (Initial: 20% A; linear rise over 5 min to 60% A; linear rise from 5–15 min to 80% A; 15–25 min steady 80% A; linear decrease from 80% to 20% A between 25–27 min and from 27–30 min steady 20% A)	• Fluorescence: Excitation 250 nm, emission 395 nm • Positive ion mode, mass range m/z 100–2000 Ionization parameters: capillary temperature 300°C ± 1°C, spray voltage 4.5 kV, sheath gas 20 mL/min, aux. gas 5 mL/min. • Detection of bicharged ion m/z 1362.7 $[M+2Na]^{2+}$ • Loss of m/z 327 fragment	PLTX standard: 7.5 ng LOQ = 20 ng	Not reported	Not reported	[39]

LC-ESI-MS	PLTX, OST	Reference PLTX + *Ostreopsis ovata* cultures	5 μm Xterra C18 (150 × 2.1 mm) Temperature: 35°C	A: MeOH B: [MeOH: 0.1 M ammonium acetate, pH = 4.0, (58:42)]	0.1 mL/min Gradient (Initial) 100% B for 16 min; 16–18 min linear rise to 100% A; 18–22 min steady 100% A; 22–25 min linear decrease to 100% B; 25–30 min 100% B)	Positive ion mode, mass range *m/z* 200–1500. Ionization parameters: capillary temperature 300°C ± 1°C, spray voltage 4.5 kV, sheath gas 20 mL/min, aux. gas 5 mL/min	Not reported	Not reported	Not reported	[37]
Micro-LC-ESI-MS/MS	PLTX, OST (McTX-A and McTX-B)	Reference PLTX + *Ostreopsis mascarenensis* cultures	5 μm RP Equisil BDS C18 silica (100 × 1 mm) or 5 μm RP Hypersil C18 (250 × 1 mm) Temperature: not reported	A: Water + trifluoroacetic acid (pH 2.5) B: Acetonitrile	0.05 mL/min, Gradient (30%–70% B over 45 min)	Positive ion mode, SRM (*m/z* 912 → 327), Tricharged ions. Collision energy: 100 eV	Not reported	1 μL	PLTX standard: Not reported McTX-A: SRM (*m/z* 327): 9.9 McTX-b: SRM (*m/z* 327): 10.25	[35]
HR-LC–MS and MS^{n}	PLTX p-PLTX, OVTXs a-f	Reference PLTX + *Ostreopsis ovata* extracts (cultures and field samples)	3 μm Gemini C18 (150 × 2 mm) Temperature: Ambient	A: Water + 30 mM acetic acid B: 95% Acetonitrile/water + 30 mM acetic acid	0.2 mL/min, Gradient (20%–50% B over 20 min, 50%–80% B over 10 min, 80%–100% B in 1 min, and hold for 5 min)	Positive ion mode/HR full MS experiments, range: *m/z* 800–1400 and *m/z* 2000–3000 (see Table 24.6 for principal ions used)	Not reported	5 μL	p-PLTX: TIC: 10.95 XIC: 10.56 OVTX-a: TIC: 11.30 XIC: 11.24 OVTX-b: TIC: 10.95 XIC: 10.98	[67,133,135]

(continued)

TABLE 24.5 (continued)

Comparative Table of Most Important Quantitative Chemical Analysis Methods for Palytoxin and Analogs

Method	Toxin	Matrix	Column Details	Mobile Phase	Flow Rate	Detection Details	Limit of Detection (LOD)	Injection Volume	Retention Time (min)	References
									OVTX-c: TIC: 10.95 XIC: 10.65 OVTX-d+e: TIC: 10.95 XIC: 10.89 OVTX-f: TIC: 11.30 XIC: 11.32	
LC/TOF/MS	PLTX, OST	Reference PLTX + *Ostreopsis ovata* extracts	3μm HILIC Luna 200A (150 × 2 mm)	A: Water + 0.1% formic acid B: 95% Acetonitrile/ water + 0.1% formic acid	0.3 mL/min, Gradient [from the beginning to 2 min steady to 10% A; linear rise over 3 min rising to 50% B; from 5 to 10 steady at 50% B; then a linear fall from 50% B to 10% A (initial conditions)]	Positive ion mode/ mass range set at m/z 100–3000 μ	Not reported	5 μL	Not reported	[68]

Technique	Toxins	Sample	Column	Mobile phase	Flow/Gradient	Detection	LOD/LOQ	Injection volume	Notes	References
LC-ESI-MS/MS	PLTX	Reference PLTX and seafood tissue (mussels, sea urchins, anchovies)	3 µm Gemini C18 (150 × 2 mm) Temperature: Ambient	A: Water + 30 mM acetic acid B: 95% Acetonitrile/water + 30 mM acetic acid	0.2 mL/min Gradient (20%–100% B over 10 min and hold 4 min)	Positive ion mode, MRM (m/z 1340.7 → 327.1 and 1331.7 → 327.1)	LOQ (corrected for recovery): • Mussels: 228 µg/kg • Sea urchins: 343 µg/kg; • Anchovies: 500 µg/kg	5 µL	Not reported	[52,152]
LC-ESI-MS/MS	PLTX, OVTX-a	Reference PLTX, *Ostreopsis* extracts and seafood tissue (mussels, wedge clams, Manila clams, sea urchins)	5 µm Gemini C18 (150 × 2 mm) Temperature: 20°C	A: Water + 2 mM ammonium formate and 50 mM formic acid B: 95% Acetonitrile/water + 2 mM ammonium formate and 50 mM formic acid	0.2 mL/min, Gradient (20%–100% B over 10 min and hold 4 min)	Positive ion mode, MRM (PLTX: m/z 1340 → 327 and 1332 → 327 and OVTX-a: 1324 → 327 and 1315 → 327)	LOD and LOQ (not corrected for recovery): • Mussels: 9 and 23 µg PLTX/kg whole tissue • Sea urchins: 10 and 25 µg PLTX/kg whole tissue	5 µL	Not reported	[53]
HPLC–UV HPLC–UV-DAD	PLTX, OST	Reference PLTX + *Ostreopsis ovata* cultures	5 µm Xterra C18 (150 × 4.6 mm) Temperature: 35°C	A: MeOH B: [MeOH: 0.1 M ammonium acetate, pH = 4.0, (58:42)]	0.75 mL/min Gradient (Initial: 100% B for 16 min; 16–18 min linear rise to 100% A; 18–22 min steady 100%)	UV @ 230 and 263 nm	1–2 µg injected quantity	Injected quantity 1.25 µg PLTX standard (50 µL from 25 µg/mL)	PLTX standard and *O. ovata* toxin: ≅ 9	[37,39, Riobó P. (personal communication)]

(continued)

TABLE 24.5 (continued)

Comparative Table of Most Important Quantitative Chemical Analysis Methods for Palytoxin and Analogs

Method	Toxin	Matrix	Column Details	Mobile Phase	Flow Rate	Detection Details	Limit of Detection (LOD)	Injection Volume	Retention Time (min)	References
HPLC–UV–DAD	PLTX, OST (McTX-A and McTX-B)	Reference PLTX + *Ostreopsis mascarenensis* cultures	5 μm Hypersil ODS C18 (250 × 4.6 mm) Temperature: not reported	A: Water + trifluoroacetic acid (pH 2.5) B: Acetonitrile	1 mL/min, Gradient (linear 30%–70% B over 45 min) A; 22–25 min linear decrease to 100% B; 25–30 min 100% B)	UV @ 230 nm	Not reported	Injected dose 1.25 μg	PLTX standard: 8.5 McTX-A: 8.3 McTX-B: 8.8	[35]
HPLC–UV	PLTX	Reference PLTX, toxin extracted from *Palythoa* aff. *margaritae*	Cosmosil 5PE (250 × 4.6 mm) Temperature: not reported	25% aqueous MeCN with 0.1% AcOH	1 mL/min Isocratic	UV @ 263 nm	PLTX standard and toxin *P.* aff *margaritae*: Aliquots of 7.5 mg sample	Not reported	PLTX standard: 8 min 55 s Toxin *P.* aff *margaritae*: 8 min 58 s	[17]
HPLC–UV	PLTX	Reference PLTX	BIO-SIL 5 ODS (250 × 4 mm) Temperature: not reported	52:48 water: acetonitrile with 0.1% trifluoroacetic acid	1 mL/min, Isocratic	UV @ 230 nm	125 ng/ injection (≅ 2.5 μg/mL)	50 μL from 2.5 μg/mL	PLTX standard: 9.8	[149]

HPLC–UV	PLTX	Reference PLTX, toxins extracted from *L. pictor* and *D. alcalai* crabs	(i) ERC ODS-1282 (250 × 6 mm) (ii) ERC ODS-1282 (250 × 6 mm) (iii) TSK G3000SW (600 × 7.5 mm)	(i) MeOH: 0.1N acetic acid (8:2) (ii) MeOH: 0.1N acetic acid (5:5) (iii) 0.03N acetic acid	0.9 mL/min, Isocratic in all (i)–(iii)	UV @ 263 nm	Not reported	Not reported	PLTX standard and crab toxins: (i) ≈ 13–14 (ii) ≈ 5–6 (iii) ≈ 17–18	[44]
HPLC-FLD	HPLC–FLD PLTX, OST	Reference PLTX + *Ostreopsis ovata* and *O. cf. siamensis* cultures	5 μm Xterra C18 (150 × 4.6 mm) Temperature: 35°C	A: MeOH B: 2 mM aqueous ammonium acetate pH = 5.8	0.75 mL/min Gradient (Initial: 100% B for 16 min; 16–18 min linear rise to 100% A; 18–22 min steady 100% A; 22–25 min linear decrease to 100% B; 25–30 min 100% B)	• Derivatization with 6-aminoquinolyl-*N*-hyroxysuccinimidyl-carbamate • SPE cleanup • Fluorescence: Excitation 250 nm, emission 395 nm	PLTX standard (derivatized): 0.75 ng Recovery: 95.13% ± 7.80% (S.D.) LOQ = 2 ng	Not reported	PLTX standard: ≈13.5 OST (derivatized extract): ≈13.5	[39]

(continued)

TABLE 24.5 (continued)

Comparative Table of Most Important Quantitative Chemical Analysis Methods for Palytoxin and Analogs

Method	Toxin	Matrix	Column Details	Mobile Phase	Flow Rate	Detection Details	Limit of Detection (LOD)	Injection Volume	Retention Time (min)	References
HPCE HPCE-UV	PLTX	Reference PLTX and toxin extracted from *L. pictor* crab	50 cm × 50 μm, uncoated Voltage: 15 kV cross 50 cm Temperature: not reported	Electrolyte solution: 25 mM borate buffer at pH 8.5	—	UV @ 230 and 263 nm	Not reported	PLTX standard: 16,720 MU/mL *L. pictor* toxin: 14,400 MU/mL Inj. pressure: 20 psi/s	PLTX standard and *L. pictor* toxin: ≅ 3.5	[139]
HPCE-UV	PLTX	Reference PLTX	50 cm × 75 μm Voltage: 15 kV cross 50 cm Temperature: 25°C	Electrolyte solution: 25 mM borate buffer at pH 8.5	—	UV @ 230 and 263 nm	0.5 pg/ injection (≅ 100 ng/mL)	5 nL from 100 ng/mL	PLTX standard: 9.0	[149]

PLTX, Palytoxin; OST, Analogues produced from *Ostreopsis* spp.; OVTX, Ovatoxin; LC-MS, Liquid chromatography—Mass spectrometry; TIC, Total ion chromatogram; XIC, Extracted ion chromatogram; SIM, Single ion monitoring; MRM, Multiple reaction monitoring; LOQ, Limit of quantification; HPLC, High performance liquid chromatography; HPCE, High performance capillary electrophoresis.

whereas MS data strongly indicative regarding their presence in a matrix include (1) the fragment ion at or near $m/z = 327$ in the bivalent and trivalent positive ion MS/MS spectra; (2) the presence of peaks at or near $m/z = 1340$ and $m/z = 912$, corresponding to the bicharged ion $[M + 2H]^{2+}$ and the tricharged ion $[M + 2H + NH_4]^{3+}$, the usual precursor ions used in multiple reaction monitoring (MRM) experiments that are able to yield the product ion $m/z = 327$ (transitions m/z $1340 \rightarrow 327$ and $912 \rightarrow 327$); (3) multiple water molecule losses from the $[M + 2H]^{2+}$ ion, attributed to the numerous hydroxyl moieties contained in PLTX and PLTX-like substances; and (4) a molecular mass around 2600 Da.[35,37,38] As previously pointed out, however, the possibility of a PLTX-like substance cannot be excluded by the absence of the $m/z = 327$ fragment ion, as this could indicate a PLTX analog differing in the A-moiety of the molecule, responsible for the formation of the $m/z = 327$ fragment ion.[45]

24.4.2.4 High-Performance Capillary Electrophoresis

Identification and detection of PLTX can be achieved with significant sensitivity by means of high-performance capillary electrophoresis (HPCE) (Table 24.5). HPCE with UV detection at 230 and 263nm using an open-capillary and a voltage of 15 kV across a 50 cm × 75 μm column (column temperature: 25°C; conducting buffer solution: 25 mM sodium borate/pH 8.5) has been successfully applied for PLTX detection, with a detection limit of 0.5 pg and a twofold detection sensitivity at 230 vs. 263 nm.[149] Similarly, HPCE has been used for PLTX derived from *L. pictor* crab.[141] The advantage of HPCE vs. other methods is that it can measure PLTX at low concentrations and in small volumes as well as its applicability for PLTX determination in biological fluids.[149]

24.4.2.5 Thin Layer Chromatography

TLC is applicable in both PLTX detection and extracted PLTX homogeneity tests.[14,141,150] One of the reported TLC methods involved the use of silica gel plates developed with pyridine–water–n-butanol–acetic acid at a ratio 10:12:15:13; toxin was stained purple with ninhydrin in ethanol, and Rf of PLTX was 0.55.[14] The same solvent mixture with cellulose plates was applied in another method, in which two close ninhydrin positive spots were observed, at Rf 0.67 for the major and Rf 0.75 for the minor spot.[150] TLC was also carried out for the comparison of pure PLTX with toxins extracted from the crabs *L. pictor* and *D. alcalai*,[44] on silica gel 60 and NH_2F_{254}s plates using two different solvent systems: (A) pyridine–water–n-butanol–acetic acid (10:12:15:13) and (B) 1-pentanol–pyridine–water (7:7:6). For toxin detection, the silica gel plates were heated after spraying with H_2SO_4, while on the NH_2F_{254}s plates, detection was achieved by exposure to UV light (254 nm). In the silica gel 60 plates, the Rfs recorded for pure PLTX were 0.50 with solvent A and 0.35 and 0.60 (two spots) for solvent B, while respective Rfs for the NH_2F_{254}s plates were 0.76 with solvent A and 0.19 and 0.20 for solvent B. Regardless of plate type and solvent mixture used, the toxins extracted from both crab species had identical Rfs with pure PLTX. In another work, comparison of the toxin extracted from the triggerfish *M. vidua* was conducted using a similar but slightly modified method.[47] The same types of plates were used, combined with solvent A and a modified solvent B (1-propanol–pyridine–water, 7:7:6), detection involved spraying the plates with a sulfuric acid–methanol (1:1) solution and subsequent charring at 150°C, whereas measured Rfs were slightly different. A fluorescent PLTX congener was isolated by employing a two-dimensional TLC; solvents used were n-butanol–acetic acid–water (9:3:8) followed by n-propanol–water (7:3) in the first dimension followed by n-propanol–25% ammonia in the second dimension.[141] The fluorescent spot observed with this method also stained yellow with exposure to iodine vapor in a chamber and purple with ninhydrin.[59]

24.4.2.6 Liquid Chromatography

LC has been a technique of significant importance regarding the purification of PLTX extracted from its sources. Additionally, a number of LC methods have been employed over the years in purpose of PLTX and analogs' identification, detection, and quantification. Most of the existing methods involve HPLC with ultraviolet detection (HPLC–UV), based on the characteristic UV spectrum (230 and 263 nm) of PLTX. Interferences, however, are very often the cause of remarkable sensitivity reduction of HPLC–UV methods, thus resulting in poor performance characteristics and/or high detection limits, especially in the case of analyzing biological matrices (e.g., phytoplankton cells, marine animal tissues). In this context, the applicability of these methods for regulatory purposes is hindered. In order to overcome such sensitivity issues, a number of LC methods combined with fluorescence detection (HPLC–FLD) or MS detection (LC–MS) have been set up in the last few years.

24.4.2.6.1 HPLC–UV

Chromatographic separation of PLTX and its analogs in purpose of studying reference PLTX and toxin identification in matrices related to food poisoning incidents has significantly relied on HPLC–UV methods. PLTX extracted from two species of xanthid crabs was analyzed and identified by HPLC together with reference PLTX by use of three different combinations of analytical column and mobile phases.[44] In all three combinations, retention times of crab toxins were comparable to those of reference PLTX (Table 24.5). Similar but slightly modified methods have been employed for the identification of the triggerfish *M. vidua* toxin (column: TSK G3000SW [600 × 7.5 mm]; mobile phase 0.1 M acetic acid; flow rate: 1.0 mL/min; detection: UV absorption at 263 nm)[47] and for the identification of the toxin contained in the crab species *D. reynaudii* (column: ERC-ODS [250 × 6 mm]; mobile phase acetonitrile: 0.05N acetic acid (1:1); flow rate: 0.9 mL/min; detection: UV absorption at 263 nm).[56] Reference PLTX detection was achieved by use of a Bio-Sil 5 ODS column at a level of 125 ng/injection[149] (Table 24.5), whereas analysis of Caribbean PLTX by HPLC has also been conducted using a Novapak C18 reversed phase column (75 × 3.9 mm) by gradient elution with 80% acetonitrile:water (4:1) and detection at 230 nm.[141] Similarly, Caribbean PLTX has also been analyzed by reversed-phase HPLC with a lower tracing quantity of 10 μg [column: Lichrospher 300 RP-8; mobile phase 0.1% TFA and 80% acetonitrile; linear gradient; detection: UV absorption at 230 nm].[19] PLTX detection by other HPLC methods with different combinations of columns and solvent mixtures has also been reported.[17,34]

A number of HPLC–UV methods have also been developed for the determination of PLTX analogs obtained from extracts of *Ostreopsis* cells. The toxically active n-BSF extracted from *O. mascarenensis* cells obtained from a natural bloom in the Southwestern Indian Ocean was compared with reference PLTX by HPLC–UV analysis with diode array detection (Table 24.5); the presence of two different PLTX analogs, namely, McTX-A and McTX-B, with similar retention times and identical UV spectra to those of reference PLTX was reported.[35] The same HPLC–UV method (Table 24.5) has been employed for the detection of PLTX-like substances with the same UV spectra and retention times compared to reference PLTX in culture extracts of *O. ovata* and *O.* cf. *siamensis* isolated from Brazil and from the western Mediterranean Sea.[37,39] In these studies, however, the minimum detectable quantity for reference PLTX was in the range of 1–2 μg/injection, while it was not always possible to detect a peak and obtain a spectrum for confirmation in the toxic *Ostreopsis* extracts.[39]

So far, there are no reports on the successful application of HPLC–UV methods for quantitative determination of PLTX and analogs in shellfish samples. Taking also into consideration the reported quality parameters, especially in terms of limits of detection (LODs), of the aforementioned HPLC–UV methods (see Table 24.5) in conjunction with the provisional limit for PLTXs of 250 μg/kg tissue, proposed by the Community Reference Laboratory for Marine Biotoxins[142] or with the tolerance limit of 30 μg/kg suggested by the European Food Safety Authority,[6] it is highly unlikely that these methods could be of routine use for regulatory monitoring of PLTX and its analogs in shellfish tissues.

24.4.2.6.2 HPLC–FLD

Sensitivity of HPLC–FLD methods is generally considered to be increased compared to that of HPLC–UV methods. Despite the fact that PLTX is not a naturally fluorescent substance,[45] a precolumn derivatization method for PLTX separation and quantification was developed, using the derivatization reagent 6-aminoquinolyl-N-hyroxysuccinimidyl carbamate (AccQ-Fluor) and taking advantage of the amino terminal group of the PLTX molecule.[39] This method was successfully applied for the determination and quantification of reference PLTX from *P. tuberculosa* as well as of toxins contained in methanolic extracts obtained from 14 different strains of cultured *Ostreopsis* cells. Cell extracts were cleaned up using SPE with two retention mechanisms: anion exchange and reverse phase without silanol groups followed by LC–FLD separation [column: C18, 5 μm, 150 × 4.6 mm i.d.; flow rate: 0.6 mL/min; excitation WL: 250 nm; emission WL: 395 nm] (Table 24.5). Detection limits for derivatized reference PLTX were as low as 0.75 ng/injection and therefore much lower compared to previously described HPLC–UV methods. Several quality data and characteristics of the method, that is, limit of quantification (LOQ; 2 ng), recovery (95.13% ± 7.80% S.D.), correlation with the hemolysis method ($r^2 = 0.9118$), stability of the fluorescent derivatives (reference PLTX and spiked samples stable for up to 2 weeks at 4°C), and lack of interferences with possible effects on quantification, point to a sufficient robustness of the method, with a potential applicability for routine use after optimization for use in shellfish extracts.

24.4.2.6.3 LC–MS

MS has been extremely useful for PLTX and analogs' identification and structure elucidation in numerous studies. Due to the low sensitivity of HPLC–UV methods when applied to PLTX analysis, it was reasonably examined as an alternative, combined with LC, for the determination of these toxins in *Palythoa* and *Ostreopsis* extracts as well as in biological tissue matrices, such as shellfish and sea urchins (Table 24.5).

LC-ESI–MS methods developed for the determination of PLTX and analogs in various biological matrices primarily rely on certain MS data (see also Sections 24.2.2.3 and 24.4.2.3 on Mass Spectrometry) denoting the presence of PLTX or its analogs: (1) presence of the $m/z = 327$ fragment ion in the bivalent and trivalent positive ion MS/MS spectra, (2) presence of peaks at or near $m/z = 1340$ and $m/z = 912$, (3) multiple losses of water molecules (18 Da) from the $[M + 2H]^{2+}$ ion, and (4) molecular mass around 2600 Da.[35,37]

24.4.2.6.3.1 Application to Reference PLTX and Plankton

Identification of PLTX and analogs in standard solutions and plankton extracts by use of LC–MS methods has been carried out in several studies.[35,37–39,52,117,131,133,135,151,152] An LC–MS method for the determination of PLTX and mascarenotoxins on an ESI-Q–TOF–MS instrument was developed employing a hypersil ODS C18 column eluted with a mixture of water acidified to pH 2.5 with trifluoroacetic acid and pure acetonitrile.[35] Toxin detection was achieved in the MRM mode by selecting the transitions m/z 864 > 327 and m/z 836 > 327 for PLTX and mascarenotoxins, respectively. The precursor ion at m/z 836 was assigned to $[M + 3H]^{3+}$ ions of McTX-A and McTX-B, and the ion at m/z 864 to $[M + 3H]^{3+}$ ion of PLTX. This appears incomprehensible since it would lead to a molecular weight of 2589 for PLTX (in place of 2679).[52] The method was applied to analyze an *O. mascarenensis* extract, but no quantitative results were provided.

An LC–FLD–MS method was also developed in which LOD and LOQ for reference PLTX by quantification of the m/z fragment were 7.5 and 20 ng, respectively.[39] Sensitivity of this method was 26-fold lower compared to the HPLC–FLD method described in the same report (Table 24.5), while correlations with hemolytic assay were also more favorable for the HPLC–FLD method (HPLC–FLD: $R^2 = 0.91$; LC–FLD–MS: $R^2 = 0.86$). The lower sensitivity of the LC–FLD–MS method in this case is likely due to instrumental limitations when using an ion trap system in MS/MS mode over a broad mass range.[52]

The majority of data on PLTX and analog quantification by use of LC–MS/MS are contributed by the numerous studies of the Ciminiello et al. group.[38,52,117,131,133,135,151,152] Four PLTX standard concentration levels [2.7, 0.9, 0.3, and 0.1 μg/mL in methanol/water (1:1 v/v) with 0.5 formic acid] were examined with regard to linearity of dose–responses by reversed phase LC-ESI–MS/MS.[38] The LC conditions selected for routine operation were a 5 μm C18 (150 × 2.00 mm) column maintained at room temperature and eluted at a flow rate of 0.2 mL/min with water (eluent A) and 95% acetonitrile/water (eluent B), both eluents containing 30 mM acetic acid; a gradient elution was required (20%–100% B over 10 min and hold 4 min). MS detection was carried out in positive ion mode; the bicharged ion at m/z 1340 and the tricharged ion at m/z 912 were monitored in selected ion monitoring (SIM) experiments, whereas the transitions m/z 1340 → 327 and m/z 912 → 327 were monitored in MRM experiments. The minimum detection levels for matrix-free toxin on column were calculated at 200 and 125 pg in SIM and MRM modes, respectively, while correlation coefficients of >0.9998 for both experiments indicated a high degree of linearity of the plots within the tested concentration range. Matrix effects were also investigated in positive MRM mode by spiking of both sample pellet and butanol extract, obtained by extraction of a seawater sample collected along Genoa coasts in a period when no *Ostreopsis* spp. was blooming in the sea, with the earlier-mentioned four PLTX standard levels.[38] LODs (S/N = 3) and LOQs (S/N = 10) were respectively 25 and 84 ng/mL for reference PLTX (matrix free standard), 39 and 131 ng/mL for PLTX-spiked butanol extract, and 38 and 127 ng/mL for spiked pellet extract. Good linearity was observed in all cases; however, the slope of the curves for matrix-matched standards indicated a slight enhancement effect (6%–8%) of the signal at low PLTX concentrations (0.1–0.3 µg/mL) and a more significant suppression effect (14%–20%) at PLTX levels higher than 0.9 µg/mL. This indicated that the matrix effect over the tested concentration range was analyte concentration dependent, suggesting that matrix-matched standards should be used for accurate quantitation. Method intraday and interday reproducibilities were also assessed, and obtained values did not exceed an RSD value of 9.6% either with pellet or butanol extracts. In the end, accuracy of the method was also tested, and recoveries were estimated to be 91%–98% for reference PLTX-spiked pellet extracts and 73%–82% for spiked butanol extracts with RSD values of <3.2% in both cases, which indicated that the extraction efficiency for PLTX was satisfactory. p-PLTX from the *Ostreopsis* cultures was also quantified using the same method and found at levels of 1.35 and 1.95 µg in the pellet and butanol extracts, respectively.

After the presence of OVTX-a was established, the earlier LC–MS/MS method was modified accordingly to allow chromatographic determination of the new PLTX analog together with p-PLTX.[131] The relative abundance of OVTX-a and p-PLTX in the plankton samples was investigated by an LC–MS experiment using the aforementioned eluents but with a slow gradient elution (20%–50% B over 20 min, 50%–80% B over 10 min, 80%–100% B in 1 min, and hold 5 min), enabling chromatographic separation of the two compounds. MS detection was accomplished in MRM mode on the triple quadrupole MS instrument by monitoring the transitions m/z 1340.7 → 327.1, 1331.7 → 327.1 for p-PLTX and m/z 1324.7 → 327.1, 1315.7 → 327.1 for OVTX-a. Assuming similar molar responses of the two compounds, due to their evident structural similarities, under these chromatographic conditions, p-PLTX eluted at the same retention time as the PLTX standard, showing a peak at 11.08 min in the ion traces at m/z 1340.7 → 327.1 and 1331.7 → 327.1, while the OVTX-a peak was at 11.48 min in the ion traces at m/z 1324.7 → 327.1 and 1315.7 → 327.1. The calculated amount of OVTX-a was in the range 1.26–3.11 pg/cell, indicating that OVTX-a was by far the predominant PLTX-like compound in the analyzed *O.* cf. *ovata* field sample, whereas quantitative analyses of the cultured strain showed p-PLTX and OVTX-a contents of 0.55 and 3.85 pg/cell, respectively.[151]

HR-LC/MS and MS[2] were later applied under similar LC conditions, for the quantitative determination of the five additional ovatoxins identified so far, that is, OVTX-b, -c, -d, -e, and –f as well as of ostreocins –b and -d in field sample extracts obtained from *O.* cf. *ovata* blooms or by cultured *O.* cf. *ovata* and *O.* cf. *siamensis* strains.[117,133,135,153] To achieve quantitative analysis, extracted ion chromatograms were obtained from full MS spectrum of the crude extract by selecting the most abundant bi- and tricharged ions of OVTXs (a–f) and PLTX (Table 24.6). An equal molar response to that of PLTX was once more assumed due to the lack of OVTX standards; a PLTX calibration curve at four[153] (25, 12.5, 6.25, and 3.13 ng/mL) or five[117,133] concentration levels (25, 12.5, 6.25, 3.13, and 1.6 ng/mL) was used to extrapolate quantitative data, while LOD and LOQ of PLTX under the used instrumental conditions were calculated at 1.6 and 3.13 ng/mL, respectively. Elemental formulae, retention times, and principal ions (m/z) of HR full MS spectra of p-PLTX, OVTX-a to –f, and ostreocins-b and -d used in the earlier quantitative analyses are presented in Table 24.6, whereas a typical chromatograph of a cultured *O.* cf. *ovata* strain containing p-PLTX and all so far identified OVTXs is shown in Figure 24.4.

Finally, another HR-LC coupled with ESI–TOF/MS method was developed for toxin pattern determination in cultured cells of *O.* cf. *ovata* from the Mediterranean Sea.[68] Sample extracts were separated on a hydrophilic interaction liquid chromatography 3 µm 150 × 2.00 mm column, and elution was accomplished with water (eluent A) and 95% acetonitrile/water (eluent B), both containing 0.1% formic acid. The flow rate was 0.3 mL/min with gradient conditions as follows: from the beginning to 2 min steady to 10% A; linear rise over 3 min rising to 50% B; from 5 to 10 steady at 50% B; then a linear fall from 50% B to 10% A (initial conditions). Sample solutions (50, 20, and 10 ppm) were prepared in MeOH/H_2O (1:1) and 5 µL were injected. Analysis was performed by LC/TOF/MS with ESI interface in positive ion

TABLE 24.6

Elemental Formula, Retention Times, and Principal Ions (*m/z*) of HR Full MS Spectra of Putative Palytoxin (p-PLTX) and Ovatoxins (OVTX-) Used in Quantitative Analyses

		p-PLTX	OVTX-a	OVTX-b	OVTX-c	OVTX-d/-e	OVTX-f
Formula		$C_{129}H_{223}N_3O_{54}$	$C_{129}H_{223}N_3O_{52}$	$C_{131}H_{227}N_3O_{53}$	$C_{131}H_{227}N_3O_{54}$	$C_{129}H_{223}N_3O_{53}$	$C_{131}H_{227}N_3O_{52}$
Rt (min)		10.56	11.24	10.98	10.65	10.89	11.32
$[M+2H-H_2O]^{2+}$	Most intense	1331.7436	1315.7498	1337.7623	1345.7584	1323.7456	1329.7650
	Monoisotopic	1331.2417	1315.2480	1337.2595	1345.2566	1323.2439	1329.2624
$[M+H+Ca]^{3+}$	Most intense	906.8167	896.1572	910.8318	916.1628	901.4884	905.4976
	Monoisotopic	906.4851	895.8255	910.4976	915.8286	901.1533	905.1632

Source: Reprinted with permission from Ciminiello, P., Dell'Aversano, C., Dello Iacovo, E., Fattorusso, E., Forino, M., Tartaglione, L., Battocchi, C., Crinelli, R., Carloni, E., Magnani, M., and Penna, A., Unique toxin profile of a Mediterranean *Ostreopsis* cf. *ovata* strain: HR LC-MS[n] characterization of ovatoxin-f, a new palytoxin congener, *Chem. Res. Toxicol.*, 25(6), 1243–1252. Copyright 2012. American Chemical Society.

mode, with mass range set at m/z 100–3000 μ. The method was applied to the determination of OVTX-a, McTX-A, and four new PLTXs in *O.* cf. *ovata* cell extracts. Concentration of the different toxins was estimated by direct comparison with the PLTX standard, and toxin quantification indicated that OVTX-a was always the most abundant compound, followed by OVTX-b and -c with comparable abundance and OVTX-d, McTX-a, and McTX-c in much lower quantity. However, no further data with regard to method performance characteristics (e.g., LOD, LOQ, linearity) are provided in this report.

24.4.2.6.3.2 Application to Seafood Samples   The serious concerns posed to human health by the occurrence of PLTX-like compounds in seafood prompted the European Community to study proper guidelines for risk assessment and monitoring of PLTXs in shellfish. Initially, a provisional limit for PLTX in seafood of 250 μg/kg shellfish[142] was proposed, which was followed by the EFSA[6] suggestion for a maximum limit of 30 μg/kg of PLTX equivalents (sum of PLTX and ostreocin-D) in shellfish, in order to avoid exceeding the ARfD for oral administration of PLTX (0.2 μg/kg body weight). In the same report, the EFSA also indicated the necessity for development both of validated chemical analyses and/or of biological assays, other than the MBA, for the detection of PLTX and analogs and of certified reference standards and reference materials for PLTX-group toxins. Finally, it was also highlighted that, although a number of extraction methods for marine toxins in shellfish were available, information lacked on their extraction efficiency for PLTXs.[6]

In purpose of complying with EFSA's requirements for the determination of PLTX in seafood, major efforts are in place with regard to optimization of the extraction and LC–MS/MS determination of PLTX and analogs from various seafood matrices for future application in routine testing.

In the last few years, the LC–MS method developed by Ciminiello et al. for combined detection of PLTX and OVTX-a[30,131] has been applied in monitoring programs of *O. ovata* for determining toxin content of seafood samples collected along the Italian coasts.[154] Application of the method in this case required mussel and sea urchin samples' extraction by the Italian official protocol for the extraction of lipophilic toxins from shellfish[155,156] with acetone and methanol and subsequent liquid–liquid partition of the crude extract between dichloromethane and MeOH/H$_2$O 6:4. With this extraction protocol, hydro-soluble toxins, such as PLTX and OVTXs, are contained in the aqueous methanol extract, which corresponds to a shellfish tissue concentration of 0.5 g tissue/mL.[52] Preliminary spiking experiments before extraction demonstrated that using the earlier procedure, recovery rates for PLTX extraction from shellfish were in the range of 49%–61%.[154] Despite the low extraction efficiency, however, this procedure was used as it provided an extract that could be officially tested by both MBA and LC–MS.

LC–MS analyses were carried out on a triple quadrupole MS in MRM mode by selecting the transitions precursor>product ion of m/z 1340.7 → 327.1 and 1331.7 → 327.1 for the detection of PLTX and m/z 1324.7 → 327.1 and 1315.7 → 327.1 for OVTX-a. A calibration curve of matrix-matched PLTX standards at four concentration levels (0.25, 0.5, 1, and 2 μg/mL) was used to calculate PLTX and OVTX-a contents. Results indicated the presence of OVTX-a in most mussel samples at levels in the range 303–625 μg/kg, which was well above the provisional limit of 250 μg/kg[142] or to the tolerance limit of 30 μg/kg,[6] whereas PLTX was not detected in any sample. On the other hand, neither PLTX nor OVTX-a was detected (or quantified) in some samples that had induced mouse death in MBA. This was attributed to the high method LOQ of 168 μg/kg (300 μg/kg, taking into account the extraction efficiency) on the used LC/MS system. This LOQ was judged as insufficient to detect PLTX in shellfish extracts taking into consideration the EFSA tolerance limit for PLTXs indicating the need for the development of more efficient extraction procedures, as well as cleanup procedures that reduce matrix effect such as SPE.[52]

In a subsequent study by Ciminiello et al.,[152] the best conditions for both PLTX extraction from seafood and quantification by using LC–MS/MS were investigated by PLTX spiking of three seafood matrices (mussels, sea urchins, and anchovies). Extraction by five different procedures was evaluated including a modified procedure based on the earlier-mentioned Italian official protocol for the extraction of lipophilic toxins (system 1) and four different methanol (MeOH) or acetonitrile (MeCN) solutions (MeOH/H$_2$O 1:1; MeOH/H$_2$O 8:2; MeCN/H$_2$O 8:2; and MeOH 100%; systems 2–5), and LC/MS analyses were carried out applying the conditions and settings of Ciminiello et al.[38] Matrix-free and matrix-matched PLTX standards at four concentration levels (2.0, 1.0, 0.5, and 0.25 μg/mL) were used to generate calibration curves that were applied for both quantitative analyses and matrix effect evaluation, while sum of MRM peak areas was used to express peak intensity. Accuracy and intraday reproducibility ($n = 3$) were evaluated for all selected matrices, but only for mussels at three spiking concentration levels including the provisional limit of 250 µg/kg, while PLTX LOQs in mussel, sea urchin, and anchovy tissues were calculated using matrix-matched standards.

Results indicated that extraction with MeOH/H$_2$O 8:2 provided the best results in mussel tissue in terms of both average PLTX recovery (92%) and matrix effect (7%–13% of ion enhancement). A matrix concentration level of 0.1 g tissue/mL was demonstrated to produce the minimum matrix effect. The same solvent mixture (MeOH/H$_2$O 8:2) provided average recoveries of 89% and 56% in sea urchins and anchovies, respectively. In both matrices, an ion enhancement effect was observed in the range 3%–19% (sea-urchins) and 7%–24% (anchovies). Irrespective of the seafood matrix tested, the measured matrix effect was concentration dependent, and, thus, the use of matrix-matched standards was strongly suggested for accurate quantification. Method LOQ including extraction and LC–MS/MS detection of PLTX in mussels, sea urchins, and anchovies was calculated at 228, 343, and 500 µg/kg, respectively.[152]

Very recently, OVTX-a and PLTX accumulation in mussels and sea urchins in relation to *O.* cf. *ovata* blooms on the French Mediterranean coast was investigated by the use of an optimized LC–MS/MS method.[53] PLTX analyses were carried out using an LC system (coupled to a hybrid triple quadrupole/ion trap mass spectrometer) according to a modified method based on Ciminiello et al.,[38] using a 5 µm C18 column (150 × 2.0 mm) maintained at 20°C and eluted at 0.2 mL/min. Eluent A was water and eluent B was 95% acetonitrile/water; both eluents contained 2 mM ammonium formate and 50 mM formic acid with the gradient in B being increased from 20% to 100% over 10 min and held for 4 min before lowering back to the initial conditions. MS detection was operated in positive mode using the MRM mode, and the transitions monitored were m/z 1340 → 327 and m/z 1332 → 327 for PLTX and m/z 1324 → 327 and m/z 1315 → 327 for OVTX-a.[53]

A number of different solvents were tested on homogenates of mussel digestive glands (DG) spiked with PLTX (in the absence of certified reference materials): (1) acetone; (2) methanol/water (50/50), acidified with 0.2% acetic acid; (3) ethanol/water (80/20); and (4) three other solvents, using increasing proportions of methanol: 80%, 90%, and 100%. Only methanol/water (50/50) showed a very low extraction efficiency (55%) compared with the recoveries obtained using the other solvents (79%–95%), while methanol/water (90/10) was the most effective solvent, since it allowed the most PLTX (95%) to be extracted. Recovery rates were also investigated in terms of the type of tissue extracted [DG of blue mussels (*Mytilus edulis*); DG of wedge clams (*Donax cuneatus*); whole tissue of Manila clam (*Tapes philippinarum*); and whole tissue of sea urchin (*Paracentrotus lividus*)] and were found to be dependable on the matrix nature, ranging from 75% to 115%. The average recovery rate of PLTX varied depending on the tissue source: Manila clam (82%), wedge clam (90%), sea urchins (92%), and mussels (97%). Results on optimization of PLTX quantification were in general agreement to those of Ciminiello et al.,[152] in terms of extraction solvent efficiency and recovery rates in seafood tissues.[53]

Furthermore, detection and quantification limits (LOD and LOQ) of the optimized method were assessed for whole tissues of sea urchin and blue mussels spiked with standard PLTX solutions of known concentration and were calculated using serial dilutions not taking into account recovery of the extraction procedure.[53] The LOD (signal/noise, S/N = 3) and LOQ (S/N = 10) obtained were equal for both matrices: (1) 10 and 25 µg PLTX/kg whole tissue of sea urchins and (2) 9 and 23 µg PLTX/kg whole tissue of mussels. The method was successfully applied to mussels and sea urchins collected from the French coasts, and toxin levels found in sea urchins were generally higher than those found in mussels, with maxima of 360 µg and 217 µg eq. PLTX/kg total body, respectively,[53] thus exceeding by far the threshold value of 30 µg PLTX/kg shellfish flesh suggested by the EFSA.[6]

Despite the fact that LC–MS has shown a good potential in the determination of PLTX and its analogs from various sources in a research setting, from the regulatory point of view, routine LC–MS analysis of PLTXs is still at a very preliminary stage. The LOQ currently achieved in seafood analysis appears insufficient to detect PLTXs in shellfish extracts at levels close to the proposed tolerance limit for PLTXs.[6] Additionally, the lack of certified reference PLTX standards and tissue materials and consequently that of validation studies for the proposed LC–MS methods represents important issues that should be faced for future routine application of LC–MS techniques in regulatory monitoring programs.[52]

24.5 Conclusion

PLTX is one of the most potent marine natural toxins so far known, and evidence suggests that species of the genus *Ostreopsis* are its potential production sources. Despite the fact that the connection between PLTX seafood poisoning and the presence of toxic *Ostreopsis* sp. has been long suspected, it has still not been established with certainty. In view of the lack of documented food poisoning incidents in humans in connection with *Ostreopsis* spp. presence and contamination of seafood until today, and of the inconclusive EFSA report[6] with regard to human risk associated with PLTXs, further research is needed to elucidate the effects of *Ostreopsis*-derived PLTX analogs when they enter the human food chain. Until this issue is clarified, however, vigilance is required regarding this dinoflagellate species, as toxic *Ostreopsis* sp. in the past decade occurred abundantly in temperate waters all over the world. It is therefore essential that routine monitoring of these benthic species in susceptible areas should be adopted, whereas improvement of chemical analysis methods to obtain sufficient sensitivity for the quantitative determination of PLTX in seafood at levels well below the proposed limits should be a priority, in order to reevaluate the potential risk posed to humans together with the necessity for regulatory limits for PLTX and PLTX analogs in seafood.

REFERENCES

1. Moore, R.E. and Scheuer, P.J. 1971. Palytoxin: A new marine toxin from a coelenterate. *Science*, 172, 495–498.
2. Ito, E., Ohkusu, M., and Yasumoto, T. 1996. Intestinal injuries caused by experimental palytoxicosis in mice. *Toxicon*, 34, 643–652.
3. Sosa, S., Del Favero, G., De Bortoli, M. et al. 2009. Palytoxin toxicity after acute oral administration in mice. *Toxicol Lett*, 191, 253–259.
4. Wiles, J.S., Vick, J.A., and Christensen, M.K. 1974. Toxicological evaluation of palytoxin in several animal species. *Toxicon*, 12, 427–433.
5. Uemura, D. 1991. Bioactive polyethers. In *Bioorganic Marine Chemistry*, Vol. 4, ed. P.J. Scheuer, pp. 1–31, Berlin, Germany: Springer-Verlag.
6. European Food Safety Authority. 2009. EFSA Panel on Contaminants in the Food Chain (CONTAM). Scientific opinion on marine biotoxins in shellfish—Palytoxin group. *EFSA J*, 7, 1393, 1–38.
7. Uemura, D., Ueda, K., Hirata, Y. et al. 1981. Further studies on palytoxin. II. Structure of palytoxin. *Tetrahedron Lett*, 22, 2781–2784.
8. Moore, R.E. and Bartolini, G. 1981. Structure of palytoxin. *J Am Chem Soc*, 103, 2491–2494.
9. Patockaa, J. and Stredab, L. 2002. Brief overview of natural non-protein neurotoxins. *ASA Newslett*, 89, 16–23.
10. Armstrong, R.W., Beau, J.-M., Cheon, S.H. et al. 1972. Total synthesis of a fully protected palytoxin carboxylic acid. *J Am Chem Soc*, 111, 7525–7530.
11. Kimura, S., Hashimoto, Y., and Yamazato, K. 1972. Toxicity of the zoanthid *Palythoa tuberculosa*. *Toxicon*, 10, 611–617.
12. Quinn, R.J., Kashiwagi, M., Moore, R.E. et al. 1974. Anticancer activity of zoanthids and the associated toxin, palytoxin, against Ehrlich ascites tumor and P-388 lymphocytic leukemia in mice. *J Pharm Sci*, 63, 257–260.
13. Attaway, D.H. and Ciereszko, L.S. 1974. Isolation and partial characterization of Caribbean palytoxin. In *Proceedings of the 2nd International Symposium for Coral Reefs I*, pp. 497–504, Brisbane, Australia: Great Barrier Reef Community.
14. Béress, L., Zwick, J., Kolkenbrock, H.J. et al. 1983. A method for the isolation of the Caribbean palytoxin (C-PTX) from the coelenterate (Zoanthid) *Palythoa caribaeorum*. *Toxicon*, 21, 285–290.
15. Moore, R.E., Woolard, F.X., and Bartolini, G. 1980. Periodate oxidation of N-(p-bromobenzoyl) palytoxin. *J Am Chem Soc*, 102, 7370–7372.
16. Uemura, D., Hirata, Y., Iwashita, T. et al. 1985. Studies on palytoxins. *Tetrahedron*, 41, 1007–1017.
17. Oku, N., Sata, N.U., Matsunaga, S. et al. 2004. Identification of palytoxin as a principle which causes morphological changes in rat 3Y1 cells in the zoanthid *Palythoa* aff. *margaritae*. *Toxicon*, 43, 21–25.

18. Uemura, D. 2006. Bioorganic studies on marine natural products—Diverse chemical structures and bioactivities. *Chem Rec*, 6, 235–248.
19. Gleibs, S., Mebs, D., and Werding, B. 1995. Studies on the origin and distribution of palytoxin in a Caribbean coral reef. *Toxicon*, 33, 1531–1537.
20. Deeds, J.R. and Schwartz, M.D. 2010. Human risk associated with palytoxin exposure. *Toxicon*, 56, 150–162.
21. Deeds, J.R., Handy, S.M., White, K.D. et al. 2011. Palytoxin found in *Palythoa* sp. zoanthids (Anthozoa, Hexacorallia) sold in the home aquarium trade. *PLoS ONE*, 6, e18235, doi:10.1371/journal.pone.0018235.
22. Mebs, D. 1998. Occurrence and sequestration of toxins in the food chains. *Toxicon*, 36, 1519–1522.
23. Gleibs, S. and Mebs, D. 1999. Distribution and sequestration of palytoxin in coral reef animals. *Toxicon*, 37, 1521–1527.
24. Moore, R.E., Helfrich, P., and Patterson, G.M.L. 1982. The deadly seaweed of Hana. *Oceanus*, 25, 54–63.
25. Carballeira, N.M., Emiliano, A., Sostre, A. et al. 1998. Fatty acid composition of bacteria associated with the toxic dinoflagellate *Ostreopsis lenticularis* and with Caribbean *Palythoa* species. *Lipids*, 33, 627–632.
26. Frolova, G.M., Kuznetsova, T.A., Michailov, V.V. et al. 2000. An enzyme linked immunosorbent assay for detecting palytoxin-producing bacteria. *Russ J Bioorg Chem*, 26, 315–320.
27. Seemann, P., Gernert, C., Schmitt, S. et al. 2009. Detection of hemolytic bacteria from *Palythoa caribaeorum* (Cnidaria, Zoantharia) using a novel palytoxin-screening assay. *A van Leeuw J Microb*, 96, 405–411.
28. Kerbrat, A.S., Amzil, Z., Pawlowiez, R. et al. 2011. First evidence of palytoxin and 42-hydroxy-palytoxin in the marine cyanobacterium *Trichodesmium*. *Mar Drugs*, 9, 543–560.
29. Nakamura, K., Asari, T., Ohizumi, Y. et al. 1993. Isolation of zooxanthellatoxins, novel vasoconstrictive substances from zooxanthella *Symbiodinium* sp. *Toxicon*, 31, 371–376.
30. Maeda, M., Kodama, T., Tanaka, T. et al. 1985. Structures of insecticidal substances isolated from a red alga, *Chondria armata*. In *Proceedings of the 27th Symposium on the Chemistry of Natural Products*, pp. 616–623, Hiroshima, Japan: Symposium Organizing Committee.
31. Usami, M., Satake, M., Ishida, S. et al. 1995. Palytoxin analogues from the dinoflagellate *Ostreopsis siamensis*. *J Am Chem Soc*, 117, 5389–5390.
32. Ukena, T., Satake, M., Usami, M. et al. 2001. Structure elucidation of ostreocin-D, a palytoxin analog isolated from the dinoflagellate *Ostreopsis siamensis*. *Biosci Biotechnol Biochem*, 65, 2585–2588.
33. Taniyama, S., Arakawa, O., Terada, M. et al. 2003. *Ostreopsis* sp., a possible origin of palytoxin (PTX) in parrotfish *Scarus ovifrons*. *Toxicon* 42, 29–33.
34. Onuma, Y., Satake, M., Ukena, T. et al. 1999. Identification of putative palytoxin as the cause of clupeotoxism. *Toxicon*, 37, 55–65.
35. Lenoir, S., Ten-Hage, L., Turquet, J. et al. 2004. First evidence of palytoxin analogues from an *Ostreopsis mascarenensis* (Dinophyceae) benthic bloom in southwestern Indian Ocean. *J Phycol*, 40, 1042–1051.
36. Riobó, P., Paz, B., Fernandez, M.L. et al. 2004. Lipophylic toxins of different strains of Ostrepsidaceae and Gonyaulaceae. In *Harmful Algae 2002, Proceedings of the Xth International Conference on Harmful Algae*, eds. K.A. Steidinger, J.H. Landsberg, C.R. Thomas, and G.A. Vargo, pp. 119–121, St. Pete Beach, FL: Florida Fish and Wildlife Conservation Commission, Florida Institute of Oceanography, and Intergovernmental Oceanographic Commission of UNESCO.
37. Penna, A., Vila, M., Fraga, S. et al. 2005. Characterization of *Ostreopsis* and *Coolia* (Dinophyceae) isolates in the western Mediterranean sea based on morphology, toxicity and internal transcribed spacer 5.8S rDNA sequences. *J Phycol*, 41, 212–225.
38. Ciminiello, P., Dell'Aversano, C., Fattorusso, E. et al. 2006. The Genoa 2005 outbreak. Determination of putative palytoxin in Mediterranean *Ostreopsis ovata* by a new liquid chromatography tandem mass spectrometry method. *Anal Chem*, 78, 6153–6159.
39. Riobó, P., Paz, B., and Franco, J.M. 2006. Analysis of palytoxin-like in *Ostreopsis* cultures by liquid chromatography with precolumn derivatization and fluorescence detection. *Anal Chim Acta*, 566, 217–223.
40. Aligizaki, K., Katikou, P., Nikolaidis, G. et al. 2008. First episode of shellfish contamination by palytoxin-like compounds from *Ostreopsis* species (Aegean Sea, Greece). *Toxicon*, 51, 418–427.
41. Bellocci, M., Ronzitti, G., Milandri, A. et al. 2008. A cytolytic assay for the measurement of palytoxin based on a cultured monolayer cell line. *Anal Biochem*, 374, 48–55.
42. Bellocci, M., Ronzitti, G., Milandri, A. et al. 2008. Addendum to "A cytolytic assay for the measurement of palytoxin based on a cultured monolayer cell line". *Anal Biochem*, 381, 178.

43. Taniyama, S., Mahmud, Y., Terada, M. et al. 2002. Occurrence of a food poisoning incident by palytoxin from a serranid *Epinephelus* sp. in Japan. *J Nat Toxins*, 11, 277–282.

44. Yasumoto, T., Yasumura, D., Ohizumi, Y. et al. 1986. Palytoxin in two species of xanthid crab from the Philippines. *Agric Biol Chem*, 50, 163–167.

45. Lau, C.O., Tan, C.H., Khoo, H.E. et al. 1995. *Lophozozymus pictor* toxin: A fluorescent structural isomer of palytoxin. *Toxicon*, 33, 1373–1377.

46. Hashimoto, Y., Fusetani, N., and Kimura, S. 1969. Aluterin: A toxin of filefish, *Alutera scripta*, probably originating from a zoantharian *Palythoa tuberculosa. Bull Jpn Soc Sci Fish*, 35, 1086–1093.

47. Fukui, M., Murata, M., Inoue, A. et al. 1987. Occurrence of palytoxin in the trigger fish *Melichtys vidua. Toxicon*, 25, 1121–1124.

48. Fukui, M., Yasumura, D., Murata, M. et al. 1988. The occurrence of palytoxin in crabs and fish. *Toxicon*, 26, 20–21.

49. Kodama, A.M., Hokama, Y., Yasumotc, T. et al. 1989. Clinical and laboratory findings implicating palytoxin as cause of ciguatera poisoning due to *Decapterus macrosoma* (mackerel). *Toxicon*, 27, 1051–1053.

50. Mahnir, V.M., Kozlovskaya, E.P., and Kalinovsky, A.I. 1992. Sea anemone *Radianthus macrodactylus*— A new source of palytoxin. *Toxicon*, 30, 1449–1456.

51. Aligizaki, K., Katikou, P., Milandri, A. et al. 2011. Occurrence of palytoxin-group toxins in seafood and future strategies to complement the present state of the art. *Toxicon*, 57, 390–399.

52. Ciminiello, P., Dell'Aversano, C., Dello Iacovo, E. et al. 2011. LC-MS of palytoxin and its analogues: State of the art and future perspectives. *Toxicon*, 57, 376–389.

53. Amzil, Z., Sibat, M., Chomerat, N. et al. 2012. Ovatoxin-a and palytoxin accumulation in seafood in relation to *Ostreopsis* cf. *ovata* blooms on the French Mediterranean coast. *Mar Drugs*, 10, 477–496.

54. Gonzales, R.B. and Alcala, A.C. 1977. Fatalities from crab poisoning on Negros island, Philippines. *Toxicon*, 15, 169–170.

55. Alcala, A.C. 1983. Recent cases of crab, cone shell and fish intoxication on southern Negros island, Philippines. *Toxicon*, 21, Suppl. 3, 1–3.

56. Alcala, A.C., Alcala, L.C., Garth, J.S. et al. 1988. Human fatality due to ingestion of the crab *Demania reynaudii* that contained a palytoxin-like toxin. *Toxicon*, 28, 105–107.

57. Noguchi, T., Hwang, D.F., Arakawa, G. et al. 1988. Palytoxin as the causative agent in parrotfish poisoning. *Toxicon*, 26, 34.

58. Okano, H., Masuoka, H., Kamei, S. et al. 1998. Rhabdomyolysis and myocardial damage induced by palytoxin, a toxin of blue humphead parrotfish. *Intern Med*, 37, 330–333.

59. Tan, C.H. and Lau, C.O. 2000. Palytoxin: Chemistry and detection. In *Seafood and Freshwater Toxins: Pharmacology, Physiology and Detection*, ed. L.M. Botana, pp. 533–548, New York: Marcel Dekker Inc.

60. Inuzuka, T., Fujisawa, T., Arimoto, H. et al. 2007. Molecular shape of palytoxin in aqueous solutions. *Org Biomol Chem*, 5, 897–899.

61. Inuzuka, T., Uemura, D., and Arimoto, H. 2008. The conformational features of palytoxin in aqueous solution. *Tetrahedron*, 64, 7718–7723.

62. Katikou, P. 2008. Palytoxin and analogues: Ecobiology and origin, chemistry, metabolism and chemical analysis. In *Seafood and Freshwater Toxins. Pharmacology, Physiology and Detection* (2nd edn.), ed. L.M. Botana, pp. 631–663, Boca Raton, FL: CRC Press.

63. Uemura, D., Ueda, K., Hirata, Y. et al. 1980. Structural studies on palytoxin, a potent coelenterate toxin. *Tetrahedron Lett*, 21, 4857–4860.

64. Uemura, D., Ueda, K., Hirata, Y. et al. 1980. Structures of two oxidation products obtained from palytoxin. *Tetrahedron Lett*, 21, 4861–4864.

65. Uemura, D., Ueda, K., Hirata, Y. et al. 1981. Further studies on palytoxin. I. *Tetrahedron Lett*, 22, 1909–1912.

66. Macfarlane, R.D., Uemura, D., Ueda, K. et al. 1980. ^{252}Cf plasma desorption mass spectrometry of palytoxin. *J Am Chem Soc*, 102, 875–876.

67. Ciminiello, P., Dell'Aversano, C., Dello Iacovo, E. et al. 2009. Stereostructure and biological activity of 42-hydroxy-palytoxin: A new palytoxin analogue from Hawaiian *Palythoa* subspecies. *Chem Res Toxicol*, 22, 1851–1859.

68. Rossi, R., Castellano, V., Scalco, E. et al. 2010. New palytoxin-like molecules in Mediterranean *Ostreopsis* cf. *ovata* (dinoflagellates) and in *Palythoa tuberculosa* detected by liquid chromatography-electrospray ionization time-of-flight mass spectrometry. *Toxicon*, 56, 1381–1387.

69. Cha, J.K., Christ, W.J., Finan, J.M. et al. 1982. Stereochemistry of palytoxin. 4. Complete structure. *J Am Chem Soc*, 104, 7369–7371.

70. Moore, R.E., Bartolini, G., and Barchi, J. 1982. Absolute stereochemistry of palytoxin. *J Am Chem Soc*, 104, 3776–3779.

71. Klein, L.L., McWhorter Jr., W.W., Ko, S.S. et al. 1982. Stereochemistry of palytoxin. 1. C85-C115 segment. *J Am Chem Soc*, 104, 7362–7364.

72. Ko, S.S., Finan, J.M., Yonaga, M. et al. 1982. Stereochemistry of palytoxin. 2. C1-C6, C47-C74 and C77-C83 segments. *J Am Chem Soc*, 104, 7364–7367.

73. Fujioka, H., Christ, W.J., Cha, J.K. et al. 1982. Stereochemistry of palytoxin. 3. C7-C51 segment. *J Am Chem Soc*, 104, 7367–7379.

74. Ciminiello, P., Dell'Aversano, C., Fattorusso, E. et al. 2011. A 4-decade-long (and still ongoing) hunt for palytoxins chemical architecture. *Toxicon*, 57, 362–367.

75. Hirata, Y., Uemura, D., Ueda, K. et al. 1979. Several compounds from *Palythoa tuberculosa* (coelenterata). *Pure Appl Chem*, 51, 1875–1883.

76. Moore, R.E., Dietrich, R.F., Hatton, B. et al. 1975. The nature of the λ 263 chromophore in the palytoxins. *J Org Chem*, 40, 540–542.

77. Moore, R.E., Woolard, F.X., Sheikh, M.Y. et al. 1978. Ultraviolet chromophores of palytoxins. *J Am Chem Soc*, 100, 7758–7759.

78. Hewetson, J.F., Rivera, V.F., Poli, M.A. et al. 1990. Modification of palytoxin activity and structure by visible and ultraviolet light. *Toxicon*, 28, 612.

79. Kan, Y., Uemura, D., Hirata, Y. et al. 2001. Complete NMR signal assignment of palytoxin and N-acetylpalytoxin. *Tetrahedron Lett*, 42, 3197–3202.

80. Ciminiello, P., Dell'Aversano, C., Dello Iacovo, E. et al. 2012. Isolation and structure elucidation of ovatoxin-a, the major toxin produced by *Ostreopsis ovata*. *J Am Chem Soc*, 134, 1869–1875.

81. Armstrong, R.W., Beau, J.-M., Cheon, S.H. et al. 1989. Total synthesis of palytoxin carboxylic acid and palytoxin amide. *J Am Chem Soc*, 111, 7530–7533.

82. Kishi, Y. 1989. Natural products synthesis: Palytoxin. *Pure Appl Chem*, 61, 313–324.

83. Suh, E.M. and Kishi, Y. 1994. Synthesis of palytoxin from palytoxin carboxylic acid. *J Am Chem Soc*, 116, 11205–11206.

84. Li, C.J. 2005. Challenges and opportunities of Green Chemistry. Green Chemistry round table, Chemistry Division Conference, Special Libraries Association, Toronto, Ontario, Canada, http://www.sla.org/division/dche/2005/li.pdf.

85. Higelmann, D. 2003. From a pump to a pore: How palytoxin opens the gates. *PNAS*, 100, 386–388.

86. Miura, D., Kobayashi, M., Kakiuchi, S. et al. 2006. Enhancement of transformed foci and induction of prostaglandins in Balb/c 3T3 cells by palytoxin: In vitro model reproduces carcinogenic responses in animal models regarding the inhibitory effect of indomethacin and reversal of indomethacin's effect by exogenous prostaglandins. *Toxicol Sci*, 89, 154–163.

87. Fujiki, H., Suganuma, M., Nakayasu, M. et al. 1986. Palytoxin is a non-12-O-tetradecanoylphorbol-13-acetate type tumor promoter in two-stage mouse skin carcinogenesis. *Carcinogenesis*, 7, 707–710.

88. Nakajima, L., Oshima, Y., and Yasumoto, T. 1981 Toxicity of benthic dinoflagellates found in coral-reef. 2. Toxicity of the benthic dinoflagellates in Okinawa. *Bull Jpn Soc Sci Fish*, 47, 1029–1033.

89. Tindall, D.R., Miller, D.M., and Tindall, P.M. 1990. Toxicity of *Ostreopsis lenticularis* from the British and United States Virgin Islands. In *Toxic Marine Phytoplankton*, eds. E. Granéli, B. Sundström, L. Edler, and D.M. Anderson, pp. 424–429, New York: Elsevier.

90. Quod, J.P. 1994. *Ostreopsis mascarenensis* sp. nov (Dinophyceae), dinoflagelle toxique associé à la ciguatéra dans l'Ocean Indien. *Cryptogamie Algol*, 15, 243–251.

91. Shears, N.T. and Ross, P.M. 2009. Blooms of benthic dinoflagellates of the genus *Ostreopsis*; an increasing and ecologically important phenomenon on temperate reefs in New Zealand and worldwide. *Harmful Algae*, 8, 916–925.

92. Fukuyo, Y. 1981. Taxonomical study on benthic dinoflagellates collected in coral reefs. *Bull Jpn Soc Sci Fish*, 47, 967–978.

93. Rhodes, L., Towers, N., Briggs, L. et al. 2002. Uptake of palytoxin-like compounds by shellfish fed *Ostreopsis siamensis* (Dinophyceae). *New Zeal J Mar and Fresh*, 36, 631–636.

94. Pearce, I., Marshall, J., and Hallegraeff, G.M. 2001. Toxic epiphytic dinoflagellates from East Coast Tasmania, Australia. In *Harmful Algal Blooms 2000*, eds. G. Hallegraeff, S.I. Blackburn, C.J. Bolch, and R.J. Lewis, pp. 54–57, Hobart, Australia: Intergovernmental Oceanographic Commission of UNESCO.

95. Granéli, E., Ferreira, C.E.L., Yasumoto, T. et al. 2002. Sea urchins poisoning by the benthic dinoflagellate *Ostreopsis ovata* on the Brazilian Coast. In *Book of Abstracts, 10th International Conference on Harmful Algae*, p. 113, St. Pete Beach, FL.

96. Faust, M.A. 1999. Three new *Ostreopsis* species (Dinophyceae): *O. marinus* sp. nov., *O. belizeanus* sp. nov. and *O. caribbeanus* sp. nov. *Phycologia*, 38, 92–99.

97. Ballantine, D.L., Tosteson, C.G., and Bardales, A.T. 1998. Population dynamics and toxicity of natural populations of benthic dinoflagellates in southwestern Puerto Rico. *J Exp Mar Biol Ecol*, 119, 201–212.

98. Aligizaki, K. and Nikolaidis, G. 2006. The presence of the potentially toxic genera *Ostreopsis* and *Coolia* (Dinophyceae) in the North Aegean Sea, Greece. *Harmful Algae*, 5, 717–730.

99. Totti, C., Accoroni, S., Cerino, F. et al. 2010. *Ostreopsis ovata* bloom along the Conero Riviera (northern Adriatic Sea): Relationships with environmental conditions and substrata. *Harmful Algae*, 9, 233–239.

100. Vila, M., Garcés, E., and Masó, M. 2001. Potentially toxic epiphytic dinoflagellate assemblages on macroalgae in the NW Mediterranean. *Aquat Microb Ecol*, 26, 51–60.

101. Sansoni, G., Borghini, B., Camici, G. et al. 2003. Fioriture algali di *Ostreopsis ovata* (Gonyaulacales: Dinophyceae): Un problema emergente. *Biol Ambient*, 17, 17–23.

102. Turki, S. 2005. Distribution of toxic dinoflagellates along the leaves of seagrass *Posidonia oceanica* and *Cymodocea nodosa* from the Gulf of Tunis. *Cah Biol Mar*, 46, 29–34.

103. Monti, M., Minocci, M., Beran, A. et al. 2007. First record of *Ostreopsis* cf. *ovata* on macroalgae in the Northern Adriatic Sea. *Mar Pollut Bull*, 54, 598–601.

104. Mangialajo, L., Ganzin, N., Accoroni, S. et al. 2011. Trends in *Ostreopsis* proliferation along the Northern Mediterranean coasts. *Toxicon*, 57, 408–420.

105. Cohu, S., Thibaut, T., Mangialajo, L. et al. 2011. Occurrence of the toxic dinoflagellate *Ostreopsis* cf. *ovata* in relation with environmental factors in Monaco (NW Mediterranean). *Mar Pollut Bull*, 62, 2681–2691.

106. Brescianini, C., Grillo, C., Melchiorre, N. et al. 2006. *Ostreopsis ovata* algal blooms affecting human health in Genova, Italy, 2005 and 2006. *Eurosurveillance*, 11, 36, pii=3040. http://www.eurosurveillance.org/ViewArticle.aspx?ArticleId=3040 (accessed September 28, 2013).

107. Ramos, V. and Vasconcelos, V. 2010. Palytoxin and analogs: Biological and ecological effects. *Mar Drugs*, 8, 2021–2037.

108. Faust, M.A., Morton, S.L., and Quod, J.P. 1996. Further SEM study of marine dinoflagellates: The genus *Ostreopsis* (Dinophyceae). *J Phycol*, 32, 1053–1065.

109. Mercado, J.A., Viera, M., Escalona de Motta, G. et al. 1994. An extraction procedure modification changes the toxicity, chromatographic profile and pharmacologic action of *Ostreopsis lenticularis* extracts. *Toxicon*, 32, 256.

110. Meunier, F.A., Mercado, J.A., Molgó, J. et al. 1997. Selective depolarization of the muscle membrane in frog nerve-muscle preparations by a chromatographically purified extract of the dinoflagellate *Ostreopsis lenticularis*. *Brit J Pharmacol*, 121, 1224–1230.

111. Norris, D.R., Bomber, J.W., and Balech, E. 1985. Benthic dinoflagellates associated with ciguatera from the Florida Keys. I. *Ostreopsis heptagona* sp. nov. In *Toxic Dinoflagellates*, eds. D.M. Anderson, A.W. White, and D.G. Baden, pp. 39–44, New York: Elsevier Scientific.

112. Schmidt, J. 1902. Flora of Koh Chang. Contribution to the knowledge of the vegetation in the Gulf of Siam. Part IV. Peridiniales. *Bot Tidsskr*, 23, 212–218.

113. Yasumoto, T., Seino, N., Murakami, Y. et al. 1987. Toxins produced by benthic dinoflagellates. *Biol Bull*, 172, 128–131.

114. Chang, F.H., Shimizu, Y., Hay, B. et al. 2000. Three recently recorded *Ostreopsis* spp. (Dinophyceae) in New Zealand: Temporal and regional distribution in the upper North Island from 1995 to 1997. *New Zeal J Mar Fresh*, 34, 29–39.

115. Rhodes, L., Adamson, J., Suzuki, T. et al. 2000. Toxic marine epiphytic dinoflagellates, *Ostreopsis siamensis* and *Coolia monotis* (Dinophyceae), in New Zealand. *New Zeal J Mar Fresh*, 34, 371–383.

116. Rhodes, L. 2011. World-wide occurrence of the toxic dinoflagellate genus *Ostreopsis* Schmidt. *Toxicon*, 57, 400–407.

117. Ciminiello, P., Dell'Aversano, C., Dello Iacovo, E. et al. 2013. Investigation of toxin profile of Mediterranean and Atlantic strains of *Ostreopsis* cf. *siamensis* (Dinophyceae) by liquid chromatography–high resolution mass spectrometry. *Harmful Algae*, 23, 19–27.

118. Holmes, M.J., Gillepsie, N.C., and Lewis, R.J. 1988. Toxicity and morphology of *Ostreopsis* cf. *siamensis* cultured from a ciguatera endemic region of Queensland, Australia. In *Proceedings of the 6th International Coral Reef Symposium: Vol. 3: Contributed Papers*, eds. J.H. Choat, D. Barnes, M.A. Borowitzka et al., pp. 49–54, Townsville, Australia.

119. Ukena, T., Satake, M., Usami, M. et al. 2002. Structural confirmation of ostreocin-D by application of negative-ion fast-atom bombardment collision-induced dissociation tandem mass spectrometric methods. *Rapid Commun Mass Spectrom*, 16, 2387–2393.

120. Ukena, T. 2001. Chemical studies on ostreocins, palytoxin analogs, isolated from the dinoflagellate *Ostreopsis siamensis*. PhD thesis, Graduate School of Life Sciences, Tohoku University, Sendai, Japan (cited in Ciminiello et al., Ref. [117]).

121. Hansen, G., Turquet, J., Quod, J.P. et al. 2001. *Potentially Harmful Microalgae of the Western Indian Ocean—A Guide Based on a Preliminary Survey.* Intergovernmental Oceanographic Commission Manuals and Guides N° Series No. 41, 105p., Paris, France: UNESCO.

122. Turquet, J., Quod, J.P., Couté, A. et al. 1998. Assemblage of benthic dinoflagellates and monitoring of harmful species in Réunion island (SW Indian Ocean) during the 1993–1996 period. In *Harmful Algae*, eds. B. Reguera, J. Blanco, M.L. Fernandez, and T. Wyatt, pp. 44–47, Vigo, Spain: Xunta de Galicia and Intergovernmental Oceanographic Commission of UNESCO.

123. Turquet, J., Lenoir, S., Quod, J.P. et al. 2002. Toxicity and toxin profiles of a bloom of *Ostreopsis mascarensis*, Dinophyceae, from the SW Indian Ocean. In *Book of Abstracts, 10th International Conference on Harmful Algae*, p. 286, St. Pete Beach, FL.

124. Yasumoto, T. 1998. Fish poisoning due to toxins of microalgal origins in the Pacific. *Toxicon*, 36, 1515–1518.

125. David, D., Laza-Martínez, A., Orive, E. et al. 2012. First bloom of *Ostreopsis* cf. *ovata* in the continental Portuguese coast. *Harmful Algae News*, 45, 12–13.

126. Nascimento, S.M., França, J.V., Gonçalves, J.E.A. et al. 2012. *Ostreopsis* cf. *ovata* (Dinophyta) bloom in an equatorial island of the Atlantic Ocean. *Mar Pollut Bull*, 64, 1074–1078.

127. Tognetto, L., Bellato, S., Moro, I. et al. 1995. Occurrence of *Ostreopsis ovata* (Dinophyceae) in the Tyrrhenian Sea during summer 1994. *Bot Mar*, 38, 291–295.

128. Simoni, F., Gaddi, A., Di Paolo, C. et al. 2003. Harmful epiphytic dinoflagellate on Tyrrhenian Sea reefs. *Harmful Algae News*, 24, 13–14.

129. Simoni, F., Gaddi, A., Di Paolo, C. et al. 2004. Further investigation on blooms of *Ostreopsis ovata*, *Coolia monotis*, *Prorocentrum lima* on the macroalgae of artificial and natural reefs in the Northern Tyrrhenian Sea. *Harmful Algae News*, 26, 5–7.

130. Paddle, B.M. 2003. Therapy and prophylaxis of inhaled biological toxins. *J Appl Toxicol*, 23, 139–170.

131. Ciminiello, P., Dell'Aversano, C., Fattorusso, E. et al. 2008. Putative palytoxin and its new analogue, ovatoxin-a, in *Ostreopsis ovata* collected along the Ligurian coasts during the 2006 toxic outbreak. *J Am Soc Mass Spectrom*, 19, 111–120.

132. Ciminiello, P., Dell'Aversano, C., Dello Iacovo, E. et al. 2012. Stereochemical studies on ovatoxin-a. *Chem Eur J*, 18, 16836–16843.

133. Ciminiello, P., Dell'Aversano, C., Dello Iacovo, E. et al. 2010. Complex palytoxin-like profile of *Ostreopsis ovata*. Identification of four new ovatoxins by high-resolution liquid chromatography/mass spectrometry. *Rapid Commun Mass Spectrom*, 24, 2735–2744.

134. Ciminiello, P., Dell'Aversano, C., Dello Iacovo, E. et al. 2012. High resolution LC–MS^n fragmentation pattern of palytoxin as template to gain new insights into ovatoxin-a structure. The key role of calcium in MS behavior of palytoxins. *J Am Soc Mass Spectrom*, 23, 952–963.

135. Ciminiello, P., Dell'Aversano, C., Dello Iacovo, E. et al. 2012. The unique toxin profile of a Mediterranean *Ostreopsis* cf. *ovata* strain HR LC–MS^n characterization of ovatoxin-f, a new palytoxin congener. *Chem Res Toxicol*, 25, 1243–1252.

136. Sato, S., Nishimura, T., Uehara, K. et al. 2011. Phylogeography of *Ostreopsis* along west Pacific coast, with special reference to a novel clade from Japan. *PLoS ONE*, 6, e27983, doi:10.1371/journal.pone.0027983.

137. Suzuki, T., Watanabe, R., Uchida, H. et al. 2012. LC-MS/MS analysis of novel ovatoxin isomers in several *Ostreopsis* strains collected in Japan. *Harmful Algae*, 20, 81–91.

138. Honsell, G., De Bortoli, M., Boscolo, S. et al. 2011. Harmful dinoflagellate *Ostreopsis* cf. *ovata* Fukuyo: Detection of ovatoxins in field samples and cell immunolocalization using antipalytoxin antibodies. *Environ Sci Technol*, 45, 7051–7059.

139. Lau, C.O., Tan, C.H., Khoo, H.E. et al. 1995. Ethanolic extraction, purification, and partial characterization of a fluorescent toxin from the coral reef crab, *Lophozozymus pictor. Nat Toxins*, 3, 87–90.

140. Teh, Y.F. and Gardiner, J.E. 1974. Partial purification of *Lophozozymus pictor* toxin. *Toxicon*, 12, 603–610.

141. Lau, C.O., Khoo, H.E., Yuen, R. et al. 1993. Isolation of a novel fluorescent toxin from the coral reef crab, *Lophozozymus pictor. Toxicon*, 31, 1341–1345.

142. CRLMB (Community Reference Laboratory for Marine Biotoxins). 2005. *Minutes of the 1st Meeting of Working Group on Toxicology of the National Reference Laboratories (NRLs) for Marine Biotoxins.* Cesenatico, Italy, October 24–25, 2005. Available on request from http://www.aesan.msps.es

143. Yasumoto, T., Fukui, M., Sasaki, K. et al. 1995. Determinations of marine toxins in foods. *J AOAC Int*, 78, 574–582.

144. Espiña, B., Cagide, E., Louzao, M.C. et al. 2009. Specific and dynamic detection of palytoxins by in vitro microplate assay with human neuroblastoma cells. *Bioscience Rep*, 29, 13–23.

145. Louzao, M.C., Espiña, B., Cagide, E. et al. 2010. Cytotoxic effect of palytoxin on mussel. *Toxicon*, 56, 842–847.

146. Bignami, G.S. 1993. A rapid and sensitive hemolysis neutralization assay for palytoxin. *Toxicon*, 31, 817–820.

147. Bignami, G.S., Raybould, T.J.G., Sachinvala, N.D. et al. 1992. Monoclonal antibody-based enzyme-linked immunoassays for the measurement of palytoxin in biological samples. *Toxicon*, 30, 687–700.

148. Alfonso, A., Fernández-Araujo, A., Alfonso, C. et al. 2012. Palytoxin detection and quantification using the fluorescence polarization technique. *Anal Biochem*, 424, 64–70.

149. Mereish, K.A., Morris, S., Mc Cullers, G. et al. 1991. Analysis of palytoxin by liquid chromatography and capillary electrophoresis. *J Liq Chromatogr*, 14, 1025–1031.

150. Habermann, E., Ahnert-Hilger, G., Chhatwal, G.S. et al. 1981. Delayed haemolytic action of palytoxin. General characteristics. *Biochim Biophys Acta*, 649, 481–486.

151. Ciminiello, P., Dell'Aversano, C., Fattorusso, E. et al. 2010. Palytoxins: A still haunting Hawaiian curse. *Phytochem Rev*, 9, 491–500.

152. Ciminiello, P., Dell'Aversano, C., Dello Iacovo, E. et al. 2011. Palytoxin in seafood by liquid chromatography tandem mass spectrometry: Investigation of extraction efficiency and matrix effect. *Anal Bioanal Chem*, 401, 1043–1050.

153. Accoroni, S., Romagnoli, T., Colombo, F. et al. 2011. *Ostreopsis* cf. *ovata* bloom in the northern Adriatic Sea during summer 2009: Ecology, molecular characterization and toxin profile. *Mar Pollut Bull*, 62, 2512–2519.

154. ARPAC. 2008. Il monitoraggio dell'*Ostreopsis ovata* lungo il litorale della Campania (giugno-agosto 2007), http://www.arpacampania.it/documents/30626/52633/Relazione+finale3.pdf (accessed September 28, 2013).

155. Yasumoto, T., Oshima, Y., and Yamaguchi, M. 1978. Occurrence of a new type of shellfish poisoning in Tohoku district. *Bull Jpn Soc Sci Fish*, 44, 1249–1255.

156. Gazzetta Ufficiale della Repubblica Italiana, 2002. Tenori massimi e metodiche di analisi delle biotossine algali nei molluschi bivalvi vivi, echinodermi, tunicati e gasteropodi marini. Italian Ministrerial Decree (Decreto Ministeriale) dated May 16, 2002. Serie Generale no. 165, July 16, 2002, pp. 15–23.

25

Palytoxin and Analogues: Biological Effects and Detection

Aurelia Tubaro, Giorgia del Favero, Marco Pelin, Gary Bignami, and Mark Poli

CONTENTS

25.1 Introduction

The early work of Drs. Philip Helfrich, Paul Scheuer, Alfred Banner, and others at the University of Hawaii in the early 1960s on their newly discovered compound that was soon to be known as "palytoxin" (PLTX) was stimulated by an early Hawaiian legend. According to this legend, in a certain rocky tide pool on the island of Maui, in the district of Hana, there lived an alga the locals called "*limu-make-o-Hana*," roughly translated as "the deadly seaweed of Hana." The location of the pool was known to only a few, and visiting it was considered taboo by the Hawaiian native population. Locating the pool was challenging, but their efforts were rewarded in 1961 by the discovery of a new species of zoanthid soft coral, *Palythoa toxica*, and the toxin it produced. Although the literature contains references to toxins from samples of zoanthids prior to this (Hashimoto et al., 1969), the seminal paper by Moore and Scheuer (1971) described PLTX as a new marine natural product for the first time and is generally considered the beginning of research in this area. Since then, PLTX has fascinated researchers for the complexity of its structure, its extreme potency, and its intriguing mechanism of action.

25.1.1 Sources

PLTX has been identified in a variety of sources and from diverse positions in the ecosystem. It is of global dimension, as it is found in tropical, subtropical, and temperate regions. As noted earlier, the original source of PLTX was a soft coral, *P. toxica*, collected in Hawaii. It has since been identified in other species of *Palythoa*, including *P. tuberculosa* (Kimura and Hashimoto, 1973; Ishida et al., 1983), *P.* aff. *margaritae* (Oku et al., 2004), *P. caribaeorum* (Attaway and Ciereszko, 1974; Béress et al., 1983), and *P. mammillosa* (Attaway and Ciereszko, 1974), the latter two collected from coral reefs of the Caribbean. PLTX and its analogue 42-OH-PLTX have been isolated from species of *P. heliodiscus* and *P. mutuki* (Deeds et al., 2011). Moreover, PLTX has also been isolated from other zoanthid species, such as *Zoanthus solanderi* and *Z. sociatus*, competitors of *Palythoa* species in the coral reef (Gleibs et al., 1995). Zoanthids *Anthozoa* and *Hexacorallia* were found to contain considerable amounts of PLTX (ranging from 0.5 to 3.5 mg of crude toxin/g zoanthid), as well. Other organisms such as sea anemones (*Radianthus macrodactylus*) may contain PLTX-like substances (Mahnir et al., 1992). Finally, PLTX and an array of analogues have been identified in various coral reef animals, including fish (Gleibs and Mebs, 1999).

  In 1995, the presence of PLTX-like molecules was discovered in benthic dinoflagellates of the genus *Ostreopsis*. This compound was named ostreocin-D (OST-D) and was isolated from *Ostreopsis siamensis* (Usami et al., 1995; Ukena et al., 2001). Other strains of *Ostreopsis*, such as *O. mascareniensis* (Lenoir et al., 2004; Rossi et al., 2011) and *O. ovata* (Ciminiello et al., 2006, 2008, 2011, 2012a; Honsell et al., 2011), were later found to contain PLTX-like molecules as well.

The presence of such structurally similar molecules in species so phylogenetically diverse is a curious phenomenon. Looking for a possible common ancestor for toxin production, some authors proposed bacteria; the literature offers some support for this hypothesis. Soon after the discovery of the molecule, Moore and coworkers isolated from *Palythoa* bacteria that seemed to contain PLTX-related molecules (Moore et al., 1982). Unfortunately, this idea was not further developed and, to our knowledge, no other studies were carried out for nearly 20 years. In 2000, Frolova and coworkers (2000) with the use of anti-PLTX antibodies detected in bacteria PLTX-like substances. Further support to this hypothesis came in 2009 when it was demonstrated that bacteria isolated from *P. caribaeorum* exerted PLTX-like hemolytic activity (Seemann et al., 2009). In addition, PLTX and its 42-hydroxyl derivative were isolated from the marine cyanobacterium *Trichodesmium* (Kerbrat et al., 2011).

25.1.2 Entrance into Ecosystems and Food Webs

In addition to those that produce it, PLTX and congeners have been found in several other organisms, including crustaceans, fish, gastropods, bivalve mollusks, and echinoderms (Aligizaki et al., 2011). They are found in a variety of habitats, either around coral reefs near *Palythoa* (Gleibs et al., 1995) or in habitats supporting microalgae preferred by *Ostreopsis* (Onuma et al., 1999; Aligizaki et al., 2008).

In one of the first descriptions of PLTX entering the food web, Hashimoto et al. (1969) found fragments of *P. tuberculosa* polyps in the gut of the toxic filefish *Alutera scripta*. Both the flesh and the zoanthids contained a toxin with very similar biological properties.

PLTX has often been reported in crustaceans. Specimens of crabs (*Demania alcalai*, *D. reynaudii*, and *Lophozozymus pictor*) collected in the Philippines were found to contain PLTX in all tissues tested (Yasumoto et al., 1986; Alcala et al., 1988). Polychaete worms (Gleibs and Mebs, 1999), fishes (Fukui et al., 1987; Gleibs and Mebs, 1999), and predators that eat zoanthid corals appear to accumulate the toxin(s) (Gleibs et al., 1995; Mebs, 1998). Similar toxin bioaccumulation probably occurs in small crustaceans (*Platypodiella spectabilis*) living in close contact with *Palythoa* corals (Mebs, 1998).

The possibility of PLTX accumulation in the food web via *Ostreopsis* has also been explored. The presence of bottom sediments in the viscera of sardines involved in a lethal case of intoxication has been considered key in the hypothesis that benthic microalgae could be related to the accumulation of the toxin in fish (Onuma et al., 1999). The possible mechanisms of toxin uptake in mollusks were explored by Rhodes et al. (2002). Shellfish were actively fed *O. siamensis* and some oyster and scallop hepatopancreas contained detectable amounts of toxin, suggesting accumulation of the toxin into the food web. Moreover, wild shellfish collected during *Ostreopsis* blooms in the Aegean Sea were found to contain PLTX-like compounds (Aligizaki et al., 2008), suggesting that toxin uptake could occur even in the wild.

25.1.3 Epidemiology

A primary concern related to the entrance of biotoxins into the ecosystem is the potential human exposure via ingestion of contaminated seafood. The presence of PLTX or PLTX-like compounds has been associated with several cases of seafood intoxications (recently reviewed by Tubaro et al., 2011a). In general, exposure routes to PLTX-containing organisms may be by (1) ingestion, (2) dermal exposure, (3) inhalational exposure, or (4) ocular exposure. In all cases, confirmation or quantification of the toxin is rarely possible. In the majority of cases, PLTX was hypothesized as a causative agent on the basis of clinical symptoms and case history, in particular when PLTX-producing and/or PLTX-containing organisms, such as *Palythoa* corals and *Ostreopsis* microalgae, were involved (Tubaro et al., 2011a).

Oral intoxications by PLTX or related toxins have been described from tropical and subtropical regions after the ingestion of contaminated fish and crustaceans (Noguchi et al., 1987; Alcala et al., 1988; Onuma et al., 1999; Taniyama et al., 2002). These intoxications can be characterized by initial gastrointestinal involvement, typically with nausea, vomiting, and diarrhea (Alcala et al., 1988; Onuma et al., 1999). In addition, myalgia and spasms (Noguchi et al., 1987; Taniyama et al., 2002) and, in lethal cases, convulsions and delirium followed prior to death (Alcala et al., 1988; Onuma et al., 1999). Other cases are described in the literature and, even though quantification of toxin in these cases was not performed in the leftovers, they occurred after ingestion of potentially PLTX-containing seafood. In these cases, symptoms were in good agreement with those already described, thus strengthening the likelihood that PLTX (or PLTXs) were the causative agent (Alcala and Halstead, 1970; Gonzales and Alcala, 1977; Fusetani et al., 1985; Ichida et al., 1988; Tan and Lee, 1988; Kodama et al., 1989; Tabata et al., 1989; Okano et al., 1998; Mahmud et al., 2000; Yoshimine et al., 2001; Taniyama et al., 2001, 2003).

Dermal toxicity has been associated with skin contact by PLTX-containing zoanthid corals or seawater containing *Ostreopsis* cells. In the former, intoxications occurred primarily in aquarium hobbyists who accidentally came into contact with *Palythoa* while cleaning aquaria. Intoxications were associated with handling of corals with both intact skin (Deeds and Schwarz, 2010; Nordt et al., 2011) and damaged skin (Hoffmann et al., 2008). In addition to local effects in the site of contact, such as edema and erythema (Nordt et al., 2011), systemic symptoms were also observed. Among these, perioral paresthesia and dysgeusia were the most common and, in the most severe cases, transitory alterations of cardiac function were noted (Hoffmann et al., 2008; Deeds and Schwarz, 2010). Probably more numerous, but less severe, was dermatitis associated with contact with seawater/microalgae during *Ostreopsis* blooms (Durando et al., 2007; Tubaro et al., 2011a). Although underreported, Durando and coworkers suggested that 5% of people seeking medical help during *Ostreopsis* blooms presented with dermatitis (Durando et al., 2007; Tichadou et al., 2010; Tubaro et al., 2011a).

The occurrence of respiratory irritation and malaise related to aerosol exposure during *O. ovata* blooms, both documented and anecdotal, suggests at least an association between the two events. Unlike cases of foodborne intoxications (as mentioned earlier), cases of inhalational toxicity related to *Ostreopsis* proliferation occurred mainly in temperate climates. In particular, the Italian coasts have seen several occurrences (Sansoni et al., 2003; Gallitelli et al., 2005; Durando et al., 2007; Tubaro et al., 2011a), as have other Mediterranean coasts (Barroso Garcia et al., 2008; Kermarec et al., 2008; Tichadou et al., 2010). Recurrent symptoms were severe rhinorrhea, cough, sore throat, fever occasionally associated with dyspnea, mucosal irritation, and conjunctivitis. In most severe cases, systemic symptoms were also recorded, such as nausea, vomiting, headache, and fever over 38°C (Durando et al., 2007).

Ocular exposure is one of the less predictable exposure routes for algal biotoxins. Nevertheless, cases of ocular irritation/conjunctivitis have been described after inhalational exposure to *Ostreopsis* blooms (Di Turi et al., 2003; Durando et al., 2007; Barroso Garcia et al., 2008; Kermarec et al., 2008; Tichadou et al., 2010). In 1982, Moore and colleagues reported anecdotally a severe eye injury with edema of the cornea lasting several weeks, associated with the contact with a mucous secretion of *P. tuberculosa* described by a physician in Hilo, Hawaii (Moore et al., 1982). In addition, two cases of keratoconjunctivitis have been described in two patients after handling zoanthid soft corals in home aquaria. Even though the presence of PLTX or congeners was not confirmed, the severity of the lesions could be ascribed to a toxin such as PLTX (Moshirfar et al., 2010).

25.2 In Vivo Effects

To fully understand the toxicological risk of PLTX in the food web, in vivo studies are required. A wide variety of animal species and exposure routes appear in the literature. Unfortunately, some studies were carried out before structural elucidation of PLTX, and chemical information regarding the test articles, especially molecular weights, is not always available or consistent (Wiles et al., 1974). Therefore, these data should be regarded with caution.

In general, the data suggest that PLTXs are much more potent by parenteral administration than by the oral route. However, the study of the toxicological effects of PLTX after oral exposure is highly relevant to understanding the risks of PLTX as a food contaminant.

25.2.1 Rodent Studies

25.2.1.1 Toxicity after Single Oral Administration

Studies describing the oral effects of PLTX in rodents are limited. The first study was performed by Vick and Wiles in 1974, who used extracts of *P. vestitus* (PLTX with reported MW 3300), and found no effects of extracts dosed up to 40 µg/kg in rats. Many years later, after increasing evidence of PLTX accumulation in the food chain, Munday and coworkers revisited the issue and estimated the median lethal dose (LD_{50}) of PLTX at 510 µg/kg in mice (data obtained according to OECD 425; Munday, 2008). This work was confirmed and expanded by Sosa and coworkers (calculated LD_{50} 767 µg/kg; 95% confidence limits: 549–1039 µg/kg), who evaluated hematology, clinical chemistry, and histology after oral administration of commercial PLTX. Animals treated with doses higher than 600 µg/kg presented scratching, jumping, dyspnea, and limb paralysis. Hematochemical analysis demonstrated dose-dependent increases in circulating levels of LDH, CPK, AST, and ALT. Histological analysis revealed inflammation of the forestomach, consistent with the irritating properties of PLTX (Sosa et al., 2009). Similarly, Ito and Yasumoto (2009) described erosion and slight fluid accumulation in the stomach after oral administration of doses up to 500 µg/kg PLTX.

Studies on PLTX congeners are even fewer and limited to OST-D (Ito and Yasumoto, 2009) and 42-OH-PLTX (Tubaro et al., 2011b). OST-D exhibits effects similar to that of PLTX, but somewhat less severe at similar doses. Dose-dependent stomach erosion and minor injury to the small intestine, lung, and kidney were observed 2 h after oral administration to mice (200 and 500 µg/kg). Acute toxicity studies with 42-OH-PLTX suggested an LD_{50} similar to that of PLTX (650 µg/kg confidence intervals 384–1018 µg/kg, mice) and increased circulating levels of LDH, CPK, AST, ALT, and K^+. Also noted were dose-dependent symptoms such as jumping, loss of righting reflex, and hind limb paralysis (Tubaro et al., 2011b).

25.2.1.2 Toxicity after Single Parenteral Administration

Studies describing parenteral administration of PLTXs (intraperitoneal [i.p.]; intravenous [i.v.]; intramuscular [i.m.]) represent the majority of the toxicity data available for this family of compounds. The most commonly used paradigm is i.p. administration to mice, often used also for the detection of the toxin with the mouse bioassay (MBA). The literature contains several studies performed on purified toxin preparations, as well as with toxic extracts. In general, toxicity values obtained from commercial PLTX or purified samples are quite consistent. Rhodes and coworkers calculated an LD_{50} after i.p. administration of 0.72 µg/kg (confidence intervals 0.64–0.80 µg/kg; Rhodes et al., 2002), and Riobò and coworkers estimated an LD_{50} of 294.6 ng/kg (±5.38 ng/kg; Riobò et al., 2008a) for commercial PLTX. In the first study, animals presented abnormal gait, hind limbs splayed backward, cessation of spontaneous movement, and slowed rate of respiration with occasional gasps before death (Rhodes et al., 2002). Similarly, in the second study, stretching of hind limbs and lower backs, curvature of spinal column, possible blindness, convulsion, and gasping before death were observed (Riobò et al., 2008a). Studies performed in mice after i.p. administration of PLTX allowed also the identifications of the main pathological effects of the toxin. Administration of 2 µg/kg of PLTX isolated from *L. pictor* resulted in severe cardiac alterations with single cell necrosis in the ventricular and septal myocardium, rounded mitochondria with increased matrix density, and separation of intracellular organelles. At the renal level, the formation of autophagic vacuoles and lysosomes beneath the brush border of convoluted urinary tubules was observed accompanied by occasional destruction of microvilli. The formation of autophagic vacuoles in the pancreas acinar cells was also observed (Terao et al., 1992). The administration of similar doses (1 µg/kg) of the toxin extracted from a crab of *D. alcalai* showed that surviving animals presented decreased body weight and paralysis of hind limbs and decreased thymus, spleen, and liver weight. At the histological level, the intestine was severely compromised with reddening, congestion, bleeding in the intestinal lumen, and degeneration and loss of epithelial cells. Congestion of jejunum and duodenum was observed 2–6 h postinjection (Ito et al., 1996).

Intraperitoneal administration of PLTX extracted from *P. vestitus* (MW 3300) resulted in an LD_{50} for rats of 0.63 µg/kg (confidence intervals 0.44–0.91 µg/kg), suggesting sensitivity similar to mice for i.p. administration of the toxin (Wiles et al., 1974).

Some studies performed in mice describe the effects of i.p. administration of PLTX-containing extracts isolated from several matrices, such as fish, crustaceans, and microalgae. In these cases, the likelihood that the observed effects derive from PLTX or congeners is very high, although the effects of co-occurring substances cannot be ruled out and should be anticipated. In addition, the varying degrees of purity make dose comparisons problematic. Symptoms described in these cases were generally motor incoordination and/or paralysis, dyspnea occasionally accompanied by cyanosis, and convulsions (Carumbana et al., 1976; Fukui et al., 1987; Chia et al., 1993; Wachi et al. 2000; Taniyama et al., 2003). In agreement with these data, Lenoir et al. described the administration of extracts of *O. mascareniensis* that resulted in hind limb paralysis and convulsions with an observed LD_{50} of 0.9 mg/kg (Lenoir et al., 2004).

Very few data describe the toxicity of PLTX analogues: OST-D purified from *O. siamensis* seems to be lethal after i.p. administration in mice above a dose of 5 µg/kg with limb paralysis and gastric erosions (Ito and Yasumoto, 2009). Ovatoxin-a isolated from *O. ovata* at a dose of 7 µg/kg caused limb paralysis and death within 30 min of administration (Ciminiello et al., 2012).

The i.v. administration of PLTX and related molecules in rodents gives results very similar to that obtained after i.p. dosing. Intravenous administration of partially purified PLTX (from *P. vestitus*, MW 3300) into mice resulted in initial drowsiness, followed by convulsions and dyspnea resulting in death with an LD_{50} of 0.45 µg/kg (confidence interval 0.33–0.62 µg/kg; Wiles et al., 1974). These data were consistent with those obtained by Deguchi after the administration of PLTX extracted from *P. tuberculosa*, thus 0.53 µg/kg (confidence interval 0.38–0.73 µg/kg; Deguchi et al., 1976). The same experiment performed in rats gave similar results, with an estimated LD_{50} of 0.089 µg/kg (confidence interval 0.080–0.098 µg/kg) and initial drowsiness and prostration followed by dyspnea and convulsions occurring prior to death (Wiles et al., 1974).

Intravenous administration of the same extract from *P. vestitus* into male and female guinea pigs (*Cavia porcellus*) also resulted in dyspnea and convulsions, followed by death (LD_{50} = 0.11 µg/kg).

Intramuscular administration of PLTX extracted from *P. vestitus* (MW 3300) in rats presented toxicity similar to that of i.v. administration, even if the onset of symptoms and lethality was slower and local irritation and swelling occurred at the site of injection (LD_{50} = 0.24 µg/kg confidence intervals 0.21–0.28 µg/kg; Wiles et al., 1974).

25.2.1.3 Toxicity after Single Administration through Other Exposure Routes

During the first characterization of the PLTX extracted form *P. vestitus* (MW 3300), toxicity of the compound was observed in rodents following administrations through different routes. Among these, subcutaneous administration in rats of the compound resulted in toxicity similar to that elicited after parenteral administration (Wiles et al., 1974). Intradermal injection of the toxin in rats and guinea pig resulted in severe vasoconstriction at the injection site, followed by local edema and erythema (Wiles et al., 1974).

The literature also offers little information regarding intratracheal (i.t.) administration of PLTXs in rodents. Intratracheal administration of toxic extracts from *P. vestitus* to rats elicited symptoms similar to i.v. administration and an LD_{50} of 0.63 µg/kg (Wiles et al., 1974). Similarly, Ito and Yasumoto (2009) observed death in mice within 2 h after i.t. administration at doses starting at 2 µg/kg. These doses were 100-fold lower than those resulting in death from gastric gavage. Symptoms included paralysis, alveolar bleeding, and gastrointestinal erosion. The same paper described i.t. evaluation of OST-D at doses of 1, 2, 4.5, 7, 9, 11, and 13 µg/kg. At the highest dose, death occurred 1 h post-administration with lung and gastric bleeding.

Lung bleeding and interstitial inflammation were also observed after sublingual administration of PLTX or OST-D, accompanied by gastrointestinal erosion and glomerular atrophy (Ito and Yasumoto, 2009).

25.2.1.4 Toxicity after Repeated Administration

Studies describing the effects of repeated PLTX administration deserve special consideration because they allow the identification of target organs in a situation mimicking a characteristic type of human exposure. Unfortunately, such studies are rare.

One of the first studies describing the effects of PLTX after repeated administration was carried out to evaluate tumor promotion activity of the toxin; in this case, 0.5 µg PLTX was applied on the mice skin two times per week for 30 weeks. PLTX exposure after initiation with 7,12-dimethylbenz[a]anthracene resulted in the development of tumors in 62.5% of the treated animals (Fujiki et al., 1986; for further details Section 25.4.3).

Few years later, Vick and Wiles (1990) described the variation of the toxicity of PLTX when rats were treated with a nonlethal dose of the toxin (5 µg/kg PLTX either *per os* or intra rectal) before the lethal one (0.25 µg/kg i.m.). The experiment resulted in a decrease mortality fraction if the second treatment took place between 24 and 48 h after the first one. Similarly, the protection was observed when the administration of 10 µg/kg PLTX *per os* was followed by 0.20 µg/kg i.v. (after 24 h; Vick and Wiles, 1990).

Repeated i.p. administration (29 injections, 0.25 µg/kg) to mice of PLTX isolated from crabs (*D. alcalai*) induced thymus weight loss, although the animals recovered after cessation of dosing (Ito et al., 1997). Histological analysis after the 5th and 10th injections revealed necrosis of lymphocytes. Spleen weight increased during the dosing period, associated with an increase in the number of megakaryocytic cells. Lymphocytes with condensed nuclei were also observed in the red pulp, as were fibrinous exudates and inflammatory cells such as granulocytes and monocytes. At the end of the treatment regimen, decreased numbers of circulating T cells and B cells and increased numbers of circulating granulocytes and monocytes were observed. At the end of the dosing period, animals presented with ascites and ventral organ adhesions that were still observable at the end of the recovery period (Ito et al., 1997).

Repeated sublingual administration of PLTX (up to 3 days of treatment, cumulative dosage up to 495 µg/kg) and OST-D (up to 5 days of treatment, cumulative dosage up to 1000 µg/kg) caused pulmonary congestion and mild alveolar destruction accompanied by stomach ulcers and erosion of the gut. These effects were more severe in mice treated with PLTX than those treated with OST-D (Ito and Yasumoto, 2009).

25.2.2 Toxicity in Nonrodent Species

25.2.2.1 Toxicity after Single Oral Administration

To our knowledge, no oral studies on purified PLTX have been performed on nonrodent species, even though lethality in cats has been reported to confirm toxicity of specimens of crabs collected in the Philippines, *D. alcalai* and *L. pictor* (Carumbana et al., 1976).

25.2.2.2 Toxicity after Single Parenteral Administration

A considerable amount of work has been performed in dogs, as this species is considered extremely sensitive to PLTX. Lethality was recorded starting from an i.v. dose of 0.06 µg/kg for PLTX extracted from *P. tuberculosa* (Ito et al., 1982). At higher doses (0.5 µg/kg), the i.v. administration of the toxin isolated from *P. mammillosa* and *P. caribaeorum* was lethal within 10 min (Kaul et al., 1974). The toxin extracted from *P. vestitus* (MW 3300) seems to be very toxic as well, with a calculated LD_{50} of 0.03 and 0.08 after i.v. and i.m. administration, respectively (Wiles et al., 1974). Intravenous administration of toxic extracts of *P. mammillosa* (Kaul et al., 1974; Munday, 2008), *P. caribaeorum* (Kaul, 1981; Munday, 2008), and *P. tuberculosa* (Ito et al., 1982) causes severe abnormalities in blood pressure and ECG profile that in most severe cases leads to cardiac arrest. In addition to the experiments performed with dogs, some information is available for other nonrodent species, even if the purity of the testing material was uncertain. For instance, alterations in blood pressure and ECG abnormalities were observed in cats after i.v. administration of toxic extracts of *P. tuberculosa* (Deguchi et al., 1974). Wiles et al. (1974) reported a comparison between species administrated with the PLTX extracted from *P. vestitus* (MW 3300); early signs of toxicity of the compound administrated to monkeys were ataxia, drowsiness, and weakness of the limbs followed by collapse and death (LD_{50} 0.078 µg/kg, confidence interval 0.060–0.090 µg/kg). In the same experimental conditions, rabbits were reported to be the most sensitive animal to i.v. administration of PLTX with an LD_{50} of 0.025 µg/kg (confidence interval 0.024–0.026 µg/kg; Wiles et al., 1974).

25.2.2.3 Toxicity after Single Administration through Other Exposure Routes

During the toxicological characterization of the *P. vestitus* PLTX extracts (MW 3300), rabbits were used to investigate the toxicity of the compound following intradermal, percutaneous, and ocular administration. The toxin was very toxic even through these exposure routes. In particular, intradermal

(0.11 and 0. 55 µg PLTX) administration resulted in severe vasoconstriction, edema, erythema, and inflammation in the site of injection. Similarly, percutaneous application of 0.1–0.5 mL of PLTX in aqueous solution (5 µg/mL) resulted in swelling and necrosis within 4–5 after application. Ocular instillation of PLTX (0.1–0.2 and 0.4 µg/kg) resulted in tearing, irritation, edema, and conjunctivitis within 4 h and severe conjunctivitis up to corneal ulceration and opacity after 24 h (Wiles et al., 1974).

25.2.2.4 Toxicity after Repeated Administration

Experiments that describe the effects of repeated administration of PLTX in nonrodent species are very limited. In spite of that, even if classical repeated toxicity studies are lacking, studies were performed to investigate if an initial sublethal dose of the toxin could prevent or reduce the toxicity of a second higher dose. In rabbits, the administration of a single nonlethal dose *per os* or intraocular seemed to reduce mortality in animals administered with a second lethal i.v. injection of PLTX after 48 and 24 h, respectively. Similarly, dogs resulted protected from the second challenge injection, when treated 48–72 h after the initial i.v. injection and monkeys were protected when treated 48 h after the first injection. With this study, the authors meant to provide information for the definition of a possible pharmacologic treatment of PLTX intoxications: they correlated the reduction in lethality with an increased blood steroid concentration detectable in the treated animals in the postinjection period and mimicked the protective effect also with injection of hydrocortisone before the administration of the toxin (Vick and Wiles, 1990).

25.2.2.5 Toxicity in Invertebrates

During blooms of *Ostreopsis* spp. along the Mediterranean coast, effects on marine invertebrates are common. Mortality and abnormalities in mussels, sea urchins, and starfish have been observed during large blooms (Sansoni et al., 2003), and dead animals (e.g., octopi) have been shown to contain significant concentrations of PLTXs or ovatoxins (Aligizaki et al., 2011). Test performed on toxic samples of *O. siamensis* (positive for PLTX to hemolysis assay performed with anti-PLTX antibodies) revealed that the microalgae can be toxic for brine shrimps and cause morbidity in paua larvae (Rhodes et al., 2000). Toxicity of PLTX evaluated with the FETAX assay revealed increased mortality, teratogenesis of the embryos at the concentrations of 37 and 370 nM. Histological examination of the surviving larvae (PLTX 37 nM) revealed structural modification at muscular and neuronal level (Franchini et al., 2008, 2010). Laboratory studies suggest PLTX can alter the physiology of mussels (*Mytilus galloprovincialis*), especially the immunocyte signaling transduction pathway (Malagoli et al., 2008). Further, analysis of *M. galloprovincialis* during different stages of the bloom revealed significant inhibition of the Na^+/K^+-ATPase and of acetylcholine esterase (Gorbi et al., 2012). During the initial phase of toxin accumulation, granulocyte numbers increased and lysosomal membrane stability decreased, suggesting a primary immune response. Moreover, in primary cultures of hepatopancreas cells and mantle cells isolated from uncontaminated *M. galloprovincialis*, PLTX reduced the metabolic rate in a time- and concentration-dependent manner (Louzao et al., 2010).

25.2.3 Conclusions

Although human poisonings, with some lethalities, were ascribed to the ingestion of PLTXs-contaminated seafood, the lack of accurate PLTX quantification in the leftovers doesn't allow to define a no observed adverse effect level (NOAEL) or a lowest observed adverse effect level (LOAEL) for the tolerable daily intake (TDI) or acute reference dose (ARfD) definition. Experimental toxicity studies indicate that the oral acute toxicity of PLTX is lower than its parenteral toxicity, although with $LD_{50} < 1$ mg/kg in mice. Studies after repeated oral administration are urgently necessary due to widespread presence of PLTXs in different seafood, which can suggest a chronic exposure to these compounds. Also, the potential toxicity of PLTXs after aerosol exposure needs to be urgently addressed due to increasing blooms of *Ostreopsis* associated with respiratory and eyes problems as well as dermotoxicity in people exposed both for recreational and working activities.

25.3 Mechanism of Action

The investigation of the mechanism of action of PLTX and its congeners has represented one of the most active fields of research regarding the molecule. In fact, the strong toxicity of this family of compounds, which can be observed in a wide variety of cellular models and tissues, as well as in vivo, seems to be related to its ability to block one of the crucial transporters of the cellular membrane, thus the Na^+/K^+-ATPase.

25.3.1 Molecular Target

The commonly accepted mechanism of action of PLTX is transformation of the Na^+/K^+-ATPase into a non-selective ionic pore. This followed the observation that PLTX induced an efflux of K^+ from erythrocytes, leading to hemolysis (Haberman et al., 1981). Use of the glycoside ouabain to inhibit PLTX-induced hemolysis confirmed the primary biological target as the Na^+/K^+-ATPase on the plasma membrane (Habermann and Chatwal, 1982). The Na^+/K^+-ATPase is a transmembrane pump belonging to the family of P-type ATPases, which are essential for maintaining cellular homeostasis. It serves to transfer three Na^+ ions out of the cell in trade for two K+ ions into the cell in a cyclic process that exploits the hydrolysis of ATP (Figure 25.1).

It has been well documented that binding of PLTX to the α-β heterodimer of the ATPase changes it from a transmembrane pump to a nonspecific cationic channel that induces a consistent ionic imbalance at the cellular level (Hilgemann, 2003; Artigas and Gadsby, 2004). The affinity of PLTX for the E_2P conformational state of the pump is extremely high (Figure 25.1; Artigas and Gadsby, 2004; Harmel and Apell, 2006; Rodrigues et al., 2008). Its binding results in substitution of cysteines for several residues in the putative fifth and sixth transmembrane helices (Guennoun and Horisberger, 2000, 2002). As a consequence, the α-helices in the membrane domain are rearranged, allowing the opening of the cytoplasmic gate of

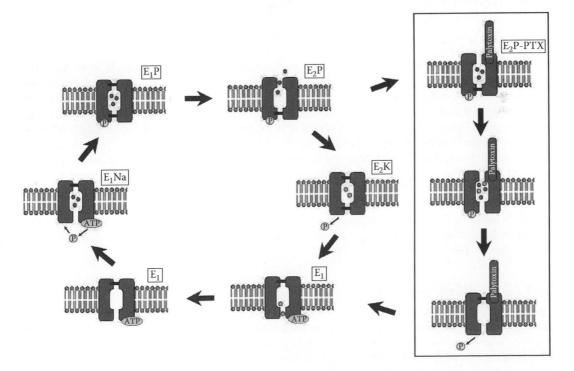

FIGURE 25.1 Albert–Post model for Na^+/K^+-ATPase pump. The pump alternates cyclically in two principal conformational states E_1 and E_2. In the state E_2P, the pump is phosphorylated; this conformation allows the binding of PLTX, which induces changes in the α-helices resulting in the opening of the intracellular gate. Toxin binding also impairs the dephosphorylation of the pump, resulting in prolonged opening of the so constituted nonspecific cationic channel. Eventually, the pump is dephosphorylated and returns into its normal physiological state.

the pump. Indeed, the channels that are formed by PLTX might arise as a consequence of a perturbation in the ATPase structure, leading to the loss of control of the gates of the enzyme and, hence, to uncoupling of the ion transports (Tosteson et al., 2003). Moreover, since in the E_2P conformational state the extracellular gate is physiologically open, the contemporary opening of the intracellular gate induces the formation of the open channel as long as the pump is phosphorylated. The dephosphorylation of the pump allows its conformational change into the E_1 state. However, PLTX binding also reduces the rate of pump dephosphorylation, protracting the opening of the channel (Artigas and Gadsby, 2004; Harmel and Apell, 2006; Rodrigues et al., 2008). Once dephosphorylated, the pump returns to its normal function. There is no agreement in the literature on whether the dephosphorylation event causes dissociation of PLTX. However, computational simulations suggest a crucial role for Na^+/K^+-ATPase phosphorylation in increasing PLTX affinity for the pump. These data are supported by the fact that even submicromolar concentrations of ATP could enhance the apparent affinity of PLTX for mammalian Na^+/K^+-ATPase, probably by supporting pump phosphorylation (Rakowski et al., 2007). On the other hand, K^+ occlusion reduces the pump affinity for PLTX, blocks the induced channels, and impedes the pump phosphorylation (Rodrigues et al., 2009). These data are in line with the idea that K^+ is able to reduce Na^+/K^+-ATPase affinity to PLTX by reducing the toxin-binding stability and, therefore, to increase its dissociation rate (Rodrigues et al., 2008).

Many studies report the ability of the cardioactive glycoside ouabain to inhibit PLTX effects in vitro (Habermann and Chhatwall, 1982; Schilling et al., 2006; Vale-Gonzalez et al., 2007a; Pelin et al., 2011, 2012) and thus support this mechanism of action. However, incomplete abolishment of PLTX biological activity in the presence of ouabain suggests that ouabain does not completely compete with PLTX on the binding sites. Indeed, Artigas and Gadsby (2004) demonstrated that PLTX and ouabain can simultaneously bind to Na^+/K^+-ATPase, suggesting the possibility of two different binding sites on the pump, as subsequently observed in vitro on skin keratinocytes, where ouabain seems to act as a negative allosteric modulator against sub-micromolar PLTX concentrations and as a non-competitive antagonist against sub-nanomolar PLTX concentrations (Pelin et al., 2013a).

25.3.2 Other Potential Targets

In the last decade, scientists have investigated other potential molecular targets of PLTX. Hypothetically, the toxin could also interfere with other P-type ATPases such as the sarcoplasmic–endoplasmic reticulum Ca^{2+} pump (SERCA) (Coca et al., 2008; Kockskämper et al., 2004) and the nongastric H^+/K^+ ATPase pump (Scheiner-Bobis et al., 2002; Qiu et al., 2006). However, despite the close structural homology among members of the P-type ATPases, PLTX did not transform the SERCA into a channel as it does on the Na^+/K^+-ATPase. Indeed, it appears that the effects of PLTX on the Na^+/K^+-ATPase and SERCA occur through different mechanisms. It seems that channel formation induced by PLTX is related to the α/β-oligomeric composition of the ATPases, rather than to the primary structure of the protein (Coca et al., 2008). The Na^+/K^+-ATPase appears to be sensitive to PLTX only when both α and β subunits are co-expressed (Scheiner-Bobis et al., 1994). Furthermore, PLTX also affects the epithelial H^+/K^+-ATPase, which has a two-subunit composition as well, in the same way (Scheiner-Bobis et al., 2002). Interestingly, α subunit of Na^+/K^+-ATPase can form functional pump complexes with the β subunit of the H^+-pump (Horisberger et al., 1991) and this hybrid between the two pumps is still sensitive to PLTX (Farley et al., 2001).

25.3.3 Role of Ionic Imbalance

The transformation of Na^+/K^+-ATPase into a nonselective cationic channel results in an upset of cellular ion homeostasis. The first event consists of an intracellular overload of Na^+ causing a depolarization of the cellular membrane that is increased by the massive efflux of K^+ and influx of Ca^{2+} (Wu, 2009). Ca^{2+} influx seems to be mediated by reverse functioning of the Na^+/Ca^{2+} exchanger (NCE) caused by increased Na^+ concentration and, depending on the cellular model, by voltage-dependent L-type Ca^{2+}-channels. Although not yet completely understood, the increase in intracellular Ca^{2+} levels may induce opening of K^+ or Cl^- channels, further impairing cell ionic balance. Moreover, the intracellular increase in Na^+ appears to induce an acidification of the cytoplasm, probably due to the reverse functioning of the Na^+/H^+ exchanger (NHE) (Rossini and Bigiani, 2011).

It is widely accepted that the cytotoxic effects of PLTX are strictly dependent on this ionic imbalance. Indeed, the increased concentrations of Ca^{2+} may trigger Ca^{2+}-dependent cytotoxic effects (Ares et al., 2005; Sheridan et al., 2005; Schilling et al., 2006; Del Favero et al., 2012) and the increased level of Na^+ itself is believed to directly cause cell toxicity (Dubois and Cohen, 1977; Muramatsu et al., 1984; Sheridan et al., 2005). The fact that Na^+ overload is the first and crucial step in mediating PLTX-induced early cell damage has been recently demonstrated on human keratinocytes: removal of Na^+ ions from the extracellular medium completely prevents PLTX effects. Moreover, in Ca^{2+}-free/Na^+-containing medium, a partial reversal of PLTX activity was observed, indicating that the initial Na^+ overload is required as an essential condition for the contribution of Ca^{2+} in mediating PLTX effects (Pelin et al., 2011). This finding is consistent with previous observations regarding Na^+ dependency on PLTX effects (Wattenberg et al., 1989; Kuroki et al., 1997; Ciminiello et al., 2009; Pérez-Gómez et al., 2010).

25.4 In Vitro Effects

The in vitro effects of PLTX seem to be strictly linked to the ionic imbalance conditions described earlier. Following PLTX interaction with the pump, the initial intracellular overload of Na^+ increases intracellular Ca^{2+} and H^+ levels. These events have direct consequences on cell viability, with different effects depending on the cellular model.

25.4.1 Effects on Excitable Cells and Tissues

25.4.1.1 Smooth Muscle

From the first evidence that PLTX caused severe alterations in ionic homeostasis and electric membrane properties, models of excitable tissues have been widely used to characterize the mechanism of action of the toxin. Among these, ex vivo preparations of smooth muscle tissue and cell culture have been extensively used. Unfortunately, early studies were often performed on semipurified material available at that time, with reported molecular weight of 3300 Da (Ito et al., 1979). It is now accepted that PLTXs have molecular weights in the range of 2659–2680 Da, depending on the source (Moore and Bartolini, 1981; Riobò and Franco, 2011), nearly 500 Da lower than that used in early studies. PLTXs induce a sustained contraction of smooth muscle that can be observed in a variety of cell models, including vascular, intestinal, tracheal, and papillary smooth muscles (Deguchi et al., 1974; Ito et al., 1976, 1977; Ozaki et al., 1983; Ishida et al., 1985). This effect is detectable after incubation of cells with PLTX in the picomolar range (Deguchi et al., 1974; Robinson and Franz, 1991; Robinson et al., 1992). PLTX (concentration above 1.0×10^{-10} g/mL) can trigger muscular tension in aorta smooth muscle, persistent even hours after toxin removal (Ito et al., 1977). Contraction appears to be dependent on external Ca^{2+} but is insensitive to several compounds that commonly modulate muscle contraction, such as atropine, tetrodotoxin, and phentolamine (Ito et al., 1976; Ozaki et al., 1983). Electrical membrane properties of smooth muscle are also impaired by PLTX (from 1.0×10^{-9} g/mL), which is known to cause increase of spiking frequency and depolarization in guinea pig tenia coli (Ito et al., 1976). Similarly, Sheridan and coworkers (2005) described an increase in Ca^{2+} spike frequency after incubation with PLTX (2 nM) and progressive membrane depolarization in cultured aortic smooth muscle cells. In porcine coronary arteries, the toxin (1 pM and 10 nM) induces contraction and PLTX-dependent intracellular Ca^{2+} increase ($[Ca^{2+}]_i$), which seems to be both dependent on extracellular Na^+ (Ozaki et al., 1983; Ishii et al., 1997). These data suggest that the initial Na^+ influx could activate voltage-dependent Ca^{2+} channels, the NCE, and Ca^{2+} release from intracellular stores, causing an $[Ca^{2+}]_i$ increase (Ishii et al., 1997). A direct effect of the toxin on muscular contractile properties was also supported by data obtained in vascular muscle (rat tail artery) preincubated with reserpine. The latter induced presynaptic release of norepinephrine but did not alter the contractile effects of PLTX, suggesting for the toxin a mechanism of action independent from the release of endogenous neurotransmitters (Karaki et al., 1988). In agreement with the proposed mechanism of action of PLTX on the Na^+/K^+-ATPase (Section 25.3), the toxin induces K^+ efflux from guinea pig ileal longitudinal smooth muscle leading to a progressive depletion of the ion from the tissue (half maximal effective concentration $(EC_{50}) = 1.8 \times 10^{-8}$ M; Hori et al., 1988). In addition to the impairment of electrical and mechanical properties of cultured smooth muscle cells, PLTX is also highly cytotoxic on cultured aortic smooth muscle cells: LDH release, measured after 15 min of incubation with the toxin and 2 h of recovery in toxin-free medium, allowed a calculation of EC_{50} of 4.1 nM at 37°C and 14.3 nM at 25°C. Cytotoxicity is also influenced by the presence of extracellular Na^+ and Ca^{2+}, supporting the importance of the two ions in the mechanism of action of the toxin. PLTX-induced cytotoxicity is accompanied by morphologic changes, such as rounding and development of granulation on the cell surface (concentration of 10 nM PLTX and above; Sheridan et al., 2005).

25.4.1.2 Skeletal Muscle

In skeletal muscle cells, PLTX seems to be able to trigger an irreversible Na^+-dependent membrane depolarization (Deguchi et al., 1974; Ecault and Sauviat, 1991), similar to that induced in other muscle models (Sections 25.4.1.1 and 25.4.1.3). These effects are nearly insensitive to typical blockers of voltage-dependent Na^+ channels, such as tetrodotoxin (TTX) (Deguchi et al., 1974; Ecault and Sauviat, 1991) and amiloride (Ecault and Sauviat, 1991). PLTXs are also able to trigger a ouabain-sensitive $[Ca^{2+}]_i$ increase in primary cultures of mouse skeletal muscle cells (Ciminiello et al., 2009). The presence of Na^+ in the extracellular environment is also crucial in mediating PLTX-induced $[Ca^{2+}]_i$ increase, in fact, in its absence, both PLTX and its analogue 42-OH-PLTX (both 6 nM) fail to trigger $[Ca^{2+}]_i$ increase. When experiments are performed in normal external solution, both toxins trigger a persistent and long-lasting $[Ca^{2+}]_i$ that is detectable up to 30 min post exposure (Ciminiello et al., 2009). The kinetics of the Ca^{2+} unbalance triggered by PLTX is usually biphasic. A transient $[Ca^{2+}]_i$ increase is usually sustained in the first phase by the activation of voltage-activated Ca^{2+} channels, the NCE (reverse mode), and Ca^{2+} release from intracellular stores. This is followed by a second phase sustained by the entrance of Ca^{2+} from the extracellular compartment, mediated by the activation of stretch-activated channels, and is of crucial importance for the development of the PLTX muscular toxicity (Del Favero et al., 2012).

25.4.1.3 Cardiac Muscle

A primary effect of PLTX on cardiac muscle is membrane depolarization, very likely mediated by Na^+ influx (Ito et al., 1979; Sauviat et al., 1987; Muramatsu et al., 1988; Artigas and Gadsby, 2002). In addition to muscular contraction and induction of spontaneous action potentials, PLTX $(3.0 \times 10^{-8}$ g/mL) seems to be able to induce also arrhythmias in guinea pig papillary muscle, insensitive to the block of β adrenergic signaling (Ito et al., 1979); Na^+ conductances triggered by PLTXs are likely linked to the interaction of PLTX with the Na^+/K^+ pump and its consequent transformation into a cationic pore (Frelin et al., 1991; Frelin and Van Renterghem, 1995; Artigas and Gadsby, 2002). PLTX is also known to trigger an outward K^+ current, independent of the presence of Na^+ in the extracellular solutions (Kinoshita et al., 1991). The connection between the mechanism of action of PLTX at the Na^+/K^+-ATPase and the alteration of the electrical properties of cellular membranes were strengthened by the work of Kockskämper et al. (2004), who demonstrated that PLTX also disrupted excitation–contraction in a cultured cat atrial myocytes when used in the nanomolar range. Van Renterghem and Freling (1993) demonstrated that Ca^{2+} was required for the elicitation of Na^+ current, which is consistent with the theory that divalent cations are critical for PLTX binding (Ecault and Sauviat, 1991; Del Favero et al., 2012). The ionic imbalance caused by PLTX in cardiac cells may also be linked to the intracellular acidification induced in this cell type (Frelin et al., 1990).

25.4.1.4 Neurons

As previously described for other excitable cell models, PLTXs are also highly cytotoxic for neuronal cells, inducing neuronal death in the picomolar range after 24 h of incubation (Pérez-Gómez et al., 2010). PLTX is also known to trigger membrane depolarization at neuronal level (Kudo and Shibata,

1980; Muramatsu et al., 1984; Louzao et al., 2006; Kagiava et al., 2012). This depolarization is at best minimally sensitive to TTX and dependent upon external Na^+ (Muramatsu et al., 1984). In agreement with the effect on the membrane potential, PLTX (100 nM) induces in primary cultures of neurons of the suprachiasmatic nucleus a transient increase in spontaneous firing possibly related to the initial phase of depolarization, followed by progressive disappearance of spontaneous spiking activity (Wang and Huang, 2006).

Moreover, PLTX (10 nM) also triggers an increase in $[Ca^{2+}]_i$ in primary cultures of cerebellar granule neurons (Vale et al., 2006). This increase seems to be sensitive to the presence of extracellular Ca^{2+} and to nifedipine (a blocker of voltage-dependent Ca^{2+} channels) and saxitoxin (a blocker of voltage-dependent Na^+ channels), when the two are both applied to the extracellular medium before PLTX (Vale et al., 2006). The homeostasis of $[Ca^{2+}]_i$ is of crucial importance for the cellular survival and the perturbation induced by PLTX influences the cell at several levels. PLTX-induced $[Ca^{2+}]_i$ increase seems to be related to intracellular acidification induced by the toxin (1–10 nM); in fact, this effect seems to be sustained by the activation of plasma membrane calcium ATPase, possibly as a secondary consequence of the $[Ca^{2+}]_i$ increase triggered by the toxin (Vale-Gonzáles et al., 2007). In the same cell model, PLTX-induced $[Ca^{2+}]_i$ increase, intracellular acidification, and cytotoxicity are probably mediated by the activation of the extracellular signal-regulated kinase ERK-2, suggesting a role for the mitogen-activated protein kinases (MAPKs) in the neurotoxic effect of PLTX (Vale et al., 2007). Further, PLTX seems to be able to disrupt at several levels the signal transduction pathways between the neurons; in the nanomolar range, the toxin triggers the release of excitatory amino acids from synaptic vesicles in cerebellar granule neurons (Vale et al., 2006). Similarly, PLTX (100 nM; 3 h exposure) induces depletion of aminergic transmitters from the innervation of the anococcygeus muscle (Amir et al., 1997). In addition to previous considerations, PLTX is also able to increase toxicity of other neurotoxins, such as domoic acid. The combination of nontoxic concentrations of these two compounds (PLTX 100–300 pM and domoic acid 5 μM) results in a synergistic toxicity sustained by the presence of Na^+ in the extracellular environment, raising serious concern about the possibility of their co-occurrence as seafood contaminants (Pérez-Gómez et al., 2010). An uncontrolled increase in $[Ca^{2+}]_i$ is often related to the development of cytotoxic events and that induced by PLTXs is no exception.

Neuroblastoma cells are another tool for the investigation of the effects of PLTX at the neuronal level. In this model, as previously described for cerebellar granule neurons (Vale et al., 2006), PLTX and its analogue OST-D were able to trigger an $[Ca^{2+}]_i$ increase (Louzao et al., 2007). Moreover, the two toxins also induced morphologic alterations through disorganization of different cytoskeletal components, such as filamentous actin (Louzao et al., 2007) and globular actin (Ares et al., 2009). The involvement of typical apoptotic markers was also evaluated in neuroblastoma cells, but the only parameter influenced by picomolar concentrations of PLTX was the mitochondrial membrane potential (Valverde et al., 2008a). In later studies, Sagara and coworkers (2011) hypothesized that the major pathway of toxicity triggered by PLTX on PC12 rat pheochromocytoma cells is nonoxidative necrotic damage, thus suggesting minimal importance of the apoptotic pathway in PLTX-induced neurotoxicity.

25.4.2 Effects on Nonexcitable Cells

As in excitable cells, the toxic effects of PLTX in nonexcitable cells are dependent upon ionic imbalances. In these models, the initial intracellular Na^+ overload is directly involved in PLTX-induced cell toxicity. This overload can trigger a secondary Ca^{2+} overload, thus inducing secondary toxic effects resulting in cell death. The primary difference between excitable and nonexcitable cells is that intracellular signaling in excitable cells is strictly regulated by Ca^{2+}-dependent pathways, making these cells overly sensitive to the effects of Ca^{2+} overload. In contrast, nonexcitable cells seem more susceptible to general ionic imbalances and are therefore more susceptible to the initial Na^+ overload. Thus, transformation of the Na^+/K^+-ATPase to a nonselective pore may have different intracellular effects mediated by different intracellular pathways, depending upon the cell model used. Therefore, the following review of in vitro intracellular effects of PLTX has been grouped according to cell model used.

25.4.2.1 Intestinal Cells

The data most relevant to human oral intoxication by PLTX have been derived using Caco-2 cells. This cell line is commonly used as a predictive model of intestinal absorption because they express morphological and functional properties typical of mature enterocytes. Valverde and coworkers (2008b) observed that PLTX decreased cell proliferation with an EC_{50} of 10^{-10} M, showing dramatic cell alterations such as cell rounding and F-actin depolymerization. Loss of the enterocyte microfilament network had been previously observed by Ares et al. (2005) in rabbit intestinal cells, presumably through a Ca^{2+}-dependent mechanism. More recently, Pelin et al. (2012) investigated the effects of PLTX on undifferentiated Caco-2 cells, which turned out to be very sensitive to PLTX, inducing cytotoxic effects at mitochondrial level with EC_{50} values of $\sim9 \times 10^{-12}$ M after 4 h exposure.

25.4.2.2 Erythrocytes

The effects of PLTX on erythrocytes are quite well characterized, since the hemolytic activity of the toxin has been exploited to develop detection assays for PLTX (see succeeding text). These assays are based on its delayed hemolytic properties. Indeed, PLTX is a potent but slow hemolysin in human, mouse, rat, rabbit, sheep, guinea pig, and hog erythrocytes (Habermann et al., 1981). Hemolysis is strictly dependent on interaction with Na^+/K^+-ATPase, as demonstrated by the inhibition of hemolysis in presence of ouabain (Ozaki et al., 1984, 1985; Habermann, 1989; Tosteston et al., 1991, 1995; Wachi et al., 2000). Indeed, PLTX-induced hemolysis causes a massive K^+ release from rabbit erythrocytes. This release is dependent on the extracellular Ca^{2+} concentrations (Nagase et al., 1986), via a possible calmodulin-dependent mechanism (Nagase et al., 1984).

The observation that PLTX toxicity resulted from binding to the Na^+/K^+-ATPase was confirmed through inhibition by ouabain, thus making erythrocytes a good tool to investigate PLTX binding. Indeed, in early work, a ^{125}I-radiolabeled PLTX bound quickly and reversibly to intact human erythrocytes with a Kd of 2×10^{-11} M (Böttinger et al., 1986). Consistent data were later derived by Tosteston et al. (1994), who, using monoclonal antibodies against PLTX, estimated an apparent dissociation constant of 2×10^{-10} M in the same model. Binding is promoted by divalent cations and by borate and inhibited by the presence of K^+ and ouabain, the latter showing a competitive behavior with PLTX on Na^+/K^+-ATPase (Böttinger et al., 1986). Despite the use of ouabain as inhibitor/displacer of PLTX on erythrocytes, it has been reported that the ouabain binding site on Na^+/K^+-ATPase may not be exactly identical to that of PLTX (Ozaki et al., 1985; Habermann, 1989).

More recently, a study performed by Ficarra et al. (2011) widely characterized PLTX effects on red blood cells. PLTX strongly affects anionic fluxes and seriously compromises both CO_2 transport and the metabolic modulation centered on the oxy–deoxy cycle of hemoglobin. The observed inhibition of the anion flux in the presence of PLTX may be related to the significant imbalance between Cl^- and HCO_3^- concentrations. Based on the anion kinetics obtained in the presence of PLTX with and without orthovanadate and ouabain, the authors hypothesize an indirect action of PLTX on the functionality of B3, the major transmembrane glycoprotein on red blood cells that mediates the electroneutral exchange of Cl^- and HCO_3^- across the plasma membrane and playing an essential role in the transport mechanism of CO_2.

25.4.2.3 Immune Cell Models

The effects of PLTX on immune cells have been assessed in neutrophils, macrophages, lymphocytes, and mast cells. In neutrophils, the major effect appears to be the induction of superoxide anions (Kano et al., 1987). However, the toxin concentration required is an EC50 value of approximately 10^{-8} M, and the relatively weak effect compared to phorbol esters raises questions of physiological relevance (Gabrielson et al., 1992). In isolated human lymphocytes, PLTX showed maximal cytotoxic effects at 10^{-8} M (Falciola et al., 1994), again suggesting low potency in these cells.

However, use of immune cell models has been pivotal in assessing the mediation of the inflammatory response induced by PLTX. This role has been demonstrated in both mast cells and macrophages.

For instance, PLTX has been demonstrated to stimulate both the metabolism of arachidonic acid and prostaglandin E_2 (PGE_2) in peritoneal rat macrophages at concentrations down to 10^{-12} M (Ohuchi et al., 1985). These features are likely related to the tumor promotion properties ascribed to the toxin (see succeeding text).

In monocyte-derived human macrophages, nuclear transcription factor-κB (NF-κB) is activated after PLTX exposure along with reduced levels of the inhibitory protein IκB-α. In this scenario, the MAPK cascade plays a crucial role in mediating the inflammatory intracellular pathway. Indeed, both PLTX and *O.* cf *ovata* extracts phosphorylated p38 MAPK, supporting the hypothesis that the activation of the MAPK cascade is probably involved in the toxin-induced transcription and accumulation of COX-2, TNF-α, and IL-8 transcripts (Crinelli et al., 2012).

Histamine may be another potential mediator of PLTX-induced inflammation. Indeed, it has been demonstrated that PLTX is a potent releaser of histamine from rat mast cells with a maximal effect at 50 ng/mL (Chhatwal et al., 1982). Furthermore, histamine release was synergistic with the presence of 10 ng/mL TPA (Ohuchi et al., 1986).

25.4.2.4 Skin Cells

The study of the effects of PLTX on skin cells was initially stimulated by the hypothesis that it may be a tumor promoter. The ability of PLTX to stimulate arachidonic acid metabolism, thus inducing release of PGE_2 from primary cultures of mouse epidermal cells, was initially observed by Aizu et al. (1990). During the following decades, the strong correlation of arachidonic acid metabolism to the mechanism(s) of tumor promotion propelled them to focus on the intracellular signaling of skin tumor promotion. These studies will be discussed more in detail in the following section.

Only recently, in view of the increasing incidence of dermatitis and irritation ascribed to PLTX exposure, an in vitro study was performed with the aim to characterize toxin effects on skin cells. Using the human keratinocyte HaCaT cell line, cytotoxicity was evaluated after a short duration exposure (4 h) by different techniques assessing different cellular endpoints. PLTX reduced mitochondrial activity, cell viability, and plasma membrane integrity with different EC_{50} values (6×10^{-11}, 5×10^{-10} M, and 2×10^{-8} M, respectively). On the basis of these EC_{50} values, it has been suggested that among the chain of intracellular events following the interaction of PLTX with the Na^+/K^+-ATPase the earliest is mitochondrial damage. This damage serves to reduce cell viability by several routes, including plasma membrane rupture with leakage of LDH (Pelin et al., 2011). Moreover, it seems that mitochondrial dysfunction could be correlated to oxidative stress induction, leading to a novel approach to investigate the intracellular pathway leading to cell death. Indeed, the intracellular H^+ overload that follows PLTX-induced Na^+ intracellular accumulation, could enhance ΔpH across mitochondrial inner membrane, mediating O_2^- production by reversing mitochondrial electron transports (Pelin et al., 2013b).

25.4.2.5 Other Cell Models

Several studies have investigated PLTX effects on cell lines derived from other tissues. In the renal LLC-PK1 cell line, PLTX induced an irreversible cytotoxic effect characterized by pronounced cell swelling and ionic imbalance, even without any specific effect on tight junctions between epithelial cells (Mullin et al., 1991). In the same study, analyzing Na^+ and K^+ fluxes using $^{22}Na^+$ and $^{86}Rb^+$, the authors reported a pronounced depolarization of the cell sheet when PLTX is exposed to the basolateral cell surface and a pronounced hyperpolarization when exposed apically.

The characterization of PLTX cytotoxicity has been further studied on the human osteoblast-like Saos-2 cell line. PLTX induced a rise in the cytosolic-free Na^+ concentration and a concentration-dependent biphasic rise in the cytosolic-free Ca^{2+} concentration, both ouabain-sensitive events (Monroe and Tashjian, 1995). Both Na^+ and Ca^{2+} fluxes were dependent upon the persistent decrease of intracellular pH as observed after 8×10^{-9} M PLTX exposure (Monroe and Tashjian, 1996).

Similarly, ion fluxes, especially Ca^{2+} intracellular overload, was investigated in mouse spleen cells. Using a Ca^{2+} fluorescent indicator, it was found that PLTX induced a concentration-dependent rise in intracellular levels of Ca^{2+}, greatly inhibited by Ni^{2+} and partially inhibited by ouabain (Satoh et al., 2003).

25.4.3 Tumor Promotion

In the early 1980s, PLTX was first identified as a skin tumor promoter using a two-stage mouse carcinogenesis model (Fujiki et al., 1986). In 2006, these results in mice were confirmed in vitro by a two-stage transformation assay using Balb/c 3T3 cells (Miura et al., 2006). Treatment with 1.9×10^{-12} M PLTX was sufficient to increase the number of transformed foci after initiation by 3-methylcholan-threne (MCA). It was postulated that the mechanism of tumor promotion was related to PGE_2 release, since the ability of PLTX to stimulate the metabolism of arachidonic acid and prostaglandin production, common effects of many tumor promoters, had been widely established previously on different cell models. However, the mechanism of PLTX tumor promotion is significantly different from other typical tumor promoters such as 12-*O*-tetradecanoylphorbol-13-acetate (TPA). Indeed, PLTX does not activate protein kinase C (PKC) or increase ornithine decarboxylase (ODC) activity in mouse skin (Fujiki et al., 1986). As such, the toxin has been defined as a non-TPA-type tumor promoter. Cell culture studies have provided further evidence that PLTX stimulates signaling pathways that do not require PKC activation. Both PLTX and TPA cause a reduction in binding of epidermal growth factor (EGF). However, whereas downregulation of PKC blocks the effect of TPA on the EGF receptor, PKC loss does not inhibit the effects of PLTX (Wattenberg et al., 1987).

Further studies have demonstrated that the mechanism leading to tumor promotion seems to involve the activation of the MAPK cascade. The most studied are the extracellular signal-regulated kinases 1 and 2 (ERK1/2), c-Jun N-terminal kinase (JNK)/stress-activated protein kinase, and p38. The kinase ERK5 is a MAP kinase family member that is less well characterized but is receiving increasing attention as a mediator of signals stimulated by both mitogens such as EGF and by stress, including ionic imbalance conditions. Data from these studies suggest that the intracellular pathway and the MAPK cascade activated by PLTX may vary with the cellular model used. Indeed, it has been demonstrated that PLTX stimulates JNK activation in Swiss 3T3 fibroblasts, with a Na^+-dependent but Ca^{2+}-independent mechanism (Kuroki et al., 1996). In addition, PLTX activates p38 in a variety of cell models. However, the intracellular signaling involved in p38 activation is different among cell types, as demonstrated by Li and Wattenberg (1999) on HeLa and COS7 cells. Further studies evaluating the effects on ERK1/2 have confirmed the dependency of the PLTX-stimulated MAPK cascade on cell type. The most surprising result was seen in the 308 cell line, an initiated mouse keratinocyte model. Unlike several other cell types, both PLTX and TPA stimulated the activation of ERK1/2 (Warmka et al., 2002; Zeliadt et al., 2004). Furthermore, PLTX increased ERK1/2 activity through a mechanism that was quite distinct from the mechanisms by which it stimulated JNK and p38 activation. Whereas PLTX-stimulated JNK and p38 through the activation of upstream MAPKs, PLTX increased ERK1/2 activity in 308 kerati-nocytes by decreasing the activity of ERK1/2 phosphatases, mainly mitogen-activated protein kinase phosphatase 3 (MKP-3), a dual-specificity phosphatase highly selective for dephosphorylation and inac-tivation of ERK1/2 (Wattenberg, 2011). PLTX-stimulated signals can also be mediated by ERK5, which is strongly linked to the mechanism of action, since ERK5 can be activated by osmotic stress such as ionic imbalance conditions. PLTX-stimulated ERK5 activation was demonstrated in HeLa and 308 cells by a mechanism dependent on Na^+/K^+-ATPase interaction (Charlson et al., 2009). However, the mecha-nism by which PLTX modulates ERK5 differs from those by which it modulates the three major MAP kinases (Wattenberg, 2011).

25.4.4 Conclusions

Generally, it can be postulated that PLTX effects observed in vitro are strictly dependent on its most quoted molecular target. Indeed, the interaction with the Na^+/K^+-ATPase and the subsequent transfor-mation in a cationic unselective pore induce a sustained imbalance of Na^+, K^+, Ca^{2+}, and H^+. The main-tenance of ionic homeostasis is essential to allow the correct cell functionalities; indeed, it is easy to understand how the sustained perturbation in cationic intracellular levels induced by the toxin could result in high cytotoxic effects. PLTX has been demonstrated to induce, in fact, high cytotoxicity on almost all the cell models so far considered. Moreover, these effects occur very rapidly and are often irreversible.

Lots of studies have been performed to characterize PLTX cytotoxicity with the aim to elucidate the intracellular pathways leading to cell death. In general, a conclusive point resides in the high dependency on the overload of Na^+ and Ca^{2+} in both excitable and nonexcitable cell models. However, excitable cell models seem to be more dependent on the intracellular increase of Ca^{2+}, which is able to trigger to dramatic Ca^{2+}-dependent cytotoxic effects. In addition, nonexcitable cell models seem to be more dependent on the general ionic imbalance conditions, mainly controlled by the intracellular overload of Na^+. Furthermore, the close dependency of PLTX effects on ionic imbalance has been demonstrated also evaluating in vitro the mechanism of tumor promotion induced by the toxin, which is able to activate MAPK cascade regulated by osmotic stress.

In conclusion, the data collected so far from in vitro studies helped to characterize the mechanism of cytotoxicity induced by PLTX, even if some points still remain to be clarified.

25.5 Detection

Detection methods have been developed for PLTX and its analogues based upon animal toxicity, cytotoxicity, receptor binding, and antibody binding. These can play an important role as preliminary screens prior to applying definitive instrumental techniques or when instrumental methods are unavailable or impractical due to sample limitations. While none of the available detection methods have been fully validated for PLTX in fish, shellfish, or microalgal samples, efforts continue toward this goal.

The expanding distribution of toxic *Ostreopsis* species into temperate regions such as the Mediterranean Sea increases the potential impact to human health through the food chain and direct exposure. *Ostreopsis* blooms have been associated with dermatitis and respiratory distress in beachgoers (Ciminiello et al., 2006; Tichadou et al., 2010; Accoroni et al., 2011; Honsell et al., 2011) and contaminated fish, sea urchins, and shellfish in temperate and intratropical areas (Onuma et al., 1999; Taniyama et al., 2003; Aligizaki et al., 2008; Amzil et al., 2012). These factors dictate an increasing need for suitable detection methods to monitor and screen for PLTX and its analogues in various sample matrices. Although no countries currently regulate PLTX in seafood, the European Food Safety Authority Panel on Contaminants in the Food Chain has recommended a limit of 30 µg (PLTX + OST-D)/kg in shellfish meat (EFSA, 2009).

25.5.1 Biological Methods

25.5.1.1 Mouse Bioassay

The MBA remains a standard method for detecting marine biotoxins in seafood and other sample matrices (APHA, 1970; Yasumoto et al., 1985). PLTX is among the most potent nonprotein animal toxins known, but its toxicity is route dependent; LD_{50}s in mice range from 0.45 µg/kg (intravenous) to >200 µg/kg (oral) (Wiles et al., 1974; Sosa et al., 2009; Munday, 2011). Time to death is dose dependent (Moore and Scheuer, 1971; Teh and Gardiner, 1974; Riobò et al., 2008b) with typical signs of lethal intoxication including stretching of the hind limbs, ataxia, paralysis, cyanosis, gasping for breath, convulsions, and death (Munday, 2011). When PLTX is administered by the i.p. route, as typically employed in the MBA, the reported LD_{50} in mice ranges between 0.15 and 0.72 µg/kg (Levine et al., 1987; Rhodes et al., 2002; Taniyama et al., 2002; Riobò et al., 2008b). Differences in mouse characteristics (strain, age, sex, diet, etc.) and post-dose observation times contribute to the observed variability in reported values. At doses four to five times greater than the i.p. LD_{50}, death may occur in an hour or less, while death following lower doses may occur 24 or more hours later (Riobò et al., 2008b). Riobò et al. (2008b), have proposed a standardized protocol employing a 24 h observation period following i.p. dosing in order to minimize MBA variability.

Sample extraction methods vary in efficiency and may impact the outcome of the MBA. Several techniques have been reported, including two methods commonly employed for PLTX sample extraction in seafood samples. The first involves acetone extraction of tissue followed by evaporation and resuspension of the residue in 1% Tween 60 (Yasumoto et al., 1978). This general method, designed primarily for extracting lipophilic marine biotoxins, is incorporated into the EU harmonized protocol for the MBA (Yasumoto et al., 1985) and is less efficient in extracting the relatively polar PLTX and analogues. Because of this, samples tested by MBA using this extraction method may be subject to interferences from other marine biotoxins, such as saxitoxin, yessotoxin, and okadaic acid (Aligizaki et al., 2008; EC, 2011). An alternate method has been applied to *Scarus ovifrons* (parrotfish) muscle and liver (Taniyama et al., 2002) or shellfish whole flesh (Aligizaki et al., 2008) and uses an initial extraction with 75% aqueous ethanol followed by defatting with diethyl ether and partitioning between water and 1-butanol. The aqueous and 1-butanol layers are dried and resuspended in water for injection. This polar extraction method reduces interference by lipophilic toxins but may still be subject to interference from co-occurring water-soluble toxins. Other techniques include extracting shellfish tissue or *Ostreopsis* spp. samples with methanol/water (50/50) acidified with 0.2% acetic acid (Rhodes et al., 2002) or extracting fish tissue with 100% ethanol, followed by partitioning between hexane and 80% aqueous ethanol, drying, and partitioned between water and 1-butanol (Onuma et al., 1999). In the latter case, the water layer was positive in the MBA for presumptive PLTX analogues. Methanol/water (50/50) is a common initial extraction medium for *Ostreopsis* spp. samples used in the MBA (Taniyama et al., 2003).

One advantage of the MBA is the ability to estimate the total animal toxicity in a sample, which may be proportional to expected toxicity in humans. This is important because the PLTX group of toxins comprises numerous congeners that may coexist in biological samples and vary in potency (Moore and Scheuer, 1971; Uemura et al., 1985; Corpuz et al., 1994; Lau et al., 1995; Usami et al., 1995; Ukena et al., 2001; Lenoir et al., 2004; Ciminiello et al., 2008, 2009, 2010; Rossi et al., 2011). However, in complex samples, the MBA cannot differentiate among PLTX congeners and identify the contributions of individual toxins to total toxicity. While the MBA does not require complex instrumentation, access to an animal facility is necessary, and disadvantages include ethical considerations, variability in interlaboratory results, and poor specificity. These limitations justify efforts to develop and validate alternate methods that do not require animal use. Consistent with this need, the European Commission has adopted liquid chromatography–mass spectrometry (LC–MS) as a standard method to detect lipophilic toxins in bivalve mollusks and mandated a phase out of the MBA by December 31, 2014 (EC, 2011).

25.5.1.2 Hemolytic Assay

Hemolysis assays detect PLTX and its cytotoxic analogues based on the characteristic delayed hemolysis observed in erythrocytes of sensitive species (Habermann et al., 1981). Hemolysis is a consequence of PLTX binding to the Na$^+$/K$^+$-ATPase, resulting in conversion of the ion pump into a nonselective pore, followed by osmotic lysis and hemoglobin release (Artigas and Gadsby, 2003a,b; Hilgemann, 2003). The observed hemolysis is time and temperature dependent, with an optimal detection limit in the low picomolar range. PLTX-specific neutralizing antibodies (Levine et al., 1987; Hewetson et al., 1989; Bignami, 1993; Taniyama et al., 2001) or PLTX pharmacologic antagonists such as ouabain can be used to improve specificity (Taniyama et al., 2003; Riobò et al., 2006, 2008a; Malagoli, 2007). In its simplest form, the method provides a visual readout that does not require laboratory instrumentation (Bignami, 1993), enabling use in low resource or even field settings. More commonly, hemoglobin release is measured spectrophotometrically using multi-well plate readers.

Hemolytic assays have the advantages of being very sensitive and capable of detecting all biologically active PLTX congeners. However, the technique as originally reported is based on a PLTX reactive monoclonal antibody (73D3) that is not commercially available and that has not been fully characterized for the ability to neutralize all cytotoxic PLTX analogues (Bignami et al., 1992). Others have used anti-PLTX rabbit polyclonal antibodies, which suffer similar shortcomings (Taniyama et al., 2001). An alternative approach employs the readily available cardiac glycoside, ouabain, as a pharmacologic competitive inhibitor of PLTX binding to its Na$^+$/K$^+$-ATPase-associated receptor (Habermann and Chhatwal, 1982). Seemann et al., adapted the ouabain hemolysis inhibition assay to a blood agar plate format using human erythrocytes and a visual readout in an investigation of possible PLTX-producing bacteria from *P. caribaeorum* (Seemann et al., 2009). Riobó and coworkers conducted a detailed study to optimize hemolytic assay parameters using sheep erythrocytes and ouabain in a tube or multi-well format (Riobò et al., 2008a).

The hemolysis assay has been applied to a variety of natural samples, including a zoanthid, *P. tuberculosa* (Bignami, 1993); fish (Onuma et al., 1999; Taniyama et al., 2001, 2002); shellfish (Aligizaki et al., 2008); and *Ostreopsis* spp. dinoflagellates (Taniyama et al., 2003; Aligizaki et al., 2008). On *O. cf ovata*, a comparison between a hemolysis neutralization assay and high-resolution (HR) LC–MS showed a good correlation between hemolytic effect and total toxin content measured through HR LC–MS (Pezzolesi et al., 2012). Aligizaki and coworkers detected putative PLTX in shellfish extracts corresponding to 0.016 µg/kg shellfish tissue, using a hemolysis assay developed with sheep erythrocytes in combination with ouabain (Aligizaki et al., 2008). This assay distinguished between shellfish extracts known to contain okadaic acid and those containing putative PLTX and also detected PLTX analogues produced by cultured and field samples of *Ostreopsis*. The high sensitivity of the hemolysis neutralization assay enabled Onuma et al., to successfully investigate a human fatality resulting from consumption of a toxic clupeid fish (blue stripe herring, *Herklotsichthys quadrimaculatus*), often associated with a severe intoxication syndrome known as clupeotoxism. Applied to a very limited sample comprising a single fish head, a presumptive PLTX-positive hemolysis assay result enabled a focused confirmatory analysis by LC–MS demonstrating the presence of a PLTX analogue (Onuma et al., 1999).

25.5.1.3 Cytotoxicity Assay

Owing to the ubiquitous nature of the Na$^+$/K$^+$-ATPase-associated PLTX receptor in animal cells, PLTX is active against numerous excitable and nonexcitable cell types of various species (see Section 25.4). The Na$^+$/K$^+$-ATPase is an integral membrane protein found in the cells of all higher eukaryotes and is responsible for translocation of K$^+$ and Na$^+$ ions across the cell membrane, utilizing ATP hydrolysis as the driving force (Lingrel and Kuntzweiler, 1994). Early cellular responses to PLTX exposure, such as K$^+$ efflux, are followed by a cascade of cellular processes ultimately leading to cytolysis (Bellocci et al., 2011; Prandi et al., 2011). Cell death, or earlier events such as depolarization (Cagide et al., 2009), may be exploited to develop functional PLTX cytotoxicity assays. Although assays that rely upon established cell lines require cell culture facilities, they offer advantages in reproducibility and not requiring live animal use.

The ability to simultaneously detect several classes of seafood toxins using a cell culture system could provide a cost-effective means to monitor seafood contamination and improve consumer protection. Manger and coworkers developed an assay using the murine neuroblastoma cell line Neuro-2a, incorporating ouabain and veratridine (a sodium channel activator) as a means to detect voltage-gated sodium channel-dependent neurotoxins, such as saxitoxins, brevetoxins, and ciguatoxins (Manger et al., 1993). Cañete and Diogène conducted a comparative study of Neuro-2a and the mouse-rat hybrid NG108-15 neuroblastoma glioma cell line in an effort to extend a neuronal cell assay to include quantification of PLTX (Cañete and Diogene, 2008). Assay parameters, such as concurrent exposure to ouabain and veratridine, toxin exposure time, and post-cell seeding time prior to initiating toxin exposure, were varied to identify conditions selective for PLTX, sodium channel toxins, and others. An endpoint was determined by the MTT [3-(4,5-dimethylthiazol-2-yl)-2,5-diphenyltetrazolium] method that measures mitochondrial reductase activity as a surrogate for cell number (Mosmann, 1983). When tested 1 h post-cell seeding, sensitivity to a 24 h PLTX exposure depended upon the presence of ouabain and veratridine in both the NG108-15 and Neuro-2a systems. Cells cultured for 24 h after seeding were insensitive to a 3 h exposure to PLTX, with or without concurrent ouabain and veratridine treatment. The relative insensitivity to PLTX following 3 h toxin exposure and a requirement for ouabain/veratridine under selected assay conditions are unique aspects of this study (Cañete and Diogene, 2008). In contrast, Ledreaux et al. reported potent PLTX cytotoxicity (MTT endpoint) against Neuro-2a cells (IC$_{50}$ 42.9 ± 3.8 pM), following a 19 h toxin exposure in the absence of veratridine (Ledreux et al., 2009). This cytotoxicity could be inhibited by pretreatment with 500 µM ouabain but was enhanced by concurrent ouabain exposure. Ledreaux et al. applied the Neuro-2a assay to detect PLTX in spiked shellfish tissue samples and PLTX-like activity in *O. ovata* extracts. They proposed assay conditions for selectively detecting and differentiating PLTX and sodium channel phycotoxins based on Neuro-2a viability following toxin exposure with or without appropriately timed ouabain or ouabain/veratridine treatment.

Espiña et al. (2009) developed a microplate-based assay to detect PLTX using BE (2)-M17 human neuroblastoma cells with or without ouabain pretreatment. The assay utilized Alamar blue, a noncytotoxic fluorescent (or colorimetric) indicator, to measure mitochondrial oxidoreductase activity. The nontoxic metabolic probe enabled the toxin exposure time to be extended in order to increase assay sensitivity. They reported detection limits of 150 pM PLTX after a 4 h incubation and 75 pM after 72 h incubation. The BE (2)-M17 assay was applied to detecting PLTX in clonal culture extracts of *O.* cf. *siamensis* derived from samples collected in Andalusian coastal waters. It was also shown to differentially detect okadaic acid and PLTX in mussel extracts, based on selective inhibition by ouabain.

The MCF-7 human breast adenocarcinoma cell line was used by Bellocci et al. (2008a) to develop a novel cytotoxicity assay for PLTX based on the cytolytic release of lactate dehydrogenase (LDH). Following a 1 h PLTX exposure, with or without ouabain pretreatment, culture medium was replaced by phosphate-buffered saline for 1 h, after which cytolysis was determined by measuring supernatant LDH activity. Prandi et al. (2011) proposed a two-step process for the PLTX-mediated cytolysis observed in MCF-7 cells. The first step was toxin dependent and osmolyte sensitive. The second step did not require the presence of the toxin and was osmolyte insensitive, but accompanied by reorganization of the cytoskeleton and cell membrane. In the MCF-7 cytolytic assay, PLTX- and OST-D–mediated cytolysis could be inhibited by ouabain, with an IC_{50} for PLTX and OST-D of approximately 50 pM and 3 nM, respectively. Maitotoxin, tetrodotoxin, okadaic acid, and yessotoxin were not cytolytic (Bellocci et al., 2008a,b). The MCF-7 cytolytic assay was compared to LC–MS for determining PLTX in naturally contaminated mussels (*M. galloprovincialis*), sea urchins (*Paracentrotus lividus*), and *O. ovata* algal samples. As originally reported, the MCF-7 cytolytic assay detected significantly higher levels of PLTX activity in the sample extracts compared to LC–MS (Bellocci et al., 2008b). However, a revision based on a higher quality PLTX standard indicated that determinations made by cytolytic or LC–MS methods were similar (Bellocci et al., 2008a).

25.5.2 Immunoassays

25.5.2.1 Radioimmunoassay

Levine and coworkers were the first to obtain PLTX-specific polyclonal antibodies (Levine et al., 1987). Immunogenic conjugates were prepared by forming amide bonds between the *N*-terminus of PLTX and carboxylic acid residues of bovine serum albumin in the presence of carbodiimide. Fortuitously, the PLTX amino group is not only synthetically accessible, but also *N*-acyl PLTX derivatives were shown to be at least 100-fold less toxic than the parent toxin (Hirata et al., 1979; Moore et al., 1980; Ohizumi and Shibata, 1980), thus providing immunogens with tolerable toxicity. In addition to neutralizing several PLTX biological activities, Levine's antibodies were used to develop a competitive radioimmunoassay employing an ^{125}I-labeled PLTX derivative (Levine et al., 1988). Although highly sensitive, the requirement for a radioiodine-labeled PLTX antigen makes this method impractical in terms of cost, antigen stability, and radioactivity. Nevertheless, Levine's radioimmunoassay established the feasibility of immunoassay techniques for detecting and measuring PLTX.

25.5.2.2 Enzyme Immunoassay

Enzyme immunoassays are widely used diagnostic tools that are easy to use, have nonradioactive labels, and are amenable to high throughput and automation. PLTX enzyme immunoassays have been reported based on both competitive inhibition and immunometric principles (i.e., "sandwich" immunoassays) (Bignami et al., 1992; Frolova et al., 2000; Garet et al., 2010; Boscolo et al., 2013). Competitive immunoassays are commonly used for low molecular weight analytes that cannot simultaneously bind two antibodies, yielding signal readouts that are inversely proportional to the analyte concentration. These typically require preparation of antigen conjugates, either as a solid-phase antigen (labeled antibody liquid phase) or a labeled liquid phase antigen (antibody solid phase). For PLTX, synthesis of these conjugates is challenging, due to the limited commercial availability, high cost, and sophisticated laboratory requirements needed for handling bulk amounts of PLTX. A competitive immunoassay format employing unmodified purified PLTX as the solid-phase antigen overcomes some of these issues (Frolova et al., 2000).

Double antibody "sandwich" immunoassays incorporate a solid-phase capture antibody and a second solution phase labeled detector antibody, thereby avoiding the need for toxin conjugates and yielding a signal that is proportional to analyte concentration. Remarkably, PLTX, a nonpeptide with a molecular weight of 2678.5 Da, is capable of forming a double antibody sandwich when two antibodies recognizing distinct epitopes are used (Bignami et al., 1992; Boscolo et al., 2013).

Bignami and coworkers developed both competitive and sandwich immunoassays based upon a murine monoclonal antibody, 73D3 (isotype IgG1, κ) (Bignami et al., 1992). This monoclonal antibody was raised against an *N*-terminal hapten conjugate of PLTX purified from Hawaiian *P. tuberculosa*. Later studies demonstrated that the purified PLTX preparation used in these studies comprised at least two congeners, PLTX and 42-hydroxy PLTX (Corpuz et al., 1994; Ciminiello et al., 2009). By surface plasmon resonance (SPR), the affinity (Kd) toward PLTX has been estimated to range between 2.14×10^{-9} and 2.46×10^{-10} M (Yakes et al., 2011; Zamolo et al., 2012). Immunoassay and/or hemolysis assay results indicate that 73D3 binds PLTX, 42-hydroxy PLTX, OST-D, and various nontoxic *N*-acyl PLTX and inactivated PLTX preparations (Bignami et al., 1992; Onuma et al., 1999; Boscolo et al., 2013). Immunofluorescence data suggest that 73D3 may also bind at least some *O.* cf. *ovata* toxins, such as ovatoxin-a (Honsell et al., 2011). It does not bind other marine toxins, including amphidinol, maitotoxin, prymnesin-2, okadaic acid, tetrodotoxin, lyngbyatoxin A, yessotoxin, domoic acid, brevetoxin-3, pectenotoxin, dinophysistoxin-1, or saxitoxin (Bignami et al., 1992; Onuma et al., 1999; Yakes et al., 2011; Boscolo et al., 2013). In a preliminary study, 73D3 was shown to be incapable of forming a homogeneous double antibody sandwich with biotinylated-73D3, suggesting that only a single PLTX epitope is accessible to 73D3 (Raybould, 1991). This apparent inconsistency with Inuzuka's dimer hypothesis (Inuzuka et al., 2007) may be due to the lower PLTX concentrations used in the immunoassay or steric factors. All of the reported PLTX-specific antibodies obtained by animal immunization used immunogens formed via conjugation of the C-115 terminal amino group (Levine et al., 1987; Raybould, 1991; Bignami et al., 1992; Frolova et al., 2000; Boscolo et al., 2013), a functional group that can be readily derivatized to form well-defined *N*-acyl haptens. There are no reports of selective conjugation through one of the 42 PLTX primary or secondary hydroxyl groups, which might yield antibodies recognizing the terminal amino group known to be essential for conferring toxicity. As evidenced by the ability to form antibody complexes between 73D3 and rabbit polyclonal antibodies, *N*-terminal conjugates elicit antibodies to at least two distinct epitopes. To date, however, no monoclonal antibodies that bind a second epitope distinct from the 73D3 site have been reported. The desired monoclonal antibody pair would reduce or eliminate the need to immunize rabbits and provide a ready source of antibodies for further development of various antibody-based methods.

Garet et al. reported the isolation of recombinant human anti-PLTX single-chain (scFv) antibodies via phage display techniques and the development of an indirect competitive enzyme immunoassay utilizing scFv phage and PLTX directly absorbed to the solid phase (Garet et al., 2010). Recombinant antibodies are advantageous because they can be produced cheaply and are amenable to genetic construction of fusion proteins that facilitate purification or detection. Garet's method was reported to be extraordinarily sensitive, with a working range of 0.0005–500 ng/mL and a PLTX detection limit of 0.5 pg/mL. Of note, a representative calibration curve achieved only partial inhibition of phage binding over a 6-log PLTX standard analyte range. Despite this, the authors reported a mean recovery rate of 90% in shellfish extracts spiked with PLTX. The cross-reactivity profile of the scFv against PLTX congeners and other marine toxins was not reported, nor were the scFv tested in a sandwich format against other phage antibodies or 73D3. Therefore, it is unknown whether this library contains scFv recognizing multiple complementary PLTX epitopes.

Enzyme immunoassays have well recognized advantages in terms of ease of use and sample throughput. However, the reported PLTX antibodies are not commercially available and are incompletely characterized. In the case of monoclonal antibody 73D3, there is limited enzyme immunoassay data available on its utility for detecting PLTX-group toxins in seafood or *Ostreopsis* spp. samples. However, cross-reactivity data suggest that enzyme immunoassays based on 73D3 cannot differentiate closely related congeners or inactive analogues. Future work could be directed to selecting antibodies that would enable an enzyme immunoassay to better correlate with total toxicity.

25.5.2.3 Biosensors

Yakes et al. (2011) reported a SPR-based immunoassay incorporating monoclonal antibody 73D3. The immunoassay utilized a Biacore T100 instrument and a solid-phase chip displaying covalently linked 73D3. Assay conditions such as running buffer, flow rate, binding time, and regeneration solutions were optimized to provide a PLTX detection limit of 0.52, 2.8, and 1.4 ng/mL in buffer, 10% spiked grouper extract, and 10% spike clam extract, respectively. The authors suggest that "matrix matching" will be required to avoid matrix interferences in natural samples. As expected, the 73D3-based SPR method was specific for PLTX and did not detect unrelated marine toxins. Although SPR methods are rapid and sensitive, the instrumentation is expensive and not widely available.

Zamolo et al. reported a very sensitive biosensor based on a sandwich immunoassay with electroche-miluminescence (ECL) detection (Zamolo et al., 2012). The sensitivity of the immunosensor was signifi-cantly increased by covalently linking a solid-phase capture antibody (73D3) to the optically transparent transduction electrode through functionalized multiwalled carbon nanotubes (CNTs), thus conferring greater antibody loading and improved conductance. A rabbit polyclonal antibody-ruthenium conjugate served as the ECL signal generating detector antibody. The biosensor had a PLTX limit of detection and quantitation in buffer of 0.07 and 0.24 ng/mL, respectively. Mussel (*M. galloprovincialis*) and complex (multispecies) microalgal extracts spiked with PLTX showed no matrix effect when diluted 1:10, and PLTX detection and quantitation limits were similar to those observed in buffer. The limit of quantita-tion in spiked mussel extract corresponded to 2.2 µg/kg meat, approximately 15-fold lower than the EFSA recommended cutoff.

25.5.2.4 Immunofluorescence

Honsell et al. (2011) reported an indirect immunofluorescence technique to detect PLTX analogues in *O.* cf. *ovata* cells using either monoclonal antibody 73D3 or rabbit polyclonal antibodies. *O.* cf. *ovata* cells harvested from the Gulf of Trieste and stained with PLTX antibodies showed cytoplasmic immunofluo-rescence, while *Coolia monotis* cells and *Ostreopsis* cells treated with pre-immune rabbit sera did not. Closer examination by confocal microscopy revealed PLTX immunofluorescence patterns seemingly associated with a cytoplasmic filament network as well as surrounding chloroplasts and other organelles. While no parent PLTX was detected by HR LC–MS in these *Ostreopsis* samples, ovatoxin-a, ovatoxin-b, ovatoxin-c, ovatoxin-d, and ovatoxin-e were present, with ovatoxin-a predominant. The distribution of PLTX-like immunofluorescence was distinct from chloroplast autofluorescence, again demonstrating a specific antibody-mediated PLTX immunolocalization. PLTX immunofluorescence offers a straightfor-ward means to qualitatively identify and monitor toxic *Ostreopsis* blooms, guide algal sampling cam-paigns, and inform public health strategies to limit the impact of toxic alga blooms to the public and seafood industry.

25.5.3 Fluorescence Polarization Assay

Alfonso et al. (2012) reported development of a fluorescence polarization (FP) assay based on carboxy-fluorescein-labeled purified Na+/K+-ATPase. FP is a spectroscopic technique that measures the change between plane-polarized excitation and emitted light as a function of molecular interaction in solution. The polarization angle of emitted light and corresponding sensitivity of FP assays is proportional to the change in mass resulting from such molecular interactions. It is a homogenous, solution phase technique that does not require separation (washing) steps, unlike most immunoassays. The method is rapid, and multiple samples could be tested in a 20 min assay with a detection limit of 2 nM PLTX determined by linear regression. Interestingly, the same group previously observed that PLTX does not bind to purified Na+/K+-ATPase immobilized on an SPR solid phase (Vale-Gonzalez et al., 2007b). To avoid matrix interferences, *Ostreopsis* and shellfish samples were subjected to rigorous cleanup methods prior to analysis by FP. Three *Ostreopsis* culture extracts tested positive for PLTX, while non-PLTX-producing *Protoceratium* and *Lingulodinium* microalgae culture extracts were negative. When applied to spiked or naturally contaminated mussel extracts, the FP assay was shown to correlate with MBA results.

25.5.4 Conclusion

The detection methods described earlier each offer certain advantages in terms of cost, ease of use, assay time, specificity, or sensitivity. A significant limitation common to all of the methods is the complex and varied chemical and biological activity of the PLTX family of toxins. Most of these are available in very limited quantities, and in many cases, structural definition is lacking. Thus, certified standards and reference materials needed for method validation are largely unavailable. Nevertheless, progress has been made toward detection and screening methods that should aid in monitoring seafood and environmental samples for the PLTX family of toxins. The chemical methods of PLTXs detection will be described in Chapter 26.

ACKNOWLEDGMENTS

This work was partially supported by Regione Friuli Venezia-Giulia, Direzione Risorse Rurali, Agroalimentari e Forestali (Progetto "Kit e biosensori di elevata sensibilità per la determinazione delle tossine di alghe nelle acque e nei prodotti ittici del Friuli Venezia-Giulia—Senstox"), and partially by a grant of the Italian Ministry of Education, University and Research (MIUR).

REFERENCES

Accoroni, S., Romagnoli, T., Colombo, F. et al. 2011. Ostreopsis cf. ovata bloom in the northern Adriatic Sea during summer 2009: Ecology, molecular characterization and toxin profile. *Mar Pollut Bull* 62: 2512–2519.

Aizu, E., Yamamoto, S., Nakadate, T., Kato, R. 1990. Differential effects of various skin tumor-promoting agents on prostaglandin E2 release from primary cultures of mouse epidermal cells. *Eur J Pharmacol* 182: 19–28.

Alcala, A.C., Alcala, L.C., Garth, J.S., Yasumura, D., Yasumoto, T. 1988. Human fatality due to ingestion of the crab *Demania reynaudii* that contained a palytoxin-like toxin. *Toxicon* 26: 105–107.

Alcala, A.C., Halstead, B.W. 1970. Human fatality due to ingestion of the crab *Demania* sp. in the Philippines. *J Toxicol Clin Toxicol* 3: 609–611.

Alfonso, A., Fernández-Araujo, A., Alfonso, C., Caramés, B., Tobio, A., Louzao, M.C., Vieytes, M.R., Botana, L.M. 2012. Palytoxin detection and quantification using the fluorescence polarization technique. *Anal Biochem* 424: 64–70.

Aligizaki, K., Katikou, P., Milandri, A., Diogène, J. 2011. Occurrence of palytoxin-group toxins in seafood and future strategies to complement the present state of the art. *Toxicon* 57: 390–399.

Aligizaki, K., Katikou, P., Nikolaidis, G., Panou, A. 2008. First episode of shellfish contamination by palytoxin-like compounds from *Ostreopsis* species (Aegean Sea, Greece). *Toxicon* 51: 418–427.

Amir, I., Harris, J.B., Zar, M.A. 1997. The effect of palytoxin on neuromuscular junctions in the anococcygeus muscle of the rat. *J Neurocytol* 26: 367–376.

Amzil, Z., Sibat, M., Chomerat, N. et al. 2012. Ovatoxin-a and palytoxin accumulation in seafood in relation to Ostreopsis cf. ovata blooms on the French Mediterranean coast. *Mar Drugs* 10: 477–496.

APHA. 1970. *Recommended Procedures for the Examination of Sea Water and Shellfish*. American Public Health Association, New York.

Ares, I.R., Cagide, E., Louzao, M.C. et al. 2009. Ostreocin-D impact on globular actin of intact cells. *Chem Res Toxicol* 22: 374–381.

Ares, I.R., Louzao, M.C., Vieytes, M.R., Yasumoto, T., Botana, L.M. 2005. Actin cytoskeleton of rabbit intestinal cells is a target for potent marine phycotoxins. *J Exp Biol* 208: 4345–4354.

Artigas, P., Gadsby, D.C. 2002. Ion channel-like properties of the Na$^+$/K$^+$ pump. *Ann NY Acad Sci* 976: 31–40.

Artigas, P., Gadsby, D.C. 2003a. Ion occlusion/deocclusion partial reactions in individual palytoxin-modified Na/K pumps. *Ann NY Acad* 986: 116–126.

Artigas, P., Gadsby, D.C. 2003b. Na$^+$/K$^+$-ligands modulate gating of palytoxin-induced ion channels. *Proc Natl Acad Sci USA* 100: 501–505.

Artigas, P., Gadsby, D.C. 2004. Large diameter of palytoxin-induced Na/K pump channels and modulation of palytoxin interaction by Na/K pump ligands. *J Gen Physiol* 123: 357–376.

Attaway, D.H., Ciereszko, L.S. 1974. Isolation and partial characterization of Caribbean palytoxin. In: *Proceedings of the Second International Coral Reef Symposium*, Brisbane, Australia, pp. 497–504.

Barroso García, P., Rueda de la Puerta, P., Parrón Carreño, T., Marín Martínez, P., Guillén Enríquez, J. 2008. Brote con síntomas respiratorios en la provincia de Almería por una posible exposición a microalgas tóxicas. *Gac Sanit* 22: 578–584.

Bellocci, M., Ronzitti, G., Milandri, A. et al. 2008a. A cytolytic assay for the measurement of palytoxin based on a cultured monolayer cell line. *Anal Biochem* 374: 48–55.

Bellocci, M., Ronzitti, G., Milandri, A. et al. 2008b. Addendum to "A cytolytic assay for the measurement of palytoxin based on a cultured monolayer cell line" [*Anal Biochem* 374 (2008) 48–55]. *Anal Biochem* 381: 178.

Bellocci, M., Sala, G.L., Prandi, S. 2011. The cytolytic and cytotoxic activities of palytoxin. *Toxicon* 57: 449–459.

Béress, L., Zwick, J., Kolkenbrock, H.J., Kaul, P.N., Wassermann, O. 1983. A method for the isolation of the Caribbean palytoxin (C-PTX) from the coelenterate (zoanthid) *Palythoa caribaeorum*. *Toxicon* 21: 285–290.

Bignami, G.S. 1993. A rapid and sensitive hemolysis neutralization assay for palytoxin. *Toxicon* 31: 817–820.

Bignami, G.S., Raybould, T.J., Sachinvala, N.D. et al. 1992. Monoclonal antibody-based enzyme-linked immunoassays for the measurement of palytoxin in biological samples. *Toxicon* 30: 687–700.

Boscolo, S., Pelin, M., De Bortoli, M. et al. 2013. Sandwich ELISA assay for the quantitation of palytoxin and its analogs in natural samples. *Environ Sci Technol* 47:2034–2042.

Böttinger, H., Beress, L., Habermann, E. 1986. Involvement of (Na+/K+)-ATPase in binding and actions of palytoxin on human erythrocytes, *Biochim Biophys Acta* 861: 165–176.

Cagide, E., Louzao, M.C., Espiña, B. et al. 2009. Production of functionally active palytoxin-like compounds by Mediterranean *Ostreopsis* cf. *siamensis*. *Cell Physiol Biochem* 23: 431–440.

Cañete, E., Diogène, J. 2008. Comparative study of the use of neuroblastoma cells (Neuro-2a) and neuroblastomaxglioma hybrid cells (NG108-15) for the toxic effect quantification of marine toxins. *Toxicon* 52: 541–550.

Carumbana, E.E., Alcala, A.C., Ortega E.P. 1976. Toxic marine crabs in Southern Negros, Philippines. *Silliman J* 23, 265–278.

Charlson, A.T., Zeliadt, N.A., Wattenberg, E.V. 2009. Extracellular signal regulated kinase 5 mediates signals triggered by the novel tumor promoter palytoxin. *Toxicol Appl Pharmacol* 241: 143–153.

Chhatwal, G.S., Ahnert-Hilger, G., Beress, L., Habermann, E. 1982. Palytoxin both induces and inhibits the release of histamine from rat mast cells. *Int Arch Allergy Appl Immunol* 68: 97–100.

Chia, D.G., Lau, C.O., Ng, P.K., Tan, C.H. 1993. Localization of toxins in the poisonous mosaic crab, *Lophozozymus pictor* (Fabricius, 1798) (Brachyura, Xanthidae). *Toxicon* 31: 901–904.

Ciminiello, P., Dell'Aversano, C., Dello Iacovo, E. et al. 2009. Stereostructure and biological activity of 42-hydroxy-palytoxin: A new palytoxin analogue from Hawaiian *Palythoa* subspecies. *Chem Res Toxicol* 22: 1851–1859.

Ciminiello, P., Dell'Aversano, C., Dello Iacovo, E. et al. 2010. Complexpalytoxin-like profile of Ostreopsisovata. Identification off our new ovatoxins by high-resolution liquid chromatography/massspectrometry. *Rapid Commun Mass Spectrom* 24: 2735–2744.

Ciminiello, P., Dell'Aversano, C., Dello Iacovo, E., Fattorusso, E., Forino, M., Tartaglione, L. 2011. LC-MS of palytoxin and its analogues: State of the art and future perspectives. *Toxicon* 57: 376–389.

Ciminiello, P., Dell'Aversano, C., Dello Iacovo, E. et al. 2012a. Isolation and structure elucidation of Ovatoxin-a, the major toxin produced by *Ostreopsis ovata*. *J Am Chem Soc* 134: 1869–1875.

Ciminiello, P., Dell'aversano, C., Dello Iacovo, E. et al. 2012b. High resolution LC-MS(n) fragmentation pattern of palytoxin as template to gain new insights into ovatoxin-a structure. The key role of calcium in MS behavior of palytoxins. *J Am Soc Mass Spectrom*. DOI: 10.1007/s13361-012-0345-7.

Ciminiello, P., Dell'Aversano, C., Fattorusso, E. et al. 2006. The Genoa 2005 outbreak. Determination of putative palytoxin in Mediterranean *Ostreopsis ovata* by a new liquid chromatography tandem mass spectrometry method. *Anal Chem* 78: 6153–6159.

Ciminiello, P., Dell'Aversano, C., Fattorusso, E. et al. 2008. Putative palytoxin and its new analogue, ovatoxin-a, in Ostreopsis ovata collected along the Ligurian coasts during the 2006 toxic outbreak. *J Am Soc Mass Spectrom* 19: 111–120.

Coca, R., Soler, F., Fernández-Belda, F. 2008. Characterization of the palytoxin effect on Ca^{2+}-ATPase from sarcoplasmic reticulum (SERCA). *Archives Biochem Biophys* 478: 36–42.

Corpuz, G.P., Grothaus, P.G. et al. 1994. An HPLC method for rapid analysis of palytoxin congeners and prodrugs. In: *International Symposium on Ciguatera and Marine Natural Products*, Kona, Hawaii, Asian-Pacific Research Foundation, Honolulu, HI.

Crinelli, R., Carloni, E., Giacomini, E., Penna, A., Dominici, S., Battocchi, C., Ciminiello, P. et al. 2012. Palytoxin and an ostreopsis toxin extract increase the levels of mRNAs encoding inflammation-related proteins in human macrophages via p38 MAPK and NF-κB. *PLoS One* 7: e38139.

Deeds, J.R., Handy, S.M., White, K.D., Reimer, J.D. 2011. Palytoxin found in palythoa sp. zoanthids (Anthozoa, Hexacorallia) sold in the home aquarium trade. *PLOS One* 6: 1–9.

Deeds, J.R., Schwartz, M. 2010. Human risk associated with palytoxin exposure. *Toxicon* 56: 150–162.

Deguchi, T., Aoshima, S., Sakai, Y., Takamatsu, S., Urakawa, N. 1974. Pharmacological actions of palythoatoxin isolated from the zoanthid, *Palythoa tuberculosa*. *Jpn J Pharmacol* 24(suppl.): 116p.

Deguchi, T., Urakawa, N., Takamatsu, S. 1976. Some pharmacological properties of palythoatoxin isolated from the zoanthid, *Palythoa tuberculosa*. *Animal, Plant, and Microbial Toxins* 2: 379–394.

Del Favero, G., Florio, C., Codan, B. et al. 2012. The stretch-activated channel blocker gd(3+) reduces palytoxin toxicity in primary cultures of skeletal muscle cells. *Chem Res Toxicol* 25: 1912–1920.

Di Turi, L., Lo Caputo, S., Marzano, M.C. et al. 2003. Ostropsidiaceae (Dynophyceae) presence along the coastal area of Bari. *Biol Mar Mediterr* 10: 675–678.

Dubois, J.M., Cohen, J.B. 1977. Effect of palytoxin on membrane potential and current of frog myelinated fibers. *J Pharmac Exp Ther* 201: 148–155.

Durando, P., Ansaldi, F., Oreste, P. et al. 2007. *Ostreopsis ovata* and human health: Epidemiological and clinical features of respiratory syndrome outbreaks from a two year syndromic surveillance, 2005–2006, in north-west Italy. *Euro Surveill* 12(23):pii=3212.

(EC), E.C. 2011. COMMISSION REGULATION (EU) No 15/2011 of January 10, 2011 amending Regulation (EC) No 2074/2005 as regards recognised testing methods for detecting marine biotoxins in live bivalve molluscs. *Official J Euro Union* 54(L6): 3–6.

Ecault, E., Sauviat, M.P. 1991. Characterization of the palytoxin-induced sodium conductance in frog skeletal muscle. *Br J Pharmacol* 102: 523–529.

EFSA Panel on Contaminants in the Food Chain (CONTAM). 2009. Scientific opinion on marine biotoxins in shellfish—Palytoxin group. *EFSA J* 7(12): 1393. [38pp.]. doi:10.2903/j.efsa.2009.1393.

Espiña, B., Cagide, E., Louzao, M.C., Fernandez, M.M., Vieytes, M.R., Katikou, P., Villar, A., Jaen, D., Maman, L., Botana, L.M. 2009. Specific and dynamic detection of palytoxins by in vitro microplate assay with human neuroblastoma cells. *Biosci Rep* 29: 13–23.

Falciola, J., Volet, B., Anner, R.M., Moosmayer, M., Lacotte, D., Anner, B.M. 1994. Role of cell membrane Na,K-ATPase for survival of human lymphocytes in vitro. *Biosci Rep* 14: 189–204.

Farley, R.A., Schreiber, S., Wang, S.G., Scheiner-Bobis, G. 2001. A hybrid between Na^+/K^+ ATPase and H^+/K^+ ATPase is sensitive to palytoxin, ouabain and SCH28080. *J Biol Chem* 276: 2608–2615.

Ficarra, S., Russo, A., Stefanizzi, F. et al. 2011. Palytoxin induces functional changes of anion transport in red blood cells: Metabolic impact. *J Membr Biol* 242: 31–39.

Franchini, A., Casarini, L., Ottavini, E. 2008. Toxicological effects of marine palytoxin evaluated by fetax assay. *Chemosphere* 73: 267–271.

Franchini, A., Malagoli, D., Ottavini, E. 2010. Targets and effects of yessotoxin, okadaic acid palytoxin: A differential review. *Marine Drugs* 8:658–677.

Frolova, G.M., Kuznetsova, T.A., Mikhailov, V.V., Eliakov, G.B. 2000. Immunoenzyme method for detecting microbial producers of palytoxin. *Bioorg Khim* 26: 315–320.

Frelin, C., Van Renterghem, C. 1995. Palytoxin. Recent electrophysiological and pharmacological evidence for several mechanisms of action. *Gen Pharm* 26: 33–37.

Frelin, C., Vigne, P., Breittmayer, J.P. 1990. Palytoxin acidifies chick cardiac cells and activate the Na/H antiporter. *FEBS Lett* 264: 63–66.

Frelin, C., Vigne, P., Breittmayer, J.P. 1991. Mechanism of cardiotoxic action of palytoxin. *Mol Pharmacol* 38: 904–909.

Fujiki, H., Suganuma, M., Nakayasu, M. et al. 1986. Palytoxin is a non-12-*O*-tetradecanoylphorbol-13-acetate type tumor promoter in two stage mouse skin carcinogenesis. *Carcinogenesis* 7: 707–710.

Fukui, M., Murata, M., Inoue, A., Gawel, M., Yasumoto, T. 1987. Occurrence of palytoxin in the trigger fish *Melichthys vidua. Toxicon* 25: 1121–1124.

Fusetani, N., Sato, S., Hashimoto, K. 1985. Occurrence of a water soluble toxin in a parrotfish (*Ypsiscarus ovifrons*) which is probably responsible for parrotfish liver poisoning. *Toxicon* 23: 105–112.

Gabrielson, E.W., Kuppusamy, P., Povey, A.C., Zweier, J.L., Harris, C.C. 1992. Measurement of neutrophil activation and epidermal cell toxicity by palytoxin and 12-O-tetradecanoylphorbol-13-acetate. *Carcinogenesis* 13: 1671–1674.

Gallitelli, M., Ungaro, N., Addante, L.M., Gentiloni Silver, M., Sabbà, C. 2005. Respiratory illness as a reaction to tropical algal blooms occurring in a temperate climate. *JAMA* 293: 2599–2600.

Garet, E., Cabado, A.G., Vieites, J.M., González-Fernández, A. 2010. Rapid isolation of single-chain antibodies by phage display technology directed against one of the most potent marine toxins: Palytoxin. *Toxicon* 55: 1519–1526.

Gleibs, S., Mebs, D. 1999. Distribution and sequestration of palytoxin in coral reef animals. *Toxicon* 37: 1521–1527.

Gleibs, S., Mebs, D., Werding, B. 1995. Studies on the origin and distribution of palytoxin in a Caribbean coral reef. *Toxicon* 33: 1531–1537.

Gonzales, R.B., Alcala, A.C. 1977. Fatalities from crab poisoning on Negros Island, Philippines. *Toxicon* 15, 169–170.

Gorbi, S, Bocchetti, R, Binelli, A. et al. 2012. Biological effects of palytoxin-like compounds from Ostreopsis cf. ovata: A multibiomarkers approach with mussels *Mytilus galloprovincialis. Chemosphere* 89: 623–632.

Guennoun, S., Horisberger, J.D. 2000. Structure of the 5th transmembrane segment of the Na,K-ATPase alpha subunit: A cysteine-scanning mutagenesis study. *FEBS Lett* 482: 144–148.

Guennoun, S., Horisberger, J.D. 2002. Cysteine-scanning mutagenesis study of the sixth transmembrane segment of the Na,K-ATPase alpha subunit. *FEBS Lett* 513: 277–281.

Habermann, E. 1989. Palytoxin acts through Na^+, K^+-ATPase. *Toxicon* 27: 1175–1187.

Habermann, E., Ahnert-Hilger, G., Chhatwal, G.S., Beress, L. 1981. Delayed haemolytic action of palytoxin. General characteristics. *Biochim Biophys Acta* 649: 481–486.

Habermann, E., Chhatwal, G.S. 1982. Ouabain inhibits the increase due to palytoxin of cation permeability of erythrocytes. *Naunyn Schmiedebergs Arch Pharmacol* 319: 101–107.

Harmel, N., Apell, H.J. 2006. Palytoxin-induced effects on partial reaction of the Na,K-ATPase. *J Gen Physiol* 128: 103–118.

Hashimoto, Y., Fusetani, N., Kimuta, S. 1969. Aluterin: A toxin of filefish *Alutera scripta*, probably originating from a zoantharian. *Bull Jpn Soc Scient Fish* 35: 1086–1093.

Hewetson, J.F., Bignami, G., Vann, D.C. et al. 1989. In vitro and in vivo protection by monoclonal antibody against palytoxin exposure. *FASEB J* 3: A1191.

Hilgemann, D.W. 2003. From a pump to a pore: How palytoxin opens the gates. *PNAS* 100: 386–388.

Hirata, Y., Uemura, D., Ueda, K., Takano, S. 1979. Several compounds from *Palythoa tuberculosa* (Coelenterata). *Pure Appl Chem* 51: 1875–1883.

Hoffmann, K., Hermanns-Clausen, M., Buhl, C. et al. 2008. A case of palytoxin poisoning due to contact with zoanthid corals through skin injury. *Toxicon* 51: 1535–1537.

Honsell, G., De Bortoli, M., Boscolo, S. et al. 2011. Harmful dinoflagellate ostreopsis cf. ovata Fukuyo: Detection of ovatoxins in field samples and cell immunolocalization using antipalytoxin antibodies. *Env Sci Tech* 45: 7051–7059.

Hori, M., Shimizu, K., Nakajyo, S., Urakawa, N. 1988. Palytoxin-induced K^+ efflux from ileal longitudinal smooth muscle of guinea-pig. *Japan J Pharmacol* 46: 285–292.

Horisberger, J.D., Jaunin, P., Reuben, M.A. et al. 1991. The H,K-ATPase beta-subunit can act as a surrogate for the beta-subunit of Na,K-pumps. *J Biol Chem* 266: 19131–19134.

Ichida, S., Tawada, E., Watanebe, Y., Minami, S., Horiba, M. 1988. Two cases of rhabdomyolysis induced by parrotfish liver poisoning. *Kidney & Dialysis (Japan)* 25: 541–544.

Inuzuka, T., Fujisawa, T., Arimoto, H., Uemura, D. 2007. Molecular shape of palytoxin in aqueous solution. *Org Biomol Chem* 5: 897–899.

Ishida, Y., Kajiwara, A., Takagi, K., Ohizumi, Y., Shibata, S. 1985. Dual effect of ouabain on the palytoxin-induced contraction and norepinephrine release in guinea-pig vas deferens. *J Pharm Exp Ther* 232: 551–556.

Ishida, Y., Takagi, K., Takahashi, M., Satake, N., Shibata, S. 1983. Palytoxin isolated from marine coelenterates the inhibitory action on the (Na,K)-ATPase.1983. *J Biol Chem* 258: 7900–7902.

Ishii, K., Ito, K.M., Uemura, D., Ito, K. 1997. Possible mechanism of palytoxin-induced Ca^{2+} mobilization in porcine coronary artery. *J Pharm Exp Ther* 281: 1077–1084.

Ito, E., Ohkusu, M., Terao, K., Yasumoto, T. 1997. Effects of repeated injections of palytoxin on lymphoid tissues in mice. *Toxicon* 35: 679–688.

Ito, E., Ohkusu, M., Yasumoto, T. 1996. Intestinal injuries caused by experimental palytoxicosis in mice. *Toxicon* 34: 643–652.

Ito, E., Yasumoto, T. 2009. Toxicological studies on palytoxin and ostreocin-D administered to mice by three different routes. *Toxicon* 54: 244–251.

Ito, K., Karaki, H., Ishida, Y., Urakawa, N., Deguchi, T. 1976. Effects of palytoxin on isolated intestinal and vascular smooth muscles. *Jpn J Pharmacol* 26: 683–692.

Ito, K., Karaki, H., Urakawa, N. 1977. The mode of contractile action of palytoxin on vascular smooth muscles. *Jpn J Pharmacol* 46: 9–14.

Ito, K., Karaki, H., Urakawa, N. 1979. Effects of palytoxin on mechanical and electrical activities of guinea pig papillary muscle. *Jpn J Pharmacol* 29: 467–476.

Ito, K., Urakawa, N., Koike, H. 1982. Cardiovascular toxicity of palytoxin on anesthetized dogs. *Arch Int Pharmacodyn* 258: 146–154.

Kagiava, A., Aligizaki, K., Katikou, P., Nikolaidis, G., Theophilidis, G. 2012. Assessing the neurotoxic effects of palytoxin and ouabain, both Na$^+$/K$^+$-ATPase inhibitors, on the myelinated sciatic nerve fibres of the mouse: An ex vivo electrophysiological study. *Toxicon* 59: 416–426.

Kano, S., Iizuka, T., Ishimura, Y., Fujiki, H., Sugimura, T. 1987. Stimulation of superoxide anion formation by the non-TPA type tumor promoters palytoxin and thapsigargin in porcine and human neutrophils. *Biochem Biophys Res Commun* 143: 672–677.

Karaki, H., Nagase, H., Ohizumi, Y., Satake, N., Shibata, S. 1988. Palytoxin-induced contraction and release endogenous noradrenaline in rat tail artery. *Br J Pharmacol* 95: 183–188.

Kaul, P.N. 1981. Compounds from the sea with actions on the cardiovascular and central nervous system. *Pharmacol Mar Nat Prod Fed Proc* 40: 10–14.

Kaul, P.N., Farmer, M.R., Ciereszko, L.S. 1974. Pharmacology of palytoxin: The most potent marine toxin known. *Proc West Pharmacol Soc* 17: 294–301.

Kerbrat, A.S., Amzil, Z., Pawlowiez, R. et al. 2011. First evidence of palytoxin and 42-hydroxy-palytoxin in the marine cyanobacterium *Trichodesmium. Mar Drugs* 9: 543–560.

Kermarec, F., Dor, F., Armengaud, A. et al. 2008. Health risks related to *Ostreopsis ovata* in recreational waters. *Env Risques Santé* 7: 357–363.

Kimura, S, Hashimoto, Y. 1973. Purification of toxin in a zoanthid *Palythoa tuberculosa. Publs Seto Mar biol Lab* 20: 713–718.

Kinoshita, K., Ikeda, M., Ito, K. 1991. Properties of palytoxin induced whole current in single rat ventricular myocytes. *Naunyn Schmiedebergs Arch Pharmacol* 344: 247–251.

Kockskämper, J., Ahmmed, G.U., Zima, A.V., Sheehan, K.A., Glitsch, H.G., Blatter, L.A. 2004. Palytoxin disrupts excitation-contraction coupling through interactions with P-type ion pumps. *Am J Physiol Cell Physiol* 287: 527–538.

Kodama, A.M., Hokama, Y., Yasumoto, T., Fukui, M., Manea, S.J., Sutherland, N. 1989. Clinical and laboratory findings implicating palytoxin as cause of ciguatera poisoning due to *Decapterus macrosoma* (mackerel). *Toxicon* 27: 1051–1053.

Kudo, Y., Shibata, S. 1980. The potent depolarizing action of palytoxin isolated from *Palythoa tubercurosa* on the isolated spinal cord of the frog. *Br J Pharmacol* 71: 575–579.

Kuroki, D.W., Bignami, G.S., Wattenberg, E.V. 1996. Activation of stress-activated protein kinase/c-Jun N-terminal kinase by the non-TPA-type tumor promoter palytoxin. *Cancer Res* 56: 637–644.

Kuroki, D.W., Minden, A., Sánchez, I., Wattenberg, E.V. 1997. Regulation of a c-Jun amino-terminal kinase/stress-activated protein kinase cascade by a sodium-dependent signal transduction pathway. *J Biol Chem* 272: 23905–23911.

Lau, C.O., Tan, C.H., Khoo, H.E. et al. 1995. *Lophozozymus pictor* toxin: A fluorescent structural isomer of palytoxin. *Toxicon* 33: 1373–1377.

Ledreux, A., Krys, S., Bernard, C. 2009. Suitability of the Neuro-2a cell line for the detection of palytoxin and analogues (neurotoxic phycotoxins). *Toxicon* 53: 300–308.

Lenoir, S., Ten-Hage, L., Turquet, J., Quod, P.J., Bernard, C., Hennion, M.C. 2004. First evidence of palytoxin analogues from an *Ostreopsis mascarenensis* (Dinophyceae) benthic bloom in southwestern Indian Ocean. *J Phycol* 40: 1042–1051.

Levine, L., Fujiki, H., Gjika H.B., Van Vunakis, H. 1987. Production of antibodies to palytoxin: Neutralization of several biological properties of palytoxin. *Toxicon* 25: 1273–1282.

Levine, L., Fujiki, H., Gjika, H.B., Van Vunakis, H. 1988. A radioimmunoassay for palytoxin. *Toxicon* 26: 1115–1121.

Li, S., Wattenberg, E.V. 1999. Cell-type-specific activation of p38 protein kinase cascades by the novel tumor promoter palytoxin. *Toxicol Appl Pharmacol* 160: 109.

Lingrel, J.B., Kuntzweiler, T. 1994. Na+/K(+)-ATPase. *J Biol Chem* 269: 19659–19662.

Louzao, M.C., Ares, I.R., Vieytes, M.R. et al. 2007. The cytoskeleton, a structure that is susceptible to the toxic mechanism activated by palytoxins in human excitable cells. *FEBS J* 274: 1991–2004.

Louzao, M.C., Espiña, B., Cagide, E. et al. 2010. Cytotoxic effect of palytoxin on mussels. *Toxicon* 56: 842–847.

Louzao, M.C., Vieytes, M.R., Yasumoto, T., Yotsu-Yamashita, M., Botana, L.M. 2006. Changes in membrane potential: An early signal triggered by neurologically active phycotoxins. *Chem Res Toxicol* 19: 788–793.

Mahmud, Y., Arakawa, O., Noguchi, T. 2000. An epidemic survey on the freshwater puffer poisoning in Bangladesh. *J Nat Toxins* 9: 319–326.

Mahnir, V.M., Kozlovskaya, E.P., Kalinovsky, A.I. 1992. Sea anemone *Radianthus macrodactylus*—A new source of palytoxin. *Toxicon* 30: 1449–1456.

Malagoli, D. 2007. A full-length protocol to test hemolytic activity of palytoxin on human erythrocytes. *ISJ* 4: 92–94.

Malagoli, D., Casarini, L., Ottaviani, E. 2008. Effect of the marine toxins okadaic acid and palytoxin on mussel phagocytosis. *Fish Shellfish Immunol* 24: 180–186.

Manger, R.L., Leja, L.S., Lee, S.Y. et al. 1993. Tetrazolium-based cell bioassay for neurotoxins active on voltage-sensitive sodium channels: Semiautomated assay for saxitoxins, brevetoxins, and ciguatoxins. *Anal Biochem* 214: 190–194.

Mebs, D. 1998. Occurrence and sequestration of toxins in food chains. *Toxicon* 36: 1519–1522.

Miura, D., Kobayashi, M., Kakiuchi, S., Kasahara, Y., Kondo, S. 2006. Enhancement of transformed foci and induction of prostaglandins in Balb/c 3T3 cells by palytoxin: In vitro model reproduces carcinogenic responses in animal models regarding the inhibitory effect of indomethacin and reversal of indomethacin's effect by exogenous prostaglandins. *Toxicol Sci* 89: 154–163.

Monroe, J.J., Tashjian, A.H. Jr. 1995. Actions of palytoxin on Na+ and Ca2+ homeostasis in human osteoblast-like Saos-2 cells. *Am J Physiol* 269: C582–C589.

Monroe, J.J., Tashjian, A.H. Jr. 1996. Palytoxin modulates cytosolic pH in human osteoblast-like Saos-2 cells via an interaction with Na(+)-K(+)-ATPase. *Am J Physiol* 270: C1277–C1283.

Moore, R.E., Bartolini, G. 1981. Structure of palytoxin. *J Am Chem Soc* 103: 2491.

Moore, R.E., Helfrich, P., Patterson, G.M.L. 1982. The deadly seaweed of Hana. *Oceanus* 25: 54–63.

Moore, R.E., Scheuer, P.J. 1971. Palytoxin: A new marine toxin from a coelenterate. *Science* 172: 495–498.

Moore, R.E., Woolard, F.X., Bartolini, G. 1980. Periodate oxidation of N-(p-bromobenzoyl)palytoxin. *J Am Chem Soc* 102: 7370–7372.

Moshirfar, M., Khalifa, Y.M., Espandar, L., Mifflin, M.D. 2010. Aquarium coral keratoconjunctivitis. *Arch Ophthalmol* 128: 1360–1362.

Mosmann, T. 1983. Rapid colorimetric assay for cellular growth and survival: Application to proliferation and cytotoxicity assays. *J Immunol Methods* 65: 55–63.

Mullin, J.M., Snock, K.V., McGinn, M.T. 1991. Effects of apical vs. basolateral palytoxin on LLC-PK1 renal epithelia. *Am J Physiol* 260: C1201–C1211.

Munday, R. 2008. Occurrence and toxicology of palytoxin. In: *Seafood and Freshwater Toxins. Pharmacology, Physiology and Detection*. Ed. L.M. Botana, pp. 693–713. CRC Press, Boca Raton, FL.

Munday, R. 2011. Palytoxin toxicology: Animal studies. *Toxicon* 57: 470–477.

Muramatsu, I., Nishio, M., Kigoshi, S., Uemura, D. 1988. Single ionic channels induced by palytoxin in guinea-pig ventricular myocytes. *Br J Pharmacol* 93: 811–816.

Muramatsu, I., Uemura, D., Fujiwara, M., Narahashi, T. 1984. Characteristics of palytoxin-induced depolarization in squid axons. *J Pharm Exp Ther* 231: 488–494.

Nagase, H., Ozaki, H., Karaki, H., Urakawa, N. 1986. Intracellular Ca2+-calmodulin system involved in the palytoxin-induced K+ release from rabbit erythrocytes. *FEBS Lett* 195: 125–128.

Nagase, H., Ozaki, H., Urakawa, N. 1984. Inhibitory effect of calmodulin inhibitors on palytoxin-induced K+ release from rabbit erythrocytes. *FEBS Lett* 178: 44–46.

Noguchi, T., Hwang, D.F., Arakawa, O. et al. 1987. Palytoxin as the causative agent in the parrotfish poisoning. In *Progress in Venom and Toxin Research: Proceedings of the first Asia-Pacific Congress on Animal, Plant and Microbial Toxins*, Eds. P. Gopalakrishnakone and C.K. Tan, pp. 325–335. Faculty of Medicine, National University of Singapore, Singapore.

Nordt, S.P., Wu, J., Zahller, S., Clark, R.F., Cantrell, F.L. 2011. Palytoxin poisoning after dermal contact with zoanthid coral. *J Emerg Med* 40: 397–399.

Ohizumi, Y., Shibata, S. 1980. Mechanism of the excitatory action of palytoxin and N-acetylpalytoxin in the isolated guinea-pig vas deferens. *J Pharm Exp Ther* 214: 209–212.

Ohuchi, K., Hirasawa, N., Takahashi, C. et al. 1986. Synergistic stimulation of histamine release from rat peritoneal mast cells by 12-O-tetradecanoylphorbol 13-acetate (TPA)-type and non-TPA-type tumor promoters. *Biochim Biophys Acta* 887: 94–99.

Ohuchi, K., Watanabe, M., Yoshizawa, K. et al. 1985. Stimulation of prostaglandin E2 production by 12-O-tetradecanoylphorbol 13-acetate (TPA)-type and non-TPA-type tumor promoters in macrophages and its inhibition by cycloheximide. *Biochim Biophys Acta* 834: 42–47.

Okano, H., Masuoka, H., Kamei, S., Seko, T., Koyabu, S., Tsuneoka, K., Tamai, T. et al. 1998. Rhabdomyolysis and myocardial damage induced by palytoxin, a toxin of blue humphead parrotfish. *Int Med* 37: 330–333.

Oku, N., Sata, N.U., Matsunaga, S., Uchida, H., Fusetani, N. 2004. Identification of palytoxin as a principle which causes morphological changes in rat 3Y1 cells in the zoanthid *Palythoa* aff. *margaritae*. *Toxicon* 43: 21–25.

Onuma, Y., Satake, M., Ukena, T. et al. 1999. Identification of putative palytoxin as the cause of clupeotoxism. *Toxicon* 37: 55–65.

Ozaki, H., Nagase, H., Urakawa, N. 1984. Sugar moiety of cardiac glycosides is essential for the inhibitory action on the palytoxin-induced K+ release from red blood cells. *FEBS Lett* 173: 196–198.

Ozaki, H., Nagase, H., Urakawa, N. 1985. Interaction of palytoxin and cardiac glycosides on erythrocyte membrane and (Na+ + K+) ATPase. *Eur J Biochem* 152: 475–480.

Ozaki, H., Tomono, J., Nagase, H., Ito, K., Urakawa, N. 1983. The mechanism of contractile action of palytoxin on vascular smooth muscle of guinea-pig aorta. *Jpn J Pharmacol* 33: 1155–1162.

Pelin, M., Sosa, S., Della Loggia, R. et al. 2012. The cytotoxic effect of palytoxin on Caco-2 cells hinders their use for in vitro absorption studies. *Food Chem Toxicol* 50: 206–211.

Pelin, M., Zanette, C., De Bortoli, M. et al. 2011. Effects of the marine toxin palytoxin on human skin keratinocytes: Role of ionic imbalance. *Toxicology* 282: 30–38.

Pelin, M., Boscolo, S., Poli, M. et al. 2013a. Characterization of palytoxin binding to HaCaT cells using a monoclonal anti-palytoxin antibody. *Mar Drugs* 11:584–598.

Pelin, M., Ponti, C., Sosa, S. et al. 2013b. Oxidative stress induced by palytoxin in human keratinocytes is mediated by a H+-dependent mitochondrial pathway. *Toxicol Appl Pharmacology* 266:1–8.

Pérez-Gómez, A., Novelli, A., Fernández-Sánchez, M.T. 2010. Na+/K+-ATPase inhibitor palytoxin enhances vulnerability of cultured cerebellar neurons to domoic acid via sodium-dependent mechanisms. *J Neurochem* 114: 28–38.

Pezzolesi, L., Guerrini, F., Ciminiello, P. et al. 2012. Influence of temperature and salinity on Ostreopsis cf. ovata growth and evaluation of toxin content through HR LC-MS and biological assays. *Water Res* 46: 82–92.

Prandi, S., Sala, G.L., Bellocci, M. et al. 2011. Palytoxin induces cell lysis by priming a two-step process in MCF-7 cells. *Chem Res Toxicol* 24: 1283–1296.

Qiu, L.Y., Swarts, H.G., Tonk, E.C. et al. 2006. Conversion of the low affinity Ouabain-binding site of non-gastric H,K ATPase into a high affinity binding site by substitution of only five amino acids. *J Biol Chem* 281: 13533–13539.

Rakowski, R.F., Artigas, P., Palma, F., Holmgren, M., De Weer, P., Gadsby, D.C. 2007. Sodium flux ratio in Na/K pump-channels opened by palytoxin. *J Gen Physiol* 130: 41–54.

Raybould, T.J. 1991. Toxin production and immunoassay development. 1. Palytoxin. Report of the Hawaii Biotechnology Group Inc Aiea, pp. 1–163. Hawaii Biotechnology Group Inc Aiea: Aiea (Hawaii).

Rhodes, L., Adamson, J., Suzuki, T., Briggs, L., Garthwaite, I. 2000. Toxic marine epiphytic dinoflagellates, *Ostreopsis siamensis* and *Coolia monotis* (Dynophyceae), in New Zealand. *N Z J Mar Freshw Res* 34: 371–383.

Rhodes, L., Towers, N., Briggs, L., Munday, R., Adamson, J. 2002. Uptake of palytoxin-like compounds by shellfish fed *Ostreopsis siamensis* (Dinophyceae). *N Z J Mar Freshw Res* 36: 631–636.

Riobò, P., Franco, J.M. 2011. Palytoxins: Biological and chemical determination. *Toxicon* 57: 368–375.

Riobò, P., Paz, B., Franco, J.M. 2006. Analysis of palytoxin-like in Ostreopsis cultures by liquid chromatography with precolumn derivatization and fluorescence detection. *Anal Chim Acta* 566: 217–223.

Riobò, P., Paz, B., Franco, J.M. 2008b. Analysis of palytoxin-like in *Ostreopsis* cultures by liquid chromatography with precolumn derivatization and fluorescence detection. *Anal Chim Acta* 566: 217–223.

Riobò, P., Paz, B., Franco J.M., Vázquez, J.A., Murado, M.A., Cacho, E. 2008a. Mouse bioassay for palytoxin. Specific symptoms and dose response against dose-death time relationship. *Food Chem Toxicol* 46: 2639–2647.

Robinson, C.P., Franz, D.R. 1991. Effects of palytoxin on guinea pig tracheal strips. *Pharm Res* 8: 859–864.

Robinson, C.P., Franz, D.R., Bondura, M.E. 1992. Effects of palytoxin on porcine coronary artery rings. *J Appl Toxicol* 12: 185–189.

Rodrigues, A.M., Almeida, A.C., Infantosi, A.F., Teixeira, H.Z., Duarte, M.A. 2008. Model and simulation of Na^+/K^+ pump phosphorylation in the presence of palytoxin. *Comput Biol Chem* 32: 5–16.

Rodrigues, A.M., Infantosi, A.F., de Almeida, A.C. 2009. Palytoxin and the sodium/potassium pump-phosphorylation and potassium interaction. *Phys Biol* 6: 036010.

Rossi, R., Castellano, V., Scalco, E., Serpe, L., Zingone, A., Soprano, V. 2011. New palytoxin-like molecules in Mediterranean Ostreopsis cf. ovata(dinoflagellates) and in *Palythoa tuberculosa* detected by liquid chromatography-electrospray ionization time-of-flight mass spectrometry. *Toxicon* 56: 1381–1387.

Rossini, G.P. and Bigiani, A. 2011. Palytoxin action on the Na(+),K(+)-ATPase and the disruption of ion equilibria in biological systems. *Toxicon* 57: 429–439.

Sagara, T., Nishibori, N., Itoh, M., Morita, K., Her, S. 2011. Palytoxin causes non oxidative necrotic damage to PC12 cells in culture. *J Appl Toxicol.* 33: 120–124.

Sansoni, G., Borghini, B., Camici, G., Casotti, M., Righini, P., Rustighi, C. 2003. Fioriture algali di *Ostreopsis ovata* (Gonyaulacales: Dinophyceae): Un problema emergente. *Biol Ambientale* 17: 17–23.

Satoh, E., Ishii, T., Nishimura, M. 2003. Palytoxin-induced increase in cytosolic-free Ca(2+) in mouse spleen cells. *Eur J Pharmacol* 465: 9–13.

Sauviat, M.P., Pater, C., Berton, J. 1987. Does palytoxin open a sodium-sensitive channel in cardiac muscle? *Toxicon* 25: 695–704.

Scheiner-Bobis, G., Hübschle, T., Diener, M. 2002. Action of palytoxin on apical H^+/K^+ ATPase in rat colon. *Eur J Biochem* 269: 3905–3911.

Scheiner-Bobis, G. Meyer zu Heringdorf, D., Christ, M., Habermann, E. 1994. Palytoxin induces K^+ efflux from yeast cells expressing the mammalian sodium pump. *Mol pharmacol* 45: 1132–1136.

Schilling, W.P., Snyder, D., Sinkins, W.G., Estacion, M. 2006. Palytoxin-induced cell death cascade in bovine aortic endothelial cells. *Am J Physiol Cell Physiol* 291: C657–C667.

Seemann, P., Gernert, C., Schmitt, S., Mebs, D., Hentschel, U. 2009. Detection of hemolytic bacteria from *Palythoa caribaeorum* (Cnidaria, Zoantharia) using a novel palytoxin-screening assay. *Antonie van Leeuwenhoek* 96: 405–411.

Sheridan, R.E., Deshpande, S.S., Adler, M. 2005. Cytotoxic action of palytoxin on aortic smooth muscle cells in culture. *J Appl Toxicol* 25: 365–373.

Sosa, S., Del Favero, G., De Bortoli, M. et al. 2009. Palytoxin toxicity after acute oral administration in mice. *Tox Lett* 191: 253–259.

Tabata, H., Nanjo, K., Kokuoka, H., Machida, K., Miyamura, K. 1989. Two cases of fish poisoning caused by ingesting parrot fish. *Int Med* 64: 974–977.

Tan, C.T.T., Lee, E.J.D. 1988. A fatal case of crab toxin (*Lophozozymus pictor*) poisoning. *Asia Pac J Pharmacol* 3: 7–9.

Taniyama, S., Arakawa, O., Terada, M. et al. 2003. *Ostreopsis* sp., a possible origin of palytoxin (PTX) in parrotfish *Scarus ovifrons*. *Toxicon* 42: 29–33.

Taniyama, S., Mahmud, Y., Tanu, M.B., Takatani, T., Arakawa, O., Noguki, T. 2001. Delayed haemolytic activity by the freshwater puffer *Tetraodon* sp. toxin. *Toxicon* 39: 725–727.

Taniyama, S., Mahmud, Y., Terada, M., Takatani, T., Arakawa, O., Noguki, T. 2002. Occurrence of a food poisoning incident by PLTX from a serranid *Epinephelus sp.* in Japan. *J Nat Toxin* 11: 277–282.

Teh, Y.F., Gardiner, J.E. 1974. Partial purification of Lophozozymus pictor toxin. *Toxicon* 12: 603–610.

Terao, K., Ito, E., Yasumoto, T. 1992. Light and electron microscopic observation of experimental palytoxin poisoning in mice. *Bull Soc Path Ex* 85: 494–496.

Tichadou, L., Glaizal, M., Armengaud, A. et al. 2010. Health impact of unicellular algae of the *Ostreopsis* genus blooms in the Mediterranean Sea: Experience of the French Mediterranean coast surveillance network from 2006 to 2009. *Clin Toxicol* 48: 839–844.

Tosteson, M.T., Bignami, G.S., Scriven, D.R., Bharadwaj, A.K., Tosteson, D.C. 1994. Inhibition of the actions of palytoxin on the K+ efflux from red cells and on the Na/K-ATPase activity by a monoclonal antibody. *Biochim Biophys Acta* 1191: 371–374.

Tosteson, M.T., Halperin, J.A., Kishi, Y., Tosteson, D.C. 1991. Palytoxin induces an increase in the cation conductance of red cells. *J Gen Physiol* 98: 969–985.

Tosteson, M.T., Scriven, D.R., Bharadwaj, A.K., Kishi, Y., Tosteson, D.C. 1995. Interaction of palytoxin with red cells: Structure-function studies. *Toxicon* 33: 799–807.

Tosteson, M.T., Thomas, J., Arnadottir, J., Tosteson, D.C. 2003. Effects of palytoxin on cation occlusion and phosphorylation of the (Na+,K+)-ATPase. *J Membr Biol* 192: 181–189.

Tubaro, A., Del Favero, G., Beltramo, D. et al. 2011b. Acute oral toxicity in mice of a new palytoxin analog: 42-Hydroxy-palytoxin. *Toxicon* 57: 755–763.

Tubaro, A., Durando, P., Del Favero, G. et al. 2011a. Case definitions for human poisonings postulated to palytoxins exposure. *Toxicon* 57: 478–495.

Uemura, D., Hirata, Y., Iwashita, T., Naoki, H. 1985. Studies on palytoxins. *Tetrahedron* 41: 1007–1017.

Ukena, T., Satake, M., Usami, T. et al. 2001. Structure elucidation of Ostreocin-D, a palytoxin analog isolated from the dinoflagellate *Ostreopsis siamensis*. *Biosci Biotechnol Biochem* 65: 2585–2588.

Usami, M., Satake, M., Ishida, S., Inoue, A., Kan, Y., Yasumoto, T. 1995. Palytoxin analogs from the dinoflagellate *Ostreopsis siamensis*. *J Am Chem Soc* 117: 5389–5390.

Vale, C., Alfonso, A., Suñol, C., Vieytes, M.R., Botana, L.M. 2006. Modulation of calcium entry and glutamate release in cultured cerebellar granule cells by palytoxin. *J Neurosci Res* 83: 1393–1406.

Vale, C., Gómez-Limia, B., Vieytes, M.R., Botana, L.M. 2007. Mitogen-activated protein kinases regulate palytoxin-induced calcium influx and cytotoxicity in cultured neurons. *Br J Pharmacol* 152: 256–266.

Vale-Gonzáles, C., Gómez-Lima, B., Vieytes, M.R., Botana, L.M. 2007a. Effects of the marine phycotoxin palytoxin in neuronal pH in primary cultures of cerebellar granule cells. *J Neurosci Res* 85: 90–98.

Vale-Gonzalez, C., Pazos, M.J., Alfonso, A., Vieytes, M.R., Botana, L.M. 2007b. Study of the neuronal effects of ouabain and palytoxin and their binding to Na,K-ATPases using an optical biosensor. *Toxicon* 50: 541–552.

Valverde, I., Lago, J., Reboreda, A., Vieites, J.M. Cabado, A.G. 2008a. Characteristics of palytoxin-induced cytotoxicity in neuroblastoma cells. *Toxicol In Vitro* 22: 1432–1439.

Valverde, I., Lago, J., Vieites, J.M. Cabado, A.G. 2008b. In vitro approaches to evaluate palytoxin-induced toxicity and cell death in intestinal cells. *J Appl Toxicol* 28: 294–302.

Van Renterghem, C., Frelin, C. 1993. 3,4-Dichlorobenzamil-sensitive, monovalent cation channel induced by palytoxin in cultured aortic myocytes. *Br J Pharmacol* 109: 859–865.

Vick, J.A., Wiles, J.S. 1990. Pharmacological and toxicological studies of palytoxin. In *Marine Toxins: Origin, Structure and Molecular Pharmacology*. Eds. S. Hall and G. Strichartz, Chapter 19, pp. 241–254. American Chemical Society: Washington, DC.

Wachi, K.M., Hokama, Y., Haga, L.S. et al. 2000. Evidence for palytoxin as one of the sheep erythrocyte lytic in lytic factors in crude extracts of ciguateric and non-ciguateric reef fish tissue. *J Nat Toxins* 9: 139–146.

Wang, Y.C., Huang, R.C. 2006. Effects of the sodium pump activity on spontaneous firing in neurons of the rat suprachiasmatic nucleus. *J Neurophysiol* 96: 109–118.

Warmka, J.K., Winston, S.E., Zeliadt, N.A., Wattenberg, E.V. 2002. Extracellular signal-regulated kinase transmits palytoxin-stimulated signals leading to altered gene expression in mouse keratinocytes. *Toxicol Appl Pharmacol* 185: 8–17.

Wattenberg, E.V. 2011. Modulation of protein kinase signaling cascades by palytoxin. *Toxicon* 57: 440–448.

Wattenberg, E.V., Byron, K.L., Villereal, M.L., Fujiki, H., Rosner, M.R. 1989. Sodium as a mediator of non-phorbol tumor promoter action. Down-modulation of the epidermal growth factor receptor by palytoxin. *J Biol Chem* 264: 14668–14673.

Wattenberg, E.V., Fujiki, H., Rosner, M.R. 1987. Heterologous regulation of the epidermal growth factor receptor by palytoxin, a non-12-O-tetradecanoylphorbol-13-acetate-type tumor promoter. *Cancer Res* 47: 4618–4622.

Wiles, J.S., Vick, J.A., Christenson, M.K. 1974. Toxicological evaluation of palytoxin in several animal species. *Toxicon* 12: 427–433.

Wu, C.H. 2009. Palytoxin: Membrane mechanism of action. *Toxicon* 54: 1183–1189.

Yakes, B.J., DeGrasse, S.L., Poli, M., Deeds, J.R. 2011. Antibody characterization and immunoassays for palytoxin using an SPR biosensor. *Anal Bioanal Chem* 400: 2865–2869.

Yasumoto, T., Murata, M., Oshima, Y. et al. 1985. Diarrhetic shellfish toxins. *Tetrahedron* 41: 1019–1025.

Yasumoto, T., Oshima, Y, Yamaguchi, M. 1978. Occurrence of a new type of shellfish poisoning in the Tohoku district. *Bull Jpn Soc Sci Fish* 44: 1249–1255.

Yasumoto, T., Yasumura, D., Ohizumi, Y., Takahashi, M., Alcala, A.C., Alcala, L.C. 1986. Palytoxin in two species of xanthid crab from the Philippines. *Agric Biol Chem* 50: 163–167.

Yoshimine, K., Orita, S., Okada, S., Sonoda, K., Kubota, K., Yonezawa, T. 2001. Two cases of parrotfish poisoning with rhabdomyolysis. *J Jpn Soc Int Med* 90: 1339–1341.

Zamolo, V.A., Valenti, G., Venturelli, E. et al. 2012. Highly sensitive electrochemiluminescent nanobiosensor for the detection of palytoxin. *ACS Nano* 6: 7989–7997.

Zeliadt, N.A., Warmka, J.K., Winston, S.E. et al. 2004. Tumor promoter-induced MMP-13 gene expression in a model of initiated epidermis. *Biochem Biophys Res Commun* 317: 570–577.

26

AZA: The Producing Organisms—Biology and Trophic Transfer

Urban Tillmann, Rafael Salas, Thierry Jauffrais, Philipp Hess, and Joe Silke

CONTENTS

26.1 Introduction

Compared to the knowledge on toxin structure, detection methods, and toxicology, convincing clarification of the etiology of azaspiracid poisoning (AZP) was seriously lacking behind for quite a long time. Based upon the seasonal and episodic accumulation of azaspiracid (AZA) toxins in suspension-feeding bivalve molluscs—a situation similar to several other marine biotoxins—a planktonic source has been suspected from the outset. Furthermore, due to their polyether structural features, AZA has ab initio been suspected to be a dinoflagellate metabolite. Thus, it was no surprise that it was a dinoflagellate species that was first claimed to be the source of AZA. Based upon chemical analysis by liquid chromatography coupled to mass spectrometry (LC–MS) of manually collected phytoplankton specimens from net hauls, Yasumoto[1] first indicated that a species of the dinoflagellate genus *Protoperidinium* was the primary source of AZA. This work was later published in detail by James et al.[2] with the culprit species described as *Protoperidinium crassipes*. The link between AZA and *P. crassipes*, however, remained controversial because production of AZA by *P. crassipes* could not be verified in spite of numerous attempts based upon field surveys[3] and laboratory investigations of cultured and isolated cells.[4] Moreover, in contrast to other proven producers of phycotoxins, which are all primarily phototrophic, *P. crassipes*

TABLE 26.1

Morphological Features for Species of *Azadinium* and *Amphidoma languida*

Feature	*Azadinium spinosum* (Tillmann et al. 2009)	*Azadinium obesum* (Tillmann et al. 2010)	*Azadinium poporum* (Tillmann et al. 2011; Krock et al. 2012)	*Azadinium caudatum* (Nezan et al. 2012)		*Azadinium polongum* (Tillmann et al. 2012b)	*Azadinium dexteroporum* (Percopo et al. 2013)	*Amphidoma languida* (Tillmann et al. 2012a)
				var. *margalefii*	var. *caudatum*			
Size (length × width)	13.8 × 8.8	15.3 × 11.7	13.0 × 9.8	31.3 × 22.4[a]	41.7 × 28.7[a]	13.0 × 9.7	8.5 × 6.2	13.9 × 11.9
Length/width ratio	1.6	1.3	1.3	1.2[b]	1.2[b]	1.3	1.4	1.2
Stalked pyrenoid(s)	1, central episome	No	Several (up to four)	No	No	No	1	1, central episome
Apical and intercalary plates	4 apicals, 3 intercalaries	4 apicals, 3 intercalaries	4 apicals, 3 intercalaries	4 apicals, 3 intercalaries	4 apicals, 3 intercalaries	4 apicals, 3 intercalaries	4 apicals, 3 intercalaries	6 apicals, 0 intercalaries
Antapical projection	Small spine	No	No	Short horn, long spine	Long horn, short spine	Small spine	Small spine	Antapical pore (pore field of small pores)
Location "ventral" pore	Left side of 1' (median position)	Left side of 1' (median position)	Left side of Po	Right side of Po	Right side of 1' (posterior position)	Left side, suture of 1' and 1" (slightly posterior)	Right side and at the end of Po	Right side of 1' (anterior position)
Shape of Po	Round/ellipsoid	Round/ellipsoid	Round/ellipsoid	Round/ellipsoid	Round/ellipsoid	Distinctly elongated	Round/ellipsoid	Round/ellipsoid
Contact of ventral precingulars with intercalaries	Ventral 1" in contact to 1a	No	Ventral 1" in contact to 1a	Ventral 1" in contact to 1a Ventral 6" in contact to 3a	Ventral 1" in contact to 1a Ventral 6" in contact to 3a	Ventral 1" in contact to 1a	Ventral 1" in contact to 1a	Not applicable (no intercalaries)
Shape of plate 4"	Similar size as other precingular, in contact to 3a	Similar size as other precingular, in contact to 3a	Similar size as other precingular, in contact to 3a	Smaller than other precingulars, no contact to 3a	Smaller than other precingulars, no contact to 3a	Similar size as other precingular, in contact to 3a	Similar size as other precingular, in contact to 3a	Similar size as other precingular
Shape of 2a	Convex	Convex	Convex	Convex	Convex	Convex	Concave	Convex
AZAs	AZA1, AZA2, AZA33	Not detected	Large strain variability, AZA36, AZA37, AZA2, AZA11	Not fully tested	No culture available, not analyzed yet	Not detected	Tentatively AZA3, AZA7 LC–MS confirmation needed	AZA34, AZA38

[a] Cell length including antapical projection (horn and spine).

[b] Length excluding antapical projection.

is a heterotrophic dinoflagellate, known to prey upon other dinoflagellates as food.[5] The likelihood, therefore, that another dinoflagellate may produce AZA, which then accumulates in *P. crassipes* through normal feeding processes, could not be neglected.

During a research cruise with RV Poseidon in the North Sea, this issue became quite evident when toxin analysis of fractionated plankton samples clearly showed that high amount of AZAs was found even when *P. crassipes* was absent, that AZA could be found in isolated cells of the predatory ciliate *Favella ehrenbergii*, and that in fractionated plankton samples, the largest AZA quantities were found in the small-size (<20 μm) classes.[6] All these hints then led to the isolation of a small dinoflagellate, which was shown to produce AZA1 and AZA2 in axenic culture[6] and which was identified as a new species *Azadinium spinosum* in a newly erected genus.[7] Considering the short interval since this first identification of *Azadinium*, the diversity of the genus has rapidly increased and now comprises six species (Table 26.1 and Figure 26.1), some of which are available as multiple strains. These species are *A. spinosum*, *A. obesum*, *A. poporum*, *A. polongum*, *A. caudatum* (which occurs in two distinct varieties: var. *margalefii* and var. *caudatum*), and *A. dexteroporum*. Moreover, with the description of *Amphidoma languida*, a closely related genus could be identified.[8] Whereas multiple strains of the type *A. spinosum* from different location have consistently been found to produce AZA1, AZA2, and AZA33, other new species have initially been described as nontoxigenic, as none of the known AZAs could be found.[9,10] However, with the recent detection of four new AZAs in a number of different species, it became evident that the species diversity within this group is also reflected by a high chemical diversity, with AZA production even found in the related genus *Amphidoma*.[11] The presence of AZAs (AZA3 and AZA7) has also been tentatively described for the most recently identified species *A. dexteroporum*,[12] but this needs to be confirmed by LC–MS analysis. In particular, *A. poporum* turned out to be a rich source of different AZA compounds,[11,13] but with a large variability of AZA profile among different strains. Three species (*A. obesum*, *A. caudatum* var. *margalefii* and *A. polongum*) still have been negative in AZA detection, but we cannot exclude the presence of yet unknown and thus undetectable AZA-related compounds. In any case, in view of the diversity of AZA-producing species, it is important to appreciate the commonalities and differences of the species as a fundamental basis for species identification, "early warning" monitoring, and bloom prediction.

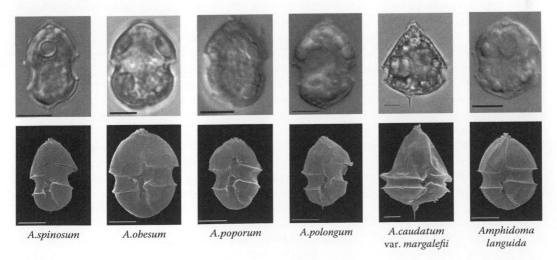

| A.spinosum | A.obesum | A.poporum | A.polongum | A.caudatum var. *margalefii* | Amphidoma languida |

FIGURE 26.1 Light microscopy (upper panel) and electron microscopy (lower panel) micrographs of species of *Azadinium* and *Amphidoma languida*. Scale bars = 5 μm. For micrographs of the most recently described species, *A. dexteroporum*, see Percopo et al. (Ref. [12]).

26.2 Morphology–Taxonomy–Phylogeny

26.2.1 General Morphology and Taxonomy

Gross morphology and a compilation of distinctive features of the species are compiled in Table 26.1 and Figure 26.1. Most species of *Azadinium* (and *Amphidoma languida*) are small (size of about 10–15 µm) and ovoid to elliptical in shape with a hemispherical hyposome. *A. caudatum* (both varieties) are distinctly larger and, with a characteristic biconical outline, significantly different in shape as well. In all species, the episome is larger than the hyposome, with slightly convex sides ending in a distinctly pointed apex. For all small species, the cingulum is deep and wide, accounting for roughly 1/5 to 1/4 of the cell length (1/6 for the larger *A. caudatum*). A central or more posteriorly located large nucleus is visible, which generally is round to elliptical but may become distinctly elongated in shape close to cell division.[8,14] All species are photosynthetic and possess a presumably single chloroplast that is parietally arranged and lobed and normally extends into both the epi- and hyposome. For a number of species, a stalked pyrenoid is visible in the light microscope because of a distinct starch cup. The presence/absence, location, number, and types of pyrenoids have been regarded as useful taxonomic characters between genera[9,15] and have in particular been discussed as a potential feature visible in light microscopy to differentiate species of *Azadinium*.[9] However, more detailed information (including ultrastructure) related to pyrenoids of *Azadinium* is needed before this feature can be unambiguously used for species determination. *Azadinium* spp. have delicate thecal plates difficult to detect in light microscopy so that live cells are sometimes difficult to differentiate from small athecate gymnodinoid species. Generally, the surface of the plates is smooth but irregularly covered by small pores. These pores are either numerous and arranged randomly (*A. caudatum*), more rare and scattered (small *Azadinium* species) or particularly concentrated on the apical plates in *Amphidoma languida*. A distinct row of pores located below the lower cingulum list may be present. All species of *Azadinium* consistently show the Kofoidean plate pattern of pore plate (Po), cp, X, 4′, 3 a, 6″, C6, 5S, 6‴, 2⁗ (Figure 26.2a through c), whereas *Amphidoma languida* has six apical plates and no intercalaries. A very characteristic feature among the AZA-relevant species is the prominent apical pore complex composed of a Po with a central round pore covered by a cover plate, and an X-plate. The pore plate (Po) is round to slightly ellipsoid, or distinctly elongated (exceptional for *A. polongum*), or markedly asymmetric, with a finger-like protrusion on the left side (exceptional for *A. dexteroporum*). The Po is always bordered by a conspicuous rim that is of slightly different run among species. A small X-plate is located where the Po abuts the first apical plate and occupies about 1/3 of the connection between Po and 1′. The X-plate shows some differences in arrangement across species; it invades the first apical plate in *A. spinosum*, *A. obesum*, *A. poporum*, and *Amphidoma languida* but abuts the first apical plate in *A. polongum* and *A. caudatum*. From the outside, the X-plate consistently among all species has a very characteristic 3D structure with fingerlike protrusions contacting the apical cover plate.

The epitheca of *Azadinium* spp. consists of four apical plates and a row of six precingular plates. Three intercalary plates are located dorsally. The median plate 2a very characteristically is the smallest of the intercalaries and is four sided (Figure 26.2a). The hypothecal plate arrangement with a row of six postcingular and two differently sized antapical plates is consistent for all the species (Figure 26.2b). The second antapical plate may bear a small spine (*A. spinosum*, *A. polongum*, *A. dexteroporum*), a distinct horn with a spine (*A. caudatum*), or a prominent antapical pore (*Amphidoma languida*). The cingulum is composed of six plates of similar size. The sulcal plate arrangement generally is difficult to analyze due to a distinct 3D shape of the sulcal area that obscures some of the small plates from view. Nevertheless, the arrangement of the five sulcal plates is very characteristic for all AZA-relevant species and is characterized by a large plate Sa invading the epitheca and a peculiar and conservative Ss plate running from C1 to C6 plates (Figure 26.2c).

All species of *Azadinium* and *Amphidoma languida* have a distinct pore located in the ventral area that is thus designated as a "ventral pore." Generally, the location of the ventral pore seems to be quite variable in *Azadinium* species (Figure 26.2d), either on the left margin of plate 1′ (*A. spinosum*, *A. obesum*), on the left side of the Po (*A. poporum*),[7,9,10] or at the right posterior end of the markedly asymmetric Po plate (*A. dexteroporum*).[12] In *A. caudatum* var. *margalefii*, this pore is located on the right margin of the Po, whereas for the second variety, *A. caudatum* var. *caudatum*, a similar pore is situated near the

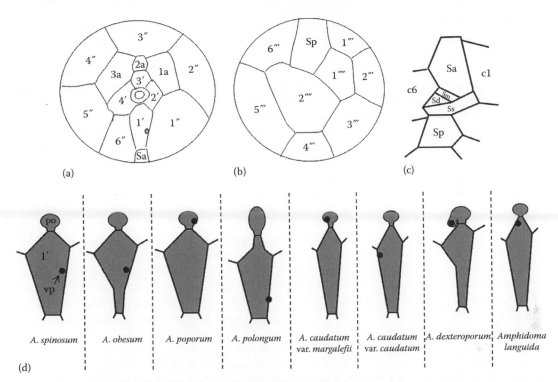

FIGURE 26.2 (a–c) General plate pattern in Kofoidean nomenclature of the genus *Azadinium* for (a) epithecal, (b) hypothecal, and (c) sulcal plates (Sa, anterior sulcal plate; Sp, posterior sulcal plate; Ss, left sulcal plate; Sm, median sulcal plate; Sd, right sulcal plate). (d) Schematic drawings (not drawn to scale) of the ventral epitheca of different species indicating the variable shape of the Po, first apical plate (1′), and the variable position of the ventral pore (vp).

posterior right margin of plate 1′.[16] In *Amphidoma languida*, it is located on the anterior right margin of 1′.[8] Very rarely, the position of the ventral pore has been observed to vary even within a culture. For one specimen of *A. languida*, the ventral pore was located in the right side of the Po[8] (as in *A. caudatum* var. *margalefii*), and for one specimen of *A. poporum* isolated from Korean waters, it was located on the left side of plate 1′.[17] As the function (if any) of these pores is completely unknown, we cannot speculate on the potential consequences of the apparent variability in pore location among the Amphidomataceae. The plate overlap pattern (imbrications pattern), which may reflect functional aspects of ecdysis and/or cysts archeopyle type, may be a useful aid in determining plate homologies.[18] It has been elucidated in details for *A. spinosum*,[19] *A. languida*,[8] *A. caudatum*,[16] and *A. polongum*.[20] The pattern is consistent among the species and identified an uncommon but stable imbrication pattern of the most dorsal apical plate (3′ in *Azadinium* or 4′ in *Amphidoma*), which characterized these two genera and might be helpful for a revision of the description of the family *Amphidomataceae*.

For most of the cultured strains of *Azadinium* analyzed so far, a distinct variability in plate patterns has been noted. Such variations from the usual plate pattern in terms of number and/or arrangement appear most often for apical and intercalary plates, but more rarely have been observed for hypothecal plates as well. However, it is unknown whether the presence and/or degree of variability is an inherited feature of the genus *Azadinium*, distinct at the strain or species level, or is simply a culture artifact. Clearly, detailed morphological investigations of field populations are needed to answer these questions.

26.2.2 Introduction to the Species

Azadinium spinosum (Figure 26.1a), the type of the genus, was first isolated from the North Sea off Scotland, and this isolate was confirmed to be a proximal source for AZA.[6] *A. spinosum* was shown to produce AZA1 and AZA2 in axenic cultures and thus AZAs are of dinoflagellate origin and unrelated to bacteria.[6]

A detailed morphological analysis supplemented by sequence information then described this strain as the new species *Azadinium spinosum*.[7] With a Kofoidean thecal tabulation of APC, 4′, 3a, 6″, 6C, 5?S, 6‴, 2‴′, the species was identified as distinctly different from other described dinoflagellate genera, and consequently, the new genus *Azadinium* was erected to comprise this novel taxon. *A. spinosum* is a small (12–16 μm length and 7–11 μm width) and slender thecate, photosynthetic dinoflagellate with a wide and descending cingulum, which is displaced by about half of its width. Eponymous for the species is the presence of a single, small, and delicate antapical spine located slightly asymmetrically at the right side of the cell. A distinct ventral pore is located on the left margin of plate 1′. In the light microscope, one large pyrenoid located in the episome is visible. Different strains have been isolated from the North Sea (Scotland,[7] Denmark,[9] Shetland Islands[20]) and from Ireland.[21] Multiple strains of *A. spinosum* from different locations have consistently been found to produce AZA1, AZA2, and AZA33 (an AZA with the molecular mass of 715 Da).[20]

Azadinium obesum (Figure 26.1b): The second species of the genus was isolated as clone 2E10 from the North Sea along the Scottish east coast, the same locality as for *A. spinosum*, the type for this genus.[10] *Azadinium obesum* also is small (13–18 μm length; 10–14 μm width) and similar in shape, but there are a number of morphological differences compared to *A. spinosum*, including a larger mean cell size (the epithet refers to the obese, corpulent appearance of the species when compared to the more slender shape of the type, *A. spinosum*), the consistent absence of an antapical spine, the lack of a stalked pyrenoid, and several details of the plate configuration. Among these thecal features, the first precingular (1″) plate of *A. obesum* does not touch the first epithecal intercalary plate and is four sided, rather than five sided as in all other *Azadinium* species reported so far. Furthermore, very different to other *Azadinium* species, the lower half of the first apical (1′) plate of *A. obesum* is very narrow and tonguelike. *A. obesum* is one of the *Azadinium* species where up to now no AZAs have been detected.[10,11]

Azadinium poporum (Figure 26.1c) was initially described from three clones isolated from the southern North Sea off the Danish coast.[9] Like other *Azadinium* species, *A. poporum* is a small (11–16 μm length, 8–12 μm width) photosynthetic dinoflagellate with exactly the Kofoidean plate tabulation of the genus. In contrast to *A. spinosum* (one pyrenoid) and *A. obesum* (no pyrenoid), there may be several pyrenoids (up to four) visible in the light microscope. The most important morphological characteristic of *A. poporum* is the conspicuous arrangement of the ventral pore, which is located at the junction of the Po and the first two apical plates. This latter feature also distinguishes *A. poporum* from *A. obesum*. As in *A. spinosum*, but different from *A. obesum*, the first precingular (1″) plate of *A. poporum* touches the first epithecal intercalary plate 1a. In *A. poporum*, a number of different AZAs toxins (see Chapter 27) have been detected, with a large variability among strains and with nontoxigenic strains present.[11,13]

Azadinium polongum (Figure 26.1d) is another very recently described species of *Azadinium*. Up to now, it has only been reported from the Shetland Islands, which are located in the northernmost part of the North Sea and are largely influenced by the Atlantic Ocean. In the light microscope, it is very similar to the other small species of *Azadinium* (*A. spinosum*, *A. obesum*, *A. poporum*) and it has an antapical spine. The presence of an antapical spine in small *Azadinium* species was hitherto restricted to *A. spinosum*. With *A. polongum* also exhibiting an antapical spine, the identification of *A. spinosum* only by light microscopy is unfortunately no longer convenient. The most obvious morphological feature (but only visible at the scanning electron microscope [SEM] level) of *A. polongum* is the shape of the Po that allows a clear separation of *A. polongum* (elongated Po) from other *Azadinium* species (round to slightly ellipsoid Po). Other features useful for species delimitation of *A. polongum* are the shape of the X-plate, the location of the ventral pore, and the absence of a distinct pyrenoid with starch sheath. No AZAs have been detected in *A. polongum*.

Azadinium caudatum (Figure 26.1e): The dinoflagellate species described in 1953 by Halldal as *Amphidoma caudata* had a somewhat checkered taxonomic history. The first plate details provided by Dodge and Saunders indicated that this species has the same basic plate pattern as *Azadinium*.[35] It was thus concluded by Tillmann et al.[9] that, notwithstanding some differences that remained to be elucidated, *Amphidoma caudata* might be transferred to the genus *Azadinium*, pending further morphological and phylogenetic studies. Consequently, a new study using field samples and cultures of "*A. caudata*" used morphological and molecular data to clarify the systematic situation and transferred the species to the genus *Azadinium* as *Azadinium caudatum*.[16] Both sequence and morphometric data clearly showed that the species occurred with two distinct varieties, var. *caudatum* and var. *margalefii*, which are easily distinguished by the different shape of the antapical projection. *Azadinium caudatum* is quite easy to distinguish from other species of *Azadinium* on the light microscopy level due to its larger size, its characteristic triangular shape, and its clearly visible antapical projection. The basic plate patter is the same as for other *Azadinium* species; nevertheless, there are a couple of minor morphological differences visible at the SEM level. The first precingular plate (1″) is in contact with the first intercalary plate (1a) (similar to all other *Azadinium* species except *A. obesum*). However, in *A. caudatum,* there is also contact between plate 6″ and 3a, which is unique among other *Azadinium* species. Another remarkable difference to other species of *Azadinium* is that the 4″ is distinctly smaller than the other precingular plates and also three sided. Other differences include the shape of the conspicuous rim around the apical Po (extending on the dorsal side alongside the anterior margins of plate 3′ for *A. caudatum*), the contact between the X-plate and the first apical plate (X-plate abuts 1′ in *A. caudatum* and invades it in other *Azadinium* species), and an unusual and unique deep depression present in the largest sulcal plate (Sp plate). Presence of AZAs in *A. caudatum* have either not been fully tested yet[16] (var. *margalefii*) or is completely lacking due to lack of cultures (var. *caudatum*).

Azadinium dexteroporum: This is the most recently described and the smallest (8.5 × 6.2 μm) species of *Azadinium* found in the Mediterranean Sea. It differs from all other *Azadinium* species for the position of the ventral pore, which is located at the right posterior end of the markedly asymmetrical Po plate, and for a pronounced concavity of the small middle intercalary plate. Like *A. spinosum* and *A. polongum,* it has a small antapical spine. The presence of AZA3 and AZA7 has been claimed,[12] but exact structures need to be confirmed by LC–MS and NMR analysis.

Other species potentially related to Azadinium: There are a few other species described in the literature that potentially are related to the genus *Azadinium* and need to be reanalyzed in more depth. A small dinoflagellate species has been described in 1959 as *Gonyaulax parva*.[22] The plate patter of this species, however, is quite different from the genus *Gonyaulax* and in fact corresponds to the plate tabulation of *Azadinium*.[7] As such, this species should probably be transferred to *Azadinium*, awaiting reinvestigation of the cingular and sulcal plates, as well as the results of molecular taxonomic studies. "*Gonyaulax gracilis*" is a second example of a *Gonyaulax* species that probably belongs to the genus *Azadinium*. Although *Gonyaulax gracilis* Schiller[23] was not validly described (ICBN ART. 32.1), Bérard-Therriault et al.[24] provided figures (pl. 90) under that name showing dinoflagellates with a distinct similarity to *Azadinium*, one specimen with a spine characteristic of *A. spinosum* and one without a spine. Other details are not given so it remains uncertain whether the dinoflagellates they reported from eastern Canada in fact represent species of *Azadinium*.

Amphidoma languida (Figure 26.1f) has been isolated concurrently with the Irish strain of *A. spinosum* from Bantry Bay, Ireland.[8] The strain SM1 was initially identified as a potential *Azadinium* species because of similarities with respect to size, shape, and swimming pattern. A detailed morphological and phylogenetic study then clearly showed that it represents a new species in the genus *Amphidoma*. The Kofoidean plate formula (Po, cp, X, 6′, 0a, 6″, 6C, 5(?) S, 6‴, 2⁗) indicates a major difference in the epithecal configuration to the genus *Azadinium*: *Amphidoma* has six apical plates and no apical intercalary plate, whereas *Azadinium* has only four apical plates but three apical intercalary plates. Nevertheless, a number of morphological similarities, such as cingular and hypothecal plates, the number and arrangement of sulcal plates, and the characteristic apical pore complex with a small X-plate centrally invading the first apical plate, indicated a close relationship between *Amphidoma* and *Azadinium*. This was supported by a phylogenetic tree based on concatenated ribosomal RNA sequence data of the small (SSU) and large subunit (LSU) of a large taxon sample, which retrieved *Azadinium* and *Amphidoma* as sister groups distinct from all established taxonomic units of Dinophyceae.[8] As a unique feature among *Amphidomataceae*, *A. languida* has a large antapical pore located at the dorsal side of the large antapical plate 2⁗. This "pore" in fact is a depressed field of a number of small pores (about 15). Another pore clearly differentiated in size and substructure from the numerous pores on the other apical plates, and which is referred to as a "ventral pore," is located at the anterior right side of plate 1′ on the suture to plate 6′. *A. languida* has been found to produce two AZAs (AZA34, AZA38) with molecular masses of 815 and 829 Da.

26.2.3 Phylogeny

Studying the phylogeny of a group of organisms (e.g., genus, species, population) aims at clarifying the evolutionary history of that group and can be based on morphology and/or sequence information. Reconstruction of the evolutionary origin of toxic dinophytes such as *Azadinium* is of considerable scientific interest and may provide information for understanding toxin production. Furthermore, phylogenetic information may be useful to identify other potential yet unidentified AZA-producing species. However, the capacity to produce phycotoxins is generally scattered on the phylogenetic tree of Dinophyceae, indicating that there is no clear trend in the evolution of this trait and that toxin production has appeared and disappeared multiple times during dinoflagellate evolution.[25] Nevertheless, for certain toxins (e.g., yessotoxins), it could be shown that its production is confined to the order Gonyaulacales within the Dinophyceae so that species within this taxonomic order should be given priority for future testing and field collections associated with monitoring for YTX contamination events.[26] Finally, phylogenetic trees and the underlying molecular database could also enhance the development of robust detection probes for monitoring AZA-producing species.

Morphology and in particular the plate tabulation with five different rows of plates undoubtedly classified the genus *Azadinium* as a member of the dinophycean subclass Peridiniphycidae.[7] This subclass is subdivided into two orders, the Peridiniales and Gonyaulacales,[27] with a number of differences discussed in detail by Fensome et al.[27] (Figure 26.3). *Azadinium* clearly exhibits morphological characteristics of both of these orders (Figure 26.3). The hypothecal plate arrangement and the presence of six precingular, six postcingular, and six cingular plates suggest a relationship to the Gonyaulacales. The epithecal plate arrangement with four apical and three intercalary plates, however, implies an affinity to the Peridiniales. Moreover, the composition of the apical pore complex with a Po, a cover plate, and the presence of an X-plate is typical for the Peridiniales. In contrast, however, to most species of the Peridiniales, the X-plate does not separate completely the first apical plate (1′) from the Po but invades plate 1′, giving broad contact of plate 1′ to the Po, each right and left, respectively, from the X-plate. The only examples of a direct contact are represented in the *Heterocapsa* Stein–*Cachonina* Loeblich species complex. In these species, the X-plate is displaced to the right side, consequently allowing direct contact of plate 1′ and the Po at the left side from the X-plate.[28] Other general features including the mode of cell division, the plate suture and growth band structure, and the presence of a ventral pore in *Azadinium* seem to be more related to the Gonyaulacales. Morphology thus did not allow for a clear order affiliation and leaves *Azadinium* in the order "uncertain." With the description of *Amphidoma languida*, the taxonomic affiliation of *Azadinium* on a family level was recently clarified. *A. languida* was found to be closely related to *Azadinium* with possible

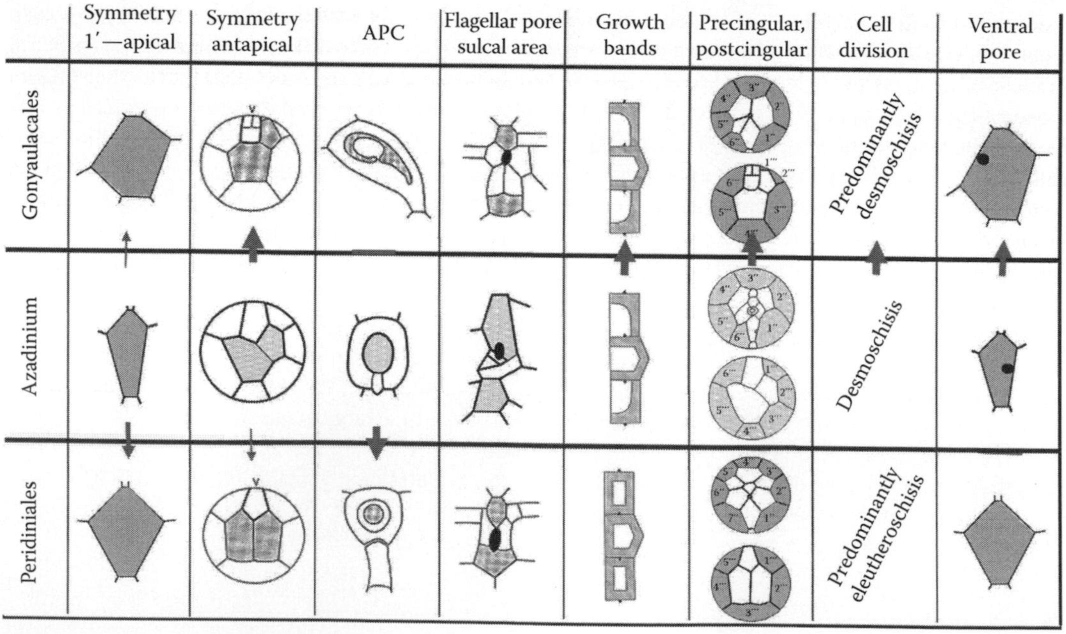

FIGURE 26.3 Schematic representation of morphological features used to characterize the two dinoflagellate orders Gonyaulacales and Peridiniales and the corresponding feature of the genus *Azadinium*. Arrows indicate a tentative affinity to the orders. (Adapted from Fensome, R.A. et al., *Micropaleontology*, Special Publication, 7, 1, 1993.)

morphological synapomorphies including the cingular and hypothecal plate arrangement, the number and arrangement of sulcal plates, and the characteristic APC with a small X-plate centrally invading the first apical plate. *Amphidoma* and *Azadinium* were thus placed in the family Amphidomataceae[29] by Tillmann et al.[8] The presence or absence of intercalary plates (present in *Azadinium* but absent in *Amphidoma*) is regarded as distinctive at the genus level. However, there is only one epithecal plate difference between the two genera that does not preclude assignment to the same family.

Molecular phylogenies based on ribosomal rDNA support the morphological considerations and likewise are not able to fully resolve the position of the genus *Azadinium* within dinoflagellate phylogeny. The first phylogenetic trees based on SSU, LSU, or ITS (internal transcribed spacer) sequence data of *A. spinosum* did not show any particularly close affiliation within the Peridiniales or Gonyaulacales nor to any other dinoflagellate order represented in molecular databases,[7] and this view has not been changed by adding new and more *Azadinium* species/strains.[20] Using a concatenated alignment of LSU and SSU, the Amphidomataceae including *Amphidoma* and *Azadinium* were an independent lineage among other monophyletic major groups of the dinophytes such as the Suessiales, Prorocentrales, Gonyaulacales, and Peridiniales.[8] Thus, the phylogenetic position of the Amphidomataceae at present cannot be identified reliably, although they have been placed on the peridinean branch remote from the Gonyaulacales. It remains to be determined whether they are part of the Peridiniales or represent a distinct lineage that would deserve the recognition at higher taxonomic level. On the family level, the tree provided by Tillmann et al.[20] clearly showed that *Amphidoma languida* and *Azadinium* together form the monophyletic and highly supported Amphidomataceae. *Amphidoma* was situated in a basal position of the maximum supported *Azadinium* clade with all five species described at that time (*A. spinosum*, *A. obesum*, *A. poporum*, *A. caudatum*, and *A. polongum*).[20] Molecular phylogeny of *A. dexteroporum* confirmed the attribution of the species to the genus and suggested a position basal to other small *Azadinium* species.[12]

In contrast to rDNA sequence data, available data on conservative proteins such as cytochrome oxidase subunit 1 (COI) indicate a general lack of base substitutions in the COI gene among species of *Azadinium*, with variation restricted only to deletions/insertions, and this might reflect the slower rate of gene evolution in the COI gene relative to the sequences from the ribosomal cistron.[7] Within *Azadinium*, there is a considerable variation of sequence data/morphology within the species as they are currently defined. *A. caudatum* has been shown to occur with two distinct varieties clearly different in terms of general size, the shape of the antapical projection, and the position of the ventral pore. Moreover, both varieties showed a considerable degree of differences in sequence data.[16] Likewise, there are considerable differences in ITS and LSU gene sequences among Asian and European strains of *A. poporum*. Minor differences in shape of the 3′ plate, which initially was hypothesized to morphologically support these molecular differences,[17] have subsequently been shown to vary among other Asian strains.[13] Nevertheless, in an LSU/ITS tree, all available strains of *Azadinium poporum* comprise three well supported clades, one of them including multiple strains originating from the coast of China as well as a Korean strain. The second clade included strains from the East China Sea and South China Sea, and the third one consisted of strains from Europe. There thus is a considerable cryptic diversity within *A. poporum* with even sympatric occurrence of two distinct ribotypes in China. Interestingly, this diversity seems to be reflected by the considerable diversity within this species in terms of toxin profile (Hess et al., this book).

26.3 Distribution

26.3.1 Global Distribution

Although initially described from the North Sea, there is increasing evidence that the genus *Azadinium* probably is distributed worldwide (Figure 26.4). In the North Sea area, five currently described species have been observed. The occurrence of *Azadinium* along the Scottish coast and the Irish Atlantic coast,[21] as well as a report of AZA in mussels from the North coast of Norway[30] and a recent record from the Shetland Islands,[20] implies distribution of the genus into more northern North Atlantic/arctic areas as well. This could be confirmed by light microscope observations of *Azadinium* spp. in plankton samples taken in the Irminger Sea between Greenland and Iceland in 2012 (unpublished information, Urban Tillmann,

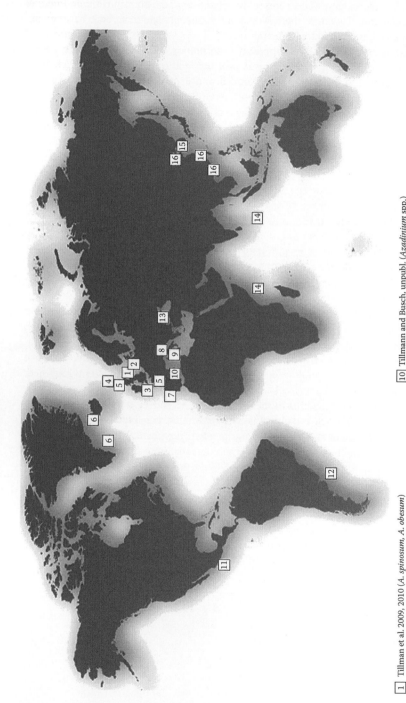

1 Tillman et al. 2009, 2010 (*A. spinosum, A. obesum*)

2 Tillmann et al. 2011 (*A. spinosum, A. poporum*)

3 Salas et al. 2011, Tillmann et al. 2012a (*A. spinosum, Amphidoma languida*)

4 Tillmann et al.2012b (*A. spinosum, A. polongum*)

5 Nezan et al. 2012 (*A. caudatum, both varieties.*)

6 Tillmann 2012, unpubl. (*Azadinium sp.*)

7 Margalef et al. 1954 (*A. caudatum var margalefii, as Oxytoxum* sp.)

8 Rampi 1969 (*A. caudatum var margalefii, as Oxytoxum margalefii*)

9 Percopo et al., 2013 (*Azadinium dexteroporum*)

10 Tillmann and Busch, unpubl. (*Azadinium* spp.)

11 Hernandez-Becerril et al. 2012 (*A. spinosum*)

12 Akselman and Negri 2012 (*A. cf. spinosum*)

13 Checklist Black Sea phytoplankton, http://phyto.bss.ibss.org.ua/wiki/Azadinium_spinosum

14 Consuelo Carbonel Moore, pers. com. (*Azadinium* sp. and *Amphidoma languida*)

15 Potvin et al. 2012 (*A. cf. poporum*)

16 Gu et al. 2013 (*A. poporum*)

FIGURE 26.4 Global records of the genus *Azadinium* and *Amphidoma languida*.

AWI). Which species are present here still need to be determined. A number of different *Azadinium* species obviously are present in French Atlantic coastal waters; in addition to *Azadinium caudatum* (see in the following text), *A. poporum* and five additional organisms have been identified by molecular analysis or SEM; taxonomic identification is underway (personal communication, Elisabeth Nezan, Ifremer, France).

The type of the genus, *A. spinosum*, has been isolated off the Scottish coast, the coast off Denmark, the Shetland Islands, and from coastal Atlantic waters in Ireland.[7,9,20,21] SEM images of Hernandez-Becerril et al.[31] depicted a species of *Azadinium* most likely *A. spinosum* from coastal pacific waters off Mexico and thus indicate a much wider distribution of that species. However, sequence information from that region supporting the preliminary species identification are not available. *A. obesum* has yet been reported only from the Scottish coast[10] but probably is also present in Ireland (unpublished information, Rafael Salas, Marine Institute). Due to its easy recognition by light microscopy, the biogeography of *Azadinium caudatum* (as *Amphidoma caudata*) is slightly better known. It has been reported from the North Sea off the Norwegian coast,[32] in a Portuguese lagoon,[33] around the British Isles and the west coast of Ireland,[34,35] at the Spanish coast of Castellón,[36] from the Ligurian Sea (Mediterranean),[37] and, most recently, all around the French Atlantic coast.[16] *Azadinium polongum* up to now has only been reported from the Shetland Islands.[20] Preliminary growth experiments of this species showed poor growth at temperatures above 10°C[20] and thus indicate that the core distribution area of *A. polongum* is more to the northern boreal/arctic waters. *Azadinium poporum* is the only species for which strains outside Europe have been obtained. As a first record of *Azadinium* in Pacific waters, *A. poporum* has been isolated from Shiwa Bay in Korea.[17] In terms of morphology, the strain designated as *A. cf. poporum* by Potvin et al.[17] is almost identical to the European *A. poporum*, but differs significantly in terms of sequence data. *A. poporum* obviously is quite widely distributed in the Asian Pacific. Gu et al.[13] succeeded in isolating 25 different strains of *A. poporum* originating from China covering Bohai Sea and East and South China Sea. The AZA-producing species *Amphidoma languida* has only been isolated from one bay in Ireland but probably has a much wider distribution: Lewis and Dodge[38] depicted the epitheca of a cell (their Figure 11)—most probably being *A. languida*—from the east Atlantic. Sequence data from plankton samples of the Skagerrak area indicate the presence of *A. languida* in the North Sea as well (personal communication, Kerstin Toebe, AWI, Germany). Furthermore, *Azadinium* sp. has been reported to form blooms in the southern Atlantic Ocean off the coast of Argentina.[39] As shown by LM and SEM, the species in question clearly had the *Azadinium* plate tabulation pattern and possessed a spine and was thus designated as *A. cf. spinosum*. However, for a final species designation, a few yet unresolved morphological details (e.g., presence of a ventral pore) of the Argentinean species need to be clarified; likewise, DNA samples and toxin measurements from that area are needed to verify the presence of toxigenic *A. spinosum*. *Azadinium* species other than *A. caudatum* mentioned previously are definitely present in the Mediterranean: The most recently described species *A. dexteroporum* has been isolated from Naples.[12] Fixed phytoplankton samples taken at Alfacs Bay, a coastal lagoon area close to the Ebro delta, undoubtedly revealed the presence of *Azadinium*, despite low abundances (unpublished information, Urban Tillmann, AWI). *Azadinium* also has been included in the check list of Black Sea phytoplankton (http://phyto.bss.ibss.org.ua/wiki/Azadinium_spinosum). The depicted species, which clearly belongs to the genus *Azadinium*, is listed as *A. spinosum*, but except the general shape and the presence of a spine, no supportive detail for that species designation is visible, and thus this record needs confirmation. Finally, and in remarkable contrast to the majority of coastal records, cells representing *Azadinium* sp. and *A. languida* have been seen in SEM preparations from samples collected at the open west Indian Ocean (personal communication, Consuelo Carbonell-Moore, Oregon State University).

This compilation clearly shows that knowledge on the biogeography of the genus currently is rather limited and patchy. It is either based on the troublesome procedure of isolating, cultivating, and fully characterizing local strains (in terms of morphology and sequence information) or based on a very few records of single specimens detected by scanning plankton samples by electron microscopy. Nevertheless, due to an increased awareness of the genus, the availability of fluorescence in situ hybridization (FISH) and quantitative polymerase chain reaction (qPCR) as species-specific detection methods[40] as well as the increasingly used "next-generation" high-throughput sequencing of environmental samples, it is expected that our knowledge on the biogeography of the Amphidomataceae will increase rapidly.

26.3.2 Temporal and Spatial Distribution

In the recent years since its first discovery, few studies on the temporal distribution of *Azadinium spinosum* have been carried out. Data sets of *Azadinium* occurrence extracted from monitoring programs are not generally reliable due to the difficulty of identification under light microscopy. Some clues as to its temporal distribution can be obtained from the presence of AZA toxins in shellfish, and in particular Irish shellfish toxicity data have long suggested that the causative species arrives in the mid to late summer months. This phenomenon was examined in detail by a study conducted on plankton samples from 2012 (unpublished information, Dave Clarke, Marine Institute) during one of the largest (both in terms of concentration and geographical distribution) AZA events observed to occur in Ireland. The event was prolonged, occurring in the majority of sites from the southwest, west, and northwest coasts from June through to November, reaching its peak during September and October, with some sites lasting into the first quarter of 2013. During this event, weekly phytoplankton samples from Killary Harbour on the West coast taken from May through to September were compared to qPCR gene probe[40] results for the identification of *Azadinium spinosum* and LC–MS/MS results for AZAs in shellfish.

The key finding of this study was that increases in *A. spinosum* cell concentration resulted in an associated rapid uptake of AZAs in mussels. *Azadinium* concentration was not consistent in the location through the test period but appears to be present in pulses, possibly associated with sea water intrusions from deeper offshore locations. These pulses were reflected in both the cell concentration and ensuing toxin peaks in the shellfish (Figure 26.5). A second set of samples from 2006 from southwest Ireland (significant year in terms of a major AZA event) were also analyzed via molecular methods, and again as in the Killary data set, there was a presence of *A. spinosum* corresponding with rapid increases in AZA intoxication in mussels in the same locality. This has also been observed in earlier laboratory feeding experiments[21,41] where toxin levels rose rapidly in test shellfish in response to consumption of a diet of *A. spinosum* cells (see Section 26.5.2).

Due to the short period of time between blooms of *A. spinosum* occurring and detection of AZAs in shellfish, observations of AZA in shellfish would be considered a useful indicator for the temporal distribution of *Azadinium*. The temporal distribution of AZA observed from 11 years of Irish shellfish monitoring shows some interesting patterns that gives us an indication of the temporal and spatial distribution of *A. spinosum*. Figure 26.6 shows a predominance of higher levels, more frequent occurrence, and longer outbreaks in the south than the rest of the country. Interannual variability is also observed; while most areas

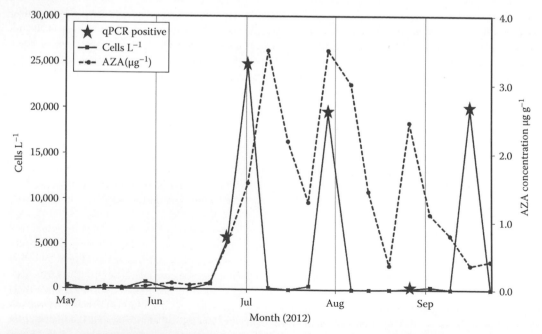

FIGURE 26.5 Cell counts, qPCR data, and AZA concentrations May to September 2012, Killary Harbour, Ireland.

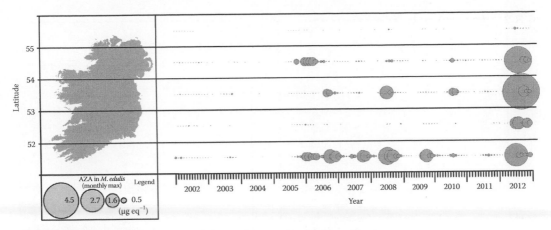

FIGURE 26.6 Distribution and concentration of AZA toxins (AZA1 µg eq g⁻¹) in Irish farmed mussels (*Mytilus* sp.) between 2002 and 2012.

show some occurrence nearly every year, there are some years (e.g., 2004 and 2005) when there is very little toxin observed anywhere. The evidence points toward an offshore factor controlling the levels observed within the bays where shellfish are produced that results in this intermittent occurrence. It is not known whether continuous intoxication over winter or the inability of shellfish to depurate AZAs is responsible for extended winter toxicity. A less frequent intoxication can also take place in early summer (May–June), but this tends to happen more intermittently. Toxin accumulation seems to oscillate during these events where toxicity increases and decreases creating a yo-yo effect over a number of weeks suggesting that shellfish is not getting intoxicated in a single incident from *A. spinosum*, but rather in consecutive waves over time perhaps from offshore pulses of toxic plankton being advected inshore by coastal processes.

This is also observed in other species in Irish waters including *Dinophysis* sp. that was shown to impact inshore shellfisheries in the southwest when oceanographic factors result in intrusions of offshore water containing high cell counts.[42] Physical circulating forces during the summer months and wind-driven exchange in a thermally stratified water column allow for phytoplankton species in the water mass to be transported into the bays in the southwest of Ireland. This could go some way toward explaining how harmful phytoplankton that are growing in the shelf waters around the southwestern coast of Ireland can penetrate into the bays and concentrate in coastal locations. These wind-driven HAB events in the southwest coast could be used as a proxy for the movement, temporal, and spatial distribution of *Azadinium* around the coast, as the inshore coastal current move clockwise around the Irish coast.

Other recent information gathered in offshore water during the month of August suggests that offshore populations of *A. spinosum* observed to occur in moderately stratified water in the Celtic Sea may pool there and await oceanographic currents to either dissipate the bloom or concentrate them into a highly toxic front that can be transported into the shellfish production areas in the southwestern bays of Ireland. The offshore presence of *Azadinium* is suggested also in earlier observations of AZA present in offshore locations during the month of July (Figure 26.7).

Outside of Ireland, there have also been indications regarding the offshore presence of *Azadinium*. During the month long survey in 2007 on the RV Poseidon around the eastern Scottish coast and Skagerrak, AZAs were found at a large number of offshore stations.[6] Taking the presence of the toxins as a proxy for the spatial distribution of the producing species, this was the first reliable information we have on the organism and its biogeographical distribution in the North Sea.

Cell densities of *Azadinium* of the magnitude reported from Argentinian waters in Akselman and Negri[39] have not been observed elsewhere. Two blooms in consecutive years in shelf breakwaters of the coast of Argentina in Austral spring time (September–November) in 1990–1991 showed the presence of a small armored dinoflagellate in large numbers (9×10^6 cells L⁻¹). The cells were characterized as *A.* cf. *spinosum*, but molecular or toxicity studies to confirm this preliminary identification were not carried out at the time. Nevertheless, the surveys carried out in Argentina showed that the distribution of this *Azadinium* species is also found in shelf breakwaters off the coast of Argentina and that it is

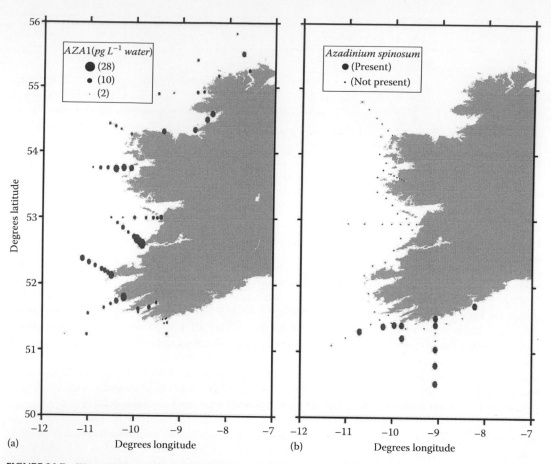

FIGURE 26.7   Western Ireland offshore AZA (2001) and *Azadinium spinosum* (2012). (a) Distribution of AZA measured by LC–MS from particulate residues from plankton net haul (20 μm) samples at 100 offshore locations in July 2001. (b) Distribution of the presence of *A. spinosum* measured by PCR from net haul samples taken at 69 stations in August 2012.

probably widely distributed, at least spatially. However, in Ireland, blooms of this magnitude have not yet been reported despite regular toxicity in shellfish at a scale not reported elsewhere.

The cosmopolitan nature of the *Azadinium* genus is shown by its presence in the Pacific Ocean,[17] where for the first time, qPCR results show *A.* cf. *poporum* temporal populations dynamics in Shiwa Bay, South Korea.[43] These populations were found every year during a 3-year study period albeit in low cell concentrations (peak concentrations of about 5 cells mL^{-1}), and the authors concluded that a combination of predation on *A.* cf. *poporum* and their physiology may contribute to these low numbers. Densities of this order of magnitude are more like the concentration of blooms observed so far of *Azadinium* and other *Azadinium* like species in Irish waters.

There remain many questions regarding the spatial and temporal distribution of *Azadinium*. These include whether or not they originate solely from offshore areas and what type of blooms they form. The cell densities that are observed so far do not fully explain observed toxicity events; more information regarding the depths at which they may form thin layers would help explain their ecology and intoxification dynamics in the sea, for instance, are they autochthonous populations wintering in our bays, encysting and excysting at different times of the year, or are they advected into them by oceanographic processes? All these questions and others have not been answered yet, and future research will have to be broadened to answer some of them. Our knowledge on their distribution is compounded by their small size and the difficulty in positive identification using light microscopy alone. Gene probes for the species have been generated,[40] and these tools will be useful in the next few years to unravel some of the mysteries surrounding these organisms.

26.4 Biology and Physiology

26.4.1 Biology

Compared to the relatively well-studied morphology, little is known on the biology and ecology of the AZA-producing species. Without doubt, all species of Amphidomataceae are photosynthetic and, as has been shown for *A. spinosum*, can grow in axenic cultures.[6] Nevertheless, most, if not all, photosynthetic dinoflagellates are believed to have mixotrophic capabilities[44,45]; however, nothing is known on potential mixotrophy of *Azadinium*. Preliminary trials offering small cyanobacteria as food failed to detect any particle uptake of *Azadinium* (unpublished information, Urban Tillmann, AWI), but this needs to be studied in much more detail. For a number of bloom forming photosynthetic dinoflagellates, the uptake of heterotrophic bacteria has been proposed.[44] For *Azadinium* grown in non-axenic culture in the presence of bacteria, transmission electron microscopy thin sectioning failed to detect intracellular food vacuoles (personal communication, Michael Schweikert, Uni Stuttgart, Germany) so that mixotrophic uptake of bacteria seems unlikely, at least at non-limiting nutrient conditions. Likewise, ultrastructural investigation failed to detect signs of intracellular/symbiotic bacteria (personal communication, Michael Schweikert, Uni Stuttgart, Germany), which is additional evidence that bacteria are not involved in AZA synthesis, neither extra- nor intracellular.

All species of Amphidomataceae have been described to exhibit a conspicuous swimming behavior. Cells normally swim at low speed (quantified for the Korean strain of *A. poporum* as 400 μm s^{-1}),[43] interrupted by short, high-speed "jumps" in various directions. *A. languida* is particularly slow in its general movement, which is reflected in its name (languida [lat.] = lazy, slow). For all species, the jumps are interspersed but regularly observed when cells approach other objects, for example, when they reach the glass bottom of the observation chamber. Rarely, larger distances may be travelled at high speed. The ability to jump is generally assumed to be a direct escape mechanism involved in predator/prey interactions.[46–48] Related jumping behavior might be observed among species of gymnodinoid dinoflagellates or within the genus *Heterocapsa*,[49] but the characteristic swimming behavior of *Azadinium/Amphidoma* still is helpful to be used at low microscope magnification as a distinguishing mark in species isolation.[13,17]

Knowledge on the life cycle of *Azadinium/Amphidoma* is quite incomplete. In culture, all species grow vegetatively by simple binary fission, as has been described in detail for *A. spinosum*[14] and *A. languida*.[8] Dividing cells keep their motility throughout the whole mitotic and cytokinetic process. As a first sign of mitosis, the normally round nucleus enlarges, considerably changes its shape, and becomes elongated stretching across almost the whole cell length in a slightly oblique manner. The nucleus then divides along its longitudinal axis. Cytokinesis is started slightly before nuclear division is finished and is of the desmoschisis type, that is, the parent theca is shared between both sister cells. The left side of the parent cell keeps the cell's apex including the apical pore complex and all apical and epithecal intercalary plates, whereas the right side of the parent cell keeps, among others, both antapical plates. Divided cells completely segregate well before thecal plates are fully renewed. When cells of *Azadinium* are stressed, the protoplasts can leave their theca (ecdysis), a common reaction among dinoflagellates to adverse conditions that is often related to temporary cyst formation.[50] This type of dinoflagellate cyst normally is round and surrounded by a cell wall. However, this has not yet been observed for *A. spinosum*. Nevertheless, ecdysis of *A. spinosum* might be of importance as it has been related to an increase of extracellular toxins after sample handling.[51] However, the reason for the increase in extracellular toxins is not clear; shedding of the cell's outer layer including thecal plates and their membrane vesicles might be associated with a pulsed toxin loss or extruded protoplasts may have a higher exudation rate.

A number of dinoflagellates are known to produce cysts, mainly as a dormant, zygotic stage of their life cycle.[50] Such cysts can accumulate in the sediment, hatch after a dormant period, and may thus act as "seed banks" with great ecological importance for bloom initiation. Among Amphidomataceae, cysts have up to now been observed for two species: *A. polongum*[20] and *A. poporum*.[13] Successful isolation of *A. poporum* by incubating sediment samples[13,17] made the presence of cysts quite likely for that species, and that has been confirmed by Gu et al.[13]: in 1 out of 25 cultured strains, they observed the presence of a few distinct cysts. These cysts are ellipsoid, around 15 μm long and 10 μm wide, and are filled with pale granules and a yellow accumulation body. Likewise, *A. polongum* has been described to produce cysts in culture, round cells of 10–16 μm in diameter and with pale white inclusion. SEM failed to detect any external cyst structures like paratabulation and/or archeopyle, and hatching was not observed. A reduced chlorophyll fluorescence of these cysts and a long persistence in an apparently unaltered state indicated that they might allow long-term survival (hypnocysts), rather than serving as temporary cysts. If true, these hypnocysts might be part of the vegetative cycle as has been observed for *Scrippsiella hangoei*,[52] or part of a sexual life cycle. Clearly, more data and observations are needed to clarify the whole life cycle of *Azadinium*.

26.4.2 Physiology (Growth and Toxin Production)

With the availability of cultures of *A. spinosum*, first laboratory experiments related to growth and toxin production could be performed. Initial studies mainly aimed at investigating the effect of environmental and nutritional factors on growth and toxin production to allow and subsequently improve large-scale AZA production for toxin isolation.[53] Here, the focus was set on some of the main environmental factors such as temperature, salinity, irradiance, turbulence, and nutrients.

26.4.2.1 Growth

Small and delicate dinoflagellates like species of *Azadinium* automatically impose the suggestion of being difficult to grow in culture. However, *A. spinosum* was found to be fairly easy to grow at a wide range of different conditions, to grow to rather high cell densities, and to be unaffected by high levels of turbulence (e.g., caused by aeration) and thus turned out to be suited for large-scale, high-density culturing in photobioreactors.[54]

Like many dinoflagellates,[55–57] *A. spinosum* is able to divide approximately once per day at optimal conditions, but of course growth is gradually affected by different environmental conditions. When exposed to different temperatures ranging from 10°C to 26°C, *A. spinosum* was able to grow at all temperatures so upper and lower temperature limits for positive growth of *A. spinosum* are not yet precisely defined. Nevertheless, growth was optimal at 22°C, with slightly lower growth at higher temperature (26°C) but significantly reduced growth at the lowest temperature tested (10°C). *A. spinosum* was isolated from different coastal locations including an inshore location in Ireland (Bantry Bay) known for their fluctuations in freshwater influence, so some flexibility of *A. spinosum* to different salinities was expected. When suddenly exposed to various salinities (10–40 psu) without an adaptation period, *A. spinosum* preadapted to 35 psu was able to grow between 30 and 40 psu, survived fairly well at 20 psu but rapidly declined at 10 psu. Although *A. spinosum* thus probably cannot be considered as fully euryhaline, at least surviving a sudden drop to 20 psu indicates that the species is adapted to grow along the Irish coast where fairly large variations of salinity frequently occur in bays due to heavy rainfall. The potential of *A. spinosum* to actively grow at lower salinities after a gentler adaptation period still needs to be determined. In attempts to achieve maximal toxin yield, the highest cell concentration of *A. spinosum* of more than 300×10^3 cells mL^{-1} was found in batch cultures with aeration compared to cultures without aeration (90×10^3 cell mL^{-1}), and turbulence/aeration was found not to reduce *A. spinosum* growth. An increase in final cell yield through turbulence/aeration has been observed for other dinoflagellates[58] and is most probably due to enhancing gas and nutrient mixing,[59] and consequently controlling pH and/or improving carbon and light availability. Growth response of *A. spinosum* to different light levels gave no signs of photoinhibition at higher light levels (tested up to 400 μmol m^{-2} s^{-1}). Growth was almost saturated down to the lowest light level tested (50 μmol m^{-2} s^{-1}), where a slight decrease in growth was noticed.[53] The response of *A. spinosum* photosynthesis to light (P/I curves) is not known yet as is growth behavior at lower light (e.g., light compensation point), so a general classification of *A. spinosum* as a "low-light" or "high-light" adapted species is currently not possible.

Although the nutritional requirements of *A. spinosum* in terms of macronutrients and trace metals/vitamins have not yet been defined precisely, culture work performed so far showed that *A. spinosum* is easy to grow on a number of different standard culture media. These include K-medium of various strengths (but with omission of ammonium),[7] F/2 medium,[21] or L1 medium with or without addition of soil extract,[53] indicating no unusual nutrient requirements. The use of different media, including the addition of soil extract, did not significantly affect growth and toxin cell quota.[53] In terms of major nutrient, *A. spinosum* is able to use different sources of nitrogen (nitrate, urea, ammonium)[53] for growth in batch cultures and chemostat bioreactors. Addition of ammonium, however, reduced growth and thus confirmed the initial observation that omitting ammonium from the standard K-recipe improved growth.[7] Nothing is known about the potential use of dissolved organic compounds by *A. spinosum* or of any other form of mixotrophy.

26.4.2.2 Toxin Production

As it has been shown for a number of other dinoflagellates producing other polyether toxins,[60,61] AZA production of *A. spinosum* seems to be constitutive (i.e., toxins are found in significant amount in the cells at all stages of growth) and stable (i.e., the strains have kept their toxin production potential now for at least 5 years in culture). Moreover, the toxin profile of *A. spinosum* consisting of AZA1, AZA2, and AZA33 (see Chapter 27) has been shown to be consistently stable at all environmental conditions tested and thus most probably is under genetic control. The vast majority of toxins (roughly 99%) are intracellular,[51] although significant amounts of dissolved toxins in cultures can be found after handling stress (e.g., extended time after centrifugation)[51] or during late senescent phase when cells start to decay.[53]

Nevertheless, despite the stability of toxin production potential and toxin profile, quantitative differences in the toxin cell quota may be large. Summarizing all available data indicates a tremendous influence of culture and environmental conditions on AZA cell quotas, which were found to vary more than 40-fold, from ca 5 to more than 200 fg/cell. Available evidence indicates that much of this variability is due to toxins accumulating in cells when growth rate declines or completely stops. Generally, when comparing growth and AZA cell quota at different environmental conditions, lower growth rate was constantly coupled with higher toxin cell quota[53] underlining the notion that toxin production is not strictly coupled to growth. This can exemplarily be illustrated with Figure 26.8 showing growth and AZA cell quota of 10 L aerated batch cultures. These cultures showed a maximum growth rate of 0.57 day^{-1} and a

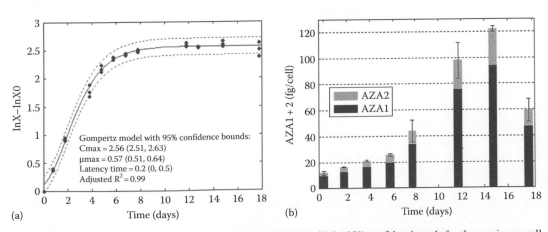

FIGURE 26.8 (a) Gompertz model fitted to the cell concentration with its 95% confident bounds for the maximum cell concentration (Cmax), growth rate (μmax), latency time, and its adjusted R^2 and (b) AZA1+2 cell quota as a function of time (error bars = SD, n = 3). (Reprinted from *Harmful Algae*, 27, Jauffrais, T., Séchet, V., Herrenknecht, C. et al., Effect of environmental and nutritional factors on growth and azaspiracid production of the dinoflagellate *Azadinium spinosum*, 138–148, Copyright 2013 with permission from Elsevier.)

maximum cell concentration of 302×10^3 cell mL^{-1}. Whereas AZA2/AZA1 ratio was quite stable during all growth phases (0.3 ± 0.02), AZA cell quota significantly increased with decreasing growth rate during the transition from the initial maximum exponential increase to growth cessation and peaked during stationary phase. The final decrease in cell quota, when cell concentration started to decline (senescent phase), coincided with a significant release of toxin into the medium (35% of total toxins compared to about 1% during all sampling points before).

The detailed role of light and nutrients for toxin production and accumulation is not clear. When grown in batch cultures at different light levels, AZA cell quota was found to be unaffected by light although growth was clearly light saturated.[53] This might indicate that under these conditions, surplus light could not be used for toxin production. However, in stirred photobioreactors operated as chemostats at high cell densities and a fixed dilution rate, light intensity under this potentially nutrient-limiting chemostat conditions had a major effect on the AZA cell quota. An increase by a factor of 3 (from 21 to 69 fg/cell) was observed between the lowest photon flux density and the highest one,[53] indicating that under nutrient-limiting growth, surplus light energy leads to an increased AZA accumulation.

In terms of nutrients, the nitrogen source (nitrate, urea, ammonium) was found not to influence toxin cell quota, neither in batch nor in continuous culture.[53] Nevertheless, nutrient limitation as a potential cause of growth cessation in batch culture is suspected to increase toxin cell quota. In terms of potential nutrient limitation, in these experiments using K-medium, which has a high surplus of nitrogen, phosphorous is expected to become the main limiting element. Such a role of P-limitation for an increase in toxin accumulation has been found for other toxin dinoflagellates.[62–67] There are more indications on factors important for promoting toxin accumulation at reduced/stagnant growth. Stationary phase cultures without aeration had a 3-fold lower cell yield and a 10-fold lower toxin cell quota compared to aerated cultures. This may indicate that carbon limitation in the unaerated cultures (reduced gas exchange) had limited toxin production, but enhanced nutrient limitation in the aerated cultures due to the substantially higher biomass also could have been important here.

In addition to accumulation of toxin in stagnant cells when toxins are continuously produced at an unchanged rate, increase in the absolute toxin production rate at certain conditions may contribute to elevated cell quota. It still needs to be tested if such an increase of toxin production rate can be found under nutrient limitation. Nevertheless, this could especially be the case for *A. spinosum* at low temperature. Here, toxin cell quota at stationary phase was about 30 times higher when grown at 10°C compared to when grown at 22°C. Even accounting for a slightly higher cell volume and for the different growth rate, a roughly five times higher absolute AZA production rate was needed to explain these large differences. The maximum cell quota of >200 fg/cell in the stationary phase when grown at 10°C may help to explain the rather unexpected but repeated AZA problems in Irish mussels during winter months.[53]

26.4.2.3 Pilot Scale Mass Culturing for Toxin Harvesting

All available data and observations from small-scale culture experiments were used to develop and optimize culture conditions to increase cell yield and AZA cell quota for large-scale toxin harvesting. As a final approach, a pH-controlled and stirred bioreactor (R1) in continuous culture mode was connected in series to a second one (R2) to induce a phase of maturation (growth stagnation but continuing toxin production) in the second bioreactor.[54] Consequently, at steady state, the total AZA cell quota increased between R1 and R2. The increase in toxin per cell from R1 to R2 reached its maximum at a dilution rate of 0.3 day^{-1} (ratio of 2.6 between cell quota in R2 compared to R1). Thus, as cell production increased with dilution rate and as AZA cell quota decreased, AZA production reached an optimum of 475 ± 17 µg day^{-1} at a flow rate of 25 L day^{-1} with 100 L bioreactors connected in series (Table 26.2).[54]

This culture method coupled to extraction and isolation procedures allowed for a sustained production of significant amounts of AZA1 and AZA2 from *A. spinosum* for toxicological studies and reference materials.[54]

TABLE 26.2

A. spinosum Concentration (cell mL^{-1}), Toxin Content (fg/cell), and Cell and Toxin Production (cell/day and µg/day, Respectively) at the Dilution Rates Studied (0.15, 0.2, 0.25, 0.3 per Day) in the Two Bioreactors in Series (R1 and R2)

A. spinosum	0.15 Day^{-1}		0.2 Day^{-1}		0.25 Day^{-1}		0.3 Day^{-1}	
	R1	R2	R1	R2	R1	R2	R1	R2
Concentration (×10^3 cell mL^{-1})	193 ± 6	214 ± 3	194 ± 8	214 ± 7	190 ± 6	221 ± 5	187 ± 5	220 ± 4
AZA1+2 (fg cell^{-1})	67 ± 3	98 ± 5	44 ± 13	95 ± 16	38 ± 2	86 ± 3	24 ± 1	63 ± 5
Cell production (×10^3 cell day^{-1})	2.90 ± 0.09	3.21 ± 0.05	3.9 ± 0.2	4.3 ± 0.1	4.8 ± 0.2	5.5 ± 0.1	5.6 ± 0.2	6.6 ± 0.1
Toxin production AZA1+2 (µg day^{-1})	193 ± 9	314 ± 15	170 ± 50	406 ± 64	180 ± 10	475 ± 17	134 ± 5	415 ± 33

Source: Adapted from Jauffrais, T. et al., Production and preparative isolation of azaspiracid-1 and -2 from *Azadinium spinosum* culture in pilot scale photobioreactors, *Marine Drugs*, 10, 1360, 2012.

Note: Standard deviations were calculated from sequential repeat measurements of each culture.

26.5 Food Web Transfer

With respect to *Azadinium*, both bloom dynamics and transfer kinetics and pathways of AZAs into bivalve molluscs are just getting started to be explored. Maxima and persistence of AZA toxins in bivalve shellfish could not yet been correlated in time and space to blooms of *Azadinium* species, but this may reflect observational deficiencies in toxic plankton and toxin monitoring programs. However, this also opens the possibility of alternative AZA sources (i.e., cryptic AZA-producing species) or toxin vectors, for example, transfer via the pelagic food web. For a number of toxic algae, grazing within the plankton community is generally viewed as the initial pathway through which algal toxins become vectored into pelagic food webs. Subsequent accumulation and trophic transfer can then intoxicate higher-trophic-level consumers such as fish, sea birds, and marine mammals.[68] For algal toxins accumulating in mussels, two transfer routes must be taken into account: AZAs could accumulate in bivalve shellfish following feeding upon AZA bound to suspended particulates or via plankton vectors (e.g., copepods, tintinnids, or other microplankton grazers) that have fed upon toxigenic *Azadinium* cells.

26.5.1 Planktonic Food Webs

Without doubt, AZAs can be present in plankton size classes larger than the size of the known producing species and also have been detected in a few grazer species. With respect to the latter, AZAs have been detected in manually picked specimens of the heterotrophic dinoflagellate *Protoperidinium crassipes*.[2] In view of the identification of *Azadinium* as a primary source of AZAs, a de novo AZA production of this heterotrophic dinoflagellate as initially claimed now seems unlikely but rather reflects a trophic accumulation.[6] Calculated cell quota of *P. crassipes* was in the range of 1.5 pg AZA per cell.[2] Compared to an AZA cell quota of *Azadinium*, this would correspond to an accumulation factor of roughly 15–150, depending on an assumed cell quota of 10–100 fg cell^{-1}.[51] However, direct microscopical observations of a mixed culture of *P. crassipes* and *A. spinosum*, which was feasible for a short time frame before the *P. crassipes* culture unfortunately was lost, made a direct trophic transfer from *A. spinosum* to *P. crassipes* unlikely: in these mixtures, ingestion was never observed; again this needs to be confirmed by more detailed observations and measurements once new *Protoperidinium* cultures are available.

Nevertheless, this grazing failure corresponds to more general observations on the feeding mode of large *Protoperidinium* species, which are characterized by a complex handling process[69,70] seemingly unsuited to handle small and jumping prey species like *Azadinium*. Likewise, the toxin profile detected in *P. crassipes* with substantial amounts of AZA3 present does not reflect the profile of known AZA producers, as AZA3 has not yet been detected here. Nevertheless, we currently can neither exclude a metabolic AZA3 formation in planktonic grazers nor exclude the involvement of a yet undetected plankton source with AZA3 in its toxin spectrum.

As a second grazer species, specimens of the large tintinnid ciliate *Favella ehrenbergii* collected from field samples have been identified to contain AZAs.[6] Estimated cell quotas were in the range of 0.7 pg per ciliate, which is about half of the quantities detected in *P. crassipes* and thus would correspond to a potential accumulation factor of 7–70 for an *A. spinosum* cell quota of 10–100 fg cell^{-1}.

Beside this detection of AZA in identified grazer species, there have been a number of reports on AZA in various plankton size fractions. During a research cruise of RV Poseidon in 2007, AZA1 was detected over the entire North Sea in plankton samples collected with a plankton net (20 μm), which is assumed not to retain the small species of *Azadinium*.[6] AZA was mostly evenly distributed among three size fractions (20–55, 50–200, and >200 μm) subsequently prepared from these net tows, but at two stations with the highest amount of AZA in net samples, the majority of AZA was found in the 50–200 μm fractions (corresponding to a high abundance of *F. ehrenbergii*). However, using pumped water samples and subsequent size fractionation, >90% of total AZA1 was found in the 3–8 and 8–10 μm fractions, which clearly corresponded to the size class of the identified AZA-producing species. It is important to note that in quantitative terms, AZAs found in larger size fractions were orders of magnitude lower. Although it is difficult to directly compare Niskin bottle samples and net tows, absolute AZA amounts in the small fraction (assumed to be due to *A. spinosum*) were approximately two to three orders of magnitude higher than the low pg L^{-1} range estimated in net tow samples (assumed to be the result of trophic transfer).

Similar results were obtained on the subsequent cruise in Danish coastal areas of the North Sea.[71] Again, AZA1 was present in a number of net tow (20 μm) samples, albeit in low amounts, with only traces found in the >200 μm fraction. AZA1 concentrations as measured in the small-size fraction (<20 μm), however, were much higher with maximum concentrations of ca 2 ng AZA1 L^{-1}. This is roughly five orders of magnitude higher than amounts found in corresponding net tow samples. Maximum AZA1 concentrations in net samples were in the range of 50 pg per net tow, which would correspond (assuming 2.5 m^3 water filtered) to a concentration of just 20 fg L^{-1} (which corresponds to typical cell quota of 20 fg for *A. spinosum*). These traces of AZA in larger-sized plankton despite of relatively high concentrations of AZA in small-size fractions are indicative of a negligible trophic transfer, at least under this particular field situation. Assuming the same cell quota of 20 fg/cell, AZA1 found in the small-size plankton with peak concentrations of 2 pg L^{-1} would correspond to an *A. spinosum* concentration of 10^5 L^{-1}.

In any case, a cell concentration of 10^5 L^{-1} is an order of magnitude lower than *Azadinium* concentrations reported from Argentina,[39] where two blooms with peak densities of 10^6 L^{-1} were observed. However, it needs to be kept in mind that it is not clear which species of *Azadinium* was responsible for these blooms. Morphology of the species in question showed some similarities with *A. spinosum*, but there also are some differences and additional morphological observations are needed.[39] Furthermore, DNA sequence data and toxin measurements from these blooms are not available, and thus, it is quite unclear if indeed the toxigenic *A. spinosum* was present. In any case, field samples of these blooms showed a high diversity and density of heterotrophic protists so that protistan grazing was discussed as an important loss factor for *Azadinium*.[39] However, just two species (*Gyrodinium fusus* and *Amphidoma* sp.) from a very diverse grazer community were reported to contain ingested *Azadinium* cells indicating that just a few but specialized grazers may have a large influence as loss factor of *Azadinium* blooms.

There is an urgent need for detailed laboratory studies analyzing grazer interaction of a broad range of different plankton grazers and different species of Amphidomataceae. The only study published so far[43] analyzed plankton grazing on the Korean strain of *A. poporum*. These authors showed that a number of protistan grazers are able to ingest cells of *Azadinium*, but just two out of nine species were able to achieve sustained growth with this food. Moreover, for these two species (the heterotrophic dinoflagellate *Oxyrrhis marina* and the ciliate *Strobilidium* sp.), maximum growth rate was much slower when compared to other prey species, indicating that *A. poporum* is of rather poor food quality. Unfortunately, this study did not include measurement of AZAs produced by *A. poporum,* and thus nothing is known with respect to potential toxin accumulation/transformation.

Other than that, there are a number of preliminary and unpublished studies using *A. spinosum* as food for other planktonic grazers (unpublished information, Urban Tillmann, AWI). As has been observed by Potvin et al.[43] for *A. poporum,* certain grazers such as *Polykrikos kofoidii* and *Amphidinium crassum* failed to ingest *A. spinosum* most probably because of prey size limitation (for *P. kofoidii*) or due to their peduncle feeding mode (for *A. crassum*). In contrast, laboratory cultures of *Favella ehrenbergii* clearly ingested *A. spinosum* with initial and substantial toxin accumulation, but failed to achieve a sustained positive growth with just *A. spinosum* as food. *Peridiniella danica*, a small heterotrophic thecate dinoflagellate, has been identified as a promising potential grazer as well, but quantitative grazing experiments have not yet been performed. For other small heterotrophic dinoflagellates as *O. marina* and *Gyrodinium dominans*, ingestion of *A. spinosum* was observed, but only rarely, and no positive growth of these grazers was observed when offered *A. spinosum.* As discussed before, swimming behavior of *Azadinium* might be involved in grazer interactions. Direct observations under the microscope show that *Azadinium* can escape by sudden jumps when attacked by these small dinoflagellates, which start feeding by first attaching a tow filament to its prey. However, the ingestion of *Azadinium* by these predators rapidly decreased from initial higher values even when immobilized prey was offered as food (unpublished information, Urban Tillmann, AWI), so it is likely that other factors than motility are involved as well. Clearly much more detailed studies are needed to test the hypothesis that AZA and/or other chemical compounds are involved in grazing interactions of *Azadinium.*

Preliminary and yet unpublished experiments with copepods indicated a minor grazing impact and AZA accumulation in this important group of plankton grazers. Cultured *A. spinosum* were added to either field plankton samples or copepods (various species) picked from field samples for 24 h, but we failed to detect any substantial grazing or significant AZA accumulation in larger size fractions and copepods, respectively.

Whereas these preliminary experiments do not contradict the possibility of vectorial transfer of AZAs to bivalves, they tend not to provide strong support for this mechanism, at least for prey–predator combinations thus far selected. Generally, predator–prey interactions are known to be species specific, and this may be even more important for toxic species where specific chemical compounds might play a role.[68,72] Furthermore, certain plankton predators have been shown to be extremely selective in their prey preferences[48] so that any generalization about a potential trophic transfer of AZA within planktonic food webs is difficult if not impossible. The few data available so far do at least not support a view of a universal and rapid spread of AZA among planktonic grazers, but may be indicative that certain (specialized) grazers at times may play an important role in food web transfer of *Azadinium* and AZAs. In any case, much more detailed investigations and experiments are needed to clarify this issue.

26.5.2 Direct Transfer to Mussels

In Ireland, AZA accumulation by bivalve molluscs occurs frequently since the 1990s and may affect many shellfish species. Among them, blue mussels were found to accumulate by far the highest concentration.[21] In Ireland, for all other species of bivalves including razor clams (*Ensis arcuatus* and *Ensis siliqua*), dog cockle (*Glycymeris glycymeris*), abalone (*Haliotis discus hannai*), common limpet (*Patella vulgata*), periwinkles (*Littorina littorea*), pullet carpet shell (*Venerupis senegalensis*), Venus clam (*Venus verrucosa*), and gastropods, AZAs were present at much lower concentrations. The toxin was also found in Chile in the two commercially important clam species Macha (*Mesodesma donacium*) and *Mulinia edulis* (Coquimbo Bay) as well as in scallops (*Argopecten purpuratus*) and mussels (*Mytilus chilensis*) (from two other areas in Chile) and in Japan, where a marine sponge *Echinoclathria sp.* was contaminated with AZA2.[73–75] In 2005 and 2006, AZAs were for the first time detected in gastropods, followed by their detection in brown crabs (*Cancer pagurus*) from the west coast of Sweden and the north and northwest coast of Norway.[30]

With the availability of *A. spinosum* cultures, a direct link between AZA accumulations by blue mussels and *A. spinosum* could recently be demonstrated.[21] Blue mussels were able to directly feed on *A. spinosum*, and the presence of AZA1 and AZA2 and of some metabolites (AZA3, -17 and -19) was detected following 24 h exposure to the microalga. AZA17 was the major metabolite (ratio of AZA17 to AZA1 toxin was 5:1) and was mainly found in the remaining flesh of mussels compared to AZA1 and AZA2, which were found in the digestive gland. This indicates that there is an active biotransformation of the toxins in the digestive system of the mussels. These observations were subsequently confirmed, and AZA17 and AZA19 were highlighted as two major metabolites of AZA1 and AZA2, respectively, over a week of contamination using *A. spinosum* at different cell concentrations.[41] These bioconversions pose a public health problem as AZA17 and AZA19 are currently not regulated (see Twiner et al., this book). The speed of accumulation (within less than 6 h of exposure to high concentrations of *A. spinosum* $(5–10 \times 10^3$ cell mL$^{-1})$, mussels exceeded the regulatory limit) was also demonstrated by the second study.[41] For mussels fed *A. spinosum* for 24 h, the following distribution of toxins was found: 73% in the digestive gland, 11% in the remaining flesh, and 8% in the gills. The other tissues (foot, labial palps, mantle, and adductor muscle) showed minor amounts of toxins with values below 3% of the total toxin accumulated. AZA accumulation was also observed at the same rate when mussels were simultaneously fed *A. spinosum* and *Isochrysis* aff. *galbana*, indicating that mussels were not able to select a nontoxic food source and did not avoid *A. spinosum*. Nevertheless, the initial and short period of fast AZA accumulation was soon displaced by a period of reduced or even without accumulation, which led the authors to subsequently evaluate the effect of *A. spinosum* on mussel feeding behavior.[76] *Azadinium spinosum* was found to have a significant, negative effect on mussel feeding behavior compared to *Isochrysis* aff. *galbana*. Clearance rate, feeding time activity, total filtration rate, and absorption were significantly lowered after a few hours of exposure. This study[76] thus clearly showed a negative effect of high concentrations of *A. spinosum* on blue mussel feeding activity and also indicated a possible regulation of AZA uptake by decreasing filtration and increasing the production of pseudo-feces. It is important to note that these experiments were carried out with mussels collected from French sites not known to be AZA contaminated. In any case, it remains to be determined if these negative effects are directly related to AZA toxins or other chemical and/or nutritional properties of *A. spinosum*.

Since the concentrations of AZAs found in mussels during short-term laboratory exposures are still ca 10-fold lower than the maximum concentrations encountered in the field, several hypotheses may be considered and need to be tested experimentally:

1. Long-term exposure to relatively low concentrations of *A. spinosum* in mixed diets is needed to avoid direct short-term negative effects of high *A. spinosum* densities and to result in high toxin accumulation.

2. Additional food web components play a role in the accumulation (e.g., planktonic grazers like small metazoans, heterotrophic dinoflagellates, or ciliates; see Section 26.5.1).

3. The short-term toxin dose in nature may be much higher, because AZA cell quota of field populations may be higher and/or environmental conditions may result in higher cell concentrations at bloom events.

4. Mussels in Ireland may have adapted to continuous exposure to *Azadinium* and thus may react differently compared to French mussels.

5. Uptake of toxins may additionally occur through the dissolved phase.

To verify the last hypothesis, we investigated the possibility of an uptake from the dissolved phase. Mussels were found to accumulate dissolved AZAs (applied at 0.75 and 7.5 μg L^{-1}) from the aqueous phase to significant levels, that is, above regulatory limits.[77] Interestingly, the toxin distribution in the mussel tissue was different: when fed *A. spinosum*, mussels mainly accumulated AZAs in digestive glands, but mussels exposed to dissolved AZAs accumulated a significant proportion of toxins in the gills. Other dissolved lipophilic toxins like brevetoxins[78] also have been shown to accumulate in bivalves or fish, apparently through the gills and by ingestion.[79,80] Dissolved AZAs were found but could not be quantified using passive sampling techniques both along the Irish[81] and Norwegian[82] coasts, indicating that this potential route of mussel intoxication should be evaluated quantitatively.

REFERENCES

1. Yasumoto, T., 2001. The chemistry and biological function of natural marine toxins. *The Chemical Record*, 1, 228–242.
2. James, K. J., Moroney, C., Roden, C. et al., 2003. Ubiquitous "benign" alga emerges as the cause of shellfish contamination responsible for the human toxic syndrome, azaspiracid poisoning. *Toxicon*, 41, 145–154.
3. Moran, S., Silke, J., Salas, R. et al., 2005. Review of phytoplankton monitoring 2005. In *6th Irish Shellfish Safety Scientific Workshop*. Ed. Marine Institute, Galway, Ireland, pp. 4–10.
4. Gribble, K. E., 2006. The ecology, life history, and phylogeny of the marine heterotrophic dinoflagellates *Protoperidinium* and *Diplopsalidaceae* (Dinophyceae), PhD thesis, Woods Hole Oceanographic Institute, Woods Hole, MA, 296p.
5. Gribble, K. E. and Anderson, D. M., 2006. Molecular phylogeny of the heterotrophic dinoflagellates, *Protoperidinium*, *Diplopsalis* and *Preperidinium* (Dinophyceae), inferred from large subunit rDNA. *Journal of Phycology*, 42, 1081–1095.
6. Krock, B., Tillmann, U., John, U., and Cembella, A. D., 2009. Characterization of azaspiracids in plankton size-fractions and isolation of an azaspiracid-producing dinoflagellate from the North Sea. *Harmful Algae*, 8, 254–263.
7. Tillmann, U., Elbrächter, M., Krock, B., John, U., and Cembella, A., 2009. *Azadinium spinosum* gen. et sp. nov. (Dinophyceae) identified as a primary producer of azaspiracid toxins. *European Journal of Phycology*, 44, 63–79.
8. Tillmann, U., Salas, R., Gottschling, M., Krock, B., O'Drisol, D., and Elbrächter, M., 2012. *Amphidoma languida* sp. nov. (Dinophyceae) reveals a close relationship between *Amphidoma* and *Azadinium*. *Protist*, 163, 701–719.
9. Tillmann, U., Elbrächter, M., John, U., and Krock, B., 2011. A new non-toxic species in the dinoflagellate genus *Azadinium*: *A. poporum* sp. nov. *European Journal of Phycology*, 46, 74–87.
10. Tillmann, U., Elbrächter, M., John, U., Krock, B., and Cembella, A., 2010. *Azadinium obesum* (Dinophyceae), a new nontoxic species in the genus that can produce azaspiracid toxins. *Phycologia*, 49, 169–182.
11. Krock, B., Tillmann, U., Voß, D. et al., 2012. New azaspiracids in Amphidomataceae (Dinophyceae): Proposed structures. *Toxicon*, 60, 830–839.
12. Percopo, I., Siano, R., Rossi, R., Soprano, V., Sarno, D., and Zingone, A., 2013. A new potentially toxic *Azadinium* species (Dinophyceae) from the Mediterranean Sea, *A. dexteroporum* sp. nov. *Journal of Phycology*, 49, 950–966.
13. Gu, H., Luo, Z., Krock, B., Witt, M., and Tillmann, U., 2013. Morphology, phylogeny and azaspiracid profile of *Azadinium poporum* (Dinophyceae) from the China Sea. *Harmful Algae*, 21–22, 64–75.
14. Tillmann, U. and Elbrächter, M., 2013. Mode of cell division in *Azadinium spinosum*. *Botanica Marina*. doi: 10.1515/bot-2013-0022.
15. Schnepf, E. and Elbrächter, M., 1999. Dinophyte chloroplasts and phylogeny—A review. *Grana*, 38, 81–97.
16. Nézan, E., Tillmann, U., Bilien, G. et al., 2012. Taxonomic revision of the dinoflagellate *Amphidoma caudata*: Transfer to the genus *Azadinium* (Dinophyceae) and proposal of two varieties, based on morphological and molecular phylogenetic analyses. *Journal of Phycology*, 48, 925–939.
17. Potvin, E., Jeong, H. J., Kang, N. S. T., Tillmann, U., and Krock, B., 2012. First report of the photosynthetic dinoflagellate genus *Azadinium* in the Pacific Ocean: Morphology and molecular characterization of *Azadinium* cf. *poporum*. *Journal of Eukaryotic Microbiology*, 59, 145–156.
18. Netzel, H. and Dürr, G., 1984. Dinoflagellate cell cortex. In *Dinoflagellates*, Spector, D. L., Ed. Academic Press Inc., Orlando, FL, pp. 43–105.
19. Tillmann, U. and Elbrächter, M., 2010. Plate overlap pattern of *Azadinium spinosum* Elbrächter et Tillmann (Dinophyceae), the newly discovered primary source of azaspiracid toxins. In *Proceedings of the 13th International Conference on Harmful Algae*, Ho, K. C., Zhou, M. J., and Qi, Y. Z., Eds. Environmental Publication House, Hong Kong, China, pp. 42–44.
20. Tillmann, U., Soehner, S., Nézan, E., and Krock, B., 2012. First record of *Azadinium* from the Shetland Islands including the description of *A. polongum* sp. nov. *Harmful Algae*, 20, 142–155.
21. Salas, R., Tillmann, U., John, U. et al., 2011. The role of *Azadinium spinosum* (Dinophyceae) in the production of azaspiracid shellfish poisoning in mussels. *Harmful Algae*, 10, 774–783.

22. Ramsfjell, E., 1959. Two new phytoplankton species from the Norwegian Sea, the diatom *Coscinosira poroseriata*, and the dinoflagellate *Gonyaulax parva*. *Nytt Magasin for Botanikk*, 7, 175–177.

23. Schiller, J., 1935. Dinoflagellatae (Peridineae) in monographischer Behandlung. In *Dr. L. Rabenhorst's Kryptogamen-Flora von Deutschland, Österreich und der Schweiz*, Rabenhorst, L., Ed. Akademische Verlagsgesellschaft, Leipzig, pp. 161–320.

24. Bérard-Therriault, L., Poulin, M., and Bossé, L., 1999. Guide d´identification du phytoplancton marin de l´estuaire et du golfe de Saint-Laurent incluant également certaines protozoaires. *Publication spéciale canadienne des sciences halieutiques et aquatiques*, 128, 1–387.

25. Zhang, H., Bhattacharya, D., and Lin, S., 2007. A three-gene dinoflagellate phylogeny suggests monophyly of prorocentrales and a basal position for *Amphidinium* and *Heterocapsa*. *Journal of Molecular Evolution*, 65, 463–474.

26. Howard, M. D. A., Smith, G. J., and Kudela, R. M., 2009. Phylogenetic relationships of yessotoxin-producing dinoflagellates, based on the large subunit and internal transcribed spacer ribosomal DNA domains. *Applied and Environmental Microbiology*, 75, 54–63.

27. Fensome, R. A., Taylor, F. J. R., Norris, G., Sarjeant, W. A. S., Wharton, D. I., and Williams, G. L., 1993. A classification of living and fossil dinoflagellates. *Micropaleontology*, Special Publication, 7, 1–351.

28. Dodge, J. D. and Hermes, H. B., 1981. A scanning electron microscopical study of the apical pores of marine dinoflagellates (Dinophyceae). *Phycologia*, 20, 424–430.

29. Sournia, A., 1984. Classification at nomenclature de divers dinoflagellates marines (classe des Dinophyceae). *Phycologia*, 23, 345–355.

30. Torgersen, T., Bruun Bremmens, N., Rundberget, T., and Aune, T., 2008. Structural confirmation and occurrence of azaspiracids in Scandinavian brown crabs (*Cancer pagurus*). *Toxicon*, 51, 93–101.

31. Hernández-Becerril, D. U., Barón-Campis, S. A., and Escobar-Morales, S., 2012. A new record of *Azadinium spinosum* (Dinoflagellata) from the tropical Mexican Pacific. *Revista de Biología Marina y Oceanografía*, 47, 553–557.

32. Halldal, P., 1953. Phytoplankton investigations from Weather Ship M in the Norwegian Sea, 1948–1949. *Hvalrådets Skrifter*, 38, 1–91.

33. Silva, E. S., 1968. Plancton da lagoa de Óbidos (III). Abundância, variações sazonais e grandes "blooms." *Notas e estudos di Instituto de Biologia Marítima*, 34, 1–79, 7 pl.

34. Dodge, J. D., 1982. *The Dinoflagellates of the British Isles*. Her Majesty´s Stationery Office, London, U.K.

35. Dodge, J. D. and Saunders, R. D., 1985. An SEM study of *Amphidoma nucula* (Dinophyceae) and description of the thecal plates in *A. caudata*. *Archiv für Protistenkunde*, 129, 89–99.

36. Margalef, R., Herrera, J., Rodiguez-Roda, J., and Larrañeta, M., 1954. Plancton recogido por los laboratorios costeros, VIII. Fitoplancton de las costas de Castellón durante el año 1952. *Publicaciones del Instituto de Biología Aplicada*, 17, 87–100.

37. Rampi, L., 1969. Su alcuni elementi fitoplanctonici (Peridinee, Silicococcales ed Heterococcales) rari o nuovi raccolti nelle acque del Mare Ligure. *Natura (Milano)*, 60, 49–56.

38. Lewis, J. and Dodge, J. D., 1990. The use of the SEM in dinoflagellate taxonomy. In *Scanning Electron Microscopy in Taxonomy and Functional Morphology*, Claugher, D., Ed. The Systematics Association, Special Vol. 41, Clarendon Press, Oxford, U.K., pp. 125–148.

39. Akselman, R. and Negri, A., 2012. Blooms of *Azadinium* cf. *spinosum* Elbrächter et Tillmann (Dinophyceae) in northern shelf waters of Argentina, Southwestern Atlantic. *Harmful Algae*, 19, 30–38.

40. Toebe, K., Joshi, A. R., Messtorff, P., Tillmann, U., Cembella, A., and John, U., 2013. Molecular discrimination of taxa within the dinoflagellate genus *Azadinium*, the source of azaspiracid toxins. *Journal of Plankton Research*, 35, 225–230.

41. Jauffrais, T., Marcaillou, C., Herrenknecht, C. et al., 2012. Azaspiracid accumulation, detoxification and biotransformation in blue mussels experimentally fed *Azadinium spinosum* (Dinophyceae). *Toxicon*, 60, 582–595.

42. Raine, R., McDermott, G., Silke, J., Lyons, K., Nolan, G., and Cusack, C., 2010. A simple short range model for the prediction of harmful algal events in the bays of Southwestern Ireland. *Journal of Marine Systems*, 83, 150–157.

43. Potvin, E., Hwang, Y. J., Yoo, Y. D., Kim, J. S., and Jeong, H. J., 2013. Feeding by heterotrophic protists and copepods on the photosynthetic dinoflagellate *Azadinium* cf. *poporum* from Western Korean waters. *Aquatic Microbial Ecology*, 68, 143–158.

44. Jeong, H. J., Yoo, Y. D., Kim, J. S., Seong, K. A., Kang, N. S., and Kim, T. H., 2010. Growth, feeding, and ecological roles of the mixotrophic and heterotrophic dinoflagellates in marine planktonic food webs. *Ocean Science Journal*, 45, 65–91.

45. Hansen, P. J., 2011. The role of photosynthesis and food uptake for the growth of mixotrophic dinoflagellates. *Journal of Eukaryotic Microbiology*, 58, 203–214.

46. Jakobsen, H. H., 2002. Escape of protists in predator-generated feeding currents. *Aquatic Microbial Ecology*, 26, 271–281.

47. Jakobsen, H. H., 2001. Escape response of planktonic protists to fluid mechanical signals. *Marine Ecology Progress Series*, 214, 67–78.

48. Tillmann, U., 2004. Interactions between planktonic microalgae and protozoan grazers. *Journal of Eukaryotic Microbiology*, 51, 156–168.

49. Iwataki, M., 2002. *Taxonomic Study on the Genus Heterocapsa (Peridiniales, Dinophyceae)*, PhD Thesis. Graduate School of Agricultural and Life Science, University of Tokyo.

50. Pfiester, L. A. and Anderson, D. M., 1987. Dinoflagellate reproduction. In *The Biology of Dinoflagellates*, Taylor, F. J. R., Ed. Academic Press, New York, pp. 611–648.

51. Jauffrais, T., Herrenknecht, C., Séchet, V. et al., 2012. Quantitative analysis of azaspiracids in *Azadinium spinosum* cultures. *Analytical and Bioanalytical Chemistry*, 403, 833–846.

52. Kremp, A. and Parrow, M. W., 2006. Evidence for asexual resting cysts in the life cycle of the marine peridinoid dinoflagellate, *Scrippsiella hangoei*. *Journal of Phycology*, 42, 400–409.

53. Jauffrais, T., Séchet, V., Herrenknecht, C. et al., 2013. Effect of environmental and nutritional factors on growth and azaspiracid production of the dinoflagellate *Azadinium spinosum*. *Harmful Algae*, 27, 138–148.

54. Jauffrais, T., Kilkoyne, J., Séchet, V. et al., 2012. Production and preparative isolation of azaspiracid-1 and -2 from *Azadinium spinosum* culture in pilot scale photobioreactors. *Marine Drugs*, 10, 1360–1382.

55. Smayda, T. J., 2002. Adaptive ecology, growth strategies and the global bloom expansion of dinoflagellates. *Journal of Oceanography*, 58, 281–294.

56. Smayda, T. J., 1997. Harmful algal blooms: Their ecophysiology and general relevance to phytoplankton blooms in the sea. *Limnology and Oceanography*, 42, 1137–1153.

57. Banse, K., 1982. Cell volumes, maximal growth rates of unicellular algae and ciliates, and the role of ciliates in the marine pelagial. *Limnology and Oceanography*, 27, 1059–1071.

58. Sullivan, J. M. and Swift, E., 2003. Effects of small-scale turbulence on net growth rate and size of ten species of marine dinoflagellates. *Journal of Phycology*, 39, 83–94.

59. Morton, S. L. and Bomber, J. W., 1994. Maximizing okadaic acid content from *Prorocentrum hoffmannianum* Faust. *Journal of Applied Phycology*, 6, 41–44.

60. Cembella, A. D., 2003. Chemical ecology of eukaryotic microalgae in marine ecosystems. *Phycologia*, 42, 420–447.

61. Cembella, A. D., 1998. Ecophysiology and metabolism of paralytic shellfish toxins in marine microalgae. In *Physiological Ecology of Harmful Algal Blooms*, Anderson, D. M., Cembella, A. D., and Hallegraeff, G. M., Eds. Springer Verlag, Berlin, Germany, pp. 381–403.

62. Anderson, D. M., Kulis, D. M., Sullivan, J. J., Hall, S., and Lee, C., 1990. Dynamics and physiology of saxitoxin production by the dinoflagellates *Alexandrium* spp. *Marine Biology*, 104, 511–524.

63. Boyer, G. L., Sullivan, J. J., Andersen, R. J., Harrison, P. J., and Taylor, F. J. R., 1987. Effects of nutrient limitation on toxin production and composition in the marine dinoflagellate *Protogonyaulax tamarensis*. *Marine Biology*, 96, 123–128.

64. Frangopulos, M., Guisande, C., deBlas, E., and Maneiro, I., 2004. Toxin production and competitive abilities under phosphorus limitation of *Alexandrium* species. *Harmful Algae*, 3, 131–139.

65. Guisande, C., Frangópulos, M., Maneiro, I., Vergara, A. R., and Riveiro, I., 2002. Ecological advantages of toxin production by the dinoflagellate *Alexandrium minutum* under phosphorus limitation. *Marine Ecology Progress Series*, 225, 169–176.

66. Siu, G. K. Y., Young, M. L. C., and Chan, D. K. O., 1997. Environmental and nutritional factors which regulate population dynamics and toxin production in the dinoflagellate *Alexandrium catenella*. *Hydrobiologia*, 352, 117–140.

67. Vanucci, S., Guerrini, F., Milandri, A., and Pistocchi, R., 2010. Effects of different levels of N- and P-deficiency on cell yield, okadaic acid, DTX-1, protein and carbohydrate dynamics in the benthic dinoflagellate *Prorocentrum lima*. *Harmful Algae*, 9, 590–599.

68. Turner, J. T., 2006. Harmful algae interactions with marine planktonic grazers. In *Ecology of Harmful Algae*, Granéli, E. and Turner, J. T., Eds. Springer, Berlin, Germany, pp. 259–270.

69. Jacobson, D. M. and Anderson, D. M., 1986. Thecate heterotrophic dinoflagellates: Feeding behavior and mechanisms. *Journal of Phycology*, 22, 249–258.

70. Hansen, P. J. and Calado, A. J., 1999. Phagotrophic mechanisms and prey selection in free-living dinoflagellates. *Journal of Eukaryotic Microbiology*, 46, 382–389.

71. Krock, B., Tillmann, U., Alpermann, T. J., Voß, D., Zielinski, O., and Cembella, A., 2013. *Phycotoxin Composition and Distribution in Plankton Fractions from the German Bight and Western Danish Coast. Journal of Plankton Research*, 35 (5), 1093–1108.

72. Turner, J. T., Tester, P. A., and Hansen, P. J., 1998. Interactions between toxic marine phytoplankton and metazoan and protistan grazers. In *Physiological Ecology of Harmful Algae Blooms*, Anderson, D. A., Cembella, A. D., and Hallegraeff, G. M., Eds. Springer, Berlin, Germany, pp. 453–474.

73. Alvarez, G., Uribe, E., Avalos, P., Marino, C., and Blanco, J., 2010. First identification of azaspiracid and spirolides in *Mesodesma donacium* and *Mulinia edulis* from Northern Chile. *Toxicon*, 55, 638–641.

74. Lopez-Rivera, A., O'Callaghan, K., Moriarty, M. et al., 2009. First evidence of azaspiracids (AZAs): A family of lipophilic polyether marine toxins in scallops (*Argopecten purpuratus*) and mussels (*Mytilus chilensis*) collected in two regions of Chile. *Toxicon*, 55, 692–701.

75. Ueoka, R., Ito, A., Izumikawa, M. et al., 2009. Isolation of azaspiracid-2 from a marine sponge *Echinoclathria* sp as a potent cytotoxin. *Toxicon*, 53, 680–684.

76. Jauffrais, T., Contreras, A., Herrenknecht, C. et al., 2012. Effect of *Azadinium spinosum* on the feeding behaviour and azaspiracid accumulation of *Mytilus edulis*. *Aqua. Toxicology*, 124–125, 179–187.

77. Jauffrais, T., Kilkoyne, J., Herrenknecht, C. et al., 2013. Dissolved azaspiracids are absorbed and metabolized by blue mussels (*Mytilus edulis*). *Toxicon*, 65, 81–89.

78. Plakas, S. M., El Said, K. R., Jester, E. L. E., Granade, H. R., Musser, S. M., and Dickey, R. W., 2002. Confirmation of brevetoxin metabolism in the Eastern oyster (*Crassostrea virginica*) by controlled exposures to pure toxins and to *Karenia brevis* cultures. *Toxicon*, 40, 721–729.

79. Bakke, M. J. and Horsberg, T. E., 2010. Kinetic properties of saxitoxin in Atlantic salmon (*Salmo salar*) and Atlantic cod (*Gadus morhua*). *Comparative Biochemistry and Physiology Part C: Toxicology & Pharmacology*, 152, 444–450.

80. Cazenave, J., Wunderlin, D. A., Bistoni, M. D. L. et al., 2005. Uptake, tissue distribution and accumulation of microcystin-RR in *Corydoras paleatus*, *Jenynsia multidentata* and *Odontesthes bonariensis*— A field and laboratory study. *Aquatic Toxicology*, 75, 178–190.

81. Fux, E., Bire, R., and Hess, P., 2009. Comparative accumulation and composition of lipophilic marine biotoxins in passive samplers and in mussels (*M. edulis*) on the west coast of Ireland. *Harmful Algae*, 8, 523–537.

82. Rundberget, T., Gustad, E., Samdal, I. A., Sandvik, M., and Miles, C. O., 2009. A convenient and cost-effective method for monitoring marine algal toxins with passive samplers. *Toxicon*, 53, 543–550.

27

Azaspiracids: Chemistry, Biosynthesis, Metabolism, and Detection

Philipp Hess, Pearse McCarron, Bernd Krock, Jane Kilcoyne, and Christopher O. Miles

CONTENTS

27.1 Introduction

This chapter describes the chemical characteristics of azaspiracids (AZAs) to complete the view on this toxin group, with two other chapters in this book dedicated to toxicological[1] and ecological aspects.[2] AZAs are a group of polyether toxins first reported to cause food poisoning in 1995.[3,4] Since then, a small number of food poisoning incidents have occurred, and it is now accepted that this group of compounds requires regulation to protect public health.[5–8] At least six risk assessments have been carried out over the last decade to determine appropriate levels for regulatory limits in order to protect public health,[1] yet all these assessments are based on a single poisoning incident in 1997 and attempt to set levels based on the presence of just three analogues: AZA1, AZA2, and AZA3. Over the last 5 years, more than 30 additional analogues have been described, with both biotransformation in shellfish and chemical interconversion shown to contribute to the chemical diversity of this toxin group.

In the following sections, we review AZAs to distinguish those analogues that are formed by the microalgae themselves from those that are formed by biotransformation or by chemical modification during extraction or sample treatment. Subsequently, chemical characteristics such as solubility and pH and thermal stability are reviewed. Methods for discovery of AZA analogues are discussed, including bioassays and chemical techniques. Finally, methodology for detection and quantitation is reviewed with consideration of quality control in routine analytical settings.

27.2 Classification

27.2.1 Naturally Biosynthesized Variants

AZAs were detected in shellfish from Killary Harbour, Ireland, harvested following the initial poisoning event.[3] Later, the most abundant variant was isolated, structurally elucidated by Japanese researchers, and named azaspiracid (now known as AZA1) after three of its chemical functions: a secondary amine (in chemical nomenclature: aza-), a trispiro assembly, and a carboxylic acid 4. Although AZAs were originally detected in contaminated shellfish, they were soon suspected to be of dinoflagellate origin because of the seasonal occurrence and the structural characteristics shared with other known phycotoxins, that is, a highly oxygenated polyether structure 4. Other structural moieties are the carboxylic acid function and a linear carbon skeleton tentatively derived from polyketide synthases (PKSs). Today, around 30 variants of AZAs are known without counting stereoisomers (Figure 27.1). AZAs have sporadically been detected in plankton[9,10] and seawater,[11,12] but no progenitor of these toxins could be assigned until 2007,[13] when a small dinoflagellate, later named *Azadinium spinosum*,[14] was unambiguously identified as an AZA1- and AZA2-producing organism (ca. 20 and 7 fg/cell, respectively). Later, Kilcoyne et al. found additional AZAs with molecular masses of 715 Da (ca. 7 fg/cell) and 816 (AZA33 and AZA34) in environmental samples and cultures of *A. spinosum*[15] (Figure 27.1).

Recently, two strains of *Azadinium poporum*, a species previously reported to be nontoxigenic,[16,17] were proven to be the producers of two previously unknown AZAs.[18] AZA37 from a North Sea isolate of

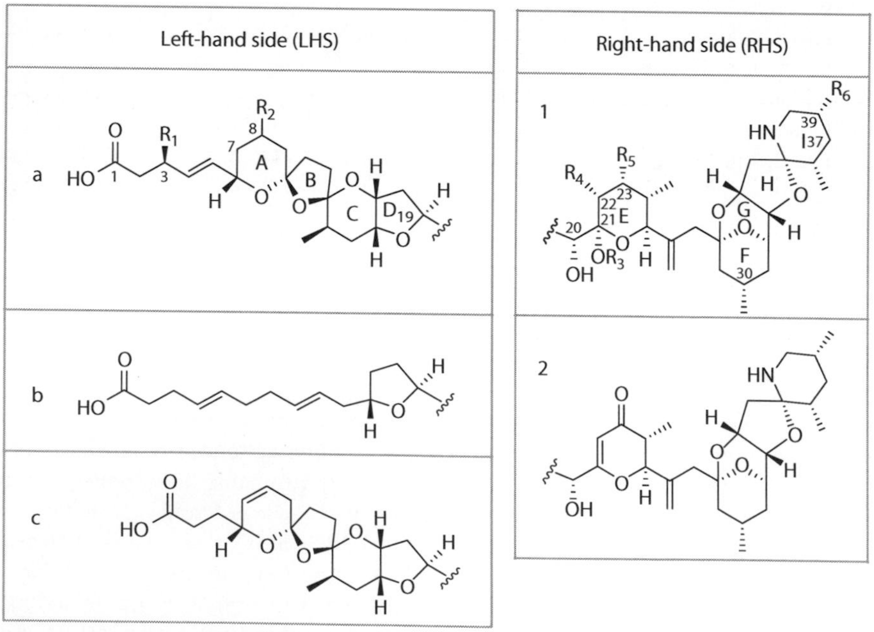

FIGURE 27.1 Structural variants of AZAs, their protonated masses, origin, and toxicity. Compounds highlighted in grey have had their structures confirmed by NMR. AZA11 has also tentatively been identified (MS) in *A. poporum*. The type refers to variations of the LHS and RHS parts of the molecule. AZA18, -20, -22, -24 and -27 proposed by Rehmann et al.[23] are now known not to exist. AZA25, -28, -31 and -35 have not had their structures well established to date.

	Type§	R_1	7,8	R_2	R_3	R_4	R_5	R_6	$[M+H]^+$	Origin	Status	Toxicity (Jurkat) EC_{50}
AZA1	a1	H	Δ	H	H	CH_3	H	CH_3	842.5	*A. spinosum*	Phycotoxin	1.1
37-*epi* AZA1	a1	H	Δ	H	H	CH_3	H	CH_3	842.5	*A. spinosum*	Artefact	0.2
AZA2	a1	H	Δ	CH_3	H	CH_3	H	CH_3	856.5	*A. spinosum*	Phycotoxin	0.3
AZA3	a1	H	Δ	H	H	H	H	CH_3	828.5	Shellfish	Metabolite	0.6
AZA4	a1	OH	Δ	H	H	H	H	CH_3	844.5	Shellfish	Metabolite	2.0
AZA5	a1	H	Δ	H	H	H	OH	CH_3	844.5	Shellfish	Metabolite	3.0
AZA6	a1	H	Δ	CH_3	H	H	H	CH_3	842.5	Shellfish	Metabolite	0.2
AZA7	a1	OH	Δ	H	H	CH_3	H	CH_3	858.5	Shellfish	Metabolite	
AZA8	a1	H	Δ	H	H	CH_3	OH	CH_3	858.5	Shellfish	Metabolite	0.3
AZA9	a1	OH	Δ	CH_3	H	H	H	CH_3	858.5	Shellfish	Metabolite	1.9
AZA10	a1	H	Δ	CH_3	H	H	OH	CH_3	858.5	Shellfish	Metabolite	3.1
AZA11	a1	OH	Δ	CH_3	H	CH_3	H	CH_3	872.5	Shellfish	Metabolite	
AZA12	a1	H	Δ	CH_3	H	CH_3	OH	CH_3	872.5	Shellfish	Metabolite	
AZA13	a1	OH	Δ	H	H	H	OH	CH_3	860.5	Shellfish	Metabolite	
AZA14	a1	OH	Δ	H	H	CH_3	OH	CH_3	874.5	Shellfish	Metabolite	
AZA15	a1	OH	Δ	CH_3	H	H	OH	CH_3	874.5	Shellfish	Metabolite	
AZA16	a1	OH	Δ	CH_3	H	CH_3	OH	CH_3	888.5	Shellfish	Metabolite	
AZA17	a1	H	Δ	H	H	COOH	H	CH_3	872.5	Shellfish	Metabolite	
AZA19	a1	H	Δ	CH_3	H	COOH	H	CH_3	886.5	Shellfish	Metabolite	
AZA21	a1	OH	Δ	H	H	COOH	H	CH_3	888.5	Shellfish	Metabolite	
AZA23	a1	OH	Δ	CH_3	H	COOH	H	CH_3	902.5	Shellfish	Metabolite	
AZA26	a2	H	Δ	H	—	—	—	—	824.5	Shellfish	Metabolite	36.6
AZA29	a1	H	Δ	H	CH_3	H	H	CH_3	842.5	Shellfish	Artefact	
AZA30	a1	H	Δ	H	CH_3	CH_3	H	CH_3	856.5	*A. spinosum*	Artefact	
AZA32	a1	H	Δ	CH_3	CH_3	CH_3	H	CH_3	870.5	*A. spinosum*	Artefact	
AZA33	b1	—	Δ	—	H	CH_3	H	CH_3	716.5	*A. spinosum*	Phycotoxin	5.2
AZA34	c1	—	Δ	—	H	CH_3	H	CH_3	816.5	*A. spinosum*	Phycotoxin	0.2
AZA36	a1	OH	Δ	CH_3	H	CH_3	H	H	858.5	*A. poporum*	Phycotoxin	
AZA37	a1	OH	—	H	H	CH_3	H	H	846.5	*A. poporum*	Phycotoxin	

FIGURE 27.1 (continued) Structural variants of AZAs, their protonated masses, origin, and toxicity. Compounds highlighted in grey have had their structures confirmed by NMR. AZA11 has also tentatively been identified (MS) in *A. poporum*. The type refers to variations of the LHS and RHS parts of the molecule. AZA18, -20, -22, -24, and -27 proposed by Rehmann et al.[23] are now known not to exist. AZA25, -28, -31 and -35 have not had their structures well established to date.

A. poporum[16] with a molecular mass of 845 Da (ca. 10 fg/cell) was determined as 39-desmethyl-7,8-dihydro-3-hydroxy-AZA1 by nuclear magnetic resonance (NMR) spectroscopy[19] (Figure 27.1). The other strain of *A. poporum*, from Shiwha Bay, Republic of Korea,[17] produced AZA36 with a molecular mass of 857 Da (ca. 2 fg/cell), which was determined as 39-desmethyl-3-hydroxy-AZA2 (Figure 27.1). Both *A. poporum*-derived AZAs have a 3-hydroxy substitution and a 39-desmethyl moiety in common. Whereas the 3-hydroxy function is also found in shellfish metabolites of AZA1 and AZA2 (e.g., AZA4 and AZA9[20]), the 39-desmethyl moiety is unique to a new class of dinoflagellate AZAs. This new class of 39-desmethyl AZAs is easily recognized in tandem mass spectrometry (MS) by a characteristic *m/z* 348 fragment, whereas all other AZAs have an *m/z* 362 fragment (Table 27.1). Two additional AZAs with *m/z* 348 fragments and molecular masses of 815 and 829 Da (ca. 11 and 6 fg/cell, respectively)[18] were also identified in a strain of *Amphidoma languida*.[21]

AZAs were also detected in isolates of *A. poporum* from Chinese coastal waters.[22] Whereas one strain did not produce any AZAs, three other strains produced exclusively AZA2 at cell quotas

TABLE 27.1

Characteristic CID Fragments of AZAs

	Group 1	Group 2	Group 3	Group 4	Group 5	Group 6
AZA1	842	672	462	362	262	168
AZA2	856	672	462	362	262	168
AZA3	828	658	448	362	262	168
AZA4	844	658	448	362	262	168
AZA5	844	674	464	362	262	168
AZA6	842	658	448	362	262	168
AZA7	858	672	462	362	262	168
AZA8	858	688	478	362	262	168
AZA9	858	658	448	362	262	168
AZA10	858	674	464	362	262	168
AZA11	872	672	462	362	262	168
AZA12	872	688	478	362	262	168
AZA13	860	674	464	362	262	168
AZA14	874	688	464	362	262	168
AZA15	874	674	478	362	262	168
AZA16	888	688	478	362	262	168
AZA17	872	702/658	492/448	362	262	168
AZA19	886	702/658	492/448	362	262	168
AZA21	888	702/658	492/448	362	262	168
AZA23	902	702/658	492/448	362	262	168
AZA25	810	658	448	362	262	168
AZA26	824	672	462	362	262	168
AZA33	716	—	462	362	262	168
AZA34	816	672	462	362	262	168
AZA35	830	672	462	362	262	168
AZA36	858	658	448	348	248	154
AZA37	846	686	448	348	248	154
AZA38	830	686	448	348	248	154
AZA39	816	—	448	348	248	154

Note: AZA1–25,[20,23,25] AZA26,[76] AZA33–35,[15] AZA36–39.[16,18]

ranging from 1.8 to 23 fg/cell. In addition, new AZAs with the *m/z* 348 fragment were detected in a fifth strain, which also produced AZA36 (1.4 fg/cell). In contrast to the Korean strains, this Chinese strain produced AZAs (with the *m/z* 348 fragment) with molecular masses of 919 and 927 Da (ca. 0.02 and 0.14 fg/cell, respectively). A sixth strain of *A. poporum* from China produced an AZA with a molecular mass of 871 Da (0.9–1.9 fg/cell) that was tentatively identified as AZA11 by comparison of retention times and CID spectra.[22] Whereas 3-hydroxylated AZAs like AZA36 and AZA37 seem to be biosynthesized by several strains of *A. poporum*, AZA11 may be the first case of an AZA being independently produced by dinoflagellate biosynthesis as well as through shellfish metabolic activity.

27.2.2 Shellfish Metabolism

To date, more than 30 AZA structural variants are known. As the exact nomenclature of AZAs according to the rules of the International Union of Pure and Applied Chemistry (IUPAC) are long and complicated, AZAs have been named by numbering in the chronological order of their detection or postulation. All AZAs up to AZA23 were originally identified or postulated from shellfish; however, AZA1 and AZA2 are of dinoflagellate origin, whereas AZA4–AZA23 have not been detected in planktonic samples and have been shown to be shellfish metabolites, with the possible exception of AZA11.[22,23]

Shellfish are known to transform AZAs by two different types of reactions: (1) hydroxylation at C3 and C23 and (2) carboxylation and subsequent decarboxylation.[23–28] Recent investigations with feeding experiments[28,29] revealed that blue mussels (*Mytilus edulis*) metabolize AZAs quickly. AZA17 and AZA19 were the most abundant metabolites of AZA1 and AZA2, respectively, suggesting that carboxylation of the methyl group at C22 is a preferred metabolic pathway.[28] Hydroxylation and decarboxylation seem to be secondary degradation routes.[25]

Hydroxylations of AZAs by shellfish metabolism occur at C3 on the carboxylic acid side chain to form 3-hydroxy-AZAs (e.g., AZA7, AZA11) as well as at C23 at the E ring of the molecule, resulting in 23-hydroxy-AZAs (AZA8, AZA12) (Figure 27.1). Furthermore, the methyl group at C22 can be oxidized to 22-carboxy-AZAs (AZA17, AZA19), which are subsequently decarboxylated to form the 22-desmethyl AZAs (AZA3, AZA6).[25,27] AZA 22-decarboxylation may be a shellfish metabolic activity; however, this reaction occurs rapidly during heating of shellfish meat and slowly in extracts stored at ambient temperature.[25] In addition, combinations of these processes are possible, to produce many of the remaining AZAs (AZA4, AZA5, AZA9, AZA10, AZA13, AZA14, AZA15, AZA16, AZA21, and AZA23). Some of the other AZAs originally detected without structural elucidation (AZA25, AZA29, AZA30, and AZA32), 23 were later identified as extraction artifacts (AZA29, AZA30, and AZA32).[30] In contrast to shellfish metabolism, phase I metabolites of AZA1 using rat liver microsomes (S9-mix) included an oxidation of the F ring of the molecule, which is not observed in shellfish metabolites. Glucuronides were found as the only phase II metabolites of AZA1 and via precursor ion experiments it could be proven that glucuronic acid is bound to AZA1 at C1 via an ester linkage.[26]

One study reported on binding of AZAs to proteins[31] finding that AZAs in mussel hepatopancreas bind to as yet unidentified proteins with molecular masses of 21.8 and 45.3 kDa.

27.2.3 Chemical Degradation Products and Artifacts

Among the modifications of AZA profiles due to extraction and/or sample processing are as follows: (1) epimerization, (2) 22-decarboxylation, and (3) formation of methyl derivatives.

Isomers of AZAs have previously been reported, which were produced as a result of the degradation of the main analogues in acidic environments.[23,32] The development of a neutral LC-MS method led to the discovery of isomers of AZAs that were not resolved at low pH.[33] These isomers recently identified as 37-*epi* AZAs are heat-induced conversion products with proportions ranging from 2% to 15% of their parent analogues.[34] As most biosynthetic processes are stereospecific, it can be assumed that only one enantiomer is produced by the organism. Similar occurrences are known from paralytic shellfish poisoning (PSP) toxins, where only the energetically less favored betamers are produced, which slowly epimerize to the more stable alphamers until equilibrium distribution.[35] The formation of the 22-desmethyl AZAs (AZA3, AZA4, AZA6, and AZA9) following heat treatment was demonstrated, and it was shown that these AZAs result from decarboxylation of their 22-carboxylated progenitors.[25] Even though it has been clearly shown that this decarboxylation is a thermally accelerated reaction, the 22-desmethyl AZAs can be detected in lower amounts in fresh, unboiled shellfish indicating that this reaction proceeds even at lower temperatures 2.[5,36]

In contrast, methyl esters and 21–methyl ketals of AZAs are clearly artifacts. The methylation of AZAs easily occurs if methanol is used for extraction of algal biomass or as a sample storage solvent for such extracts.[30] The methylation is a relatively slow process at low temperatures but is promoted by high temperatures and alkaline or acidic conditions. For instance, planktonic field samples that were extracted with methanol and stored in the same solvent at −20°C, after 5 years, displayed more than 50% of the total AZA content as methyl esters.[18] However, methyl esters can be detected in relatively fresh methanolic extracts of AZA-containing samples. For example, the reported isomer of AZA2 in *A. spinosum*[14] was later identified as AZA1 methyl ester.[30] Consequently, the use of methanol as extraction solvent may be avoided and replaced by acetone or aqueous acetonitrile, if analysis for AZAs is of special concern.[37]

27.3 Chemical Characteristics

In addition to the biotransformation and chemical reactions described earlier, chemical characteristics of AZAs contribute to the overall understanding of the behavior in the environment and in isolation studies, as well as their impact on biological systems.

27.3.1 Solubility and Uptake

To date, no formal solubility studies have been reported for AZAs, most likely due to the limited availability of the toxins. However, there are several observations from a number of studies that can, at least qualitatively, aid in the understanding of the behavior of AZAs. Studies on the isolation of AZAs have been particularly helpful in this context. As could be expected from the structure, the initial isolation of the compound confirmed the intermediate polarity of AZAs 4, demonstrating that AZA1 is easily soluble in aqueous methanol or acetone but poorly soluble in hexane. The same study also showed that AZAs tend to partition to dichloromethane or ethyl acetate rather than water or saline buffer. Several studies have demonstrated the solubility of AZAs in purely aqueous media, that is, natural seawater 11,[12] or algal culture medium.[38] The latter study in particular allowed for the estimation of a minimal solubility of AZA1 in aqueous media of approximately 5 μg/L, as this concentration was observed in filtered culture medium following tangential flow filtration; however, some of the toxin may have been protein bound and may therefore not reflect real water solubility. The pK_a of AZA1 is 5.8,[39] reflecting that the carboxylic acid group of AZA1 would be deprotonated at pH 7–8 and that the cyclic amine function would be protonated at pH values below 5. Hence, due to the two most polar functional groups of AZAs (carboxylic acid and cyclic amine), the molecule should be ionized over the whole pH range contributing to its significant solubility in water. Furthermore, this feature is likely to contribute to the observed bioavailability in the human digestive tract.

27.3.2 Thermal Stability

Thermal stability has been mostly studied for AZAs in shellfish tissue. In particular, mussel tissue has been subjected to an array of treatments.[40] The stability of the analogues differs significantly: While AZA1 and AZA2 are stable in mussel tissue up to ca. 110°C and only significantly start degrading from ca. +130°C, AZA3 transforms into isomers from ca. +90°C onward. It has been shown that AZA3 and AZA6 exhibit similar stability in mussel tissues, with equivalent degradation products formed at elevated temperatures.[41] Little is known of the toxicity of isomers and heat degradation products of AZAs in general; however, a recent study on 37-*epi*-AZA1 indicated that it is more toxic than AZA1.[34] This differential behavior of analogues to heat treatment is also known for other toxin groups, for example, okadaic acid that is stable up to +120°C while DTX2 starts degrading from ca. +90°C.[40,42] Most important though is the heat-induced decarboxylation of AZA17 and AZA19, resulting in the formation of AZA3 and AZA6, respectively, for which significant toxicity has been demonstrated.[1,20,43,44] Therefore, most AZA analogues are stable in typical cooking conditions (i.e., up to +90°C) with the exception of those analogues that have an additional carboxyl group at C22. This behavior drives the need for review of current legislation that regulates raw shellfish flesh to be analyzed.[5,6] Stability of AZAs has also been tested in shellfish tissue at lower temperatures,[36] with AZA1 showing good stability up to +40°C for a period up to 240 days. The thermal stability of most AZAs in shellfish tissue at +40°C suggests that there is little degradation at body temperature on digestion of shellfish tissues in the human digestive tract.

Thermal stability in solvents has also been tested using acidic liquid chromatography (LC)-MS/MS methods for a number of analogues. AZA1 and AZA2 were stable for up to 30 days at temperatures up to +37°C (and for 1 year when refrigerated),[45] while AZA3 and AZA6 (both lacking a methyl group at C22) were significantly less stable.[37]

27.3.3 Stability in Different pH Environments

AZAs are unstable in methanolic solution when exposed to strong acid (e.g., HCl) or to strong base (e.g., NaOH).[32] Poor stability at high pH, for example, in the conditions frequently used in the protocol for base hydrolysis, has significantly hampered the discovery of potential fatty acid esters of AZAs: still, screening for the predicted masses of such esters did not result in any positive finding 23. For all deviations from neutral pH, the treatment with weak base (50% aqueous acetonitrile with 50 mM ammonium hydroxide) resulted in the least degradation: no degradation at +20°C after 48 h and only some degradation at +45°C after 48 h.[32] In methanolic solution, AZA1 degraded almost completely within 10 min at +37°C when subjected to HCl, while weaker acids, such as 0.1% acetic acid or 40 mM formic acid, required more time or higher temperatures (e.g., +70°C) to cause significant degradation.[32] The lack of stability at low pH means that extraction procedures using strong acids should be avoided or used with care. Interestingly, there is some tolerance to HCl when AZAs are contained in naturally contaminated mussel tissue: AZA-contaminated mussel tissue exposed to either HCl alone or combined with pepsin (to mimic human digestion conditions) did not result in significant degradation of AZAs.[32] On the contrary, the acidic treatment involving pepsin as a digestive enzyme resulted in a higher yield of AZA than that obtained with extraction using methanol. This finding suggests that AZAs are to some extent protein bound in naturally contaminated shellfish matrix, an observation made in parallel by other authors.[31] This protective effect of the shellfish matrix may also contribute to the strong effect AZAs exert in the human digestive tract. Indeed, human gastric conditions appear to be an efficient extraction method for AZAs from shellfish tissues, as is seen from the toxic effects of contaminated shellfish on humans. This, combined with the minimal degradation observed in weak basic conditions (similar to the human intestine), would contribute to the overall high bioavailability.

27.4 Methods of Discovery and Isolation

27.4.1 Bioassays

Following the first poisoning incident in 1995, *M. edulis* samples were sent from Ireland to Tohoku University in Japan where the toxic compounds were isolated using mouse bioassay (MBA)-guided fractionation 4. Fractions were injected into mice and those that resulted in mouse lethalities (200 μg/kg) were identified as containing the toxins of interest. In mice, intraperitoneally (IP) injected acetone extracts of contaminated mussel tissue caused "neurotoxin-like" symptoms characterized by sluggishness, respiratory difficulties, spasms, progressive paralysis, and death within 20–90 min.[3,4,46]

The IP minimum lethal doses of AZA2 and AZA3 were 110 and 140 μg/kg, respectively, suggesting higher potency relative to AZA1.[43] Pathological changes induced by AZAs were stated to be different from those induced by diarrhetic, paralytic and amnesic shellfish poisoning toxins.[47,48]

In 2009, a study comparing the performance of the MBA with LC-MS/MS at various concentration levels found that both methods were equivalent at the regulatory limit (95% probability of MBA detecting the 160 μg/kg limit); however, sensitivity of the MBA was an issue at lower levels (5% probability of MBA detecting 80 μg/kg).[49] This limitation of the MBA in detection capability also diminishes its usefulness in the discovery of novel AZA analogues as the amount of toxin consumed by the assay is very high.

27.4.2 Isolation Procedures

The initial isolation of AZA1 was performed with contaminated mussel tissue (20 kg whole flesh) from Killary Harbour, Ireland, and involved seven purification steps: extraction with acetone, liquid–liquid partitioning with hexane and 80% aqueous methanol, silica gel chromatography, size-exclusion chromatography on Toyopearl HW-40, and ion exchange chromatography on two different materials (cationic exchanger CM650, anionic exchanger DEAE). Final purification of the toxin was achieved by further chromatography on Toyopearl HW-40 yielding 2 mg of AZA1 4.

AZA2–5 were subsequently isolated from contaminated whole flesh using a procedure that included additional cleanup steps (eight steps in total).[43,50] A second liquid–liquid partitioning with ethyl acetate and water helped to remove salts in addition to the hexane partitioning step. Low-pressure reverse-phase chromatography on C18 silica (Develosil) resulted in a cleaner sample for subsequent ion exchange steps. The most crucial change to the original isolation procedure was the substitution of a final cleanup on HW-40 with a reverse-phase C18 polymeric material (ODP-50, Asahipak). Chromatography on this material facilitated the separation of the methyl and hydroxy analogues. Purification of AZA2–5 was guided by LC-MS/MS and MBA.[43,50]

Furthermore, AZA1, AZA2, and AZA3 isolations performed as part of the ASTOX project[51] employed a modified seven-step procedure: extraction (from 500 g dissected hepatopancreas tissues) with ethanol, two partitioning steps, and four chromatography steps, silica gel (normal phase), LH20, C8 silica (reverse phase, flash), and finally, C8 silica (reverse-phase, HPLC). With this modified procedure, recoveries of approximately 23% were reported.[45] Purification was guided by LC-MS/MS and ultra-violet detection at 210 nm.

In 2008, a different procedure was used to isolate AZA1–5. Dissected hepatopancreas (2.6 kg) and whole flesh (3 kg) were extracted with acetone and methanol, followed by two partitioning steps, solid-phase extraction (SPE) on silica, and preparative HPLC guided by LC-MS/MS.[52] Overall recovery and purity of the final material were not reported in this study so it is difficult to compare with other reported isolation approaches.

Up to this point, all the AZA isolation procedures employed acidic mobile phases. In 2008, a study evaluating the stability of AZAs at various pH values found that significant degradation (due to the formation of rearrangement isomers) occurred even under slightly acidic conditions in solution. Under neutral and slightly alkaline conditions, AZAs were more stable.[32]

In 2009, isolation of AZA2 from a marine sponge collected in Japan was reported. Purification was performed by a partitioning with hexane and 80% aqueous methanol followed by C18 flash chromatography, silica gel, and four reverse-phase HPLC steps, without using acidic or inorganic additives in the mobile phase. The final purification step employed a phenyl hexyl stationary phase, removing all the sample contaminants.[53]

An improved AZA isolation procedure has recently been reported[37] based on the method by Perez et al.,[45] in which neutral and moderately alkaline conditions were employed for the final steps of the procedure with increased recoveries (50%) and increased purities. Further changes included the replacement of the C8 stationary phase in the penultimate flash step with a phenyl hexyl stationary phase (Figure 27.2). The phenyl hexyl enabled separation of AZAs leading to a more efficient final cleanup. In addition to AZA1–3, AZA6 was also purified in sufficient amounts to enable structural determination by NMR, confirming the structure postulated from LC-MS/MS data.[37] Using this same method, AZA7–10[20] and 37-*epi*-AZA1[34] were purified and their structures confirmed by NMR (Figure 27.1).

Currently, the main sources of toxins for purification work are toxin-producing organisms, cultured or harvested from natural blooms, for example, okadaic acid group toxins,[54] brevetoxins,[55] saxitoxins,[56] yessotoxins,[57] cyclic imines,[58,59] and pectenotoxins.[60] Isolation from plankton sources is preferred as extracts are considerably purer than those from shellfish. In addition, shellfish purifications are dependent on the occurrence of significant toxic episodes.

Once *A. spinosum* was identified as the producer of AZA1 and AZA2, bulk cultures were produced to facilitate the sustainable production of pure compounds for use in the production of certified reference materials (CRMs) that are critical for the accurate determination of toxins in shellfish. In 2012, the successful bulk culturing of *A. spinosum* in pilot-scale photobioreactors and subsequent purification of AZA1 and AZA2 from the culture harvest was reported.[38] Compared with the shellfish isolation procedure reported by Kilcoyne et al.,[37] only five steps were required, eliminating the hexane partitioning and the LH20 steps (Figure 27.2). Recovery improved accordingly, to more than 70%, and isolation of material from 1200 L of culture yielded 9.3 mg of AZA1 and 2.2 mg of AZA2 of >95% purity.[38]

In addition to AZA1 and AZA2, two novel AZAs were isolated with molecular masses of 715 and 815 Da (subsequently named AZA33 and AZA34, respectively). NMR revealed significant differences in the structures of these compounds compared to the hitherto known AZAs (Figure 27.1) that will provide valuable information on structure–activity relationships. The levels of AZA33 in the *A. spinosum* were similar to those of AZA2; however, in shellfish extracts, there was a significantly lower proportion, possibly due to faster metabolism. Lower levels of AZA34 were detected in the *A. spinosum* with little or none at all in the shellfish.[15]

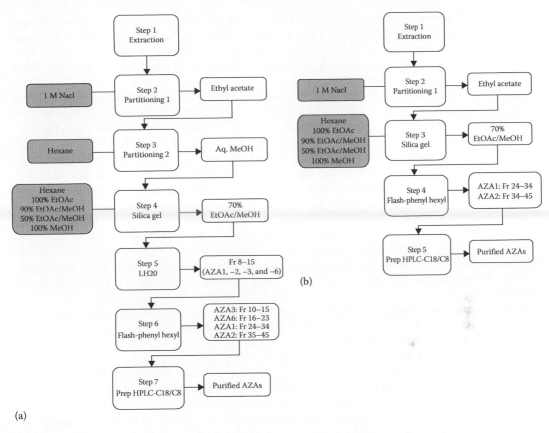

FIGURE 27.2 AZA isolation procedure from (a) shellfish and (b) phytoplankton.

The availability of purified toxins has enabled significant progress in assessing the toxicological impact of these compounds, in addition to ensuring supply of CRMs for the regulated toxins. While AZA1 and AZA2 requirements can be sustained with the availability of the *A. spinosum* cultures, the supply of AZA3 will be dependent on the availability of suitably contaminated shellfish, unless a more efficient method is developed.

27.4.3 MS Studies

The first reported analysis of AZA1–5 was performed using both positive and negative CID fast atom bombardment (FAB) MS/MS, which were used to confirm the NMR structures.[4,43,50] Numerous MS methods have been developed for the analysis of AZAs using a variety of chromatography systems.[33,61–63] Quantitative analysis is generally performed in positive ion mode and the majority of methods employ triple-quadrupole systems operating in selected reaction monitoring (SRM) mode with gradient elution. Due to the targeted nature of SRM, these methods have mostly contributed to confirmation of known AZAs and not to the discovery of novel analogues. An exception is the discovery of the 37-epimers of AZA1, AZA2, and AZA3, which was possible through the use of a neutral mobile phase.[33] The only difference in the mass fragmentation pattern between the parent analogue and the epimer was the ratio of the retro Diels–Alder (RDA) and subsequent water loss fragments. 37-*epi*-AZA1 (Figure 27.1) was consequently isolated from shellfish, differing from the parent analogue by the orientation of the methyl group at the C37 position.[34]

In 2008, the presence of 20 novel AZAs was reported using LC-MS/MS employing both quadrupole time-of-flight (QToF) and quadrupole ion trap (QTrap) MS systems operated in full and precursor ion scanning modes 23. The QToF also enabled accurate mass measurements. The novel AZAs were observed by monitoring for precursors of characteristic AZA fragments, in particular the m/z 362 ion. This led to the discovery of oxidized AZAs with an additional carboxy function. The carboxylated analogues AZA17–24 were first reported by Rehmann et al.[23] AZA17, AZA19, AZA21, and AZA23 were later identified and found to decarboxylate to form AZA3, AZA6, AZA4, and AZA9, respectively, using LC-MS/MS via heating, deuterium labelling, and kinetic experiments.[25]

Additional novel AZAs (AZA33–39)[15,18] were detected using ion trap, Orbitrap, QTrap, and QToF systems in precursor (for fragments m/z 362 and 348, mass range m/z 400–1100) or product ion modes (mass range from m/z 150–860). FTICR-MS and Orbitrap systems were used for accurate mass determination. The fragmentation pattern of the AZAs with an m/z 348 fragment suggested the lack of a methyl or methylene group at the amine end of the molecule (C24–C40), specifically the E to I rings. The mass spectrum of AZA33 showed water losses typical of AZA structures (m/z 698 and 680). Additionally, a fragment peak for the m/z 362 and 462 ions indicated that the amine end of the AZA1 compound was present. No RDA fragment was present, however, suggesting differences in the A ring of the molecule. AZA34 also displayed water loss fragments (m/z 798 and 780), an RDA fragment, in addition to the typical m/z 362 and 462 ions (Table 27.1).

The use of Orbitrap systems for high-resolution MS as a means of screening for marine biotoxins, including AZAs, has been described as allowing rapid identification with high sensitivity and selectivity.[64,65] Such methods can be used rather effectively for the detection of novel compounds and metabolites and may replace the triple-quadrupole systems in the future as the number of toxins identified and regulated increases.

Accurate quantitation of novel AZAs is hindered by the absence of standards. When sufficient amounts of purified compounds are available, quantitative NMR (qNMR) can be used to accurately determine concentrations.[66] The preparation of reference standards can subsequently be used to determine the relative molar response factors of AZAs in LC-MS/MS analysis. If qNMR is not possible, quantitation against a certified standard of a closely related AZA analogue is usually performed. The LC-MS/MS mobile-phase composition can influence the ionization efficiency; therefore, it is important to test under isocratic conditions if possible. The MS detection mode can also influence results. While selected ion monitoring (SIM) depends only on the ionization efficiency of the compounds in the ESI source, and the transport of the ions through to the quadrupole, detection in SRM can also be affected by differences in the fragmentation of compounds.[15,20] Hence, analysis using SIM with isocratic elution is preferred. Relative molar response studies following derivatization with 9-anthryldiazomethane (ADAM) is also an option for quantitation of purified AZAs, and the method was used to confirm the certified concentrations of AZA CRMs.[67]

27.4.4 Characteristics of AZA CID Mass Spectra

The mass spectral behavior of AZAs has been investigated by several research groups with high-resolution MS and tandem MS[23,68–70] as well as with hydrogen/deuterium exchange experiments[71] or with deuterium labelling at C22.[25] Electrospray ionization (ESI), which is typically used for phycotoxin analysis, is a soft ionization technique that transfers the positive charge via a proton transfer to the amine nitrogen of the AZA molecule. In this ionization mode, the charge is located at the end of the molecule and fragmentation occurs by elimination of smaller or larger parts of the molecule from its charged end. For this reason, CID mass spectra of AZAs are characterized by specific fragmentations of the molecule, which are followed by several water losses. The molecular ion usually cleaves off up to six molecules of water (group 1 fragments). The smallest cleavage other than water losses is caused by a RDA reaction of ring A (A-ring cleavage), where the bonds between C6 and the ether bridge and between C9 and C10 are cleaved. This results in the loss of C1–C9 with its substituents, followed by several water losses resulting in the group 2 fragments (Table 27.1). The second fragmentation of the carbon skeleton is the C-ring cleavage, where the bonds between C15 and C16 as well as the bond between C17 and the ether bridge of the C ring are cleaved. The remaining fragment with its water losses gives the group 3 fragments. By the C-ring cleavage, the C1–C15 part of the molecule is eliminated. The group 4 fragments are formed by the E-ring cleavage (RDA), where C1–C23 are eliminated. Before identification of the AZA-producing organisms, all published AZAs had diagnostic substituents located at C1–C23, and all shared the remaining m/z 362 fragment. The recently discovered variants form m/z 348 as the major ion in the group 4 fragments. Other fragmentations of less diagnostic value are the cleavage between C27 and C28 resulting in the group 5 fragments, with m/z 262/248 and the G-ring cleavage giving the group 6 fragments with m/z 168/154.[17,18,22]

Apart from these general fragmentation patterns, a specific fragmentation pathway exists for 3-hydroxy AZAs, which can be observed within the molecular ion cluster. In addition to the subsequent water losses from the pseudomolecular ion, which is common among all AZAs, 3-hydroxy AZAs also eliminate CO_2 followed by several water losses. The fragments resulting from the CO_2 elimination are not very abundant (typically they make up to approximately 20% of the highest peak) but are clearly visible. Another fragmentation pathway unique for 3-hydroxy AZAs is the elimination of a 78 Da fragment equivalent to $C_2H_6O_3$, which probably is caused by a cleavage between C2 and C3 combined with one water loss. Like the CO_2 elimination, this fragmentation pathway is not dominant, but the combination of a CO_2 cleavage and a 78 Da elimination is characteristic for 3-hydroxy AZAs and can be observed in AZA4, AZA11, AZA36, and AZA37 (Figure 27.3).

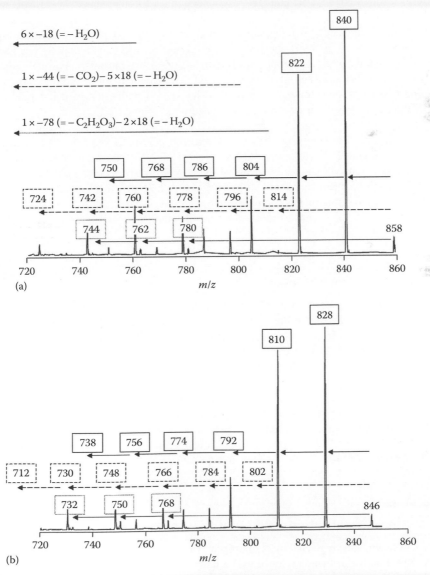

FIGURE 27.3   CID molecular ion clusters of two 3-hydroxy-AZAs: (a) AZA37 and (b) AZA36. Full arrows mark the water losses, dashed arrows mark the CO_2 elimination followed by water losses and pointes arrows mark the $C_2H_6O_3$ elimination followed by water losses.

27.4.5 NMR Studies

AZAs consist of chains of carbon atoms substituted with hydrogen atoms and connected via ether links and an amino link. The ^{1}H and ^{13}C nuclei are particularly amenable to NMR spectroscopy, and it is this method, supplemented by MS, that has primarily been used for AZA structure determination. The structure of AZA1 was established in this way and full ^{1}H and ^{13}C NMR assignments were reported in 1998.[4] Subsequent isolation of two other AZAs led to structure elucidation of AZA2 and AZA3 and presentation of their full ^{1}H- and ^{13}C-NMR assignments.[43] AZA4 and AZA5 are hydroxylated analogues and were isolated in smaller amounts, such that only ^{1}H NMR was obtained.[50] It should be noted that these NMR studies did not reveal the absolute stereochemistry of the AZAs nor even their complete relative stereochemistries. From 2000, the first syntheses of AZA substructures began to be reported. This synthetic activity[72–75] eventually led to definition of the absolute stereochemistry of AZAs.

Establishing the 2D and 3D structures of complex molecules by NMR spectroscopy requires the presence of useful through-bond [1]H–[1]H and [1]H–[13]C connectivities, through-space [1]H–[1]H NoE interactions, and coupling constant information. In complex organic molecules, some of these correlations can be absent or hard to observe due to overlapping signals or unfavorable coupling constants, preventing full structure determination from NMR spectra alone. A series of synthetic studies by Nicolaou and co-workers revealed that the originally proposed structure of AZA1 was partially incorrect[72] and eventually established the stereochemistry and structures of AZA1–3 as shown in Figure 27.1.[72–75] The structures of the remaining AZAs have been revised accordingly (Figure 27.1), with a consequent reassignment of the original NMR assignments[4,43] for resonances associated with C7 and C9.[37]

AZA6 was isolated and its structure, proposed originally from MS data, was established by NMR.[37] AZA7–10 have also been isolated, and their structures originally proposed from MS studies were confirmed by NMR[20] (Figure 27.1). However, NMR analysis of AZA26[76] showed a structure different to that originally proposed from MS studies 23. Most of the remaining AZAs (i.e., AZA11–17, –19, –23 and AZA29–32) have not yet been characterized by NMR, and their structures therefore remain tentative. Additional structural information has been derived for AZA17, AZA19, AZA21, and AZA23 following the discovery that these AZAs convert to analogues with established structures (AZA3, AZA6, AZA4, and AZA9, respectively).[25]

27.4.6 Characterization Reactions

In addition to NMR, a number of different approaches have been used to support structural hypotheses. All AZAs have a carboxyl group at the C1 position. Treatment of a sample with diazomethane, which specifically reacts with a carboxyl moiety to produce the methyl ester, has been used to confirm the presence of the carboxyl group for some AZAs.[18] This method has also been used to confirm the identity of AZA methyl derivatives.[30,37] In addition, derivatization of the free carboxyl group on AZAs with 9-ADAM[67] was used to differentiate between methyl esters of AZAs and methyl ketals.[30]

The presence of a diol at C20–C21 can also be confirmed by reaction with sodium periodate, which cleaves the *cis* diol on AZAs to produce a lactone derivative containing only C21–C40 with appended functional groups. This method was used to support structural evidence for dehydro-AZA3 23, for the conversion of AZA17–AZA3 via decarboxylation using deuterium labelling,[25] and for structural confirmation (C21–C40) of AZA6,[37] 37-*epi*-AZA1,[34] and AZA33 and AZA34.[15]

27.5 Detection, Quantitation, and Quality Control Tools

When AZAs were explicitly regulated by the European Union (EU) in 2002, the reference method was the DSP MBA (based on the method developed by Yasumoto et al., 1984), which was considered at the time to be capable of detecting the regulatory limit of 160 µg/kg AZA equivalents 5. Because fatty acid esters of the okadaic acid group appeared to require a longer time period to exert their toxicity in the MBA,[77] the observation period was set to 24 h for all lipophilic toxins. An assay was considered positive if two or three of the three mice injected had died within the 24 h period, whereas if only one or no mouse died, the sample was considered negative. A significant shortcoming of the MBA is that it is not quantitative and provides no information on AZA toxin profile.

A risk assessment carried out by the Food Safety Authority in Ireland lent credence to the set regulatory limit.[78] The Irish biotoxin monitoring program employed the MBA in parallel with LC-MS/MS from 2001 to 2011, and over that period, the agreement between the two methods was 93% (Jane Kilcoyne, unpublished data).

The qualitative qualitative nature of the MBA means it is not possible to describe the repeatability of the assay for a particular shellfish tissue without using further tests to characterize the shellfish tissue quantitatively. Additional concerns relating to specificity, accuracy, and ethics prompted substantial efforts to replace it with instrumental methods.[79] In 2011, the EU replaced the MBA with LC-MS/MS as the primary monitoring method for the analysis of lipophilic toxins in shellfish.[8]

27.5.1 Quantitative Methods

It was clear from the early days of AZA analysis that alternative methods to the bioassay were necessary for accurate and precise quantitation of AZAs. Although AZAs have a distinctive structure with spiro assemblies, carboxylic acid, and cyclic amine functionalities,[4,73] they lack a strong chromophore or fluorophore, so direct analysis by UVD or fluorescence detection (FLD) methods is not possible. Therefore, LC-MS/MS is currently the most widely used method for detection and quantitation of AZAs. The presence of the amine enables specific and sensitive detection of AZAs in positive ESI mode.

Quantitative LC-MS/MS methods for AZAs are primarily based on reverse-phase chromatography systems. Most methods employ standard bonded-phase silica columns (e.g., C8 or C18), but the use of monolithic columns has also been reported.[70] Monolithic columns allow high flow rates, enabling analysis of multiple AZA analogues with run times as fast as 30 s.[80]

The first quantitative LC-MS method for AZAs was reported in 1999[61] and included an SPE cleanup step to help remove interferences. A C18 column was used with an acidic mobile-phase and isocratic elution, detecting the molecular ions of AZA1/6 (842.5), AZA2 (856.5), and AZA3 (828.5). This SIM method had a detection limit of 50 pg. Tandem MS, in particular the use of triple-quadrupole instruments in SRM mode, allows for greater selectivity and sensitivity over methods based on SIM. With advances in instrumentation, and increased accessibility, SRM is now the predominant scanning mode used in the MS analysis of AZAs. Draisci and co-workers[81] reported a tandem MS method for SRM detection of AZA1 with a detection limit of 20 pg. Tandem MS methods were subsequently expanded for detection of AZA1–3 and 6[82] as well as a series of hydroxylated AZAs (AZA4, AZA5, AZA7–11).[24] As part of work on the identification of new AZA analogues in mussels, an LC-MS/MS method was used for profiling more than 20 AZAs simultaneously 23. The fragmentation of AZAs in positive ionization mode offers a range of ions for Q3 selection in SRM scanning. Water losses from the protonated molecules offer the best sensitivity in SRM analysis but the use of such fragments is not ideal as they lack selectivity. For this reason, SRM transitions that use Q3 ions that result from true fragmentation of the molecule are more appropriate (e.g., the A-ring fragmentation producing *m/z* 672 for AZA1).

While LC-MS/MS offers good sensitivity and selectivity, the accuracy of the technique can be influenced by matrix effects. Matrix effects are the alteration of instrument signal due to suppression or enhancement of analyte ionization in the ion source due to the presence of coextracted sample components. Possible mechanisms for matrix effects have been discussed.[83] Matrix effects associated with the analysis of AZAs are generally presented as ion suppression.[33,84,85] To alleviate the issue of matrix effects in quantitative analysis of AZAs, a number of approaches have been taken. The use of SPE has been studied for AZA-specific methods[61,86] and also for AZAs as part of multitoxin procedures.[63,87] Techniques such as flow diversion, column flushing, matrix-matched calibration, and standard addition have also been applied for the alleviation or correction of matrix effects associated with LC-MS/MS analysis of AZAs.[33,85,88]

Due to the chemical diversity of lipophilic shellfish toxins, both regulated and unregulated, multitoxin LC-MS/MS methods are preferred. Multitoxin LC-MS/MS analysis of lipophilic toxins was initially reported by Quilliam et al.[62] Subsequently, a range of multitoxin methods have been developed using acidic (pH 2.3),[89] neutral (pH 6.8),[33,90] moderately alkaline (pH 7.9),[87] and alkaline (pH 11)[63] chromatography systems. Ultra-performance liquid chromatography (UPLC) methods have also been reported.[91] Acidic systems have been used traditionally, but an issue with these methods is that toxin groups that are preferentially analyzed in opposing ionization modes frequently co-elute. This is a problem for older mass spectrometers that lack the scanning speeds required for simultaneous monitoring in positive and negative ionization modes. The issue is mitigated with modern MS systems that are capable of rapid polarity switching. A benefit of neutral and basic systems is that the selectivity of separation is controlled such that toxins can be grouped according to the preferred ionization mode. An additional advantage of the neutral method is the capability of resolving the 37 epimers of AZA1, AZA2, and AZA3. The mobile-phase pH significantly affects the chromatography of AZAs. Figure 27.4 illustrates the elution profile and peak shapes of AZAs under acidic, neutral, and basic pH conditions. Peak shapes are sharpest under acidic conditions but are frequently compromised under basic conditions, apparently due to increased interaction with the stationary phase at higher pH. In spite of the compromised peak shapes, it was reported that the basic pH systems offers comparable sensitivity to the acidic method for AZAs.[63]

An acidic multitoxin method with a total run time of 30 min was subjected to an extensive in-house validation exercise by McNabb et al.[89] As part of work by the EU Reference Laboratory for Marine Biotoxins (EURLMB), this method was shortened to achieve higher throughput and underwent a single-laboratory validation.[92] The EURLMB subsequently coordinated an interlaboratory study for the determination of lipophilic toxins, including AZAs. Study participants were allowed a choice of chromatographic conditions.[93] In 2011, These et al.[94] reported results of a separate collaborative study on the determination of lipophilic marine biotoxins, but again, LC-MS/MS parameters were not specified. The study reported a limit of detection (LOD) of 4.7 µg/kg for AZA1. Following a successful in-house validation[95] of the alkaline method reported by Gerssen et al.,[63] an interlaboratory study was organized considering AZAs and the other regulated classes of lipophilic toxins. Matrix-matched standards were used to compensate for matrix effects, and the reproducibility and trueness of the method was demonstrated.[94] A LOD of 2 µg/kg was reported for AZA1. The success of the method validation exercises has demonstrated the effectiveness of LC-MS/MS for monitoring AZAs and other lipophilic toxins.

With advances in MS instrumentation available to monitoring laboratories, and because of the requirement to monitor increasing numbers of compounds in samples, the capability of nontargeted LC-MS screening methodologies are now being utilized. Blay et al. reported a nontargeted high-resolution LC-MS approach applied for screening lipophilic toxins.[64] Mass accuracies <1 ppm for AZAs were reported, and LODs were <0.1 µg/L. To facilitate in the application of such methodology, a library of toxins has been developed.[65]

Some work has been carried out on the development of alternative methods for AZA detection and quantitation. The presence of carboxylic and amine functional groups provides potential for analysis of AZAs by UVD or FLD following chemical derivatization. A method involving derivatization of the carboxylic function of okadaic acid group toxins with ADAM has been used extensively to enable analysis by FLD,[96,97] and this procedure was successfully applied to the derivatization of AZAs.[67] Figure 27.5 shows a mixture of AZA1, AZA2, and AZA3 standards analyzed by LC-FLD and LC-MS/MS following derivatization with ADAM. Although the method is quite laborious due to the extraction and cleanup steps involved, it does offer a feasible alternative for AZA quantitation. An advantage of the method is that it does not suffer from any discernible matrix effects.

Apart from chemical analytical methodologies, work on alternative detection approaches for AZAs has been limited. Forsyth and coworkers[98] developed a fragment-specific antibody for AZAs using synthetic haptens, but the assay in its current format is not yet sensitive enough for routine analysis of shellfish.

27.5.1 Extraction Methods

Extraction procedures for AZAs are primarily based on the liquid–solid extraction (LSE) format and have been developed with various solvents, sample-to-solvent ratios (SSRs), and numbers of extraction steps. Studies examining the presence and distribution of AZAs have reported the use of acetone as an extraction solvent.[30,81,82,99–102] The extracts generally underwent a partitioning with ethyl acetate or diethyl ether

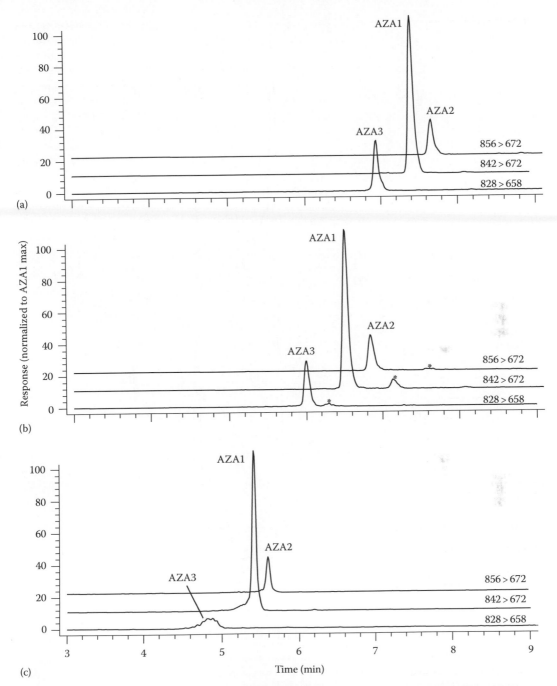

FIGURE 27.4 Effects of mobile phase pH on the chromatography of AZA1–3. Gradient elution from 25% to 100% MeCN over 8 min at 250 μL/min on a Gemini-NX C18 (3 μm, 50 × 2.1 mm) using acidic: pH 2.3 (a), neutral: pH 6.8 (b), and basic: pH 11 (c) conditions 37-epimers of AZAs resolved at neutral pH are noted with an asterisk (*).

and water prior to dissolution in methanol or aqueous acetonitrile for analysis. However, little information was provided on the efficiency of the initial acetone extraction. For screening and regulatory monitoring work, 80% methanol was used as an extraction solvent,[103,104] while 90% methanol has also been employed.[105,106] All these procedures using methanol involved a single-step dispersive extraction. The first study examining in detail the extraction of AZAs from shellfish was carried out by Hess et al.[107] Duplicate extraction with 100% methanol gave better recovery than with 100% acetone. Going from a single-step

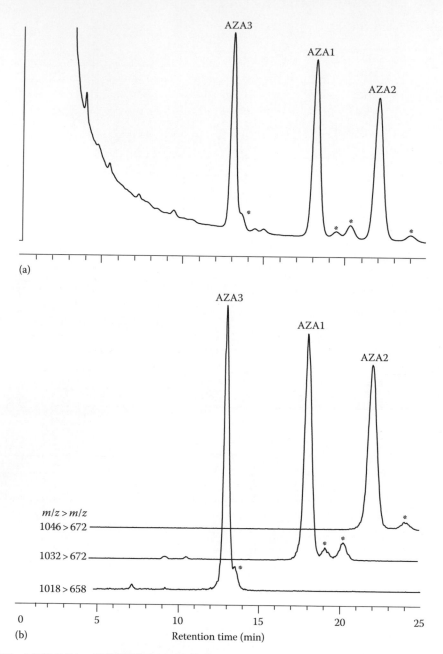

FIGURE 27.5 LC-FLD (A) and LC-MS (B) analysis of a mixture of AZA1-3 calibrant CRMs following ADAM derivatization for a relative molar response study. Isomeric AZAs are noted with an asterisk (*). (Reproduced from McCarron, P. et al., *J. Chromatogr. A*, 1218, 8089, 2011.)

extraction with 80% methanol and an SSR of 1:4 to a duplicate 100% methanol extraction with an SSR of 1:12.5 increased AZA recovery by >10%. A two-step methanol extraction is now commonly used for the extraction of AZAs as part of lipophilic toxin analysis procedures. Studies on the development of reference materials (RMs) for lipophilic toxins showed >99% recovery of AZA1–3 and AZA6 when using a three-step extraction with methanol.[33] For certification of an AZA RM, a fully exhaustive four-step extraction procedure with methanol was used (McCarron Pearse, NRCC, unpublished data); however, these extensive procedures are generally not necessary for screening and monitoring purposes.

27.5.2 Quality Control Tools

With the shift toward chemical monitoring methods for lipophilic toxins, including AZAs, it is important that appropriate RMs are available. RMs are essential for the development, validation, and quality control of analytical methods[108] and can generally be classified in two categories: Pure standard RMs are necessary for instrument calibration, while matrix RMs are designed to assess the performance of entire analytical methods, including testing of the extraction step, assessing matrix effects, and evaluating the accuracy of measurement or determination steps.

As part of the ASTOX project, significant work was performed on the isolation and purification of AZAs for the preparation of AZA calibrant RMs.[51] Work was also carried out by the National Research Council of Canada (NRCC) in collaboration with the UK Food Safety Authority.[109] These efforts led to the production of CRMs for AZA1, AZA2, and AZA3,[51] which are commercially available from the NRCC.[110] Certified values were assigned using qNMR,[66] with confirmation through a relative molar response study based on LC-FLD analysis following ADAM derivatization. Isolation procedures for AZAs have been further improved to ensure continued supply of pure AZAs for production of calibrant CRMs.[37] Noncertified AZA standards are available from CIFGA.[111]

AZA matrix RMs were also developed as part of the ASTOX project.[51] Studies were aimed at the production of homogeneous and stable materials, primarily prepared from mussel tissues. A variety of stabilization techniques were studied, including gamma irradiation and freeze-drying.[36,112] This extensive feasibility work led to the production and certification of a mussel matrix CRM with assigned values for AZA1–3.[113] Certified values were assigned using direct analysis by LC-MS/MS and confirmed by LC-FLD following ADAM derivatization. Recently, as part of an international collaboration, a multi-toxin CRM containing AZAs was prepared as a freeze-dried mussel powder,[114] and this has been utilized in method validation exercises.

In addition to the availability of calibrant and matrix RMs for AZAs, a proficiency testing exercise for lipophilic toxins, including AZAs, is provided by QUASIMEME.[115] This scheme allows laboratories who test for AZAs to assess their performance in comparison with peer laboratories.

27.6 Summary and Outlook

Major advances have been made in the area of LC-MS/MS analysis of AZAs in terms of monitoring, discovery, and characterization. A number of validated methods for monitoring of AZAs in shellfish have been described detailing ways of overcoming issues with matrix interferences. In addition to the bioassay tools for discovery of AZAs, the use of LC-MS/MS in the discovery of novel analogues has been invaluable, with previously proposed structures based on fragmentation patterns being corroborated by NMR. Both the temperature-dependent degradation of AZA17 and AZA19 into AZA3 and AZA6, respectively, and the discovery of a new family of analogues, which have one methyl group less in the amino ring, suggest that monitoring methods should be amended to include several additional analogues. For the novel AZAs, significant research is required to determine their toxicity. The advance of high-speed high-resolution MS systems also paves the way for enhanced monitoring and detection programs in the future.

REFERENCES

1. Twiner, M. J., Hess, P., and Doucette, G. J., 2013. Azaspiracids: Toxicology, pharmacology, and risk assessment, in *Seafood and Freshwater toxins*, 3rd edn., Botana, L., Ed., Chapter 28, CRC Press, Boca Raton, FL.
2. Tillmann, U., Salas, R., Jauffrais, T., Hess, P., and Silke, J., 2013. Azaspiracids; the producing organisms: Biology and food web transfer, in *Seafood and Freshwater Toxins*, 3rd edn., Botana, L., Ed., Chapter 26, CRC Press, Boca Raton, FL.
3. McMahon, T. and Silke, J., 1996. Winter toxicity of unknown aetiology in mussels. *Harmful Algae News*, 14, 2.

4. Satake, M., Ofuji, K., Naoki, H. et al., 1998. Azaspiracid, a new marine toxin having unique spiro ring assemblies, isolated from Irish mussels, *Mytilus edulis*. *Journal of the American Chemical Society*, 120, 9967–9968.

5. Anonymous, 2002. Commission decision 2002/225/EC of 15 March 2002 laying down detailed rules for the implementation of council directive 91/492/EEC as regards the maximum levels and the methods of analysis of certain marine biotoxins in bivalve molluscs, echinoderms, tunicates and marine gastropods. *Official Journal*, L75, 62–64.

6. Anonymous, 2004. Regulation (EC) No 853/2004 of the European parliament and of the council of 29 April 2004 laying down specific hygiene rules for food of animal origin. *Official Journal*, L139, 55–205.

7. Anonymous, 2004. Regulation (EC) No 854/2004 of the European parliament and of the council of 29 April 2004 laying down specific rules for the organisation of official controls on products of animal origin intended for human consumption. *Official Journal*, L139, 206–320.

8. Anonymous, 2011. Commission regulation (EU) No 15/2011 of 10 January 2011 amending regulation (EC) No 2074/2005 as regards recognised testing methods for detecting marine biotoxins in live bivalve molluscs. *Official Journal*, L6, 3–6.

9. James, K. J., Moroney, C., Roden, C. et al., 2003. Ubiquitous 'benign' alga emerges as the cause of shellfish contamination responsible for the human toxic syndrome, azaspiracid poisoning. *Toxicon*, 41, 145–151.

10. Krock, B., Tillman, U., John, U., and Cembella, A. D., 2008. LC-MS/MS aboard ship: Tandem mass spectrometry in the search for phycotoxins and novel toxigenic plankton from the North Sea. *Analytical and Bioanalytical Chemistry*, 392, 797–803.

11. Rundberget, T., Sandvik, M., Larsen, K. et al., 2007. Extraction of microalgal toxins by large-scale pumping of seawater in Spain and Norway, and isolation of okadaic acid and dinophysistoxin-2. *Toxicon*, 50, 960–970.

12. Fux, E., Bire, R., and Hess, P., 2009. Comparative accumulation and composition of lipophilic marine biotoxins in passive samplers and in mussels (*M. edulis*) on the West Coast of Ireland. *Harmful Algae*, 8, 523–537.

13. Krock, B., Tillmann, U., John, U., and Cembella, A. D., 2009. Characterization of azaspiracids in plankton size-fractions and isolation of an azaspiracid-producing dinoflagellate from the North Sea. *Harmful Algae*, 8, 254–263.

14. Tillmann, U., Elbrachter, M., Krock, B., John, U., and Cembella, A. D., 2009. *Azadinium spinosum* gen. et sp nov (Dinophyceae) identified as a primary producer of azaspiracid toxins. *European Journal of Phycology*, 44, 63–79.

15. Kilcoyne, J., Nulty, C., Jauffrais, T. et al., 2013. Isolation, structural elucidation and toxicity of two novel azaspiracids from *Azadinium spinosum*. Manuscript in preparation.

16. Tillmann, U., Elbrachter, M., John, U., and Krock, B., 2011. A new non-toxic species in the dinoflagellate genus *Azadinium*: *A. poporum* sp. nov. *European Journal of Phycology*, 46, 74–87.

17. Potvin, E., Jeong, H. J., Kang, N. S., Tillmann, U., and Krock, B., 2012. First report of the photosynthetic dinoflagellate genus *Azadinium* in the pacific ocean: Morphology and molecular characterization of *Azadinium cf. poporum*. *Journal of Eukaryotic Microbiology*, 59, 145–156.

18. Krock, B., Tillmann, U., Voss, D. et al., 2012. New azaspiracids in *Amphidomataceae* (Dinophyceae). *Toxicon*, 60, 830–839.

19. Krock, B., Tillmann, U., Potvin, E., et al., 2013. Structural elucidation of new azaspiracids isolated from *A. poporum*. Manuscript in preparation.

20. Kilcoyne, J., Twiner, M., McCarron, P. et al., 2013. Isolation, structural determination, relative molar response and toxicity of AZA7-10. Manuscript in preparation.

21. Tillmann, U., Salas, R., Gottschling, M., Krock, B., O'Driscoll, D., and Elbrächter, M., 2012. *Amphidoma languida* sp. nov. (Dinophyceae) reveals a close relationship between *Amphidoma* and *Azadinium*. *Protist*, 163, 701–719.

22. Gu, H., Luo, Z., Krock, B., Witt, M., and Tillmann, U., 2013. Morphology, phylogeny and azaspiracid profile of *Azadinium poporum* (Dinophyceae) from the China Sea. *Harmful Algae*, 21–22, 64–75.

23. Rehmann, N., Hess, P., and Quilliam, M. A., 2008. Discovery of new analogs of the marine biotoxin azaspiracid in blue mussels (*Mytilus edulis*) by ultra-performance liquid chromatography/tandem mass spectrometry. *Rapid Communications in Mass Spectrometry*, 22, 549–558.

24. James, K. J., Sierra, M. D., Lehane, M., Magdalena, A. B., and Furey, A., 2003. Detection of five new hydroxyl analogues of azaspiracids in shellfish using multiple tandem mass spectrometry. *Toxicon*, 41, 277–283.

25. McCarron, P., Kilcoyne, J., Miles, C. O., and Hess, P., 2009. Formation of azaspiracids-3,-4,-6, and -9 via decarboxylation of carboxyazaspiracid metabolites from shellfish. *Journal of Agricultural and Food Chemistry*, 57, 160–169.

26. Kittler, K., Preiss-Weigert, A., and These, A., 2010. Identification strategy using combined mass spectrometric techniques for elucidation of phase I and phase II in vitro metabolites of lipophilic marine biotoxins. *Analytical Chemistry*, 82, 9329–9335.

27. O'Driscoll, D., Skrabakova, Z., O'Halloran, J., van Pelt, F., and James, K. J., 2011. Mussels increase xenobiotic (azaspiracid) toxicity using a unique bioconversion mechanism. *Environmental Science and Technology*, 45, 3102–3108.

28. Jauffrais, T., Marcaillou, C., Herrenknecht, C. et al., 2012. Azaspiracid accumulation, detoxification and biotransformation in blue mussels (*Mytilus edulis*) experimentally fed *Azadinium spinosum. Toxicon*, 60, 582–595.

29. Salas, R., Tillmann, U., John, U. et al., 2011. The role of *Azadinium spinosum* (Dinophyceae) in the production of azaspiracid shellfish poisoning in mussels. *Harmful Algae*, 10, 774–783.

30. Jauffrais, T., Herrenknecht, C., Sechet, V. et al., 2012. Quantitative analysis of azaspiracids in *Azadinium spinosum* cultures. *Analytical and Bioanalytical Chemistry*, 403, 833–846.

31. Nzoughet, K. J., Hamilton, J. T. G., Floyd, S. D. et al., 2008. Azaspiracid: first evidence of protein binding in shellfish. *Toxicon*, 51, 1255–1263.

32. Alfonso, C., Rehmann, N., Hess, P. et al., 2008. Evaluation of various pH and temperature conditions on the stability of azaspiracids and their importance in preparative isolation and toxicological studies. *Analytical Chemistry*, 80, 9672–9680.

33. McCarron, P., Giddings, S., and Quilliam, M., 2011. A mussel tissue certified reference material for multiple phycotoxins. Part 2: Liquid chromatography–mass spectrometry, sample extraction and quantitation procedures. *Analytical and Bioanalytical Chemistry*, 400, 835–846.

34. Kilcoyne, J., McCarron, P., Twiner, M. et al., 2013. Epimers of azaspiracids: isolation, structural elucidation and relative response of 37-*epi*-azaspiracid 1. Manuscript in preparation.

35. Cembella, A. D., 1998. Ecophysiology and metabolism of paralytic shellfish toxins in marine microalgae. In *Physiological Ecology of Harmful Algal Blooms*. Volume NATO-Advanced study institute series, Vol. 41, Anderson, D. M., Cembella, A. D., Hallegraeff, G. M., Eds., Springer Verlag Berlin, Heidelberg, Germany, pp. 381–403.

36. McCarron, P., Emteborg, H., and Hess, P., 2007. Freeze-drying for the stabilisation of shellfish toxins in mussel tissue (*Mytilus edulis*) reference materials. *Analytical and Bioanalytical Chemistry*, 387, 2475–2486.

37. Kilcoyne, J., Keogh, A., Clancy, G. et al., 2012. Improved isolation procedure for azaspiracids from shellfish, structural elucidation of azaspiracid-6, and stability studies. *Journal of Agricultural and Food Chemistry*, 60, 2447–2455.

38. Jauffrais, T., Kilcoyne, J., Sechet, V. et al., 2012. Production and isolation of azaspiracid-1 and -2 from *Azadinium spinosum* culture in pilot scale photobioreactors. *Marine Drugs*, 10, 1360–1382.

39. Fux, E., 2008. PhD-thesis. Development and evaluation of passive sampling and LC-MS based techniques for the detection and monitoring of lipophilic marine toxins in mesocosms and field studies, Dublin Institute of Technology, Ireland.

40. McCarron, P., 2007. PhD-thesis: Studies on the development of reference materials for phycotoxins, with a focus on azaspiracids, University College Dublin, Dublin, Ireland.

41. McCarron, P., Emteborg, H., Giddings, S. D., Wright, E., and Quilliam, M. A., 2011. A mussel tissue certified reference material for multiple phycotoxins. Part 3: Homogeneity and stability. *Analytical and Bioanalytical Chemistry*, 400, 847–858.

42. McCarron, P., Kilcoyne, J., and Hess, P., 2008. Effects of cooking and heat treatment on concentration and tissue distribution of okadaic acid and dinophysistoxin-2 in mussels (*Mytilus edulis*). *Toxicon*, 51, 1081–1089.

43. Ofuji, K., Satake, M., McMahon, T. et al., 1999. Two analogs of azaspiracid isolated from mussels, *Mytilus edulis*, involved in human intoxication in Ireland. *Natural Toxins*, 7, 99–102.

44. Twiner, M. J., El-Ladki, R., Kilcoyne, J., and Doucette, G. J., 2012. Comparative effects of the marine algal toxins azaspiracid-1, -2, and -3 on Jurkat T lymphocyte cells. *Chemical Research in Toxicology*, 25, 747–754.

45. Perez, R., Rehmann, N., Crain, S. et al., 2010. The preparation of certified calibration solutions for aza-spiracid1, -2, and -3, potent marine biotoxins found in shellfish. *Analytical and Bioanalytical Chemistry*, 398, 2243–2252.

46. McMahon, T. and Silke, J., 1998. Re-occurrence of winter toxicity. *Harmful Algae News*, 17, 12.

47. Flanagan, A. F., Callanan, K. R., Donlon, J., Palmer, R., Forde, A., and Kane, M., 2001. A cytotoxicity assay for the detection and differentiation of two families of shellfish toxins. *Toxicon*, 39, 1021–1027.

48. Twiner, M. J., Rehmann, N., Hess, P., and Doucette, G. J., 2008. Azaspiracid shellfish poisoning: a review on the chemistry, ecology, and toxicology with an emphasis on human health impacts. *Marine Drugs*, 6, 39–72.

49. Hess, P., Butter, T., Petersen, A., Silke, J., and McMahon, T., 2009. Performance of the EU-harmonised mouse bioassay for lipophilic toxins for the detection of azaspiracids in naturally contaminated mussel (*Mytilus edulis*) hepatopancreas tissue homogenates characterised by liquid chromatography coupled to tandem mass spectrometry. *Toxicon*, 53, 713–722.

50. Ofuji, K., Satake, M., McMahon, T. et al., 2001. Structures of azaspiracid analogs, azaspiracid-4 and azaspiracid-5, causative toxins of azaspiracid poisoning in Europe. *Bioscience Biotechnology and Biochemistry*, 65, 740–742.

51. Hess, P., McCarron, P., Rehmann, N. et al., 2007. Isolation and purification of AZAs from naturally con-taminated materials, and evaluation of their toxicological effects (ASTOX). Marine Institute, Galway, Ireland, Marine Environment & Health Series Report 28, 128p.

52. Alfonso, C., Alfonso, A., Otero, P. et al., 2008. Purification of five azaspiracids from mussel samples contaminated with DSP toxins and azaspiracids. *Journal of Chromatography B-Analytical Technologies in the Biomedical and Life Sciences*, 865, 133–140.

53. Ueoka, R., Ito, A., Izumikawa, M. et al., 2009. Isolation of azaspiracid-2 from a marine sponge *Echinoclathria* sp as a potent cytotoxin. *Toxicon*, 53, 680–684.

54. Miles, C. O., Wilkins, A. L., Hawkes, A. D. et al., 2006. Isolation and identification of a *cis*-C-8-diol-ester of okadaic acid from *Dinophysis acuta* in New Zealand. *Toxicon*, 48, 195–203.

55. Abraham, A., Plakas, S. M., Wang, Z. H. et al., 2006. Characterization of polar brevetoxin derivatives isolated from *Karenia brevis* cultures and natural blooms. *Toxicon*, 48, 104–115.

56. Laycock, M. V., Thibault, P., Ayer, S. W., and Walter, J. A., 1994. Isolation and purification procedures for the preparation of paralytic shellfish poisoning toxin standards. *Natural Toxins*, 2, 175–183.

57. Loader, J. I., Hawkes, A. D., Beuzenberg, V. et al., 2007. Convenient large-scale purification of yes-sotoxin from *Protoceratium reticulatum* culture and isolation of a novel furanoyessotoxin. *Journal of Agricultural and Food Chemistry*, 55, 11093–11100.

58. Miles, C. O., Wilkins, A. L., Stirling, D. J., and MacKenzie, A. L., 2003. Gymnodimine C, an isomer of gymnodimine B, from *Karenia selliformis*. *Journal of Agricultural and Food Chemistry*, 51, 4838–4840.

59. Torigoe, K., Murata, M., Yasumoto, T., and Iwashita, T., 1988. Prorocentrolide, a toxic nitrogenous mac-rocycle from a marine dinoflagellate, *Prorocentrum lima*. *Journal of the American Chemical Society*, 110, 7876–7877.

60. Miles, C. O.; Wilkins, A. L.; Munday, R. et al., 2004. Isolation of pectenotoxin-2 from *Dinophysis acuta* and its conversion to pectenotoxin-2 seco acid, and preliminary assessment of their acute toxicities. *Toxicon*, 43, 1–9.

61. Ofuji, K., Satake, M., Oshima, Y., McMahon, T., James, K. J., and Yasumoto, T., 1999. A sensitive and specific determination method for azaspiracids by liquid chromatography mass spectrometry. *Natural Toxins*, 7, 247–250.

62. Quilliam, M. A., Hess, P., and Dell'Aversano, C., 2001. Recent developments in the analysis of phy-cotoxins by liquid chromatography–mass spectrometry. Chapter 11 in *Mycotoxins and Phycotoxins in Perspective at the Turn of the Millenium*, Willem J. de Koe, Robert A. Samson, Hans P. van Egmond, John Gilbert and Myrna Sabino, Eds., *Proceedings of the Xth International IUPAC Symposium on Mycotoxins and Phycotoxins*, Guaruja, Brazil, May 21–25, 2000, pp. 383–391.

63. Gerssen, A., Mulder, P. P. J., McElhinney, M. A., and de Boer, J., 2009. Liquid chromatography-tandem mass spectrometry method for the detection of marine lipophilic toxins under alkaline conditions. *Journal of Chromatography A*, 1216, 1421–1430.

64. Blay, P., Hui, J. P. M., Chang, J. M., and Melanson, J. E., 2011. Screening for multiple classes of marine biotoxins by liquid chromatography-high-resolution mass spectrometry. *Analytical and Bioanalytical Chemistry*, 400, 577–585.

65. Gerssen, A., Mulder, P. P. J., and de Boer, J., 2011. Screening of lipophilic marine toxins in shellfish and algae: Development of a library using liquid chromatography coupled to orbitrap mass spectrometry. *Analytica Chimica Acta*, 685, 176–185.

66. Burton, I. W., Quilliam, M. A., and Walter, J. A., 2005. Quantitative H-1 NMR with external standards: Use in preparation of calibration solutions for algal toxins and other natural products. *Analytical Chemistry*, 77, 3123–3131.

67. McCarron, P., Giddings, S. D., Miles, C. O., and Quilliam, M. A., 2011. Derivatization of azaspiracid biotoxins for analysis by liquid chromatography with fluorescence detection. *Journal of Chromatography A*, 1218, 8089–8096.

68. Brombacher, S., Edmonds, S., and Volmer, D. A., 2002. Studies on azaspiracid biotoxins. II. Mass spectral behavior and structural elucidation of azaspiracid analogs. *Rapid Communications in Mass Spectrometry*, 16, 2306–2316.

69. Hamilton, B., Díaz Sierra, M., Lehane, M., Furey, A., and James, K. J., 2004. The fragmentation pathways of azaspiracids elucidated using positive nanospray hybrid quadrupole time-of-flight (QqTOF) mass spectrometry. *Spectroscopy: An International Journal*, 18, 355–362.

70. Volmer D. A., Brombacher, S., Whitehead B., 2002. Studies of azaspiracid biotoxins. I. Ultrafast high-resolution liquid chromatography/mass spectrometry separations using monolithic columns. *Rapid Communications in Mass Spectrometry*, 16, 2298–2305.

71. Diaz Sierra, M., Furey, A., Hamilton, B., Lehane, M., and James, K. J., 2003. Elucidation of the fragmentation pathways of azaspiracids, using electrospray ionisation, hydrogen/deuterium exchange, and multiple-stage mass spectrometry. *Journal of Mass Spectrometry*, 38, 1178–1186.

72. Nicolaou, K. C., Vyskocil, S., Koftis, T. V. et al., 2004. Structural revision and total synthesis of azaspiracid-1, part 1: Intelligence gathering and tentative proposal. *Angewandte Chemie-International Edition*, 43, 4312–4318.

73. Nicolaou, K. C., Chen, D. Y. K., Li, Y. W. et al., 2003. Total synthesis of the proposed azaspiracid-1 structure, part 2: Coupling of the C1-C20, C21-C27, and C28-C40 fragments and completion and synthesis. *Angewandte Chemie-International Edition*, 42, 3649–3653.

74. Nicolaou, K. C., Koftis, T. V., Vyskocil, S. et al., 2004. Structural revision and total synthesis of azaspiracid-1, part 2: Definition of the ABCD domain and total synthesis. *Angewandte Chemie-International Edition*, 43, 4318–4324.

75. Nicolaou, K. C., Frederick, M. O., Petrovic, G., Cole, K. P., and Loizidou, E. Z., 2006. Total synthesis and confirmation of the revised structures of azaspiracid-2 and azaspiracid-3. *Angewandte Chemie-International Edition*, 45, 2609–2615.

76. Kilcoyne, J., Twiner, M., McCarron, P., Giddings, S. D., Hess, P., and Miles, C. O., 2013. Structural elucidation and toxicity of a unique azaspiracid isolated from shellfish (*Mytilus edulis*). Manuscript in preparation.

77. Yanagi, T., Murata, M., Torigoe, K., and Yasumoto, T., 1989. Biological activities of semisynthetic analogs of dinophysistoxin-3, the major diarrhetic shellfish toxin. *Agriculture and Biological Chemistry*, 53, 525–529.

78. FSAI, 2006. Risk assessment of azaspiracids (AZAs) in shellfish. A Report of the Scientific Committee of the Food Safety Authority of Ireland (FSAI), Dublin, Ireland, August 2006, 39 pp.

79. Hess, P., Grune, B., Anderson, D. B. et al., 2006. Three Rs approaches in marine biotoxin testing—The report and recommendations of a joint ECVAM/DG SANCO workshop (ECVAM workshop 55). *Alternatives to Laboratory Animals*, 34, 193–224.

80. Volmer, D. A., Brombacher, S., and Whitehead, B., 2002. Studies on azaspiracid biotoxins. I. Ultrafast high-resolution liquid chromatography/mass spectrometry separations using monolithic columns. *Rapid Communications in Mass Spectrometry*, 16, 2298–2305.

81. Draisci, R., Palleschi, L., Ferretti, E. et al., 2000. Development of a method for the identification of azaspiracid in shellfish by liquid chromatography-tandem mass spectrometry. *Journal of Chromatography*, 871, 12–21.

82. Furey, A., Brana-Magdalena, A., Lehane, M. et al., 2002. Determination of azaspiracids in shellfish using liquid chromatography/tandem electrospray mass spectrometry. *Rapid Communications in Mass Spectrometry*, 16, 238–242.

83. King, R., Bonfiglio, R., Fernandez-Metzler, C., Miller-Stein, C., and Olah, T., 2000. Mechanistic investigation of ionization suppression in electrospray ionization. *Journal of the American Society for Mass Spectrometry*, 11, 942–950.

84. Fux, E., Rode, D., Bire, R., and Hess, P., 2008. Approaches to the evaluation of matrix effects in the liquid chromatography-mass spectrometry (LC-MS) analysis of three regulated lipophilic toxin groups in mussel matrix (*Mytilus edulis*). *Food Additives and Contaminants Part A-Chemistry Analysis Control Exposure & Risk Assessment*, 25, 1024–1032.

85. Kilcoyne, J. and Fux, E., 2010. Strategies for the elimination of matrix effects in the liquid chromatography tandem mass spectrometry analysis of the lipophilic toxins okadaic acid and azaspiracid-1 in molluscan shellfish. *Journal of Chromatography A*, 1217, 7123–7130.

86. Moroney, C., Lehane, M., Magdalena, A., Furey, A., and James, K. J., 2002. Comparison of solid-phase extraction methods for the determination of azaspiracids in shellfish by liquid chromatography-electrospray mass spectrometry. *Journal of Chromatography A*, 963, 353–361.

87. These, A., Scholz, J., and Preiss-Weigert, A., 2009. Sensitive method for the determination of lipophilic marine biotoxins in extracts of mussels and processed shellfish by high-performance liquid chromatography-tandem mass spectrometry based on enrichment by solid-phase extraction. *Journal of Chromatography A*, 1216, 4529–4538.

88. Gerssen, A., van Olst, E. H. W., Mulder, P. P. J., and de Boer, J., 2010. In-house validation of a liquid chromatography tandem mass spectrometry method for the analysis of lipophilic marine toxins in shellfish using matrix-matched calibration. *Analytical and Bioanalytical Chemistry*, 397, 3079–3088.

89. McNabb, P., Selwood, A. I., and Holland, P. T., 2005. Multiresidue method for determination of algal toxins in shellfish: Single-laboratory validation and interlaboratory study. *Journal of AOAC International*, 88, 761–772.

90. Stobo, L. A., Lacaze, J., Scott, A. C., Gallacher, S., Smith, E. A., and Quilliam, M. A., 2005. Liquid chromatography with mass spectrometry—Detection of lipophilic shellfish toxins. *Journal of AOAC International*, 88, 1371–1382.

91. Fux, E., McMillan, D., Bire, R., and Hess, P., 2007. Development of an ultra-performance liquid chromatography-mass spectrometry method for the detection of lipophilic marine toxins. *Journal of Chromatography A*, 1157, 273–280.

92. Villar-Gonzalez, A., Rodriguez-Velasco, M. L., and Gago-Martinez, A., 2011. Determination of lipophilic toxins by LC/MS/MS: single-laboratory validation. *Journal of AOAC International*, 94, 909–922.

93. EURL, 2011. EU Reference Laboratory Marine Biotoxins, website, http://www.aesan.msssi.gob.es/en/CRLMB/web/procedimientos_crlmb/crlmb_standard_operating_procedures.shtml (last accessed on February 21, 2013).

94. These, A., Klemm, C., Nausch, I., and Uhlig, S., 2011. Results of a European interlaboratory method validation study for the quantitative determination of lipophilic marine biotoxins in raw and cooked shellfish based on high-performance liquid chromatography-tandem mass spectrometry. Part I: Collaborative study. *Analytical and Bioanalytical Chemistry*, 399, 1245–1256.

95. Van den Top, H. J., Gerssen, A., McCarron, P., and van Egmond, H. P., 2011. Quantitative determination of marine lipophilic toxins in mussels, oysters and cockles using liquid chromatography-mass spectrometry: Inter-laboratory validation study. *Food Additives and Contaminants Part a-Chemistry Analysis Control Exposure & Risk Assessment*, 28, 1745–1757.

96. Lee, J. S., Yanagi, T., Kenma, R., and Yasumoto, T., 1987. Fluorometric determination of diarrhetic shellfish toxins by high-performance liquid chromatography. *Agriculture and Biological Chemistry*, 51, 877–881.

97. Quilliam, M. A., Gago-Martinez, A., and Rodriguez-Vazquez, J. A., 1998. Improved method for preparation and use of 9-anthryldiazomethane for derivatization of hydroxycarboxylic acids—Application to diarrhetic shellfish poisoning toxins. *Journal of Chromatography A*, 807, 229–239.

98. Forsyth, C. J., Xu, J. Y., Nguyen, S. T. et al., 2006. Antibodies with broad specificity to azaspiracids by use of synthetic haptens. *Journal of the American Chemical Society*, 128, 15114–15116.

99. Furey, A., Moroney, C., Magdalena, A., Fidalgo Saez, M. J., Lehane, M., and James, K. J., 2003. Geographical, temporal, and species variation of the polyether toxins, azaspiracids, in shellfish. *Environmental Science and Technology*, 37, 3078–3084.

100. Magdalena, A. B., Lehane, M., Moroney, C., Furey, A., and James, K. J., 2003. Food safety implications of the distribution of azaspiracids in the tissue compartments of scallops (*Pecten maximus*). *Food Additives and Contaminants*, 20, 154–160.

101. James, K. J., Furey, A., Lehane, M. et al., 2002. First evidence of an extensive northern European distribution of azaspiracid poisoning (AZP) toxins in shellfish. *Toxicon*, 40, 909–915.

102. Lehane, M., Brana-Magdalena, A., Moroney, C., Furey, A., and James, K. J., 2002. Liquid chromatography with electrospray ion trap mass spectrometry for the determination of five azaspiracids in shellfish. *Journal of Chromatography A*, 950, 139–147.

103. Hess, P., Swords, D., Clarke, D., Silke, J., and Mc Mahon, T., 2004. Confirmation of azaspiracids, okadaic acid and dinophysistoxins in phytoplankton samples from the West coast of Ireland by liquid chromatography-tandem mass spectrometry, in Steidinger, K. A., Landsberg, J. H., Tomas, C. R., and Vargo, G. A., Eds., *Proceedings of the 10th International Conference Harmful Algal Blooms*, St. Pete Beach, FL, October 21–25, 2002, pp. 252–254.

104. Vale, P., 2004. Is there a risk of human poisoning by azaspiracids from shellfish harvested at the Portuguese coast? *Toxicon*, 44, 943–947.

105. Taleb, H., Vale, P., Amanhir, R., Benhadouch, A., Sagou, R., and Chafik, A., 2006. First detection of azaspiracids in mussels in north west Africa. *Journal of Shellfish Research*, 25, 1067–1070.

106. Aasen, J. A. B., Torgersen, T., Dahl, E., Naustvoll, L.-J., and Aune, T., 2006. Confirmation of azaspiracids in mussels in Norwegian coastal areas, and full profile at one location, in Henshilwood, K., Deegan, B., McMahon, T. et al., Eds., *Proceedings of the 5th International Conference on Molluscan Shellfish Safety*, Galway, Ireland, June 14–18, 2004. The Marine Institute, Rinville, Oranmore, Galway, Ireland, pp. 162–169.

107. Hess, P., Nguyen, L., Aasen, J. et al., 2005. Tissue distribution, effects of cooking and parameters affecting the extraction of azaspiracids from mussels, *Mytilus edulis*, prior to analysis by liquid chromatography coupled to mass spectrometry. *Toxicon*, 46, 62–71.

108. Hess, P., McCarron, P., and Quilliam, M. A., 2007. Fit-for-purpose shellfish reference materials for internal and external quality control in the analysis of phycotoxins. *Analytical and Bioanalytical Chemistry*, 387, 2463–2474.

109. Quilliam, M. A., Reeves, K., MacKinnon, S. et al., 2004. Preparation of reference materials for azaspiracids, in *5th International Conference of Molluscan Shellfish Safety*, Galway, Ireland, June 14–18, 2004. Deegan, B., Butler, C., Cusack, C. K. et al., Eds., Marine Institute, Galway, Ireland, pp. 111–115.

110. NRCC, NRCC—Website on biotoxin CRMs—Overview, http://www.nrc-cnrc.gc.ca/eng/solutions/advisory/crm/biotoxin_index.html (accessed November 8, 2012.)

111. CIFGA, CIFGA-website: Marine biotoxin certified reference materials, http://www.cifga.es/index.php (accessed October 12, 2008.)

112. McCarron, P., Kotterman, M., de Boer, J., Rehmann, N., and Hess, P., 2007. Feasibility of gamma irradiation as a stabilisation technique in the preparation of tissue reference materials for a range of shellfish toxins. *Analytical and Bioanalytical Chemistry*, 387, 2487–2493.

113. McCarron, P., Giddings, S. D., Reeves, K., and Quilliam, M. A., 2011. NRC CRM-AZA-Mus, mussel tissue certified reference material for AZA toxins, CRMP Technical Report CRM-AZA-Mus-200603, National Research Council Canada, Halifax, Nova Scotia, Canada, NRCC publication # 54053.

114. McCarron, P., Emteborg, H., Nulty, C. et al., 2011. A mussel tissue certified reference material for multiple phycotoxins. Part 1: Design and preparation. *Analytical and Bioanalytical Chemistry*, 400, 821–833.

115. QUASIMEME, QUASIMEME-website: Laboratory performance studies, http://www.quasimeme.org/ (accessed November 8, 2012.)

28

Azaspiracids: Toxicology, Pharmacology, and Risk Assessment

Michael J. Twiner, Philipp Hess, and Gregory J. Doucette

CONTENTS

28.1 Introduction

Azaspiracids (AZAs) are a group of marine algal toxins produced by the small dinoflagellate *Azadinium spinosum*[1,2] that is closely related to *Amphidoma*.[3] This relatively new class of toxins was first identified in the 1990s following an outbreak of human illness in the Netherlands that was associated with ingestion of contaminated shellfish originating from Killary Harbour, Ireland. Although the symptoms were typical of diarrhetic shellfish poisoning (DSP) toxins such as okadaic acid (OA) and dinophysistoxins (DTXs), the levels of DSP toxins in these shellfish were well below the regulatory level. Over the next few years, it was established that the shellfish were contaminated with a unique marine toxin, originally named "Killary toxin" or KT-3.[4] Shortly thereafter, the toxin was renamed to AZA to more appropriately reflect its chemical structure: a cyclic amine, or aza group, with a tri-spiro assembly and carboxylic acid group.[4,5]

To date, over 20 AZA analogues have been identified in phytoplankton and shellfish.[5–12] Over the last 15 years, AZAs have been reported in shellfish from many coastal regions of western Europe,[13–19] northern Africa,[20,21] South America,[22,23] and North America[24] (M. Quilliam, pers. comm.). In addition, AZAs have been found in Japanese sponges[25] and Scandinavian crabs.[26] Not surprisingly, the global distribution of AZAs appears to correspond to the apparent widespread occurrence of *Azadinium*.[27–29] Empirical evidence is now available that unambiguously demonstrates the accumulation of AZAs in shellfish via direct feeding on AZA-producing *A. spinosum*.[30,31]

Whereas extensive study of this toxin class has been historically constrained by limited availability of purified material, these restraints are now less of an impediment due to advances in isolation and purification of AZAs from naturally contaminated shellfish[32] and to identification of the toxigenic organism *A. spinosum* coupled with its mass culture in bioreactors.[7] As such, certified reference standards of naturally produced AZA1–3 are now commercially available.[33] Although not yet realized for commercial purposes, limits on toxin supply may be further alleviated by advances in the organic total synthesis of AZA1[34] and AZA3 (C. Forsyth, pers. comm.). Accessibility to purified AZAs has led to rapid progress with respect to understanding AZA toxicology over the last few years. While certain characteristics of these toxins and their pharmacological effects have been summarized previously,[17,35–37] we feel the timing is appropriate to critically review the advances in AZA research with an emphasis on their toxicology, pharmacology, and risk assessment.

28.2 Human Health Effects

Unlike many of the other well-described marine phycotoxins, much less is known about the AZA toxin class. Similar to DSP toxins, human consumption of AZA-contaminated shellfish can result in severe acute symptoms that include nausea, vomiting, diarrhea, and stomach cramps.[17] To date, six human AZA poisoning (AZP) events have been confirmed (Table 28.1), but it is quite possible, due to the similarity of

TABLE 28.1

Confirmed Cases of AZP

Event	Location of AZP	Date	Implicated Food Source	Amount Consumed	Area of Production	Number of Illnesses Recorded	[AZA$_{total}$] (µg/g)	[AZA1] (µg/g)	[AZA2] (µg/g)	[AZA3] (µg/g)	Comments	References
Confirmed AZP	The Netherlands	Nov-95	Mussels (*M. edulis*)	Not recorded	Killary Harbour, Ireland	8	1.43[a,b]	1.14[a,b]	0.23[a,b]	0.06[a,b]		[17,37,39]
Confirmed AZP	Arranmore, Ireland	Sep/Oct-97	Mussels (*M. edulis*)	"As few as 10–12 mussels"	Arranmore Island, Ireland	Estimated 20–24 (8 seen by a doctor)	30[c]	Present	Present	Present	Equivalent to ~6 µg/g whole mussel meat; AZA4,5 were also present.	[17,37]
Confirmed AZP	Ravenna, Italy	Sep-98	Mussels (*M. edulis*)	Not recorded	Clew Bay, Ireland	10	1.0[c]	0.5[c]	0.06[c]	0.44[c]		[17,37]
Confirmed AZP	France	Sep-98	Mussels (*M. edulis*)	Not recorded	Bantry Bay, Ireland	Estimated 20–30	1.1–1.5[a]	Present	Present	Present	Were tested for DSP toxins using MBA and deemed "safe."	[17,37]
Confirmed AZP	United Kingdom	Aug-00	Frozen mussels (*M. edulis*)	Not recorded	Bantry Bay, Ireland	12–16	0.85[a]	Present	Present	Present		[17,37]
Confirmed AZP	France	Apr-08	Frozen mussels (*M. edulis*)	Not recorded	Ireland	"Large outbreak"	>0.16[a]					[37,40]
Confirmed AZP	United States	Jul-08	Frozen mussels (*M. edulis*)	*ca.* 113 and 340 grams	Bantry Bay, Ireland	2	0.086–0.244[a]	Present	Present	Present	~150 tonnes were voluntarily destroyed; AZA6 was also present.	[41]

[a] Whole mussel meat.

[b] Sampled in April 1996 (5 months after event).

[c] Digestive glands/hepatopancreas.

symptoms observed for people with DSP or other types of food poisoning (e.g., bacterial enteritis), that many more undocumented events have occurred. Coincidently, each of the confirmed AZP events have been traced to contaminated Irish shellfish (*Mytilus edulis*).

The first confirmed AZP event occurred in November 1995. Mussels harvested from Killary Harbour, Ireland, were exported to the Netherlands, resulting in eight people falling ill with DSP-like symptoms of gastrointestinal (GI) illness, including nausea, vomiting, severe diarrhea, and stomach cramps.[4,5,37,38] The absence of known DSP toxins OA and DTX-2 led to the discovery and identification of a novel etiological agent, temporarily called KT-3 before being renamed to AZA1.[5] Mussels collected from the same area 5 months after the event were shown to contain (in µg/g whole meat) AZA1 (1.14), AZA2 (0.23), and AZA3 (0.06).[11,39]

In September/October 1997, as few as 10–12 AZA-contaminated mussels were consumed by individuals in the Arranmore Island region of Donegal, Ireland. At least 20–24 people were believed to have been exposed to AZAs in this event, but only 8 sought medical attention. Symptoms included nausea, vomiting, and diarrhea for 2–5 days prior to full recovery. Analysis of the shellfish revealed five AZA analogues, AZA1–5, with most of the toxin concentrated in the digestive glands[10,11] at levels exceeding 30 µg/g (estimated at 6 µg/g whole mussel meat).[37] The AZAs persisted in the mussels at elevated levels for at least 8 months.[37]

In September 1998, mussels exported from Clew Bay, Ireland, to Ravenna, Italy, were consumed and 10 people fell victim to AZP with typical GI symptoms. Digestive glands were shown to contain ~1 µg/g AZA_{total} with three AZA analogues present (in µg/g digestive gland): AZA1 (0.5), AZA2 (0.06), and AZA3 (0.44).[37]

Also in September 1998, a large shipment of mussels from Bantry Bay, Ireland, was sent to France, resulting in an estimated 20–30 human illnesses due to AZP. Ironically, these shellfish had been tested ahead of time and deemed safe according to the DSP mouse bioassay (MBA); however, it was later determined that the DSP MBA is susceptible to false negatives for the AZA toxins. Coincidently, the French government imposed an embargo on the import of Irish shellfish for most of 1999. Follow-up analysis of the shellfish by liquid chromatography coupled to mass spectrometry (LC/MS) determined that high levels of AZA were present (up to 1.5 µg/g whole meat).[37]

In August 2000, between 12 and 16 people from various regions (Warrington, Aylesbury, Isle of Wight, Sheffield) of the United Kingdom were intoxicated following the consumption of frozen, precooked mussels that originated from Bantry Bay, Ireland. Symptoms included nausea, diarrhea, abdominal pain, and cramps.[39] These mussels were also deemed safe for human consumption based on results from MBAs; however, LC/MS analysis determined the presence of AZA1–3 in an uneaten portion from this same batch. Toxin concentrations were 0.85 µg/g shellfish meat (not including the digestive gland), which likely represented an underestimation of the total concentration.[37]

No other AZP events occurred until 2008 when there were two events. In April 2008, many people in France fell ill due to AZP following the consumption of contaminated frozen, precooked mussels from Ireland. This event was categorized by the French government as a "large outbreak" that paralleled a separate incident of salmonellosis.[40] Unfortunately, these contaminated shellfish were accidently released onto the consumer market after being identified as containing unsafe levels of AZA toxins and stored in quarantine.[37]

The second 2008 AZP event occurred in the United States in July. Frozen, precooked mussels from Bantry Bay, Ireland, were exported and intoxicated two people. It is estimated that each person ate between 113 and 340 g of shellfish. Within 5 h following the meal, each person experienced abdominal heaviness, vomiting (5–15 times), and diarrhea for up to 30 h. Analysis of similar products with the same lot number revealed the presence of AZA1–3 with up to 0.244 µg AZA_{total}/g tissue.[41] As a result of this event, over 150 tonnes of commercial product were removed from the market and voluntarily destroyed by the manufacturer (R. Dickey, pers. comm.).

Due to the limited epidemiological data available from the previously mentioned human AZP events, nearly all information regarding AZA toxicology has been obtained from controlled in vitro and in vivo experiments. Many of these efforts have been directed towards assessing the risk of AZA consumption in contaminated shellfish and accompanied by intensive, wide-ranging studies aimed at identifying the molecular target(s) of AZA.

28.3 Organismal Effects

28.3.1 Clinical and Behavioral Effects

28.3.1.1 Intraperitoneal Exposure

During the initial AZP intoxication event in 1995 involving shellfish from Killary Harbour, Ireland (see Table 28.1), mussel extracts tested highly positive in the DSP rat bioassay and the DSP MBA.[38] However, in the absence of significant levels of OA or DTX2, and mouse symptomatology atypical of DSP or YTX toxins,[4,42] AZA1 was subsequently identified in these samples.[5] Mice exposed to mussel extracts containing AZA via intraperitoneal (i.p.) injection exhibited "neurotoxin-like" symptoms characterized by sluggishness, respiratory difficulties, spasms, progressive paralysis, and death within 20–90 min.[4,38,43]

More recently, conjugates of AZA1 bound to the carrier protein keyhole limpet hemocyanin (KLH) were i.p. injected into mice as a part of an immunization protocol for antibody development and all animals (*n* = 4) died unexpectedly within ~24 h.[44] This result was dose dependent but could not be explained as a function of unbound AZA1 or the KLH carrier protein itself. Bovine serum albumin (BSA) conjugated to AZA1 did not induce lethality. Future structure–activity relationship (SAR), metabolism, and/or degradation studies may help explain this phenomenon.

28.3.1.2 Oral Exposure

Mice receiving moderate oral doses of AZA1 (100–300 µg/kg) generally display little to no signs of clinical disease.[45,46] However, mice surviving higher doses (420–780 µg/kg) developed dose- and time-dependent signs of clinical disease (i.e., depression and reduced movement) but without indications of diarrhea. After 24 h, all surviving mice were greatly depressed and did not move from sternal recumbency (i.e., remained lying down on chest).[47] Similarly, many mice receiving small (20 or 50 µg/kg), repeated (>30) doses of AZA1 exhibited extreme weakness that necessitated them being sacrificed in order to prevent further suffering. Repeated doses of 1 or 5 µg/kg did not induce weakness or illness.[48]

28.3.2 Weight Changes

Body and organ weight changes appear to be common in mice exposed to AZA1. Following a single oral dose of AZA1 (420–780 µg/kg), loss of total body weight over 24 h in treated mice ranged from −3% to −9%, whereas control mice gained 2%.[47] Concurrently, stomach weight (including the contents) increased four-fold over controls, suggesting prolonged food retention possibly due to reduced GI tract mobility.[47] Similarly, in mice repeatedly exposed to low doses of AZA1, there were reductions in the weight of various individual tissues (heart, liver, kidney, spleen, thymus) that were manifested as a 33.5%–31.4% whole body weight loss.[48] At 24 h following exposure to higher concentrations of AZA1 (500 µg/kg), mouse livers had increased in weight by 38%.[49]

28.3.3 Toxicokinetics

28.3.3.1 Absorption and Distribution

Until recently, it was not known whether the AZAs were absorbed from the GI tract and systemically distributed.[17] Indications in shellfish suggested that the molecules were biologically mobile, possibly due to their zwitterionic properties[50] and all pathological indications in previous in vivo studies suggested that an active molecule was inducing toxicological effects towards multiple internal organs.[48,49] These suspicions have now been confirmed via murine uptake and distribution studies that definitively demonstrate that AZA1 is absorbed and systemically distributed (Figure 28.1).[45–47] Animal sacrifices at 1 day following a single dose (100–300 µg/kg) illustrate that most of the AZA (AZA1 was used for exposure and AZA1–3 were analyzed by LC–MS/MS) was retained within the tissues of the various sections of the GI tract (i.e., stomach > duodenum > jejunum > ileum > colon) with internal organs receiving smaller

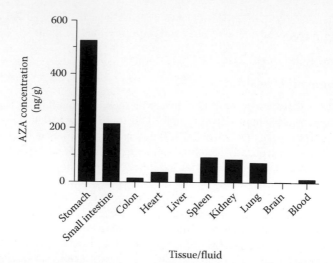

FIGURE 28.1   The uptake and distribution of AZA1 in mice at one day following oral exposure. (Data kindly provided by Aasen, J.A. et al., *Toxicon*, 57, 909, 2011; Norwegian School of Veterinary Science, Oslo, Norway.)

proportions of the AZA dose (spleen > kidney > lung > heart > liver > blood > brain (trace)) (Figure 28.1). After 7 days, the tissues of the GI tract contained low amounts of AZA, whereas levels in the kidneys, spleen, and lungs were still elevated.

   Absorption and distribution of AZAs following oral exposure (~240 µg AZA/kg body weight) has also been demonstrated in a minipig study. Twenty-four hours post-exposure, a minipig was sacrificed and tissues were quantitatively assessed for AZAs by LC–MS/MS analysis. The highest concentrations of known AZA analogues were found in the stomach and colon contents with detectable levels in the blood, feces, and liver (J. Geraghty, unpubl. data).

28.3.3.2 Metabolites

To date, very little is known about AZA metabolism in vivo. However, some progress has been made through a recent minipig study. The orally exposed minipig absorbed and distributed (see earlier) the AZAs with some indication of metabolism. Most notably, the AZA toxin ratio in the colon contents had changed whereby the administered analogues, AZA1–3, only made up ~50% of the profile with the other 50% predominantly AZA8 and AZA10. Furthermore, additional evidence suggested the presence of phase II conjugation metabolites (J. Geraghty, unpubl. data).

28.3.3.3 Half-Lives and Bioavailability

As noted in Section 28.3.3.1, AZA1 absorption and systemic distribution following ingestion have been confirmed in murine and minipig models. Nonetheless, there are few, if any, published data available on the half-life of AZAs in mammalian blood following oral exposure. A recent preliminary experiment involving oral administration of 230 µg AZA_{total} (AZA1:AZA2:AZA3 = 1.0:0.8:0.6)/kg to a single minipig has provided some initial insights over the first 24 h post-exposure (G. Doucette, unpubl. data). Results demonstrated rapid uptake of AZAs into blood, with toxin detected within 30 min (first time point) of consuming AZA-contaminated feed. In contrast, elimination of AZAs from the blood was considerably slower, with toxin remaining near initially measured (i.e., 30 min) levels at the final 24 h time point. This level was about half the maximum concentration reported, which was achieved at 4 h. Toxicokinetic/toxicodynamic modeling demonstrated that the rate of AZA1 entry into blood was ~55-fold the rate of elimination over this 24 h experiment. The half-life estimated for elimination of AZA1 from blood was ~24 h, although a considerably longer time course will be required to determine the time required for complete elimination. Interestingly, the AZA1:AZA2 ratio in blood was almost three-fold higher than in the contaminated feed, suggesting that AZA1 and AZA2 appear to be differentially absorbed from the GI tract and/or eliminated from blood.

In terms of bioavailability, the evidence presented earlier for murine and minipig models confirms that purified AZAs presented orally by either gavage or contaminated feed, respectively, are indeed absorbed into the bloodstream for distribution to various tissues and organs. However, in the case of naturally AZA-contaminated shellfish, questions of bioavailability following ingestion still remain. Specifically, the shellfish matrix appears to protect AZAs from acidic pH and enzyme activity (i.e., pepsin) reflective of the stomach's conditions,[51] presumably as a result of the toxins being bound to matrix components (e.g., proteins, liposomes). In fact, AZA–protein interactions in naturally contaminated blue mussel were confirmed recently by Nzoughet et al.,[52] who documented the presence of four proteins in the hepatopancreas of AZA-contaminated material but not of nontoxic controls.[53] Notably, AZAs (>10 ng/mL AZA1) were detected in native PAGE gel slices containing several of these proteins (~10 μg total protein loaded; slices eluted in 0.15 mL MeOH). Three of these proteins shared respective homologies with superoxide dismutase, cathepsin D, and glutathione S-transferase P, enzymes associated with response to xenobiotics or carcinogenic agents. Clearly, additional experiments involving ingestion of AZA-contaminated shellfish material will be required to more accurately assess toxin bioavailability *in matrix*, as well as subsequent metabolism in mammalian systems.

28.3.4 Lethal Doses

28.3.4.1 Intraperitoneal Injection

The i.p. minimum lethal dose of partially purified AZA1 (i.e., KT-3) was originally determined to be 150 μg/kg.[4] The i.p. minimum lethal doses of AZA2 (8-methylazaspiracid) and AZA3 (22-demethyl-AZA) were 110 and 140 μg/kg, respectively,[11] suggesting higher potency relative to AZA1. On the other hand, the more polar AZA4 and AZA5 (hydroxylated versions of AZA3) were less potent with lethal dose values of 470 and < 1000 μg/kg, respectively.[10] Assuming equivalent degrees of purity, the order of AZA analogue potency by i.p. injection appears to be AZA2 > AZA3 > AZA1 > AZA4 > AZA5, which has since been used for toxic equivalence factor (TEF) determination and application for regulatory purposes.[54]

28.3.4.2 Acute Oral

Much progress has been made on assessing the in vivo effects of AZA. In the original studies, crude extracts of AZA1 (>900 μg/kg) were given orally to mice via gastric intubation.[55] At six-fold the i.p. injected dose that induced 100% mortality, all mice survived with no clinical signs after 24 h. Subsequent studies using purified material have further detailed the effects of AZA1 on mice following oral exposure.[45–47,49] Studies by Ito[49] using male ICR mice orally administered single doses of AZA1 ranging from 300 to 900 μg/kg demonstrated the lethal nature of AZA1, whereby all mice receiving 900 μg/kg AZA1 had to be sacrificed prior to the end of the 24 h experiment. Although there was not a clear dose–response, likely due to insufficient experimental replicates, an approximate oral minimum lethal dose with purified AZA1 was estimated at 500 μg/kg. Similarly, separate studies by Aasen et al.[45] and Aune et al.[47] using female NMRI mice demonstrated that doses of 100–540 μg/kg were insufficient to kill any of the tested animals but doses above 600 μg/kg resulted in some mortality. The experimentally determined LD_{10} and LD_{50} levels (with 95% confidence intervals) were 570 (435–735) and 775 (596–1055) μg/kg, respectively.[47]

28.3.4.3 Repeated Oral

In another series of in vivo exposure studies, mice were orally administered low, repeated doses of AZA1 (1–50 μg/kg) and then monitored for recovery.[48] Ten percent of the mice survived the 40 repeated injections at the highest dose (50 μg/kg), as the other 90% were sacrificed due to extreme weakness, and 30% of the mice in the 20 μg/kg treatment group were also sacrificed early. In separate experiments, severe injuries were induced by two repeated doses of 250, 300, 350, or 450 μg/kg, 2 days apart, and recovery was monitored for up to 90 days. Of the 16 mice receiving 450 μg/kg, 11 died prior to the second dose, suggesting a revised minimum oral lethal dose of <450 µg/kg. In fact, some mice died at 250 and 300 µg/kg, but only two replicate mice were available for each dose.

28.3.5 Histological/Pathological

28.3.5.1 Intraperitoneal Exposure

I.p. injection of mice with a lethal dose (>150 µg/kg) caused swelling of the stomach and liver concurrent with reduction in size/weight of the thymus and spleen.[55] There were vacuole formation and fatty acid accumulation in the hepatocytes, parenchymal cell pyknosis in the pancreas, dead lymphocyte debris in the thymus and spleen, and erosion and bleeding in the stomach. The pathological changes induced by AZA were stated to be unique from those induced by DSP, PSP, and amnesic shellfish poisoning (ASP) toxins. This was an important observation at the time before the AZAs were identified as a new toxin class.

28.3.5.2 Acute Oral

The most common pathological effect of AZA1 following oral exposure is degradation of the lining surrounding the upper small intestine.[45,47–49] Single-dose studies in mice examined 24 h following oral intubation of AZA1 (100–300 µg/kg) clearly demonstrated shortened villi, elongated crypts, and exfoliation of epithelial layer in villi along the lumen of the duodenum[45] (Figure 28.2). In addition, there were indications of edema, hyperemia, infiltration of neutrophils (>five-fold more than controls), and single-cell necrosis/apoptosis with apoptotic bodies in the lamina propria (Figure 28.2c).[45,47] These pathological effects were dose dependent but were completely healed after 7 days recovery.

Similarly, Ito et al.[49] observed sporadic degeneration and erosion of the small intestinal microvilli, vacuole degeneration in epithelial cells, and atrophy of the lamina propria at 4 h following exposure to 300 µg/kg AZA1. Higher doses of AZA1 (500–700 µg/kg) revealed progressive intestinal erosion at 8 h and continued atrophy of the lamina propria at 24 h. However, at 24 h, there were fewer degenerating epithelial cells in the microvilli, suggesting some signs of recovery. Compared to mice orally exposed to OA, the damage elicited by AZA1 was slower in onset with much longer times required for recovery.[49] Many of these same effects were also observed in mice treated with synthetic AZA1 but with slightly reduced potency (i.e., minimum lethal dose >700 µg/kg vs. ~500 µg/kg with natural AZA1).[56] Unfortunately, percent purities were not available.

Despite known uptake and systemic distribution of AZA1 following oral exposure, only limited and less severe histopathological changes have been observed in other internal organs/tissues. The stomach, which has consistently been shown to contain the highest AZA concentrations following oral exposure,[45] was pathologically normal. However, there was a dramatic increase in food retention suggesting localized constipation.[45,47] Moderate doses of AZA1 (100–300 µg/kg) resulted in the liver being abnormally pale in coloration,[47] which may be the result of fatty acid droplet accumulation.[49] Higher doses (500–700 µg/kg)

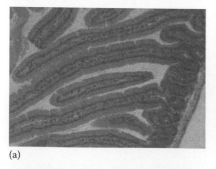 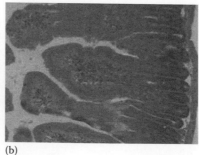 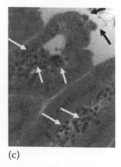

(a)   (b)   (c)

FIGURE 28.2 Representative micrographs of duodenum from mice orally exposed to (a) vehicle or (b and c) AZA1 (300 µg/kg) examined at 24 h. (b) In exposed animals, the villi of the small intestine were shortened and broader than normal and with an increased number of cells in the lamina propria. (c) A large fraction of these cells were neutrophils and some apoptotic cells were also detected (white arrows). There was increased exfoliation of epithelial cells in the tips of the villi (black arrows) and subepithelial vacuolation. (Images kindly provided by Aasen, J. and Espenes, A., Norwegian School of Veterinary Science, Oslo, Norway.)

increased liver weight by 38%. There were time- and dose-dependent effects on the number of necrotic lymphocytes in the thymus, spleen, and the Peyer's patches of the small intestine, which was supported by quantification of the number of non-granulocytes (lymphocytes, monocytes, macrophages) in the spleen. AZA1 treatments of 600 and 700 µg/kg resulted in a 33% decrease in the number of non-granulocytes, which were primarily T and B lymphocytes.[49] There were no reported histological changes associated with the kidney, heart, lung, and brain.[45,47,49]

28.3.5.3 Repeated Oral

Limited data are available for repeated oral exposures to AZA. In the study by Ito et al.,[48] mice that were orally administered repeated doses of AZA1 exhibited pathological effects similar, only more dramatic, to those outlined earlier for single oral doses. Reductions in the weight of various tissues (heart, liver, kidney, spleen, thymus) appeared to be manifested by up to a 35% whole body weight loss. These effects were likely due to reduced nutrient absorption in the eroded GI tract. Similar to the effects of higher oral AZA1 doses,[45,47–49] the GI tract displayed obvious signs of erosion (i.e., edema, shortened and damaged microvilli) and an accumulation of gas.[48] As well, there were typical effects on the spleen and thymus. However, low-dose repeated exposures of AZA1 caused mild liver inflammation with virtually no effects on liver fatty acid content. Lung tissue displayed signs of interstitial inflammation and bleeding. Although not observed in a dose-dependent manner, there was a low incidence of lung tumor formation (20% incidence; 4 out of 20 mice in the 20 and 50 µg/kg treatment groups) and hyperplasia (enlargement of the tissue due to accumulation of cells) in the stomach (60% incidence; 6 out of 10 mice in the 20 µg/kg treatment group). Lung tumors were only observed after 2–3 months into the recovery phase and were S-100 reactive.[48] S-100 proteins are biomarkers of many cancerous and inflamed tissues[57] and coincidently the gene for these proteins was shown to be differentially expressed in T lymphocytes following exposure to AZA1.[58]

Similar pathological effects were observed in mice orally administered two doses of AZA1 and then monitored for recovery.[48] Recovery times for each tissue were as follows: liver = 7 days, lymphoid = 10 days, lung = 56 days, and the stomach = >12 weeks. During the recovery, there were also signs of bacterial infection in the stomach lining. Although these findings of protracted recovery times are likely a function of tissue-specific turnover time and the rates of AZA1 metabolism and elimination, they correspond with the in vitro findings of the irreversible nature of AZA1-induced cytotoxicity[59] and persistence in various internal organs.[45] It is interesting that these recovery time data slightly contrast with the pathological data presented by Aune et al.[47] and Aasen et al.[45]; however, these more recent studies only assessed the animals after a single dose (100–300 µg/kg) of AZA1.

Repeated treatments of mice with 1 or 5 µg/kg displayed significant GI effects, suggesting that the lowest observable adverse effect level (LOAEL) for AZA1 is on the order of 1 µg/kg in mice. This is comparable with the LOAELs estimated in humans of *ca.* 0.4–2 µg/kg body weight in the two risk assessments that were conducted by the Food Safety Authority of Ireland (FSAI).[60,61]

28.3.6 Structure–Activity Relationship Studies

Limited in vivo SAR data are available for the AZAs. From the initial i.p. experiments, whereby minimum lethal doses were used as the endpoint, it was determined that the relative order of AZA analogue potency was AZA2 > AZA3 > AZA1 > AZA4 > AZA5.[5,10,11] These data suggest that methylation at C8 and C22 plays a minor role in determining relative potency; however, hydroxylation of the AZA molecule, thereby increasing its polarity, results in a more dramatically reduced potency. Future studies are necessary to determine the oral LD_{50} values for at least AZA1, AZA2, and AZA3.

Studies utilizing products from the organic synthesis of AZA1[34,62] have also yielded very valuable SAR information. Twelve truncated AZA1 analogues and one AZA1 diastereomer (C_1-C_{20}-*epi*-AZA1) were tested in mice via oral and/or i.p. exposure.[56] The truncated AZA1 analogues exhibited no signs of toxicity, whereas the diastereomer was at least a three- to four-fold less potent (*ca.* > 3000 µg/kg) relative to the parent AZA1. These synthetic AZA analogues induced virtually no morphological effects on the GI system, suggesting that stereospecific orientation and the full length of the AZA molecule are required for toxicity.[56,63]

28.3.7 Effects of Toxin Mixtures

When assessing toxin profiles in shellfish, it is not uncommon to find the presence of multiple algal toxin classes in the same animal. As such, there is escalating concern about the potential toxicological effects of mixtures of these various toxins towards human and environmental health—particularly if these toxin combinations prove to behave synergistically. Regarding the AZA class, it is not uncommon to find these toxins in shellfish that are also contaminated with pectenotoxins, yessotoxin (YTX), and/or the DSP toxins OA and DTX-2.

The first attempts to address these questions were performed in vivo using orally exposed mice. Although combined exposures of PTX2 (5 mg/kg) and AZA1 (200 µg/kg) did not elicit any clinical symptoms in mice, there was a substantial increase in the absorption/distribution of PTX2 in mice exposed to PTX2/AZA1 versus PTX2 alone. This was particularly evident in the lung, blood, spleen, kidney, and liver.[64] The combination also induced a slightly greater degree of pathological change in the small intestine (i.e., enhanced edema in the lamina propria and fusion of villi) but not in any other tissue/organ. However, the recent European Food Safety Authority (EFSA) opinion suggests this enhanced effect is of low concern.[65]

Combination studies with YTX and AZA were particularly warranted since YTX has low oral toxicity (but is highly toxic when exposed via i.p. injection) and AZA1 is well known to disrupt the epithelial barrier of the GI tract, potentially resulting in enhanced YTX absorption. However, this hypothesis was not experimentally supported as levels of YTX in the various organs were not affected by the presence of AZA1 with the lone exception of the stomach tissues, which far exceeded (up to 117-fold more) the levels observed in mice exposed to YTX alone.[46] Similarly, the combined exposure of AZA1 with YTX did not enhance the absorption of AZA1. Combined exposures of YTX (1 or 5 mg/kg) with AZA1 (200 µg/kg) did not elicit any clinical symptoms or cause any enhanced pathological changes in the small intestine and other organs including the heart.[46] As such, the most current EFSA opinion suggests that this combination is also of low concern.[66]

The combined effects of OA (780–880 µg/kg) and AZA1 (570 µg/kg) were assessed in vivo. These combinations did not enhance acute toxicity (lethality) or observable pathological changes in the small intestine beyond the effects that these toxins elicit on their own.[47] Furthermore, there were no significant pathological changes in various internal organs. Interestingly, absorption and distribution of the toxins when provided in combinations were altered. Most notably, each toxin reduced the absorption[47] of the other, suggesting an antagonistic effect of this toxin combination.

As a caveat, it should be noted that in all of the earlier cases, only acute toxicity was determined and these studies did not address the long-term effects of these toxin mixtures. For instance, OA is a known tumor promoter,[67] while the AZAs have shown both teratogenic[68] and carcinogenic potential[48] that may result in enhanced downstream teratogenicity and/or carcinogenicity over time.

28.3.8 Effects of AZAs and *Azadinium* on Various Organisms

28.3.8.1 Japanese Medaka

A few studies have been conducted using nonmammalian model organisms. As a model for maternal transfer of lipophilic substances, Japanese medaka fish were microinjected with small (pg) quantities of AZA1 and monitored throughout embryonic development.[68] Most notably, doses as small as 40 pg AZA1/egg delayed development, causing dose-dependent growth retardation, bradycardia, and reduced hatching success.

28.3.8.2 Crustaceans

Some toxicological studies have been performed using brine shrimp (*Artemia salina*). These crustaceans are commonly used for toxicological assessments of wastewater effluents. In this study, AZA1 was directly applied to the aqueous medium containing *A. salina* and observed over 24 h. At the end of the experiment, the surviving crustaceans were noticeably twitching and exhibited greatly reduced vertical mobility. AZA1 was shown to be moderately toxic to these organisms with a determined LD_{50} (at 24 h) of 178 ± 22 nM (mean $\pm$ SE) (Figure 28.3).

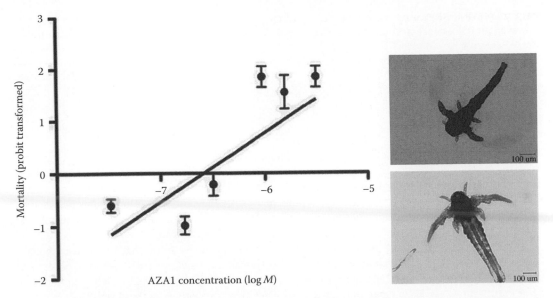

FIGURE 28.3 The effects of AZA1 the viability of brine shrimp (*A. salina*) after 24 h of continuous exposure. The calculated (mean ± SE) LD_{50} value was 178 ± 22 nM (unpubl. data). (Photo courtesy of S. Butler.)

28.3.8.3 Protozoa

Preliminary studies have also been performed on two strains of the protozoan parasite, *Plasmodium falciparum*, one of the species known to cause malaria in humans. AZA1 was shown to be highly potent towards both protozoan strains (D6 and W2) with a toxicity IC_{50} value of ~0.8 nM (unpubl. data).

28.3.8.4 Bacteria

During a study of protein biomarkers in naturally AZA-contaminated blue mussels (*M. edulis*), Nzoughet et al.[53] discovered the presence of a protein with homology to *Methylobacterium* or *Agrobacterium* flagellar proteins that were not detected in uncontaminated mussels. This finding led to the recent isolation of two *Methylobacterium* strains, one from AZA-contaminated mussels and the other from nontoxic mussels.[69] A *Hyphomicrobium* strain was also isolated from the toxic mussels using the same methanol-containing selective growth medium. Interestingly, supplementing growth medium of the two bacteria isolated from the toxic mussels with AZAs (AZA1, 356.5 nM; AZA2, 38.6 nM) significantly elevated biomass yields above those of control cultures receiving no AZAs. Conversely, yields of the strain originating from the nontoxic mussels were significantly depressed by AZAs relative to the same controls. In all cases, upon termination of the experiment, AZA-supplemented cultures contained ~1% of the total toxin added at the outset. The mechanism(s) by which AZAs specifically promote or depress the growth of these bacteria remains to be elucidated.

28.3.8.5 Shellfish

Recent experiments related to AZA accumulation in blue mussels (*M. edulis*) upon direct feeding with *A. spinosum* revealed slightly increased mussel mortality and negative effects on the thickness of mussel digestive gland tubules compared to nontoxic diet based on *Isochrysis* aff. *galbana* (*T-iso*).[31] A second experiment showed *A. spinosum* to have a significant effect on mussel feeding behavior compared to *T-iso*. Clearance rate was lowered by a factor of 6, feeding time activity by a factor of 5, total filtration rate by a factor of 3, and absorption rate decreased to negative values for the last day of exposure. These results show a negative effect of *A. spinosum* on blue mussel feeding activity and indicate a possible regulation of AZA uptake by decreasing filtration and increasing pseudofeces production. Consistent with physiological observations, AZA accumulation was observed during the first hours of the trial as less than 6 h of feeding were required to reach AZA concentration in mussel above the regulatory level. However, an AZA concentration of about 200 µg/kg did not increase further until the end of the study.[70]

28.4 Cellular Effects

28.4.1 Cytotoxicity

The AZAs are well-known cytotoxins with the original observations performed by Flanagan et al.[42,71,72] using HepG2 hepatoblastoma cells and human bladder carcinoma cells (ECV-304) exposed to contaminated crude mussel extracts. A multitude of additional studies have since confirmed these findings and shown that AZA1 is a strong cytotoxin that is capable of killing many different cell types from various mammalian sources in a time- and concentration-dependent manner. More recently, studies have also shown that AZA2 and AZA3 are also cytotoxins. A comprehensive list of tested cells is shown in Table 28.2.

Despite the fact that most of the cell lines tested are highly sensitive to the AZA toxins, a few have been identified as being relatively insensitive to AZA. Human mastocytoma cells displayed no signs of cytotoxicity to AZA1 or AZA2 at concentrations in excess of 1000 nM,[77] and HeLa cells were shown to be insensitive to AZA2 at concentrations up to 2300 nM.[24] The insensitivity of these cells lines may provide important clues pertaining to the mechanism of action of the AZA toxin class. The effects of AZA on the human colonic Caco-2 cell line are less clear. Caco-2 cells are often used as a model for studying intestinal drug transport[87] and/or transepithelial electrical resistance (TEER)[88] and were putatively chosen as an in vitro model to parallel the extensive intestinal effects that AZAs are known to have on mammals when tested in vivo.[45,46,48,49] Two investigations suggested that AZA1 has little to no effect on Caco-2 cells,[14,74] whereas two separate investigations have shown AZA1 to be somewhat cytotoxic.[59,76] Despite these different findings regarding cytotoxic endpoints, monolayers of Caco-2 cells exposed to AZA1 have shown significant reductions in TEER assays when exposed to low concentrations of AZA1 (i.e., 5 nM)[14,75] suggesting altered permeability and/or cellular function. Visual confirmation has demonstrated monolayer perturbations that result in a loss of electrical resistance across the epithelial cells, suggesting that even if the Caco-2 cells are not susceptible to an AZA1-induced cytotoxic response, they are sensitive to the effects of AZA1 on monolayer integrity. These observations are certainly corroborated by in vivo observations.[45,47–49]

One cell line in particular has been shown to particularly sensitive to the AZA toxins. Jurkat T lymphocyte cells are highly sensitive to the AZAs (AZA1, AZA2, and AZA3), demonstrating the time- and concentration-dependent effects as well as differences in AZA analogue potencies (Figure 28.4).[79] As such, this in vitro model has been helpful in ascertaining the SAR of the various AZA analogues.

During the many cytotoxicity experiments listed in Table 28.2, a variety of morphological effects have been observed. T lymphocytes cells initially responded to AZA1 by a reduction in membrane integrity, organelle protrusion concurrent with flattening of cells, and a retraction of their pseudopodia or lamellipodia.[73,79] This was followed by protracted cell lysis. Intriguingly, unique morphological differences were observed in T lymphocytes exposed to AZA1 versus AZA2 and AZA3. AZA1 caused a time- and concentration-dependent retraction of pseudopodia, whereas pseudopodia were not affected by AZA2 and AZA3 when tested at cytotoxic EC$_{50}$ concentrations. In leukemia cells, AZA2 caused DNA synthesis phase arrest.[24] In neuroblastoma cells, AZA1 induced cell rounding and detachment from adjacent cells.[59] At the subcellular level, disruption of the Golgi complex and an accumulation of vesicles have been reported.[78] At the cellular level, AZA1, AZA2, and two other semisynthetic analogues of AZA2 all induced gross morphological changes.[77] AZA1 is a potent cytotoxin towards primary cerebellar granular cells (CGCs),[80] neocortical cells,[85] and spinal cord neurons.[84] In CGCs, AZA-induced cytotoxicity was related to the activation of the c-Jun-N-terminal kinase (JNK),[81,83] whereby AZA1 exposure resulted in decreased neuronal volume that was protected by preincubation of the neurons with a JNK inhibitor (SP 600125), a chloride channel blocker (4,4-diisothiocyanatostilbene-2,2-disulfonic acid [DIDS]), and a Na$^+$–K$^+$-ATPase blocker (amiloride).[81,82] The effects of AZA1 and AZA2 on cytotoxicity (and other cellular indices) appear to be irreversible.[59,77,84,89] Experiments using human breast cancer cells and

TABLE 28.2

Overview of AZA Cytotoxicity

Cell Type	Cell Line	Source	Cytotoxic	EC$_{50}$ (nM)[a]			Method of Analysis[b]	References
				AZA1	AZA2	AZA3		
Bladder carcinoma	ECV-304	Human	Yes	Unknown			MTT	[40,71,72]
B lymphocyte	Raji	Human	Yes	1.6*			MTT	[73]
Breast cancer	MCF-7	Human	Yes	>1*			DNA content; cell number	[74]
Cervical carcinoma	HeLa	Human	No		>2300*		MTT	[24]
Cervical carcinoma	KB	Human	Yes	0.22*			MTT	M. Geiger and P. Hess, unpubl. data
Colon adenocarcinoma	Caco-2	Human	No	nd			DNA content	[74]
Colon adenocarcinoma	Caco-2	Human	No	nd			alamarBlue®	[14,75]
Colon adenocarcinoma	Caco-2	Human	Yes	2.3–2.6*			MTS	[76]
Embryonic kidney	HEK-293	Human	Yes	4.6*			MTT	[73]
Hepatoblastoma	HepG2	Human	Yes	Unknown			MTT	[42,71,72]
Lung epithelial	A547	Human	Yes	1.5*			MTT	[73]
Lung carcinoma	NCI-H460	Human	Yes	220*			Sulforhodamine B	[59]
Mastocytoma	HMC-1	Human	No	>1000*	>1000*		alamarBlue®	[77]
Monocyte	THP-1	Human	Yes	2.4*			MTT	[73]
Neuroblastoma	BE(2)-M17	Human	Yes	n.d.			Morphological	[59]
Neuroblastoma	BE(2)-M17	Human	Yes	<1*	<1*		alamarBlue®	[77]
Neuroblastoma	BE(2)-M17	Human	Yes	7.4–7.5*			MTS	[76]
Neuroblastoma	SH-SY5Y	Human	Yes	nd			Morphological	[78]
T lymphocyte	Jurkat E6–1	Human	Yes	1.1			G6PH	[58]
T lymphocyte	Jurkat E6–1	Human	Yes	3.5			MTT	[73]
T lymphocyte	Jurkat E6–1	Human	Yes	1.4–2.1	0.38	0.44	MTS	[76,79]
Cerebellar granule cells	Primary	Mouse	Yes	0.87			MTT	[80]
Cerebellar granule cells	Primary	Mouse	Yes	~3–5			MTT	[81]
Cerebellar granule cells	Primary	Mouse	Yes	nd			LDH	[80]
Cerebellar granule cells	Primary	Mouse	Yes	5.2–9.2			MTT	[82]
Cerebellar granule cells	Primary	Mouse	Yes		2.4–5.8		MTT	[83]

(continued)

TABLE 28.2 (continued)

Overview of AZA Cytotoxicity

Cell Type	Cell Line	Source	Cytotoxic	EC_{50} (nM)[a]			Method of Analysis[b]	References
				AZA1	AZA2	AZA3		
Frontal cortex	Primary	Mouse	No	>10			Action potentials	[84]
Leukemia cells	P388	Mouse	Yes		0.84*		MTT	[24]
Neocortical neurons	Primary	Mouse	Yes	42.7*	48*		LDH	[85]
Neuroblastoma	Neuro-2A	Mouse	Yes	2.3*		9.88*	MTT	[73]
	NG108–15	Mouse/rat	Yes	2–10.6			MTT	[86]
	Primary	Mouse	Yes	>10			DNA content	[74]
	Primary	Mouse	Yes	nd			Action potentials	[84]
	Clone-9	Rat	Yes	<1*	~1*		alamarBlue®	[77]
Neuroblastoma x glioma hybrid	GH$_4$C1	Rat	Yes	16.8			MTT	[7]
Skin fibroblasts								

Note: nd = values not determined and "unknown" indicates cytotoxicity induced by crude mussel extracts. Values designated with an asterisk (*) are EC_{50} values at 48 h or later.

[a] Effective concentration that results in 50% cell death at 24 h.

[b] MTT, MTS, and alamarBlue® are mitochondrial enzyme-dependent viability assays. Glucose-6-phosphate dehydrogenase (G6PH) and Lactose dehydrogenase (LDH) assays are based on the release of these cytosolic enzymes from intact cells.

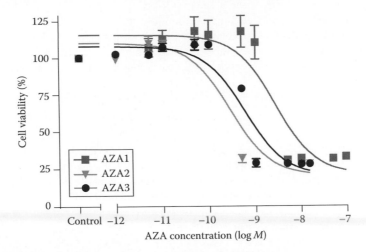

FIGURE 28.4   The cytotoxic effects of various AZA analogues on T lymphocyte cells.

mouse fibroblasts exposed to AZA1 have also demonstrated that the reductions in cellular proliferation and density are not unlike the actions elicited by YTX, raising the possibility of similar mechanisms of action for these two phycotoxin classes.[73,89]

28.4.2 Cytoskeletal Effects

The initial study documenting a link between the effects of AZA toxins and the cytoskeleton was performed by Roman et al.[91] and this topic has been recently reviewed.[92] In the initial study, AZA1 was shown to quantitatively decrease the levels of F-actin in neuroblastoma cells following AZA1 exposure. However, the concentrations of AZA1 required to induce these effects were very high ($\geq$7.5 μM), approximately 3 orders of magnitude higher than those required to induce cytotoxicity. Nonetheless, AZA exposure to a variety of cell types has been shown to induce various cytoskeletal effects. AZA1 has been shown to cause cytoskeletal disarrangement in T lymphocytes coincident with the retraction of the actin-filled pseudopodial structures.[73,79] Although actin levels were not quantified, it appeared as though F-actin was reorganized following AZA1 exposure. AZA2 and AZA3 also appeared to affect the intracellular organization of actin; however, the effects on the pseudopodia were unique to AZA1.[79] In neuroblastoma cells, AZA1 and an enantiomer of AZA1 induced distinguishable morphological and cytoskeletal (i.e., F-actin) effects following 24–48 h exposures.[59,89] Low concentrations of AZA1 appeared to induce retraction of the neurites (cellular projections) and cell rounding with simultaneous actin cytoskeleton disarrangement.[77] Stress fibers (actin microfilament bundles), which spread all over the cell cytosol in control cells, became concentrated in thick cell prolongations in AZA1-treated cells.[59] Proteomic profiling in neuroblastoma cells also revealed the plethora of cytoskeletal proteins that were differentially expressed as a result of AZA1 exposure.[78]

28.4.3 Cell Signaling

Many AZA analogues have been shown to cause a variety of effects on intracellular signaling molecules. In mammalian cells, cytosolic calcium is an important secondary messenger for a variety of pathways, including cell death,[93,94] and many marine toxins are known to modulate cytosolic calcium.[95–99] Human lymphocytes exposed to AZA1 (200 nM) were shown to elevate cytosolic calcium levels by *ca*. 50% above basal.[91] This response was shown to be sensitive to extracellular calcium, protein kinase C (PKC) activation, protein phosphatase (PP) inhibition, and cyclic adenosine monophosphate (cAMP) elevation. In addition, elevations in cAMP were sensitive to adenylate cyclase inhibition but insensitive to PP inhibition and extracellular calcium. cAMP is a second messenger that responds to membrane receptor activation and often functions to activate kinases. Similarly, AZA2 and AZA3 also elevated cytosolic calcium and cAMP,[100] whereas AZA4 did not affect basal cytosolic calcium levels but did have an inhibitory effect on calcium uptake from the extracellular medium.[101] In neocortical neurons, AZA1–3 each caused a concentration-dependent suppression of Ca^{2+} oscillations with EC_{50} values (in nM) of 445, 325, and 138, respectively.[85]

28.4.4 Apoptosis

Other phycotoxins such as the DSP toxins and ichthyotoxic compounds from *Heterosigma* are known inducers of apoptosis.[99,102] In vivo, there is an indication that mice orally exposed to AZA1 exhibited pyknosis (chromatin condensation indicative of apoptosis) in dead and dying lymphocyte cells within the spleen and thymus.[56] However, initial in vitro studies were inconclusive and suggestive of necrotic lysis. These observations were made based on cytotoxic morphological observations,[73] the absence of mitochondrial membrane potential changes in neuroblastoma cells,[91] and the absence of a sub-G1 population in leukemia cells exposed to AZA2. However, more recent evidence suggests that AZA1 does indeed induce apoptosis. In neuroblastoma cells, caspases were shown to be activated as determined using caspase-specific fluorescently tagged peptides,[89] which was recently confirmed in three cell types (T lymphocytes, neuroblastoma, and intestinal Caco-2).[76] In the most sensitive cell type, T lymphocytes, the initiator caspases 2 and 10 were upregulated, as were the effector caspases 3/7. Caspase activation appeared to be reversible through the use of a pan-caspase inhibitor. Furthermore, T lymphocyte cells were shown to have elevated levels of solubilized intracellular cytochrome c and fragmented DNA—both indicators of apoptosis.[76]

In neuroblastoma cells, cleavage of poly (ADP-ribose) polymerase (PARP) by activated caspases was detected with an antibody specific for a caspase-cleaved PARP fragment following protracted exposure to AZA1 and AZA2.[77] In a different neuroblastoma cell line, cellular ATP depletion and Bax protein upregulation by AZA1 are also supportive of an apoptotic mechanism.[78] In neocortical neurons, nuclear condensation was clearly evident and the percentage of apoptotic cells increased from 7% to 63% following 24 h exposure to 1 µM AZA1.[85] Caspase 3 activity was also upregulated by AZA1, AZA2, and AZA3. In CGCs, the cytoprotective effect of ouabain against AZA1-induced cytotoxicity suggests that the cytoprotective effect of anion channel blockers against AZA-induced cytotoxicity is mainly due to the preventive effect of these compounds against apoptosis.[82] Collectively, it is believed that the AZA toxins can induce both necrotic and apoptotic cell death.[76,85]

28.4.5 Membrane Changes

In addition to the growing body of literature on the effects of AZAs on cellular actin cytoskeleton and intracellular signaling pathways, there are many new and novel insights being generated by investigations into the effects of AZAs on membrane proteins such as claudins and cadherins. Claudins are integral membrane proteins involved in tight junction cell adhesion and are pivotal in paracellular transport of epithelial and endothelial cells,[103] with at least 24 claudin types known.[104] Caco-2 epithelial cells exposed to AZA1 exhibited an increase in soluble and insoluble fractions of claudin-2 protein expression and a decrease in insoluble claudin-3.[14] These responses appeared to be reversibly mediated by ERK 1,2, members of the mitogen-activated protein kinase (MAPK) family of proteins that commonly respond to extracellular stressors or signals.[105] Epithelial cadherins, or E-cadherins, are transmembrane adherens proteins that are involved in cell-to-cell adhesion.[104] In Caco-2 cells, a fragment representing an extracellular domain of E-cadherin was upregulated following exposure to AZA1.[74] Not unlike latrunculin A, AZA1 was shown to inhibit endocytosis of plasma membrane proteins, specifically E-cadherin, in three different cell types.[106] The membrane protein low-density lipoprotein receptor (LDLR) gene and protein were shown to be upregulated in T lymphocytes by as much as 3.5- and 2.5-fold, respectively.[58] This LDLR effect appears to be in response to decreased levels of intracellular cholesterol caused by AZA1. LDLR is a well-described membrane protein that internalizes via endocytosis cholesterol bound to low-density lipoproteins into the cell. Cholesterol is required to maintain membrane integrity and function and is intricately involved with tight junction and adherens proteins.[107]

28.4.6 Metabolism Studies

There are very few data available regarding in vitro metabolism of AZAs. In a study by Vilariño et al.,[77] various AZA analogues were confirmed to rapidly ($\leq$10 min) translocate into neuroblastoma cells and in the case of AZA2-methyl ester was progressively metabolized to AZA2. Biotinylated AZA2 was much more slowly metabolized back to AZA2.

28.4.7 Structure–Activity Relationships

Discerning the SARs for the AZA toxins has benefited tremendously from the recent availability of natural[33] and synthetic[62,108,109] AZA analogues. Although many structural fragments have been tested for their cytotoxicity and effects on cell signaling molecules (i.e., Ca^{2+}), it appears that most/all of the parent structure is necessary for conserved biological activity. Cytotoxicity experiments using a lung carcinoma cell line demonstrated that no AZA fragment or stereoisomer had any activity except for ABCD-*epi*-AZA-1 (where the ABCD domain is enantiomeric to AZA1), which conserved toxicity.[59] Similarly, two open E-ring AZA1 analogues and 12 fragments of AZA1 with varying stereochemistry tested for cytoskeletal effects and cytotoxicity were found to be inactive.[59,80,89] The full AZA molecule was also shown to be necessary for maintained cytotoxic activity and induction of caspase-3 in primary neocortical neurons; however, AZA analogues containing the FGHI domain attached to a phenyl glycine methyl ester moiety were inhibitors of Ca^{2+} oscillations (albeit at higher concentrations than those necessary to induce cytotoxicity), raising the possibility of multiple biological targets.[85]

Synthetic AZA1, AZA2, and AZA2 methyl ester each induced cytotoxicity, caused cytoskeletal alterations, and stimulated PARP in neuroblastoma cells with similar potencies and kinetics. As well, biotinylation at C1 of AZA2 also displayed similar toxicities in neuroblastoma cells collectively, suggesting that small (i.e., methylation) and large (i.e., biotin) moiety alterations at the C8 (AZA2) and C1 (AZA2 methyl ester and biotin AZA2) positions do not significantly alter the toxic potential of the AZAs.[77] However, as the authors point out, these data may be complicated by the metabolism of these analogues back to AZA2.

Corroborating in vivo data, the relative cytotoxic potencies of naturally isolated AZA1–3 towards T lymphocytes were AZA2 > AZA3 > AZA1,[79] providing further evidence that methylation at the C8 and C22 positions plays a role in the determining toxicity. To further support this trend, preliminary data suggest that AZA6 is equipotent with AZA2 (M. Twiner, unpubl. data). However, these relative potencies contradict those of Cao et al. (i.e., AZA3 > AZA2 ~ AZA1) in neocortical neurons[85] and require further clarification. Although the toxicophore of the AZA molecule has not yet been identified, in the T lymphocyte cytotoxicity model, the A/B/C ring region of the AZA molecule is highly important for maintained cytotoxicity. In this model, the AZA fragment *m/z* 716 (AZA1 missing A/B/C rings) was significantly less potent than AZA1 (~5-fold), whereas AZA *m/z* 816 (AZA1 missing C4/C5 alkene) was 5.5-fold more potent than AZA1.[110] Similarly, an AZA1 isomer (21-*epi*-AZA1) was 5.1-fold more potent than AZA1.[111] Semisynthetic hydrogenated AZA1 analogues, 4,5-dihydroAZA1 and 4,5,7,8-tetrahydroAZA1, were also tested. Both compounds were found to be approximately equipotent to AZA1 (M. Twiner, unpubl. data), suggesting that the C4/C5 alkene and the C7/C8 olefin bonds are not necessary for toxicological activity.

28.5 Molecular Effects

The molecular toxicology of the AZA toxins is an area of active research that seeks to ultimately identify the pharmacologic target(s) and mechanism(s) of action. Since the biological activities of AZAs and YTX appear to have some similar features, it has been proposed that the target(s) and/or biological effectors may be similar, thus mediating common responses with identical endpoints and cross talk at multiple levels.[90] Nonetheless, many potential targets for the AZA toxins have been investigated and these findings are outlined in the following texts.

28.5.1 Protein Phosphatase (PP) Inhibitors

Due to the similarities in GI symptoms that AZAs have in common with the DSP toxins (OA and DTXs), AZAs were originally classified together with the DSP toxins.[17] It was first postulated, with sound reasoning, that the most likely mechanism of action, similar to OA, was PP inhibition.[71] PPs are well-described regulators of cell signaling pathways where they act in a manner opposite to that of kinases by removing phosphate groups from proteins. The serine/threonine PPs are known to be inhibited by OA.[112] However, the effects of crude blue mussel extracts containing AZAs demonstrated no indication of PP1 enzyme inhibition[72] and a subsequent study utilizing the same assay format but with PP2A also found no effects of purified AZA1 on enzyme activity.[73] Furthermore, the AZAs have been subsequently tested against a non-receptor phospho-tyrosine PP (PTP-1B) and a T cell protein tyrosine phosphatase (TC-PTP) with no change in enzyme activity (M. Twiner, unpubl. data). Collectively, these data suggest that the AZA toxins are not PP inhibitors.

28.5.2 Actin Inhibition

Pectenotoxins are another class of phycotoxins that are known actin inhibitors.[113–115] Considering the extensive effects that AZAs are known to elicit on the cytoskeleton of various cell lines, the ability of AZAs to alter actin polymerization and/or depolymerization has been considered and shown to have no inhibitory effect on the polymerization or depolymerization of purified actin (M. Twiner, unpubl. data). This finding suggests that intracellular cytoskeletal rearrangements mediated by the AZA toxins are likely an indirect or downstream effect of a toxicological response.

28.5.3 Kinases

Not unlike PPs, kinases play a very important role in cell communication, signaling, metabolism, and death. In particular, MAPKs are present a multitude of different pathways and play crucial roles in the regulation of cell death and survival induced by several mechanisms. Although the AZA cytotoxicity response was not altered by inhibitors of extracellular signal-regulated kinase (ERK) or p38 MAPK, cytotoxicity was reduced in the presence of a JNK inhibitor[81,83] that corresponds to JNK activation.[82] However, this phenomenon may only be restricted to CGCs as it was not observed in neocortical neurons.[85] In a similar manner, the cAMP pathway and PKC and phosphatidylinositol 3-kinase were ruled out as possible targets.[81]

In a set of screening assays, a mixture of AZA1–3 (348 nM total) was tested against 40 different human kinases for changes in enzyme activity. These kinases were Abl, AMPKα1, CaMKIIβ, CaMKIIγ, CaMKIIδ, CaMKIV, CDK1/cyclinB, CDK2/cyclinA, CDK2/cyclinE, CDK3/cyclinE, CDK5/p25, CDK5/p35, CDK7/cyclinH/MAT1, CDK9/cyclin T1, Flt3, GSK3β, IR, LKB1, Lyn, MAPK1, MAPK2, p70S6K, PhKγ2, PKA, PKBβ, PKCα, PKCβI, PKCβII, PKCγ, PKCδ, PKCε, PKCη, PKCι, PKCμ, PKCθ, PKCζ, PKG1α, PKG1β, ROCK-II, and SAPK2a. Since enzyme activity was not altered, AZAs were ruled out as kinase inhibitors.

28.5.4 Neurotransmitter Release and G-Protein-Coupled Receptors

In cultured neurons, AZA was tested for its effects on neurotransmitter release. AZA1 did not have any effect on cholinergic, purinergic, or inotropic receptors (i.e., gamma-aminobutyric acid [GABA$_A$]).[82] However, the effects of AZA1 on bioelectrical activity of spinal cord neurons were enhanced in the presence of a GABA$_A$ inhibitor.[84] AZAs were also tested for agonistic (348 nM) and antagonistic (436 nM) activities towards 76 G-protein-coupled receptors (GPCRs) (M. Twiner, unpubl. data). The GPCRs tested were 5-HT1A, 5-HT2A, 5-HT2B, 5-HT2C, A1, A3, ADRA1A, ADRA1D, ADRA2A, ADRB1, ADRB2, AT1, BB2, BDKR2, BLT1, C5aR, CB1, CB2, CCK2, CCR1, CCR2B, CGRP1, CRF1, CX3CR1, CXCR1, CysLT1, D1, D2, D5, DP, EP2, EP3, ETA, ETB, FP, FPR1, GAL1, GnRH, GPR109a, GPR14, H1, H2, H3, IP1, LPA1, LPA3, M1, M2, M3, MC5, motilin, NK1, NK3, NMU1, NTR1, OPRD1, OPRK1, OPRM1, OT, OX1, P2Y1, PAC1, PAF, PK1, PRP, PTH1, S1P3, SST4, thrombin-activated PARs, TP, TSH, V1A, V2, VPAC1, VPAC2, and Y2. Since none of the GPCR activities were stimulated or inhibited, AZAs were ruled out as GPCR agonists or antagonists.

28.5.5 Ion Channels

There are ample data available that suggest the AZA toxins alter ion flux in various cell types. The AZAs have been shown to alter intracellular calcium flux,[85,91,100,116] proton homeostasis,[101] and membrane hyperpolarization.[82] In CGCs, anion channel blockers and ouabain greatly ameliorated the cytotoxic effect of AZA1 in immature neurons and completely eliminated it in older cultures.[82] Furthermore, short exposures of cultured neurons to AZA1 caused a significant decrease in neuronal volume that was reduced by preincubation of the neurons with DIDS (a chloride channel blocker) or amiloride (Na^+–K^+-ATPase blocker).[82] In neocortical neurons, voltage-gated sodium channels (VGSCs), N-methyl-D-aspartic acid (NMDA), glutamate receptors, and L-type Ca^{2+} channels were ruled out as potential targets for AZA1-induced neurotoxicity, which is consistent with earlier reports that demonstrated AZA1 did not affect VGSC or voltage-gated calcium channel currents.[84] Although AZA1 did not alter membrane potential in SH-SY5Y neuroblastoma cells, a plethora of proteins related to ion/anion channels were differentially expressed.[78]

Recently, a series of screening experiments was performed whereby the effects of AZA1 towards various ion channels were directly monitored. Although there was no effect of the AZAs (AZA1–3 mixture at 348 nM total concentration) towards a VGSC (Nav1.5), voltage-gated L-type calcium channel (Cav1.2), inward-rectifying voltage-gated potassium channel (Kir2.1), hyperpolarization-activated cyclic nucleotide-gated potassium channel (HCN4), or three voltage-gated potassium channels (Kv4.3/KChIP2, Kv1.5, KCNQ1/mink) (M. Twiner, unpubl. data), there was a distinct and significant inhibition of the human *ether-à-go-go*-related gene (hERG) potassium channel. Further exploration of this phenomenon has demonstrated that AZA1–3 were open state blockers of hERG potassium channels.[117] hERG channels are important in the cardiac action potential by mediating the "rapid" delayed rectifier current (I_{Kr}).[118] hERG K^+ channels are transcriptionally expressed in a broad array of cell/tissue types including the heart (differentially expressed across the four chambers), brain, liver, kidney, breast, pancreas, and colon, with the highest levels of expression in heart and brain tissue.[119] Expression is cell cycle dependent, involved in apoptosis,[120] and commonly upregulated in cancerous cells.[121] Considering that the concentrations of AZA necessary to inhibit hERG channels (IC_{50} range: 640–840 nM) are at least two orders of magnitude higher than those capable of causing cytotoxicity and cytoskeletal effects, it is likely that yet another target and mechanism of action exists for the AZA toxin class.

28.6 Human Concerns, Risk Assessment, and Management

Codex has laid down working principles for the risk analysis of food stuffs in a guideline[122] to clarify the approach proposed to governments. In these guidelines, a clear role is attributed to each of the following three integral components of the process:

1. Risk assessment or evaluation
2. Risk management
3. Risk communication

This three-pronged approach to risk analysis should be applied consistently in an open, transparent, and documented manner (Figure 28.5). In addition, risk analysis should be evaluated and reviewed in light of newly generated scientific data. There should be a functional separation of risk assessment and risk management to the degree practicable in order to ensure the scientific integrity of the risk assessment, to avoid confusion over the functions to be performed by risk assessors and risk managers, and to reduce any conflict of interest. Risk communication is required for the sake of consumers and food producers but also to improve understanding between risk assessors and risk managers, for instance, to clarify elements of uncertainty in a risk assessment to risk managers. Risk assessment should be structured as a process including the elements of hazard identification and characterization, exposure assessment, and risk characterization. Risk management also

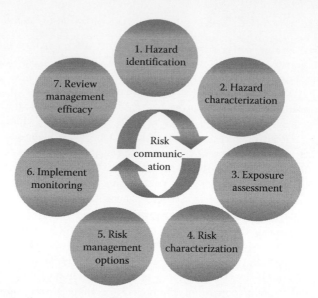

FIGURE 28.5 Steps involved in risk analysis: risk assessment includes steps 1–4; risk management includes steps 5–7. Risk communication ensures understanding of all steps by all stakeholders. The process is considered iterative as new information becomes available.

follows a structured approach including specific steps, such as preliminary activities, evaluation of risk management options, implementation, monitoring, and review of the decisions taken. While these general principles make the Codex approach very clear, it must be noted that specific risk analyses are far from trivial, in particular because of the frequent lack of data on toxin analogues, relative toxicities, exposure, and epidemiology. This lack of data often makes risk assessments provisional and requires frequent review of the assessment and the management options derived. This fact has also been recognized by Codex and, therefore, the iterative character of the risk analysis process has been stressed in the guidelines.

28.6.1 Risk Assessment

28.6.1.1 Human Health Risk

Hazard identification of novel toxins may, in principle, be carried out using different triggers: (1) human illness, (2) biological surveillance using animal or cellular assays, or (3) analytical discovery of analogues of existing toxins. In the case of AZAs, even though there are only seven poisoning events recorded, human illness following shellfish consumption has clearly been the main driver for identifying the hazard,[38,43] with subsequent identification of AZAs as a novel compound group causing the poisoning. In all of those cases, acute shellfish poisoning was observed within hours of shellfish consumption (see sections earlier for description of symptoms). To date, no effects other than GI disorder have been described in humans. In contrast to other algal toxins (e.g., ciguatoxins), symptoms of AZP clearly disappear after a few days and complete recovery of patients has been reported in all of the few cases reported to date. Thus, no chronic ill effect of AZAs has been reported in humans so far. This may be due to several factors: (1) due to the acute poisoning effects, medical doctors have focused on the symptoms associated with the acute poisoning and may have neglected long-term effects; (2) the detection of subacute effects following chronic exposure is typically very difficult since it is usually underreported and convoluted with many other environmental factors; (3) the mode of action of AZAs is not yet known, and hence the detection of effects at molecular or cellular level is not easily followed; and (4) no biomarkers have been developed for human exposure to AZAs and hence no epidemiological studies can use such tools to actually trace exposure.

Still, a number of studies on animals suggest that there is a potential for subacute effects. An early study by Ito et al.[48] on chronic exposure of mice to AZA suggested that more tumors were observed in AZA-exposed mice compared to the control population. Unfortunately, the study was not considered conclusive as the number of animals used was quite low and there was no clear dose–response relationship (i.e., more lung tumors were observed at the lower dose of 20 µg/kg twice weekly [3/10 mice] than at the higher dose of 50 µg/kg twice weekly [1/10 mice]). Still, 9 out of 10 mice at the higher dose level were sacrificed along the study due to extreme weakness, and the lung tumor that was observed at the highest dose level was the earliest tumor observed (the other two tumors being observed at the lower dose level during the period of recovery post exposure). Hence, a tumorigenic effect of AZAs cannot be completely ruled out at this stage. The study by Colman et al.,[68] even though only based on a single-dose exposure, also showed strong subacute effects on embryonic development of Japanese medaka fish. This study suggests a teratogenic potential of AZAs at subacute levels in this model, and transfer across the placental barrier in pregnant women should be considered a hazard that needs to be investigated further. This hazard appears of particular importance in light of the facile uptake observed for AZA1 across the intestinal barrier in small rodents.[45] Initial observations of AZA-exposed mice had also suggested that AZA should be considered a neurotoxin as symptoms had included jumping behavior in mice.[38] A further indication of neurotoxicity was found by Kulagina et al.[84] who detected effects of AZA1 on neuronal cells. Hence, further confirmation of neurotoxic effects should be made once the mechanism(s) of action is (are) clarified in case subacute effects in humans may be caused.

28.6.1.2 Synergistic Effects with Other Algal Toxins

Co-exposure of humans to toxicants of anthropogenic origin is a common phenomenon; however, overall, the science of the toxicology of mixtures is still in its infancy and evaluation of the combined effects of algal toxins is at a similar stage. Due to the fact that many algal blooms typically occur during summer, combined with rapid accumulation of various toxins by bivalve mollusks, co-exposure is a relatively likely phenomenon. Several countries (e.g., Japan, Ireland, and Norway) have reported co-occurrence of toxin groups. In Japan, YTXs were found to co-occur with OA-group toxins during the event that led to the discovery of YTXs.[123] Both YTXs and AZAs have been observed in shellfish from the same location in several countries.[17,19,124] In Ireland, AZAs also frequently co-occur with OA-group toxins[125–127] and in Norway co-occurrence of AZAs has been observed for both OA- and YTX-group toxins[46] (Norwegian National Surveillance Program, 2000–2010, unpubl. data). While it had been clearly established that AZA has a different mode of action than OA through the absence of PP1 and PP2a inhibition by AZA,[72,73] the proximal target site of AZAs and OA in humans is the GI tract. As animal studies have shown damage at tissue level[45,49] upon exposure to AZA, it might be possible that such effects were additive or even synergistic. Also, toxins that have not been shown to exert acute human illness but otherwise have a great toxic potential, such as YTX, might pass more easily the intestinal barrier if the intestine is damaged by AZAs.

Hence, a number of studies have been carried out to investigate the possibility of additive or synergistic effects. A first study established levels of orally administered doses that would cause damage to the intestinal tract of mice without killing the animals.[45] These dose levels were in the range from 100 to 300 µg/kg body weight and effects were only detectable in the upper part of the small intestine (duodenum). Moreover, the animals recovered totally after 7 days without exposure. A follow-up study combining these dose levels of AZA with sublethal doses of YTX established that the effects of AZA on the GI tract of mice did neither lead to increased absorption of YTX into the systemic blood stream nor did they allow orally dosed YTX to exert the ill effects it causes through i.p. administration.[46] Thus, additive or synergistic effects between these two toxin groups (i.e., AZA and YTX) appear very unlikely to play a major role in the toxicology of mixtures. Obviously, human physiology is somewhat different than that of mice, and if noninvasive biomarkers of exposure can be identified for the two toxin groups, it would still be important to verify that there are no such effects in humans. Interestingly, the two toxin groups that do separately cause ill effects in humans, OA and AZA, also did not show any tendency to enhance the effects of each other in mice orally exposed to sublethal doses of both groups.[47] Although the number of mice was small due to low availability of AZA1, the results indicate no additive or synergistic effect on lethality when AZA1 and OA were given together. Similar lack of increased toxicity was observed concerning pathological effects that were restricted to the GI tract. OA and AZA1 were absorbed from the GI tract to a very low degree, and when given together, uptake was reduced. Taken together, these results indicate that the present practice of regulating toxins from the OA and AZA group individually does not present an unwanted increased risk for consumers of shellfish.

28.6.2 Risk Assessment and AZA Analogues to Be Regulated

After hazard identification, a central part of any quantitative risk assessment for acute poisoning is the establishment of an acute reference dose (ARfD) (i.e., a dose of compound that may be considered safe). The ARfD is derived from the LOAEL by applying a safety factor. Ideally in the sense of risk assessment, the LOAEL should be from a human poisoning event and safety factors would be 10 for interindividual variability and 10 for extrapolation of LOAEL to the no observable adverse effect level (NOAEL). The NOAEL is then divided by 60 (to account for a standard 60 kg person) to yield the ARfD.

Interestingly, even though there have been a number of poisoning events reported (see Table 28.1), all of the six formal risk assessments for AZAs have been based on the 1997 event, initially reported by McMahon and Silke[43] (Table 28.3).

Very different results have been found in the different exercises, with recommended levels ranging from as little as 6.3 to as much as 161 µg/kg shellfish meat. These differences are due to the fact that different mathematical models were used (deterministic or probabilistic) and due to the fact that different consumption of shellfish was assumed. Also, there were different assumptions made in different risk assessments (e.g., on heat stability of AZAs and the ratio of hepatopancreas [HP] vs. whole flesh [WF] in mussels). The two more recent tendencies for using probabilistic assessment on the one hand and assuming higher consumption on the other compensate for each other to some extent: probabilistic assessment leads to higher recommended limits while higher portion sizes result in lower recommended limits. The lowest portion size used in any assessment was in the Irish risk assessment in 2001 (93 g whole shellfish meat); however, this was cooked flesh and is thus

TABLE 28.3

Overview of the Six Formal Risk Evaluation Exercises for AZAs from 2001 to 2008

Risk Assessment	Method of Quantitative Assessment	LOAEL (µg/Person)	Safety Factor	NOAEL (µg/Person)	ARfD (µg/kg Human Body Weight)	Consumption (kg Shellfish)	Proposed Limit (µg/kg Shellfish)
2001 FSAI	Deterministic	6.7	1	7.7	n.e.g	0.093[c]	97
	Probabilistic	Distribution[a]	1	15	n.e.g.	0.093[c]	161
2001 EURL-MB-WG	Deterministic	23	3	7.7	0.13	0.1	80
2005 FAO/IOC/WHO	Deterministic	23	10	2.3	0.04	0.250–0.380	6.3–9.6
2005 EURL-MB-WG	Deterministic	23	3	7.7	0.13	0.25	32
2006 FSAI	Probabilistic	Distribution[b]	—	38	0.63	0.25	151.4
2008 EFSA	Probabilistic	113	9	12.6	0.2	0.4	30

Notes: n.e.g. = not explicitly given; 2001 FSAI risk assessment assumed 70% reduction in levels of AZAs upon cooking; 2006 FSAI risk assessment did not make this assumption; 2006 FSAI risk assessment had new information on distribution of ratios of hepatopancreas (HP) to whole flesh (WF).

[a] Range = 6.7–24.9.

[b] Minimum = 23.

[c] Applies to cooked mussel flesh and safety factor derives from the recommendation that this level should be applied to raw mussel tissue.

not directly comparable to the other estimates. Three major differences between the two Irish risk assessments from 2001 to 2006 were as follows:

1. The tissue distribution of HP in WF: Statistically more valid data were available from continued routine monitoring in Ireland.
2. Ratios of AZAs were refined based on more monitoring data.
3. Effects of cooking on the stability of AZAs (2-fold increase instead of 70-fold reduction).

Interestingly, these changes have more or less compensated for each other, since the probabilistic estimates are within 10% of each other. The lowest recommended limits are derived from the FAO/IOC/WHO and the EFSA expert groups, both of which use high portion sizes and high safety factors. An evaluation of portion sizes for shellfish consumption has been formalized in the framework of the EFSA.[128]

A somewhat complex issue also concerns the number of analogues that should be regulated for appropriate protection of public health. While the causative organism, *A. spinosum*, only produces AZA1 and AZA2, mussels biotransform these analogues rapidly into 18 additional compounds.[9,12,30,31] Whereas all the risk evaluations have been based on the estimation of concentrations of AZA1, AZA2, and AZA3 that were present in the mussels that made Irish consumers sick in 1997, it is now clear that other analogues must have also been present at the time. In principle, one could argue that the presence of additional analogues would simply lead to an increased total amount of AZA equivalents, which in turn would result in an increase in the limit recommended. Such a higher limit would then be compensated for by including the additional analogues in the monitoring requirements, yet de facto, there would be no change in practice for shellfish area management. Still, the assessment of the initial concentrations was made on the basis of ratios of AZA1, AZA2, and AZA3 to be present (as the early determinations had been carried out on cooked shellfish), while the legislation is based on the analysis of raw shellfish. Hence, current monitoring practice is heavily biased towards underestimation of the actual concentrations present and thus presents the consumer with undue risks. As the concentrations of AZA3 and AZA6 are negligible in raw mussels, yet will dramatically increase through decarboxylation of AZA17 and AZA19 during the cooking of mussels,[9] the overall concentrations are underestimated by methods used according to current legislation (see Section 28.6.4). The risk managers have been made formally aware of these phenomena through the EFSA opinion on the effects of processing.[129]

28.6.3 Risk Management

28.6.3.1 Regulatory Limits

After the two poisoning events in 1995 and 1997, and the subsequent product rejects in other European Union (EU) countries, it became apparent that explicit regulation was a matter for both health protection and sustainable growth of the aquaculture activity in Ireland. Hence, the first country worldwide to establish regulation for AZAs in shellfish was Ireland in 2000. Even though the initial risk assessment of the Irish Food Safety Authority (FSAI[61]) suggested a limit of 100 µg/kg, there was no certified calibrant available to implement that limit. Hence, a more pragmatic approach of using the MBA for DSP was applied in practice. Still, an additional effort was made by the Irish authorities through the decision to implement a parallel, toxin-specific testing regime based on the technique of LC/MS for the toxins of the OA and the AZA toxin groups.[125] This dual approach for official control has been quite unique and the chemical analysis[130] was accredited in 2003 by the Irish National Accreditation Board (INAB).

The historical developments of regulations for biotoxins in Europe have recently been reviewed.[131] Briefly, at the EU level, AZAs have been regulated de facto since 1991, since the introduction of the DSP MBA as reference method for the detection of OA and analogues.[132,133] Following the 2001 European Union Reference Laboratory for Marine Biotoxins (EURL-MB) working group on toxicology[134] in 2002, this regulation was amended by Commission Decision 2002/225[135] to explicitly include AZAs into the EU regulation of lipophilic toxins, with a limit of 160 µg/kg being implemented. Incidentally, that working group also reviewed the 2001 risk assessment of the IFSA,[61] coming to similar conclusions on the basis of the few available data. In 2004, the previous regulation and decisions were amalgamated into a single legislative package, the Food Hygiene Package,[136,137] without making any change to limits or methods. Following the three major recent risk assessments by

1. The FAO/IOC/WHO working group,[138] also reviewed by the EURL-MB working group on toxicology[139]
2. The IFSA[60]
3. The EFSA[54]

the EU regulatory limit has remained at 160 µg/kg, even if the most recent amendment to legislation[140] led to a change in the reference method for the determination of AZAs from MBA to the LC–MS method as developed by Villar-Gonzalez et al.[141] Interestingly, two out of three of the risk assessments (FAO/IOC/WHO and EFSA) had recommended lower levels of AZAs than the current regulatory levels to be appropriate as safe levels. Still the level of 160 µg/kg had de facto been implemented since 1991, and there were no reports of illness when either the MBA or chemical testing (e.g., Ireland 2001–2008) was implemented and results of monitoring respected by the shellfish producers.

In the United States, the Food and Drug Administration has established an action level for AZP of 0.16 ppm (i.e., 160 µg/kg) AZA equivalents.[142] This action level is consistent with that currently employed in the EU.

In Japan and several other Asian countries, the MBA is still in use and the detection limit of this method has been shown to be around 160 µg AZA1 equivalent/kg whole shellfish flesh.[143] Hence, the regulatory limit can be considered equivalent to the value in the EU.

As in the Irish national context, a full circle of risk assessment and management has also been carried out in the international framework of the Codex Alimentarius. The Codex Committee on Fish and Fisheries Products (CCFFP) had asked for review of toxin levels and methods in 2003, leading to the expert group in 2004, the report of which was published in 2005.[138] Subsequently, negotiations took place in the CCFFP and executive subcommittees, leading to the Codex Standard 292/2008. A full report on the assessment and management practices was communicated in 2011.[144]

28.6.4 Implementation Process

Following a joint EU workshop between the EU government directorate for Food Safety and Consumer Protection (DG Sanco) and the European Centre for the Validation of Alternative Methods (ECVAM) in 2005,[145] many efforts were undertaken to review and validate alternative methods.[54,128,129,141] These efforts have now led to a revised legislation,[140] yet the limit implemented is de facto the same as the one set in 1991 through the use of the DSP MBA. The performance of the MBA (in its harmonized version) has been evaluated by Hess et al.[143] Clearly, the MBA detects AZA levels of 160 µg/kg with a probability of around 95% and may thus serve the implementation of this limit. However, the inconvenience of the assay is that it is neither specific to AZAs (interference is caused by YTX and other compounds) nor quantitative. The same study also showed that the probability to detect a level at half the current regulatory limit, that is, 80 µg/kg, is only 5%. That means that the MBA cannot be used to detect low, albeit rising, levels of toxicity and hence monitoring may lose 1 week of advance warning and thus protect less efficiently the consumer (from illness) and the producer (from economic losses). Detection methods, and the validation thereof, rely on the availability of reference calibrants.[124] As mentioned earlier, according to the tool box approach of the NRCC, certified standards and tissue reference materials have now been prepared and characterized for AZA1, AZA2, and AZA3, the three analogues currently regulated in the EU.[33,127] With these advances in both detection methodology and quality control tools, the EU has now efficient tools to implement routine monitoring for AZAs in the management of shellfish areas.

In Japan, official control of diarrhetic shellfish toxins in shellfish has been carried out using the MBA since 1979, and this assay has allowed for safe shellfish to be placed on the market with no records of human poisoning due to DSP since the introduction of the assay in 1979.[146] Indirectly, this assay also detects AZA-group toxins, although only effective at the current EU regulatory level of 160 µg/kg.[143] Other Asian countries either base their monitoring of lipophilic toxins on the MBA (Philippines) or use LC–MS/MS (Korea and Singapore) or a combination of both (Thailand and Vietnam).

In the United States, only recently have DSP and AZP been acknowledged as a public health threat. In 2008, OA levels exceeding the 0.16 ppm action level were recorded for the first time in the Gulf of Mexico along the Texas coast, and in 2011 the first cases of DSP from shellfish originating in US waters were reported from Washington State.[24] In the case of AZP, two intoxications linked to consumption of imported Irish mussels containing above 0.16 ppm AZAs occurred in 2008.[147] No AZP intoxications have yet been caused by shellfish harvested in the United States. According to the USFDA, methods validated through the US National Shellfish Sanitation Program (NSSP) should be employed for regulatory purposes in the United States; however, there is currently no NSSP-validated method for AZAs. As a result, it is understood that a method(s) based on the best available science (e.g., LC–MS/MS) should be adopted until an NSSP-validated method is in place.

At the international level, methodological discussions are still continuing due to the ease of use of the MBA on one hand and the complexity of toxin profiles and the cost of chemical analysis on the other. A Codex working group is attempting to establish method criteria for the most transparent and coherent implementation of official control methods globally.

28.7 State of the Science

AZAs and their contamination of shellfish resources continue to be recognized as a public health as well as an economic issue in many countries (e.g., western Europe), whereas this toxin group has more recently emerged to pose a new threat in other regions not previously affected (e.g., N. and S. America). Our ability to monitor AZAs has benefited tremendously from the development, refinement, and validation of analytical techniques (see chapter on Azaspiracids: chemistry, metabolism, and detection) as well as the commercial availability of certified reference material required for calibrating these methods. The latter is a direct result of advances in toxin isolation and purification protocols and will likely benefit in the future from material sourced from organic synthesis of AZAs and mass culture of toxigenic *Azadinium*. The availability of purified toxins has also fueled efforts to better understand the toxicology and pharmacology of AZAs through wide-ranging in vitro and in vivo studies. Whereas our knowledge of AZAs and their toxic effects at the organismal, cellular, and molecular levels has expanded considerably over the past decade, identification of the primary mode(s) of action and pharmacologic receptor(s) for the main AZA analogues remains elusive. In fact, several lines of evidence suggest that the various analogues examined to date may exhibit unique modes of action and/or receptors.

In the near term, there is clearly a need to expand and focus on studies aimed at elucidating the mode of action and pharmacologic receptor for at least AZA1–3 and, optimally, for additional analogues such as AZA6, AZA17, and AZA19, which are known to also be present at elevated levels in contaminated shellfish (in certain cases, after cooking). The finding that AZA1–3 are open state blockers of hERG potassium channels[117] is intriguing, yet the elevated IC_{50} values (i.e., 640–840 nM) suggest that this is not the primary mode of action or receptor. Various laboratories are exploring the potential for synthesizing radiolabeled AZA as a probe for determining the toxin receptor and label-free techniques (e.g., surface plasmon resonance) may also be useful in identifying a proximate binding site. Expanded screening for effects on diverse molecular targets, such as that which led to the discovery of the hERG potassium channel interaction, may also provide new insights in the search for the toxin receptor(s) and mode of action. These critical pieces of information are essential not only for elucidating the molecular basis for AZP but may also lead to the development of therapeutic measures for treatment following exposure to AZAs as well as serving as the basis for establishing rapid, receptor-based toxin screening assays.

With the increasing availability of purified toxins, a wider range of in vivo studies in various animal models using multiple AZA analogues is becoming more tractable. The vast majority of in vivo work has employed a murine model as the quantity of toxin required to achieve desired dose rates is minimal compared with larger animals; however, commercial availability of toxin standards, although costly, will permit studies using alternative models that may be more appropriate to address specific questions or hypotheses. For example, the preliminary minipig in vivo oral exposure experiment noted earlier was designed to take advantage of the fact that this species is considered to have a digestive system closely resembling that of humans, potentially yielding data more representative of consumers' response to AZA exposure. Use of additional rodent models such as the rat, which is generally acknowledged as a preferred system for toxicology studies, should also be considered. In addition, detailed in vivo experiments should be expanded to include both i.p. and oral exposures for all sufficiently available AZA analogues, especially those of relevance to potential human exposure. Such an effort will provide accurate LD_{50} determinations and allow comparative evaluation of toxicokinetic/toxicodynamic (see in the following texts) properties.

In vivo experiments employing different animal models will provide exciting opportunities to address important topics such as the toxicokinetics/toxicodynamics of exposure to AZA analogues, which includes the processes of toxin absorption, distribution, metabolism, and excretion. In particular, verification of the so-called "phase II" metabolites (i.e., the result of conjugation reactions generally converting lipophilic to more polar compounds more easily excreted as part of the detoxification process) and evaluation of their distribution and toxicity is a critical need. Efforts to implement toxicokinetic/toxicodynamic (i.e., TK/TD) modeling of in vivo exposure data will yield a more complete conceptual framework of how organisms process and eliminate AZAs following exposure, with the potential for interspecies extrapolation (including humans). Application of '-omics-based strategies (i.e., genomics, transcriptomics, proteomics) in concert with in vivo experiments (as well as in vitro models) will provide additional insights into the response of organisms to AZA exposure and may lead to the identification of biomarkers of toxin exposure potentially useful in epidemiological studies.

An important question with potential human health implications that remains to be fully addressed is whether one or more of the AZA analogues should be classified as tumor promoters. There is some indication from studies in mice described earlier that lung tumor formation may result following chronic, low-dose exposure; however, this response was not dose dependent. Nonetheless, since a mutagenic and/or tumorigenic effect of AZAs cannot be completely ruled out, further targeted in vivo and in vitro studies (e.g., Ames test, comet assay) are warranted to critically examine the genotoxic potential of this toxin group.

From the standpoint of risk assessment and risk management, there is a clear need for additional epidemiological data given that all of the information available to date is based on only seven human poisoning events. Additionally, it should be noted that all six risk assessments have been based on a single, albeit well-described, poisoning incident—the 1997 incident on Arranmore Island, Ireland. This incident comprised only 11 described cases. For all assessments, and in particular the four formal exercises, a high degree of uncertainty due to the lack of epidemiological data has been emphasized. Owing to the most recent incidents in France and the United States in 2008 (Table 28.1), it is quite clear that the low safety factors result in a very tight margin between the regulatory level and the level making people sick. More specifically, with regard to the AZA analogues that are regulated, further consideration should be given to including other analogues in addition to AZA1–3 as is currently the case. The EFSA opinion on the effects of processing[129] makes clear that although a raw shellfish product may be considered safe, processing (e.g., cooking) the material can lead to a ~2-fold increase in toxin concentration that may cause the product to exceed the regulatory limit and thus be unsafe for human consumption. Specifically, we now know that AZA3 and AZA6 levels are negligible in raw mussels but increase markedly with cooking (via decarboxylation of AZA17 and AZA19)[9]; therefore, under the current regulatory legislation, total AZA levels will likely be underestimated. We thus recommend that AZA6, AZA17, and AZA19 be formally included in legislation and official monitoring programs for the AZA group of toxins. The earlier findings also support the recommended lowering of regulatory action levels outlined by the two international risk assessments (FAO, 2005 #862, and EFSA, 2009 #1751).

Overall, the many recent advances in the toxicology, pharmacology, and risk assessment related to the AZA toxin group have significantly improved our understanding of how and to what extent AZAs may affect consumers, as well as our ability to protect public health. Nonetheless, we have identified earlier several critical issues and questions that remain to be addressed in order to meet the challenges associated with evaluating the short- and long-term human health implications of AZP and with better protecting consumers, as well as economic interests, as the global distribution of AZP incidents continues to expand.

REFERENCES

1. Tillmann, U., Elbrächter, M., Krock, B., John, U., and Cembella, A. 2009. *Azadinium spinosum* gen. et sp. nov. (Dinophyceae) identified as a primary producer of azaspiracid toxins. *Eur. J. Phycol.*, 44, 63–79.

2. Krock, B., Tillmann, U., John, U., and Cembella, A. D. 2009. Characterization of azaspiracids in plankton size-fractions and isolation of an azaspiracid-producing dinoflagellate from the North Sea. *Harmful Algae*, 8, 254–263.

3. Tillmann, U., Salas, R., Gottschling, M., Krock, B., O'Driscoll, D., and Elbrächter, M. 2012. *Amphidoma languida* sp. nov. (Dinophyceae) reveals a close relationship between *Amphidoma* and *Azadinium*. *Protist*, 163, 701–719.

4. Satake, M., Ofuji, K., James, K. J., Furey, A., and Yasumoto, T. 1998. New toxic event caused by Irish mussels. In: Reguera, B., Blanco, J., Fernandez, M. L. et al. (eds.) *Harmful Algae, Proceedings of the VIII International Conference on Harmful Algae*, June 1999, Vigo, Spain. Santiago de Compostela, Spain: Xunta de Galicia and Intergovernmental Oceanographic Commission of UNESCO.

5. Satake, M., Ofuji, K., Naoki, H., James, K. J., Furey, A., McMahon, T. et al. 1998. Azaspiracid, a new marine toxin having unique spiro ring assemblies, isolated from Irish mussels, *Mytilus edulis. J. Am. Chem. Soc.*, 120, 9967–9968.

6. James, K. J., Sierra, M. D., Lehane, M., Braña Magdalena, A., and Furey, A. 2003. Detection of five new hydroxyl analogues of azaspiracids in shellfish using multiple tandem mass spectrometry. *Toxicon*, 41, 277–283.

7. Jauffrais, T., Kilcoyne, J., Séchet, V., Herrenknecht, C., Truquet, P., Hervé, F. et al. 2012. Production and isolation of azaspiracid-1 and -2 from *Azadinium spinosum* culture in pilot scale photobioreactors. *Mar. Drugs*, 10, 1360–1382.

8. Lehane, M., Braña Magdalena, A., Moroney, C., Furey, A., and James, K. J. 2002. Liquid chromatography with electrospray ion trap mass spectrometry for the determination of five azaspiracids in shellfish. *J. Chromatogr. A*, 950, 139–147.

9. McCarron, P., Kilcoyne, J., Miles, C. O., and Hess, P. 2009. Formation of azaspiracids-3, -4, -6, and -9 via decarboxylation of carboxyazaspiracid metabolites from shellfish. *J. Agric. Food Chem.*, 57, 160–169.

10. Ofuji, K., Satake, M., McMahon, T., James, K. J., Naoki, H., Oshima, Y. et al. 2001. Structures of azaspiracid analogs, azaspiracid-4 and azaspiracid-5, causative toxins of azaspiracid poisoning in Europe. *Biosci. Biotechnol. Biochem.*, 65, 740–742.

11. Ofuji, K., Satake, M., McMahon, T., Silke, J., James, K. J., Naoki, H. et al. 1999. Two analogs of azaspiracid isolated from mussels, *Mytilus edulis*, involved in human intoxication in Ireland. *Nat. Toxins*, 7, 99–102.

12. Rehmann, N., Hess, P., and Quilliam, M. 2008. Discovery of new analogs of the marine biotoxin azaspiracid in blue mussels (*Mytilus edulis*) by ultra-performance liquid chromatography/tandem mass spectrometry. *Rapid Commun. Mass Spectrom.*, 22, 549–558.

13. Braña Magdalena, A., Lehane, M., Krys, S., Fernandez, M. L., Furey, A., and James, K. J. 2003. The first identification of azaspiracids in shellfish from France and Spain. *Toxicon*, 42, 105–108.

14. Hess, P., McCarron, P., Rehmann, N., Kilcoyne, J., McMahon, T., Ryan, G. et al. 2007. Isolation and purification of azaspiracids from naturally contaminated materials, and evaluation of their toxicological effects. Final project report ASTOX (ST/02/02). Galway, Ireland: Marine Institute—Marine Environment & Health Series.

15. James, K. J., Furey, A., Lehane, M., Ramstad, H., Aune, T., Hovgaard, P. et al. 2002. First evidence of an extensive northern European distribution of azaspiracid poisoning (AZP) toxins in shellfish. *Toxicon*, 40, 909–915.

16. James, K. J., Furey, A., Satake, M., and Yasumoto, T. 2001. Azaspiracid poisoning (AZP): A new shellfish toxic syndrome in Europe. In: Hallegraeff, G. M., Blackburn, S. I., Bolch, C. J. et al. (eds.) *Harmful Algal Blooms 2000*. Paris, France: Intergovernmental Oceanographic Commission of UNESCO.

17. Twiner, M. J., Rehmann, N., Hess, P., and Doucette, G. J. 2008. Azaspiracid shellfish poisoning: A review on the chemistry, ecology, and toxicology with an emphasis on human health impacts. *Mar. Drugs*, 6, 39–72.

18. Furey, A., Moroney, C., Braña Magdalena, A., Saez, M. J. F., Lehane, M., and James, K. J. 2003. Geographical, temporal, and species variation of the polyether toxins, azaspiracids, in shellfish. *Environ. Sci. Technol.*, 37, 3078–3084.

19. Amzil, Z., Sibat, M., Royer, F., and Savar, V. 2008. First report on azaspiracid and yessotoxin groups detection in French shellfish. *Toxicon*, 52, 39–48.

20. Elgarch, A., Vale, P., Rifai, S., and Fassouane, A. 2008. Detection of diarrheic shellfish poisoning and azaspiracid toxins in Moroccan mussels: Comparison of the LC-MS method with the commercial immunoassay kit. *Mar. Drugs*, 6, 587–594.

21. Taleb, H., Vale, P., Amanhir, R., Benhadouch, A., Sagou, R., and Chafik, A. 2006. First detection of azaspiracids in mussels in north west Africa. *J. Shellfish Res.*, 25, 1067–1070.

22. Álvarez, G., Uribe, E., Ávalos, P., Mariño, C., and Blanco, J. 2010. First identification of azaspiracid and spirolides in *Mesodesma donacium* and *Mulinia edulis* from Northern Chile. *Toxicon*, 55, 638–641.

23. López-Rivera, A., O'Callaghan, K., Moriarty, M., O'Driscoll, D., Hamilton, B., Lehane, M. et al. 2010. First evidence of azaspiracids (AZAs): A family of lipophilic polyether marine toxins in scallops (*Argopecten purpuratus*) and mussels (*Mytilus chilensis*) collected in two regions of Chile. *Toxicon*, 55, 692–701.

24. Trainer, V. L., Moore, L., Bill, B. D., Adams, N. G., Harrington, N., Borchert, J., da Silva, D. A. M., and Eberhart, B.-T. L. 2013. Diarrhetic shellfish toxins and other lipohilic toxins of human health concern in Washington State. *Mar. Drugs*, 11, 1815–1835.

25. Ueoka, R., Ito, A., Izumikawa, M., Maeda, S., Takagi, M., Shin-Ya, K. et al. 2009. Isolation of azaspiracid-2 from a marine sponge *Echinoclathria* sp. as a potent cytotoxin. *Toxicon*, 53, 680–684.

26. Torgersen, T., Bruun Bremmes, N., Rundberget, T., and Aune, T. 2008. Structural confirmation and occurrence of azaspiracids in Scandinavian brown crabs (*Cancer pagurus*). *Toxicon*, 51, 93–101.

27. Akselman, R. and Negri, R. M. 2012. Blooms of Azadinium cf. spinosum Elbrächter et Tillmann (Dinophyceae) in northern shelf waters of Argentina, Southwestern Atlantic. *Harmful Algae*, 19, 30–38.

28. Tillmann, U., Elbrachter, M., John, U., and Krock, B. 2011. A new non-toxic species in the dinoflagellate genus Azadinium: *A. poporum* sp. nov. *European J. Phycol.*, 46, 74–87.

29. Tillmann, U., Elbrächter, M., John, U., Krock, B., and Cembella, A. 2010. *Azadinium obesum* (Dinophyceae), a new nontoxic species in the genus that can produce azaspiracid toxins. *Phycologia*, 49, 169–182.

30. Salas, R., Tillmann, U., John, U., Kilcoyne, J., Burson, A., Cantwell, C. et al. 2011. *The role of Azadinium spinosum* (Dinophyceae) in the production of azaspiracid shellfish poisoning in mussels. *Harmful Algae*, 10, 774–783.

31. Jauffrais, T., Marcaillou, C., Herrenknecht, C., Truquet, P., Séchet, V., Nicolau, E. et al. 2012. Azaspiracid accumulation, detoxification and biotransformation in blue mussels (*Mytilus edulis*) experimentally fed *Azadinium spinosum*. *Toxicon*, 60, 582–595.

32. Kilcoyne, J., Keogh, A., Clancy, G., Le Blanc, P., Burton, I., Quilliam, M. et al. 2012. Improved isolation procedure for azaspiracids from shellfish, structural elucidation of azaspiracid-6, and stability studies. *J. Agric. Food Chem.*, 60, 2447–2455.

33. Perez, R., Rehmann, N., Crain, S., Leblanc, P., Craft, C., Mackinnon, S. et al. 2010. The preparation of certified calibration solutions for azaspiracid-1, -2, and -3, potent marine biotoxins found in shellfish. *Anal. Bioanal. Chem.*, 398, 2243–2252.

34. Nicolaou, K. C., Koftis, T. V., Vyskocil, S., Petrovic, G., Tang, W., Frederick, M. O. et al. 2004. Total synthesis and structural elucidation of azaspiracid-1. Final assignment and total synthesis of the correct structure of azaspiracid-1. *J. Am. Chem. Soc.*, 128, 2859–2872.

35. Vilariño, N. 2007. Biochemistry of azaspiracid poisoning toxins. In: Botana, L. M. (ed.) *Phycotoxins Chemistry and Biochemistry*. Oxford, U.K.: Blackwell Publishing.

36. James, K. J., Fidalgo Saez, M. J., Furey, A., and Lehane, M. 2004. Azaspiracid poisoning, the food-borne illness associated with shellfish consumption. *Food Addit. Contam.*, 21, 879–892.

37. Furey, A., O'Doherty, S., O'Callaghan, K., Lehane, M., and James, K. J. 2010. Azaspiracid poisoning (AZP) toxins in shellfish: Toxicological and health considerations. *Toxicon*, 56, 173–190.

38. McMahon, T. and Silke, J. 1996. Winter toxicity of unknown aetiology in mussels. *Harmful Algae News*, 14, 2.

39. Ryan, G., Cunningham, K., and Ryan, M. P. 2008. Pharmacology and epidemiological impact of azaspiracids. In: Botana, L. M. (ed.) *Seafood and Freshwater Toxins: Pharmacology, Physiology, and Detection*, 2nd edn. Boca Raton, FL: CRC Press (Taylor & Francis Group).

40. Rasff. 2008. The Rapid Alert System for Food and Feed (RASFF) Annual Report 2008. http://ec.europa.eu/food/food/rapidalert/report2008_en.pdf (accessed September 27, 2013).

41. Klontz, K. C., Abraham, A., Plakas, S. M., and Dickey, R. W. 2009. Mussel-associated azaspiracid intoxication in the United States. *Ann. Intern. Med.*, 150, 361.
42. Flanagan, A. F. 2002. Detection and biochemical studies on the novel algal toxin, azaspiracid. PhD, National University of Ireland, Galway, Ireland.
43. McMahon, T. and Silke, J. 1998. Re-occurrence of winter toxicity. *Harmful Algae News*, 17, 12.
44. Frederick, M. O., De Lamo Marin, S., Janda, K. D., Nicolaou, K. C., and Dickerson, T. J. 2009. Monoclonal antibodies with orthogonal azaspiracid epitopes. *ChemBioChem*, 10, 1625–1629.
45. Aasen, J. A., Espenes, A., Hess, P., and Aune, T. 2010. Sub-lethal dosing of azaspiracid-1 in female NMRI mice. *Toxicon*, 56, 1419–1425.
46. Aasen, J. A., Espenes, A., Miles, C. O., Samdal, I. A., Hess, P., and Aune, T. 2011. Combined oral toxicity of azaspiracid-1 and yessotoxin in female NMRI mice. *Toxicon*, 57, 909–917.
47. Aune, T., Espenes, A., Aasen, J. A., Quilliam, M. A., Hess, P., and Larsen, S. 2012. Study of possible combined toxic effects of azaspiracid-1 and okadaic acid in mice via the oral route. *Toxicon*, 60, 895–906.
48. Ito, E., Satake, M., Ofuji, K., Higashi, M., Harigaya, K., McMahon, T. et al. 2002. Chronic effects in mice caused by oral administration of sublethal doses of azaspiracid, a new marine toxin isolated from mussels. *Toxicon*, 40, 193–203.
49. Ito, E., Satake, M., Ofuji, K., Kurita, N., McMahon, T., James, K. et al. 2000. Multiple organ damage caused by a new toxin azaspiracid, isolated from mussels produced in Ireland. *Toxicon*, 38, 917–930.
50. James, K. J., Lehane, M., Moroney, C., Fernandez-Puente, P., Satake, M., Yasumoto, T. et al. 2002. Azaspiracid shellfish poisoning: Unusual toxin dynamics in shellfish and the increased risk of acute human intoxications. *Food Addit. Contam.*, 19, 555–561.
51. Hess, P. and Rehmann, N. 2008. Pharmacological concepts and chemical studies relevant to evaluating the toxicity of azaspiracids. *Mar. Environ. Health Ser.*, 33, 55–64.
52. Nzoughet, K. J., Hamilton, J. T. G., Floyd, S. D., Douglas, A., Nelson, J., Devine, L. et al. 2008. Azaspiracid: First evidence of protein binding in shellfish. *Toxicon*, 51, 1255–1263.
53. Nzoughet, J. K., Hamilton, J. T. G., Botting, C. H., Douglas, A., Devine, L., Nelson, J. et al. 2009. Proteomics identification of azaspiracid toxin biomarkers in blue mussels, *Mytilus edulis. Mol. Cell. Proteomics*, 8(8), 1811–1822.
54. EFSA. 2008. Marine biotoxins in shellfish—Azaspiracid group: Scientific opinion of the panel on contaminants in the food chain. *EFSA J.*, 723, 1–52.
55. Ito, E., Terao, K., McMahon, T., Silke, J., and Yasumoto, T. 1998. Acute pathological changes in mice caused by crude extracts of novel toxins isolated from Irish mussels. In: Reguera, B., Blanco, J., Fernandez, M. L. et al. (eds.) *Harmful Algae*. Santiago de Compostela, Spain: Xunta de Galicia and Intergovernmental Oceanographic Commission of UNESCO.
56. Ito, E., Frederick, M. O., Koftis, T. V., Tang, W., Petrovic, G., Ling, T. et al. 2006. Structure toxicity relationships of synthetic azaspiracid-1 and analogs in mice. *Harmful Algae*, 5, 586–591.
57. Donato, R. 2003. Intracellular and extracellular roles of S100 proteins. *Microsc. Res. Tech.*, 60, 540–551.
58. Twiner, M. J., Ryan, J. C., Morey, J. S., Smith, K. J., Hammad, S. M., Van Dolah, F. M. et al. 2008. Transcriptional profiling and inhibition of cholesterol biosynthesis in human lymphocyte T cells by the marine toxin azaspiracid. *Genomics*, 91, 289–300.
59. Vilariño, N., Nicolaou, K. C., Frederick, M. O., Cagide, E., Ares, I. R., Louzao, M. C. et al. 2006. Cell growth inhibition and actin cytoskeleton disorganization induced by azaspiracid-1 structure-activity studies. *Chem. Res. Toxicol.*, 19, 1459–1466.
60. FSAI. 2006. *Risk Assessment of Azaspiracids (AZAs) in Shellfish, August 2006—A Report of the Scientific Committee of the Food Safety Authority of Ireland (FSAI)*. Dublin, Ireland: Food Safety Authority of Ireland (FSAI), 39pp.
61. Anderson, W. A., Whelan, P., Ryan, M., McMahon, T., and James, K. J. 2001. *Risk Assessment of Azaspiracids (AZAs) in Shellfish*. Dublin, Ireland: Food Safety Authority of Ireland.
62. Nicolaou, K. C., Koftis, T. V., Vyskocil, S., Petrovic, G., Ling, T., Yamada, T. M. A. et al. 2004. Structural revision and total synthesis of azaspiracid-1, Part 2: Definition of the ABCD domain and total synthesis. *Angew. Chem. Int. Ed.*, 43, 4318–4324.
63. Ito, E. 2008. Toxicology of azaspiracid-1: Acute and chronic poisoning, tumorigenicity, and chemical structure relationship to toxicity in a mouse model. In: Botana, L. M. (ed.) *Seafood and Freshwater Toxins: Pharmacology, Physiology, and Detection*, 2nd edn. Boca Raton, FL: CRC Press (Taylor & Francis Group).

64. Aune, T. 2009. Oral toxicity of mixtures of lipophilic marine algal toxins in mice. In: Lassus, P. (ed.) *7th International Conference on Molluscan Shellfish Safety*, Nantes, France, June 14–19, 2009 (Abstract). Versailles, France: Quae Publishing.

65. EFSA. 2009. Marine biotoxins in shellfish—Pectenotoxin group: Scientific opinion of the panel on contaminants in the food chain. *EFSA J.*, 1109, 1–47.

66. EFSA. 2008. Marine biotoxins in shellfish—Yessotoxin group: Scientific opinion of the panel on contaminants in the food chain. *EFSA J.*, 907, 1–62.

67. Suganuma, M., Fujiki, H., Suguri, H., Yoshizawa, S., Hirota, M., Nakayasu, M. et al. 1988. Okadaic acid: An additional non-phorbol-12-tetradecanoate-13-acetate-type tumor promoter. *Proc. Natl. Acad. Sci. U S A*, 85, 1768–1771.

68. Colman, J. R., Twiner, M. J., Hess, P., McMahon, T., Satake, M., Yasumoto, T. et al. 2005. Teratogenic effects of azaspiracid-1 identified by microinjection of Japanese medaka (*Oryzias latipes*) embryos. *Toxicon*, 45, 881–890.

69. Nzoughet, J. K., Grant, I. R., Prodöhl, P. A., Hamilton, J. T. G., Botana, L. M., and Elliott, C. T. 2011. Evidence of *Methylobacterium* spp. and *Hyphomicrobium* sp. in azaspiracid toxin contaminated mussel tissues and assessment of the effect of azaspiracid on their growth. *Toxicon*, 58, 619–622.

70. Jauffrais, T., Contreras, A., Herrenknecht, C., Truquet, P., Séchet, V., Tillmann, U. et al. 2012. Effect of *Azadinium spinosum* on the feeding behaviour and azaspiracid accumulation of *Mytilus edulis*. *Aquatic Toxicol.*, 124–125, 179–187.

71. Flanagan, A. F., Kane, M., Donlon, J., and Palmer, R. 1999. Azaspiracid, detection of a newly discovered phycotoxin *in vitro*. *J. Shellfish Res.*, 18, 716.

72. Flanagan, A. F., Callanan, K. R., Donlon, J., Palmer, R., Forde, A., and Kane, M. 2001. A cytotoxicity assay for the detection and differentiation of two families of shellfish toxins. *Toxicon*, 39, 1021–1027.

73. Twiner, M. J., Hess, P., Bottein Dechraoui, M.-Y., McMahon, T., Samons, M. S., Satake, M. et al. 2005. Cytotoxic and cytoskeletal effects of azaspiracid-1 on mammalian cell lines. *Toxicon*, 45, 891–900.

74. Ronzitti, G., Hess, P., Rehmann, N., and Rossini, G. P. 2007. Azaspiracid-1 alters the E-cadherin pool in epithelial cells. *Toxicol. Sci.*, 95, 427–435.

75. Ryan, G. E., Hess, P., and Ryan, M. P. 2006. Development of a functional in vitro bioassay for azaspiracids (AZA) using human colonic epithelial cells. In: Henshilwood, K., Deegan, B., McMahon, T. et al. (eds.) *Proceedings of the 5th International Conference on Molluscan Shellfish Safety, Galway, Ireland*, June 14–18, 2004. Galway, Ireland: The Marine Institute.

76. Twiner, M. J., Hanagriff, J. C., Butler, S. C., Madhkoor, A. K., and Doucette, G. J. 2012. Induction of apoptosis pathways in several cell lines following exposure to the marine algal toxin azaspiracid-1. *Chem. Res. Toxicol.*, 25, 1493–1501.

77. Vilariño, N., Nicolaou, K. C., Frederick, M. O., Cagide, E., Alfonso, C., Alonso, E. et al. 2008. Azaspiracid substituent at C1 Is relevant to in vitro toxicity. *Chem. Res. Toxicol.*, 21, 1823–1831.

78. Kellmann, R., Schaffner, C. A., Grønset, T. A., Satake, M., Ziegler, M., and Fladmark, K. E. 2009. Proteomic response of human neuroblastoma cells to azaspiracid-1. *J. Proteomics*, 72, 695–707.

79. Twiner, M. J., El-Ladki, R., Kilcoyne, J., and Doucette, G. J. 2012. Comparative effects of the marine algal toxins azaspiracid-1, -2, and -3 on Jurkat T lymphocyte cells. *Chem. Res. Toxicol.*, 25, 747–754.

80. Vale, C., Nicolaou, K. C., Frederick, M. O., Gomez-Limia, B., Alfonso, A., Vieytes, M. R. et al. 2007. Effects of azaspiracid-1, a potent cytotoxic agent, on primary neuronal cultures. A structure-activity relationship study. *J. Med. Chem.*, 50, 356–363.

81. Vale, C., Gomez-Limia, B., Nicolaou, K. C., Frederick, M. O., Vieytes, M. R., and Botana, L. M. 2007. The c-Jun-N-terminal kinase is involved in the neurotoxic effect of azaspiracid-1. *Cell Physiol Biochem.*, 20, 957–966.

82. Vale, C., Nicolaou, K. C., Frederick, M. O., Vieytes, M. R., and Botana, L. M. 2010. Cell volume decrease as a link between azaspiracid-induced cytotoxicity and c-Jun-N-terminal kinase activation in cultured neurons. *Toxicol. Sci.*, 113, 158–168.

83. Vale, C., Wandscheer, C., Nicolaou, K. C., Frederick, M. O., Alfonso, C., Vieytes, M. R. et al. 2008. Cytotoxic effect of azaspiracid-2 and azaspiracid-2-methyl ester in cultured neurons: Involvement of the c-Jun N-terminal kinase. *J. Neurosci. Res.*, 86, 2952–2962.

84. Kulagina, K. V., Twiner, M. J., Hess, P., McMahon, T., Satake, M., Yasumoto, T. et al. 2006. Azaspiracid-1 inhibits bioelectrical activity of spinal cord neuronal networks. *Toxicon*, 47, 766–773.

85. Cao, Z., Lepage, K. T., Frederick, M. O., Nicolaou, K. C., and Murray, T. F. 2010. Involvement of caspase activation in azaspiracid-induced neurotoxicity in neocortical neurons. *Toxicol. Sci.*, 114, 323–334.

86. Cañete, E. and Diogene, J. 2010. Improvements in the use of neuroblastomaxglioma hybrid cells (NG108–15) for the toxic effect quantification of marine toxins. *Toxicon*, 55, 381–389.

87. Artursson, P., Palm, K., and Luthman, K. 2001. Caco-2 monolayers in experimental and theoretical predictions of drug transport. *Adv. Drug Deliv. Rev.*, 46, 27–43.

88. Narai, A., Arai, S., and Shimizu, M. 1997. Rapid decrease in transepithelial electrical resistance of human intestinal caco-2 cell monolayers by cytotoxic membrane perturbents *Toxicol. Vitro*, 11, 347–354.

89. Vilariño, N., Nicolaou, K. C., Frederick, M. O., Vieytes, M. R., and Botana, L. M. 2007. Irreversible cytoskeletal disarrangement is independent of caspase activation during in vitro azaspiracid toxicity in human neuroblastoma cells. *Biochem. Pharmacol.*, 74, 327–335.

90. Rossini, G. P. and Hess, P. 2010. Phycotoxins: Chemistry, mechanisms of action and shellfish poisoning. In: Luch, A. (ed.) *Molecular, Clinical and Environmental Toxicology*. Basel, Switzerland: Birkhäuser Basel.

91. Roman, Y., Alfonso, A., Louzao, M. C., De La Rosa, L. A., Leira, F., Vieites, J. M. et al. 2002. Azaspiracid-1, a potent, nonapoptotic new phycotoxin with several cell targets. *Cell. Signal.*, 14, 703–716.

92. Vilariño, N. 2008. Marine toxins and the cytoskeleton: Azaspiracids. *FEBS J.*, 275, 6075–6081.

93. McConkey, D. J. 1998. Biochemical determinants of apoptosis and necrosis. *Toxicol. Lett.*, 99, 157–168.

94. Hengartner, M. D. 1992. The biochemistry of apoptosis. *Nature*, 407, 770–776.

95. De La Rosa, L. A., Alfonso, A., Vilariño, N., Vieytes, M. R., Yasumoto, T., and Botana, L. M. 2001. Maitotoxin-induced calcium entry in human lymphocytes: Modulation by yessotoxin, Ca^{2+} channel blockers and kinases. *Cell. Signal.*, 13, 711–716.

96. De La Rosa, L. A., Alfonso, A., Vilariño, N., Vieytes, M. R., and Botana, L. M. 2001. Modulation of cytosolic calcium levels of human lymphocytes by yessotoxin, a novel marine phycotoxin. *Biochem. Pharmacol.*, 61, 827–833.

97. Perovic, S., Tretter, L., Brummer, F., Wetzler, C., Brenner, J., Donner, G. et al. 2000. Dinoflagellates from marine algal blooms produce neurotoxic compounds: Effects on free calcium levels in neuronal cells and synaptosomes. *Environ. Toxicol. Pharmacol.*, 8, 83–94.

98. Xi, D. and Ramsdell, J. S. 1996. Glutamate receptors and calcium entry mechanisms for domoic acid in hippocampal neurons. *Neuroreport*, 7, 1115–1120.

99. Twiner, M. J., Chidiac, P., Dixon, S. J., and Trick, C. G. 2005. Extracellular organic compounds from the ichthyotoxic red tide alga *Heterosigma akashiwo* elevate cytosolic calcium and induce apoptosis in Sf9 cells. *Harmful Algae*, 4, 789–800.

100. Roman, Y., Alfonso, A., Vieytes, M. R., Ofuji, K., Satake, M., Yasumoto, T. et al. 2004. Effects of azaspiracids 2 and 3 on intracellular cAMP, $[Ca^{2+}]$, and pH. *Chem. Res. Toxicol.*, 17, 1338–1349.

101. Alfonso, A., Vieytes, M. R., Ofuji, K., Satake, M., Nicolaou, K. C., Frederick, M. O. et al. 2006. Azaspiracids modulate intracellular pH levels in human lymphocytes. *Biochem. Biophys. Res. Commun.*, 346, 1091–1099.

102. Rossini, G. P., Sgarbi, N., and Malaguti, C. 2001. The toxic responses induced by okadaic acid involve processing of multiple caspase isoforms. *Toxicon*, 39, 763–770.

103. Gonzalez-Mariscal, L., Tapia, R., and Chamorro, D. 2008. Crosstalk of tight junction components with signaling pathways. *Biochim. Biophys. Acta*, 1778, 729–756.

104. Hartsock, A. and Nelson, W. J. 2008. Adherens and tight junctions: Structure, function and connections to the actin cytoskeleton. *Biochim. Biophys. Acta*, 1778, 660–669.

105. Cowan, K. J. and Storey, K. B. 2003. Mitogen-activated protein kinases: New signaling pathways functioning in cellular responses to environmental stress. *J. Exper. Biol.*, 206, 1107–1115.

106. Bellocci, M., Sala, G. L., Callegari, F., and Rossini, G. P. 2010. Azaspiracid-1 inhibits endocytosis of plasma membrane proteins in epithelial cells. *Toxicol. Sci.*, 117, 109–121.

107. Lambert, D., O'Neill, C. A., and Padfield, P. J. 2005. Depletion of Caco-2 cell cholesterol disrupts barrier function by altering the detergent solubility and distribution of specific tight-junction proteins. *Biochem. J.*, 387(Pt 2), 553–560.

108. Frederick, M. O., Cole, K. P., Petrovic, G., Loizidou, E., and Nicolaou, K. C. 2007. Structural assignment and total synthesis of azaspiracid-1. In: Botana, L. M. (ed.) *Phycotoxins Chemistry and Biochemistry*. Ames, IA: Blackwell Publishing.

109. Nicolaou, K. C., Frederick, M. O., Petrovic, G., Cole, K. P., and Loizidou, E. Z. 2006. Total synthesis and confirmation of the revised structures of azaspiracid-2 and azaspiracid-3. *Angew. Chem. Int. Ed.*, 45, 2609–2615.

110. Kilcoyne, J., Nulty, C., Jauffrais, T., McCarron, P., Herve, F., Wilkins, A. L. et al. 2013. Isolation, structural elucidation and toxicity of two novel azaspiracids from *Azadinium spinosum*. Manuscript in preparation.

111. Kilcoyne, J., McCarron, P., Twiner, M. J., Nulty, C., Crain, S., Rise, F. et al. 2013. Epimers of azaspiracids: isolation, structural elucidation, relative LCMS response, and *in vitro* toxicity of 37-*epi*-azaspiracid-1. Manuscript in preparation.

112. Cohen, P. 1989. The structure and regulation of protein phosphatases. *Annu. Rev. Biochem.*, 58, 453–508.

113. Allingham, J. S., Miles, C. O., and Rayment, I. 2007. A structural basis for regulation of actin polymerization by pectenotoxins. *J. Molec. Biol.*, 371, 959–970.

114. Butler, S. C., Miles, C. O., Karim, A., and Twiner, M. J. 2012. Inhibitory effects of pectenotoxins from marine algae on the polymerization of various actin isoforms. *Toxicol. In Vitro*, 26, 493–499.

115. Hori, M., Matsuura, Y., Yoshimoto, R., Ozaki, H., Yasumoto, T., and Karaki, H. 1999. Actin depolymerizing action by marine toxin, pectenotoxin-2. *Nippon Yakurigaku Zasshi*, 114, 225P–229P.

116. Alfonso, A., Roman, Y., Vieytes, M. R., Ofuji, K., Satake, M., Yasumoto, T. et al. 2005. Azaspiracid-4 inhibits Ca^{2+} entry by stored operated channels in human T lymphocytes. *Biochem. Pharmacol.*, 69, 1627–1636.

117. Twiner, M. J., Doucette, G. J., Rasky, A., Huang, X.-P., Roth, B. L., and Sanguinetti, M. C. 2012. The marine algal toxin azaspiracid is an open state blocker of hERG potassium channels. *Chem. Res. Toxicol.*, 25, 1975–1984.

118. Sanguinetti, M. C. and Tristani-Firouzi, M. 2006. hERG potassium channels and cardiac arrhythmia. *Nature*, 440, 463–469.

119. Luo, X., Xiao, J., Lin, H., Lu, Y., Yang, B., and Wang, Z. 2008. Genomic structure, transcriptional control, and tissue distribution of HERG1 and KCNQ1 genes. *Am. J. Physiol. Heart Circ. Physiol.*, 294, H1371–H1380.

120. Jehle, J., Schweizer, P., Katus, H., and Thomas, D. 2011. Novel roles for hERG K^+ channels in cell proliferation and apoptosis. *Cell Death Dis.*, 2, e193.

121. Pardo, L. A., Del Camino, D., Sanchez, A., Alves, F., Bruggemann, A., Beckh, S. et al. 1999. Oncogenic potential of EAG K^+ channels. *EMBO J.*, 18, 5540–5547.

122. Codex Alimentarius. 2007. CAC/GL 62–2007: Working principles for risk analysis for food safety for application by governments. Rome, Italy: FAO, 4pp.

123. Murata, M., Kumagai, M., Lee, J. S., and Yasumoto, T. 1987. Isolation and structure of yessotoxin, a novel polyether compound implicated in diarrhetic shellfish poisoning. *Tetrahedron Lett.*, 28, 5869–5872.

124. Hess, P. 2010. Requirements for screening and confirmatory methods for the detection and quantification of marine biotoxins in end-product and official control. *Anal. Bioanal. Chem.*, 397, 1683–1694.

125. Hess, P., McMahon, T., Slattery, D., Swords, D., Dowling, G., McCarron, M. et al. 2003. Use of LC-MS testing to identify lipophilic toxins, to establish local trends and interspecies differences and to test the comparability of LC-MS testing with the mouse bioassay: An example from the Irish biotoxin monitoring programme 2001. In: Villalba, A., Reguera, B., Romalde, J. L. et al. (eds.) *Molluscan Shellfish Safety, Proceedings of 4th International Conference Molluscan Shellfish Safety*. Santiago de Compostela, Spain: Consellería de Pesca e Asuntos Marítimos da Xunta de Galicia and Intergovernmental Oceanographic Commission of UNESCO.

126. McCarron, P., Emteborg, H., and Hess, P. 2007. Freeze-drying for the stabilisation of shellfish toxins in mussel tissue (*Mytilus edulis*) reference materials. *Anal. Bioanal. Chem.*, 387, 2475–2486.

127. McCarron, P., Emteborg, H., Nulty, C., Rundberget, T., Loader, J. I., Teipel, K. et al. 2011. A mussel tissue certified reference material for multiple phycotoxins: Part 1. Design and preparation. *Anal. Bioanal. Chem.*, 400, 821–833.

128. EFSA. 2009. Marine biotoxins in shellfish—Summary opinion, scientific opinion of the panel on contaminants in the food chain, Adopted on August 13, 2009. *EFSA J.*, 1306, 1–23.

129. EFSA. 2009. Influence of processing on the levels of lipophilic marine biotoxins in bivalve molluscs, Statement of the Panel on Contaminants in the Food Chain (Question No EFSA-Q-2009–00203), Adopted on March 25, 2009. *EFSA J.*, 1016, 1–10.

130. Hess, P., Nguyen, L., Aasen, J., Keogh, M., Kilcoyne, J., McCarron, P. et al. 2005. Tissue distribution, effect of cooking and parameters affecting the extraction of azaspiracids from mussels, *Mytilus edulis*, prior to analysis by liquid chromatography coupled to mass spectrometry. *Toxicon*, 46, 62–71.

131. Hess, P. 2012. Phytoplankton and biotoxin monitoring programmes for the safe exploitation of shellfish in Europe. In: Cabado, A. G. and Vieites, J. M. (eds.) *New Trends in Marine and Freshwater Toxins*: *Food Safety Concerns*. Hauppauge, New York: Nova Publishers.

132. Anon. 1991. Council directive 91/492/EEC of 15 July 1991, laying down the health conditions for the production and the placing on the market of live bivalve molluscs. *J. Eur. Commun.*, L268, 34, 24/09/1991, 1–14.

133. Anon. 1991. Council Directive 91/493/EEC of 22 July 1991 laying down the health conditions for the production and the placing on the market of fishery products. *Journal of the European Communities*, L268, 34, 24/09/1991, 15–34.

134. Anon. 2001. Report of the meeting of the EU working group on toxicology of DSP and AZP. May 21–23, 2001, Brussels, Belgium.

135. Anon. 2002. Commission decision 2002/225/CE of 15 March 2002, laying down detailed regulations for the application of Council Directive 91/492/EEC. *J. Eur. Commun.*, L75, 62–64.

136. Anon. 2004. Regulation (EC) No 853/2004 of the European Parliament and of the Council of 29 April 2004 laying down specific hygiene rules for food of animal origin. *J. Eur. Commun.*, April 30, 2004, 55–205.

137. Anon. 2004. Regulation (EC) No 854/2004 of the European Parliament and of the Council of 29 April 2004 laying down specific rules for the organisation of official controls on products of animal origin intended for human consumption. *OJEC*, L139, 30/4/2004, 206–320.

138. FAO. 2005. *Report of the Joint FAO/IOC/WHO ad hoc Expert Consultation on Biotoxins in Molluscan Bivalves* (Oslo, Norway, September 26–30, 2004). Rome, Italy: Food and Agriculture Organization, 31pp.

139. Anon. 2005. CRLMB report of the meeting of the working group on toxicology. October 24–25, 2005, Cesenatico, Italy.

140. Anon. 2011. Commission Regulation (EU) No 15/2011 of 10 January 2011 amending Regulation (EC) No 2074/2005 as regards recognised testing methods for detecting marine biotoxins in live bivalve molluscs. *OJEC*, L6, January 11, 2011, 3–6.

141. Villar-Gonzalez, A., Luisa Rodriguez-Velasco, M., and Gago-Martinez, A. 2011. Determination of lipophilic toxins by LC/MS/MS: Single-laboratory validation. *J. AOAC Int.*, 94, 909–922.

142. Anon. 2011. *Fish and Fisheries Products Hazards and Controls Guidance*, 4th edn. Washington, DC: Department of Health and Human Services, Public Health Service, US Food and Drug Administration, Center for Food Safety and Applied Nutrition, 468p.

143. Hess, P., Butter, T., Petersen, A., Silke, J., and McMahon, T. 2009. Performance of the EU-harmonised mouse bioassay for lipophilic toxins for the detection of azaspiracids in naturally contaminated mussel (*Mytilus edulis*) hepatopancreas tissue homogenates characterised by liquid chromatography coupled to tandem mass spectrometry. *Toxicon*, 53, 713–722.

144. Lawrence, J., Loreal, H., Toyofuku, H., Hess, P., Karunasagar, I., and Ababouch, L. 2011. Assessment and management of biotoxin risks in bivalve molluscs. FAO Fisheries and Aquaculture Technical Paper No. 551. Rome, Italy: FAO, 337pp.

145. Hess, P., Grune, B., Anderson, D., Aune, T., Botana, L. M., Caricato, P. et al. 2006. Three Rs approaches in marine biotoxin testing: The report and recommendations of a joint ECVAM/DG SANCO workshop (ECVAM Workshop 55). *Altern. Lab. Anim. (ATLA)*, 32, 193–224.

146. Suzuki, T. and Watanabe, R. 2012. Shellfish toxin monitoring system in Japan and some Asian countries. In: Cabado, A. G. and Vieites, J. M. (eds.) *New Trends in Marine and Freshwater Toxins*: *Food Safety Concerns*. Hauppauge, New York: Nova Publishers.

147. U.S. Food and Drug Administration. 2011. *Fish and Fishery Products Hazards and Controls Guidance*, 4th edn., Rockville, MD, 468pp.

29

Polycavernosides and Other Scarce New Toxins

M. Carmen Louzao, Natalia Vilariño, and Mari Yotsu-Yamashita

CONTENTS

29.1 Polycavernosides

29.1.1 Chemistry

29.1.1.1 Introduction

Polycavernoside A (PA, Figure 29.1) and its minor analog, polycavernoside B (PB), were isolated by Yasumoto and his colleagues as the causative toxin of the human fatal poisoning occurred in Guam in 1991, resulting from the ingestion of the red alga *Gracilaria edulis*.[1,2] Three out of thirteen patients were killed in that case. PA was also identified in the same alga that caused the poisoning, killing 8 out of 36 patients in the Philippines in 2002–2003.[3] The planar structures of PA[2] and four minor analogs, polycavernoside A2 (PA2), A3 (PA3), B (PB), and B2 (PB2)[4] (Figure 29.1), were determined. All these polycavernosides possess the same macrolide aglycone containing a five-member cyclohemiacetal adjacent to a ketone at C9. Structural variation among these analogs are in the conjugated diene (PB, PB2) or triene (PA, PA2, PA3) side chain at C15, and in *O*-methylated or *O*-acetylated L-fucosyl-D-xylose sugar unit at C5. Yotsu-Yamashita et al. also isolated other two minor analogs, polycavernoside C (PC) and polycavernoside C2 (PC2), and their structures were determined as shown in Figure 29.1.[5] PC and PC2 have a common aglycone structure that is distinctly different from PA and other analogs. In this chapter, the chemistry of PC and PC2 is mainly described.

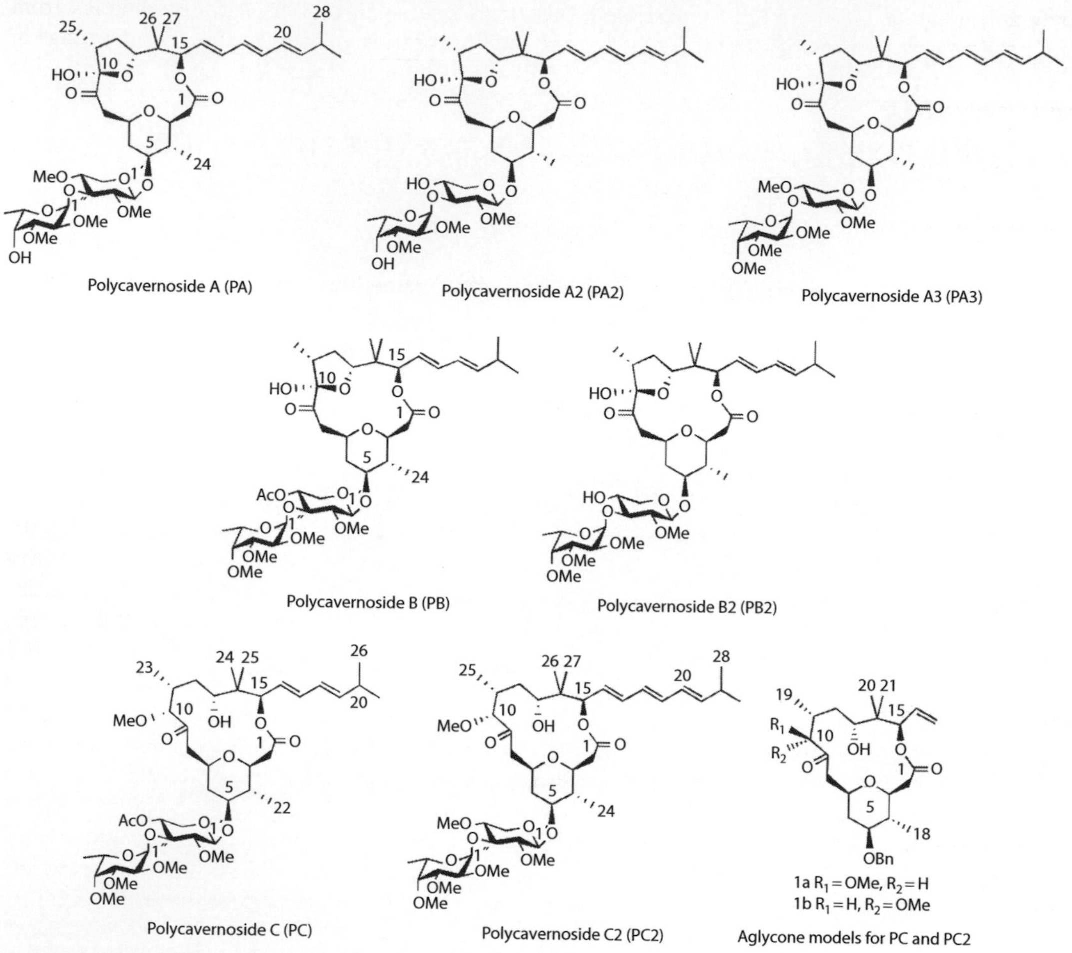

FIGURE 29.1 Structures of polycavernosides and aglycone models for PCs. (From Yotsu-Yamashita, M. et al., *J. Am. Chem. Soc.*, 115, 1147, 1993; Yotsu-Yamashita, M. et al., *Tetrahedron Lett.*, 36, 5563, 1995; Yotsu-Yamashita, M. et al., *Tetrahedron Lett.*, 48, 2255, 2007.)

29.1.1.2 Polycavernoside C and C2

29.1.1.2.1 Isolation

PC (0.1–0.2 mg) was isolated together with PA (0.2 mg) and PB (0.1 mg), from *G. edulis* (4 kg) collected on June 25, 1991, in Guam.[5] *G. edulis* was extracted with acetone three times, and the solvent was evaporated *in vacuo.* The residue was partitioned between H_2O and CH_2Cl_2, and the residue from CH_2Cl_2 layer was applied to column chromatography on silica gel 60 using CH_2Cl_2–MeOH [1:0,99:1 (PB, PC) and 9:1 (PA)]. Each residue from the eluate with CH_2Cl_2–MeOH 99:1 and 9:1 was purified by successive chromatography on ODS-Q3 (H_2O–MeCN 15:85), Develosil ODS-7 (H_2O–MeCN 1:4), and Cosmosil 5C18AR (H_2O–MeCN 1:4). Throughout the purification, elution of polycavernosides was monitored by mouse assays and with a diode array ultraviolet (UV) detector. For final separation of PC from PB, Capcell pack CN (H_2O–MeCN from 1:1 to 0:10) was used, and PC was eluted before PB. PC2 (0.1–0.2 mg) was isolated from the same alga (2 kg, collected on June 11, 1992, in Guam) with PA (0.4 mg), PA2 (0.1 mg), PA3 (0.4 mg), and PB2 (0.1 mg).[5] The alga was extracted with CH_2Cl_2–MeOH 2:1 three times. After solvent evaporating, the residue was successively partitioned between H_2O–MeOH 1:4 and hexane (toxins in the H_2O–MeOH 1:4) and between CH_2Cl_2 and H_2O. The residue from CH_2Cl_2 phase was applied to column chromatography on ODS-Q3 (H_2O–MeCN 1:3) and then on Develosil ODS-5 (H_2O–MeCN 1:3). PA2, PB2, PA, PC2, and PA3 were sequentially eluted from the last column in this order and further purified on the same column by gradient elution (H$_2$O–MeCN from 35:65 to 0:100).[4] PC2 was eluted after PA2, PB2, and PA from this column and further purified on the same column. PC2 has been kept intact until now after storage in CD$_3$CN at −20°C for more than 10 years, while PC was decomposed in pyridine-d$_5$. For this reason, PC2 was mainly used for the structural analysis of the aglycone of PC and PC2.

29.1.1.2.2 Chemical Properties and Detection

PC was found to have a molecular weight 856 as determined from FABMS [M-H$_2$O+H]$^+$ *m/z* 839, [M+Na]$^+$ *m/z* 879, [M+K]$^+$ *m/z* 895. PC2 was found to have a molecular formula of C$_{45}$H$_{74}$O$_{15}$ by HR-FAB MS ([M+Na]$^+$ 877.4930, Δ +0.5 mmu).[5] ^{1}H NMR spectra and ^{1}H–^{1}H COSY of PC and PC2 (CD$_3$CN), and UV absorption (λ_{max} 220 nm for PC, 259, 270, 280 nm for PC2, MeCN) suggested the presence of conjugated diene for PC and conjugated triene for PC2. UV absorption of PA, PA2, and PA3 (λ_{max} 259, 269, 280 nm, MeCN)[4] was almost the same as that of PC2. The $^3J_{HH}$ values (16 Hz for PC, 15.4 Hz for PC2) indicated *E, E* and *E, E, E* geometry for PC and PC2, respectively.

The relative stereostructures of PC and the absolute structure of PC2 were determined by spectroscopic analysis and synthesis of the models of their aglycone (**1a**, **1b** in Figures 29.1 and 29.2). The NMR data of synthesized **1b** were compared with those of PC2. The difference of the ^{1}H NMR chemical shifts of H2–H15, H24–27, 10-OMe, and 13-OH of PC2 from those of H2–H15, H18–21, 10-OMe, and 13-OH of **1b**, respectively, was less than 0.1 ppm, except H5 (0.15 ppm), H6a (0.14 ppm), and H6b (0.10 ppm), which were probably due to difference of the substituents at C5. The differences of the ^{13}C NMR chemical shifts of C2–C15, C24–C27, and 10-OMe of PC2 from C2–C15, C18–C21, and 10-OMe of **1b**, respectively, were not more than 1 ppm except at C5 (2 ppm). In addition, $^3J_{H10/H11}$ value of PC2 (10.2 Hz) was close to that of **1b** (10.6 Hz). According to these data, the planar structure of the aglycone of PC and PC2 was confirmed, and the relative stereostructures of PC and PC2 (10*R**, 13*R**) were determined as shown in Figure 29.1. To determine the absolute configuration of PC2, CD spectra of PC2 and **1b** were measured. Both of these CD spectra showed a similar characteristic single Cotton effect of negative sign in the region of the transition of ketone (n-π*) around 300 nm, which was also shown in the CD spectrum of PA.[6] Based on these data, the absolute configuration of PC2 was determined as same as those of **1b** and PA.

The total synthesis of (−)-PA was achieved by six groups: Fujiwara/Murai et al.,[6] Paquette et al.,[7,8] White/Blakemore et al.,[9,10] Woo and Lee,[11] and Kasai/Sasaki et al.[12] and Brewitz/Fürstner et al.[79] Further synthetic efforts for PA were reported by Perez-Balado and Marko,[13,14] Barry et al.,[15] and Pierre et al.[16]

The structures of PC and PC2 provide information for the biosynthetic pathway or metabolism of polycavernosides, which is necessary for monitoring the occurrence of these human lethal toxins. Cyanobacterium was proposed for the origin of polycavernosides,[3,17] and the study on the details of this issue is now in progress.

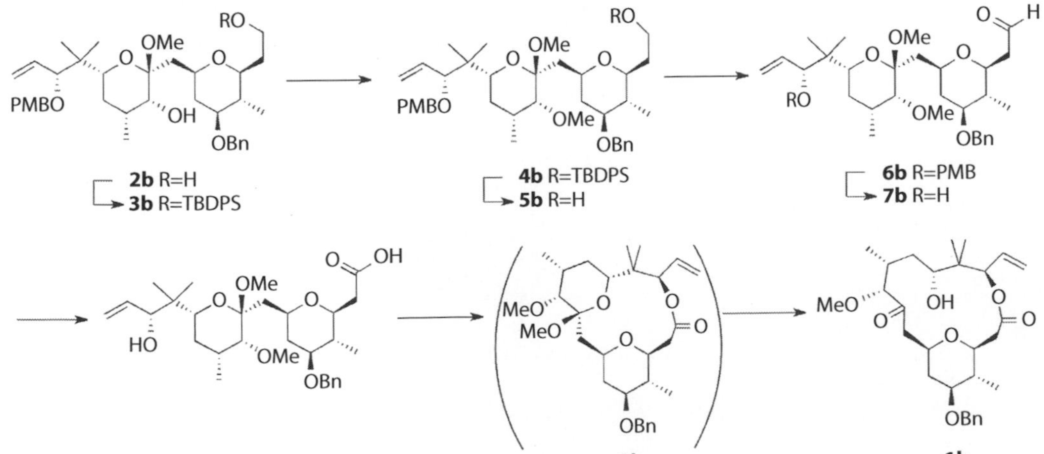

FIGURE 29.2 Synthesis of aglycone model for PCs (**1b**) from **2b**. (From Yotsu-Yamashita, M. et al., *Tetrahedron Lett.*, 48, 2255, 2007.)

29.1.2 Structure–Activity Relationship

Barriault et al. determined the toxicities of derivatives of PA and PB to male mice by intraperitoneal (i.p.) injection observing the mice for 24 h (Figure 29.3).[18] Results suggest that macrocyclic core and triene side chain are required for toxicity.[6] The PA analogs with aglycone structure showed reduced activity; however, the symptoms that caused in mice were rapid, severe, and with lethal effects. Also, the analogs that possess an isopropyl group in the side chain showed high-level toxicity.[18] Analogs sharing the same structure as aglycone including the C15 side chain have differences in the toxicity levels that may arise because of the availability of a free hydroxyl substituent in the sugar component.[19] Therefore, based on the symptoms elicited by the active compounds, Barriault et al. suggested that the active form is the aglycone, the disaccharide being important for the transportation/absorption to the target tissues and for biostability. This hypothesis assumes that the polycavernosides are activated by hydrolysis of the disaccharide in vivo; therefore, the expression of toxicity requires a longer onset period than that for the aglycone. Accordingly, oral administration of polycavernosides may cause much more damage than intraperitoneal injection because the sugars undergo hydrolysis to the aglycone in the strongly acidic environment of the stomach.[3,18]

29.1.3 Pharmacology

Pharmacology of polycavernosides was poorly investigated due to the limitation of sample supply. The complete mechanism of action and molecular targets of these new phycotoxins have not been characterized.

Yotsu-Yamashita's group determined the cytotoxicity of natural PA and synthetic analogs in mouse neuroblastoma cells, Neuro-2a.[20] The cytotoxicities were tested only at 12 μM by counting the viable cells after treatment with toxins for 24 h. Barriault et al. synthesized[18] two analogs of PA with an isopropyl group in the side chain and high-level mouse toxicity, analogs **4** and **5** (Figure 29.3), which showed no cytotoxicity and more than 90% cell death, respectively. Those results suggest that cytotoxicity is not always comparable to the toxicity to mice. They proved that 24 h treatment with 12 μM analog **5** induced

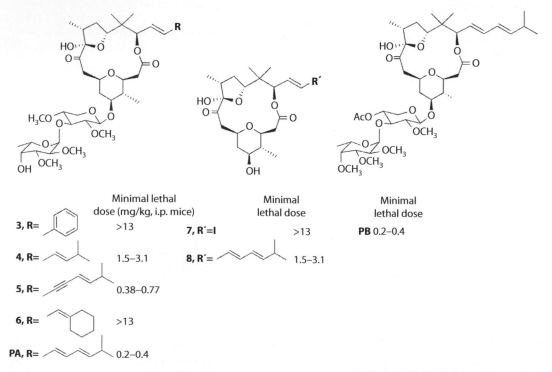

FIGURE 29.3 Structure–activity relationships of polycavernosides. (From Barriault, L. et al., *Bioorg. Med. Chem. Lett.*, 9, 2069, 1999.)

apoptosis in Neuro-2a by activation of caspase-3/7, nucleosomal DNA fragmentation, and TUNEL (TdT-mediated dUTP-biotin nick-end labeling) staining.[20] Therefore, analog **5** turned out to be a potent cytotoxin as confirmed by Cagide et al.[21] It produced a significantly high reduction in the metabolic activity of human neuroblastoma cells as shown in Figure 29.4, which could be indicative of the impact produced by the natural PA.[21]

This synthetic analog has a minimal lethal dose very similar to the natural toxin. Also, the symptoms were the same as those observed for PA, with paralysis 30 min after injection and death occurring within 24 h. Based on the neurological symptoms observed in mice, Louzao et al. performed initial studies by using 4 µg/mL analog **5** on a suspension of human neuroblastoma cell line BE(2)M-17 and found no change in membrane potential.[22] Following previous experiments, Cagide et al.[23] continued studying the mechanism of action of polycavernosides with the same analog **5** (Figure 29.4). In this case, a different approach was chosen; changes in membrane potential were measured with bis-oxonol on human neuroblastoma plated cells, and variations in intracellular calcium levels were monitored with fura-2 in an imaging system. Results showed that a higher concentration of analog **5** than the one tested before (12 µM) induced a membrane depolarization (Figure 29.4) and also enhanced the cytosolic calcium level (Figure 29.4). This toxin triggers an initial extracellular calcium entry not produced across L-type

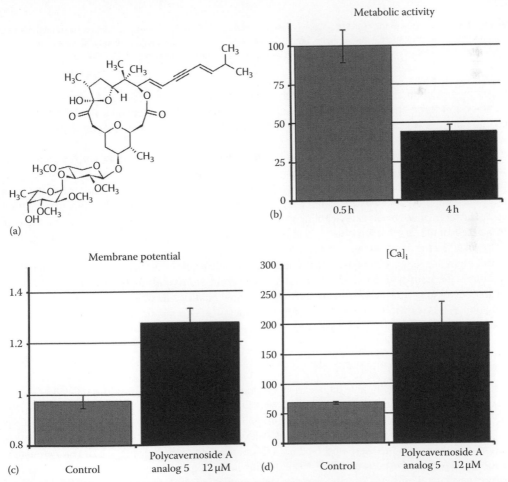

FIGURE 29.4 Effects of 12 µM polycavernoside A analog 5 (a) on metabolism, membrane potential, and intracellular free calcium of human neuroblastoma cells. Cellular metabolism was quantified by using the Alamar Blue bioassay where the toxin produces a time-dependent reduction in cell viability (b). Toxin-treated cells show an increase in bis-oxonol fluorescence indicating a membrane potential depolarization (c). The toxin also stimulates a fluorescence rise in fura-loaded neuroblastoma cells, which is indicative of a cytosolic calcium increment (d). Mean ± S.E.M. of 3 experiments. (From Cagide, E. et al., *Chem. Res. Toxicol.*, 24, 835, 2011; Cagide, E. et al., *Cell Physiol. Biochem.*, 19, 185, 2007.)

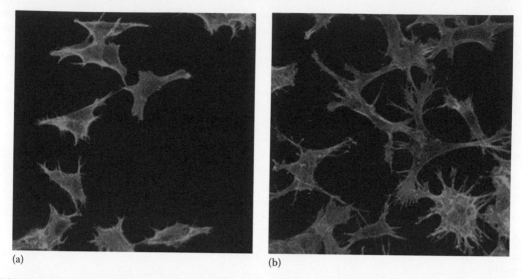

FIGURE 29.5　Evaluation of the effect of polycavernoside A analog 5 in F-actin of neuroblastoma cells stained with fluorescent phalloidin. Representative photographs showing actin cytoskeletons of untreated cells (a) and cells incubated with 4.8 μM polycavernoside A analog 5 (b). (From Cagide, E. et al., *Cell Physiol. Biochem.*, 19, 185, 2007.)

voltage-gated calcium channels, confirmed by the lack of inhibitory effect of nifedipine, a commonly used blocker of those channels.[19] Depolarization is a secondary effect induced by the extracellular calcium entry since it was abolished in a Ca^{2+}-free medium. These results provide the first insight into the mode of action of PA.[23]

PA possibly has a cyanobacterial origin, basing on its chemical structure and the sudden and transient occurrence of toxicity of the alga *Polycavernosa tsudai*.[2,17] Some of the toxins produced by cyanobacteria are neurotoxins that block neurotransmission by acting on cholinergic receptors. Also, the symptoms of intoxication induced by PA in mice are similar to a stimulation of the parasympathetic nervous system. However, muscarinic acetylcholine receptors are not the pharmacological target for the toxin. This is based on the fact that atropine, a muscarinic receptor antagonist, did not modify the increment in $[Ca^{2+}]_i$ evoked by the synthetic analog 5 of PA.[23]

In the literature, other compounds that induce neurological and/or gastrointestinal disorders cause alterations in the actin cytoskeleton.[24–27] Nevertheless, neuroblastoma cells incubated with 4.8 μM of analog **5** at 37°C for long time periods (up to 24 h) did not show modifications in the amount of F-actin or its distribution as it is shown in Figure 29.5. Cytomorphology was also maintained unaltered (Figure 29.5). These findings suggest that actin cytoskeleton is not an early target for PA analog 5.[23]

29.1.4 Toxicology

The first reported case of human intoxication resulting from the ingestion of the red alga *G. edulis* (*P. tsudai*) occurred in Guam in 1991. This is a widely consumed alga that had no potential risk registered before. In this incident, 13 people became ill and 3 of them died.[2] Two toxins were isolated from the alga: PA and PB. The toxicities of polycavernosides to mice were determined by intraperitoneal (i.p.) injection, and the symptoms were observed until 24 h after injection. The LD_{99} dose was estimated to be 200–400 μg/kg for both PA and PB.[2,18] Both toxins induced gastrointestinal and neurological disorders in experimental animals, causing diarrhea, hypersalivation, lachrymation effects, muscle spasms, and cyanosis. These symptoms are comparable to those observed in the human patients involved in the Guam case, according to Dr. R. Roos, Guam Memorial Hospital.[2] The similarity of the symptoms in experimental animals and human patients supports that PA and PB were responsible for this poisoning.[2] Toxicity of PC2 was also analyzed; however, the mice did not show any symptoms and survived, suggesting that the value of LD_{99} for PC2 was more than 0.2 mg/kg.[5]

Outbreaks of poisoning due to polycavernosides were not reported again until 2002–2003 in Philippines. Three fatal human intoxications occurred from ingestion of the same red alga *G. edulis*, besides another one, *Acanthophora spicifera*.[3] Although the toxicity of the Philippines' alga to mice was considerably lower than that of Guam, the number of deaths and symptoms of the patients were quite similar to each other.[19]

29.1.5 Biological Detection

29.1.5.1 In Vivo Bioassays

In order to prevent food intoxications due to the ingestion of these red algae, screening methods are required. The mouse bioassay is a simple and inexpensive method for monitoring the level of toxicity. The test consists of injecting intraperitoneally toxic extracts into mice (12–15 g body weight) and observing the symptoms over 24 h, although in this case, the low sensitivity of mice to some poly-cavernoside analogs must be considered.[3] In order to improve the sample preparation process for the mouse bioassay, a partition between $CHCl_3$ and MeOH–water 2:3 (v/v) was necessary to remove the large amount of salt from the sample. Lyophilization of seaweed is recommended before extraction with organic solvent. The organic extraction would reduce the amount of inorganic salt in the extracts. In addition, after extraction, the organic layer ($CHCl_3$ layer, for example) containing toxins should be washed with water or MeOH–water 2:3 (v/v) to remove the salts. These processes are very important because inorganic salt from seaweed can kill mice at relatively low doses when injected intraperitoneally.[19]

29.1.5.2 In Vitro Assays

Polycavernosides are cytotoxic compounds at least against neuroblastoma cells. Yotsu-Yamashita et al.[20] first discovered this effect with several analogs of PA on the neuroblastoma cell line Neuro-2a, and Cagide et al.[23] confirmed this effect with analog 5 on a different neuroblastoma cell line, BE(2)M-17. Taking these preliminary experiments into account, a cytotoxic assay for the detection of polycavernosides could be developed.[19]

29.2 Other Scarce New Toxins

Research groups are doing considerable effort in order to perform investigations that follow new or scarce toxin episodes. There are many compounds newly emerging of which little information is available. Some other toxins are well known but, for human or environmental reasons, appear in new locations as different analogs. On the other hand, the lack of toxic material from natural sources severely hampers the structure elucidation as well as the study of the biological properties of these compounds. This chapter will highlight some examples that might fit these characteristics.

29.2.1 Goniodomin

Goniodomin is a polyether macrolide first obtained from the dinoflagellate *Goniodoma* sp. by Sharma et al.[28] Later on, goniodomin A (Figure 29.6) was isolated as a potent antifungal agent from the dino-flagellate *G. pseudogoniaulax* collected in the rock pool at Jogashima in Japan in 1988.[29] It was also reported that the dinoflagellate *Alexandrium monilatum* produced goniodomin A.[30] On the basis of the NMR studies, the gross planar structure of goniodomin A was established by Murakami and coworkers to be a novel polyether macrolide, which contains a spiroacetal ring, an additional 4 oxacycles, and 17 stereogenic centers embedded within a 36-carbon chain.[29] The absolute configuration of goniodomin A was defined on the basis of detailed 2D NMR studies and degradation experiments of the natural product, the synthesis of suitable model compounds for NMR spectroscopic comparisons, and the correlation with synthetic reference compounds.[30]

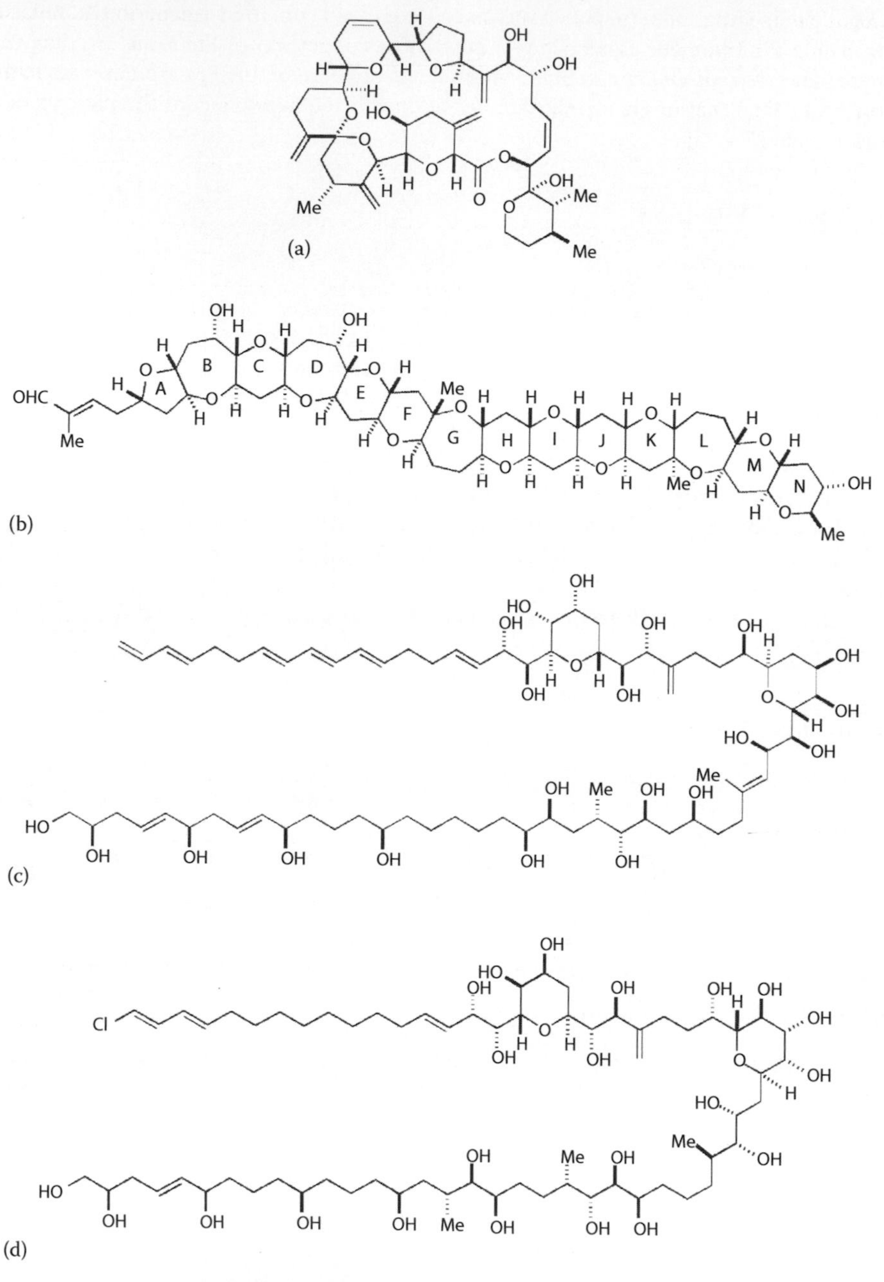

FIGURE 29.6 Structures of (a) goniodomin A, (b) gymnocin-A, (c) amphidinol 3, and (d) karlotoxin 2.

From a toxicological perspective, goniodomins are responsible for killing fish. It is also poisonous for mammals; the i.p. LD$_{50}$ values of goniodomin A in male mice were 1.2 and 0.7 mg/kg at 24 and 48 h, respectively. This toxin induced morphological changes in the liver and thymus of male mice. Histopathological studies indicated perihepatitis, nonfatty vacuoles in the hepatocytes, central necrosis of the liver, and massive necrosis of lymphocytes, in the cortical layer of the thymus.[31]

From a pharmacological point of view, the progress on the mechanism of action of this toxin is quite recent. Goniodomin A inhibits cell division in the fertilized sea urchin.[29] It has been demonstrated that the toxin modifies the rabbit skeletal actomyosin ATPase activity.[32] Goniodomin A binds to actin and causes its conformational change to modulate actomyosin ATPase activity. These findings suggest that this conformational change of actin molecules may modify the interaction between actin and myosin.[33] The marked enhancement of the skeletal muscle actomyosin ATPase activity by goniodomin A may be physiologically significant because it appears to be highly sensitive to the regulatory protein system, troponin/tropomyosin complex.[34] Moreover, goniodomin A affects actin to modify cardiac actomyosin ATPase activity, and this modulation differs between ventricular and atrial muscles.[35] Therefore, this toxin is a valuable pharmacological tool for studies on cardiac muscle contraction. It has also been reported that goniodomin A causes morphological changes in human astrocytoma, a nonmuscle cell, by increasing the content of filamentous actin (F-actin).[36] In 2002, goniodomin A was reported to inhibit angiogenesis in vivo, suppressing endothelial cell migration and basic fibroblast growth factor-induced tube formation. Those effects were mediated at least in part through the inhibition of actin reorganization.[37] These results indicated that goniodomin A might provide a selective modulator of actin for the study of not only the relationship between the structure and the function of actin but also the molecular mechanism of the activation of actomyosin ATPase.

29.2.2 Gymnocin

Gymnocins are a series of marine polycyclic ether toxins, produced by the dinoflagellate *Karenia* (formerly *Gymnodinium*) *mikimotoi*. This is a dinoflagellate close to the producer of brevetoxins, *K. brevis*.[38] The dinoflagellate *K. mikimotoi* is one of the most notorious red tide species that cause devastating damages to aquaculture and marine ecosystems worldwide. Gymnocin-A (Figure 29.6) has been isolated from *K. mikimotoi* by Satake et al.[39] Structure was elucidated by 2D-NMR analysis and FAB collision-induced MS/MS experiments; 14 contiguous saturated ether rings and a 2-methyl-2-butenal side chain at 5-position of A ring characterized it.[17] The absolute configuration of gymnocin-A was also determined by applying the modified Mosher method at the 50-OH group. Sasaki and coworkers have achieved the total synthesis of this complex molecule.[38]

Though its mechanism of action has not been determined, gymnocin-A exhibits potent in vitro cytotoxicity against a murine P388 lymphocytic leukemia cell line with EC_{50} value of 1.3 μg/mL.[38] Several congeners of gymnocin-A were also isolated, and some of them displayed cytotoxicity far stronger than this toxin.[40] Gymnocin-B was isolated from the dinoflagellate *K. mikimotoi*.[41,42] On the basis of extensive NMR and MS analysis, the structure and the relative configuration of gymnocin-B were elucidated. Similar to gymnocin-A, this new toxin contains 15 contiguous polyether skeletons and a 2-methyl-2-butenal side chain at the C-5 position. The structure of gymnocin-A is related to ciguatoxins (CTXs), brevetoxins (PbTxs), and gambierol.[40,41,43–45] These molecules generally present a great diversity in size, with widely varying functional groups and different toxicological and chemical characteristics, and potent biological activities. In fact, gambierol, CTX-3C, and PbTx-3 and -9 have been reported to be successful in producing a membrane depolarization and a subsequent calcium influx.[22,46] However, gymnocin-A was unable to modify any of those parameters in neuroblastoma cells.[21] In addition, the actin cytoskeleton seems not to be an early target for any of these toxins since none of them induced morphological changes or alterations in the actin assembly in neuroblastoma cells. Interestingly, the cells showed a slight reduction in the metabolism of the cells with gambierol, while the metabolic rate showed no decrease when incubating with CTX-3C, PbTx-3, or gymnocin-A.[21] According to this, sharing the same polycyclic ether backbone is not enough to produce the same effects on neuroblastoma cells.

29.2.3 Amphidinols

Amphidinols (AMs) comprise a family of architecturally unique marine metabolites isolated from the dinoflagellate *Amphidinium klebsii* and *A. carterae* that belong to the order Gymnodiniales.[47–49] AM structures are characterized by long carbon chain encompassing multiple hydroxyl groups and polyolefins. The lopsided distribution of these hydrophilic and hydrophobic moieties may be reminiscent of polyene macrolides such as amphotericin B and endow amphiphilic nature to the molecules. The middle portion containing the two tetrahydropyran rings is highly conserved among the AM congeners, and structural diversity arises from the polyol and polyene moieties.[50] However, unlike other natural or synthetic antifungal agents, neither nitrogenous polycycles nor macrocyclic structures are present in the structure. Amphidinol 1 (AM1) was reported by Satake et al. in 1991 as the first member of a new class of long-chain polyhydroxyl polyene natural compounds.[47] Since then, nearly 20 AMs have been reported so far.[47–49,51,52] The isolation of amphidinol 2 (AM2) was reported in 1995.[48] The structure of amphidinol 3 (AM3) was elucidated by mass spectroscopic analysis and NMR spectroscopy using a potentially powerful new *J*-based method, modified Mosher method, and HPLC analysis of the degradation products via oxidative cleavage.[49,53] The intriguing complexity of the structure of AM3 arises in part from the 67-carbon backbone that contains 25 stereocenters, a highly oxygenated bis-tetrahydropyran core (C31–C51), a heavily unsaturated region featuring a unique (*E,E,E*)-triene (C52–C67), and a polyol domain consisting of repeating 1,5-diol moieties (C1–C30). Since Murata's assignment of the AM3 absolute configuration appeared in 1999, a number of synthetic studies have been disclosed, including reports from Flamme and Roush,[54] de Vicente et al.,[55] and Paquette and Chang.[56] In 2008, Murata et al. published a revised structure in which the absolute configuration at C2 had been changed to *R* by comparing synthetic specimens with a fragment of AM3,[57] the absolute configuration at C45 has been recently confirmed by Manabe et al.,[58] and the absolute configuration at C51 was revised by Ebine et al.[78]) (Figure 29.6).

AMs have shown antifungal activity that substantially exceeds that of commercial drugs such as amphotericin B.[51,59] Besides the antifungal activity against *Aspergillus niger*, AMs possess potent toxicity against diatoms, implying the allelochemical roles against other epiphytic microbes in marine ecosystems.[51] AMs also possess potent hemolytic activity against human erythrocytes.[48] AM2 is toxic to primary rat hepatocytes with IC_{50} values of 6.4 μM. AM2 caused a rapid mitochondrial swelling and leakage of Ca^{2+}, underlying the change in the permeability of mitochondria.[60] However, the mitochondrial actions of AM2 are not involved in the plasma membrane permeabilizing effects, which might account for its cytotoxicity.

AM3 is the key member of the family and one of the most biologically active. AM3 enhances the permeability of the biological membrane by direct interaction with the membrane lipids, which is thought to be responsible for their potent antifungal activity.[51,59,61] Their powerful membrane-disrupting activity is originated from a channel-like assemblage.[51] The molecular mode of action has been proposed on the basis of the conformation of AM3 in sodium dodecyl sulfate micelles as follows: (1) AMs bind to bilayer membrane chiefly with the polyene part (C52–C67 of AM3); (2) the polyhydroxyl chain (C1–C20 of AM3) is responsible for formation of the pore/lesion across membrane; (3) the central region (C20–C51 of AM3) takes hairpin-shaped conformation that is stabilized by hydrogen bonds under amphipathic environments.[59,62] The structure–activity relations have been examined using naturally occurring AMs and chemically modified AM derivatives. It has been found that (1) hydrophobicity of the polyene chain of AMs dramatically affects the membrane activities, (2) the polyhydroxyl chain moderately modulates the biological activities, and (3) substitution of the sulfate group is generally inhibitory to antifungal and hemolytic activities, while giving rise to an insignificant effect on the size of pores/lesions.[61,62] Besides, the conformation and location of AM3 in a membrane environment were also determined using isotropic bicelles, a more natural membrane model than micelles, showing that AM3 takes turn structures at the two tetrahydropyran rings. Most of the hydrophilic region of the molecule is predominantly present in the surface, while the hydrophobic polyolefin penetrates in the bicelle interior. This conformational and positional preference of AM3 is considered to play a crucial role for pore formation in biological membranes.[62]

The efficacies of AM2 and AM3 have been measured by fluorescent-dye leakage experiments for liposomes with various cholesterol and ergosterol contents, indicating the significant enhancement of the membrane permeability with increasing concentrations of the sterol.[61] Moreover, AM3 has 1000 and 5300 times higher affinity for cholesterol- and ergosterol-containing liposomes, respectively, than those without sterol.[51,63] The interaction is composed of two steps, which correspond to binding to the membrane and internalization to form stable complexes.[63] Their activity was not affected by membrane thickness; therefore, AMs permeabilized membrane by a different mechanism from that of polyene macrolide antibiotics.[61] Also there is a potentiation of action by Glycophorin A, or membrane integral peptides may be due to a higher affinity of AMs to protein-containing membranes than that to pure lipid bilayers.[64] Therefore, AM3 is one of few nonionic compounds that possess potent sterol-dependent membrane-permeabilizing activity with nondetergent mechanism.[59]

29.2.4 Karlotoxin

Analogs related to AMs such as the luteophanols, lingshuiol, and karatungiol have been reported displaying cytotoxic and antifungal activity, respectively. Another closely related toxic compounds were first described from *Karlodinium veneficum* following an investigation of a large mortality event at HyRock fish farm, Maryland, USA, in 1996.[65] More recently, the structure of those compounds, called karlotoxins (KmTxs) and classified as ichthyotoxins, was determined.[66] The producer organism *K. veneficum*, first named as *Gymnodinium veneficum* and collected from the English Channel in 1950,[67] has been associated with fish kills worldwide.[68]

The karlotoxins, like the AMs, have a hairpin-like structure with three distinct regions: a polyol arm that exhibits variable hydroxylation and methylation; a hinge region containing two ether rings; and a lipophilic arm that, in karlotoxins, contains a terminal diene that gives these compounds their distinctive UV spectra. The length of the lipophilic arm is an important determinant for potency of the karlotoxins, and sulfonation might provide an effective means of reducing toxicity.[69]

Two families of karlotoxins, the KmTx 1 and KmTx 2, have been described, which differ from one another in UV absorbance maxima, potency, and geographic distribution.[69] In recent years, the structure and absolute configuration of KmTx 2 (Figure 29.6) have been reported.[70] KmTx 2, found in isolates and fish kill waters from outside of the Chesapeake Bay watershed, Maryland, USA, was recently reported to be a linear polyketide with a molecular weight of 1344.8 Da.[66,71] The difference between KmTx1 and KmTx 2 in carbon chain structure is localized to the length of the lipophilic side chain. In KmTx 1, the side chain is two carbons longer. Moreover, it is possible for KmTx 1-like and KmTx 2-like compounds to occur in the same organism. So far, only three KmTx compounds have been published with complete mass and UV data, but up to six structures have been identified by LC-MS.[71]

KmTxs display a variety of interesting effects on biological systems including cytotoxic and hemolytic activities and kill fish through damage to sensitive gill epithelial tissues and immobilization of prey organisms.[72,73] Those effects are reproducible from toxin produced in culture as well as from the environment.[66] There is growing evidence that the karlotoxins support a number of ecological roles for *K. veneficum* including deterring predation and assisting prey capture. The mechanism of toxicity of KmTx is based on the membrane pore formation increasing the ionic permeability of biological membranes destroying the osmotic balance of the cell and leading to cell death.[73] The cytolytic activity of the karlotoxins is modulated by membrane sterol composition, which also appears to be responsible for the apparent immunity of *K. veneficum* to the membrane-disrupting properties of its own toxins.[66,74,75] Cells containing 4α-methyl sterols are immune, whereas cells containing 4-desmethyl sterols (like cholesterol) are susceptible to KmTx. This may play an important role in prey immobilization since the principal source of food possesses mainly these sterols in their membranes while *K. veneficum* possesses in majority 4α-methyl sterols.[76]

Karlotoxins provide an interesting opportunity to create a nontoxic cholesterol pharmacophore that could potentially transport cholesterol from the arteries to the liver or kidneys for excretion. Therefore, karlotoxins are intriguing molecules for the design and synthesis of novel cholesterol-targeted drug leads for the treatment of severe human health issues including heart disease and cancer.[77]

REFERENCES

1. Haddock, R. L.; Cruz, O. L. 1991. Foodborne intoxication associated with seaweed. *Lancet*, 338, 195–196.
2. Yotsu-Yamashita, M.; Haddock, R. L.; Yasumoto, T. 1993. Polycavernoside A: A novel glycosidic macrolide from the red alga *Polycavernosa tsudai* (*Gracilaria edulis*). *J. Am. Chem. Soc.*, 115, 1147–1148.
3. Yotsu-Yamashita, M.; Yasumoto, T.; Yamada, S.; Bajarias, F. F. A., Formelozsa, M. A., Romero, M. L., Fukuyo, Y. 2004. Identification of polycavernoside A as the causative agent of the fatal food poisoning resulting from ingestion of the red alga *Gracilaria edulis* in the Philippines. *Chem. Res. Toxicol.*, 17, 1265–1271.
4. Yotsu-Yamashita, M.; Seki, T.; Paul, V. J.; Naoki, H.; Yasumoto, T. 1995. Four new analogs of polycavernoside A. *Tetrahedron Lett.*, 36, 5563–5566.
5. Yotsu-Yamashita, M.; Abe, K.; Seki, T.; Fujiwara, K.; Yasumoto, T. 2007. The structures of polycavernoside C and C2, the new analogs of the human lethal toxin polycavernoside A, from the red alga, *Gracilaria edulis*. *Tetrahedron Lett.*, 48, 2255–2259.

6. Fujiwara, K.; Murai, A.; Yotsu-Yamashita, M.; Yasumoto, T. 1998. Total synthesis and absolute configuration of polycavernoside A. *J. Am. Chem. Soc.*, 120, 10770–10771.

7. Paquette, L. A.; Barriault, L.; Pissarnitski, D. 1999. A convergent total synthesis of the macrolactone disaccharide toxin (-)-polycavernoside A. *J. Am. Chem. Soc.*, 121, 4542–4543.

8. Paquette, L. A.; Barriault, L.; Pissarnitski, D.; Johnston, J. N. 2000. Stereocontrolled elaboration of natural (-)-polycavernoside A, a powerfully toxic metabolite of the red alga *Polycavernosa tsudai*. *J. Am. Chem. Soc.*, 122, 619–631.

9. White, J. D.; Blakemore, P. R.; Browder, C. C.; Hong, J.; Lincoln, C. M.; Nagornyy, P. A.; Robarge, L. A.; Wardrop, D. J. 2001. Total synthesis of the marine toxin polycavernoside A via selective macrolactonization of a trihydroxy carboxylic acid. *J. Am. Chem. Soc.*, 123, 8593–8595.

10. Blakemore, P. R.; Browder, C. C.; Hong, J.; Lincoln, C. M.; Nagornyy, P. A.; Robarge, L. A.; Wardrop, D. J.; White, J. D. 2005. Total synthesis of polycavernoside A, a lethal toxin of the red alga *Polycavernosa tsudai*. *J. Org. Chem.*, 70, 5449–5460.

11. Woo, S. K.; Lee, E. 2010. Polycavernoside A: The prins macrocyclization approach. *J. Am. Chem. Soc.*, 132, 4564–4565.

12. Kasai, Y.; Ito, T.; Sasaki, M. 2012. Total synthesis of (-)-polycavernoside A: Suzuki-Miyaura coupling approach. *Org. Lett.*, 14, 3186–3189.

13. Perez-Balado, C.; Marko, I. E. 2005. A connective approach to the tetrahydropyran subunit of polycavernoside A via a novel 1,1-dianion equivalent. *Tetrahedron Lett.*, 46, 4887–4890.

14. Perez-Balado, C.; Marko, I. E. 2006. 1-Iodo-1-seleno-alkenes as versatile alkene 1,1-dianion equivalents. Novel connective approach towards the tetrahydropyran subunit of polycavernoside A. *Tetrahedron*, 62, 2331–2349.

15. Barry, C. S.; Bushby, N.; Harding, J. R.; Willis, C. L. 2005. Stereoselective synthesis of the tetrahydropyran core of polycavernoside A. *Org. Lett.*, 7, 2683.

16. Pierre, J.; Freddi, P.; Raphael, D.; Istvan, E. M. 2009. Pentadienyl sulfoxide in triene synthesis. Efficient assembly of the Northern fragment of polycavernoside. *Tetrahedron Lett.*, 50, 3366–3370.

17. Yasumoto, T. 2001. The chemistry and biological function of natural marine toxins. *Chem. Rec.*, 1, 228–242.

18. Barriault, L.; Boulet, S. L.; Fujiwara, K.; Murai, A.; Paquette, L. A.; Yotsu-Yamashita, M. 1999. Synthesis and biological evaluation of analogs of the marine toxin polycavernoside A. *Bioorg. Med. Chem. Lett.*, 9, 2069–2072.

19. Louzao, M. C.; Cagide, E.; Yotsu-Yamashita, M.; Sasaki, M. 2008. Polycavernosides and gambierol: Chemistry, pharmacology, toxicology and detection. In Botana, L. M. (Ed.) *Seafood and Freshwater Toxins: Pharmacology, Physiology and Detection*. Boca Raton, FL: CRC Press.

20. Yotsu-Yamashita, M.; Abe, K.; Taya, Y.; Yasumoto, T.; Seki,T.; Yamada, S.; Bajarias, F. F. A.; Formelozsa, M.; Fukuyo, Y. 2004. Identification of polycavernoside A as the causative agent of the fatal food poisoning resulting from ingestion of the red alga *Gracilaria edulis* in Philippines: Origin, biological activity and the structures of new analogs of polycavernosides. In Hirata, T. (Ed.) *Proceedings of the 46th Symposium on the Chemistry of Natural Products*. Hiroshima, Japan.

21. Cagide, E.; Louzao, M. C.; Espina, B. et al. 2011. Comparative cytotoxicity of gambierol versus other marine neurotoxins. *Chem. Res. Toxicol.*, 24, 835–842.

22. Louzao, M. C.; Vieytes, M. R.; Yasumoto, T.; Yotsu-Yamashita, M.; Botana, L. M. 2006. Changes in membrane potential: An early signal triggered by neurologically active phycotoxins. *Chem. Res. Toxicol.*, 19, 788–793.

23. Cagide, E.; Louzao, M. C.; Ares, I. R. et al. 2007. Effects of a synthetic analog of polycavernoside A on human neuroblastoma cells. *Cell Physiol. Biochem.*, 19, 185–194.

24. Ares, I. R.; Louzao, M. C.; Vieytes, M. R.; Yasumoto, T.; Botana, L. M. 2005. Actin cytoskeleton of rabbit intestinal cells is a target for potent marine phycotoxins. *J. Exp. Biol.*, 208, 4345–4354.

25. Espiña, B.; Louzao, M. C.; Ares, I. R. et al. 2008. Cytoskeletal toxicity of pectenotoxins in hepatic cells. *Br. J. Pharmacol.*, 155, 934–944.

26. Louzao, M. C.; Ares, I. R.; Cagide, E. 2008. Marine toxins and the cytoskeleton: A new view of palytoxin toxicity. *FEBS J.*, 275, 6067–6074.

27. Louzao, M. C.; Ares, I. R.; Cagide, E. et al. 2010. Palytoxins and cytoskeleton: An overview. *Toxicon*, 57, 460–469.

28. Sharma, G. M.; Michaelis, L.; Burkholder, P. R. 1968. Goniodomin, a new antibiotic from a dinoflagellate. *J. Antibiot.*, 21, 659–664.

29. Murakami, M.; Makabe, K.; Yamaguchi, S.; Konosu, S.; Walchli, R. 1988. Goniodomin A, a novel polyether macrolide from the dinoflagellate *Goniodoma pseudogoniaulax*. *Tetrahedron Lett.*, 29, 1149.

30. Takeda, Y.; Shi, J.; Oikawa, M.; Sasaki, M. 2008. Assignment of the absolute configuration of goniodomin A by NMR spectroscopy and synthesis of model compounds. *Org. Lett.*, 10, 1013–1016.

31. Terao, K.; Ito, E.; Murakami, M.; Yamaguchi, K. 1989. Histopathological studies on experimental marine toxin poisoning—III. Morphological changes in the liver and thymus of male ICR mice induced by goniodomin A, isolated from the dinoflagellate *Goniodoma pseudogoniaulax*. *Toxicon*, 27, 269–271.

32. Furukawa, K. I.; Sakai, K.; Watanabe, S. et al. 1993. Goniodomin A induces modulation of actomyosin ATPase activity mediated through conformational change of actin. *J. Biol. Chem.*, 268, 26026–26031.

33. Ohizumi, Y. 1997. Application of physiologically active substances isolated from natural resources to pharmacological studies. *Jpn. J. Pharmacol.*, 73, 263–289.

34. Matsunaga, K.; Nakatani, K.; Murakami, M.; Yamaguchi, K.; Ohizumi, Y. 1999. Powerful activation of skeletal muscle actomyosin ATPase by goniodomin A is highly sensitive to troponin/tropomyosin complex. *J. Pharmacol. Exp. Ther.*, 291, 1121–1126.

35. Yasuda, M.; Nakatani, K.; Matsunaga, K.; Murakami, M.; Momose, K.; Ohizumi, Y. 1998. Modulation of actomyosin ATPase by goniodomin A differs in types of cardiac myosin. *Eur. J. Pharmacol.*, 346, 119–123.

36. Mizuno, K.; Nakahata, N.; Ito, E.; Murakami, M.; Yamaguchi, K.; Ohizumi, Y. 1998. Goniodomin A, an antifungal polyether macrolide, increases the filamentous actin content of 1321N1 human astrocytoma cells. *J. Pharm. Pharmacol.*, 50, 645–648.

37. Abe, M.; Inoue, D.; Matsunaga, K. et al. 2002. Goniodomin A, an antifungal polyether macrolide, exhibits antiangiogenic activities via inhibition of actin reorganization in endothelial cells. *J. Cell. Physiol.*, 190, 109–116.

38. Sasaki, M.; Tsukano, C.; Tachibana, K. 2002. Studies toward the total synthesis of gymnocin A, a cytotoxic polyether: A highly convergent entry to the F-N ring fragment. *Org. Lett.*, 4, 1747–1750.

39. Satake, M.; Shoji, M.; Oshima, Y.; Naoki, H.; Fujita, T.; Yasumoto, T. 2002. Gymnocin-A, a cytotoxic polyether from the notorious red tide dinoflagellate, *Gymnodinium mikimotoi*. *Tetrahedron Lett.*, 43, 5829–5832.

40. Tsukano, C.; Ebine, M.; Sasaki, M. 2005. Convergent total synthesis of gymnocin-A and evaluation of synthetic analogues. *J. Am. Chem. Soc.*, 127, 4326–4335.

41. Tanaka, K.; Itagaki, Y.; Satake, M.; H. Naoki; T. Yasumoto; K. Nakanishi; Berova, N. 2005. Three challenges toward the assignment of absolute configuration of gymnocin-B. *J. Am. Chem. Soc.*, 127, 9561–9570.

42. Satake, M.; Tanaka, Y.; Ishikura, Y.; Oshima, Y.; Naoki, H.; Yasumoto, T. 2005. Gymnocin-B with the largest contiguous polyether rinds from the red tide dinoflagellate, Karenia (formerly Gymnodinium) mikimotoi. *Tetrahedron Lett.*, 46, 3537–3540.

43. Tsukano, C.; Sasaki, M. 2003. Total synthesis of gymnocin-A. *J. Am. Chem. Soc.*, 125, 14294–14295.

44. Sasaki, M.; Fuwa, H. 2008. Convergent strategies for the total synthesis of polycyclic ether marine metabolites. *Nat. Prod. Rep.*, 25, 401–426.

45. Van Dyke, A. R.; Jamison, T. F. 2009. Functionalized templates for the convergent assembly of polyethers: Synthesis of the HIJK rings of gymnocin A. *Angew. Chem. Int. Ed. Engl.*, 48, 4430–4432.

46. Louzao, M. C.; Cagide, E.; Vieytes, M. R. et al. 2006. The sodium channel of human excitable cells is a target for gambierol. *Cell Physiol. Biochem.*, 17, 257–268.

47. Satake, M.; Murata, M.; Yasumoto, T.; Fujita, H.; Naoki, M. 1991. Amphidinol, a polyhydroxy-polyene antifungal agent with an unprecedented structure, from a marine dinoflagellate, *Amphidinium klebsii*. *J. Am. Chem. Soc.*, 113, 9859–9861.

48. Paul, G. K.; Matsumori, N.; Murata, M.; Tachibana, K. 1995. Isolation and chemical structure of amphidinol 2, a potent hemolytic compound from marine dinoflagellate *Amphidinium klebsii*. *Tetrahedron Lett.*, 36, 6279–6282.

49. Murata, M.; Matsuoka, S.; Matsumori, N.; Paul, G. K.; Tachibana, K. 1999. Absolute configuration of amphidinol 3, the first complete structure determined from amphidinol homologues: Application of a new configuration analysis based on carbon-hydrogen spin-coupling constants. *J. Am. Chem. Soc.*, 121, 870–871.

50. Kanemoto, M.; Murata, M.; Oishi, T. 2009. Stereoselective synthesis of the C31-C40/C43-C52 unit of amphidinol 3. *J. Org. Chem.*, 74, 8810–8813.

51. Paul, G. K.; Matsumori, N.; Konoki, K.; Murata, M.; Tachibana, K. 1997. Chemical structures of amphidinols 5 and 6 isolated from marine dinoflagellate *Amphidinium klebsii* and their cholesterol-dependent membrane disruption. *J. Mar. Biotechnol.*, 5, 124–128.

52. Fürstner, A.; Bouchez, L. C.; Morency, L. et al. 2009. Total syntheses of amphidinolides B1, B4, G1, H1 and structure revision of amphidinolide H2. *Chem. Eur. J.*, 15, 3983–4010.

53. Matsumori, N.; Kaneno, D.; Murata, M.; Nakamura, H.; Tachibana, K. 1999. Stereochemical determination of acyclic structures based on carbon-proton spin-coupling constants. A method of configuration analysis for natural products. *J. Org. Chem.*, 64, 866–876.

54. Flamme, E. M.; Roush, W. R. 2002. Enantioselective synthesis of 1,5-anti- and 1,5-syn-diols using a highly diastereoselective one-pot double allylboration reaction sequence. *J. Am. Chem. Soc.*, 124, 13644–13645.

55. de Vicente, J.; Betzemeier, B.; Rychnovsky, S. D. 2005. A C-Glycosidation approach to the central core of amphidinol 3: Synthesis of the C39-C52 fragment. *Org. Lett.*, 7, 1853–1856.

56. Paquette, L. A.; Chang, S. K. 2005. The polyol domain of amphidinol 3. A stereoselective synthesis of the entire C(1)-C(30) sector. *Org. Lett.*, 7, 3111–3114.

57. Oishi, T.; Kanemoto, M.; Swasono, R.; Matsumori, N.; Murata, M. 2008. Combinatorial synthesis of the 1,5-polyol system based on cross metathesis: Structure revision of amphidinol 3. *Org. Lett.*, 10, 5203–5206.

58. Manabe, Y.; Ebine, M.; Matsumori, N.; Murata, M.; Oishi, T. 2012. Confirmation of the absolute configuration at C45 of amphidinol 3. *J. Nat. Prod.*, 75, 2003–2006.

59. Houdai, T.; Matsuoka, S.; Matsumori, N.; Murata, M. 2004. Membrane-permeabilizing activities of amphidinol 3, polyene-polyhydroxy antifungal from a marine dinoflagellate. *Biochim. Biophys. Acta*, 1667, 91–100.

60. Qi, X. M.; Yu, B.; Huang, X. C.; Guo, Y. W.; Zhai, Q.; Jin, R. 2007. The cytotoxicity of lingshuiol: A comparative study with amphidinol 2 on membrane permeabilizing activities. *Toxicon*, 50, 278–282.

61. Morsy, N.; Houdai, T.; Konoki, K.; Matsumori, N.; Oishi, T.; Murata, M. 2008. Effects of lipid constituents on membrane-permeabilizing activity of amphidinols. *Bioorg. Med. Chem.*, 16, 3084–3090.

62. Houdai, T.; Matsumori, N.; Murata, M. 2008. Structure of membrane-bound amphidinol 3 in isotropic small bicelles. *Org. Lett.*, 10, 4191–4194.

63. Swasono, R. T.; Mouri, R.; Morsy, N.; Matsumori, N.; Oishi, T.; Murata, M. 2010. Sterol effect on interaction between amphidinol 3 and liposomal membrane as evidenced by surface plasmon resonance. *Bioorg. Med. Chem. Lett.*, 20, 2215–2218.

64. Morsy, N.; Konoki, K.; Houdai, T.; Matsumori, N.; Oishi, T.; Murata, M.; Aimoto, S. 2008. Roles of integral protein in membrane permeabilization by amphidinols. *Biochim. Biophys. Acta*, 1778, 1453–1459.

65. Deeds, J. R.; Terlizzi, D. E.; Adolf, J. E.; Stoecker, D. K.; Place, A. R. 2002. Hemolytic and ichthyotoxic activity from cultures of *Karlodinium micrum* (Dinophyceae) associated with fish mortalities in an estuarine aquaculture facility. *Harmful Algae*, 1, 169–189.

66. Van Wagoner, R. M.; Deeds, J. R.; Satake, M.; Ribeiro, A. A.; Placed, A. R.; Wright, J. L. C. 2008. Isolation and characterization of karlotoxin 1, a new amphipathic toxin from *Karlodinium veneficum*. *Tetrahedron Lett.*, 49, 6457–6461.

67. Ballantine, D. 1956. Two new marine species of Gymnodinium isolated from the Plymouth area. *J. Mar. Biol. Assoc. U.K.*, 35, 467–474.

68. Kempton, J. W.; Lewitus, A. J.; Deeds, J. R.; Law, J. M.; Place, A. R. 2002. Toxicity of *Karlodinium micrum* (Dinophyceae) associated with a fish kill in a South Carolina brackish retention pond. *Harmful Algae*, 1, 223–241.

69. Van Wagoner, R. M.; Deeds, J. R.; Tatters, A. O.; Place, A. R.; Tomas, C. R.; Wright, J. L. C. 2010. Structure and relative potency of several karlotoxins from *Karlodinium weneficum*. *J. Nat. Prod.*, 73, 1360–1365.

70. Peng, J.; Place, A. R.; Yoshida, W.; Clemens, A.; Hamann, M. T. 2010. Structure and absolute configuration of Karlotoxin-2, an ichthyotoxin from the marine dinoflagellate *Karlodinium veneficum*. *J. Am. Chem. Soc.*, 132, 3277–3279.

71. Bachvaroff, T. R.; Adolf, J. E.; Squier, A. H.; Harvey, H. R.; Place, A. R. 2008. Characterization and quantification of karlotoxins by liquid chromatography-mass spectrometry. *Harmful Algae*, 7, 473–484.

72. Deeds, J. R.; Reimschuessel, R.; Place, A. R. 2006. Histopathological effects in fish exposed to the toxins from *Karlodinium micrum*. *J. Aquat. Anim. Health*, 18, 136–148.

73. Sheng, J.; Malkiel, E.; Katz, J.; Adolf, J. E.; Place, A. R. 2010. A dinoflagellate exploits toxins to immobilize prey prior to ingestion. *Proc. Natl. Acad. Sci.*, 107, 2082–2087.

74. Adolf, J. E.; Bachvaroff, T. R.; Krupatkina, D. N. et al. 2006. Species specificity and potential roles of *Karlodinium micrum* toxin. *Afr. J. Mar. Sci.*, 28, 415–419.

75. Adolf, J. E.; Krupatkina, D.; Bachvaroff, T.; Place, A. R. 2007. Karlotoxin mediates grazing by *Oxyrrhis marina* on strains of *Karlodinium veneficum*. *Harmful Algae*, 6, 400–412.

76. Place, A. R.; Bai, X.; Kim, S.; Sengco, M. R.; Coats, D. W. 2009. Dinoflagellate host-parasite sterol profiles dictate karlotoxin sensitivity. *J. Phycol.*, 45, 375–385.

77. Waters, A. L.; Hill, R. T.; Place, A. R.; Hamann, M. T. 2010. The expanding role of marine microbes in pharmaceutical development. *Curr. Opin. Biotechnol.*, 21, 780–786.

78. Ebine, M.; Kanemoto, M.; Manabe, Y.; Knno, Y.; Sakai, K.; Matsumori, N.; Murata, M.; Oishi, T. 2013. Synthesis and structure revision of the C43-C67 part of amphidinol 3. *Org. Lett.*, 15, 2846–2649.

79. Brewitz, L.; Llaveria, J.; Yada, A.; Frstner, A.; 2013. Formal total synthesis of the algal toxin (-)-polycavernoside A. *Chem. Eur. J.*,19, 4532–4537.

Part V

Marine Neurotoxins

30

Domoic Acid: Chemistry and Pharmacology

Carmen Vale

CONTENTS

30.1 Introduction

The excitatory amino acid domoic acid is a naturally occurring potent excitotoxin produced by various marine algae and diatoms. The toxin and its isomers are responsible for a human illness known as amnesic shellfish poisoning (ASP). The main symptoms of ASP in humans are gastrointestinal alterations including vomiting, diarrhea or abdominal cramps, and/or neurological symptoms characterized by confusion, loss of memory, or other alterations such as seizure or coma. In humans, the symptoms of ASP develop within 24–48 h after consuming contaminated shellfish. The toxicity mechanisms of domoic acid have been extensively investigated since an incident in 1987 in Eastern Canada, where several hundred people experienced serious health problems after ingesting mussels.[1] This first documented outbreak of ASP occurred in persons who had eaten cultivated mussels and affected 107 patients. The most common symptoms of the illness were vomiting (in 76% of the patients), abdominal cramps (which affected 50% of the patients), diarrhea (42%), incapacitating headache (in 43% of the patients), and loss of short-term memory (which affected 25% of the patients). In this ASP outbreak, 19 patients were hospitalized, of whom 12 required intensive care to treat seizures, coma, profuse respiratory secretions, or unstable blood pressure. In addition, three patients died. This first confirmed outbreak of ASP was related to the consumption of mussels affected by a bloom of the *Pseudo-nitzschia pungens*.[1]

Domoic acid is a water-soluble cyclic amino acid that acts as a partial agonist of some types of glutamate receptors. Domoic acid isomers have also been detected in shellfish in the United States and in a number of European countries. Although several isomers of domoic acid (diastereoisomer epidomoic acid and isodomoic acids) have been identified, data on the occurrence only of domoic acid and epidomoic acid (expressed as sum DA) have been reported to establish the current regulatory limits for domoic acid in the European Union.[2]

The molecular mechanisms involved in the toxicity elicited by domoic acid have been extensively investigated since the poisoning incident in 1987 in Eastern Canada. The chemistry, pharmacology, and toxicology of domoic acid is the basis of this chapter, which reviews the main characteristics of excitatory neurotransmission, the interaction of domoic acid with glutamate receptors, and the pharmacology of domoic acid and its isomers.

30.2 Excitatory Neurotransmission

L-glutamate (L-Glu) is the principal excitatory neurotransmitter in the central nervous system (CNS), where it regulates learning and memory, synaptic activity, neuronal plasticity, cell survival, and other relevant functions. L-glutamate mediates the majority of excitatory neurotransmission in the brain and spinal cord, and recent evidence suggests that glutamatergic receptors are also expressed by immune cells, regulating the degree of cell activation.[3]

Glutamate receptors mediate fast excitatory synaptic transmission in the CNS and are localized on neuronal and nonneuronal cells. These receptors regulate multiple functions in the brain, spinal cord, retina, and peripheral nervous system and play important roles in numerous neurological diseases: schizophrenia, stroke, epilepsy, Alzheimer's disease, and Parkinson's.[4,5] Initial pharmacological studies showed that glutamate receptors were not homogeneous. Glutamate receptor agonists are generally α-amino acids with one or more stereogenic centers due to strict requirements in the agonist binding pocket of the activated state of the receptor.[6]

Glutamate receptors are divided into two major subclasses: metabotropic glutamate receptors (mGluRs) coupled to guanosine 5′-triphosphate-binding proteins and the production of second messengers and ionotropic glutamate receptors (iGluRs), which form cation-specific ion channels and regulate fast excitatory transmission.[7] Since ionotropic glutamate receptors are the target of domoic acid and related isomers, this section reviews the main characteristics of these receptors.

30.2.1 Ionotropic Glutamate Receptors

The ionotropic class of glutamate receptors are integral membrane proteins composed of four subunits (>900 residues) that assemble to form a central ion channel pore. These receptors assemble as tetrameric complexes of subunits, and functional receptors are formed exclusively by the assembling of subunits within the same receptor class.[5]

The development of selective agonists for the different glutamate receptors led to the classification of the ionotropic glutamate receptors in three different groups: N-methyl-D-aspartate (NMDA), α-amino-3-hydroxy-5-methylisoxazoleproprionic acid (AMPA), and kainate receptors on the basis of the preferred agonist for each subtype.[8] Recently, the International Union of Basic and Applied Pharmacology (IUPHAR) has reviewed the subunit nomenclature of ionotropic glutamate receptors,[9,10] and this nomenclature will be followed through this chapter.

In the subunit nomenclature proposed by the IUPHAR, AMPA receptors are formed by coassembly of GluA1–4 subunits, while kainate receptors are composed of GluK1–5 subunits and NMDA receptors by coassembly of GluN1 with GluN2A–D and GluN3A–B.[9,10] Two additional members of a fourth ionotropic glutamate receptor gene family (GluD1 and GluD2) have also been described and are widely distributed in the rat cerebellum, but apparently, they do not generate functional glutamate ion channels.[11] Table 30.1 summarizes the current nomenclature of ionotropic receptor subunits as proposed by the IUPHAR as well as their common names.[9,10]

The current carried through most glutamate receptor channels is a mixture of monovalent cations (K^+ and Na^+) and Ca^{2+}. However, receptors containing the edited forms of GluA2, GluK1, or GluK2 are impermeable to calcium.[5] Moreover, the influx of Ca^{2+} through NMDA and Ca^{2+}-permeable AMPA receptors contributes to synaptic plasticity, gene regulation, neuropathology, and neurotransmitter release.[12]

TABLE 30.1

Ionotropic Glutamate Receptor Subunits

	IUPHAR Name	Common Names
AMPA receptors		
	GluA1	GluR1, GluRA
	GluA2	GluR2, GluRB
	GluA3	GluR3, GluRC
	GluA4	GluR4, GluRD
Kainate receptors		
	GluK1	GluR5
	GluK2	GluR6
	GluK3	GluR7
	GluK4	KA1
	GluK5	KA2
NMDA receptors		
	GluN1	NMDAR1, NR1, GluRε1
	GluN2A	NMDAR2A, NR2A, GluRε1
	GluN2B	NMDAR2B, NR2B, GluRε2
	GluN2C	NMDAR2C, NR2C, GluRε3
	GluN2D	NMDAR2D, NR2D, GluRε4
	GluN3A	NR3A
	GluN3B	NR3B
Delta receptors		
	GluD1	δ1, GluR delta-1
	GluD2	δ2, GluR delta-2

30.2.1.1 AMPA Receptors

AMPA receptors are one type of ionotropic glutamate receptors involved in rapid excitatory synaptic transmission. AMPA receptors have been increasingly implicated in long-term potentiation, thus regulating learning and memory, and participate in disorders affecting the nervous system. AMPA receptors are formed by the assembly of either homomeric or heteromeric GluA1–GluA4 subunits and present distinct functional properties. Native AMPA receptor channels are impermeable to calcium, a function controlled by the GluA2 subunit. The calcium permeability of the GluA2 subunit is determined by the posttranscriptional editing of the GluA2 mRNA, which changes the glutamine residue of the second transmembrane region to arginine; this is the so-called Q/R editing site. Glu2 subunits containing glutamine (Q) are calcium permeable, while GluA2 subunits containing arginine (R) are calcium impermeable. Almost all the GluA2 protein expressed in the CNS is in the GluA2(R) form, giving rise to calcium-impermeable AMPA receptors.[13]

AMPA receptors can be distinguished from other ionotropic glutamate receptors by the fast desensitization induced by the agonist AMPA. AMPA itself shows a good selectivity for AMPA receptors over kainate receptors (10- to 20-fold higher affinity for GluA1–4 over a representative kainate receptor subunit, GluK1). However, it shows no selectivity for different AMPA receptor subunits. Selective antagonists for AMPA receptors include the competitive antagonist NBQX (6-nitro-7-sulfamoylbenzo[f]quinoxaline-2,3-dione) and the noncompetitive antagonist GYKI53655 (1-(4-Aminophenyl)-3-methylcarbamyl-4-methyl-3,4-dihydro-7,8-methylenedioxy-5H-2,3-benzodiazepine hydrochloride). The latter is widely used to isolate kainate receptor responses from a mixed AMPA/kainate receptor-mediated response.[5,14,15]

30.2.1.2 Kainate Receptors

Activation of kainate receptors can induce postsynaptic responses, presynaptic regulation of neurotransmitter release, and generation of seizure activity. Like the other ionotropic glutamate receptors, they possess an extracellular N-terminus that, together with a loop between the transmembrane segments II and IV, forms the ligand-binding domain and a reentrant loop at the second transmembrane region (TMII) that forms the lining of the pore region of the ion channel.

Distinct populations of the kainate-type ionotropic glutamate receptors have been described in different cell types and subcellular compartments. Moreover, the diverse downstream signaling mechanisms activated by kainate receptors represent a complex system with large capacity for modulatory effects ranging from actions specific at the synapse to alterations in the excitability of large neuronal populations.

As mentioned earlier, kainate receptors are composed of the GluK1–GluK5 subunits according to the current IUPHAR nomenclature.[9] The kainate receptor subunits GluK1–GluK3 form both homo- and heteromers, but GluK4 and GluK5 form functional receptors only when coexpressed with GluK1 to GluK3.[5] Although the research on the physiological actions of kainate receptors has been initially slowed by the lack of specific kainate receptor modulators, early studies showed that recovery from desensitization after glutamate activation was 10-fold slower for kainate receptors than for AMPA receptors.[16]

Nowadays it is well established that kainate receptors regulate the activity of neuronal networks through yet incompletely understood mechanisms[17] that include postsynaptic depolarization, presynaptic modulation of both excitatory and inhibitory neurons, and increase in the neuronal excitability, thus affecting the equilibrium between neuronal excitation and inhibition. Moreover, recent evidences indicate that kainate receptors contribute to network regulation during development and are involved in the formation and maturation of glutamatergic synapses.[18]

Among ionotropic glutamate receptors, the relevance of kainate receptors to pathophysiology has been least explored. However, it is now well established that kainate receptors are located both pre- synaptically and postsynaptically. At the presynaptic location, kainate receptors encoded by GluK1 regulate glutamate and GABA release, and thus excitability, and participate in short-term plasticity. At the postsynaptic level, activation of kainate receptors encoded by GluK1 contributes to synaptic integration.[19]

Kainate receptors are distributed throughout the brain, but differ from the other two groups of iono- tropic glutamate receptors by the fact that kainate receptors are not predominantly found in excitatory postsynaptic complexes.[17] In addition to act as conventional ionotropic receptors, kainate receptors link to metabotropic signaling pathways modulating GABA release in the hippocampus through a mecha- nism involving a pertussis toxin-sensitive G-protein and protein kinase C, although the mechanistical aspects of this signaling are not yet fully understood but probably involve accessory proteins and neu- romodulators released in response to kainate receptor activation.[17] The diverse physiological roles of kainate receptors are summarized in Figure 30.1.[17]

Recent findings indicate that subunit-specific antagonists of kainate receptors have therapeutic potential in neurodegenerative and psychiatric diseases as well as in epilepsy and pain.[20] Thus, kainic acid activates nociceptors, and kainic acid antagonists have analgesic activity.[21] Moreover, antagonists of GluK1 containing receptors prevent epileptiform activity in hippocampal slices and seizures in vivo elicited by pilocarpine or electrical stimulation.[22,23] These observations as well as the alterations in kainate receptors in diverse neuro- degenerative and psychiatric disorders[20] have, lately, placed kainate receptors as relevant therapeutic targets.

30.2.1.3 NMDA Receptors

NMDA is the selective agonist that binds to NMDA receptors but not to other types of glutamate recep- tors. Functional NMDA receptors require assembly of two GluN1 subunits together with either two GluN2 subunits or a combination of GluN2 and GluN3 subunits together with the simultaneous binding of glutamate and glycine for activation. The glycine binding site is located at the GluN1 and GluN3 sub- units while the glutamate binding site is located in the GluN2 subunit.[5] Activation of NMDA receptors

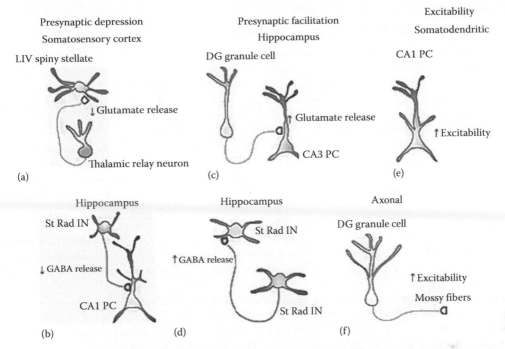

FIGURE 30.1 Physiological effects of kainate receptor activation. At the presynaptic level, kainate receptors depress (a) glutamate release between thalamic neurons and layer IV neurons (LIV neurons) or facilitate (c) glutamate release at synapses between dentate gyrus neurons (DG) and CA3 pyramidal cells (PC). In addition, kainate receptors inhibit (b) GABA release (between stratum radiatum interneurons—ST INs—and CA1 pyramidal cells) and increase (d) GABA release (between stratum radiatum interneurons). Nonsynaptic kainate receptors participate in the modulation of excitability at different subcellular compartments including the somatodendritic compartment of pyramidal cells in the CA1 region of the hippocampus (e) and the axons of granule cells in the dentate gyrus of the hippocampus (f). (Reprinted from *Trends Neurosci.*, 34, Contractor, A., Mulle, C., and Swanson, G.T., Kainate receptors coming of age: Milestones of two decades of research, 154–163, Copyright 2011, with permission from Elsevier.)

results in the opening of an ion channel nonselective to cations. One particularity of this receptor is the blockade of the receptor by extracellular magnesium; therefore, NMDA receptors are considered to be sensitive voltage and ligand complexes.

Since glutamate-induced neuronal damage is mainly caused by overactivation of NMDA receptors while normal physiological brain function and neuronal survival require adequate activation of NMDA receptors, this type of receptors is the subtype of glutamate receptors that have attracted much attention in the literature to data. Studies have revealed that NMDA receptor-induced neuronal death or survival is mediated through distinct subset of NMDA receptors triggering different intracellular signaling pathways. The NMDAR subunits are differentially expressed throughout the CNS with localization patterns that change during development. In the adult brain, GluN1 and GluN2A are expressed ubiquitously, while expression of GluNB is confined to the forebrain and striatum. GluN2C is predominantly expressed in cerebellum. GluN2D is mainly expressed early in development and is restricted to brainstem, midbrain, and thalamus. In addition, GluN3A is expressed in the CA1 pyramidal cell layer. NMDA receptors assemble as obligate heteromers that may be formed by GluN1, GluN2A, GluN2B, GluN2C, GluN2D, GluN3A, and GluN3B subunits. Alternative splicing can generate eight isoforms of GluN1 with differing pharmacological properties. Depending on the subunit composition and presence or absence of intracellular binding partners along the postsynaptic membrane, these NMDAR subtypes are allocated to distinct synaptic inputs converging onto a neuron or are distributed differentially among synaptic or extrasynaptic sites.[24] It is widely accepted that these receptors modulate glutamate excitotoxicity in the brain and are characterized by slow gating characteristics, high permeability to calcium ions, and voltage-dependent magnesium blockade.

30.3 Ecobiology and Chemistry of Domoic Acid

Domoic acid is a tricarboxylic acid, with an anhydrous molecular weight of 311.14, very similar to the glutamatergic agonist kainate and to the amino acid glutamate. Its IUPAC name is (2S,3S,4S)-4-[(2Z,4E,6R)-6-carboxyhepta-2,4-dien-2-yl]-3-(carboxymethyl)pyrrolidine-2-carboxylic acid and its chemical formula $C_{15}H_{21}NO_6$. At physiological conditions, domoic acid is deprotonated at the three carboxyl groups and protonated at the amino group, thus bearing a negative charge of 2.[25] The stability of domoic acid in solution is compromised at high temperatures and/or extreme pH.[26]

Domoic acid is a naturally occurring excitatory amino acid used originally for traditional and medicinal purposes in Japan and was consequently called after the Japanese word for seaweed, which is "doumoi."[27] In Japan, domoic acid was known as a folk medicine and used to treat intestinal pinworm infestations when used in very small doses and after that forgotten until the outbreak of ASP in Canada.[28] After the Canadian human poisoning produced by domoic acid, the primary source of the toxin was attributed to the diatom *P. multiseries*.[29] Since then, several *Pseudo-nitzschia* diatoms have been identified as major producers of domoic acid, among them *P. multiseries, P. australis*, and *P. seriata* produce high levels (>10 pg/cell) of domoic acid.[30] Furthermore, the diatoms *Nitzschia navis-varingica* and the red alga *Chondria armata* have also been reported separately as producers of domoic acid (see [30] for review).

Domoic acid belongs to the kainoid class of compounds. The compound is a water-soluble potent neurotoxin that has at least nine geometrical isomers named 5'-epi-domoic acid and isodomoic acids A–H. Isodomoic acid A, B, and C have been found in seaweed but not detected in extracts of plankton or shellfish tissue, while isodomoic acids D, E, and F and 5'-domoic acid have been found in plankton cells and shellfish tissue.[31] Formation of the geometrical isomers of domoic acid can be achieved by exposure of domoic acid solutions to UV light, while heating favors the conversion of domoic acid to 5'-domoic acid.[31] Moreover, the isomers of isodomoic acid A, B, E, F, G, and H were also found in small amounts in the red alga *C. armata*.[32] The chemical structures of domoic acid and some of its isomers are shown in Figure 30.2.

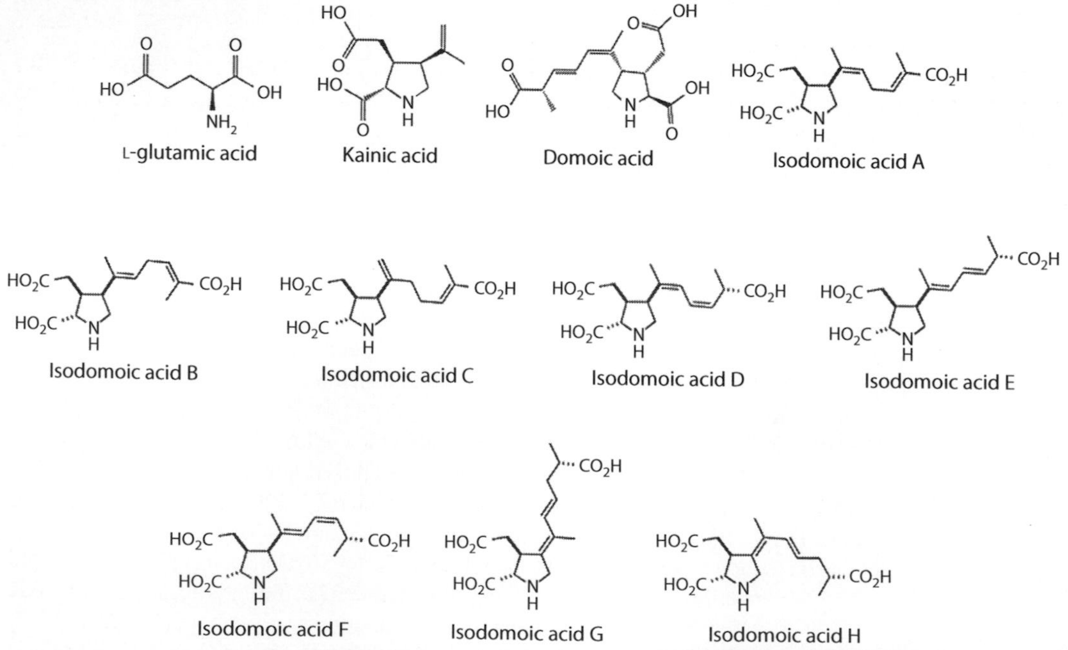

FIGURE 30.2 Chemical structures of L-glutamate, kainic acid, domoic acid, and related isomers.

30.4 Mechanism of Action of Domoic Acid and Its Isomers

Domoic acid is defined as a "non-NMDA" receptor agonist that activates both kainate and AMPA subtypes of glutamate receptors.[33] Initial studies on the effect of kainate and domoic acids on the right anterior pallial neuron of the African snail showed similar excitatory activity of domoic acid and kainic acid.[34] Soon after, it was also shown that both kainate and domoic acids had similar potencies in several types of giant neurons of the African giant snail *Achatina fulica Ferussac*.[35] However, it was not until the poisoning incident in Canada in 1987, when a detailed report on the activity of domoic acid stated by three different techniques the similarity of the action of domoic acid and kainic acid, the prototype agonist of the kainate receptor. The authors demonstrated that the neuroexcitatory properties of domoic acid in vitro (cultured hippocampal neurons) and its neurotoxic properties both in vitro (chick embryo retina) and in vivo (adult rat) were similar to those of kainic acid. First, they evaluated the currents induced in hippocampal neurons by domoic acid and kainic acid and found that both currents were identical, displayed a linear current/voltage relationship and were nondesensitizing. In addition, the domoic acid–elicited currents were not blocked by NMDA antagonists but were blocked by CNQX, an antagonist of non-NMDA receptors. Second, they demonstrated that lesions caused by domoic acid and kainic acid in the chick embryo retina were similar and blocked by CNQX but not by NMDA antagonists. And third, they showed that subcutaneous administration of domoic acid (2.5–3 mg/kg) to adult rats caused seizures identical to the ones induced by kainic acid at a dose four times higher (12 mg/kg), and similar neurotoxicity observed in poisoned victims of the Canada outbreak of ASP.[36]

Nowadays it is widely demonstrated that domoic acid acts as a high potent partial agonist at kainate receptors at both native and recombinant kainate receptors.[16,37] Moreover, although the response of kainate receptors to domoate is characterized by large steady-state currents and slow inactivation kinetics,[16,38] domoic acid and kainic acid displayed similar inhibition constant at the [^{3}H]-kainic acid binding sites (IC_{50} = 5 and 7 nM, respectively). Moreover, in brain synaptosomes, domoic acid displaced radiolabeled kainate with and IC_{50} of 0.37 nM.[39]

The specificity of domoic acid for the different kainate receptor subunits was also assessed, and radioligand-binding experiments showed an affinity constant of 2 nM for domoic acid at the GluK1 subunit and 9–11 nM at the GluK2 subunit.[40,41] In both GluK1 and GluK2 subunits, the desensitizing currents elicited by domoic acid were characterized by long steady-state currents much larger than those evoked either by kainic acid or by glutamate.[37,41] Further studies determined the glycosylated ligand-binding domain of the kainate receptor in complex with domoic acid and demonstrated that the binding of domoic acid to the GluK2 subunit of kainate receptors showed a similar orientation to that of glutamate and kainic acid with the side arm pointing out of the binding cleft,[19,42] but it showed a lower degree of cleft closure than the glutamate complex, a fact in agreement with the partial agonist action of domoic acid on kainate receptors.[38]

Although domoic acid is known to bind with high affinity to the GluK1 and GluK2 subunits (formerly GluR5 and GluR6) of kainate receptors, it also interacts at higher doses with the GluK4 and GluK5 subunits of these receptors (formerly KA1 and KA2) as reviewed previously by Doucette and Ramsdell.[26,27] As mentioned earlier, kainate receptor responses to domoic acid are characterized by large steady-state currents. In fact, kainate receptor currents evoked by domoic acid (400 µM) in naive kainate receptor exhibited an incomplete and slower desensitization in the order of 160 ms, and a very slow current decay after domoic acid washout (715 ms) than the currents elicited by kainic acid. In the same cells, cultured hippocampal neurons, kainic acid at 300 µM evoked faster inward responses that showed a faster decay than domoic acid currents.[16] The slower desensitization of domoic acid–induced currents in GluK1 and GluK2 receptors[16,37] contrast to the responses of GluK1 receptors to kainic acid, which desensitize slowly in the presence of kainic acid, while GluK2 receptors have a rapid and almost complete desensitization.[41] However, the GluK3 subunits (formerly GluR7) of the kainate receptor were insensitive to 100 µM domoic acid.[41] In addition, it was also demonstrated that the GluK1 receptor binding site has a high affinity for domoic acid (K_D approximately 2 nM) and kainate (K_D approximately 70 nM) as reported in recombinant GluK1 receptors.[37] By radioligand-binding assays, it was demonstrated that domoic acid activated GluK1 receptors with an affinity constant of 2 nM and GluK2 receptors with an affinity constant of 9–11 nM.[40]

The high affinity of domoic acid for GluK1 and GluK2 subunits of the kainate receptor seems to be important for its pharmacological effects since at presynaptic sites, kainate receptors encoded by the GluK1 subunit modulate neurotransmitter release, while at postsynaptic sites, these receptors encoded by GluK2 evoke slow synaptic responses.[19] The structure of the GluK2 agonist binding domain complexed with domoic acid, as well as the mutations that affect domoic acid binding to this kainate receptor subunit have been recently elucidated.[38,42] In agreement with the partial agonism of domoic acid at kainate receptors, the ligand-binding core of the GluK1 complex is stabilized by domoic acid in a conformation that is more open than that obtained at the complex of the full agonist glutamic acid with the GluK1 subunit.[43]

Furthermore, in neurons, kainate evokes larger steady-state AMPA receptor currents than domoic acid, although kainate has been shown to exhibit a lower potency to activate heterologous expressed AMPA receptors.[44,45] Neuronal AMPA receptors contain a transmembrane AMPA receptor-regulatory protein auxiliary subunit (TARP) for which five isoforms (γ-2 (or stargazin), γ-3, γ-4, γ-7, and γ-8) have been identified and shown a differential pattern of expression through the brain.[46,47] It has been shown that the transmembrane AMPA receptor-associated proteins γ-2 (or stargazin) and γ-8 increase the efficacy and potency of domoic acid as AMPA receptor agonist.[47] This issue is interesting, but it needs further studies because compounds that enhance TARP interactions may have therapeutic applications since drugs that potentiate AMPA receptor responses are emerging as novel therapeutics for the treatment of cognitive and mental diseases.[48,49]

Initial radioligand-binding experiments indicated that domoic acid isomers were less potent than domoic acid at both kainic and AMPA binding sites and suggested that the conjugated double bond in the cis configuration at the C1–C2 position of the side chain was necessary for strong binding of domoic acid isomers at AMPA–kainate receptors and for their seizurogenic activity.[50] These initial studies showed that the key feature leading to strong glutamate receptor binding of domoic acid and its analogs is a double bond in the side chain at C1–C2 with a Z (cis) configuration.[50]

By measuring the acute intraperitoneal toxicity and the behavioral changes caused in mice by intraperitoneal injection of domoic acid, isodomoic acid A, or isodomoic acid C, the group of Munday demonstrated that at the dose of 5 mg/kg, isodomoic acid A and isodomoic acid B were about 95% and 100% less effective than domoic acid, while isodomoic acid C lacked an effect at this dose, needed doses being three times higher (15 mg/kg) to elicit some behavioral effects similar to those evoked by isodomoic acid A at 5 mg/kg. Taking into account that the severities of the behavioral changes induced by isodomoic acids A, B, and C were all much lower than that of domoic acid itself, the authors concluded that these substances were of relatively little risk to human or animal health and that the regulation of monitoring for these compounds was not required.[51] This observation was in agreement with the fact that the affinity of isodomoic acid C at GluK2 receptors was 240-fold lower than that of domoic acid.[52] By comparing the effect of domoic acid and its natural isomers isodomoic acid A and isodomoic acid C on synaptically evoked population spikes in the CA1 region of the hippocampus, the authors found that isodomoic acid A and isodomoic acid C caused transient neuronal excitability followed by a dose-dependent spike suppression and were 4 and 20 times, respectively, less potent than the parent compound domoic acid. Interestingly, the authors also showed that both isomers failed to induce tolerance to subsequent domoic acid treatments.[53] Therefore, this study suggested that the neuroexcitatory effects of isodomoic acid A in the CA1 region of the hippocampus may involve both AMPA and kainate receptors, while the neuroexcitatory effects of isodomoic acid C likely involved the activation of AMPA receptors alone.[53]

Competitive binding studies using homomeric GluR6 kainate receptors showed that the affinity of isodomoic acid A (130 nM) was about 40-fold lower than the affinity of domoic acid, which was 3.35 nM.[53] As reported later by the same group, domoic acid, isodomoic acid A, isodomoic acid B, and isodomoic acid C produced significant dose-dependent increases in seizure activity following intrahippocampal administration. The doses producing half maximal cumulative seizure scores (ED_{50}) were 137 pmol for domoic acid, 171 pmol for isodomoic acid A, 13,000 pmol for isodomoic acid B, and 3,150 pmol for isodomoic acid C.[54] In the same study, preconditioning with low dose of domoic acid or isodomoic acid A, 60 min before a high test dose of domoic acid, produced a significant reduction in seizure scores. In contrast, isodomoic acid B and isodomoic acid C failed to induce any detectable tolerance to high doses of domoic acid. The same work showed that isodomoic acid B lacked seizurogenic activity even at an intrahippocampal dose of 8000 pmol. Moreover, the potential of domoic acid analogs to induce seizures correlated well with their

TABLE 30.2

Inhibition Constants for the Binding to Kainate and
AMPA Receptors by Domoic Acid and Its Isomers

	Kainate Receptors (nM)	AMPA Receptors (μM)
Domoic acid	2.4	24
Isodomoic acid A	4.4	113
Isodomoic acid B	4990	1100
Isodomoic acid C	171	110
Isodomoic acid D	600	53
Isodomoic acid E	600	300
Isodomoic acid F	67	14

IC_{50} for inhibiting kainate binding in rat brain membranes, which were 4.3 nM for domoic acid, 7.9 nM for isodomoic acid A, 9 μM for isodomoic acid B, and 300 nM for isodomoic acid C, therefore, indicating that domoic acid and isodomoic acid A are functionally equipotent in seizure induction by direct intrahippocampal administration and kainate binding, while isodomoic acid B and isodomoic acid C were less potent.[54]

Further studies addressed also the acute seizurogenic potencies of the isomers D, E, and F of domoic acid and their binding affinities at kainate and AMPA receptors from rat cerebrum finding that the seizurogenic potency of isodomoic F (E-configuration) closely correlated with its affinities at both kainate (IC_{50}: 1.2 μM, 1 μM, and 120 nM for isomers D, E, and F, respectively) and AMPA receptors for which isomers F and D showed affinities in the micromolar range while isomers B, C, and E showed affinities in the millimolar range.[55] Again, the seizurogenic potencies of domoic acid isomers correlated well with their binding affinities at kainate receptors. Moreover, the authors also reported that acute preconditioning with low dose of isodomoic acid D, E, or F before high dose of domoic acid failed to impart behavioral tolerance.[55] The same report indicates that domoic acid and isodomoic acids A, B, C, D, E, and F inhibited [³H]-AMPA binding to AMPA receptors in a concentration-dependent manner, although all the isomers of domoic acid were much less potent inhibiting [³H]-AMPA binding than [³H]-kainate binding. The binding of domoic acid to AMPA receptors was fitted by a two-site binding model with IC_{50} values of 6.6 nM at the high-affinity site and 24 μM at the low-affinity site. Isodomoic acid A also showed two binding affinities with IC_{50} values of 178 nM at the high-affinity site and 113 μM at the low-affinity site. Isomers F and D had a single binding site with IC_{50} values of 14 and 53 μM respectively, while isodomoic acids C, E, and B had IC_{50} values of 110, 300, and 1100 μM, respectively.[55] Thus, these recent studies on the activity of domoic acid isomers at kainate and AMPA receptors corroborate earlier data on the lower toxicity of domoic acid isomers after intraperitoneal injection.[51] Table 30.2 summarizes the binding affinity of domoic acid and its isomers to AMPA and kainate receptors as reported by [53,55]

Although the initial radioligand competition studies indicated that the structural requirement leading to strong glutamate receptor binding by domoic acid and its analogs was a double bond in the side chain at C1–C2 with a Z (cis) configuration,[50] an alternative structure–activity relationship for the binding of domoic acid isomers to kainate receptors has been proposed recently.[55] In the new structural model for the binding of domoic acid isomers to kainate receptors, domoic acid isomers with opposite stereochemistry of side chain double bonds (domoic acid (Z,E), isodomoic acid A (Z,E), and isodomoic acid F (E,Z)) exhibited higher seizurogenic potencies and binding affinities at kainate receptors than isomers with the same stereochemistry (isodomoic acid D (Z,Z), isodomoic acid E (E,E), and isodomoic acid B (E,E)).

30.5 Toxicokinetics of Domoic Acid

Together with human poisonings by domoic acid, seabird and marine mammal deaths are of major relevance for the penetration and persistence of domoic acid in the marine food chain. In vertebrates such as birds and mammals, domoic acid seems to be very little metabolized. Furthermore, the excretion of the toxin appears to occur primarily by urinary elimination.[56–58]

In spite of the fact that oral ingestion of contaminated food is the primary route for ASP in humans, there is limited information on the gastrointestinal absorption of domoic acid. Since early reports in the toxicokinetics of domoic acid have been extensively reviewed by [26,27] this section will focus mainly on the toxicokinetic data appeared during the last 5 years.

Following oral administration, domoic acid is poorly absorbed at the gastrointestinal tract. Absorbed domoic acid is rapidly excreted by renal elimination,[2] and renal clearance of domoic acid occurs mainly by glomerular filtration.[56] Recent studies by the Ramsdell group indicate that about 6% of the domoic acid dose administered intravenously reaches the brain, about 5% reaches the cerebrospinal fluid, and domoic acid levels remained nearly identical in brain and cerebrospinal fluid for 12 h, being above the amount needed to activate hippocampal neurons for 2 h.[59] In order to obtain a model for the gastrointestinal absorption of domoic acid, an in vitro model employing Caco-2 cells was employed. The transcellular transport of domoic acid from the apical to the basolateral membrane of Caco-2 cells was sodium independent and suggest that in these cells, the transcellular transport of domoic acid is mediated by a sensitive anion transport system.[60] As mentioned earlier, domoic acid is known to reach the rat brain.[59,61] The recent study by the Ramsdell group clearly demonstrates that domoic acid levels decrease rapidly in the cerebrospinal fluid as previously shown by the same group for the plasma.[59] In addition, during gestation, domoic acid crosses the placenta, reaches the brain tissue of the fetus, accumulates in the amniotic fluid and is transferred to neonates through the milk.[61,62]

30.6 In Vitro and In Vivo Effects of Domoic Acid Exposure

While the neurotoxic activity of domoic acid has been extensively investigated, there is little information on the toxicity of domoic acid isomers. This is an important point, in order to include the natural domoic acid isomers on monitoring programs. The neurobiological effects of chronic exposure to low amounts of domoic acid are currently unknown; however, in recent years, several research papers have evaluated the risk of continued exposure to nontoxic doses of domoic acid. Most of the studies aiming to characterize the excitatory effect of domoic acid have employed rodents as model species.[63] The available data indicate that humans are between 10 and 20 times more sensitive than mice and rats, respectively, to low doses of domoic acid.[63]

The most important risk of exposure of humans and marine wildlife to domoic acid is the dietary consumption of contaminated filter-feeding marine organisms such as shellfish and finfish.[63] Affected brain regions of mice after exposure to an intraperitoneal dose of 4 mg/kg of domoic acid during 72 h included the olfactory bulb, septal area, and limbic system.[64] Although human exposure to domoic acid is limited to oral exposure, most of the studies on the neurotoxic effects of domoic acid have been conducted using intravenous or intraperitoneal administrations, a fact that limits the extrapolation of the data since it is known that the intravenous and intraperitoneal routes cause clinical symptoms at lower doses than the oral route.

The main clinical symptoms caused by domoic acid at low doses are hyperactivity and stereotypical scratching, while mild doses of the toxin cause memory alterations and behavioral hyperreactivity. At higher doses, domoic acid produces neurotoxicity with seizures, status epilepticus, and even death.[65] An issue of rising concern in domoic acid toxicity is the analysis of the effect of chronic exposure to nontoxic doses of the toxin. A recent paper evaluating the human domoic exposure in Belgium indicates that for a daily intake of 56–108 g/day, 1% of the population will be at risk for human intoxication, while 5%–6% of the population will have chronic exposure to domoic acid doses exceeding the tolerable daily intake.[66] In Europe, the acute reference dose established by the European Food Safety Authority for domoic acid is 30 µg DA/kg body weight due to the presence of domoic acid in food together with the isomer epidomoic acid.[2] This report establishes that the intake of a 400 g portion of shellfish containing domoic acid at the actual European Union limit of 20 mg of domoic acid per kilogram of shellfish meat would result to a daily exposure of about 130 µg of domoic acid per kilogram of body weight and a risk of exposure for 1% of the population.[2,67]

Although domoic acid–induced toxicity has been studied initially, mainly in adult animals, developmental and chronic effects of domoic acid exposure have also been recently reported.[62,68–71] Based on these experiments, neonates have been shown to be more sensitive to domoic acid toxicity than adults, and this effect has been attributed to the reduced serum clearance of the toxin in neonates,[71] the activation of the neonatal brain microglia,[72] a greater access of domoic acid through the undeveloped blood–brain barrier,[59,61] and the transfer of the toxin from the milk to the plasma of nursing neonatal animals.[62]

Prenatal exposure to domoic acid is associated with neuron loss and damage in different brain regions, although the mechanism of neurotoxicity is not entirely clear. Some studies suggest that domoic acid decreases the levels of brain gamma-amino butyric acid (GABA) and increases glutamate levels,[73] while other reports show an increase in GABA release after domoic acid treatment in chick retina,[74] which was completely abolished in the presence of the non-NMDA glutamate receptor antagonist CNQX.

Another important issue in domoic acid exposure is the induction of delayed central nervous toxicity. Recently, it was described that domoic acid altered neuronal activities in the developing brain after administration of a single intraperitoneal dose of domoic acid (1 mg/kg) to pregnant female,[75] an effect suggested to be due in part to the increase in the expression of glutamate receptors during brain development.[76] Similarly, a single injection of 20 µg/kg of domoic acid from postnatal days 8 to 14 to rat pups caused changes in cognition and emotionality in adult rats of 120 days, providing additional evidences indicating that perinatal treatment of rats with low doses of domoic acid results in permanent changes in brain function manifested by modifications in spatial cognition and altered response to emotional challenges.[69] Using the same experimental procedure and low doses of domoic acid in neonatal rats, altered prepulse inhibition and alterations in the acoustic startle response in adult rats were observed, a paradigm altered also in schizophrenia.[77] In addition, low-dose injections of domoic acid (20 µg/kg) over postnatal days 8–14 caused long-lasting alterations on learning and memory in adolescent and adult rats as evaluated by two spatial memory tasks: the radial 8-arm maze and the Morris water maze, respectively. In this study, adolescent animals treated with domoic acid, regardless of sex, demonstrated superior choice accuracy over 7 days of testing in the 8-arm baited version of the radial maze. As adults, the same animals manifested improvements in performance measures in the water maze, indicating that the administration of low doses of domoic acid causes lasting changes in learning and memory in rats.[77] Using the same experimental paradigm, the same group described that the administration of low doses of domoic acid to rat pups caused alterations in the novelty-related behavior in a novelty trial in adult rats, increasing the time spent exploring familiar objects during the novelty trial of the playground maze. In the nicotine-induced conditioned place preference, domoic acid–treated females developed a conditioned place preference for the nicotine-paired compartment of the test arena.[78] The same authors described that 7 days of postnatal exposure to domoic acid eliminates the nicotine-induced conditioned place preference; after exposure of neonates to low nonconvulsive doses of domoic acid and tested as adolescents in a nicotine-induced conditioned place preference paradigm, in contrast to control animals, nicotine-induced conditioned place preference paradigm was absent in the domoic acid–treated animals.[79]

After the establishment of a regulatory limit for domoic acid (20 µg/g) estimated to produce half the no-observed-adverse-effect-level[80] for harvested shellfish, most humans have been protected from high-level domoic exposure. Therefore, consequences of low-level exposure to domoic acid are of greatest relevance to human health.[63] However, sex differences must also be taken into account since a recent study indicates that male rats exposed to low doses of domoic acid as adults may be more susceptible to severe neurological alterations while females seem to be affected more quickly.[81] Therefore, the developmental and adult effects of chronic exposure to low doses of domoic acid need to be further studied both in vivo and in vitro to determine its potential neurotoxic/beneficial effects.

As most studies on domoic acid using experimental animals have focused on the mechanisms of neurotoxicity, limited information is available on the intestinal absorption, distribution, metabolism, and excretion of domoic acid after ingestion. In monkeys and rats, domoic acid is rapidly excreted after intravenous dosage with a plasma half life of 114.5 min in monkeys and 21.6 min in rats,[57] and in rats, domoic acid is completely recovered in the urine after 160 min of intravenous dosing, being cleared from plasma mainly through the kidney and renal glomerular filtration.[56] However, the absorption of domoic acid in rats after 30 days of oral administration was very small as evaluated by urinary excretion (1.8% in rats), but it was the double in monkeys (4%–7%).[82,83]

The low pKa value of domoic acid favors its rapid absorption as a neutral acid in the stomach, although absorption after oral administration is very low.[25] A recent report on the intestinal absorption of domoic acid using Caco-2 cells, an in vitro system, which is morphologically and functionally similar to small intestinal epithelial cells and used widely as a model to "in vivo" oral absorption in humans, describes the transcellular transport mechanism of domoic acid using Caco-2 cell monolayers cultured on permeable membranes. The transcellular transport of domoic acid from the apical to the basolateral side was about twofold the transport in the opposite direction. Moreover, the transport of domoic acid from the apical side was both temperature and Cl^- dependent and optimal at neutral pH, but was Na^+ independent and decreased by about 50% by coincubation with 4,4'-diisothiocyanostilbene-2,2'-disulfonic acid (DIDS). In this system, coincubation with probenecid (a nonspecific anion transport inhibitor) significantly decreased the transport of domoic acid by 31%. In contrast, coincubation with glutamic acid, succinic acid (a dicarboxylic acid), or citric acid (a tricarboxylic acid) did not decrease the transport of domoic acid. These results suggest that the transcellular transport of domoic acid is mediated by DIDS-sensitive anion transport systems[60] and not by the same transporter as that for glutamic acid, which seems to be sodium dependent.[84]

Several reports indicate that domoic acid exposure primarily affects the hippocampus and is associated with seizures and alterations in cognitive processes, including transient and permanent changes in the brain that are similar to human anterograde amnesia.[65] In fact, brain histological alterations after acute domoic acid poisoning showed neuronal death in several brain regions including the hippocampus, nucleus accumbens, thalamus, and cortical areas (reviewed by [85]).

The current data on domoic acid–induced neurotoxicity support that the main cause of neuronal loss induced by the toxin is the activation of glutamate ionotropic receptors and the increase in the release of endogenous glutamate that will activate the cellular cascade leading to neuronal damage.[58,85] Since glutamate is the main excitatory transmitter in the CNS, the increase in released glutamate elicited by domoic acid is of key importance in the neuronal damage induced by the toxin. Thus, activation of presynaptic and postsynaptic kainate receptors by domoic acid causes an integrative action of the compound at both sides of the synapse that, together with its nondesensitizing effect on ion channels, compromises neuronal survival.

At the presynaptic site, kainate receptor activation by domoic acid leads to increase in glutamate release, which in turn activates also NMDA receptors, which have lost their physiological blockade by magnesium due to the depolarization elicited as a consequence of the activation of postsynaptic kainate receptors by domoic acid. As a consequence, there is an increase in the intracellular calcium concentration, which eventually causes the activation of proapoptotic cascades as well as alterations in ion homeostasis leading to excitotoxicity-mediated cell death. As a consequence of the activation of kainate and AMPA receptors, domoic acid (50 nM) elevates the cytosolic free calcium, and initial reports indicated that this effect was prevented by 6-cyano-7-nitroquinoxaline-2,3-dione (CNQX, an antagonist of non-NMDA receptors), but not 2-amino-5-phosphonovaleric acid (AP-5, an antagonist of NMDA receptors), while at higher concentrations of domoic acid (5 μM), the calcium rise elicited by domoic acid was only partially inhibited by 100 μM CNQX. The voltage-dependent calcium channel antagonist, nimodipine given at 300 nM, prevented the elevation in $[Ca^{2+}]_i$ caused by 50 nM and 5 μM domoic acid, indicating that domoic acid induced Ca^{2+} entry through type L voltage-dependent calcium channels. These results provided the initial evidence for at least two domoic acid–sensitive non-NMDA receptor subtypes in primary cultures of neonatal hippocampal pyramidal cells.[86]

Further reports demonstrated that the calcium increase caused by domoic acid in cultured cerebellar neurons was mediated by the secondary activation of NMDA receptors, L-type voltage-sensitive calcium channels, and the reversed mode of operation of the Na^+/Ca^{++} exchanger, signals that are activated secondarily as a consequence of the stimulation of the AMPA/kainate receptors by domoate and the consequent increase in excitatory neurotransmitter release.[87] The primary effect of domoic acid in cultured cortical neurons is the activation of kainate and AMPA receptors that cause neuronal depolarization, increase in action potential firing, ionic alterations, and neuronal swelling due to prolonged activation of the receptors. As a consequence, the increase in excitatory amino acid release causes activation of NMDA receptors, which leads to the rise in cytosolic calcium and neuronal death.[88]

Interestingly, chronic treatment of mixed cortical and glial cultures with domoic acid decreased the mRNA levels of neuronal cytoskeleton proteins and the mRNA levels of NMDA receptors and GABA_A receptors thus affecting both the excitatory and inhibitory transmissions.[89] Although the chronic effects

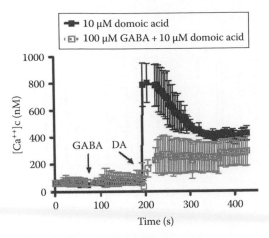

FIGURE 30.3 Calcium increase in cerebellar granule cells exposed to domoic acid is decreased in the presence of the neurotransmitter GABA.

of domoic acid on the inhibitory transmission are not known in detail, the toxin has been reported to decrease the levels of GABA in vivo,[90] and the neurotoxicity of domoic acid in vitro was also ameliorated by the neurotransmitter GABA.[89] In our laboratory, we have also described that domoic acid increases the cytosolic calcium concentration in primary cultures of cerebellar neurons,[91] and the cytosolic calcium increase elicited by glutamate was diminished by the addition of GABA. As shown in Figure 30.3, in single cultured cerebellar granule cells loaded with the fluorescent dye fura-2 acetoxymethyl ester (Fura-2 AM), 10 μM domoic acid elicited a rapid rise in the intracellular calcium concentration, which was decreased by coincubation of the cells with 100 μM GABA.

In the same in vitro system, domoic acid elicited an increase in the release of excitatory amino acids aspartate and glutamate that was dependent on the time of exposure of the cells to the toxin and on the domoic acid concentration. Primary cultures of cultured cortical neurons were exposed to 10 μM domoic acid during 5, 15, or 30 min, and the released levels of glutamate and aspartate were measured by high-performance liquid chromatography fluorometric analysis. As shown in Figure 30.4, 30-min exposure of cerebellar neurons caused a significant increase in the release of glutamate although the effect of domoic acid in aspartate levels did not reach significance.

Interestingly, the concentration-dependent increase in intracellular calcium produced by domoic acid caused a calcium- and concentration-dependent intracellular acidification that was suggested to exacerbate the cell death caused by the toxin.[91] The changes in intracellular pH in primary

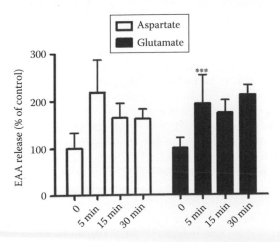

FIGURE 30.4 Effect of domoic acid in aspartate and glutamate release in primary cultures of cerebellar granule cells exposed to domoic acid.

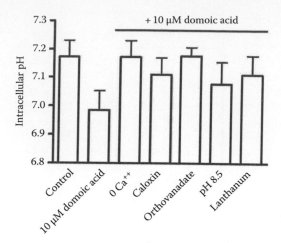

FIGURE 30.5 Effect of domoic acid on intracellular pH. In primary cultures of cerebellar granule cells, domoic acid causes a rapid decrease in intracellular pH, which is calcium dependent and reverted by inhibitors of the plasma membrane adenosine triphosphatase.

cultures of cerebellar granule cells were analyzed by loading the cells with the pH-sensitive dye 2′,7′-bis(carboxyethyl)-5(6)-carboxyfluorescein acetoxymethyl ester (BCECF-AM). In this system, 10 μM domoic acid caused an intracellular acidification that was prevented in calcium-free medium, in the presence of the AMPA/kainate receptor antagonist CNQX and by inhibition of the plasma membrane calcium adenosine triphosphatase (ATPAse) (PMCA), including orthovanadate, lanthanum, extracellular pH of 8.5, and by the specific inhibitor caloxin 2A-1, as summarized in Figure 30.5. Therefore, our results indicate that the PMCA is involved in the intracellular acidification caused by domoic acid in primary cultured cerebellar granule cells. In addition, by simultaneous determination of the cytosolic calcium concentration and intracellular pH, we further suggest that the increase in intracellular calcium caused by domoic acid will activate the calcium extrusion mechanisms by the calcium pump, which in turn will decrease the intracellular pH by counter transport of H^+ ions.

30.7 Impact of Low-Level Domoic Acid Exposure

Nowadays, domoic acid–producing diatom blooms are increasing in frequency worldwide and therefore increasing the threat to wildlife and human health.[63] Besides this fact, while most studies have focused on the in vivo and in vitro toxic effects of domoic acid, less studies have addressed the physiological effects of low-level domoic acid intake, although recent evidences reviewed in this section indicate that even nontoxic doses of domoic acid may produce persistent changes in brain systems. As mentioned, domoic acid toxicity is most likely attributed to the activation of AMPA/kainate receptors by the compound, which increases intracellular calcium levels, and this in turn causes glutamate release that subsequently activates NMDA receptors.[87,92] This may produce both necrotic and apoptotic neuronal death, which depends on the concentration of domoic acid.[89]

The neurotoxicity produced by domoic acid is caused by the activation of both AMPA/kainate and NMDA receptors. These receptors are involved in the neurotoxicity caused by domoic acid at higher doses (10 μM) and the consequent release of glutamate, which activates NMDA receptors,[88,93] while the apoptotic effect of domoic acid is mediated only by NMDA receptors.[94] Thus, low doses of domoic acid (100 nM) applied to primary cultures of cerebellar granule cells induced apoptosis mainly due to the selective stimulation of AMPA/kainate receptors and mediated by the generation of oxidative stress and stimulation of caspase 3.[94,95] At low doses, treatment of cerebellar granule cells for 1 h with 100 nM domoic acid induced apoptosis related with an increase in the phosphorylation of some mitogen-activated protein kinases (MAPK), including the c-Jun NH2-terminal kinase (JNK) and the p38 MAPK, while it decreased the phosphorylation of the Erk1/2 kinase (extracellular signal-regulated kinase), with a maximal effect at 3 h after treatment, while the total level of these kinases was not modified by the toxin. The AMPA/kainate receptor antagonist NBQX, but not the NMDA receptor antagonist MK-801 ((+)-5-methyl-10,11-dihydro-5*H*-dibenzo[a, d] cyclohepten-5,10-imine-maleate), prevented the activation of p38 and the JNK kinases by domoic acid. Moreover, several antioxidants (glutathione ethyl ester, catalase, and phenylbutylnitrone) also decreased the phosphorylation of JNK and p38 MAP kinases by domoic acid. Inhibitors of p38 (SB203580) and JNK (SP600125) used alone or in combination also prevented the apoptosis induced by low doses of domoic acid.[95] From these results, the authors remark the importance of oxidative stress–activated JNK and p38 MAP kinase pathways in the apoptosis induced by domoic acid, which was also inhibited by the activation of the muscarinic receptor with carbachol as the same authors reported later.[96] In the same in vitro model, higher doses of domoic acid (10 µM) induced necrosis through the increase in glutamate release and secondary activation of NMDA receptors.[94]

In primary cultures of cortical neurons, it has been described that the neurotoxicity of domoic acid was higher than that elicited by kainic acid. Exposure of cortical neurons at low doses of domoic acid ranging from 0.1 to 100 µM decreased neuronal viability with an EC_{50} of 4.2 µM when applied for 24 h. Moreover, the domoic acid toxicity was reduced by antagonists of AMPA/kainate receptors and NMDA receptors but not by antagonist of metabotropic glutamate receptors.[88] In addition, the authors showed that the maximum neuronal death caused by high doses of domoic acid ($\geq$10 µM) occurred after 2 h of exposure, while at doses lower than 10 µM, the death occurred even after 22 h of washout of the toxin. Although the toxicity of domoic acid has been studied mainly in neuronal tissues, it has also been described that domoic acid induces apoptosis, DNA damage, alterations in cell membrane integrity, and damage to lysosomes and mitochondria in Caco-2 cells after 24 h of exposure of the cells to domoic acid doses of 0.3, 0.6, and 0.9 µM.[97]

Although in vivo neonates seem to be more sensitive to domoic acid toxicity, in vitro, the developmental neurotoxic effect of domoic acid has also been recently evaluated in immature and mature cortical neurons.[88,89] The recent paper by Hoeberg and coauthors evaluated the toxicity of domoic acid in vitro exposing mixed glia and neuronal cultures from rat cerebellum to domoic acid at nontoxic concentrations of domoic acid (5–20 µM) from 1 to 10 days in vitro or from 7 to 10 div and showed that mature cultures were more sensitive to the toxin since the effects were observed at lower concentrations and shorter exposure times than in immature neurons. Interestingly, a recent paper showed that longtime exposure (10 days) to low nontoxic concentrations of domoic acid (5 nM) did not cause toxicity and in contrast reduced the oxidative stress–mediated apoptotic cell death induced by the exposure of the neurons to an intermediate concentration of domoic acid (100 nM for 24 h) and the acute toxicity of several oxidants.[98]

30.8 Conclusions

The acute toxicity of domoic acid has been widely studied in different species with few species differences in the symptoms elicited by the toxin. However, the recent indication that nontoxic doses of domoic acid decrease the acute toxicity of the toxin opens the door to further studies about the effect of exposure to low doses of the compounds as beneficial tools to analyze the potential therapeutic effect of kainate receptors. However, perinatal exposure to nontoxic concentrations of the toxin may cause neurological deficits. Although some studies have addressed the action of domoic acid analogs, more research needs to be performed in order to analyze the effects of the combination of domoic acid with its isomers. The increase in models to analyze the physiological effects of kainate receptors such as genetic-modified mice and the description of kainate and AMPA receptors accessory proteins will improve the knowledge of the exact interaction of each domoic acid isomer with its molecular target.

REFERENCES

1. Perl, T. M., Bedard, L., Kosatsky, T., Hockin, J. C., Todd, E. C., and Remis, R. S., 1990. An outbreak of toxic encephalopathy caused by eating mussels contaminated with domoic acid. *N Engl J Med*, 322, 1775–1780.
2. EFSA, E. F. S. A., 2009. Marine biotoxins in shellfish-Domoic acid. Scientific opinion of the panel on contaminants in the food chain. *EFSA J*, 1181, 1–61.
3. Volpi, C., Fazio, F., and Fallarino, F., 2012. Targeting metabotropic glutamate receptors in neuroimmune communication. *Neuropharmacology*, 63, 501–506.
4. Bowie, D., 2010. Ion-dependent gating of kainate receptors. *J Physiol*, 588, 67–81.
5. Traynelis, S. F., Wollmuth, L. P., McBain, C. J. et al., 2010. Glutamate receptor ion channels: Structure, regulation, and function. *Pharmacol Rev*, 62, 405–496.
6. Vogensen, S. B., Greenwood, J. R., Bunch, L., and Clausen, R. P., 2011. Glutamate receptor agonists: Stereochemical aspects. *Curr Top Med Chem*, 11, 887–906.
7. Ozawa, S., Kamiya, H., and Tsuzuki, K., 1998. Glutamate receptors in the mammalian central nervous system. *Prog Neurobiol*, 54, 581–618.
8. Watkins, J. C., Krogsgaard-Larsen, P., and Honore, T., 1990. Structure-activity relationships in the development of excitatory amino acid receptor agonists and competitive antagonists. *Trends Pharmacol Sci*, 11, 25–33.
9. Peters, J. A., Peineau, S., Collingridge, G. L., and Wenthold, R. J., 2009. Ionotropic glutamate receptors. http://www.iuphar-db.org/DATABASE/FamilyMenuForward?familyId = 75.
10. Collingridge, G. L., Olsen, R. W., Peters, J., and Spedding, M., 2009. A nomenclature for ligand-gated ion channels. *Neuropharmacology*, 56, 2–5.
11. Kumar, J. and Mayer, M. L., 2013. Functional insights from glutamate receptor ion channel structures. *Annu Rev Physiol*, 75, 313–337.
12. Malenka, R. C. and Bear, M. F., 2004. LTP and LTD: An embarrassment of riches. *Neuron*, 44, 5–21.
13. Greger, I. H., Khatri, L., Kong, X., and Ziff, E. B., 2003. AMPA receptor tetramerization is mediated by Q/R editing. *Neuron*, 40, 763–774.
14. Kristensen, A. S., Jenkins, M. A., Banke, T. G. et al., 2011. Mechanism of Ca2+/calmodulin-dependent kinase II regulation of AMPA receptor gating. *Nat Neurosci*, 14, 727–735.
15. Lodge, D., 2009. The history of the pharmacology and cloning of ionotropic glutamate receptors and the development of idiosyncratic nomenclature. *Neuropharmacology*, 56, 6–21.
16. Lerma, J., Paternain, A. V., Naranjo, J. R., and Mellstrom, B., 1993. Functional kainate-selective glutamate receptors in cultured hippocampal neurons. *Proc Natl Acad Sci U S A*, 90, 11688–11692.
17. Contractor, A., Mulle, C., and Swanson, G. T., 2011. Kainate receptors coming of age: Milestones of two decades of research. *Trends Neurosci*, 34, 154–163.
18. Lauri, S. E. and Taira, T., 2011. Role of kainate receptors in network activity during development. *Adv Exp Med Biol*, 717, 81–91.
19. Mayer, M. L., 2005. Crystal structures of the GluR5 and GluR6 ligand binding cores: Molecular mechanisms underlying kainate receptor selectivity. *Neuron*, 45, 539–552.
20. Matute, C., 2011. Therapeutic potential of kainate receptors. *CNS Neurosci Ther*, 17, 661–669.
21. Pinheiro, P. and Mulle, C., 2006. Kainate receptors. *Cell Tissue Res*, 326, 457–482.
22. Smolders, I., Bortolotto, Z. A., Clarke, V. R. et al., 2002. Antagonists of GLU(K5)-containing kainate receptors prevent pilocarpine-induced limbic seizures. *Nat Neurosci*, 5, 796–804.
23. Barton, M. E., Peters, S. C., and Shannon, H. E., 2003. Comparison of the effect of glutamate receptor modulators in the 6 Hz and maximal electroshock seizure models. *Epilepsy Res*, 56, 17–26.
24. Körh, G., 2006. NMDA receptor function: Subunit composition versus spatial distribution. *Cell Tissue Res*, 326, 439–496.
25. Ramsdell, J. S., 2010. Neurological disease rises from ocean to bring model for human epilepsy to life. *Toxins (Basel)*, 2, 1646–1675.
26. Doucette, T. A. and Tasker, A., 2008. Domoic acid: Detection, methods, pharmacology and toxicology, in *Seafood and Freshwater Toxins, Pharmacology, Physiology and Detection*. Botana, L. M., ed., CRC Press, Boca Raton, FL, pp. 383–396.
27. Ramsdell, J., 2007. The molecular and integrative basis to domoic acid toxicity, in *Phycotoxins: Chemistry and Biochemistry*. Botana, L., ed. Wiley-Blackwell, Cambridge, MA, pp. 223–250.

28. Mos, L., 2001. Domoic acid: A fascinating marine toxin. *Environ Toxicol Pharmacol*, 9, 79–85.
29. Bates, S. S., Bird, C. J., Freitas, A. S. W. et al., 1989. Pennate diatom nitzschia pungens as the primary source of domoic acid, a toxin in shellfish from eastern Prince Edward Island, Canada. *Can J Fish Aquat Sci*, 46, 1203–1215.
30. Kotaki, Y., 2008. Ecobiology of amnesic shellfish producing diatoms, in *Seafood and Freshwater Toxins. Pharmacology, Physiology, and Detection*, 2nd edn. Botana, L. M., ed. CRC Press, Boca Raton, FL, pp. 383–396.
31. He, Y., Fekete, A., Chen, G. et al., 2010. Analytical approaches for an important shellfish poisoning agent: Domoic acid. *J Agric Food Chem*, 58, 11525–11533.
32. Zaman, L., Arakawa, O., Shimosu, A. et al., 1997. Two new isomers of domoic acid from a red alga, *Chondria armata*. *Toxicon*, 35, 205–212.
33. Bettler, B. and Mulle, C., 1995. Review: Neurotransmitter receptors. II. AMPA and kainate receptors. *Neuropharmacology*, 34, 123–139.
34. Takeuchi, H., Watanabe, K., Nomoto, K., Ohfune, Y., and Takemoto, T., 1984. Effects of alpha-kainic acid, domoic acid and their derivatives on a molluscan giant neuron sensitive to beta-hydroxy-L-glutamic acid. *Eur J Pharmacol*, 102, 325–332.
35. Nakajima, T., Nomoto, K., Ohfune, Y. et al., 1985. Effects of glutamic acid analogues on identifiable giant neurones, sensitive to beta-hydroxy-L-glutamic acid, of an African giant snail (*Achatina fulica* Ferussac). *Br J Pharmacol*, 86, 645–654.
36. Stewart, G. R., Zorumski, C. F., Price, M. T., and Olney, J. W., 1990. Domoic acid: A dementia-inducing excitotoxic food poison with kainic acid receptor specificity. *Exp Neurol*, 110, 127–138.
37. Sommer, B., Burnashev, N., Verdoorn, T. A., Keinanen, K., Sakmann, B., and Seeburg, P. H., 1992. A glutamate receptor channel with high affinity for domoate and kainate. *EMBO J*, 11, 1651–1656.
38. Zhang, Y., Nayeem, N., and Green, T., 2008. Mutations to the kainate receptor subunit GluR6 binding pocket that selectively affect domoate binding. *Mol Pharmacol*, 74, 1163–1169.
39. Crawford, N., Lang, T. K., Kerr, D. S., and de Vries, D. J., 1999. High-affinity [3H] kainic acid binding to brain membranes: A re-evaluation of ligand potency and selectivity. *J Pharmacol Toxicol Methods*, 42, 121–125.
40. Lomeli, H., Wisden, W., Kohler, M., Keinanen, K., Sommer, B., and Seeburg, P. H., 1992. High-affinity kainate and domoate receptors in rat brain. *FEBS Lett*, 307, 139–143.
41. Swanson, G. T., Gereau, R. W. 4th., Green, T., and Heinemann, S. F., 1997. Identification of amino acid residues that control functional behavior in GluR5 and GluR6 kainate receptors. *Neuron*, 19, 913–926.
42. Nanao, M. H., Green, T., Stern-Bach, Y., Heinemann, S. F., and Choe, S., 2005. Structure of the kainate receptor subunit GluR6 agonist-binding domain complexed with domoic acid. *Proc Natl Acad Sci U S A*, 102, 1708–1713.
43. Hald, H., Naur, P., Pickering, D. S. et al., 2007. Partial Agonism and Antagonism of the Ionotropic Glutamate Receptor iGLuR5: Structures of the ligand-binding core in complex with domoic acid and 2-amino-3-[5-tert-butyl-3-(phosphonomethoxy)-4-isoxazolyl]propionic acid. *J Biol Chem*, 282, 25726–25736.
44. Jonas, P. and Sakmann, B., 1992. Glutamate receptor channels in isolated patches from CA1 and CA3 pyramidal cells of rat hippocampal slices. *J Physiol*, 455, 143–171.
45. Kiskin, N. I., Krishtal, O. A., and Tsyndrenko, A., 1986. Excitatory amino acid receptors in hippocampal neurons: Kainate fails to desensitize them. *Neurosci Lett*, 63, 225–230.
46. Kato, A. S., Zhou, W., Milstein, A. D. et al., 2007. New transmembrane AMPA receptor regulatory protein isoform, gamma-7, differentially regulates AMPA receptors. *J Neurosci*, 27, 4969–4977.
47. Tomita, S., Byrd, R. K., Rouach, N. et al., 2007. AMPA receptors and stargazin-like transmembrane AMPA receptor-regulatory proteins mediate hippocampal kainate neurotoxicity. *Proc Natl Acad Sci USA*, 104, 18784–18788.
48. O'Neill, M. J., Murray, T. K., Whalley, K. et al., 2004. Neurotrophic actions of the novel AMPA receptor potentiator, LY404187, in rodent models of Parkinson's disease. *Eur J Pharmacol*, 486, 163–174.
49. Goff, D. C., Leahy, L., Berman, I. et al., 2001. A placebo-controlled pilot study of the ampakine CX516 added to clozapine in schizophrenia. *J Clin Psychopharmacol*, 21, 484–487.
50. Hampson, D. R., Huang, X. P., Wells, J. W., Walter, J. A., and Wright, J. L., 1992. Interaction of domoic acid and several derivatives with kainic acid and AMPA binding sites in rat brain. *Eur J Pharmacol*, 218, 1–8.

51. Munday, R., Holland, P. T., McNabb, P., Selwood, A. I., and Rhodes, L. L., 2008. Comparative toxicity to mice of domoic acid and isodomoic acids A, B and C. *Toxicon*, 52, 954–956.
52. Holland, P. T., Selwood, A. I., Mountfort, D. O. et al., 2005. Isodomoic acid C, an unusual amnesic shellfish poisoning toxin from Pseudo-nitzschia australis. *Chem Res Toxicol*, 18, 814–816.
53. Sawant, P. M., Weare, B. A., Holland, P. T. et al., 2007. Isodomoic acids A and C exhibit low KA receptor affinity and reduced in vitro potency relative to domoic acid in region CA1 of rat hippocampus. *Toxicon*, 50, 627–638.
54. Sawant, P. M., Holland, P. T., Mountfort, D. O., and Kerr, D. S., 2008. In vivo seizure induction and pharmacological preconditioning by domoic acid and isodomoic acids A, B and C. *Neuropharmacology*, 55, 1412–1418.
55. Sawant, P. M., Tyndall, J. D., Holland, P. T., Peake, B. M., Mountfort, D. O., and Kerr, D. S., 2010. In vivo seizure induction and affinity studies of domoic acid and isodomoic acids-D, -E and -F. *Neuropharmacology*, 59, 129–138.
56. Suzuki, C. A. and Hierlihy, S. L., 1993. Renal clearance of domoic acid in the rat. *Food Chem Toxicol*, 31, 701–706.
57. Truelove, J. and Iverson, F., 1994. Serum domoic acid clearance and clinical observations in the cynomolgus monkey and Sprague-Dawley rat following a single i.v. dose. *Bull Environ Contam Toxicol*, 52, 479–486.
58. Watanabe, K. H., Andersen, M. E., Basu, N. et al., 2011. Defining and modeling known adverse outcome pathways: Domoic acid and neuronal signaling as a case study. *Environmental Toxicology and Chemistry*, 30, 9–21.
59. Maucher Fuquay, J., Muha, N., Wang, Z., and Ramsdell, J. S., 2012. Elimination kinetics of domoic Acid from the brain and cerebrospinal fluid of the pregnant rat. *Chem Res Toxicol*, 25, 2805–2809.
60. Kimura, O., Kotaki, Y., Hamaue, N., Haraguchi, K., and Endo, T., 2011. Transcellular transport of domoic acid across intestinal Caco-2 cell monolayers. *Food Chem Toxicol*, 49, 2167–2171.
61. Maucher, J. M. and Ramsdell, J. S., 2007. Maternal-fetal transfer of domoic acid in rats at two gestational time points. *Environ Health Perspect*, 115, 1743–1746.
62. Maucher, J. M. and Ramsdell, J. S., 2005. Domoic acid transfer to milk: Evaluation of a potential route of neonatal exposure. *Environ Health Perspect*, 113, 461–464.
63. Lefebvre, K. A. and Robertson, A., 2010. Domoic acid and human exposure risks: A review. *Toxicon*, 56, 218–230.
64. Colman, J. R., Nowocin, K. J., Switzer, R. C., Trusk, T. C., and Ramsdell, J. S., 2005. Mapping and reconstruction of domoic acid-induced neurodegeneration in the mouse brain. *Neurotoxicol Teratol*, 27, 753–767.
65. Grant, K. S., Burbacher, T. M., Faustman, E. M., and Grattan, L., 2010. Domoic acid: Neurobehavioral consequences of exposure to a prevalent marine biotoxin. *Neurotoxicol Teratol*, 32, 132–141.
66. Andjelkovic, M., Vandevijvere, S., Van Klaveren, J., Van Oyen, H., and Van Loco, J., 2012. Exposure to domoic acid through shellfish consumption in Belgium. *Environ Int*, 49, 115–119.
67. Paredes, I., Rietjens, I. M., Vieites, J. M., and Cabado, A. G., 2011. Update of risk assessments of main marine biotoxins in the European Union. *Toxicon*, 58, 336–354.
68. Bernard, P. B., MacDonald, D. S., Gill, D. A., Ryan, C. L., and Tasker, R. A., 2007. Hippocampal mossy fiber sprouting and elevated trkB receptor expression following systemic administration of low dose domoic acid during neonatal development. *Hippocampus*, 17, 1121–1133.
69. Doucette, T. A., Ryan, C. L., and Tasker, R. A., 2007. Gender-based changes in cognition and emotionality in a new rat model of epilepsy. *Amino Acids*, 32, 317–322.
70. Marriott, A. L., Ryan, C. L., and Doucette, T. A., 2012. Neonatal domoic acid treatment produces alterations to prepulse inhibition and latent inhibition in adult rats. *Pharmacol Biochem Behav*, 103, 338–344.
71. Xi, D., Peng, Y. G., and Ramsdell, J. S., 1997. Domoic acid is a potent neurotoxin to neonatal rats. *Nat Toxins*, 5, 74–79.
72. Mayer, A. M., 2000. The marine toxin domoic acid may affect the developing brain by activation of neonatal brain microglia and subsequent neurotoxic mediator generation. *Med Hypotheses*, 54, 837–841.
73. Dakshinamurti, K., Sharma, S. K., Sundaram, M., and Watanabe, T., 1993. Hippocampal changes in developing postnatal mice following intrauterine exposure to domoic acid. *J Neurosci*, 13, 4486–4495.
74. Alfonso, M., Duran, R., Duarte, C. B., Ferreira, I. L., and Carvalho, A. P., 1994. Domoic acid induced release of [3H]GABA in cultured chick retina cells. *Neurochem Int*, 24, 267–274.
75. Tanemura, K., Igarashi, K., Matsugami, T.-R., Aisaki, K.-I., Kitajima, S., and Kanno, J., 2009. Intrauterine environment-genome interaction and Children's development (2): Brain structure impairment and behavioral disturbance induced in male mice offspring by a single intraperitoneal administration of domoic acid (DA) to their dams. *J Toxicol Sci*, 34, SP279–SP286.

76. Lujan, R., Shigemoto, R., and Lopez-Bendito, G., 2005. Glutamate and GABA receptor signalling in the developing brain. *Neuroscience*, 130, 567–580.

77. Adams, A. L., Doucette, T. A., James, R., and Ryan, C. L., 2009. Persistent changes in learning and memory in rats following neonatal treatment with domoic acid. *Physiol Behav*, 96, 505–512.

78. Burt, M. A., Ryan, C. L., and Doucette, T. A., 2008. Altered responses to novelty and drug reinforcement in adult rats treated neonatally with domoic acid. *Physiol Behav*, 93, 327–336.

79. Burt, M. A., Ryan, C. L., and Doucette, T. A., 2008. Low dose domoic acid in neonatal rats abolishes nicotine induced conditioned place preference during late adolescence. *Amino Acids*, 35, 247–249.

80. Kumar, K. P., Kumar, S. P., and Nair, G. A., 2009. Risk assessment of the amnesic shellfish poison, domoic acid, on animals and humans. *J Environ Biol*, 30, 319–325.

81. Baron, A. W., Rushton, S. P., Rens, N., Morris, C. M., Blain, P. G., and Judge, S. J., 2013. Sex differences in effects of low level domoic acid exposure. *Neuro Toxicol*, 34, 1–8.

82. Truelove, J., Mueller, R., Pulido, O., and Iverson, F., 1996. Subchronic toxicity study of domoic acid in the rat. *Food Chem Toxicol*, 34, 525–529.

83. Truelove, J., Mueller, R., Pulido, O., Martin, L., Fernie, S., and Iverson, F., 1997. 30-day oral toxicity study of domoic acid in cynomolgus monkeys: Lack of overt toxicity at doses approaching the acute toxic dose. *Nat Toxins*, 5, 111–114.

84. Mordrelle, A., Jullian, E., Costa, C. et al., 2000. EAAT1 is involved in transport of L-glutamate during differentiation of the Caco-2 cell line. *Am J Physiol Gastrointest Liver Physiol*, 279, G366–G373.

85. Pulido, O., 2008. Domoic acid toxicologic pathology: A review. *Marine Drugs*, 6, 180–219.

86. Xi, D. and Ramsdell, J. S., 1996. Glutamate receptors and calcium entry mechanisms for domoic acid in hippocampal neurons. *Neuroreport*, 7, 1115–1120.

87. Berman, F. W., LePage, K. T., and Murray, T. F., 2002. Domoic acid neurotoxicity in cultured cerebellar granule neurons is controlled preferentially by the NMDA receptor Ca2+ influx pathway. *Brain Res*, 924, 20–29.

88. Qiu, S. and Currás-Collazo, M. C., 2006. Histopathological and molecular changes produced by hippocampal microinjection of domoic acid. *Neurotoxicol Teratol*, 28, 354–362.

89. Hogberg, H. T. and Bal-Price, A. K., 2011. Domoic acid-induced neurotoxicity is mainly mediated by the AMPA/KA receptor: Comparison between immature and mature primary cultures of neurons and glial cells from rat cerebellum. *J Toxicol*, 2011, 543512.

90. Dakshinamurti, K., Sharma, S. K., and Geiger, J. D., 2003. Neuroprotective actions of pyridoxine. *Biochim Biophys Acta*, 1647, 225–229.

91. Vale-González, C., Alfonso, A., Suñol, C., Vieytes, M. R., and Botana, L. M., 2006. Role of the plasma membrane calcium adenosine triphosphatase on domoate-induced intracellular acidification in primary cultures of cerebellar granule cells. *J Neurosci Res*, 84, 326–337.

92. Berman, F. W. and Murray, T. F., 1997. Domoic acid neurotoxicity in cultured cerebellar granule neurons is mediated predominantly by NMDA receptors that are activated as a consequence of excitatory amino acid release. *J Neurochem*, 69, 693–703.

93. Giordano, G., White, C. C., McConnachie, L. A., Fernandez, C., Kavanagh, T. J., and Costa, L. G., 2006. Neurotoxicity of domoic acid in cerebellar granule neurons in a genetic model of glutathione deficiency. *Mol Pharmacol*, 70, 2116–2126.

94. Giordano, G., White, C. C., Mohar, I., Kavanagh, T. J., and Costa, L. G., 2007. Glutathione levels modulate domoic acid–induced apoptosis in mouse cerebellar granule cells. *Toxicol Sci*, 100, 433–444.

95. Giordano, G., Klintworth, H. M., Kavanagh, T. J., and Costa, L. G., 2008. Apoptosis induced by domoic acid in mouse cerebellar granule neurons involves activation of p38 and JNK MAP kinases. *Neurochem Int*, 52, 1100–1105.

96. Giordano, G., Li, L., White, C. C. et al., 2009. Muscarinic receptors prevent oxidative stress-mediated apoptosis induced by domoic acid in mouse cerebellar granule cells. *J Neurochem*, 109, 525–538.

97. Carvalho Pinto-Silva, C. R., Moukha, S., Matias, W. G., and Creppy, E. E., 2008. Domoic acid induces direct DNA damage and apoptosis in Caco-2 cells: Recent advances. *Environ Toxicol*, 23, 657–663.

98. Giordano, G., Kavanagh, T. J., Faustman, E. M., White, C. C., and Costa, L. G., 2013. Low-level domoic Acid protects mouse cerebellar granule neurons from acute neurotoxicity: Role of glutathione. *Toxicol Sci*, 132, 399–408.

31

Gambierol: Synthetic Aspects

Haruhiko Fuwa

CONTENTS

31.1 General Introduction

Marine polycyclic ether natural products are known to be the secondary metabolites of unicellular algae, mainly dinoflagellates (Murata and Yasumoto, 2000; Yasumoto and Murata, 1993). Following the structure elucidation of brevetoxin B by Nakanishi, Clardy, and coworkers (Lin et al., 1981), marine polycyclic ether metabolites have been attracting the attention of numerous chemists and biologists because of their extraordinarily complex molecular architecture, highly potent biological activities, and limited availability from natural sources (Figure 31.1). A common structural motif is shared among the family of marine polycyclic ether metabolites: six- to nine-membered cyclic ethers are disposed in a ladderlike array with strict regularity, in which the oxygen atoms are placed alternately on the two sides of the molecule (Figure 31.2). Furthermore, the molecular length of this class of natural products reaches several nanometers in general. Despite these structural similarities, it is particularly intriguing that marine polycyclic ethers elicit diverse biological activities, such as neurotoxicity, cytotoxicity, hemolytic activity, and antifungal activity. The mechanism of the biosynthesis of marine polycyclic ethers has also been a long-standing mystery. Nakanishi and Shimizu have independently proposed a hypothetical biosynthetic pathway that involves a cascade cyclization of polyepoxides (Figure 31.3a) (Nakanishi, 1985; Shimizu, 1986). Jamison and coworkers recently showed that such a powerful cascade reaction could be reproduced in a laboratory setting, simply by heating a suitably designed synthetic polyepoxide in H_2O at 70°C (Figure 31.3b) (Vilotijevic and Jamison, 2007). The cascade reaction reported by Jamison et al. is in line with the Nakanishi–Shimizu hypothesis and might account for the biosynthetic mechanism of marine polycyclic ethers.

The structural and biological aspects of marine polycyclic ether metabolites make them particularly attractive and challenging target molecules for the synthetic community (Inoue, 2005; Nakata, 2005; Nicolaou et al., 2008). Nicolaou and coworkers have developed a number of powerful methodologies for the stereoselective synthesis of medium-sized cyclic ethers, and they completed the total synthesis of brevetoxins A and B in the mid- to late 1990s (Nicolaou et al., 1995a,b,c, 1998, 1999a,b,c,d). A few years later, Hirama and colleagues accomplished the total synthesis of CTX3C, a natural congener of ciguatoxin (Hirama etal., 2001). Undoubtedly, these total syntheses are landmark achievements in modern

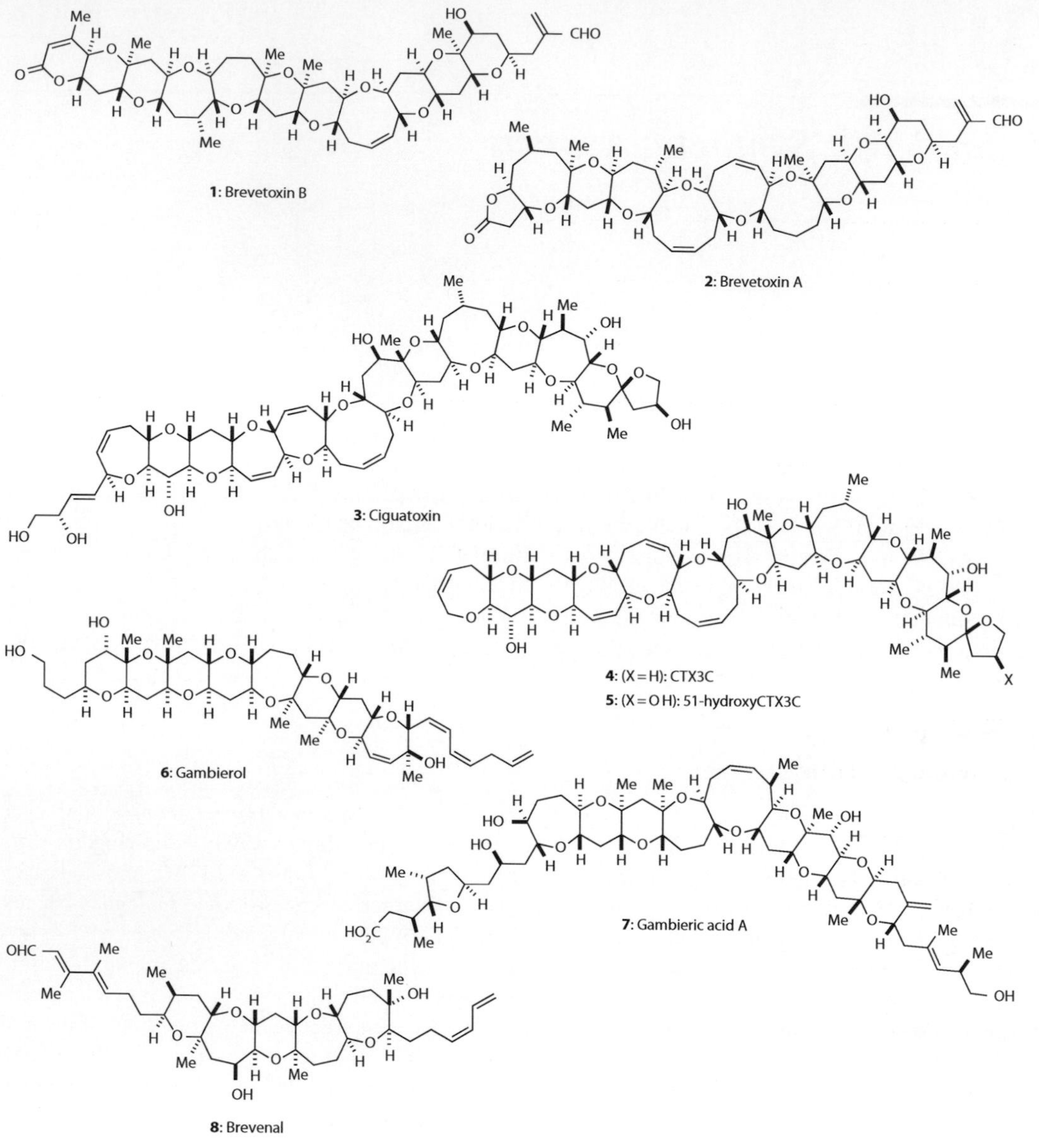

FIGURE 31.1 Structures of representative marine polycyclic ether natural products.

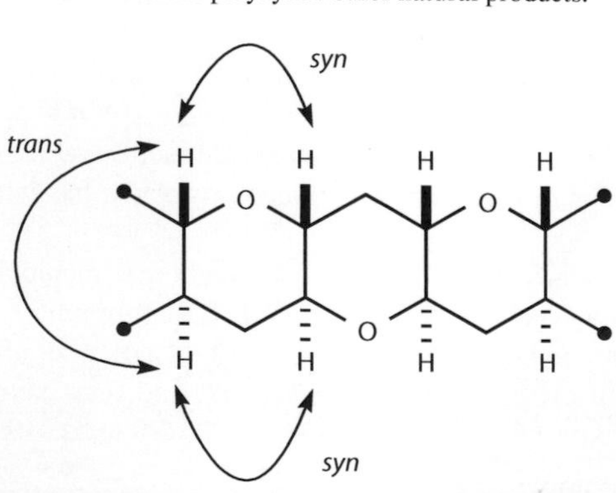

FIGURE 31.2 Common structural motif found in marine polycyclic ether natural products.

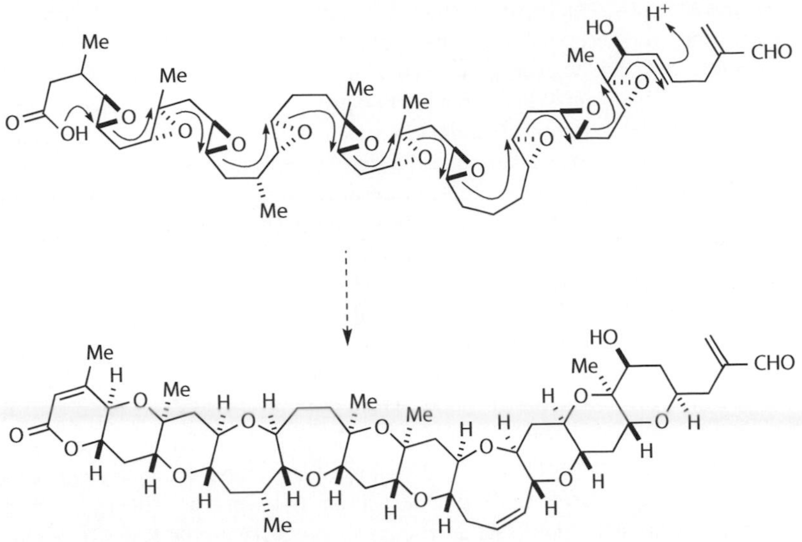

FIGURE 31.3 Polyepoxide cyclization cascade.

organic synthesis. After the dawn of the twenty-first century, the availability of convergent strategies for the synthesis of large polycyclic skeletons greatly improved our ability to synthesize marine polycyclic ether metabolites. Indeed, the total syntheses of ciguatoxin (Inoue et al., 2006), 51-hydroxyCTX3C (Inoue et al., 2006), brevetoxin B (Kadota et al., 2005; Matsuo et al., 2004), brevetoxin A (Crimmins et al., 2009a,b,c), gambierol (Furuta et al., 2009, 2010; Fuwa et al., 2002a,b; Johnson et al., 2005, 2006; Kadota et al., 2003a,b; Majumder et al., 2006), gymnocin-A (Tsukano and Sasaki, 2003; Tsukano et al., 2005), brevenal (Ebine et al., 2008, 2011; Fuwa et al., 2006a,b), and gambieric acid A (Fuwa et al., 2012) have been reported within the past decade.

Importantly, total synthesis has afforded a practical supply of material for accelerating in-depth biological investigations of marine polycyclic ether metabolites. For example, using material from total synthesis, Bigiani and coworkers successfully identified voltage-gated potassium channels (VGPCs) as the primary target biomolecule of gambierol (Ghiaroni et al., 2005). Chemical synthesis has also paved the way to unnatural structural analogues by exploiting the concept of "diverted total synthesis" (Njardarson et al., 2004). Such unnatural analogues can be used to explore structure–activity relationships (SARs), as accomplished for gambierol (Fuwa et al., 2003, 2004), gymnocin-A (Tsukano and Sasaki, 2006), and ciguatoxins (Inoue et al., 2008). Moreover, artificially designed polycyclic ethers with intriguing biological functions have been described (Alonso et al., 2012; Oguri et al., 2006; Oishi et al., 2012; Torikai et al., 2008). Thus, total synthesis is not merely an intellectual challenge for organic chemists; it is a powerful means of facilitating biological investigations and the discovery of biologically functional molecules based on naturally occurring substances. In the following sections, we will provide an overview of the total synthesis of gambierol.

31.2 Gambierol

31.2.1 Introduction

In 1993, Satake, Yasumoto, and coworkers reported the isolation of gambierol (**6**, Figure 31.1) from the cultured cells of the ciguatera causative dinoflagellate *Gambierdiscus toxicus* (Satake et al., 1993). The gross structure and relative stereochemistry of gambierol were established through extensive 2D NMR spectroscopic analyses. Subsequently, the same group determined the absolute configuration by applying the modified Mosher analysis (Morohashi et al., 1998). The structural features of this natural product include the ladder-shaped octacyclic polyether skeleton consisting of six- and seven-membered cyclic ethers and a partially skipped triene side chain attached at the end of the molecule. Satake et al. have reported that gambierol exhibits potent lethal toxicity in mice (LD_{99} 50 μg/kg, i.p.), and the neurological symptoms induced in the mice resemble those shown by ciguatoxins. These observations point to the possibility that gambierol is also implicated in ciguatera seafood poisoning. However, further investigations into the biological activity of gambierol had been precluded for almost a decade because of the lack of available material from natural sources.

The Sasaki/Tachibana group was the first to accomplish the total synthesis of gambierol (Fuwa et al., 2002a,b). Significantly, their synthetic material contributed to the elucidation of the primary target biomolecule of gambierol. Thus, Bigiani and coworkers in a collaborative work with Sasaki et al. have identified that this natural product inhibits VGPCs (Kv channels) in mouse taste cells at low nanomolar concentrations (Ghiaroni et al., 2005, 2006). Subsequently, the synthetic material prepared by the Rainier group (Johnson et al., 2005, 2006) enabled Snyders and coworkers to demonstrate that this natural product selectively inhibits Kv1 and Kv3 subfamilies and binds to the previously undescribed binding site present between the S5 and S6 segments of Kv3.1 channels (Kopljar et al., 2009). The Sasaki group also collaborated with Botana and coworkers to show that gambierol is a weak partial agonist of voltage-gated sodium channels in human neuroblastoma cells (Louzao et al., 2006). They have also shown that gambierol induces extracellular calcium ion-dependent calcium oscillations in cerebellar granule neurons (Alonso et al., 2010).

The Sasaki group has also made significant contributions to clarifying the SARs of gambierol. To systematically explore SARs, they exploited the concept of "diverted total synthesis" (Njardarson et al., 2004) and prepared 18 totally synthetic structural analogues of gambierol starting from a synthetic intermediate of their total synthesis (Fuwa et al., 2003, 2004). Evaluation of the lethal toxicity of the synthetic analogues in mice has elucidated that the H-ring double bond and the length and the unsaturated (Z,Z)-diene system of the side chain are essential for the potent toxicity, while the A-ring hydroxy groups only seem to be relevant to the pharmacokinetic properties of the natural product (Figure 31.4). Although it has long been believed that the molecular length is essential for the biological activity of marine polycyclic ether metabolites, these results led to the hypothesis that the left end of the molecule can potentially be truncated without affecting the biological potency. Accordingly, the Sasaki group designed and synthesized truncated analogues **9** and **10** and demonstrated that both of these analogues showed low nanomolar inhibitory activity against Kv channels, being equipotent to the natural product (Alonso et al., 2012) (Figure 31.5). Notably, compounds **9** and **10** represent the first successful truncation of marine polycyclic ether metabolites.

It is now clear that chemical synthesis has afforded significant advances in our understanding of the biological mode of action of gambierol and enabled systematic SAR investigations and elaboration of novel truncated analogues. The following sections will summarize the total syntheses of gambierol that have been reported to date (Mori, 2010).

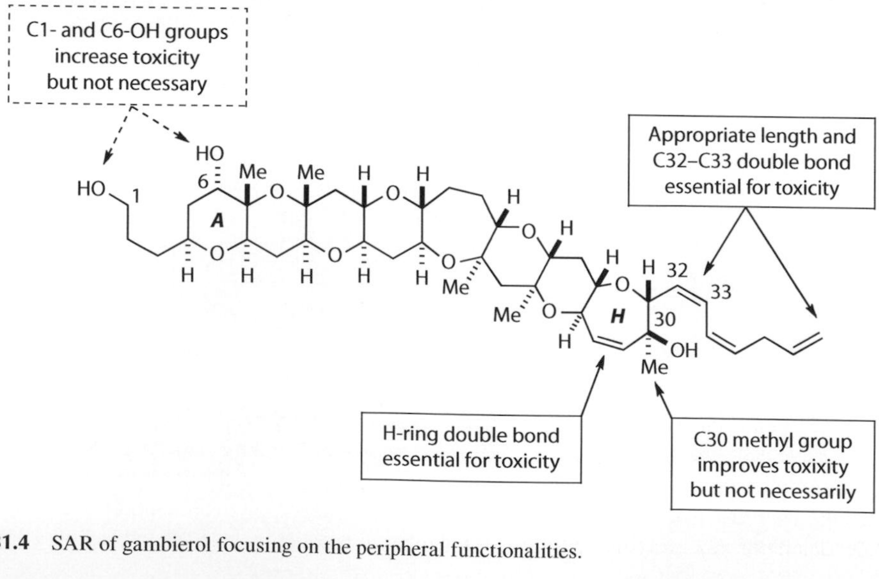

FIGURE 31.4 SAR of gambierol focusing on the peripheral functionalities.

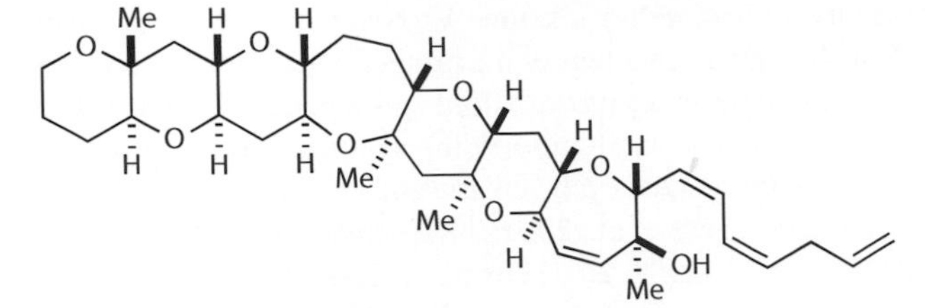

9: Heptacyclic analogue

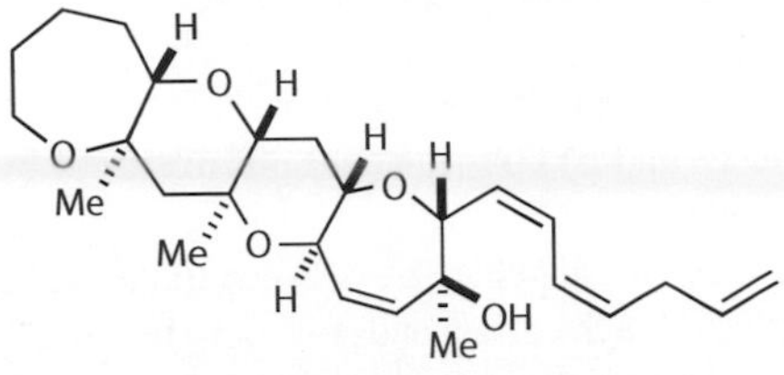

10: Tetracyclic analogue

FIGURE 31.5 Truncated analogues of gambierol with potent Kv channel inhibitory activity.

31.2.2 Total Synthesis of Gambierol by the Sasaki Group

The Sasaki group has developed a convergent strategy for the synthesis of polycyclic ether arrays by exploiting the Suzuki–Miyaura reaction (Miyaura and Suzuki, 1995; Suzuki, 2011), outlined in Figure 31.6. Stereoselective hydroboration of exocyclic enol ether **I** with 9-borabicyclo[3.3.1] nonane (9-BBN-H) generates the corresponding alkylborane **II**, which reacts with lactone-derived enol triflate or phosphate **III** in the presence of a base and a palladium catalyst to provide endocyclic enol ether **IV**. Usually, lactone-derived enol phosphates are superior to their triflate counterparts in terms of ease of handling and chromatographic purification (Fuwa, 2011). Stereoselective hydroboration of **IV** followed

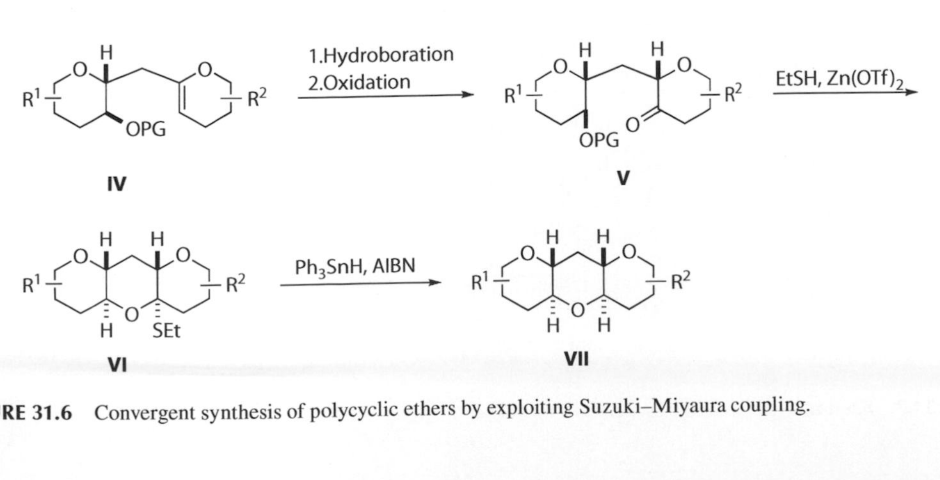

FIGURE 31.6 Convergent synthesis of polycyclic ethers by exploiting Suzuki–Miyaura coupling.

by oxidation of the resultant alcohol delivers ketone **V** (Nicolaou et al., 1996). Mixed thioacetalization (Fuwa et al., 2001) of **V** with concomitant loss of the protective group (PG) and ensuing reduction of the derived mixed thioacetal (Nicolaou et al., 1989a) affords polycyclic ether **VI**. The strategy established by the Sasaki group allows for a practical and high-yielding synthesis of complex polycyclic ether skeletons containing various sizes of medium-sized cyclic ethers, and its feasibility has been well demonstrated by the total syntheses of gambierol (Fuwa et al., 2002a,b), gymnocin-A (Tsukano et al., 2005; Tsukano and Sasaki 2003), brevenal (Ebine et al., 2008, 2011; Fuwa et al., 2006a,b), and gambieric acid A (Fuwa et al., 2012), wherein Suzuki–Miyaura coupling has been utilized in a spectacular manner for the convergent assembly of the entire polyether framework of these natural products.

Toward the total synthesis of gambierol, the Sasaki group planned their synthesis as illustrated in Figure 31.7. The apparently sensitive triene side chain was to be introduced at the final stage of the total synthesis using a Stille reaction of (Z)-vinyl bromide **11** and (Z)-vinyl stannane **12** (Matsukawa et al., 1999; Shirakawa et al., 1999). The polycyclic ether skeleton of **11** was considered to be accessible from the ABC-ring exocyclic enol ether **13** and EFGH-ring enol phosphate **14** by means of a Suzuki–Miyaura coupling and a mixed thioacetalization.

The synthesis of the ABC-ring exocyclic enol ether **13**, outlined in Figure 31.8, started from the known tetrahydropyran **15** (Nicolaou et al., 1990), which corresponds to the B-ring, and the rings were constructed in the order of B → AB → ABC. Oxidative cleavage of the double bond of **15**, Horner–Wadsworth–Emmons (HWE) olefination of the derived aldehyde, and subsequent reduction with diisobutylaluminum hydride (DIBALH) gave allylic alcohol **16**. The C6 stereogenic center was introduced by Sharpless asymmetric epoxidation of **16** (Gao et al., 1987), and the resultant epoxy alcohol was regioselectively reduced with Red-Al® (Finan and Kishi, 1982) to provide 1,3-diol **17**. This diol was transformed to alcohol **18** via *p*-methoxybenzylidene acetal formation and regioselective DIBALH reduction. Oxidation of **18** followed by a Wittig reaction and ensuing

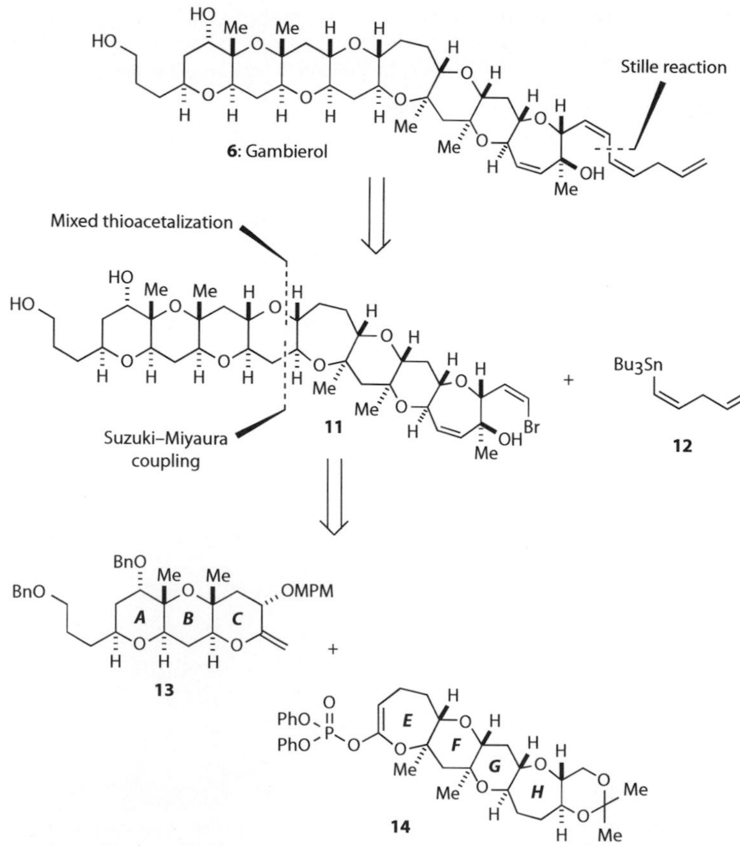

FIGURE 31.7 Synthesis plan toward gambierol (**6**) by the Sasaki group.

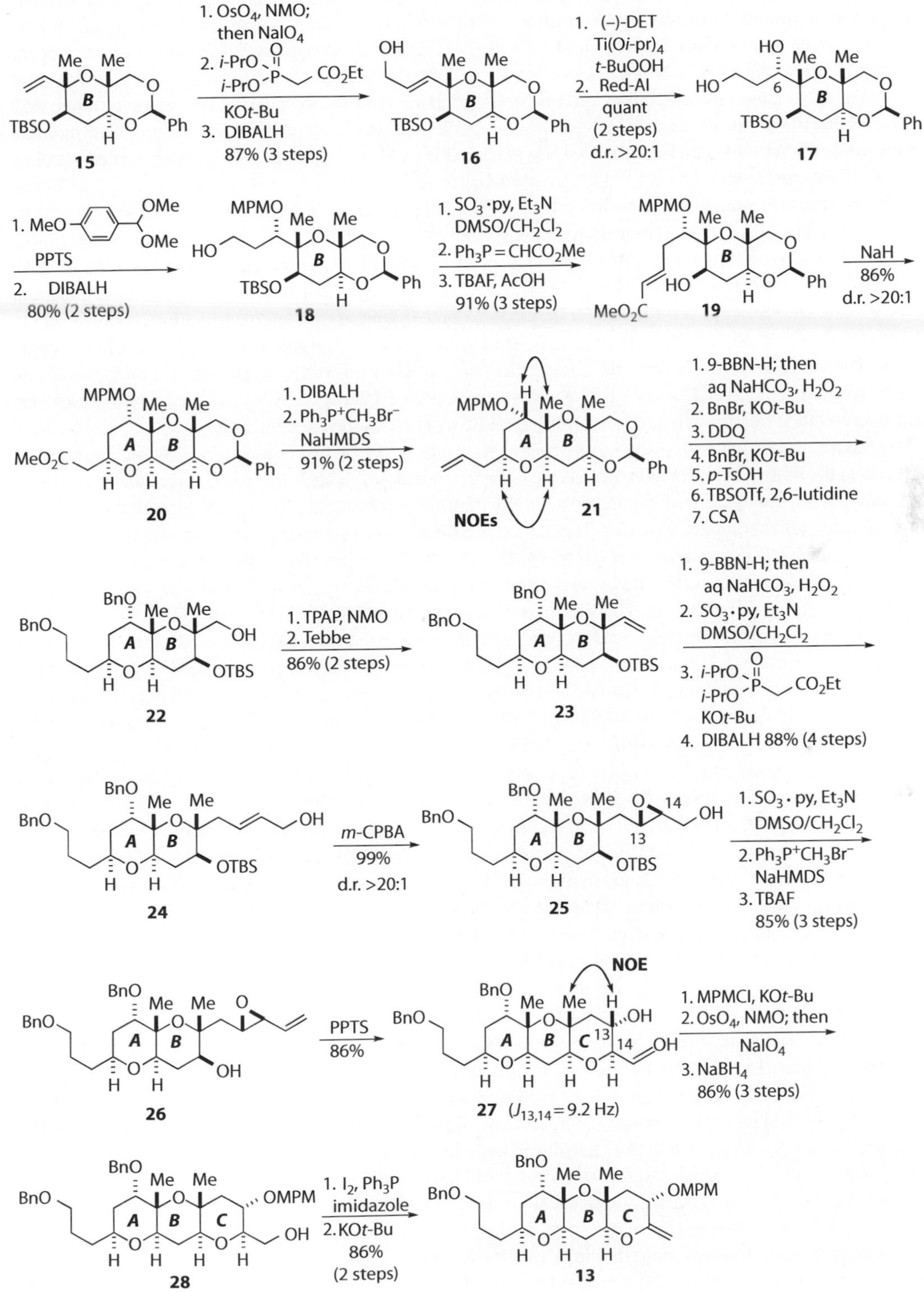

FIGURE 31.8 Synthesis of the ABC-ring exocyclic enol ether **13**.

cleavage of the silyl ether with tetra-*n*-butylammonium fluoride (TBAF) buffered with acetic acid delivered alcohol **19**. The A-ring was stereoselectively forged by means of an intramolecular oxa-conjugate cyclization. Thus, the exposure of **19** to NaH in tetrahydrofuran (THF) at room temperature afforded ester **20** in 86% yield as a single stereoisomer. Reduction of **20** with DIBALH and subsequent Wittig methylenation of the resultant aldehyde gave olefin **21**. The stereochemistry of the C4 stereogenic center was secured at this stage by a nuclear Overhauser effect (NOE) experiment. Olefin **21** was transformed to suitably protected alcohol **22** in seven steps mainly using standard PG chemistry. Alcohol **22** was oxidized with tetra-*n*-propylammonium perruthenate (TPAP)/*N*-methylmorpholine (NMM) *N*-oxide (NMO) (Ley et al., 1994) and then methylenated using the Tebbe reagent (Tebbe et al., 1978) to afford olefin **23**. Toward the construction of the C-ring, allylic alcohol **24** was efficiently elaborated from **23** via a four-step sequence involving hydroboration, oxidation, HWE olefination, and DIBALH reduction. Stereoselective epoxidation of **24** was optimally performed with *m*-chloroperoxybenzoic acid (*m*-CPBA) to provide epoxy alcohol **25** as a single stereoisomer, setting the C13 and C14 stereogenic centers. Epoxy alcohol **25** was oxidized and then methylenated to give, after desilylation, vinyl epoxide **26**. The stage was thus set for the closure of the C-ring via a 6-*endo* cyclization (Nicolaou et al., 1989b); treatment of **26** with pyridinium *p*-toluenesulfonate (PPTS) furnished tricycle **27** as a single stereoisomer. The stereochemistry around the C-ring was established by an NOE experiment and a $^3J_{H,H}$ value, as shown. The double bond of **27** was oxidatively cleaved and reduced with NaBH$_4$ to give alcohol **28**, which was iodinated and then treated with a base to afford the ABC-ring exocyclic enol ether **13**.

The Sasaki group synthesized the EFGH-ring enol phosphate **14** by two completely different approaches. Outlined in the following text (Figure 31.9) is the second-generation synthesis that has been performed in a linear fashion by exploiting the SmI$_2$-promoted reductive cyclization (Hori et al., 1999a,b, 2002; Nakata, 2010) and vinyl epoxide cyclization methodologies (Nicolaou et al., 1989b). The synthesis of **14** commenced with ozonolysis of the known α,β-unsaturated ester **29** (Nicolaou et al., 1999b), which, after reductive workup with NaBH$_4$, gave alcohol **30**. Iodination of **30**, alkylation of the derived iodide **31** with 2-lithio-1,3-dithiane, and cleavage of the silyl ether delivered alcohol **32**. This alcohol was reacted with ethyl propiolate and NMM, and the dithio-acetal was removed to afford aldehyde **33**. According to the Nakata reductive cyclization protocol, aldehyde **33** was exposed to SmI$_2$ in the presence of MeOH in THF at room temperature to furnish the H-ring lactone **34** in 70% yield as a single stereoisomer, after purification by silica gel column chromatography. Reduction of lactone **34** with DIBALH followed by Wittig olefination provided α,β-unsaturated ester **35**. Protection of the resultant hydroxy group gave silyl ether **36**. DIBALH reduction of the ester functionality of **36** and Sharpless asymmetric epoxidation of the resultant allylic alcohol gave epoxy alcohol **37** as a single stereoisomer, which was oxidized and then methylenated to deliver vinyl epoxide **38**. After the removal of the silyl group from **38**, the G-ring was constructed via an acid-catalyzed 6-*endo* cyclization to furnish alcohol **39** as a single stereoisomer. The newly generated stereogenic centers around the G-ring were unambiguously established by NOE experiments and a $^3J_{H,H}$ analysis, as shown. Silylation of **39** was followed by the replacement of the benzylidene acetal with an isopropylidene acetal to give olefin **40**, which was transformed to methyl ketone **41** in a four-step sequence involving hydroboration, oxidation, methylation, and oxidation. The silyl group of **41** was cleaved and the liberated alcohol was reacted with ethyl propiolate/NMM to deliver α,β-unsaturated ester **42**, setting the stage for the formation of the F-ring. Thus, **42** was treated with SmI$_2$ in the presence of MeOH in THF at 0°C to afford alcohol **43** in 87% yield as a single stereoisomer. Protection of alcohol **43** as its trimethylsilyl (TMS) ether, half reduction of the ester functionality, Wittig olefination of the derived aldehyde, and removal of the TMS group led to α,β-unsaturated ester **43**. Hydrogenation of the double bond of **43** with concomitant hydrogenolysis of the benzyl ester, followed by Yamaguchi lactonization (Inanaga et al., 1979) of the resultant seco-acid, afforded a lactone, which was enolized with potassium hexamethyldisilazide (KHMDS) in the presence of (PhO)$_2$P(O)Cl (Nicolaou et al., 1997) to furnish the EFGH-ring enol phosphate **14**.

The ABC- and EFGH-ring fragments (**13** and **14**, respectively) were next assembled via a Suzuki–Miyaura reaction (Figure 31.10). Stereoselective hydroboration of **13** with 9-BBN-H followed by the coupling of the resultant alkylborane with **14** by the action of aqueous Cs$_2$CO$_3$ and dichloro[1,1′-bis(diphenylphosphino)ferrocene]palladium dichloromethane complex [PdCl$_2$(dppf)·CH$_2$Cl$_2$] in *N,N*-dimethylformamide (DMF) at 50°C provided endocyclic enol ether **45** in 86% yield. Stereoselective hydroboration of **45** using BH$_3$·THF and oxidative workup gave an alcohol, which was oxidized with TPAP/NMO to deliver ketone **46** as a single stereoisomer. The C16 stereogenic center was established through an NOE experiment. After the cleavage of the *p*-methoxyphenylmethyl (MPM) ether of **46**,

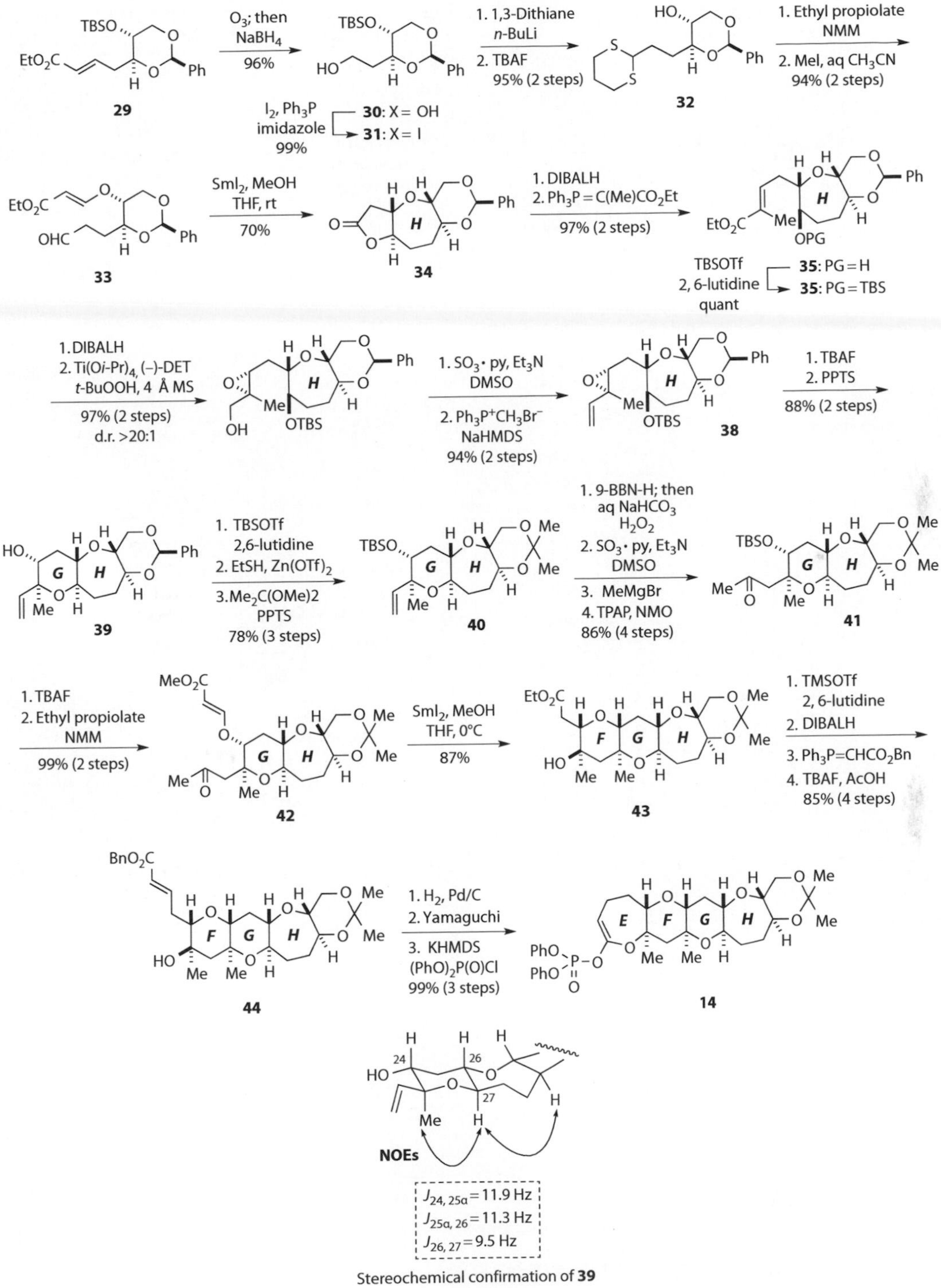

FIGURE 31.9 Synthesis of the EFGH-ring enol phosphate **14**.

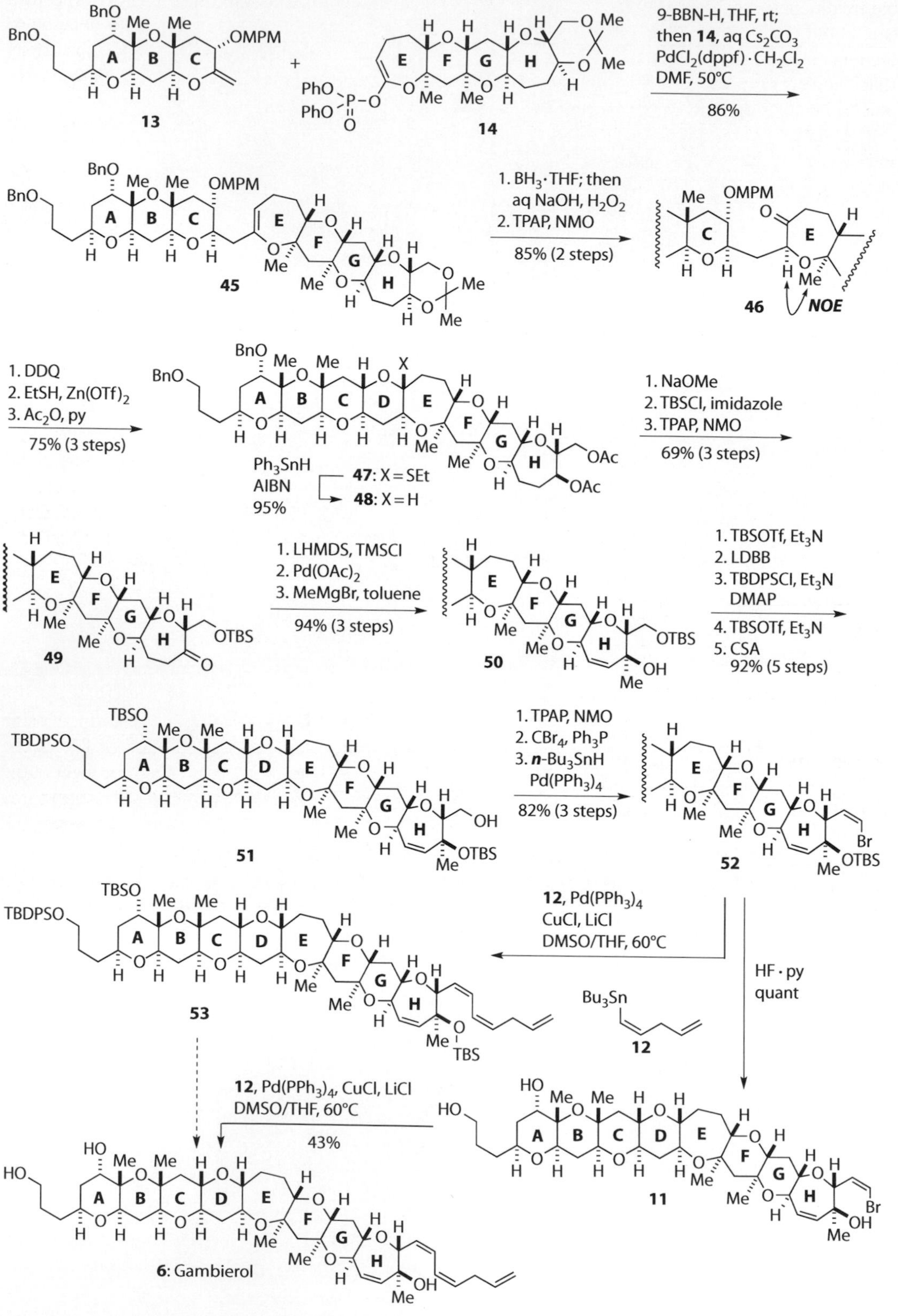

FIGURE 31.10 Completion of the total synthesis by the Sasaki group.

the treatment of the resultant product with EtSH and zinc trifluoromethanesulfonate [Zn(OTf)$_2$] (Fuwa et al., 2001) brought about spontaneous removal of the isopropylidene acetal. Subsequent acetylation of the unmasked hydroxy groups led to mixed thioacetal **47**. Reduction of **47** under tin hydride conditions (Nicolaou et al., 1989a) furnished octacycle **48**. Thus, the Sasaki group successfully assembled the entire polycyclic ether framework of gambierol in a highly convergent manner.

The Sasaki group next elaborated the H-ring functionalities. Methanolysis of the acetyl groups of **48** followed by selective silylation of the liberated primary alcohol and oxidation of the remaining secondary alcohol gave ketone **49**. The H-ring double bond was introduced to **49** by the Ito–Saegusa method (Ito et al., 1978). Thus, ketone **49** was converted to the corresponding enol silyl ether and then exposed to palladium acetate [Pd(OAc)$_2$] in acetonitrile at room temperature to provide an enone, which was reacted with methylmagnesium bromide in toluene at −78°C (Feng and Murai, 1992) to afford tertiary alcohol **50** as a single stereoisomer. After completing the functionalization of the H-ring, the PGs within **50** were suitably modified via a five-step sequence to deliver alcohol **51**. The (Z)-vinyl bromide moiety, required for the introduction of the triene side chain, was introduced by the oxidation of alcohol **51** followed by dibromoolefination and stereoselective reduction of the derived dibromoolefin by using n-Bu$_3$SnH in the presence of tetrakis(triphenylphosphine)palladium [Pd(PPh$_3$)$_4$] (Uenishi et al., 1996, 1998). The (Z)-vinyl bromide **52** thus obtained was coupled with (Z)-vinyl stannane **12** under Corey's modified conditions [Pd(PPh$_3$)$_4$, CuCl, LiCl, DMSO/THF, 60°C] (Han et al., 1999) to afford tris-silyl gambierol **53**. However, all attempts to deprotect the silyl groups in the presence of the fragile triene side chain were unsuccessful. Accordingly, the Sasaki group removed all the silyl groups before introducing the triene side chain. Thus, exposure of **52** to excess HF·pyridine provided triol **11**, which was coupled with **12** under Corey's conditions to furnish gambierol (**6**) in 43% yield. The spectroscopic data (IR, ^{1}H, ^{13}C NMR, HRMS, CD) and optical rotation value of the synthetic material matched those of the authentic sample, thereby confirming the complete stereostructure of the natural product for the first time. Most importantly, the Sasaki group has synthesized more than 100 mg of gambierol for extensive biological investigations (Sasaki and Fuwa, 2008).

31.2.3 Total Synthesis of Gambierol by the Kadota/Yamamoto Group

The Kadota/Yamamoto group relied on intramolecular alkylation of α-acyloxy ethers and ring-closing metathesis (RCM) for the synthesis of polycyclic ethers (Kadota et al., 2001) (Figure 31.11). Cyclic ether fragments **VIII** and **IX** are coupled through an esterification to give ester **X**. After elaborating the γ-alkoxy allylstannane moiety (Kadota et al., 1996), α-acyloxy ether **XII** is conveniently prepared from the corresponding ester **XI** by DIBALH reduction and in situ acylation, according to the method developed by Rychnovsky and coworkers (Dahanukar and Rychnovsky, 1996; Kopecky and Rychnovsky, 2000). Treatment of the resultant α-acyloxy ether **XII** with an appropriate Lewis acid (e.g., BF$_3$·OEt$_2$, MgBr·OEt$_2$) promotes an intramolecular alkylation to afford O-linked cyclic ether **XIII**. As described in the following discussion, in some cases, the choice of the acyl group is found to be important for the stereochemical outcome of the cyclization. Subsequent RCM (Gradillas and Pérez-Castells, 2006; Hoveyda and Zhugralin, 2007; Nicolaou et al., 2005) completes the synthesis of polycyclic ether **XIV**. The Kadota/Yamamoto strategy has been successfully applied to their total syntheses of gambierol (Kadota et al., 2003a,b), brevetoxin B (Kadota et al., 2005), and brevenal (Takamura et al., 2009, 2010).

The Kadota/Yamamoto group devised their synthetic approach toward gambierol as summarized in Figure 31.12. They envisioned that the D- and E-rings could be successively constructed by means of an intramolecular alkylation of α-acyloxy ether **54** followed by RCM of the resultant diene and that **54** could be obtained from the ABC-ring carboxylic acid **55** and FGH-ring alcohol **56**.

The synthesis of the ABC-ring carboxylic acid **55**, illustrated in Figure 31.13, started with the known AB-ring olefin **23**, which was previously prepared by the Sasaki group (Fuwa et al., 2002b). The Kadota/ Yamamoto group made use of the SmI$_2$-mediated reductive cyclization methodology reported by the Nakata group (Hori et al., 1999a,b, 2002; Nakata, 2010) for the construction of the C-ring. Hydroboration of olefin **23** gave alcohol **57**. The alcohol **57** was oxidized and then reacted with 1,3-propanedithiol and BF$_3$·OEt$_2$ to provide, after desilylation with TBAF, dithioacetal **58**. Introduction of a β-alkoxy acrylate moiety to **58** was followed by removal of the dithioacetal, leading to aldehyde **57**, which upon treatment with SmI$_2$ (methanol, THF, 0°C) furnished tricyclic ether **58** as a single stereoisomer. Silylation of the

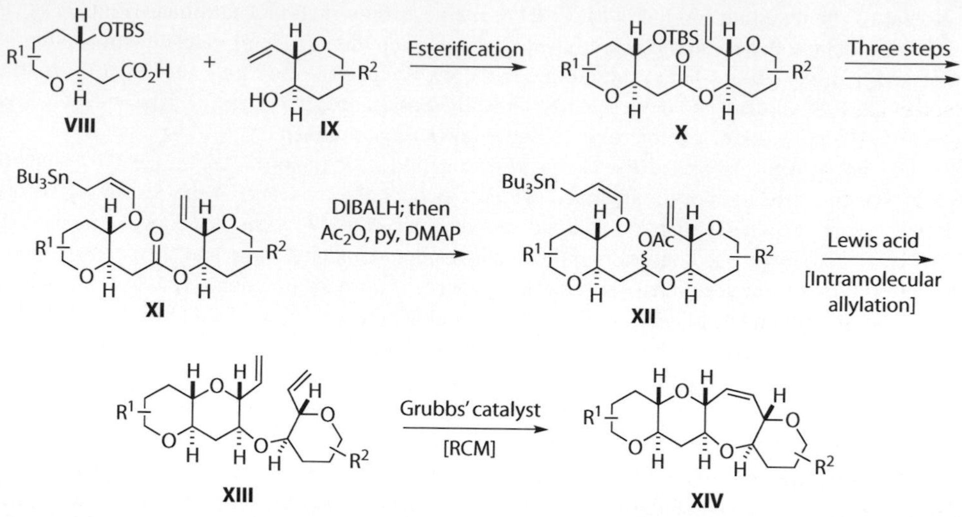

FIGURE 31.11   Convergent synthesis of polycyclic ethers via intramolecular alkylation.

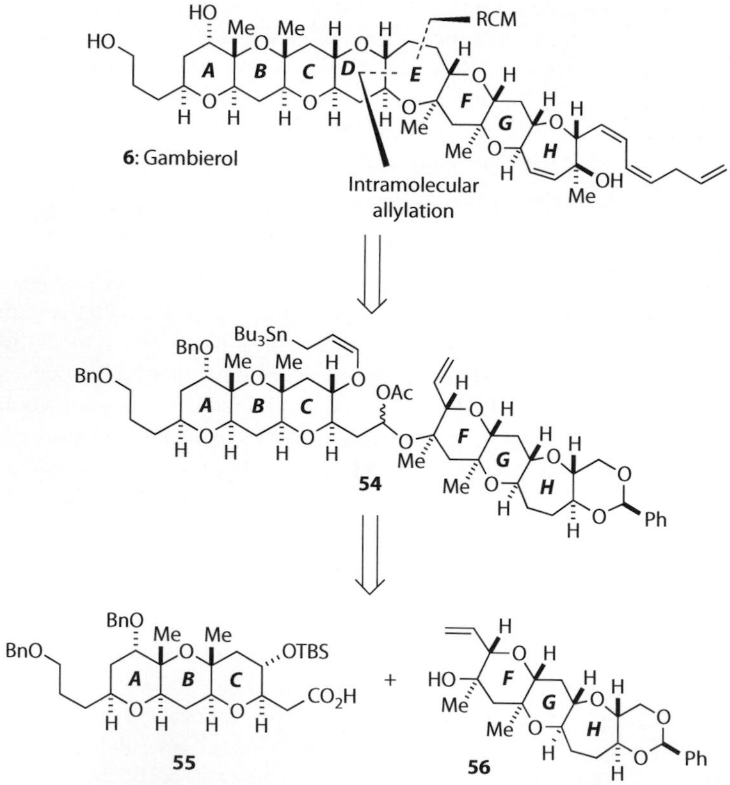

FIGURE 31.12   Synthesis plan toward gambierol (**6**) by the Kadota/Yamamoto group.

hydroxy group within **58** and subsequent reduction of the ester functionality gave alcohol **59**, which was uneventfully oxidized to the ABC-ring carboxylic acid **55**.

The synthesis of the FGH-ring alcohol **56**, summarized in Figure 31.14, utilized the FG-ring ester **62**, whose preparation was previously reported by the Nakata group (Sakamoto et al., 2001). The Kadota/Yamamoto group constructed the H-ring via the intramolecular alkylation methodology developed within their group (Kadota et al., 1997; Yamada et al., 1990). Reduction of **62** with LiAlH₄ followed

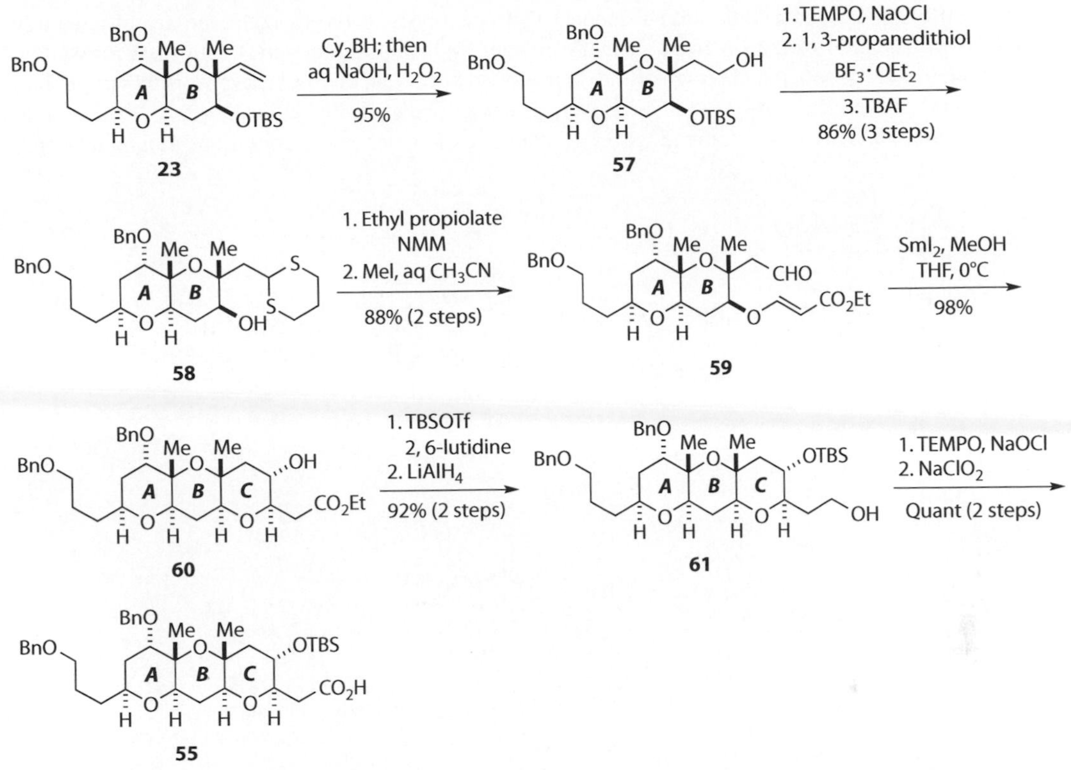

FIGURE 31.13 Synthesis of the ABC-ring carboxylic acid **55**.

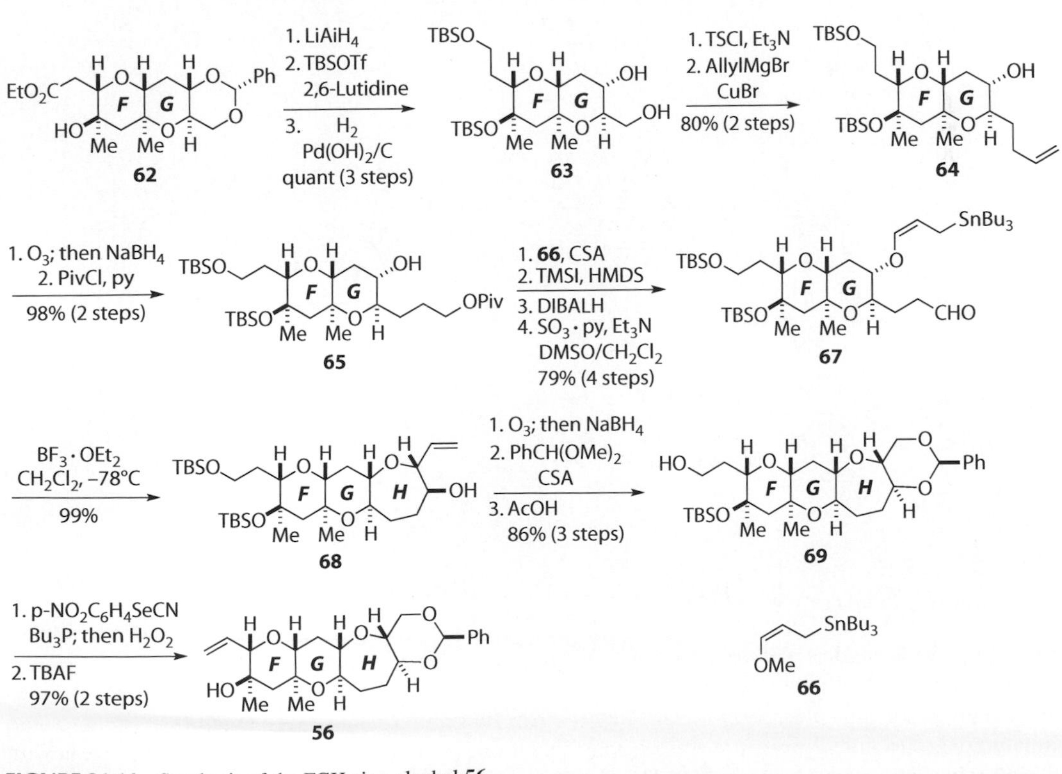

FIGURE 31.14 Synthesis of the FGH-ring alcohol **56**.

by silylation of the resultant diol, and subsequent hydrogenolysis of the benzylidene acetal gave diol **63**. Selective tosylation of the liberated primary alcohol, followed by copper(I)-catalyzed alkylation, delivered olefin **64**. Ozonolytic cleavage of the double bond within **64** and reductive workup gave a diol, whose primary hydroxy group was then selectively protected with pivaloyl chloride (PivCl)/pyridine to produce alcohol **65**. This was acetalized with allylstannane **66** under acidic conditions and then treated

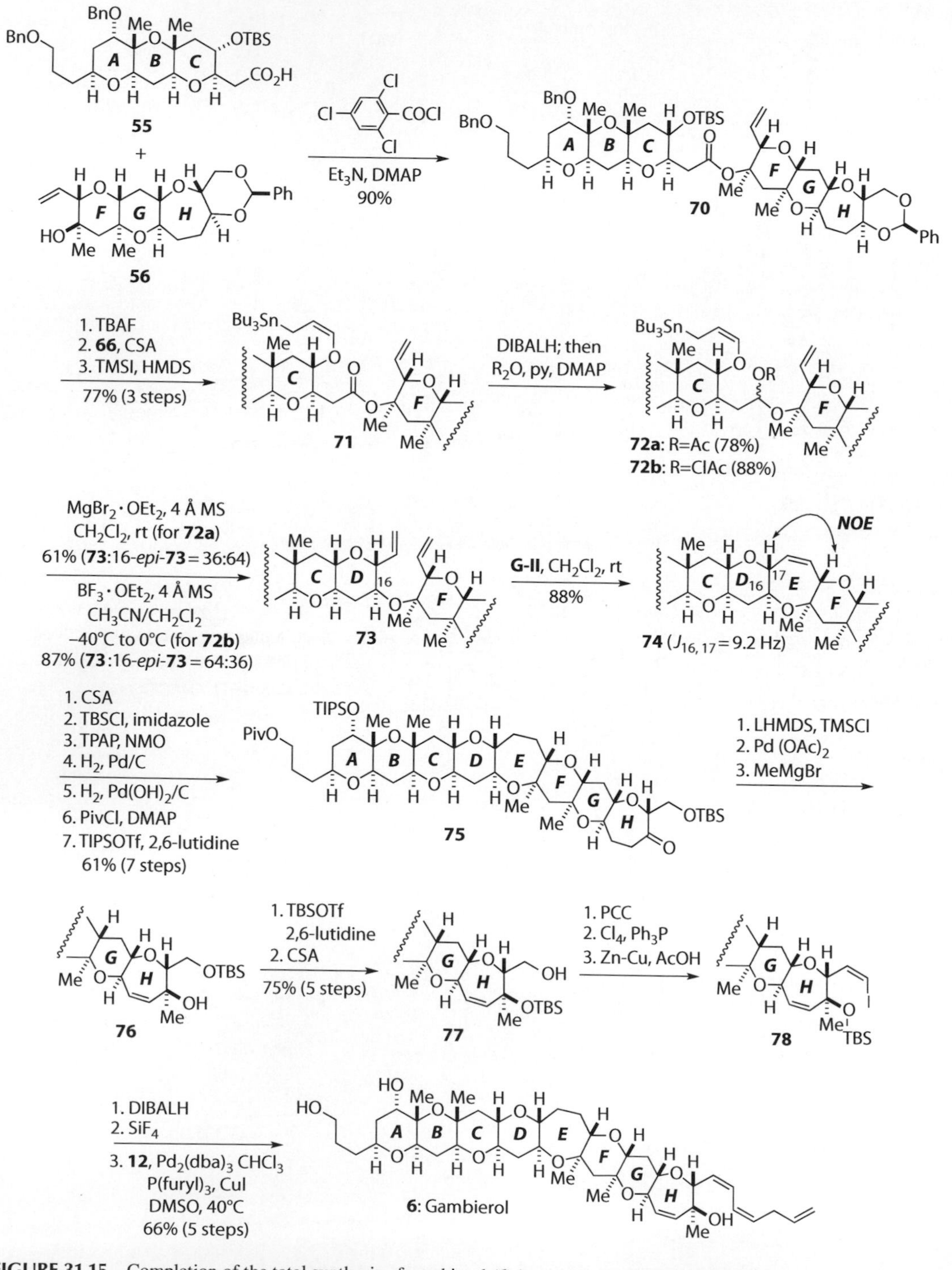

FIGURE 31.15   Completion of the total synthesis of gambierol (**6**) by the Kadota/Yamamoto group.

with hexamethyldisilazane (HMDS)/TMS iodide (TMSI) to afford a γ-alkoxy allylstannane (Kadota et al., 1996). Reductive removal of the pivaloyl group and oxidation of the resultant alcohol led to aldehyde **67**. Intramolecular alkylation of **67** promoted by BF₃·OEt₂ proceeded to afford tricyclic ether **68** in 99% yield as a single stereoisomer. Ozonolysis of the double bond of **68** followed by benzylidene acetal protection of the derived diol and selective desilylation gave alcohol **69**. The liberated primary alcohol **69** was dehydrated according to the Grieco–Nishizawa protocol (Grieco et al., 1976), and the remaining silyl group was removed to furnish the FGH-ring alcohol **56**.

The Kadota/Yamamoto group next coupled the ABC- and FGH-ring fragments (i.e., **55** and **56**, respectively) and completed the octacyclic skeleton of gambierol by exploiting their intramolecular alkylation/RCM methodology (Figure 31.15). Esterification of **55** and **56** under Yamaguchi conditions (Inanaga et al., 1979) provided ester **70**. Deprotection of the silyl group of **70** followed by the acid-catalyzed mixed acetalization, and the elimination of methanol (HMDS, TMSI) delivered allylic stannane **71**. Here, the Kadota/Yamamoto group initially examined the intramolecular alkylation of α-acetoxy ether **72a**. However, treatment of **72a** with MgBr·OEt₂ in CH₂Cl₂ at −40°C to 0°C delivered diene **73** and its C16 epimer (i.e., 16-*epi*-**73**) in a 36:64 diastereomeric ratio (61% combined yield), favoring the undesired stereoisomer. After several experiments, they found that intramolecular alkylation of α-chloroacetoxy ester **72b** upon treatment with BF₃·OEt₂ in CH₃CN/CH₂Cl₂ (20:1) at −40°C to 0°C gave diene **73** in 87% yield with 64:36 diastereoselectivity. The reversal of the observed diastereoselectivity could be ascribed, in part, to the greater potential of the chloroacetoxy group as a leaving group, which should allow the reaction to proceed through a cationic S_N1 mechanism. Furthermore, it is likely that the use of acetonitrile, a solvent with a high dielectronic constant, should help stabilize an intermediate oxocarbenium cation, further facilitating the S_N1 process. Finally, diene **73** was exposed to the Grubbs' second-generation catalyst to afford octacycle **74**. The stereogenic centers around the E-ring were established through an NOE experiment and a coupling constant analysis.

The final stage of the Kadota/Yamamoto synthesis basically followed that of the Sasaki synthesis. At this stage, the PGs for the A-ring hydroxy functionalities were suitably exchanged. The H-ring double bond was next introduced to ketone **75** using the Ito–Saegusa method (Ito et al., 1978), and the resultant enone was reacted with methylmagnesium iodide in toluene at −78°C (Feng and Murai, 1992) to provide tertiary alcohol **76**. After a two-stage PG manipulation, the derived alcohol **77** was transformed to (Z)-vinyl iodide **78** via stereoselective reduction of a diiodoolefin with Zn(Cu). Removal of the pivaloyl and silyl groups within **78** and then coupling with (Z)-vinyl stannane **12** by the action of Pd₂(dba)₃·CHCl₃, tri(2-furyl)phosphine and CuI (DMSO, 40°C) completed the total synthesis of gambierol (**6**).

31.2.4 Total Synthesis of Gambierol by the Rainier Group

In 2005, Rainier and colleagues reported the third total synthesis of gambierol, which relied on stereoselective alkylation of glycal epoxides and RCM of olefinic esters.

As outlined in Figure 31.16, the Rainier group has reported an efficient strategy for the stereoselective functionalization of endocyclic enol ethers (Allwein et al., 2002; Rainier and Allwein, 1998), which makes use of the chemistry of glycal epoxides (i.e., 1,2-anhydro sugars) (Evans et al., 1998; Halcomb and Danishefsky, 1989). Stereoselective epoxidation of endocyclic enol ether **XV** generates unstable glycal epoxide **XVI**, where the stereochemical outcome is controlled by the local structure of the starting material. A density functional theory analysis of the stereoselective epoxidation of endocyclic enol ethers with dimethyldioxirane (DMDO) has been described (Orendt et al., 2006). Addition of a nucleophile to **XVI** takes place via an S_N2 mechanism to afford alcohol **XVII**. Rainier and coworkers have found that

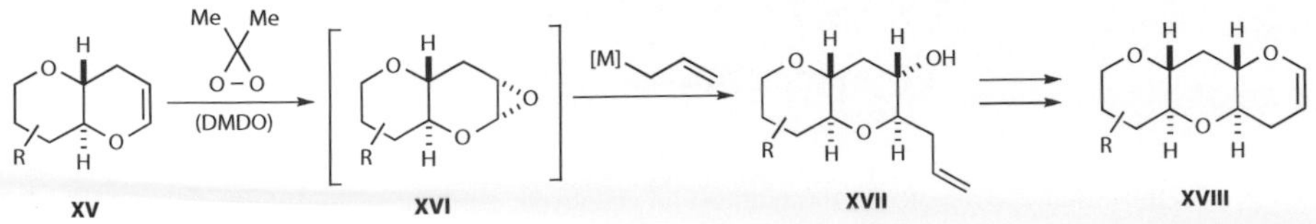

FIGURE 31.16 Synthesis of cyclic ethers via glycal epoxides.

both the nature of the nucleophile and the reaction temperature used in the addition step are important for selective β-C-glycosidation. Alcohol **XVII** in turn is elaborated to endocyclic enol ether **XVIII** by means of RCM or an acid-mediated annulation reaction. Iterative application of this "C-glycoside centered" strategy allows for the synthesis of polycyclic ethers in a linear fashion (Rainier et al., 2001).

Subsequently, Rainier and coworkers developed RCM of olefinic esters involving Takai–Utimoto-type titanium alkylidene complexes (Takai et al., 1994) for the construction of endocyclic enol ethers. Rainier's methodology is basically built upon the concept of a domino methylenation/RCM reaction of olefinic esters described by Nicolaou and coworkers (Nicolaou et al., 1996). An example is shown in Figure 31.17a. Ester **79** initially reacted with the Tebbe reagent at room temperature to give enol ether **80**. The formation of **80** was fully supported by its isolation and spectroscopic characterization. The olefin of **80** then reacted with a second molecule of the Tebbe reagent to generate metallacyclobutane **81**, which collapsed to deliver titanium alkylidene **82**. Finally, RCM of **82** afforded endocyclic enol ether **83**. Rainier et al. favored the use of the Takai–Utimoto reduced titanium alkylidenes because of their ease of preparation, their increased reactivity relative to the Petasis reagent, and their low Lewis acidic character relative to the Tebbe reagent. Importantly, Rainier found that while treatment of olefinic

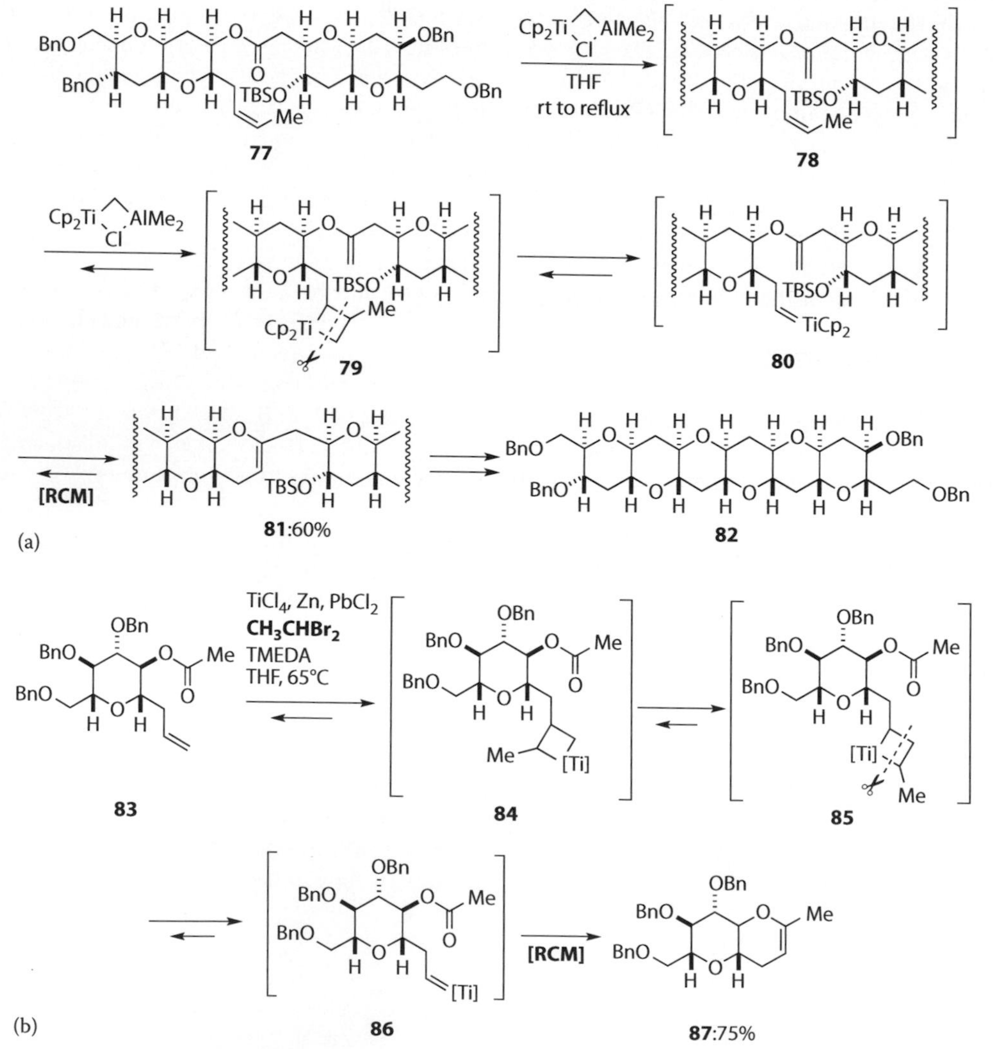

FIGURE 31.17 Olefinic ester cyclizations for the synthesis of endocyclic enol ethers. (a) Domino methylenation/RCM of olefinic esters by using the Tebbe reagent. (From Nicolaou, K.C. et al., *J. Am. Chem. Soc.*, 118, 1565, 1996.) (b) RCM of olefinic esters by using a reduced titanium ethylidene. (From Iyer, K. and Rainier, J.D., *J. Am. Chem. Soc.*, 129, 12604, 2007.)

esters with the Takai–Utimoto titanium *methylidene* gave acyclic enol ethers as the major product, the use of the Takai–Utimoto titanium *ethylidene* predominantly produced endocyclic enol ethers (Roberts and Rainier, 2007). An example is shown in Figure 31.17b. The RCM of olefinic esters proceeds via the intermediacy of titanium alkylidene complex **88**, whose formation is a prerequisite for the productive RCM pathway. It appears that the equilibrium between **86** and **87** shifts toward **87** when the titanium ethylidene was used in place of the titanium methylidene (Iyer and Rainier, 2007). The Rainier group has also demonstrated the RCM of olefinic amides and lactams by using a reduced titanium ethylidene (Zhou and Rainier, 2009).

Rainier et al. planned their synthesis of gambierol as illustrated in Figure 31.18. They envisioned that the polycyclic ether framework of gambierol could be derived from endocyclic enol ether **90**, which in turn could be obtained from olefinic ester **91** via RCM. Olefinic ester **91** could be derived from the ABC-ring carboxylic acid **92** and FGH-ring alcohol **93**.

The synthesis of **92** started with an asymmetric hetero-Diels–Alder cycloaddition of aldehyde **94** and enol silyl ether **95** by the action of the Jacobsen tridentate chromium(III) catalyst **96** (Dossetter et al., 1999) to provide dihydropyrone **97** in 90% yield with 94% ee (Figure 31.19). Luche reduction of **97** followed by protection of the derived alcohol gave MPM ether **98**. The unnatural C6 configuration was important for controlling the C7 and C8 stereogenic centers in subsequent transformations. The A-ring endocyclic enol ether **98** was functionalized through alkylation of a glycal epoxide. Stereoselective

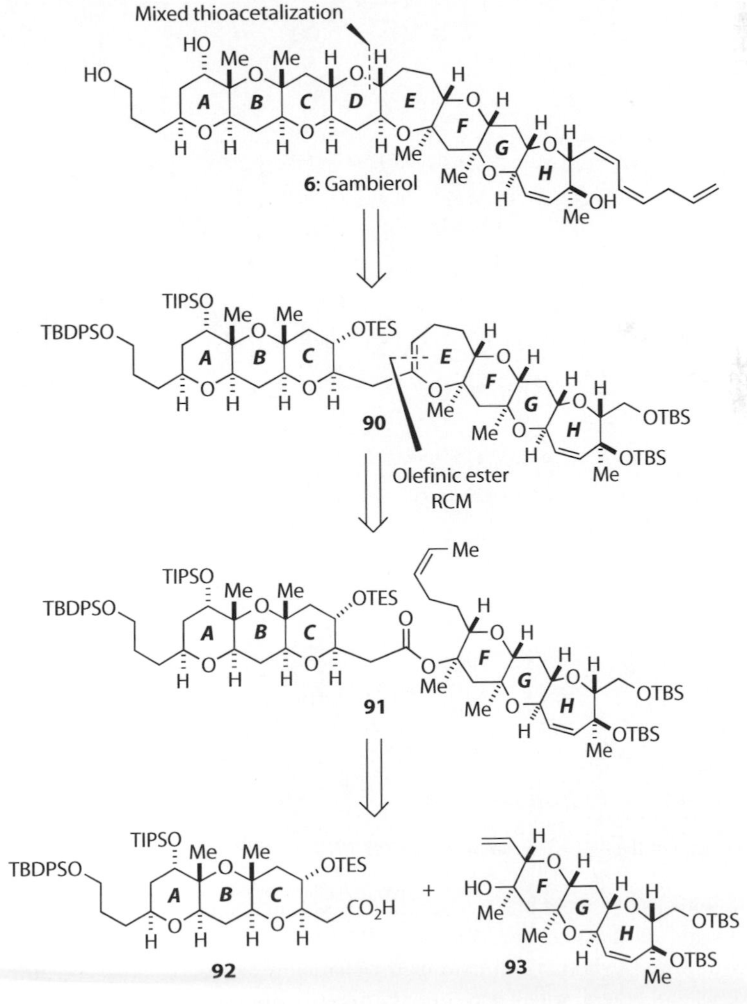

FIGURE 31.18 Synthesis plan toward gambierol (**6**) by the Rainier group.

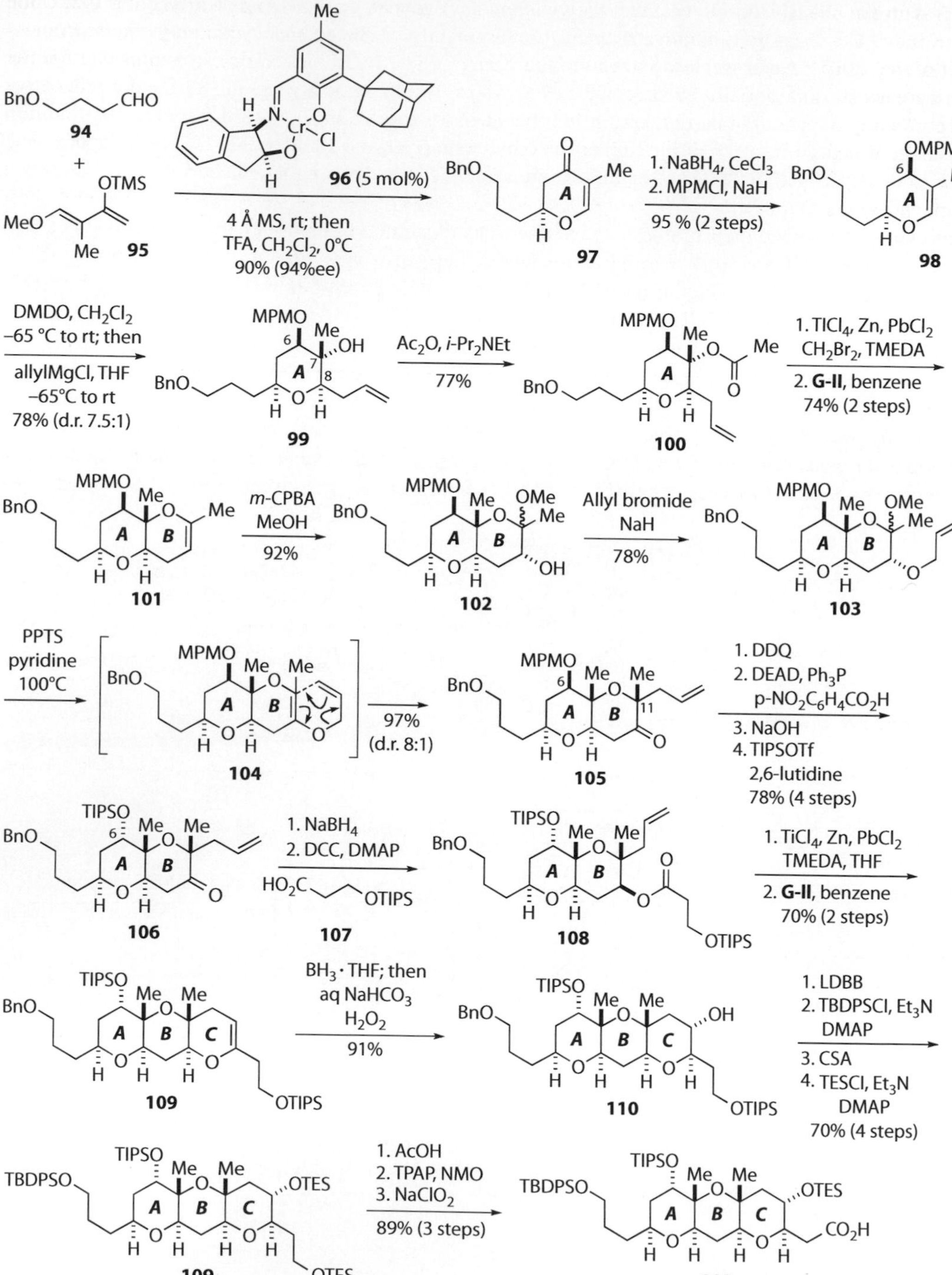

FIGURE 31.19 Synthesis of the ABC-ring carboxylic acid **92**.

epoxidation of **98** with DMDO and one-pot addition of allylmagnesium chloride afforded a 7.5:1 mixture of alcohol **99** and its diastereomer, 7,8-di-*epi*-**99** (structure not shown) in 78% combined yield. Acetylation of **99** followed by Takai–Utimoto methylenation of the derived acetate **100** gave a mixture of acyclic and cyclic enol ethers, which was directly treated with the **G-II** catalyst to cyclize the acyclic enol ether affording dihydropyran **101**. Exposure of **101** to *m*-CPBA in MeOH led to methyl acetal **102** as a mixture of diastereomers, which was allylated with allyl bromide/NaH to give allyl ether **103**. Upon treatment of **103** with PPTS in pyridine at 100°C, elimination of MeOH from **103** and in situ rearrangement of the resultant enol ether **104** occurred to afford an 8:1 mixture of ketone **105** and its C11 epimer (structure not shown) in 97% combined yield. At this stage, the configuration of the C6 stereogenic center was corrected to that of the natural product by means of Mitsunobu inversion (Mitsunobu, 1981), giving rise to ketone **106**. Stereoselective reduction of **106** followed by esterification with carboxylic acid **107** provided ester **108**. Takai–Utimoto methylenation of **108** and ensuing RCM afforded endocyclic enol ether **109** in 80% yield for the two steps. Stereoselective hydroboration of **109** followed by alkaline peroxide workup furnished alcohol **110**, which was elaborated to the ABC-ring carboxylic acid **92** in seven steps via standard chemistry.

The synthesis of the FGH-ring alcohol **93** is summarized in Figure 31.20. The starting material, D-glucal (**112**), was sequentially protected with di-*t*-butylsilylene and *t*-butyldiphenylsilyl (TBDPS) groups and then methylated at the C23 position with *t*-BuLi/MeI to give endocyclic enol ether **113**, which corresponds to the G-ring. Stereoselective epoxidation of **113** with DMDO followed by one-pot epoxide opening using 2-methallylmagnesium bromide delivered alcohol **114** in 92% yield (d.r. >95:5). Importantly, the bulky TBDPS ether played an important role in defining the C23 and C24 stereogenic centers. However, the bulkiness of the C25 TBDPS ether within **114** was found to be detrimental to the subsequent esterification of the C24 hydroxy group. Thus, the TBDPS ether was cleaved under basic conditions, and the resultant C25 hydroxy group was tentatively protected as its TMS ether before the C24 hydroxy group was esterified with carboxylic acid **115**. Subsequent desilylation under mild acidic conditions provided alcohol **116**. This alcohol was carefully converted to the corresponding xanthate under controlled conditions and then deoxygenated using *n*-Bu$_3$SnH/AIBN to afford ester **117**. Takai–Utimoto methylenation of **117** gave acyclic enol ether **118** in 83% yield, which underwent RCM in the presence of **G-II** (45 mol%) to furnish endocyclic enol ether **119** in 83% yield. Stereoselective epoxidation of **119** and in situ reductive opening of the derived epoxide with DIBALH afforded tertiary alcohol **121** in 93% yield. The latter process involves an intramolecular hydride delivery in the aluminum ate complex **120**. Tertiary alcohol **121** was converted to olefinic ester **123** in six steps by standard chemistry. This ester was exposed to the Takai–Utimoto methylenation conditions and then treated with the Schrock molybdenum catalyst (Schrock, 1999) to deliver endocyclic enol ether **124** in 62% yield for the two steps. Stereoselective DMDO epoxidation/DIBALH reduction of **124** provided alcohol **126** in a stereoselective manner, presumably via the intermediacy of the aluminum ate complex **125**. Installation of the H-ring double bond and C30 methyl group was performed in the same manner as that reported by the Sasaki group (Fuwa et al., 2002a,b). The resultant tertiary alcohol **127** was elaborated to the FGH-ring alcohol **93** in six standard steps.

Esterification of the ABC-ring carboxylic acid **92** and FGH-ring alcohol **93** provided olefinic ester **91** (Figure 31.21). Upon exposure of **91** to the Takai–Utimoto reduced ethylidene, endocyclic enol ether **90** was isolated in 60% yield along with acyclic enol ether **128** in 30% yield. Acyclic enol ether **128** could be transformed to endocyclic enol ether **90** in 65% yield by first effecting ethenolysis of the less hindered olefin followed by RCM of the in situ generated diene. Stereoselective DMDO epoxidation/DIBALH reduction of **90** and subsequent oxidation gave ketone **129** with 10:1 diastereoselectivity. The minor diastereomer was separated by flash chromatography on silica gel. The stereochemical outcome of the DMDO epoxidation was in line with that observed for **124**. Acidic removal of the silyl groups, mixed thioacetalization [EtSH, Zn(OTf)$_2$], and radical reduction of the resultant mixed thioacetal furnished octacycle **130**. The total synthesis of gambierol (**6**) was completed following the sequence developed by the Kadota/Yamamoto group (Kadota et al., 2003a,b). Thus, octacycle **130** was converted to (Z)-vinyl iodide **131** via oxidation, diiodoolefination, and stereoselective reduction with Zn(Cu). All the silyl groups were removed with SiF$_4$, and subsequent Stille coupling with (Z)-vinyl stannane **12** furnished gambierol (**6**).

31.2.5 Total Synthesis of Gambierol by the Mori Group

The Mori group has developed an iterative, linear strategy for the synthesis of polycyclic ethers by using alkylative coupling of oxiranyl anions, as shown in Figure 31.22 (Furuta et al., 2003; Mori et al., 1996). Thus, triflate **XX**, obtained from diol **XIX** by one-pot triflation/silylation, is alkylated with a

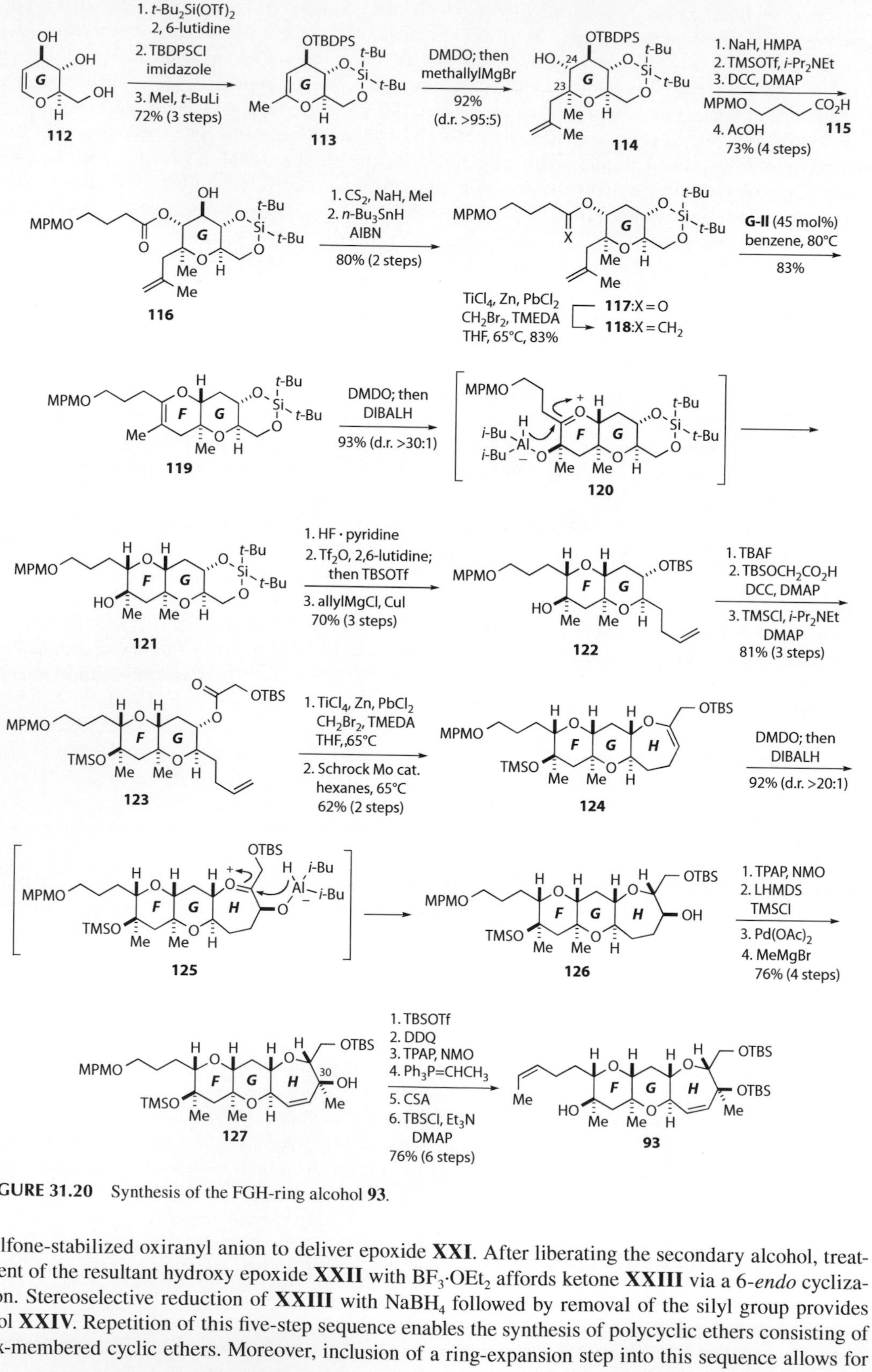

FIGURE 31.20   Synthesis of the FGH-ring alcohol **93**.

sulfone-stabilized oxiranyl anion to deliver epoxide **XXI**. After liberating the secondary alcohol, treatment of the resultant hydroxy epoxide **XXII** with BF₃·OEt₂ affords ketone **XXIII** via a 6-*endo* cyclization. Stereoselective reduction of **XXIII** with NaBH₄ followed by removal of the silyl group provides diol **XXIV**. Repetition of this five-step sequence enables the synthesis of polycyclic ethers consisting of six-membered cyclic ethers. Moreover, inclusion of a ring-expansion step into this sequence allows for

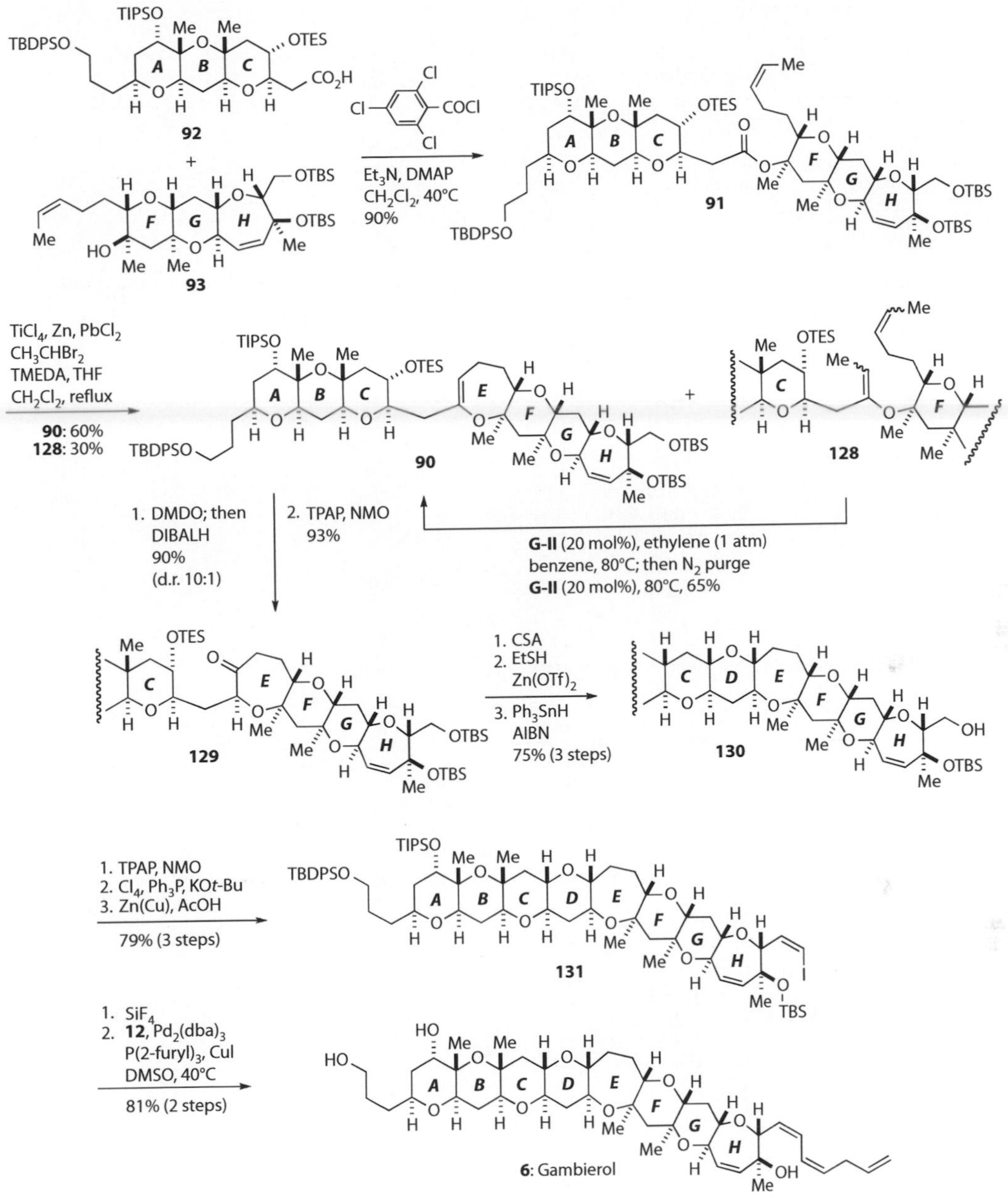

FIGURE 31.21 Completion of the total synthesis of gambierol (**6**) by the Rainier group.

the synthesis of polycyclic ethers incorporating seven-membered cyclic ethers. Thus, the ring expansion of ketone **XXIII** by the action of TMSCHN$_2$ and BF$_3$·OEt$_2$ (Maruoka et al., 1994; Mori et al., 1997a,b,c) gives, after acidic treatment, ketone **XXV**, which is desilylated and then stereoselectively reduced with Me$_4$NBH(OAc)$_3$ (Evans et al., 1988) to afford diol **XXVI**. The feasibility of the oxiranyl anion strategy has been demonstrated by a formal synthesis of hemibrevetoxin B (Mori et al., 1997a,b). Very recently, the Mori group has successfully applied the oxiranyl anion chemistry to a convergent synthesis of polycyclic ethers (Sakai et al., 2011).

In contrast to the previous syntheses, the Mori group has designed their synthesis of gambierol (**6**) in a completely linear manner (Figure 31.23). They planned to construct the octacyclic polyether skeleton in the following order: ABCD → ABCDE → ABCDEF → ABCDEFG → ABCDEFGH. The E-, G-, and

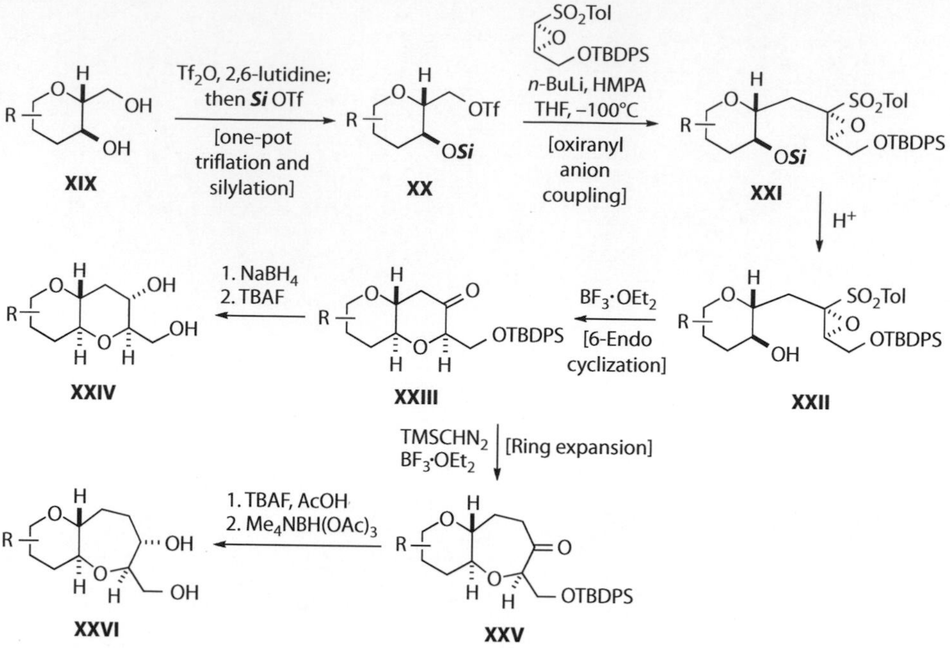

FIGURE 31.22 Iterative synthesis of polycyclic ethers by using oxiranyl anions.

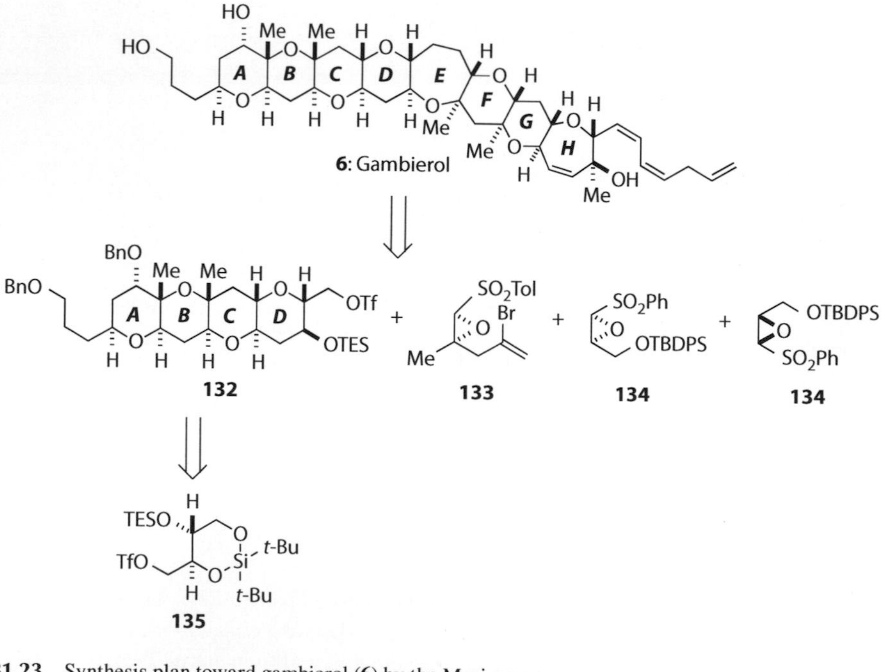

FIGURE 31.23 Synthesis plan toward gambierol (**6**) by the Mori group.

H-rings were to be forged by exploiting the oxiranyl anion chemistry. The ABCD-ring fragment **132** was in turn traced to the known triflate **135** (Mori and Hayashi, 2001) by considering well-established methodologies, including the SmI$_2$-induced reductive cyclization (Hori et al., 1999a,b, 2002; Nakata, 2010) and 6-*endo* vinyl epoxide cyclization (Nicolaou et al., 1989b).

The synthesis of the ABCD-ring triflate **132** commenced by the alkylation of triflate **135** with an oxiranyl anion generated by the lithiation of racemic sulfone **136**. Subsequent removal of the TES group

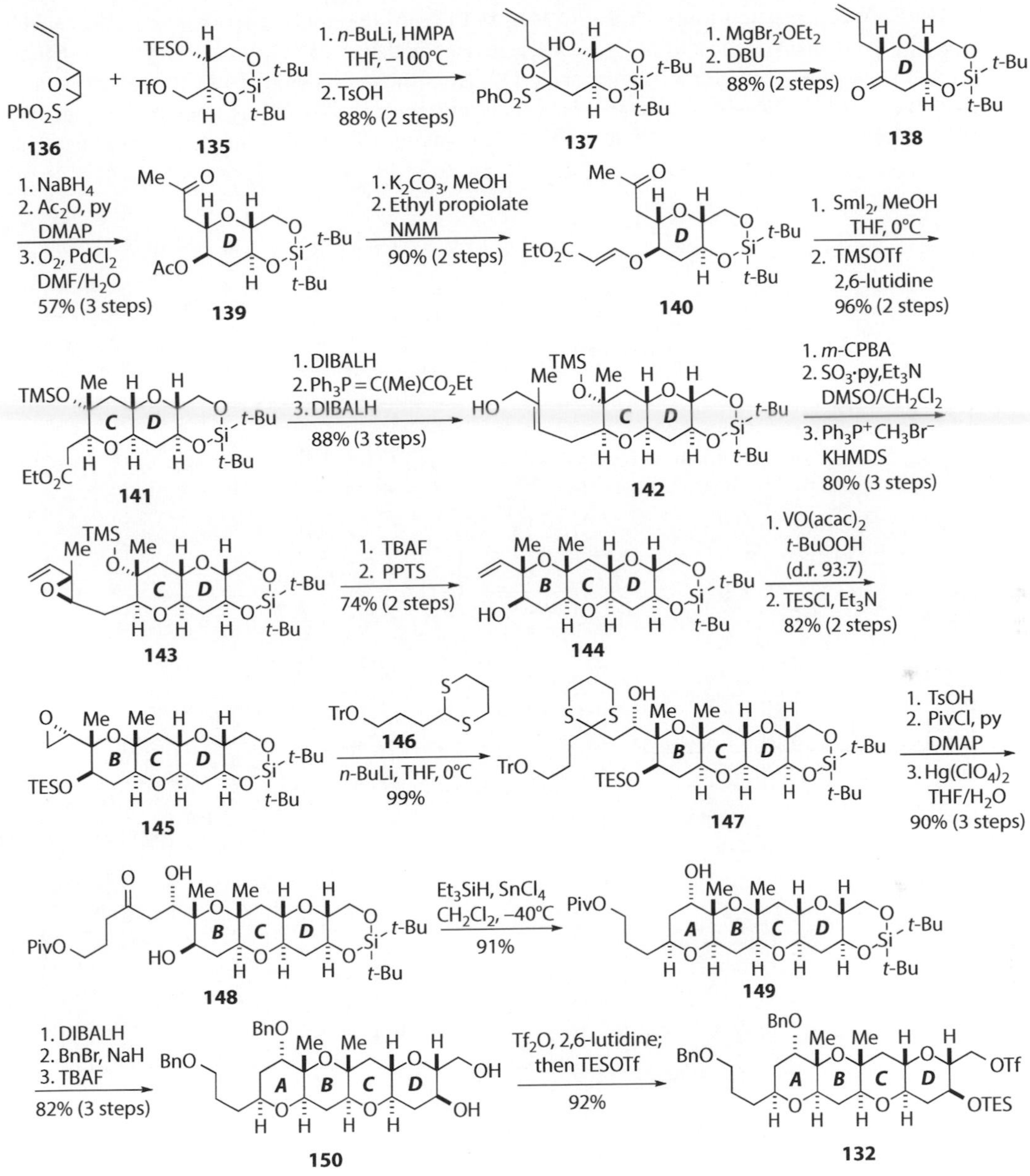

FIGURE 31.24 Synthesis of the ABCD-ring **132**.

under acidic conditions gave alcohol **137** as a mixture of diastereomers (Figure 31.24). Exposure of **137** to MgBr$_2$·OEt$_2$ and cyclization of the resultant diastereomeric α-bromo ketones using 1,8-diazabicyclo[5.4.0]undec-7-ene (DBU) provided ketone **138** as a single stereoisomer (Mori et al., 1999). The use of racemic sulfone **136** for alkylation of **135** was of no consequence, because the DBU-mediated cyclization conditions also promoted epimerization of the undesired 13-*epi*-**138** (structure not shown) to **138**. Stereoselective reduction of **138** with NaBH$_4$, acetylation of the derived alcohol, and Wacker oxidation of the terminal olefin afforded methyl ketone **139**, which corresponds to the D-ring. Next, the C-ring was efficiently forged by means of the SmI$_2$-induced reductive cyclization. The β-alkoxy acrylate **140**, obtained from **139** by transesterification and hetero-Michael addition, was treated with SmI$_2$ (MeOH, THF, 0°C) to deliver, after silylation (TMSOTf, 2,6-lutidine), the CD-ring ester **141** in 96% yield. The B-ring was then constructed using the vinyl epoxide cyclization methodology. Half reduction of **141** with DIBALH, Wittig reaction using $Ph_3P = C(Me)CO_2Et$, and subsequent DIBALH reduction of the derived ester provided allylic alcohol **142**. Stereoselective epoxidation of **142** with *m*-CPBA, oxidation, and Wittig methylenation gave rise to vinyl epoxide **143**. After the desilylation of **143**, the resultant alcohol was exposed to PPTS to afford alcohol **144**, which represents the BCD-ring domain. To complete the construction of the ABCD-ring fragment **132**, the A-ring was formed via reductive etherification.

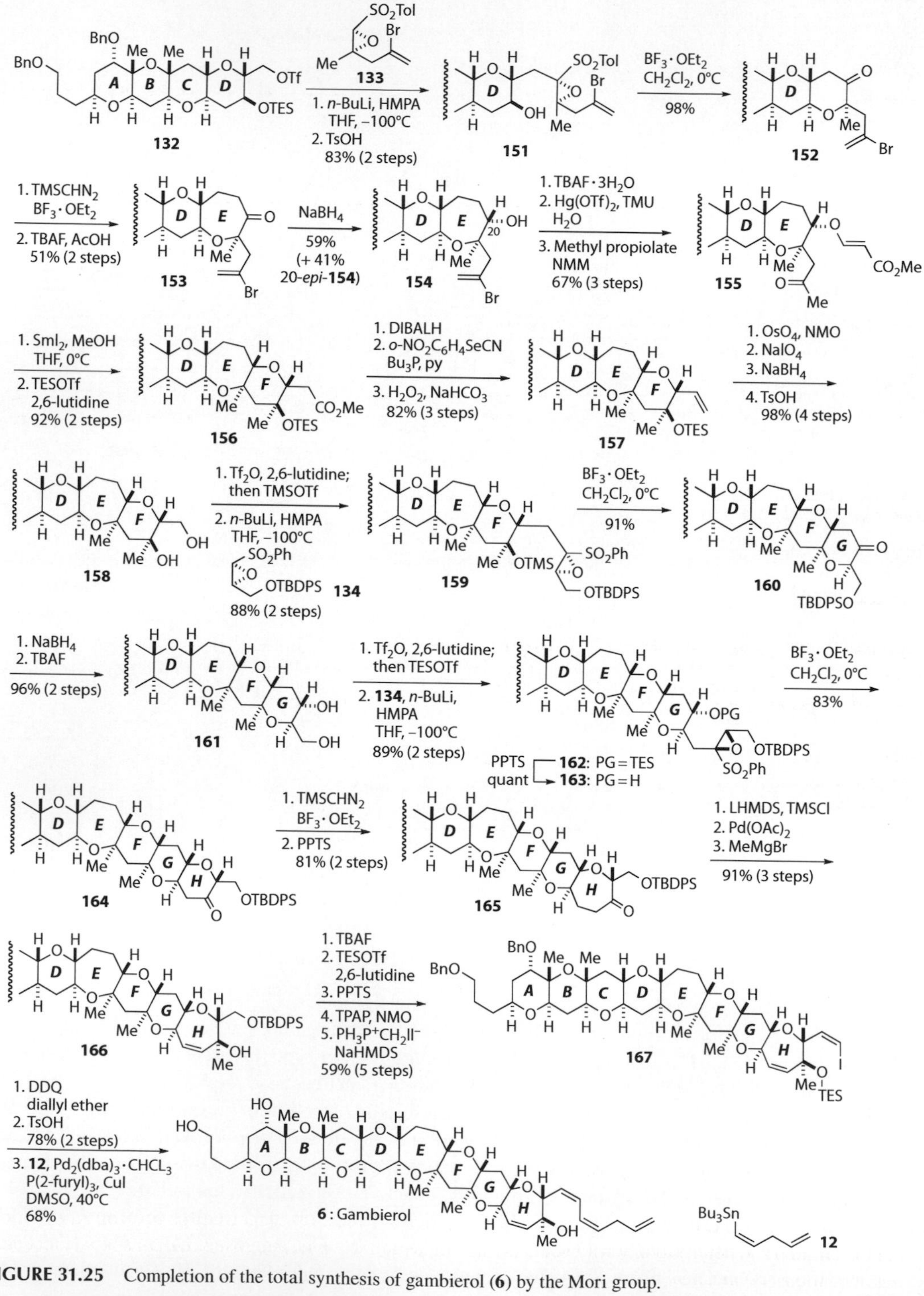

FIGURE 31.25 Completion of the total synthesis of gambierol (**6**) by the Mori group.

VO(acac)$_2$-catalyzed epoxidation of **144** followed by silylation led to **145**, which was alkylated with the 2-lithio-1,3-dithiane derivative generated from **146** to deliver alcohol **147**. Subsequent routine PG manipulations gave rise to dihydroxy ketone **148**, which was reduced with Et$_3$SiH/SnCl$_4$ to furnish alcohol **149** in 91% yield. This alcohol was transformed into diol **150** via removal of the pivaloyl group, benzylation, and desilylation. Sequential triflation/silylation of **150** then afforded the ABCD-ring triflate **132**.

Construction of the EFGH-ring domain and completion of the total synthesis are depicted in Figure 31.25. The ABCD-ring triflate **132** was alkylated with an oxiranyl anion generated from **133** to give, after cleaving the silyl group, epoxide **151**. Treatment of **151** with BF$_3$·OEt$_2$ delivered ketone **152** via a 6-*endo* cyclization. Ring expansion of **152** using TMSCHN$_2$/BF$_3$·OEt$_2$, followed by desilylation of the derived α-TMS ketone, afforded ketone **153**. Reduction of **153** with NaBH$_4$ to give alcohol **154** proceeded with a low diastereoselectivity (d.r. 59:41). However, the mixture could be separated, and the undesired diastereomer, 20-*epi*-**154** (structure not shown), was recycled to ketone **153** via oxidation. Dehydrobromination of **154** (*n*-Bu$_4$NF·3H$_2$O, DMF, 60°C), oxymercuration (Nishizawa et al., 2002) of the resultant alkyne, and introduction of a β-alkoxyacrylate moiety delivered methyl ketone **155**. SmI$_2$-induced reductive cyclization of **155** followed by silylation of the derived alcohol provided ester **156**. This ester was reduced with DIBALH to give the corresponding alcohol, which was dehydrated by a two-step sequence involving selenylation and oxidative elimination of a selenide to afford olefin **157**. The terminal olefin within **157** was oxidatively cleaved and then reduced with NaBH$_4$ to provide, after desilylation, diol **158**. Sequential triflation/silylation of **158** followed by coupling with an oxiranyl anion derived from **134** afforded epoxide **159** in 88% yield (two steps). Direct cyclization of **159** upon treatment with BF$_3$·OEt$_2$ led to ketone **160** in 91% yield. Reduction of **160** with NaBH$_4$ and ensuing desilylation provided diol **161**. One-pot triflation/silylation of **161** followed by alkylation with a sulfonyl-stabilized oxiranyl anion generated from **134** gave epoxide **162** in 89% yield (two steps). Removal of the silyl group of **162** under mild acidic conditions and subsequent cyclization of epoxy alcohol **163** (BF$_3$·OEt$_2$, CH$_2$Cl$_2$, 0°C to room temperature) gave rise to ketone **164**. Treatment of **164** with TMSCHN$_2$/BF$_3$·OEt$_2$ successfully delivered ring-expanded ketone **165**. The H-ring was then functionalized following the Sasaki precedent (Fuwa et al., 2002a,b). Thus, Ito–Saegusa oxidation and stereoselective methylation (Feng and Murai, 1992) afforded tertiary alcohol **166**. A three-step sequence of PG manipulations was required for masking the C30 alcohol and liberating the C32 alcohol. The resultant alcohol was oxidized and then reacted with Stork's ylide [Ph$_3$PCH$_2$I]$^+$I$^-$/NaHMDS (Stork and Zhao, 1989) to provide (Z)-vinyl iodide **167**. The benzyl and triethylsilyl groups were sequentially removed, and finally, Stille coupling with (Z)-vinyl stannane **12** under the conditions established by the Kadota/Yamamoto group (Kadota et al., 2003a,b) completed the fourth total synthesis of gambierol (**6**).

31.3 Summary and Outlook

As recently as the 1990s, it was a formidable challenge for organic chemists to synthesize marine polycyclic ether natural products with anomalous structural complexity. To overcome these challenges, organic chemists have devoted their efforts to the development of new and efficient methodologies for the stereoselective synthesis of cyclic ethers and enabled the assembly of architecturally complex polycyclic ether derivatives. As described in this chapter, the first decade of the twenty-first century has witnessed four total syntheses of gambierol, each featuring unique synthetic methodologies for the construction of the polycyclic ether skeleton. Supported by chemical synthesis as a reliable source of material supply, it is becoming possible to extensively investigate the biological mode of actions of marine polycyclic ether natural products. The future challenge for organic chemists will be the synthesis of new designer biofunctional molecules inspired by such complex natural products.

REFERENCES

Allwein SP, Cox JM, Howard BE, Johnson HWB, and Rainier JD (2002) *C*-Glycosides to fused polycyclic ethers. *Tetrahedron* **58**: 1997–2009.

Alonso E, Fuwa H, Vale C et al. (2012) Design and synthesis of skeletal analogues of gambierol: Attenuation of amyloid β and tau pathology with voltage-gated potassium channel and *N*-methyl-D-aspartate receptor implications. *J Am Chem Soc* **134**: 7467–7479.

Alonso E, Vale C, Sasaki M et al. (2010) Calcium oscillations induced by gambierol in cerebellar granule cells. *J Cell Biochem* **110**: 497–508.

Crimmins MT, Ellis JM, Emmitte KA et al. (2009a) Enantioselective total synthesis of brevetoxin A: Unified strategy for the B, E, G, and J subunits. *Chem Eur J* **15**: 9223–9234.

Crimmins MT, Zuccarello JL, Ellis JM et al. (2009b) Total synthesis of brevetoxin A. *Org Lett* **11**: 489–492.

Crimmins MT, Zuccarello JL, McDougall PJ, and Ellis JM (2009c) Enantioselective total synthesis of brevetoxin A: Convergent coupling strategy and completion. *Chem Eur J* **15**: 9235–9244.

Dahanukar VH and Rychnovsky SD (1996) General synthesis of α-acetoxy ethers from esters by DIBALH reduction and acetylation. *J Org Chem* **61**: 8317–8320.

Dossetter AG, Jamison TF, and Jacobsen EN (1999) Highly enantio- and diastereoselective hetero-Diels–Alder reactions catalyzed by new chiral tridentate chromium(III) catalysts. *Angew Chem Int Ed* **38**: 2398–2400.

Ebine M, Fuwa H, and Sasaki M (2008) Total synthesis of (–)-brevenal: A concise synthetic entry to the pentacyclic core. *Org Lett* **10**: 2211–2214.

Ebine M, Fuwa H, and Sasaki M (2011) Total synthesis of (–)-brevenal: A streamlined strategy for practical synthesis of polycyclic ethers. *Chem Eur J* **17**: 13754–13761.

Evans DA, Chapman KT, and Carreira EM (1988) Directed reduction of β-hydroxy ketones employing tetramethylammonium triacetoxyborohydride. *J Am Chem Soc* **110**: 3560–3578.

Evans DA, Trotter BW, and Côté B (1998) Addition of allylstannanes to glycal epoxides. A diastereoselective approach to β-C-glycosidation. *Tetrahedron Lett* **39**: 1709–1712.

Feng F and Murai A (1992) Synthesis of the C- and D-ring system of hemibrevetoxin-B. *Chem Lett* 1587–1590.

Finan JM and Kishi Y (1982) Reductive ring openings of allyl-alcohol epoxides. *Tetrahedron Lett* **23**: 2719–2722.

Furuta H, Hasegawa Y, Hase M, and Mori Y (2010) Total synthesis of gambierol by using oxiranyl anions. *Chem Eur J* **16**: 7586–7595.

Furuta H, Hasegawa Y, and Mori Y (2009) Total synthesis of gambierol. *Org Lett* **11**: 4382–4385.

Furuta H, Takase T, Hayashi H, Noyori R, and Mori Y (2003) Synthesis of trans-fused polycyclic ethers with angular methyl groups using sulfonyl-stabilized oxiranyl anions. *Tetrahedron* **59**: 9767–9777.

Fuwa H (2011) Palladium-catalyzed synthesis of N- and O-heterocycles starting from enol phosphates. *Synlett* 6–29.

Fuwa H, Ebine M, Bourdelais AJ, Baden DG, and Sasaki M (2006b) Total synthesis, structure revision, and absolute configuration of (–)-brevenal. *J Am Chem Soc* **128**: 16989–16999.

Fuwa H, Ebine M, and Sasaki M (2006a) Total synthesis of the proposed structure of brevenal. *J Am Chem Soc* **128**: 9648–9650.

Fuwa H, Ishigai K, Hashizume K, and Sasaki M (2012) Total synthesis and complete stereostructure of gambieric acid A. *J Am Chem Soc* **134**: 11984–11987.

Fuwa H, Kainuma N, Satake M, and Sasaki M (2003) Synthesis and biological evaluation of gambierol analogues. *Bioorg Med Chem Lett* **13**: 2519–2522.

Fuwa H, Kainuma N, Tachibana K, and Sasaki M (2002b) Total synthesis of (–)-gambierol. *J Am Chem Soc* **124**: 14983–14992.

Fuwa H, Kainuma N, Tachibana K, Tsukano C, Satake M, and Sasaki M (2004) Diverted total synthesis and biological evaluation of gambierol analogues: Elucidation of critical structural elements for potent toxicity. *Chem Eur J* **10**: 4894–4909.

Fuwa H, Sasaki M, Satake M, and Tachibana K (2002a) Total synthesis of gambierol. *Org Lett* **4**: 2981–2984.

Fuwa H, Sasaki M, and Tachibana K (2001) Synthetic studies on a marine polyether toxin, gambierol: Stereoselective synthesis of the EFGH ring system via B-alkyl Suzuki coupling. *Tetrahedron* **57**: 3019–3033.

Gao Y, Hanson RM, Klunder JM, Ko SY, Masamune H, and Sharpless KB (1987) Catalytic asymmetric epoxidation and kinetic resolution: Modified procedures including in situ derivatization. *J Am Chem Soc* **109**: 5765–5780.

Ghiaroni V, Fuwa H, Inoue M et al. (2006) Effect of ciguatoxin 3C on voltage-gated Na+ and K+ currents in mouse taste cells. *Chem Senses* **31**: 673–680.

Ghiaroni V, Sasaki M, Fuwa H et al. (2005) Inhibition of voltage-gated potassium currents by gambierol in mouse taste cells. *Toxicol Sci* **85**: 657–665.

Gradillas A and Pérez-Castells J (2006) Macrocyclization by ring-closing metathesis in the total synthesis of natural products: Reaction conditions and limitations. *Angew Chem Int Ed* **45**: 6086–6101.

Grieco PA, Gilman S, and Nishizawa M (1976) Organoselenium chemistry. A facile one-step synthesis of alkyl aryl selenides from alcohols. *J Org Chem* **41**: 1485–1486.

Halcomb RL and Danishefsky SJ (1989) On the direct epoxidation of glycals: Application of a reiterative strategy for the synthesis of β-linked oligosaccharides. *J Am Chem Soc* **111**: 6661–6666.

Han X, Stolz BM, and Corey EJ (1999) Cuprous chloride accelerated Stille reactions. A general and effective coupling system for sterically congested substrates and for enantioselective synthesis. *J Am Chem Soc* **121**: 7600–7605.

Hirama M, Oishi T, Uehara H et al. (2001) Total synthesis of ciguatoxin CTX3C. *Science* **294**: 1904–1907.

Hori N, Matsukura H, Matsuo G, and Nakata T (1999a) An efficient strategy for the iterative synthesis of polytetrahydropyran ring system via SmI$_2$-induced reductive intramolecular cyclization. *Tetrahedron Lett* **40**: 2811–2814.

Hori N, Matsukura H, Matsuo G, and Nakata T (2002) Efficient strategy for the iterative synthesis of *trans*-fused polycyclic ether via SmI$_2$-induced reductive intramolecular cyclization. *Tetrahedron* **58**: 1853–1864.

Hori N, Matsukura H, and Nakata T (1999b) Efficient synthesis of *trans*-fused polycyclic ethers including tetrahydropyrans and oxepanes based on SmI$_2$-induced reductive cyclization. *Org Lett* **1**: 1099–1101.

Hoveyda AH and Zhugralin AR (2007) The remarkable metal-catalysed olefin metathesis reaction. *Nature* **450**: 243–251.

Inanaga J, Hirata K, Saeki H, Katsuki T, and Yamaguchi M (1979) A rapid esterification by means of mixed anhydride and its application to large-ring lactonization. *Bull Chem Soc Jpn* **52**: 1989–1993.

Inoue M (2005) Convergent strategies for syntheses of *trans*-fused polycyclic ethers. *Chem Rev* **105**: 4379–4405.

Inoue M, Lee N, Miyazaki K, Usuki T, Matsuoka S, and Hirama M (2008) Critical importance of the nine-membered F ring of ciguatoxin for potent bioactivity: Total synthesis and biological evaluation of F-ring-modified analogues. *Angew Chem Int Ed* **47**: 8611–8614.

Inoue M, Miyazaki K, Ishihara Y et al. (2006) Total synthesis of ciguatoxin and 51-hydroxyCTX3C. *J Am Chem Soc* **128**: 9352–9354.

Ito Y, Hirao T, and Saegusa T (1978) Synthesis of α,β-unsaturated carbonyl compounds by palladium(II)-catalyzed dehydrosilylation of silyl enol ethers. *J Org Chem* **43**: 1011–1013.

Iyer K and Rainier JD (2007) Olefinic ester and diene ring-closing metathesis using a reduced titanium alkylidene. *J Am Chem Soc* **129**: 12604–12605.

Johnson HWB, Majumder U, and Rainier JD (2005) The total synthesis of gambierol. *J Am Chem Soc* **127**: 848–849.

Johnson HWB, Majumder U, and Rainier JD (2006) Total synthesis of gambierol: Subunit coupling and completion. *Chem Eur J* **12**: 1747–1753.

Kadota I, Kawada M, Gevorgyan V, and Yamamoto Y (1997) Intramolecular reaction of (γ-alkoxyallyl)stannane with aldehyde: Origin of the stereoselectivities. *J Org Chem* **62**: 7439–7446.

Kadota I, Sakaihara T, and Yamamoto Y (1996) A general and efficient method for the preparation of γ-alkoxyallylstannanes via an acetal cleavage. *Tetrahedron Lett* **37**: 3195–3198.

Kadota I, Takamura H, Nishii H, and Yamamoto Y (2005) Total synthesis of brevetoxin B. *J Am Chem Soc* **127**: 9246–9250.

Kadota I, Takamura H, Sato K et al. (2003b) Convergent total syntheses of gambierol and 16-*epi*-gambierol and their biological activities. *J Am Chem Soc* **125**: 11893–11899.

Kadota I, Takamura H, Sato K, Ohno A, Matsuda K, and Yamamoto Y (2003a) Total synthesis of gambierol. *J Am Chem Soc* **125**: 46–47.

Kopecky DJ and Rychnovsky SD (2000) Improved procedure for the reductive acetylation of acyclic esters and a new synthesis of ethers. *J Org Chem* **65**: 191–198.

Kopljar I, Labro AJ, Cuypers E et al. (2009) A polyether biotoxin binding site on the lipid-exposed face of the pore domain of Kv channels revealed by the marine toxin gambierol. *Proc Natl Acad Sci USA* **106**: 9896–9901.

Ley SV, Norman J, Griffith WP, and Marsden SP (1994) Tetrapropylammonium perruthenate, Pr$_4$N$^+$RuO$_4^-$: A catalytic oxidant for organic synthesis. *Synthesis*: 639–666.

Lin YY, Risk M, Ray SM et al. (1981) Isolation and structure of brevetoxin B from the "red tide" dinoflagellate *Ptychodiscus brevis* (*Gymnodinium breve*). *J Am Chem Soc* **103**: 6773–6775.

Louzao MC, Cagide E, Vieytes MR et al. (2006) Sodium channel of human excitable cells is a target for gambierol. *Cell Physiol Biochem* **17**: 257–268.

Majumder U, Cox JM, Johnson HWB, and Rainier JD (2006) Total synthesis of gambierol: The generation of the A–C and F–H subunits by using a *C*-glycoside centered strategy. *Chem Eur J* **12**: 1736–1746.

Maruoka K, Concepcion AB, and Yamamoto H (1994) Organoaluminum-promoted homologation of ketones with diazoalkanes. *J Org Chem* **59**: 4725–4726.

Matsukawa Y, Asao N, Kitahara H, and Yamamoto Y (1999) Lewis acid catalyzed allylstannylation of unactivated alkynes. *Tetrahedron* **55**: 3779–3790.

Matsuo G, Kawamura K, Hori N, Matsukura H, and Nakata T (2004) Total synthesis of brevetoxin-B. *J Am Chem Soc* **126**: 14374–14376.

Mitsunobu O (1981) The use of diethyl azodicarboxylate and triphenylphosphine in synthesis and transformation of natural products. *Synthesis* 1–28.

Miyaura N and Suzuki A (1995) Palladium-catalyzed cross-coupling reactions of organoboron compounds. *Chem Rev* **95**: 2457–2483.

Mori Y (2010) Total synthesis of gambierol. *Heterocycles* **81**: 2203–2228.

Mori Y and Hayashi H (2001) Practical synthesis of 1,3-*O*-di-*tert*-butylsilylene-protected D- and L-erythritols as a four-carbon chiral building block. *J Org Chem* **66**: 8666–8668.

Mori Y, Yaegashi K, and Furukawa H (1996) A new strategy for the reiterative synthesis of *trans*-fused tetrahydropyrans via alkylation of oxiranyl anion and 6-*endo* cyclization. *J Am Chem Soc* **118**: 8158–8159.

Mori Y, Yaegashi K, and Furukawa H (1997a) Oxiranyl anions in organic synthesis: Application to the synthesis of hemibrevetoxin B. *J Am Chem Soc* **119**: 4557–4558.

Mori Y, Yaegashi K, and Furukawa H (1997b) Formal total synthesis of hemibrevetoxin B by an oxiranyl anion strategy. *J Org Chem* **63**: 6200–6209.

Mori Y, Yaegashi K, and Furukawa H (1997c) Stereoselective synthesis of the 6,7,6- and 6,7,7-ring systems of polycyclic ethers by 6-*endo* cyclization and ring expansion. *Tetrahedron* **53**: 12917–12932.

Mori Y, Yaegashi K, and Furukawa H (1999) Synthesis of trans-fused tetrahydropyrans via intramolecular cyclization of α-bromo-γ'-hydroxy ketones. *Tetrahedron Lett* **40**: 7239–7242.

Morohashi A, Satake M, and Yasumoto T (1998) The absolute configuration of gambierol, a toxic marine polyether from the dinoflagellate, *Gambierdiscus toxicus. Tetrahedron Lett.* **39**: 97–100.

Murata M and Yasumoto T (2000) The structure elucidation and biological activities of high molecular weight algal toxins: maitotoxin, prymnesins and zooxanthellatoxins. *Nat Prod Rep* **17**: 293–314.

Nakanishi K (1985) The chemistry of brevetoxins: a review. *Toxicon* **23**: 473–479.

Nakata T (2005) Total synthesis of marine polycyclic ethers. *Chem Rev* **105**: 4314–4347.

Nakata T (2010) SmI$_2$-induced reductive cyclizations for the synthesis of cyclic ethers and applications in natural product synthesis. *Chem Soc Rev* **39**: 1955–1972.

Nicolaou KC, Bulger PG, and Sarlah D (2005) Metathesis reactions in total synthesis. *Angew Chem Int Ed* **44**:4490–4527.

Nicolaou KC, Bunnage ME, McGarry DG et al. (1999a) Total synthesis of brevetoxin A: Part 1: First generation strategy and construction of BCD ring system. *Chem Eur J* **5**: 599–617.

Nicolaou KC, Frederick MO, and Aversa RJ (2008) The continuing saga of the marine polyether biotoxins. *Angew Chem Int Ed* **47**: 7182–7225.

Nicolaou KC, Gunzner JL, Shi GQ, Agrios KA, Gärtner P, and Yang Z (1999d) Total synthesis of brevetoxin A: Part 4: Final stages and completion. *Chem Eur J* **5**: 646–658.

Nicolaou KC, Hwang CK, Duggan ME et al. (1995a) Total synthesis of brevetoxin B. 1. First generation strategies and new approaches to oxepane systems. *J Am Chem Soc* **117**: 10227–10238.

Nicolaou KC, Nugiel DA, Couladouros E, and Hwang C-K (1990) Stereocontrolled second generation syntheses of the ABC and FG ring systems of brevetoxin B. *Tetrahedron* **46**: 4517–4552.

Nicolaou KC, Postema MHD, and Claiborne CF (1996) Olefin metathesis in cyclic ether formation. Direct conversion of olefinic esters to cyclic enol ethers with Tebbe-type reagents. *J Am Chem Soc* **118**: 1565–1566.

Nicolaou KC, Prasad CVC, Hwang CK, Duggan ME, and Veale CA (1989a) Cyclizations of hydroxy dithioketals. New synthetic technology for the construction of oxocenes and related medium-ring systems. *J Am Chem Soc* **111**: 5321–5330.

Nicolaou KC, Prasad CVC, Somers PK, and Hwang CK (1989b) Activation of 6-*endo* over 5-*exo* hydroxy epoxide openings. Stereoselective and ring selective synthesis of tetrahydrofuran and tetrahydropyran systems. *J Am Chem Soc* **111**: 5330–5334.

Nicolaou KC, Rutjes FPJT, Theodrakis EA, Tiebes J, Sato M, and Untersteller E (1995c) Total synthesis of brevetoxin B. 3. Final strategy and completion. *J Am Chem Soc* **117**: 10252–10263.

Nicolaou KC, Shi GQ, Gunzner JL et al. (1999c) Total synthesis of brevetoxin A: Part 3: Construction of GHIJ and BCDE ring systems. *Chem Eur J* **5**: 628–645.

Nicolaou KC, Shi GQ, Gunzner JL, Gärtner P, and Yang Z (1997) Palladium-catalyzed functionalization of lactones via their cyclic ketene acetal phosphates. Efficient new synthetic technology for the construction of medium and large cyclic ethers. *J Am Chem Soc* **119**: 5467–5468.

Nicolaou KC, Theodrakis EA, Rutjes FPJT et al. (1995b) Total synthesis of brevetoxin B. 2. Second generation strategies and construction of the dioxepane region [DEFG]. *J Am Chem Soc* **117**: 10239–10251.

Nicolaou KC, Wallace PA, Shi S et al. (1999b) Total synthesis of brevetoxin A: Part 2: Second generation strategy and construction of EFGH model system. *Chem Eur J* **5**: 618–627.

Nicolaou KC, Yang Z, Shi GQ, Gunzner JL, Agrios KA, and Gärtner P (1998) Total synthesis of brevetoxin A. *Nature* **392**: 264–269.

Nishizawa M, Skwarczynski M, Imagawa H, and Sugihara T (2002) Mercuric triflate-TMU catalyzed hydration of terminal alkyne to give methyl ketone under mild conditions. *Chem Lett* 12–13.

Njardarson JT, Gaul C, Shan D, Huang X-Y, and Danishefsky SJ (2004) Discovery of potent cell migration inhibitors through total synthesis: Lessons from structure–activity studies of (+)-migrastatin. *J Am Chem Soc* **126**: 1038–1040.

Oguri H, Tanabe S, Oomura A, Umetsu M, and Hirama M (2006) Synthesis and evaluation of α-helix mimetics based on a *trans*-fused polycyclic ether: Sequence selective binding to aspartate pairs in α-helical peptides. *Tetrahedron Lett* **47**: 5801–5805.

Oishi T, Konoki K, Tamate R et al. (2012) Artificial ladder-shaped polyethers that inhibit maitotoxin-induced Ca^{2+} influx in rat glioma C6 cells. *Bioorg Med Chem Lett* **22**: 3619–3622.

Orendt AM, Roberts SW, and Rainier JD (2006) The role of asynchronous bond formation in the diastereoselective epoxidation of cyclic enol ethers: A density functional theory study. *J Org Chem* **71**: 5565–5573.

Rainier JD and Allwein SP (1998) An iterative approach to fused ether ring systems. *J Org Chem* **63**: 5310–5311.

Rainier JD, Allwein SP, and Cox JM (2001) *C*-Glycosides to fused polycyclic ethers. A formal synthesis of (±)-hemibrevetoxin B. *J Org Chem* **66**: 1380–1386.

Roberts SW and Rainer JD (2007) Synthesis of an A–E gambieric acid subunit with use of a *C*-glycoside centered strategy. *Org Lett* **9**: 2227–2230.

Sakai T, Sugimoto A, and Mori Y (2011) A convergent strategy for the synthesis of polycyclic ethers by using oxiranyl anions. *Org Lett* **13**: 5850–5853.

Sakamoto Y, Matsuo G, Matsukura H, and Nakata T (2001) Stereoselective syntheses of the C'D'E'F'-ring system of maitotoxin and FG-ring system of gambierol. *Org Lett* **3**: 2749–2752.

Sasaki M and Fuwa H (2008) Convergent strategies for the total synthesis of polycyclic ether marine metabolites. *Nat Prod Rep* **25**: 401–426.

Satake M, Murata M, and Yasumoto T (1993) Gambierol: A new toxic polyether compound isolated from the marine dinoflagellate Gambierdiscus toxicus. *J Am Chem Soc* **115**: 361–362.

Schrock RR (1999) Olefin metathesis by molybdenum imido alkylidene catalysts. *Tetrahedron* **55**: 8141–8153.

Shimizu Y (1986) *Natural Toxins: Animal, Plant and Microbial*. Ed. Harris JB, Clarendon Press, Oxford, U.K., p. 115.

Shirakawa E, Yamasaki K, Yoshida H, and Hiyama T (1999) Nickel-catalyzed carbostannylation of alkynes with allyl-, acyl-, and alkynylstannanes: Stereoselective synthesis of trisubstituted vinylstannanes. *J Am Chem Soc* **121**: 10221–10222.

Stork G and Zhao K (1989) A stereoselective synthesis of (Z)-1-iodo-1-alkenes. *Tetrahedron Lett* **30**: 2173–2174.

Suzuki A (2011) Cross-coupling reactions of organoboranes: An easy way to construct C–C bonds (Nobel Lecture). *Angew Chem Int Ed* **50**: 6722–6737.

Takai K, Kakiuchi T, Kataoka Y, and Utimoto K (1994) A novel catalytic effect of lead on the reduction of a zinc carbenoid with zinc metal leading to a geminal dizinc compound. Acceleration of the Wittig-type olefination with the $RCHX_2$-$TiCl_4$-Zn systems by addition of lead. *J Org Chem* **59**: 2668–2670.

Takamura H, Kikuchi S, Nakamura Y et al. (2009) Total synthesis of brevenal. *Org Lett* **11**: 2531–2534.

Takamura H, Yamagami Y, Kishi T et al. (2010) Total synthesis of brevenal. *Tetrahedron* **66**: 5329–5344.

Tebbe FN, Parshall GW, and Reddy GS (1978) Olefin homologation with titanium methylene compounds. *J Am Chem Soc* **100**: 3611–3613.

Torikai K, Oishi T, Ujihara S et al. (2008) Design and synthesis of ladder-shaped tetracyclic, heptacyclic, and decacyclic ethers and evaluation of the interaction with transmembrane proteins. *J Am Chem Soc* **130**: 10217–10226.

Tsukano C, Ebine M, and Sasaki M (2005) Convergent total synthesis of gymnocin-A and evaluation of synthetic analogues. *J Am Chem Soc* **127**: 4326–4335.

Tsukano C and Sasaki M (2003) Total synthesis of gymnocin-A. *J Am Chem Soc* **125**: 14294–14295.

Tsukano C and Sasaki M (2006) Structure -activity relationship studies of gymnocin-A. *Tetrahedron Lett.* **47**: 6803–6807.

Uenishi J, Kawahama R, Yonemitsu O, and Tsuji J (1996) Palladium-catalyzed stereoselective hydrogenolysis of conjugated 1,1-dibromo-1-alkenes to (Z)-1-bromo-1-alkenes. An application to stepwise and one-pot synthesis of enediynes and dienynes. *J Org Chem* **61**: 5716–5717.

Uenishi J, Kawahama R, Yonemitsu O, and Tsuji J (1998) Stereoselective hydrogenolysis of 1,1-dibromo-1-alkenes and stereospecific synthesis of conjugated (Z)-alkenyl compounds. *J Org Chem* **63**: 8965–8975.

Vilotijevic I and Jamison TF (2007) Epoxide-opening cascades promoted by water. *Science* **317**: 1189–1192.

Yamada J, Asano T, Kadota I, and Yamamoto Y (1990) A new approach to the construction of β-alkoxy-substituted cyclic ethers via the intramolecular cyclization of ω-trialkylplumbyl and ω-trialkylstannyl ether acetals. *J Org Chem* **55**: 6066–6068.

Yasumoto T and Murata M (1993) Marine toxins. *Chem Rev* **93**: 1897–1909.

Zhou J and Rainier JD (2009) Olefinic-amide and olefinic-lactam cyclizations. *Org Lett* **11**: 3774–3776.

32

Ciguatera Toxins: Pharmacology, Toxicology, and Detection

Irina Vetter, Katharina Zimmermann, and Richard J. Lewis

CONTENTS

32.1 Introduction

Ciguatera is a form of ichthyosarcotoxism caused by consumption of many species of tropical and subtropical fishes from the Indo-Pacific Oceans and Caribbean Sea that have become contaminated by ciguatoxins, orally effective polyether sodium channel activator toxins that cause characteristic neurological, gastrointestinal, and cardiovascular symptoms in humans. Arguably, ciguatera is the most significant form of fish toxicoses in terms of the number and severity of poisoning episodes. The increased harvesting of tropical marine resources together with an increase in incidence has meant that fish consumption is associated with an increasing incidence of human intoxication, making ciguatera the most common nonbacterial seafood poisoning and a significant health concern globally.

The causative agents implicated in the clinical presentation of ciguatera, the ciguatoxins, arise from blooms of certain strains of benthic dinoflagellates of the genus *Gambierdiscus*. In addition to *G. toxicus*, additional toxic strains including *G. polynesiensis*, *G. belizeanus*, *G. australes*, and *G. caribbaeus* have been implicated in the biosynthesis of ciguatoxin precursors, which are then metabolized and bioaccumulated in fish through the marine food chain.[1-3] Environmental degradation may play a role in the increased incidence of ciguatera, though the precise factors involved remain to be elucidated.[1] Degrading reef health is known to be associated with increases in the occurrence of ciguatera, as climatic disturbances/disruptions of reef areas result in overgrowth of species of the dinoflagellate *Gambierdiscus*, with subsequent increases in fish toxicity and ciguatera incidence in endemic areas as well as increased spread of ciguatera to currently non-endemic areas.[4] Increased incidence of ciguatera can also be expected to adversely affect human nutrition, with fish species currently considered as relatively safe to eat increasingly becoming toxic for human consumption. Thus, of the marine toxin diseases, ciguatera has the greatest public health and economic impact. The role played by other marine toxins in ciguatera, including those produced by other toxic benthic dinoflagellates, has not been clearly demonstrated, although mild cases of palytoxin poisoning may be mistaken for ciguatera.[1] With climate change likely to cause increases in the incidence of ciguatera,[3,4] it is now more important than ever to understand the mechanisms and impact of ciguatera on human health in order to devise rational treatment and mitigation approaches and minimize its detrimental effects to human health.

The ciguatoxins are a family of temperature-stable, lipid-soluble, highly oxygenated, cyclic polyether molecules that were first isolated from moray eel in 1967.[5-8] Several ciguatoxins have been isolated from biodetritus containing wild *G. toxicus*,[7,9-11] from toxic strains of cultured dinoflagellate isolated from different parts of the world,[11-13] or from various ciguateric fish.[9,14-18] The ciguatoxin family is comprised of several closely related structural variants that are, according to their origin, denoted as Caribbean, Indian, or Pacific ciguatoxins (C-CTX, I-CTX, and P-CTX, respectively). Using NMR techniques, the chemical structures of a number of Pacific ciguatoxins from fish and *G. toxicus* have been elucidated.[7,10,12,13,19-21] Of these, P-CTX-1 is considered most toxic and along with closely related congeners is responsible for the neurological symptoms in the Pacific. The structures of C-CTX-1 and C-CTX-2, the major ciguatoxins from Caribbean fish, have been elucidated,[8] and additional C-CTX congeners have been described but were not structurally characterized.[22-24] In addition, several ciguatoxins from the Indian Ocean (I-CTX-1–4) have been isolated and characterized.[25,26]

All ciguatoxins isolated to date have a structural framework that is reminiscent of the brevetoxins (PbTx), another family of potent lipid-soluble polyether toxins produced by the marine dinoflagellate *Gymnodinium breve* (*Ptychodiscus brevis*) that include PbTx-1 to PbTx-10.[27,28] From our knowledge of the chemical structure of ciguatoxins found at different trophic levels, it is evident that P-CTX-1, the dominant and most potent ciguatoxin extracted from the moray eel *Gymnothorax javanicus*, arises from the acid-catalyzed spiroisomerization and oxidative modification of P-CTX-4A produced by the dinoflagellate *G. toxicus*.[1,7,21] The chemical structures of known ciguatoxins are compared with PbTx-2 in Figure 32.1.

At the molecular level, the ciguatoxins are the most potent sodium channel toxins known (see Table 32.1). Despite their potency, ciguatoxins rarely accumulate in fish flesh to levels that are lethal to humans; however, organs, especially the liver, may concentrate much higher levels of ciguatoxin. The pathophysiological effects of the ciguatoxins are defined by their ability to cause the persistent activation of voltage-sensitive sodium channels (Na_v) and to inhibit neuronal potassium channels, leading to increased neuronal excitability and neurotransmitter release, impaired synaptic vesicle recycling, and modified Na^+-dependent mechanisms in numerous cell types. It is these effects that are believed to underlie the complex of symptoms associated with ciguatera. Ciguatera can be distinguished from scombroid fish poisoning, a preventable intoxication that results mainly from consumption of *Scombridae* fish containing unusually high levels of histamine due to inappropriate storage or handling of fish, based on symptomatology. Ciguatera also differs from tetrodotoxin intoxication, one of the most lethal seafood toxins associated with the consumption of most puffer fish species (family *Tetraodontidae*). Even though puffer fish are easily recognized, there are still many cases of tetrodotoxin poisoning reported yearly. Interestingly, puffer fish toxins selectively block sodium channels in excitable membranes, an action that antagonizes the action of ciguatoxin. This blockade of sodium channels prevents action potentials from propagating along axons, nerve terminals, and muscle fibers, which leads to inhibition of nerve impulse-evoked neurotransmitter release at chemical synapses.

In this review, we provide an update on the pharmacology and toxicology of ciguatoxins and their detection provided in the original edition of this book.[29]

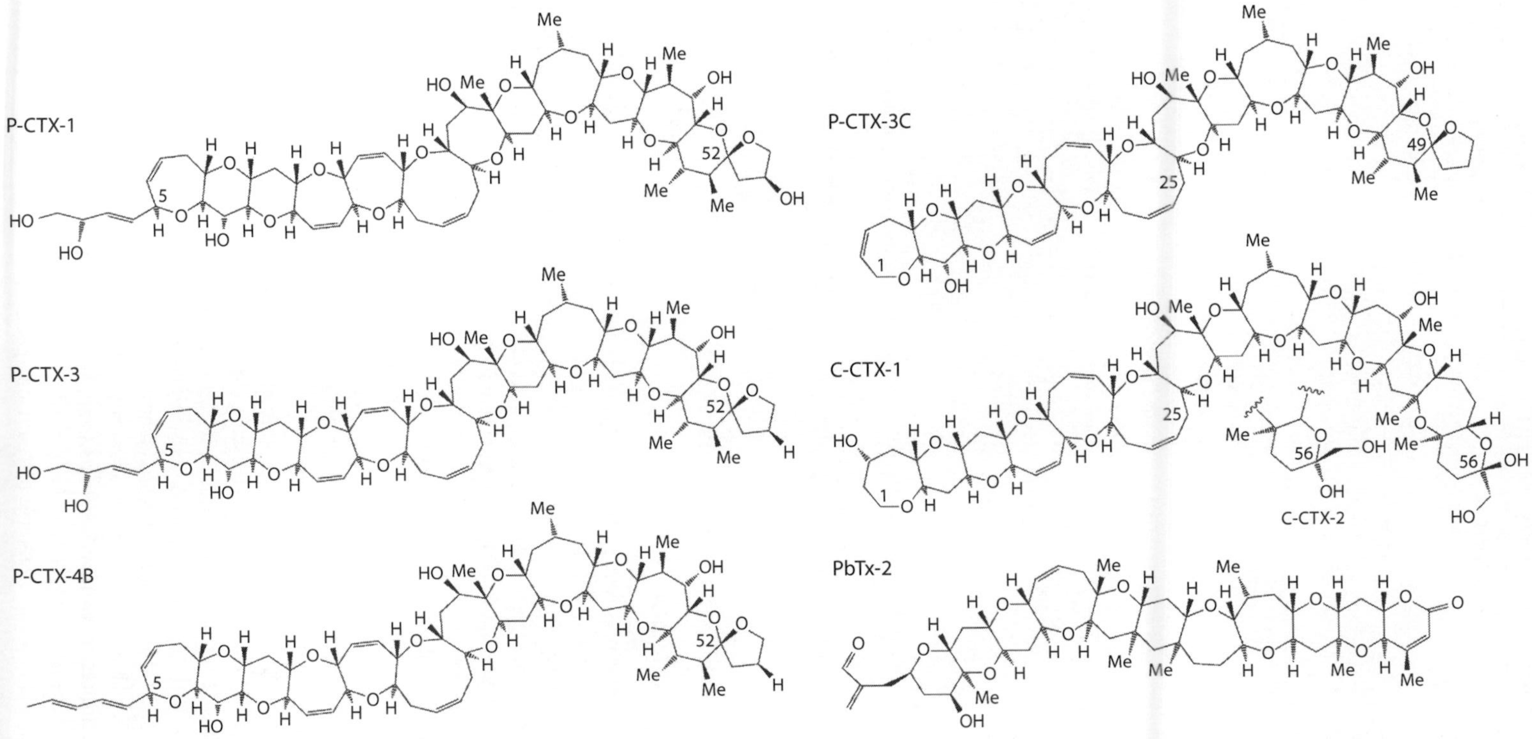

FIGURE 32.1 Structures of ciguatoxins from the Pacific Ocean and Caribbean Sea. Shown are P-CTX-1,[8,9] P-CTX-3,[20] CTX-4B,[8] P-CTX-3C,[13] and C-CTX-1 (the less energetically favorable epimer C-CTX-2 is shown in the inset).[9,17] Similarly, P-CTX-2 is the C52 epimer of C-CTX-3. Brevetoxin (PbTx-2) is shown for comparison.

TABLE 32.1

Characteristics[a] of Structurally Defined Ciguatoxins Found in Fish and *G. toxicus*

Name	Alternative Name	Source	[M + H]+	Potency (μg/kg)	References
P-CTX-1	CTX CTX-1B	Carnivore	1111	0.25	[8,9]
P-CTX-2		Carnivore	1095	2.3	[21]
P-CTX-3		Carnivore	1095	0.9	[20]
P-CTX-3C		*G. toxicus*	1045	—	[13]
2,3-DihydroxyCTX-3C	CTX-2A1	Carnivore	1057	1.8	[22]
51-HydroxyCTX-3C		Carnivore	1039	0.27	[22]
CTX-4A		*G. toxicus* Herbivore	1061	2	[14]
CTX-4B	GT-4B	*G. toxicus* Herbivore	1061	4	[8]
C-CTX-1		Carnivore	1141	3.6	[9,17]
C-CTX-2		Carnivore	1141	1	[9,17]
I-CTX-1		Carnivore	1141	~0.4[b]	[26,27]
I-CTX-2		Carnivore	1141	~0.4[b]	[26,27]
I-CTX-3		Carnivore	1157	~1.2[b]	[26,27]
I-CTX-4		Carnivore	1157	~1.2[b]	[26,27]

[a] The protonated molecular mass ([M + H]+) and potency following intraperitoneal injection are given.

[b] Based on in vitro potency compared to P-CTX-1 in brevetoxin binding assay.

32.2 Effects of Ciguatoxins in Humans and Animals

32.2.1 Ciguatera in Humans

Ciguatera is becoming an increasingly global health concern with climate change and associated predicted increases in ocean temperatures causing a rise in the incidence of ciguatera.[4,30,31] The global incidence of ciguatera is estimated to be as high as 50,000–500,000 cases annually.[4,32] Ciguatera is endemic in tropical and subtropical regions of the Pacific, Atlantic, and Indian Ocean, including the Caribbean and Australia. In addition, the increased export of potentially ciguateric fish due to global trade has led to increasing numbers of ciguatera cases in non-endemic areas.[4] Despite increased awareness, the true incidence of ciguatera remains a topic of much debate, as ciguatera remains underreported in endemic areas and under-recognized in non-endemic areas. Nonetheless, several lines of evidence support an increase in ciguatera globally, including reports of ciguatoxin fish from the eastern Atlantic[14,33] and the eastern Mediterranean.[34] In the Pacific, a 60% increase in the incidence of ciguatera between 1998–2008 and 1973–1983 was reported.[35]

While ciguateric fish can occur globally between latitudes 35° north and 35° south, the occurrence of the disease is both spatially and temporally unpredictable.[36,37] Interestingly, toxic dinoflagellates have been found recently in temperate waters, suggesting their range may increase with global warming.[38] More than 400 species of warm water marine fishes may be poisonous to humans after ingestion, with most being associated with ciguatera. Many of these ciguateric fish species, but not all, are found in coral reef waters. Usually, their distribution is highly localized, often restricted to a given island or side of an island, as is the case for the southern reef of Tarawa and the western reef of Maraki in the Republic of Kiribati, which are at high risk, while adjacent reefs are low risk.[37] Most ciguateric fish are nonmigratory reef fish and can be either herbivores or carnivores. Some fish species, in some locations, are toxic at all times,[39] while in most risk areas, ciguateric fish of each species may comprise 10% to <0.01% of those captured. Ciguatera in the Pacific has its greatest impact in communities inhabiting atoll islands, where fish are the primary source of dietary protein.[40]

TABLE 32.2

Clinical Symptoms of Ciguatera Fish Poisoning

Symptoms	Frequency (%)
Neurological	
Paresthesias	64–100
Cold allodynia	76–94
Arthralgia, myalgia	56–85
Pruritus	42–76
Headache	50–62
Fatigue, asthenia	60–100
Dental pain	21–37
Dysuria	13–33
Perspiration	49–60
Gastrointestinal	
Diarrhea	50–77
Nausea/vomiting	26–82
Abdominal pain	43–75
Cardiovascular	
Hypotension	12
Bradycardia	16

Sources: Gillespie, N.C. et al., *Med. J. Aust.*, 145, 584, 1986; Bagnis, R. et al., *Am. J. Trop. Med. Hyg.*, 28, 1067, 1979; Baumann, F. et al., *Toxicon*, 56, 662, 2010; Arena, P. et al., *Harmful Algae*, 3, 51, 2004; Bagnis, R. and Legrand, A.-M., Clinical features on 12,890 cases of ciguatera (fish poisoning) in French Polynesia, in *Progress in Venom and Toxin Research*, Gopalakrishnakone, P. and Tan, C. K. (Eds.), National University of Singapore and International Society of Toxinology, Asia-Pacific Section, Singapore, pp. 372–384, 1987; Schnorf, H. et al., *Neurology*, 58, 873, 2002.

Note: Reported range of occurrence (%) of clinical symptoms of ciguatera at time of diagnosis.

Epidemiological characterization of ciguatera has been limited by the lack of laboratory tests to confirm the presence of ciguatoxins, leaving diagnosis purely symptomatic based on detailed anamnesis. While the pathophysiological features and symptoms of the disease in different areas of the world have been extensively examined,[36,41–49] ciguatera can present with a perplexing array of gastrointestinal, neurological, and, to a lesser extent, cardiovascular symptoms (Table 32.2). The duration, severity, and number of ciguatera symptoms depend on the quantity of ciguatoxin consumed, the type of fish (herbivore, carnivore), and the ocean in which the fish was caught.[35,50]

Gastrointestinal symptoms of ciguatera are apparent shortly after ingestion of ciguateric fish and consist predominantly of nausea and vomiting, diarrhea, and abdominal pain. These symptoms tend to be short lived and generally precede the neurological symptoms that tend to be the most distinctive and enduring features of ciguatera. The predominant symptomatology associated with ciguatera includes sensory changes such as generalized pruritus, circumoral numbness, long-lasting weakness and fatigue, blurred vision or reduced visual contrast sensitivity, and a distinctive phenomenon referred to as paradoxical "temperature reversal," with cold temperatures eliciting a sensation of hot or burning.[51,52] This symptom is more correctly known as cold allodynia rather than an inability to distinguish temperatures, with patients reporting intense burning pain when exposed to usually innocuous cool stimuli.[51] A recent study has identified that this occurs due to activation of peripheral sensory neurons expressing the cold sensor TRPA1.[53] As this symptom has been reported to occur in up to 95% of ciguatera sufferers but is not usually associated with related marine toxin disease, cold allodynia is generally considered pathognomonic for ciguatera. More generalized or neuropsychiatric symptoms of ciguatera include anxiety, depression, and fatigue. These symptoms can in rare cases become chronic and may persist for weeks, months, or even years. In addition, mental state changes such as hallucinations, giddiness, ataxia, and coma appear to occur more frequently in the Indian and Pacific Ocean.[41,49,54–56] Such regional differences in the clinical presentation of ciguatera presumably arise from the chemically distinct ciguatoxin isoforms that occur in fish captured in the Caribbean Sea, Pacific Ocean, and Indian Ocean.

Ciguatera is also associated with autonomic neuronal dysfunction, leading to hypotension, bradycardia, and hypersalivation in severe cases. Patients with bradycardia and/or hypotension may require urgent care because cardiovascular symptoms may indicate a poor prognosis.[57,58] However, cardiac symptoms usually occur only in severe poisoning and do not contribute significantly to the clinical presentation in the majority of ciguatera sufferers.

Although the symptoms associated with ciguatera are well documented, the disease often goes unreported and misdiagnosed. Early symptom recognition has improved the identification and clinical management of ciguatera in endemic and non-endemic areas. However, there is still a need for better diagnostic, preventive, and reporting protocols to more accurately study and understand this diverse clinical syndrome. Though difficult to implement, preventive strategies remain the best defense against ciguatera. Prevention of intoxication, at present, depends upon the avoidance of potential vectors. Immunoassays and bioassays, as well as methods based on mass spectrometry, are being developed to detect sub-ppb levels of ciguatoxins in suspect fish flesh prior to consumption.

32.2.2 Treatment of Ciguatera

Despite significant advances in our understanding of the pathophysiology of ciguatera, treatment remains predominantly supportive in nature. Based on the pharmacological effect of ciguatoxins on Na_v, treatment with a wide range of clinically available adjunct analgesics with activity at neuronal Na_v or Ca_v channels has been reported. However, in the absence of systematic clinical trials, evidence for the efficacy of these agents remains anecdotal. Case reports of efficacy in treating ciguatera exist for the tricyclic antidepressant amitriptyline[59–62]; the L-type calcium channel inhibitor nifedipine[61]; gabapentin[63]; and the sodium channel inhibitor tocainide.[64] Symptomatic improvement of chronic fatigue associated with ciguatera has also been observed with the selective serotonin reuptake inhibitor fluoxetine.[65] In addition, a range of other treatments have also been reported to give benefit to sufferers of ciguatera in isolated instances. Traditional remedies for ciguatera may also provide benefit,[66–69] but as with most other potential therapies, there is a paucity of evidence to confirm efficacy, and systematic evaluation of clinical efficacy of these drugs remains lacking.

Symptoms associated with ciguatera generally resolve spontaneously, albeit with a highly variable time course. Intravenous D-mannitol has been advocated as a unique remedy for patients with acute poisoning from Pacific and Caribbean fish for many years.[70–73] The therapeutic effect of mannitol was postulated to arise from a reversal of the striking edema of the circumaxonal Schwann cell cytoplasm observed in severe ciguatera as well as other neuroprotective effects observed in vitro.[72,74–76] Despite a number of case reports as well as an open-label clinical trial supporting the use of mannitol,[70,73,77–79] a lack of consistent efficacy in treating ciguatera was attributed to timing of administration, severity of poisoning, and individual variations in response to ciguatoxin and/or mannitol.[77] However, rat and mouse models of ciguatera failed to show the expected benefits of mannitol,[80,81] and a lack of efficacy, particularly in more prevalent milder forms of the disease, was recently reported in a double-blind, placebo-controlled trial.[82] Since the study only used a small mildly poisoned population of ciguatera sufferers that did not appear to be randomly separated from the control group, recommendations that it should not be used routinely[83] may have been premature. As the molecular basis of the disease improves, novel small molecule treatments and potentially even monoclonal antibodies may become available in the future.[84] Interestingly, cholestyramine, a bile acid sequestrant acting in the gastrointestinal tract to prevent bile reabsorption, was recently suggested to be of benefit in ciguatera.[85] In ciguatera, cholestyramine is thought to function as an ion exchange resin that enables faster elimination of ciguatoxins via the gastrointestinal tract and apparently reduces the duration of neurological symptoms. Efficacy of cholestyramine remains to be assessed in a double-blind, placebo-controlled trial.

32.2.3 Toxicokinetics of Ciguatoxins

While the gastrointestinal symptoms of ciguatera generally subside within days, the acute neurological symptoms of ciguatera can persist for several weeks, and in about 5% of cases, chronic disease characterized by prolonged fatigue, weakness, and depression can develop. The pathophysiological basis of the prolonged duration of ciguatera symptoms in some patients remains to be elucidated. It has been suggested that long-term effects may be the result of permanent neurological damage associated with neuronal edema or may be a reflection of slow detoxification or caused by a chronic systemic inflammatory reaction.[85] Indeed, the toxicokinetics of ciguatoxin after oral administration are consistent with the relatively fast onset of gastrointestinal effects, which can most likely be attributed to local effects due to high gastrointestinal concentrations. The delayed onset and prolonged duration of neurological effects likely reflect slower distribution to the systemic circulation as well as a slow biphasic elimination with a terminal half-life of approximately 4 days.[86] While ciguatoxin appears to be cleared predominantly through hepatic routes, some urinary excretion was also observed, and this may account for the occurrence of genitourinary effects including painful urination reported in ciguatera patients.[86]

32.2.4 In Vivo Effects of Ciguatoxin in Animals

Ciguatoxins have been found to be toxic in a range of animal species, especially mammals (see Gillespie et al.[36] for a review of earlier literature). The in vivo effects in mice are well characterized and mimic the symptoms of human ciguatoxin poisoning to some degree.[87,88] Intraperitoneal administration of single sublethal dose of ciguatoxin is associated with diarrhea, hypothermia, salivation, lacrimation, muscle weakness, decreased motor activity, and cyanosis.[87,88] In addition, systemic exposure to ciguatoxin causes decreased nerve conduction velocity and decreased corneal and nociceptive withdrawal reflexes and rarely ataxia, convulsions, or paralysis.[87,88] The systemic effects of ciguatoxin were accompanied by morphological changes evident at the light and electron microscopic level, including cardiac myocyte necrosis and vacuolation in the cytoplasm and a decrease in the number of secretory granules in medullary cells.[89] However, although severe diarrhea was elicited by the administration of ciguatoxins, no morphological alterations were seen in the mucosa and muscle layers of the small intestine, except in autonomic nerve fibers and synapses.[89] Ciguatoxin also accelerated mucus secretion from goblet cells and peristalsis in the colon and stimulated defecation at the rectum, while epithelial cell damage was observed only in the upper portion of the large intestine.[90]

One of the most prominent effects of ciguatoxins in mice is the rapidly developing hypothermia.[81] This symptom, which has also been observed in human ciguatera sufferers, most likely arises from neuroexcitatory effects in regions of the brain stem receiving vagal afferent inputs as well as activation of ascending pathways associated with visceral and thermoregulatory responses.[91] Transcriptional changes in the brain of mice systemically exposed to P-CTX-1 were consistent with activation of pathways protective against neuroinflammation.[92] Similarly, genomic changes in the blood and liver from mice suffering from ciguatoxicosis showed increased expression of genes involved in detoxification pathways, cytokine signaling, proteasome complex, and ribosomal function.[93–95]

Consistent with an effect of ciguatoxin on neuronal voltage-gated sodium channels (VGSCs), a significant reduction of mixed and motor nerve conduction velocities and nerve amplitudes was demonstrated in the rat ventral tail nerve following intraperitoneal injection of ciguateric fish extracts.[96] Both absolute and supernormal periods were significantly prolonged, together with an exaggeration of the supernormal response. The predominant action of ciguatoxin to increase neuronal excitability is believed to give rise to the multitude of sensory disturbances associated with ciguatera. Accordingly, a novel animal model of ciguatoxin-induced peripheral sensory disturbances demonstrated that local intraplantar injection of P-CTX-1 was able to elicit spontaneous nocifensive behavior including lifting, licking, and flinching of the paw, as well as increased withdrawal responses upon exposure to a cooled surface.[53] These findings are consistent with the clinical picture of ciguatoxin-induced pain and corroborate cold allodynia as a characteristic consequence of activation of specific subsets of peripheral sensory neurons by P-CTX-1.

32.3 In Vitro Pharmacology of Ciguatoxin

Pharmacological studies have revealed that ciguatoxins act on VGSCs (Na_v). These ion channels are large membrane-spanning proteins (Figure 32.2) that mediate the rapid increase in membrane Na^+ conductance responsible for the depolarizing phase of action potentials in many excitable cells. To date, nine isoforms termed $Na_v1.1$ to $Na_v1.9$ have been described. These isoforms are expressed in a spatially and temporally controlled manner in various tissues. Most notably, $Na_v1.1$, $Na_v1.2$, $Na_v1.3$, and $Na_v1.6$ are the predominant isoforms expressed in the CNS,[97] while $Na_v1.7$, $Na_v1.8$, and $Na_v1.9$ are restricted to the peripheral nervous system, $Na_v1.4$ is expressed in skeletal muscle, and $Na_v1.5$ is the cardiac isoform. Ciguatoxins directly affect Na_v in excitable cells and induce many cellular and physiological effects as a consequence, including increased membrane excitability, spontaneous action potential discharge, release of neurotransmitters, increase of intracellular Ca^{2+}, and axonal and Schwann edema.

32.3.1 Ciguatoxins Bind to Site 5 of the Na_v Channel

In addition to having similar polyether structures (Figure 32.1), ciguatoxins and brevetoxins both selectively target a common binding site on Na_v.[19,27,28,98–100] Ligand binding studies have revealed more than 12 distinct classes of biologically active neurotoxins that interact with at least 6 specific receptor sites identified on the α-subunit of neuronal sodium channels. Brevetoxins bind with high affinity to neurotoxin receptor site 5 of the sodium channel (Figure 32.2), as revealed by direct binding studies using radiolabeled [³H]PbTx-3 and by binding assays that show noncompetitive interactions between site 5 and a variety of toxin probes specific for sites 1–4.[99,101–103] Functional studies, such as increasing the potency of batrachotoxin-induced Na^+ influx into cells, further show that ciguatoxin does not act as a competitor at sites 1–4 of the VGSC.[101]

Ciguatoxins are not available as radiolabeled analogues for direct investigation of their specific binding; therefore, [³H]PbTx-3 has been used in homologous and heterologous displacement experiments to define site 5 toxins. Competition studies between purified ciguatoxin[104] or pure P-CTX-1, P-CTX-2, or P-CTX-3[19,98,105,106] and [³H]PbTx-3 indicate that the ciguatoxins are competitive inhibitors of brevetoxin binding and thus have overlapping binding at site 5 on the sodium channel (see Figure 32.2). Using a photolabeled derivative of PbTx-3 and site-directed antibody mapping, the partial localization of the receptor site 5 of voltage-dependent Na^+ channels (from rat brain) has been suggested to be in the region of interaction of segments S6 and S5 of domains I and IV, respectively[105] (Figure 32.2).

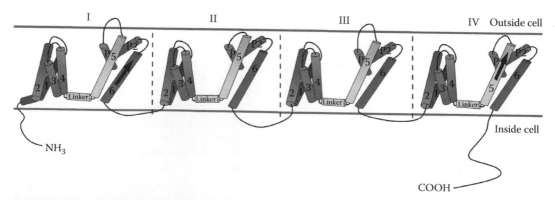

FIGURE 32.2 Ciguatoxin binding site (site 5) on the neuronal voltage-sensitive sodium channel. The sodium channel comprises the α-subunit of about 240–280 kDa (~2000 amino acids) organized in four repeated homologous domains (I–IV), each containing six putative transmembrane spanning α-helical segments (S1–S6). Site 5 (arrows) is formed by critical residues in S6 of domain I and S5 of domain IV.

32.3.2 Mode(s) of Activation of Sodium Channels by Ciguatoxin

As a consequence of ciguatoxin binding to the sodium channel, there is a shift in the voltage dependence of activation that results in Na$^+$ influx through the channel at membrane potentials where usually less sodium channels can be activated (Figure 32.3). Nanomolar concentrations of ciguatoxin alter the electrical properties of excitable cells of various tissues, causing increased Na$^+$ permeability and spontaneous action potential firing (reviewed by[107]). Although it is clear that ciguatoxin affects the biophysical properties of sodium channels, the pharmacological properties of toxin-modified Na$^+$ channels remain largely unaffected.[108,109] For example, both peak Na$^+$ current (i.e., unmodified Na$_v$) and late Na$^+$ current

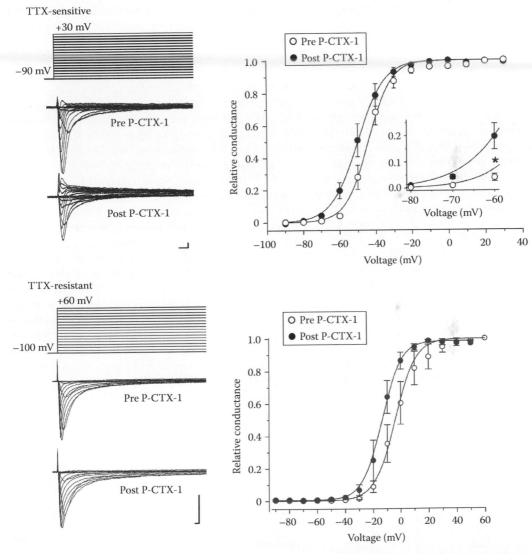

FIGURE 32.3 Effect of P-CTX-1 (1 nM) on the voltage-conduction relationship of TTX-sensitive and TTX-resistant Na$^+$ currents. TTX-sensitive: representative current traces recorded from TTX-sensitive VGSC of large-sized mouse dorsal root ganglion neurons (42.9 ± 1.4 μm). Upper lane: voltage protocol, middle: sample traces before, and lower: traces after perfusion with P-CTX-1 (1 nM). P-CTX-1 shifted the voltage dependence of activation of TTX-sensitive channels to more negative potentials and induced significant channel activation at −60 mV. TTX-resistant: representative recording of current traces recorded from ND7/23 cells heterologously expressing Na$_v$1.8. Upper lane: voltage protocol, middle: sample traces before, and lower: traces after perfusion with P-CTX-1 (1 nM). P-CTX-1 also elicited a 10 mV hyperpolarizing shift of the voltage dependence of Na$_v$1.8. Scale bars represent 1 ms and 1 nA. (Adapted from Vetter, I. et al., *EMBO J.*, 31, 3795, 2012.)

(i.e., toxin-modified Na_v) were inhibited in a similar manner by the local anesthetic lidocaine or the Na_v blocker tetrodotoxin, by increasing the external Ca^{2+} concentration or by increasing the external osmolality with D-mannitol, tetramethylammonium, or sucrose.

To gain a clearer understanding of how ciguatoxins increase neuronal excitability, the action of P-CTX-1 was examined on single VGSCs in parasympathetic neurons using patch-clamp recording techniques.[101] Under current clamp, bath application of 1–10 nM P-CTX-1 caused a gradual membrane depolarization and tonic action potential firing that ceased as the membrane became depolarized beyond approximately −35 mV. Similar effects were observed in cultured dorsal root ganglion neurons.[53] P-CTX-1 was found to increase the opening probability of TTX-sensitive sodium channels in response to depolarizing voltage steps but did not alter the channel conductance or reversal potential. Some P-CTX-1 modified channels opened spontaneously and did not close, even at hyperpolarized membrane potentials.[101] Thus, P-CTX-1 increases neuronal excitability through effects on the voltage dependence of activation and the induction of persistent Na^+ current.

Using whole-cell patch-clamp recording techniques, the effects of P-CTX-1 (0.2–20 nM) were examined on TTX-sensitive and TTX-resistant VGSCs present in dissociated rodent dorsal root ganglion neurons.[53,110] P-CTX-1 had no effect on the time course of activation and inactivation; however, a concentration-dependent reduction in peak current amplitude was observed for both channel types. For TTX-sensitive sodium channels, P-CTX-1 caused a hyperpolarizing shift in the voltage dependence of activation, a hyperpolarizing shift in steady-state inactivation (h), and a TTX-sensitive leakage current that also arose from ciguatoxin-modified TTX-sensitive sodium channels that presumably arose from persistent channel openings. In contrast, the major effect of P-CTX-1 on TTX-resistant sodium channels was to increase the rate of recovery from sodium channel inactivation.[110] These results were confirmed in a recent study, which showed that P-CTX-1 modifies VGSCs present in peripheral sensory neurons to increase nerve excitability[53] (Figure 32.3). P-CTX-1 depolarized the membrane potential of cultured DRG neurons (Figure 32.4), and this was frequently followed by spontaneous action potential firing[53] (Figure 32.5). In heterologous expression systems, another Pacific ciguatoxin, CTX3C, caused a hyperpolarizing shift in the threshold of activation for $rNa_v1.2$, $rNa_v1.4$, and $rNa_v1.5$ and significantly accelerated the time to peak current particularly for $rNa_v1.2$ and also for $rNa_v1.4$ and $rNa_v1.5$ at higher concentrations.[111] In addition, CTX3C shifted the inactivation potential for all isoforms in the negative direction and markedly delayed recovery from slow inactivation.[111] At less negative holding potentials, a lower concentration of CTX3C was required to achieve comparable effects on $rNa_v1.2$, and even more pronounced effects were observed on $rNa_v1.8$ heterologously expressed in ND7/23 neuroblastoma cells,[113] where CTX-3C elicited background currents and shifted the voltage dependence of activation and fast inactivation to more negative potentials.[112] Similar effects were observed with P-CTX-1, which shifted the voltage dependence of activation of

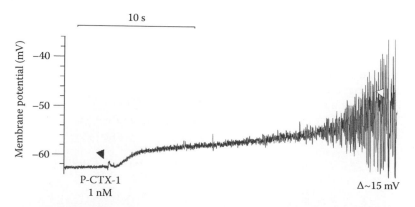

FIGURE 32.4 Effect of 1 nM P-CTX-1 on resting membrane potential and action potential firing in dorsal root ganglion neurons. Application of P-CTX-1 (black arrow) caused depolarization of the membrane potential recorded in current-clamp mode by 10 mV on average. Shown is a representative example of P-CTX-1-induced depolarization. (Adapted from Vetter, I. et al., *EMBO J.*, 31, 3795, 2012.)

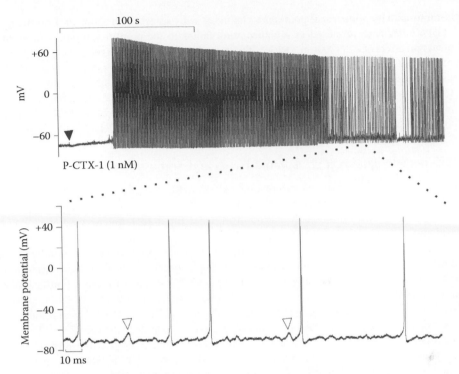

FIGURE 32.5 P-CTX-1 causes spontaneous action potential firing in cultured dorsal root ganglion neurons. Upper panel: membrane depolarization induced by P-CTX-1 (1 nM) rapidly leads to series of action potentials. Detail expanded in lower panel: P-CTX-1 (1 nM) induced membrane oscillations that were frequently followed by action potentials. (Adapted from Vetter, I. et al., *EMBO J.*, 31, 3795, 2012.)

heterologously expressed $Na_v1.8$ to more hyperpolarized potentials, albeit at much lower concentrations than those needed to observe an effect with CTX-3C.[53] These ciguatoxin-induced effects on sodium channels, resulting in increased activation at the resting membrane potential and accumulation of intracellular Na^+,[113] are responsible for numerous Na^+-dependent effects observed experimentally ([114] reviewed by[107]).

32.3.3 Ciguatoxins Inhibit Neuronal Potassium Channels

In addition to their pronounced effects on neuronal Na_vs, ciguatoxins and the related precursor toxin gambierol were also shown to inhibit potassium channels in frog myelinated axons, rat cerebellar granule and dorsal root ganglion neurons, and skeletal muscle cells.[115–118] In dorsal root ganglion neurons, P-CTX-1 caused a significant block of K_v channels, in particular, delayed-rectifier and "A-type" potassium currents with an IC_{50} of approximately 20 nM.[117] This effect, in conjunction with modification of Na_v activation, contributes to the increased neuronal excitability observed in DRG neurons, the prolonged action potential and afterhyperpolarization (AHP) duration, and influences the firing threshold and the resting membrane potential of dorsal root ganglion neurons.[117] A similar effect was also observed for P-CTX-4B in frog myelinated axons; however, while P-CTX-4B was more effective than P-CTX-1B at inhibiting potassium channels, it was approximately 50-fold less potent at Na_v channels in axonal membranes.[118] In contrast, P-CTX-1B was more effective than P-CTX-3C and 51-OH-CTX-3C at inhibiting potassium currents in cerebellar granule neurons. While the precise potassium channel isoforms contributing to the in vivo effects of ciguatoxin remain poorly defined, gambierol, a related polyether produced by *G. toxicus*, was found to be potent at $K_v1.2$ and $K_v3.1$, while no activity was found at K_v2, K_v4, $K_v1.6$, hERG, and *Shaker*IR,[119,120] suggesting that[116] polyether toxins including ciguatoxins are likely to be K_v subtype selective.

In addition to activity at neuronal potassium channels, a direct action of gambierol on the capsaicin receptor TRPV1 has been proposed as a contributing factor to the painful symptoms of ciguatera.[121] Given that no that effect of P-CTX-1 on TRPV1, TRPA1 or TRPM8 was observed in heterologous expression systems,[53] and that gambierol has no proven role in ciguatera, TRPV1 is unlikely to contribute to ciguatera symptomatology. However, enhanced neuronal excitability induced by ciguatoxin is sufficient to drive TRPA1-dependent calcium influx in response to mild cooling that is responsible for the development of cold allodynia, as evidenced by a large reduction of excitatory effect of P-CTX-1 on TRPA1-deficient nociceptive C-fibers and of ciguatoxin-induced cold allodynia in TRPA1-null mutant mice.[53]

32.3.4 Effects of Ciguatoxin on Isolated Heart and Smooth Muscle

Ciguatoxin causes a transient negative inotropy (reduced strength of contraction), followed by a dominant positive inotropic effect in the left atria, and positive inotropic effects in papillary muscle, by stimulating the release of excitatory and/or inhibitory neurotransmitters from innervating nerves.[114,122–125] A second, slower-developing phase of P-CTX-1 effect on guinea pig atria and papillary muscle resulted from an additional direct action of P-CTX-1 on the myocardium.[123,126] The link between P-CTX-induced increase of intracellular concentration of Na^+ and the positive inotropic response can be explained as follows. The enhanced Na^+ influx reduces the effectiveness of the Na^+–Ca^{2+} exchanger to remove intracellular Ca^{2+}, leading to enhanced Ca^{2+}-induced Ca^{2+} release from intracellular calcium stores (the major source of Ca^{2+} for cardiac contraction) and stronger contractions.[123] At high doses, P-CTX-1 additionally causes negative inotropic and arrhythmic effects in guinea pig atria and papillary muscles.[126]

P-CTX-1 also causes a large, sustained, and concentration-dependent positive inotropy in human atrial trabeculae. However, in this tissue, the inotropic effects arise through stimulation of intrinsic nerves, resulting in the release of noradrenaline.[123] The addition of mannitol (50 mM) was unable to reverse the positive inotropic effects of P-CTX-1 in human atrial trabeculae. In frog atria, C-CTX-1 does not affect membrane potential but caused a TTX-sensitive reduction in cardiac action potential duration,[127] possibly by stimulating the release of acetylcholine from intrinsic nerves.

P-CTX-1 (0.001–1 nM) causes a sustained, dose-dependent contraction of the longitudinal smooth muscle of the guinea pig ileum.[125,128] At high doses of P-CTX-1, P-CTX-2, and P-CTX-3, these contractions last for over 20 min[125] and are associated with bursts of contractile activity. The response to P-CTX-1 is completely blocked by atropine, and low extracellular Na^+ bath solution is enhanced by the acetylcholinesterase inhibitor eserine, but is unaffected by hexamethonium or mepyramine.[128] Repeated doses of P-CTX-1 are tachyphylactic, and responses to nicotine are irreversibly reduced by prior exposure to P-CTX-1, P-CTX-2, or P-CTX-3.[125,128] P-CTX-1 does not alter ileal responses to histamine, acetylcholine, and 5-hydroxytryptamine. These results indicate that P-CTX-1 causes the release of acetylcholine from cholinergic nerve terminals via the excitation of postganglionic nerves in the ilea. The tachyphylactic nature of the action of ciguatoxin suggests that nerve stimulation is followed by nerve blockade, probably as a consequence of further nerve depolarization.

P-CTX-1 also induces a contraction of isolated guinea pig vas deferens that is inhibited or abolished by treatment with TTX, procaine, cold storage, incubation in a low Na^+ bath solution, phentolamine, or guanethidine, but is not affected by atropine or mecamylamine.[129] From these results and the observation that P-CTX-1 caused a TTX-sensitive release of noradrenaline from the adrenergic nerves, it was determined that P-CTX-1-induced contractions occur via the release of noradrenaline from adrenergic nerve terminals. P-CTX-1 also markedly potentiates contraction of vas deferens induced by noradrenaline, acetylcholine, or high-K^+, but inhibits contractile responses arising from electrically stimulated neural elements. In a subsequent study, P-CTX-induced potentiation was shown to be inhibited or abolished by TTX and Na^+-deficient bath solution and suggested that P-CTX-1 may potentiate vas deferens contractile responses through a direct action on smooth muscle sodium channels.[130] However, subsequent studies have failed to confirm this result, instead indicating that P-CTX-1 caused potentiation only through the effects of neurally released noradrenaline (Lewis and Wong Hoy, unpublished results).

The effects of P-CTX-1 have also been examined on the membrane potential of smooth muscle cells of isolated rat proximal tail arteries.[131] P-CTX-1 (≥10 pM) increased the frequency of spontaneous excitatory junction potentials, while 100–400 pM P-CTX-1 additionally caused a maintained depolarization of up to

20 mV. Although the threshold and latency of the excitatory junction potential were not affected by these concentrations of P-CTX-1, propagated impulses were blocked ≥100 pM P-CTX-1. Spontaneous activity and the depolarization produced by P-CTX-I were reduced by adding 0.1 mM Ca^{2+}, 25 mM Mg^{2+}, or 6 mM Ca^{2+} to the bath solution or in the presence of 300 nM TTX, 100 nM ω-conotoxin GVIA, or 0.1 mM Cd^{2+}. Subsequent addition of 1 μM phentolamine (an α-adrenoceptor inhibitor) repolarized the membrane, while 1 mM suramin (a nonselective inhibitor of purinergic receptors) selectively abolished excitatory junction potentials caused by P-CTX-1. Thus, P-CTX-1 releases noradrenaline and ATP by initiating the asynchronous discharge of postganglionic perivascular nerves. Applied at concentrations of 100–400 pM, P-CTX-1 depolarized the smooth muscle to levels resembling those recorded in vivo, indicating that P-CTX-1 may be used to produce models of smooth muscle activity that are reminiscent of the in vivo situation.[131]

32.3.5 Ciguatoxin Mobilizes Intracellular Ca^{2+} in Nerve Cells

Intracellular Ca^{2+} plays a key second messenger role in numerous physiological processes in excitable cells.[132,133] Low concentrations of P-CTX-1 (2.5–25 nM) increase the intracellular Ca^{2+} concentration in cultured differentiated NG108–15 mouse neuroblastoma cells.[133,134] The increase of intracellular Ca^{2+} concentration, assessed by fura-2-based microfluorometric recordings, occurred either in cells bathed in a standard medium containing Ca^{2+} or after exposure to a Ca^{2+}-free medium supplemented with the Ca^{2+} chelator EGTA. Blockade of sodium channels by TTX completely prevented the P-CTX-1-induced increase in intracellular Ca^{2+} concentration, suggesting that the effect of the toxin on Ca^{2+} mobilization depends upon Na^+ influx through sodium channels.

A Na^+-dependent mobilization of Ca^{2+} from inositol 1,4,5-trisphosphate ($InsP_3$–)-sensitive stores could explain the increase in asynchronous quantal neurotransmitter release from motor nerve terminals that have been exposed to P-CTX-1 in a Ca^{2+}-free bath solution.[135,136] Indeed, in rat myotubules, P-CTX-1 (10 nM) caused a transient increase of intracellular $InsP_3$, which was blocked by TTX. The Ca^{2+} response elicited by P-CTX-1 was maintained in the absence of extracellular Ca^{2+}, suggesting release from $InsP_3$-sensitive stores, activated by P-CTX-1-induced membrane depolarization as the likely source of Ca^{2+} in these cells.[113]

In cultured rat dorsal root ganglion neurons, P-CTX-1 (1 nM) elicited Ca^{2+} responses in 51% of cells, with immunohistochemical characterization of the responding cell population showing that the majority of ciguatoxin-sensitive neurons were peptidergic, IB4-negative, TRPA1-expressing cells[53] (Figure 32.6).

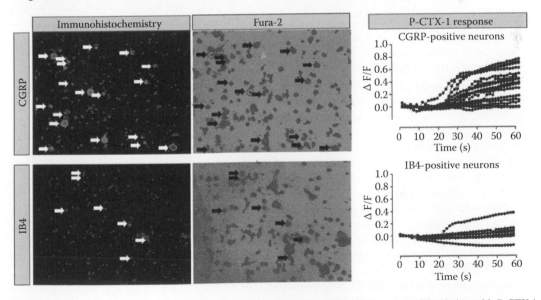

FIGURE 32.6 P-CTX-1 induces Ca^{2+} responses in cultured dorsal root ganglion neurons. Stimulation with P-CTX-1 (1 nM) caused an increase in intracellular Ca^{2+} responses, measured using the fluorescent Ca^{2+} dye Fura-2, in CGRP-positive neurons. In contrast, the majority of IB4-positive neurons did not respond to P-CTX-1. (Adapted from Vetter, I. et al., *EMBO J.*, 31, 3795, 2012.)

Consistent with preferential activation of dorsal root ganglion neurons expressing the cold-sensing ion channel TRPA1, treatment with P-CTX-1 induced cold-evoked Ca^{2+} responses in previously cold-insensitive mouse dorsal root ganglion neurons. In addition, neurons with functional responses to the TRPA1 agonist allyl isothiocyanate showed the largest Ca^{2+} increase in response to P-CTX-1.[53]

32.3.6 Role of Na+–Ca2+ Exchange in the Action of Ciguatoxin

One transporter that plays a critical role in the control of Ca^{2+} homeostasis in many cells is the Na^+–Ca^{2+} exchanger, which harnesses the Na^+ gradient developed by the Na^+/K^+-ATPase to lower intracellular Ca^{2+} concentration. The plasma membrane Na^+–Ca^{2+} exchanger acts in concert with the plasma membrane ATP-driven Ca^{2+} pumps, Ca^{2+} channels, and intracellular Ca^{2+} sequestration systems to control cytoplasmic Ca^{2+} levels. The Na^+–Ca^{2+} exchanger is an electrogenic transporter, the operation of which depends on the prevailing ionic conditions, allowing it to act normally as a Ca^{2+} efflux pathway or, under certain conditions, may even promote Ca^{2+} influx. Through the activation of sodium channels and subsequent reduction of the Na^+ gradient, ciguatoxin reduces the ability of the Na^+–Ca^{2+} exchanger to extrude Ca^{2+} ions.

Exposure of cholinergic synaptosomes isolated from the electric organ of the fish *Torpedo marmorata* to P-CTX-1 (0.1 pM–10 nM) revealed that the toxin increases Na^+ influx into synaptosomes, thus enhancing acetylcholine release triggered by Ca^{2+}.[137] This action does not result from P-CTX-1-induced depolarization of the synaptosomal membrane to levels above those needed to activate Ca^{2+} channels, because simultaneous blockade of Ca^{2+} channel subtypes by Gd^{3+}, ω-conotoxin GVIA, and FTX (a low-molecular-weight toxin purified from the venom of the American funnel-web spider *Agelenopsis aperta*) did not prevent acetylcholine release caused by P-CTX-1 upon addition of Ca^{2+}. In addition, little transmitter release was detected when Na^+ was replaced by Li^+, consistent with the fact that Li^+ cannot replace Na^+ in the Na^+–Ca^{2+} exchanger.[138] Furthermore, inhibitors of the Na^+–Ca^{2+} exchanger, such as bepridil and cetiedil, completely prevented the Ca^{2+}-dependent acetylcholine release induced by P-CTX-1.[139] Therefore, P-CTX-1 appears to cause an increase in Na^+ levels in synaptosomes that leads to an elevation of cytoplasmic Ca^{2+} via the Na^+–Ca^{2+} exchanger and, as a consequence, promotes Ca^{2+}-dependent neurotransmitter release.

32.3.7 Ciguatoxin Induces Swelling of Nerve Cells

Another consequence of the persistent activation of voltage-dependent Na^+ channels induced by ciguatoxins at the resting membrane potential is the swelling of nerve cells. Swelling has been observed during the action of the P-CTX-1, P-CTX-4B, or P-CTX-3C on myelinated axons, motor nerve terminals, and on perisynaptic Schwann cells in situ, as determined by confocal laser scanning microscopy.[75,108,140–142] These toxins induced a marked nodal swelling of single myelinated axons and spontaneous action potentials, without apparent modification of the morphology of the internodal parts of nerve fibers characterized by the presence of myelin sheath layers. Similarly, motor nerve terminals innervating skeletal muscle fibers, as well as perisynaptic Schwann cells in situ, swelled when exposed to either P-CTX-1 or P-CTX-4B. Quantification of the swelling revealed that Pacific ciguatoxins cause a approximately two-fold increase in the nodal volume of myelinated axons and in motor nerve terminal area per unit length. These effects were reversed increasing the osmolality of the external solution by ~50% either with 100 mM D-mannitol, 50 mM tetramethylammonium chloride, or with 100 mM sucrose. Although the hyperosmolar external solutions almost completely reversed the nodal swelling of myelinated axons induced by ciguatoxin, the solutions only partially decreased the nerve terminal swelling, which results from both the incorporation of synaptic vesicle membranes into the nerve terminal axolemma during stimulated neurotransmitter release and from osmotic changes.

In the continuous presence of TTX, ciguatoxins did not cause significant changes in the nodal volume of myelinated axons or in the motor nerve terminal area per unit length. Thus, it is likely that ciguatoxins promote the entry of Na^+ through ciguatoxin-modified sodium channels that are permanently activated at the resting membrane potential and through unmodified sodium channels that open during ciguatoxin-induced spontaneous action potential discharges. The resulting increase in intracellular Na^+

concentration directly and indirectly disturbs the osmotic equilibrium between the intra- and extracellular medium and is associated with an influx of water that acts to restore both the osmotic equilibrium and the intracellular Na^+ concentration to basal levels. The cellular basis for the beneficial action of hyperosmotic D-mannitol in the treatment of ciguatera thus likely involves its ability to both shrink nerve cells swollen by ciguatoxins and inhibit sodium channels activated by ciguatoxin.[108]

32.3.8 Ciguatoxin Enhances Excitability of Nerves

As a consequence of the persistent activation of sodium channels at the resting membrane potential, ciguatoxins increase the excitability of nerve membranes. P-CTX-1 evokes a membrane depolarization, which in turn causes spontaneous and/or repetitive action potential discharges at high frequencies (60–100 Hz) in myelinated axons and motor nerve terminals.[107,108,135,142,143] In neuroblastoma cells and rat parasympathetic neurons, P-CTX-1 also induces membrane depolarization and, under appropriate conditions, induces spontaneous oscillations in the resting membrane potential and repetitive action potentials[101,109] (Figures 32.4 and 32.5). Research on the other ciguatoxins is less extensive, mainly due to difficulties in obtaining purified toxin. P-CTX-4B, from the dinoflagellate *Gambierdiscus toxicus*, has effects on myelinated nerve fibers that are similar to those of P-CTX-1, but is ~50-fold less effective than P-CTX-1.[144] In contrast to P-CTX-1, P-CTX-4B decreases the amplitude and increases the duration of spontaneous action potentials, consistent with block of K^+ channels. The physiological consequence of any K^+ channel blocking action of ciguatoxins remains to be elucidated. The ability of ciguatoxins to increase membrane excitability is consistent with studies on nerve conduction, which show that partially purified extracts of ciguateric fish increase and prolong the supernormal period of the nerve excitability.[96,145,146]

It is noteworthy that in myelinated axons, the local anesthetic lidocaine (50 µM), an increase in external Ca^{2+} concentration (1.8–5.4 mM), or an increase in external osmolality with D-mannitol (100 mM), tetramethylammonium chloride (50 mM), or sucrose (100 mM) first decrease the frequency of spontaneous and repetitive action potentials induced by either P-CTX-1 or P-CTX-4B and then progressively suppress these action potentials.[108,143,144] However, in the presence of these inhibitors, the action potentials evoked by depolarizing stimuli are still maintained, suggesting these agents act to specifically reverse the effects of ciguatoxin on VGSCs nerves.

32.3.9 Effects of Ciguatoxin on Synaptic Transmission

Membrane depolarization and increased excitability of presynaptic nerve terminals induced by P-CTX-1 and C-CTX-1 markedly alter neurotransmission efficacy in various chemical synapses and secretory terminals. As a consequence of the changes in presynaptic excitability induced by ciguatoxins, volleys of action potentials can reach nerve terminals either spontaneously or in response to a single stimulus. Voltage-gated calcium channels open during each presynaptic action potential, and the ensuing rise of intracellular Ca^{2+} concentration triggers the exocytosis of synaptic vesicles resulting in synchronous spontaneous or repetitive multi-quantal neurotransmitter release.[147]

At vertebrate neuromuscular junctions, nanomolar concentrations of Pacific and Caribbean CTX-1 trigger spontaneous or repetitive end plate potentials at frequencies of up to 40 and 100 Hz, respectively, in response to a single nerve stimulus.[135,148] Such synaptic activity at neuromuscular junctions is transient and probably due to ciguatoxin-induced depolarization of motor nerve terminals. In neuromuscular junctions equilibrated with low Ca^{2+}–high Mg^{2+} bath solution, P-CTX-1 first increases the mean quantal content of end plate potentials, then reduces before finally blocking nerve-evoked transmitter release in an irreversible manner. It is likely that the increase in the averaged number of quanta released during P-CTX-1 action is not due to an enhanced Ca^{2+} influx through voltage-dependent calcium channels, but due to the reversed-mode operation of the Na^+/Ca^{2+} exchanger, which allows Ca^{2+} entry in exchange for intracellular Na^+ as reported in isolated nerve endings.[135,137,139]

Studies of guinea pig sympathetic ganglia using intracellular recording techniques showed that low concentrations of P-CTX-1 (0.2–0.8 nM) generated a marked increase in the frequency of spontaneous

TABLE 32.3

Modes of Action of Ciguatoxins

Activate sodium channels of excitable and nonexcitable cells
Inhibit neuronal potassium channels
Induce membrane depolarization and spontaneous and repetitive action potential firing in excitable cells
Lead to elevation of intracellular Ca^{2+} due to alteration of the cellular Na^+ gradient and subsequent recruitment of the Na^+–Ca^{2+} exchanger
Induce repetitive, synchronous, and asynchronous neurotransmitter release
Produce a transient increase and decrease in the quantal content of synaptic responses
Cause spontaneous fasciculations and tetanic muscle contractions
Impair synaptic vesicle recycling that exhausts neurotransmitter available for release
Cause swelling of axons, nerve terminals, and perisynaptic Schwann cells
Elicit cold allodynia by enhancing excitability of TRPA1-expressing peripheral sensory neurons

excitatory synaptic potentials, which often occurred in bursts (15–66 Hz) of similar amplitudes.[149] However, the passive electrical properties, the amplitude and threshold of action potentials evoked by depolarizing current, and the threshold, latency, and form of the initial responses to nerve stimulation were not affected by P-CTX-1. Single stimuli to incoming nerves produced long-lasting repetitive synaptic responses arising from preganglionic axons. All activity generated by P-CTX-1 was significantly reduced or abolished by (+)-tubocurarine, hexamethonium (10 µM), TTX (≥0.1 µM), ω-conotoxin GVIA (100 nM), reduced Ca^{2+} (0.1 mM Ca^{2+})/10 mM Mg^{2+} Ringer), and elevated Ringer Ca^{2+} (6 mM) or Mg^{2+} (25 mM). The results of this study suggest that P-CTX-1 activates preganglionic axons by activating a subpopulation of sodium channels.[149] These effects occurred at lower concentrations in unmyelinated than myelinated axons, suggesting that many of the symptoms of ciguatera poisoning may be explained by activity at unmyelinated nerves.

Ciguatoxins also increase spontaneous quantal acetylcholine release from motor nerve terminals, detected as an increase in miniature end plate potential (MEPP) frequency. The increase in MEPP frequency occurred even in a Ca^{2+}-free medium supplemented with the calcium chelator, EGTA, and leads to an exhaustion of neurotransmitter stores. Ultrastructural examination of these motor nerve terminals revealed both a marked depletion of synaptic vesicles and an increase in the nerve terminal perimeter, suggesting that the synaptic vesicle recycling process is impaired during the action of CTX-1.[136] The activation of VGSCs by ciguatoxins, and the subsequent entry of Na^+ ions into nerve terminals, appears to be responsible for the enhancement of asynchronous neurotransmitter release and the depletion of synaptic vesicles, since blockade of Na^+ influx into the terminals by TTX prevents these effects. These results further suggest that ciguatoxin-induced increases in intracellular Na^+ concentration in motor nerve endings can (1) mobilize Ca^{2+} from intracellular stores, (2) directly activate the asynchronous neurotransmitter release process in motor nerve terminals, and (3) impair the synaptic vesicle recycling process that is crucial for the maintenance of a functional population of synaptic vesicles during prolonged periods of transmitter release.

Table 32.3 summarizes our present understanding of the mode of action of ciguatoxins.

32.4 Detection Methods

As no clinically validated treatments for ciguatera are currently available, prevention of intoxication and identification of ciguateric fish remains a primary management strategy. Thus, significant efforts have been made toward developing assays for the rapid, inexpensive, and accurate quantification of ciguatoxins in fish flesh. Based on data from human intoxication incidents and toxicological data obtained in in vitro and in vivo laboratory tests, a minimum permitted level of 0.01 ng/g P-CTX-1, or 0.1 ng/g C-CTX-1, has been proposed for fish caught in the Pacific and Caribbean, respectively.[18,150,151] Detection methods should thus be able to accurately quantify ciguatoxins at these levels in order to provide estimates of safety (reviewed in[152]). In addition, ciguatoxin detection assays with sufficient specificity and sensitivity could see applications in the diagnosis of ciguatera, and some efforts toward the isolation and identification of ciguatoxins from the blood of patients have already been made.[153–155]

Development of a universal ciguatoxin detection assay has been hampered not only by the exquisite potency of ciguatoxins, necessitating very low levels to cause human illness, but also by the high diversity and structural complexity of ciguatoxin congeners present in ciguateric fish and, as a consequence, in biological samples from ciguatera sufferers. Depending on the intended application of ciguatoxin detection methods, different assay characteristics may be required. Factors that need to be taken into consideration include the time required for assay results, cost, sensitivity, specificity and accuracy, interference from matrix, and the need for specialized laboratory equipment and expertise.

32.4.1 Animal Assays for Ciguatoxins

Since ciguatoxins are odorless and tasteless, feeding tests in animals have been traditionally used to monitor suspected or toxic fish samples. These tests are based on feeding cats, mongoose, chicken, crayfish, or insects (mosquito and Diptera larvae) with flesh or viscera of suspect fish. Observations of symptoms, behavior, growth, body temperature, and survival time of the animals over time are used to characterize and quantify toxin levels.[87,156–160] Of the 37 animal species tested by Banner et al.,[161] only 5 were found to be sensitive to the oral administration of ciguateric fish. In these studies, the cat was rejected because it often regurgitated the tested fish sample, but this may be most problematic when highly toxic samples are tested.

A mosquito assay for ciguatoxins in crude fish extracts has been reported.[156] Intrathoracic injection of serial dilutions of extract allowed the toxicity of the fishes to be established. A significant correlation between the mosquito bioassay and the mouse bioassay performed on the same extracts was shown, with correct detection of 96% of the toxic fishes, while 91% of fish extracts nontoxic to mice were nontoxic to mosquitoes. The following year, Vernoux et al.[157] reported a chick feeding assay for testing toxic fish tissues or extracts. Symptoms included internal hypersalivation, a decrease in weight, and acute motor ataxia. Detoxification was slow, with repeated administration leading to toxin accumulation. The liver, which is typically the most toxic tissue, gave a roughly quantitative response to toxin level, indicating that the chick assay may be a useful screening test in ciguatera-endemic regions. Perhaps the simplest animal assay to be developed for ciguatoxins is the fly assay.[160] The meat-eating *Parasarcophaga argyrostoma* (Diptera, Sarcophagidae) larvae were able to detect ciguatoxin at > ~0.2 ng/g in fish flesh or liver. Despite its ability to detect medium and highly toxic fish, the test has not gained widespread acceptance, and the mouse bioassay has remained a widely used assay to establish levels of ciguatoxin in extracts of fish for many years (reviewed in [159]). The method quantifies lethal and sublethal doses of ciguatoxin in crude extracts administered intraperitoneally to mice. The signs of intoxication are well described, and include hypothermia, hypersalivation, lacrimation, penile erection, hind limb paralysis for certain ciguatoxins, respiratory difficulties, and asphyctic convulsions preceding death that is the result of respiratory failure.[87] The establishment of dose-time-to-death relationship for the major toxins allows the numbers of mice required for quantitation to be reduced to as few as two per sample and avoids testing LD_{50} doses that are lethal at ~24 h.[159] Despite these considerations, ethical concerns remain with the use of mice for toxicity testing. In addition, the assay is not sufficiently sensitive to detect low-toxicity fish in crude extracts and may give false-positive results if high doses of lipid are administered (>20 mg per mouse).[17] Ciguatoxins are also potent fish toxins, but differ from the brevetoxins that are more potent on fish than mammals.[162]

32.4.2 Sodium Channel Assays for Ciguatoxin

Based on the pharmacological action of ciguatoxins on Na_v, several in vitro assays for the detection of ciguatoxins have been developed. These assays detect ciguatoxin-induced Na^+ influx in Na_v-expressing cells through a variety of end points, including cell cytotoxicity, metabolic activity, or fluorescent detection of membrane potential changes. The sensitivity of sodium channel assays for ciguatoxin is often enhanced by concomitant exposure to the site 2 toxin veratridine and the Na^+/K^+-ATPase inhibitor ouabain. Synergistic effects of ciguatoxins and veratridine lead to enhanced activation of Na_v channels endogenously expressed in various cell lines of neuronal origin, such as the N2a mouse neuroblastoma or BE(2)-M17 human neuroblastoma cell lines. Activation of Na_v at resting membrane potential, in conjunction with inhibition of Na^+ efflux by ouabain, leads to accumulation of intracellular Na^+. This in turn leads to cellular toxicity, manifested through decreased metabolic activity and cellular viability, which in turn is assessed by colorimetric assays, most commonly the 3-(4,5-dimethylthiazol-2-yl)-2,5-diphenyltetrazolium] MTT assay. Several groups have demonstrated that these in vitro assays can be developed as simple and sensitive methods to detect sodium channel-specific marine toxins including ciguatoxins.[86,88,106,153,163–166]

The assay responds in a dose-dependent manner to ciguatoxins, brevetoxins, and saxitoxins, and delineates the toxic activity as either sodium channel enhancing or sodium channel blocking toxins. Within several hours, CTX can be detected at subpicogram levels.[164,166] A sensitive cell-based assay for brevetoxins, saxitoxins, and ciguatoxins has also been reported that employs a *c-fos*-luciferase reporter gene stably expressed in cells.[167] [^{3}H]PbTx-3 binding to brain membrane can also be used to detect ciguatoxins in crude extracts[99] and can be developed into high-throughput assays. The results obtained from cell bioassay of ciguateric fish extracts correlate with those obtained by mouse bioassay; however, cell-based toxicity assays cannot distinguish between ciguatoxins and other sodium channel activator toxins that are not orally active.

32.4.3 Immunoassays and Physicochemical Analysis

Immunoassays can provide a rapid, cost-effective, highly sensitive method of detecting ciguatoxins based on the ability of ciguatoxin-specific antibodies to react with their antigens. However, due to the high toxicity, scarcity, and chemical complexity of ciguatoxins, this approach has proven challenging. Nonetheless, several groups have successfully generated antibodies to various ciguatoxin congeners, and these have found application in enzyme immunoassays, which generally correlate very well with cell-based or in vivo ciguatoxin assays.[168–174]

An immunobead assay test kit, Cigua-Check, was available commercially for several years; however, in the absence of information on its validation, production has since been halted. Thus, there are currently no commercially available immunoassay-based kits available for the detection of ciguatoxin, although work in this area is progressing rapidly. The limit of detection of ciguatoxins using immunoassay approaches was initially inferior to the mouse bioassay or sodium channel assays; however, recent developments have seen significant improvements, with detection of ciguatoxins in the sub-nanomolar range now feasible.[168,171,172,174,175]

Chromatography and mass spectrometry assays have been instrumental in the isolation and characterization of various ciguatoxins from the Pacific, Caribbean, and Indian Oceans. Such assays can accordingly also find applications in the detection of ciguatoxins from fish or biological samples, and significant advances have been made in recent years, which continually improve the performance of these techniques. Recently, improved HPLC-MS/MS detection following a ciguatoxin rapid extraction method was described, which achieved a limit of quantification of 0.1 ng/g.[176] Similarly, a method for detection of ciguatoxins by gradient reversed-phase HPLC/tandem mass spectrometry with a limit of detection of 40 pg/g P-CTX-1 and 100 pg/g C-CTX-1 was reported.[177] Such assays are well on the way to replacing animal testing for ciguatoxins and warrant further validation to determine the potential of such assays to be developed into rapid screens for public health protection.

32.5 Conclusions

Considerable progress has been made in determining the chemical structures of the principal toxins involved in ciguatera and in characterizing their cellular modes of action. However, only rarely are diagnoses based on the identification of the bioactive agents present in the remains of the fish implicated in the poisoning. This is a concern, since differential diagnosis of the various types of fish poisoning depends on clinical recognition of specific signs and symptoms, but is complicated by difficulties distinguishing ciguatera from other forms of seafood poisoning and other illnesses. For most types of fish poisoning described here, treatment remains nonspecific, symptomatic, and supportive. Various substances and herbal remedies have been used for the treatment of ciguatera, including local anesthetics, calcium gluconate, vitamins, antidepressants, and glucose. However, the efficacy of these therapeutic agents remains uncertain, and antagonists effective at specifically reversing the pathophysiological basis of ciguatoxin action remain elusive. The development of specific tests that detect the presence of ciguatoxin and related toxins in fish prior to consumption will significantly improve the management of ciguatera and overcome present limitations of diagnosis and existing therapies.

The action of ciguatoxin is to increase cell Na^+ permeability through Na_v that open at normal resting membrane potentials. As a consequence, ciguatoxins affect various Na^+-dependent mechanisms to enhance membrane excitability, activate Na^+–Ca^{2+} exchange, induce mobilization of intracellular Ca^{2+}, and produce cell swelling. The effects of ciguatoxin are most prominent in nerves. These neurocellular actions of ciguatoxin are consistent with the generalized disturbance of nerve conduction, synaptic transmission, and cellular morphology observed in intoxicated patients.[145]

ACKNOWLEDGMENTS

This work was supported by funding from the National Health and Medical Research Council Australia Research Fellowship to RJL and the Australian Biomedical Research Fellowship to IV.

REFERENCES

1. Lewis, R. J. and Holmes, M. J., 1993. Origin and transfer of toxins involved in ciguatera. *Comp Biochem Physiol C,* 106, 615–628.
2. Chinain, M., Darius, H. T., Ung, A. et al., 2010. Growth and toxin production in the ciguatera-causing dinoflagellate Gambierdiscus polynesiensis (Dinophyceae) in culture. *Toxicon,* 56, 739–750.
3. Litaker, R. W., Vandersea, M. W., Faust, M. A. et al., 2010. Global distribution of ciguatera causing dinoflagellates in the genus Gambierdiscus. *Toxicon,* 56, 711–730.
4. Llewellyn, L. E., 2010. Revisiting the association between sea surface temperature and the epidemiology of fish poisoning in the South Pacific: Reassessing the link between ciguatera and climate change. *Toxicon,* 56, 691–697.
5. Scheuer, P. J., Takahashi, W., Tsutsumi, J., and Yoshida, T., 1967. Ciguatoxin: Isolation and chemical nature. *Science,* 155, 1267–1268.
6. Tachibana, K., Nukina, M., Joh, Y., and Scheuer, P., 1987. Recent developments in the molecular structure of ciguatoxin. *Biol Bull,* 172, 122–127.
7. Murata, M., Legrand, A., Ishibashi, Y., Fukui, M., and Yasumoto, T., 1990. Structures and configurations of ciguatoxin from the Moray eel Gymnothorax-javanicus and its likely precursor from the dinoflagellate Gambierdiscus-toxicus. *J Am Chem Soc,* 112, 4380–4386.
8. Lewis, R. J., Vernoux, J. P., and Brereton, I. M., 1998. Structure of Caribbean ciguatoxin isolated from Caranx latus. *J Am Chem Soc,* 120, 5914–5920.
9. Legrand, A. M., Fukui, M., Cruchet, P., Ishibashi, Y., and Yasumoto, T., Characterization of ciguatoxins from different fish species and wild *Gambierdiscus toxicus,* in *Proceedings of the Third International Conference on Ciguatera Fish Poisoning,* Tosteson, T. R., Ed. Polyscience Publications, Montreal, Quebec, Canada, 1992, pp. 25–32.
10. Murata, M., Legrand, A. M., Ishibashi, Y., and Yasumoto, T., 1989. Structures and configurations of ciguatoxin and its congener. *J Am Chem Soc,* 111, 8929–8931.
11. Holmes, M. J., Lewis, R. J., Poli, M. A., and Gillespie, N. C., 1991. Strain dependent production of ciguatoxin precursors (gambiertoxins) by *Gambierdiscus toxicus* (Dinophyceae) in culture. *Toxicon,* 29, 761–775.
12. Satake, M., Murata, M., and Yasumoto, T., 1993. The structure of CTX3c, a ciguatoxin congener isolated from cultured *Gambierdiscus toxicus. Tetraheron Lett,* 34, 1975–1978.

13. Satake, M., Ishibashi, Y., Legrand, A. M., and Yasumoto, T., 1996. Isolation and structure of ciguatoxin-4A, a new ciguatoxin precursor, from cultures of dinoflagellate *Gambierdiscus toxicus* and parrotfish Scarus gibbus. *Biosci Biotechnol Biochem*, 60, 2103–2105.

14. Otero, P., Perez, S., Alfonso, A. et al., 2010. First toxin profile of ciguateric fish in Madeira Arquipelago (Europe). *Anal Chem*, 82, 6032–6039.

15. Legrand, A. M., Litaudon, M., Genthon, J. N., Bagnis, R., and Yasumoto, T., 1989. Isolation and some properties of ciguatoxin. *J Appl Phycol* 1, 183–188.

16. Vernoux, J. P. and Lewis, R. J., 1997. Isolation and characterisation of Caribbean ciguatoxins from the horse-eye jack (Caranx latus). *Toxicon*, 35, 889–900.

17. Lewis, R. J. and Sellin, M., 1993. Recovery of ciguatoxin from fish flesh. *Toxicon*, 31, 1333–1336.

18. Lewis, R. J. and Jones, A., 1997. Characterization of ciguatoxins and ciguatoxin congeners present in ciguateric fish by gradient reverse-phase high-performance liquid chromatography/mass spectrometry. *Toxicon*, 35, 159–168.

19. Lewis, R. J., Sellin, M., Poli, M. A., Norton, R. S., MacLeod, J. K., and Sheil, M. M., 1991. Purification and characterization of ciguatoxins from moray eel (*Lycodontis javanicus*, Muraenidae). *Toxicon*, 29, 1115–1127.

20. Lewis, R. J., Norton, R. S., Brereton, I. M., and Eccles, C. D., 1993. Ciguatoxin-2 is a diastereomer of ciguatoxin-3. *Toxicon*, 31, 637–643.

21. Satake, M., Fukui, M., Legrand, A. M., Cruchet, P., and Yasumoto, T., 1998. Isolation and structures of new ciguatoxin analogs, 2,3-dihydroxyCTX3C and 51-hydroxyCTX3C, accumulated in tropical reef fish. *Tetrahedron Lett*, 39, 1197–1198.

22. Pottier, I., Hamilton, B., Jones, A., Lewis, R. J., and Vernoux, J. P., 2003. Identification of slow and fast-acting toxins in a highly ciguatoxic barracuda (*Sphyraena barracuda*) by HPLC/MS and radiolabelled ligand binding. *Toxicon*, 42, 663–672.

23. Pottier, I., Vernoux, J. P., Jones, A., and Lewis, R. J., 2002. Analysis of toxin profiles in three different fish species causing ciguatera fish poisoning in Guadeloupe, French West Indies. *Food Addit Contam*, 19, 1034–1042.

24. Pottier, I., Vernoux, J. P., Jones, A., and Lewis, R. J., 2002. Characterisation of multiple Caribbean ciguatoxins and congeners in individual specimens of horse-eye jack (*Caranx latus*) by high-performance liquid chromatography/mass spectrometry. *Toxicon*, 40, 929–939.

25. Hamilton, B., Hurbungs, M., Jones, A., and Lewis, R. J., 2002. Multiple ciguatoxins present in Indian Ocean reef fish. *Toxicon*, 40, 1347–1353.

26. Hamilton, B., Hurbungs, M., Vernoux, J. P., Jones, A., and Lewis, R. J., 2002. Isolation and characterisation of Indian Ocean ciguatoxin. *Toxicon*, 40, 685–693.

27. Baden, D. G., 1989. Brevetoxins: Unique polyether dinoflagellate toxins. *FASEB J*, 3, 1807–1817.

28. Gawley, R. E., Rein, K. S., Kinoshita, M., and Baden, D. G., 1992. Binding of brevetoxins and ciguatoxin to the voltage-sensitive sodium channel and conformational analysis of brevetoxin B. *Toxicon*, 30, 780–785.

29. Lewis, R. J., Molgo, J., and Adams, D. J., 2000. Ciguatera toxins: Pharmacology of toxins involved in ciguatera and related fish poisonings, in *Seafood and Freshwater Toxins: Pharmacology, Physiology, and Detection*, 1st edn. Botana, L. M., Ed. Marcel Dekker, New York. pp. 419–447.

30. Tester, P. A., Feldman, R. L., Nau, A. W., Kibler, S. R., and Wayne Litaker, R. 2010. Ciguatera fish poisoning and sea surface temperatures in the Caribbean Sea and the West Indies. *Toxicon*, 56, 698–710.

31. Hall, G. and Kirk, M., 2005. Food-borne illness in Australia. Annual incidence circa 2000. *Australian Government Department of Health and Ageing*.

32. Chateau-Degata, M.-L., Chinainb, M., Cerfc, N., Gingrasa, S., Hubertc, B., and Dewaillya, E., 2005. Seawater temperature, Gambierdiscus spp. variability and incidence of ciguatera poisoning in French Polynesia. *Harmful Algae*, 4, 1053–1062.

33. Perez-Arellano, J. L., Luzardo, O. P., Perez Brito, A. et al., 2005. Ciguatera fish poisoning, Canary Islands. *Emerg Infect Dis*, 11, 1981–1982.

34. Bentur, Y. and Spanier, E., 2007. Ciguatoxin-like substances in edible fish on the eastern Mediterranean. *Clin Toxicol (Phila)*, 45, 695–700.

35. Skinner, M. P., Brewer, T. D., Johnstone, R., Fleming, L. E., and Lewis, R. J., 2011. Ciguatera fish poisoning in the Pacific Islands (1998 to 2008). *PLoS Negl Trop Dis*, 5, e1416.

36. Gillespie, N. C., Lewis, R. J., Pearn, J. H. et al., 1986. Ciguatera in Australia. Occurrence, clinical features, pathophysiology and management. *Med J Aust*, 145, 584–590.

37. Lewis, R. J., 2006. Ciguatera: Australian perspectives on a global problem. *Toxicon*, 48, 799–809.
38. Jeong, H. J., Lim, A. S., Jang, S. H. et al., 2012. First report of the epiphytic dinoflagellate *Gambierdiscus caribaeus* in the temperate waters off Jeju Island, Korea: Morphology and molecular characterization. *J Eukaryot Microbiol*, 59, 637–650.
39. Chan, W. H., Mak, Y. L., Wu, J. J. et al., 2011. Spatial distribution of ciguateric fish in the Republic of Kiribati. *Chemosphere*, 84, 117–123.
40. Lewis, R. J., 1992. Socioeconomic impacts and management ciguatera in the Pacific. *Bull Soc Pathol Exot*, 85, 427–434.
41. Bagnis, R., Kuberski, T., and Laugier, S., 1979. Clinical observations on 3,009 cases of ciguatera (fish poisoning) in the South Pacific. *Am J Trop Med Hyg*, 28, 1067–1073.
42. Lawrence, D. N., Enriquez, M. B., Lumish, R. M., and Maceo, A., 1980. Ciguatera fish poisoning in Miami. *JAMA*, 244, 254–258.
43. Stewart, I., Lewis, R. J., Eaglesham, G. K., Graham, G. C., Poole, S., and Craig, S. B., 2010. Emerging tropical diseases in Australia. Part 2. Ciguatera fish poisoning. *Ann Trop Med Parasitol*, 104, 557–571.
44. Gollop, J. H. and Pon, E. W., 1992. Ciguatera: A review. *Hawaii Med J*, 51, 91–99.
45. Dickey, R. W. and Plakas, S. M., 2010. Ciguatera: A public health perspective. *Toxicon*, 56, 123–136.
46. Friedman, M. A., Fleming, L. E., Fernandez, M. et al., 2008. Ciguatera fish poisoning: Treatment, prevention and management. *Mar Drugs*, 6, 456–479.
47. Swift, A. E. and Swift, T. R., 1993. Ciguatera. *J Toxicol Clin Toxicol*, 31, 1–29.
48. Lange, W. R., 1994. Ciguatera fish poisoning. *Am Fam Physician*, 50, 579–584.
49. Quod, J. P. and Turquet, J., 1996. Ciguatera in Reunion Island (SW Indian Ocean): Epidemiology and clinical patterns. *Toxicon*, 34, 779–785.
50. Baumann, F., Bourrat, M. B., and Pauillac, S., 2010. Prevalence, symptoms and chronicity of ciguatera in New Caledonia: Results from an adult population survey conducted in Noumea during 2005. *Toxicon*, 56, 662–667.
51. Cameron, J. and Capra, M. F., 1993. The basis of the paradoxical disturbance of temperature perception in ciguatera poisoning. *J Toxicol Clin Toxicol*, 31, 571–579.
52. Pearn, J., 2001. Neurology of ciguatera. *J Neurol Neurosurg Psychiatry*, 70, 4–8.
53. Vetter, I., Touska, F., Hess, A. et al., 2012. Ciguatoxins activate specific cold pain pathways to elicit burning pain from cooling. *EMBO J*, 31, 3795–3808.
54. Friedman, M. A., Arena, P., Levin, B. et al., 2007. Neuropsychological study of ciguatera fish poisoning: A longitudinal case-control study. *Arch Clin Neuropsychol*, 22, 545–553.
55. Arena, P., Levin, B., Fleming, L. E., Friedman, M. A., and Blythe, D. G., 2004. A pilot study of the cognitive and psychological correlates of chronic ciguatera poisoning. *Harmful Algae*, 3, 51–60.
56. Bagnis, R. and Legrand, A.-M., 1987. Clinical features on 12,890 cases of ciguatera (fish poisoning) in French Polynesia, in *Progress in Venom and Toxin Research*, Gopalakrishnakone, P. and Tan, C. K., (Eds.), National University of Singapore and International Society of Toxinology, Asia-Pacific Section, Singapour, pp. 372–384.
57. Chan, T. Y. and Wang, A. Y., 1993. Life-threatening bradycardia and hypotension in a patient with ciguatera fish poisoning. *Trans R Soc Trop Med Hyg*, 87, 71.
58. Miller, R. M., Pavia, S., and Keary, P., 1999. Cardiac toxicity associated with ciguatera poisoning. *Aust N Z J Med*, 29, 373–374.
59. Bowman, P. B., 1984. Amitriptyline and ciguatera. *Med J Aust*, 140, 802.
60. Davis, R. T. and Villar, L. A., 1986. Symptomatic improvement with amitriptyline in ciguatera fish poisoning. *N Engl J Med*, 315, 65.
61. Calvert, G. M., Hryhorczuk, D. O., and Leikin, J. B., 1987. Treatment of ciguatera fish poisoning with amitriptyline and nifedipine. *J Toxicol Clin Toxicol*, 25, 423–428.
62. Ruprecht, K., Rieckmann, P., and Giess, R., 2001. Ciguatera: Clinical relevance of a marine neurotoxin. *Dtsch Med Wochenschr*, 126, 812–814.
63. Perez, C. M., Vasquez, P. A., and Perret, C. F., 2001. Treatment of ciguatera poisoning with gabapentin. *N Engl J Med*, 344, 692–693.
64. Lange, W. R., Kreider, S. D., Hattwick, M., and Hobbs, J., 1988. Potential benefit of tocainide in the treatment of ciguatera: Report of three cases. *Am J Med*, 84, 1087–1088.
65. Berlin, R. M., King, S. L., and Blythe, D. G., 1992. Symptomatic improvement of chronic fatigue with fluoxetine in ciguatera fish poisoning. *Med J Aust*, 157, 567.

66. Kumar-Roine, S., Taiana Darius, H., Matsui, M. et al., 2011. A review of traditional remedies of ciguatera fish poisoning in the Pacific. *Phytother Res*, 25, 947–958.

67. Matsui, M., Kumar-Roine, S., Darius, H. T., Chinain, M., Laurent, D., and Pauillac, S., 2009. Characterisation of the anti-inflammatory potential of Vitex trifolia L. (Labiatae), a multipurpose plant of the Pacific traditional medicine. *J Ethnopharmacol*, 126, 427–433.

68. Kumar-Roine, S., Matsui, M., Reybier, K. et al., 2009. Ability of certain plant extracts traditionally used to treat ciguatera fish poisoning to inhibit nitric oxide production in RAW 264.7 macrophages. *J Ethnopharmacol*, 123, 369–377.

69. Bourdy, G., Cabalion, P., Amade, P., and Laurent, D., 1992. Traditional remedies used in the western Pacific for the treatment of ciguatera poisoning. *J Ethnopharmacol*, 36, 163–174.

70. Palafox, N. A., 1992. Review of the clinical use of intravenous mannitol with ciguatera fish poisoning from 1988 to 1992. *Bull Soc Pathol Exot*, 85, 423–424.

71. Palafox, N. A., Jain, L. G., Pinano, A. Z., Gulick, T. M., Williams, R. K., and Schatz, I. J., 1988. Successful treatment of ciguatera fish poisoning with intravenous mannitol. *JAMA*, 259, 2740–2742.

72. Pearn, J. H., Lewis, R. J., Ruff, T. et al., 1989. Ciguatera and mannitol: Experience with a new treatment regimen. *Med J Aust*, 151, 77–80.

73. Blythe, D. G., De Sylva, D. P., Fleming, L. E., Ayyar, R. A., Baden, D. G., and Shrank, K., 1992. Clinical experience with i.v. Mannitol in the treatment of ciguatera. *Bull Soc Pathol Exot*, 85, 425–426.

74. Birinyi-Strachan, L. C., Davies, M. J., Lewis, R. J., and Nicholson, G. M., 2005. Neuroprotectant effects of iso-osmolar D-mannitol to prevent Pacific ciguatoxin-1 induced alterations in neuronal excitability: A comparison with other osmotic agents and free radical scavengers. *Neuropharmacology*, 49, 669–686.

75. Mattei, C., Molgo, J., Marquais, M., Vernoux, J., and Benoit, E., 1999. Hyperosmolar D-mannitol reverses the increased membrane excitability and the nodal swelling caused by Caribbean ciguatoxin-1 in single frog myelinated axons. *Brain Res*, 847, 50–58.

76. Allsop, J. L., Martini, L., Lebris, H., Pollard, J., Walsh, J., and Hodgkinson, S., 1986. Neurologic manifestations of ciguatera. 3 cases with a neurophysiologic study and examination of one nerve biopsy. *Rev Neurol (Paris)*, 142, 590–597.

77. Bagnis, R., Spiegel, A., Boutin, J. P. et al., 1992. Evaluation of the efficacy of mannitol in the treatment of ciguatera in French Polynesia. *Med Trop (Mars)*, 52, 67–73.

78. Mitchell, G., 2005. Treatment of a mild chronic case of ciguatera fish poisoning with intravenous mannitol, a case study. *Pac Health Dialog*, 12, 155–157.

79. Schwarz, E. S., Mullins, M. E., and Brooks, C. B., 2008. Ciguatera poisoning successfully treated with delayed mannitol. *Ann Emerg Med*, 52, 476–477.

80. Purcell, C. E., Capra, M. F., and Cameron, J., 1999. Action of mannitol in ciguatoxin-intoxicated rats. *Toxicon*, 37, 67–76.

81. Lewis, R. J., Hoy, A. W., and Sellin, M., 1993. Ciguatera and mannitol: In vivo and in vitro assessment in mice. *Toxicon*, 31, 1039–1050.

82. Schnorf, H., Taurarii, M., and Cundy, T., 2002. Ciguatera fish poisoning: A double-blind randomized trial of mannitol therapy. *Neurology*, 58, 873–880.

83. Isbister, G. K. and Kiernan, M. C., 2005. Neurotoxic marine poisoning. *Lancet Neurol*, 4, 219–228.

84. Inoue, M., Lee, N., Tsumuraya, T., Fujii, I., and Hirama, M., 2009. Use of monoclonal antibodies as an effective strategy for treatment of ciguatera poisoning. *Toxicon*, 53, 802–805.

85. Shoemaker, R. C., House, D., and Ryan, J. C., 2010. Defining the neurotoxin derived illness chronic ciguatera using markers of chronic systemic inflammatory disturbances: A case/control study. *Neurotoxicol Teratol*, 32, 633–639.

86. Bottein, M. Y., Wang, Z., and Ramsdell, J. S., 2011. Toxicokinetics of the ciguatoxin P-CTX-1 in rats after intraperitoneal or oral administration. *Toxicology*, 284, 1–6.

87. Hoffman, P. A., Granade, H. R., and McMillan, J. P., 1983. The mouse ciguatoxin bioassay: A dose-response curve and symptomatology analysis. *Toxicon*, 21, 363–369.

88. Bottein Dechraoui, M. Y., Rezvani, A. H., Gordon, C. J., Levin, E. D., and Ramsdell, J. S., 2008. Repeat exposure to ciguatoxin leads to enhanced and sustained thermoregulatory, pain threshold and motor activity responses in mice: Relationship to blood ciguatoxin concentrations. *Toxicology*, 246, 55–62.

89. Terao, K., Ito, E., Oarada, M., Ishibashi, Y., Legrand, A. M., and Yasumoto, T., 1991. Light and electron microscopic studies of pathologic changes induced in mice by ciguatoxin poisoning. *Toxicon*, 29, 633–643.

90. Ito, E., Yasumoto, T., and Terao, K., 1996. Morphological observations of diarrhea in mice caused by experimental ciguatoxicosis. *Toxicon*, 34, 111–122.

91. Peng, Y. G., Taylor, T. B., Finch, R. E., Moeller, P. D., and Ramsdell, J. S., 1995. Neuroexcitatory actions of ciguatoxin on brain regions associated with thermoregulation. *Neuroreport*, 6, 305–309.

92. Ryan, J. C., Morey, J. S., Bottein, M. Y., Ramsdell, J. S., and Van Dolah, F. M., 2010. Gene expression profiling in brain of mice exposed to the marine neurotoxin ciguatoxin reveals an acute anti-inflammatory, neuroprotective response. *BMC Neurosci*, 11, 107.

93. Matsui, M., Kumar-Roine, S., Darius, H. T., Chinain, M., Laurent, D., and Pauillac, S., 2010. Pacific ciguatoxin 1B-induced modulation of inflammatory mediators in a murine macrophage cell line. *Toxicon*, 56, 776–784.

94. Ryan, J. C., Bottein Dechraoui, M. Y., Morey, J. S. et al., 2007. Transcriptional profiling of whole blood and serum protein analysis of mice exposed to the neurotoxin Pacific Ciguatoxin-1. *Neurotoxicology*, 28, 1099–1109.

95. Morey, J. S., Ryan, J. C., Bottein Dechraoui, M. Y. et al., 2008. Liver genomic responses to ciguatoxin: Evidence for activation of phase I and phase II detoxification pathways following an acute hypothermic response in mice. *Toxicol Sci*, 103, 298–310.

96. Cameron, J., Flowers, A. E., and Capra, M. F., 1991. Effects of ciguatoxin on nerve excitability in rats (Part I). *J Neurol Sci*, 101, 87–92.

97. Vacher, H., Mohapatra, D. P., and Trimmer, J. S., 2008. Localization and targeting of voltage-dependent ion channels in mammalian central neurons. *Physiol Rev*, 88, 1407–1447.

98. Poli, M. A., Mende, T. J., and Baden, D. G., 1986. Brevetoxins, unique activators of voltage-sensitive sodium channels, bind to specific sites in rat brain synaptosomes. *Mol Pharmacol*, 30, 129–135.

99. Poli, M. A., Lewis, R. J., Dickey, R. W., Musser, S. M., Buckner, C. A., and Carpenter, L. G., 1997. Identification of Caribbean ciguatoxins as the cause of an outbreak of fish poisoning among U.S. soldiers in Haiti. *Toxicon*, 35, 733–741.

100. Sharkey, R. G., Jover, E., Couraud, F., Baden, D. G., and Catterall, W. A., 1987. Allosteric modulation of neurotoxin binding to voltage-sensitive sodium channels by Ptychodiscus brevis toxin 2. *Mol Pharmacol*, 31, 273–278.

101. Hogg, R. C., Lewis, R. J., and Adams, D. J., 1998. Ciguatoxin (CTX-1) modulates single tetrodotoxin-sensitive sodium channels in rat parasympathetic neurones. *Neurosci Lett*, 252, 103–106.

102. Cestele, S., Sampieri, F., Rochat, H., and Gordon, D., 1996. Tetrodotoxin reverses brevetoxin allosteric inhibition of scorpion alpha-toxin binding on rat brain sodium channels. *J Biol Chem*, 271, 18329–18332.

103. Lombet, A., Bidard, J. N., and Lazdunski, M., 1987. Ciguatoxin and brevetoxins share a common receptor site on the neuronal voltage-dependent Na+ channel. *FEBS Lett*, 219, 355–359.

104. Dechraoui, M. Y., Naar, J., Pauillac, S., and Legrand, A. M., 1999. Ciguatoxins and brevetoxins, neurotoxic polyether compounds active on sodium channels. *Toxicon*, 37, 125–143.

105. Trainer, V. L., Baden, D. G., and Catterall, W. A., 1994. Identification of peptide components of the brevetoxin receptor site of rat brain sodium channels. *J Biol Chem*, 269, 19904–19909.

106. Manger, R. L., Leja, L. S., Lee, S. Y., Hungerford, J. M., and Wekell, M. M., 1993. Tetrazolium-based cell bioassay for neurotoxins active on voltage-sensitive sodium channels: Semiautomated assay for saxitoxins, brevetoxins, and ciguatoxins. *Anal Biochem*, 214, 190–194.

107. Molgó, J., Benoit, E., Comella, J. X., and Legrand, A. M., 1992. Ciguatoxin: A tool for research on sodium-dependent mechanisms, in *Methods in Neuroscience*. Conn, P. M., Ed. Academic Press, New York. pp. 149–164.

108. Benoit, E., Juzans, P., Legrand, A. M., and Molgo, J., 1996. Nodal swelling produced by ciguatoxin-induced selective activation of sodium channels in myelinated nerve fibers. *Neuroscience*, 71, 1121–1131.

109. Bidard, J. N., Vijverberg, H. P., Frelin, C. et al., 1984. Ciguatoxin is a novel type of Na+ channel toxin. *J Biol Chem*, 259, 8353–8357.

110. Strachan, L. C., Lewis, R. J., and Nicholson, G. M., 1999. Differential actions of pacific ciguatoxin-1 on sodium channel subtypes in mammalian sensory neurons. *J Pharmacol Exp Ther*, 288, 379–388.

111. Yamaoka, K., Inoue, M., Miyahara, H., Miyazaki, K., and Hirama, M., 2004. A quantitative and comparative study of the effects of a synthetic ciguatoxin CTX3C on the kinetic properties of voltage-dependent sodium channels. *Br J Pharmacol*, 142, 879–889.

112. Yamaoka, K., Inoue, M., Miyazaki, K. et al., 2009. Synthetic ciguatoxins selectively activate Nav1.8-derived chimeric sodium channels expressed in HEK293 cells. *J Biol Chem*, 284, 7597–7605.

113. Hidalgo, J., Liberona, J. L., Molgo, J., and Jaimovich, E., 2002. Pacific ciguatoxin-1b effect over Na+ and K+ currents, inositol 1,4,5-triphosphate content and intracellular Ca2+ signals in cultured rat myotubes. *Br J Pharmacol*, 137, 1055–1062.

114. Legrand, A. M. and Bagnis, R., 1984. Effects of ciguatoxin and maitotoxin on isolated rat atria and rabbit duodenum. *Toxicon*, 22, 471–475.

115. Perez, S., Vale, C., Alonso, E. et al., 2012. Effect of gambierol and its tetracyclic and heptacyclic analogues in cultured cerebellar neurons: A structure-activity relationships study. *Chem Res Toxicol*, 25, 1929–1937.

116. Perez, S., Vale, C., Alonso, E. et al., 2011. A comparative study of the effect of ciguatoxins on voltage-dependent Na+ and K+ channels in cerebellar neurons. *Chem Res Toxicol*, 24, 587–596.

117. Birinyi-Strachan, L. C., Gunning, S. J., Lewis, R. J., and Nicholson, G. M., 2005. Block of voltage-gated potassium channels by Pacific ciguatoxin-1 contributes to increased neuronal excitability in rat sensory neurons. *Toxicol Appl Pharmacol*, 204, 175–186.

118. Schlumberger, S., Mattei, C., Molgo, J., and Benoit, E., 2010. Dual action of a dinoflagellate-derived precursor of Pacific ciguatoxins (P-CTX-4B) on voltage-dependent K(+) and Na(+) channels of single myelinated axons. *Toxicon*, 56, 768–775.

119. Cuypers, E., Abdel-Mottaleb, Y., Kopljar, I. et al., 2008. Gambierol, a toxin produced by the dinoflagellate *Gambierdiscus toxicus*, is a potent blocker of voltage-gated potassium channels. *Toxicon*, 51, 974–983.

120. Kopljar, I., Labro, A. J., Cuypers, E. et al., 2009. A polyether biotoxin binding site on the lipid-exposed face of the pore domain of Kv channels revealed by the marine toxin gambierol. *Proc Natl Acad Sci U S A*, 106, 9896–9901.

121. Cuypers, E., Yanagihara, A., Rainier, J. D., and Tytgat, J., 2007. TRPV1 as a key determinant in ciguatera and neurotoxic shellfish poisoning. *Biochem Biophys Res Commun*, 361, 214–217.

122. Lewis, R. J. and Endean, R., 1986. Direct and indirect effects of ciguatoxin on guinea-pig atria and papillary muscles. *Naunyn Schmiedebergs Arch Pharmacol*, 334, 313–322.

123. Lewis, R. J., Hoy, A. W., and McGiffin, D. C., 1992. Action of ciguatoxin on human atrial trabeculae. *Toxicon*, 30, 907–914.

124. Seino, A., Kobayashi, M., Momose, K., Yasumoto, T., and Ohizumi, Y., 1988. The mode of inotropic action of ciguatoxin on guinea-pig cardiac muscle. *Br J Pharmacol*, 95, 876–882.

125. Lewis, R. J. and Hoy, A. W., 1993. Comparative action of three major ciguatoxins on guinea-pig atria and ilea. *Toxicon*, 31, 437–446.

126. Lewis, R. J., 1988. Negative inotropic and arrhythmic effects of high doses of ciguatoxin on guinea-pig atria and papillary muscles. *Toxicon*, 26, 639–649.

127. Sauviat, M. P., Marquais, M., and Vernoux, J. P., 2002. Muscarinic effects of the Caribbean ciguatoxin C-CTX-1 on frog atrial heart muscle. *Toxicon*, 40, 1155–1163.

128. Lewis, R. J. and Endean, R., 1984. Mode of action of ciguatoxin from the Spanish Mackerel, Scomberomorus commerson, on the guinea-pig ileum and vas deferens. *J Pharmacol Exp Ther*, 228, 756–760.

129. Ohizumi, Y., Shibata, S., and Tachibana, K., 1981. Mode of the excitatory and inhibitory actions of ciguatoxin in the guinea-pig vas deferens. *J Pharmacol Exp Ther*, 217, 475–480.

130. Ohizumi, Y., Ishida, Y., and Shibata, S., 1982. Mode of the ciguatoxin-induced supersensitivity in the guinea-pig vas deferens. *J Pharmacol Exp Ther*, 221, 748–752.

131. Brock, J. A., McLachlan, E. M., Jobling, P., and Lewis, R. J., 1995. Electrical activity in rat tail artery during asynchronous activation of postganglionic nerve terminals by ciguatoxin-1. *Br J Pharmacol*, 116, 2213–2220.

132. Verkhratsky, A. J. and Petersen, O. H., 1998. Neuronal calcium stores. *Cell Calcium*, 24, 333–343.

133. Kostyuk, P. and Verkhratsky, A., 1994. Calcium stores in neurons and glia. *Neuroscience*, 63, 381–404.

134. Molgo, J., Shimahara, T., and Legrand, A. M., 1993. Ciguatoxin, extracted from poisonous morays eels, causes sodium-dependent calcium mobilization in NG108–15 neuroblastoma x glioma hybrid cells. *Neurosci Lett*, 158, 147–150.

135. Molgo, J., Comella, J. X., and Legrand, A. M., 1990. Ciguatoxin enhances quantal transmitter release from frog motor nerve terminals. *Br J Pharmacol*, 99, 695–700.

136. Molgo, J., Comella, J. X., Shimahara, T., and Legrand, A. M., 1991. Tetrodotoxin-sensitive ciguatoxin effects on quantal release, synaptic vesicle depletion, and calcium mobilization. *Ann N Y Acad Sci*, 635, 485–488.

137. Molgo, J., Gaudry-Talarmain, Y. M., Legrand, A. M., and Moulian, N., 1993. Ciguatoxin extracted from poisonous moray eels Gymnothorax javanicus triggers acetylcholine release from Torpedo cholinergic synaptosomes via reversed Na(+)-Ca2+ exchange. *Neurosci Lett*, 160, 65–68.

138. Hermoni, M., Barzilai, A., and Rahamimoff, H., 1987. Modulation of the Na+-Ca2+ antiport by its ionic environment: The effect of lithium. *Isr J Med Sci*, 23, 44–48.

139. Gaudry-Talarmain, Y. M., Molgo, J., Meunier, F. A., Moulian, N., and Legrand, A. M., 1996. Reversed mode Na(+)-Ca2+ exchange activated by ciguatoxin (CTX-1b) enhances acetylcholine release from Torpedo cholinergic synaptosomes. *Ann N Y Acad Sci*, 779, 404–406.

140. Molgo, J., Juzans, P., and Legrand, A. M., 1994. Confocal laser scanning microscopy: A new tool for studying the effects of ciguatoxin (CTX-1b) and mannitol at motor nerve terminals of the neuromuscular junction in situ. *Memoirs of the Queensland Museum* 34, 577–585.

141. Mattei, C., Benoit, E., Juzans, P., Legrand, A. M., and Molgo, J., 1997. Gambiertoxin (CTX-4B), purified from wild *Gambierdiscus toxicus* dinoflagellates, induces Na(+)-dependent swelling of single frog myelinated axons and motor nerve terminals in situ. *Neurosci Lett*, 234, 75–78.

142. Mattei, C., Dechraoui, M. Y., Molgo, J., Meunier, F. A., Legrand, A. M., and Benoit, E., 1999. Neurotoxins targetting receptor site 5 of voltage-dependent sodium channels increase the nodal volume of myelinated axons. *J Neurosci Res*, 55, 666–673.

143. Benoit, E. and Legrand, A. M., 1992. Purified ciguatoxin-induced modifications in excitability of myelinated nerve fibre. *Bull Soc Pathol Exot*, 85, 497–499.

144. Benoit, E. and Legrand, A. M., 1994. Gambiertoxin-induced modifications of the membrane potential of myelinated nerve fibres. *Memoirs of the Queensland Museum*, 34, 461–464.

145. Cameron, J., Flowers, A. E., and Capra, M. F., 1991. Electrophysiological studies on ciguatera poisoning in man (Part II). *J Neurol Sci*, 101, 93–97.

146. Cameron, J., Flowers, A. E., and Capra, M. F., 1993. Modification of the peripheral nerve disturbance in ciguatera poisoning in rats with lidocaine. *Muscle Nerve*, 16, 782–786.

147. Molgo, J., Meunier, F. A., Dechraoui, M. Y., Benoit, E., Mattei, C., and Legrand, A. M., 1998. Sodium-dependent alterations of synaptic transmission mechanisms by brevetoxins and ciguatoxins, in *Harmful Microalgae.*, Reguera, B., Blanco, J., Fernández, M. L., and Wyatt, T., (Eds.), Santiago De Compostella: Xunta de Galicia and Intergovernmental Oceanographic Commission of UNESCO, pp. 594–597.

148. Marquais, M., Vernoux, J. P., Molgo, J., Sauviat, M. P., and Lewis, R. J., 1998. Isolation and electrophysiological characterisation of a new ciguatoxin extracted from Caribbean fish, in *Harmful Microalgae.*, Reguera, B., Blanco, J., Fernández, M. L., and Wyatt, T., (Eds.), Santiago De Compostella: Xunta de Galicia and Intergovernmental Oceanographic Commission of UNESCO, pp. 476–477.

149. Hamblin, P. A., McLachlan, E. M., and Lewis, R. J., 1995. Sub-nanomolar concentrations of ciguatoxin-1 excite preganglionic terminals in guinea pig sympathetic ganglia. *Naunyn Schmiedebergs Arch Pharmacol*, 352, 236–246.

150. Lehane, L., 2000. Ciguatera update. *Med J Aust*, 172, 176–179.

151. Lehane, L. and Lewis, R. J., 2000. Ciguatera: Recent advances but the risk remains. *Int J Food Microbiol*, 61, 91–125.

152. Caillaud, A., de la Iglesia, P., Darius, H. T. et al., 2010. Update on methodologies available for ciguatoxin determination: Perspectives to confront the onset of ciguatera fish poisoning in Europe. *Mar Drugs*, 8, 1838–1907.

153. Bottein Dechraoui, M. Y., Wang, Z., and Ramsdell, J. S., 2007. Optimization of ciguatoxin extraction method from blood for Pacific ciguatoxin (P-CTX-1). *Toxicon*, 49, 100–105.

154. Bottein Dechraoui, M. Y., Wang, Z., Turquet, J. et al., 2005. Biomonitoring of ciguatoxin exposure in mice using blood collection cards. *Toxicon*, 46, 243–251.

155. Matta, J., Navas, J., Milad, M., Manger, R., Hupka, A., and Frazer, T., 2002. A pilot study for the detection of acute ciguatera intoxication in human blood. *J Toxicol Clin Toxicol*, 40, 49–57.

156. Chungue, E., Bagnis, R., and Parc, F., 1984. The use of mosquitoes (Aedes aegypti) to detect ciguatoxin in surgeon fishes (Ctenochaetus striatus). *Toxicon*, 22, 161–164.

157. Vernoux, J. P., Lahlou, N., Magras, L. P., and Greaux, J. B., 1985. Chick feeding test: A simple system to detect ciguatoxin. *Acta Trop*, 42, 235–240.

158. Labrousse, H., Pauillac, S., Jehl-Martinez, C., Legrand, A. M., and Avrameas, S., 1992. Techniques de détection de la ciguatoxine in vivo et in vitro. *Océanis*, 18, 189–191.
159. Lewis, R. J., 1995. Detection of ciguatoxins and related benthic dinoflagellate toxins: In vivo and in vitro methods, in *Manual on Harmful Marine Microalgae IOC Manuals and Guides UNESCO*. Hallegraph, G. M., Anderson, D. M., and Cembella, A. D., Eds., Paris, France. pp. 135–161.
160. Labrousse, H. and Matile, L., 1996. Toxicological biotest on Diptera larvae to detect ciguatoxins and various other toxic substances. *Toxicon*, 34, 881–891.
161. Banner, A. H., Sasaki, S., Helfrich, P., Alender, C. B., and Scheuer, P. J., 1961. Bioassay of ciguatera toxin. *Nature*, 189, 229–230.
162. Lewis, R. J., 1992. Ciguatoxins are potent ichthyotoxins. *Toxicon*, 30, 207–211.
163. Manger, R. L., Leja, L. S., Lee, S. Y. et al., 1995. Detection of sodium channel toxins: Directed cytotoxicity assays of purified ciguatoxins, brevetoxins, saxitoxins, and seafood extracts. *J AOAC Int*, 78, 521–527.
164. Caillaud, A., Eixarch, H., de la Iglesia, P. et al., 2012. Towards the standardisation of the neuroblastoma (neuro-2a) cell-based assay for ciguatoxin-like toxicity detection in fish: Application to fish caught in the Canary Islands. *Food Addit Contam Part A Chem Anal Control Expo Risk Assess*, 29, 1000–1010.
165. Louzao, M. C., Vieytes, M. R., Yasumoto, T., and Botana, L. M., 2004. Detection of sodium channel activators by a rapid fluorimetric microplate assay. *Chem Res Toxicol*, 17, 572–578.
166. Dechraoui, M. Y., Tiedeken, J. A., Persad, R. et al., 2005. Use of two detection methods to discriminate ciguatoxins from brevetoxins: Application to great barracuda from Florida Keys. *Toxicon*, 46, 261–270.
167. Fairey, E. R., Edmunds, J. S., and Ramsdell, J. S., 1997. A cell-based assay for brevetoxins, saxitoxins, and ciguatoxins using a stably expressed c-fos-luciferase reporter gene. *Anal Biochem*, 251, 129–132.
168. Campora, C. E., Hokama, Y., and Ebesu, J. S., 2006. Comparative analysis of purified Pacific and Caribbean ciguatoxin congeners and related marine toxins using a modified ELISA technique. *J Clin Lab Anal*, 20, 121–5.
169. Empey Campora, C., Dierking, J., Tamaru, C. S., Hokama, Y., and Vincent, D., 2008. Detection of ciguatoxin in fish tissue using sandwich ELISA and neuroblastoma cell bioassay. *J Clin Lab Anal*, 22, 246–253.
170. Tsumuraya, T., Fujii, I., and Hirama, M., 2010. Production of monoclonal antibodies for sandwich immunoassay detection of Pacific ciguatoxins. *Toxicon*, 56, 797–803.
171. Tsumuraya, T., Takeuchi, K., Yamashita, S., Fujii, I., and Hirama, M., 2012. Development of a monoclonal antibody against the left wing of ciguatoxin CTX1B: Thiol strategy and detection using a sandwich ELISA. *Toxicon*, 60, 348–357.
172. Empey Campora, C., Hokama, Y., Yabusaki, K., and Isobe, M., 2008. Development of an enzyme-linked immunosorbent assay for the detection of ciguatoxin in fish tissue using chicken immunoglobulin Y. *J Clin Lab Anal*, 22, 239–245.
173. Hokama, Y., Abad, M. A., and Kimura, L. H., 1983. A rapid enzyme-immunoassay for the detection of ciguatoxin in contaminated fish tissues. *Toxicon*, 21, 817–824.
174. Oguri, H., Hirama, M., Tsumuraya, T. et al., 2003. Synthesis-based approach toward direct sandwich immunoassay for ciguatoxin CTX3C. *J Am Chem Soc*, 125, 7608–7612.
175. Hokama, Y., Asahina, A. Y., Hong, T. W., Shang, E. S., and Miyahara, J. T., 1990. Evaluation of the stick enzyme immunoassay in Caranx sp. and Seriola dumerili associated with ciguatera. *J Clin Lab Anal*, 4, 363–366.
176. Lewis, R. J., Yang, A., and Jones, A., 2009. Rapid extraction combined with LC-tandem mass spectrometry (CREM-LC/MS/MS) for the determination of ciguatoxins in ciguateric fish flesh. *Toxicon*, 54, 62–66.
177. Lewis, R. J., Jones, A., and Vernoux, J. P., 1999. HPLC/tandem electrospray mass spectrometry for the determination of Sub-ppb levels of Pacific and Caribbean ciguatoxins in crude extracts of fish. *Anal Chem*, 71, 247–250.

33

Cyclic Imine Toxins: Chemistry, Origin, Metabolism, Pharmacology, Toxicology, and Detection

Jordi Molgó, Rómulo Aráoz, Evelyne Benoit, and Bogdan I. Iorga

CONTENTS

33.1 Introduction

Bioactive cyclic imine toxins constitute a growing family of structurally related marine neurotoxins of dinoflagellate origin contaminating shellfish (for reviews, see Refs. [1–11]). Over the past 20 years, there has been an important research expansion on cyclic imine toxins. This has been possible since vast efforts have been dedicated to the isolation and chemical characterization of these toxins, as well as in determining their natural origin, toxicity, and mode and mechanisms of actions. Moreover, important progress in the chemical synthesis and in analytical methods has been obtained for these toxins, driven by technology improvement.

In this review chapter, we consider the chemistry of cyclic imine toxins, their origin, metabolism, toxicology, pharmacology, and methods developed for their detection.

33.2 Chemistry of Cyclic Imine Toxins

A number of reference studies not only reviewed the chemistry of cyclic imines in a general manner[1] but also focused on specific families (pinnatoxins,[2–6] spirolides,[7,8] and gymnodimines[9]). A general overview of available studies related to structural features, identification, and synthetic efforts within the cyclic imine phycotoxins family is presented later, and for a more in-depth description, the reader is invited to consult the cited references.

33.2.1 Structural Features

The main characteristic of this class of phycotoxins is represented by an imine moiety as a part of a bicyclic ring system. This system can be of hexahydroisoquinoline type, as found in prorocentrolides, but the vast majority of these toxins contain a cyclic spiroimine motif, present in gymnodimines, spirolides, pinnatoxins, pteriatoxins, and spiro-prorocentrimine (Figure 33.1). The spiroimine ring system can be either 6:6 (gymnodimines, spiro-prorocentrimine) or 6:7 (spirolides, pinnatoxins, pteriatoxins).

The cyclic imine fragment is part of a macrocyclic system, featuring one (gymnodimines, spirolides, pinnatoxins, pteriatoxins) or two (spiro-prorocentrimine, prorocentrolides) macrocycles (Figure 33.1). This global arrangement confers to the toxin a globular form and a great stability.[10]

Another feature of this toxin family is the presence of a trispiroketal ring system, with either a 5:5:6 arrangement, specific for spirolides, or 6:5:6 arrangement, specific for pinnatoxins. There are a few exceptions to this rule, for example, a 5:6:6 arrangement for spirolide G and bispiroketal 5:6 ring system for spirolides H and I. The spiroketal fragment is replaced by a tetrahydrofuran ring in the gymnodimine family, and has no direct equivalent in the spiro-prorocentrimine and prorocentrolides structure (Figure 33.1).

More generally, the structure of these toxins can be represented by rigid building blocks connected by flexible linkers. The nature, size, and substitution pattern of these fragments are variable, conferring to these naturally occurring compounds a wide range of biological activity and selectivity against different receptors, and eventually, at a more detailed level, against the receptor subtypes. The specific structural features for each subclass of the cyclic imine toxins family will be presented in more detail in the following sections.

33.2.2 Identification, Structure, and Stereochemistry Assignment

33.2.2.1 Gymnodimines

Gymnodimine A was isolated for the first time in 1995 from New Zealand oysters and the dinoflagellate, *Gymnodinium* sp. and its structure elucidated by spectroscopic methods.[11,12] The complete stereochemistry and absolute configuration were assigned 2 years later starting from the crystal structure of the *p*-bromobenzamide derivative of the reduced form of gymnodimine A.[13] Two analogs belonging to this family, called gymnodimines B[14] and C,[15] were later isolated in small quantities from *Karenia selliformis*

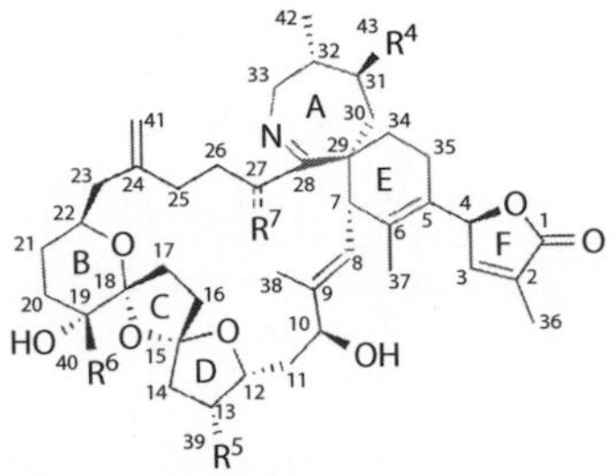

Spirolide A : R^4 = H, R^5 = CH_3, R^6 = CH_3, R^7 = H,H
Spirolide C : R^4 = CH_3, R^5 = CH_3, R^6 = CH_3, R^7 = H,H
13-Desmethyl spirolide C : R^4 = CH_3, R^5 = H, R^6 = CH_3, R^7 = H,H
13,19-Desmethyl spirolide C : R^4 = CH_3, R^5 = H, R^6 = H, R^7 = H,H
27-Hydroxy-13-desmethyl spirolide C : R^4 = CH_3, R^5 = H, R^6 = CH_3, R^7 = H,OH
27-Hydroxy-13,19-didesmethyl spirolide C : R^4 = CH_3, R^5 = H, R^6 = H, R^7 = H,OH
27-Oxo-13,19-didesmethyl spirolide C : R^4 = CH_3, R^5 = H, R^6 = H, R^7 = O

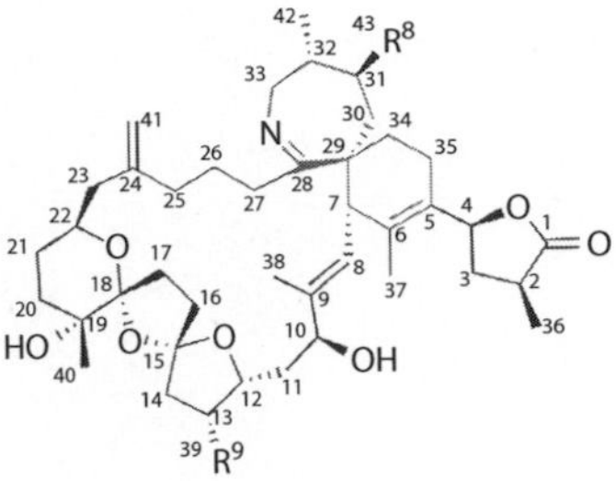

Spirolide B : R^8 = H, R^9 = CH_3
Spirolide D : R^8 = CH_3, R^9 = CH_3
13-Desmethyl spirolide D : R^8 = CH_3, R^9 = H

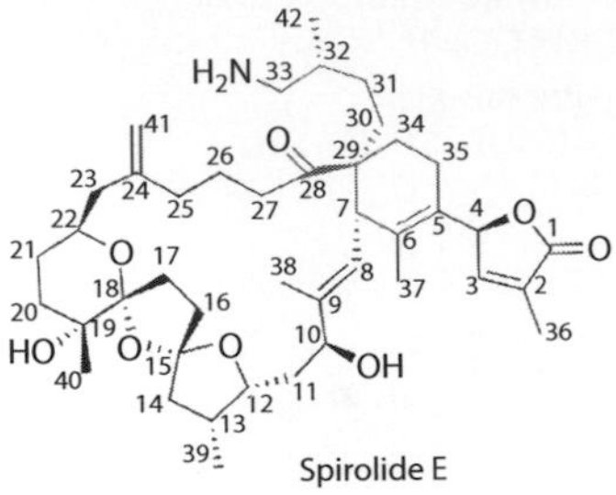

Spirolide E

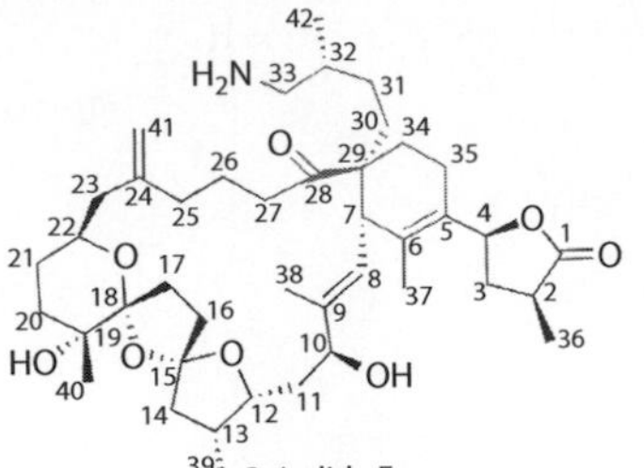

Spirolide F

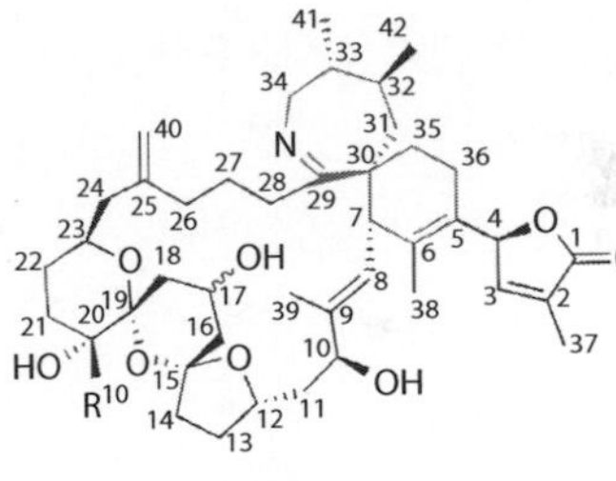

Spirolide G : R^{10} = H
20-Methyl spirolide G : R^{10} = CH_3

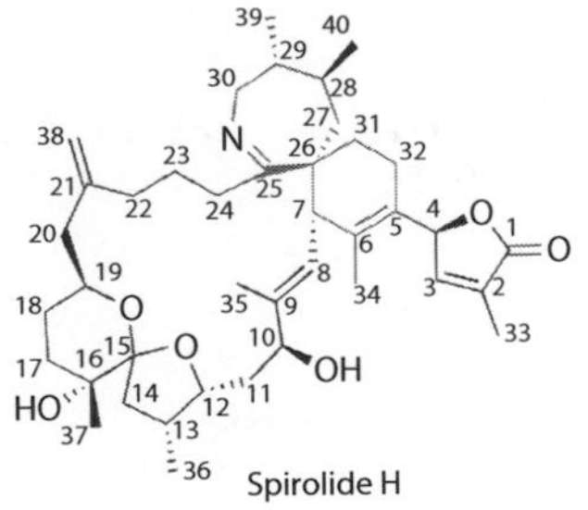

Spirolide H

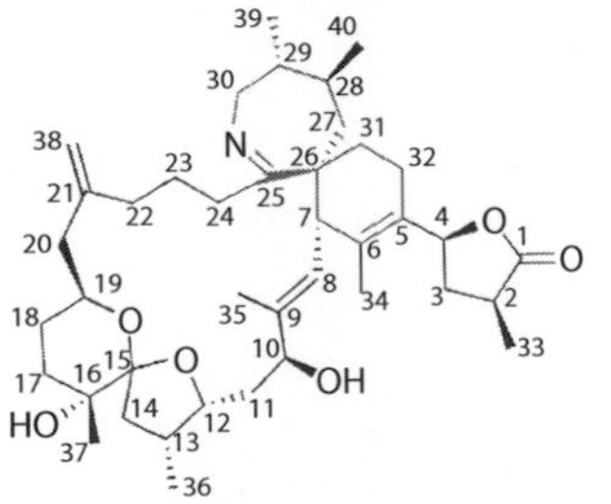

Spirolide I

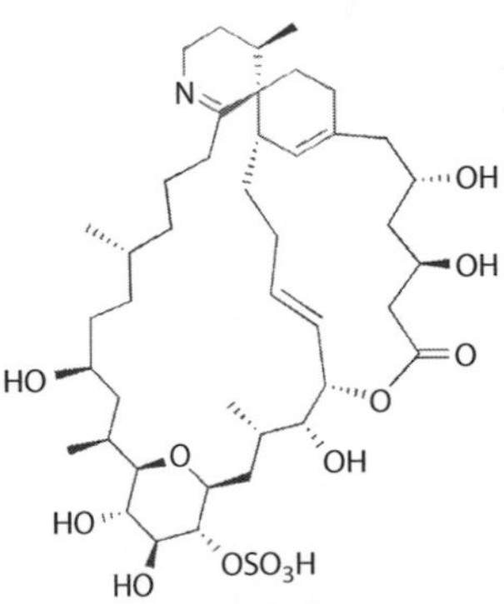

Spiro-prorocentrimine

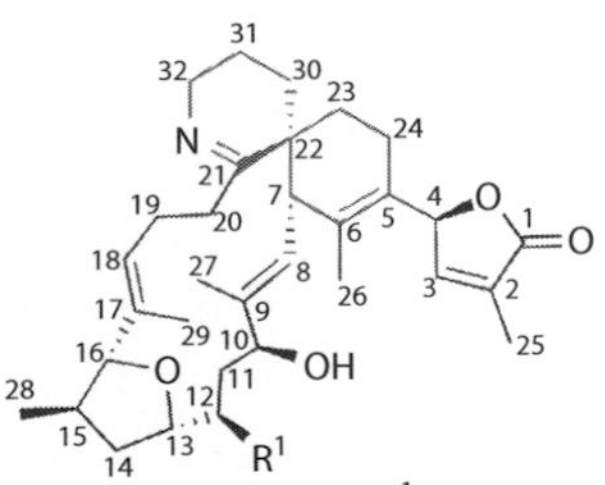

Gymnodimine A : R^1 = H
12-Methyl gymnodimine A : R^1 = CH_3

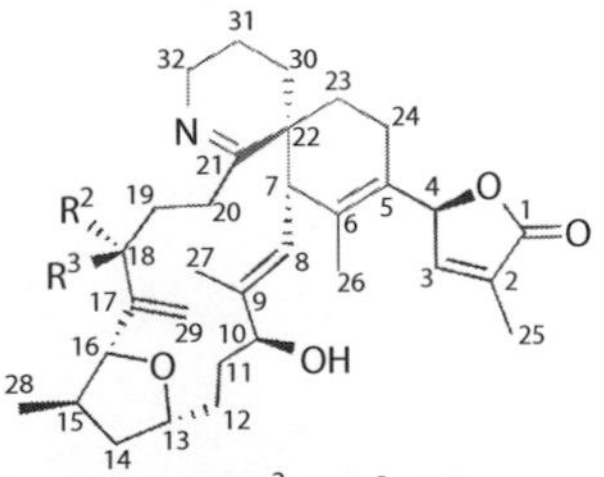

Gymnodimine B : R^2 = H, R^3 = OH
Gymnodimine C : R^2 = OH, R^3 = H

FIGURE 33.1   Chemical structures of known cyclic imine toxins.

(continued)

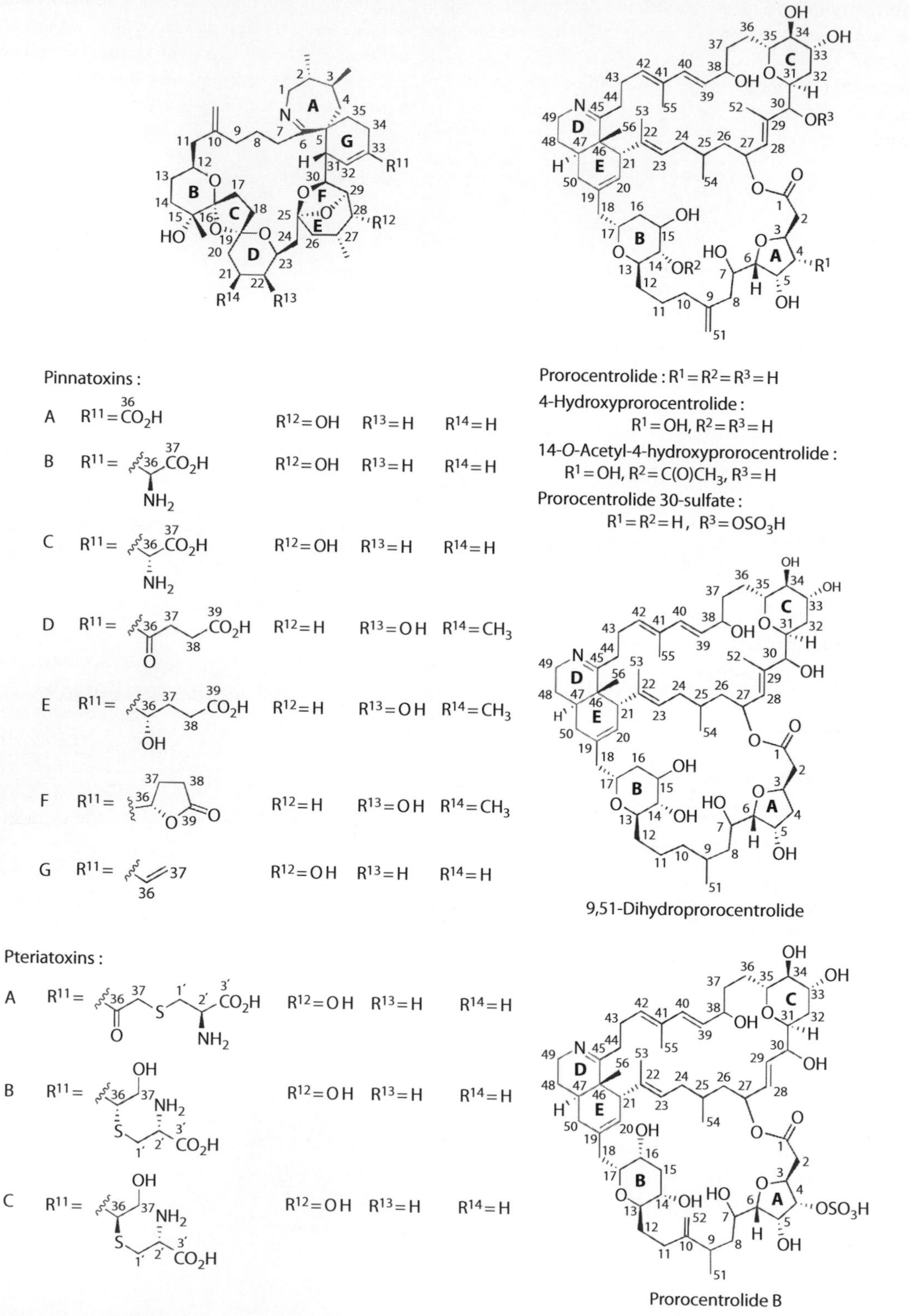

Pinnatoxins:

A $R^{11} = \overset{36}{CO_2H}$ $R^{12} = OH$ $R^{13} = H$ $R^{14} = H$

B $R^{11} = \overset{36}{}\overset{37}{CO_2H}$, NH_2 $R^{12} = OH$ $R^{13} = H$ $R^{14} = H$

C $R^{11} = \overset{36}{}\overset{37}{CO_2H}$, NH_2 $R^{12} = OH$ $R^{13} = H$ $R^{14} = H$

D $R^{11} = \overset{36}{}\overset{37}{}\overset{39}{CO_2H}$ (38, O) $R^{12} = H$ $R^{13} = OH$ $R^{14} = CH_3$

E $R^{11} = \overset{36}{}\overset{37}{}\overset{39}{CO_2H}$ (38, OH) $R^{12} = H$ $R^{13} = OH$ $R^{14} = CH_3$

F $R^{11} = $ (lactone 36, 37, 38, O 39, O) $R^{12} = H$ $R^{13} = OH$ $R^{14} = CH_3$

G $R^{11} = \overset{37}{\diagup}$ 36 $R^{12} = OH$ $R^{13} = H$ $R^{14} = H$

Pteriatoxins:

A $R^{11} = \overset{36}{}\overset{37}{}\overset{O}{}S\overset{1'}{}\overset{2'}{}\overset{3'}{CO_2H}$, NH_2 $R^{12} = OH$ $R^{13} = H$ $R^{14} = H$

B $R^{11} = \overset{36}{}\overset{37}{}$ OH, NH_2, $S\overset{1'}{}\overset{2'}{}\overset{3'}{CO_2H}$ $R^{12} = OH$ $R^{13} = H$ $R^{14} = H$

C $R^{11} = \overset{36}{}\overset{37}{}$ OH, NH_2, $S\overset{1'}{}\overset{2'}{}\overset{3'}{CO_2H}$ $R^{12} = OH$ $R^{13} = H$ $R^{14} = H$

Prorocentrolide: $R^1 = R^2 = R^3 = H$

4-Hydroxyprorocentrolide:
   $R^1 = OH$, $R^2 = R^3 = H$

14-*O*-Acetyl-4-hydroxyprorocentrolide:
   $R^1 = OH$, $R^2 = C(O)CH_3$, $R^3 = H$

Prorocentrolide 30-sulfate:
   $R^1 = R^2 = H$, $R^3 = OSO_3H$

9,51-Dihydroprorocentrolide

Prorocentrolide B

FIGURE 33.1 (continued)   Chemical structures of known cyclic imine toxins.

(formerly known as *Gymnodinium selliforme*). These oxidized analogs contain an exocyclic methylene at C17, a feature shared with the pinnatoxins and spirolides but not with gymnodimine, and an allylic hydroxyl group at C18 (18S and 18R configurations for the B and C derivatives, respectively).[14,15] The presence of gymnodimine A, but not of the gymnodimine B and C derivatives, could also be evidenced in several batches of contaminated clams harvested in Tunisia.[16] Recently, a 12-methyl gymnodimine A congener was isolated from a North Carolina sample of the dinoflagellate *Alexandrium peruvianum*.[17]

33.2.2.2 Spirolides

The first four members of this family, spirolides A–D, were isolated from digestive glands of mussels (*Mytilus edulis*) and scallops (*Placopecten magellanicus*) harvested in Nova Scotia, Canada. Spirolides B and D were the two major components, first characterized by nuclear magnetic resonance (NMR) and mass spectrometry (MS) studies.[18] Several years later, the structures of the remaining spirolides A and C were determined as well, along with a new derivative, 13-desmethyl spirolide C.[19] Molecular modeling studies using distance constraints generated from nuclear Overhauser effect spectroscopy (NOESY) and rotating frame nuclear Overhauser effect spectroscopy (ROESY) data led to the assignment of relative stereochemistry for these spirolides, except for one center, at C4.[20] Later on, a number of spirolides C and D derivatives were isolated and characterized, including 13-desmethyl spirolide D,[21,22] 13,19-dides-methyl spirolide C,[23,24] 27-hydroxy-13,19-didesmethyl spirolide C,[25] 27-hydroxy-13-desmethyl spirolide C,[26] and 27-oxo-13,19-didesmethyl spirolide C.[26] Some of these derivatives can be isolated in relatively large amounts using an improved protocol that was recently described.[27] The study of biosynthetic pathway for 13-desmethyl spirolide C revealed that most carbons of the macrocycle are polyketide-derived and that glycine is incorporated as an intact unit into the cyclic imine moiety.[28,29]

Two new spirolide derivatives, E and F, possessing a ketoamine form instead of the characteristic cyclic imine, were isolated from shellfish extracts and characterized using standard NMR and MS techniques. Unlike all other spirolides known at that time, they proved to be inactive in the mouse bioassay. This result, corroborated with the inactivity of the reduced form (secondary amine) of spirolide B, led to the conclusion that the cyclic spiroimine group is the main pharmacophore, essential for biological activity.[30]

An interesting member of the spirolide family, named spirolide G, contains a 5:6:6-trispiroketal ring system instead of the usual 5:5:6 one. It was isolated from Danish strains of the toxigenic dinoflagellate *Alexandrium ostenfeldii* and characterized using infrared (IR), NMR, and MS.[23] The 20-desmethyl spirolide G as well as the fatty acid ester metabolites of spirolide G were evidenced by liquid chromatography (LC)/tandem MS from cultured mussels sampled on the Western coast of Norway, without being fully characterized.[31]

A new subclass of spirolide toxins, containing spirolides H and I, were isolated from the marine dinoflagellate *A. ostenfeldii*. The distinctive feature of this subclass is represented by the 5:6 dispiroketal ring system, which replaces the 5:5:6 trispiroketal ring characteristic for the spirolides family. Surprisingly, although they possess the conserved cyclic spiroimine pharmacophore, spirolides H and I were reported to show no toxicity in the mouse assay, suggesting that the presence of the cyclic imine moiety is not the only structural requirement for toxicity.[32]

The 13-desmethyl spirolide C has been extensively characterized by MS[33] and compared to other spirolides;[34] this approach was very useful in the characterization of known and unknown spirolides and other related compounds. A full stereochemistry assignment was reported for 13,19-didesmethyl spirolide C, using a combined NMR and molecular modeling approach.[24] However, the R-configuration at C4 assigned in this study is in contradiction with the S-configuration at C4 determined by NMR for spirolides H and I[32] and by x-ray crystallography for a gymnodimine A derivative.[13] Although more in-depth investigations are required to formally assign the configuration of this chiral center, the S-configuration seems to be more probable from the experimental data available to date.

33.2.2.3 Pinnatoxins and Pteriatoxins

Pinnatoxin was first reported in 1990, isolated from *Pinna attenuate* collected in the South China Sea.[35] A few years later, four members of this family, pinnatoxins A–D, were isolated from the Okinawan *Pinna muricata* and characterized,[36] with full assignment of the relative stereochemistry for pinnatoxin

A[37,38] and D.[39] The relative stereochemistry of pinnatoxins B and C, which could not be separated by reversed-phase HPLC, proved to be more difficult to assign and required chemical transformations to allow the direct comparison with a pinnatoxin A derivative.[40,41] The absolute stereochemistry of chiral centers in pinnatoxins could be assigned only after the completion of Kishi's total synthesis of (–)-pinnatoxin A, which proved to be inactive, in contrast with the natural (+)-pinnatoxin A.[42]

Three new members of this class, pinnatoxins E, F, and G, were recently isolated from Pacific oysters (*Crassostrea gigas*) collected from South Australia. Structural assignment showed that pinnatoxins E and F are more related to pinnatoxin D, whereas pinnatoxin G shares most of its structural features with pinnatoxins A–C.[43]

The three toxins belonging to the pteriatoxin family known to date, pteriatoxins A–C, were isolated from the Okinawan bivalve *Pteria penguin*. Their structures were determined from NMR and MS/MS spectra, showing a common scaffold with pinnatoxins A–C. The only structural differences were evidenced at the level of C33 substituent, suggesting that these spirotoxins may be synthesized by common symbionts in both *Pinna* sp. and *Pteria* sp.[41,44] The absolute stereochemistry of C33 substituents in pteriatoxins A–C could be assigned by the synthesis of all possible stereoisomers and comparison of ^{1}H-NMR spectra with natural samples.[45]

33.2.2.4 Spiro-Prorocentrimine and Prorocentrolides

Spiro-prorocentrimine, a polar lipid-soluble toxin isolated from a laboratory-cultured benthic *Prorocentrum* species of Taiwan,[46] presents a very different structure compared to the other classes of cyclic spiroimines. Although it contains the characteristic 6:6 spiroimine ring system, similar to gymnodimines, the substitution pattern is somewhat different and the macrolide feature is similar to the one found in prorocentrolides. Structural features and stereochemistry assignments for the chiral centers of this toxin were obtained from ultraviolet (UV), IR, NMR, and HR-FABMS spectral analysis, but the major contribution came from the x-ray diffraction crystal structure of spiro-prorocentrimine that could be obtained, which undoubtedly confirmed its absolute stereochemistry. Despite the presence of the cyclic spiroimine moiety, considered as a required feature for the activity of this family of marine biotoxins, spiro-prorocentrimine showed much less toxicity (LD$_{99}$ of 2.5 mg/kg mouse) compared to other known marine cyclic spiroimine toxins (LD$_{99}$ in the range 0.18–0.45 mg/kg mouse).[46]

Prorocentrolides represent the only family among the cyclic imine toxins not containing the spiroimine ring system, which in this case is replaced by a hexahydroisoquinoline fragment. The first member of this family was isolated in 1988 from a benthic dinoflagellate, *Prorocentrum lima*,[46–48] followed by a number of derivatives (9,51-dihydroprorocentrolide,[47,49] 4-hydroxyprorocentrolide,[46] 14-*O*-acetyl-4-hydroxyprorocentrolide,[46] prorocentrolide 30-sulfate[49]). The biosynthesis of prorocentrolide was studied by culturing *P. lima* in media containing [1-^{13}C], [2-^{13}C], and [1,2-^{13}C] acetic acid, which led to the labeling of only 44 out of 56 carbons. Interestingly, two carbons (C43, C50) could be labeled by either [13]CH$_3$COOH or CH$_3$[13]COOH. The biosynthesis of prorocentrolide seems to involve polyketides, succinic acid, and hydroxymethyl glutaric acid, but the whole biosynthetic pathway is still unknown.[50] Another member of this family, prorocentrolide B, was isolated from a tropical dinoflagellate, *Prorocentrum maculosum* Faust.[51] Compared to the parent prorocentrolide, this new structure presents some significant differences: the substitution pattern of hydroxyl groups on ring B, the substituents of C9 and C10, the presence of a sulfonate group at C4, and a methyl substituent missing on C29.[51]

33.2.3 Synthetic Studies

Synthetic strategies have been developed over the time to bring solutions for the important challenges associated with the complex structure of cyclic spirotoxins. Some of them are targeting common fragments and consequently have wider applications, whereas others are dedicated to very specific structural features, found only in a few members of this marine toxin family.

In the gymnodimine series, methodological studies were devoted to the preparation of tetrahydrofuran,[52–57] and spirocyclic system fragments,[52,53,56,58–63] and, to a lesser extent, to macrocyclic ring closure approaches.[55,56] During these studies, an unexpected bromine-induced ring expansion of the spiroimine group was observed.[64] Within the spirolides family, a number of synthetically useful methods for the preparation of CD-[65] and BCD-spiroacetal ring systems[66–73] and spiroimine fragments[74–79] were reported, as well as a strategy for the formation of the 23-membered all-carbon macrocyclic framework.[80] Some of these studies can be applied in both gymnodimines and spirolides series, since they are focused on their common scaffold. Relevant examples are the preparation of the butenolide fragment[81] and of the bicyclic spiroimine system with variable imine ring size.[82–84] Methodological developments aimed toward the synthesis of pinnatoxins were focused on the synthesis of tricyclic 6:5:6 BCD-dispiroketal fragment,[85–88] EF-bicyclic ketal,[89] spiroimine AG-bicyclic system,[90–96] and the more advanced BCDEF-pentacyclic fragment.[59,97–100] Additionally, the natural form of the BCD-dispiroketal system was found to be the most favored among all the possible isomers,[101] and an unusual stability to hydrolysis of the imine ring in pinnatoxin A was also recently reported.[10] During these studies, the crystal structure of a pinnatoxin A fragment containing the BCD spiroketal ring system was reported, allowing the assignment of stereochemistry for five chiral centers in the pinnatoxin A structure.[102]

The ultimate aim of the studies mentioned earlier is the total synthesis of these toxins, an achievement of greatest importance allowing the assignment of relative and absolute stereochemistry in difficult cases, providing larger quantities required for more advanced biological evaluation. The great majority of total syntheses reported to date were focused on pinnatoxins. The unnatural (−)-pinnatoxin A was synthesized for the first time in 1998, using a biomimetic intramolecular Diels–Alder reaction.[42,103,104] As this form proved to be biologically inactive, it was concluded that the natural compound is (+)-pinnatoxin A, which was subsequently synthesized using a similar approach.[103,104] In a later study, the use of an exoselective Diels–Alder reaction, followed by a Ru-catalyzed cycloisomerization of the 27-membered carbocyclic ring as key steps, provided (+)-pinnatoxin A in 53 steps and 0.21% overall yield.[105] A highly convergent formal total synthesis of (+)-pinnatoxin A was also reported.[106] A robust and scalable, enantioselective total synthesis of (+)-pinnatoxin A based on a Ireland–Claisen rearrangement was recently described, with an overall yield of 1.4%,[107,108] and a similar synthetic sequence allowed the completion of the first total synthesis of (+)-pinnatoxin G.[108] The stereochemically controlled total synthesis of pinnatoxins B and C allowed the unambiguous assignment of stereochemistry at C36 (see Figure 33.1 for numbering scheme),[109] and the same unified synthetic strategy gave a straightforward access to the pteriatoxins A–C.[45,110] A single total synthesis of (−)-gymnodimine and of its C4-*epi*-diastereoisomer is available to date, which was accomplished using a synthetic sequence involving a intermolecular Nozaki–Hiyama–Kishi reaction, a Barbier-type macrocyclization and a vinylogous Mukaiyama aldol addition as key steps.[111,112]

33.3 Origin of Cyclic Imine Toxins

With the exception of prorocentrolide congeners and spiro-prorocentrimine, most of the cyclic imine toxins were first discovered in contaminated shellfish before the producers were identified as being dinoflagellates. It is well known that dinoflagellates, a very large and diverse group of eukaryotic microalgae in the marine ecosystem, are not only important marine primary producers and grazers, but also the major causative agents of harmful algal blooms. In the past few decades, extensive studies have been devoted to dinoflagellate toxins, and five major seafood poisoning syndromes caused by toxins have been identified from dinoflagellates (for a recent review, see Ref. [113]): paralytic shellfish poisoning (PSP), neurotoxic shellfish poisoning (NSP), amnesic shellfish poisoning (ASP), diarrhetic shellfish poisoning (DSP), and ciguatera fish poisoning (CFP). Although many dinoflagellate species can produce various natural toxins that impact humans, those involved in the production of cyclic imine toxins are limited to mainly *Prorocentrum*, *Karenia* (formerly *Gymnodinium*), *Alexandrium*, and *Vulcanodinium* sp. (see Table 33.1).

33.3.1 Prorocentrolides and Spiro-Prorocentrimine

Prorocentrolide A is the first cyclic imine discovered as originating from dinoflagellates. Hence, as soon as 1988, this cyclic imine was reported to be produced by cultures of *P. lima* isolated 3 years before at Sesoko Island, Okinawa, Japan, and previously known as producer of DSP toxins.[48] Interestingly, no prorocentrolide or congener was observed in two strains of *P. lima* obtained from the colder waters of

TABLE 33.1

Cyclic Imine Toxins Known to be Produced by Dinoflagellate Species

Cyclic Imine Toxins	Dinoflagellate Species	Localization	References
Prorocentrolide A	*Prorocentrum lima*	Japan (Okinawa)	[48]
		Taiwan	[46]
Prorocentrolide B	*Prorocentrum maculosum*	Tropical waters	[51]
4-Hydroxy prorocentrolide	*Prorocentrum lima*	Taiwan	[46]
14-*O*-Acetyl-4-hydroxy Prorocentrolide	*Prorocentrum lima*	Taiwan	[46]
Spiro-prorocentrimine	*Prorocentrum* sp.	Taiwan	[46]
Gymnodimine A	*Karenia* (formerly *Gymnodinium) mikimotoi*	New Zealand	[12]
	Karenia selliformis	Australia (Queensland)	[114]
Gymnodimine B	*Karenia* (formerly *Gymnodinium)* sp.	New Zealand	[14]
Gymnodimine C	*Karenia selliformis*	New Zealand	[15]
12-Methyl gymnodimine	*Alexandrium peruvianum*	USA (North Carolina)	[17,115]
		USA (Rhode Island)	[116]
Spirolide A	*Alexandrium ostenfeldii*	Canada (Nova Scotia)	[19,117,118]
Spirolide B	*Alexandrium ostenfeldii*	Canada (Nova Scotia)	[117,118]
	Alexandrium peruvianum	Mediterranean Sea	[119]
Spirolide C	*Alexandrium ostenfeldii*	Canada (Nova Scotia)	[19,33,34,117,118,120]
		Canada (Atlantic estuarine)	[121]
		Scotland	[122,123]
		Ireland (Bantry Bay)	[124]
	Alexandrium peruvianum	Mediterranean Sea	[119]
Spirolide C2 (a spirolide C isomer)	*Alexandrium ostenfeldii*	Canada (Nova Scotia)	[118]
Spirolide C3 (a spirolide C isomer)	*Alexandrium ostenfeldii*	Canada (Nova Scotia)	[33,34]
		Canada (Atlantic estuarine)	[121]
Spirolide D	*Alexandrium ostenfeldii*	Canada (Nova Scotia)	[33,34,117,118,120]
		Canada (Atlantic estuarine)	[121]
		Italy (Emilia-Romagna coasts)	[22]
		Denmark (Limfjord)	[125]
		Ireland (Bantry Bay)	[124]
	Alexandrium peruvianum	Mediterranean Sea	[119]
		USA (North Carolina)	[126]
Spirolide D2 (a spirolide D isomer)	*Alexandrium ostenfeldii*	Canada (Nova Scotia)	[117,118]
Spirolide D3 (a spirolide D isomer)	*Alexandrium ostenfeldii*	Canada (Nova Scotia)	[33,34]
Spirolide G	*Alexandrium ostenfeldii*	Denmark (Limfjord)	[23]
Spirolide H	*Alexandrium ostenfeldii*	Canada (Nova Scotia)	[32]
Spirolide I	*Alexandrium ostenfeldii*	Canada (Nova Scotia)	[32]

TABLE 33.1 (continued)

Cyclic Imine Toxins Known to be Produced by Dinoflagellate Species

Cyclic Imine Toxins	Dinoflagellate Species	Localization	References
13-Desmethyl spirolide C	*Alexandrium ostenfeldii*	Canada (Nova Scotia)	[19,33,34,117,118,120]
		Canada (Atlantic estuarine)	[121]
		Denmark (Limfjord)	[23,28,125,127]
		Italy (Emilia-Romagna coasts)	[22,25]
		Ireland (Cork Harbour)	[128]
	Alexandrium peruvianum	Mediterranean Sea	[119]
		Ireland (Lough Swilly)	[124]
		USA (North Carolina)	[17,115,126]
		USA (Rhode Island)	[116]
13-Desmethyl spirolide D	*Alexandrium ostenfeldii*	Canada (Nova Scotia)	[19,33,34]
		Canada (Atlantic estuarine)	[121]
		Italy (Emilia-Romagna coasts)	[22]
		Denmark (Limfjord)	[125]
	Alexandrium peruvianum	Mediterranean Sea	[119]
		Ireland (Lough Swilly)	[124]
		USA (North Carolina)	[126]
20-Methyl spirolide G	*Alexandrium ostenfeldii*	Norway (Sognefjord)	[129]
		Ireland (Cork Harbour)	[128]
13,19-Didesmethyl spirolide C	*Alexandrium ostenfeldii*	Denmark (Limfjord)	[23,125,127]
		Italy (Emilia-Romagna coasts)	[25]
27-Hydroxy-13-desmethyl Spirolide C	*Alexandrium ostenfeldii*	Italy (Emilia-Romagna coasts)	[26]
27-Hydroxy-13,19-didesmethyl Spirolide C	*Alexandrium ostenfeldii*	Italy (Emilia-Romagna coasts)	[25]
27-Oxo-13,19-didesmethyl Spirolide C	*Alexandrium ostenfeldii*	Italy (Emilia-Romagna coasts)	[26]
Pinnatoxin A	Scrippsielloid dinoflagellates	Australia (South)	[130]
	Vulcanodinium rugosum	Australia (South)	[131]
Pinnatoxin E	Peridinoid dinoflagellate	New Zealand (Northland)	[132]
	Scrippsielloid dinoflagellates	Australia (South)	[130]
	Vulcanodinium rugosum	New Zealand (Northland)	[131]
		Australia (South)	[131]
Pinnatoxin F	Peridinoid dinoflagellate	New Zealand (Northland)	[132]
	Scrippsielloid dinoflagellates	Australia (South)	[130]
	Vulcanodinium rugosum	New Zealand (Northland)	[131]
		Australia (South)	[131]
Pinnatoxin G	Scrippsielloid dinoflagellates	Australia (South)	[130]
	Peridinoid dinoflagellate	Japan (Okinawa)	[133]
	Vulcanodinium rugosum	France (Mediterranean lagoons)	[134,135]
		Australia (South)	[131]
		Japan (Okinawa)	[131]

various localities in Eastern Canada.[51] Eight years after the discovery of prorocentrolide A, a structurally related cyclic imine—prorocentrolide B—was isolated and characterized from a tropical strain of *P. maculosum*.[51] More recently, two prorocentrolide analogs—4-hydroxy and 14-*O*-acetyl-4-hydroxy prorocentrolides—were found in a Taiwanese (PL01) strain of *P. lima*, and, in addition to prorocentrolide A, a novel macrocyclic imine, denoted spiro-prorocentrimine, was obtained from another Taiwanese unidentified (PM08) strain of *Prorocentrum* sp.[46] To date, it thus appears that the occurrence of prorocentrolide congeners and spiro-prorocentrimine is restricted to primarily benthic or epiphytic *Prorocentrum* sp. that, unlike their pelagic counterparts, tend not to form dense blooms. Moreover, the benthic habitat of these dinoflagellates may account for the absence of reports regarding the presence of cyclic imine toxins in shellfish.

33.3.2 Gymnodimines

In 1995, the dinoflagellate *Gymnodinium* cf. *mikimotoi* was shown to produce gymnodimine A,[12] responsible for the high levels of toxicity found in 1994 in New Zealand oysters and associated with concurrent blooms of this dinoflagellate species.[136] Five years later, gymnodimine B, an oxidized analog of gymnodimine A, was also isolated from cells recovered by filtration from cultures of *Gymnodinium* sp.[14] Then, in 2003, gymnodimine C, found to be isomeric with gymnodimine B, was isolated from extracts of *K. selliformis* cells.[15] It is worth noting that the culprit species of gymnodimines production in New Zealand was first identified as being *Gymnodinium* sp., described as closely related morphologically to *Gymnodinium mikimotoi*, and was then, following subsequent taxonomic revision, assigned to a new dinoflagellate species *K. selliformis* (formerly *G. selliforme*). More recently, gymnodimine A, which has been detected in shellfish from the Moreton bay region in Australia, also appeared to be associated with *K. selliformis*, as in New Zealand.[114] The production of gymnodimines was thus exclusively attributed to *K. selliformis* until three recent reports revealing that a novel gymnodimine congener, 12-methyl gymnodimine, originates from another dinoflagellate, *A. peruvianum* isolated from North Carolina[17,115] and Rhode Island[116] in the United States (Table 33.1).

33.3.3 Spirolides

These three latter reports are of great interest because, since 1998, some members of the dinoflagellate genus *Alexandrium* are well recognized as producers of spirolides (Table 33.1). It is worth noting that the global distribution of this genus and its impacts on marine systems and human health were recently reviewed by Anderson et al.[137] who listed 31 species along with toxin types, most of them being those responsible for PSP. Hence, 3 years after the discovery of spirolides in the digestive glands of both mussels and scallops from aquaculture sites in Nova Scotia, Canada,[18] the planktonic origin of these spirolides was identified.[138] Then *A. ostenfeldii* from Nova Scotia was confirmed as the biological source of spirolides A, B, C, and D as well as two spirolide C isomers (spirolides C2 and C3), two spirolide D isomers (spirolides D2 and D3), and two desmethyl spirolide derivatives, identified as 13-desmethyl spirolides C and D.[19,21,33,34,117,118,120] Recently, a new subclass of spirolides—spirolides H and I—was characterized from the *A. ostenfeldii* strain AOSH2, clonally isolated from Nova Scotia.[32] Indeed, a cDNA library was established to gain a general overview of the transcriptome of this spirolide-producing *A. ostenfeldii* strain.[139] It is worth noting that the spirolide profile (content and composition) varies widely both in field samples and in cultures of *A. ostenfeldii* between different sites in Nova Scotia and, at a given site, between years (see Ref. [118]). Similarly, an estuarine isolate of *A. ostenfeldii* from Atlantic Canada was also reported to produce some spirolide congeners such as spirolides C, C3, and D as well as 13-desmethyl spirolides C and D.[121]

In addition to Canadian waters, the spirolide-producing *A. ostenfeldii* has also been found widely distributed in European coasts, and crude extracts from its different strains collected from different coastal regions have shown important and, in some cases, dramatic differences in toxicity and toxin profile (see Table 33.1). Interestingly, some spirolide congeners that had not been reported so far in other strains of the dinoflagellate were detected. In particular, 20-methyl spirolide G was found in algal samples dominated by *A. ostenfeldii* in Sognefjord, Norway.[129] Similarly, in addition to 13-desmethyl spirolide C, two new spirolides—13,19-didesmethyl spirolide C and spirolide G—were detected in two clonal isolates of *A. ostenfeldii* from Limfjord, Denmark.[23,28] However, some divergences in the type of spirolides produced by different strains of this Danish dinoflagellate were recently reported, pointing out the effects of environmental factors on the toxin profile. Hence, whereas the major components of the cultured CCMP1773 strain were 13-desmethyl spirolide C and 13,19-didesmethyl spirolide C,[127] similar levels of spirolide D and 13-desmethyl spirolide D were also found.[125] In Italy, a strain of *A. ostenfeldii* collected along the Emilia-Romagna coasts was shown to contain three novel desmethyl derivatives—27-hydroxy-13,19-didesmethyl spirolide C, 27-oxo-13,19-didesmethyl spirolide C, and 27-hydroxy-13-desmethyl spirolide C—in addition to spirolide D, 13-desmethyl spirolides C and D, and 13,19-didesmethyl spirolide C.[22,25,26] A large-scale sampling effort along the East coast of Scotland revealed the presence of a wide variety of spirolides in plankton tow samples taken from different locations.[140] However, the presence of these toxins had not been conclusively linked to *A. ostenfeldii*, despite the high coincidence of this dinoflagellate species with spirolide occurrence. A direct relationship between Scottish spirolides, dominated by spirolide C, and *A. ostenfeldii* was established later.[122,123] Finally, in Ireland, a cyst-derived culture of *A. ostenfeldii* from Bantry Bay was reported to mainly produce spirolides C and D,[124] whereas 13-desmethyl spirolide C and 20-methyl spirolide G, with dynamics generally congruent with those of *A. ostenfeldii*, were identified from Cork Harbour.[128] Here again, this points out differences in toxin profiles between geographically separated populations that remain unclear. To further support this, no spirolide congener has been found in *A. ostenfeldii* strains isolated from New Zealander and Northern Baltic (Åland Archipelago) seawaters which were shown to produce, instead, toxins belonging to the PSP group, such as gonyautoxins and saxitoxins.[141,142] In contrast, only spirolides but not PSP toxins were detected in the Canadian, Adriatic, Danish, and Irish strains of this dinoflagellate.[21,22,118,124,127] More complex is that certain *A. ostenfeldii* populations, notably from Scandinavia and Scotland, produce both spirolides and PSP toxins, but at very low levels.[120,123]

A. ostenfeldii was recognized as the sole spirolide-producing dinoflagellate until another *Alexandrium* species, *A. peruvianum*, was also pointed out as a spirolide producer, during the past 6 years (see Table 33.1). Hence, a clone of *A. peruvianum* from Northwestern Mediterranean Sea waters was reported as the first indication of spirolides (mainly 13-desmethyl spirolide C, but also spirolides B and D, 13-desmethyl spirolide D, and traces of spirolide C) in that region.[119] Two years later, an investigation regarding the diversity of *Alexandrium* species in Irish coastal waters revealed that, in addition to *A. ostenfeldii* from Cork Harbour, a cyst-derived culture of *A. peruvianum* from Lough Swilly also produced spirolides, notably 13-desmethyl spirolides C and D.[124] Finally and very recently, the presence of a spirolide-producing (mainly 13-desmethyl spirolides C and D and spirolide D) species *A. peruvianum* was confirmed for the first time in the US coastal waters.[17,115,116,126] Very interestingly, the US species was proven to also contain 12-methyl gymnodimine[17,115,116] as well as PSP and undefined hemolytic toxins,[126] whereas only spirolides were detected in the Irish species.[124] In contrast, in Malaysian waters, *A. peruvianum* was shown to contain PSP toxins only with no mention of spirolides.[143] These observations emphasize the intraspecific variability that has been also reported for other dinoflagellates such as *A. ostenfeldii* (see earlier). It is worth noting that spirolides E and F were not detected in dinoflagellates since these two spirolide congeners were observed to be degradation products in shellfish.[30]

33.3.4 Pinnatoxins

Analysis of surface sediment samples from mangrove habitats in both New Zealand and South Australia, where shellfish were reported positive for pinnatoxins,[43,144] resulted in the discovery of peridinoid or scrippsielloid dinoflagellates producing pinnatoxins E and F in New Zealand[132] and pinnatoxins A, E, F, and/or G in South Australia.[130] Similar studies on surface sediment samples obtained from Okinawa, Japan, have also reported the presence of a peridinoid dinoflagellate containing only pinnatoxin G.[133] Interestingly, New Zealander, Australian, and Japanese strains were shown to be identical, based on large subunit (LSU) rDNA and internal transcribed spacer (ITS) region sequence data[130] and on light and scanning electron microscopy.[133] Moreover, morphological and phylogenetic similarities were observed between these strains and a more recently described new peridinoid dinoflagellate, named *Vulcanodinium rugosum*, obtained from water samples of Mediterranean lagoons in the coast of France.[131,145]

Thus, _V. rugosum_ is responsible for the production of pinnatoxins in New Zealand, South Australia, Japan, and France. Indeed, although shellfish (mussels and clams) contamination by pinnatoxins and the link to the dinoflagellate _V. rugosum_ have been first reported in France in 2011, retroanalysis indicates high levels of pinnatoxin G since 2006.[134,135]

33.4 Metabolism of Cyclic Imine Toxins

Phytoplanktons are primary producers that sustain marine food web, and they are responsible for ~40% of the photosynthetic carbon fixation in the biosphere. Phytoplankton's growth is characterized by seasonal blooming (~100,000 to 1,000,000 cells/L). Harmful algal blooms are dominated by toxic phytoplankton species.[146] The ecoclimatic reasons why a toxic phytoplankton species episodically bloom during some days or weeks are not well understood.[147] Shellfish that filter feed on harmful phytoplankton is able to accumulate toxins in their digestive glands and edible tissues constituting a primary vector for the transfer of marine phycotoxins to humans.[146,148,149]

33.4.1 Biomagnification

Phycotoxin biomagnification implies that shellfish are "resistant" to the action of such harmful compounds. A well-illustrated example is the molecular mechanism behind the resistance to saxitoxin in soft shell clam (_Mya arenaria_) populations.[150] Saxitoxin prevents siphon retraction and burrowing capacity due to muscle paralysis; filter-feeding rate is also dramatically impaired with high mortality in sensitive clams. The mutation of a single amino acid residue in domain II of the Na^+ channel pore region of _M. arenaria_ confers to the Na^+ channel a 1000-fold decreased affinity to saxitoxin. As a result, resistant soft shell clams show an increased accumulation capacity for saxitoxin that may contribute to the risk of human PSP.[150] Similar mechanisms of resistance were described for saxitoxin and tetrodotoxin in puffer fish.[151]

Biomagnification of cyclic imine toxins by shellfish is not well understood yet. Gymnodimine A was observed to persist for several years in oyster samples from Foveaux Strait (New Zealand) following a toxic bloom dominated by _K. selliformis_ in 1995.[12,152] Since then, the endemic character of gymnodimine A in shellfish samples monitored in New Zealand coasts was shown.[153] Gymnodimine A is retained by shellfish for longer periods than other phycotoxins following a toxic algal bloom. Intriguingly, the concentration of gymnodimine A in other tissues outside the digestive glands remained constant over a period of 5 months.[152]

In vitro contamination/detoxification studies, using _K. selliformis_ cultures as source of gymnodimine A, showed that filtration rate was heavily impaired in the grooved carpet shell clams fed with the toxic phytoplankton. In average, 40% of the clams evidenced siphon opening and no mortality was reported. At the end of the 7 day intoxication period, 97% of the gymnodimine A was concentrated in the digestive glands. Detoxification rates were faster from the digestive glands than from other tissues, and after 5–7 days toxin clearance, mouse bioassay was negative. Detoxification was enhanced by feeding the clams with the nontoxic algae _Isochrysis galbana_.[154]

A similar in vitro study to assess the detoxification rate of spirolides used triploid oysters (_C. gigas_) fed by a culture of _A. ostenfeldii_ producing 13,19-didesmethyl spirolide C, 13-desmethyl spirolide C, and 13-desmethyl spirolide D.[155] Following a contamination period of 4 days, 83% of the spirolides were accumulated in the digestive glands of oysters. Histological studies showed inflammatory responses in the intestinal tract of the mollusks. However, no oyster mortality was reported. Spirolides detoxification from digestive glands decreased exponentially. At the end of the 7-day detoxification period, the concentrations of spirolides (10% of the initial values) were similar in the digestive glands and the remaining tissues. Detoxification rates of spirolides were improved by feeding the oysters with nontoxic algae. Like gymnodimine A, spirolides remained longer time in other tissues outside the digestive gland.[155]

The blockage of voltage-gated sodium channels by saxitoxin prevents the generation of a proper action potential in nerves and muscle fibers leading to neuromuscular paralysis and 26%–42% mortality of sensitive clams exposed 14 days to _Alexandrium tamarense_ (60–98 pg saxitoxin equivalent per cell).[150] The shorter exposure time to cyclic imines did not provoke shellfish mortality.[154,155] In contrast, the blockade of nicotinic acetylcholine receptors (nAChRs) by cyclic imines at the neuromuscular junction of mice leads to death by respiratory arrest. In mollusks, the neuromuscular transmission is not exclusively cholinergic but also glutamatergic. It is known that in the herbivorous marine gastropod *Aplysia*, most of the motoneurons innervating the buccal muscles are cholinergic,[156,157] and a small number of motoneurons are glutamatergic.[158,159] How could shellfish mollusks accumulate high concentrations of cyclic imines is not known yet, but it may be potentially harmful for public health.

33.4.2 Metabolism in Shellfish

The finding of the ketoamine derivatives of spirolides A and B, namely, spirolides E and F in the digestive glands of scallops, indicated that shellfish are able to transform spirolides into nontoxic molecules by hydrolyzing the spiroimine ring.[30] Oxalic acid hydrolysis of spirolide B confirmed the opening of the imine ring giving spirolide F as final product.[30] However, spirolide C, 13-desmethyl spirolide C, and spirolide D were shown to be resistant to oxalic acid hydrolysis suggesting that the double methylation of the spiroimine ring confers chemical resistance to the latter spirolides.[19] It is important to quote that with the exception of spirolides A and B, all the remaining spirolides including pinnatoxins and pteriatoxins described to date, possess a double-methylated spiroimine ring (see Figure 33.1).

To approach the question whether the opening of the spiroimine ring is enzymatically mediated, protein extracts of different shellfish species were incubated with cellular extracts of *A. ostenfeldii*, producer of 13-desmethyl spirolide C, 13,19-didesmethyl spirolide C, and spirolide G. Under the conditions tested, no evidence for a possible spirolide metabolism was detected, leading the authors to hypothesize that the double-methylated spirolides tested were resistant to the enzymatic hydrolysis by shellfish protein extracts.[160] However, more studies are needed in order to confirm this hypothesis.

Shellfish metabolic transformation of pinnatoxins was hypothesized based on the characterization of the toxin profile of toxic Pacific oysters (*C. gigas*) and razor fish (*Pinna bicolor*) bivalves and the analysis of sediments and phytoplankton, all collected from the Franklin Harbour area in South Australia.[43] The close structural features of pinnatoxins and pteriatoxins may support these observations. Pinnatoxin F was proposed as progenitor of pinnatoxins D and E, while pinnatoxin G was proposed to be at the origin of pinnatoxins A–C and pteriatoxins A–C via metabolic transformations within the shellfish.[43] Chemical interconversion of pinnatoxins was also reported.[40,43] However, pinnatoxins G and E were shown to be resistant to alkaline hydrolysis.[43] Further, a study to assess the stability of pinnatoxin A showed that this particular toxin was stable at acidic pH (1.5 and 4.1) even after heating at 100°C for 72 h in deuterium oxide. Only after heating pinnatoxin A at 100°C for 24 h in KH_2PO_4 buffer at pH 7.3, 20% of pinnatoxin A was hydrolyzed to give the aminoketone derivative of pinnatoxin A.[10]

Shellfish developed a common strategy for the metabolism of an array of phycotoxins, which consists in the acylation of bioactive molecules (i.e., okadaic acid, DSP toxins) to reduce their biological activity.[161–163] Esterification of cyclic imine toxins by toxic shellfish was also reported. Thus, a high number of fatty acid acyl esters derivatives of 20-methyl spirolide G (21; C12:0–C22:6),[31] and pinnatoxin G (26; C14:0–C24:6)[164] were found in Canadian cultured mussels (*M. edulis*) following toxic blooms. Recently, 47 fatty acid ester metabolites of gymnodimine A (C12:2–C14:6) were described in contaminated grooved carpet shells clams (*Ruditapes decussatus*) collected in the Gulf of Gabes of Tunisia.[165] To estimate the amount of sterified phycotoxins, shellfish extracts are subject to alkaline hydrolysis.[161,166] As a result, the phycotoxin is released and quantified subsequently. While gymnodimine A- and 20-methyl spirolide G-acyl derivatives were reported to be degraded by alkaline hydrolysis,[163,165] pinnatoxin G-acyl derivatives are resistant to this chemical treatment.[164] The amount of pinnatoxin G stored in the form of acyl derivatives was in some cases three times higher than free pinnatoxin G in contaminated mussel samples.[164] It would be important to assess the toxicity of acylated esters of cyclic imine toxins.

33.4.3 Metabolism in Mammals

Specific information on the absorption, distribution, metabolism, and excretion of cyclic imine toxins in laboratory animals or humans is not available from the literature. However, systemic mouse toxicity observed following oral administration of several of these compounds (see later) clearly indicates that they are absorbed from the intestinal tract. Moreover, recent results show that 13-desmethyl spirolide C and 13,19-didesmethyl spirolide C can be detected in blood, urine, and feces of mice as soon as 30–60 min after oral administration of sublethal doses of toxins, while no quantifiable levels were found after 1–24 h.[172] These results strongly suggest that a rapid excretion of the toxins occurs in mammals.

33.5 Toxicology of Cyclic Imine Toxins

From a general point of view, the toxicological studies of cyclic imines classify these toxins as "fast-acting" ones since they induce rapid onset of neurological symptoms similar to those reported for the acute toxicity of PSP toxins, followed by death within minutes (3–50 min) upon intraperitoneal (i.p.) injection into mice. This indicates rapid absorption of the cyclic imines from the peritoneum. With some exceptions, the onset of symptoms is delayed and death occurs later when the cyclic imines are orally administrated (gavage, with food or by voluntary feeding). It is worth noting that, in any cases, animals either die rapidly or make a full recovery with no perceptible long-term effects.

The symptoms of intoxication are the same for all the cyclic imines and for all routes of administration. In particular, when injected intraperitoneally to mice, prorocentrolide congeners,[46,48,51] spiro-prorocentrimine,[46] gymnodimines A and B,[12,153,167,173] some forms of spirolides such as spirolides A–D, G, 13-desmethyl spirolide C, and 20-methyl spirolide G[18,19,21,160,168–170,172] as well as pinnatoxins A–G[37,39,40,42,43,171] have been reported to produce neurological symptoms that include hyperactivity, pilo-erection, hyperextension of the back, stiffening and arching of the tail toward the head, tremors progressing to spam, paralysis and extension of the hind limbs, respiratory distress with marked abdominal breathing, tremors of the whole body, and respiratory arrest.

The 50% lethal doses (LD_{50}) of some cyclic imines by i.p. injection into mice are shown in Table 33.2. By this route of administration and according to the group of Munday,[43,170,171] 13-desmethyl spirolide C, spirolide C, and 20-methyl spirolide G are highly toxic (while spirolides A and B are about 5 and 13 times lower), closely followed by pinnatoxin F (while pinnatoxins E and G are also significantly less so) and finally by gymnodimine A. However, higher LD_{50} values, that is, 0.028 and >0.063 mg/kg mouse, were determined by Otero et al.[172] for 13-desmethyl spirolide C and 20-methyl spirolide G, respectively (Table 33.2), showing lower levels of toxicity for these two spirolides than those reported by Munday et al.[170] Such differences may be attributable to the purity of the test compound, or differences in animal strains or sex used in the studies. Gymnodimine A is 10-fold more toxic than gymnodimine B with mean LD_{50} values after i.p. injection of 0.080 and 0.800 mg/kg mouse, respectively (Table 33.2).[173] Prorocentrolide has a mouse lethality of 0.4 mg/kg mouse,[48] while spiro-prorocentrimine exhibits much less toxicity than other known marine cyclic imine toxins.[46] Interestingly, all the above molecules contain an imine moiety, suggesting that this functionality may be important for toxicological activity. Indeed, when the imine group is destroyed by ring opening, as in spirolides E and F which are supposed to be metabolites in shellfish, the toxicity is greatly decreased.[30,168,169] However, it is not the only structural requirement for toxicity since spirolide H, although containing the imine function, was reported of low toxicity to mice by i.p. injection, with only transient effects being observed at a dose of 2.000 mg/kg mouse.[32] In addition, a toxicological study performed by MacKinnon et al.[23] reveals that the loss of the methyl group at C19 in 13-desmethyl spirolide C, giving the 13,19-didesmethyl spirolide C, results in a fivefold loss of toxicity. Similarly, the fact that 13-desmethyl spirolide C, spirolide C, and 20-methyl spirolide G are more toxic than spirolides A and B[170,172] strongly suggests that the cyclic imine ring C31 methyl group, which is present in 13-desmethyl spirolide C, spirolide C, and 20-methyl spirolide G but not in spirolides A and B, could have a significant influence on the toxic response.

It is considered critical that, for regulating a toxin, i.p. studies must be complemented by oral studies, with voluntary intake taking priority over gavage. The spirolide derivatives are also toxic to mice, with the same trend in toxic response, after oral administration via gavage, although the LD_{50} by this route is between 15 and 23 times lower than those by i.p. injection in fed mice. However, by gavage, there is a marked effect of state of alimentation, with fasted mice being significantly more susceptible, by factors of between 1.3 and 3.3 than fed animals (Table 33.2). It is likely that an increase in the rate of passage of cyclic imine toxins from the stomach to the small intestine is responsible for the higher toxicity observed

TABLE 33.2

Fifty Percent Lethal Doses (LD$_{50}$) of Cyclic Imine Toxins according to their Administration Route

Cyclic Imine Toxins	Administration Routes	LD$_{50}$ (mg/kg Mouse)	References
Gymnodimine A	Intraperitoneal injection	0.096	[167]
	Intraperitoneal injection	0.080	[173]
	Intracerebroventricular injection	0.003	[173]
	Gavage	0.755	[167]
	With food	4.057	[167]
	Voluntarily feeding	>7.500	[167]
Gymnodimine B	Intraperitoneal injection	0.800	[173]
Spirolide A	Intraperitoneal injection	0.037	[170]
	Gavage (fed)	0.550	[170]
	Gavage (fasted)	0.240	[170]
	Voluntarily feeding (fed)	1.300	[170]
	Voluntarily feeding (fasted)	1.200	[170]
Spirolide B	Intraperitoneal injection	0.099	[170]
	Gavage (fasted)	0.440	[170]
Spirolide C	Intraperitoneal injection	0.008	[170]
	Gavage (fed)	0.180	[170]
	Gavage (fasted)	0.053	[170]
	Voluntarily feeding (fed)	0.780	[170]
	Voluntarily feeding (fasted)	0.500	[170]
13-Desmethyl spirolide C	Intraperitoneal injection	0.007	[170]
	Intraperitoneal injection	0.028	[172]
	Gavage (fed)	0.160	[170]
	Gavage (fasted)	0.130	[170]
	Voluntarily feeding (fed)	1.000	[170]
	Voluntarily feeding (fasted)	0.500–0.630	[170]
13,19-Didesmethyl spirolide C	Intraperitoneal injection	0.032	[172]
27-Hydroxy-13-desmethyl spirolide C	Intraperitoneal injection	>0.027	[26]
27-Oxo-13,19-didesmethyl spirolide C	Intraperitoneal injection	>0.035	[26]
Spirolide E	Intraperitoneal injection	>1.000	[30]
Spirolide F	Intraperitoneal injection	>1.000	[30]
20-Methyl spirolide G	Intraperitoneal injection	0.008	[170]
	Intraperitoneal injection	>0.063	[172]
	Gavage (fed)	0.160	[170]
	Gavage (fasted)	0.088	[170]
	Voluntarily feeding (fed)	0.630	[170]
	Voluntarily feeding (fasted)	0.500	[170]
Pinnatoxin E	Intraperitoneal injection	0.045–0.057	[43,171]
	Gavage (fed)	2.800	[171]
Pinnatoxin F	Intraperitoneal injection	0.013–0.016	[43,171]
	Gavage (fed)	0.025	[171]
	Gavage (fasted)	0.030	[171]
	Voluntarily feeding (fed)	0.050	[171]
	Voluntarily feeding (fasted)	0.050–0.077	[171]
Pinnatoxin G	Intraperitoneal injection	0.043–0.050	[43,171]
	Gavage (fed)	0.150	[171]
	Voluntarily feeding (fed)	0.400	[171]

in fasted mice. The toxicities of the spirolides are even lower when administered by feeding (Table 33.2). It is worth noting that administration by feeding may be a more relevant method of dosing toxins since the test material becomes uniformly distributed through the stomach contents of mice and is gradually released into the small intestine, thus more closely reproducing the situation in the human. In contrast, gavage may give an artifactually high estimate of the risk of such compounds to human health. In comparative studies with 13-desmethyl spirolide C, it was shown that the vehicle employed for administration (dry mousefood, moist mousefood, or cream cheese) had no significant effect on the acute toxicity of this substance[170] and, again, fasted mice are more sensitive than fed animals (Table 33.2). Similar results are obtained for gymnodimine A and some pinnatoxin congeners (Table 33.2). The lower toxicity of pure cyclic imines when ingested compared to that when i.p. injected may explain that these compounds are of low risk to humans, a conclusion that is consonant with anecdotal evidence for the absence of harmful effects in individuals consuming shellfish contaminated with cyclic imines. Hence, human toxicity is still unknown, even if gastric distress and tachycardia, following consumption of contaminated shellfish, were reported in the period during which spirolides were detected in Nova Scotian shellfish. However, the LD_{50} of lipophilic shellfish extracts, comprising mostly 13-desmethyl spirolide C, was determined to be higher after i.p. injection than after oral administration into mice, that is, 40 and 1 mg/kg mouse, respectively.[168] Moreover, extracts of mass cultures of New Zealand dinoflagellate containing pinnatoxin congeners (E and F) were evaluated for toxicity in mice by i.p. injection, gavage, and voluntary consumption, giving LD_{50} values of 1.330, 2.330, and 5.950 mg/kg mouse, respectively.[132] The acute toxicity of pinnatoxin-containing microalgae extracts by i.p. injection was therefore similar to that by gavage. The similarity for these two routes of administration is unusual among pure cyclic imines and other algal toxins. The extracts were also highly toxic by voluntary intake, with LD_{50} by this route being only 4.5 times higher than that by i.p. injection. This is again unusual since pure cyclic imines are more than 60 times less toxic by feeding than by injection (see Table 33.2). Similar results were obtained with crude extracts of mass cultures of Australian isolates containing pinnatoxin congeners (E, F, and G or G and small amounts of F).[130]

Finally, the LD_{50} for gymnodimine A is remarkably low after intracerebroventricular (i.c.) injection (i.e., 0.003 mg/kg mouse, Table 33.2) to mice.[173] The observation that this compound is about 30 times more toxic when administered by i.c. than by i.p. injection indicates that it acts with high affinity on the mouse central nervous system (see later). In addition, histopathological examination of the brains of mice injected with 13-desmethyl spirolide C reveals that the neurological mode of action of this spirolide involves the hippocampus and brain stem as the primary affected organs.[169] These findings strongly suggest that accumulation of cyclic imine toxins in shellfish could pose a potential human health hazard vectored through seafood.

33.6 Pharmacology of Cyclic Imine Toxins

33.6.1 Cellular and Molecular Targets of Cyclic Imine Toxins: nAChRs

The main targets of cyclic imine toxins are the muscle and neuronal types of nAChRs, which are members of the pentameric Cys-loop ligand-gated ion channel superfamily.[108,173–175] The nAChR mediating skeletal neuromuscular transmission was the first to be purified and characterized. The muscle nAChR comprises five subunits (pentamer) designated $(\alpha)_2$, β, γ, and δ, arranged around a central pore. At mature skeletal muscle endplates, the γ-subunit is replaced by the ε-subunit. The binding sites for ACh are located on amino acids forming the α-subunits, and amino acid residues from the other subunit also contribute to the ACh or agonist-binding site and also influence agonist affinity, so that the two binding sites in skeletal muscle nAChR are not identical.

33.6.1.1 Cyclic Imine Toxins on Embryonic and Mature Muscle Types of nAChRs

Gymnodimine A in the nanomolar range was shown to block nerve-evoked twitch tension in isolated frog and mouse skeletal nerve–muscle preparations, without affecting directly elicited contractions, as shown

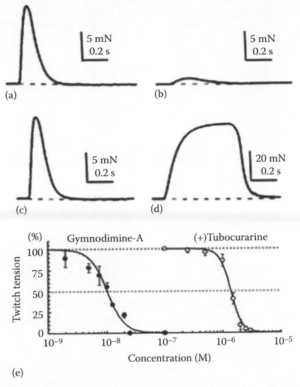

FIGURE 33.2 Block of nerve-evoked twitch tension in isolated mouse hemidiaphragm preparations by gymnodimine A. (a) Control tension recording. (b) Tension recording after 30 min exposure to gymnodimine A (20 nM). Note the decreased amplitude of the twitch response. Lack of effect of gymnodimine A (25 nM) on twitch (c) and tetanic contractions (80 Hz, d) evoked by direct muscle stimulation of the same mouse hemidiaphragm preparation as shown in (a) and (b). (e) Concentration-inhibition curves expressed as percent of the maximal twitch response for gymnodimine A (filled circles, $EC_{50} = 10.2 \pm 0.7$ nM) and (+) tubocurarine (open circles, $EC_{50} = 1.3 \pm 0.1$ μM). The dashed line indicates the effective concentration inhibiting 50% twitch height (EC_{50}). Points are mean values ± standard error of the mean (SEM) obtained in 4–6 different hemidiaphragm nerve–muscle preparations. (Modified from Kharrat, R. et al., *J. Neurochem.*, 107, 952, 2008.)

in Figure 33.2. In addition, gymnodimine A reduced and blocked miniature endplate potentials amplitude and endplate potentials, without altering the resting membrane potential of muscle fibers as determined in recordings performed in single neuromuscular junctions. Such actions are due to the block of endplate nAChRs. The block of the endplate potential amplitudes by the toxin prevents these potentials from reaching the threshold for action potential generation in muscle fibers leading to the block of muscle contraction.[173] Similar actions were observed with the 13-desmethyl spirolide C.[176] Notably, gymnodimine A and 13-desmethyl spirolide C were, on equimolar basis, much more potent than (+)-tubocurarine, a classical blocker of endplate nAChR of the neuromuscular junction, as shown in Figure 33.2.

Pinnatoxin F and crude pinnatoxins E and F dinoflagellate extracts (strain CAWD167, Cawthron Institute Culture Collection of Micro-algae) were also reported to block extracellularly recorded compound muscle action potentials evoked by phrenic nerve stimulation without altering electrically elicited compound action potentials.[177]

Available evidence indicates that not only the mature muscle-type $\alpha 1_2 \beta 1 \delta \varepsilon$ nAChR is an important target for cyclic imine toxins, but also the embryonic muscle-type $\alpha 1_2 \beta 1 \gamma \delta$ nAChR. Indeed, gymnodimine A was shown to block inward nicotinic currents evoked by iontophoretic ACh pulses in skeletal myocytes derived from *Xenopus laevis* embryos (Figure 33.3), and the block was unaffected by changing the holding membrane potential, as revealed by patch-clamp recordings. Furthermore, gymnodimine A when applied alone had no agonist action on the embryonic muscle-type nAChRs.[173] Similar results were also obtained with 13-desmethyl spirolide C, indicating that the block induced by these cyclic imine toxins exhibits no voltage dependency.

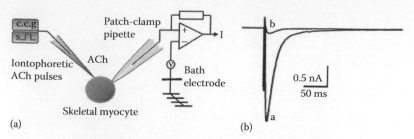

FIGURE 33.3 (a) Schematic representation of the strategy used to deliver ACh to the surface of *Xenopus* skeletal myocytes to record nicotinic currents with the patch-clamp technique[178] and to study the action of cyclic imine toxins. Iontophoretic ACh pulses were delivered to the myocyte surface through a high-resistance pipette (150 MΩ) made with borosilicate glass and filled with 1 M ACh hydrochloride. The ACh-filled micropipette was positioned as close as possible to the cell membrane. The ACh efflux was induced by cationic current pulses of constant intensity and duration (1 ms) (s) applied to the ACh-filled micropipette using a constant current generator (c.c.g), allowing the use of breaking currents to prevent spontaneous ACh efflux and avoid nAChR desensitization. The iontophoretic pulses were applied before and after perfusion with an external solution containing the cyclic imine toxin. (b) A representative example of inward nicotinic currents induced by ACh pulses recorded in the whole-cell configuration, under voltage-clamp conditions, at a holding potential of −90 mV, before (a) and after 100 nM gymnodimine A perfusion (b). Each nicotinic current trace represents the average of 10 constant iontophoretic ACh pulses.

It is well known that the muscle-type nAChR comprising $\alpha 1_2 \beta 1 \gamma \delta$ subunits is also present in the electric organs of some fish such as *Torpedo marmorata*. The microinjection of purified electrocyte membranes from the *Torpedo* electric organ into *Xenopus* oocytes leads to the incorporation of the embedded native $\alpha 1_2 \beta 1 \gamma \delta$ nAChR to the oocyte membrane, with their own glycosylation and together with any ancillary proteins they may have.[179,180] With this approach, it has been possible to study the actions of gymnodimine A, 13-desmethyl spirolide C, and pinnatoxin A on $\alpha 1_2 \beta 1 \gamma \delta$ nAChR, using the two-microelectrode voltage-clamp technique. These cyclic imine toxins blocked in a concentration-dependent manner ACh-elicited nicotinic currents indicating an antagonist action on the $\alpha 1_2 \beta 1 \gamma \delta$ nAChR. All the cyclic imines toxins studied so far have no agonist action on the nAChR. The 13-desmethyl spirolide C was the most potent and exhibited slower reversibility, when compared to gymnodimine A and pinnatoxin A. Competition binding studies revealed that the three cyclic imines studied interact with high affinity with the $\alpha 1_2 \beta 1 \gamma \delta$ nAChR, and in a concentration-dependent manner totally displaced [125I]α-bungarotoxin from the binding site.[108,173,174]

Synthetic 6,6-spiroimine analogs of gymnodimine A have also been shown to block ACh-evoked currents in *Xenopus* oocytes having incorporated the $\alpha 1_2 \beta 1 \gamma \delta$ nAChR.[63] Although the synthetic analogs are much less active than gymnodimine A, the 6,6-spiroimine moiety represents an essential structural factor for the blockade of nAChRs. Interestingly, the tetrahydrofuran component of gymnodimine A was unable to inhibit the binding of biotinylated α-bungarotoxin to the $\alpha 1_2 \beta 1 \gamma \delta$ nAChR.[57] The study of a synthetic pinnatoxin A analog containing an open form of the imine ring was also reported to be inactive on the various nAChR subtypes investigated,[108] indicating the structural importance of the seven-membered cyclic imine in pinnatoxins. Overall, these studies point out on the prominent role the six- or seven-membered imine ring of cyclic imine toxins plays for their powerful interaction with nAChRs.

33.6.1.2 Cyclic Imine Toxins on Neuronal Type of nAChRs

In the peripheral and central nervous system, different subtypes of neuronal nAChRs coexist (for reviews, see Refs. [181–183]). Neuronal nAChRs are encoded by nine α (α2–α10) and three β (β2–β4) subunit genes and form pentameric arrangement of homogeneous (homopentamer), for example, α7, α9, or α10, or heterogeneous combination of subunits (heteropentamer), for example, the α4β2 (reviewed in Ref. [184]), which exhibit distinct biophysical and pharmacological properties. A characteristic feature of neuronal nAChRs is their prominent heterogeneity, based on their different subunit composition and stoichiometry.[184]

In autonomic mammalian ganglia neurons, for example, superior cervical ganglion, the main nAChR is the heteromeric α3β4 subtype, and there are a number of combinations with α5 and/or β2 subunits.[185] In the mammalian brain, α7 and α4β2 nAChRs play an important role in the control of synaptic transmission mediated by γ-aminobutyric acid (GABA) and glutamate. Interestingly, nAChRs are also expressed in a number of nonneuronal cells and tissues.[186,187]

Acute toxicological studies with 13-desmethyl spirolide C performed in rats revealed an upregulation of M1, M4, and M5 muscarinic acetylcholine receptor (mAChR) genes and nAChR α2 and β4 genes, suggesting that the spirolide may have an action on cholinergic receptors from the central nervous system.[169] Indeed, the cyclic imine toxins gymnodimine A, 13-desmethyl spirolide C, and pinnatoxin A have been shown to interact with the major neuronal nAChRs, as revealed by functional and competition ligand-binding studies.[108,173–176]

Functional electrophysiological studies using the two-microelectrode voltage-clamp technique in oocytes expressing the human homomeric α7 (Figure 33.4) or the human heteromeric α4β2 nAChR subtype revealed that neither gymnodimine A and 13-desmethyl spirolide C nor pinnatoxin A by itself have an agonist action on these receptors. However, all three cyclic imine toxins individually blocked the ACh-elicited currents in a concentration-dependent manner.[173,174,176] The antagonist activity of gymnodimine A on both human α7 and α4β2 nAChR subtypes was promptly reversible, while that of 13-desmethyl spirolide C was slowly reversible,[174] as that reported for pinnatoxin A on the human α7 nAChR.[108]

The use of a fluorescence calcium mobilization assay, with the calcium-sensitive dye FLIPR calcium 4 and a FLIPR tetra fluorometric imaging plate reader, revealed that neither gymnodimine nor 13-desmethyl spirolide C, up to 10 μM concentration, displayed by itself any calcium activity on cell lines expressing specific nAChR subtypes. In contrast, preincubation of gymnodimine or 13-desmethyl spirolide C with those cells inhibited the nicotine-induced calcium responses in a dose-dependent manner.[175] The rank order of potency for gymnodimine was low sensitivity form of α4β2 > human α3β4 > α7 > high sensitivity

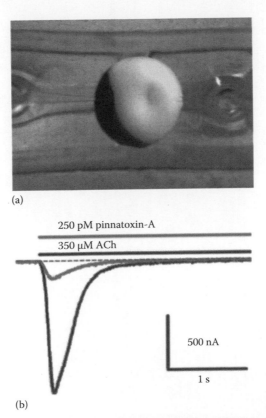

(a)

250 pM pinnatoxin-A

350 μM ACh

500 nA

1 s

(b)

FIGURE 33.4 (a) *Xenopus* oocyte previously transfected with the cDNA for the human α7 nAChR and impaled with two microelectrodes for voltage clamping in the experimental chamber perfused with a modified Ringer solution containing either the agonist or the cyclic imine studied. (b) Typical ACh-evoked current recordings at a holding potential of −60 mV before (black tracing) and after (gray tracing) the action of 250 pM pinnatoxin A. The lines above the current tracing indicate the time ACh or pinnatoxin A was perfused on to the medium.

TABLE 33.3

Affinity (K_i) Constants for Gymnodimine A, 13-Desmethyl Spirolide C, and Pinnatoxin A on Different Neuronal nAChR Subtypes

Gymnodimine

nAChR subtype	Chick α7-5HT3	Human α7/RIC3	Rat α4β2	Human α4β4	Human α4β2	Human α3β2	Rat α3β4	Human α6β3β4α5 cells
Membrane source	HEK-293 cells	HEK-293 cells	Rat cortex	SH-EP1 cells	SH-EP1 cells	HEK-293 cells	PC12 cells	SH-EP1 cells
Radioligand used	[125I]α-Bungarotoxin	[3H]Epibatidine	[3H]Epibatidine	[3H]Epibatidine	[3H]Nicotine	[3H]Epibatidine	[3H]Epibatidine	[3H]Epibatidine
K_i ± SEM (nM)	0.33 ± 0.08[a]	1.0 ± 0.1	68 ± 18	36 ± 8	70 ± 19	0.24 ± 0.09[a]	8 ± 3	1.0 ± 0.3
Reference	[173]	[175]	[175]	[175]	[175]	[173]	[175]	[175]

13-Desmethyl spirolide C

nAChR subtype	Human α7/RIC3	Human α4β2	Human α3β2	Rat α3β4
Membrane source	HEK-293 cells	HEK-293 cells	HEK-293 cells	PC12 cells
Radioligand used	[3H]Epibatidine	[3H]Epibatidine	[3H]Epibatidine	[3H]Epibatidine
K_i ± SEM (nM)	0.7 ± 0.2	0.58 ± 0.07	0.021 ± 0.005	24 ± 11
Reference	[175]	[174]	[174]	[175]

Pinnatoxin A

nAChR subtype	Chick α7-5HT3	Human α4β2	Human α3β2
Membrane source	HEK-293 cells	HEK-293 cells	HEK-293 cells
Radioligand used	[125I]α-Bungarotoxin	[3H]Epibatidine	[3H]Epibatidine
K_i ± SEM (nM)	0.35 ± 0.04	15.6 ± 5.2	9.4 ± 1.9
Reference	[108]	[108]	[108]

Note: $K_i = IC_{50}/(1+L*/K_d)$.

[a] Calculated from IC_{50} values, determined by fitting the competition data to a binding isotherm and conversion to K_i constants using the Cheng and Prusoff[188] equation.

form of α4β2 > human α4β4 > rat α3β4 nAChRs, while for 13-desmethyl spirolide C, it was α7 > low sensitivity form of α4β2 > human α3β4 > high sensitivity form of α4β2 > human α4β4 > rat α3β4 nAChR.

Also, gymnodimine A and 13-desmethyl spirolide C were shown to inhibit nicotine-mediated dopamine release from rat striatal synaptosomes with IC_{50} of 0.3 and 0.2 nM, respectively, indicating a similar potency.[175]

Competition binding studies, performed at equilibrium, on membranes from cells expressing different neuronal nAChR subtypes, revealed that gymnodimine A totally displaced, in a concentration-dependent manner, [^{125}I]α-bungarotoxin binding to the chicken chimeric α7-5HT3 nAChR and [^{3}H]epibatidine binding to human α3β2 and α4β2 nAChRs. The order of potency for gymnodimine A was chicken α7-5HT3 > mouse α1$_2$β1γδ > human α3β2 > human α4β2 nAChR.[173] A comparable broad specificity on neuronal nAChR subtypes was reported for 13-desmethyl spirolide C.[174] Notably, pinnatoxin A exhibited higher affinity for the human α7 compared to the human α3β2 and α4β2 nAChRs.[108] Table 33.3 summarizes affinity constants (K_i) for some of the cyclic imine toxins studied on an extended range of neuronal nAChR subtypes.

33.6.2 Cyclic Imine Toxins on Muscarinic Acetylcholine Receptors

The mAChRs are G protein–coupled receptors expressed on most target organs of the parasympathetic branch of the autonomic nervous system controlling diverse vegetative functions and in the central nervous system where they modulate cognitive, sensory, and motor functions and contribute to important and complex processes such as learning and memory.[189–192] The mAChRs comprise a family of five distinct subtypes, denoted M1–M5, and each subtype is the product of a separate gene.[193] The use of transgenic mice lacking one or more genes strongly suggests that all mAChR subtypes have a well-defined function in both peripheral and central nervous systems.[194,195] The M1, M3, and M5 mAChR subtypes are coupled to Gαq proteins leading to the activation of phospholipase Cβ, and subsequent calcium release from intracellular stores, and the stimulation of protein kinase C. The M2 and M4 mAChRs couple predominantly to Gαi/o proteins to inhibit adenylate cyclase, causing a decrease in intracellular cAMP levels.[196,197]

Available evidence indicates that cyclic imine toxins also interact with some mAChRs subtypes. Thus, in human neuroblastoma BE(2)-M17 cells, loaded with the Ca^{2+}-sensitive dye fura-2, exposure to 0.1 μM 13-desmethyl spirolide C for 1 h was reported to inhibit ACh-induced Ca^{2+} signals. The inhibitory effect of the spirolide on the ACh-induced calcium signal was significantly reduced when incubated simultaneously with 100 μM atropine, suggesting a competition between atropine and 13-desmethyl C spirolide for the same binding site. The spirolide at a concentration of 0.5 μM inhibited by about 50% [^{3}H]*N*-methyl scopolamine specific binding to the cells. A similar inhibition of [^{3}H]quinuclidynyl benzilate binding (59%) was observed under the same conditions. The human neuroblastoma BE(2)-M17 cells used in those studies were shown to express M3 mAChRs, and the inhibition of the 13-desmethyl spirolide C effect on [^{3}H]quinuclidynyl benzilate binding by atropine suggested that the spirolide binds to the orthosteric binding site of the mAChR.[198] In the neuroblastoma BE(2)-M17 cells, the total protein content of M3 mAChR did not change significantly after exposure to 0.1 μM 13-desmethyl spirolide C, as revealed by Western blot of whole-cell lysates.[198]

The interaction of gymnodimine and 13-desmethyl spirolide C with mAChRs was also reported in membrane preparations from rat cortices and the human clonal cell line TE671/RD in competition binding assays with [^{3}H]quinuclidynyl benzilate. Gymnodimine A at the highest concentration tested (100 μM) did not exhibit a substantial interaction with mAChRs (M1 and M2 subtypes), as deduced by the weak displacement (<25%) of [^{3}H]quinuclidynyl benzilate specifically bound to rat cortical membranes. Similar results were obtained with 13-desmethyl spirolide C, which displaced <10% of [^{3}H]quinuclidynyl benzilate binding to rat cortices. In the human clonal line TE671/RD membranes, expressing M3 mAChRs, gymnodimine A, and 13-desmethyl spirolide C displaced [^{3}H]quinuclidynyl benzilate specifically bound by <50% and <20%, respectively.[175] Further studies in Chinese hamster ovary (CHO) cells stably expressing the five human mAChRs subtypes revealed that pinnatoxin A at a concentration of 1 μM had no significant action on [^{3}H]*N*-methyl scopolamine binding to M1, M2, M3, and M4 mAChR subtypes, but induced a 35% radiotracer displacement in the M5 mAChR. Interestingly, this effect was lost when a pinnatoxin A analog with an open form of the imine ring A was studied.[108]

TABLE 33.4

Binding Assay Data for Synthetic Pinnatoxin A (10 μM) Screened with More than 40 Receptors, Ion Channels, and Transporters

Receptor	Receptor Subtype	Source	^{3}H-Ligand	Mean % Inhibition
	Alpha1A	Human, cloned	Prazosin/^{125}I-heat	27.8
	Alpha1B	Human, cloned	Prazosin/^{125}I-heat	8.7
	Alpha1D	Human, cloned	^{3}H-Prazocin	4.3
	Alpha2A	Human, cloned	Clonidine (2 nM)/^{125}Iodoclonidine	1.7
Adrenergic	Alpha2B	Human, cloned	Clonidine (2 nM)/^{125}iodoclonidine	4.0
	Alpha2C	Human, cloned	Clonidine (2 nM)/^{125}iodoclonidine	12.6
	Beta1	Human, cloned	Dihydroalprenolol/^{125}iodopindolol	−1.8
	Beta2	Human, cloned	Dihydroalprenolol/^{125}iodopindolol	−4.0
	Beta3	Human, cloned	Dihydroalprenolol/^{125}iodopindolol	−7.6
BZP rat brain site	—	Rat brain	Flunitrazepam	−0.9
Calcium channel	—	Rat heart	[^{3}H]Nitrendipine (0.1 nM)	$K_i > 10{,}000$ nM
	D1	Human, cloned	SCH23390	
	D2	Human, cloned	*N*-Methylspiperone, NMSP	−5.9
Dopamine	D3	Human, cloned	*N*-Methylspiperone, NMSP	6.4
	D4	Human, cloned	*N*-Methylspiperone, NMSP	63.4
	D5	Human, cloned	SCH23390	12.9
Dopamine transporter	DAT	Human, cloned	WIN35428	5.9
GABAergic	GABA$_A$	Rat, forebrain	Muscimol	39.5
Histamine	H1	Human, cloned	Pyrilamine	51.2
	H2	Human, cloned	Tiotidine	12.2
	M1	Human, cloned	[^{3}H]QNB (0.5 nM)	−11.7
	M2	Human, cloned	[^{3}H]QNB (0.5 nM)	8.5
Muscarinic (ACh)	M3	Human, cloned	[^{3}H]QNB (0.5 nM)	27.9
	M4	Human, cloned	[^{3}H]QNB (0.5 nM)	5.0
	M5	Human, cloned	[^{3}H]QNB (0.5 nM)	−0.6
Norepinephrine transporter	NET	Human, cloned	Nisoxetine	11.7
Opioid	Sigma1	GP rat brain	[^{3}H]Pentazocine (3 nM)	26.6
	Sigma2	PC12	[^{3}H]DTG (3 nM)	−14.7
δ-Opioid	DOR	Human, cloned	DADL	10.0
κ-Opioid	KOR	Rat, cloned	U69593	6.7
μ-Opioid	MOR	Human, cloned	DAMGO	−10.3
	5HT1A	Human, cloned	8-OH-DPAT	−2.5
	5HT1B	Human, cloned	GR-125743/5CT	−5.4
	5HT1D	Human, cloned	GR-125743/5CT	−5.9
	5HT1E	Human, cloned	5HT	−0.5
	5HT2A	Human, cloned	Ketanserin	0.9
Serotonin	5HT2B	Human, cloned	LSD	−14.5
	5HT2C	Rat, cloned	Mesulergine	38.7
	5HT3	Human, cloned	LY 278,584	2.4
	5HT5A	Human, cloned	LSD	−6.9
	5HT6	Human, cloned	LSD	−18.3
	5HT7	Human, cloned	LSD	0.0
Serotonin transporter	SERT	Human, cloned	Citalopram	12.2

Source: Modified with permission from Aráoz, R., Servent, D., Molgó, J. et al., Total synthesis of pinnatoxins A and G and revision of the mode of action of pinnatoxin A, *J. Am. Chem. Soc.*, 133, 10499–10511, 2011. Copyright 2011, American Chemical Society.

Further ligand-binding studies performed with synthetic pinnatoxin A on other selected G protein–coupled neurotransmitter receptors, transporters, and channels revealed, as shown in Table 33.4, that pinnatoxin A at 10 μM concentration had no specific action on >40 receptors, channels, and transporters that were screened at this high toxin concentration.[108]

Overall, cyclic imine toxins interact with low affinity with mAChR subtypes, and further work is needed to determine whether other members of this family may have a higher affinity for these G protein–coupled receptors.

33.6.3 Molecular Interactions

Experimental evidence was brought in 2010, using x-ray crystallography, for the interaction between *Aplysia californica* acetylcholine-binding protein (AChBP) and two representative spiroimine toxins, gymnodimine A and 13-desmethyl spirolide C.[174] These toxins are located within the orthosteric site, at the interface between two subunits, and present characteristic hydrogen bonds between the backbone carbonyl of Trp147 and the iminium group, between the Lys143 side chain and the lactone ring, and between Tyr195 side chain and the spiroketal ring system (Figure 33.5a).[174] Homology modeling (Figure 33.5b) and docking calculations (Figure 33.5c) provided insight into the interaction mode of these two toxins

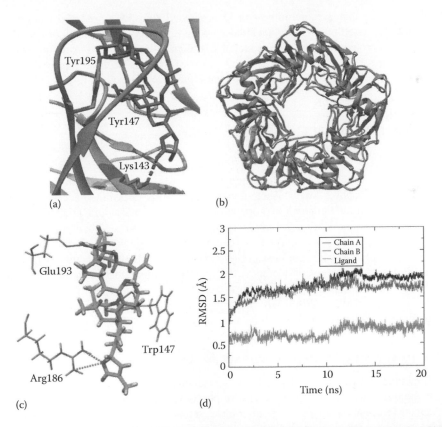

FIGURE 33.5 Selected techniques used for the study of the interaction between spiroimine toxins and nAChRs or their analogs: (a) X-ray diffraction structure of 13-desmethyl spirolide C in complex with *A. californica* acetylcholine-binding protein (From Bourne, Y. et al., *Proc. Natl. Acad. Sci. USA*, 107, 6076, 2010); (b) homology model of α7 nAChR superimposed with its template, *A. californica* acetylcholine-binding protein; (c) docking complex of 13-desmethyl spirolide C (cyan) with α7 nAChR; and (d) root-mean-square distance (RMSD) plot from a molecular dynamics simulation of the complex between 13-desmethyl spirolide C and *A. californica* acetylcholine-binding protein. (From Aráoz, R. et al., Molecular dynamics studies of acetylcholine binding protein with spiroimine toxins, in *Advances and New Technologies in Toxicology*, Barbier, J., Benoit, E., Marchot, P., Mattei, C., and Servent, D., eds., French Society of Toxinology, Paris, France, pp. 109–114, 2010.)

with AChBP and three nAChR subtypes (human α7, human α4β2, and *Torpedo* α1₂β1γδ). Subsequent molecular dynamics simulations (Figure 33.5d) of these receptor–ligand complexes evidenced specific conformational changes of the receptor induced by the toxins, as well as a limited amount of conformational flexibility of the toxins within the binding site.[199,200] Docking calculations of gymnodimine and 13-desmethyl spirolide C with the α7 nAChR reported later on showed that in addition to the previously described cation-π and hydrogen-bond interactions, hydrophobic enclosures play a significant role in driving the binding affinity.[175] Docking of pinnatoxin A with three nAChR subtypes (human α7, human α4β2, and *Torpedo* α1₂β1γδ), built by homology modeling, allowed the identification of key residues responsible for the affinity and the subtype selectivity determined experimentally for this toxin. The currently available docking software were found to be unable to deal directly with the ligand flexibility in macrocyclic systems, and a two-step protocol was employed for the fully flexible docking of pinnatoxin A with nAChRs.[108] Moreover, these studies could evidence a particular conformer of the aminoketone form of pinnatoxin A, strongly stabilized by ionic interactions between the ammonium and carboxylate groups, that is unable to bind into the receptor-binding site, thus explaining the absence of activity against nAChRs observed for this derivative.[108,201]

33.6.4 Cyclic Imine Toxins In Vivo

Recent studies revealed that gymnodimine and 13-desmethyl spirolide C reduced glutamate-induced neurotoxicity and decreased both the intracellular amyloid-β peptide and the level of hyperphosphorylated isoforms of tau protein in an in vitro model of Alzheimer disease.[202,203] A similar neuroprotective action and improvement of amyloid-β peptide and neuronal markers was detected with 13-desmethyl spirolide C in vivo treatment in a triple transgenic mouse model of Alzheimer disease.[204]

33.7 Detection Methods of Cyclic Imine Toxins

33.7.1 Mouse Bioassay

Traditionally, cyclic imine toxins were detected using the mouse bioassay protocol developed by Yasumoto et al.[205] for lipophilic toxins. Acute toxicity is currently determined according to the guidelines of the Organisation for Economic Co-operation and Development (OECD).[206] Cyclic imine toxins, at lethal doses, kill mice 3 min after intraperitoneal injection preceded by hyperactivity, jumping, paralysis of the hind legs, and severe dyspnea. Cyclic imine toxins are not internationally regulated and they are often considered as a source of false positives for lipophilic toxins detection by mouse bioassay.

The mouse bioassay, long time considered as the "golden method" for marine biotoxin monitoring, needs to be replaced in Europe because of ethical concerns.[207] The European Commission has established that LC coupled to MS (LC/MS) will be the reference method for monitoring marine lipophilic toxins and that mouse bioassay could be still be used until December 2014 for the same purpose.[207]

33.7.2 Physicochemical Detection Methods for Cyclic Imine Toxins

LC–MS/MS methods provide sensitivity, selectivity, structural, and quantitative information for unambiguous and simultaneous monitoring of an array of phycotoxins, based on the elution profile of a given toxin, the exact determination of its the molecular mass, and the determination of its mass fragmentation.

The fragmentation pathway proposed for gymnodimines, spirolides, pinnatoxins, and pteriatoxins begins with the intramolecular retro-Diels–Alder ring opening of their six-membered monounsaturated ring (named C, D, E, or G according to the type of cyclic imine toxin; see Figure 33.1), followed by water molecules losses and bond cleavage of the carbocycles leading to the formation of base fragment ions in the range of *m/z* 378–460 (for references, see Table 33.5).

A particular signature of mass fragmentation of the cyclic imine toxins is a daughter ion fragment associated with the cyclic imine ring A, that is, *m/z* 121 for gymnodimine[17] and *m/z* 164 for pinnatoxins[40] and pteriatoxins.[44] In the case of spirolides A and B, a fragment of *m/z* 150 is obtained because their

TABLE 33.5

Mass Fragmentation Data of Cyclic Imine Toxins

	Cyclic Imine Toxin	Molecular Formula	[M + H]+ (*m/z*)	Water Losses Fragments (*m/z*)	Carbocycle Fragments (*m/z*)	References
1	Gymnodimine A	$C_{32}H_{45}NO_5$	508.3405	490	410/392/202/174/ 160/136/121	[173,211]
2	Gymnodimine B	$C_{32}H_{45}NO_5$	523.3277	506/488	408/390/216/202/ 174/160/136/122	[15,173]
3	Gymnodimine C	$C_{32}H_{45}NO_5$	523.3298			[15]
4	12-Methyl gymnodimine	$C_{33}H_{47}NO_4$	522.3584	504	406/246/216/202/ 174/162/136/121	[17]
5	Spirolide A	$C_{42}H_{61}NO_7$	692.4503		462/444/426/150	[19]
6	Spirolide B		694	676/658/640	444/426/150/95	[30]
7	Spirolide C	$C_{43}H_{63}NO_7$	706.4698	688/670/652	458/440/230/204/164	[19,33]
8	13-Desmethyl spirolide C	$C_{42}H_{61}NO_7$	692.4569	674/656/638	462/444/426/ 342/204/177/164	[19,33,210, 211]
9	27-Hydroxy-13-desmethyl spirolide C	$C_{42}H_{61}NO_8$	708.4466	690/672	478/460/442/180/164	[26]
10	13,19-Didesmethyl spirolide C	$C_{41}H_{59}NO_7$	678.4375	660/642/624	430/412/348/ 246/206/164	[23,211]
11	27-Hydroxy-13,19-didesmethyl spirolide C	$C_{41}H_{59}NO_8$	694.43179	676, 658,640/622	464/446/428/ 410/180/164	[26]
12	27-Oxo-13,19-didesmethyl spirolide C	$C_{41}H_{57}NO_8$	692.4148	674/656	444/178/165	[26]
13	Spirolide D	$C_{43}H_{66}NO_7$	708	690/672/654	442/302/164	[210]
14	13-Desmethyl spirolide D	$C_{42}H_{64}NO_7$	694	676/658/640	446/428/206/164	[210]
15	Spirolide G	$C_{42}H_{61}NO_7$	692.4564	675/656	378/360/334/332/164	[23,211]
16	20-Methyl spirolide G	$C_{43}H_{63}NO_7$	706.465	688/670/652	392/374/346/258/164	[129,211]
17	Spirolide H	$C_{40}H_{60}NO_6$	650.4407	632/614	402/384/206/164	[32]
18	Spirolide I	$C_{40}H_{62}NO_6$	652.4570	634/616	402/384/206/164	[32]
19	Pinnatoxin A	$C_{41}H_{61}NO_9$	712.4444	694/676/658	458/440/432/249/ 230/206/177/164	[37,43,211]
20	Pinnatoxin B	$C_{42}H_{64}N_2O$	741.4707		697/668/458/432/320/ 258/220/177/164	[40]
21	Pinnatoxin C	$C_{42}H_{64}N_2O$	741.4707		697/668/458/432/320/ 258/220/177/164	[40]
22	Pinnatoxin D	$C_{45}H_{67}NO_{10}$	782.4845	764/746/728/710	488/470/452/446/230/ 220/206/177/164	[43]
23	Pinnatoxin E	$C_{45}H_{69}NO_{10}$	784.5008	766/748/730/712	488/470/452/446/230/ 220/206/177/164	[43]
24	Pinnatoxin F	$C_{45}H_{67}NO_9$	766.4889	748/730/712/694	488/470/452/446/230/ 220/206/177/164	[43]
25	Pinnatoxin G	$C_{42}H_{63}NO_7$	694.4683	676/658/640	572/458/440/342/258/ 220/206/177/164	[43]
26	Pteriatoxin A	$C_{45}H_{70}N_2O_{10}S$	831.4824	342/258/230	787/744/694/542/458/ 320/220/177/164	[44]
27	Pteriatoxin B	$C_{45}H_{70}N_2O_{10}S$	831.4824	342/258/230	787/744/712/710/542/ 458/320/177/164	[44]
28	Pteriatoxin C	$C_{45}H_{70}N_2O_{10}S$	831.4813	342/258/230	787/744/712/710/542/ 458/320/177/164	[44]
29	Prorocentrolide A	$C_{56}H_{85}NO_{13}$	980.6168			[48]
30	Prorocentrolide B	$C_{56}H_{85}NO_{17}S$	1076		759/679/633/553/ 361/249	[48]
31	Spiro-prorocentrimine	$C_{42}H_{69}NO_{13}S$	828.4576			[46]

imine ring A shows only one methyl substitution, while in the case of spirolide C, D, G, I, and H and their corresponding derivatives, a fragment ion of *m/z* 164 is obtained due to the double methylation of the imine ring A (Figure 33.1). Spirolides E and F, which are ketoamine derivative of spirolides A and B, respectively, lack the fragment *m/z* 150 denoting the opening of the imine moiety in these nontoxic derivatives.[30]

Numerous cyclic imine toxins possess the same molecular formula, similar mass but different structure and thus different elution profile from the chromatographic column and different mass fragmentation which is the case for spirolide A, 13-desmethyl spirolide C, and spirolide G[19,23] or for spirolide C and 20-methyl spirolide G[19,129] or pinnatoxins A and B[40] or pteriatoxins A and B.[44] Another group of cyclic imines are isomers, that is, gymnodimines A and B,[15] pinnatoxins B and C,[40] or pteriatoxins B and C.[44]

Reversed-phase LC coupled to MS detection was shown to be useful for multitoxin analysis of lipophilic phycotoxins worldwide. A 21 min LC–MS run in the single ion monitoring mode led to the detection of spirolide C and 13-desmethyl spirolide C among 11 other lipophilic toxins in phytoplankton samples collected in the East coast of Scotland.[208] An LC–MS/MS method developed for the simultaneous detection of 10 lipophilic toxins in the multiple reaction monitoring (MRM) mode led to the detection of gymnodimine A in mussel samples collected in New Zealand coasts.[152] The capacity of LC–MS/MS methods for simultaneous detection of lipophilic toxins including gymnodimine A was demonstrated by a full single laboratory validation work in New Zealand and limited interlaboratory study between laboratories in eight countries.[209]

Matrix-assisted laser desorption ionization–time of flight MS (MALDI–TOF/MS) was applied directly on *A. ostenfeldii* extracts providing exact *m/z* measurements that supported the identification and characterization of 13-desmethyl spirolide C, 13-desmethyl spirolide D, spirolide C, and spirolide D.[210] However, the sensitivity of MALDI–TOF for the analysis of cyclic imine toxins is poor compared to other LC/MS/MS methods.[211]

Cyclic imine toxins lack chromophores in the UV region. Nonetheless, an HPLC method with UV detection at 210 nm was developed for the quantitative detection of gymnodimine A (LOQ: 8 μg GYM A/kg digestive gland).[212]

As a part of interlaboratory validation programs to replace mouse bioassay, a series of LC–MS/MS methods for simultaneous detection of lipophilic phycotoxins were developed in Europe.[213–221] Toxin detection was performed using tandem quadrupole MS in the MRM mode, one of the most suitable methods for optimal quantitative and analytical analysis of bioactive molecules, using one, two, and sometimes three specific ion transitions.

The LC–MS/MS methods developed for routine monitoring of lipophilic phycotoxins were focused on the detection of 13 lipophilic toxins that were regulated by the European Commission that included some cyclic imine toxins for which certified standards are commercially available. A cruise ship equipped with an LC–MS/MS device monitored in a near real-time manner 23 lipophilic toxins in a 25 min run detecting 13-desmethyl spirolide C and 20-methyl spirolide G in some phytoplankton samples from the North Sea in 2007.[215] By exploiting the capacity of ultraperformance LC–MS/MS (UPLC–MS/MS) to fast switching between transitions improving the dwell times used and the amount of data points obtained over one peak, 21 lipophilic phycotoxins that included gymnodimine A and 13-desmethyl spirolide C were monitored in a 6.6 min chromatographic run.[214] In Spain, extracts from mussels, oysters, cockles, clams, small clams, edible whelks, and scallops collected from different shellfish farms were monitored by LC–MS/MS for the presence of seven lipophilic toxins that included 13-desmethyl spirolide C, which was not found.[216] LC under alkaline conditions improved the separation and sensitivity of detection by MS/MS of 28 lipophilic toxins in a single run. Under alkaline conditions, negatively charged lipophilic toxins eluted early in the chromatogram and were best analyzed under negative ESI mode, while another group of toxins that included spirolides and gymnodimine A eluted later and were best analyzed under positive ESI mode.[213]

The concerted effort to develop LC–MS/MS protocols for detecting cyclic imine toxins among other lipophilic toxins allowed the detection of pinnatoxin G, spirolide C, 13-desmethyl spirolide C, 13,19-didesmethyl spirolide C, and 20-methyl spirolide G in Norway coasts;[219] the detection of 13-desmethyl spirolide C, 13,19-didesmethyl spirolide C, and 27-hydroxy-13,19-didesmethyl spirolide C in mussel samples collected from natural banks and breeding areas located along Emilia-Romagna coasts in Italy;[220] or the detection of gymnodimine A in shellfish collected in Chinese and Tunisian shellfish farms.[221,222]

Although cyclic imine toxins are highly characterized, LC/MS/MS-based detection methods depend on certified toxin standards for determining (1) the chromatographic elution profile under a given mobile phase of a cyclic imine toxin, (2) the optimal conditions for mass fragmentation of a given cyclic imine toxin for determining its corresponding MRM transitions, (3) the effect of a given matrix on the elution and/or mass fragmentation profile of a cyclic imine toxin, and (4) the limits of detection (LOD) and limits of quantification (LOQ) for the detection of a cyclic imine toxin by a LC–MS/MS method.

To circumvent the lack of certified standards, some research groups used purified phycotoxins[152,208,219,220] or shellfish extracts rich in determined cyclic imine toxins.[208,213,219] To enlarge the number of monitored cyclic imine toxins, theoretical MRM transitions were also used.[213,215] An alternative LC/MS technique to accurately and simultaneously detect unexpected cyclic imine toxins in a sample is the use of high-resolution MS. A set of 10 lipophilic toxins that included gymnodimine A and 13-desmethyl spirolide C were analyzed with a benchtop Orbitrap system, and their corresponding molecular masses were determined with a error ranging between 0.47 and 4.7 ppm using toxin standards and toxic shellfish extracts.[223] However, accurate mass alone is not enough for the identification of certain cyclic imine toxins (see Table 33.5). Synthetic chemistry efforts toward the synthesis of cyclic imine toxins are of paramount importance for unambiguous detection and risk assessment to the exposition to this family of toxins. Recently, the availability of synthetic pinnatoxin A and G allowed the development of an UPLC–MS/MS method for simultaneous monitoring of six cyclic imine toxins.[211]

Prior to LC–MS/MS analysis, the shellfish samples are homogenized, and the lipophilic toxins, if any, are extracted with methanol. The samples are also spiked with certified toxin standards during the homogenization step or following methanol extraction.[217] Methanolic shellfish extracts constitute, however, a complex mixture of biomolecules that can exert the so-called matrix effect (ion suppression or ion enhancement). In order to overcome the matrix effect, cleanup procedures by solid-phase extraction,[224,225] heat treatment of the sample,[214] chromatographic conditions, and the pH of the solvents[213] were considered to reduce and/or avoid the matrix effect.

An interesting approach to monitor the exposure of shellfish to toxic phytoplankton in shellfish farms is the use of passive sampling disks that were proven to accumulate azaspiracids, okadaic acid analogs, pectenotoxins, yessotoxins, and spirolides. The toxins retained by a solid-phase adsorption resin can be easily recovered and analyzed by LC–MS/MS.[226]

The monitoring of toxic mussels contaminated with 20-methyl spirolide G following a toxic *A. ostenfeldii* bloom showed persistent mouse toxicity for several weeks. Knowing that shellfish can metabolize a series of phycotoxins such as dinophysistoxins, a LC–MS/MS device coupled with an API 4000 triple quadrupole MS system equipped with a turbo ion-spray source was used to identify acylated derivatives that are stored in edible tissues.[31] Precursor ion spectra were acquired in the positive ion mode using a Q1 scan range of *m/z* 800–1100, the trapped ions were fragmented with N_2 in Q2, and the product ion *m/z* 164 was monitored in Q3. The product ion spectra of acyl esters were acquired by selecting precursor [M + H]⁺ ions in Q1, fragmenting in Q2, and scanning from *m/z* 100 to 1000 in Q3. As a result, 21 fatty acid methyl esters of 20-methyl spirolide G were detected in toxic shellfish but not in toxic *A. ostenfeldii*–cultured cells.[31] In a similar manner, 26 acyl esters of pinnatoxin G were discovered in mussel samples harvested on the Atlantic coast of Canada contaminated with pinnatoxin G.[227] The biological activity of acyl derivatives of cyclic imine toxins needs to be studied.

LC–MS/MS is a robust and sensitive detection method for lipophilic toxins including gymnodimine A and 13-desmethyl spirolide C (Table 33.5). Notwithstanding the lack of certified standards and the requirement of costly equipment and highly trained personnel for routine monitoring of lipophilic toxins, the European Union Reference Laboratory for Marine Biotoxins (EURLMB) promoted the implementation and validation of in-house LC–MS/MS methods for simultaneous monitoring of lipophilic toxins in Europe that included gymnodimine A and 13-desmethyl spirolide C,[217,218] in order to definitively replace mouse bioassay by 2015.[207,228,229]

33.7.3 Functional Assays for Detection of Cyclic Imine Toxins

The European Commission has regulated the use of LC/MS and mouse bioassay for monitoring internationally regulated marine biotoxins. LC/MS is the reference method for lipophilic toxin detection and mouse bioassay could be still used until December 2014 for this purpose. Although LC/MS methods provide high levels of accuracy, sensitivity, and reliability for the simultaneous detection of an array of phycotoxins including cyclic imine toxins, novel functional assays are needed to replace mouse bioassay for rapid detection of unknown and unanticipated neurotoxins related to harmful algal blooms and seafood safety that could facilitate LC/MS analysis.[211,230,231]

A series of functional methods based on the mechanism of action of cyclic imine toxins were developed using *Torpedo* electrocyte membranes enriched in nAChR of muscle type.

First, filtration radioactive ligand-binding assay using *Torpedo* electrocyte membranes and [^{125}I] α-bungarotoxin as tracer was used to characterize the affinity of cyclic imine toxins for muscle and neuronal types of nAChR.[108,173,174] Radioactive methods are currently being used for high-throughput screening of natural and synthetic ligands of nAChR with a high sensitivity and robustness especially because of the extreme affinity of [^{125}I]α-bungarotoxin for the *Torpedo* nAChR ($K_d = 50$ pM).[174] However, radioactive debris and radiodecomposition are serious drawbacks limiting the use of radioactive ligand-binding assays to specialized laboratories.

A fluorescence polarization-binding assay to detect cyclic imine toxins was developed using *Torpedo*-nAChR and α-bungarotoxin Alexa Fluor 488 conjugate as nonradioactive tracer. Upon excitation by plane polarized light, a given fluorophore will emit fluorescence in the same plane as the exciting light. Small fluorophore dyes, such as α-bungarotoxin Alexa Fluor 488 conjugate, tumbles rapidly (4.1 ns fluorescent lifetime), as a result it will be randomly oriented and when excited by plane polarized light, its emission fluorescence will be low. The binding of α-bungarotoxin Alexa Fluor 488 to *Torpedo*-nAChR dramatically slows fluorophore's rotation and when excited by plane polarized light, the resultant emission fluorescence will be high. The presence of nanomolar concentrations of cyclic gymnodimine A and 13-desmethyl spirolide C in the reaction mixture inhibits the binding of fluorescent α-bungarotoxin to nAChR in a concentration-dependent manner. The marine phycotoxins okadaic acid, yessotoxin, and brevetoxin-2 did not interfere with this assay.[232] The matrix effect of mussels, clams, cockles, and scallops on the competitive fluorescence polarization assay was also assessed.[232,233]

A solid-phase receptor-based assay for the detection of cyclic imines was also developed. The solid-phase assay is based on the immobilization of the complex [biotin–α-bungarotoxin–*Torpedo*-nAChR] on streptavidin-coated microplates. *Torpedo*-nAChRs are detected subsequently by using an anti-nAChR primary antibody. The use of secondary antibody conjugated to horseradish peroxidase allowed the detection of binding inhibition by chemiluminescence, fluorescence, or colorimetry. The presence of gymnodimine A or 13-desmethyl spirolide C inhibits the binding of biotin–α-bungarotoxin to the *Torpedo*-nAChR.[234]

A microplate receptor–binding assay based on the immobilization of *Torpedo* electrocyte membranes on the surface of 96-well plastic microplates and on the mechanism of action of competitive agonists and antagonists of nAChRs was recently developed. This functional assay is a high-throughput method for the rapid detection of cyclic imines and cyanobacterial anatoxins directly in environmental samples with minimal sample handling, high sensitivity, reduced matrix effect, and low cross-reactivity.[211] The microplate receptor–binding assay was shown to be highly sensitive and specific for the detection of six cyclic imine toxins. However, this functional method cannot identify a given cyclic imine toxin in a shellfish sample. To tackle this drawback, the receptor-affinity binding was coupled to MS. The cyclic imine toxins tightly bound to the coated *Torpedo*-nAChRs were eluted from the wells and analyzed by MS shortening the time between screening and toxin characterization.[211]

An innovative microsphere receptor-based assay for the sensitive detection of cyclic imines by using a flow cytometry for detection was recently developed. *Torpedo*-nAChR or AChBP from *Lymnaea stagnalis* were immobilized on the surface of carboxylated microspheres. Following incubation of the coated microspheres with cyclic imines and with biotinylated α-bungarotoxin, the mixture was filtrated and streptavidin-R–phycoerythrin conjugate was added for the detection of competitive binding by flow cytometry luminex system. The advantage of this methodology is the use of microsphere beads possessing different intrinsic fluorescence meaning that more than one nAChR subtype could be simultaneously analyzed.[235]

Although less sensitive, because of the lower affinity of nonradioactive tracers, (K_d of biotinylated α-bungarotoxin for *Torpedo*-nAChR is 3.5 nM, compared to 50 pM for [^{125}I]α-bungarotoxin),[174] most of the nonradioactive methods are less expensive and can be used for routine monitoring of toxins targeting nAChRs in the subnanomolar to nanomolar range directly on contaminated shellfish samples.[211,232,233] These functional methods based on the mechanism of action of cyclic imine toxins toward nAChRs could be used as an alternative to mouse bioassay for the survey of known and unknown neurotoxins targeting nAChRs.

33.8 Conclusion

Considerable progress has been obtained during the last 20 years on cyclic imine toxins as reviewed herein, due to important advances in chemical synthesis and analytical approaches for these toxins. Furthermore, the natural sources for those toxins have been identified. However, we still have a lack of basic knowledge on the natural pathways that lead to the biosynthesis of cyclic imine toxins in the distinct dinoflagellates species, on the genes implicated in their production, and on the ecological factors that favor the dinoflagellate blooming. Furthermore, the apparent expansion of the dinoflagellate producing microorganisms worldwide offers good opportunities to compare commonalities existing in the various ecosystems involved in the production of cyclic imine toxins. Traditional vectors as shellfish have been analyzed, but further work needs to be done on depuration rates, compartmentalization, and biotransformations in filter-feeding bivalves, and also in nontraditional vectors that have been little explored.

One of the distinguishing features of cyclic imine toxins is the presence of a six- or seven-membered imine ring in their structure that plays an essential role in the high-affinity interaction with muscle and neuronal nAChR subtypes. Although cyclic imine toxins are at present not regulated, there is consensus that further studies on chronic exposure need to be performed to assess the risk these toxins may have for human health, and assure both public safety and shellfish consumer's confidence.

ACKNOWLEDGMENTS

Work performed in the laboratory of authors was funded by the European 7th Frame Program grants STC-CP2008-1-555612 (Atlantox), Interreg IVB Trans-national 2009-1/117 (Pharmatlantic), grant Aquaneurotox ANR-12-ASTR-0037-01 from the Agence Nationale de la Recherche (France), and by National Institutes of Health (USA, NIGMS R01 GM077379 to A.Z., with subcontract KK1036 to J.M.).

REFERENCES

1. O'Connor, P. D. and Brimble, M. A., 2007. Synthesis of macrocyclic shellfish toxins containing spiroimine moieties. *Nat. Prod. Rep.* 24: 869–885.
2. Kita, M. and Uemura, D., 2006. Shellfish poisons. *Prog. Mol. Subcell. Biol.* 43: 25–51.
3. Kincta, M. and Uemura, D., 2006. Bioactive heterocyclic alkaloids of marine origin, in *Bioactive Heterocycles I*. Eguchi, S., ed. Springer, Berlin, Germany, pp. 157–179.
4. Kiyota, H., 2006. Synthesis of marine natural products with bicyclic and/or spirocyclic acetals. *Top. Heterocycl. Chem.* 5: 65–95.
5. Nakamura, K., Kitamura, M., and Uemura, D., 2009. Biologically active marine natural products. *Heterocycles* 78: 1–17.
6. Beaumont, S., Ilardi, E. A., Tappin, N. D. C., and Zakarian, A., 2010. Marine toxins with spiroimine rings: Total synthesis of pinnatoxin A. *Eur. J. Org. Chem.* 5743–5765.
7. Guéret, S. M. and Brimble, M. A., 2010. Spiroimine shellfish poisoning (SSP) and the spirolide family of shellfish toxins: Isolation, structure, biological activity and synthesis. *Nat. Prod. Rep.* 27: 1350–1366.
8. Sperry, J., Liu, Y.-C. W., and Brimble, M. A., 2010. Synthesis of natural products containing spiroketals via intramolecular hydrogen abstraction. *Org. Biomol. Chem.* 8: 29–38.
9. Liu, R.-Y. and Liang, Y.-B., 2009. Cyclic imine toxin gymnodimine: A review. *Chin. J Appl. Ecol. (Yingyong Shengtai Xuebao)* 20: 2308–2313.
10. Jackson, J. J., Stivala, C. E., Iorga, B. I., Molgó, J., and Zakarian, A., 2012. Stability of cyclic imine toxins: Interconversion of pinnatoxin amino ketone and pinnatoxin A in aqueous media. *J. Org. Chem.* 77: 10435–10440.

11. Satake, M., Seki, T., Murata, K. et al., 1995. Structures of new brevetoxin analogs and gymnodimine found in shellfish from New Zealand. *Tennen Yuki Kagobutsu Toronkai Koen Yoshishu* 37: 684–689.

12. Seki, T., Satake, M., Mackenzie, L., Kaspar, H. F., and Yasumoto, T., 1995. Gymnodimine, a new marine toxin of unprecedented structure isolated from New Zealand oysters and the dinoflagellate, *Gymnodinium* sp. *Tetrahedron Lett.* 36: 7093–7096.

13. Stewart, M., Blunt, J. W., Munro, M. H. G., Robinson, W. T., and Hannah, D. J., 1997. The absolute stereochemistry of the New Zealand shellfish toxin gymnodimine. *Tetrahedron Lett.* 38: 4889–4890.

14. Miles, C. O., Wilkins, A. L., Stirling, D. J., and MacKenzie, A. L., 2000. New analogue of gymnodimine from a *Gymnodinium* species. *J. Agric. Food Chem.* 48: 1373–1376.

15. Miles, C. O., Wilkins, A. L., Stirling, D. J., and MacKenzie, A. L., 2003. Gymnodimine C, an isomer of gymnodimine B, from *Karenia selliformis*. *J. Agric. Food Chem.* 51: 4838–4840.

16. Biré, R., Krys, S., Frémy, J.-M., Dragacci, S., Stirling, D., and Kharrat, R., 2002. First evidence on occurrence of gymnodimine in clams from Tunisia. *J. Nat. Toxins* 11: 269–275.

17. Van Wagoner, R. M., Misner, I., Tomas, C. R., and Wright, J. L. C., 2011. Occurrence of 12-methylgymnodimine in a spirolide-producing dinoflagellate *Alexandrium peruvianum* and the biogenetic implications. *Tetrahedron Lett.* 52: 4243–4246.

18. Hu, T., Curtis, J. M., Oshima, Y. et al., 1995. Spirolides B and D, two novel macrocycles isolated from the digestive glands of shellfish. *J. Chem. Soc., Chem. Commun.* 2159–2161.

19. Hu, T., Burton, I. W., Cembella, A. D. et al., 2001. Characterization of spirolides A, C, and 13-desmethyl C, new marine toxins isolated from toxic plankton and contaminated shellfish. *J. Nat. Prod.* 64: 308–312.

20. Falk, M., Burton, I. W., Hu, T., Walter, J. A., and Wright, J. L. C., 2001. Assignment of the relative stereochemistry of the spirolides, macrocyclic toxins isolated from shellfish and from the cultured dinoflagellate *Alexandrium ostenfeldii*. *Tetrahedron* 57: 8659–8666.

21. Cembella, A. D., Lewis, N. I., and Quilliam, M. A., 1999. Spirolide composition of micro-extracted pooled cells isolated from natural plankton assemblages and from cultures of the dinoflagellate *Alexandrium ostenfeldii*. *Nat. Toxins* 7: 197–206.

22. Ciminiello, P., Dell'Aversano, C., Fattorusso, E. et al., 2006. Toxin profile of *Alexandrium ostenfeldii* (Dinophyceae) from the Northern Adriatic Sea revealed by liquid chromatography–mass spectrometry. *Toxicon* 47: 597–604.

23. MacKinnon, S. L., Walter, J. A., Quilliam, M. A. et al., 2006. Spirolides isolated from Danish strains of the toxigenic dinoflagellate *Alexandrium ostenfeldii*. *J. Nat. Prod.* 69: 983–987.

24. Ciminiello, P., Catalanotti, B., Dell'Aversano, C. et al., 2009. Full relative stereochemistry assignment and conformational analysis of 13,19-didesmethyl spirolide C via NMR- and molecular modeling-based techniques. A step towards understanding spirolide's mechanism of action. *Org. Biomol. Chem.* 7: 3674–3681.

25. Ciminiello, P., Dell'Aversano, C., Fattorusso, E. et al., 2007. Spirolide toxin profile of Adriatic *Alexandrium ostenfeldii* cultures and structure elucidation of 27-hydroxy-13,19-didesmethyl spirolide C. *J. Nat. Prod.* 70: 1878–1883.

26. Ciminiello, P., Dell'Aversano, C., Iacovo, E. D. et al., 2010. Characterization of 27-hydroxy-13-desmethyl spirolide C and 27-oxo-13,19-didesmethyl spirolide C. Further insights into the complex Adriatic *Alexandrium ostenfeldii* toxin profile. *Toxicon* 56: 1327–1333.

27. Otero, P., Alfonso, A., Alfonso, C. et al., 2010. New protocol to obtain spirolides from *Alexandrium ostenfeldii* cultures with high recovery and purity. *Biomed. Chromatogr.* 24: 878–886.

28. MacKinnon, S. L., Cembella, A. D., Burton, I. W., Lewis, N., LeBlanc, P., and Walter, J. A., 2006. Biosynthesis of 13-desmethyl spirolide C by the dinoflagellate *Alexandrium ostenfeldii*. *J. Org. Chem.* 71: 8724–8731.

29. Kellmann, R., Svendsen, H. M., Stueken, A., Jakobsen, K. S., and Orr, R. J. S., 2010. Biosynthesis and molecular genetics of polyketides in marine dinoflagellates. *Marine Drugs* 8: 1011–1048.

30. Hu, T., Curtis, J. M., Walter, J. A., and Wright, J. L. C., 1996. Characterization of biologically inactive spirolides E and F: Identification of the spirolide pharmacophore. *Tetrahedron Lett.* 37: 7671–7674.

31. Aasen, J. A. B., Hardstaff, W., Aune, T., and Quilliam, M. A., 2006. Discovery of fatty acid ester metabolites of spirolide toxins in mussels from Norway using liquid chromatography/tandem mass spectrometry. *Rapid Commun. Mass Spectrom.* 20: 1531–1537.

32. Roach, J. S., LeBlanc, P., Lewis, N. I., Munday, R., Quilliam, M. A., and MacKinnon, S. L., 2009. Characterization of a dispiroketal spirolide subclass from *Alexandrium ostenfeldii*. *J. Nat. Prod.* 72: 1237–1240.

33. Sleno, L., Windust, A. J., and Volmer, D. A., 2004. Structural study of spirolide marine toxins by mass spectrometry. Part I. Fragmentation pathways of 13-desmethyl spirolide C by collision-induced dissociation and infrared multiphoton dissociation mass spectrometry. *Anal. Bioanal. Chem.* 378: 969–976.

34. Sleno, L., Chalmers, M. J., and Volmer, D. A., 2004. Structural study of spirolide marine toxins by mass spectrometry. Part II. Mass spectrometric characterization of unknown spirolides and related compounds in a cultured phytoplankton extract. *Anal. Bioanal. Chem.* 378: 977–986.

35. Zheng, S., Huang, F., Chen, S. et al., 1990. The isolation and bioactivities of pinnatoxin. *Zhongguo Haiyang Yaowu (Chin. J. Mar. Drugs)* 9: 33–35.

36. Chou, T., Haino, T., Nagatsu, A. et al., 1994. Structure of pinnatoxins, potent shellfish poisons. *Tennen Yuki Kagobutsu Toronkai Koen Yoshishu* 36: 57–64.

37. Uemura, D., Chou, T., Haino, T. et al., 1995. Pinnatoxin A: A toxic amphoteric macrocycle from the Okinawan bivalve *Pinna muricata*. *J. Am. Chem. Soc.* 117: 1155–1156.

38. Chou, T., Kamo, O., and Uemura, D., 1996. Relative stereochemistry of pinnatoxin A, a potent shellfish poison from *Pinna muricata*. *Tetrahedron Lett.* 37: 4023–4026.

39. Chou, T., Haino, T., Kuramoto, M., and Uemura, D., 1996. Isolation and structure of pinnatoxin D, a new shellfish poison from the Okinawan bivalve *Pinna muricata*. *Tetrahedron Lett.* 37: 4027–4030.

40. Takada, N., Umemura, N., Suenaga, K. et al., 2001. Pinnatoxins B and C, the most toxic components in the pinnatoxin series from the Okinawan bivalve *Pinna muricata*. *Tetrahedron Lett.* 42: 3491–3494.

41. Takada, N., Umemura, N., Suenaga, K. et al., 2001. Nano-mole-order structure determination of pinnatoxins and pteriatoxins, extremely minor toxins from the Okinawan bivalves. *Tennen Yuki Kagobutsu Toronkai Koen Yoshishu* 43: 377–382.

42. McCauley, J. A., Nagasawa, K., Lander, P. A., Mischke, S. G., Semones, M. A., and Kishi, Y., 1998. Total synthesis of pinnatoxin A. *J. Am. Chem. Soc.* 120: 7647–7648.

43. Selwood, A. I., Miles, C. O., Wilkins, A. L. et al., 2010. Isolation, structural determination and acute toxicity of pinnatoxins E, F and G. *J. Agric. Food Chem.* 58: 6532–6542.

44. Takada, N., Umemura, N., Suenaga, K., and Uemura, D., 2001. Structural determination of pteriatoxins A, B and C, extremely potent toxins from the bivalve *Pteria penguin*. *Tetrahedron Lett.* 42: 3495–3498.

45. Hao, J., Matsuura, F., Kishi, Y. et al., 2006. Stereochemistry of pteriatoxins A, B, and C. *J. Am. Chem. Soc.* 128: 7742–7743.

46. Lu, C.-K., Lee, G.-H., Huang, R., and Chou, H.-N., 2001. Spiro-prorocentrimine, a novel macrocyclic lactone from a benthic *Prorocentrum* sp. of Taiwan. *Tetrahedron Lett.* 42: 1713–1716.

47. Torigoe, K., Murata, M., Yasumoto, T., and Iwashita, T., 1988. Prorocentrolide, a toxic nitrogenous macrocycle from a marine dinoflagellate, *Prorocentrum lima. Tennen Yuki Kagobutsu Toronkai Koen Yoshishu* 30: 41–48.

48. Torigoe, K., Murata, M., Yasumoto, T., and Iwashita, T., 1988. Prorocentrolide, a toxic nitrogenous macrocycle from a marine dinoflagellate, *Prorocentrum lima. J. Am. Chem. Soc.* 110: 7876–7877.

49. Hu, W., Xu, J., Sinkkonen, J., and Wu, J., 2010. Polyketides from marine dinoflagellates of the genus *Prorocentrum*, biosynthetic origin and bioactivity of their okadaic acid analogues. *Mini Rev. Med. Chem.* 10: 51–61.

50. Schmitz, F. J. and Yasumoto, T., 1991. The 1990 United States—Japan seminar on bioorganic marine chemistry, meeting report. *J. Nat. Prod.* 54: 1469–1490.

51. Hu, T., deFreitas, A. S. W., Curtis, J. M., Oshima, Y., Walter, J. A., and Wright, J. L. C., 1996. Isolation and structure of prorocentrolide B, a fast-acting toxin from *Prorocentrum maculosum. J. Nat. Prod.* 59: 1010–1014.

52. Ishihara, J., Miyakawa, J., Tsujimoto, T., and Murai, A., 1997. Synthetic study on gymnodimine. Highly stereoselective construction of substituted tetrahydrofuran and cyclohexene moieties. *Synlett* 1417–1419.

53. Yang, J., Cohn, S. T., and Romo, D., 2000. Studies toward (−)-gymnodimine: Concise routes to the spirocyclic and tetrahydrofuran moieties. *Org. Lett.* 2: 763–766.

54. White, J. D., Wang, G., and Quaranta, L., 2003. Studies on the synthesis of gymnodimine. Stereocontrolled construction of the tetrahydrofuran subunit. *Org. Lett.* 5: 4109–4112.

55. Johannes, J. W., Wenglowsky, S., and Kishi, Y., 2005. Biomimetic macrocycle-forming Diels-Alder reaction of an iminium dienophile: Synthetic studies directed toward gymnodimine. *Org. Lett.* 7: 3997–4000.

56. White, J. D., Quaranta, L., and Wang, G., 2007. Studies on the synthesis of (−)-gymnodimine. Subunit synthesis and coupling. *J. Org. Chem.* 72: 1717–1728.

57. Toumieux, S., Beniazza, R., Desvergnes, V., Aráoz, R., Molgó, J., and Landais, Y., 2011. Synthesis of the gymnodimine tetrahydrofuran core through a Ueno-Stork radical cyclization. *Org. Biomol. Chem.* 9: 3726–3732.

58. Ahn, Y., Cardenas, G. I., Yang, J., and Romo, D., 2001. Studies toward gymnodimine: Development of a single-pot Hua reaction for the synthesis of highly hindered cyclic imines. *Org. Lett.* 3: 751–754.

59. Murai, A., Fujiwara, K., Ishihara, J. et al., 2001. Studies toward total syntheses of shellfish toxins. *Tennen Yuki Kagobutsu Toronkai Koen Yoshishu* 43: 235–240.

60. Tsujimoto, T., Ishihara, J., Horie, M., and Murai, A., 2002. Asymmetric construction of the azaspiro[5.5] undec-8-ene system towards gymnodimine synthesis. *Synlett* 399–402.

61. White, J. D., Wang, G., and Quaranta, L., 2003. Studies on the synthesis of gymnodimine. Construction of the spiroimine portion via Diels–Alder cycloaddition. *Org. Lett.* 5: 4983–4986.

62. Kong, K., Moussa, Z., and Romo, D., 2005. Studies toward a marine toxin immunogen: Enantioselective synthesis of the spirocyclic imine of (−)-gymnodimine. *Org. Lett.* 7: 5127–5130.

63. Duroure, L., Jousseaume, T., Aráoz, R. et al., 2011. 6,6-Spiroimine analogs of (−)-gymnodimine A: Synthesis and biological evaluation on nicotinic acetylcholine receptors. *Org. Biomol. Chem.* 9: 8112–8118.

64. Brimble, M. A., Robinson, J. E., Merten, J. et al., 2006. A novel bromine-induced ring expansion of the spiroimine moiety of the shellfish toxin gymnodimine. *Synlett* 1610–1612.

65. Brimble, M. A., Fares, F. A., and Turner, P., 2000. Synthesis of an oxaspirolactone intermediate for the synthesis of spirolides. *Aust. J. Chem.* 53: 845–852.

66. Caprio, V., Brimble, M. A., and Furkert, D. P., 2001. Synthesis of the novel 1,7,9-trioxadispiro[4.1.5.2] tetradecane ring system present in the spirolides. *Tetrahedron* 57: 4023–4034.

67. Furkert, D. P. and Brimble, M. A., 2002. Synthesis of the C10–C22 bis-spiroacetal domain of spirolides B and D via iterative oxidative radical cyclization. *Org. Lett.* 4: 3655–3658.

68. Brimble, M. A., 2004. Radical oxidative cyclization of spiroacetals to bis-spiroacetals: An overview. *Molecules* 9: 394–404.

69. Brimble, M. A. and Furkert, D. P., 2004. Synthesis of the 1,6,8-trioxadispiro[4.1.5.2]tetradec-11-ene ring system present in the spirolide family of shellfish toxins and its conversion into a 1,6,8-trioxadispiro[4.1.5.2]-tetradec-9-en-12-ol via base-induced rearrangement of an epoxide. *Org. Biomol. Chem.* 2: 3573–3583.

70. Ishihara, J., Ishizaka, T., Suzuki, T., and Hatakeyama, S., 2004. Enantio- and stereocontrolled formation of the bis-spiroacetal core of spirolide B. *Tetrahedron Lett.* 45: 7855–7858.

71. Meilert, K. and Brimble, M. A., 2005. Synthesis of the bis-spiroacetal moiety of spirolides B and D. *Org. Lett.* 7: 3497–3500.

72. Meilert, K. and Brimble, M. A., 2006. Synthesis of the bis-spiroacetal moiety of the shellfish toxins spirolides B and D using an iterative oxidative radical cyclization strategy. *Org. Biomol. Chem.* 4: 2184–2192.

73. Brimble, M. A. and Halim, R., 2007. Synthetic studies toward shellfish toxins containing spiroacetal units. *Pure Appl. Chem.* 79: 153–162.

74. Brimble, M. A., Crimmins, D., and Trzoss, M., 2005. Synthesis of spirolactams via Diels-Alder addition of 1,3-butadienes to an α-methylene lactam. *ARKIVOC* 39–52.

75. Stivala, C. E. and Zakarian, A., 2009. Studies toward the synthesis of spirolides: Assembly of the elaborated E-ring fragment. *Org. Lett.* 11: 839–842.

76. Guéret, S. M., Furkert, D. P., and Brimble, M. A., 2010. Synthesis of a functionalized 7,6-bicyclic spiroimine ring fragment of the spirolides. *Org. Lett.* 12: 5226–5229.

77. Guéret, S. M. and Brimble, M. A., 2011. Synthetic studies toward the spiroimine unit of the spirolides. *Pure Appl. Chem.* 83: 425–433.

78. Zhang, Y. C., Furkert, D. P., Guéret, S. M., Lombard, F., and Brimble, M. A., 2011. Gold(I)-catalysed intramolecular hydroamination of α-quaternary alkynes: Synthetic studies towards spiroimine marine toxins. *Tetrahedron Lett.* 52: 4896–4898.

79. Jousseaume, T., Retailleau, P., Chabaud, L., and Guillou, C., 2012. Studies on the asymmetric Birch reductive alkylation to access spiroimines. *Tetrahedron Lett.* 53: 1370–1372.

80. Stivala, C. E., Gu, Z., Smith, L. L., and Zakarian, A., 2012. Studies toward the synthesis of spirolide C: Exploration into the formation of the 23-membered all-carbon macrocyclic framework. *Org. Lett.* 14: 804–807.

81. Kong, K. and Romo, D., 2006. Diastereoselective, vinylogous Mukaiyama aldol additions of silyloxy furans to cyclic ketones: Annulation of butenolides and γ-lactones. *Org. Lett.* 8: 2909–2912.

82. Trzoss, M. and Brimble, M. A., 2003. Synthesis of spirocyclic imines: Key pharmacophores in the shellfish toxins spirolides and gymnodimine. *Synlett* 2042–2046.

83. Brimble, M. A. and Trzoss, M., 2004. A double alkylation-ring closing metathesis approach to spiroimines. *Tetrahedron* 60: 5613–5622.

84. Marcoux, D., Bindschadler, P., Speed, A. W. H. et al., 2011. Effect of counterion structure on rates and diastereoselectivities in α,β-unsaturated iminium-ion Diels–Alder reactions. *Org. Lett.* 13: 3758–3761.

85. Sugimoto, T., Ishihara, J., and Murai, A., 1997. The first construction of the B,C,D-ring fragment of pinnatoxins via highly stereocontrolled acetallization. *Tetrahedron Lett.* 38: 7379–7382.

86. Noda, T., Ishiwata, A., Uemura, S., Sakamoto, S., and Hirama, M., 1998. Synthetic study of pinnatoxin A. Stereoselective synthesis of the BCD-ring unit, a novel 6,5,6-bis-spiroketal system. *Synlett* 298–300.

87. Nakamura, S., Inagaki, J., Kudo, M. et al., 2002. Studies directed toward the total synthesis of pinnatoxin A: Synthesis of the 6,5,6-dispiroketal (BCD ring) system by double hemiketal formation/hetero-Michael addition strategy. *Tetrahedron* 58: 10353–10374.

88. Lu, C.-D. and Zakarian, A., 2007. Studies toward the synthesis of pinnatoxins: The B,C,D-dispiroketal fragment. *Org. Lett.* 9: 3161–3163.

89. Suthers, B. D., Jacobs, M. F., and Kitching, W., 1998. Synthesis and NMR profiling of dioxabicyclo[3.2.1]octanes related to pinnatoxin D. Confirmation of the relative stereochemistry about rings E and F. *Tetrahedron Lett.* 39: 2621–2624.

90. Ishiwata, A., Sakamoto, S., Noda, T., and Hirama, M., 1999. Synthetic study of pinnatoxin A. Intramolecular Diels–Alder approach to the AG-ring. *Synlett* 692–694.

91. Nitta, A., Ishiwata, A., Noda, T., and Hirama, M., 1999. Synthetic study of pinnatoxin A. Intramolecular alkylation approach to the G-ring. *Synlett* 695–696.

92. Wang, J., Sakamoto, S., Kamada, K. et al., 2003. Construction of the AG-ring unit of pinnatoxin A via intramolecular alkylation and aza-Wittig reaction. *Synlett* 891–893.

93. Pelc, M. J. and Zakarian, A., 2005. An approach to the imine ring system of pinnatoxins. *Org. Lett.* 7: 1629–1631.

94. Pelc, M. J. and Zakarian, A., 2006. Synthesis of the A,G-spiroimine of pinnatoxins by a microwave-assisted tandem Claisen–Mislow–Evans rearrangement. *Tetrahedron Lett.* 47: 7519–7523.

95. Stivala, C. E. and Zakarian, A., 2007. Studies toward the synthesis of pinnatoxins: The spiroimine fragment. *Tetrahedron Lett.* 48: 6845–6848.

96. Nakamura, S., Kikuchi, F., and Hashimoto, S., 2008. Stereoselective synthesis of a C1–C6 fragment of pinnatoxin A via a 1,4-addition/alkylation sequence. *Tetrahedron: Asymmetry* 19: 1059–1067.

97. Sugimoto, T., Ishihara, J., and Murai, A., 1999. Synthesis of the B,C,D,E,F-ring fragment of pinnatoxins. *Synlett* 541–544.

98. Ishihara, J., Tojo, S., Kamikawa, A., and Murai, A., 2001. One-step assembling reaction to the pentacyclic acetal of pinnatoxins. *Chem. Commun.* 1392–1393.

99. Nakamura, S., Inagaki, J., Sugimoto, T., Kudo, M., Nakajima, M., and Hashimoto, S., 2001. A stereoselective synthesis of the C10–C31 (BCDEF ring) portion of pinnatoxin A. *Org. Lett.* 3: 4075–4078.

100. Nakamura, S., Inagaki, J., Sugimoto, T., Ura, Y., and Hashimoto, S., 2002. A highly stereoselective synthesis of the C10–C31 (BCDEF ring) portion of pinnatoxin A. *Tetrahedron* 58: 10375–10386.

101. Ishihara, J., Sugimoto, T., and Murai, A., 1998. Studies on the stability of the 1,7,9-trioxadispiro[5.1.5.2] pentadecane system. The common tricyclic acetal moiety in pinnatoxins. *Synlett* 603–606.

102. Ito, T., Yamada, K., Midorikawa, M., and Noda, T., 2006. (3S,2′S,5,5′S,6′R,8′R,10′R)-3-hydroxy-4-(5′-hydroxy-10′-hydroxymethyl-5′-methyl-1′,7′,9′-trioxadispiro[5.1.5.2]pentadec-2′-yl)but-1-ene. *Acta Crystallogr., Sect. E: Struct. Rep. Online* E62: o3968–o3969.

103. Nagasawa, K., McCauley, J. A., Lander, P. A. et al., 1999. Total synthesis of pinnatoxin A. *Tennen Yuki Kagobutsu Toronkai Koen Yoshishu* 41: 19–24.

104. Nagasawa, K., 2000. Total synthesis of pinnatoxin A. *Yuki Gosei Kagaku Kyokaishi* 58: 877–886.

105. Nakamura, S., Kikuchi, F., and Hashimoto, S., 2008. Total synthesis of pinnatoxin A. *Angew. Chem. Int. Ed.* 47: 7091–7094.

106. Sakamoto, S., Sakazaki, H., Hagiwara, K. et al., 2004. A formal total synthesis of (+)-pinnatoxin A. *Angew. Chem. Int. Ed.* 43: 6505–6510.

107. Stivala, C. E. and Zakarian, A., 2008. Total synthesis of (+)-pinnatoxin A. *J. Am. Chem. Soc.* 130: 3774–3776.

108. Aráoz, R., Servent, D., Molgó, J. et al., 2011. Total synthesis of pinnatoxins A and G and revision of the mode of action of pinnatoxin A. *J. Am. Chem. Soc.* 133: 10499–10511.

109. Matsuura, F., Hao, J., Reents, R., and Kishi, Y., 2006. Total synthesis and stereochemistry of pinnatoxins B and C. *Org. Lett.* 8: 3327–3330.

110. Matsuura, F., Peters, R., Anada, M., Harried, S. S., Hao, J., and Kishi, Y., 2006. Unified total synthesis of pteriatoxins and their diastereomers. *J. Am. Chem. Soc.* 128: 7463–7465.

111. Kong, K., Romo, D., and Lee, C., 2009. Enantioselective total synthesis of the marine toxin (–)-gymnodimine employing a Barbier-type macrocyclization. *Angew. Chem. Int. Ed.* 48: 7402–7405.

112. Kong, K., Moussa, Z., Lee, C., and Romo, D., 2011. Total synthesis of the spirocyclic imine marine toxin (–)-gymnodimine and an unnatural C4-epimer. *J. Am. Chem. Soc.* 133: 19844–19856.

113. Wang, D. Z., 2008. Neurotoxins from marine dinoflagellates: A brief review. *Mar. Drugs* 6: 349–371.

114. Takahashi, E., Yu, Q., Eaglesham, G. et al., 2007. Occurrence and seasonal variations of algal toxins in water, phytoplankton and shellfish from North Stradbroke Island, Queensland, Australia. *Mar. Environ. Res.* 64: 429–442.

115. Tatters, A. O., Van, W. R. M., Wright, J. L. C., and Tomas, C. R., 2012. Regulation of spiroimine neurotoxins and hemolytic activity in laboratory cultures of the dinoflagellate *Alexandrium peruvianum* (Balech & Mendiola) Balech & Tangen. *Harmful Algae* 19: 160–168.

116. Borkman, D. G., Smayda, T. J., Tomas, C. R., York, R., Strangman, W., and Wright, J. L. C., 2012. Toxic *Alexandrium peruvianum* (Balech and de Mendiola) Balech and Tangen in Narragansett Bay, Rhode Island (USA). *Harmful Algae* 19: 92–100.

117. Cembella, A. D., Bauder, A. G., Lewis, N. I., and Quilliam, M. A., 2001. Association of the gonyaulacoid dinoflagellate *Alexandrium ostenfeldii* with spirolide toxins in size-fractionated plankton. *J. Plankton Res.* 23: 1413–1419.

118. Gribble, K. E., Keafer, B. A., Quilliam, M. A. et al., 2005. Distribution and toxicity of *Alexandrium ostenfeldii* (Dinophyceae) in the Gulf of Maine, USA. *Deep-Sea Res II* 52: 2745–2763.

119. Franco, J., Paz, B., Riobo, P. et al., 2006. First report of the production of spirolides by *Alexandrium peruvianum* (Dinophyceae) from the Mediterranean Sea, in *12th International Conference on Harmful Algae*, Copenhagen, Denmark, pp. 174–175.

120. Cembella, A. D., Lewis, N. I., and Quilliam, M. A., 2000. The marine dinoflagellate *Alexandrium ostenfeldii* (Dinophyceae) as the causative organism of spirolide shellfish toxins. *Phycologia* 39: 67–74.

121. Maclean, C., Cembella, A. D., and Quilliam, M. A., 2003. Effects of light, salinity and inorganic nitrogen on cell growth and spirolide production in the marine dinoflagellate *Alexandrium ostenfeldii* (Paulsen) Balech et Tangen. *Bot. Mar.* 46: 466–476.

122. John, U., Cembella, A., Hummert, C., Elbrächter, M., Groben, R., and Medlin, L., 2003. Discrimination of the toxigenic dinoflagellates *Alexandrium tamarense* and *A. ostenfeldii* in co-occurring natural populations from Scottish coastal waters. *Eur. J. Phycol.* 38: 25–40.

123. Brown, L., Bresnan, E., Graham, J., Lacaze, J.-P., Turrell, E., and Collins, C., 2010. Distribution, diversity and toxin composition of the genus *Alexandrium* (Dinophyceae) in Scottish waters. *Eur. J. Phycol.* 45: 375–393.

124. Touzet, N., Franco, J. M., and Raine, R., 2008. Morphogenetic diversity and biotoxin composition of *Alexandrium* (dinophyceae) in Irish coastal waters. *Harmful Algae* 7: 782–797.

125. Medhioub, W., Sechet, V., Truquet, P. et al., 2011. *Alexandrium ostenfeldii* growth and spirolide production in batch culture and photobioreactor. *Harmful Algae* 10: 794–803.

126. Tomas, C. R., van Wagoner, R., Tatters, A. O., White, K. D., Hall, S., and Wright, J. L. C., 2012. *Alexandrium peruvianum* (Balech and Mendiola) Balech and Tangen a new toxic species for coastal North Carolina. *Harmful Algae* 17: 54–63.

127. Otero, P., Alfonso, A., Vieytes, M. R., Cabado, A. G., Vieites, J. M., and Botana, L. M., 2010. Effects of environmental regimens on the toxin profile of *Alexandrium ostenfeldii*. *Environ. Toxicol. Chem.* 29: 301–310.

128. Touzet, N., Lacaze, J. P., Maher, M., Turrell, E., and Raine, R., 2011. Summer dynamic of *Alexandrium ostenfeldii* (Dinophyceae) and spirolide toxins in Cork Harbour, Ireland. *Mar. Ecol. Prog. Ser.* 425: 21–33.

129. Aasen, J., MacKinnon, S. L., LeBlanc, P. et al., 2005. Detection and identification of spirolides in Norwegian shellfish and plankton. *Chem. Res. Toxicol.* 18: 509–515.

130. Rhodes, L., Smith, K., Selwood, A. et al., 2011. Production of pinnatoxins E, F and G by scrippsielloid dinoflagellates isolated from Franklin Harbour, South Australia. *N. Z. J. Mar. Freshwater Res.* 45: 703–709.

131. Rhodes, L., Smith, K., Selwood, A. et al., 2011. Dinoflagellate *Vulcanodinium rugosum* identified as the causative organism of pinnatoxins in Australia, New Zealand and Japan. *Phycologia* 50: 624–628.
132. Rhodes, L., Smith, K., Selwood, A. et al., 2010. Production of pinnatoxins by a peridinoid dinoflagellate isolated from Northland, New Zealand. *Harmful Algae* 9: 384–389.
133. Smith, K. F., Rhodes, L. L., Suda, S., and Selwood, A. I., 2011. A dinoflagellate producer of pinnatoxin G, isolated from sub-tropical Japanese waters. *Harmful Algae* 10: 702–705.
134. Hess, P., 2011. First report of pinnatoxin in mussels and a novel dinoflagellate, *Vulcanodinium rugosum*, from France, in *8th International Conference on Molluscan Shellfish Safety*, Charlottetown, Prince Edwards Island, Canada, June 12–17, 2011.
135. Hess, P., Abadie, E., Hervé, F. et al., 2013. Pinnatoxin G is responsible for atypical toxicity in mussels (*Mytilus galloprovincialis*) and clams (*Venerupis decussata*) from Ingril, a French Mediterranean lagoon. *Toxicon* 75: 16–26.
136. MacKenzie, L., 1994. More blooming problems: Toxic algae and shellfish biotoxins in the South Island. *Seafood New Zealand* 2: 47–50.
137. Anderson, D. M., Alpermann, T. J., Cembella, A. D., Collos, Y., Masseret, E., and Montresor, M., 2012. The globally distributed genus *Alexandrium*: Multifaceted roles in marine ecosystems and impacts on human health. *Harmful Algae* 14: 10–35.
138. Cembella, A. D., A., Q. M., Lewis, N. I., Bauder, A. G., and Wright, J. L. C., 1998. Identifying the planktonic origin and distribution of spirolides in coastal Nova Scotian waters, in *Harmful Algae*. Reguera, B., Blanco, J., Fernandez, M. L., and Wyatt, T., eds. Xunta de Galicia and IOC/UNESCO, Santiago de Compostela, Spain, pp. 481–484.
139. Jaeckisch, N., Yang, I., Wohlrab, S. et al., 2011. Comparative genomic and transcriptomic characterization of the toxigenic marine dinoflagellate *Alexandrium ostenfeldii*. *PLoS One* 6: e28012.
140. Rühl, A., Hummert, C., Reinhardt, K., Gerdts, G., and Luckas, B., Determination of new algal neurotoxins (spirolides) near the Scottish east coast, International Council for the Exploration of the Sea, Copenhagen, Denmark, CM 2001/S:09.
141. MacKenzie, L., White, D., Oshima, Y., and Kapa, J., 1996. The resting cyst and toxicity of *Alexandrium ostenfeldii* (Dinophyceae) in New Zealand. *Phycologia* 35: 148–155.
142. Hakanen, P., Suikkanen, S., Franzén, J., Franzén, H., Kankaanpää, H., and Kremp, A., 2012. Bloom and toxin dynamics of *Alexandrium ostenfeldii* in a shallow embayment at the SW coast of Finland, northern Baltic Sea. *Harmful Algae* 15: 91–99.
143. Lim, P. T., Usup, G., Leaw, C. P., and Ogata, T., 2005. First report of *Alexandrium taylori* and *Alexandrium peruvianum* (Dinophyceae) in Malaysia waters. *Harmful Algae* 4: 391–400.
144. McNabb, P., Rhodes, L., and Selwood, A., 2008. Cawthron Report No. 1453 18.
145. Nézan, E. and Chomérat, N., 2011. *Vulcanodinium rugosum* gen. et sp. nov. (Dinophyceae), un nouveau dinoflagellé marin de la côte méditerranéenne française. *Cryptogamie, Algologie* 32: 3–18.
146. Van Egmond, H. P., Van Apeldoorn, M. E., and Speijers, G. J. A., 2004. *Marine Biotoxins*. FAO, Rome, Italy.
147. Scholin, C. A., Gulland, F., Doucette, G. J. et al., 2000. Mortality of sea lions along the central California coast linked to a toxic diatom bloom. *Nature* 403: 80–84.
148. James, K. J., Carey, B., O'Halloran, J., van Pelt, F., and Skrabáková, Z., 2010. Shellfish toxicity: Human health implications of marine algal toxins. *Epidemiol. Infect.* 138: 927–940.
149. Van Dolah, F. M., 2000. Marine algal toxins: Origins, health effects, and their increased occurrence. *Environ. Health Perspect.* 108: 133–141.
150. Bricelj, V. M., Connell, L., Konoki, K. et al., 2005. Sodium channel mutation leading to saxitoxin resistance in clams increases risk of PSP. *Nature* 434: 763–767.
151. Jost, M. C., Hillis, D. M., Lu, Y., Kyle, J. W., Fozzard, H. A., and Zakon, H. H., 2008. Toxin-resistant sodium channels: Parallel adaptive evolution across a complete gene family. *Mol. Biol. Evol.* 25: 1016–1024.
152. MacKenzie, L., Holland, P., McNabb, P., Beuzenberg, V., Selwood, A., and Suzuki, T., 2002. Complex toxin profiles in phytoplankton and Greenshell mussels (*Perna canaliculus*), revealed by LC-MS/MS analysis. *Toxicon* 40: 1321–1330.
153. Stirling, D. J., 2001. Survey of historical New Zealand shellfish samples for accumulation of gymnodimine. *N. Z. J. Mar. Freshwater Res.* 35: 851–857.

154. Medhioub, W., Gueguen, M., Lassus, P. et al., 2010. Detoxification enhancement in the gymnodimine-contaminated grooved carpet shell, *Ruditapes decussatus* (Linne). *Harmful Algae* 9: 200–207.

155. Medhioub, W., Lassus, P., Truquet, P. et al., 2012. Spirolide uptake and detoxification by *Crassostrea gigas* exposed to the toxic dinoflagellate *Alexandrium ostenfeldii*. *Aquaculture* 358–359: 108–115.

156. Elliott, C. J. H. and Susswein, A. J., 2002. Comparative neuroethology of feeding control in molluscs. *J. Exp. Biol.* 205: 877–896.

157. Cohen, J. L., Weiss, K. R., and Kupfermann, I., 1978. Motor control of buccal muscles in *Aplysia*. *J. Neurophysiol.* 41: 157–180.

158. Fox, L. E. and Lloyd, P. E., 1999. Glutamate is a fast excitatory transmitter at some buccal neuromuscular synapses in *Aplysia*. *J. Neurophysiol.* 82: 1477–1488.

159. Keating, C. and Lloyd, P. E., 1999. Differential modulation of motor neurons that innervate the same muscle but use different excitatory transmitters in *Aplysia*. *J. Neurophysiol.* 82: 1759–1767.

160. Christian, B., Below, A., Dressler, N., Scheibner, O., Luckas, B., and Gerdts, G., 2008. Are spirolides converted in biological systems? A study. *Toxicon* 51: 934–940.

161. Suzuki, T., Ota, H., and Yamasaki, M., 1999. Direct evidence of transformation of dinophysistoxin-1 to 7-*O*-acyl-dinophysistoxin-1 (dinophysistoxin-3) in the scallop *Patinopecten yessoensis*. *Toxicon* 37: 187–198.

162. Vale, P. and de Sampayo, M. A., 2002. Esterification of DSP toxins by Portuguese bivalves from the Northwest coast determined by LC-MS—A widespread phenomenon. *Toxicon* 40: 33–42.

163. Doucet, E., Ross, N. N., and Quilliam, M. A., 2007. Enzymatic hydrolysis of esterified diarrhetic shellfish poisoning toxins and pectenotoxins. *Anal. Bioanal. Chem.* 389: 335–342.

164. McCarron, P., Rourke, W. A., Hardstaff, W., Pooley, B., and Quilliam, M. A., 2012. Identification of pinnatoxins and discovery of their fatty acid ester metabolites in mussels (*Mytilus edulis*) from Eastern Canada. *J. Agric. Food Chem.* 60: 1437–1446.

165. de la Iglesia, P., McCarron, P., Diogene, J., and Quilliam, M. A., 2013. Discovery of gymnodimine fatty acid ester metabolites in shellfish using liquid chromatography/mass spectrometry. *Rapid Commun. Mass Spectrom.* 27: 643–653.

166. Villar-González, A., Rodríguez-Velasco, M. L., Ben-Gigirey, B., and Botana, L. M., 2007. Lipophilic toxin profile in Galicia (Spain): 2005 toxic episode. *Toxicon* 49: 1129–1134.

167. Munday, R., Towers, N. R., Mackenzie, L., Beuzenberg, V., Holland, P. T., and Miles, C. O., 2004. Acute toxicity of gymnodimine to mice. *Toxicon* 44: 173–178.

168. Richard, D., Arsenault, E., Cembella, A., and Quilliam, M., 2001. Investigations into the toxicology and pharmacology of spirolides, a novel group of shellfish toxins, in *Harmful Algal Blooms 2000*. Hallegraeff, G. M., Blackburn, S. I., Bolch, C. J., and Lewis, R. J., eds. Intergovernmental Oceanographic Commission of UNESCO, Paris, France, pp. 383–386.

169. Gill, S., Murphy, M., Clausen, J. et al., 2003. Neural injury biomarkers of novel shellfish toxins, spirolides: A pilot study using immunochemical and transcriptional analysis. *Neurotoxicology* 24: 593–604.

170. Munday, R., Quilliam, M. A., LeBlanc, P. et al., 2012. Investigations into the toxicology of spirolides, a group of marine phycotoxins. *Toxins* 4: 1–14.

171. Munday, R., Selwood, A. I., and Rhodes, L., 2012. Acute toxicity of pinnatoxins E, F and G to mice. *Toxicon* 60: 995–999.

172. Otero, P., Alfonso, A., Rodríguez, P. et al., 2012. Pharmacokinetic and toxicological data of spirolides after oral and intraperitoneal administration. *Food Chem. Toxicol.* 50: 232–237.

173. Kharrat, R., Servent, D., Girard, E. et al., 2008. The marine phycotoxin gymnodimine targets muscular and neuronal nicotinic acetylcholine receptor subtypes with high affinity. *J. Neurochem.* 107: 952–963.

174. Bourne, Y., Radic, Z., Aráoz, R. et al., 2010. Structural determinants in phycotoxins and AChBP conferring high affinity binding and nicotinic AChR antagonism. *Proc. Natl. Acad. Sci. USA* 107: 6076–6081.

175. Hauser, T. A., Hepler, C. D., Kombo, D. C. et al., 2012. Comparison of acetylcholine receptor interactions of the marine toxins, 13-desmethylspirolide C and gymnodimine. *Neuropharmacology* 62: 2239–2250.

176. Aráoz, R., Servent, D., Ouanounou, G., Benoit, E., and Molgó, J., 2009. The emergent marine dinoflagellate toxins spirolides and gymnodimines target nicotinic acetylcholine receptors. *Biol. Res.* 42(Suppl. A): R-118.

177. Hellyer, S. D., Selwood, A. I., Rhodes, L., and Kerr, D. S., 2011. Marine algal pinnatoxins E and F cause neuromuscular block in an in vitro hemidiaphragm preparation. *Toxicon* 58: 693–699.

178. Hamill, O. P., Marty, A., Neher, E., Sakmann, B., and Sigworth, F. J., 1981. Improved patch-clamp techniques for high-resolution current recording from cells and cell-free membrane patches. *Pflugers Arch.* 391: 85–100.

179. Eusebi, F., Palma, E., Amici, M., and Miledi, R., 2009. Microtransplantation of ligand-gated receptor-channels from fresh or frozen nervous tissue into *Xenopus* oocytes: A potent tool for expanding functional information. *Prog. Neurobiol.* 88: 32–40.

180. Krieger, F., Mourot, A., Aráoz, R. et al., 2008. Fluorescent agonists for the *Torpedo* nicotinic acetylcholine receptor. *ChemBioChem* 9: 1146–1153.

181. Corringer, P. J., Le Novère, N., and Changeux, J. P., 2000. Nicotinic receptors at the amino acid level. *Annu. Rev. Pharmacol. Toxicol.* 40: 431–458.

182. Dani, J. A. and Bertrand, D., 2007. Nicotinic acetylcholine receptors and nicotinic cholinergic mechanisms of the central nervous system. *Annu. Rev. Pharmacol. Toxicol.* 47: 699–729.

183. Albuquerque, E. X., Pereira, E. F., Alkondon, M., and Rogers, S. W., 2009. Mammalian nicotinic acetylcholine receptors: From structure to function. *Physiol. Rev.* 89: 73–120.

184. Gotti, C., Clementi, F., Fornari, A. et al., 2009. Structural and functional diversity of native brain neuronal nicotinic receptors. *Biochem. Pharmacol.* 78: 703–711.

185. David, R., Ciuraszkiewicz, A., Simeone, X. et al., 2010. Biochemical and functional properties of distinct nicotinic acetylcholine receptors in the superior cervical ganglion of mice with targeted deletions of nAChR subunit genes. *Eur. J. Neurosci.* 31: 978–993.

186. Bschleipfer, T., Schukowski, K., Weidner, W. et al., 2007. Expression and distribution of cholinergic receptors in the human urothelium. *Life Sci.* 80: 2303–2307.

187. Wessler, I. and Kirkpatrick, C. J., 2008. Acetylcholine beyond neurons: The non-neuronal cholinergic system in humans. *Br. J. Pharmacol.* 154: 1558–1571.

188. Cheng, Y. and Prusoff, W. H., 1973. Relationship between inhibition constant (K_i) and concentration of inhibitor which causes 50 per cent inhibition (IC_{50}) of an enzymatic reaction. *Biochem. Pharmacol.* 22: 3099–3108.

189. Hulme, E. C., Birdsall, N. J., and Buckley, N. J., 1990. Muscarinic receptor subtypes. *Annu. Rev. Pharmacol. Toxicol.* 30: 633–673.

190. Wess, J., 1996. Molecular biology of muscarinic acetylcholine receptors. *Crit. Rev. Neurobiol.* 10: 69–99.

191. Eglen, R. M., 2005. Muscarinic receptor subtype pharmacology and physiology. *Prog. Med. Chem.* 43: 105–136.

192. Langmead, C. J., Watson, J., and Reavill, C., 2008. Muscarinic acetylcholine receptors as CNS drug targets. *Pharmacol. Ther.* 117: 232–243.

193. Wess, J., 2003. Novel insights into muscarinic acetylcholine receptor function using gene targeting technology. *Trends Pharmacol. Sci.* 24: 414–420.

194. Wess, J., 2004. Muscarinic acetylcholine receptor knockout mice: Novel phenotypes and clinical implications. *Annu. Rev. Pharmacol. Toxicol.* 44: 423–450.

195. Wess, J., Eglen, R. M., and Gautam, D., 2007. Muscarinic acetylcholine receptors: Mutant mice provide new insights for drug development. *Nat. Rev. Drug Discov* 6: 721–733.

196. Caulfield, M. P., 1993. Muscarinic receptors—Characterization, coupling and function. *Pharmacol. Ther.* 58: 319–379.

197. Caulfield, M. P. and Birdsall, N. J., 1998. International Union of Pharmacology. XVII. Classification of muscarinic acetylcholine receptors. *Pharmacol. Rev.* 50: 279–290.

198. Wandscheer, C. B., Vilariño, N., Espina, B., Louzao, M. C., and Botana, L. M., 2010. Human muscarinic acetylcholine receptors are a target of the marine toxin 13-desmethyl C spirolide. *Chem. Res. Toxicol.* 23: 1753–1761.

199. Aráoz, R., Chabaud, L., Guillou, C., Molgó, J., and Iorga, B. I., 2010. Molecular dynamics studies of acetylcholine binding protein with spiroimine toxins, in *Advances and New Technologies in Toxicology*. Barbier, J., Benoit, E., Marchot, P., Mattei, C., and Servent, D., eds. French Society of Toxinology, Paris, France, pp. 109–114.

200. Aráoz, R., Chabaud, L., Guillou, C., Molgó, J., and Iorga, B. I., 2011. Spiroimine toxins in complex with nicotinic acetylcholine receptors: Structure and dynamics. *Biophys. J.* 100: 347a.

201. Aráoz, R., Zakarian, A., Molgó, J., and Iorga, B. I., 2011. Insights into the interaction of pinnatoxin A with nicotinic acetylcholine receptors using molecular modeling, in *Toxins and Ion Transfers*. Barbier, J., Benoit, E., Gilles, N. et al., eds. French Society of Toxinology, Paris, France, pp. 49–54.

202. Alonso, E., Vale, C., Vieytes, M. R., Laferla, F. M., Gimenez-Llort, L., and Botana, L. M., 2011. The cholinergic antagonist gymnodimine improves Aβ and tau neuropathology in an in vitro model of Alzheimer disease. *Cell. Physiol. Biochem.* 27: 783–794.

203. Alonso, E., Vale, C., Vieytes, M. R., Laferla, F. M., Gimenez-Llort, L., and Botana, L. M., 2011. 13-Desmethyl spirolide C is neuroprotective and reduces intracellular Aβ and hyperphosphorylated tau in vitro. *Neurochem. Int.* 59: 1056–1065.

204. Alonso, E., Otero, P., Vale, C. et al., 2013. Benefit of 13-desmethyl spirolide C treatment in triple transgenic mouse model of Alzheimer disease: β-Amyloid and neuronal markers improvement. *Curr. Alzheimer Res.* 10: 279–289.

205. Yasumoto, T., Oshima, Y., and Yamaguchi, M., 1978. Occurrence of a new type of shellfish poisoning in Tohoku district. *Bull. Jpn. Soc. Sci. Fish.* 44: 1249–1255.

206. OECD, 2001. *OECD Guideline for Testing of Chemicals 425. Acute Oral Toxicity—Up and Down Procedure*. Organisation for Economic Co-operation and Development, Paris, France (http://www.epa. gov/oppfead1/harmonization/docs/E425guideline.pdf).

207. 2011. Commission Regulation (EU) No. 15/2011 of January 10, 2011, amending Regulation (EC) No. 2074/2005 as regards recognised testing methods for detecting marine biotoxins in live bivalve molluscs. *Off. J. Eur. Union* 54: 3–7.

208. Hummert, C., Ruhl, A., Reinhardt, K., Gerdts, G., and Luckas, B., 2002. Simultaneous analysis of different algal toxins by LC-MS. *Chromatographia* 55: 673–680.

209. McNabb, P., Selwood, A. I., and Holland, P. T., 2005. Multiresidue method for determination of algal toxins in shellfish: Single-laboratory validation and interlaboratory study. *J. AOAC Int.* 88: 761–772.

210. Sleno, L. and Volmer, D. A., 2005. Toxin screening in phytoplankton: Detection and quantitation using MALDI triple quadrupole mass spectrometry. *Anal. Chem.* 77: 1509–1517.

211. Aráoz, R., Ramos, S., Pelissier, F. et al., 2012. Coupling the *Torpedo* microplate-receptor binding assay with mass spectrometry to detect cyclic imine neurotoxins. *Anal. Chem.* 84: 10445–10453.

212. Marrouchi, R., Dziri, F., Belayouni, N. et al., 2010. Quantitative determination of gymnodimine A by high performance liquid chromatography in contaminated clams from Tunisia coastline. *Mar. Biotechnol.* 12: 579–585.

213. Gerssen, A., Mulder, P. P. J., McElhinney, M. A., and de Boer, J., 2009. Liquid chromatography–tandem mass spectrometry method for the detection of marine lipophilic toxins under alkaline conditions. *J. Chromatogr. A* 1216: 1421–1430.

214. Fux, E., McMillan, D., Biré, R., and Hess, P., 2007. Development of an ultra-performance liquid chromatography–mass spectrometry method for the detection of lipophilic marine toxins. *J. Chromatogr. A* 1157: 273–280.

215. Krock, B., Tillmann, U., John, U., and Cembella, A., 2008. LC-MS-MS aboard ship: Tandem mass spectrometry in the search for phycotoxins and novel toxigenic plankton from the North Sea. *Anal. Bioanal. Chem.* 392: 797–803.

216. Chapela, M. J., Reboreda, A., Vieites, J. M., and Cabado, A. G., 2008. Lipophilic toxins analyzed by liquid chromatography–mass spectrometry and comparison with mouse bioassay in fresh, frozen, and processed molluscs. *J. Agric. Food Chem.* 56: 8979–8986.

217. Gerssen, A., van, O. E. H. W., Mulder, P. P. J., and de Boer, J., 2010. In-house validation of a liquid chromatography tandem mass spectrometry method for the analysis of lipophilic marine toxins in shellfish using matrix-matched calibration. *Anal. Bioanal. Chem.* 397: 3079–3088.

218. García-Altares, M., Diogène, J., and de la Iglesia, P., 2013. The implementation of liquid chromatography tandem mass spectrometry for the official control of lipophilic toxins in seafood: Single-laboratory validation under four chromatographic conditions. *J. Chromatogr. A* 1275: 48–60.

219. Rundberget, T., Aasen, J. A. B., Selwood, A. I., and Miles, C. O., 2011. Pinnatoxins and spirolides in Norwegian blue mussels and seawater. *Toxicon* 58: 700–711.

220. Ciminiello, P., Dell'Aversano, C., Fattorusso, E. et al., 2010. Complex toxin profile of *Mytilus galloprovincialis* from the Adriatic sea revealed by LC-MS. *Toxicon* 55: 280–288.

221. Naila, I. B., Hamza, A., Gdoura, R., Diogène, J., and de la Iglesia, P., 2012. Prevalence and persistence of gymnodimines in clams from the Gulf of Gabes (Tunisia) studied by mouse bioassay and LC-MS/MS. *Harmful Algae* 18: 56–64.

222. Liu, R., Liang, Y., Wu, X., Xu, D., Liu, Y., and Liu, L., 2011. First report on the detection of pectenotoxin groups in Chinese shellfish by LC-MS/MS. *Toxicon* 57: 1000–1007.

223. Blay, P., Hui, J. P. M., Chang, J., and Melanson, J. E., 2011. Screening for multiple classes of marine biotoxins by liquid chromatography–high-resolution mass spectrometry. *Anal. Bioanal. Chem.* 400: 577–585.

224. Gerssen, A., McElhinney, M. A., Mulder, P. P. J., Biré, R., Hess, P., and de Boer, J., 2009. Solid phase extraction for removal of matrix effects in lipophilic marine toxin analysis by liquid chromatography–tandem mass spectrometry. *Anal. Bioanal. Chem.* 394: 1213–1226.

225. Regueiro, J., Rossignoli, A. E., Alvarez, G., and Blanco, J., 2011. Automated on-line solid-phase extraction coupled to liquid chromatography–tandem mass spectrometry for determination of lipophilic marine toxins in shellfish. *Food Chem.* 129: 533–540.

226. Rundberget, T., Gustad, E., Samdal, I. A., Sandvik, M., and Miles, C. O., 2009. A convenient and cost-effective method for monitoring marine algal toxins with passive samplers. *Toxicon* 53: 543–550.

227. McCarron, P., Emteborg, H., Giddings, S. D., Wright, E., and Quilliam, M. A., 2011. A mussel tissue certified reference material for multiple phycotoxins. Part 3: Homogeneity and stability. *Anal. Bioanal. Chem.* 400: 847–858.

228. These, A., Klemm, C., Nausch, I., and Uhlig, S., 2011. Results of a European interlaboratory method validation study for the quantitative determination of lipophilic marine biotoxins in raw and cooked shellfish based on high-performance liquid chromatography–tandem mass spectrometry. Part I. Collaborative study. *Anal. Bioanal. Chem.* 399: 1245–1256.

229. van den Top, H. J., Gerssen, A., McCarron, P., and van Egmond, H. P., 2011. Quantitative determination of marine lipophilic toxins in mussels, oysters and cockles using liquid chromatography–mass spectrometry: Inter-laboratory validation study. *Food Addit. Contam. A* 28: 1745–1757.

230. Botana, L. M., Alfonso, A., Botana, A. et al., 2009. Functional assays for marine toxins as an alternative, high-throughput-screening solution to animal tests. *TrAC-Trend Anal. Chem.* 28: 603–611.

231. Aráoz, R., Vilariño, N., Botana, L. M., and Molgó, J., 2010. Ligand-binding assays for cyanobacterial neurotoxins targeting cholinergic receptors. *Anal. Bioanal. Chem.* 397: 1695–1704.

232. Vilariño, N., Fonfría, E. S., Molgó, J., Aráoz, R., and Botana, L. M., 2009. Detection of gymnodimine A and 13-desmethyl C spirolide phycotoxins by fluorescence polarization. *Anal. Chem.* 81: 2708–2714.

233. Fonfría, E. S., Vilariño, N., Espina, B. et al., 2010. Feasibility of gymnodimine and 13-desmethyl C spirolide detection by fluorescence polarization using a receptor-based assay in shellfish matrixes. *Anal. Chim. Acta* 657: 75–82.

234. Rodríguez, L. P., Vilariño, N., Molgó, J. et al., 2011. Solid-phase receptor-based assay for the detection of cyclic imines by chemiluminescence, fluorescence, or colorimetry. *Anal. Chem.* 83: 5857–5863.

235. Rodríguez, L. P., Vilariño, N., Molgó, J. et al., 2013. Development of a solid-phase receptor-based assay for the detection of cyclic imines using a microsphere-flow cytometry system. *Anal. Chem.* 85: 2340–2347.

34

Saxitoxin and Analogs: Ecobiology, Origin, Chemistry, and Detection

Paulo Vale

CONTENTS

34.1 Historical Perspective

The severity of a kind of seafood poisoning, today attributed to saxitoxin (STX) and its analogs (the paralytic shellfish poisoning [PSP] toxins or PSTs), attracted early scientific attention to its study since the dawn of the twentieth century. Native North American populations for centuries were used to this type of occasional food poisoning after bivalve consumption. But it was only in the 1920s that it was understood how sea mussels (*Mytilus californianis*) would become unsafe to eat: toxicity appeared only when a certain microalgae species (*Gonyaulax catenella*) occurred in seawater at higher concentrations than usual (Schantz 1984). At that time the syndrome was known as "mytilism," later to be replaced by the acronym PSP.

Mild symptoms of PSP include a tingling sensation or numbness around the lips, gradually spreading to the face and neck, a prickly sensation in fingertips and toes, headache, dizziness, and nausea (FAO 2004). Moderately severe symptoms are incoherent speech, progression of prickly sensation to arms and legs, stiffness and non-coordination of limbs, general weakness and feeling of lightness, slight respiratory difficulty, and rapid pulse plus backache as a late symptom. In extremely severe cases, symptoms include muscular paralysis, pronounced respiratory difficulty, and a choking sensation. In fatal cases, death is caused by respiratory paralysis (FAO 2004).

In the following decades, efforts were carried out to purify the poison responsible for "mytilism." Its purification from mussel digestive glands was very difficult due to the sporadic feature of its natural occurrence in high concentrations. It was observed that the Alaska butter clam (*Saxidomus giganteus*) would maintain toxicity in its siphons for long periods of time. The poison was finally purified mainly from these clams collected year-round and named after its Latin name: "saxitoxin."

In the 1950s, this concentrated poison was used to standardize a mouse bioassay (MBA) carried out routinely for food safety in US laboratories (Schantz et al. 1958) and donated also for physiology studies, which determined its blocking action of the inward sodium current in nerve and muscle cell membranes

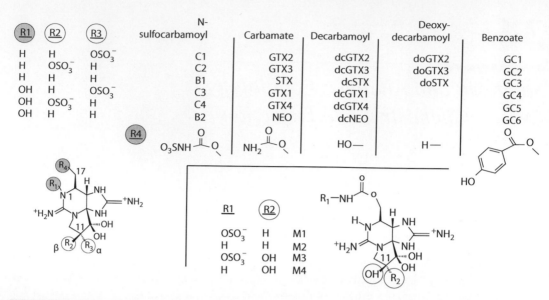

R1	R2	R3	N-sulfocarbamoyl	Carbamate	Decarbamoyl	Deoxy-decarbamoyl	Benzoate
H	H	OSO₃⁻	C1	GTX2	dcGTX2	doGTX2	GC1
H	OSO₃⁻	H	C2	GTX3	dcGTX3	doGTX3	GC2
H	H	H	B1	STX	dcSTX	doSTX	GC3
OH	H	OSO₃⁻	C3	GTX1	dcGTX1		GC4
OH	OSO₃⁻	H	C4	GTX4	dcGTX4		GC5
OH	H	H	B2	NEO	dcNEO		GC6

R1	R2	
OSO₃⁻	H	M1
H	H	M2
OSO₃⁻	OH	M3
H	OH	M4

FIGURE 34.1 Upper scheme: structures of saxitoxin analogs grouped according to variations in the side chain R₄. (From Oshima, Y., Chemical and enzymatic transformation of paralytic shellfish toxins in marine organisms, in: Lassus, P., Arzul, G., Erard, E., Gentien, P., and Marcaillou, C. Eds., *Harmful Marine Algal Blooms*, Lavoisier Science Publishers, Paris, France, pp. 475–480, 1995a; Negri, A. et al., *Chem. Res. Toxicol.*, 16(8), 1029, 2003; Vale, P., *J. Chromatogr. A*, 1195, 85, 2008b.) The first three groups are commonly found in marine dinoflagellates and bivalves. Deoxydecarbamoyl and benzoate analogs were only reported in the marine dinoflagellate *G. catenatum*. Lower scheme: exclusive bivalve metabolites, derived from successive oxidations of B1 and STX at C11. (From Dell'Aversano, C. et al., *J. Nat. Products*, 71(9), 1518, 2008.)

(Schantz 1984). This same MBA (Anon 2005a), despite its ethical drawback of animal testing, is still commonly used in the twenty-first century by regulatory bodies in many countries worldwide.

During the 1960s and 1970s, STX composition and later its full structure elucidation were achieved (Schantz et al. 1975). Its structural features include a tetrahydropurine moiety with a five-membered ring fused at an angular position and a ketone hydrate stabilized by two neighboring electron-withdrawing guanidinium groups (Figure 34.1). The first total synthesis of D,L-STX and decarbamoyl STX was published in 1977 (Tanino et al. 1977). Until recently, other research groups have continued to pursue its synthesis by different approaches (Jacobi et al. 1984; Fleming and Du Bois 2006; Bhonde and Looper 2011).

Along the 1970s and 1980s, researchers became aware that STX was not the single alkaloid involved in PSP chemistry (Figure 34.1). In cultures of toxic marine dinoflagellates, other analogs were named "gonyautoxins" (GTXs) after the genus where these were purified from (*Gonyaulax* spp.) (Shimizu et al. 1975). Today the toxic species of this genus are grouped under genus *Alexandrium* (Hallegraeff 1993), but toxin nomenclature was left unchanged.

34.2 Distribution of Producing Microorganisms

Two dinoflagellate species (*Pyrodinium bahamense* and *Gymnodinium catenatum*) and several species belonging to a single genus (*Alexandrium* spp.) have been linked to marine PSTs production (Figure 34.2) and shellfish contamination outbreaks.

P. bahamense is a tropical/subtropical species that strongly impacts PSP occurrence in the Southeast Asia and is also an important source of toxicity on both the Pacific and Atlantic coasts of Central America, including Florida (reviewed in Usup et al. 2012). It has also been found in the Caribbean Sea, the Persian Gulf, and the Red Sea.

G. catenatum has a warm-temperate to tropical distribution (Hallegraeff et al. 2012). Some coastal areas strongly affected are South Australia/Tasmania, West Iberian coast, Gulf of California, among others.

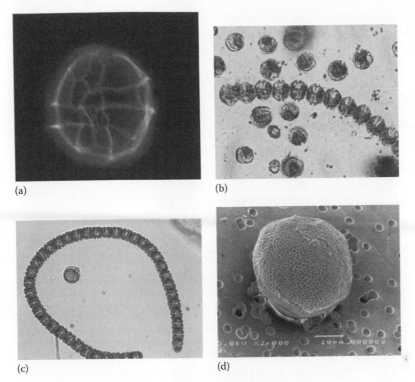

(a) (b)

(c) (d)

FIGURE 34.2 Depending on the species, dinoflagellates that produce PSTs exist in nature from single cells to medium or to long chain formations. (a) *A. minutum* from Galícia (Biaona Ria Spain, courtesy of Dr. I. Bravo); (b) *A. catenella* from the Mediterranean (Tarragona harbor, Spain; courtesy of Dr. M. Fernandez-Tejedor); (c) *G. catenatum* (Bahia de la Paz, Mexico, courtesy of Dr. J. Bustillos-Guzman); (d) a G. catenatum cyst (Portugal, courtesy of Dr. A. Amorim).

Members of the genus *Alexandrium* are widespread globally, with species present in waters of subarctic, temperate, and tropical regions of the Northern and Southern Hemispheres (Taylor et al. 1995). The *Alexandrium tamarense* species complex (comprising *A. catenella, A. tamarense*, and *A. fundyense*) appears to be the most widely dispersed and occurs in many regions worldwide, except from the tropic equatorial region (Lilly et al. 2007).

At least half of the more than 30 species in genus *Alexandrium* are known to be toxic or have otherwise harmful effects (reviewed in Anderson et al. 2012). In addition to PSTs, some species produce spirolides (*A. ostenfeldii*), and others are ichthyotoxic (e.g., *A. monilatum, A. tamarense*). Some species can present multiple toxins. For instance, *A. peruvianum* from North Carolina (United States) can present simultaneously spirolides, PSTs, and strong hemolytic activity (Tomas et al. 2012).

Common to all PSP-producing dinoflagellates is the production of a resting cyst. World distribution of resting cysts can be larger than the currently known distribution of the vegetative cells (Usup et al. 2012). This could be attributed to the species rare occurrence that has remained undetected in the water column so far. The cysts could also have been advected to and deposited at locations far from where they were formed.

Although the scientific interest in the study of PSP started a century ago in North America due to its recurrent nature, this global occurrence of producing microalgae was responsible along the twentieth century for other numerous human poisoning outbreaks from high latitudes to equatorial regions (FAO 2004). Some countries without monitoring programs were sometimes stroke with an unexpected outbreak of paralysis and even fatalities, such as in Guatemala in 1987, with an official counting of 176 poisonings and 26 fatalities (Rosales-Loessener et al. 1989). In other cases, surveillance programs existed, but there was a deficient detailed coverage (in time and/or space) of coastal areas where bivalves are available for picking. Sometimes only the official production areas are monitored, while wild mussels, for instance, can be picked at low tide in a much wider variety of locations without any specialized harvesting techniques.

In general, shellfish toxicities higher than those recorded in both the Pacific and the Atlantic coasts of North America have only been registered in the Patagonian fjords of South America (reviewed in Bricelj and Shumway 1998). Fatal poisonings still have been recorded at the twenty-first century (García et al. 2004). In very extensive coastlines, such as in Chile, where a detailed surveillance is impractical, harvesting is forbidden all year-round, but locals often disregard this ban, taking chances and putting themselves sometimes at risk.

34.3 PSTs Chemistry Defines Relative Potencies

There are several ways to group the oldest known STX analogs (depending on their substituents). Two variations are common to all STX analogs: (1) the presence or absence of an N1-hydroxyl group at N1 position and the presence or absence of an epimeric 11-hydroxysulfate group at C11 position (Figure 34.1). Additional variations in the side chain (R4) define the carbamate group, which could additionally contain an N-sulfate at the N21 position (N21-sulfocarbamoyl group), or the carbamate group could be absent (decarbamoylation into a hydroxyl function at the C17 position, or still deoxydecarbamoylation at the C17 position) (Oshima 1995b).

One mouse unit (MU), the amount of toxin administered by intraperitoneal (i.p.) injection that kills a 20 g mouse in 15 min, has been calculated as 0.18 μg of STX (Schantz 1984). Variations in the side chain (R4) are the major determinant to the relative toxicity among STX analogs, as determined by the i.p. route in mice (Oshima 1995b). The carbamoyl analogs are the most toxic, decarbamoyl analogs have intermediate toxicity, and the N-sulfocarbamoyl analogs are the least toxic, while for the deoxydecarbamoyl analogs, there is no information (Table 34.1).

The data originally supplied by Oshima (1995b) was later updated (Quilliam 2007). A recent work evaluated the relative toxicity with certified toxin standards, and the relative toxicity of dc-STX seems to be underestimated in Oshima's work compared to that of Vale et al. (2008). In order to replace biological testing by analytical testing, a recent Panel on Contaminants in the Food Chain under the auspices of the European Food Safety Authority reviewed data on toxicity and proposed toxicity equivalent factors (TEFs) for individual PSTs (EFSA 2009). These are meant to be used to express total toxicity in seafood in relation to STX (Table 34.1).

The human safety level was initially established as 400 MU/100 g shellfish meat. This is equivalent to 80 μg STX/100 g (Anon 2005a). Toxin levels above this limit are considered hazardous and

TABLE 34.1

Specific Toxicity (Expressed in MU/μmol) for Some Commonly Studied PSTs, Initially Reported by Oshima (1995b), and Toxicity Equivalent Factors (TEFs) in Relation to STX Recently Proposed by the EFSA Panel on Contaminants in the Food Chain

Toxin	Toxicity	TEF	Toxin	Toxicity	TEF
STX	2483	1.0	dcGTX2	382[a]	0.2
NeoSTX	2295	1.0	dcGTX3	935[a]	0.4
GTX1	2468	1.0	B1 (GTX5)	160	0.1
GTX2	892	0.4	B2 (GTX6)	NS	0.1
GTX3	1584	0.6	C1	15	NS
GTX4	1803	0.7	C2	239	0.1
dcSTX	1274	1.0[b]	C3	33	NS
dcNEO	NS	0.4	C4	143	0.1

Source: EFSA, *EFSA J.*, 1019, 1, 2009.

Note: NS, Not supplied.

[a] Updated by Oshima in Quilliam (2007).

[b] According to recent studies by Vale et al. (2008).

unsafe for human consumption around the world (Toyofuku 2006). Human case reports from around the world indicate a lowest-observed-adverse-effect level for PSP of around 1.5 µg STX equivalents/kg body weight (EFSA 2009). Severe cases have been reported to occur after ingestion of as low as 5.6 µg STX equivalents/kg body weight.

The lack of commercial certified standards for all known toxins (and the subsequent lack for the corresponding individual toxicities) is not the only challenge for replacing live animal testing for analytical determination of PSTs (NRC-CRMP 2012). The complex chemistry of PSTs has also been a major challenge. Nevertheless, replacing live mammal assays is imperative, not only for ethical, but also for technical reasons.

The classic MBA has several drawbacks. The sensitivity is only about half of the current regulatory limit, but this can depend on the bivalve species tested. A good correlation has been obtained when comparing LC results with MBA for some species (mussels, cockles, and clams), but a poor correlation for oysters, where the LC results were found to be on average more than double the values determined by MBA (Turner et al. 2011). These effects have been attributed to the high concentration of zinc and manganese commonly present in oysters (Turner et al. 2012). Transitional metal ions interact with the voltage-gated sodium channels, with IC_{50} for zinc and cadmium in much lower concentrations than for other divalent cations, such as manganese, calcium, or magnesium (Doyle et al. 1993). The opposite can happen with oysters from polluted areas, where high levels of zinc can result in false-positive bioassays in the absence of PSTs (McCulloch et al. 1989; Aune et al. 1998; Vale and Sampayo 2001).

34.4 Analytical Challenges of Chromatographic Methods

STX and its analogs do not exhibit natural ultraviolet absorption or fluorescence. These properties are only obtained after their conversion into purine derivatives, conducted in alkaline media (Figure 34.3a and b). Hydrogen peroxide was initially proposed as an oxidant for STX (Bates and Rapoport 1975), but toxins hydroxylated at N1 position cannot be oxidized by this reactive *tert*-butyl hydroperoxide (Oshima et al. 1984) and periodic acid has been used instead (Oshima et al. 1989).

Gradient separation was first proposed to separate the main toxins known in the early 1980s (the carbamate group) (Sullivan and Wekell 1984), but this strategy revealed inadequate for separating toxins from the groups later discovered (N-sulfocarbamoyl and decarbamoyl). Separate isocratic runs based on their net charge have been the preferred methodology for research purposes of naturally occurring PSTs in microalgae and bivalves (Oshima et al. 1989; Oshima 1995b).

Both of these methods were based on postcolumn oxidation of toxins separated chromatographically. The difficulty of running in a single day all the isocratic runs without resorting to three HPLC systems prompted the gradual perfection of an alternative methodology based on precolumn oxidation, followed by chromatographic separation of the oxidation products (Lawrence et al. 1991).

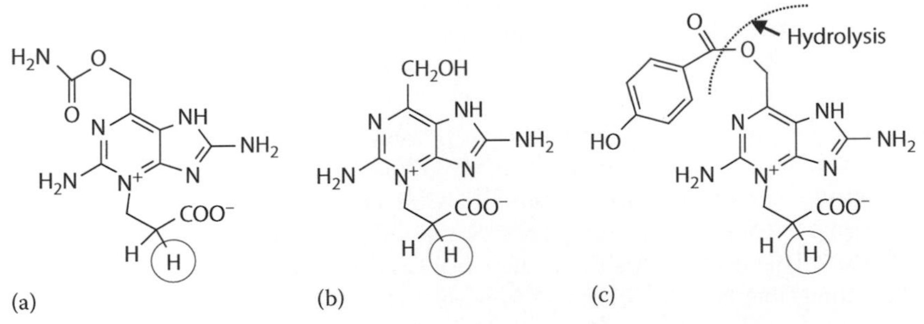

FIGURE 34.3 Proposed structures of major oxidation products of selected toxins: (a) saxitoxin, (b) decarbamoylsaxitoxin. (From Quilliam, M.A. et al., *Rapid Commun. Mass Spectrom.*, 7, 482, 1993.) (c) GC3. During oxidation, hydroxybenzoate analogs can produce simultaneously the oxidized original molecule and oxidized decarbamoyl analogs, resulting from ester hydrolysis in the strong alkalinizing reaction media. The C11-hydroxysulfate analogs also maintain the hydroxysulfate group at the position signaled by a circle.

In order to overcome superposition of different toxins (each with different toxicity) that produce the same oxidation product(s), the method refining strategies later incorporated a separation carried out by solid-phase extraction with a cation-exchange resin based on their net charges (Lawrence et al. 2005). In order to obtain the toxin profiles, the original reverse-phase cleaned extract is oxidized by both peroxide and periodate reagents, and the cation-exchange fractions are oxidized by periodate. The peroxide oxidation is used to determine the N1-hydrogen group, while the periodate is used to calculate the remaining N1-hydroxyl group (Figure 34.1).

This method was submitted to an interlaboratory collaborative study and is now the AOAC Official Method 2005.06 (Anon 2005b). Nevertheless, it is time-consuming, and the automation of the cleanup steps was later proposed by another group (Turner et al. 2009). For algae with complex toxin profiles, such as *G. catenatum*, application of this method was found to be troublesome (Ben-Gigirey et al. 2007).

Meanwhile, novel improvements to the gradient postcolumn oxidation approach were also achieved (Rourke et al. 2008), and after a collaborative study, this new method is now the AOAC Official Method 2011.02 (Anon 2011). Postcolumn oxidation methods are able to separate the C11 hydroxysulfate epimers, while precolumn methods are not. Poor column resolution in postcolumn methods can lead to superposition between STX and dcSTX or between NEO and dcNEO. This has raised the question of whether some reported profiles showing a high content of STX or NEO were correct (Luckas 1990; Bustillos-Guzman et al. 2011).

Not only toxin identification but also quantitative determination by HPLC-based methods have been strongly restricted by availability of standards, as these toxins possess quite different fluorescent responses (Franco and Fernández-Vila 1993). In addition, fluorescence detection might suffer interference problems. When studying the production of PSTs by bacteria associated with dinoflagellates, several PSTs impostors were found (Baker et al. 2003). For confirmation of PSTs, it is recommendable to use a modern detector with spectra capabilities (Baker et al. 2003; Vale 2008a,b). Interferents are commonly found in bivalves and other seafood matrices (such as crustaceans). Solid-phase extraction with C18 resins can eliminate these to a certain extent (Vale and Taleb 2005). Injection of unoxidized samples is helpful in ruling out toxin presence. This is expeditious in precolumn methods, but complicated in postcolumn methods (Vale and Sampayo 2001).

Modern detectors have been used to discover several new STX analogs along the 2000s. Strains of *G. catenatum* from several Pacific and Atlantic coasts are the only known to date to produce hydrophobic STX analogs with a *p*-hydroxybenzoate side chain, coined GC toxins from the name of its producing microalgae (Figure 34.1) (Negri et al. 2003, 2007; Vale 2008b; Bustillos-Guzman et al. 2011). Their hydrophobic nature requires higher percentage of organic solvent in the mobile phase for elution (Figure 34.5a) (Vale 2008b).

The oxidation products of these toxins differ from the "classic" PSTs mainly in their UV absorption and fluorescence spectra (Vale 2008b). The first fluorescence excitation maximum is similar to other PSTs, but the second maximum is shifted toward higher wavelengths, reflecting absorption by the benzoate side chain (Figures 34.3 and 34.4a,b; Table 34.2). The study of the oxidation products of classical PSTs by mass spectrometry has revealed that these could maintain their R4 side chain (Figure 34.3a), such as the carbamoyl moiety in STX or the N-sulfocarbamoyl moiety in C-toxins (Quilliam et al. 1993). This seems to be also the case with GC toxins as pointed by its ultraviolet and fluorescence excitation spectra (Figure 34.4b; Vale 2008b).

Upon oxidation, 11-hydroxysulfate PST analogs also maintain their hydroxysulfate group, producing another set of oxidation products (Quilliam et al. 1993). With GC toxins, two major oxidation peaks are observable, one resulting from the 11-hydroxysulfate GC1/2 and the other from the non-11-hydroxysulfate analog GC3 (Figure 34.5a). Fluorescence spectra can supply additional information regarding the hydroxysulfation at C11 (Figure 34.4c). Either classic or GC toxins with a hydroxysulfate at C11 position (designated here altogether as the GTX analogs) present both excitation and emission maxima shifted about 2 nm or more from the corresponding analogs where it is absent (designated altogether as the STX analogs) (Table 34.2). This is a typical blue shift resulting from the influence of the nonbonded extra electron pairs from the sulfate group (Miyawa and Schulman 2001).

The toxins bearing an N1-hydroxyl do produce the same oxidation products as their N1-hydrogen counterparts, but produce additionally a set of other secondary oxidation products whose structure has

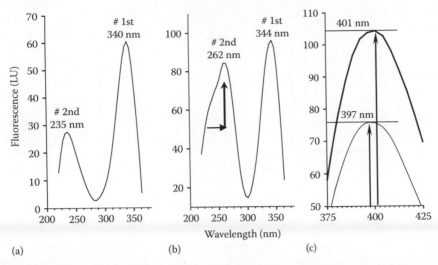

FIGURE 34.4 Flourescence spectra from classic PSTs and hydroxybenzoate PSTs after pre-column peroxide oxidation: (a) excitation spectra of second peak from dcGTX2/3, (b) excitation spectra of major peak from GCs-GTX (arrows highlight benzoate moiety contribution), (c) blue shift difference in emission maxima between major peak of GCs-STXs (397 nm) versus GCs-GTXs (401 nm).

TABLE 34.2

Selected Examples of Wavelength Differences in Fluorescence Maxima between Gonyautoxin-Type and Saxitoxin-Type PSTs

Toxin Peak Number	Type of Maxima	GTXs Analog	STXs Analog	λ Difference (nm)
Excitation				
DCs—1st peak	2nd maxima	235	233	+2
	1st maxima	340	338	+2
DCs—2nd peak	2nd maxima	235	233	+2
	1st maxima	338	333	+5
GCs—major peak	2nd maxima	262	260	+2
	1st maxima	344	341	+3
Emission				
DCs—1° peak	Single	389	386	+3
DCs—2° peak	Single	393	392	+1
GCs—major peak	Single	401	397	+4

Notes: Upon precolumn oxidation, DC analogs produce two major peaks, while a mixture of GCs produces a major peak and several minor ones. Data were obtained with an Agilent 1200 Series fluorescence detector.

Abbreviations: GC, benzoate analogs; DC, decarbamoyl analogs.

not been so well characterized (Quilliam et al. 1993). Minor oxidation products were also noted in chromatograms of GC toxins, which are probably related to the respective N1-hydroxyl counterparts found by LC-MS (Vale 2008b).

Another strategy is to use a confirmatory wavelength to detect imposters, resorting to wavelength ratios (between absorption maxima and another arbitrary wavelength). Imposters can have reverted ratios and are easily distinguished. Slight changes in this ratio might be related to different analogs not listed under the 21 classic analogs or the GC toxins. Changes in wavelength ratio associated with minor differences in retention time led to the supposition of new analogs in bivalves from Angola, but their structure remains unknown (Vale et al. 2009).

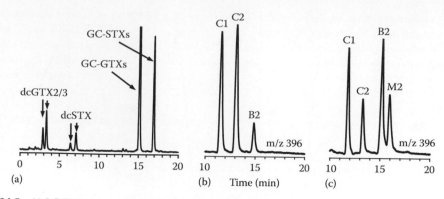

FIGURE 34.5 (a) LC-FLD chromatogram obtained after pre-column oxidation of C18 cleaned *G. catenatum* extract evidentiating GC toxins, and their hydrolysis products: decarbamoyl gonyautoxins and decarbamoylsaxitoxins. HILIC-MS chromatograms obtained in selected ion monitoring mode of: (b) cultured *G. catenatum*, (c) mussel digestive glands with M toxins. Dinoflagellate cells produce more of the β epimer (e.g., C2 in (b) is more preeminent than in (c)).

A new GTX analog was reported from a Vietnamese *Alexandrium minutum* strain, but its structure has not been elucidated until now (Lim et al. 2007). A real-time comparison study carried out by the Canadian Food Inspection Agency between testing bivalves with the AOAC MBA and the newest post-column oxidation method (Rourke et al. 2008) showed a clear methodology discrepancy during analysis of some shipments of scallops (*Zygochlamys patagonica*) imported from Argentina. Elucidation of the compound involved pointed to a decarbamoyl STX analog: 13-nor-decarbamoyl STX (13-nor-dcSTX) (Gibbs et al. 2009). Its toxicity is about six times less than STX.

Mass spectrometry detection for routine screening of marine biotoxins has been extended to the PSTs during the 2000s. The mobile phase modifiers used in common HPLC are not compatible with mass spectrometry detection. Dell'Aversano et al. (2005) experimented successfully the use of an HILIC stationary phase without the use of these ion pair modifiers. Nevertheless, detection levels that can be achieved were inferior to traditional fluorescence detection. With the TSK-gel Amide-80 column used, GTX1 coelutes with GTX2. Furthermore, inconstant retention times for PSP toxins in different seafood matrices were observed. This was overcome by other researchers using a zwitterionic (ZIC)-HILIC column (Diener et al. 2007). The detection limits were also improved with this column (Turrell et al. 2008). Additional preparative procedures could be used for the isolation and concentration of PSP toxins prior to MS analysis. The use of ZIC-HILIC SPE cartridges presented recoveries ranging from 70% to 112% (Turrell et al. 2008).

New analogs that were never detected previously by fluorescence were discovered by HILIC-MS (Dell'Aversano et al. 2008). These were designated M1 through M5 due to their presence in mussels but not in microalgae extracts. These result from single or double hydroxylation at C11 (Figure 34.1). Their presence has been extended to other bivalves, such as the estuarine common cockle and both estuarine and offshore clams (Figure 34.5b and c) (Vale 2010a).

34.5 Other Detection Methods

Besides MBA and several liquid chromatography methods, other methodologies have been developed over the years, but none has been successfully collaboratively validated to the same extent as those described earlier. While chromatography methods are time-dependent on sequential analysis, the advantage of some biomolecular methods is that several samples can be processed simultaneously in a microplate format with a short response time.

Despite the tendency to move away from live animal assays (in particular, the mammal assays), detection methods for these neurotoxins based on live invertebrates, mainly insects (cockroaches and locusts), have been refined until recent years (Cook et al. 2006; Ruebhart et al. 2011). One advantage of using insects is that statistical robustness can be increased by using larger numbers of test organisms without the legal and ethical constraints of using mammals. Among other practical advantages, insects are less expensive than mice and can be easily transported to the field. These bioassays are quicker than cell assays and could provide an alternative for the identification of new toxic fractions from column chromatography, requiring less toxin amount than MBAs. Nevertheless, when using non-pretreated shellfish matrices, the desert locust bioassay may suffer interferences, making it difficult to achieve low levels of detection (Cook et al. 2006).

Cell assays for PSTs rely on the dose-dependent reversal of the combined cytotoxic effects caused by veratridine (a sodium channel opener) and ouabain (an inhibitor of Na^+, K^+-ATPase) that lead to neuroblastoma death. Jellett et al. (1992) modified cytotoxicity assays developed by previous researchers into a colorimetric assay, avoiding individual cell counting. A major disadvantage is that adequate facilities are needed for maintenance and handling of cell cultures. An alternative, using commercial neuroblastoma preparations produced by Jellett Biotek, was collaboratively tested, but with little success due to large variations in cell viability mostly associated with transportation.

Methods based on toxin receptors have been developed using preparations of sodium channels from several sources, such as semipurified brain homogenates. Unlike chemical methods, these provide toxicity equivalent results, but the most advanced assays require the use of radioactivity-labeled isotopes, which restricts its use to specially equipped laboratories (EFSA 2009). Assays with the circulatory protein saxiphilin are more selective toward STX analogs, while sodium channel assays can detect simultaneously other neurotoxins such as tetrodotoxins (TTXs) (Negri and Llewellyn 1998).

Methods based on antibodies are very sensitive, but their main problem resides in their lack of good cross reactivity to all the members of the PSTs group. As these methods do not provide a toxicity equivalent result, and PSTs can present large discrepancy in their specific toxicities (Table 34.1), these methods can present both underestimation (due to lack of adequate cross reactivity, reported, e.g., for N1-OH analogs) and overestimation (due to low toxic N-sulfocarbamoyl derivatives being accounted as the more toxic STX). This kind of extreme scenarios will depend much on the toxin profile, which in turn is dependent on the producing microalgae and its ulterior biotransformation by shellfish (Section 34.6).

A few approaches reached commercial scale, and some results were reported in the scientific literature. The competitive enzyme-linked immunosorbent assay (ELISA) developed by Usleber et al. (1991) has been able to quantify toxins in different matrices (Usleber et al. 1997; Garet et al. 2010).

The method able to supply the quickest result is based on lateral flow immunochromatography (LFIC) testing (Jellett et al. 2002). These kinds of assays do not supply quantitative information, as required in a monitoring program, but its yes/no type information can prove quite interesting in a few situations. One is aboard fishing vessels where time until testing is a crucial step. Another is in remote regions, where subsistence bivalve gathering represents an important food source. And third, in monitoring programs has been used to reduce animal testing (Mackintosh et al. 2002), when alternatives to whole animal testing had not yet been officially approved within the European Union. However, the high percentage of false positives requires subsequent retesting via officially approved methods to prevent unnecessary closures (Costa et al. 2009).

More recently, optical biosensor technology, which uses the phenomenon of surface plasmon resonance (SPR), was also developed for the detection of PSTs (Campbell et al. 2007). These biosensor-based assays measure the competition between the interactions of a specific biological binder with the target analyte (e.g., toxin) immobilized onto the sensor chip surface and in the sample. In a similar fashion to ELISA assays, it is difficult to detect these low-molecular-weight toxins, with analogs differing at four chemical substitution sites, using a single binder (Campbell et al. 2011). Although successful comparisons with MBA- and HPLC-based methods were achieved (Campbell et al. 2009), SPR has not yet reached a commercial scale.

34.6 From Dinoflagellates to Bivalves: Changes in Toxin Profiles

Toxic dinoflagellates usually produce a few, but not all, of the known STX analogs listed in Figure 34.1. The complexity varies even within the same species among the same or separate geographic areas. The simplest toxin profiles are found in some *A. minutum* populations, which produce only GTX2/3 (Touzet et al. 2007), while others produce mainly GTX1/4 (Chou et al. 2004). Other *Alexandrium* members present more complex toxin profiles, although all decarbamoyl derivatives and the N21-sulfocarbamoyl analogs C3 and C4 are rarely found (Anderson et al. 2012). Toxin profiles of *P. bahamense* contain carbamate analogs, but might also present dcSTX, B1 and B2 (Usup et al. 2012).

The most complex profiles to date were found in *G. catenatum*. It can produce all the six N-sulfocarbamoyl analogs; several decarbamoyl and deoxydecarbamoyl analogs, GC analogs, and toxins from the carbamate group can also be found in trace levels (Oshima et al. 1993; Negri et al. 2003; Ordás et al. 2004; Vale 2008b). The benzoate analogs were initially reported to be only three, none belonging to the N1-hydroxyl group (Figure 34.1) (Negri et al. 2003). Detailed analysis revealed later that three additional N1-hydroxyl variants were also produced (Figure 34.1), and two additional GC families are also present in a Portuguese strain, differing one by an extra hydroxyl in the side chain, and the other probably by the replacement of the hydroxyl group by a sulfate group in the benzoate side chain (Vale 2008b). So far, GC analogs were only reported in *G. catenatum* and are produced by strains from around the world (Negri et al. 2007; Bustillos-Guzman et al. 2011).

In bivalves, toxin profiles are changed, sometimes to such an extreme that it is difficult to trace the origin of the toxins to the causative microalgae. During a toxic bloom, bivalve's toxin profiles usually display the full array of PSTs produced by the blooming microalgae, but these gradually change due to several species-specific chemical and enzymatic transformations (Oshima 1995a).

The most common are due to the chemical properties of toxins like epimerization that occurs spontaneously in toxins having a 11-hydroxysulfate, and it goes until it reaches equilibrium (Figure 34.6).

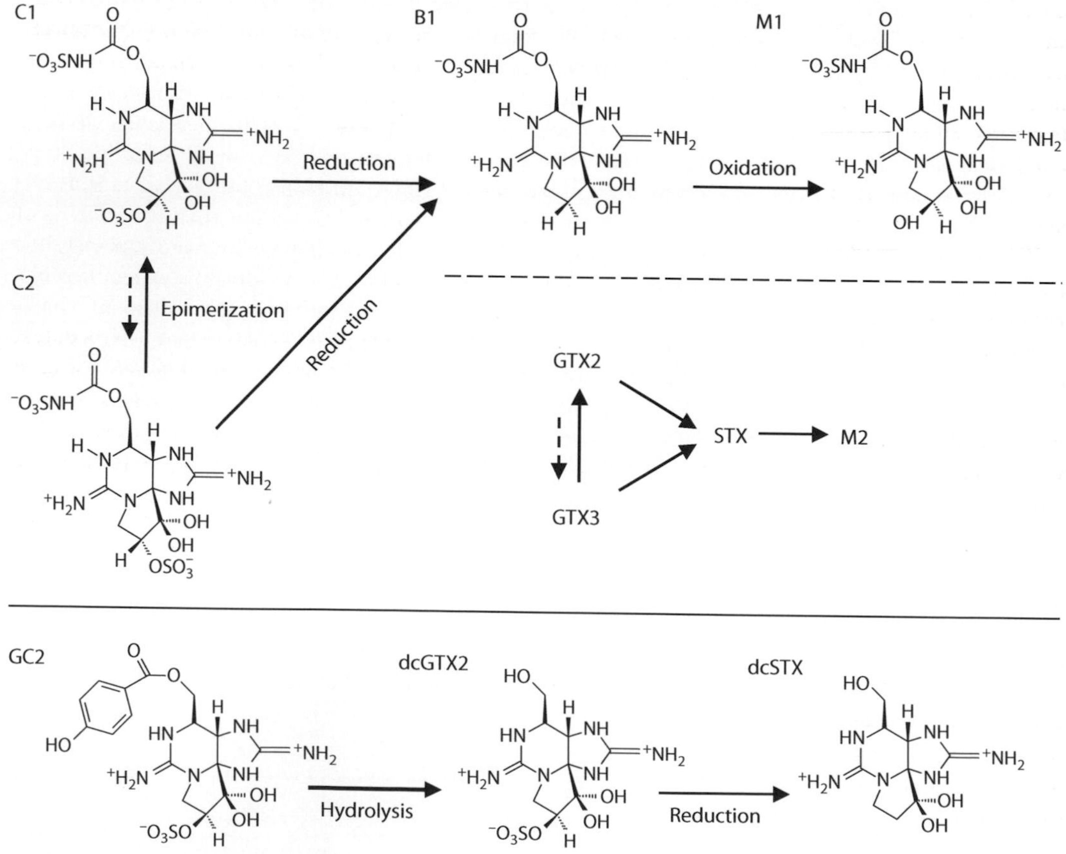

FIGURE 34.6 Examples of some PSTs biotransformation in bivalves. The hydroxysulfate group at C11 suffers spontaneous epimerization either in purified algal extracts or shellfish (upper and middle schemes). It is also quite labile both in vivo and in vitro, and in long-term retention reduction of hydroxysulfate takes places (all schemes). In bivalves with strong carbamoylase activity all carbamate, *N*-sulfocarbamoyl or benzoate toxins are rapidly hydrolyzed into decarbamoyl derivatives (lower scheme).

Dinoflagellates usually produce more of the β-epimer than of the α-epimer (Ordás et al. 2004; Dell'Aversano et al. 2005; Touzet et al. 2007), but the most stable is the α-epimer (Oshima 1995a). These epimeric pairs are sold commercially only as a mixture with an α:β ratio close to 3:1 (NRC-CRMP 2012).

Toxins having an N-sulfocarbamoyl moiety can be rapidly converted to their carbamate counterparts at low pH during boiling in hydrochloric acid for the preparation of shellfish matrices for food safety testing. This is seen as an artifact and acetic acid extraction is used instead for keeping the profiles unaltered for research purposes. This has been kept throughout the decades also with the intention of releasing cryptic toxicity of N-sulfocarbamoyl toxins, by imitating the gastric juice action. However, the common 0.1 M HCl boiling causes only partial hydrolysis, and much cryptic toxicity remains, unless 1.0 M extraction is used (Botelho et al. 2008). Nonetheless, in a human poisoning incident from bivalves containing abundant N-sulfocarbamoyl toxins, the presence in urine of the corresponding carbamate counterparts was not detected (Rodrigues et al. 2012). Aside the ease of laboratorial chemical conversation, rapid enzymatic hydrolysis of N-sulfocarbamoyl toxins has also been described in clams such as *Tapes japonica* (Samsur et al. 2006).

Carbamoylase enzymes catalyze hydrolysis of the carbamate or N-sulfocarbamoyl moiety, rendering them into the corresponding decarbamoyl analogs (Figure 34.6). Strong carbamoylase activity is uncommon among bivalves and has been demonstrated in a few clam species (Oshima 1995a). Substrate specificity varies among species.

In *Protothaca staminea* and *Spisula solidissima* from the North American coast, transformation of N-sulfocarbamoyl analogs is very extensive, while for carbamate analogs it is of lesser importance (Buzy et al. 1994; Bricelj and Cembella 1995). In *Mactra chinensis* from Japan, both N-sulfocarbamoyl and carbamate analogs are transformed, while in *Peronidia venulosa,* carbamate analogs are not transformed at all (Oshima 1995a). In *Spisula solida* from Portugal, all PSTs are rapidly biotransformed, in vivo and in vitro, including the GC analogs. This occurs to such a rapid extent that in nature the *S. solida* profile is dominated solely by decarbamoyl analogs, even during the *G. catenatum* blooming phase (Artigas et al. 2007; Vale 2008a).

Carbamoylase I from *M. chinensis* was purified and characterized by Lin et al. (2004), and sulfocarbamoylase I from *P. venulosa* was purified and characterized by Cho et al. (2008). While the activity of carbamoylase I, comprised from two ionically bound 150 kDa subunits, was restricted to the digestive gland, sulfocarbamoylase I activity, comprised from two 94 kDa subunits bound through S–S linkage, was found in all tissues.

Despite the high abundance of GC toxins in *G. catenatum*, these PSTs analogs seem to represent a minor contribution to the toxin profiles found in bivalves. Vale (2008a,b) hypothesized that a generalized metabolization into decarbamoyl analogs can exist for these toxins for the majority of Portuguese commercial bivalves. So far, this hypothesis has not been tested in bivalves from other world regions. This might indeed be a ubiquitous reaction, because a specialized hydrolysis of the carbamoyl group is not required (it is absent in these toxins), and probably could involve a broader esterase activity.

Chemical transformation by natural reductants commonly found in shellfish, such as glutathione and cysteine, can cause elimination of the N1-hydroxyl and/or elimination of the 11-hydroxysulfate (Figure 34.6) (Oshima 1995a). Many dinoflagellate strains commonly produce an abundant proportion of 11-hydroxysulfate analogs. However, after the blooming phase, the bivalves tend to gradually present a toxin profile dominated by analogs without the 11-hydroxysulfate group. In bivalves contaminated by *G. catenatum*, the C-toxins (C1–C4) gradually are replaced by the B-toxins (B1 and B2) (Figure 34.7). Bivalves contaminated with *A. tamarense* rich in C2 will also present in a few days a rapid enrichment in B1 (Choi et al. 2003), while bivalves contaminated with GTXs (e.g., from *A. minutum*) will gradually present STX (Taleb 2005).

Not only the 11-hydroxysulfate group is lost, but further successive oxidations can take place at the C11 position leading to formation of the M-toxins. This was confirmed at least for B1 and STX (Dell'Aversano et al. 2008). Due to the recent discovery of the M-toxins and its absence of fluorescence, scarce data is available until now on time-course metabolization. Vale (2011) hypothesized if B2 could also be oxidized, but sensitivity and limitation of the spectral capabilities of the mass spectrometry system used hampered further confirmation.

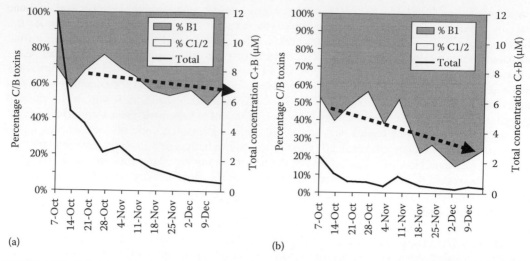

FIGURE 34.7 Relative toxin composition for selected toxins during the detoxification phase from a bloom of *G. catenatum*: (a) blue mussel (*Mytilus galloprovincialis*), (b) common cockle (*Cerastoderma edule*). Wild populations from Ria de Aveiro, Portugal. Cockles presented the fastest disappearance of the hydroxysulfate group from C1/2.

Extreme biotransformation is usually found in bivalves that retain longer the toxins, such as the giant cockle *Acanthocardia tuberculata* in the Mediterranean. After bloom contamination with *G. catenatum*, decarbamoyl GTX and C-toxins abundant in this microalgae disappear, and the profile is dominated by decarbamoyl STX, STX, and B1 (Burdaspal et al. 1998; Vale and Sampayo 2002; Sagou et al. 2005). *S. giganteus* is another example, which initially mislead the researchers to attribute PSP to a single poison STX (Schantz 1984).

Biotransformation and elimination rates are species-specific and have profound implications for the shellfish industry. In the case of the rapid carbamoylase activity present in *S. solida*, it greatly increases the mammalian toxicity by hydrolyzing the low-potency N-sulfocarbamoyl analogs abundant in *G. catenatum* to the most toxic decarbamoyl analogs (Table 34.1). The slow release and also the gradual biotransformation into the most toxic dcSTX analog render *A. tuberculata* unfit for direct human consumption for many months, almost year-round (Márquez 1993; Taleb et al. 2001). For this reason, a particular European legislation was put in force allowing harvesting of this bivalve for industrial processing in southern Spain (Anon 1996).

The binding of toxins has not been much studied so far. It is estimated that protein binding can play an important role in toxin sequestering (Takati et al. 2007). When comparing blue mussel (*Mytilus galloprovinciallis*) with common cockle (*Cerastoderma edule*), the first one has been found on several occasions to biotransform the 11-hydroxysulfate toxins slower than the other, as exemplified in Figure 34.7. The possible role of toxin sequestering in the bioavailability for enzyme conversion is poorly understood at the moment. Despite a few bivalve species, which display prolonged retention of PSTs, the blue mussel is noteworthy for sequestering to higher levels and for longer periods a larger array of marine biotoxins in comparison with other commercial estuarine bivalves (Vale 2011).

34.7 Nonbivalve Vectors

The main focus of PSP studies has been placed in bivalves due to their greater relevance in recorded human food-poisoning outbreaks. But a variety of marine organisms in different trophic levels can accumulate these marine toxins, and represent transfer vectors of these toxins not only to man but also to other susceptible animals (Deeds et al. 2008). Mortalities of marine birds and mammals have been linked to toxic blooms (Geraci et al. 1989; Reyero et al. 1999; Shumway et al. 2003; Doucette et al. 2006). But some animals can display avoidance feeding behaviors: for example, sea otters switch from their preferred prey (such as *S. giganteus*) to other less-contaminated bivalves during HAB events (Kvitek and Bretz 2004).

Among gastropods consumed by humans, a few species can present recurrent contamination. Abalone (*Haliotis* sp.) contamination is a common problem for its safe marketing in Spain and South Africa. While dcSTX was the most abundant toxin, followed by low concentrations of STX, in abalone from Spain, only STX was detected in abalone from South Africa (Bravo et al. 1999; Pitcher et al. 2001).

Toxicity generally increases with increasing abalone size and age, leading to a puzzling mystery about its origin. Depuration of toxin in the Galician abalone did not occur after a few months in culture and fed a variety of macroalgae (Bravo et al. 1996). Controlled feeding experiments using juvenile abalone demonstrated that depuration was low when abalone were either fed kelp or starved. However, toxin reduction to half when abalone was fed artificial feed was observed after 2 weeks (Etheridge et al. 2004).

Anatomical distribution showed higher toxicity in the foot when compared to the muscle, in particular in the epithelium (Bravo et al. 1999). Toxins were found predominantly in the foot side epithelium, rather than the foot sole epithelium. An endosymbiotic origin for the toxins was hypothesized, but no relationship between photosynthetic pigment granules and PSTs was found (Bravo et al. 2001).

PSTs not only have been detected in crabs from several world regions, but have also been involved in a few fatal human poisonings (Koyama et al. 1983; Shumway 1995; Negri and Llewellyn 1998). Among the species in which toxins have been found, xanthid crabs such as *Atergatis floridus* and *Zosimus aeneus* are quite remarkable for presenting levels well above the regulatory limit.

In crabs, toxicity can be attributed to the simultaneous presence of PSTs and TTXs. These are structurally unrelated to the PSTs and are commonly associated with puffer fish but believed to be primarily produced by bacteria (Noguchi et al. 1987). Aside animal predation, another origin for the toxins has been attributed to the macroalgae *Jania* sp. (Kotaki et al. 1983). The presence of saxiphilin, a hemolymph protein that binds STX, may explain why some xanthid crab species appear to tolerate exceptionally high levels of toxins (Llewellyn 1997).

Toxin transformation has been observed similar to that found in bivalves. For instance, in *Telmessus acutidens*, N1-OH toxins (GTX1+4) were reduced to N1-H (GTX2+3), changing the toxin proportion found in its blue mussel prey (Oikawa et al. 2004). Consumption of lobster's hepatopancreas also poses a food safety risk. Holding lobsters in tanks does not promote significant detoxification (Desbiens and Cembella 1995).

Usually finfish, unlike shellfish, are unable to accumulate these toxins in their flesh, and there seems to be little problem in terms of the suitability of fish for human consumption, except possibly in instances where whole fish are consumed without processing (White 1984). So far, the exception is only known in puffers, which typically can present TTXs, but often have been found to contain also PSTs (Sato et al. 2000).

An outbreak of human food poisoning with puffer fish *Sphoeroides nephelus* harvested along the coast of Florida (United States) in 2002 was attributed exclusively to STX (Quilliam et al. 2004). Subsequent research by Landsberg et al. (2006) proposed characterizing this food-poisoning syndrome as STX puffer fish poisoning (SPFP) to distinguish it from puffer fish poisoning (PFP), which is traditionally associated with TTXs, and from PSP caused by PSTs in shellfish. *P. bahamense* was pointed as the putative toxin source.

34.8 PSTs Role in the Marine Ecosystem

Due to their specific blockage of voltage-gated sodium channels, these neurotoxins have played an important role among the scientific community for the detailed study of these types of channels (Penzotti et al. 1998). More recently, it was described how these toxins might also modify potassium channel gating (Wang et al. 2003) and partially block calcium currents (Su et al. 2004). But what is their real advantage for the producing dinoflagellate itself remains to be fully understood.

Many eukaryotes (cnidarians, mollusks, and vertebrates), particularly those that are routinely exposed to algal toxins, have toxin-insensitive or toxin-resistant Na$^+$ channels (reviewed by Anderson et al. 2004). What was the role of these and other marine neurotoxins in the evolution of voltage-gated sodium channels remains an interesting subject (Anderson et al. 2004).

The role of PSTs as allelochemicals against grazers and competitors has been postulated for some time. However, this role against copepods and protozoa has been questioned and attributed to other extracellular exudates (Tillmann and John 2002). Loss of motility and cell lysis can be caused by several *Alexandrium* strains, either PST producers or not (Tillmann and John 2002). More recently, it was hypothesized that membrane sterols serve as molecular targets of these lytic compounds and that differences in sterol composition among donor and target cells may cause the insensitivity of *Alexandrium* cells and sensitivity of targets to lytic compounds (Ma et al. 2011). The lytic compounds increased permeability of the cell membrane for Ca^{2+} ions. Nevertheless, *A. minutum* exposed to copepod cues could contain up to 2.5 times more PSTs than controls and was more resistant to further copepod grazing (Selander et al. 2006).

Intracellular location of STX was established in *A. tamarensis* resorting to immunocytochemical techniques using a polyclonal antibody and epifluorescence microscopy (Anderson and Cheng 1988). Although the location of the labeled antigen at the outer edge of starch grains remains speculative, the distinct labeling in the nuclear region suggests that PSTs, with its two positively charged guanidinium groups, may bind to nucleic acids or nuclear proteins in a manner analogous to the polyamines and other cations. This data suggested that PSTs may not simply be secondary metabolites but instead could be important compounds involved in the structure and function of the *A. tamarensis* genome (Anderson and Cheng 1988). Another role hypothesized has been that of pheromones involved in chemical communication for assisting in gamete encounter during sexual reproduction (Wyatt and Jenkinson 1997).

As regards to the few STX-producing cyanobacterial strains known, their "sxt" gene cluster appears to have been largely vertically inherited and was therefore likely present early in the divergence of the Nostocales, at least 2100 Ma, the earliest reliably dated appearance of a secondary metabolite (Murray et al. 2011). The strong sequence conservation in the sxt cluster shows that it has maintained a vital adaptive role in cyanobacteria since its initial divergence. The increase in STX with increased Na^+ levels led to hypothesize its role in cyanobacterial homeostasis, which could be related to the production of other amine osmolytes, such as proline (Pomati et al. 2004).

34.9 Concluding Remarks

Although a lot on the study of PSP chemistry and detection was slowly discovered along the twentieth century, in just the first decade after the turn of the century, the number of known PSTs doubled, largely due to the spread of mass spectrometry detection (Vale 2010b). The toxicity of many of these analogs remains unknown.

Commercial availability of standards has been progressing slowly. For the most studied groups (carbamate, decarbamoyl, and N-sulfocarbamoyl), full availability is still lacking. Currently, 13 compounds from these 18 are available (NRC-CRMP 2012). For the M-toxins, the benzoate and deoxydecarbamoyl groups, none are available. These facts restrict scientific research and can pose a problem for routine chemical detection of these newest compounds, particularly in seafood imports where uncommon toxin profiles might exist. Although only recently TEFs were established by the European Food Safety Authority (EFSA 2009), these only take into account the carbamate, decarbamoyl, and N-sulfocarbamoyl groups.

The ecobiology of these compounds is not yet fully understood. With the discovery of new analogs and the known increased distribution of PSTs, not only in marine but also in freshwater/terrestrial habitats, the complexity of STX ecobiology has increased. Other STX analogs apart from those described in Figure 34.1 with an acetate R4 side chain are known in the freshwater filamentous cyanobacterium *Lyngbya wollei* (Figure 34.8a), but so far not in the marine environment (Onodera et al. 1997). Additionally, evidence that STX is produced by certain facultative anaerobic bacteria (belonging to *Enterobacter* and *Klebsiella*) has been reported by Sevcik et al. (2003). Such bacteria were proposed to cause the bovine paraplegic syndrome.

An unusual STX analog was isolated from the skin of a rare South American frog: zetekitoxin (Figure 34.8b). This compound differs from STX in having a chain bearing a pentacyclic ring connecting carbons 6 and 11 (Yotsu-Yamashita et al. 2004). This is becoming more and more similar to the widest distribution of TTX analogs in nature (Miyazawa and Noguchi 2001).

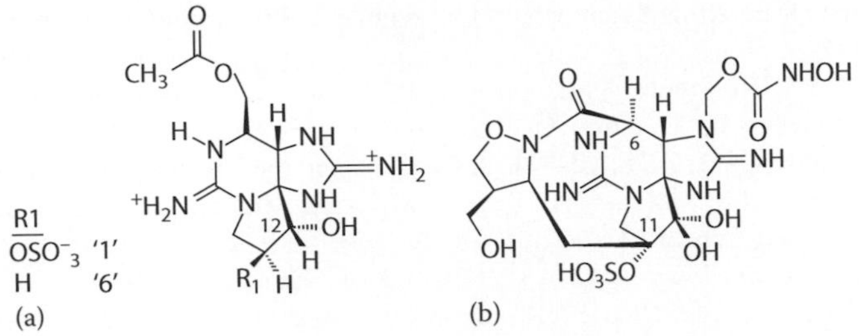

FIGURE 34.8 Structures of some of the STX analogs produced by *Lyngbya wollei*. (From Onodera, H., *Nat. Toxins*, 5, 146, 1997.) (b) Structures of zetekitoxin AB. (From Yotsu-Yamashita, M. et al., *Proc. Natl. Acad. Sci. USA*, 101, 4346, 2004.)

STX, which was first described as a marine dinoflagellate metabolite, is now known to occur in a much wider variety of habitats and is produced also by cyanobacteria and possibly several bacteria. Coexistence between STXs and TTXs is already known to occur in puffers and frogs. Additionally, dinoflagellates from genus *Alexandrium* can produce simultaneously several STXs, spirolides, and hemolytic compounds.

REFERENCES

Anderson, D.M., Alpermann, T.J., Cembella, A.D., Collos, Y., Masseret, E., and Montresor, M., 2012. The globally distributed genus *Alexandrium*: Multifaceted roles in marine ecosystems and impacts on human health. *Harmful Algae*, 14, 10–35.

Anderson, D.M. and Cheng, T.P.-O., 1988. Intracellular localization of saxitoxins in the dinoflagellate *Gonyaulax tamarensis*. *J. Phycol.*, 24, 17–22.

Anderson, P.A.V., Roberts-Misterly, J., and Greenberg, R.M., 2004. The evolution of voltage-gated sodium channels: Were algal toxins involved? *Harmful Algae*, 4(1), 95–107.

Anon, 1996. Commission Decision 96/77/EC of 18 January 1996 establishing the conditions for the harvesting and processing of certain bivalve molluscs coming from areas where the paralytic shellfish poison level exceeds the limit laid down by Council Directive 91/492/EEC. *Off. J. Eur. Commun.*, L15, 46–47.

Anon, 2005a. AOAC official method 959.08. Paralytic Shellfish Poison. Biological method. Final action. In: Truckses, M.W. (Ed.), *Natural Toxins*, 18th edn. AOAC Official Methods for Analysis AOAC International, Gaithersburg, MD, pp. 79–80 (Chapter 49).

Anon, 2005b. AOAC Official Method 2005.06, *Quantitative Determination of Paralytic Shellfish Poisoning Toxins in Shellfish using Prechromatographic Oxidation and Liquid Chromatography with Fluorescence Detection*. AOAC International, Gaithersburg, MD.

Anon, 2011. AOAC Official Method 2011.02, *Determination of Paralytic Shellfish Poisoning Toxins in Mussels, Clams, Oysters and Scallops. Post-Column Oxidation Method (PCOX)*. First action 2011. AOAC International, Gaithersburg, MD.

Artigas, M.L., Vale, P., Gomes, S.S., Botelho, M.J., Rodrigues, S.M., and Amorim, A., 2007. Profiles of PSP toxins in shellfish from Portugal explained by carbamoylase activity. *J. Chromatogr. A*, 1160(1–2), 99–105.

Aune, T., Ramstad, H., Heinenreich, B., Landsverk, T., Waaler, T., Eggas, E., and Julshamn, K., 1998. Zinc accumulation in oysters giving mouse deaths in paralytic shellfish poisoning bioassay. *J. Shell Res.*, 17(4), 1243–1246.

Baker, T.R., Doucette, G.J., Powell, C.L., Boyer, G.L., and Plumley, F.G., 2003. GTX4 imposters: Characterization of fluorescent compounds synthesized by *Pseudomonas stutzeri* SF/PS and *Pseudomonas/Alteromonas* PTB-1, symbionts of saxitoxin-producing *Alexandrium* spp. *Toxicon*, 41(3), 339–347.

Bates, H.A. and Rapoport, H., 1975. Chemical assay for saxitoxin, the paralytic shellfish poison. *J. Agric. Food Chem.*, 23(2), 237–239.

Ben-Gigirey, B., Rodríguez-Velasco, M.L., Villar-González, A., and Botana, L.M., 2007. Influence of the sample toxic profile on the suitability of a high performance liquid chromatography method for official paralytic shellfish toxins control. *J. Chromatogr. A*, 1140(1–2), 78–87.

Bhonde V.R. and Looper, R.E., 2011. A stereocontrolled synthesis of (+)-saxitoxin. *J. Am. Chem. Soc.*, 133(50), 20172–20174.

Botelho, M.J., Gomes, S.S., Rodrigues, S.M., and Vale, P., 2008. Studies on cryptic PSP toxicity depends on the extraction procedure. In: Moestrup, Ø. et al. (Eds.), *Proceedings of 12th International Conference on Harmful Algae*. ISSHA and IOC of UNESCO, Copenhagen, the Netherlands, pp. 338–340.

Bravo, I., Cacho, E. Franco, J.M., Miguez, A., Reyero, M.I., and Martinez, A., 1996. Study of PSP toxicity in *Haliotis tuberculata* from the Galician coast. In: Yasumoto, T., Oshima, Y., and Fukuyo, Y. (Eds.), *Harmful and Toxic Algal Blooms*. IOC of UNESCO, Paris, France, pp. 421–424.

Bravo, I., Franco, J.M., Alonso, A., Dietrich, R., and Molist, P., 2001. Cytological study and immunohisto-chemical location of PSP toxins in foot skin of the ormer, *Haliotis tuberculata*, from the Galician coast (NW Spain). *Mar. Biol.*, 138, 709–715.

Bravo, I., Reyero, M.I., Cacho, E., and Franco, J.M., 1999. Paralytic shellfish poisoning in *Haliotis tuberculata* from the Galician coast: Geographical distribution, toxicity by lengths and parts of the mollusc. *Aquat. Toxicol.*, 46, 79–85.

Bricelj, V.M. and Cembella, A.D., 1995. Fate of gonyautoxins in surfclams, *Spisula solidissima*, grazing upon toxigenic *Alexandrium*. In: Lassus, P., Arzul, G., Erard, E., Gentien, P., and Marcaillou, C. (Eds.), *Harmful Marine Algal Blooms*. Lavoisier Science Publishers, Paris, France, pp. 413–418.

Bricelj, V.M. and Shumway, E., 1998. Paralytic shellfish toxins in bivalve molluscs: Occurrence, transfer kinetics, and biotransformation. *Rev. Fish. Sci.*, 6, 315–383.

Burdaspal, P.A., Bustos, J., Legarda, T.M., Olmedo, J.B., Vigo, M., Gonzalez, L., and Berenguer, J.A. 1998. Commercial processing of *Acanthocardia tuberculatum* L. naturally-contaminated with PSP: Evaluation after one year industrial experience. In: Reguera, B., Blanco, J., Fernández, M.L., and Wyatt, T. (Eds.), *Harmful Algae*. Xunta de Galicia and IOC of UNESCO, Spain, pp. 241–244.

Bustillos-Guzman, J., Vale, P., and Band-Schmidt, C., 2011. Presence of benzoate-type toxins in *Gymnodinium catenatum* Graham isolated from the Mexican Pacific. *Toxicon*, 57(6), 922–926.

Buzy, A., Thibault, P., and Laycock, M.V., 1994. Development of a capillary electrophoresis method for the characterization of enzymatic products arising from the carbamoylase digestion of paralytic shellfish poisoning toxins. *J. Chromatogr. A*, 688, 301–316.

Campbell, K., Huet, A.-C., Charlier, C., Higgins, C., Delahaut, P., and Elliott, C.T., 2009. Comparison of ELISA and SPR biosensor technology for the detection of paralytic shellfish poisoning toxins. *J. Chromatogr. B*, 877(32), 4079–4089.

Campbell, K., Rawn, D.F.K., Niedzwiadek, B., and Elliott, C.T., 2011. Paralytic shellfish poisoning (PSP) toxin binders for optical biosensor technology: Problems and possibilities for the future: A review. *Food Addit. Contam. Pt A*, 28(6), 711–725.

Campbell, K., Stewart, L.D., Fodey, T.L., Haughey, S.A., Doucette, G.J., Kawatsu, K., and Elliott, C.T., 2007. Assessment of specific binding proteins suitable for the detection of paralytic shellfish poisons using optical biosensor technology. *Anal. Chem.*, 79, 5906–5914.

Cho, Y., Ogawa, N., Takahashi, M., Lin, H.-P., and Oshima, Y., 2008. Purification and characterization of paralytic shellfish toxin transforming enzyme, sulfocarbamoylase I, from Japanese bivalve, *Peronidia venulosa*. *Biochim. Biophys. Acta*, 1784, 1277–1285.

Choi, M.C., Hsieh, D.P.H., Lam, P.K.S., and Wang, W.X., 2003. Field depuration and biotransformation of paralytic shellfish toxins in scallop *Chlamys nobilis* and green-lipped mussel *Perna viridis*. *Mar. Biol.*, 143(5), 927–934.

Chou, H.N., Chen, Y.M., and Chen, C.Y., 2004. Variety of PSP toxins in four culture strains of *Alexandrium minutum* collected from southern Taiwan. *Toxicon*, 43, 337–340.

Cook, A.C., Morris, S., Reese, R.A., and Irving, S.N., 2006. Assessment of fitness for purpose of an insect bioassay using the desert locust (*Schistocerca gregaria* L.) for the detection of paralytic shellfish toxins in shellfish flesh. *Toxicon*, 48, 662–671.

Costa, P.R., Baugh, K.A., Wright, B., RaLonde, R., Nance, S.L., and Tatarenkova, N., Etheridge, S.M., and Lefebvre, K.A., 2009. Comparative determination of paralytic shellfish toxins (PSTs) using five different toxin detection methods in shellfish species collected in the Aleutian Islands, Alaska. *Toxicon*, 54, 313–320.

Deeds, J.R., Landsberg, J.H., Etheridge, S.M., Pitcher, G.C., and Longan, S.W., 2008. Non-traditional vectors for paralytic shellfish poisoning. *Marine Drugs*, 6(2), 308–348.

Dell'Aversano, C., Hess, P., and Quilliam, M.A., 2005. Hydrophilic interaction liquid chromatography–mass spectrometry for the analysis of paralytic shellfish poisoning (PSP) toxins. *J. Chromatogr. A*, 1081, 190–201.

Dell'Aversano, C., Walter, J.A., Burton, I.W., Stirling, D.J., Fattorusso, E., and Quilliam, M.A., 2008. Isolation and structure elucidation of new and unusual saxitoxin analogues from mussels. *J. Nat. Products*, 71(9), 1518–1523.

Desbiens, M. and Cembella, A.D., 1995. Occurrence and elimination kinetics of PSP toxins in the American lobster (*Homarus americanus*). In: Lassus, P., Arzul, G., Erard-Le-Denn, E., Gentien, P., and Marcaillou-Le-Baut, C. (Eds.), *Harmful Marine Algal Blooms*. Technique et Documentation, Lavoisier, Paris, France, pp. 433–438.

Diener, M., Erler, K., Christian, B., and Luckas, B., 2007. Application of a new zwitterionic hydrophilic interaction chromatography column for determination of paralytic shellfish poisoning toxins. *J. Sep. Sci.*, 30, 1821–1826.

Doucette, G.J., Cembella, A.D., Martin, J.L., Michaud, J., Cole, T.V.N., and Rolland, R.M., 2006. Paralytic shellfish poisoning (PSP) toxins in North Atlantic right whales *Eubalaena glacialis* and their zooplankton prey in the Bay of Fundy, Canada. *Mar. Ecol. Prog. Ser.*, 306, 303–313.

Doyle, D.D., Guo, Y., Lustig, S.L., Satin, J., Rogart, R.B., and Fozzard, H.A., 1993. Divalent cation competition with [3H] saxitoxin binding to tetrodotoxin-resistant and sensitive sodium channels. *J. Gen. Physiol.*, 101, 153–182.

EFSA, 2009. Marine biotoxins in shellfish—Saxitoxin Group. Scientific Opinion of the Panel on Contaminants in the Food Chain. *EFSA J.*, 1019, 1–76.

Etheridge, S.M., Pitcher, G.C., and Roesler, C.S., 2004. Depuration and transformation of PSP toxins in the South African abalone *Haliotis midae*. In: Steidinger, K.A., Landsberg, J.H., Thomas, C.R., and Vargo, G.A. (Eds.), *Harmful Algae 2002*. Florida Fish and Wildlife Conservation Commission, Florida Institute of Oceanography, and Intergovernmental Oceanographic Commission of UNESCO, pp. 175–177.

FAO, 2004. *Marine Biotoxins*, FAO Food and Nutrition Paper, 80. Food and Agriculture Organization of the United Nations, Rome, Italy, 278 pp.

Fleming, J.J. and Du Bois, J., 2006. A synthesis of (+)-saxitoxin. *J. Am. Chem. Soc.*, 128, 3926–3927.

Franco, J.M. and Fernández-Vila, P., 1993. Separation of paralytic shellfish toxins by reversed phase high performance liquid chromatography, with post-column reaction and fluorimetric detection. *Chromatographia*, 35(9–12), 613–620.

García, C., Bravo, M.C., Lagos, M., and Lagos, N., 2004. Paralytic shellfish poisoning: Post-mortem analysis of tissue and body fluid samples from human victims in the *Patagonia fjords. Toxicon*, 43, 149–158.

Garet, E., González-Fernández, A., Lago, J., Vieites, J.M., and Cabado, A.G., 2010. Comparative evaluation of enzyme-linked immunoassay and reference methods for the detection of shellfish hydrophilic toxins in several presentations of seafood. *J. Agric. Food Chem.*, 58, 1410–1415.

Geraci, J.R., Anderson, D.M., Timperi, R.J., St. Aubin, D.J., Early, G.A., Prescott, J.H., and Mayo, C.A., 1989. Humpback whales (*Megaptera novaeangliae*) fatally poisoned by dinoflagellate toxin. *Can. J. Fish. Aquat. Sci.*, 46, 1895–1898.

Gibbs, R.S., Thomas, K., Rourke, W.A., Murphy, C.J., McCarron, P., Burton, I., Walter, J., van de Riet, J.M., and Quilliam, M.A., 2009. Detection and identification of a novel saxitoxin analogue in Argentinean scallops (*Zygochlamys patagonica*). In: *Proceedings of the 7th International Conference on Molluscan Shellfish Safety*, Nantes, 2009. http://www.symposcience.org//exl-doc//colloque//ART-00002577.pdf (accessed April 24, 2012).

Hallegraeff, G.M. 1993. A review of harmful algal blooms and their apparent global increase. *Phycologia*, 32, 79–99.

Hallegraeff, G.M., Blackburn, S.I., Doblin, M.A., and Bolch, C.J.S., 2012. Global toxicology, ecophysiology and population relationships of the chain-forming PST dinoflagellate *Gymnodinium catenatum*. *Harmful Algae*, 14, 130–143.

Jacobi, P.A., Martinelli, M.J., and Polanc, S., 1984. Total synthesis of (+)-saxitoxin. *J. Am. Chem. Soc.*, 106, 5594–5598.

Jellett, J., Marks, L., Stewart, J., Dorey, M., Watson-Wright, W., and Lawrence, J.F., 1992. Paralytic shellfish poison (saxitoxin family) bioassays: Automated endpoint determination and standardization of the in vitro tissue culture bioassay, and comparison with the standard mouse bioassay. *Toxicon*, 30(10), 1143–1156.

Jellett, J.F., Roberts, R.L., Laycock, M.V., Quilliam, M.A., and Barrett R.E., 2002. Detection of paralytic shellfish poisoning (PSP) toxins in shellfish tissue using MIST Alert™, a new rapid test, in parallel with the regulatory AOAC® mouse bioassay. *Toxicon*, 40(10), 1407–1425.

Kotaki, Y., Tajiri, Y., Oshima, Y., and Yasumoto, T., 1983. Identification of a calcareous red alga as the primary source of paralytic shellfish toxins in coral reef crabs and gastropods. *Bull. Jap. Soc. Sci. Fish.*, 49, 283–286.

Koyama, K., Noguchi, T., Uzu, A., and Hashimoto, K., 1983. Individual, local, and size-dependent variations in toxicity of the xanthid crab *Zosimus aeneus*. *Nippon Suis. Gakk.*, 49, 1273–1279.

Kvitek, R.G. and Bretz, C., 2004. Harmful algal bloom toxins protect bivalve populations from sea otter predation. *Mar. Ecol. Prog. Ser.*, 271, 233–234.

Landsberg, J.H., Hall, S., Johannessen, J.N. et al., 2006. Saxitoxin puffer fish poisoning in the United States, with the first report of *Pyrodinium bahamense* as the putative toxin source. *Environ. Health Perspect.*, 114(10), 1502–1507.

Lawrence, J.F., Ménard, C., Charbonneau, C., and Hall, S., 1991. A study of ten toxins associated with paralytic shellfish poison using prechromatographic oxidation and liquid chromatography with fluorescence detection. *J. Assoc. Offic. Anal. Chem.*, 74(2), 404–409.

Lawrence, J.F., Niedzwiadek, B., and Menard, C., 2005. Quantitative determination of paralytic shellfish poisoning toxins in shellfish using prechromatographic oxidation and liquid chromatography with fluorescence detection: Collaborative study. *J. AOAC Int.*, 88(6), 1714–1732.

Lilly, E.L., Halanych, K.M., and Anderson, D.M., 2007. Species boundaries and global biogeography of the *Alexandrium tamarense* complex (Dinophyceae). *J. Phycol.*, 43, 1329–1338.

Lim, P.T., Sato, S., Thuoc, C.V., Tu, P.T., Huyen, N.T.M., Takata, Y., Yoshida, M., Kobiyama, A., Koike, K., and Ogata, T., 2007. Toxic *Alexandrium minutum* (Dinophyceae) from Vietnam with new gonyautoxin analogue. *Harmful Algae*, 6(3), 321–331.

Lin, H.-P., Cho, Y., Yashiro, H., Yamada, T., and Oshima, Y., 2004. Purification and characterization of paralytic shellfish toxin transforming enzyme from *Mactra chinensis*. *Toxicon*, 44, 657–668.

Llewellyn, L.E., 1997. Haemolymph protein in xanthid crabs: Its selective binding of saxitoxin and possible role in toxin bioaccumulation. *Mar. Biol.*, 128, 599–606.

Luckas, B., 1990. The occurrence of decarbamoyl saxitoxin in canned mussels. In: Bernoth, E.M. (Ed.), *Public Health Aspects of Seafood-Borne Zoonotic Diseases*, *Vet. Med. Hefte*, WHO, Geneva, pp. 89–97.

Ma, H., Krock, B., Tillmann, U., Bickmeyer, U., Graeve, M., and Cembella, A., 2011. Mode of action of membrane-disruptive lytic compounds from the marine dinoflagellate *Alexandrium tamarense*. *Toxicon*, 58, 247–258.

Mackintosh, F.H., Gallacher, S., Shanks, A.M., and Smith, E.A., 2002. Assessment of MIST Alert™, a commercial qualitative assay for detection of paralytic shellfish poisoning toxins in bivalve molluscs. *J. AOAC Int.*, 85(3), 632–641.

Márquez, I., 1993. Presencia de PSP en el corruco (*Acanthocardia tuberculata*) en el litoral de la provincia marítima de Malaga y distritos maritimos de la linea y Algeciras. In: Mariño, J. and Maneiro, J.C. (Eds.), *III Reunión Iberica sobre Fitoplancton Tóxico y Biotoxinas*. Consejería de Agricultura y Pesca, Xunta de Galicia, pp. 27–33.

McCulloch, A.W., Boyd, R.K., de Freitas, A.S.W. et al., 1989. Zinc from oyster tissue as causative factor in mouse deaths in Official Bioassay for Paralytic Shellfish Poison. *J. Assoc. Offic. Anal. Chem.*, 72(2), 384–386.

Miyawa, J.H. and Schulman, S.G., 2001. Ultraviolet–visible spectrophotometry. In: Ohannesian, L. and Streeter, A.J. (Eds.), *Handbook of Pharmaceutical Analysis*. Marcel Dekker, New York, 585pp.

Miyazawa, K. and Noguchi, T., 2001. Distribution and origin of tetrodotoxin. *Toxin Rev.*, 20(1), 11–33.

Murray, S.A., Mihali, T.K., and Neilan, B.A., 2011. Extraordinary conservation, gene loss, and positive selection in the evolution of an ancient neurotoxin. *Mol. Biol. Evol.*, 28(3), 1173–1182.

Negri, A. and Llewellyn, L., 1998. Comparative analyses by HPLC and the sodium channel and saxiphilin ^{3}H-saxitoxin receptor assays for paralytic shellfish toxins in crustaceans and molluscs from tropical North West Australia. *Toxicon*, 36, 283–298.

Negri, A., Stirling, D., Quilliam, M., Blackburn, S., Bolch, C., Burton, I., Eaglesham, G., Thomas, K., Walter, J., and Willis, R., 2003. Three novel hydroxybenzoate saxitoxin analogues isolated from the dinoflagellate *Gymnodinium catenatum*. *Chem. Res. Toxicol.*, 16(8), 1029–1033.

Negri, A.P., Bolch, C.J.S., Geier, S., Green, D.H., Park, T.G., and Blackburn, S.I., 2007. Widespread presence of hydrophobic paralytic shellfish toxins in *Gymnodinium catenatum*. *Harmful Algae*, 6(6), 774–780.

Noguchi, T., Hwang, D.F., Arakawa, O., Sugita, H., Deguchi, Y., Shida, Y., and Hashimoto, K., 1987. *Vibrio alginolyticus*, a tetrodotoxin-producing bacterium, in the intestines of the fish *Fugu vermicularis* vermicularis. *Mar. Biol.*, 94, 625–630.

NRC-CRMP, 2012. Certified Reference Materials Program. http://www.nrc-cnrc.gc.ca/eng/solutions/advisory/crm/biotoxin/list_products.html (accessed August 29, 2012).

Oikawa, H., Fujita, T., Saito, K., Watabe, S., and Yano, Y., 2004. Comparison of paralytic shellfish toxin between carnivorous crabs (*Telmessus acutidens* and *Charybdis japonica*) and their prey mussel (*Mytilus galloprovincialis*) in an inshore food chain. *Toxicon*, 43, 713–719.

Onodera, H., Satake, M., Oshima, Y., Yasumoto, T., and Carmichael, W.W., 1997. New saxitoxin analogues from the freshwater filamentous cyanobacterium *Lyngbya wollei*. *Nat Toxins*, 5, 146–151.

Ordás, M.C., Fraga, S., Franco, J.M., Ordás, A., and Figueras, A. 2004. Toxin and molecular analysis of *Gymnodinium catenatum* (Dinophyceae) strains from Galicia (NW Spain) and Andalucia (S Spain). *J. Plankt. Res.*, 26(3), 341–349.

Oshima, Y., 1995a. Chemical and enzymatic transformation of paralytic shellfish toxins in marine organisms. In: Lassus, P., Arzul, G., Erard, E., Gentien, P., and Marcaillou, C. (Eds.), *Harmful Marine Algal Blooms*. Lavoisier Science Publishers, Paris, France, pp. 475–480.

Oshima, Y., 1995b. Postcolumn derivatization liquid chromatographic method for paralytic shellfish toxins. *J. AOAC Int.*, 78(2), 528–532.

Oshima, Y., Blackburn, S.I., and Hallegraeff, G.M., 1993. Comparative study on paralytic shellfish toxin profiles of the dinoflagellate *Gymnodinium catenatum* from three different countries. *Mar. Biol.*, 116, 471–476.

Oshima, Y., Machida, M., Sasaki, K., Tamaoki, Y., and Yasumoto, T., 1984. Liquid chromatographic–fluorometric analysis of paralytic shellfish toxins. *Agric. Biol. Chem.*, 48(7), 1707–1711.

Oshima, Y., Sugino, K., and Yasumoto, T., 1989. Latest advances in HPLC analysis of paralytic shellfish toxins. In: Natori, S., Hashimoto, K., and Ueno, Y. (Eds.), *Mycotoxins and Phycotoxins '88*. Elsevier Science, Amsterdam, the Netherlands, pp. 319–326.

Penzotti, J.L., Fozzard, H.A., Lipkind, G.M., and Dudley, S.C. Jr., 1998. Differences in saxitoxin and tetrodotoxin binding revealed by mutagenesis of the Na⁺ channel outer vestibule. *Biophys. J.*, 75, 2647–2657.

Pitcher, G.C., Franco, J.M., Doucette, G.J., Powell, C.L., and Mouton, A., 2001. Paralytic shellfish poisoning in the abalone *Haliotis midae* on the west coast of South Africa. *J. Shellfish Res.*, 20, 895–904.

Pomati, F., Rossetti, C., Manarolla, G., Burns, B.P., and Neilan, B.A., 2004. Interactions between intracellular Na⁺ levels and saxitoxin production in *Cylindrospermopsis raciborskii* T3. *Microbiology*, 150, 455–461.

Quilliam, M.A., 2007. National Research Council of Canada—Certified Reference Materials Programme: Supplemental information for PSP toxin CRMs. 5pp.

Quilliam, M.A., Janecek, M., and Lawrence, J.F., 1993. Characterization of the oxidation products of paralytic shellfish poisoning toxins by liquid chromatography/mass spectrometry. *Rapid Commun. Mass Spectrom.*, 7, 482–487.

Quilliam, M.A., Wechsler, D., Marcus, S., Ruck, B., Wekell, M., and Hawryluk, T., 2004. Detection and identification of paralytic shellfish poisoning toxins in Florida pufferfish responsible for incidents of neurologic illness. In: Steidinger, K.A., Landsberg, J.H., Tomas, C.R., and Vargo, G.A. (Eds.), *Harmful Algae 2002*. Florida Fish and Wildlife Conservation Commission of UNESCO, St. Petersburg, FL, pp. 116–118.

Reyero, M., Cacho, E., Martinez, A., Vásquez, J., Marina, A., Fraga, S., and Franco, J.M., 1999. Evidence of saxitoxin derivatives as causative agents in the 1997 mass mortality of monk seals in the Cape Blanc Peninsula. *Nat. Toxins*, 7, 311–315.

Rodrigues, S.M., de Carvalho, M., Mestre, T., Ferreira, J.F., Coelho, M., Peralta, R., and Vale, P., 2012. Paralytic shellfish poisoning due to ingestion of *Gymnodinium catenatum* contaminated cockles—Application of the AOAC HPLC Official Method. *Toxicon*, 59(5), 558–566.

Rosales-Loessener, F., Porras, E., and Dix, M.W., 1989. Toxic shellfish in Guatemala. In: Okaichi, T., Anderson, D.M., and Nemoto, T. (Eds.), *Red Tides: Biology, Environmental Science and Toxicology*. Elsevier, New York, pp. 113–116.

Rourke, W.A., Murphy, C.J., Pitcher, G., Van Deriet, J.M., Burns, B.G., Thomas, K.M., and Quilliam, M.A., 2008. Rapid postcolumn methodology for determination of paralytic shellfish toxins in shellfish tissue. *J. AOAC Int.*, 91(3), 589–597.

Ruebhart, D.R., Radcliffe, W.L., and Eaglesham, G.K., 2011. Alternative bioassay for the detection of saxitoxin using the speckled cockroach (*Nauphoeta cinerea*). *J. Toxicol. Environ. Health, Part A*, 74(10), 621–637.

Sagou, R., Amanhir, R., Taleb, H., Vale, P., Blaghen, M., and Loutfi, M., 2005. Comparative study on differential accumulation of PSP between cockle (*Acanthocardia tuberculatum*) and sweet clam (*Callista chione*). *Toxicon*, 46(6), 612–618.

Samsur, M., Yamaguchi, Y., Sagara, T., Takatani, T., Arakawa, O., and Noguchi, T., 2006. Accumulation and depuration profiles of PSP toxins in the short-necked clam *Tapes japonica* fed with the toxic dinoflagellate *Alexandrium catenella*. *Toxicon*, 48(3), 323–330.

Sato, S., Ogata, T., Borja, V., Gonzales, C., Fukuyo, Y., and Kodama, M., 2000. Frequent occurrence of paralytic shellfish poisoning toxins as dominant toxins in marine puffer from tropical water. *Toxicon*, 38, 1101–1109.

Schantz, E.J., 1984. Historical perspective on paralytic shellfish poison. *Seafood Toxins*. American Chemical Society, Washington, DC, pp. 99–111.

Schantz, E.J., Ghazarossian, V.E. Schnoes, H.K., Strong, F.M., Springer, J.P., Pezzanite, J.O., and Clardy, J., 1975. Structure of saxitoxin. *J. Am. Chem. Soc.*, 97(5), 1238–1239.

Schantz, E.J., McFarren, E.F., Schaffer, M.L., and Lewis, K.H., 1958. Purified shellfish poison for bioassay standardization. *J. Assoc. Offic. Anal. Chem.*, 41(1), 160–168.

Selander, E., Thor, P., Toth, G., and Pavia, H., 2006. Copepods induce paralytic shellfish toxin production in marine dinoflagellates. *Proc. R. Soc. B*, 273, 1673–1680.

Sevcik, C., Noriega, J., and D'Suze, G., 2003. Identification of *Enterobacter* bacteria as saxitoxin producers in cattle's rumen and surface water from Venezuelan savannahs. *Toxicon*, 42, 359–366.

Shimizu, Y., Alam, M., Oshima, Y., and Fallon, W.E., 1975. Presence of four toxins in red tide infested clams and cultured *Gonyaulax tamarensis* cells. *Biochem. Biophys. Res. Commun.*, 66(2), 731–737.

Shumway, S.E., 1995. Phycotoxin-related shellfish poisoning: Bivalve molluscs are not the only vectors. *Rev. Fish. Sci.*, 3, 1–31.

Shumway, S.E., Allen, S.M., and Boersma, P.D., 2003. Marine birds and harmful algal blooms: Sporadic victims or under-reported events? *Harmful Algae*, 2(1), 1–17.

Su, Z., Sheets, M., Ishida, H., Li, F., and Barry, W.H., 2004. Saxitoxin blocks L-Type I_{Ca}. *J. Pharmacol. Exp. Ther.*, 308, 324–329.

Sullivan, J.J. and Wekell, M.M., 1984. Determination of paralytic shellfish poisoning toxins by high pressure liquid chromatography. In: Ragelis, E.P. (Ed.), *Seafood Toxins*. ACS Symposium Series 262 American Chemical Society, Washington, DC, pp. 197–205.

Takati, N., Mountassif, D., Taleb, H., Lee, K., and Blaghen M., 2007. Purification and partial characterization of paralytic shellfish poison-binding protein from *Acanthocardia tuberculatum*. *Toxicon*, 50(3), 311–321.

Taleb, H., 2005. Phycotoxines paralysantes (PSP) et diarrhéiques (DSP) le long des cotes marocaines: évolution spatio-temporelle, profil toxinique et cinétique de décontamination. Thèse pour Docteur d'Etat (PhD), Université Hassan II, Faculté des Sciences Ain Chok, Casablanca, Morocco, pp. 159.

Taleb, H., Vale, P., Jaime, E., and Blaghen, M., 2001. Study of paralytic shellfish poisoning toxin profile in shellfish from the Mediterranean shore of Morocco. *Toxicon*, 39(12), 1855–1861.

Tanino, H., Nakata, T., Kaneko, T., and Kishi Y., 1977. A stereospecific total synthesis of DL-saxitoxin. *J. Am. Chem. Soc.*, 99(8), 2818–2819.

Taylor, F.J.R., Fukuyo, Y., and Larsen, J., 1995. Taxonomy of harmful dinoflagellates. In: Hallegraeff, G.M., Anderson, D.M., and Cembella, A.D. (Eds.), *Manual on Harmful Marine Microalgae*. IOC Manuals and Guides No. 33, UNESCO, Paris, France, pp. 283–317.

Tillmann, U. and John, U., 2002. Toxic effects of *Alexandrium* spp. on heterotrophic dinoflagellates: An allelo-chemical defense mechanism independent of PSP-toxin content. *Mar. Ecol. Prog. Ser.*, 230, 47–58.

Tomas, C.R., van Wagoner, R., Tatters, A.O., White, K.D., Hall, S., and Wright, J.L.C., 2012. *Alexandrium peruvianum* (Balech and Mendiola) Balech and Tangen a new toxic species for coastal North Carolina. *Harmful Algae*, 17, 54–63.

Touzet, N., Franco, J.M., and Raine, R., 2007. Influence of inorganic nutrition on growth and PSP toxin production of *Alexandrium minutum* (Dinophyceae) from Cork Harbour, Ireland. *Toxicon*, 50(1), 106–119.

Toyofuku, H., 2006. Joint FAO/WHO/IOC activities to provide scientific advice on marine biotoxins (research report). *Mar. Pollut. Bull.*, 52(12), 1735–1745.

Turner, A.D., Dhanji-Rapkova, M., Algoet, M., Suarez-Isla, B.A., Cordova, M., Caceres, C., Murphy, C.J., Casey, M., and Lees, D.N., 2012. Investigations into matrix components affecting the performance of the official bioassay reference method for quantitation of paralytic shellfish poisoning toxins in oysters. *Toxicon*, 59, 215–230.

Turner, A.D., Hatfield, R.G., Rapkova, M., Higman, W., Algoet, M., Suarez-Isla, B.A., Cordova, M., Caceres, C., van de Riet, J., Gibbs, R., Thomas, K., Quilliam, M., and Lees, D.N., 2011. Comparison of AOAC 2005.06 LC official method with other methodologies for the quantitation of paralytic shellfish poisoning toxins in UK shellfish species. *Anal. Bioanal. Chem.*, 399, 1257–1270.

Turner, A.D., Norton, D.M., Hatfield, R.G., Morris, S., Reese, A.R., Algoet, M., and Lees, D.N., 2009. Refinement and extension of AOAC method 2005.06 to include additional toxins in mussels: Single-laboratory validation. *J. AOAC Int.*, 92(1), 190–207.

Turrell, E., Stobo, L., Lacaze, J.-P., Piletsky, S., and Piletska, E., 2008. Optimization of hydrophilic interaction liquid chromatography/mass spectrometry and development of solid-phase extraction for the determination of paralytic shellfish poisoning toxins. *J. AOAC Int.*, 91(6), 1372–1386.

Usleber, E., Donald, D., Straka, M., and Martlbauer, E., 1997. Comparison of enzyme immunoassay and mouse bioassay for determining paralytic shellfish poisoning toxins in shellfish. *Food Addit. Contam.*, 14(2), 193–198.

Usleber, E., Schneider, E., and Terplan, G., 1991. Direct enzyme immunoassay in microtitration plate and test strip format for the detection of saxitoxin in shellfish. *Lett. Appl. Microbiol.*, 13, 275–277.

Usup, G., Ahmad, A., Matsuoka, K., Lim, P.T., and Leaw, C.P., 2012. Biology, ecology and bloom dynamics of the toxic marine dinoflagellate *Pyrodinium bahamense*. *Harmful Algae*, 14, 301–312.

Vale, C., Alfonso, A., Vieytes, M.R., Romarís, X.M., Arévalo, F., Botana, A.M., and Botana, L.M., 2008. In vitro and in vivo evaluation of paralytic shellfish poisoning toxin potency and the influence of the pH of extraction. *Anal. Chem.*, 80(5), 1770–1776.

Vale, P., 2008a. Fate of benzoate paralytic shellfish poisoning toxins from *Gymnodinium catenatum* in shellfish and fish detected by pre-column oxidation and liquid chromatography with fluorescence detection. *J. Chromatogr. A*, 1190(1–2), 191–197.

Vale, P., 2008b. Complex profile of hydrophobic paralytic shellfish poisoning compounds in *Gymnodinium catenatum* detected by liquid chromatography with fluorescence and mass spectrometry detection. *J. Chromatogr. A*, 1195, 85–93.

Vale, P., 2010a. Metabolites of saxitoxin analogues in bivalves contaminated by *Gymnodinium catenatum*. *Toxicon*, 55(1), 162–165.

Vale, P., 2010b. Saxitoxin analogues: Developments in toxin chemistry, detection and biotransformation during the 2000's. *Phytochem. Rev.*, 9(4), 525–535.

Vale, P., 2011. Marine biotoxins and blue mussel: One of the most troublesome species during harmful algal blooms. In: McGevin, L.E. (Ed.), *Mussels: Anatomy, Habitat and Environmental Impact*. Nova Science Publishers, Hauppauge, New York, pp. 413–428.

Vale, P., Rangel, I., Silva, B., Coelho, P., and Vilar, A., 2009. Atypical profiles of paralytic shellfish poisoning toxins in shellfish from Luanda and Mussulo bays, Angola. *Toxicon*, 53, 176–183.

Vale, P. and Sampayo, M.A.M., 2001. Determination of paralytic shellfish toxins in Portuguese shellfish by automated pre-column oxidation. *Toxicon*, 39(4), 561–571.

Vale, P. and Sampayo, M.A.M., 2002. Evaluation of marine biotoxin's accumulation by *Acanthocardia tuberculatum* from Algarve, Portugal. *Toxicon*, 40(5), 511–517.

Vale, P. and Taleb, H., 2005. Assessment of quantitative determination of paralytic shellfish poisoning toxins by pre-column derivatization and elimination of interfering compounds by SPE extraction. *Food Addit. Contam.*, 22(9), 838–846.

Wang, J., Salata, J.J., and Bennett, P.B., 2003. Saxitoxin is a gating modifier of hERG K+ channels. *J. Gen. Physiol.*, 121, 583–598.

White, A.W., 1984. Paralytic shellfish toxins and finfish. In: Ragelis, E.P. (Ed.), *Seafood Toxins*. ACS Symposium Series 262, American Chemical Society, Washington, DC, pp. 171–180.

Wyatt, T. and Jenkinson, I.R., 1997. Notes on *Alexandrium* population dynamics. *J. Plankton Res.*, 19(5), 551–575.

Yotsu-Yamashita, M., Kim, Y.H., Dudley, S.C. Jr., Choudhary, G., Pfahnl, A., Oshima, Y., and Daly, J.W., 2004. The structure of zetekitoxin AB, a saxitoxin analog from the Panamanian golden frog *Atelopus zeteki*: A potent sodium-channel blocker. *Proc. Natl. Acad. Sci. USA*, 101, 4346–4351.

Part VI

Cyanobacterial Toxins

35

Cyanobacterial Toxins in Aquaculture

Paul T. Smith

CONTENTS

35.1 Link between Cyanobacteria and Aquaculture

Aquaculture and cyanobacteria are not usually discussed in the same forum even though it is an important topic and the relationship is at an important interface. It is representative of the anthropogenic pressures that are currently impacting on all species and every environment. Population growth, climate change, diminishing resources, energy demand, and environmental pollution are all accelerating at rates that were hardly imagined a century ago. Today, we find that aquaculture and cyanobacteria are intimately linked by these contemporary drivers. This chapter builds on previous examinations of this topic (Smith 2000, 2008). In this section, we will explore the link between cyanobacteria and aquaculture. In the following sections, we will examine the current scientific understanding in this multidisciplinary field and make an assessment of the level of risk posed by cyanobacterial toxins to seafood as well as consider possible future directions for research.

Total production of seafood from wild fisheries and aquaculture has grown by an average rate of 3.2% per year in the last 50 years. This is a faster rate than that of the global population of 1.7% per year. In the same period, world per capita fish usage increased from an average of 9.9 kg per person in the 1960s to 18.6 kg per person in 2009 (FAO 2012). Currently, fisheries and aquaculture provide livelihoods and income for an estimate 54.8 million people as well as employment in ancillary activities for 660–820 million people (FAO 2012).

Production by capture fisheries plateaued at 90 million tonnes per annum in 1990, mainly because of anthropogenic impacts of overexploitation, pollution, and habit loss (Ye et al. 2012). Although wild fisheries production has been at a steady level for more than two decades, the statistics hide the fact that most fish stocks have been declining during this period due to intensification of fishing effort. In recognition of this situation, the 2002 World Summit on Sustainable Development (WSSD) agreed to urgent actions to restore wild fish stocks to more sustainable levels by 2015. Many countries have implemented programs for increasing fish and shellfish stocks that include restocking waterways, providing aquatic reserves, limiting fishing quotas, and establishing size limits. For example, China has focused on fish stock enhancement programs, whereby hatcheries are used to breed and to restock water bodies with juvenile animals, plus applied a range of other approaches to improve inland fisheries (Chen et al. 2012). However, global fisheries have continued to significantly decline and pressures on wild fisheries have increased. Now it is estimated that the global fish catch needs to be cut by an unachievable level of 36%–48% in order to meet WSSD goals (Ye et al. 2012).

In contrast to the progressive deterioration in wild fisheries, aquaculture has expanded to meet the increase in demand for seafood. In the last 50 years, aquaculture production has increased by an average of 7% per annum and now represents 42% of total world fisheries production. In fact, recent data shows that the annual rate of growth of global aquaculture production appears to be accelerating, with an increase from 47.3 million tons in 2006 to 63.6 million tons in 2011 (De Silva 2012; FAO 2012).

Aquaculture is a diverse primary industry that produces a range of finfish, shrimp, prawns, oysters, mussels, seaweed, as well as smaller quantities of other species (i.e., reptiles, sea urchins, frogs). Its history can be traced back at least 4000 years in Asia, and the first known book on fish culture was written by Fan Li in 473 BC (see pp. 3–4, Tapiador et al. 1977). The integration of rice and fish farming can be dated to the Han Dynasty (206_{BC}–225_{BC}) in China (FAO 2012).

The modern era of aquaculture began approximately 50 years ago when it became commercially viable to farm aquatic animals through innovations such as the use of aerators to increase stocking densities and the use of dry formulated feeds to improve the diet. Nevertheless, one-third of global food fish production in 2010 was produced without the use of feed (i.e., by farming bivalves and filter-feeding carps). Also when aquatic plants and nonfood products are included, the global aquaculture production in 2010 was 79 million tonnes, with a value of US$125 billion (FAO 2012). Asia's aquaculture production accounted for 89% of the volume of global aquaculture production in 2010, of which China contributed 61.4%.

In developed countries, aquaculture tends to focus on highly valued species (i.e., salmon, shrimp, oysters), but in developing countries, the focus is on producing highly valued products for export (e.g., shrimp) and high-quality food (e.g., carp species) to supplement the diets of rural people (Anderson and Valderrama 2013). The dominant forms of aquaculture in 2010 (FAO 2012) were farming of several species of carps (24.2 million tons), tilapia (3.5 million tons), oysters/molluscs (14.2 million tons), and shrimp/crustaceans (5.7 million tons).

The importance of freshwater aquaculture to people in developing countries cannot be overestimated. The key concerns of inland rural communities are food security, poverty reduction, and socioeconomic development (UNFPA 2008). Protein is usually deficient in the diet of most communities, and small-scale aquaculture is recognized as an important component in alleviating rural poverty, improving health as well as providing income and employment. To illustrate this point, we can consider the situation in Papua New Guinea, a tropical nation of 6.5 million people with more than 85% of the population living in remote rural communities (Smith 2007; Smith and Mufuape 2013). In PNG, the rural people suffer with severe problems that are demonstrated by key indicators of low life expectancy, high maternal birthing mortalities, high birth rates, high infant mortality, high levels of illiteracy, high rate of HIV, high levels of malnutrition, and low per capita income (UNFPA 2008).

In light of these issues, PNG has listed the relatively new rural activity of freshwater fish farming as a priority for developing household food security and income (NADP 2007). In the last decade, the number of small-scale fish farms has increased from 5,400 to more than 15,000, which has helped improve nutrition for families, reduced the burden on rural women, and provided new forms of employment for youths and communities (Smith and Mufuape 2013). Training and technical support has been a major bottleneck, so 1450 small-scale farmers were trained in 2006–2008 on using local homegrown ingredients and agricultural waste to feed common carp and tilapia in small earthen ponds (Smith 2007, 2010; Smith and Mufuape 2013). Also, farmers have been encouraged to use pond effluent to irrigate crops and vegetable gardens. The training workshops for women empowered them by providing opportunities to earn extra income and provide high-quality food for their families (Smith and Mufuape 2013). Women were found to be more likely to train other women and children; they effectively became skilled extension workers. Also, they were found to be more consistent than men with fish husbandry and economics (i.e., feeding, breeding, marketing) because these tasks fit with their everyday tasks. Nevertheless, the situation is grim in PNG as well as in other developing countries and it will take much more effort to overcome chronic socioeconomic problems.

Globally, aquaculture is most commonly carried out in earthen ponds with freshwater or brackish water (Anderson and Valderrama 2013; FAO 2012). This inevitably leads to environmental impacts on water bodies (Jegatheesan et al. 2011) and encourages the growth of toxic cyanobacteria. The most important negative impacts of aquaculture are summarized as follows:

1. Eutrophication of water bodies as a result of the discharge of pond effluent that often contains elevated levels of nutrients
2. Increased levels of dissolved organic nutrients because of a general reliance on commercial feeds that are based on fishmeal and have high levels of protein (25%–45% dry weight)
3. Hydrological changes due to very high levels of water use, salt intrusion, and waste disposal
4. Other changes that include impacts on wild species through spread of disease and changes in habitat

In addition, 10%–15% of the global sources of fishmeal (i.e., anchovies, sardines) are used to make aquaculture feeds, though there are efforts to replace fish-based proteins with vegetable proteins (De Silva 2012). Unfortunately, well-meaning research can have poor outcomes by encouraging unnecessary use of fishmeal. We use the example of PNG again, long-term research programs that have been funded by international aid agencies (JICA of Japan and ACIAR of Australia), and advocate the use of 25%–35% fishmeal in diets for farmed fish. This has encouraged subsistence fish farmers to buy commercial feeds with high levels of protein to grow carp and tilapia in ponds and cages (Hair et al. 2006). This type of farming produces a feed conversion ratio of 2:1 (dry feed to wet fish) and a cost of feed of approximately half of the sale price of farmed fish. It is evident that the best the farmer can expect is to come out even at the end of the crop. When mortalities, cost of fingerlings, and other factors are considered, the farmer can never make a profit. Further, this method of farming has been identified as causing unnecessary eutrophication of ponds and water bodies (Smith and Mufuape 2013) and this can lead to blooms of benthic cyanobacteria in ponds (Figure 35.1). Hence, not only is the use of fishmeal by these subsistence farmers economically unviable, it causes eutrophication of water bodies.

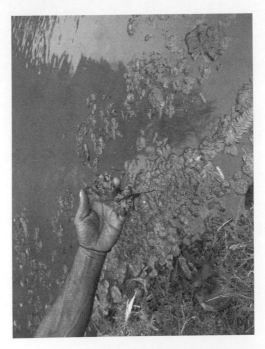

FIGURE 35.1 Image of benthic blooms of cyanobacteria in fish ponds in PNG. Benthic blooms consist of *Oscillatoria* spp. that are carried to the surface by gas bubbles in the daytime. The use of feeds with high levels of fishmeal protein and phosphates encourages the development of cyanobacterial blooms.

Blooms of benthic cyanobacteria have a place in traditional forms of fish farming in Asian countries, where organic fertilizers are applied to shallow earthen ponds in early stages of the crop to encourage benthic mats (known as *lablab*). The benthos is a complex community of filamentous and unicellular cyanobacteria as well as diatoms and invertebrates. These benthic communities are acknowledged to have nutritional value for early stages in the traditional culture of milk fish, carp, tilapia, and shrimp

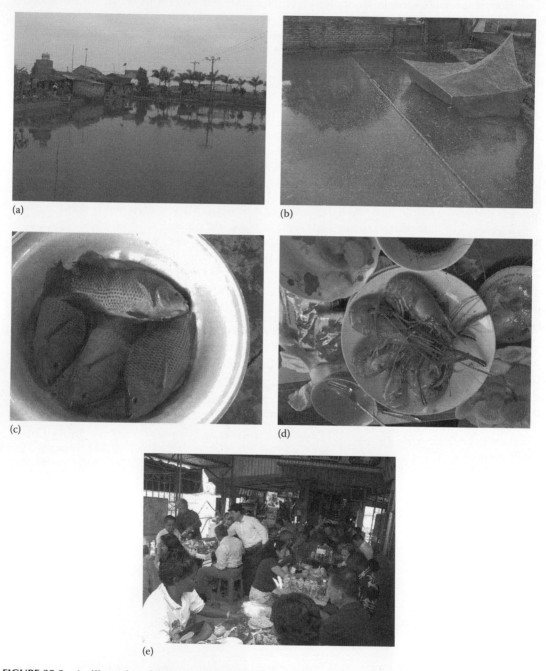

FIGURE 35.2   An illustration of the link between cyanobacteria and aquaculture. (a) Tilapia and freshwater prawns are cultured in earthen ponds that are beside a family's seafood restaurant. Blooms of *Microcystis* sp. are present. (b) The nursery pond for raising juvenile tilapia fish has a thick algal blooms that is dominated by *Microcystis* sp. (c) Freshly harvested tilapia are ready for immediate cooking. (d) Giant freshwater prawns from the ponds are cooked and ready for the customers. (e) Tourists and locals consume the freshly prepared tilapia and prawns.

(Smith 2008). However, benthic blooms are not sufficient for growth and so they are usually replaced after the early stages of the crop, by increasing the water level so that microalgal blooms and zooplankton can develop.

The occurrence of cyanobacterial blooms during later stages of culture can be detrimental because it is associated with reduced productivity, off-flavors, and mortalities (Tucker 2000, 2005; Yusoff et al. 2001; Howgat 2004). Nevertheless, in spite of efforts by farmers to minimize cyanobacterial blooms, it is common for noxious and toxic cyanobacterial blooms of species such as *Nodularia*, *Microcystis*, and *Oscillatoria* to still occur (Smith 2003).

To illustrate the strong link between cyanobacteria and aquaculture, a montage is given of photographs taken in 2010 of a typical farm near Hanoi, Vietnam (Figure 35.2). Earthen ponds are used to culture tilapia fish, *Oreochromis niloticus*, and giant freshwater prawns, *Macrobrachium* sp. (Figure 35.2A). Blooms of *Microcystis* are common and normally of no concern to the farmer (Figure 35.2B). It is quite common for farms to also sell their fresh produce (Figure 35.2C) directly to locals or to sell cooked meals of fish and prawns (Figure 35.2D) to tourists and travellers at the farm's restaurant (Figure 35.2E). The farm that is illustrated in Figure 35.2 is typical of the many thousands of fish farms that operate in this way in Asian countries, providing high-quality protein and essential oils for millions and perhaps billions of people.

In summary, this section has demonstrated that aquaculture has been expanding at a phenomenal rate for 50 years and that this trend is predicted to continue as output from wild fisheries either stabilize or diminish. Also, we have seen that aquaculture, and effluent from aquaculture, produces conditions that are conducive to the development of cyanobacteria. Hence, the link between aquaculture, cyanobacteria, and seafood is clearly established. This chapter will now explore this relationship.

35.2 Cyanobacterial Toxins

Cyanobacteria are photosynthetic bacteria that were once thought to be a type of alga. So even today, they are often referred to as blue-green algae, and cyanobacterial blooms are often categorized as hazardous algal blooms (HABs). Cyanobacteria play important roles in many aquatic ecosystems by producing oxygen, generating organic matter, and fixing nitrogen. The occurrence of toxic blooms of cyanobacteria in freshwater and brackish water environments has increased noticeably in frequency and severity in recent decades (Codd et al. 2005). Cyanobacteria are the most diverse types of prokaryotes in terms of structure and development. They can also cause problems by producing noxious odors and forming dense blooms and scums that lower the dissolved oxygen concentration and increase pH. Many species are capable of producing secondary metabolites by nonribosomal processes that include cyanobacterial toxins or cyanotoxins (Neilan et al. 1999; Wiegand and Plugmacher 2005). These toxins are generally categorized as liver toxins (hepatotoxins), nerve toxins (neurotoxins), cytotoxins, and endotoxins. This is worrying because cyanotoxins are known to cause morbidity and mortalities in birds and mammals (Carmichael 1988, 1994, 2007). This section examines the cyanobacterial toxins that have been discovered and their mechanism of action.

Many cyanobacterial toxins, including microcystins and hepatotoxins, are made of unique amino acids and are produced by cellular processes rather than by ribosomal activity. Molecular techniques have been developed to identify the genes that are responsible for toxin production in cyanobacteria (Neilan et al. 1997, 1999). These techniques have been used to show that up to 2% of the cell's machinery can be devoted to the production of cyanobacterial toxins. Also, these types of molecular techniques have enabled researchers to use primers that target microcystin-producing genes, to differentiate between toxigenic and nontoxigenic genotypes in *Microcystis*, *Nostoc*, *Anabaena*, and *Planktothrix* (Neilan et al. 1997; Dittman and Borner 2005). Several studies have found that the proportion of toxic cyanobacterial cells ranges from >1% to 55% and that global warming appears to be linked to more intense and more toxic *Microcystis* blooms (Paerl and Huisman 2008; Te and Gin 2011).

The various types of cyanobacterial toxins are microcystins, nodularins, cylindrospermopsins, anatoxin-a, anatoxin-a(S), lyngbyatoxin-a, saxitoxins, lipopolysaccharides, and aplysiatoxins (Table 35.1). Generally, microcystins are the most frequently identified cyanobacterial toxins in freshwater habitats,

TABLE 35.1

Toxins Produced by Cyanobacteria

Cyanobacterial Toxin	Genera of Cyanobacteria	Mode of Action
1. Cyclic peptides		
Microcystins	*Microcystis, Anabaena, Anabaenopsis, Nostoc, Planktothrix* (previously known as *Oscillatoria*)	Hepatotoxin
Nodularins	*Nodularia*	Hepatotoxin
2. Alkaloids		
Cylindrospermopsins	*Cylindrospermopsis, Aphanizomenon, Umezakia*	Cytotoxin, Hepatotoxin
Anatoxin-a	*Anabaena, Aphanizomenon, Planktothrix* (previously known as *Oscillatoria*)	Neurotoxin
Anatoxin-a(S)	*Anabaena*	Neurotoxin
Saxitoxins	*Anabaena, Aphanizomenon,*	Neurotoxin
Lyngbyatoxin-a	*Lyngbya, Cylindrospermopsis Lyngbya*	Epidermal irritant
3. Others		
Lipopolysaccharides	All genera	Epidermal irritant
Aplysiatoxins	*Lyngbya, Schizothrix, Planktothrix* (previously known as *Oscillatoria*)	Epidermal irritant

while nodularins are the most commonly found cyanobacterial toxins in habitats where brackish water and freshwater interact. There are at least 75 different chemical forms of microcystins and more seem to be found as techniques develop. For example, a study of Lake Chao in Anhui Province, China, revealed that some isolated strains of *Microcystis* were capable of producing up to 11 variants of microcystins with concentrations of up to 4.8 mg g/DW (Krüger et al. 2010).

Microcystins are small proteins (polypeptides) having seven amino acids and their structure is either cyclic or ringed. Nodularins have a similar structure to microcystin but have only five amino acids. The naming of microcystins reflects the fact that the toxin was first discovered in members of the genera *Microcystis*, but they have since been found in many genera of cyanobacteria (Table 35.1).

Microcystins and nodularins are the most commonly found toxins in toxic cyanobacterial blooms and they pose a risk to human health when waters are used by people for drinking (Falconer et al. 1988; Falconer 2005). Nodularin and microcystin are absorbed into the blood through epithelial membranes of the intestines, gills, and lungs (Runnegar et al. 1995). They generally accumulate in hepatocytes (liver cells) where they inhibit protein phosphatases and cause an imbalance in cellular reactions that involve phosphorylation/dephosphorylation. Also, hepatocytes can no longer maintain their shape because of the collapse of the cytoskeleton (Runnegar and Falconer 1986). As a consequence, hepatocytes shrink and leave spaces between cells (i.e., sinusoids). Blood seeps from capillaries into these spaces and blood accumulates there. This leads to local tissue damage in the liver and shock as well as death if the toxin concentration is high enough. When an animal has died from ingesting these hepatotoxins, the liver and kidney are enlarged because of the internal bleeding (i.e., hemorrhage) and they are heavily mottled (i.e., surface patches of blood). These hepatotoxins also cause oxidative stress by increasing the concentration of harmful reactive oxygen species. This effectively decreases the antioxidant capability of the cell that can result in DNA degradation and cell death as well as tumor promotion (Smith et al. 2008).

Cylindrospermopsins was initially found about 20 years ago in a bloom of *Cylindrospermopsis raciborskii* in the drinking water on Palm Island, Queensland Australia. Since then, it has been found in several genera of cyanobacteria (Table 35.1). Cylindrospermopsin and its analogs are hepatotoxins, but because they also affect many other organs of animals, they are classified as cytotoxins. Toxicity to cells occurs through irreversible inhibition of protein synthesis, DNA fragmentation, tumor initiation, and irreversible inhibition of protein synthesis (Smith et al. 2008).

Saxitoxins are water-soluble neurotoxins that are also commonly known as paralytic shellfish poison (PSP). Saxitoxins have been found in a range of cyanobacteria (Table 35.1) though they were initially found in the butter calm (*Saxidomus giganteus*) and later found in puffer fish and marine dinoflagellates. There are at least 26 forms of saxitoxins and act by binding to Na⁺ channels in animal cells and cause cellular membrane potentials to remain hyperpolarized (i.e., cells are unable to depolarize and incapable of transmitting an action potential). The most toxic forms of saxitoxins are the carbamate moieties and they include saxitoxin, neosaxitoxin, and gonyautoxins (Oshima et al. 1993; Smith 2000; Etheridge 2010).

Another group of alkaloid neurotoxins includes anatoxin-a, homo-anatoxin-a, and anatoxin-a(S) and have been isolated from various genera (Table 35.1). Anatoxin-a and homoanatoxin-a mimic acetylcholine in nerve and muscle synapses of mammals. Anatoxin-a(S) blocks acetylcholinesterase activity in neurons of mammals, thus causing overstimulation of muscles, fatigue, and paralysis. The account by Smith (2000) provides a more complete description of the toxicology and pharmacology of neurotoxins.

Cyanobacterial lipopolysaccharides are located on the surface of the outer cell layer of all cyanobacteria (Table 35.1). Lipopolysaccharides are composed of a carbohydrate polymer, an oligosaccharide, and a glycolipid. Toxic cyanobacterial lipopolysaccharides cause inflammation, liver damage, and septic shock syndrome. Lyngbyatoxins and aplysiatoxins act as irritants (dermatoxins) as well as tumor promoters (Ito et al. 2002).

35.3 Evidence of Cyanobacterial Toxins in Aquaculture

The beginning of this chapter described the clear and intensifying link between cyanobacteria and aquaculture. Previous examinations of this topic (Smith 2000, 2008) have provided evidence for the existence in aquaculture of many genera of cyanobacteria and a range of cyanobacterial toxins. Three other relatively recent reviews can assist the reader in exploring aspects of this topic (Ibelings and Chorus 2007; Smith et al. 2008; Amado and Monserrat 2010). We start with the interesting proposition based on anecdotal evidence as well as historical evidence that blooms of cyanobacteria are common in aquaculture, yet there are relatively few cases of either (1) clearly defined toxic effects caused by cyanobacteria on the cultured species or (2) toxic effects of cyanobacterial toxins on consumers of seafood. This leads to a null hypothesis, which will be examined here. (It is hoped that the reader will tolerate the author's indulgence in describing some relevant findings from his research in the area of shrimp farming.)

As a reference, we note that the World health Organization (WHO) set a guideline for a maximum concentration of 1 µg/L microcystin-LR in drinking water and a tolerable daily intake in the diet of 0.04 g/kg body weight (Falconer et al. 1999).

35.3.1 Cyanobacterial Toxins in Shrimp Farms

Wild shrimp (also known as prawns) have been shown to accumulate microcystins from toxic blooms of cyanobacteria in freshwater lakes in China (Chen and Xie 2005). *Macrobrachium* and *Palaemon* accumulated microcystins in the hepatopancreas (0.43 and 4.29 µg/g DW, respectively) as well as the gonad (0.48 and 1.17 µg/g DW, respectively). In 31% of samples, shrimp muscle was also above the WHO tolerable daily intake level (0.04 µg/kg/day), which enabled the authors to conclude that consumers were at risk when eating contaminated wild shrimp from these lakes and other water bodies that have been impacted by recent eutrophication.

In contrast, traditional farming of shrimp encouraged blooms of microalgae and cyanobacteria. In more recent times, modern shrimp farming has taken a new direction of controlling blooms. Also, a new method of encouraging bacterial bioflocs is used by some farmers. Shrimp can be raised at higher densities and the protein content of the feed can be lowered because the microbial community provides shrimp with a source of proteins (Baloi et al. 2013). However, when shrimp are cultured in brackish water that is affected by persistent cyanobacterial blooms, there is relatively low productivity for species such as the black tiger shrimp, *Penaeus monodon* (see Smith 2000, 2008;

Alonso-Rodríguez and Paez-Osuna 2003). Shrimp in affected ponds have relatively slow growth rates, darker coloration of body and hepatopancreas, and a greater susceptibility to diseases. On the face of it, these observations suggest that either cyanobacteria are a poorer source of nutrition than microalgal blooms or compounds produced by cyanobacteria may increase the stress on shrimp and render them more susceptible to viruses and pathogenic bacteria. On rare occasions, cyanobacterial blooms are associated with mortalities.

From a marketing point of view, shrimp in ponds with cyanobacterial blooms usually have musty off-flavors. Also, cooked shrimp occasionally have blackened heads. It appears that cyanobacterial pigments are released from ruptured hepatopancreas, and the spreading of the dark pigments postharvest causes a blackening of the shrimp's head.

The oldest reports of cyanobacterial toxicity in shrimp farms indicated that cyanobacteria could cause morbidity or mortalities in shrimp. Lightner (1978) reported a pathology known as hemocytic enteritis of the intestines of *P. stylirostris* that was associated with a bloom of *Spirulina* sp. The identity of the toxin/s was not determined in that incident. Lightner also encountered a similar problem in an investigation of hemocytic enteritis in *P. stylirostris* that was associated with a bloom of *Lyngbya* sp. (originally identified as *Spirulina* sp.). In Australia, planktonic and benthic cyanobacterial blooms of *Planktothrix* sp. (formerly *Oscillatoriales*) were found to have neurotoxic effects on *P. monodon*, *P. japonicus*, and *Artemia salina* (Smith 1996). In that report, it was noted that cyanobacterial species were ubiquitous in shrimp farms. The toxins that caused mortalities in those incidents were not identified.

In a more recent study, nodularin was detected in blooms of *Nodularia* in Australian shrimp ponds at concentrations of 30 μg/L in pond water and 1000 mg/kg dry wt. algae (Smith and Kankaanpää 2001; Kankaanpää et al. 2005). Mouse bioassay was performed by intraperitoneal (i.p.) injection of freeze-dried *Nodularia* bloom that was resuspended in physiological saline. The pellet was sublethal and hepatotoxic, while supernatant was hepatotoxic and lethal in 54 min. Necropsy of mice tested with supernatant revealed that their livers were heavily mottled, patchy, dark, and enlarged. Kidneys were also heavily mottled. However, nodularin was not as toxic to shrimp. When shrimp were injected with pure nodularin (10, 100 μg/kg) or supernatant from the *Nodularia* bloom, there were no mortalities after 7 days (P.T. Smith unpublished).

To quantify the types of phytoplankton in shrimp ponds, a weekly survey was carried out at four farms growing *P. monondon* in Far North Queensland, Australia (D. Ivanoff and P.T. Smith unpublished). Cyanobacteria were the second most abundant form of phytoplankton (Table 35.2). The main genera of cyanobacteria were filamentous, including *Planktothrix* sp. (found in 14% of samples) followed by *Pseudanabaena* sp. and *Anabaena* sp. (in 7% of samples). On rare occasions, other forms of cyanobacteria were observed, and these included *Microcystis* sp. and *Nodularia* sp. It was found that planktonic forms of cyanobacteria started to occur in some ponds approximately 60 days after stocking and from then onward, ponds either had high numbers (>400,000 cells/mL) or were relatively free of planktonic

TABLE 35.2

Results of a Survey of Phytoplankton in 214 Shrimp Ponds in Far North Queensland, Australia (2000–2001)[a]

Plankton	Cell count/mL (mean ± s.e.m.)
Nonmotile green algae	278,000 ± 19,000
Cyanobacteria	131,400 ± 9,000
Flagellates	56,100 ± 3,800
Diatoms	35,600 ± 2,400
Dinoflagellates	6,060 ± 410
Protozoans	830 ± 60

[a] By Daniel Ivanoff and P.T. Smith (unpublished).

cyanobacteria. In general, the other species of algae tended to be present in varying densities in most ponds throughout the crop of approximately 5–6 months.

A similar survey of shrimp ponds was carried out in the following season (2001–2002) at *P. monodon* farms in Northern NSW, Australia (P.T. Smith unpublished). Benthic blooms were common in the first 4 weeks of the crop, after which the pattern was similar to the earlier survey in Queensland. However, blooms of *Nodularia spumigena* were more frequent, occurring in 5% of ponds in the final 3 months of the crop. *Anabaenopsis* sp. and *Microcystis* sp. also occurred during these times. This period also corresponded to increased rainfall and decreased river salinity (i.e., from 28–30 to 12–15 ppt).

The presence of cyanobacterial toxins was investigated by collecting samples of cyanobacterial blooms from shrimp ponds. Samples were separated into pellet and supernatant, then freeze dried and tested for toxicity by biotoxicity tests with mice, biotoxicity tests with shrimp, and LC-MS. The results are summarized in Table 35.3. Four types of known microcystins were present in the samples, and there were three other microcystins that were present but not identified (P.T. Smith and Ambrose Furey, unpublished).

Some six separate biotoxicity tests with shrimp were carried out with the cyanobacterial blooms of Table 35.3. Healthy shrimp were injected (intramuscular [i.m.]) with filtered extracts and sacrificed within 24 h following injection. Histopathology revealed that the microcystins caused damage to the hepatopancreas of shrimp. Hepatopancreatic tubules contained cells that appeared to have sloughed off into the lumen (i.e., broken away from the basement membrane). The parenchyma tissue between the tubules is often lost. In extreme cases, the hepatopancreatic cells of the tubules "rounded up" and the structure of the tubules were severely damaged (Smith 2003). These findings are consistent with the action of microcystin on mammalian liver tissue. However, it was clear from these tests that the cyanobacteria were not as toxic to farmed shrimp as they were to mice (Table 35.3).

TABLE 35.3

Detection of Microcystins in Blooms from Shrimp Farms in Australia[a]

Sample Number	Type of Cyanobacteria Bloom	Fraction of Freeze-Dried Extract	Result of Mouse Toxicity Test	MC Detected
1	*Spirulina* sp. and *Planktothrix* sp.	Pellet	Livers and kidneys were patchy—possible toxic.	No MC detected
		Supernatant	Livers and kidneys were patchy—possible toxic.	MC-RR
2	*Microcystis aeruginosa* and *Microcystis flos-aquae*	Pellet	Livers and kidneys were mottled—possible toxic.	MC-LR, MC-LA
		Supernatant	Mice appeared ill and livers slightly enlarged, heavily mottled and kidneys mottled—sublethal hepatotoxin.	MC-YR, MC-LR, MC-LA
3	*Planktothrix* sp.	Pellet	Mice appeared very ill and livers were heavily mottled and kidneys were mottled—possible toxic.	MC-RR, MC-YR, and 2 other unknown microcystins
		Supernatant	Liver patchy but close to normal—possible toxic.	MC-YR, MC-LR, MC-LA, and 1 other unknown microcystin

[a] By P.T. Smith and Ambrose Furey (unpublished).

35.3.2 Cyanobacterial Toxins in Fish Farms

An early study of cyanobacteria in fish ponds (Sevrin-Reyssac and Pletikosic 1990) described reports of cyanobacteria inhibiting nutrition and reproduction of rotifers as well as reports of mortalities of carp and other freshwater fish in blooms of *Microcystis* sp. and *Anabaena flos-aquae*. However, the study concluded on the weight of evidence that most fish mortalities in ponds and aquatic habitats are not caused by cyanobacterial toxins. Instead, most instances of morbidity and mortalities could be explained by either the poor nutritional value of cyanobacterial blooms or their impacts on water quality (i.e., dissolved oxygen, pH, and ammonia). Nevertheless, there are some older reports that suggested that mortalities of trout were caused by toxic cyanobacterial blooms (Phillips et al. 1985; Rodger et al. 1994).

The review of the effect of microcystins on oxidative stress in aquatic animals by Amado and Monserrat (2010) listed 17 reports in which aquatic animals (i.e., polychaeta, crustaceans, and fish) showed alterations in the antioxidant system as a result of exposure to microcystins. In those reports, the aquatic animals were exposed to microcystins by a number of methods that are summarized as follows (with the number of reports in brackets):

1. Eleven studies reported on exposure to extracts of *Microcystis* bloom by bathing (3), feeding (6), or injection (2).
2. Six studies reported on exposure to pure microcystin by irrigation of tissue culture (2), bathing (1), feeding (1), or injection (2).

The summary by Amado and Monserrat (2010) reveals that there are a wide range of methods that have been used to investigate cyanobacterial toxicity in aquatic animals. Also, the testing may be carried out on representative fish, such as zebrafish, rather than farmed fish (Kist et al. 2012).

A research paper by Gélinas et al. (2012) provided a summary table of reports of microcystins from toxic cyanobacterial blooms affecting a range of species of farmed fish (i.e., *Cyprinus carpio, Anguilla anguilla, Hypophthalmichthys molitrix, O. niloticus*). Various methods were used to expose fish to microcystins (including bathing, feeding, and injection) and doses ranged widely for each technique. For instance, i.p. doses ranged from 176 to 1000 µg/kg and feeding doses varied in rates and units (i.e., 50 µg/fish/day, 50 µg/kg). The differences in methodology and expression of dose rates are clear problems for comparative analysis of the findings.

It is apparent that in recent times, the evidence is building that fish do experience hepatotoxic effects from cyanobacteria (Magalhaes et al. 2003; Malbrouck and Krestemont 2006). Also, there is evidence that saxitoxins can accumulate in farmed freshwater tilapia, *O. niloticus* (Galvão et al. 2009). It has been suggested that although fish such as tilapia, *O. niloticus*, can have a high rate of accumulation of microcystins from toxic cyanobacterial blooms, these fish have a high depuration rate (Deblois et al. 2011). The efficient elimination system of tilapia may explain the tolerance of these fish to toxic blooms.

35.3.3 Cyanobacterial Toxins in Oyster Farms and Other Forms of Aquaculture

PSP is a well-known worldwide problem for consumers of seafood that occurs because of eating bivalves, molluscs, and other shellfish that have accumulated saxitoxins and other neurotoxins (Etheridge 2010). Toxic microalgal blooms are the most common source of the toxins; however, there is growing evidence that saxitoxins are also produced by freshwater and brackish water cyanobacteria (Deeds et al. 2008). Oyster industries and mussel industries in many countries have responded by introducing quality assurance programs in which samples of water and shellfish are routinely gathered and tested for the presence of toxic microalgae and toxic cyanobacteria.

Oysters, mussels, and freshwater gastropods have been shown to bioaccumulate microcystins by ingesting toxic cyanobacteria or by absorbing dissolved microcystins from the surrounding water (Gérard et al. 2009; Zhang et al. 2012). Also, sediment-dwelling bivalves and amphipods have been shown to accumulate nodularin from toxic cyanobacterial blooms in the Baltic Sea (Karlson and Mozūraitis 2011). Nodularin concentrations in tissue samples were 50–120 ng/g DW, and it was concluded that the macrofauna may contribute to transfer of nodularin in food webs.

35.4 Future Directions for Research into Cyanobacterial Toxins in Aquaculture

So far, it has not been necessary to introduce similar quality assurance programs to test for cyanobacterial toxins in fish farming or shrimp farming. This difference with the oyster and mussel industries is interesting and puzzling, especially since many of the toxins produced by microalgae are also found in cyanobacteria. It may be argued that this situation occurs because oysters and mussels are herbivorous filter feeders. However, fish species (i.e., carps, tilapias) that account for much of the global production of fish farms are herbivores or omnivores. Similarly, many of the farmed crustaceans (i.e., *Penaeus* sp.) are omnivores that can consume cyanobacteria.

There is a need for more research into the effects of cyanobacterial toxins on farmed aquatic animals, rather than extrapolating findings from cyanobacterial research with mice or nonfarmed aquatic species. Also, there needs to be more research into the mode of uptake of cyanobacterial toxins, as well as the depuration and detoxification processes by farmed aquatic animals. For example, research is often carried out on fish or invertebrates that are either cultured in an aquarium or collected from the wild, rather than on farmed aquatic animals. But this research is not sufficient because we need to know about animals that are food sources. Also, at a pragmatic level, farmers and farmer organizations are the ones who ultimately invest funds and resources into this type of research. Hence, they should expect that the research projects should focus on their animals and their farms. Lessons can be learned from the way oyster farmers and mussel farmers in countries such as New Zealand have worked collaboratively with research projects to develop quality assurance programs for microalgal toxin testing. During this process, researchers have developed new procedures and made discoveries that have been possible because scientists and farmers worked in a partnership.

In addition, there is a need to standardize the methods for testing cyanobacterial blooms in aquaculture. Standard methods should include pond-side observations of the water quality, condition of the bloom, and the health of farmed aquatic animals. The testing of toxicity should include simple protocols for toxin testing by feeding, immersion, and injection as well as agreed protocols for histopathology. For example, a simple protocol for biotoxicity tests on farmed shrimp or fish that has been successfully used is as follows:

> Samples of chilled cyanobacterial bloom from the farm were centrifuged and separated into pellet or supernatant upon arrival. Measured quantities of subsample (0.2 g) were reconstituted in 5 mL Millipore water. The subsamples were sonicated and filter-sterilized. Animals were held appropriately while 1 mL was delivered by i.p. or i.m. injection (duplicates per test). Animals were maintained in appropriate aquatic conditions and observed for 24 hrs or until death, then livers and kidneys from each animal were examined and processed for histopathology and electron microscopy.

Obviously, the protocol needs to take into account the size of the animal, the types of tissues and organs that need to be examined, the range of concentrations of extracts, and other factors such as consistency of units and doses. By using farmed animals and applying consistent protocols, it should be possible to obtain comparative parameters, which are of benefit to aquaculture industries and researchers. This type of approach should assist in increasing scientific understanding of the interaction between toxic cyanobacteria and farmed species. Farmers, agencies, and consumers also need such information on the types of cyanobacterial toxins that occur, the rate of bioaccumulation of toxins, the rate of elimination or depuration of cyanobacterial toxins, as well as the health risks of farmed seafood.

35.5 Conclusion

Modern aquaculture is the world's most rapidly growing rural industry and it is set to replace wild fisheries as the main supplier of seafood. In less than 50 years, the industry has grown, particularly in developing counties, at a rate that was beyond expectations. Nevertheless, the industry and scientific research on aquaculture both have a long way to go before they catch up with terrestrial forms of agriculture in terms of animal husbandry, selective breeding, disease management, and environmental protection. Similarly, research on cyanobacterial toxins has progressed from a position 50 years ago when blue-green algae were reclassified as cyanobacteria, to today's position of using advanced tools of molecular genetics and instrumentation to better understand the cellular production of cyanobacterial toxins and their chemical nature and toxicology.

The link between aquaculture and cyanobacteria will continue to grow because of anthropogenic demands on the environment and seafood production. The findings presented in this chapter show that cyanobacterial blooms are rarely found to be the direct cause of mortalities in aquaculture; however, the findings also suggest that the occurrence of toxic cyanobacterial blooms in aquaculture should be avoided. The literature and anecdotal evidence from farms suggest that cyanobacterial blooms cause reduced growth rates and impair farm productivity. Also, postharvest observations reveal that cyano-bacterial blooms cause farmed fish and shrimp to have musty off-flavors or an unattractive appearance. Moreover, there is a growing body of evidence that suggests that many cyanobacterial blooms can contain a variety of cyanotoxins. It appears that many aquatic species are capable of dealing with or recovering from these cyanotoxins by detoxification or depuration. Nevertheless, some aquatic species accumulate cyanobacterial toxins (e.g., molluscs and herbivorous species), and other aquatic species can have elevated levels of cyanotoxins in certain organs (liver and hepatopancreas).

It is concluded that toxic cyanobacterial blooms pose a risk for consumers, workers at aquaculture farms, and farm profitability. It is fortunate that aquatic animals appear to be able to better cope with the occurrence of cyanobacterial toxins than terrestrial animals and humans. This aspect may lower the level of risk to consumers. Nevertheless, aquaculture industries need education, awareness, and vigilance in order to reduce the occurrence of cyanobacterial blooms and to be able to act appropriately if toxicity is suspected. Also, researchers need to work cooperatively with farmers in order to be able to access blooms on farms and carry out scientific investigations at this important interface.

ACKNOWLEDGMENTS

The author is thankful for funding from the Australian Centre for International Agricultural Research (ACIAR) and Fisheries Research and Development Corporation (FRDC), which facilitated research in the Australia–Asia-Pacific region.

REFERENCES

Alonso-Rodríguez, R. and Paez-Osuna, F. 2003. Nutrients, phytoplankton and harmful algal blooms in shrimp ponds: A review with special reference to the situation in the Gulf of California. *Aquaculture*, 219, 317–336.

Amado, L.L. and Monserrat, J.M. 2010. Oxidative stress generation by microcystins in aquatic animals: Why and how? A review in: *Environmental International*, 36, 226–235.

Anderson, J. and Valderrama, D. 2013. Production: global shrimp review. Global Aquaculture Advocate, Global Aquaculture Alliance, St. Louis, MO, January/February, pp. 12–13.

Baloi, M., Arantes, R., Scheitzer, R., Magnotti, C., and Vinatea, L. 2013. Performance of pacific white shrimp *Litopenaeus vannamei* raised in biofloc systems with varying levels of light exposure. *Aquaculture Engineering*, 52, 39–44.

Carmichael, W.W. 1988. Toxins of freshwater algae, In: *Handbook of Natural Toxins. Vol. 3: Marine Toxins and Venoms*. Ed. A.T. Tu, Marcel Dekker, New York, p. 121.

Carmichael, W.W. 1994. The toxins of cyanobacteria. *Scientific American*, 270, 78–86.

Carmichael, W.W. 2007. A world overview—One hundred and seventy-five years of research on toxic cyanobacteria: Where do we go from here? In: *Proceedings of the Interagency Symposium on Cyanobacterial Harmful Algal Blooms, Advances in Experimental Medicine and Biology*. Ed. H.K. Hudnell, New York, pp. 95–115.

Chen, D., Shijian, L., and Wang, K. 2012. Enhancement and conservation of inland fisheries resources in China. *Environmental Biology of Fishes*, 93, 531–545.

Chen, J. and Xie, P. 2005. Tissue distribution and seasonal dynamics of the hepatotoxic microcystins-LR and -RR in two freshwater shrimps, *Palaemon modestus* and *Machrobrachium nipponensis*, from a large shallow, eutrophic lake of the subtropical China, *Toxicon*, 45, 615–625.

Codd, G.A., Azevedo, S.M.F.O., Bagchi, S.N., Burch, M.D., Carmichael, W.W., Harding, W.R., Kaya, K., and Utkilen, H.C. 2005. *Executive Summary, Cyanonet a Global Network for Cyanobacterial Bloom and Toxin Risk Management: Initial Situation Assessment and Recommendations*, International Hydrological Program of UNESCO, Paris, France, p. 1.

Deblois, C.P., Giani, A., and Bird, D.F. 2011. Experimental model of microcystin accumulation in the liver of *Oreochromis niloticus* exposed subchronically to a toxic bloom of Microcystis sp. *Aquatic Toxicology*, 103, 63–70.

De Silva, S.S. 2012. Aquaculture: A newly emergent food production sector—and perspectives of its impacts on biodiversity. *Biodiversity and Conservation*, 21, 3187–3220.

Deeds, J.R., Landsberg, J.H., Etheridge, S.M., Pitcher, G.C., and Longan, S.W. 2008. Non-traditional vectors for paralytic shellfish poisoning. *Marine Drugs*, 6, 308–348.

Dittmann, E. and Borner, T. 2005. Genetic contributions to the risk assessment of microcystin in the environment. *Toxicology and Applied Pharmacology*, 2003, 192–200.

Etheridge, S.M. 2010. Paralytic shellfish poisoning: Seafood safety and human health perspectives. *Toxicon*, 56, 108–122.

Falconer, I.R. 2005. Is there a human health hazard from microcystins in the drinking water supply. *Acta Hydrochimica et Hydrobiologica*, 33, 64–71.

Falconer, I.R., Bartram, J., Kuiper-Goodman, T., Utkilen, H., Burch, M., and Codd, G.A. 1999. Safe levels and safe practices. In: *Toxic Cyanobacteria in Water: A Guide to Their Public Health Consequences, Monitoring and Management*. Eds. I. Chorus and J. Bartram, World Health Organization, Taylor and Francis, London, U.K. and New York, pp. 155–178.

Falconer, I.R., Smith, J.V., Jackson, A.R.B., Jones, A., and Runnegar, M.T.C. 1988. Oral toxicity of a bloom of the cyanobacterium *Microcystis aeruginosa* administered to mice over periods up to 1 year. *Journal of Toxicology and Environmental Health*, 24, 291–305.

FAO. 2012. *State of World Fisheries and Aquaculture*. Fisheries and Aquaculture Department, Food and Agricultural Organization of the United Nations, Rome, Italy, p. 209.

Galvão, J.A., Oetterer, M., Bittencourt-Oliveira, M., Gouêa-Barros, S., Hiller, S., Erler, K., Lucas, B. et al. 2009. Saxitoxins accumulated by freshwater tilapia (*Oreochromis niloticus*) for human consumption. *Toxicon*, 54, 891–894.

Gélinas, M., Juneau, P., and Gagné, F. 2012. Early biochemical effects of *Microcystis aeruginosa* on juvenile rainbow trout (*Oncorhynchus mykiss*). *Comparative Biochemistry and Physiology, Part B*, 161, 261–267.

Gérard, C., Poullain, V., Lance, E., Acou, A., Brient, L., and Carpentier, A. 2009. Influence of toxic cyanobacteria on community structure and microcystin accumulation of freshwater molluscs. *Environmental Pollution*, 157, 609–617.

Hair, C., Wani, J., Minimulu, P., and Solato, W. 2006. Improved feeding and stocking density for intensive cage culture of GIFT tilapia, *Oreochromis niloticus*, in Yonki reservoir. Final Report on ACIAR Miniproject, ACIAR, Canberra, Australia, 15pp.

Howgate, P. 2004. Tainting of farmed fish by geosmin and 2-methyl-iso-borneol: A review of sensory aspects and of uptake/depuration. *Aquaculture*, 234, 155.

Ibelings, B.W. and Chorus, I. 2007. Accumulation of cyanobacterial toxins in freshwater "seafood" and its consequences for public health: A review. *Environmental Pollution*, 150, 177–192.

Ito, E., Satake, M., and Yasumoto, T. 2002. Pathological effects of lyngbyatoxin A upon mice. *Toxicon*, 40, 551–556.

Jegatheesan, V., Shu, L., and Visvanathan, C. 2011. *Aquaculture Effluent: Impacts and Remedies for Protecting the Environment and Human Health*. Elsevier B.V., Burlington, VT, pp. 123–135.

Kankaanpää, H.T., Holliday, J., Schröder, H., Goddard, T.J., Fister, R.V., and Carmichael, W.W. 2005. Cyanobacteria and prawn farming in Northern New South Wales, Australia—A case study on cyanobacteria diversity and hepatotoxin bioaccumulation. *Toxicology and Applied Pharmacology*, 203, 243–255.

Karlson, A.M.L. and Mozūraitis, R. 2011. Deposit-feeders accumulate the cyanobacterial toxin nodularin. *Harmful Algae*, 12, 77–81.

Kist, L.W., Rosemberg, D.B., Pereira, T.C.B. et al. 2012. Microcystin-LR acute exposure increases ACHE activity via transcriptional *ache* activation in zebrafish (*Danio rerio*) brain. *Comparative Biochemistry and Physiology, Part C*, 155, 247–252.

Krüger, T., Wiegand, C., Kun, L., Luckas, B., and Pflugmacher, S. 2010. More and more toxins around—analysis of cyanobacterial strains isolated from Lake Chao (Anhui Province, China). *Toxicon*, 56, 1520–1524.

Lightner, D.V. 1978. Possible toxic effects of the marine blue-green alga, *Spirulina subsalsa*, on the blue shrimp *Penaeus stylirostris. Journal of Invertebrate Pathology*, 32, 139–150.

Magalhaes, V.F., Marinho, M.M., Domingos, P., Olivera, A.C., Costa, S.M., Azevedo, L.O., and Azevedo, S.M. 2003. Microcystins (cyanobacteria hepatotoxins) bioaccumulation in fish and crustaceans from Sepetiba Bay (Brasil RJ). *Toxicon*, 42, 289–295.

Malbrouck, C. and Krestemont, P. 2006. Effects of microcystins on fish. *Environmental Toxicology and Chemistry*, 25, 72–86.

NADP. 2007. National Agriculture and Development Plan 2007–2016. Vol. 1: Policies and Strategies. Vol. 2: Implementation Plan. PNG Ministry of Agriculture and Livestock. Downloaded from www.acair.gov.au/node/2406

Neilan, B.A., Dittmann, E., Rouhianen, L., Bass, R.A., Schaub, V., Sivonen, K., and Borner, T. 1999. Nonribosomal peptide synthesis and toxigenicity of cyanobacterial. *Journal of Bacteriology*, 181, 4089–4097.

Neilan, B.A., Jacobs, D., Therese, D.D, Blackall, L.L., Hawkins, P.R., Cox, P.T., and Goodman, A.E. 1997. rRNA sequences and evolutionary relationships among toxic and nontoxic cyanobacteria of the genus *Microcystis. International Journal of Systematic Bacteriology*, 47, 693–697.

Oshima, Y., Blackburn, S.I., and Hallegraeff, G.M. 1993. Comparative study on paralytic shellfish toxin profiles of the dinoflagellate *Gymnodinium catenatum* from three different countries. *Marine Biology*, 116, 471–476.

Paerl, H.W. and Huisman, J. 2008. Blooms like it hot. *Science*, 320, 57–58.

Phillips, M.J., Roberts, R.J., Stewart, J.A., and Codd, G.A. 1985. The toxicity of the cyanobacterium, microcystis aeruginosa to rainbow trout, Salmo gairdneri Richardson. *Journal of Fish Diseases*, 8, 339–344.

Rodger, H.D., Turnbull, T., Edwards, C., and Codd, G.A. 1994. Cyanobacterial (blue-green algal) bloom associated pathology in brown trout, Salmo trutta L., in Loch Leven, Scotland. *Journal of Fish Diseases*, 17, 177–181.

Runnegar, M., Berndt, N., and Kaplowitz, N. 1995. Microcystin uptake and inhibition of protein phosphatases: Effects of chemoprotectants and self-inhibition in relation to known hepatic transporters. *Toxicology and Applied Pharmacology*, 134, 264–272.

Runnegar, M.T.C. and Falconer, I.R. 1986. Effect of toxin from the cyanobacterium *Microcystis aeruginosa* on ultrastructure, morphology and actin polymerization in isolated hepatocytes. *Toxicon*, 24, 109–115.

Sevrin-Reyssac, J. and Pletikosic, M. 1990. Cyanobacteria in fish ponds. *Aquaculture*, 88, 1–20.

Smith, P.T. 1996. Toxic effects of blooms of marine species of Oscillatoriales on farmed prawns (*Penaeus monodon, Penaeus japonicus*) and brine shrimp (*Artemia salina*). *Toxicon*, 34(8), 857–869.

Smith, P.T. 2000. Freshwater neurotoxins: Mechanisms of action, pharmacology, toxicology, and impacts on aquaculture. Chapter 27. In: *Seafood and Freshwater Toxins: Pharmacology, Physiology, and Detection*. Ed. L.M. Botana, Marcel Dekker Inc., New York, pp. 583–602.

Smith, P.T. 2003. *Final Report: Application of Extracellular Enzyme Techniques to Studying the Role of Bacteria in the Ecology of Prawn Ponds and Disease of Penaeus monodon*. Published by FRDC, Canberra, Australia, p. 168.

Smith, P.T. 2007. *Aquaculture in Papua New Guinea: Status of Freshwater Fish Farming*. ACIAR Monograph No. 125, Canberra, Australia, 112pp.

Smith, P.T. 2008. Cyanobacterial toxins in aquaculture. Chapter 37. In: *Seafood and Freshwater Toxins: Pharmacology, Physiology, and Detection*, 2nd edn. Ed. L.M. Botana, CRC Press, Boca Raton, FL, UWS, pp. 787–806.

Smith, P.T. 2010. Raun Raun Pisman: The Travelling Fishman, Film produced by Wok Didiman, Sydney Australia, 95 minutes.

Smith, J.L., Boyer, G.L., and Zimba, P.V. 2008. A review of cyanobacterial odorous and bioactive metabolites: Impacts and management alternatives in aquaculture. *Aquaculture*, 280, 5–20.

Smith, P.T. and Kankaanpää, H.T. 2001. Toxic blooms of *Nodularia* sp. in prawn farms that culture *Penaeus monodon*. In: *Abstracts of Fifth International Conference on Toxic Cyanobacteria*, Noosa, Queensland.

Smith, P.T. and Mufuape, K. 2013. Small-scale aquaculture in Papua New Guinea: Examination of entry points for international aid donors. In: *Proceedings FAO Expert Workshop on Enhancing the Contribution of Small-Scale Aquaculture to Food Security, Poverty Alleviation and Socio-Economic Development*, April 21–24, 2010, Hanoi, Viet Nam, Ed. M. Reantaso, FAO, Rome, Italy, pp. 49–60.

Tapiador, D.D., Henderson, H.F., Delmendo, M.N., and Tsutui, H. 1977. *Background Information: Freshwater Fisheries and Aquaculture in China, A Report of the FAO Fisheries (Aquaculture) Mission to China*, April 21–May 12, 1976, FAO, Rome, Italy.

Te, S.H. and Gin, K.Y.-H. 2011. The dynamics of cyanobacteria and microcystin production in a tropical reservoir of Singapore. *Harmful Algae*, 10, 319–329.

Tucker, C.S. 2000. Off-flavor problems in aquaculture. *Reviews in Fisheries Science*, 8(1), 45.

Tucker, C.S. 2005. Limits of catfish production in ponds. *Global Aquaculture Advocate*, 8(6), 59.

UNFPA. 2008. *State of the World Population 2008*. United Nations, Rome, Italy.

Weigand, C. and Plugmacher, S. 2005. Ecotoxicological effects of selected cyanobacterial secondary metabolites: A short review. *Toxicology and Applied Pharmacology*, 203, 201–218.

Ye, Y., Cochrane, K., Bianchi, G., Willmann, R., Majkowski, J., Tandstad, M., and Carocci, Y. 2012. Rebuilding global fisheries: The world summit goal, costs and benefits. *Fish and Fisheries*, 14, 174–185.

Yusoff, F.M., Matias, H.B., Khalid, A.Z., and Phang, F-M. 2001. Culture of microalgae using interstitial water extracted from shrimp pond bottom sediments, *Aquaculture*, 201, 263–270.

Zhang, J., Wang, Z., Song, Z., Xie, Z., Li, L., and Song, L. 2012. Bioaccumulation of microcystins in two freshwater gastropods from a cyanobacteria-bloom plateau lake, Lake Dianchi. *Environmental Pollution*, 164, 227–234.

36

Cylindrospermopsin: Chemistry, Origin, Metabolism, Effects, and Detection

Ambrose Furey, Vaishali P. Bane, Mary Lehane,
Christopher T. Elliott, and Clare H. Redshaw

CONTENTS

36.1 Introduction

Cylindrospermopsin (CYN) was first discovered on Palm Island (Queensland, Australia) in 1979 following the intoxication of 148 people, mainly children, who required hospitalization after consuming drinking water from a reservoir infiltrated by the toxin progenitor *Cylindrospermopsis raciborskii* (Bourke et al., 1983; Byth, 1980). Subsequently, it was found that CYN and several of its analogues are hepatotoxic, nephrotoxic, neurotoxic, and possibly carcinogenic (Griffiths and Saker, 2003; Kiss et al., 2002; Runnegar et al., 1994, 1995, 2002). It has been shown that upwards of ten algal species produce the CYN toxins including *C. raciborskii* (Hawkins et al., 1985, 1997), *Umezakia natans* (Terao et al., 1994), *Aphanizomenon ovalisporum* (Banker et al., 1997; Shaw et al., 1999), *Anabaena bergii* (Schembri et al., 2001), *Raphidiopsis curvata* (Li et al., 2001a), *Anabaena lapponica* (Spoof et al., 2006), *Aphanizomenon flos-aquae* (Preußel et al., 2006), *Lyngbya wollei* (Seifert et al., 2007), *Oscillatoria* sp. (Mazmouz et al., 2010), and *Raphidiopsis mediterranea* (McGregor et al., 2011) (Table 36.1).

CYN presents a risk to human and animal health worldwide as it has been found in regions as diverse as Australia, Europe, America, and Asia (Hardy, 2011; Moreira et al., 2012). It has been postulated that the apparent spread of CYN-producing algae is attributable to global warming and increased eutrophication of formerly clean water bodies and by the algae's ability to adapt to changing environments (Kling, 2009). In addition, CYN is often found to co-occur with other known algal-borne toxins (Barón-Sola et al., 2012; Messineo et al., 2009; Oehrle et al., 2010), and many freshwater invertebrates have a natural propensity to concentrate CYN in their tissues (e.g., crustaceans, redclaw crayfish (Saker and Eaglesham, 1999), freshwater mussels, *Anodonta cygnea* (Saker et al., 2004), gastropod (*Melanoides tuberculata*)

(White et al., 2006), and tegogolo snail (*Pomacea patula catemacensis*) (Berry and Lind, 2010). The CYN toxin family has also been shown to be capable of accumulation in certain aquatic and terrestrial plants (e.g., duckweed [*Lemna punctata*] [Seifert, 2007] and brassica vegetables [Kittler et al., 2012]), which raises some environmental concerns regarding the potential impact on ecological systems.

As most of the earth's population relies heavily on surface waters as a source of drinking water (WHO/UNICEF, 2011), it is necessary for the regulatory authorities to ensure the implementation of fully validated analytical, instrumental-based monitoring programs to protect human and animal health from the threat posed by the CYN toxin class.

36.1.1 Cylindrospermopsin, the Toxin

CYN is an alkaloid toxin of cyanobacterial origin that is hepatotoxic, cytotoxic, and genotoxic (Bain et al., 2008). CYN has the ability to cause irreversible inhibition of protein synthesis, cellular necrosis, deoxyribonucleic acid (DNA) fragmentation, and mutagenesis (Smith et al., 2008). CYN intoxication cannot be relieved by any known antidote. It is believed that in vivo metabolism of the toxin by cytochrome P450 (CYP) may produce bioconversion products that exacerbate the toxicity of CYN (Runnegar et al., 1995). Cyanobacterial blooms that produce CYN can occur in surface waters used for bathing, recreation, and drinking water, and they therefore present a threat to human and animal users (Bain et al., 2008; Bownik, 2010; Codd et al., 2005).

Structurally, the CYN molecule possesses a tricyclic guanidine moiety combined with hydroxymethyluluracil (Figure 36.1, Table 36.1), and the toxin is found both intra- and extracellularly to the cyanobacteria that produce it (Wormer et al., 2008). The toxin is a relatively stable compound (Carson, 2000; Chiswell et al., 1999) and it has been shown to persist in even contaminated water bodies for up to 40 days (Wormer et al., 2008). However, in a recent study, CYN was shown to exhibit the following biodegradability ranking: microcystin-LR (MC-LR) > CYN > geosmin > saxitoxins (Ho et al., 2012). There are several known CYN analogues such as the naturally produced deoxycylindrospermopsin (deoxy-CYN) (Jiang et al., 2012; Kubo et al., 2005; Li et al., 2001a,b; McGregor et al., 2011; Seifert et al., 2007), 7-epicylindrospermopsin (7-epi-CYN) (Banker et al., 2000), the chlorination by-products cylindrospermic acid (Looper et al., 2005, 2006), and 5-chlorocylindrospermopsin (5-chloro-CYN) (Rodríguez et al., 2007); all these analogues possess variable toxic potency relative to CYN.

Human exposure to CYN is most likely to occur from drinking water (Poniedzialek et al., 2012) or following the consumption of fish that have ingested the toxin progenitor (Saker and Eaglesham, 1999). Gutierrez-Praena et al. have recently written a review of the data available on the possible CYN (and microcystin) exposure risks from edible aquatic organisms, plants, and food supplements (based on algae) and on the influence of different cooking procedures on these levels in food (Gutierrez-Praena et al., 2012). Intoxication may also occur via swimming or bathing in contaminated waters (Codd et al., 2005; Griffiths and Saker, 2003).

The results of CYN exposure studies on mice indicated (by extrapolation) that the tolerable daily intake (TDI) for CYN ought not to exceed 0.02 g/kg body weight per day with significantly lower levels advised for children and infants (Banker et al., 2000, 2001; Carson, 2000; Griffiths and Saker, 2003).

36.1.2 Cylindrospermopsin and Its Derivatives

Table 36.1 provides a comprehensive summary of the key structural features of CYN and its main analogues and related compounds. The structure of CYN (Figure 36.1) together with its relative

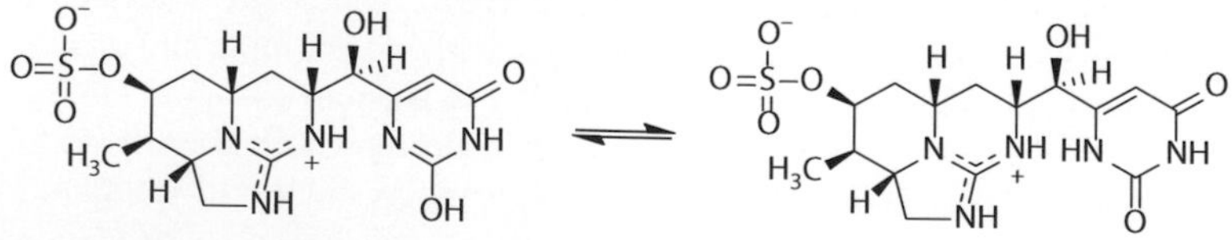

FIGURE 36.1 The structure of CYN; $C_{15}H_{21}N_5O_7S$, molecular weight (MW) 415.43. CAS: 143545-90-8. *Note*: The positive charge is shared between 3 N atoms (not C as shown).

TABLE 36.1

CYN Analogues, Molecular Formula, Structures, Exact Molar Mass, Identified MRM Transitions, and Source Organisms

No.	Name of the Analogue	Molecular Formula	Structure	Exact Molar Mass	Exact Molar Mass [M + H]⁺	MRM	Source Organism	References
1	CYN	$C_{15}H_{21}N_5O_7S$		415.116172	416.123997	416.3/194.2 (Mazmouz et al., 2010) 416.1/194.1 and 416.1/336.1 (Kittler et al., 2012) 416/194 and 416/176 (Oehrle et al., 2010) 414 in negative mode (Kikuchi et al., 2007)	*C. raciborskii, Raphidiopsis mediterranea skuja, U. natans, L. wollei* (Farlow ex Gomont) Speziale and Dyck, *Anabaena bergii, Aphanizomenon flos-aquae, Aphanizomenon gracile, Anabaena lapponica, Anabaena bergii, Anabaena planctonica, Oscillatoria sp.,* and *Aphanizomenon klebahnii*	Bláhováet al. (2009), Looper et al. (2006), Mazmouz et al. (2010), McGregor et al. (2011), Ohtani et al. (1992), Pearson et al. (2010), Poniedzialek et al. (2012), Seifert (2007), Spoof et al. (2006)
2	7-epi-CYN	$C_{15}H_{21}N_5O_7S$		415.116172	416.123997	416.3/194.2 (Mazmouz et al., 2010)	*Aphanizomenon ovalisporum*	Banker et al. (2000), Mazmouz et al. (2010)
3	deoxy-CYN	$C_{15}H_{21}N_5O_6S$		399.121257	400.129082	400.3/194.2 (Mazmouz et al., 2010) 400/194 (Oehrle et al., 2010)	*C. raciborskii, R. curvata, Raphidiopsis mediterranea skuja,* and *L. wollei* (Farlow ex Gomont) Speziale and Dyck	McGregor et al. (2011), Seifert et al. (2007), Mazmouz et al. (2010)

(continued)

TABLE 36.1 (continued)

CYN Analogues, Molecular Formula, Structures, Exact Molar Mass, Identified MRM Transitions, and Source Organisms

No.	Name of the Analogue	Molecular Formula	Structure	Exact Molar Mass	Exact Molar Mass $[M + H]^+$	MRM	Source Organism	References
4	5-chloro-CYN	$C_{15}H_{20}ClN_5O_7S$		449.077200	450.085025	NR	Chlorination product of CYN	Merel et al. (2010)
5	CYN-acid	$C_{12}H_{19}N_3O_7S$		349.094374	350.102199	NR	Chlorination product of CYN	Merel et al. (2010)

Abbreviations: CYN, cylindrospermopsin; 7-epi-CYN, 7-epicylindrospermopsin; deoxy-CYN, deoxycylindrospermopsin; 5-chloro-CYN, 5-chlorocylindrospermopsin; CYN-acid, cylindrospermic acid; NR, not reported.

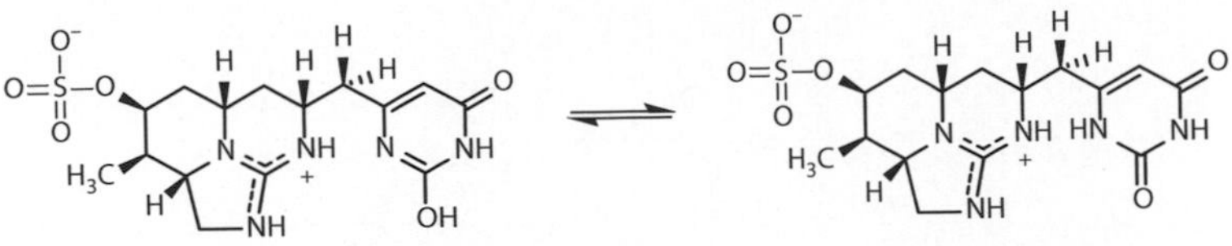

FIGURE 36.2   The structure of deoxycylindrospermopsin (deoxy-CYN); $C_{15}H_{21}N_5O_6S$, MW 399.

stereochemistry was first elucidated by Ohtani et al. who also noted the possibility of keto-enol tautomerism (shifts observed around pH 7), with the enol form favored (probably due to uracil and guanidine units being coplanar with 18(N)-H hydrogen bonded to N-1). CYN possesses a zwitterionic tricyclic guanidine moiety ($NH_2C(=NH)NH_2$) with a sulfate ester functionality that is combined with a hydroxymethyluracil (Ohtani et al., 1992). This sulfated-guanidinium alkaloid with 5-substituted-2,4-dioxypyrimidine (uracil) moiety, CYN, is highly water soluble. CYN is a relatively stable compound that exhibits no significant degradation at 100°C sustained for 15 min (Carson, 2000; Chiswell et al., 1999). The compound displays only slow decomposition on storage (4°C–50°C in aqueous solution) to form another compound thought to be a CYN isomer. CYN is pH stable (approximately 25% degradation at pH 4, 7, and 10 over an 8-week period) (Carson, 2000). CYN tends to photodegrade in natural algal extract; however, ultraviolet (UV) degradation of CYN is not observed in pure water (Chiswell et al., 1999) suggesting degradation occurs via indirect photolysis and that the presence of photosensitizers is necessary.

C. raciborskii is the dominant (or most well-known producer) of CYN, and some isolates of this cyanobacteria have been found to additionally produce saxitoxin and gonyautoxins, for example, Brazilian isolates (Bernard et al., 2003). *C. raciborskii* also produces deoxycylindrospermopsin (deoxy-CYN; Figure 36.2). *R. curvata* is another species of cyanobacteria that produces the deoxy-CYN analogue (Li et al., 2001a).

Aphanizomenon ovalisporum produces CYN and the toxic variant 7-epicylindrospermopsin (7-epi-CYN). This toxic minor metabolite, 7-epi-CYN (Figure 36.3), was isolated from *Aphanizomenon ovalisporum* by Banker et al. (2000). The 7-epi diastereomer shows similar potency to CYN by the mouse toxicity assay (Banker et al., 2000; Griffiths and Saker, 2003). In common with *C. raciborskii,* this species from the *Aphanizomenon* family have been shown to produce saxitoxin (Berry et al., 2009; Griffiths and Saker, 2003). *Anabaena flos-aquae* strains produce CYN as well as anatoxin-a (Messineo et al., 2009).

The deoxy-CYN variant lacks the OH group (replaced by H) on the uracil bridge (H-7), and therefore, it has a slightly lower polarity and is less water soluble than CYN (Senogles et al., 2000). The *Raphidiopsis* strain HB1 (*R. curvata*) in fact produces more deoxy-CYN than CYN (deoxy-CYN 1.3 mg/g; CYN 0.56 mg/g (dry wt. cells) (Li et al., 2001a,b). Deoxy-CYN is believed to be nontoxic based on results from mouse bioassays (Griffiths and Saker, 2003; Li et al., 2001a,b; Senogles et al., 2000). However, there is some controversy over the toxicity of the deoxy-CYN analogues, as it has also been found to be a potent protein synthesis inhibitor in vitro (using a rabbit reticulocyte system; 12 µM for complete inhibition) and in whole cells (10 µM for complete inhibition). Deoxy-CYN also exhibits inhibition of glutathione synthesis. There is uncertainty and debate as to whether tautomers of deoxy-CYN exist (Figure 36.2) or whether the toxin remains predominantly in the keto form (Looper et al., 2005).

Mono- and di-chlorinated uracil-CYN (chlorination at C5) are formed during the chlorination of drinking water producing 5-chlorocylindrospermopsin (5-chloro-CYN) and cylindrospermic acid (CYN-acid; Figure 36.4) (Griffiths and Saker, 2003; Looper et al., 2006).

In order to investigate the toxic effects of chlorinated CYN compounds, pure CYN and cell-free extracts were chlorinated and mice were dosed (via drinking water). The study was carried out on male mice, 40% of whom developed fatty vacuolation in the liver (but only when treated with the cell-free

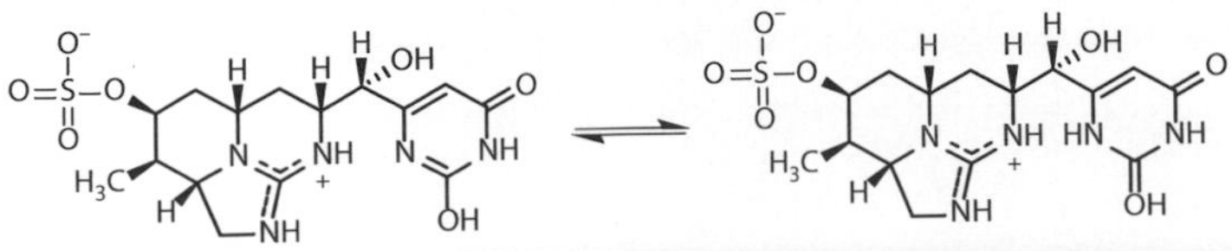

FIGURE 36.3   The structure of 7-epicylindrospermopsin (7-epi-CYN); $C_{15}H_{21}N_5O_7S$, MW 415.43.

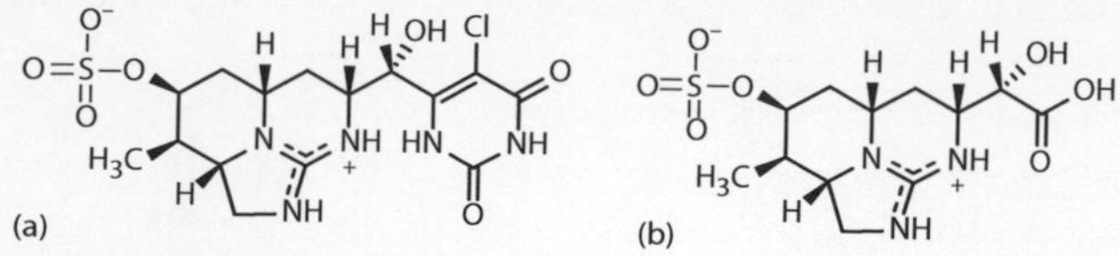

FIGURE 36.4   Structures of (a) 5-chlorocylindrospermopsin (5-chloro-CYN); $C_{15}H_{20}ClN_5O_7S$, MW 449 and (b) cylin-drospermic acid (CYN-acid); $C_{12}H_{19}N_3O_7S$, MW 349.

extract). However, this toxic effect cannot be directly attributed to the formation of 5-chloro-CYN or CYN-acid, as the presence of these compounds was not measured by any analytical means, and the researchers measured only the decrease in CYN levels (Senogles-Derham et al., 2003).

36.2 Toxin Production/Biosynthesis In Vivo (Including Associated Genes)

As previously stated, the cyanobacterium *Cylindrospermopsis raciborskii* is believed to be the main source of CYN, and this species has been found worldwide: in Australia (Hawkins et al., 1985; Shaw et al., 1999; Smith et al., 1998), Israel (Banker et al., 1997), Thailand (Li et al., 2001b), Brazil (Azevedo et al., 2002), Germany (Fastner et al., 2003; Preußel et al., 2006), New Zealand (Stirling and Quilliam, 2001; Wood and Stirling, 2003), Portugal (Saker et al., 2003), Greece (Cook et al., 2004), Spain (Quesada et al., 2006), Finland (Spoof et al., 2006), Florida (Yilmaz et al., 2008), France (Brient et al., 2009), Czech Republic (Bláhová et al., 2008, 2009), Italy (Messineo et al., 2009), Poland (Kokociński et al., 2009), Slovakia, Mexico (Berry and Lind, 2010), and Hungary (Antal et al., 2011).

CYN has been found in samples containing *C. catemaco* and *C. philippinensis* from Mexico; however, further confirmation is required in order to unequivocally determine if these species are the culprits (Berry and Lind, 2010). The species *Aphanizomenon flos-aquae* has been shown to produce CYN in Germany (Preußel et al., 2006), France (Brient et al., 2009), and Italy (Messineo et al., 2009), and *Aphanizomenon ovalisporum* has been implicated as the main toxin producer in Israel (Banker et al., 1997), Spain (Quesada et al., 2006), and Florida (Yilmaz et al., 2008). *Aphanizomenon gracile* is suspected as another source of CYN in Germany and France (Brient et al., 2009). The alga *Anabaena planctonica* has also been shown to be a source of the toxin in France (Brient et al., 2009). In Finland, *Anabaena lapponica* is a suspected CYN progenitor. In Australia, *Anabaena bergii* and *Lyngbya wollei* have been deemed responsible for CYN contamination (Seifert et al., 2007). In China and Japan, *R. curvata* and *U. natans* produce the toxin (Jiang et al., 2012; Li et al., 2001a).

The cyanobacteria that produce CYN are, in common with most other cyanobacteria, nitrogen-fixing species; the presence of nitrate or ammonium in their vicinity will enhance their growth rates. However, CYN production is greatest in the absence of nitrogen (Griffiths and Saker, 2003). In fact, there exists a negative correlation between CYN content and cyanobacterial growth rate (when light or nitrogen is limited) (Griffiths and Saker, 2003). A negative correlation between CYN content in cyanobacteria and ambient water temperature has also been demonstrated. Cyanobacteria are prone to photoinhibition at high light intensities (especially at low temperatures); this susceptibility is mainly due to changes in the saturation level of fatty acids in thylakoid membranes, which affects the function of membrane-bound enzymes (Griffiths and Saker, 2003; Preußel et al., 2009). About 80%–90% of the CYN toxin is intracellular during the active (exponential) growth phase of the cyanobacterial cycle. CYN production matches the rate of cyanobacterial cell division (i.e., when the exponential growth rate involves one doubling per day), but during the stationary growth phase (where growth rate involves 0.04 doublings per day), the toxin production doubles giving rise to a toxin production equivalent to the rate of 0.08 doublings per day (Griffiths and Saker, 2003). Extracellular toxin loading also increases during the stationary phase (approximately 50% extracellular). The levels of intracellular CYN at different growth rate stages range from 0.002 to 0.005 × 10^{-6} μg/cell, with extracellular CYN accounting for 19%–98% of total toxin during different growth stages (Griffiths and Saker, 2003).

The biosynthesis of CYN in *C. raciborskii* is thought to progress through a number of distinct stages:

- Initiation via amidinotransfer onto glycine (Mihali et al., 2008).
- Guanidoacetic acid acts as the starter unit for the polyketide structure (Griffiths and Saker, 2003).
- The polyketide is derived from five acetate units to make up C4–C13 (Griffiths and Saker, 2003).
- Oxygen atoms present in C4–C12 are derived directly from the acetate (Griffiths and Saker, 2003).
- C1 and C2 of glycine become C14 and C15 of CYN, with glycine incorporated as an intact unit into the C14, C15, and N16 (Griffiths and Saker, 2003).
- The origin of the amidino group in the starter unit, and uracil ring, is not known (Griffiths and Saker, 2003).
- A novel pyrimidine biosynthesis mechanism is proposed for the uracil ring formation, along with tailoring reactions (including sulfation and hydroxylation) to complete the biosynthesis (Mihali et al., 2008).

A gene-encoding amidinotransferase from *Aphanizomenon ovalisporum* is the first reported amidinotransferase gene in cyanobacteria. This gene is likely to be involved in the formation of guanidinoacetic acid (the biosynthesis starter unit). Aminooxyacetic acid (*aoaA*) is located in a genomic region bearing genes encoding a polyketide synthase (PKS) (type I PKS) and a peptide synthetase (PS), further supporting its putative role in CYN biosynthesis (Shalev-Alon et al., 2002). A genetic method utilizing the base sequences of a PKS and a PS gene demonstrated a direct link between the presence of these two genes and CYN production in *C. raciborskii* isolates. In total, 13 strains of algae were tested, 10 of the species that produced CYN possessed both genes, and in all nontoxin-producing strains of the cyanobacterium, both of these genes were absent (Griffiths and Saker, 2003; Schembri et al., 2001).

Additionally, polymerase chain reaction (PCR) tests were able to simultaneously identify PKS and PS determinants (i.e., two genes associated with CYN production) (Schembri et al., 2001) while also being able to distinguish *C. raciborskii* from other CYN-producing cyanobacteria (*Anabaena bergii* and *Aphanizomenon ovalisporum*), by targeting the *rpoCl* gene (Fergusson and Saint, 2003).

The deployment of 16S ribosomal ribonucleic acid (RNA) (16S rRNA) sequencing has confirmed similarity between *C. raciborskii* and CYN-producing strains of *Aphanizomenon ovalisporum* (93.3%) and *Anabaena bergii* (93.3%). A similar correlation has been shown with other Nostocalean genera (Nostocales are nitrogen fixing) that do not produce CYN. The *C. raciborskii* genetic relationship with CYN-producing *U. natans* is 84.6% (Griffiths and Saker, 2003). In fact, 16S rRNA phylogenetic trees involving three clusters of CYN-producing cyanobacteria in European, American, and Australian isolates were observed to be very closely related. Studies also revealed that straight and coiled forms of *C. raciborskii* are genetically identical (Griffiths and Saker, 2003). It has also been established that toxin production profiles vary between species; the production of deoxy-CYN has been reported to be approximately 10% of total CYN production for certain species. However, *L. wollei* produced approximately 300 times more deoxy-CYN than CYN (Seifert et al., 2007).

Extensive investigations have been undertaken to determine the effect of temperature and light on CYN production (Preußel et al., 2009) in toxic cyanobacteria; the results may be summarized as follows:

- Increased temperature leads to a decrease in the intracellular concentration of CYN and an increase in extracellular CYN.
- The effect of light intensity upon CYN concentration depends upon the ambient temperature.
- The concentration of CYN does not appear to be related to the growth rate of the cyanobacterial progenitor.
- Contrived temperature–light regimes that have been employed to mimic physiological stressed conditions appear to trigger CYN production and induce the release of the toxin from the cyanobacterial cells. Authors conclude that CYN release is therefore active, rather than just due to leaky cells (Preußel et al., 2009).

Experiments conducted on samples from a freshwater river found that the *C. raciborskii* doubling time during the bloom phase was 3.5 days. The *C. raciborskii* river bloom was initiated during windy conditions with the first movement of the thermocline into an anoxic hypolimnion (dense, bottom layer [below the thermocline] of water in a thermally stratified lake that is depleted of dissolved oxygen). It was found that the *C. raciborskii* exponential growth and bloom formation coincided with the arrival and retention of wet-season inflows into the river (Banker et al., 2001). Additionally, it has also been demonstrated that *C. raciborskii* produces akinetes (resting spores), and these have been linked with bloom initiation, that is, seeding from sediment (Fabbro and Duivenvoorden, 1996).

36.3 Detection in Environmental Samples

Some organisms that feed on cyanobacteria have the ability to concentrate high levels of toxins in vivo. Redclaw crayfish (*Cherax quadricarinatus*) accumulate CYN in the hepatopancreas (4.3 mg/g freeze-dried tissue) and muscle (0.9 mg/g freeze-dried muscle tissue), but subsequent bioavailability to consumers is not known (Griffiths and Saker, 2003; Saker and Eaglesham, 1999). CYN has also been detected in rainbow fish (*Melanotaenia*), but location of the tissue of maximum accumulation was not identified, and therefore, the risk to consumers cannot be quantitated (Griffiths and Saker, 2003). A freshwater mussel (swan mussel: *Anodonta cygnea*) exposed to *C. raciborskii* for 16 days accumulated up to 2.52 mg/g tissue dry weight; the distribution of the toxin was hemolymph (68.1%), viscera (23.3%), foot and gonad (7.7%), and mantle (0.9%). After a 2-week depuration period, approximately 50% of the toxin persisted in the tissues (Saker et al., 2004). Cane toad tadpoles (*Bufo marinus*) exposed to *C. raciborskii* extracts did not bioaccumulate CYN, but those exposed to live cells did (maximum average tissue concentrations of 895 mg free-CYN/kg fresh weight); this implies uptake is via feeding (White et al., 2007). *Daphnia magna* fed on *C. raciborskii* resulted in a 90% mortality rate within 48 h exposure, with levels of CYN found in tissues at 0.025 ng/animal (Saker et al., 2003).

Lake Lago Catemaco, Mexico, is dominated by *C. catemaco* and *C. philippinensis* species, and raw water was found to contain 0.68 ng/L of CYN (enzyme-linked immunosorbent assay (ELISA), liquid chromatography (LC)–mass spectrometry (MS), and high-performance liquid chromatography (HPLC)–UV were used for confirmation); the algal material was found to contain 21.34 ng/L. Snails (*Pomacea patula catemacensis*; used for human consumption) were found to bioaccumulate CYN (the bioaccumulation factor was found to be 157; 3.35 ng/g; established by ELISA) (Berry and Lind, 2010).

CYN was first detected in Europe in the late 1990s (Kabziński et al., 2000; Messineo et al., 2009). CYN was found in a well that was used for drinking water supply in Italy (126 µg/L) (Messineo et al., 2009). CYN was detected in tissues from two *Salmo trutta* trouts (with levels of up to 2.7 ng/g) taken from a lake in Italy; the toxin was distributed in viscera (2.7 ng/g) and in muscle (0.8 ng/g). Analysis of an ovary sample also showed the presence of CYN in the eggs (0.07 ng/g). From 1989 to 2006, 28 Italian lakes were sampled and CYN was detected (0.3–126 ng/mL extracellular; 21.1 and 175.1 ng/mg intracellular) in the surface water of some lakes, dominated or co-dominated by two alga species: *C. raciborskii* and *Aphanizomenon ovalisporum* (Messineo et al., 2009).

Testing of reservoirs in the Czech Republic showed that in surface water samples, *Aphanizomenon* or *Cylindrospermopsis* species were present (Bláhová et al., 2009).

C. raciborskii blooms generally occur in warm summer waters; the optimal growth conditions for this algae species are considered to be 25+°C. *C. raciborskii* does not form a floating surface scum; it is usually concentrated several meters below the surface of the water body (Carson, 2000).

In Hervey Bay, Queensland, at height of the *C. raciborskii* bloom, CYN concentrations of 63 g/L, which correlated to 2 million cells/mL, were recorded (Carson, 2000).

CYN has frequently been detected in German water bodies with a maximal concentration of 12 µg/L (Brient et al., 2009).

In Florida, treated waters have had concentrations of CYN of up to 90 µg/L. A study that examined five lakes in Florida found *C. raciborskii* at cell densities of 88,000–176,000 cells/mL (Brient et al., 2009; Carson, 2000).

CYN was detected by LC–MS–MS (intracellular concentration of 1.55–1.95 µg/L) in 6 of 11 tested water bodies in Western France, in the presence of the alga *Aphanizomenon flos-aquae* or *Anabaena planctonica* (Brient et al., 2009).

36.4 CYN Toxic Effects

Human intoxication can occur after drinking contaminated domestic water (Bourke et al., 1983; Byth, 1980; Griffiths and Saker, 2003; Hawkins et al., 1985) and from eating contaminated fish (see the previous section). Other exposure pathways (i.e., recreational contact) through swimming, jet/water skiing, and wind surfing have also been considered as a likely route to intoxication (Hardy, 2011). CYN is a potent hepatotoxin and the pyrimidine ring is essential for toxicity (Griffiths and Saker, 2003).

Human intoxication produces various gastrointestinal symptoms after initial exposure, and in the case of exposure to high toxin levels, kidney malfunction and death may occur (Griffiths and Saker, 2003). Acute exposure can also affect adversely the liver, heart, thymus, spleen, and intestine (Brient et al., 2009; Falconer et al., 1999). It is also thought that the sulfate group in the CYN molecule plays a role in toxicity (Runnegar et al., 2002). Deoxy-CYN is nontoxic using the mouse bioassay (toxin delivered by oral intubation)—therefore, it is likely that the hydroxyl on the uracil bridge or the keto-enol status of uracil moiety is critical for hepatotoxic action. However, as previously outlined (Section 36.1.2), the toxicity risk to humans of deoxy-CYN is a topic of debate (Griffiths and Saker, 2003; Looper et al., 2006; Senogles et al., 2000).

Toxicology studies with mice that have been conducted by intraperitoneal (i.p.) injection (Griffiths and Saker, 2003) of cell extract indicate that CYN can induce devastating effects including the following:

- Centrilobular to massive hepatocyte necrosis
- Injury to kidneys (including glomerulus abnormalities and the accumulation of proteinaceous material in distal tubules)
- Damage to adrenal glands, lungs, and intestines
- Damage to the liver (destruction of the hepatocytes, cellular vacuolation, enlarged intercellular spaces, necrosis, and foamy lipid vacuolation due to the inhibition of protein synthesis and interference with conversion of triglyceride to lipoproteins)

Extrapolations of these results have led to the assignation of an LD_{50} of 0.2 mg total CYN/kg for mice (Looper and Williams, 2001). It has been found that *C. raciborskii* cell lysates are more toxic than pure CYN, therefore suggesting additional unidentified toxic compounds are present in the lysate. Oral exposure of mice to freeze-dried *C. raciborskii* produced similar histological damage as that observed by i.p., together with some esophageal mucosa ulceration. In a dose of cell-free culture extract administered to mice, the median lethal concentration of CYN was estimated to be 6.0 mg/kg. There was no observable adverse effect in mice following oral administration in drinking water at a level of 0.15 mg CYN/kg/day (Griffiths and Saker, 2003). The toxicity of 7-epi-CYN by mouse bioassay LD_{50} (i.p.) for 5 days was 200 µg/kg (i.e., same as CYN). In addition, the assessment of the toxicity of 5-chloro-CYN and cylindrospermic acid (Figure 36.4) by mouse bioassay LD_{50} (i.p.) for 5 days was >10,000 µg/kg, that is, both compounds showed no toxic effects even at doses 50 times higher than the LD_{50} of CYN (Banker et al., 2001).

The toxicity of CYN at the LD_{50} over 72 h for rat hepatocytes was 40 ng/mL (Chong et al., 2002).

The results of animal assays indicate that there is some evidence to suggest that CYN is capable of mutagenicity. In vivo studies showed that mice fed with *C. raciborskii* extract developed tumors (5 of 53). In vitro studies showed micronucleus formation and whole chromosome loss in a human lymphoblastoid cell line (Falconer and Humpage, 2001).

The TDI for the toxin is 0.3 µg CYN/kg/day and the guidance value for human consumption is set at 10.5 µg CYN/day (based on 70 kg adult, drinking 2 L water/day). This guidance value would be reached at *C. raciborskii* cell densities of 404×10^3 cells/mL (based on 0.02 pg/cell intracellular CYN), which are not uncommon in raw water samples. Additionally, there may also be an extracellular CYN input, therefore validating public health concerns (Griffiths and Saker, 2003). The oral no-observed effect exposure limit (NOAEL) was estimated to be 30 µg/g/day, and the lowest-observed-adverse-effect level (LOAEL) was 60 µg/g/day (Bláhová et al., 2009). NOAEL was used to calculate the TDI of 0.03 µg/g/day; this value was used to calculate a maximum allowable intake of total CYN for a 2-week period of 252 µg, and this in turn along with typical fortnightly consumption patterns of shellfish was used to calculate the following health alert levels:

- Fish 158 µg/kg/wet wt.
- Prawns 720 µg/kg/wet wt.
- Mussels 933 µg/kg/wet wt. (Saker et al., 2004)

A drinking water guideline of 1 µg/L has already been stipulated in the regulations in Brazil, Australia, and New Zealand (Bláhová et al., 2009; Burch, 2008). France has set the maximum concentration of CYN allowable in drinking water at 0.3 µg/L (Brient et al., 2009). In Washington, the Department of Health has proposed a recreational guidance value for CYN (4.5 µg/L); this value will be applied in lake management protocols. Provisional recreational guidance value for microcystins, anatoxin-a, and saxitoxin were also calculated at 6, 1, and 75 µg/L, respectively. These values are being adapted into a management protocol (referred to as the "three-tiered approach") to manage Washington's water bodies during cyanobacterial blooms (Hardy, 2011).

To establish teratogenic effects, studies were conducted on CYN exposed to zebra fish embryos (*Danio rerio*). The results showed that CYN was only toxic (lethal) when embryos were injected with the toxin (dose dependent; $LC_{50} = 4.50$ fmol CYN/embryo for 1 day post-fertilization). No consistent developmental defects were observed, thus suggesting that CYN does not inhibit specific developmental pathways (Berry and Lind, 2010).

However, studies involving the immersion of zebra fish embryos in extracts of isolates (i.e., non-pure CYN) resulted in mortality and consistent developmental dysfunctions (twisted body axis, impairment of eye formation, and edemas); therefore, there are other unidentified compounds produced by *C. raciborskii* and *Aphanizomenon ovalisporum* that do interfere with developmental pathways (Berry et al., 2009). In fact, lipophilic extracts (chloroform, which would not contain CYN) were more consistently potent in the production of developmental abnormalities than the polar (30% methanol) extract (Berry and Lind, 2010).

Experiments on subacute toxicity revealed that mice exposed to drinking water that contained low levels of CYN had a significant reduction in red blood cell count, followed by deformation of red blood cells. Fetal toxicity in mice was observed upon chronic parental exposure to CYN during late gestation (Griffiths and Saker, 2003). Injection of fish, *Rutilus rutilus* L., with pure CYN or *C. raciborskii* extract, resulted in liver damage and inhibited respiration (Carson, 2000).

In the investigation of cane toad (*B. marinus*) tadpoles exposed to freeze-thawed *C. raciborskii* whole cell extracts or live *C. raciborskii* containing CYN, the following were observed:

- Damage to multiple organs, but most severe in liver, intestine, nephric ducts, and gill epithelia. The extent of cellular damage was similar in both exposures (aqueous and cell-bound toxins), despite unequal toxin concentrations being present in each. The authors concluded that the presence of cell-bound toxin plays a crucial role in the exertion of histological effects in *B. marinus* (Kinnear, 2010).
- Live culture treatment solutions resulted in up to 66% mortality, but exposure to aqueous extracts caused no mortality. Decreases in relative growth rates and in time spent swimming were observed in both treatments (White et al., 2007).

Inhibition of white mustard seedling growth (*Sinapis alba*) resulted from exposure to CYN, IC_{50} of 18.2 µg/mL (Beyer et al., 2009). A *C. raciborskii* extract (containing 0.4 µg/mL CYN) stimulated growth in an aquatic plant, *Hydrilla verticillata*, while decreasing its chlorophyll content (Beyer et al., 2009). *Naegleria lovaniensis*, a unicellular phagotrophic protozoa that is known as being susceptible to CYN ($LD_{50} \sim 60$ µg/mL), was not affected by the toxin at environmentally relevant concentrations (Rasmussen et al., 2008).

Carson (2000) provides a series of data tables summarizing toxicity studies and guideline values (and data from which they are calculated) (Carson, 2000).

36.5 Mode of Action

To date, little is known about the mode of action of CYN. Results of studies with mice indicate that CYN interferes with protein/enzyme synthesis (Carson, 2000; Griffiths and Saker, 2003). The following events were recorded in mice cells and tissue following i.p. injection of CYN (Carson, 2000):

- First, exposure symptoms revealed the detachment of ribosomes from membranes of the rough endoplasmic reticulum and the accumulation of hepatocytes in cytoplasm.
- Twenty-four hours after CYN was administered, a decrease in CYP enzymes and membrane proliferation was observed.
- Post-24 h, an accumulation of fat droplets in the central portion of hepatic lobules was observed.
- Finally, the toxin induced the termination phase of severe hepatic necrosis.

The globin synthesis assay was used to confirm the inhibition of protein synthesis, with complete inhibition of protein synthesis in mouse hepatocytes occurring at concentrations >0.5 µM CYN (Griffiths and Saker, 2003). Other studies suggest that protein synthesis inhibition (maximum inhibition at 0.5 µM after 4 h of exposure) in mice hepatocytes was found to be irreversible (on removal of toxin-containing media). However, protein synthesis inhibition is not believed to be the primary mode of toxicity of CYN (Froscio et al., 2009). Toxicity is thought to be associated with the reduction of glutathione (GSH) concentration, that is, the reduction in the levels of GSH precedes the observation of the toxic effects. Dose-dependent cytotoxicity was observed in rat and mouse hepatocytes at concentrations of CYN 1–5 µM (Froscio et al., 2009; Griffiths and Saker, 2003).

In fact, there is also a debate as to whether the reduction in the concentration of GSH is the key mechanism for toxicity. Norris et al. suggest that the CYP enzyme system may be involved in the toxicity of CYN (Griffiths and Saker, 2003; Norris et al., 2002). The primary toxic effect occurs in the periacinar region of the liver (xenobiotic metabolism region). Pretreatment with CYP-blocking agent (alpha-napthoflavone) provided partial protection against CYN; this may indicate that the toxin is activated by CYP. This would mean that it is the metabolites of the toxin that are responsible for toxic response. Toxicity assessment studies based on the amount of lactate dehydrogenase (tissue breakdown marker, i.e., loss of cell membrane integrity) released by hepatocytes (Froscio et al., 2009; Senogles et al., 2000) indicated that there was evidence to support the theory that the formation of metabolites by CYP is important in the mechanism of CYN toxicity (to hepatocytes) (Froscio et al., 2009; Senogles et al., 2000). However, blocking CYP did not change CYN effect on protein synthesis, that is, this would mean that CYN is responsible for protein synthesis inhibition, but that CYN metabolites are responsible for cytotoxicity.

Mice studies with i.p. injection of radiolabeled CYN ($NaH^{14}CO_3$ used in cell medium) revealed the majority of CYN was excreted in the urine (along with some in the feces) within 24 h. However, radiolabeled CYN accumulated in liver—50% of this was methanol extractable and the remaining 50% of CYN was strongly bound to liver proteins—or was converted into an unidentified metabolite. Of the extractable fraction, 25% was CYN and 75% was an unknown compound more polar than CYN (i.e., perhaps a bioconversion compound of CYN) (Norris et al., 2001; Senogles et al., 2000).

Investigations into a toxicity effect associated with a DNA or RNA involvement were also conducted; the results are summarized as follows:

- CYN nucleotide structure and presence of reactive guanidine and sulfate groups may suggest the toxic effect is due to interaction with the host's DNA/RNA (Griffiths and Saker, 2003).
- CYN (plus its metabolites) may covalently bond to DNA in mice, resulting in DNA strand breakage at CYN exposure concentrations of 1–10 µg/mL (Griffiths and Saker, 2003).

- In vitro chromosomal effects may suggest CYN is a spindle poison or can damage the centromere/kinetochore function; however, the mechanisms involved are unknown (Griffiths and Saker, 2003).
- CYN can inhibit pyrimidine nucleotide synthesis in mouse liver free cell extracts (Beyer et al., 2009).

Other studies have shown that the interference in the conversion of triglyceride to lipoproteins together with the inhibition of protein synthesis results in foamy lipid vacuolation in liver (Griffiths and Saker, 2003).

In vitro studies (mouse; cell-free liver extract) show that CYN inhibits activity of uridine monophosphate (UMP) synthase complex (responsible for conversion of orotic acid to UMP), but this effect was quite slight when mice were exposed via subacute (drinking water) routes. In these circumstances, the UMP synthase complex had a low affinity for CYN (Reisner et al., 2004).

Mice exposed to CYN in drinking water had abnormal red blood cells (as acanthocytes), and there was an increase in the ratio between free cholesterol and phospholipids in the red blood cell membrane, that is, free cholesterol accumulated in red blood cell membranes (Reisner et al., 2004).

It has also been demonstrated that CYN alters plant growth (in studies using common reed, *Phragmites australis*) and anatomy through reorganization of microtubules.

Studies involving plant tissue cultures exposed to CYN (Beyer et al., 2009) caused the following:

- Decrease in root elongation and to a less extend shoot.
- Increase in root number (general stress response).
- Necrosis in root cortex.
- Formation of callus-like tissue in root cortex—radically swollen cells that correlated with reorientation of microtubules, alongside a decrease of microtubules in the elongation zone. Microtubule orientation determines the pattern and direction of plant growth.
- Increase in β-tubulin in reed plantlets, that is, whole plant. Therefore, the decrease in microtubule density seen cannot be due to a decrease in β-tubulin.
- Formation of abnormal (split or double) preprophase bands, which are the first stage in cell division.
- Disruption of mitotic spindles (tripolar spindles), which lead to incomplete sister chromatid separation and disrupted phragmoplasts in root tip meristem. Phragmoplasts (along with preprophase bands) determine the position of a maturing cell plate.

Investigations into the uptake of CYN into animal cells produced the following information:

- The mechanism by which CYN enters the intracellular environment is unclear, as the molecule size and CYNs hydrophilic nature suggest it would not readily cross the lipid bilayer. The disruption of cell growth in various mammalian cell lines (including hepatic, renal, gastric, and intestinal) would suggest that the uptake mechanism is common/generalized. Toxin uptake (Vero cell line expressing green fluorescent protein) is slow and progressive, that is, uptake continued over 24 h of incubation period (Froscio et al., 2009).
- It is likely that uracil nucleobase transporters are not involved in the uptake of the toxin (Froscio et al., 2009).
- The sulfate group at C12 in the toxin structure is not necessary for the transport of hydrophilic CYN across cell membranes (Griffiths and Saker, 2003; Runnegar et al., 2002).
- The bile transport system may have partial involvement in CYN uptake into hepatocytes; the authors also propose passive diffusion is key, as a cell line lacking the bile transport system also showed cytotoxicity, that is, there may be more than one transport system involved in CYN uptake into hepatocytes (Chong et al., 2002).

36.6 CYN Detection: Bioassay

There are several methods described for the detection and quantitation of CYN and related compounds. One of the earliest means of determining their presence has been the mouse bioassay (Griffiths and Saker, 2003; Hawkins et al., 1985). In this test, trichomes are harvested and then centrifuged from a batch culture of *C. raciborskii*; these are then freeze-dried and extracted ultrasonically with NaCl (0.9% w/v) at 4°C. The cell debris is removed and a portion of the supernatant is injected intraperitoneally into the mouse after a preselected time period (to allow the toxin to be assimilated); the mice are then sacrificed and the toxicity is then assessed by autopsy (Hawkins et al., 1997). The presence of the toxin is determined by the type of tissue damage observed, and the degree of toxicity is related to the extent of the damage to the tissue.

Another bioassay involves exposure of *Artemia salina* (brine shrimp) to CYN. With this species, there is a dose-dependent mortality rate, where levels of CYN in samples are correlated with the known levels in a pure CYN standard (LD_{50} 8.1 µg/mL, over 24 h, and LD_{50} 0.71 µg/mL, over 72 h) (Carson, 2000; Hawkins et al., 1997; Metcalf et al., 2002b).

Thamnocephalus platyurus (aquatic invertebrate, fairy shrimp) is the basis of a bioassay used in a commercial Thamnotox kit (Agrawa et al., 2012; Falconer, 2004; Griffiths and Saker, 2003; Harada et al., 1999).

Rabbit reticulocyte lysate translation systems (basic kits available from Promega Corporation—in radiochemical and non-radiochemical versions) are protein synthesis inhibition assays and generate sigmoidal dose-dependent curves in response to CYN levels. This assay works by monitoring the incorporation of ^{3}H-leucine in newly synthesized protein (or measures residual leucine if non-radiochem kit is used). The limit of detection (LOD) is 50 nM CYN with an IC_{50} of 120 nM CYN (approximately 50 ng/mL) for inhibition of protein synthesis. The working range of the assay is 0.5–3.0 µM CYN (200–1200 µg/L). It is unknown if the kit is applicable to the analysis of deoxy-CYN. It has been shown that extracts of non-CYN-producing cyanobacteria did not inhibit protein synthesis in this kit, thus raising the confidence of the specificity of this kit for the detection of CYN in samples (Froscio et al., 2009; Griffiths and Saker, 2003; Rasmussen et al., 2008).

For visual microscopic identification of *C. raciborskii* (Fabbro and Duivenvoorden, 1996), 2% Lugol's iodine is required for adequate staining (10 g pure iodine, 20 g potassium iodide, 200 mL DI, 20 g glacial acetic acid) and cell sedimentation is observed over 48 h.

36.7 CYN Detection: Chemical Assays

Table 36.2 provides a summary of the methods described in the literature to extract CYN and analogues from various matrix types, while Table 36.3 provides a summary of analytical instrumentation-based methods for CYN determination. One of the most common methods for the analysis of toxins that possess a chromophore is liquid chromatography–ultraviolet/visible (LC–UV/Vis) detection. CYN has a maximum UV absorbance of 262 nm (Griffiths and Saker, 2003; Li et al., 2001b; Welker et al., 2002). The wavelength of maximum absorption of 5-Cl-CYN is 196 and 227 nm, and the λ_{max} for CYN-acid is 195 nm.

LC–UV determination of CYN in a culture extract was employed by Welker et al. (2002) and Harada et al. (1994). An LC–UV diode array detection (DAD) method was also deployed but required a lengthy solid-phase extraction (SPE) cleanup; a polygraphite column was used but the LOD was poor (Griffiths and Saker, 2003). The main problem with UV/Vis detection (and in particular with UV/DAD) of real samples is that they are prone to a high degree of interference from co-eluting matrix constituents. Thus, time-consuming and complex extraction procedures need to be applied before analysis for the target compound. SPE-based cleanup of samples may help but extensive interference from co-eluting compounds is likely to persist where the target analyte is at µg levels in kilos of complex matrix (Wormer et al., 2008). In 2004, an interlaboratory comparison involving six laboratories from Europe, Israel, and Australia was organized to evaluate the measurement of CYN in lyophilized cyanobacterial cells. All of

TABLE 36.2

Recovery of CYN from Different Matrix

Matrix	Extraction	Analyte	Recovery (%)	References
Drinking water	C-18 and Carbon SPE, 90% MeOH	CYN	95 ± 5 (pure water) 85 ± 5 (reservoir water)	Hung-Kai et al. (2011)
Natural lake water	C-18 SPE, MeOH	CYN	>90	Bláhová et al. (2009)
C. raciborskii cell extract	50% MeOH	CYN	93.1 ± 2.3	Kikuchi et al. (2007)
C. raciborskii cell extract	5% aa followed by 0.1 M carbonate buffer, A tandem SPE system (polystyrene and anion exchange)	CYN and deoxy-CYN	75 ± 1	Kubo et al. (2005)
C. raciborskii cell extract	100% water	CYN	30	Welker et al. (2002)
Lake water	C-18 and polygraphite carbon SPE	CYN	100	Metcalf et al. (2002a)

Abbreviations: aa, acetic acid; MeOH, methanol; H$_2$O, water (distilled and HPLC grade); SPE, solid-phase extraction.

the methods used for extraction of the toxin and HPLC analysis were satisfactory on the basis of statistical evaluation, according to ISO standards 5725-1 and 5725-2; however, this study found that the most effective extraction procedure used 5% formic acid as it minimizes interference in chromatograms by contaminant compounds (Törökne et al., 2004).

LC coupled with multiple tandem MS (LC–MS/MS) is perhaps the best means of qualitatively and quantitatively determining trace toxins, contaminants, and/or residues in complex (sometimes crude), varied, and partially cleaned-up matrices. These matrices can vary from, for example, biological fluids, shellfish, milk, honey, veterinary tissues, fruit, and wastewater (Watson and Sparkman, 2007), and the analytes and their metabolites detected and quantified using LC–MS are quite extensive, for example, urine (Moriarty et al., 2011, 2012a,b), shellfish biotoxins (Díaz Sierra et al., 2003; Furey et al., 2001, 2002; Hamilton et al., 2004; Puente et al., 2004), veterinary drug residues (Kinsella et al., 2011; Power et al., 2012; Whelan et al., 2010, 2013), alkaloids (Griffin et al., 2013), lactic acid bacteria (Brosnan et al., 2012), insecticides (Soler et al., 2006, 2007), endocrine disruptors (Viglino et al., 2008), pharmaceuticals (Grabic et al., 2012; Queiroz et al., 2012), and personal care products (Gilbert-Lopez et al., 2012; Queiroz et al., 2012), to name just a few. Because of the high selectivity and specificity of LC–MS/MS, only minimum sample preparation is often required.

Table 36.3 summarizes many of the LC–MS-based methods that have been deployed for the determination of CYN and related compounds. LC–MS/MS is generally favored over LC–MS (single-stage MS) because it provides fingerprint fragmentation patterns that facilitate unambiguous identification of target analytes. An interesting LC–ESI–MS/MS method, developed by Bláhová, that deployed multiple reaction monitoring (MRM) of surface reservoir water samples from the Czech Republic is described in the literature. The MRM experiment used the following precursor–product ion transitions for CYN analysis [M + H]$^+$ *m/z* 416.2 to daughter ions *m/z* 194.2 and 176.1. Using the daughter ions for quantification, the authors quoted an LOD < 0.2 µg/L (Bláhová et al., 2008, 2009).

Another LC–MS/MS method that used MRM was developed and provided a LOD of 0.05 µg CYN/L. In this method, an MRM precursor–product ion transition pair of *m/z* 413.81–272.1 was used for quantification (Cheng et al., 2009).

Preußel et al. used LC–(turbo ion spray) MS/MS in MRM mode to determine the concentration of CYN in extracellular and intracellular fractions (Preußel et al., 2009). The LC column was a Nova Pak C18, and a gradient elution was deployed similar to that described in Saker and Eaglesham (1999).

TABLE 36.3

HPLC–PDA, LC–MS, and LC–MS/MS Analytical Methods for CYN and Its Analogues

Sample	Extraction	Column	Mobile Phase	MS	Analytes	LOD and LOQ	Linear Range	Year and References
Cyanobacteria Aphanizomenon flos-aquae 22D11	10% MeOH	Phenyl hexyl column	MP#1 = 5 mM AHC + 9 mM aa in 98% H_2O + 1% ACN + 1% MeOH MP#2 = 5 mM AHC + 9 mM aa in 40% H_2O + 30% ACN + 30% MeOH	LC–MS	CYN	LOQ = 17 pg; LOD = 6 pg	NR	Kittler et al. (2012)
Brassica oleracea var. *sabellica* and *Brassica juncea*	10% aa in H_2O	Conditions following Kittler et al. (2012)	Conditions following Kittler et al. (2012)	LC–MS	CYN	LOQ = 17 pg; LOD = 6 pg	NR	Kittler et al. (2012)
Cyanobacteria	5% FA	Conditions following Törökne et al. (2004)	Conditions following Törökne et al. (2004)	HPLC–PDA	CYN	NR	NR	Barón-Sola et al. (2012)
Non-axenic *C. raciborskii*	90% MeOH	C-18	MP#1 = 0.05% TFA in H_2O MP#2 = 0.05% TFA in ACN	HPLC–PDA and LC–MS	CYN	LOD <0.01 μg/mg freeze-dried cells	0–10 μg/mL	Antal et al. (2011)
Cyanobacteria	90% MeOH, C-18 SPE	C-18	MP#1 = 0.01 M TFA + 0.01% HFBA in H_2O MP#2 = 0.01 M TFA + 0.01% HFBA in ACN	LC–MS	CYN	LOD = 100 ng/L (pure water); LOD = 500 ng/L (reservoir water)	NR	Hung-Kai et al. (2011)
Raphidiopsis mediterranea skuja	—	C-18	MP#1 = 0.1% aa in 1% MeOH MP#2 = 0.1% aa in 95% MeOH	LC–MS	CYN and deoxy-CYN	NR	NR	McGregor et al. (2011)
Drinking water	SPE (conditions following Metcalf et al. (2002a) and Nicholson et al. (1994)	C-8	MP#1 = 0.5% FA MP#2 = ACN	LC–MS	CYN	NR	NR	Ho et al. (2011)

(continued)

TABLE 36.3 (continued)

HPLC–PDA, LC–MS, and LC–MS/MS Analytical Methods for CYN and Its Analogues

Sample	Extraction	Column	Mobile Phase	MS	Analytes	LOD and LOQ	Linear Range	Year and References
Freshwater	—	Acquity UPLC HSS T3	MP#1 = 0.1% FA in H_2O; MP#2 = 0.1% FA in ACN	LC–MS	CYN	LOD = 0.17 ppb	0.5–100 ppb	Oehrle et al. (2010)
Drinking water	—	HILIC (conditions following Kovalova et al. (2009) and Chiswell et al. (1999))	10 mM AA in 80% ACN	LC–MS	CYN, 5-chloro-CYN, CYN-acid and unnamed product	NR	NR	Merel et al. (2010)
Freshwater snail (*Pomacea patula catemacensis*)	5% FA in H_2O (conditions following Törökne et al. (2004) and Kubo et al. (2005))	C-18 (conditions following Welker et al. (2002))	0.01% TFA in MeOH	LC–MS	CYN	NR	NR	Berry and Lind (2010)
C. raciborskii	SPE with graphitized carbon cartridges	—	—	LC–MS	CYN	LOD = 0.07 µg/mL LOQ = 0.126 µg/mL	0.08–5 µg/mL	Guzmán-Guillén et al. (2012)
Oscillatoria sp.	—	C-18	MP#1 = MeOH/water (1:99) MP#2 = 5 mM AA in MeOH/H_2O (90:10)	LC–MS	CYN, 7-epi-CYN and 7-deoxy-CYN	NR	NR	Mazmouz et al. (2010)
Aphanizomenon flos-aquae	Conditions following Welker et al. (2002)	C-18	MP#1 = 5 mM AA in 1% MeOH MP#2 = 5 mM AA in 60% MeOH	LC–MS	CYN	LOD = 10 pg	NR	Preußel et al. (2009)
Water	—	RP-18e (for HPLC–UV and LC–MS)	For HPLC–UV: MP#1 = 0.05% TFA in H_2O; MP#2 = 0.05% TFA in MeOH For LC–MS; MP#1 = 0.1% FA in 1% ACN; MP#2 = 0.1% FA in ACN	HPLC–UV and LC–MS	CYN	LOD = 0.15 µg/L (lake water)	NR	Kokociński et al. (2009)

Organism	Cleanup	Column	Mobile phase	Detection	Analyte	LOD	LOQ	References
C. raciborskii	SPE C-18 and ENVI-Carb Supelclean cartridge	C-18	MP#1 = 5 mM AA in MeOH/water (1: 99) MP#2 = 5 mM AA in MeOH/H$_2$O (90: 10)	LC–MS	CYN	LOD = <0.2 µg/L	NR	Bláhová et al. (2009)
Freshwater Phytoplankton	—	Conditions following Fastner et al. (2007)	Conditions following Fastner et al. (2007)	LC–MS	CYN	NR	NR	Brient et al. (2009)
Aphanizomenon sp.	0.1% TFA (conditions following Welker et al. (2002)	Supelcosil ABZ + plus column	MP#1 = 0.05% TFA in H$_2$O MP#2 = 0.05% TFA in MeOH	HPLC–UV	CYN	NR	NR	Bláhová et al. (2008)
Freshwater cyanobacterium, *L. wollei*	—	C-18	MP#1 = 5 mM AA in 1% MeOH MP#2 = 5 mM AA in 90% MeOH	LC–MS	CYN and deoxy-CYN	NM	NM	Seifert et al. (2007)
C. raciborskii	5% aa, anion exchange cartridge	Amide-80	90%–60% aq ACN	LC–MS	CYN	NR	NR	Kikuchi et al. (2007)
Aphanizomenon flos-aquae	Conditions following Welker et al. (2002)	C-18	MP#1 = 5 mM AA in 1% MeOH MP#2 = 5 mM AA in 60% MeOH	LC–MS	CYN	NR	NR	Preußel et al. (2006)
C. raciborskii	Conditions following Metcalf et al. (2002a)	Conditions following Metcalf et al. (2002a)	Conditions following Metcalf et al. (2002a)	HPLC–PDA	CYN	NR	NR	Lindsay et al. (2006)
C. raciborskii	5% aa, 0.1 M potassium carbonate buffer (pH 10.5), styrene polymer and anion exchange cartridges	Amide-80	90%–60% aq MeCN linear gradient for 20 min, then 60% aq. MeCN held for 10 min	HPLC–PDA and LC–MS	CYN and deoxy-CYN	NR	NR	Kubo et al. (2005)
Anabaena circinalis and *C. raciborskii*	ACN/H$_2$O/FA (80:19.9:0.1)	TSK gel Amide-80	MP#1 = 2 mM AF + 3.6 mM FA (pH 3.5) in H$_2$O MP#2 = 2 mM AF + 3.6 mM FA (pH 3.5) in ACN: H$_2$O (95: 5)	LC–MS	CYN and deoxy-CYN	NR	NR	Dell' Aversano et al. (2004)

(continued)

TABLE 36.3 (continued)

HPLC–PDA, LC–MS, and LC–MS/MS Analytical Methods for CYN and Its Analogues

Sample	Extraction	Column	Mobile Phase	MS	Analytes	LOD and LOQ	Linear Range	Year and References
C. raciborskii	—	C-18	MP#1 = 5 mM AA in 1% MeOH MP#2 = 5 mM AA in 60% MeOH	LC–MS	CYN and deoxy-CYN	NR	NR	Saker et al. (2003)
C. raciborskii	—	Conditions following Welker et al. (2002)	Conditions following Welker et al. (2002)	HPLC–PDA	CYN	Conditions following Welker et al. (2002)	Conditions following Welker et al. (2002)	Fastner et al. (2003)
Aphanizomenon ovalisporum (Forti)	90% MeOH, Toyopearl size exclusion column	C-18	TFA in MeOH (pH 3.5)	HPLC–PDA	CYN	NR	NR	Vasas et al. (2002)
C. raciborskii	—	RP-18	0.05% TFA in H_2O, MeOH, and ACN	HPLC–PDA	CYN	NR	1–300 ng	Welker et al. (2002)
C. raciborskii	C-18 SPE	C-18	MP#1 = H_2O MP#2 = MeOH	HPLC–PDA	CYN	NR	NR	Metcalf et al. (2002a)
C. raciborskii	—	C-18	MP#1 = H_2O MP#2 = MeOH	HPLC–PDA	CYN	NR	NR	Harada et al. (1994), Lawton et al. (1994), and Metcalf et al. (2002a)
C. raciborskii	ODS YMC GEL (120A)	C-8	10% MeOH	HPLC–NMR	CYN and 7-epi-CYN	NR	NR	Runnegar et al. (2002)

Species	SPE	Column	Mobile phase	Method	Analyte	LOD	LOQ	References
C. raciborskii	MeOH and C-18 SPE	C-18 (For HPLC–PDA and LC–MS)	For HPLC–PDA MP#1 = 0.1% TFA in H$_2$O MP#2 = 0.1% TFA in ACN For LC–MS 5 mM AA in MeOH	HPLC–PDA and LC–MS	CYN (HPLC–PDA) CYN and deoxy-CYN (LC–MS)	LOD = 0.2 µg/L (LC–MS)	NR	Eaglesham et al. (1999), Li et al. (2001a,b), and Norris et al. (1998)
Cylindrospermum sp.	—	C-18	MP#1 = 50 mM FA + 2 mM AF in H$_2$O MP#2 = 50 mM FA + 2 mM AF in ACN: H$_2$O (95:5)	LC–MS	CYN	NR	NR	Eaglesham et al. (1999), Stirling and Quilliam (2001)
C. raciborskii	5% aa	C-18	5% MeOH	LC–MS	CYN	NR	NR	Humpage et al. (2000)
C. raciborskii	—	Conditions following Eaglesham et al. (1999)	Conditions following Eaglesham et al. (1999)	LC–MS	CYN	NR	NR	Eaglesham et al. (1999), Senogles et al. (2000)
C. raciborskii	—	C-18	5 mM AA in MeOH	LC–MS	CYN	LOD = 0.2 µg/L water	NR	Eaglesham et al. (1999), Saker and Eaglesham (1999)

Abbreviations: aa, acetic acid; AA, ammonium acetate; AF, ammonium formate; AHC, ammonium hydrogen carbonate; aq, aqueous; MeOH, methanol; ACN, acetonitrile; H$_2$O, water (distilled and HPLC grade); MP#1, mobile phase 1; MP#2, mobile phase 2; CYN, cylindrospermopsin; AHC, ammonium hydrogen carbonate; FA, formic acid; NM, not mentioned; deoxy-CYN, deoxycylindrospermopsin; 7-epi-CYN, 7-epicylindrospermopsin; 5-chloro-CYN, 5-chlorocylindrospermopsin; CYN-acid, cylindrospermic acid; LC–MS, liquid chromatography–mass spectrometry; HPLC–PDA, high-performance liquid chromatography–photodiode array detector; HPLC–UV, high-performance liquid chromatography–ultraviolet spectrometry; UPLC, ultrahigh-performance liquid chromatography; HILIC, hydrophilic interaction liquid chromatography; SPE, solid-phase extraction; LOD, limit of detection; LOQ, limit of quantitation; NMR, nuclear magnetic resonance; TFA, triflouroacetic acid; HFBA, heptafluorobutyric acid; MeCN, methyl cyanide.

The MRM transitions used to determine CYN were m/z 416.1–194 and 176. The product ion at m/z 194 was used for quantification and the ion at m/z 176 used for confirmation.

Quadrupole ion trap (QIT) MS techniques facilitate the acquisition of multigenerational fragmentation ion spectra. This is made possible by sequential trapping and controlled fragmentation of target ions, to produce what are known as MS^n spectra; this approach facilitates a high degree of specificity. An LC–ESI-ion trap MS, with single reaction monitoring (SRM), was applied to the analysis of CYN in a range of sample types including water samples, fish tissues, and suspended cells following individual sample extraction procedures (Gallo et al., 2009). Water samples were subjected to an SPE cleanup involving an Oasis HLB SPE cartridge, with a mean recovery of 65%–76%. Fish muscle was extracted by liquid–liquid extraction with a mean recovery of 64%, and suspended cells were analyzed by cell destruction and centrifugation. The SRM MS method was conducted in positive ion mode where the CYN $[M + H]^+$ ion at m/z 416.0 underwent MS/MS to produce two fragmentation pathways. The first fragmentation pathway yielded two ions, the first ion resulting from the cleavage of sulfate group $[M–SO_3 + H]^+$ m/z 336.2 (base peak ion, used for quantification), followed by loss of water $[M–SO_3–H_2O + H]^+$ m/z 318.2. The second fragmentation pathway consisted of cleavage of the uracil group (ring D) and uracil bridge hydroxyl functionality from the tricyclic guanidine, that is, cleavage across the uracil bridge between the hydroxyl group and the tricyclic guanidine $[M–C_5H_6N_2O_3 + H]^+$ m/z 274.2, subsequent cleavage of the sulfate group, $[M–C_5H_6N_2O_3 –SO_3 + H]^+$, at m/z 194, and finally the production of the water loss ion $[M–C_5H_6N_2O_3–SO_3–H_2O + H]^+$ at m/z 176. The limit of quantitation (LOQ) for water samples was 0.1 ng/mL, and the LOQ for fish muscle was 1.0 ng/g. Some matrix ion suppression was caused by components in the fish tissues; the use of matrix-matched calibration series was deployed to correct this.

Li et al. optimized a method using an LC-turbo spray MS with MRM for deoxy-CYN analysis (Li et al., 2001a). The precursor ion $[M + H]^+$ at m/z 400.2 was chosen for analysis and two different fragmentation pathways were also observed. The first fragmentation pathway consisted of sulfate group cleavage ($[M–SO_3 + H]^+$; m/z 320.2; base peak ion, used for quantification), followed by a loss of water ($[M–SO_3–H_2O + H]^+$; m/z 302.2). In the second fragmentation, pathway cleavage of the uracil group (ring D) and uracil bridge hydroxyl functionality away from the tricyclic guanidine was observed ($[M–C_5H_6N_2O_2 + H]^+$; m/z 274.2), prior to cleavage of the sulfate group ($[M–C_5H_6N_2O_2–SO_3 + H]^+$; m/z 194.2) and subsequent loss of water ($[M–C_5H_6N_2O_2–SO_3–H_2O + H]^+$; m/z 176).

Ultra-performance (UP) LC–MS/MS with MRM was applied to the analysis of CYN (Oehrle et al., 2010). A Waters Acquity UP LC system was hyphenated with a triple quadrupole MS/MS. The LC column was an Acquity UPLC HSST3 column and the sample was separated by a gradient elution. Confirmation of the presence of CYN was determined by the MRM transition from m/z 416 to 176, and the m/z 416 to 194 base peak transition was used for quantification purposes. These transitions were selected based upon their prior usage by other mass spectrometrists, including Li et al. (2001a,b). However, the authors of this chapter highlight that although the m/z 194 and 176 product ions are generated by other CYN congeners (Hiller et al., 2007), any (currently unknown) congeners in which structural modification has occurred at the guanidinyl residue will not generate these fragments and therefore will not be identified. The authors therefore illustrate the potential for false positives to occur by referring to their own river water sampling data.

A fast atom bombardment MS was used to determine related analogues of CYN (Banker et al., 2001). The ion monitored for the determination of 5-Cl-CYN was the sodiated adduct ion $[M + Na]^+$. This method had high-mass-accuracy capabilities and determined a chemical formula of $C_{15}H_{20}{}^{35}ClN_5NaO_7S$ from the pertinent ion at 472.0692 m/z in the mass spectrum. Another CYN-related compound, CYN-acid, displayed a prominent sodiated adduct ion at 394 m/z in its mass spectrum along with a molecular ion at 350 m/z. The high-mass-accuracy data for the molecular ion designated a chemical formula of $C_{12}H_{20}N_3O_7S^+$ from the peak at 350.1040 m/z.

Other analytical methods for the detection of CYN include a DNA biosensor (Valerio et al., 2008). Work on this sensor is at a very early stage. The premise of this approach is that it is possible to use 4-ATP (as a self-assembled monolayer) terminal NH_2 groups to immobilize a single strand of DNA (with a modified 5′-phosphate) from a CYN-producing strain, via the use of N-(3-dimethylaminopropyl)-N'-ethylcarbodiimide hydrochloride/N-hydroxy-succinimide. Use of a self-assembled monolayer ensures that the DNA probe is in the correct orientation. Electrochemical detection can then occur based upon the different electrochemical behavior of compounds that interact with the DNA, for example, methylene blue, which binds reversibly and turns blue in color when oxidized. This information could be used in the development of an electrochemical DNA hybridization biosensor.

Immunoassays and immunosensors are deployed for the detection of toxins, due to their relatively low-cost, high-throughput, rapid analysis capabilities (Van Apeldoorn et al., 2007; Vilarino et al., 2009). Commercially available ELISAs, such as that produced by Abraxis, are able to quantitatively detect both CYN and deoxy-CYN, but cannot however differentiate between the two, due to the specific cross-reactivity of the antibodies used (Abraxis kit LOD 0.04 μg/L; CYN specificity 100%, deoxy-CYN 112%). These ELISA kits are designed for use with water samples, and no/limited sample preparation is required, thus making them amenable to high-throughput applications. Even more rapid (and often portable) analysis can be achieved when these antibodies are incorporated into immunosensor formats, which take advantage of electrochemical, optical, piezoelectric, and magnetic-based sensing (Hodnik and Anderluh, 2009; Holford et al., 2012). Recently produced monoclonal and polyclonal antibodies, raised against CYN and with low deoxy-CYN cross-reactivity, have proven to be highly sensitive and appropriate for use in an optical biosensor and in a competitive indirect ELISA format (sensitivity, ELISA 27 to 131 pg/mL; surface plasmon resonance 4.4–11.1 ng/mL; (Elliott et al., 2012), thus providing another approach for CYN detection.

A proteomic method involving 2D-PAGE (Plominsky et al., 2009) has been developed for the analysis of *C. raciborskii* water-soluble proteins (which should include 9 of the 15 enzymes hypothesized to be involved in CYN production); 500–700 clear protein spots were found. Comparison of CYN-producing and nonproducing strains revealed many unique protein spots. Actually so many that it was not possible to interpret the data, once *C. raciborskii* complete genome has been sequenced (currently underway), comparison/predictions will allow these proteins to be identified and toxicity of strains confirmed. Another advantage of this proteomic approach is that the use of non-axenic strains is not problematic for this assay format.

36.8 Water Body Management/Treatment Strategies

Several treatment strategies have been suggested for the management of CYN-producing strains of cyanobacteria including filtration (Griffiths and Saker, 2003). Slow sand filtration may be a feasible and inexpensive option; this involves the mechanical removal of particles of cells/filaments. However, gentle filtration is required to prevent cell lysis. Unfortunately, filtration alone does *not* remove dissolved toxins.

Sediment filtration, for purification of drinking water (Klitzke et al., 2010, 2011), has been evaluated. It was found that CYN in sandy sediments had a tracer-like behavior, that is, it was not retained. In closed-loop column degradation experiments (using non-preconditioned sediments), a lag of 20 days was seen; after 40 days, >92% of CYN was degraded.

The effect of chlorination of drinking water on CYN levels was also investigated. CYN was found to convert to two chlorination products 5-chloro-CYN and CYN-acid (Banker et al., 2001), with a 1:1 molar ratio of CYN/chlorine yielding predominantly 5-Cl-CYN (some CYN-acid also seen), whereas a 1:2 molar ratio of CYN/chlorine yields CYN-acid. It has been postulated that CYN-acid is formed from further chlorination of 5-Cl-CYN (Merel et al., 2010).

Griffiths (Griffiths and Saker, 2003) also investigated chlorination effects on CYN. The addition of chlorine at 2 mg/L, 30 min, reduced the concentration of CYN below the LOD (0.2 μg/L), and the treatment was most effective at a pH 6+. However, this chlorination approach induced the formation of mono- and di-chlorinated CYN. Chlorine addition is thought to occur at C5 of the uracil ring to give 5-chlorouracil CYN.

Another treatment involving the addition of chlorine, permanganate, and ozone to the water along with UV irradiation (Cheng et al., 2009) has shown that free Cl and ozone together were the most effective combination for the removal of CYN from water. Treatment with chlorine dioxide, monochloramine, permanganate, and UV irradiation had very little effect on CYN levels.

Rodriquez et al. studied the reaction kinetics of CYN and Cl, applied as sodium hypochlorite (in excess by eightfold; in phosphate buffer, pH modified with NaOH; thiosulfate used to stop reaction), and found that the reaction followed second-order reaction kinetics (first-order in respect to each reactant) (Merel et al., 2010; Rodríguez et al., 2007). Maximum reactivity was achieved at pH 7 (rate constant = 1265 M/s), and by 50 s, all CYN was converted to 5-chloro-CYN (7.2 μM CYN + 64 μM Cl; 20°C; pH 7.1). Further degradation of 5-chloro-CYN then continued to occur at a rate of 10–20 more slowly than CYN. The authors did not state what this compound degraded to.

A chlorination study by Senogles et al. using relatively low chlorine doses (<1 mg/L; NaHOCl; acetic acid used to quench reaction prior to LC–MS) resulted in the concentration of CYN decreasing by 99% within 1 min (pH 6–9). A residual concentration of chlorine of 0.5 mg/L (i.e., at the end of 1 min) was required for this degradation to occur. This would imply that higher Cl doses are required when dissolved oxygen concentration is high. Less degradation is seen at low pH, which indicates that substitution and oxidation reaction processes are key in CYN degradation (Senogles et al., 2000).

The effectiveness of activated carbon in CYN removal has yet to be demonstrated (Ho et al., 2011). However, preliminary results using powdered activated carbon in laboratory studies demonstrated that activated carbon was less effective than chlorination (Griffiths and Saker, 2003).

Photocatalysis (Griffiths and Saker, 2003) using UV irradiation, with a metal oxide catalyst (TiO_2 that produces hydroxyl radicals that modify oxidation conditions), has been shown to be very effective for CYN removal: 100 μg/L CYN solution had a $t_{1/2}$ of 0.7 min. The catalyst does require periodic regeneration using distilled water or weak acid wash.

Vertical mixing of the water column (Griffiths and Saker, 2003) was tested to evaluate its effect on CYN levels. The rationale behind this approach is based on the fact that buoyant cyanobacteria have their greatest competitive advantage when water columns are stabile, that is, stratified. Therefore, artificial destratification may reduce the likelihood of a bloom occurring.

Biocontrol (Griffiths and Saker, 2003) measures involve a bio-manipulation (modification of food web) approach that may control the proliferation of cyanobacterial blooms. Silver carp (*Hypophthalmichthys molitrix*) appears to be able to reduce standing stock of *C. raciborskii*—however, there are some doubts as to whether this is suitable biocontrol.

An entire fish stock was removed from a hypertrophic fish pond in Hungary and prevented the usual summer *C. raciborskii* bloom. It was postulated that the removal of the fish led to increased grazing pressure from the increased zooplankton population, resulting in depletion of the toxin bearing bloom. However, no reliable data on the population dynamics of this experiment were presented.

Another potential biocontrol approach is via the use of probiotic bacteria. Nybom et al. tested several *Lactobacillus rhamnosus* and *Bifidobacterium* spp. for their ability to remove cyanotoxins from aqueous solutions (Nybom et al., 2008). All strains were able to remove CYN within 24 h (20%–30% removal), with *Bifidobacterium longum* strain 46 providing the greatest removal (31.6% of pure CYN from 100 μg/L solution; 37°C; 24 h) from aqueous solution. The removal of other cyanobacterial toxins (microcystin-LR, microcystin-LF, and microcystin-RR) was greater still with *L. rhamnosus* strains GG and LC-705 removing 45%–80%.

36.9 Conclusion

CYN toxins can exert a profound negative effect on the health of humans and animals and on the quality of drinking and recreational waters. Moreover, the ubiquity of progenitor algal species that produce these toxins, together with the toxin resilience to common detoxification protocols and their persistence in water bodies, presents a daunting challenge to scientists, regulators, and public health authorities. The fact that the CYN toxins may co-occur with other algal-borne toxins like the microcystins and the anatoxins further exacerbates the problem. At this juncture, the only logical approach to the protection of water consumers is the implementation of a highly sensitive, selective, and multicomponent analysis program. One of the most versatile and accurate methods for detecting multiple target analytes in various matrices is LC–MS/MS. The strength of LC–MS/MS is that not only can the technology identify known toxins but MS/MS fragmentation studies can be deployed to identify unknown analogues by elucidating moiety fragments that are characteristic of the main toxin group. Given the widespread dispersion of algal-borne toxins, it is good practice for the regulatory authorities to implement regular screening of water bodies as part of their health protection programs.

ACKNOWLEDGMENTS

The authors acknowledge the funding obtained under the EU/INTERREG IIIB Atlantic Area Programme for projects titled ATLANTOX "Advanced Tests about New Toxins Occurring in the Atlantic Area due to Climate Change" and PHARMATLANTIC "Knowledge Transfer Network for Prevention of Mental Diseases and Cancer in the Atlantic Area." The authors also acknowledge the European Cooperation in Science and Technology, COST Action ES 1105 "CYANOCOST—Cyanobacterial blooms and toxins in water resources: Occurrence, impacts and management" for adding value to this study through networking and knowledge sharing with European experts and researchers in the field.

REFERENCES

Agrawa, M., Yadav, S., Patel, C., Raipuria, N., Agrawal, M.K., 2012. Bioassay methods to identify the presence of cyanotoxins in drinking water supplies and their removal strategies. *European Journal of Experimental Biology* 2: 321–336.

Antal, O., Karisztl-Gacsi, M., Farkas, A., Kovacs, A., Acs, A., Toro, N., Kiss, G. et al., 2011. Screening the toxic potential of *Cylindrospermopsis raciborskii* strains isolated from Lake Balaton, Hungary. *Toxicon* 57: 831–840.

Azevedo, S.M., Carmichael, W.W., Jochimsen, E.M., Rinehart, K.L., Lau, S., Shaw, G.R., Eaglesham, G.K., 2002. Human intoxication by microcystins during renal dialysis treatment in Caruaru-Brazil. *Toxicology* 181–182: 441–446.

Bain, P., Burcham, P., Falconer, I., Fontaine, F., Froscio, S., Humpage, A., Neumann, C., Patel, B., Shaw, G., Wickramasinghe, W., 2008. Cylindrospermopsin mechanism of toxicity and genotoxicity—Research Report No 61, pp. 1–75.

Banker, R., Carmeli, S., Hadas, O., Teltsch, B., Porat, R., Sukenik, A., 1997. Identification of cylindrospermopsin in *Aphanizomenon ovalisporum* (Cyanophyceae) isolated from lake Kinneret, Israel. *Journal of Phycology* 33: 613–616.

Banker, R., Carmeli, S., Teltsch, B., Sukenik, A., 2000. 7-Epicylindrospermopsin, a toxic minor metabolite of the cyanobacterium *Aphazomenon ovalisporum* from Lake Kinneret, Israel. *Journal Natural Products* 63: 387–389.

Banker, R., Carmeli, S., Werman, M., Teltsch, B., Porat, R., Sukenik, A., 2001. Uracil moiety is required for toxicity of the cyanobacterial hepatotoxin cylindrospermopsin. *Journal of Toxicology Environmental Health: Part A* 62: 281–288.

Barón-Sola, A., Ouahid, Y., del Campo, F.F., 2012. Detection of potentially producing cylindrospermopsin and microcystin strains in mixed populations of cyanobacteria by simultaneous amplification of cylindrospermopsin and microcystin gene regions. *Ecotoxicology and Environmental Safety* 75: 102–108.

Bernard, C., Harvey, M., Biré, R., Krys, S., Fontaine, J.J., 2003. Toxicological comparison of diverse *Cylindrospeermopsis raciborskii* strains: Evidence of liver damage cuased by a French C. Raciborskii strain. *Environmental Toxicology* 18: 176–186.

Berry, J.P., Gibbs, P.D.L., Schmale, M.C., Saker, M.L., 2009. Toxicity of cylindrospermopsin, and other apparent metabolites from Cylindrospermopsis raciborskii and *Aphanizomenon ovalisporum*, to the zebrafish (*Danio rerio*) embryo. *Toxicon* 53: 289–299.

Berry, J.P., Lind, O., 2010. First evidence of "paralytic shellfish toxins" and cylindrospermopsin in a Mexican freshwater system, Lago Catemaco, and apparent bioaccumulation of the toxins in "tegogolo" snails (*Pomacea patula catemacensis*). *Toxicon* 55: 930–938.

Beyer, D., Suranyi, G., Vasas, G., Roszik, J., Erdodi, F., M-Hamvas, M., Bacsi, I. et al. 2009. Cylindrospermopsin induces alternatives of root histology and microtubule organization in common reed (*Phragmites australis*) plantlets cultured *in vitro*. *Toxicon* 54: 440–449.

Bláhová, L., Babica, P., Adamovský, O., Kohoutek, J., Maršálek, B., Bláha, L., 2008. Analyses of cyanobacterial toxins (microcystins, cylindrospermopsin) in the reservoirs of the Czech Republic and evaluation of health risks. *Environmental Chemistry Letters* 6: 223–227.

Bláhová, L., Oravec, M., Marsálek, B., Sejnohová, L., Simek, Z., Bláha, L., 2009. The first occurrence of the cyanobacterial alkaloid toxin cylindrospermopsin in the Czech Republic as determined by immunochemical and LC/MS methods. *Toxicon* 53: 519–524.

Bourke, A.T.C., Hawes, R.B., Neilson, A., Stallman, N.D., 1983. An outbreak of hepato-enteritis (the Palm Island mystery disease) possibly caused by algal intoxication. *Toxicon* 21(Supplement 3): 45–48.

Bownik, A., 2010. Harmful algae: Effects of alkaloid cyanotoxins on animal and human health. *Toxin Reviews* 29: 99–114.

Brient, L., Lengronne, M., Bormans, M., Fastner, J., 2009. First occurrence of cylindrospermopsin in freshwater in France. *Environmental Toxicology* 24: 415–420.

Brosnan, B., Coffey, A., Arendt, E.K., Furey, A., 2012. Rapid identification, by use of the LTQ Orbitrap hybrid FT mass spectrometer, of antifungal compounds produced by lactic acid bacteria. *Analytical Bioanalytical Chemistry* 403: 2983–2995.

Burch, M.D., 2008. Chapter 36: Effective doses, guidelines and regulations. in: Hudnell, H.K. (ed.), *Cyanobacterial Harmful Algal Blooms: State of the Science and Research Needs*, New York: Springer. http://link.springer.com/chapter/10.1007/978-0-387-75865-7_36.

Byth, S., 1980. Palm Island mystery disease. *Medical Journal of Australia* 2: 40–42.

Carson, B., 2000. *Cylindrospermopsin: Review of Toxicological Literature*, National Institute of Envrionmental Health Sciences, Research Traiange Park, NC, Contract No. N01-ES-65402, p. 37.

Cheng, X., Shi, H., Adams, C.D., Timmons, T., Ma, Y., 2009. Effects of oxidative and physical treatments on inactivation of *Cylindrospermopsis raciborskii* and removal of cylindrospermopsin. *Water Science and Technology* 60: 689–697.

Chiswell, R.K., Shaw, G.R., Eaglasham, G.K., Smith, M.J., Norris, R.L., Seawright, A.A., Moore, M.R., 1999. Stability of cylindrospermopsin, the toxin from the cyanobacterium, *Cylindrospermopsis raciborskii*: Effects of pH, temperature and sunlight on decomposition. *Environmental Toxicology* 14: 155–161.

Chong, M.W.K., Wong, B.S.F., Lam, P.K.S., Shaw, G.R., Seawright, A.A., 2002. Toxicity and uptake mechanism of cylindrospermopsin and lophyrotomin in primary rat hepatocytes. *Toxicon* 40: 205–211.

Codd, G.A., Morrison, L.F., Metcalf, J.S., 2005. Cyanobacterial toxins: Risk management for health protection. *Toxicology and Applied Pharmacology* 203: 264–272.

Cook, C.M., Vardaka, E., Lanaras, T., 2004. Toxic cyanobacteria in Greek freshwaters, 1987–2000: Occurrence, toxicity, and impacts in the Mediterranean region. *Acta Hydrochimica Et Hydrobiologica* 32: 107–124.

Dell'Aversano, C., Eaglesham, G.K., Quilliam, M.A., 2004. Analysis of cyanobacterial toxins by hydrophilic interaction liquid chromatography-mass spectrometry. *Journal of Chromatography A* 1028: 155–164.

Díaz Sierra, M., Furey, A., Hamilton, B., Lehane, M., James, K.J., 2003. Elucidation of the fragmentation pathways of azaspiracids, using electrospray ionisation, hydrogen/deuterium exchange, and multiple-stage mass spectrometry. *Journal of Mass Spectrometry* 38: 1178–1186.

Eaglesham, G., Norris, R., Shaw, G., Smith, M.J., Chiswell, R., David, B.C., Neville, G.R., Seawright, A.A., Moore, M.R., 1999. Use of HPLC-MS/MS to monitor cylindrospermopsin, a blue-green algal toxin, for public health purposes. *Environmental Toxicology* 14: 151–154.

Elliott, C.T., Redshaw, C.H., George, S.E., Campbell, K., 2013. First development and characterization of polyclonal and monoclonal antibodies to the emerging fresh water toxin cylindrospermopsin. *Harmful Algae* 24: 10–19.

Fabbro, L.D., Duivenvoorden, L.J., 1996. Profile of the bloom of cyanobacterium *Cylindrospermopsis racibor-skii* (Woloszynska) Seenaya and Subba Raju in the Fitzroy river in tropical central Queensland. *Marine and Freshwater Research* 47: 685–694.

Falconer, I.R., 2004. Chapter 10: Detection and analysis of cylindrospermopsins and microcystins. *Cyanobacterial Toxins of Drinking Water Supplies*, Boca Raton, FL: CRC Press, pp. 185–211.

Falconer, I.R., Hardy, S.J., Humpage, A.R., Froscio, S.M., Tozer, G.J., Hawkins, P.R., 1999. Hepatotoxicity and renal toxicity of the blue-green alga (Cyanobacterium) *Cylindrospermopsis raciborskii* in male Swiss albino mice. *Environmental Toxicology* 14: 143–150.

Falconer, I.R., Humpage, A.R., 2001. Preliminary evidence for in vivo tumor initiation by oral administration of extracts of blue-green alga *Cylindrospermopsis raciborskii* containing the toxin cylindrospermopsin. *Environmental Toxicology* 16: 192–195.

Fastner, J., Heinze, R., Humpage, A.R., Mischke, U., Eaglesham, G.K., Chorus, I., 2003. Cylindrospermopsin occurrence in two German lakes and preliminary assessment of toxicity and toxin production of *Cylindrospermopsis raciborskii* (Cyanobacteria) isolates. *Toxicon* 42: 313–321.

Fastner, J., Rücker, J., Stüken, A., Preußel, K., Nixdorf, B., Chorus, I., Köhler, A., Wiedner, C., 2007. Occurrence of the cyanobacterial toxin cylindrospermopsin in Germany. *Environmental Toxicology* 22: 26–32.

Fergusson, K.M., Saint, C.P., 2003. Multiplex PCR assay for *cylindrospermopsis raciborskii* and cylindrospermopsin-producing cyanobacteria. *Environmental Toxicology* 18: 120–125.

Froscio, S.M., Cannon, E., Lau, H.M., Humpage, A.R., 2009. Limited uptake of the cyanobacterial toxin cylindrospermopsin by Vero cells. *Toxicon* 54: 862–868.

Furey, A., Braña-Magdalena, A., Lehane, M., Moroney, C., James, K.J., Satake, M., Yasumoto, T., 2002. Determination of azaspiracids in shellfish using liquid chromatography-tandem electrospray mass spectrometry. *Rapid Communications in Mass Spectrometry* 16: 238–242.

Furey, A., Lehane, M., Gillman, M., Fernández-Puente, P., James, K.J., 2001. Determination of domoic acid in shellfish by liquid chromatography with electrospray ionization and multiple tandem mass spectrometry. *Journal of Chromatography* 938: 167–174.

Gallo, P., Fabbrocino, S., Cerulo, M.G., Ferranti, P., Bruno, M., Serpe, L., 2009. Determination of cylindrospermopsin in freshwater and fish tissue by liquid chromatography coupled to electrospray ion trap mass spectrometry. *Rapid Communications Mass Spectrometry* 23: 3279–3284.

Gilbert-Lopez, B., Garcia-Reyes, J.F., Meyer, C., Michels, A., Franzke, J., Molina-Diaz, A., Hayen, H., 2012. Simultaneous testing of multiclass organic contaminants in food and environment by liquid chromatography/dielectric barrier discharge ionization-mass spectrometry. *The Analyst* 137: 5403–5410.

Grabic, R., Fick, J., Lindberg, R.H., Fedorova, G., Tysklind, M., 2012. Multi-residue method for trace level determination of pharmaceuticals in environmental samples using liquid chromatography coupled to triple quadrupole mass spectrometry. *Talanta* 100: 183–195.

Griffin, C.T., Danaher, M., Elliott, C.T., Kennedy, G.D., Furey, A., 2013. Detection of pyrrolizidine alkaloids in commercial honey using liquid chromatography–ion trap mass spectrometry. *Food Chemistry* 136: 1577–1583.

Griffiths, D.J., Saker, M.L., 2003. The Palm Island mystery disease 20 years on: A review of research on the cyanotoxin cylindrospermopsin. *Environmental Toxicology* 18: 78–93.

Gutierrez-Praena, D., Jos, Á., Pichardo, S., Moreno, I.M., Camean, A.M., 2013. Presence and bioaccumulation of microcystins and cylindrospermopsin in food and the effectiveness of some cooking techniques at decreasing their concentrations: A review. *Food and Chemical Toxicology* 53: 139–152.

Guzmán-Guillén, R., Prieto, A.I., González, A.G., Soria-Díaz, M.E., Cameán, A.M., 2012. Cylindrospermopsin determination in water by LC-MS/MS: Optimization and validation of the method and application to real samples. *Environmental Toxicology and Chemistry* 31: 2233–2238.

Hamilton, B., Díaz Sierra, M., Lehane, M., Furey, A., James, K.J., 2004. The fragmentation pathways of azaspiracids elucidated using positive nanospray hybrid quadrupole time-of-flight (QqTOF) mass spectrometry. *Journal of Spectroscopy* 18: 355–362.

Harada, K., Kondo, F., Lawton, L., 1999. Chapter 13: Laboratory analysis of cyanotoxins, in: Chorus, I., Bartram, J. (eds.), *Toxic Cyanobacteria in Water: A Guide to Their Public Health Consequences, Monitoring and Management*, London, U.K.: E & FN Spon, pp. 369–405.

Harada, K.-I., Ohtani, I., Iwamot, K., Suzuki, M., Watanabe, M.F., Watanabe, M., Terao, K., 1994. Isolation of cylindrosepermopsin from a cyanobacterium umezakia natans and its screening method. *Toxicon* 32: 73–84.

Hardy, J., 2011. *Washington State Provisional Recreational Guidance for Cylindrospermopsin and Saxitoxin*, Washington, DC: Washington State Department of Health, p. 36.

Hawkins, P.R., Chandrasena, N.R., Jones, G.J., Humpage, A.R., Falconer, I.R., 1997. Isolation and toxicity of *Cylindropermopsis raciborskii* from an ornamental lake. *Toxicon* 35: 341–346.

Hawkins, P.R., Runnegar, M.T., Jackson, A.R., Falconer, I.R., 1985. Severe hepatotoxicity caused by the tropical cyanobacterium (blue-green alga) *Cylindrospermopsin raciborskii* (Woloszynska) Seenaya and Subba Raju isolated from a domestic water supply reservoir. *Applied Environmental Microbiology* 50: 1292–1295.

Hiller, S., Krock, B., Cembella, A., Luckas, B., 2007. Rapid detection of cyanobacterial toxins in precursor ion mode by liquid chromatography tandem mass spectrometry. *Journal of Mass Spectrometry* 42: 1238–1250.

Ho, L., Lambling, P., Bustamante, H., Duker, P., Newcombe, G., 2011. Application of powdered activated carbon for the adsorption of cylindrospermopsin and microcystin toxins from drinking water supplies. *Water Research* 45: 2954–2964.

Ho, L., Tang, T., Monis, P.T., Hoefel, D., 2012. Biodegradation of multiple cyanobacterial metabolites in drinking water supplies. *Chemosphere* 87: 1149–1154.

Hodnik, V., Anderluh, G., 2009. Toxin detection by surface plasmon resonance. *Sensors* 9: 1339–1354.

Holford, T.R.J., Davis, F., Higson, S.P.J., 2012. Recent trends in antibody based sensors. *Biosensors and Bioelectronics*, 34: 12–24.

Humpage, A.R., Fenech, M., Thomas, P., Falconer, I.R., 2000. Micronucleus induction and chromosome loss in transformed human white cells indicate clastogenic and aneugenic action of the cyanobacterial toxin, cylindrospermopsin. *Mutation Research/Genetic Toxicology and Environmental Mutagenesis* 472: 155–161.

Hung-Kai, Y., Tsair-Fuh, L., Pao-Chi, L., 2011. Simultaneous detction of nine cyanotoxins in drinking water using dual solid-phase extraction and liquid chromatography-mass spectrometry. *Toxicon* 58: 209–218.

Jiang, Y., Xiao, P., Yu, G., Sano, T., Pan, Q., Li, R., 2012. Molecular basis and phylogenetic implications of deoxycylindrospermopsin biosynthesis in the cyanobacterium raphidiopsis curvata. *Applied and Environmental Microbiology* 78: 2256–2263.

Kabziński, A.K.M., Juszczak, R., Miękoś, E., Tarczyńska, M., Sivonen, K., Rapala, J., 2000. The first report about the presence of cyanobacterial toxins in Polish lakes. *Polish Journal of Environmental Studies* 9: 171–178.

Kikuchi, S., Kubo, T., Kaya, K., 2007. Cylindrospermopsin determination using 2-[4-(2-hydroxyethyl)-1-piperazinyl]ethanesulfonic acid (HEPES) as the internal standard. *Analytica Chimica Acta* 583: 124–127.

Kinnear, S., 2010. Cylindrospermopsin: A decade of progress on bioaccumulation research. *Marine Drugs* 8: 542–564.

Kinsella, B., Byrne, P., Cantwell, H., McCormack, M., Furey, A., Danaher, M., 2011. Determination of the new anthelmintic monepantel and its sulfone metabolite in milk and muscle using a UHPLC–MS/MS and QuEChERS method. *Journal of Chromatography B* 879: 3707–3713.

Kiss, T., Vehovszky, A., Hiripi, L., Kovacs, A., Voros, L., 2002. Membrane effects of toxins isolated from a cyanobacterium, *Cylindrospermopsis raciborskii*, on identified molluscan neurones. *Comparative Biochemistry and Physiology Part C: Toxicol and Pharmacology* 131: 167–176.

Kittler, K., Schreiner, M., Krumbein, A., Manzei, S., Koch, M., Rohn, S., Maul, R., 2012. Uptake of the cyanobacterial toxin cylindrospermopsin in Brassica vegetables. *Food Chemistry* 133: 875–879.

Kling, H., 2009. *Cylindrospermopsis raciborskii* (Nostocales, Cyanobacteria): A brief historic overview and recent discovery in the Assiniboine River (Canada). *Fottea* 9: 45–47.

Klitzke, S., Apelt, S., Weiler, C., Fastner, J., Chorus, I., 2010. Retention and degradation of the cyanobacterial toxin cylindrospermopsin in sediments—The role of sediment preconditioning and DOM composition. *Toxicon* 55: 999–1007.

Klitzke, S., Beusch, C., Fastner, J., 2011. Sorption of the cyanobacterial toxins cylindrospermopsin and anatoxin-a to sediments. *Water Research* 45: 1338–1346.

Kokociński, M., Dziga, D., Spoof, L., Stefaniak, K., Jurczak, T., Mankiewicz-Boczek, J., Meriluoto, J., 2009. First report of the cyanobacterial toxin cylindrospermopsin in the shallow, eutrophic lakes of western Poland. *Chemosphere* 74: 669–675.

Kovalova, L., McArdell, C.S., Hollender, J., 2009. Challenge of high polarity and low concentrations in analysis of cytostatics and metabolites in wastewater by hydrophilic interaction chromatography/tandem mass spectrometry. *Journal of Chromatography A* 1216: 1100–1108.

Kubo, T., Sano, T., Hosoya, K., Tanaka, N., Kaya, K., 2005. A new simply and effective fractionation method for cylindrospermopsin analyses. *Toxicon* 46: 104–107.

Lawton, L.A., Edwards, C., Codd, G.A., 1994. Extraction and high-performance liquid chromatographic method for the determination of microcystins in raw and treated waters. *The Analyst* 119: 1525–1530.

Li, R., Carmichael, W.W., Brittain, S., Eaglesham, G.K., Shaw, G.R., Liu, Y., Watanabe, M.M., 2001a. First report of the cyanotoxins cylindrospermopsin and deoxycylindrospermopsin from *Raphidiopsis Curvata* (Cyanobacteria). *Journal of Phycology* 37: 1121–1126.

Li, R., Carmichael, W.W., Brittain, S., Eaglesham, G.K., Shaw, G.R., Mahakhant, A., Noparatnaraporn, N., Yongmanitchai, W., Kaya, K., Watanabe, M.M., 2001b. Isolation and identification of the cyanotoxin cylindrospermopsin and deoxy-cylindrospermopsin from a Thailand strain of *Cylindrospermopsis raciborskii* (Cyanobacteria). *Toxicon* 39: 973–980.

Lindsay, J., Metcalf, J.S., Codd, G.A., 2006. Protection against the toxicity of microcystin-LR and cylindrospermopsin in *Artemia salina* and *Daphnia* spp. by pre-treatment with cyanobacterial lipopolysaccharide (LPS). *Toxicon* 48: 995–1001.

Looper, R.E., Runnegar, M.T.C., Williams, R.M., 2005. Synthesis of the putative structure of 7-deoxycylindrospermopsin: C7 oxygenation is not required for the inhibition of protein synthesis. *Agnewandte Chemie International Edition* 44: 3879–3881.

Looper, R.E., Runnegar, M.T.C., Williams, R.M., 2006. Syntheses of the cylindrospermopsin alkaloids. *Tetrahedron* 62: 4549–4562.

Looper, R.E., Williams, R.M., 2001. Construction of the A-ring of cylindrospermopsin via an intramolecular oxazinone-N-oxide dipolar cycloaddition. *Tetrahedron Letters* 42: 769–771.

Mazmouz, R., Chapuis-Hugon, F., Mann, S., Pichon, V., Mejean, A., Ploux, O., 2010. Biosynthesis of cylindrospermopsin and 7-epicylindrospermopsin in Oscillatoria sp. strain PCC 6506: Identification of the cyr gene cluster and toxin analysis. *Applied and Environmental Microbiology* 76: 4943–4949.

McGregor, G.B., Sendall, B.C., Hunt, L.T., Eaglesham, G.K., 2011. Report of the cyanotoxins cylindrospermopsin and deoxy-cylindrospermopsin from *Raphidiopsis mediterranea Skuja* (Cyanobacteria/Nostocales). *Harmful Algae* 10: 402–410.

Merel, S., Clement, M., Mourot, A., Fessard, V., Thomas, O., 2010. Characterization of cylindrospermopsin chlorination. *Science of the Total Environment* 408: 3433–3442.

Messineo, V., Bogialli, S., Melchiorre, S., Sechi, N., Luglie, A., Casiddu, P., Mariani, M.A. et al. 2009. Cyanobacterial toxins in Italian freshwaters. *Limnologica—Ecology and Management of Inland Waters* 39: 95–106.

Metcalf, J.S., Beattie, K.A., Saker, M.L., Codd, G.A., 2002a. Effects of organic solvents on the high performance liquid chromatographic analysis of the cyanobacterial toxin cylindrospermopsin and its recovery from environmental eutrophic waters by solid phase extraction. *FEMS Microbiology Letters* 216: 159–164.

Metcalf, J.S., Lindsay, J., Beattie, K.A., Birmingham, S., Saker, M.L., Törökné, A.K, Codd, G.A., 2002b. Toxicity of cylindrospermopsin to the brine shrimp *Artemia salina*: Comparisons with protein synthesis inhibitors and microcystins. *Toxicon* 40: 1115–1120.

Mihali, A., Mann, S., Maldiney, T., Vassiliadis, G., Lequin, O., Ploux, O., 2008. Characterization of the gene cluster responsible for cylindrospermopsin biosynthesis. *Applied and Environmental Microbiology* 74: 716–722.

Moreira, C., Azevedo, J., Antunes, A., Vasconcelos, V., 2012. Cylindrospermopsin: Occurrence, methods of detection and toxicology. *Journal of Applied Microbiology*. doi: 10.1111/jam.12048.

Moriarty, M., Lee, A., O'Connell, B., Kelleher, A., Keeley, H., Furey, A., 2011. Development of an LC-MS/MS method for the analysis of serotonin and related compounds in urine and the identification of a potential biomarker for attention deficit hyperactivity/hyperkinetic disorder. *Analytical and Bioanalytical Chemistry* 401: 2481–2493.

Moriarty, M., Lee, A., O'Connell, B., Lehane, M., Keeley, H., Furey, A., 2012a. The application and validation of hybridSPE-precipitation cartridge technology for the rapid clean-up of serum matrices (from phospholipids) for the clinical analysis of serotonin, Dopamine and Melatonin. *Chromatographia* 75: 1257–1269.

Moriarty, M., Lehane, M., O'Connell, B., Keeley, H., Furey, A., 2012b. Development of a nano-electrospray MSn method for the analysis of serotonin and related compounds in urine using a LTQ-orbitrap mass spectrometer. *Talanta* 90: 1–11.

Nicholson, B.C., Rositano, J., Burch, M., 1994. Destruction of cyanobacterial peptide hepatotoxins by chlorine and chloramine. *Water Research* 6: 1297–1303.

Norris, R.L., Eaglesham, G.K., Shaw, G.R., Chriswell, R.K., Smith, M.J., Davis, B.C., Seawright, A.A., Moore, M.R., 1998. Choice of standard material and robustness of HPLC-MS/MS assay for Cylindrospermopsin, *4th International Toxic Cyanobacteria Symposium*, Beaufort, NC.

Norris, R.L., Seawright, A.A., Shaw, G.R., Senogles, P., Eaglesham, G.K., Smith, M.J., Chiswell, R.K., Moore, M.R., 2002. Hepatic xenobiotic metabolism of cylindrospermopsin in vivo in the mouse. *Toxicon* 40: 471–476.

Norris, R.L.G., Seawright, A.A., Shaw, G.R., Smith, M.J., Chiswell, R.K., Moore, M.R., 2001. Distribution of 14C cylindrospermopsin in vivo in the mouse. *Environmental Toxicology* 16: 498–505.

Nybom, S.M.K., Salminen, S.J., Meriluoto, J.A.O., 2008. Specific strains of probiotic bacteria are efficient in removal of several different cyanobacterial toxins from solution. *Toxicon* 52: 214–220.

Oehrle, S.A., Southwell, B., Westrick, J., 2010. Detection of various freshwater cyanobacterial toxins using ultra-performance liquid chromatography tandem mass spectrometry. *Toxicon* 55: 965–972.

Ohtani, I., Moore, R., Runnegar, M., 1992. Cylindrospermopsin: A potent hepatotoxin from the blue-green alga Cylindrospermopsis raciborskii. *Journal of the American Chemical Society* 114: 7941–7942.

Pearson, L., Mihali, T., Moffitt, M., Kellmann, R., Neilan, B.A., 2010. On the chemistry, toxicology and genetics of the cyanobacterial toxins, microcystin, nodularin, saxitoxin and cylindrospermopsin. *Marine Drugs* 8: 1650–1680.

Plominsky, A.M., Soto-Liebe, K., Vasquez, M., 2009. Optimisation of 2D-PAGE protocols for proteomic analysis of two nonaxenic toxin-producing freshwater cyanobacteria: *Cylindrospermopsis raciborskii* and *Raphidiopsis sp. Letters in Applied Microbiology* 49: 332–337.

Poniedzialek, B., Rzymski, P., Kokocinski, M., 2012. Cylindrospermopsin: Water-linked potential threat to human health in Europe. *Environmental Toxicology and Pharmacology* 34: 651–660.

Power, C., Sayers, R., O'Brien, B., Bloemhoff, Y., Danaher, M., Furey, A., Jordan, K., 2012. Partitioning of nitroxynil, oxyclozanide and levamisole residues from milk to cream, skim milk and skim milk powder. *International Journal of Dairy Technology* 65: 503–506.

Preußel, K., Stüken, A., Wiedner, C., Chorus, I., Fastner, J., 2006. First report on cylindrospermopsin producing *Aphanizomenon flos-aquae* (Cyanobacteria) isolated from two German lakes. *Toxicon* 47: 156–162.

Preußel, K., Wessel, G., Fastner, J., Chorus, I., 2009. Response of cylindrospermopsin production and release in *Aphanizomenon flos-aquae* (Cyanobacteria) to varying light and temperature conditions. *Harmful Algae* 8: 645–650.

Puente, P.F., Sáez, M.J.F., Hamilton, B., Lehane, M., Ramstad, H., Furey, A., James, K.J., 2004. Rapid determination of polyether marine toxins using liquid chromatography–multiple tandem mass spectrometry. *Journal of Chromatography A* 1056: 77–82.

Queiroz, F.B., Brandt, E.M., Aquino, S.F., Chernicharo, C.A., Afonso, R.J., 2012. Occurrence of pharmaceuticals and endocrine disruptors in raw sewage and their behavior in UASB reactors operated at different hydraulic retention times. *Water Science and Technology* 66: 2562–2569.

Quesada, A., Moreno, E., Carrasco, D., Paniagua, T., Wormer, L., De Hoyos, C., Sukenik, A., 2006. Toxicity of *Aphanizomenon ovalisporum* (Cyanobacteria) in a Spanish water reservoir. *European Journal of Phycology* 41: 39–45.

Rasmussen, J.P., Cursaro, M., Froscio, S.M., Saint, C.P., 2008. An examination of the antibiotic effects of cylindrospermopsin on common gram-negative and gram-positive bacteria and the protozoan *Naegleria lovaniensis. Environmental Toxicology* 23: 36–43.

Reisner, M., Carmeli, S., Werman, M., Sukenik, A., 2004. The cyanobacterial toxin cylindrospermopsin inhibits pyrimidine nucleotide synthesis and alters cholesterol distribution in mice. *Toxicological Sciences* 82: 620–627.

Rodríguez, E., Sordo, A., Metcalf, J.S., Acero, J.L., 2007. Kinetics of the oxidation of cylindrospermopsin and anatoxin-a with chlorine, monochloramine and permanganate. *Water Research* 41: 2048–2056.

Runnegar, M.T., Kong, S.M., Zhong, Y.Z., Ge, J.L., Lu, S.C., 1994. The role of glutathione in the toxicity of a novel cyanobacterial alkaloid cylindrospermopsin in cultured rat hepatocytes. *Biochemical and Biophysical Research Communications* 201: 235–241.

Runnegar, M.T., Kong, S.M., Zhong, Y.Z., Lu, S.C., 1995. Inhibition of reduced glutathione synthesis by cyanobacterial alkaloid cylindrospermopsin in cultured rat hepatocytes. *Biochemical Pharmacology* 49: 219–225.

Runnegar, M.T., Xie, C., Snider, B.B., Wallace, G.A., Weinreb, S.M., Kuhlenkamp, J., 2002. In vitro hepatotoxicity of the cyanobacterial alkaloid cylindrospermopsin and related synthetic analogues. *Toxicological Sciences* 67: 81–87.

Saker, M.L., Eaglesham, G.K., 1999. The accumulation of cylindrospermopsin from the cyanobacterium *Cylindrospermopsis raciborskii* in tissues of the Redclaw crayfish *Cherax quadricarinatus. Toxicon* 37: 1065–1077.

Saker, M.L., Metcalf, J.S., Codd, G.A., Vasconcelos, V.M., 2004. Accumulation and depuration of the cyanobacterial toxin cylindrospermopsin in the freshwater mussel *Anodonta cygnea. Toxicon* 43: 185–194.

Saker, M.L., Nogueira, I.C., Vasconcelos, V.M., Neilan, B.A., Eaglesham, G.K., Pereira, P., 2003. First report and toxicological assessment of the cyanobacterium *Cylindrospermopsis raciborskii* from Portuguese freshwaters. *Ecotoxicology Environmental Safety* 55: 243–250.

Schembri, M.A., Neilan, B.A., Saint, C.P., 2001. Identification of genes implicated in toxin production in the cyanobacterium *Cylindrospermopsis raciborskii. Environmental Toxicology* 16: 413–421.

Seifert, M., 2007. *The Ecological Effects of the Cyanobacterial Toxin Cylindrospermopsin*. The University of Queensland, Brisbane, Queensland, Australia.

Seifert, M., McGregor, G., Eaglesham, G., Wickramasinghe, W., Shaw, G., 2007. First evidence for the production of cylindrospermopsin and deoxy-cylindrospermopsin by the freshwater benthic cyanobacterium, *Lyngbya wollei* (Farlow ex Gomont) Speziale and Dyck. *Harmful Algae* 6: 73–80.

Senogles, P., Shaw, G., Smith, M., Norris, R., Chiswell, R., Mueller, J., Sadler, R., Eaglesham, G., 2000. Degradation of the cyanobacterial toxin cylindrospermopsin, from *Cylindrospermopsis raciborskii*, by chlorination. *Toxicon* 38: 1203–1213.

Senogles-Derham, P.J., Seawright, A., Shaw, G., Wickramisingh, W., Shahin, M., 2003. Toxicological aspects of treatment to remove cyanobacterial toxins from drinking water determined using the heterozygous P53 transgenic mouse model. *Toxicon* 41: 979–988.

Shalev-Alon, G., Sukenik, A., Livnah, O., Schwarz, R., Kaplan, A., 2002. A novel gene encoding amidino-transferase in the cylindrospermopsin producing cyanobacterium *Aphanizonmeon ovalisporum*. *FFMS Microbiology Letters* 209: 87–91.

Shaw, G.R., Sukenik, A., Livne, A., Chiswell, R.K., Smith, M.J., Seawright, A.A., Norris, R.L., Eaglasham, G.K., Moore, M.R., 1999. Blooms of cylindrospermopsin containing cyanobacterium, *Aphanidizinium ovalisporum* (Forti), in newly constructed lakes, Queensland, Australia. *Environmental Toxicology* 14: 167–177.

Smith, J.L., Boyer, G.L., Zimba, P.V., 2008. A review of cyanobacterial odorous and bioactive metabolites: Impacts and management alternatives in aquaculture. *Aquaculture* 280: 5–20.

Smith, M.J., Shaw, G.R., Chriswell, R.K., Seawright, A.A., Norris, R.L., Eaglesham, G.K., Moore, M.R., 1998. *Aphanizomenon ovalisporum*, a cyanobacterium producing the toxin cylindrospermopsin in Queensland, Australia, *4th International Toxic Cyanobacteria Symposium*, Beaufort, NC.

Soler, C., Hamilton, B., Furey, A., James, K.J., Manes, J., Pico, Y., 2006. Optimisation of LC-MS/MS using triple quadrupole mass analyser for the simultaneous analysis of carbosulfan and its main metabolites in oranges. *Analytica Chimca Acta* 571: 1–11.

Soler, C., Hamilton, B., Furey, A., James, K.J., Mañes, J., Picó, Y., 2007. Liquid chromatography quadrupole time-of-flight mass spectrometry analysis of carbosulfan, carbofuran, 3-hydroxycarbofuran, and other metabolites in food. *Analytical Chemistry* 79: 1492–1501.

Spoof, L., Berg, K.A., Rapala, J., Lahti, K., Lepisto, L., Metcalf, J.S., Codd, G.A., Meriluoto, J., 2006. First observation of cylindrospermopsin in *Anabaena lapponica* isolated from the boreal environment (Finland). *Environmental Toxicology* 21: 552–560.

Stirling, D.J., Quilliam, M.A., 2001. First report of the cyanobacterial toxin cylindrospermopsin in New Zealand. *Toxicon* 39: 1219–1222.

Terao, K., Ohmori, S., Igarashi, K., Ohtani, I., Watanabe, M.F., Harada, K.I., Ito, E., Watanabe, M., 1994. Electron microscopic studies on experimental poisoning in mice induced by cylindrospermopsin isolated from blue-green alga *Umezakia Natans*. *Toxicon* 32: 883–843.

Törökne, A., Asztalos, M., Bankine, M., Bickel, H., Borbely, G., Carnmeli, S. et al., 2004. Interlaboraotry comparison trial on cylindrospermopsin measurement. *Analytical Biochemistry* 332: 280–284.

Valerio, E., Abrantes, L.M., Viana, A.S., 2008. 4-Aminothiophenol self-assembled monolayer for the development of a DNA biosensor aiming the detection of cylindrospermopsin producing cyanobacteria. *Electroanalysis* 20: 2467–2474.

Van Apeldoorn, M.E., Van Egmond, H.P., Speijers, G.J.A., Bakker, G.J.I., 2007. Toxins of cyanobacteria. *Molecular Nutrition & Food Research* 51: 7–60.

Vasas, G., Gáspár, A., Surányi, G., Batta, G., Gyémánt, G., M-Hamvas, M., Máthé, C., Grigorszky, I., Molnár, E., Borbély, G., 2002. Capillary electrophoretic assay and purification of cylindrospermopsin, a cyanobacterial toxin from *Aphanizomenon ovalisporum*, by plant test (blue-green sinapis test). *Analytical Biochemistry* 302: 95–103.

Viglino, L., Aboulfadl, K., Prévost, M., Sauvé, S., 2008. Analysis of natural and synthetic estrogenic endocrine disruptors in environmental waters using online preconcentration coupled with LC-APPI-MS/MS. *Talanta* 76: 1088–1096.

Vilarino, N., Fonfria, E.S., Louzao, M.C., Botana, L.M., 2009. Use of biosensors as alternatives to current regulatory methods for marine biotoxins. *Sensors* 9: 9414–9443.

Watson, J.T., Sparkman, O.D. 2007. *Introduction to Mass Spectrometry: Instrumentation, Applications, and Strategies for Data Interpretation*, 4th edition. Hoboken, NJ: John Wiley & Sons.

Welker, M., Bickela, H., Fastner, J., 2002. HPLC-PDA detection of cylindrospermopsin—Opportunities and limits. *Water Research* 36: 4659–4663.

Whelan, M., Kinsella, B., Furey, A., Moloney, M., Cantwell, H., Lehotay, S.J., Danaher, M., 2010. Determination of anthelmintic drug residues in milk using ultra high performance liquid chromatography–tandem mass spectrometry with rapid polarity switching. *Journal of Chromatography A* 1217: 4612–4622.

Whelan, M., O'Mahony, J., Moloney, M., Cooper, K.M., Furey, A., Kennedy, G.D., Danaher, M., 2013. Maximum residue level validation of triclabendazole marker residues in bovine liver, muscle and milk matrices by ultra high pressure liquid chromatography tandem mass spectrometry. *Journal of Chromatography A*. 1275, 41–47.

White, S.H., Duivenvoorden, L.J., Fabbro, L.D., Eaglesham, G.K., 2006. Influence of intracellular toxin concentrations on cylindrospermopsin bioaccumulation in a freshwater gastropod (*Melanoides tuberculata*). *Toxicon* 47: 497–509.

White, S.H., Duivenvoorden, L.J., Fabbro, L.D., Eaglesham, G.K., 2007. Mortality and toxin bioaccumulation in Bufo marinus following exposure to *Cylindrospermopsis raciborskii* cell extracts and live cultures. *Environmental Pollution* 147: 158–167.

WHO/UNICEF, 2011. Drinking water equity, safety and sustainability: Thematic report on drinking water 2011, JMP Thematic Report on Drinking Water WHO/UNICEF Joint Monitoring Programme for Water Supply and Sanitation (JMP), pp. 1–61.

Wood, S.A., Stirling, D.J., 2003. First identification of the cylindrospermopsin-producing cyanobacterium *Cylindrospermopsis raciborskii* in New Zealand. *New Zealand Journal of Marine and Freshwater Research* 37: 821–828.

Wormer, L., Cires, S., Carrasco, D., Quesada, A., 2008. Cylindrospermopsin is not degraded by co-occurring natural bacterial communities during a 40-day study. *Harmful Algae* 7: 206–213.

Yilmaz, M., Phlips, E.J., Szabo, N.J., Badylak, S., 2008. A comparative study of Florida strains of cylindrospermopsis and aphanizomenon for cylindrospermopsin production. *Toxicon* 51: 130–139.

37

Anatoxin: Chemistry, Effects, Source, Metabolism, and Detection

Justine Dauphard, Mary Lehane, Frank van Pelt, John O'Halloran, and Ambrose Furey

CONTENTS

37.1 Anatoxins: Cyanobacterial Neurotoxins

Several species of cyanobacteria including *Anabaena* sp. (*A. flos-aquae* [Carmichael et al., 1975; Devlin et al., 1977; Furey et al., 2003b; Gallon et al., 1994; Harada et al., 1993; Kangatharalingam and Priscu, 1993; Sivonen et al., 1989], *A. circinalis* [Sivonen et al., 1989], *A. planctonica* [Bruno et al., 1994], *A. mendotae* [Rapala et al., 1993]); *Oscillatoria* sp. (Araóz et al., 2005) (*O. agardhii* [Sivonen et al., 1989], *O. formosa* [Araóz et al., 2005; Skulberg et al., 1992]); *Microcystis* sp. (*M. aeruginosa* [Harada et al., 1993]); *Raphidiopsis* sp. (*R. mediterranea* [Namikoshi et al., 2003; Watanabe et al., 2003]); *Planktothrix* (*P. rubescens* [Viaggiu et al., 2004]); *Arthrospira* sp. (*A. fusiformes* [Ballot et al., 2004]); *Nostoc* sp. (*N. carneum* [Ghassempour et al., 2005]); *Phormidium* sp. (*P. favosum* [Gugger et al., 2005]); and *Aphanizomenon* sp. (Sivonen et al., 1989) produce potent neurotoxins that can induce severe poisoning in vivo (James et al., 2008; Osswald et al., 2007). Anatoxin-a (AN) and homoanatoxin (HMAN) are two powerful nicotinic agonists (Thomas et al., 1993; Wonnacott et al., 1992). Symptoms of AN and HMAN toxicosis include tremors, convulsions, muscle fasciculations, and rapid (within 30 min) death due to respiratory failure (Adams and Swanson, 1994; Carmichael and Gorham, 1974; Carmichael et al., 1975, 1977; Stevens and Krieger, 1991a). Postmortem investigations of animals exposed to these toxins show that extensive organ damage is not a significant feature of their toxicological effects (Gunn et al., 1992; Park et al., 1993; Sivonen et al., 1989).

There are, in fact, three main categories of cyanobacterial borne neurotoxins: (1) anatoxin-a (AN) and analogues, (2) anatoxin-a(s), and (3) saxitoxin and analogues (Anon, 2008; WHO, 1998, 1999). The focus of this review is on AN and its analogues.

37.1.1 Chemistry

AN was first detected from a bloom of *A. flos-aquae* in the 1960s (Gorham, 1964), and due to its potency it was originally called very fast death factor (VFDF) (Carmichael and Gorham, 1974). Initial studies indicated that the toxin was a low-molecular-weight amine. Devlin et al. (1977) subsequently isolated

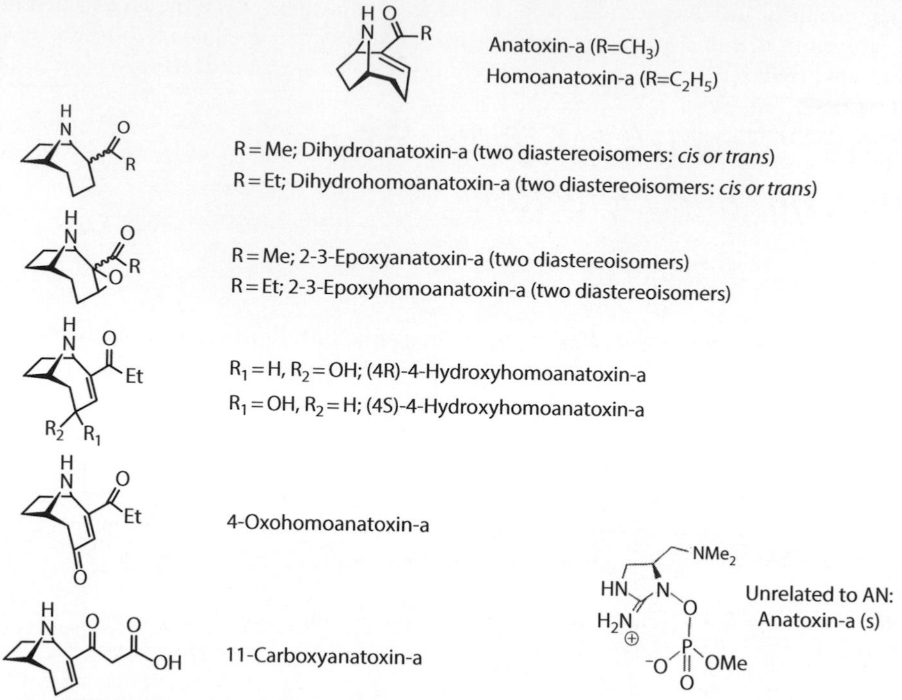

Anatoxin-a (R=CH₃)
Homoanatoxin-a (R=C₂H₅)

R = Me; Dihydroanatoxin-a (two diastereoisomers: *cis or trans*)
R = Et; Dihydrohomoanatoxin-a (two diastereoisomers: *cis or trans*)

R = Me; 2-3-Epoxyanatoxin-a (two diastereoisomers)
R = Et; 2-3-Epoxyhomoanatoxin-a (two diastereoisomers)

R₁ = H, R₂ = OH; (4R)-4-Hydroxyhomoanatoxin-a
R₁ = OH, R₂ = H; (4S)-4-Hydroxyhomoanatoxin-a

4-Oxohomoanatoxin-a

11-Carboxyanatoxin-a

Unrelated to AN:
Anatoxin-a (s)

FIGURE 37.1 Chemical structures of AN-a, HMAN-a, and their known natural derivatives. Included also is the structure of ANs. (From Kellman, R. et al., Neurotoxic alkaloids from cyanobacteria, in: Ramawat, K.G. and Merillon, J.M., eds., *Handbook of Natural Products*, Springer-Verlag, Berlin, Germany, DOI 10.1007/1978-1003-1642-22144-22146_22147, 2013.)

and determined AN to be a bicyclic secondary amine incorporating an α,β-unsaturated ketone moiety. The structure was later corroborated by x-ray crystallography (Huber, 1972). AN is a naturally occurring alkaloid with the characteristic homotropane core of 9-azabicyclo[4.2.1]non-2-ene; its full systematic name is (propan-1-oxo-1-yl)-9-azabicyclo[4.2.1]non-2-ene (Figure 37.1).

In 1992, a methylene analogue of AN designated HMAN-a was isolated from *O. formosa* in Norway by Skulberg et al. (1992). In toxicological trials, HMAN demonstrated signs of poisoning in mice consistent with AN. Like AN, HMAN is a powerful neuromuscular blocking agent with an LD₅₀ of 250 μg/kg (i.p.). HMAN exhibits the same mode of action as AN (Aas et al., 1996; Lilleheil et al., 1997).

AN and HMAN undergo rapid chemical degradation in nature, the main degradation products are dihydro and epoxy analogues (Figure 37.1) (Harada et al., 1989; Smith and Lewis, 1987; Stevens and Krieger, 1991b). In 2003, Namikoshi identified a new HMAN-a derivative assigned by spectroscopic investigation as 4-hydroxyhomoanatoxin-a from the cyanobacteria *R. mediterranea* (Namikoshi et al., 2003; Osswald et al., 2007). In 2007 Selwood et al. discovered another AN derivative, 11-carboxyl AN, in a strain of *Aph. issatschenkoi* (CAWBG02), which was cultured for AN production and which was then acidified; it is believed that this compound is a biosynthetic precursor in the production of AN (Selwood et al., 2007). This corroborated previous findings by Hemscheidt that predicted, from radiolabeled studies, that 11-carboxyl intermediates were involved in the biosynthesis of the toxin (Hemscheidt et al., 1995). Figure 37.1 shows the naturally occurring AN and HMAN derivatives identified to date. The known degradation products of AN and HMAN are not believed to be significantly toxic (James et al., 1998b, 2007; Osswald et al., 2007; Stevens and Krieger, 1991b).

The biosynthetic pathways of AN and HMAN have been studied by feeding experiments using radiolabeled precursors (Namikoshi et al., 2004). The homotropane portion of AN is thought to originate from glutamic acid or ornithine; the C1 carboxylic acid of the glutamate is retained within the carbon structure of AN. The remainder of the carbon skeleton originates from acetate, while the C12 methyl group of HMAN originates from S-methylmethionine, a derivative of the essential amino acid methionine (Gallon et al., 1990, 1994; Hemscheidt et al., 1995; Namikoshi et al., 2003; Wonnacott and Gallagher, 2006).

Animal studies of samples of cyanobacterial blooms conducted in western Canada in the 1970s identified another toxin in strains of *A. flos-aquae*. It produced several symptoms that were coincident with AN. However, in addition to the typical symptoms of AN poisoning, this new toxin also induced profuse salivation and lachrymation in mice, rats, and chicks (in rats specifically it also produced chromodacryorrhea: bloody tears). On account of the extreme salivation effects, it is abbreviated AN-a(s) (Figure 37.1). This toxin is not, in fact, structurally related to AN. AN-a(s) is a unique *N*-hydroxyguanidine methyl phosphate ester (Cook et al., 1988, 1989b, 1990; Devic et al., 2002; Dörr et al., 2010; Henriksen et al., 1997; Hyde and Carmicheal, 1991; Mahmood and Carmichael, 1986; Matsunaga et al., 1989b; Molica et al., 2005; Moore et al., 1992; Onodera et al., 1997; Villatte et al., 2002). AN and AN-a(s) are not only chemically distinct but they have different bioactivities. AN-a(s) is an acetylcholinesterase inhibitor with an LD_{50} of approximately 50 µg/kg bw (i.p. mouse) (Mahmood and Carmichael, 1986a, 1987; Matsunaga et al., 1989a). Several animal and bird deaths worldwide have been attributed to AN-a(s) (Becker et al., 2010; Cook et al., 1989a; Henriksen et al., 1997; Mahamood et al., 1988; Molica et al., 2005; Onodera et al., 1997).

37.2 Effects

AN and HMAN are potent (LD_{50} = 200–250 µg/kg: mouse, i.p.), postsynaptic, depolarizing, neuromuscular blocking agents that affect mainly the nicotinic receptors (Aas et al., 1996; Adams and Swanson, 1994; Carmichael and Gorham, 1978; Carmichael et al., 1975, 1979; Lilleheil et al., 1997).

AN acts by attaching to the nicotinic ACh receptors of Torpedo electric tissue (Aronstam and Witkop, 1981). ACh is a key cationic neurotransmitter that acts in both the peripheral nervous system (PNS), to activate muscles, and the central nervous system (CNS) where it plays a critical role in memory and sensory functions.

The protonated form of AN, (+)-AN, dominates at physiological pH; (+)-AN exerts its most lethal effects as a nicotinic agonist; it is about 20 times more potent than ACh (Fawell et al., 1999).

When ACh is released by nerve cells that control the muscle cells, it binds to postsynaptic nicotinic receptor, which is a ligand-gated ion channel. Activation of the receptor by ACh results in the opening of the ion channel causing an influx of ions that induces muscle cells to contract. ACh in the synaptic cleft is quickly degraded by the enzyme acetylcholinesterase, thus preventing overstimulation of the muscle cells. However, AN and HMAN cannot be degraded by acetylcholinesterase or by any other enzyme in eukaryotic cells so they remain active and overstimulate the muscle (Carmichael, 1994), which leads to very rapid death from respiratory failure (Beasley et al., 1989; Carmichael, 1988; Skulberg et al., 1992). It is important to highlight that there is a high degree of interspecies variability to the effects of the toxins; some species appear to have a higher tolerance than others (Osswald et al., 2007).

37.3 Sources and Metabolism

AN is known to be produced by several strains of blue-green algae: *A. flos-aquae, Aphanizomenon, Microcystis, Raphidiopsis, and Oscillatoria* (Osswald et al., 2007).

AN is unstable under natural conditions and is naturally degraded either partially or totally to the nontoxic products dihydroanatoxin-a and epoxyanatoxin-a, depending on environmental conditions (James et al., 1988a,b, 2005; Stevens and Krieger, 1991b). Studies using laboratory-cultured cyanobacteria combined with reported observations from natural blooms indicate that environmental factors (fluctuations in light, temperature, pH, and nutrients), as well as physical factors (algae buoyancy, weather conditions, and water currents), lead to significant differences in cyanobacterial composition and toxicity (Rapala et al., 1993). Other variables like the age of the cells, their tendency to break open and release toxins, high copper levels, and natural detoxification mechanisms also affect the toxicological profiles of cyanobacterial blooms (Carmichael and Gorham, 1980; Stevens and Krieger, 1991a). Therefore, AN and HMAN can disappear very quickly, sometimes within hours of a toxic occurrence (Furey et al., 2003b; Smith and Lewis, 1987; Stevens and Krieger, 1991b).

Rapala et al. compared the effects of sterilized sediments with non-sterilized sediments and observed that in vials with the sterilized sediments, AN persisted throughout the experiment, while in the vials containing the non-sterilized sediment, the AN concentration decreased significantly. The authors surmised that microbial activity also has a role to play in AN decomposition (Kiviranta et al., 1991; Rapala et al., 1994). In another experiment, a sample that was collected (and not frozen) from a lake was collected and tested directly by Gas Chromatography-Mass Spectrometry (GC-MS) and showed the presence of AN; another sample that had been frozen and analyzed some time later contained only trace quantities of AN but significant amounts of dihydro-AN (Smith and Lewis, 1987).

An HMAN derivative, 4-hydroxy-HMAN, was also identified in a strain of *R. mediterranea* (Namikoshi et al., 2003). This would suggest that analytical methods should examine water samples for the breakdown products as well as for the main precursor toxins (Furey et al., 2003a, 2005; James et al., 1998b, 2005), as this rapid degradation of the AN and HMAN may lead to underreporting of toxic incidents. Underestimation of the main toxins is a substantial risk, especially where Liquid Chromatography-Mass Spectrometry (LC-MS) is used, as toxin degradation destroys the unsaturated ketone moiety, which is the active toxin's key chromophore (Harada et al., 1989; Smith and Lewis, 1987; Stevens and Krieger, 1991b).

37.4 Incidents

AN was first discovered in Canada (Devlin et al., 1977; Gorham et al., 1964) in 1964; since then it has been found in numerous types of water bodies (including lakes, rivers, and estuaries) worldwide. ANs have been identified throughout Europe, Asia, South Africa, Australia, South America, western Canada, and Midwestern United States. A comprehensive listing and convenient tabulation of events have been published by James et al. (2007), Osswald et al. (2007), and Kellman et al. (2013). That AN and HMAN pose a threat to human and animal health from water bodies is beyond doubt (via ingestion, spray inhalation, and skin contact); these toxins also pose a threat in so-called dietary supplements (Rellán et al., 2009; Wood et al., 2007). In 2009, several dietary cyanobacterial-based nutrition supplements labeled as containing *Spirulina* (an unlikely progenitor of AN) but suspected of being contaminated with *Arthrospira* (a morphologically similar cyanobacteria and a known producer of AN) were found to contain AN (Heussner et al., 2012; Rellán et al., 2009).

37.5 Detection

Animal bioassays, in particular the mouse bioassay, have been applied to the detection of the ANs in samples and extracts. Usually, the pure toxin or the extract from a suspected toxic bloom is administered to (intraperitoneally (i.p.) or rats (oral administration) (Adeyemo and Siren, 1992; Al-Layl et al., 1988; Astrachan and Archer, 1981; Astrachan et al., 1980; Baker and Humpage, 1994; Lahti et al., 1995; Stevens and Krieger, 1988; Watanabe et al., 2003). The test relies on the observation of the classical symptoms of AN poisoning outlined in Section 37.2 of this review. In general, live animal bioassays are criticized for poor sensitivity and their inadequacy at determining actual levels of the toxin present in a given sample (this is a worry where concentrations of the toxin may be at levels dangerous to health; this test cannot discriminate between moderate and high toxin levels) and for the unnecessary suffering that they inflict on the animals involved (Al-Layl et al., 1988; Stevens and Krieger, 1988).

Methods are currently being refined to synthesize an analogue of AN for monoclonal antibody production that could be incorporated into a bioassay kit for detecting AN (Marc et al., 2009).

GC-MS was the first instrumental analytical method applied to the detection of AN and HMAN (Devlin et al., 1977). Most of the early GC-MS approaches were based on the Devlin et al. method where the toxins were determined using their N-acetyl derivatives (Devlin et al., 1977; Himberg, 1989; Ross et al., 1989; Smith and Lewis, 1987). Liquid chromatography (LC) with ultraviolet (UV) detection has also been used to determine the ANs. AN and HMAN conveniently display a strong absorbance at 227 nm (log $\varepsilon = 4.10$) as a consequence of the α,β-unsaturated ketone group. However, UV detection methods are prone to interference from extraneous materials in real samples, which can compromise sensitivity and selectivity (Harada et al., 1989). Furthermore, the dihydro- and epoxy-degradation products of AN and HMAN do not possess the unsaturated ketone chromophore in their structures so cannot be detected by UV methods. Considering the propensity of AN and HMAN to degrade and the speed with which they do degrade, this is a very serious deficiency for their analyses by methods using UV detection (Edwards et al., 1992; Furey et al., 2003b; Harada et al., 1989; James et al., 2008; Namikoshi et al., 2003; Powell, 1997; Rapala et al., 1994; Wong and Hindin, 1982; Zotou et al., 1993).

Liquid chromatography with fluorescence detection (LC-FLD) offers many advantages and has been often used to test for AN and its associated analogues (James and Furey, 2000; James and Sherlock, 1996; James et al., 1997b, 1998b; Rawn et al., 2005; Rellán et al., 2007). A highly sensitive method was developed by James et al. (James et al., 1997a, 1998b), where AN and HMAN and their degradation products were devitalized using 4-fluoro-7-nitro-2,1,3-benzoadiazole (NBD-F) before LC-FLD analysis. The advantage of this particular reagent is that NBD-F is not strongly fluorescent until it binds to the target analyte; this removes the necessity of a protracted sample cleanup step. In 2002, Namera and Pawlisayn developed an AN method based on solid-phase microextraction (SPME) coupled with high-performance LC with fluorescence detection and on-fiber derivatization (Namera et al., 2002).

Rawn et al. (2005) used NBD-F to incorporate into a SPME-based method to determine the AN and associated compounds in algal extracts. Rellán et al. (2007) found that the LODs obtained for SPME-LC-FLD were poorer than those obtained by SPME (SPE)-LC-FLD due to the lower sample volumes used with SPME. However, the primary drawback of using NBD-F for the analysis of the anatoxins and analogues is that the reagent reacts with many primary amines, which may lead to overestimation of the toxins in samples or indeed give false-positive results (Rawn et al., 2005); additionally, sample cleanup strategies may inadvertently concentrate both the toxin and matrix interferences during the extraction process (Namera et al., 2002; Rellán et al., 2007).

It is fair to assert that LC-multiple tandem MS is the best method for determining the ANs (Dahlmann et al., 2003; Furey et al., 2003a; Harada et al., 1993; Hormazábal et al., 2000; Poon et al., 1993; Takino et al., 1999). However, the LC-MS analysis of the AN has not been without its own particular difficulties; it is hampered by the ubiquitous presence of the amino acid phenylalanine (Phe), which not only has the same nominal mass as AN but also has a similar chromatographic retention profile (Furey et al., 2005). Several methods have been developed to overcome this nuisance (Dimitrakopoulos et al., 2010; Furey et al., 2005). Much work has been done by James et al. (2005) and Furey et al. (2003a) to elucidate the fragmentation pathways of the ANs using LC-quadrupole ion trap (QIT) MS and LC-quadrupole time-of-flight (QqTOF MS) to facilitate the identification of key fragmentation ions that allow for the unequivocal identification of these toxins in samples. Other more focused methods have also been deployed to overcome Phe interference (Furey et al., 2005). Similar to all analytical applications, ion suppression is also an important consideration when applying LC-MS to the analysis of lake water, bloom samples, freeze-dried algae, and tissue samples for AN, HMAN, and its degradation products. Furey et al. (2013) have just published a review paper on the causes, evaluation, and prevention of ion suppression along with suggested applications to minimize its effect.

A detailed review of selected analytical methods used to determine AN and associated compounds was published in 2008 (Anon, 2008; de la Cruz et al., 2008; James et al., 2008), which summarizes the best AN methods up to 2005. Kellman et al. (2013) and Osswald et al. (2007) have amassed and tabulated succinctly the best of the analytical methods applied to AN analysis up to 2012.

ACKNOWLEDGMENTS

The authors acknowledge the funding obtained under the EU/INTERREG IIIB Atlantic Area Programme for projects titled ATLANTOX "Advanced Tests about New Toxins Occurring in the Atlantic Area due to Climate Change" and PHARMATLANTIC "Knowledge Transfer Network for Prevention of Mental Diseases and Cancer in the Atlantic Area." The Higher Education Authority (Programme for Research in Third-Level Institutions, Cycle 4 (PRTLI IV)) National Collaboration Programme on Environment and Climate Changes: Impacts and Responses is also acknowledged for funding the PhD studies of JD. Finally, A. Furey acknowledges the European Cooperation in Science and Technology, COST Action ES 1105 "CYANOCOST—Cyanobacterial blooms and toxins in water resources: Occurrence, impacts and management" for adding value to this study through networking and knowledge sharing with European experts and researchers in the field.

REFERENCES

Aas, P., Eriksen, S., Kolderup, J., Lundy, P., Haugen, J.-E., Skulberg, O.M., Fonnum, F., 1996. Enhancement of acetylcholine release by homoanatoxin-a from *Oscillatoria formosa. Environ. Toxicol. Pharmacol.* 2: 223–232.

Adams, M.E., Swanson, G., 1994. *Trends in Neurosciences Neurotoxins Supplement.* Elsevier Science.

Adeyemo, O.M., Siren, A.L., 1992. Cardio-respiratory changes and mortality in the conscious rat induced by (±)- and (±/-)-anatoxin-a. *Toxicon* 30: 899–905.

Al-Layl, K., Poon, G., Codd, G., 1988. Isolation and purification of peptide and alkaloid toxins from Anabaena flos-aquae using high performance thin-layer chromatography. *J. Microbiol. Methods* 7: 251–258.

Anon., 2008. *Cyanobacterial Harmful Algal Blooms: State of the Sciences and Research Needs*, Springer Advances in Experimental Medicine and Biology. New York: Springer.

Araóz, R., Nghiem, H.O., Rippka, R., Palibroda, N., de Marsac, N.T., Herdman, M., 2005. Neurotoxins in axenic oscillatorian cyanobacteria: Coexistence of anatoxin-alpha and homoanatoxin-alpha determined by ligand-binding assay and GC/MS. *Microbiol.-Sgm* 151: 1263–1273.

Aronstam, R.S., Witkop, B., 1981. Anatoxin-a interactions with cholinergic synaptic molecules. *Proc. Natl. Acad. Sci.* 78: 4639.

Astrachan, N.B., Archer, B.G., 1981. Simplified monitoring of anatoxin-a by reverse phase high performance liquid chromatography and sub-acute effects of anatoxin-a in rats. In: Carmicheal, W.W. (ed.), *The Water Environment: Algal Toxins and Health*, pp. 437–446. New York: Plenum Press.

Astrachan, N.B., Archer, B.G., Hilbelink, D.R., 1980. Evaluation of the sub-acute toxicity and teratogenicity of anatoxin-a. *Toxicon* 18: 684–688.

Baker, P.D., Humpage, A.R., 1994. Toxicity associated with commonly occurring cyanobacteria in surface waters of the Murray-Darling Basin, Australia. *Aust. J. Mar. Freshwster. Res.* 45: 773–786.

Ballot, A., Krienitz, L., Kotut, K., Wiegand, C., Metcalf, J.S., Codd, G.A., Pflugmacher, S., 2004. Cyanobacteria and cyanobacterial toxins in three alkaline rift valley lakes of Kenya—Lakes Bogoria, Nakuru and Elmenteita. *J. Plankton Res.* 26: 925–935.

Beasley, V.R., Cook, W.O., Dahlem, A.M., Hooser, S.B., Lovell, R.A., Valentine, W.M., 1989. Algae intoxication in livestock and water fowl. *Clin. Toxicol.* 5: 345–361.

Becker, V., Ihara, P., Yunes, J.S., Huszar, V.L.M., 2010. Occurrence of anatoxin-a(s) during a bloom of *Anabaena crassa* in a water supply reservoir in southern Brazil. *J. Appl. Phycol.* 22: 235–241.

Bruno, M., Barbani, D., Pierdominici, E., Serse, A., Ioppolo, A., 1994. Anatoxin-a and a previously unknown toxin in *Anabaena Planctonica* blooms found in lake Mulargia (Italy). *Toxicon* 32: 369–373.

Carmichael, W.W., 1988. Toxins of freshwater algae. In: Hardegree, M.C., Tu, A.T. (eds.), *Handbook of Natural Toxins: Bacterial Toxins*, Vol. 4, pp. 121–147. New York: Marcel Dekker.

Carmichael, W.W., 1994. The toxins of cyanobacteria. *Sci. Am.* 270: 64–72.

Carmichael, W.W., Biggs, D.F., Gorham, P.R., 1975. Toxicology and pharmacological action of anabaena flos-aquae toxin. *Science* 187: 542–544.

Carmichael, W.W., Biggs, D.F., Peterson, M.A., 1979. Pharmacology of anatoxin-a, produced by freshwater cyanophyte Anabaena flos-aquae NRC-44-1. *Toxicon* 17: 229–236.

Carmichael, W.W., Gorham, P.R., 1974. An improved method for obtaining axenic clones of planktonic blue-green algae. *J. Phycol.* 10: 238–241.

Carmichael, W.W., Gorham, P.R., 1978. Anatoxins from clones of *Anabaena flos-aquae* isolated from lakes in western Canada. *Mitt. Int. Ver. Theor. Angew. Limnol.* 21: 285–295.

Carmichael, W.W., Gorham, P.R., 1980. Freshwater cyanophyte toxins: Types and their effects on the use of micro algae biomass. In: Shelef, G., Soeder, C.J. (eds.), *Algae Biomass: Production and Use*, pp. 437–438. Amsterdam, the Netherlands: Elsevier.

Carmichael, W.W., Gorham, P.R., Biggs, D.F., 1977. Two laboratory case studies on the oral toxicity to calves of the freshwater cyanocytes (blue green algae) *Anabaena flos-aquae* NRC-44-1. *Can. Vet. J.* 18: 71–75.

Cook, W., Beasley, V., Dahlem, A., Dellinger, J., Harlin, K., Carmichael, W., 1988. Comparison of effects of anatoxin-a(s) and paraoxon, physostigmine and pyridostigmine on mouse-brain cholinesterase activity. *Toxicon* 26: 750–753.

Cook, W., Beasley, V., Lovell, R., Dahlem, A., Hooser, S., Mahamood, N., Carmichael, W., 1989a. Consistent inhibition of peripheral cholinesterase by neurotoxins from the freshwater cyanobacterium *Anabaena flos-aquae*: Studies of duck, swine, mice and steer. *Environ. Toxicol. Chem.* 8: 915–922.

Cook, W.O., Dellinger, J.A., Singh, S.S., Dahlem, A.M., Carmichael, W.W., Beasley, V.R., 1989b. Regional brain cholinesterase activity in rats injected intraperitoneally with anatoxin-a(s) or paraoxon. *Toxicol. Lett.* 49(1): 29–34.

Cook, W.O., Iwamoto, G.A., Schaeffer, D.J., Carmichael, W.W., Beasley, V.R., 1990. Pathophysiologic effects of anatoxin-a(s) in anesthetized rats—The influence of atropine and artificial-respiration. *Pharmacol. Toxicol.* 67: 151–155.

Dahlmann, J., Budakowski, W.R., Luckas, B., 2003. Liquid chromatography-electrospray ionisation-mass spectrometry based method for the simultaneous determination of algal and cyanobacterial toxins in phytoplankton from marine waters and lakes followed by tentative structural elucidation of microcystins. *J. Chromatogr. A* 994: 45–57.

de la Cruz, A.A., Rublee, P., Hungerford, J.M., Zimba, P.V., Wilhelm, S., Meriluoto, J.A.O., Echols, K. et al., 2008. Analytical methods workgroup report (Chapter 20). In: Hudnell, H.K.E. (ed.), *Cyanobacterial Harmful Algal Blooms: State of the Sciences and Research Needs*, pp. 476–481. Springer Advances in Experimental Medicine and Biology, New York: Springer.

Devic, E., Li, D.H., Dauta, A., Henriksen, P., Codd, G.A., Marty, J.L., Fournier, D., 2002. Detection of ana-toxin-a(s) in environmental samples of cyanobacteria by using a biosensor with engineered acetylcholin-esterases. *Appl. Environ. Microbiol.* 68: 4102–4106.

Devlin, J.P., Edwards, O.E., Gorham, P.R., Hunter, N.R., Pike, R.K., Stavric, B., 1977. Anatoxin-a, a toxic alkaloid from *Anabaena flos-aquae* NRC-44h. *Can. J. Chem.* 55: 1367–1371.

Dimitrakopoulos, I.K., Kaloudis, T.S., Hiskia, A.E., Thomaidis, N.S., Koupparis, M.A., 2010. Development of a fast and selective method for the sensitive determination of anatoxin-a in lake waters using liquid chromatography-tandem mass spectrometry and phenylalanine-d5 as internal standard. *Anal. Bioanal. Chem.* 397: 2245–2252.

Dörr, F.A., Rodríguez, V., Molica, R., Henriksen, P., Krock, B., Pinto, E., 2010. Methods for detection of anatoxin-a(s) by liquid chromatography coupled to electrospray ionization-tandem mass spectrometry. *Toxicon* 55: 92–99.

Edwards, C., Beattie, K.A., Scrimgeour, C.M., Codd, G.A., 1992. Identification of anatoxin-a in benthic cyanobacteria (blue-green algae) and in associated dog poisonings at Loch Insh, Scotland. *Toxicon.* 30: 1165–1175.

Fawell, J.K., Mitchell, R.E., Hill, R.E., Everett, D.J., 1999. The toxicity of cyanobacterial toxins in the mouse: II anatoxin-a. *Hum. Exp. Toxicol.* 18: 168–173.

Furey, A., Crowley, J., Hamilton, B., Lehane, M., James, K.J., 2005. Strategies to avoid the mis-identifica-tion of anatoxin-a using mass spectrometry in the forensic investigation of acute neurotoxic poisoning. *J. Chromatogr. A* 1082: 91–97.

Furey, A., Crowley, J., Lehane, M., James, K.J., 2003a. Liquid chromatography with electrospray ion-trap mass spectrometry for the determination of anatoxins in cyanobacteria and drinking water. *Rapid Commun. Mass Spectrom.* 17: 583–588.

Furey, A., Crowley, J., Shuilleabhain, A.N., Skulberg, A.M., James, K.J., 2003b. The first identification of the rare cyanobacterial toxin, homoanatoxin-a, in Ireland. *Toxicon* 41: 297–303.

Furey, A., Moriarty, M., Vaishali, B., Kinsella, B., Lehane, M., 2013. Ion Suppression: A critical review on causes, evaluation, prevention and applications. *Talanta* 115: 104–122.

Gallon, J.R., Chit, K.N., Brown, E.G., 1990. Biosynthesis of the tropine-related cyanobacterial toxin anatoxin-alpha—Role of ornithine decarboxylase. *Phytochemistry* 29: 1107–1111.

Gallon, J.R., Kittakoop, P., Brown, E.G., 1994. Biosynthesis of anatoxin-a by *Anabaena flos-aquae*: Examination of primary enzymatic steps. *Phytochemistry* 35: 1195–1203.

Ghassempour, A., Najafi, N.M., Mehdinia, A., Davarani, S.S.H., Fallahi, M., Nakhshab, M., 2005. Analysis of anatoxin-a using polyaniline as a sorbent in solid-phase microextraction coupled to gas chromatography-mass spectrometry. *J. Chromatogr. A* 1078: 120–127.

Gorham, P.R., 1964. Toxic algae. In: Jackson, D.F.E. (ed.), *Algae and Man*, pp. 307–336. New York: Plenum Press.

Gorham, P.R., McLachlan, J., Hammer, U.T., Kim, W.K., 1964. Isolation and culture of toxic strains of *Anabaena flos-aquae* (Lyngb.) de Breb. *Mitt. Int. Ver. Limnol.* 15: 796–804.

Gugger, M., Lenoir, S., Berger, C., Ledreux, A., Druart, J.C., Humbert, J.F., Guette, C., Bernard, C., 2005. First report in a river in France of the benthic cyanobacterium *Phormidium favosum* producing anatoxin-a associated with dog neurotoxicosis. *Toxicon* 45: 919–928.

Gunn, G.J., Rafferty, A.G., Rafferty, G.C., Cockburn, N., Edwards, C., Beattie, K.A., Codd, G.A., 1992. Fatal canine neurotoxicosis attributed to blue-green algae (cyanobacteria). *Vet. Rec.* 130: 301–302.

Harada, K., Kimura, I., Ogawa, K., Suzuki, M., Dahlem, A.M., Beasley, V.R., Carmichael, W.W., 1989. A new procedure for the analysis and purification of naturally occurring anatoxin-a from the blue-green alga *Anabaena flos- aquae*. *Toxicon* 27: 1289–1296.

Harada, K.-I., Nagai, H., Kimura, Y., Suzuki, M., Park, H.-D., Watanabe, M., Kuukkainen, R., Sivonen, K., Carmichael, W.W., 1993. Liquid chromatography/mass spectrometric detection of anatoxin-a, a neuro-toxin from cyanobacteria. *Tetrahedron* 49: 9251–9260.

Hemscheidt, T., Rapala, J., Sivonen, K., Skulberg, O.M., 1995. Biosynthesis of anatoxin-a in *Anabaena flos-aquae* and homoanatoxin-a in *Oscillatoria formosa*. *J. Chem. Soc. Chem. Commun.* 13: 1361–1362.

Henriksen, P., Carmichael, W.W., An, J., Moestrup, O., 1997. Detection of an anatoxin-a(s)-like anticholin-esterase in natural blooms and cultures of cyanobacteria/blue-green algae from Danish lakes and in the stomach contents of poisoned birds. *Toxicon* 35: 901–913.

Heussner, A.H., Mazija, L., Fastner, J., Dietrich, D.R., 2012. Toxin content and cytotoxicity of algal dietary supplements. *Toxicol. Appl. Pharmacol.* 265: 263–271.

Himberg, K., 1989. Determination of anatoxin-a, the neurotoxin of Anabaena flos-aquae cyanobacterium, in algae and water by gas chromatography-mass spectrometry. *J. Chromatogr.* 481: 358–362.

Hormazábal, V., Østensvik, Ø., Underdal, B., Skulberg, O.M., 2000. Simultaneous determination of the cyano-toxins anatoxin-a, microcystin desmethyl-e, LR, RR, and YR in fish muscle using liquid chromatography mass spectrometry. *J. Liq. Chromatogr. Rel. Technol.* 23: 185–196.

Huber, C.S., 1972. The crystal structure and absolute configuration of 2,9-diacetyl-9-azabiocyclo(4,2,1)non-2,3-ene. *Acta Crystallogr.* 28: 2577–2582.

Hyde, E.G., Carmicheal, W.W., 1991. Anatoxin-a(s), a naturally occurring organophosphate, is an irre-versible active site directed inhibitor of acetylcholinesterase (EC 3.1.1.7). *J. Biochem. Toxicol.* 6: 195–201.

James, K.J., Crowley, J., Dauphard, J., Lehane, M., Furey, A., 2007. Anatoxin-a and analogues: Discovery, distribution and toxicology. In: Botana, L. (ed.), *Phycotoxins—Chemistry and Biochemistry*, pp. 141–158. Oxford, U.K.: Blackwell Publishing.

James, K.J., Crowley, J., Hamilton, B., Lehane, M., Skulberg, O., Furey, A., 2005. Anatoxins and degradation products, determined using hybrid quadrupole time-of-flight and quadrupole ion-trap mass spectrometry: Forensic investigations of cyanobacterial neurotoxin poisoning. *Rapid Commun. Mass Spectrom.* 19: 1167–1175.

James, K.J., Dauphard, J., Crowley, J., Furey, A., 2008. Cyanobacterial neurotoxins, anatoxin-a and analogues: Detection and analysis. In: Botana, L. (ed.), *Seafood and Freshwater Toxins—Pharmacology, Physiology and Detection*, pp. 809–822. Boca Raton, FL: CRC Press.

James, K.J., Furey, A., 2000. Neurotoxins: Chromatography. In: Wilson, I.D., Adlard, T.R., Poole, C.F., Cook, M. (eds.), *Encyclopedia of Separation Science*, pp. 3482–3490. London, U.K.: Academic Press.

James, K.J., Furey, A., Kelly, S.S., Sherlock, I.R., Stack, M.A., 1997a. The first identification of neurotoxins in freshwaters and shellfish in Ireland. *Toxicon (Abstract)* 35: 811.

James, K.J., Furey, A., Sherlock, I.R., Skulberg, O., Stack, M.A., 1998a. The analysis of the toxic and non-toxic anatoxins from cyanobacteria. In: Reguera, B., Blanco, J., Fernandez, M.L., Wyatt, T. (eds.), *Harmful Algae*, pp. 525–528. Vigo, Spain: Xunta de Galicia and Intergovernmental Oceanographic Commission of UNESCO.

James, K.J., Furey, A., Sherlock, I.R., Stack, M.A., Twohig, M., Caudwell, F.B., Skulberg, O.M., 1998b. Sensitive determination of anatoxin-a, homoanatoxin-a and their degradation products by liquid chromatography with fluorimetric detection. *J. Chromatogr.* 798: 147–157.

James, K.J., Sherlock, I.R., 1996. Determination of the cyanobacterial neurotoxin, anatoxin-a, by derivatisation using 7-fluoro-4-nitro-2,1,3-benzoxadiazole (NBD-F) and HPLC analysis with fluorimetric detection. *Biomed. Chromatogr.* 10: 46–47.

James, K.J., Sherlock, I.R., Stack, M.A., 1997b. Anatoxin-a in Irish freshwaters and cyanobacteria, determined using a new fluorimetric liquid chromatographic method. *Toxicon* 35: 963–971.

Kangatharalingam, N., Priscu, J., 1993. Isolation and verification of anatoxin-a producing clones of *Anabaena flos-aquae* (lyngb.) de Breb. from a eutrophic lake. *FEMS Microbiol. Ecol.* 12: 127–130.

Kellman, R., Ploux, O., Neilan, B., 2013. Neurotoxic alkaloids from cyanobacteria. In: Ramawat, K.G., Merillon, J.M. (eds.), *Handbook of Natural Products*, DOI 10.1007/1978-1003-1642-22144-22146_22147. Berlin, Germany: Springer-Verlag.

Kiviranta, J., Sivonen, K., Lahti, K., Luukkainen, R., Niemelae, S.I., 1991. Production and biodegradation of cyanobacterial toxins-a laboratory study. *Archiv für Hydrobiologie* 121: 281–294.

Lahti, K., Ahtiainen, J., Rapala, J., Sivonen, K., Niemela, S.I., 1995. Assessment of rapid bioassays for detecting cyanobacterial toxicity. *Lett. Appl. Microbiol.* 21: 109–114.

Lilleheil, G., Andersen, R.A., Skulberg, O.M., Alexander, J., 1997. Effects of a homoanatoxin-a-containing extract from *Oscillatoria formosa (Cyanophyceae/* cyanobacteria) on neuromuscular transmission. *Toxicon* 35: 1275–1289.

Mahmood, N.A., Carmichael, W.W., 1986. The pharmacology of anatoxin-a(s), a neurotoxin produced by the freshwater cyanobacterium Anabaena flos-aquae NRC 525-17. *Toxicon* 24: 425–434.

Mahmood, N.A., Carmichael, W.W., 1987. Anatoxin-a(s), an anticholinesterase from the cyanobacterium *Anabaena flos-aquae* NRC 525-17. *Toxicon* 25: 1221–1227.

Mahamood, N., Carmichael, W., Pfhaler, D., 1988. Anticholinesterase poisoning in dogs from a cyanobacterial (blue-green algae) bloom dominated by *Anabaena flos-aquae. Am. J. Vet. Res.* 49: 500–503.

Marc, M., Outurquin, F., Renard, P.-Y., Créminon, C., Franck, X., 2009. Synthesis of a (±)-anatoxin-a analogue for monoclonal antibodies production. *Tetrahedron Lett.* 50: 4554–4557.

Matsunaga, S., Moore, R., Niemczura, W., 1989. Anatoxin-a(s), a potent anticholinesterase from *Anabaena flos-aquae. J. Am. Chem. Soc.* 111: 8021–8023.

Molica, R.J.R., Oliveira, E.J.A., Carvalho, P.V.C., Costa, A., Cunha, M.C.C., Melo, G.L., Azevedo, S., 2005. Occurrence of saxitoxins and an anatoxin-a(s)-like anticholinesterase in a Brazilian drinking water supply. *Harmful Algae* 4: 743–753.

Moore, B.S., Ohtani, I., de Koning, C., Moore, R.E., 1992. Biosynthesis of anatoxin-a(s), origin of the carbons. *Tetrahedron Lett.* 33: 6595–6598.

Namera, A., So, A., Pawliszyn, J., 2002. Analysis of anatoxin-a in aqueous samples by solid-phase microextraction coupled to high-performance liquid chromatography with fluorescence detection and on-fiber derivatization. *J. Chromatogr. A* 963: 295–302.

Namikoshi, M., Murakami, T., Fujiwara, T., Nagai, H., Niki, T., Harigaya, E., Watanabe, M.F., Oda, T., Yamada, J., Tsujimura, S., 2004. Biosynthesis and transformation of homoanatoxin-a in the cyanobacterium *Raphidiopsis mediterranea* Skuja and structures of three new homologues. *Chem. Res. Toxicol.* 17: 1692–1696.

Namikoshi, M., Murakami, T., Watanabe, M.F., Oda, T., Yamada, J., Tsujimura, S., Nagai, H., Oishi, S., 2003. Simultaneous production of homoanatoxin-a, anatoxin-a, and a new non-toxic 4-hydroxyhomoanatoxin-a by the cyanobacterium *Raphidiopsis mediterranea* Skuja. *Toxicon* 42: 533–538.

Onodera, H., Oshima, Y., Henriksen, P., Yasumoto, T., 1997. Confirmation of anatoxin-a(s), in the cyanobacterium *Anabaena lemmermannii*, as the cause of bird kills in Danish lakes. *Toxicon* 35: 1645–1648.

Osswald, J., Rellán, S., Gago-Martinez, A., Vasconcelos, V., 2007. Toxicology and detection methods of the alkaloid neurotoxin produced by cyanobacteria, anatoxin-a. *Environ. Int.* 33: 1070–1089.

Park, H., Watanabe, M., Harada, K., Nagai, H., Suzuki, M., Watanabe, M.F., Hayashi, H., 1993. Hepatotoxin (microcystin) and neurotoxin (anatoxin-a) contained in natural blooms and strains of cyanobacteria from Japanese freshwaters. *Nat. Toxins* 1: 353–360.

Poon, G.K., Griggs, L.J., Edwards, C., Beattie, K.A., Codd, G.A., 1993. Liquid chromatography-electrospray ionization-mass spectrometry of cyanobacterial toxins. *J. Chromatogr.* 628: 215–233.

Powell, M.W., 1997. Analysis of anatoxin-a in aqueous samples. *Chromatographia*: 45: 25–28.

Rapala, J., Lahiti, K., Sivonen, K., Niemelae, S.I., 1994. Biodegradability and adsorption on lake sediments of cyanobacterial hepatotoxins and anatoxin-a. *Lett. Appl. Microbiol.* 19: 423–428.

Rapala, J., Sivonen, K., Luukkainen, R., Niemela, S., 1993. Anatoxin-a concentration in Anabaena and Aphanizomenon under different environmental conditions and comparison of growth by toxic and non-toxic Anabaena-strains—A laboratory study. *J. Appl. Phycol.* 5: 581.

Rawn, D.F.K., Lau, B.P.Y., Niedzwiadek, B., Lawrence, J.F., 2005. Improved method for the determination of anatoxin-a and two of its metabolites in blue-green algae using liquid chromatography with fluorescence detection. *J. AOAC Int.* 88: 1741–1747.

Rellán, S., Osswald, J., Saker, M., Gago-Martinez, A., Vasconcelos, V., 2009. First detection of anatoxin-a in human and animal dietary supplements containing cyanobacteria. *Food Chem. Toxicol.* 47: 2189–2195.

Rellán, S., Osswald, J., Vasconcelos, V., Gago-Martinez, A., 2007. Analysis of anatoxin-a in biological samples using liquid chromatography with fluorescence detection after solid phase extraction and solid phase microextraction. *J. Chromatogr.* 1156: 134–140.

Ross, M.M., Kidwell, D.A., Callahan, J.H., 1989. Mass spectrometric analysis of anatoxin-a. *J. Anal. Toxicol.* 13: 317–321.

Selwood, A.I., Holland, P.T., Wood, S.A., Smith, K.F., McNabb, P.S., 2007. Production of anatoxin-a and a novel biosynthetic precursor by the Cyanobacterium *Aphanizomenon issatschenkoi*. *Environ. Sci. Technol.* 41: 506–510.

Sivonen, K., Himberg, K., Luukkainen, R., Niemela, S.I., Poon, G.K., Codd, G.A., 1989. Preliminary characterization of neurotoxic cyanobacteria blooms and strains from Finland. *Toxic. Assess.* 4: 339–352.

Skulberg, O.M., Carmichael, W.W., Anderson, R.A., Matsunaga, S., Moore, R.E., Skulberg, R., 1992. Investigations of a neurotoxic oscillatorialean strain (Cyanophyceae) and its toxin. Isolation and characterisation of homoanatoxin-a. *Environ. Toxic. Chem.* 11: 321–329.

Smith, R.A., Lewis, D., 1987. A rapid analysis of water for anatoxin-a, the unstable toxic alkaloid from *Anabaena flos-aquae*, the stable non-toxic alkaloids left after bioreduction and a related amine which may be nature's precursor to anatoxin-a. *Vet. Hum. Toxicol.* 29: 153–154.

Stevens, D.K., Krieger, R.I., 1988. Analysis of anatoxin-a by GC/ECD. *J. Anal. Toxicol.* 12: 126–131.

Stevens, D.K., Krieger, R.I., 1991a. Effect of route of exposure and repeated doses on the acute toxicity in mice of the cyanobacterial nicotinic alkaloid anatoxin-A. *Toxicon* 29: 134–138.

Stevens, D.K., Krieger, R.I., 1991b. Stability studies on the cyanobacterial nicotinic alkaloid anatoxin-a. *Toxicon* 29: 167–179.

Takino, M., Daishima, S., Yamaguchi, K., 1999. Analysis of anatoxin-a in freshwaters by automated on-line derivatization-liquid chromatography-electrospray mass spectrometry. *J. Chromatogr.* 862: 191–197.

Thomas, P., Stephens, M., Wilkie, G., Amar, M., Lunt, G.G., Whiting, P., Gallagher, T. et al., 1993. (±)-Anatoxin-a is a potent agonist at neuronal nicotinic acetylcholine receptors. *J. Neurochem.* 60: 2308–2311.

Viaggiu, E., Melchiorre, S., Volpi, F., Di Corcia, A., Mancini, R., Garibaldi, L., Crichigno, G., Bruno, M., 2004. Anatoxin-A toxin in the cyanobacterium *Planktothrix rubescens* from a fishing pond in northern Italy. *Environ. Toxicol.* 19: 191–197.

Villatte, F., Schulze, H., Schmid, R.D., Bachmann, T.T., 2002. A disposable acetylcholinesterase-based electrode biosensor to detect anatoxin-a(s) in water. *Anal. Bioanal. Chem.* 372: 322–326.

Watanabe, M.F., Tsujimura, S., Oishi, S., Niki, T., Namikoshi, M., 2003. Isolation and identification of homoanatoxin-a from a toxic strain of the cyanobacterium *Raphidiopsis mediterranea* Skuja isolated from Lake Biwa, Japan. *Phycologia* 42: 364–369.

WHO, 1998. *Guidelines for Drinking Water Quality*, 2nd edn., Addendum to volume 2, health criteria and other supporting information. Geneva, Switzerland: World Health Organisation.

WHO, 1999. In: Chorus, I., Bartram, J. (eds.), *Toxic Cyanobacteria in Water: A Guide to Their Public Health Consequences, Monitoring and Management*. London, U.K.: E & FN Spon.

Wong, H.S., Hindin, E., 1982. Detecting an algal toxin by high-pressure liquid chromatography. *J. Am. Water Works Assoc.* 74: 528–529.

Wonnacott, S., Gallagher, T., 2006. The chemistry and pharmacology of anatoxin-a and related homotropanes with respect to Nicotinic Acetylcholine Receptors. *Mar. Drugs* 4: 228–254.

Wonnacott, S., Swanson, K.L., Albuguerque, E.X., Huby, N.J.S., Thomson, P., Gallaghers, T., 1992. Homoanatoxin: A potent analogue of anatoxin-a. *Biochem. Pharmacol.* 43: 419–423.

Wood, S.A., Selwood, A.I., Rueckert, A., Holland, P.T., Milne, J.R., Smith, K.F., Smits, B., Watts, L.F., Cary, C.S., 2007. First report of homoanatoxin-a and associated dog neurotoxicosis in New Zealand. *Toxicon* 50: 292–301.

Zotou, A., Jefferies, T.M., Brough, P.A., Gallagher, T., 1993. Determination of anatoxin-a and homoanatoxin in blue-green algal extracts by high-performance liquid chromatography and gas chromatography-mass spectrometry. *Analyst* 118: 753–758.

38

Marine Cyanobacterial Toxins: Source, Chemistry, Toxicology, Pharmacology, and Detection

Vitor Vasconcelos and Pedro Leão

CONTENTS

38.1 Introduction

Cyanobacterial toxins or cyanotoxins have been studied for the past decades mostly due to the fact that they may cause severe human and animal intoxications when present in freshwaters used for drinking, recreation, or dialysis (Jochimsen et al., 1998; Chorus and Bartram, 1999). Although cyanotoxins may be taken up by freshwater organisms such as mussels, crustaceans, or fish, there is now record or evidences that intake via food may cause severe human intoxications as it occurs in the marine environment with the toxins associated with harmful algal blooms (HABs). Cyanobacteria may produce a wide array of cyanotoxins, being classified, accordingly to the main effects in mammals, hepatotoxins, neurotoxins, cytotoxins, and dermatotoxins (Chorus and Bartram, 1999). Many other secondary metabolites have been described, some with allelopathic properties (Leão et al. 2010, 2012) or being active against virus, bacteria, and cancer cells (Martins et al., 2008; Herfindal et al., 2010; Lopes et al., 2011), but for most of them, no toxicity against humans has been studied or reported. So, in this chapter, we will deal with the main cyanobacterial toxins that affect the marine environment, including brackish waters in estuaries or the Baltic Sea.

In the marine environment, cyanobacterial toxins have been associated with human and animal intoxications more seldom, except with the cases of *Moorea producens* (formerly *Lyngbya majuscula*) associated toxins that may cause the "swimmer's itch" (Cardellina et al., 1979). The main toxin associated with this species is the lyngbyatoxin with severe toxicity to humans including tumor promotion.

More recently the study of blooms of the marine cyanobacteria *Trichodesmium* spp. obtained in New Caledonia revealed the occurrence of the toxin palytoxin (Kerbrat et al., 2011). This toxin was first described as being produced by a coral, later by marine dinoflagellates, and now by marine cyanobacteria.

The Baltic Sea being a large brackish water body is heavily eutrophic having severe cyanobacterial blooms with particular emphasis on the species *Nodularia spumigena* and the toxin nodularin (NOD). Cases of domestic animal poisoning are frequent and there is also the potential toxin uptake by aquatic vertebrates and invertebrates and potential human exposure via food. Microcystins (MCs) are cyclic peptides similar to NOD and frequent in freshwaters. Nevertheless, recent reports show that they may persist and be taken up in costal marine food chains, causing animal intoxications (Miller et al., 2010). These toxins have also being found in inland salt lakes showing that salinity may not be a factor preventing the synthesis of this toxin (Carmichael and Li, 2006).

Recent studies confirm that brackish water and marine cyanobacteria produce the amino acid β-N-methylamino-L-alanine (BMAA) associated with neurodegenerative diseases such as amyotrophic lateral syndrome (ALS). BMAA is accumulated in food webs of the North Atlantic, from cyanobacteria, to zooplankton, to invertebrates, and to vertebrates (fish) with increasing BMAA concentration within higher trophic levels (Brand et al., 2010; Jonasson et al., 2010).

In this chapter, we will review the main cyanobacterial toxins with importance in the marine environment with special emphasis on the main sources, chemistry, toxicology, pharmacology of the toxins, and the main detection methods.

38.2 Sources

38.2.1 Palytoxin

The polyhydroxylated secondary metabolite palytoxin (Figure 38.1) was first isolated from a Hawaiian soft coral, *Palythoa* sp. (Moore and Scheuer, 1971), and it is among these zoanthids that this toxin and some analogues are most commonly found (e.g., Gleibs and Mebs, 1999). Still, and as pointed out recently (Ramos and Vasconcelos, 2010), palytoxin and its analogues (hereafter, referred to as palytoxins) have been found in several marine invertebrates and fish. Such punctuated distribution and a seasonal variation in the toxicity that correlated with bacterial abundance in *Palythoa* pointed, since very early, toward a microbial source for these metabolites (Moore et al., 1982b). Usami et al. (1995) discovered ostreocin-D from a culture of a Japanese *Ostreopsis siamensis* strain. This established these dinoflagellates as a microbial source for palytoxins. Several palytoxin analogues, such as the mascarenotoxins (Lenoir et al., 2004) and ovatoxins (Ciminiello et al., 2008, 2010, 2012b) were also found to be produced by *Ostreopsis* spp. However, clear chemotaxonomical relationships in this genus still need to be established (Ciminiello et al., 2013).

Very recently, and justifying their inclusion in this chapter, palytoxin and its 42-hydroxylated analogue have been found in environmental samples of blooms of the filamentous marine cyanobacterium *Trichodesmium* spp. obtained in New Caledonia (Kerbrat et al., 2011). *Trichodesmium* is a globally important cyanobacterial genus belonging to the order Oscillatoriales that is known to play a pivotal role in nitrogen fixation throughout the world's oceans (Bergman et al., 2013). The toxins were detected by LC/MS/MS analyses and toxicity was evaluated by biological assays (Kerbrat et al., 2011). Even though the bloom samples contained other organisms (including dinoflagellates), the authors indicate that *Trichodesmium* spp. were the major components of the samples (Kerbrat et al., 2011). While it would be desirable to obtain proof of palytoxin production by an axenic culture of a *Trichodesmium* cyanobacterium, the aforementioned study provides strong evidence toward cyanobacterial production of these toxins.

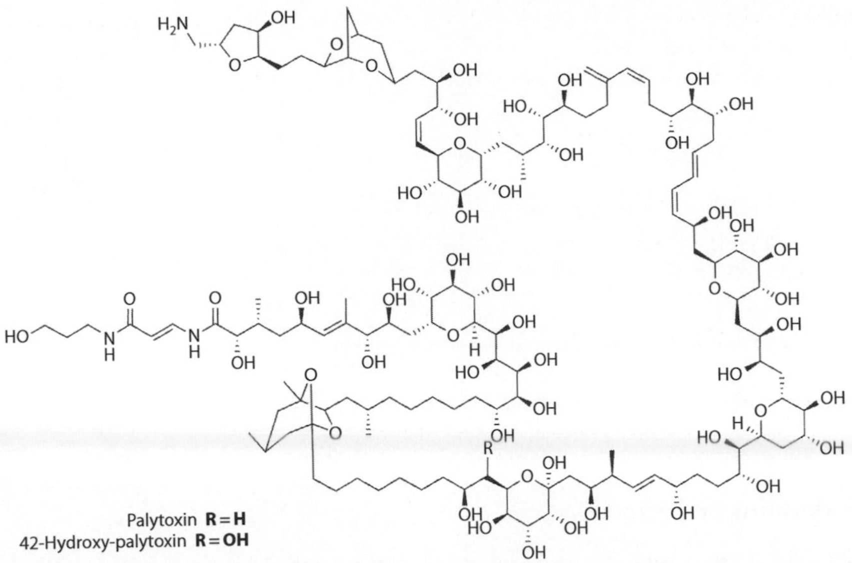

FIGURE 38.1 Chemical structure of palytoxin.

38.2.2 Lyngbyatoxin

The marine toxin lyngbyatoxin A (or simply lyngbyatoxin) (Figure 38.2) was first reported from a mat-forming *M. producens*—formerly *Lyngbya majuscula*, see Engene et al. (2012)—cyanobacterium growing in shallow water in Kahala Beach, Oahu, Hawaii (Cardellina et al., 1979). The discovery of this molecule was prompted by investigations of "swimmer's itch" reported by individuals that had come into direct contact with the cyanobacterium (Cardellina et al., 1979). Lyngbyatoxin A is structurally related to the teleocidins (teleocidin A-1 is equivalent to and teleocidin A-2 is the C-19 epimer of lyngbyatoxin A), secondary metabolites produced by *Streptomyces* bacteria (Cardellina et al., 1979; Sakai et al., 1986). A decade later, Aimi and coworkers (1990) were able to isolate and structurally characterize two other congeners, lyngbyatoxins B and C (Figure 38.2), from the same cyanobacterium. *M. producens* is a well-known rich source of secondary metabolites, found in tropical areas (Engene et al., 2012).

The genome of strain 3L from this species was recently sequenced (Jones et al., 2011) and does not include the lyngbyatoxin gene cluster, which had been reported earlier from a collection of *M. producens* from Kahala Beach (Edwards JACS, 2004). Surprisingly, a smaller-than-expected fraction of the genome of this strain is dedicated to secondary metabolism (Jones et al., 2011). The authors argue— and this has been also stressed by Engene et al. (2011)—that the perceived richness of *M. producens* in terms of secondary metabolite production is the result of the microdiversity in this species, with several

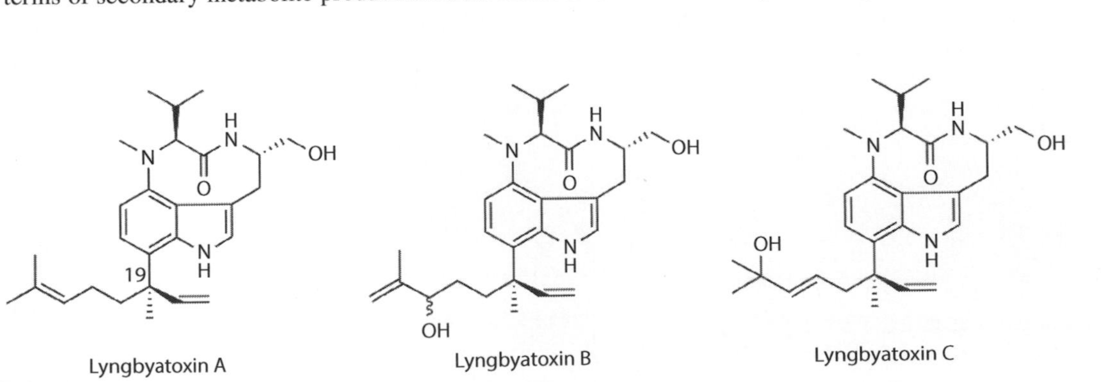

FIGURE 38.2 Chemical structures of lyngbyatoxin A, B, and C.

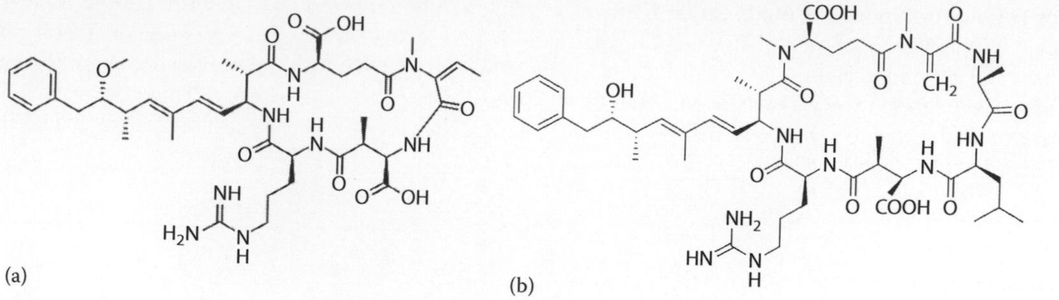

FIGURE 38.3 Chemical structure of nodularin (a) and microcystin (b).

morphologically similar cyanobacteria producing different metabolites (Jones et al., 2011). Such findings should be taken into account when considering potential lyngbyatoxin(s)-producing *M. producens* strains.

38.2.3 Nodularins and Microcystins

NOD (Figure 38.3a) are produced mainly by the brackish water cyanobacterium *N. spumigena*. The main reservoir of NOD is the Baltic Sea because due to its eutrophication, low salinity, and adequate physical conditions, it has heavy blooms of *N. spumigena* every year (Sivonen and Jones, 1999).

Concerning MC (Figure 38.3b), they were first described as being produced by *Microcystis aeruginosa* (Botes et al., 1985) but following a growing number of reports showed that MC may be produced by many genera and species of cyanobacteria (Sivonen and Jones, 1999). Most of these reports of MC occurrence are related to freshwater environments (Vasconcelos et al., 1996), estuaries (D'ors et al., 2013), or symbioses (Kaasalainen et al., 2012). Nevertheless, work done in the salt lake Salton Sea showed that MC can also occur in saline environments (Carmichael and Li, 2006). The black band disease, a pathology of marine sponges caused by cyanobacteria, has been associated with MC produced by *Leptolyngbya* and *Geitlerinema* (Gantar et al., 2009). More recently, there has been report about the occurrence of MC in coastal areas in the Pacific (Miller et al., 2010) and Mediterranean (Vareli et al., 2012), causing animal intoxication, although in these cases, the origin is continental. Nevertheless, it has been shown that freshwater cyanotoxins may persist in the marine environment and due to their uptake by aquatic organisms, increase their concentrations to levels that may be harmful.

38.2.4 BMAA

BMAA (Figure 38.4) was firstly isolated from the seeds of the cycad tree (*Cycas sp.*) in 1967, in Guam (Vega and Bell, 1967). Later, biomagnification of BMAA through trophic chains was first proposed for the Guam ecosystem and showed the presence of BMAA from the endosymbiotic *Nostoc sp.* (on the coralloid roots of *Cycas*) (Cox et al., 2003). More recently, it was reported that a large number of cyanobacteria strains could produce BMAA, either as symbionts or as free-living species in marine, brackish,

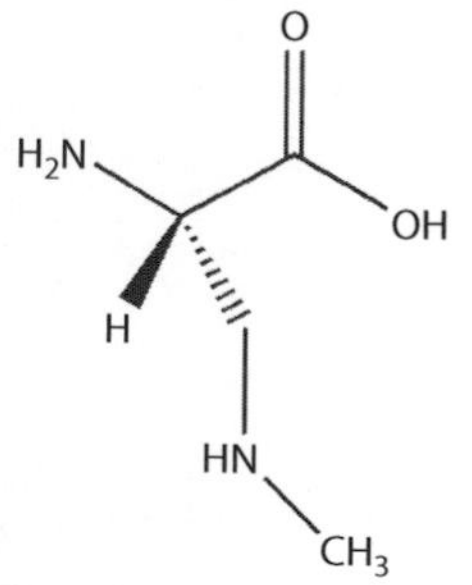

FIGURE 38.4 Chemical structure of β-methylamino-L-alanine (BMAA).

or freshwater biota (Cox et al., 2005; Bannack et al., 2007; Esterhuizen and Downing, 2008; Metcalf et al., 2008; Cianca et al., 2012). One of the main problems associated with BMAA is the fact that it can be taken up in food chains and reach humans by consumption of fish and shellfish. The biomagnification of BMAA in food webs of the North Atlantic has been shown, from cyanobacteria, to zooplankton, to invertebrates, and to vertebrates (fish) with increasing BMAA concentration within higher trophic levels (Brand et al., 2010; Jonasson et al., 2010).

38.3 Chemistry

38.3.1 Palytoxin

The remarkably complex structure of palytoxin (Figure 38.1) was fully revealed one decade after its isolation was reported by Moore and Scheuer (1971). Two groups independently published the full structure and stereochemistry (Cha et al., 1982; Moore et al., 1982a). Palytoxins are large (>2500 Da) molecules featuring a polyhydroxylated and partially unsaturated aliphatic chain, punctuated by cyclic ether moieties (Ciminiello et al., 2011c). These molecules also bear three nitrogen atoms, present as one primary amino group and two amide moieties. Over a dozen members of this group of natural products are currently known (Ciminiello et al., 2011c), the most recent being ovatoxin-f (Ciminiello et al., 2012c). The high degree of hydroxylation and the olefin moieties confer to these molecules an elevated stereogenic complexity. Palytoxin, for example, has 2^{71} possible stereoisomers (64 stereogenic centers and 7 double bonds with geometrical isomerism). This particular feature, coupled with the large size of palytoxins, has been a substantial challenge for synthetic chemists attempting syntheses of this class of compounds. The total synthesis of palytoxin was carried out from seven already-complex building blocks, in 39 steps (Armstrong et al., 1989; Suh and Kishi, 1994). The total number of steps for the synthesis is estimated at over 140 (Newhouse et al., 2009), which highlights the complexity of this endeavor. Apart from palytoxin, the only analogue tentatively produced by cyanobacteria is 42-hydroxy-palytoxin (Kerbrat et al., 2011). The structural elucidation of this analogue benefited from previous knowledge on other palytoxins and was achieved by high-resolution LC/MS analyses, coupled with Nuclear Magnetic Resonance (NMR) experiments, avoiding the resort to degradation studies (Ciminiello et al., 2009). Still, for other analogues with less homology to fully characterized palytoxins, structural elucidation remains a demanding task, in particular due to the stereogenic centers, as exemplified by ovatoxin-a (Ciminiello et al., 2006, 2012a,b).

The polyketide nature of the polyoxygenated skeleton of palytoxins could putatively occur through the action of polyketide synthase (PKS) enzymes. Still, to date, the biosynthetic pathway for palytoxin biosynthesis remains elusive, although PKS genes are known to occur in both dinoflagellates (Monroe and VanDolah, 2008; Murray et al., 2012) and cyanobacteria (Jones et al., 2009).

38.3.2 Lyngbyatoxin

Lyngbyatoxin A is an indole alkaloid featuring an indolactam V moiety with a pending linalyl group (Figure 38.2). Its structural elucidation was carried out through a combination of spectroscopic techniques, most prominently ^{1}H and ^{13}C NMR (Cardellina et al., 1979). The stereochemistry of the indolactam moiety was determined by comparison of its optical rotation data with that of the fully characterized teleocidin B (Cardellina et al., 1979). The remaining stereochemical assignment, C-19 (*R*) in the linalyl group, was achieved by Sakai et al. (1986). The first total synthesis of lyngbyatoxin A, over 11 steps, was soon reported (Muratake and Natsume, 1987). Lyngbyatoxins B and C (Aimi et al., 1990) share the indolactam substructure with their "A" congener but have modified (hydroxylated) linalyl moieties.

The biosynthetic gene cluster for the lyngbyatoxins was discovered by means of a genomic fosmid library screening. This approach sought for putative genes encoding enzyme functions associated with the predicted non-ribosomal peptide synthetase (NRPS) logic leading to the lyngbyatoxins (Edwards and Gerwick, 2004). The *ltx* gene cluster was shown to span a roughly 11 kb genome region and to contain four open reading frames coding for four proteins LtxA, B, C, and D (Edwards and Gerwick, 2004).

LtxA is a NRPS with two modules that N-methylates L-Val and catalyzes its condensation with L-Trp and reductive release of the dipeptide alcohol, this latter step via the action of a C-terminal reductase domain (Edwards and Gerwick, 2004; Read and Walsh, 2007). The dipeptide is then cyclized by LtxB, a P450 cytochrome monooxygenase, which catalyzes an intramolecular N-arylation (Edwards and Gerwick, 2004; Huynh et al., 2010). The prenyltransferase LtxC is responsible for the attachment of the linalyl group, from geranyl pyrophosphate (GPP). Finally, LtxD is thought to be involved in the conversion of lyngbyatoxin A to its B and C congeners (Edwards and Gerwick, 2004).

38.3.3 Nodularins and Microcystins

MCs are cyclic heptapeptides with a general chemical structure as cyclo (D-Ala-L-X-D-erythro-b-methyl-isoAsp-L-Y-Adda-D-isoGlu-N-methyldehydroAla) where X and Y are variable L-amino acids (Figure 38.3b). The most distinctive amino acid of MC and NOD is the (2S,3S,8S,9S,4E,6E)-3-amino-9-methoxy-2,6,8-trimethyl-10-phenyl-4,6-decadienoic acid (ADDA). There are more than 80 variants or isoforms of MC with molecular weights ranging from 800 to 1100 Da, the MC-LR being the most common (Vasconcelos et al., 1996; Sivonen and Jones, 1999; Saker et al., 2005). NODs are similar to MC but are pentapeptides (Figure 38.3a), having also ADDA as the distinctive amino acid. Due to the ring structure, MC and NOD are very stable, resistant even to boiling, freezing, and other physical treatments (Morais et al., 2008).

MC biosynthesis is done by a family of NRPSs and PKSs organized into modules (Dittman et al., 2001). Each PKS or NRPS module is made up of a set of three domains, two of which are catalytic and one that acts as a carrier, and together are responsible for the polyketide or polypeptide biosynthesis (Dittman et al., 2001). NRPS comprise three domains: (1) the adenylation-(A)- domain responsible for amino acid recognition and activation, (2) the peptidyl carrier protein for transport to the respective catalytic centers, and (3) the condensation-(C) domain for the formation of the peptide bond. Cyanobacterial NRPS and PKS are organized into gene clusters in the genome (Moreira et al., 2013). The MC biosynthetic pathway has been previously described from a *Microcystis aeruginosa* strain PCC7806. The MC gene cluster (mcy) contains 55 kb of DNA encoding 10 ORF's mcyA-mcyJ in a bidirectional operonic structure. The larger of the two putative operons (mcyD-J) encodes PKS/NRPS modules catalyzing the formation of the pentaketide-derived b-amino acid Adda and its linkage to D-glutamate, while the smaller putative operons (mcyA-C) encode the NRPS modules for the extension of the dipeptidyl intermediate to the heptapeptidyl step and subsequent peptide cyclization of MC (Tillett et al., 2000).

38.3.4 BMAA

The methylated amino acid BMAA is a nonprotein amino acid. BMAA had been reported to move as a basic amino acid on electrophoresis (Bell, 2009) and that the characterization of this amino acid showed a 1H NMR spectrum characteristic of an optically active compound, with the pKa of the two amino groups being 6.5 and 9.8 (Nunn and O'Brien, 1989). L-2,4-Diamino-n-butyric acid (DAB) is a structural isomer of BMAA that can co-elute in some detection methods with BMAA. BMAA can occur free or bound to protein; so to detect this last fraction, we need to hydrolyzed in 6 M HCl in a vacuum atmosphere (Cianca et al., 2012). So far, information regarding BMAA biosynthesis pathway is not available, and therefore, the mechanisms that might condition the production of this amino acid are not known.

38.4 Toxicology and Pharmacology

38.4.1 Palytoxin

Palytoxin is one of the most potent known toxins, with a 24 h LD_{50} in rats of 0.089 μg kg^{-1} (intravenous) (Wiles et al., 1974). A pioneering assessment of the effects of exposure to palytoxin (with unknown structure at the time) using semi-purified material (Wiles et al., 1974) allowed to evaluate its acute toxicity among different animal species. Intravenous administration caused the highest toxicity (evaluated by

24 h LD_{50}), which ranged from 0.033 to 0.45 µg kg^{-1} in dogs and mice, respectively (Wiles et al., 1974). Conversely, intrarectal administration of the semi-purified toxin caused no observable toxicity. Oral administration of palytoxin shows only moderate toxicity (Ramos and Vasconcelos, 2010; Munday, 2011). The effects associated with intoxication reported by Wiles et al. (1974) include kidney, pulmonary, and ocular damage. Altered histology was additionally observed in the liver, gastrointestinal tract, and brain. Following exposure, animals became prostrated, dyspneic, and convulsive, and eventually collapsed. Several studies have also evaluated the ecological effects of palytoxins, as reviewed by Ramos and Vasconcelos (2010). As with other known toxins, palytoxins are subject to bioaccumulation along the food chain (Gleibs and Mebs, 1999). Apart from its lethality, which can affect aquatic invertebrates and vertebrates (Simoni et al., 2004; Franchini et al., 2008), exposure to these toxins can cause developmental impairment in marine invertebrates (Ramos and Vasconcelos, 2010 and references therein). Most of the data on marine organisms originate from laboratory-based bioassays; therefore, field studies are needed to assess the potential impacts at the ecosystem level.

Deeds and Schwartz (2010) have provided an account of human risk associated with exposure to palytoxin, by reviewing several primary reports of human intoxications. The intoxication routes include direct contact with contaminated materials, inhalation of aerosols containing the toxin, and dietary ingestion of the toxin in contaminated organisms. Human intoxication with palytoxin through dermal contact has been well documented in two instances. Hoffmann et al. (2008) report the poisoning of an adult male following finger injury with a zoanthid colony while performing aquarium maintenance. The patient displayed general poisoning symptoms, altered ECG and symptoms of rhabdomyolysis, and recovered following 48 h of symptomatic treatment. The link between the intoxication and palytoxin was established by testing the zoanthids in a human red cell hemolysis assay, which indicated that 2–3 mg of palytoxin per gram (f.w.) of zoanthid sample was present. The other report concerns an intoxication of an adult woman following handling of a zoanthid coral from an aquarium (Nordt et al., 2011). In this case, no wounding was reported. The patient showed neurologic and local dermatologic symptoms and was treated with corticosteroids and antihistamines. The symptoms persisted for a few days. A palytoxin-like molecule is presumed to have been involved in this episode, although no confirmation was sought through the analysis of the zoanthid.

The Genoa 2005 outbreak, one of the best-known cases of human intoxication by palytoxins (Ciminiello et al., 2006), is an example of inhalational exposure to these toxins. About 200 people suffered of respiratory illness, with symptoms of cough, fever, and bronchoconstriction as a result of marine aerosol exposure on the seaside of Genoa, Italy. This event coincided with an *Ostreopsis ovata* bloom. Ciminiello et al. (2006) were able to establish the connection between the intoxication and a palytoxin-like molecule, found in *O. ovata* cells, through LC/MS analysis. The compound was later found to be the palytoxin analogue, ovatoxin-a (Ciminiello et al., 2008). A case report of exposure to palytoxin through inhalation was also conveyed by Majlesi et al. (2008), again with a zoanthid coral in an aquarium. An adult male poured boiling water over the *Palythoa* sp. and inadvertently inhaled the resulting fumes. Respiratory symptoms began after the inhalation and included chest pain and bronchospasm, and the patient was discharged after 24 h, following treatment and amelioration of the symptoms. No direct confirmation of the involvement of palytoxins in this episode was reported.

Intoxication with palytoxins through ingestion of contaminated food has been reported more often than the types of exposure discussed previously; some resulting in fatal outcomes and have been recently reviewed (Deeds and Schwartz, 2010). Most documented events concern the consumption of fish in tropical and subtropical areas (Deeds and Schwartz, 2010). Of particular notice is the association between clupeotoxism (intoxication from ingestion of clupeoid fish) and palytoxin, currently regarded as its causative agent (Onuma et al., 1999). This assumption arose primarily from a fatal intoxication of adult woman in Madagascar, following consumption of the herring *Herklotsichthys quadrimaculatus*. Following analysis of fish tissue, a palytoxin-like compound was found to be present by bioassay and chromatographic/mass spectrometric analysis. The authors suggest that the source of the toxin was cells from the dinoflagellate *O. siamensis* consumed by the fish (Onuma et al., 1999). Exposure to palytoxins through consumption of crustaceans has also been reported in the Philippines, as reviewed by Deeds and Schwartz (2010). The intoxications were a consequence of ingesting different species of crabs that were shown to contain palytoxins and resulted in several fatalities (e.g., Gonzales and Alcala, 1977; Alcala et al., 1988).

Accumulating evidence on electrophysiological damage caused by palytoxin, such as involuntary muscle contraction, depolarization, and K^+ efflux (Wu, 2009 and references therein), led to numerous investigations at the molecular level on the mechanism of action of palytoxin. It was soon discovered that palytoxin is only active if applied to the outer side of cells (Muramatsu et al., 1984). Blockers to voltage-gated sodium channels, potassium channels, and calcium channels were not able to antagonize the action of palytoxin, indicating a different mechanism of action from those currently known (Muramatsu et al., 1984; Wu, 2009). In fact, palytoxin binds to the Na^+/K^+-ATPase quite strongly (Bottinger et al., 1986). This binding induces conformational changes that turn the pump into a de facto ion channel, allowing the nonspecific passage of monovalent cations and corrupting the ion gradient of the cells (Habermann, 1989). Ultimate proof for this enzyme being the molecular target of palytoxin (and for its unusual mechanism of action) was provided when K^+ and Na^+ efflux were observed in yeast engineered to express functional mammalian Na^+/K^+-ATPase (Scheinerbobis et al., 1994). The Na^+/K^+-ATPase is present in the plasma membrane of all animal cells; this explains the generalized toxicity of palytoxin, as well as the wide range of effects elicited by exposure to the toxin (Frelin and Vanrenterghem, 1995; Wu, 2009). Some of the reported functional outcomes of this uncommon mechanism of action are actin filament damage (Louzao et al., 2011), tumor suppression and tumor promotion (Wu, 2009), necrotic damage to cells (Sagara et al., 2013), and upregulation of pro-inflammatory proteins (Crinelli et al., 2012).

38.4.2 Lyngbyatoxin

The severe contact dermatitis ("swimmer's itch") that motivated the discovery of lyngbyatoxin A (Cardellina et al., 1979) was studied following an epidemic that occurred in 1958 and in which over a hundred swimmers in Oahu, Hawaii, were affected (Izumi and Moore, 1987 and references therein). The causative agent had been found to be *M. producens* (Grauer and Arnold, 1961). Exposure to the cyanobacterium rapidly causes stinging and burning sensations and sometimes damage in oral and ocular mucosa. Following contact with the cyanobacterium, an erythematous dermatitis develops in the perineal, perianal, and scrotum areas (Izumi and Moore, 1987). Following the study of Cardellina and coworkers (1979), lyngbyatoxin has been implicated in "swimmer's itch." The toxin has been shown to be slightly lipophilic and to exhibit considerable skin penetration (Stafford et al., 1992), which is consistent with its cutaneous toxicity profile.

Acute toxicity of lyngbyatoxin A in mice has been studied for intraperitoneal and oral administration (Ito et al., 2002). For the latter case, no lethality was observed up to 1000 μg kg^{-1}, but several injuries and associated inflammation were reported, mainly in the gastrointestinal tract and in the lungs. Intraperitoneal administration revealed an LD_{50} of 250 μg kg^{-1} in young mice, with death occurring 3.5 h following injection, at that dosage. Injuries were observed in the small intestine (with bleeding), large intestine, and lungs (Ito et al., 2002). The toxin was also shown to cause sensitization (redness) of mice ears, after topical administration (Fujiki et al., 1983).

Fatal human intoxication with lyngbyatoxin A, following consumption of sea turtle (*Chelonia mydas*) meat, has been reported to have occurred in Madagascar (Yasumoto, 1998). The toxin was detected in the turtle meat by means of LC/MS and was deduced to originate from dietary consumption of the toxic cyanobacterium by the marine animal (Yasumoto, 1998). Gatti et al. (2008) report a similar fatal intoxication of an adult, pregnant woman from Tuamotu Archipelago (French Polynesia) after consumption of sea turtle. Gastrointestinal and then neurologic symptoms preceded coma, and a series of metabolic alterations and multiorgan failure ensued that culminated in death. Another 18 members of the woman's family developed intoxication signs, but more serious symptoms were not reported. No analysis was conducted to confirm that lyngbyatoxins were involved (Gatti et al., 2008). It is known that *C. mydas* feeds on lyngbyatoxin-producing *M. producens*, or on macroalgae in which this cyanobacterium grows epiphytically (Arthur et al., 2006, 2008). Different studies have detected the toxin in the tissue of these animals (Yasumoto, 1998; Arthur et al., 2008). In fact, such feeding behavior has been implicated in fibropapillomatosis, a neoplastic disease that causes death to many of these turtles (Arthur et al., 2008). Other marine animals are known to forage on lyngbyatoxins-containing *M. producens* and accumulate the toxin (Capper et al., 2005), and toxicity to fish (100% mortality in *Poecilia vittata* at 0.15 μg mL^{-1}) was reported with the discovery of lyngbyatoxin A (Cardellina et al., 1979). The sea hare *Stylocheilus striatus* preferred to feed on a *M. producens* strain producing only lyngbyatoxin A than on one other strain that also produced another toxin (Capper et al., 2006). Still, several other animals have been shown to avoid feeding on *Moorea* spp. (Paul et al., 2007 and references therein), including lyngbya-toxin-containing strains. In spite of the various research efforts regarding feeding on lyngbyatoxin A containing organisms, little is known regarding the trophic transfer of this toxin in the marine environment (Paul et al., 2007).

Lyngbyatoxin A and teleocidins are commonly referred to as tumor promoters (Fujiki et al., 1981). Following a two-stage protocol to evaluate tumor promoters, the cyanobacterial toxin was found to induce ornithine decarboxylase activity (prevented by 13-*cis*-retinoic acid) when applied topically on mice. The compound also promoted the adhesion of HL-60 leukemia cells and inhibited the DMSO-induced terminal differentiation of Friend erythroleukemia cells (Fujiki et al., 1981). These findings motivated the authors to study and describe the potent activity of lyngbyatoxin A as an in vivo promoter of skin carcinogenesis in mice (Fujiki et al., 1984). The structural analogue of lyngbyatoxins, teleocidin (which was actually a mixture of teleocidin A and B), was found to activate protein kinase C (PKC) (Fujiki et al., 1984), and the authors proposed that the phenotypic manifestations of exposure to this compound resulted from this biochemical event. A similar reasoning was put forward by Friedman and co-workers (1984), following studies on the phosphorylation of tyrosine of the epidermal growth factor (EGF). This reaction was inhibited by teleocidin and lyngbyatoxin A, and given the previous connection of these compounds with PKC, this latter kinase was implied in EGF tyrosine phosphorylation and carcinogenesis. A series of structure activity relationship studies with synthetic analogues of lyngbyatoxins have revealed that the lactam ring scaffold is essential for activation of PKC (Kozikowski et al., 1989) and that the hydrophobic moiety connected to the ring is important for the same effect, due to a presumed interaction with cellular membranes (Kozikowski et al., 1991). Lyngbyatoxin A and teleocidins have become important molecular tools in the study the involvement of PKC in tumor promotion (Nakagawa, 2012).

38.4.3 Nodularins and Microcystins

The hepatotoxic peptides MC and NOD are protein phosphatase inhibitors (Mackintosh et al., 1995), with a potency that varies accordingly to the variants. MC-LR is one of the most toxic ones having an intraperitoneal LD50 in rat of 50 µg kg^{-1} (Chorus and Bartram, 1999). NOD has a similar LD50 compared to MC-LR (Rinehart et al., 1988). Nevertheless, oral toxicity of these hepatotoxins is 10–100 times lower (Sivonen and Jones, 1999). Protein phosphatases catalyze the dephosphorylation of proteins in residues previously phosphorylated by the corresponding protein kinases. Some of the most important human pathologies (e.g., cancer, diabetes, and Alzheimer's disease) can be linked to an abnormal degree of phosphorylation in specific proteins (Pereira et al., 2010).

MC produces several toxic effects in humans such as acute hepatic failure and the potential development of hepatocarcinoma after chronic low-level exposure to the toxin. One of the most hazardous acute human intoxication episodes was the incident in Caruaru, Brazil (Jochimsen et al., 1998).

MC can also be ingested by humans through contaminated water or in aquatic organisms that bioaccumulate the toxin, for example, bivalves, crayfish, and fish (Vasconcelos, 1995; Amorim and Vasconcelos, 1999; Vasconcelos et al., 2001). Plants do not seem to accumulate high amounts of the toxins although they can suffer when exposed to the toxins via water used for irrigation (Saqrane et al., 2008; Pereira et al., 2009; Prieto et al., 2011; El Khalloufi et al., 2012).

38.4.4 BMAA

The hypothesis that BMAA is a neurotoxin and is involved in the etiology of amyotrophic lateral sclerosis (ALS), particularly sporadic ALS, has been raised by several authors (Rachele et al., 1998; Corcia et al., 2003; Karamyan and Speth, 2008).

BMAA binds to NMDA and AMPA/kainate receptors, being this process enhanced when the BMAA is carbamated, producing a molecule that resembles glutamate (Weiss et al., 1989; Rao et al., 2006).

BMAA induces selective motor neuron (MN) loss in dissociated mixed spinal cord cultures and may be incorporated into proteins and subsequently lead to protein misfolding. BMAA also inhibits the cystine/glutamate antiporter (system Xc(-) mediated cystine uptake, which leads to glutathione depletion and increased oxidative stress (Liu et al., 2009). BMAA has previously been shown to be acutely neurotoxic to chicks, rats, and monkeys (Bell, 2009), but there is not yet a viable animal model.

38.5 Detection Methods

38.5.1 Palytoxin

A strong motivation for the development of detection methods for palytoxin arose almost as soon as the existence of palytoxin was reported. The reason for this is naturally related to its toxicity to humans and to the various poisoning events that were attributable to it. Detection methods are important to monitor the presence of the toxin but also to push research forward. Several methodologies, based on biological or chemical detection, have since been developed. Still, to our knowledge, there are currently no official methods or regulations regarding palytoxins, in spite of the potential health and economic problems that may result from its presence in seafood (Riobo and Franco, 2011). The European Food Safety Authority (EFSA) has, nevertheless, begun working toward a guideline value of the toxin in food and bloom samples and proposed a limit of 30 µg kg^{-1} of palytoxin equivalents in shellfish (Chain, 2009).

The traditional, unspecific, mouse bioassay (Yasumoto et al., 1978) has been often used to detect palytoxin; however, a specific enzyme-linked immunosorbent assay (ELISA) was developed as early as 1992 (Bignami et al., 1992), making use of a previously developed anti-palytoxin monoclonal antibody. The ELISA showed poor sensitivity in complex samples, which prompted the development of a hemolysis assay (Bignami, 1993), making combined use of the hemolytic activity of palytoxin and of the specificity provided by the anti-palytoxin monoclonal antibody. Alternatively, ouabain (palytoxin antagonist) has been used instead of the monoclonal antibody to associate the hemolysis with palytoxin (Riobo and Franco, 2011). The (total) toxin concentration is estimated from a calibration curve using palytoxin standards, and sub-pM sensitivity was reported in the original study (Bignami, 1993). Single-chain antibodies, selected using phage display, have allowed the development an indirect ELISA method (Garet et al., 2010) with a remarkable reported sensitivity of 0.5 pg mL^{-1} (sub-picomolar). A more recent sandwich ELISA has been developed for the detection of palytoxin and its 42-hydroxy analogue in biological matrices, with sub-nanomolar sensitivity and with little cross-reactivity (Boscolo et al., 2013). Cytotoxicity assays with detection based on the widely used systems of lactate dehydrogenase (LDH) release (inMCF-7 cells, Bellocci et al., 2008) or MTT reduction to formazan (in Neuro-2a cells, Ledreux et al., 2009) have also been employed to detect palytoxin in biological samples (ouabain being also used for specificity). A recently reported surface plasmon resonance (SPR) immunoassay for the detection of palytoxin in seafood (Yakes et al., 2011) showed good sensitivity (sub-nanomolar limit of detection) and no cross-reactivity. An electrochemiluminescent sensor using anti-palytoxin antibodies was developed by Zamolo and coworkers (2012) and showed a good limit of quantification (LOQ) in mussel tissue (2.2 µg kg^{-1}). These studies may set the stage for the development of palytoxin biosensors for monitoring purposes.

Chemical detection methods, such as chromatography-based methods, have the advantage of detecting and identifying most of the different palytoxin congeners, while being usually less sensitive. While capillary electrophoresis with UV detection (Mereish et al., 1991), LC–UV (UV detection) (e.g., Lenoir et al., 2004), and LC–fluorescence detection (FLD) (e.g., Riobo et al., 2006) methodologies have been used to detect and quantify palytoxin(s), current approaches employ LC/MS instruments (now widely available) to determine palytoxin concentrations in varied matrices (Ciminiello et al., 2011b). Following the Genoa 2005 outbreak, an LC–ESI–MS/MS method was developed by Ciminiello et al. (2006) and used to detect palytoxin and ovatoxin-a in *Ostreopsis* cells (Ciminiello et al., 2008) with a limit of detection in the low-nanomolar range. This method was also applied to the quantification of palytoxins in seafood matrices (Ciminiello et al., 2011a) and allowed the quantification of as low as 228 µg kg^{-1} of palytoxin in the tissue of the mussel *Mytilus galloprovincialis*, a value and order of magnitude higher than the EFSA suggested limit. A lower LOQ (10 μg kg^{-1}) that allows the enforcement of an eventual regulation on palytoxin levels was achieved in a new LC–ESI–MS/MS method reported by Selwood and coworkers (2012). The large increase in sensitivity results from the incorporation of an on-column (solid-phase extraction [SPE]) oxidation step (with periodic acid) coupled to the sample cleanup. The oxidation step cleaves palytoxin(s) at the two vicinal diols, resulting in two nitrogen-containing aldehyde fragments, from each end of the molecule(s). As argued by the authors (Selwood et al., 2012), multiple known palytoxin variants can be quantified using a single standard by monitoring the two aldehyde fragments, and problems associated with the MS interpretation and analysis of a large molecule such as palytoxins (several multiple charged species, ^{13}C contribution) are avoided.

Recently, complementary methodologies that may aid in the early warning and risk management of palytoxin have been developed, such as quantitative PCR (qPCR) techniques applied to the detection of *Ostreopsis* cells inside predators or filter feeders (Furlan et al., 2013) and in marine aerosols (Casabianca et al., 2013).

38.5.2 Lyngbyatoxin

To our knowledge, no analytical methods have been developed for the determination of lyngbyatoxin A. Still, LC/MS has been used for detecting the presence of this toxin (Yasumoto, 1998), and an LC/MS analytical methodology has been developed for teleocidins (Sedlock et al., 1992).

38.5.3 Nodularins and Microcystins

The current methods to detect and quantify NOD and MC are chemical (high-performance liquid chromatography (HPLC), LC/MS, MALDI-TOF), immunological (ELISA), or enzymatic (protein phosphatase or acetylcholinesterase inhibition). The detection of these toxins by HPLC has some limitation due to the fact that there are not many commercially available MC standards. Whenever we are dealing with some of the most common toxins such as MC-LR, MC-RR, or MC-YR, the detection is based an the retention time compared to a standard, and the detection limits can be as low as 0.1 ppm (Martins et al., 2011). In order to have a more sensitive method, samples may be concentrated by lyophilization or by SPE cartridges. Nevertheless, this is a time-consuming method and direct analysis is advisable. Separation of the toxins is done in a C18 column, usually in an oven to stabilize and optimize the temperature, and the detection is done by UV or a diode array detector (Vasconcelos et al., 2006). The development of LC/MS methodologies allows identifying more variants of the toxins and even unknown toxins (Mayumi et al., 2006). This technique is usually more sensitive and is nowadays currently used. Allis et al. (2007) developed an LC–ESI–MS/MS with a limit of detection (LOD) of 0.27 and LOQ of 0.90 μg L^{-1}. The MALDI-TOF has been used mostly for toxin identification since it not only detects common and new variants of the toxins but also is very sensitive allowing to detect the toxins in single colonies of filaments of cyanobacteria (Saker et al., 2009).

ELISAs have been developed for the detection of cyanobacteria in the 1990s (Ann and Carmichael, 1994). Nowadays, there is a diversity of kits using monoclonal or polyclonal antibodies (Ann and Carmichal, 1994, Ueno et al., 1996), and the kits can be used not only in the laboratory in 96 well plates coated with the antibodies but also in the field. Currently, ELISAs for MC and NOD have a quantification limit of 0.1 μg L^{-1} although false positives may occur in case of samples rich in organic matter. Tippkötter et al. (2009) developed immunochromatographic lateral flow dipstick assay for the fast detection of MC-LR. This assay has a detection limit of 1–5 μg L^{-1}. The ready-to-use dipsticks were successfully tested with MC-LR-spiked samples of outdoor drinking and salt water and applied to the tissue of MC-fed mussels, which could be used for aquaculture in order to have a quick result in situ.

Since MC and NOD inhibit serine–threonine protein phosphatases, these mechanisms of action were on the base of enzyme inhibition assays with radioisotopic (Lambert et al., 1994) or colorimetric detection

(Ward et al., 1997; Rapala et al., 2002). These methods are quite sensitive but other contaminants with similar activity, for example, okadaic acid, may respond to the assay, giving false positives.

38.5.4 BMAA

This amino acid has been detected mostly by chromatographic methods such as HPLC and LC/MS. Nevertheless, some attempts have been done using capillary electrophoresis with some success (Baptista et al., 2011). A capillary electrophoretic method for the determination of the amino acid BMAA was developed using a fused-silica capillary column (50 cm, 75 mm) filled with 5 mM sodium tetraborate solution, and detection was performed by direct UV absorbance at 192 nm. The LODs and LOQs were 0.5 and 2.0 mg L^{-1}, respectively (Baptista et al., 2011).

Due to the fact that BMAA has no chromophore, there is a need for a derivatization step before the toxin is quantified by a fluorescence detector. Cianca et al. (2012) developed a method for BMAA detection and quantification by HPLC. The novelty of the method is that they have used methanol instead of acetonitrile as the eluent. The method includes extraction with 0.1 M trichloroacetic acid (free BMAA) or protein hydrolysis with 6 M hydrochloric acid (total BMAA), derivatization with AQC (6-aminoquinolyl-N-hydroxysuccinimidyl carbamate), and reversed-phase HPLC analysis with fluorescence detection (HPLC/FD). Detection limits ranged from 0.35 to 0.75 pg injected, while quantification limits ranged from 1.10 to 2.55 pg injected for total and free BMAA hydrolysis, respectively (Cianca et al., 2012).

REFERENCES

Aimi, N., Odaka, H., Sakai, S. 1990. Lyngbyatoxins B and C, two new irritants from *Lyngbya majuscula. J Nat Prod* 53: 1593–1596.

Alcala, A.C., Alcala, L.C., Garth, J.S., Yasumura, D., Yasumoto, T. 1988. Human fatality due to ingestion of the crab *Demania reynaudii* that contained a palytoxin-like toxin. *Toxicon* 26: 105–107.

Allis, O., Dauphard, J., Hamilton, B., Shuilleabhain, A., Lehane, M., James, K., Furey, A. 2007. Liquid chromatography-tandem mass spectrometry application, for the determination of extracellular hepatotoxins in Irish Lake and drinking waters. *Anal Chem* 79: 3436–3447.

Amorim, A., Vasconcelos, V. 1999. Dynamics of microcystins in the mussel *Mytilus galloprovincialis. Toxicon* 37: 1041–1052.

Armstrong, R.W., Beau, J.M., Cheon, S.H., Christ, W.J., Fujioka, H., Ham, W.H. et al. 1989. Total synthesis of palytoxin carboxylic-acid and palytoxin amide. *J Am Chem Soc* 111: 7530–7533.

Arthur, K., Limpus, C., Balazs, G., Capper, A., Udy, J., Shaw, G. et al. 2008. The exposure of green turtles (*Chelonia mydas*) to tumour promoting compounds produced by the cyanobacterium *Lyngbya majuscula* and their potential role in the aetiology of fibropapillomatosis. *Harmful Algae* 7: 114–125.

Arthur, K.E., Limpus, C.J., Roelfsema, C.M., Udy, J.W., Shaw G.R. 2006. A bloom of *Lyngbya majuscula* in Shoalwater Bay, Queensland, Australia: An important feeding ground for the green turtle (*Chelonia mydas*). *Harmful Algae* 5: 251–265.

Banack, S., Johnson, H., Chen, R., Cox, P. 2007. Production of the neurotoxin BMAA by a marine cyanobacterium. *Mar Drugs* 5: 180–196.

Baptista, M.S., Cianca, R.C.C.C., Almeida, M.R., Vasconcelos, V.M. 2011. Determination of the non protein amino acid β-N-methylamino-L-alanine in estuarine cyanobacteria by capillary electrophoresis. *Toxicon* 58: 410–414.

Bell, E.A. 2009. The discovery of BMAA, and examples of biomagnification and protein incorporation involving other non-protein amino acids. *Amyotroph Lateral Scler* 10(Suppl 2): 21–25.

Bellocci, M., Ronzitti, G., Milandri, A., Melchiorre, N., Grillo, C., Poletti R. et al. 2008. A cytolytic assay for the measurement of palytoxin based on a cultured monolayer cell line. *Anal Biochem* 374: 48–55.

Bergman, B., Sandh, G., Lin, S., Larsson, J., Carpenter, E.J. 2013. *Trichodesmium*—A widespread marine cyanobacterium with unusual nitrogen fixation properties. *FEMS Microbiol Rev* 37: 286–302.

Bignami, G.S. 1993. A rapid and sensitive hemolysis neutralization assay for palytoxin. *Toxicon* 31: 817–820.

Bignami, G.S., Raybould, T.J.G., Sachinvala, N.D., Grothaus, P.G., Simpson, S.B., Lazo, C.B. et al. 1992. Monoclonal antibody-based enzyme-linked immunoassays for the measurement of palytoxin in biological samples. *Toxicon* 30: 687–700.

Boscolo, S., Pelin, M., De Bortoli, M., Fontanive, G., Barreras, A., Berti, F. et al. 2013. Sandwich ELISA assay for the quantitation of palytoxin and its analogs in natural samples. *Environ Sci Technol* 47: 2034–2042.

Botes, D., Wessels, P., Kruger, H., Runnegar, M., Santikarn, S., Smith, R., Barna, J., Williams, D. 1985. Structural studies on cyanoginosins-LR, -YR, -YA, and -YM, peptide toxins from *Microcystis aeruginosa*. *J Chem Soc* 1: 2747–2748.

Bottinger, H., Beress, L., Habermann, E. 1986. Involvement of (Na$^+$+K$^+$)-ATPase in binding and actions of palytoxin on human-erythrocytes. *Biochim Biophys Acta* 861: 165–176.

Capper, A., Tibbetts, I.R., O'Neil, J.M., Shaw, G.R. 2005. The fate of *Lyngbya majuscula* toxins in three potential consumers. *J Chem Ecol* 31: 1595–1606.

Capper, A., Tibbetts, I.R., O'Neil, J.M., Shaw, G.R. 2006. Dietary selectivity for the toxic cyanobacterium *Lyngbya majuscula* and resultant growth rates in two species of opisthobranch mollusc. *J Exp Mar Biol Ecol* 331: 133–144.

Cardellina, J.H., Marner, F.J., Moore, R.E. 1979. Seaweed dermatitis—Structure of lyngbyatoxin-A. *Science* 204: 193–195.

Carmichael, W.W., Li, R. 2006. Cyanobacteria toxins in the Salton Sea. *Saline Sys* 2: 5.

Casabianca, S., Casabianca, A., Riobo, P., Franco, J.M., Vila, M., Penna, A. 2013. Quantification of the toxic dinoflagellate *Ostreopsis* spp. by qPCR assay in marine aerosol. *Environ Sci Technol* 47: 3788–3795.

Cha, J.K., Christ, W.J., Finan, J.M., Fujioka, H., Kishi, Y., Klein, L.L. et al. 1982. Stereochemistry of palytoxin. Part 4. Complete structure. *J Am Chem Soc* 104: 7369–7371.

Chain, E., EFSA Panel on Contaminants in the Food Chain (CONTAM). 2009. Scientific opinion on marine biotoxins in shellfish—Palytoxin group. *EFSA J* 7: 1393.

Chorus, I., Bartram, J. (eds.) 1999. *Toxic Cyanobacteria in Water*. E & FN Spon & WHO, Geneva, Switzerland.

Cianca, R.C.C., Baptista, M.S., Silva, L.P., Lopes, V.R., Vasconcelos, V.M. 2012. Reversed-phase HPLC/FD method for the quantitative analysis of the neurotoxin BMAA (β-N-methylamino-L-alanine) in cyanobacteria. *Toxicon* 59: 373–378.

Ciminiello, P., Dell'Aversano, C., Dello Iacovo, E., Fattorusso, E., Forino, M., Grauso, L. et al. 2009. Stereostructure and biological activity of 42-hydroxy-palytoxin: A new palytoxin analogue from Hawaiian *Palythoa* subspecies. *Chem Res Toxicol* 22: 1851–1859.

Ciminiello, P., Dell'Aversano, C., Dello Iacovo, E., Fattorusso, E., Forino, M., Grauso, L. et al. 2010. Complex palytoxin-like profile of *Ostreopsis ovata*. Identification of four new ovatoxins by high-resolution liquid chromatography/mass spectrometry. *Rapid Commun Mass Spectrom* 24: 2735–2744.

Ciminiello, P., Dell'Aversano, C., Dello Iacovo, E., Fattorusso, E., Forino, M., Grauso, L. et al. 2012a. Stereochemical studies on ovatoxin-a. *Chem-Eur J* 18: 16836–16843.

Ciminiello, P., Dell'Aversano, C., Dello Iacovo, E., Fattorusso, E., Forino, M., Grauso, L. et al. 2012b. Isolation and structure elucidation of ovatoxin-a, the major toxin produced by *Ostreopsis ovata*. *J Am Chem Soc* 134: 1869–1875.

Ciminiello, P., Dell'Aversano, C., Dello Iacovo, E., Fattorusso, E., Forino, M., Tartaglione, L. et al. 2011a. Palytoxin in seafood by liquid chromatography tandem mass spectrometry: Investigation of extraction efficiency and matrix effect. *Anal Bioanal Chem* 401: 1043–1050.

Ciminiello, P., Dell'Aversano, C., Dello Iacovo, E., Fattorusso, E., Forino, M., Tartaglione, L. 2011b. LC-MS of palytoxin and its analogues: State of the art and future perspectives. *Toxicon* 57: 376–389.

Ciminiello, P., Dell'Aversano, C., Dello Iacovo, E., Fattorusso, E., Forino, M., Tartaglione, L. et al. 2012c. Unique toxin profile of a mediterranean *Ostreopsis* cf. *ovata* strain: HR LC-MSn characterization of ovatoxin-f, a new palytoxin congener. *Chem Res Toxicol* 25: 1243–1252.

Ciminiello, P., Dell'Aversano, C., Dello Iacovo, E., Fattorusso, E., Forino, M., Tartaglione, L. et al. 2013. Investigation of toxin profile of Mediterranean and Atlantic strains of *Ostreopsis* cf. *siamensis* (Dinophyceae) by liquid chromatography-high resolution mass spectrometry. *Harmful Algae* 23: 19–27.

Ciminiello, P., Dell'Aversano, C., Fattorusso, E., Forino, M., Grauso, L., Tartaglione, L. 2011c. A 4-decade-long (and still ongoing) hunt for palytoxins chemical architecture. *Toxicon* 57: 362–367.

Ciminiello, P., Dell'Aversano, C., Fattorusso, E., Forino, M., Magno, G.S., Tartaglione, L. et al. 2006. The Genoa 2005 outbreak. Determination of putative palytoxin in Mediterranean *Ostreopsis ovata* by a new liquid chromatography tandem mass spectrometry method. *Anal Chem* 78: 6153–6159.

Ciminiello, P., Dell'Aversano, C., Fattorusso, E., Forino, M., Tartaglione, L., Grillo, C. et al. 2008. Putative palytoxin and its new analogue, ovatoxin-a, in *Ostreopsis ovata* collected along the Ligurian coasts during the 2006 toxic outbreak. *J Am Soc Mass Spectrom* 19: 111–120.

Corcia, P., Jafari-Schluep, H.F., Lardillier, D., Mazyad, H., Giraud, P., Clavelou, P., et al. 2003. A clustering of conjugal amyotrophic lateral sclerosis in southeastern France. *Arch Neurol* 60(4):553–557.

Crinelli, R., Carloni, E., Giacomini, E., Penna, A., Dominici, S., Battocchi, C. et al. 2012. Palytoxin and an *Ostreopsis* toxin extract increase the levels of mRNAs encoding inflammation-related proteins in human macrophages via p38 MAPK and NF-kappa B. *Plos One* 7: e38139.

D'ors, A., Bartolomé, M.C., Sánchez-Fortún, S. 2013. Toxic risk associated with sporadic occurrences of Microcystis aeruginosa blooms from tidal rivers in marine and estuarine ecosystems and its impact on *Artemia franciscana* nauplii populations. *Chemosphere* 90: 2187–2192.

Deeds, J.R., Schwartz, M.D. 2010. Human risk associated with palytoxin exposure. *Toxicon* 56: 150–162.

Dittmann, E., Neilan, B.A., Börner, T. 2001. Molecular biology of peptide and polyketide biosynthesis in cyanobacteria. *Appl Microbiol Biotechnol* 57: 467–473.

Edwards, D.J., Gerwick, W.H. 2004. Lyngbyatoxin biosynthesis: Sequence of biosynthetic gene cluster and identification of a novel aromatic prenyltransferase. *J Am Chem Soc* 126: 11432–11433.

El Khalloufi, F., El Ghazali, I., Saqrane, S., Oufdou, K., Vasconcelos, V., Oudra, B. 2012. Phytotoxic effects of a natural bloom extract containing microcystins on Lycopersicon esculentum germination, growth and biochemistry. *Ecotoxicol Environ Safety* 79:199–205.

Engene, N., Choi, H., Esquenazi, E., Rottacker, E.C., Ellisman, M.H., Dorrestein, P.C. et al. 2011. Underestimated biodiversity as a major explanation for the perceived rich secondary metabolite capacity of the cyanobacterial genus *Lyngbya*. *Environ Microbiol* 13: 1601–1610.

Engene, N., Rottacker, E.C., Kaštovský, J., Byrum, T., Choi, H., Ellisman, M.H. et al. 2012. *Moorea producens* gen. nov., sp. nov. and *Moorea bouillonii* comb. nov., tropical marine cyanobacteria rich in bioactive secondary metabolites. *Int J Syst Evol Microbiol* 62: 1171–1178.

Franchini, A., Casarini, L., Ottaviani, E. 2008. Toxicological effects of marine palytoxin evaluated by FETAX assay. *Chemosphere* 73: 267–271.

Frelin, C., Vanrenterghem, C. 1995. Palytoxin—Recent electrophysiological and pharmacological evidence for several mechanisms of action. *Gen Pharmacol* 26: 33–37.

Friedman, B.A., Frackelton, A.R., Ross, A.H., Connors, J.M., Fujiki, H., Sugimura, T. et al. 1984. Tumor promoters block tyrosine-specific phosphorylation of the epidermal growth-factor receptor. *Proc Natl Acad Sci USA-Biol Sci* 81: 3034–3038.

Fujiki, H., Mori, M., Nakayasu, M., Terada, M., Sugimura, T., Moore, R.E. 1981. Indole alkaloids— Dihydroteleocidin-B, teleocidin, and lyngbyatoxin-a as members of a new class of tumor promoters. *Proc Natl Acad Sci USA-Biol Sci* 78: 3872–3876.

Fujiki, H., Suganuma, M., Hakii, H., Bartolini, G., Moore, R.E., Takayama, S. et al. 1984. A 2-stage mouse skin carcinogenesis study of lyngbyatoxin-A. *J Cancer Res Clin Oncol* 108: 174–176.

Fujiki, H., Sugimura, T., Moore, R.E. 1983. New classes of environmental tumor promoters—Indole alkaloids and polyacetates. *Environ Health Perspect* 50: 85–90.

Furlan, M., Antonioli, M., Zingone, A., Sardo, A., Blason, C., Pallavicini, A. et al. 2013. Molecular identification of *Ostreopsis* cf. *ovata* in filter feeders and putative predators. *Harmful Algae* 21–22: 20–29.

Gantar, M., Sekar, R., Richardson, L. 2009. Cyanotoxins from black band disease of corals and from other coral reef environments. *Microb Ecol* 58:856–864.

Garet, E., Cabado, A.G., Vieites, J.M., Gonzalez-Fernandez, A. 2010. Rapid isolation of single-chain antibodies by phage display technology directed against one of the most potent marine toxins: Palytoxin. *Toxicon* 55: 1519–1526.

Gatti, C., Oelher, E., Legrand, A.M. 2008. Severe seafood poisoning in French Polynesia: A retrospective analysis of 129 medical files. *Toxicon* 51: 746–753.

Gleibs, S., Mebs, D. 1999. Distribution and sequestration of palytoxin in coral reef animals. *Toxicon* 37: 1521–1527.

Gonzales, R.B., Alcala, A.C. 1977. Fatalities from crab poisoning on Negros Island, Philippines. *Toxicon* 15: 169–170.

Grauer, F.H., Arnold, H.L. 1961. Seaweed dermatitis. *Arch Dermatol* 84: 720.

Habermann, E. 1989. Palytoxin acts through Na$^+$,K$^+$-ATPase. *Toxicon* 27: 1171–1187.

Herfindal, L., Jokela, J., Myhren, L., Permi, P., Selheim, F., Wahlsten, M., Kleppe, R. et al. 2010. A novel nostocyclopeptide inhibits microcystin and nodularin induced apoptosis in hepatocytes. *Chem Bio Chem* 11:1594–1599.

Hoffmann, K., Hermanns-Clausen, M., Buhl, C., Buchler, M.W., Schemmer, P., Mebs, D. et al. 2008. A case of palytoxin poisoning due to contact with zoanthid corals through a skin injury. *Toxicon* 51: 1535–1537.

Huynh, M.U., Elston, M.C., Hernandez, N.M., Ball, D.B., Kajiyama, S., Irie, K. et al. 2010. Enzymatic production of (-)-indolactam V by LtxB, a cytochrome P450 monooxygenase. *J Nat Prod* 73: 71–74.

Ito, E., Satake, M., Yasumoto, T. 2002. Pathological effects of lyngbyatoxin A upon mice. *Toxicon* 40: 551–556.

Izumi, A.K., Moore, R.E. 1987. Seaweed (*Lyngbya majuscula*) dermatitis. *Clin Dermatol* 5: 92–100.

Jochimsen, E.M., Carmichael, W.W., An, J.S., Cardo, D.M., Cookson, S.T., Holmes, C.E., Antunes, M.B. et al. 1998. Liver failure and death after exposure to microcystins at a hemodialysis center in Brazil. *N Engl J Med* 338:873–878.

Jones, A.C., Gu, L.C., Sorrels, C.M., Sherman, D.H., Gerwick, W.H. 2009. New tricks from ancient algae: Natural products biosynthesis in marine cyanobacteria. *Curr Opin Chem Biol* 13: 216–223.

Jones, A.C., Monroe, E.A., Podell, S., Hess, W.R., Klages, S., Esquenazi, E. et al. 2011. Genomic insights into the physiology and ecology of the marine filamentous cyanobacterium *Lyngbya majuscula*. *Proc Natl Acad Sci USA* 108: 8815–8820.

Kaasalainen, U., Fewer, D.P., Jokela, J., Wahlsten, M., Sivonen, K., Rikkinen, J. 2012. Cyanobacteria produce a high variety of hepatotoxic peptides in lichen symbiosis. *Proc Natl Acad Sci USA* 109(15): 5886–5891.

Karamyan, V.T., Speth, R.C., 2008. Animal models of BMAA neurotoxicity: A critical review. *Life Sci* 82: 233–246.

Kerbrat, A.S., Amzil, Z., Pawlowiez, R., Golubic, S., Sibat, M., Darius, H.T. et al. 2011. First evidence of palytoxin and 42-hydroxy-palytoxin in the marine cyanobacterium *Trichodesmium*. *Mar Drugs* 9: 543–560.

Kozikowski, A.P., Sato, K., Basu, A., Lazo, J.S. 1989. Synthesis and biological studies of simplified analogs of lyngbyatoxin-a—Use of an isoxazoline-based indole synthesis—Quest for protein kinase-C modulators. *J Am Chem Soc* 111: 6228–6234.

Kozikowski, A.P., Shum, P.W., Basu, A., Lazo, J.S. 1991. Synthesis of structural analogs of lyngbyatoxin-a and their evaluation as activators of protein-kinase-C. *J Med Chem* 34: 2420–2430.

Lambert, T.W., Boland, M.P., Holmes, C.F.B., Hrudey, S.E. 1994. *Environ Sci Technol* 28:753.

Leão, P.N., Engene, N., Antunes, A., Gerwick, W.H., Vasconcelos, V. 2012. The chemical ecology of cyanobacteria. *Nat Prod Rep* 29: 372–391.

Leão, P.N., Pereira, A.R., Liu, W.-T., Konig, G.M., Dorrestein, P.C., Vasconcelos, V.M., Gerwick, W.H.. 2010. Synergistic allelochemicals from a freshwater cyanobacterium. *Proc Natl Acad Sci* 107: 11183–11188.

Ledreux, A., Krys, S., Bernard, C. 2009. Suitability of the Neuro-2a cell line for the detection of palytoxin and analogues (neurotoxic phycotoxins). *Toxicon* 53: 300–308.

Lenoir, S., Ten-Hage, L., Turquet, J., Quod, J.P., Bernard, C., Hennion, M.C. 2004. First evidence of palytoxin analogues from an *Ostreopsis mascarenensis* (Dinophyceae) benthic bloom in Southwestern Indian Ocean. *J Phycol* 40: 1042–1051.

Liu, X., Rush, T., Zapata, J., Lobner, D. 2009. Beta-N-methylamino-L-alanine induces oxidative stress and glutamate release through action on system Xc(-). *Exp Neurol* 217(2): 429–433.

Lopes, V.R., Sschimtke, M., Fernandes M.H., Martins, R., Vasconcelos, V. 2011. Cytotoxicity in L929 fibroblasts and inhibition of herpes simplex virus type 1 Kupka viruses by estuarine cyanobacteria. *Toxicol In Vitro* 25: 944–950.

Louzao, M.C., Ares, I.R., Cagide, E., Espina, B., Vilarino, N., Alfonso, A. et al. 2011. Palytoxins and cytoskeleton: An overview. *Toxicon* 57: 460–469.

MacKintosh, R.W., Dalby, K.N., Campbell, D.G., Cohen, P.T.W., Cohen, P., MacKintosh, C. 1995. The cyanobacterial toxin microcystin binds covalently to to cysteine-273 on protein phosphatase 1. *FEBS Lett* 371: 236–240.

Majlesi, N., Su, M.K., Chan, G.M., Lee, D.C., Greller, H.A. 2008. A case of inhalational exposure to palytoxin. *Clin Toxicol* 46: 637–637.

Martins, J., Saker M., Moreira C., Welker, M., Fastner J., Vasconcelos, V., 2009. Peptides produced by strains of the cyanobacterium *Microcystis aeruginosa* isolated from Portuguese water supplies. *Appl Microbiol Biotechnol* 82(5): 951–961.

Martins, J.C., Machado, J.P., Martins, A., Azevedo, J., Olivateles, L., Vasconcelos, V. 2011. Dynamics of protein phosphatase gene expression in *Corbicula fluminea* exposed to microcystin-LR and to toxic *Microcystis aeruginosa* cells. *Int J Mol Sci* 12: 9172–9188.

Martins, R., Ramos, M., Herfindal, L., Sousa, J.A., Doskeland, S., Vasconcelos, V.M., 2008. Antimicrobial and cytotoxic assessment of marine cyanobacteria extracts. *Marine Drugs* 6(1): 1–11.

Mayumi, T., Kato, H., Imanishi, S., Kawasaki, Y., Hasegawa, M., Harada, K. 2006. Structural characterization of microcystins by LC/MS/MS under ion trap conditions. *J Antibiot* 59, 710–719.

Mereish, K.A., Morris, S., Mccullers, G., Taylor, T.J., Bunner, D.L. 1991. Analysis of palytoxin by liquid-chromatography and capillary electrophoresis. *J Liq Chromatogr* 14: 1025–1031.

Miller, M., Kudela, R., Mekebri, A., Crane, D., Oates, S., Tinker, M.T., Staedler, M. et al. 2010. Evidence for a novel marine harmful algal bloom: Cyanotoxin (Microcystin) transfer from land to sea otters. *PLoS One* 5(9): e12576.

Monroe, E.A., Van Dolah, F.M. 2008. The toxic dinoflagellate *Karenia brevis* encodes novel type I-like polyketide synthases containing discrete catalytic domains. *Protist* 159: 471–482.

Moore, R.E., Bartolini, G., Barchi, J., Bothnerby, A.A., Dadok, J., Ford, J. 1982a. Absolute stereochemistry of palytoxin. *J Am Chem Soc* 104: 3776–3779.

Moore, R.E., Helfrich, P., Patterson, G.M.L. 1982b. The deadly seaweed of Hana. *Oceanus* 25: 54–63.

Moore, R.E., Scheuer, P.J. 1971. Palytoxin—New marine toxin from a coelenterate. *Science* 172: 495–498.

Morais, J., Augusto, M., Carvalho, A.P., Vale, M., Vasconcelos, V.M. 2008. Microcystins—Cyanobacteria hepatotoxins- bioavailability in contaminated mussels exposed to different environmental conditions. *Eur Food Res Technol* 227: 949–952.

Munday, R. 2011. Palytoxin toxicology: Animal studies. *Toxicon* 57: 470–477.

Muramatsu, I., Uemura, D., Fujiwara, M., Narahashi, T. 1984. Characteristics of Palytoxin-induced depolarization in squid Axons. *J Pharmacol Exp Ther* 231: 488–494.

Muratake, H., Natsume, M. 1987. Total synthesis of lyngbyatoxin-a (Teleocidin-a-1) and Teleocidin-a-2. *Tetrahedron Lett* 28: 2265–2268.

Murray, S.A., Garby, T., Hoppenrath, M., Neilan, B.A. 2012. Genetic diversity, morphological uniformity and polyketide production in dinoflagellates (*Amphidinium*, Dinoflagellata). *Plos One* 7: e38253.

Nakagawa, Y. 2012. Artificial analogs of naturally occurring tumor promoters as biochemical tools and therapeutic leads. *Biosci Biotechnol Biochem* 76: 1262–1274.

Newhouse, T., Baran, P.S., Hoffmann, R.W. 2009. The economies of synthesis. *Chem Soc Rev* 38: 3010–3021.

Nordt, S.P., Wu, J., Zahller, S., Clark, R.F., Cantrell, F.L. 2011. Palytoxin poisoning after dermal contact with zoanthid coral. *J Emerg Med* 40: 397–399.

Onuma, Y., Satake, M., Ukena, T., Roux, J., Chanteau, S., Rasolofonirina, N. et al. 1999. Identification of putative palytoxin as the cause of clupeotoxism. *Toxicon* 37: 55–65.

Paul, V.J., Arthur, K.E., Ritson-Williams, R., Ross, C., Sharp, K. 2007. Chemical defenses: From compounds to communities. *Biol Bull* 213: 226–251.

Pereira, S., Saker, M., Vale, M., Vasconcelos, V.M. 2009. Comparison of sensitivity of grasses (*Lolium perenne* L. and *Festuca rubra* L.) and lettuce (*Lactuca sativa* L.) exposed to water contaminated with microcystins. *Bull Environ Contam Toxicol* 83: 81–84.

Pereira, S., Vasconcelos, V., Antunes, A., 2010. The phosphoprotein phosphatase family of Ser/Thr phosphatases as principal targets of naturally occurring toxins. *Crit Rev Toxicol* 41: 83–110.

Prieto, A., Campos A., Camean, A., Vasconcelos, V. 2011. Effects on growth and oxidative stress status of rice plants (*Oryza sativa*) exposed to two extracts of toxin-producing cyanobacteria (*Aphanizomenon ovalisporum* and *Microcystis aeruginosa*). *Ecotoxicol Environ Safety* 74: 1973–1980.

Rachele, M.G., Mascia, V., Tacconi, P., Dessi, N., Marrosu, F., Giagheddu, M. 1998. Conjugal amyotrophic lateral sclerosis: A report on a couple from Sardinia, Italy. *Ital J Neurol Sci* 19(2):97–100.

Ramos, V., Vasconcelos, V. 2010. Palytoxin and analogs: Biological and ecological effects. *Mar Drugs* 8: 2021–2037.

Rao, S.D., Banack, S.A., Cox, P.A., Weiss, J.H. 2006. BMAA selectively injures motor neurons via AMPA/kainate receptor activation. *Exp Neurol* 201(1): 244–252.

Rapala, J., Erkomaa, K., Kukkonen, J., Sivonen, K., Lahti, K., 2002. Detection of microcystins with protein phosphatase inhibition assay, high-performance liquid chromatography–UV detection and enzyme-linked immunosorbent assay. Comparison of methods. *Anal Chim Acta* 466: 213–231.

Read, J.A., Walsh, C.T. 2007. The lyngbyatoxin biosynthetic assembly line: Chain release by four-electron reduction of a dipeptidyl thioester to the corresponding alcohol. *J Am Chem Soc* 129: 15762–15763.

Rinehart, K.L., Harada, K., Namikoshi, M., Chen, C., Harvis, C.A. 1988. Nodularin, microcystin and the configuration of Adda. *J Am Chem Soc* 110(25): 8557–8558.

Riobo, P., Franco, J.M. 2011. Palytoxins: Biological and chemical determination. *Toxicon* 57: 368–375.

Riobo, P., Paz, B., Franco, J.M. 2006. Analysis of palytoxin-like in *Ostreopsis* cultures by liquid chromatography with precolumn derivatization and fluorescence detection. *Anal Chim Acta* 566: 217–223.

Sagara, T., Nishibori, N., Itoh, M., Morita, K., Her, S. 2013. Palytoxin causes nonoxidative necrotic damage to PC12 cells in culture. *J Appl Toxicol* 33: 120–124.

Sakai, S., Hitotsuyanagi, Y., Aimi, N., Fujiki, H., Suganuma, M., Sugimura, T. et al. 1986. Absolute configuration of Lyngbyatoxin-a (Teleocidin a-1) and Teleocidin a-2. *Tetrahedron Lett* 27: 5219–5220.

Saker, M.L., Fastner, J., Dittmann, E., Christiansen, G., Vasconcelos, V.M., 2005. Variation between strains of the cyanobacterium *Microcystis aeruginosa* isolated from a Portuguese river. *J Appl Microbiol* 99:749–757.

Saqrane, S., El Ghazali, I., Oudra, B., Bouarab, L., Vasconcelos, V. 2008. Effects of cyanobacteria producing microcystins on seed germination and seedling growth of several agricultural plants. *J Enviorn Sci Health- Part B* 43(5): 443–451.

Scheinerbobis, G., Heringdorf, D.M.Z., Christ, M., Habermann, E. 1994. Palytoxin Induces K^+ efflux from yeast-cells expressing the mammalian sodium-pump. *Mol Pharmacol* 45: 1132–1136.

Sedlock, D.M., Sun, H.H., Smith, W.F., Kawaoka, K., Gillum, A.M., Cooper, R. 1992. Rapid identification of teleocidins in fermentation broth using HPLC photodiode array and LC MS methodology. *J Ind Microbiol* 9: 45–52.

Selwood, A.I., van Ginkel, R., Harwood, D.T., McNabb, P.S., Rhodes, L.R., Holland, P.T. 2012. A sensitive assay for palytoxins, ovatoxins and ostreocins using LC-MS/MS analysis of cleavage fragments from micro-scale oxidation. *Toxicon* 60: 810–820.

Simoni, F., Gaddi, A., Di Paolo, C., Lepri, L., Macnino, A., Falaschi, A. 2004. Further investigation on blooms of *Ostreopsis ovata*, *Coolia monotis*, *Prorocentrum lima* on the macroalgae of artificial and natural reefs in the Northern Tyrrhenian Sea. *Harmful Algae News* 26: 5–7.

Sivonen, K., Jones, G. 1999. In toxic cyanobacteria in water. A guide to their public health consequences, monitoring and management, eds. Chorus, I., Bartram, J. E & FN Spon, London, U.K., pp. 41–111.

Stafford, R.G., Mehta, M., Kemppainen, B.W. 1992. Comparison of the partition-coefficient and skin penetration of a marine algal toxin (Lyngbyatoxin-a). *Food Chem Toxicol* 30: 795–801.

Suh, E.M., Kishi, Y. 1994. Synthesis of palytoxin from palytoxin carboxylic-acid. *J Am Chem Soc* 116: 11205–11206.

Tillett, D., Dittmann, E., Erhard, M., von Döhren H, Börner T, Neilan, B.A. 2000. Structural organization of microcystin biosynthesis in *Microcystis aeruginosa* PCC 7806: An integrated peptide-polyketide synthetase system. *Chem Biol* 7: 753–764.

Tippkötter, N., Stückmann, H., Kroll, S., Winkelmann, G., Noack, U., Scheper, T., Ulber, R. 2009. A semiquantitative dipstick assay for microcystin. *Anal Bioanal Chem* 394: 863–869.

Ueno, Y., Nagata, S., Tsutsumi, T., Hasegawa A., Yoshida, F., Suttajit, M., Pütsch, M., Vasconcelos V., 1996. *Nat Toxins* 4: 271.

Usami, M., Satake, M., Ishida, S., Inoue, A., Kan, Y., Yasumoto, T. 1995. Palytoxin analogs from the dinoflagellate *Ostreopsis siamensis*. *J Am Chem Soc* 117: 5389–5390.

Vareli, K., Zarali, E., Zacharioudakis, G., Vagenas, G., Varelis, V., Pilidis, G., Briasoulis, E., Sainis, I. 2012. Microcystin producing cyanobacterial communities in Amvrakikos Gulf (Mediterranean Sea, NW Greece) and toxin accumulation in mussels (*Mytilus galloprovincialis*). *Harmful Algae* 15: 109–118.

Vasconcelos, V., Oliveira, S., Teles, F.O. 2001. Impact of a toxic and a nontoxic strain of *Microcystis aeruginosa* on the crayfish *Procambarus clarkii*. *Toxicon* 39: 1461–1470.

Vasconcelos, V.M. 1995. Uptake and depuration of the heptapeptide toxin microcystin-LR in *Mytilus galloprovincialis*. *Aquat Toxicol* 32: 227–237.

Vasconcelos, V.M., Sivonen, K., Evans, W.R., Carmichael, W.W., Namikoshi, M. 1996. Hepatotoxic microcystin diversity in cyanobacterial blooms collected in Portuguese freshwaters. *Water Res* 30: 2377–2384.

Ward, C.J., Beattie, K.A., Lee, E.Y.C., Codd, G.A. 1997. *FEMS Microbiol Lett* 153: 465.

Weiss, J.H., Koh, J.Y., Choi, D.W. 1989. Neurotoxicity of beta-N-methylamino-L-alanine (BMAA) and beta-N-oxalylamino-L-alanine (BOAA) on cultured cortical neurons. *Brain Res* 497(1): 64–71.

Wiles, J.S., Vick, J.A., Christen, M.K. 1974. Toxicological evaluation of palytoxin in several animal species. *Toxicon* 12: 427–433.

Wu, C.H. 2009. Palytoxin: Membrane mechanisms of action. *Toxicon* 54: 1183–1189.

Yakes, B.J., DeGrasse, S.L., Poli, M., Deeds, J.R. 2011. Antibody characterization and immunoassays for palytoxin using an SPR biosensor. *Anal Bioanal Chem* 400: 2865–2869.

Yasumoto, T. 1998. Fish poisoning due to toxins of microalgal origins in the Pacific. *Toxicon* 36: 1515–1518.

Yasumoto, T., Oshima, Y., Yamaguchi, M. 1978. Occurrence of a new type of shellfish poisoning in the Tohoku district. *Bull Jpn Soc Sci Fish* 44: 1249–1255.

Zamolo, V.A., Valenti, G., Venturelli, E., Chaloin, O., Marcaccio, M., Boscolo, S. et al. 2012. Highly sensitive electrochemiluminescent nanobiosensor for the detection of palytoxin. *ACS Nano* 6: 7989–7997.

39

Calcium Channels for Exocytosis and Endocytosis: Pharmacological Modulation

Antonio M.G. de Diego, Luis Gandía, Fernando Padín, and Antonio G. García

CONTENTS

39.1 Introduction

Voltage-dependent Ca^{2+} channels (VDCCs) constitute a key element in neuronal communication, serving as transducers of membrane potential changes into intracellular Ca^{2+} transients that initiate many physiological events. The combination of patch-clamp techniques, ω-toxins, and molecular strategies has revealed a great heterogeneity of VDCCs in neurons. Up to ten members of the VDCC family have been identified in mammals, and they serve distinct roles in cellular signal transduction. Peptide toxins derived from the venoms of marine snails *Conus geographus* (ω-conotoxin GVIA), *C. magus* (ω-conotoxins MVIIA, MVIIC, and MVIID), as well as from *Agelenopsis aperta* spider venom (FTX, ω-agatoxin IVA) are powerful diagnostic pharmacological tools to discriminate between different subtypes of neuronal Ca^{2+} channels. Thus, the so-called high-voltage-activated (HVA) Ca^{2+} channels are selectively recognized by ω-conotoxin GVIA and MVIIA (N type), by low concentrations (nanomolar) of ω-agatoxin IVA (P-type), or by high concentrations of ω-agatoxin IVA (micromolar) or the ω-conotoxins MVIIC and MVIID (Q type). L-type HVA Ca^{2+} channels present in neurons, cardiovascular tissues, skeletal and smooth muscle, and endocrine cells are targeted by the so-called organic Ca^{2+} antagonists such as the 1,4-dihydropyridines (DHP) nifedipine or the agonist BayK8644, the benzylalkylamine verapamil, or the benzothiazepine diltiazem; they are also specifically blocked by snake toxins calciseptine and calcicludine. Wide-spectrum ω-toxins (ω-conotoxin MVIIC, ω-agatoxin IA, IIA, and IIIA) and organic compounds (flunarizine, dotarizine, cinnarizine, fluspirilene, R56865, lubeluzole, ITH33/IQM9.21) can block several classes of HVA Ca^{2+} channels, including the L type. A neuronal R-type HVA channel seems to be sensitive to SNX-482, a peptide from the venom of the African tarantula *Hysterocrates gigas*. Low-voltage-activated (LVA) channels (T-type) are blocked by 1-octanol, amiloride, mibefradil, and NNC 55-0396 and are more sensitive to Ni^{2+} than to Cd^{2+}; no toxins are known that recognize these channels.

It is interesting that a single cell can express different subtypes of HVA Ca^{2+} channels and that the quantitative expression of each channel subtype differs with the animal species. The example of adrenal medulla chromaffin cells is illustrative. In the bovine, P/Q type (45%) and N type (35%) are predominant; the L-type Ca^{2+} channel carries a minor component of the whole-cell current (20%). In the rat and the mouse, the L type predominates (50%), together with the N type (35%), whereas the P/Q family accounts for a minor component (15%). In cat chromaffin cells, L-type Ca^{2+} channels carry 50% of the current and N-type channels 45%; P/Q account by only 5%. In human chromaffin cells, P/Q-type Ca^{2+} channels dominate (60%), while in pig chromaffin cells, N-type channels are predominant (80%). The functional significance of this variety of Ca^{2+} channels begins to be understood.

Ca^{2+} channels basically consist of a multiple subunit protein complex with a central pore-forming α_1 subunit and several regulatory and/or auxiliary subunits, which include β subunits, γ subunits, and the disulfide-linked α_2/δ subunit. The α_1 subunit contains the Ca^{2+} conductance pore, the essential gating machinery, the receptor sites for the most prominent pharmacological agents, and modulatory sites for

G protein subunits, protein kinase–induced phosphorylation, or exocytotic machinery protein binding sites. The mammalian family of Ca^{2+} channel α_1 subunits is encoded by at least 10 genes. These subunits are grouped in three families, Ca_V1, Ca_V2, and Ca_V3, that give rise to inward Ca^{2+} currents termed HVA or L, N, P/Q, and R channels and LVA or T-type channels.

Marine toxins have been invaluable tools to recognize the role of each channel subtype in controlling the Ca^{2+}-dependent exocytotic release of a given neurotransmitter. Thus, N-type Ca^{2+} channels are highly involved in the control of norepinephrine release from sympathetic neurons, as well as acetylcholine release from the electric fish muscle end plate, the myenteric plexus, and detrusor muscle. Also, N channels partially control the nonadrenergic, noncholinergic (NANC) neurotransmission in smooth muscle, gamma-aminobutyric acid (GABA) release in cerebellar neurons, glycine release in dorsal horn neurons of the spinal cord, epinephrine release from the dog adrenal, dynorphin release in dentate gyrus, and the synaptic neurotransmission in retinal ganglion neurons and the hippocampus. P channels dominate the release of GABA from deep cerebellar neurons, glycine from dorsal horn neurons of the spinal cord, and acetylcholine from the mammalian neuromuscular junction. They also seem to participate partially in the control of the release of other neurotransmitters. Up to now, Q channels have been implicated in the control of neurotransmission in the hippocampus and in the release of catecholamines from bovine chromaffin cells. L-type Ca^{2+} channels dominate the release of catecholamines in rat and cat chromaffin cells and partially control the secretory process in bovine chromaffin cells.

A critical question is why a neurosecretory cell expresses several Ca^{2+} channel subtypes. In bovine adrenal chromaffin cells, L, N, P, Q, and R channels have been found; depending on the stimulus and the experimental conditions, all of them seem to be involved in the control of catecholamine release induced by depolarizing stimuli. It is uncertain whether a given Ca^{2+} channel subtype colocalizes more than others with the secretory machinery of chromaffin cells. Many other questions remain unanswered, for instance, to find a selective blocker for the R-type channel. A third question relates to the number of Ca^{2+} channels yet unrecognized. The functions of the Ca^{2+} channels not related to exocytosis (i.e., the neuronal L-type channels) are beginning to be discovered; thus, Ca^{2+} entry through these channels may cause gene induction, apoptosis, or preferentially activates endo- over exocytosis, in bovine chromaffin cells.[1] Finally, it is important to stress the need of finding non-peptide molecules to target specifically different channel subtypes; these compounds should cross the blood–brain barrier and thus serve as therapeutic drugs to treat different brain diseases. We will review in this chapter all these aspects, making emphasis in ω-toxins as tools to identify Ca^{2+} channels, Ca^{2+} signals, and cell function, particularly exocytosis.

39.2 ω-Toxins as Pharmacological Tools

Some static or slow animals, both terrestrial (snakes, spiders) and marine (snails), have developed a distinctive repertoire of venom peptides that are used both as a defense mechanism and also to facilitate the immobilization and digestion of prey. These peptides target a wide variety of voltage- and ligand-gated ion channels, which make them an invaluable resource for studying the properties of these ion channels in normal and diseased states, as well as being a collection of compounds of potential pharmacological use in their own right.

One of the most representative examples of venomous animals is constituted by the invertebrate cone marine snails (genus *Conus*) comprising approximately 700 species,[2] with each *Conus* species producing a distinctive repertoire of about 100–200 venom peptides.[3,4] The venom peptides are used to immobilize and digest prey as well as to defend cone snails from predators by potently and specifically targeting the voltage- and ligand-gated ion channels in the nervous systems of prey. In addition, it has been demonstrated that these *Conus* peptides also act on homologous mammalian ion channels due to the degree of structural conservation exhibited by the voltage- and ligand-gated ion channels across higher eukaryotes, providing valuable research tools for the dissection of the role played by the different ion channels in excitable cells.

Several types of conotoxins have been identified and characterized so far,[5] which target different ionic channels, such as α (alpha)-conotoxins, which inhibit nicotinic receptors at nerves and muscles[6]; δ (delta)-conotoxins, which inhibit the inactivation of voltage-dependent sodium channels[7]; κ (kappa)-conotoxins, which inhibit potassium channels[8]; μ (mu)-conotoxins, which inhibit voltage-dependent sodium channels[9]; and ω (omega)-conotoxins, which inhibit VDCCs.[3]

Of these approximately 700 *Conus* species, about 40–100 prey primarily on fish (fish-hunting species), and these species use two parallel physiological mechanisms requiring multiple neurotoxins to immobilize fish rapidly[10]: neuromuscular block and exocytotoxic shock. Fish-hunting *Conus* snails use a harpoon-like device to inject their venom in their preys. The venom contains a cocktail of neurotoxins that will cause a double-phase paralytic process (Table 39.1), with an initial phase characterized by a fast paralysis with tetanus and a second phase characterized by a flaccid paralysis. Finally, the fish will be engulfed by the snail.

The fast paralysis of the phase I is mediated by two groups of neurotoxins, the δ-conotoxins, which suppress the inactivation of the voltage-dependent Na+ channels, thus causing an increase in Na+ influx, and the κ-conotoxins, which block K+ channels, not allowing the cells to repolarize. This combination of toxins lead to hyperactivity of the fish, followed by a continuous contraction and extension of major fins, without death. The second phase consists in a flaccid state and is caused by a different cocktail of neurotoxins (see Table 39.1): The α-conotoxins, which block nicotinic acetylcholine receptors; the μ-conotoxins, which block voltage-dependent Na+ channels; the ψ-conotoxins, which also block nicotinic acetylcholine receptors; the κ-conotoxins, which cause the blockade of K+ channels; the δ-conotoxins, which suppress the inactivation of the voltage-dependent Na+ channels; and the ω-conotoxins, which block VDCCs and are the subject of this chapter.

Another example of venomous animals is the funnel-web spider *A. aperta* that has a potent venom with paralytic properties. As in the *Conus*, the venom of this spider possesses a mixture of toxins with different targets, with the polyamines and the polypeptides being the main components of such venom. The polyamines group is composed of the funnel-web toxin (FTX), which targets VDCCs,[11] and the acyl-polyamines (α-agatoxins), which are noncompetitive, use-dependent antagonists of glutamate receptor channels. The other group, the polypeptide toxins, is composed of other two agatoxins, the μ-agatoxins, which are potent activators of voltage-dependent Na+ channels, and the ω-agatoxins, which selectively block different subtypes of VDCCs.[12] This combination of toxins secures a fast and reversible paralytic effect (induced by the α- and μ-agatoxins) with a slower but irreversible paralysis of the prey, induced by the ω-agatoxins. The α-agatoxins and ω-agatoxins modify both insect and vertebrate ion channels, while the μ-agatoxins are selective for insect channels.[13]

Finally, venoms from different snakes from the *Elapidae* and *Hydrophiidae* families also contain a cocktail of different paralytic toxins, some of which are selective for VDCCs. For instance, the venom of the black mamba (*Dendroaspis polylepis polylepis*) contains a toxin termed calciseptine, which selectively blocks L-type Ca2+ channels,[14] and the venom from the green mamba (*D. angusticeps*) contains calciclu-dine, a toxin that acts as a potent blocker of most of the high VDCCs.[15] A more detailed explanation of the toxins most frequently used to characterize the various subtypes of HVA Ca2+ channels follows.

TABLE 39.1

Paralytic Process Induced by the Venom of Conus Marine Snails and Neurotoxins Involved in Their Mechanisms of Action

Phase I: Fast Paralysis with Tetanus (Rapid Immobilization)	
δ-Conotoxins	Suppression of Na+ channel inactivation (increases Na+ influx)
κ-Conotoxins	Blockade of K+ channels
Phase II: Flaccid Paralysis	
α-Conotoxins	Blockade of nicotinic acetylcholine receptors
μ-Conotoxins	Blockade of voltage-dependent Na+ channels
ψ-Conotoxins	Blockade of nicotinic acetylcholine receptors
κ-Conotoxins	Blockade of K+ channels
δ-Conotoxins	Suppression of Na+ channel inactivation
ω-Conotoxins	Blockade of voltage-dependent Ca2+ channels

39.2.1 ω-Conotoxins

ω-Conotoxins are small disulfide-bonded peptides, typically composed of 24–30 amino acid residues (Figure 39.1); they share several features, which are common to all ω-conotoxins. The more characteristic is the presence of a Cys-residue scaffolding pattern, with six Cys residues, and three intramolecular disulfide bridges, forming a structure known as "four-loop framework."[16,17] This arrangement of Cys residues is similar to that observed in δ-conotoxins, which target voltage-gated Na$^+$ channels.[18]

ω-Conotoxins with defined activity at mammalian VDCCs isoforms have so far been isolated only from piscivorous cone snails,[19] and up to 22 ω-conotoxins targeting VDCCs have been identified and functionally characterized.[5,20] Although the sequence of different ω-conotoxins has great interspecies variations, they can compete for the same Ca^{2+} binding site and show similar physiological effects. For instance, ω-conotoxin GVIA[21] and ω-conotoxin MVIIA[22] have a homology lower than 30% in the non-Cys residues, but both target N-type Ca^{2+} channels (as described in the succeeding text) and elicit similar biological effects; the major differences are that ω-conotoxin GVIA blocks N-type Ca^{2+} channels in an irreversible manner,[3,23] whereas ω-conotoxin MVIIA does it in a reversible manner.[24,25]

Other ω-conotoxins have broader Ca^{2+} channel blocking properties than ω-conotoxin GVIA and ω-conotoxin MVIIA. cDNA clones encoding a previously unknown ω-conotoxin were identified from a cDNA library made from the venom duct of *C. magus*.[26] The predicted peptides ω-conotoxin MVIIC and ω-conotoxin MVIID were chemically synthesized and characterized. Both peptides inhibit N-type Ca^{2+} channels and P-type Ca^{2+} channels, but also other Ca^{2+} channels resistant to 1,4-DHP, ω-conotoxin GVIA, and ω-agatoxin IVA,[26] and thus, they constitute actually an important tool for the characterization of P/Q types of Ca^{2+} channels, as described in the succeeding text. Some differences between the ω-conotoxins relate to the reversibility of its blocking effects, and thus, N-type Ca^{2+} channels can be blocked in an irreversible manner by ω-conotoxin MVIIC but in a reversible manner by ω-conotoxin MVIID.[27]

39.2.2 ω-Agatoxins

ω-Agatoxins derived from the venom of *A. aperta* are also a heterogeneous group of polypeptides (5–100 kD) that specifically target VDCCs. Four subtypes of ω-agatoxins have been identified up to now.[12,13,28,29] Type I ω-agatoxins (ω-Aga-IA, ω-Aga-IB, and ω-Aga-IC) are potent blockers of neuromuscular transmission in insects. Of these, the most studied is ω-agatoxin IA, which seems to block both L- and N-type Ca^{2+} channels.[30] Type II ω-agatoxins have a spectrum of action on neuronal Ca^{2+} channels

ω-Conotoxin GVIA	CKSOGSS**C**SOTSYN**CC**R.S**C**NOYTRK**C**Y
ω-Conotoxin MVIIA	CKGKGAK**C**SRLMYD**CC**TGS**C**R..SGK**C**
ω-Conotoxin MVIIC	CKGKGAP**C**RKTMYD**CC**SGS**C**.GRRGK**C**
ω-Conotoxin MVIID	CQGRGAS**C**RKTMYN**CC**SGS**C**..NRGR**C**
ω-Conotoxin CVID	CKSKGAK**C**SKLMYD**CC**SGS**C**SGTVGR**C**
ω-Conotoxin CVIE	CKGKGAS**C**RRTSYD**CC**TGS**C**R..SGR**C**
ω-Conotoxin CVIF	CKGKGAS**C**RRTSYD**CC**TGS**C**R..LGR**C**
ω-Conotoxin SVIA	CRSSGSO**C**GVTSI.**CC**.GR**C**..YRGK**C**T
Disulfide linkages	C......C......CC...C.....C

FIGURE 39.1 Upper panel shows the sequence of ω-conotoxins isolated from *C. geographus* (GVIA), *C. magus* (MVIIA, MVIIC, and MVIID), *C. catus* (CVID, CVIE, and CVIF), and *C. striatus* (SVIA). Lower panel shows the arrangement of the Cys residues that constitutes de "four-loop" structure.

in vertebrates similar to that of ω-agatoxin IA, although they may block Ca^{2+} channels by a different mechanism.[31] ω-Agatoxin IIA has been shown as a potent blocker of both L- and N-type Ca^{2+} channels.[32]

Type III ω-agatoxins (ω-Aga IIIA, ω-Aga IIIB, ω-Aga IIIC, and ω-Aga IIID) have a broader spectrum of blockade than other agatoxins and block several subtypes of VDCCs.[33,34] Of these, ω-agatoxin IIIA has been shown to be a potent inhibitor or L-, N-, and P/Q-type Ca^{2+} channels in neurons of rats and frogs[35–37]; it shows a very high potency ($IC_{50} < 1$ nM) for both inhibiting L- and N-type channels, being more potent than ω-conotoxin GVIA for blocking N-type channels.[38] Efficacy of blockade induced by ω-agatoxin IIIA is higher for L-type channels and decreases for N- and P/Q-type Ca^{2+} channels.[36] In these latter channel subtypes, ω-agatoxin IIIA seems to act as a high-affinity partial antagonist, blocking less than 50% of Ca^{2+} conductance.[36]

Type IV ω-agatoxins (ω-Aga-IVA and ω-Aga-IVB) were discovered through screening of the venomous fractions against chick and rat synaptosomes. A new toxin, ω-Aga-IVA, was found showing a high specificity for P-type Ca^{2+} channels in mammalian brain with a K_d of 2–3 nM, with no effects on T-type, L-type, or N-type currents in a variety of central and peripheral neurons.[32,39,40] Since then, ω-Aga-IVA has become a diagnostic ligand for P-type channels in mammalian brain.[13] Further screening of *A. aperta* venom fractions identified a closely related toxin called ω-Aga-IVB (also called ω-Aga-TK).[41,42] The specificity and affinity of ω-Aga-IVB for P-type channels is indistinguishable from that of ω-Aga-IVA, although the kinetics of block are significantly slower.[41] Interestingly, the concentration of ω-Aga-IVB in the venom is 10-fold higher than that of ω-Aga-IVA.

39.3 Molecular Properties of Voltage-Dependent Ca^{2+} Channels

VDCCs are oligomeric complexes composed of up to five distinct proteins (α_1, β, α_2, δ, and γ).[43–46]

The α_1 protein incorporates the conduction pore, the voltage sensor, and gating apparatus, as well as most of the known binding sites of channel regulation by second messengers, drugs, and toxins. Associated with the pore-forming α_1 subunits of the Ca_v1 and Ca_v2 channels are the cytoplasmic β subunit (encoded by 4 different genes), the membrane anchored extracellular α_2/δ subunits (4 genes known), and the transmembrane γ subunit (10 genes known). Although the α_1 subunit has been considered as the central actor in these Ca_v channel complexes, auxiliary subunits aid membrane expression and alter the biophysical properties of the α_1 subunit.[44,47–49] Figure 39.2

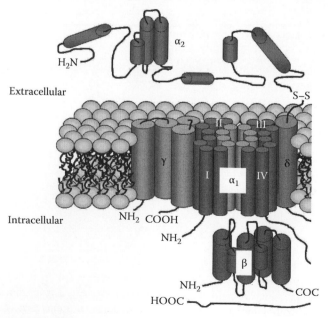

FIGURE 39.2 Subunit arrangement for a typical HVA Ca^{2+} channel.

represents the hypothetical subunit arrangement for a typical HVA Ca^{2+} channel. In contrast, the subunit composition of the Ca_v3 channels remains an open controversial issue.[50]

The α_1 subunits are large proteins with molecular weight between 212 and 273 kD. Each α_1 subunit of Ca_v channel is organized in four homologous repeats (I–IV) of the six transmembrane structures. Each repeat contains an S4 region that acts as the voltage sensor, a P-loop that forms the selective filter, and S6 segments that form the channel pore (Figure 39.2). The four domains are connected through cytoplasmic linkers, and both C- and N-termini are cytoplasmic. These regions contain sites of interaction with auxiliary subunits, binding sites for various activators and blockers, including G proteins, as well as several putative phosphorylation sites.

The β subunit of all HVA Ca_v channels is an intracellular auxiliary subunit that binds to a conserved alpha-interaction domain (AID) of the α_1 subunit to modulate channel gating properties and promote cell surface trafficking (Figure 39.2). This interaction site of both subunits was identified on the connector between I–II domains of the α_1 subunit.[51,52] Interestingly, it has been demonstrated that Gem, a small guanosine triphosphatase (GTPase) of the Rem–Gem–Kir (RGK) family, binds directly to the β subunit; this interaction inhibits the association of the β with the α_1 subunit, decreasing channel abundance by inhibiting transport to the plasma membrane.[53]

Although the aforementioned data suggest that the only function of the β subunit was to modulate the expression, targeting, gating, and activity of the main α_1 subunit, recent experimental evidence indicates that this function could represent a "part-time" job for some isoforms of the β subunit. In fact, the identification of a Src homology type (SH3) and guanylate kinase (GK) domains in the structure of the β subunit indicates that this subunit belongs to the membrane-associated guanylate kinase (MAGUK) family, thereby suggesting a role for the β subunit in scaffolding multiple signaling pathways around the channel.[52] Moreover, a recent study reveals that β_3 subunits directly reduce glucose-induced Ca^{2+} oscillations in pancreatic β cells.[54] Although far from being clearly demonstrated, two signaling pathways are proposed in this β_3 subunit-mediated effect: direct regulation of the inositol trisphosphate (IP_3) receptor and indirect reduction of phospholipase Cβ. Thus, β subunit now claims the status of independent regulatory protein.

The α_2/δ subunit is translated as a single protein but cleaved into δ (a single transmembrane-spanning helix) and α_2 (the extracellular domain), which are linked by a disulfide bond; however, its interaction site on the α_1 subunit is unknown. The γ subunit, characterized by four predicted transmembrane domains, was formerly found in skeletal muscle and later on in heart and brain Ca^{2+} channels.[49] One member of the γ subunit (γ_6) has been shown reducing the activity of a subtype of T-type Ca^{2+} channel in cardiomyocytes.[55] Even more, functional studies have suggested a dual role for another member of this family of proteins (γ_2, also known as stargazing), both as a modulatory γ subunit for Ca^{2+} channels and as a regulator of postsynaptic membrane targeting for AMPA-type glutamate receptors.[56,57]

39.3.1 Diversity of Ca^{2+} Channel α_1 Subunits

As described later, several types of VDCCs have been identified and classified based on their biophysical and pharmacological profiles as L-, N-, P-, Q-, R-, or T-types. These different types of VDCCs are primarily defined from the nature of the principal pore-forming α_1 subunit, and 10 different ones have been characterized by cDNA cloning and functional expression in mammalian cells or *Xenopus laevis*.[46]

These subunits can be divided into three structurally and functionally different families of Ca_v channel α_1 subunits.[58] The first Ca_v1 subfamily ($Ca_v1.1$-$Ca_v1.4$) includes VDCCs containing α_1 subunits that mediate L-type Ca^{2+} currents (α_{1S}, α_{1C}, α_{1D}, and α_{1F}). The second Ca_v2 subfamily ($Ca_v2.1$–$Ca_v2.3$) comprises VDCCs channels containing α_1 subunits that mediate P/Q-type (α_{1A}), N-type (α_{1B}), and R-type (α_{1E}) Ca^{2+} currents. Finally, the third Ca_v3 subfamily ($Ca_v3.1$–$Ca_v3.3$) includes LVA VDCCs channels containing α_1 subunits (α_{1G}, α_{1H}, and α_{1I}); members of this subfamily mediate T-type Ca^{2+} currents. In contrast to the Ca_v3 channels, which express by themselves as typical T-type Ca^{2+} channels in heterologous systems, Ca_v1 and Ca_v2 channels function as oligomeric complexes containing auxiliary subunits.

Table 39.2 summarizes the sequence similarity among the diverse Ca_v α_1 subunits known to date as well as the name of the gene encoding for each subunit. The amino acid alignment was constructed using the CLUSTAL program. Only the membrane-spanning regions of α_1 sequences were included into analysis.

TABLE 39.2

Calcium Channel Subtypes according to Their α_1-Containing Subunit

Calcium Channel Type					
(Novel Nomenclature)	(Traditional Nomenclature)	Type of Current	Blockers	Activators	Tissue Location
$Ca_v1.1$	α_{1S}	L	Nifedipine Nisoldipine Nitrendipine	BayK8644 FPL64176	Skeletal muscle
$Ca_v1.2$	α_{1C}	L	Nifedipine Nisoldipine Nitrendipine	BayK8644 FPL64176 PCA50941	Heart Smooth muscle Brain Pituitary Adrenal medulla
$Ca_v1.3$	α_{1D}	L	Nifedipine Calciseptine Calcicludine	BayK8644 FPL64176 PCA50941	Brain Pancreas Adrenal medulla Cochlea Kidney Ovary
$Ca_v1.4$	α_{1F}	L	Nifedipine	BayK8644 FPL64176	Retina
$Ca_v2.1$	α_{1A}	P/Q	ω-Aga-IVA ω-CTx-MVIIC ω-CTx-MVIID		Cerebellum Pituitary Cochlea Adrenal medulla
$Ca_v2.2$	α_{1B}	N	ω-CTx-GVIA ω-CTx-MVIIA ω-CTx-CVID ω-CTx-CVIE ω-CTx-CVIF	Glycerotoxin	Brain Peripheral nervous system Adrenal medulla
$Ca_v2.3$	α_{1E}	R	SNX-482		Brain Cochlea Retina Heart Pituitary Adrenal medulla
$Ca_v3.1$	α_{1G}	T	Kurtoxin Mibefradil NNC 55-0396		Brain Peripheral nervous system Adrenal medulla
$Ca_v3.2$	α_{1H}	T	Kurtoxin Mibefradil NNC 55-0396		Heart Brain Kidney Liver Adrenal glomerulosa Adrenal medulla
$Ca_v3.3$	α_{1I}	T	Mibefradil NNC 55-0396		Brain

ω-Aga-IVA, ω-agatoxin IVA; ω-CTx-GVIA, ω-conotoxin GVIA; ω-CTx-MVIIA, ω-conotoxin MVIIA; ω-CTx-MVIIC, ω-conotoxin MVIIC; ω-CTx-MVIID, ω-conotoxin MVIID.

Table 39.2 also shows the major sites of expression for each gene product. The diversity of α_1 genes found so far, together with the alternative splicing from each single gene, add a large structural diversity to the multitude of Ca^{2+} channel α_1 gene subproducts.

39.4 Calcium Currents through Voltage-Dependent Ca^{2+} Channels: Biophysical and Pharmacological Properties

Two approaches are mainly responsible for the discovery of the rich functional diversity of VDCCs. On the one hand, the characterization of the biophysical properties of Ca^{2+} channels (kinetics of activation, inactivation, and deactivation, voltage range for activation, conductance), both at the single-channel and at the whole-cell level has been possible thanks to the improvement of the patch-clamp techniques.[59] On the other hand, the isolation, purification, and synthesis of different neurotoxins have provided ligands with remarkable discrimination for different subtypes of high-threshold DHP-resistant Ca^{2+} channels.[3]

With the combination of the patch-clamp techniques and these pharmacological probes, at least five functional subtypes of VDCCs have been described up to now: T, L, N, P/Q, and R (Table 39.3). These channels can be classified according to their range of activation in two main groups: one with a low threshold for activation (LVA) and another with a high threshold for activation (HVA).

39.4.1 Low-Voltage-Activated, T-Type Ca^{2+} Channels

The first attempt to identify different subtypes of VDCCs was carried out by Carbone and Lux,[60] who identified two types of channels, those that open with small depolarizations from a hyperpolarized holding potential, so called LVA channels, and those that require higher depolarizations to open, so called HVA channels.

In addition to its low threshold for activation, LVA Ca^{2+} channels[60] are characterized by a similar permeability for Ca^{2+} and Ba^{2+}.[61,62] This channel was termed T (for "transient" or "tiny"), being the main characteristics of this channel its fast inactivation, which generates a transient current, and their inactivation when the holding potential is fixed between −60 and −50 mV. The single-channel conductance has been estimated to be around 8 pS.

In the last years, increasing attention has been focused on T-type Ca^{2+} channels and their possible physiological and pathophysiological roles. Efforts toward elucidating the exact roles of these Ca^{2+} channels have been hampered by the lack of T-type specific antagonists (there is currently no peptide toxin for T-type Ca^{2+} channels comparable to those targeting N- or P-type Ca^{2+} channels, and there are no organic molecules with potency and selectivity comparable to those of DHP for L-type Ca^{2+} channels), resulting in the subsequent use of less selective Ca^{2+} channel antagonists. In addition, the activities of these blockers often vary with cell or tissue type.

TABLE 39.3

Diversity of Voltage-Activated Ca^{2+} Channel α_1 Subunit Genes

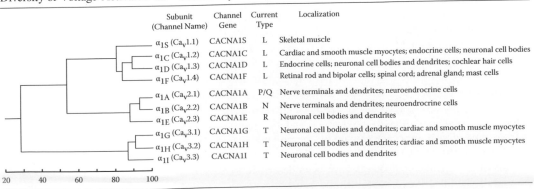

Subunit (Channel Name)	Channel Gene	Current Type	Localization
α_{1S} ($Ca_V1.1$)	CACNA1S	L	Skeletal muscle
α_{1C} ($Ca_V1.2$)	CACNA1C	L	Cardiac and smooth muscle myocytes; endocrine cells; neuronal cell bodies
α_{1D} ($Ca_V1.3$)	CACNA1D	L	Endocrine cells; neuronal cell bodies and dendrites; cochlear hair cells
α_{1F} ($Ca_V1.4$)	CACNA1F	L	Retinal rod and bipolar cells; spinal cord; adrenal gland; mast cells
α_{1A} ($Ca_V2.1$)	CACNA1A	P/Q	Nerve terminals and dendrites; neuroendocrine cells
α_{1B} ($Ca_V2.2$)	CACNA1B	N	Nerve terminals and dendrites; neuroendocrine cells
α_{1E} ($Ca_V2.3$)	CACNA1E	R	Neuronal cell bodies and dendrites
α_{1G} ($Ca_V3.1$)	CACNA1G	T	Neuronal cell bodies and dendrites; cardiac and smooth muscle myocytes
α_{1H} ($Ca_V3.2$)	CACNA1H	T	Neuronal cell bodies and dendrites; cardiac and smooth muscle myocytes
α_{1I} ($Ca_V3.3$)	CACNA1I	T	Neuronal cell bodies and dendrites

20   40   60   80   100

Pharmacologically, T-type channels can be distinguished from other subtypes because they are more sensitive to blockade by the inorganic Ca^{2+} channel blocker Ni^{2+} than to Cd^{2+}.[60-62] It has been described in various cell models how Ni^{2+}, despite the fact of blocking HVA Ca^{2+} channels, it was more sensitive for T-type Ca^{2+} channels.[63] Ni^{2+} is a selective blocker of α_{1H} channels; however, the concentrations that block the other T-subtypes (α_{1G} and α_{1I}) also inhibit HVA currents.[64] Low concentrations of Ni^{2+} (<50 μM) have been used to selectively block T-type currents in several cell types, such as sinoatrial nodal cells[65] and sensory neurons.[66] However, T-type currents in various neuronal cells require much higher concentrations of Ni^{2+} to be blocked.[66,67]

Interestingly, a scorpion toxin (kurtoxin) that binds to the α_{1G} T-type Ca^{2+} channel expressed in oocytes with high affinity was identified; it inhibits the channel by modifying voltage-dependent gating.[68] Kurtoxin inhibits the $Ca_v3.1$ and $Ca_v3.2$, but not the $Ca_v3.3$ channel in nanomolar concentrations. However, more recent studies conducted in rat central and peripheral neurons showed that kurtoxin also partially inhibited N-type and L-type Ca^{2+} currents in sympathetic and thalamic neurons.[69]

Mibefradil has been widely employed as a T-type Ca^{2+} channel antagonist, with an IC_{50} for T-type channels in rat neonate vascular muscle of approximately 100 nM.[70,71] However, other authors have shown that mibefradil, although much weaker, also inhibits L-type calcium currents in isolated cardiomyocytes[72] and others, HVA Ca^{2+} channels (α_{1A}, α_{1B}, α_{1E}) in *Xenopus* oocytes.[73] Mibefradil has been found to inhibit T-type calcium currents in several neuronal preparations, including neuroblastoma cells,[74] sensory neurons,[66] and rat spinal motoneurons where the compounds also inhibited HVA calcium currents.[75]

A mibefradil derivative, NNC 55-0396 [(1S,2S)-2-(2-(N-[(3-benzimidazol-2-yl)propyl]-N-methyl-amino)ethyl)-6-fluoro-1,2,3,4-tetrahydro-1-isopropyl-2-napthyl cyclopropanecarboxylate dihydrochloride], has also been more recently described.[76,77] NNC 55-0396 exerts no effect against HVA Ca^{2+} channels at 100 μM[76] but inhibits T-type channels in HEK293 cells with a potency comparable to that of mibefradil (IC_{50} 6.8 vs. 10.1 μM).

Several organic blockers have also been postulated to act as selective inhibitors of T-type currents. Thus, $Ca_v3.1$ channel is moderately sensitive to phenytoin. The $Ca_v3.2$ channel is sensitive to ethosuximide, amlodipine, and amiloride. Several neuroleptics and anticonvulsants inhibit all three LVA channels in clinically relevant concentrations. All three channels are also inhibited by the endogenous cannabinoid anandamide.[78]

39.4.2 High-Voltage-Activated Channels

All members of the HVA channels family share some common features, such as that they are biophysically characterized by their activation by strong depolarizing steps,[61,62] a higher permeability to Ba^{2+} than to Ca^{2+}, and a higher sensitivity to Cd^{2+} than to Ni^{2+}, in contrast to LVA channels. Up to now, five major subtypes (L, N, P, Q, and R) of HVA channels have been identified. The major differences between them are related to their inactivation kinetics and their pharmacological properties.

39.4.2.1 L-Type Ca²⁺ Channels

L-type (for "long-lasting") Ca^{2+} channels are kinetically characterized by showing little inactivation during depolarizing steps ($\tau_{inact} > 500$ ms) and their lower sensitivity to depolarized holding potentials. Single-channel conductance was estimated to be around 18–25 pS. This subtype of Ca^{2+} channel seems to be present in all excitable cells and in many non-excitable cells, and they constitute the main pathway for Ca^{2+} entry in heart and smooth muscle, serving also to control hormone and transmitter release from endocrine cells and some neuronal preparations. Four different α_1 subunits (α_{1C}, α_{1D}, α_{1F}, and α_{1S}) are responsible for L-type Ca^{2+} currents in different tissues (see Table 39.2).

Pharmacologically, L-type Ca^{2+} channels are characterized by their high sensitivity to DHPs (Table 39.2), both agonists (i.e., BayK8644) and antagonists (i.e., nifedipine, nimodipine, furnidipine). DHP agonist effects are characterized by the prolongation of the mean time for channel opening,[79,80] typically observed in whole-cell electrophysiological recordings as a prolongation of tail currents.[81]

Other small organic compounds have been described to effectively block L-type Ca^{2+} channels[82,83]: the arylalkylamines (i.e., verapamil) and benzothiazepines (i.e., diltiazem) are particularly useful in cardiac and smooth muscle cells, where they exert negative inotropic effects. Some piperazine derivatives (cinnarizine, flunarizine, dotarizine, R56865) also block L-type Ca^{2+} channels, but they block other subtypes of Ca^{2+} channels and thus have been proposed as "wide-spectrum" Ca^{2+} channel blockers.[84–86] The same is true for imidazole antimycotics.[87]

Some neurotoxins have also been shown to block L-type Ca^{2+} channels either selectively or in a nonselective manner. Thus, calciseptine, a 60-amino acid peptide isolated from the venom of the black mamba (*D. polylepis*), selectively blocks L-type Ca^{2+} channels and is totally inactive on other VDCCs such as N-type and T-type channels[14]; it seems that the channel sensitivity to calciseptine is tissue dependent and higher in cardiovascular system cells, where it has an IC_{50} of 15 nM.[14] On the other hand, calcicludine, a 60-amino acid polypeptide from the venom of the green mamba (*D. angusticeps*), appears to be a highly potent blocker of L-subtype of neuronal Ca^{2+} channels when used in the low nanomolar range, but voltage-clamp experiments on a variety of excitable cells have shown that calcicludine specifically blocks most of the high-threshold Ca^{2+} channels (L, N, or P type) when used in the 10–100 nM range.[15] Other neurotoxins such as ω-agatoxin IA, ω-agatoxin IIA, and ω-agatoxin IIIA also block L-type channels in a nonselective manner.[33,34]

39.4.2.2 N-Type Ca^{2+} Channels

N-type Ca^{2+} channels display faster inactivation kinetics (τ_{inact} 50–80 ms) than that of L-type channels. This relative fast inactivation usually leads to their inactivation when maintaining a depolarizing holding potential, although in some preparations, N-type Ca^{2+} channels can contain a noninactivating component, even at the end of long depolarizations, for instance, in bovine chromaffin cells in which N-type channels have been described as "nonclassical N type."[88] Single-channel conductance of N-type channels has been estimated to be around 13 pS.

Pharmacologically, N-type Ca^{2+} channels are well characterized by the irreversible blockade induced by the *C. geographus* toxin ω-conotoxin GVIA[3,21,79,89] and the reversible blockade induced by the *C. magus* toxin ω-conotoxin MVIIA (Table 39.2).[24,25,90]

The more recently identified ω-conotoxins CVID, CVIE, and CVIF from the venom of the piscivorous *C. catus* are the most selective ω-conotoxins for the N-type channels to date.[91,92]

Other wide-spectrum toxins such as ω-conotoxin MVIIC and ω-conotoxin MVIID[26,93] can also block N-type Ca^{2+} channels in a nonselective manner. This is also the case for ω-agatoxin IIA, ω-agatoxin IIIA,[33] and ω-grammotoxin SIA (isolated from the venom of the tarantula *Grammostola spatulata*).[94,95]

A novel 320 kDa protein toxin isolated from the venom of the sea worm *Glycera convoluta*, named glycerotoxin, has been described to be able of reversibly stimulating spontaneous and evoked neurotransmitter release at the frog neuromuscular junction acting via N-type ($Ca_V2.2$) channels. In neuroendocrine cells, it elicits a robust and transient Ca^{2+} influx sensitive to the $Ca_V2.2$ blockers ω-conotoxin GVIA and MVIIA. Moreover, glycerotoxin triggers a Ca^{2+} transient in human embryonic kidney (HEK) cells overexpressing $Ca_V2.2$ but not $Ca_V2.1$ (P/Q type).[96,97]

39.4.2.3 P-Type Ca^{2+} Channels

P-type Ca^{2+} channels were first described by Llinás et al.[98] in cerebellar Purkinje cells, in which Ca^{2+} currents were resistant to blockade by DHPs and ω-conotoxin GVIA. The toxin fraction from the venom of the funnel-web spider *A. aperta* (FTX) was found effectively to block this resistant current, and these results led these authors to suggest the existence of a new subtype of HVA Ca^{2+} channel, which was termed P (for "Purkinje").

P-type Ca^{2+} channels are characterized by their relative insensitivity to changes in the holding potential and do not inactivate during depolarizing steps[32,99,100]; multiple single-channel conductances have been described for P-type Ca^{2+} channels.[101,102]

Pharmacologically, P-type Ca^{2+} channels can be effectively blocked by FTX and its synthetic analog sFTX and by ω-agatoxin IVA at concentrations in the nanomolar range (<30–100 nM). This toxin is actually accepted to be the selective probe to identify the presence of P-type Ca^{2+} channels (see Table 39.2).[32,39,100]

P-type Ca^{2+} channels can be also blocked in a nonselective manner by ω-conotoxin MVIIC,[26,93] ω-conotoxin MVIID, and by ω-grammotoxin SVIA.[94,95,103,104]

39.4.2.4 P/Q-Type Ca²⁺ Channels

In many neuronal preparations, a significant component of the whole-cell current through Ca^{2+} channels is resistant to blockade with DHPs, ω-conotoxin GVIA, and ω-agatoxin IVA (<100 nM), suggesting the presence of a subtype of Ca^{2+} channel different from L-, N-, and P-types. The isolation, purification, and synthesis of the toxin from the marine snail *C. magus* ω-conotoxin MVIIC[26,93] led to the identification and characterization of a new subtype of HVA channel termed Q.[105,106]

Characterization of Q-type Ca^{2+} channels is mostly based on pharmacological criteria. As described, Q-type channels are resistant to blockade by DHPs, ω-conotoxin GVIA, and low doses (<100 nM) of ω-agatoxin IVA, but they are sensitive to ω-conotoxin MVIIC (1–3 μM). Increasing concentrations of ω-agatoxin IVA (up to 2 μM) can also block Q-type Ca^{2+} channels.[106] Other toxins that can also block this subtype of Ca^{2+} channel include the *C. magus* snail toxin ω-conotoxin MVIID[93] and the *G. spatulata* tarantula toxin ω-grammotoxin SIA.[94,95,103,104] It should be noted that these toxins, used to identify Q-type channels, are not selective for this subtype of channel, and they also block in a nonselective manner N- and P-types.

To date, only two specific P/Q-type blockers are known, the ω-agatoxins. Other peptidic calcium channel blockers with activity at P/Q channels are available, albeit with less selectivity. A number of low-molecular-weight compounds have shown some efficacy to modulate P/Q-type currents, and some exhibit a peculiar bidirectional pattern of modulation (for a recent review see [107]). Probably, the best-examined small molecule acting as a modulator of P/Q channels is the cyclin-dependent kinase inhibitor roscovitine, which has been shown to enhance P/Q-type calcium tail currents with an IC_{50} of about 20 μM in isolated neostriatal neurons, and effect that is the result of slowed deactivation kinetics.[108] However, subsequent studies found that roscovitine slows deactivation of all recombinantly expressed presynaptic calcium channels (P/Q, N, and R) in stably transfected cell lines.[109,110]

39.4.2.5 R-Type Ca²⁺ Channels

In neuronal tissues, a residual Ca^{2+} current, characterized by its insensitivity to blockade by DHPs, ω-conotoxin GVIA, ω-agatoxin IVA, and ω-conotoxin MVIIC, has also been described and termed "R type" (for "resistant").[105] This new subtype of Ca^{2+} channel belongs to the HVA group, is rapidly inactivating ($\tau = 22$ ms), and is more sensitive to blockade by Ni^{2+} ($IC_{50} = 66$ μM) than to Cd^{2+}. It has been further described that R-type channels may comprise multiple calcium channel subtypes.[111]

Newcomb et al.[112] described the first selective R channel blocker, SNX-482, a peptide from the venom of the African tarantula *Hysterocrates gigas*. We found, however, that this toxin also blocks P/Q channels in the bovine chromaffin cell.[113] Thus, caution should be exerted when using this toxin to target R-type currents.

39.5 Species Differences in the Expression of VDCC Subtypes

Drastic species differences in the subtypes of Ca^{2+} channels expressed by different cell types have been found. For instance, the K^+-evoked Ca^{2+} entry in brain cortex synaptosomes is controlled by N channels in the chick and by P channels in the rat.[114] On the other hand, neurotransmitter release at the muscle end plate is controlled by N channels in fish[115–117] and amphibians[118] and by P channels in mammals.[119]

Detailed comparative electrophysiological studies among six mammalian species have been performed only in adrenal medullary chromaffin cells (Figure 39.3).

T-type currents are difficult to record in chromaffin cells. Although we have detected T-type channel mRNA in bovine chromaffin cells,[120] we have been unable to record T-type currents. However, there are three studies reporting T-type Ca^{2+} currents in bovine[121] and rat chromaffin cells.[122,123] It has been suggested that T-type Ca^{2+} channels are mainly expressed in immature developing chromaffin cells,[122] where they are essential for the acute response of chromaffin cells to hypoxia.[124,125] T-type channels of the α_{1H} class have also been found to be expressed in rat chromaffin cells exposed to cAMP[126]; those channels were found to trigger a secretory response.[127] This α_{1H} T-type Ca^{2+} channel has also been identified in rat adrenal glomerulosa zone.[128]

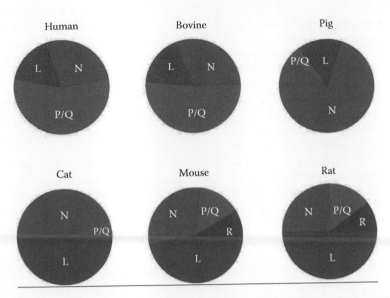

FIGURE 39.3 Species differences between the relative densities of HVA Ca^{2+} channels expressed by adrenal chromaffin cells.

L-type currents have been characterized in bovine,[88,129–133] rat,[80,134] mouse,[135] pig,[136] cat,[137] and human chromaffin cells.[138] Recent studies have presented molecular evidence that L-type currents in chromaffin cells are carried out by two different Ca^{2+} channels: α_{1C} and α_{1D}.[139] L-type Ca^{2+} channels account for near half of the whole-cell Ca^{2+} channel current in the cat,[137] rat,[80] and mouse chromaffin cells.[135] In pig,[136] bovine,[129,133] and human species,[138] L channels carry only 15%–20% of the whole-cell Ca^{2+} current.

N-channel currents have been characterized in chromaffin cells of various species including bovine,[88,140] pig,[136] cat,[137] rat,[80] mouse,[135] and human.[138] The N channel also shows a high interspecies variability. In the pig, it carries as much as 80% of the whole-cell Ca^{2+} channel current[136] and in the cat 45%[137]; in bovine,[140] rat,[80] mouse,[135] and human chromaffin cells,[138] the N-type fraction accounts for 30% of the whole-cell Ca^{2+} channel current.

P channels have proven difficult to characterize in chromaffin cells. Through the use of the synthetic funnel-web toxin sFTX,[133] 1 µM ω-agatoxin IVA,[129] or 100 nM ω-agatoxin IVA,[141] as much as 40%–55% of the whole-cell Ca^{2+} channel current was attributed to P channels. However, later on, we learned that concentrations of ω-agatoxin IVA higher than 10–20 nM in addition of P channels[100] also block Q channels.[106] Thus, nanomolar concentrations of ω-agatoxin IVA known to block fully and selectively P channels[32] cause only 5%–10% blockade of Ca^{2+} channel current in bovine chromaffin cells.[142] In cat chromaffin cells, combined ω-conotoxin GVIA plus nisoldipine blocked 90% of the current, leaving little room for P channels.[137] In rat[80] and mouse,[135] the ω-agatoxin IVA-sensitive current fraction was only 10%–15%. Thus, in all species studied, it seems that P channels are barely expressed if at all, in their chromaffin cells. This, together with the difficulty of separating the α_{1A} subunit into P and Q channels,[143] suggests the convenience of speaking of P/Q channels rather than of two separate Ca^{2+} channel subtypes.

The P/Q channel component is pharmacologically isolated by 2 µM ω-conotoxin MVIIC or ω-conotoxin MVIID or by 2 µM ω-agatoxin IVA. In bovine chromaffin cells, ω-conotoxin MVIID blocks the N current reversibly, while ω-conotoxin MVIIC does so irreversibly.[27] Thus, the use of ω-conotoxin MVIID followed by its washout can be a convenient tool to isolate the P/Q channel. The blocking effects of ω-conotoxin MVIIC are extraordinarily slowed down and decreased in the presence of excessive concentrations (i.e., more than 2 mM) of Ba^{2+}[142,144] or Ca^{2+}.[25] Taking into consideration these methodological problems, we believe that the fraction of current carried out by P/Q channels in bovine chromaffin cells amounts to 50%.[142] This fraction is even higher (60%) in human chromaffin cells.[138] The opposite occurs in pig[136] and cat chromaffin cells[137] where P/Q channels carry only 5% of the current. Finally, in rat chromaffin cells, P/Q channels contribute 20% to the current[80] and in the mouse 30%.[135] Later studies showed that this component is about 15% in mouse chromaffin cells.[145]

Differences have been reported in various laboratories concerning the expression of R-type Ca^{2+} channels in chromaffin cells, and they may be due to the configuration of the patch-clamp technique used (whole-cell vs. perforated-patch recordings). In some initial studies, an R-type component of I_{Ca} could not be detected in bovine,[129,130,133,141,142,146–148] cat,[137] human,[138] pig,[136] or mouse chromaffin cells.[135,149] In contrast, using the perforated-patch configuration instead of the whole-cell configuration of the patch-clamp technique, an R-type component was found in slices of mouse adrenal medulla and mouse chromaffin cells.[145,149] The most obvious explanation for this finding is that some soluble cytosolic factor, which is necessary for chromaffin cell R channel activity, is dialyzed with the whole-cell, but not with the perforated-patch configuration.

We do not know yet what the physiological relevance of these drastic species differences is. But surely, it has clear consequences for the fine control of the differential exocytotic release of epinephrine and norepinephrine in response to different stressors. Different autocrine/paracrine regulation by catecholamines and other co-exocytosed vesicular components of L- and non-L-types of Ca^{2+} channels might be a reason. Other regulatory mechanisms, that is, voltage-dependent[150] or Ca^{2+}-dependent inactivation of Ca^{2+} channels[151] could also explain the preferential expression of one or another channel type in a given species. Also, the selective segregation of a given channel type to exocytotic microdomains, and the uneven geographic distribution of other channel types, might also decide a given neurosecretory cell to express preferentially one or another channel type. The drastic difference of channel type expression provides different models of chromaffin cells to study the dominant role of a given Ca^{2+} channel subtype in controlling exocytosis.[152]

39.6 Modulation of VDCC Activity

39.6.1 Modulation of VDCCs by Protein Kinase–Dependent Phosphorylation

Families of Ca_v1 and Ca_v2 channels are substrates for phosphorylation by cAMP-dependent protein kinase A (PKA). Single-channel recordings have suggested that phosphorylation by PKA is necessary for the channels to become active, and once these channels are active, phosphorylation can increase their open probability. Ser1928 located in the C-terminal region of the cardiac α_1 subunit of the $Ca_v1.2$ channel is the only detectable phosphorylation site for this kinase, whereas other phosphorylation site in the intracellular loop connecting domains II and III has also been found for the $Ca_v1.1$ α_1 subunit. Interestingly, it has been proposed that PKA may be in close proximity to the Ca_v channel thanks to the A-kinase anchor protein (AKAP), an adapter protein that directs PKA to a variety of substrates and intracellular locations (see review by Felix[153]).

Protein kinase C (PKC) can also modulate Ca_v channels; moreover, this regulation is believed to be of substantial physiological importance since it mediates the effects of several hormones and intracellular messengers. It has been shown that this activated-PKC pathway mediates the regulation of L-type Ca^{2+} currents by α-adrenergic agonists, ATP, and glucocorticoids among others.[153] Residues in the N-terminal and in the intracellular loop connecting domains I and II seem to be necessary for the modulation by PKC of some members of the Ca_v1 and Ca_v2 channel families. Moreover, PKC can reverse G protein inhibition of these channels by phosphorylating the intracellular loop connecting I and II domains. This characteristic cross talk between G protein and PKC is thought to allow the α_1 subunit to integrate multiple modulatory inputs.[154]

39.6.2 Regulation of VDCCs by Ca^{2+}–Calmodulin

Ca^{2+} influx through VDCCs not only serves to generate an intracellular Ca^{2+} signal that can activate gene transcription, protein phosphorylation, neurotransmitter release, and other intracellular functions, but it also exerts a feedback regulation of the channel activity. Both Ca^{2+}-dependent facilitation (CDF) and inactivation (CDI) have been described mainly for VDCCs of the Ca_v1 and Ca_v2 families both in native cell types and heterologous expression systems.[46,155,156] CDI and some forms of CDF depend on calmodulin (CaM), a ubiquitously expressed Ca^{2+}-binding protein containing four EF hands (Ca^{2+}-binding sites), binding to the pore-forming Ca_v α_1 subunit. In fact, there is experimental evidence indicating that Ca^{2+}/CaM complex regulates $Ca_v1.2$ and $Ca_v2.1$ channels due to CaM interaction with an amino acid sequence, called the IQ motif, located in the C-terminal of the α_1 subunit.[157,158]

It is well established that Ca^{2+} binding to CaM causes the CDI cardiac L-type ($Ca_v1.2$) VCDDs,[159,160] a process that is crucial for limiting Ca^{2+} entry during long cardiac action potentials. Although CDI has also been characterized for L-type VDCCs expressed in neuronal and neuroendocrine cells (likely $Ca_v1.2$ and $Ca_v1.3$),[156] the functional significance of the CDI of L-type VDCCs in these cell types is not entirely clear. On the other hand, L-type cardiac VDCCS can also undergo a CDF process that helps amplify intracellular Ca^{2+} signals coupled to contraction of the heart. This CDF for $Ca_v1.2$ channels also depends on CaM, which activates CaM-dependent protein kinase II (CaMKII).[155]

Similar to Ca_v1 channels, CDI for Ca_v2 channels involves CaM binding to an IQ-like domain in the $\alpha1$ C-terminal domain. In addition, for Cavl.2 channels, an additional CaM-binding domain (CBD) C-terminal to the IQ-like domain seems to be also involved in this CDI process.[158,161,162] The CDF of Ca_v2 channels is also related to CaM binding; however, only the IQ motif seems to be necessary for facilitation.[46]

In contrast to the well-known regulatory mechanisms of Ca_v1 and Ca_v2 VDCCs, little is known about the regulation of the Ca_v3 family of channels. In the case of Ca^{2+}/CaM regulation, it seems to depend on the activity of the CaMKII. Thus, activation of this kinase in cells expressing recombinant $Ca_v3.2$ channels increases current amplitude at negative test potentials as the result of Ser1198 phosphorylation within the intracellular linker connecting domains II and III in the α_1 subunit.[163,164]

39.6.3 Modulation of VDCCs by G Protein–Coupled Receptors

Dunlap and Fischbach[165] were first to report that the exogenous application of norepinephrine, GABA, or serotonin onto the surface of chick sensory neurons inhibited their Ca^{2+} conductance. This observation was corroborated soon in rat sympathetic neurons[165–167] and was demonstrated to affect HVA, but not LVA calcium channels.[168] The inhibition of the current was associated to many neurotransmitters, receptors, and neurons[169–172] and was shown to be a membrane-delimited mechanism, directly coupled to G proteins.[30,173–177]

Marchetti et al.[178] first observed that the neurotransmitter-mediated inhibition of calcium channel currents is modulated by voltage. Dopamine slows down HVA channel activation and this effect is stronger at the more negative membrane potentials. Another intriguing observation was that strong depolarizing prepulses, instead of the expected voltage-dependent channel inactivation, caused an augmentation of the calcium channel current induced by milder depolarizing test pulses, the so-called facilitation.[179]

We believe that both observations have the same underlying mechanism, a membrane-delimited G protein–mediated inhibition of calcium channels that is relieved by voltage. In resting conditions, G proteins are not coupled to calcium channels, and when channels open, a large amount of Ca^{2+} flows through them, inducing a typical HVA current characterized by a fast activation and a meager inactivation. When a neurotransmitter binds to its receptor (i.e., ATP in chromaffin cells), it activates a G protein that couples negatively to the VDCC, slowing down the current activation[180] and decreasing its peak amplitude. Under these conditions, application of a strong positive depolarizing prepulse causes a change in the structural conformation of the G protein coupled to the calcium channels that uncouples the G protein from the channel and thus the current recovers its control profile (facilitation).[178,180] So, the higher the inhibition of the current produced by a given neurotransmitter, the greater the facilitation by prepulses. The facilitation depends then on the degree of inhibition of the current, and this inhibition may depend on the secretory activity of the explored cell (autocrine modulation) or neighboring cells (paracrine modulation).[152]

G protein α subunits are thought to confer specificity in neurotransmitter receptor coupling to VDCCs, but G protein $\beta\gamma$ subunits are responsible for modulation of Ca^{2+} channels.[43,46]

Voltage-induced facilitation may be significant (more than 80% at +9 mV), but it is usually partial, leaving a variable amount of residual voltage-independent depression. In neurons, voltage-dependent modulation primarily targets $Ca_v2.1$ (P/Q-type) and $Ca_v2.2$ (N-type) VDCCs.[39,181–185] Initially, it was thought that $Ca_v2.3$ (R-type) VDCCs were insensitive to G proteins, although other studies suggested that these channels were also inhibited by similar mechanisms.[186–188]

On the other hand, voltage-independent inhibition has been reported to be associated to N-type channels,[189] P-type channels,[190] but mostly to L-type channels in neurosecretory cells,[191,192] peripheral and central neurons.[186,193,194]

39.7 Regulation of Exocytosis by Different VDCC Subtypes at the Various Cells and Tissues

It has been long demonstrated that Ca^{2+} is essential for neurotransmitter release. The existence of multiple types of Ca^{2+} channels and the fact that several of them can coexist in the same cell type has raised questions about which channel (or channels) contributes to the control of the delivery of the Ca^{2+} necessary to trigger a secretory signal in a particular synapse. We will therefore review throughout this section how the different Ca^{2+} channel subtypes (defined by ω-conotoxin blockade of neurosecretion) control the release of neurotransmitters depending on the synapse, the neurotransmitter, and the animal species. Tables 39.4 through 39.7 summarize how Ca^{2+} entry through different Ca^{2+} channel subtypes control neurotransmitter release at different sites of the central and peripheral nervous system, motor nerve terminals, and chromaffin cells.

39.7.1 Brain Synaptosomes

Ca^{2+} influx and subsequent neurotransmitter release from brain synaptosomes is controlled by different Ca^{2+} channels and is greatly dependent on the animal species studied.[195,196] In chick brain synaptosomes, inositol phosphate production together with norepinephrine release is highly sensitive to ω-conotoxin GVIA.[197] Ca^{2+} transients measured in chick brain synaptosomes loaded with the Ca^{2+}-sensitive fluorescent dye fura-2 demonstrated that increases in the $[Ca^{2+}]_c$ induced by high K^+ was almost completely suppressed by ω-conotoxin GVIA.[114] On the other hand, in rat brain synaptosomes, the production of inositol phosphate and secretion of norepinephrine is insensitive to ω-conotoxin GVIA but sensitive to ω-agatoxin IVA.[198] Glutamate release from rat brain synaptosomes is blocked 56% by ω-agatoxin IVA and 23% by ω-agatoxin IIIA, an L–N–P-type Ca^{2+} channel blocker.[40] These results indicate that in chick brain synaptosomes, Ca^{2+} entry, and therefore neurotransmitter release, is predominately controlled via an N-type Ca^{2+} channel. In rat brain synaptosomes, L- and N-type Ca^{2+} channel blockers do not modify $[Ca^{2+}]_c$ levels or transmitter release; therefore, a different Ca^{2+} entry pathway seems to be involved in the control of neurotransmitter release.

Turner and Dunlap[199] measured [³H]-glutamate release from rat cortical synaptosomes as an assay for presynaptic Ca^{2+} channel activity. In this system, they observed that the blocking efficacies of ω-agatoxin IVA and ω-conotoxin GVIA and MVIIC were increased either when Ca^{2+} influx was decreased by decreasing the KCl concentration to diminish the extent of depolarization, by decreasing the external concentration of Ca^{2+} or by partially blocking Ca^{2+} influx with one of the other toxins. Using these ω-toxins, they find at least three types of pharmacologically distinct Ca^{2+} channels that participate in exocytosis. The largest fraction of glutamate release was blocked by ω-agatoxin IVA with an IC_{50} of 12.2 nM and ω-conotoxin MVIIC with an IC_{50} of 35 nM, consistent with the pharmacology of a P-type Ca^{2+} channel. The N-type Ca^{2+} channel blocker ω-conotoxin GVIA inhibited a significant portion of the release (IC_{50} less than 1 nM) but only under conditions of reduced Ca^{2+} concentrations. These results suggest that the N-type channel in nerve terminals is different to that found in hippocampal somata since it appears to be resistant to ω-conotoxin MVIIC. The combination of ω-conotoxin GVIA (100 nM) and either ω-agatoxin IVA or ω-conotoxin MVIIC (1 μM) blocked approximately 90% of release when the Ca^{2+} concentration was reduced (0.46 mM or less), but 30%–40% of release remained when the concentration of Ca^{2+} in the stimulus buffer was 1 mM or greater, indicating that a resistant channel also participates in exocytosis.

Age-related changes in the relative contribution of VDCC subtypes to depolarization-induced Ca^{2+} influx into rat brain synaptosomes have been described. It has been found that in adult rat synaptosomes, L-, N-, P-, and Q-type channels accounted for 24%, 32%, 27%, and 12%, respectively, of the total Ca^{2+}

TABLE 39.4

Control of Neurotransmitter Release by N-Type Ca^{2+} Channels

Neurotransmitter	Preparation	ω-Conotoxin GVIA (μM)	% Inhibition	Reference
Acetylcholine	Electric fish (*Torpedo marmorata*)	5	30	[116]
	Electric fish (*Gymnotus carapo*)	2.5	>95	[117]
	Myenteric plexus (guinea pig)	0.01	92	[219]
	Myenteric plexus (rat)	0.1	70	[119]
	Detrusor (guinea pig)	0.1	88	[223]
	Urinary bladder (guinea pig)	1	71	[220]
	Urinary bladder (rat)	1	25	[220]
	Urinary bladder (rat)	0.3	54	[221]
	Atria (guinea pig)	$IC_{50} = 0.42$ μM		[227]
	Phrenic nerve (rat)	0.1	47	[119]
	Brain slices (rat)	1	60	[335]
ATP	Vas deferens (rat)	$IC_{50} = 20$ nM		[226]
Epinephrine	Urethra (rabbit)	0.1	77	[223]
	Chromaffin cells (dog)	0.4 μg/min	33	[336]
Catecholamines	Chromaffin cells (bovine)	5	17	[141]
	Chromaffin cells (bovine)	1	10	[140]
	Chromaffin cells (bovine)	3	30	[241]
	Chromaffin cells (cat)	1	20	[230]
	Chromaffin cells (rat)	1	42	[249]
Dopamine	Striatum (rabbit)	0.005	39	[203]
	Striatum (rat)	1	38	[201]
	Brain slices (rat)	1	30	[335]
Dynorphin	Dentate gyrus dendrite (guinea pig)	1	79	[206]
	Dentate gyrus axon (guinea pig)	1	50	[206]
EPSCs	Retinal ganglion neurons (rat)	5	67	[216]
EPSP	Hippocampal synaptic transmission (rat)	1	46	[106]
GABA	Deep cerebellar neurons (rat)	0.1	50	[205]
5-HT	Brain slices (rat)	1	30	[335]
Glutamate	Hippocampal CA1 pyramidal cells (rat)	3	80	[205]
	Hippocampal synaptosomes (rat)	1	16	[204]
Glycine	Dorsal horn neurons of the spinal cord (rat)	3	50	[205]
Norepinephrine	Brain synaptosomes (rat)	1	>90	[197]
	Neocortex (rabbit)	0.005	46	[114]
	Sympathetic neurons (rat)	0.1	92	[213]
	Vas deferens (rat)	1	100	[220]
	Anococcygeus (guinea pig)	0.01	98	[220]
	Vas deferens (guinea pig)	0.01	97	[219]
	Atria (guinea pig)	$IC_{50} = 0.200$ μM		[25]
	Atria (guinea pig)	0.1	80	[337]
	Atria (guinea pig)	10	49	[338]
	Chromaffin cells (dog)	0.4 μg/min	32	[336]
	Mesenteric artery (rat)	0.01	92	[224]
	Right atria (mouse)	0.1	100	[224]
	Right atria (rat)	0.1	100	[224]
NANC	Detrusor (rabbit)	0.1	85	[223]
	Anococcygeus (guinea pig)	0.05	64	[220]
	Urinary bladder (guinea pig)	0.1	58	[220]

(continued)

TABLE 39.4 (continued)

Control of Neurotransmitter Release by N-Type Ca^{2+} Channels

Neurotransmitter	Preparation	ω-Conotoxin GVIA (μM)	% Inhibition	Reference
	Urethra (rabbit)	0.1	47	[223]
	Jejunum (guinea pig)	0.1	33	[219]
	Taenia caecum (guinea pig)	0.05	20	[219]
Oxytocin	Neurohypophysial terminals (bovine)	0.8	32	[210]
Vasopressin	Neurohypophysial terminals (bovine)	0.8	32	[210]

NANC, nonadrenergic, noncholinergic neurotransmission; EPSCs, excitatory postsynaptic currents; EPSPs, excitatory postsynaptic potentials.

TABLE 39.5

Control of Neurotransmitter Release by P-type Ca^{2+} Channels (Blockade with Low Concentrations of ω-Agatoxin IVA)

Neurotransmitter	Preparation	ω-Agatoxin IVA (μM)	% Inhibition	Reference
Acetylcholine	Phrenic nerve (guinea pig)	0.02	>95	[338]
	Phrenic nerve hemidiaphragm (mouse)	0.1	92	[224]
	Phrenic nerve hemidiaphragm (rat)	0.1	0	[224]
Catecholamines	Chromaffin cells (bovine)	0.1	35	[141]
GABA	Deep cerebellar neurons (rat)	0.2	98	[205]
Glutamate	Brain synaptosomes (rat)	0.2	56	[40]
	Cortex synaptosomes (rat)	$IC_{50} = 12.2$ nM		[199]
	Hippocampal synaptosomes (rat)	0.2	40	[204]
	Hippocampal CA1 pyramidal cells (rat)	0.2	25	[205]
Glycine	Dorsal horn neurons of the spinal cord (rat)	0.2	98	[205]

GABA, gamma-aminobutyric acid.

TABLE 39.6

Control of Neurotransmitter Release by Q-Type Ca^{2+} Channels

Neurotransmitter	Preparation	ω-Conotoxin MVIIC (μM)	% Inhibition	Reference
Acetylcholine	Urinary bladder (rat)	3	54	[221]
	Atria (guinea pig)	$IC_{50} = 0.28$ μM		[227]
	Phrenic nerve hemidiaphragm (mouse)	1	80	[224]
	Phrenic nerve hemidiaphragm (rat)	1	57	[224]
	Chromaffin cells (bovine)	$IC_{50} = 218$ nM		[240]
ATP	Vas deferens (rat)	$IC_{50} = 200$ nM		[226]
Catecholamines	Chromaffin cells (bovine)	3	50	[140]
Glutamate	Cortex synaptosomes (rat)	$IC_{50} = 35$ nM		[199]
EPSPs	Hippocampal synaptic transmission (rat)	5	100	[106]
Norepinephrine	Atria (guinea pig)	0.5	100	[338]
	Atria (guinea pig)	$IC_{50} = 0.19$ μM		[25]
	Atria (mouse)	1	100	[224]
	Atria (rat)	1	100	[224]
	Chromaffin cells (bovine)	$IC_{50} = 182$ nM		[240]
Vasopressin	Neurohypophysial terminals (bovine)	0.3	25	[210]

ATP, adenosine triphosphate; EPSPs, excitatory postsynaptic potentials.

TABLE 39.7

Control of Neurotransmitter Release by P/Q-Type Ca^{2+} Channels
(Blockade with High Concentrations of ω-Agatoxin IVA)

Neurotransmitter	Preparation	ω-Agatoxin IVA (μM)	% Inhibition	Reference
Acetylcholine	Urinary bladder (rat)	3	46	[221]
	Atria (guinea pig)	3	37	[227]
	Brain slices (rat)	1	50	[335]
GABA	Brain slices (rat)	1	100	[335]
Glutamate	Brain slices (rat)	1	100	[335]
Dopamine	Brain slices (rat)	1	70	[335]
5-HT	Brain slices (rat)	1	50	[335]
Norepinephrine	Atria (guinea pig)	3	21	[227]

influx, respectively. Brain aging significantly reduced the relative contributions of N- and P-type channels and increased the contribution of the channels resistant to the four blockers used. The densities of VDCC subtypes, determined by binding experiments using radiolabeled PN200-110, ω-conotoxin GVIA, and ω-conotoxin MVIIC, were found to be significantly decreased in aged synaptic plasma membranes.[200]

39.7.2 Striatum

In the striatum, neurotransmitter release is controlled by different Ca^{2+} channels. Dopamine release induced by K$^+$ is blocked around 30% by ω-conotoxin GVIA,[198,201] although dopamine release evoked by electrical stimulation is almost completely inhibited by ω-conotoxin GVIA.[201] Turner and coworkers, using subsecond measurements of glutamate and dopamine release from rat striatal synaptosomes, showed that P-type Ca^{2+} channels, which are sensitive to ω-agatoxin IVA, trigger the release of both neurotransmitters although dopamine (but not glutamate) was also partially blocked by ω-conotoxin GVIA-sensitive Ca^{2+} channels. Another interesting observation by these authors is that the blockade of neurotransmitter release is voltage dependent. With strong depolarizations (60 mM K$^+$), neither ω-agatoxin IVA nor ω-conotoxin GVIA was effective alone, although a combination of both produced a synergistic inhibition of 60%–80% of Ca^{2+}-dependent dopamine release. With milder depolarizations (30 mM K$^+$), ω-agatoxin IVA (200 nM) blocked over 80% dopamine and glutamate release, while ω-conotoxin GVIA (1 μM) blocked dopamine release by 25% and left unaffected glutamate release. The results suggest that multiple Ca^{2+} channel subtypes coexist to regulate neurosecretion under normal physiological conditions in the majority of nerve terminals, while P type and ω-conotoxin GVIA– and ω-agatoxin IVA–resistant channels coexist in glutamatergic terminals. Such an arrangement could lend a high degree of flexibility in the regulation of transmitter release under diverse conditions of stimulation and modulation.

Differences in the recruitment of VDCC subtypes in the process of controlling striatal dopamine release depending on the stimulation firing patterns have been described.[202] Thus, in dorsolateral neostriatum, a role for N-, P-, and Q-type channels was demonstrated for discrete stimulations, while at least one other unidentified channel was also involved in dopamine release on "burst" stimulations. Similarly, in the medial axis of the neostriatum, N-, P-, and Q-type channels were involved in dopamine release for discrete stimulations, and N-, Q-, and at least one other channel type for "burst" stimulations. However, blockade of P-type channels had no effect on dopamine release for "burst" stimulations in the medial axis. In both regions and stimulation paradigms, N-type channels played a greater role than P/Q-type channels. In the medial axis of the neostriatum, there was a smaller contribution by N- and P-type channels and the unidentified component, but a greater Q-type contribution to DA release. "Burst" stimulations induced a lesser involvement of N- and P-type channels than discrete stimulations and a greater role of the unidentified component.[202]

39.7.3 Hippocampus

In the hippocampus of rabbits, Doodley et al.[203] demonstrated that electrically induced release of dopamine, 5-hydroxytryptamine, and acetylcholine was similarly blocked (around 40%) by nanomolar concentrations of ω-conotoxin GVIA. Under the same experimental conditions, dopamine release from the corpus striatum and norepinephrine release from the neocortex was also blocked 40% by ω-conotoxin GVIA (5 nM). Using a superfusion system with subsecond temporal resolution, Luebke et al.[204] studied the effects of ω-conotoxin GVIA and ω-agatoxin IVA on glutamate release from rat hippocampal synaptosomes. K+-induced release of glutamate was inhibited 16% by ω-conotoxin GVIA and 40% by ω-agatoxin IVA; such blockade was increased when lower concentrations of K+ were employed to induce secretion. The amplitude of excitatory postsynaptic potentials in CA1 pyramidal neurons was reduced by ω-conotoxin GVIA and ω-agatoxin IVA, although ω-agatoxin IVA was more rapid and more efficacious.[204] Thus, at least two Ca2+ channels seem to control glutamate release from hippocampal neurons, but P-type channels seem to play a major role.

Synaptic transmission between hippocampal CA3 and CA1 neurons is mediated by N-type Ca2+ channels together with Ca2+ channels whose pharmacology differs from L- and P-type channels but resembles that of Q-type Ca2+ channels encoded by the α_{1A} subunit gene. Using rat hippocampal slices, Wheeler et al.[106] showed that ω-conotoxin GVIA blocked EPSP by 46%, while P- and L-type Ca2+ channel antagonists had no effect. In contrast, ω-conotoxin MVIIC (N–P–Q Ca2+ channel blocker) inhibited 100% of the EPSP. This suggests that hippocampal synaptic transmitter release is regulated by N and Q subtype of Ca2+ channels. Measuring excitatory postsynaptic currents (EPSCs) from hippocampal CA1 pyramidal neurons, Takahashi and Momiyama[205] demonstrated that synaptic transmission at this level is predominantly controlled by N-type Ca2+ channels (80% block of EPSPs by ω-conotoxin GVIA) and to a lesser extent by P-type Ca2+ channels (25% inhibition by ω-agatoxin IVA).

The release of the neuropeptide dynorphin is controlled by different Ca2+ channels, depending on the release site (dendrite or axon). L-type Ca2+ channels mediate dynorphin release from dendrites and N-type Ca2+ channels mediate dynorphin release from the axons of hippocampal granule cells.[206]

39.7.4 Cerebellum

Inhibitory postsynaptic currents (IPSCs) evoked in neurons of the deep cerebellar nuclei by stimulating presumptive Purkinje cell axons were reversibly abolished by bicuculline, indicating that the responses were mediated by GABA. The application of ω-agatoxin IVA (200 nM) blocked IPSCs amplitude by 50%, while the L-type Ca2+ channel blocker nicardipine had no effect[205] indicating that GABA release from Purkinje cell axons is mediated via Ca2+ entry through P-type Ca2+ channels.

In a related study by these same authors, the effects of calcium channel blockers on potassium-induced transmitter release were studied in thin slices of cerebellum from neonatal rats. Miniature inhibitory postsynaptic currents (mIPSCs) mediated by GABA were recorded from deep cerebellar nuclear neurons. The frequency of mIPSCs was reproducibly increased by a brief application of high-potassium solution. Under these stimulatory conditions, in the presence of the L-type Ca2+ channel blocker nicardipine, the potassium-induced increase in mIPSC frequency was suppressed by 49%. The N-type Ca2+ channel blocker ω-conotoxin GVIA had no effect on the frequency of potassium-induced mIPSCs, and the P-type Ca2+ channel blocker ω-Aga-IVA (200 nM) suppressed the potassium-induced increase in mIPSC frequency by 83%. Comparing these data with those of the previous study of neurally evoked transmission, authors concluded that the VDCC subtypes responsible for potassium-induced transmitter release may be different from those mediating fast synaptic transmission.[207]

39.7.5 Neurohypophysis

The neurohypophysis comprises the nerve terminals of hypothalamic neurosecretory cells, which contain arginine vasopressin (AVP) and oxytocin (OT). Neurohypophysial terminals exhibit besides L- and N-type currents,[208] another component of the Ca2+ current. This GVIA- and nicardipine-resistant component has been subclassified into two groups: one group in which this resistant current is blocked by ω-Aga-IVA (Q-type channel) and one in which is sensitive to SNX-492 (R-type channel).[209] Immunohistochemistry of isolated neurohypophysial terminals labeled with AVP or OT versus P/Q-subtype VDCCs indicates that the P/Q channel is found only in AVP terminals. Thus, Q-type channels are preferentially located on AVP-containing terminals. In agreement with these results, in the study performed by Wang and coworkers,[210] they demonstrated that secretion of vasopressin was controlled by N, L, and Q channels, while that of oxytocin was regulated mainly by N and L channels with no participation of Q channels. Similar results have been recently obtained by Tobin et al.,[211] who found that when oxytocin release was primed by prior exposure to thapsigargin, both N- and L-type channel blockers reduced release, while P/Q and R-type blockers were ineffective.

39.7.6 Sympathetic Neurons

In rat sympathetic neurons, whole-cell recordings have provided evidence for two subtypes of Ca^{2+} channels, the N and the L type,[79] although norepinephrine release is predominantly blocked by ω-conotoxin GVIA.[212,213] In contrast to sympathetic neurons, release of substance P from peripheral sensory neurons is highly dependent on Ca^{2+} entry through L-type Ca^{2+} channels. In the sympathetic nerve endings of the iris, ω-conotoxin GVIA (1 μM) blocked over 80% of norepinephrine synthesis induced by high K^+ while nicardipine had no effect, indicating that Ca^{2+} entry through N-type Ca^{2+} channels play a major role in norepinephrine synthesis.[214]

Noradrenaline release from sympathetic neurons in the rabbit isolated carotid artery evoked by electrical-field stimulation at a low frequency (2 Hz) is mediated mainly by the N-type calcium channels. At a high frequency (30 Hz), T-type Ca^{2+} channels are also involved.[215]

39.7.7 Retinal Ganglion Neurons

Glutamatergic synaptic responses in rat retinal ganglion neurons are partially sensitive to ω-conotoxin GVIA (30% block) and insensitive to ω-agatoxin IVA.[216] These results indicate that the major part of synaptic glutamate release in retinal ganglion neurons is governed by a toxin-resistant Ca^{2+} channel that could possibly be of the Q or R type.

Tamura et al. examined the properties of VDCCs mediating endogenous dopamine and acetylcholine release in the isolated rat retina. In this study, the high K^+-evoked dopamine release was largely blocked by both ω-agatoxin IVA and ω-conotoxin MVIIC and partly blocked by the L-type antagonist isradipine and ω-conotoxin GVIA. ω-Agatoxin IVA at a small dose, sufficient to block P-type channels alone, was however without effect. On the other hand, the high K^+-evoked acetylcholine release was partly blocked by ω-agatoxin IVA and ω-conotoxin MVIIC but was resistant to isradipine and ω-conotoxin GVIA. Flunarizine, a nonselective T-type calcium channel antagonist, did not inhibit the release of dopamine and acetylcholine. These results suggested that the high K^+-evoked release of retinal dopamine is largely mediated by ω-agatoxin IVA- and ω-conotoxin MVIIC-sensitive calcium channels (probably Q-type channels), while the release of retinal acetylcholine is partially mediated by ω-agatoxin IVA- and ω-conotoxin MVIIC-sensitive calcium channels but largely mediated by an uncharacterized Cd^{2+}-sensitive calcium channel.[217]

39.7.8 Intestinal Tract

Electrically evoked release of acetylcholine is predominantly controlled through N-type Ca^{2+} channels at the myenteric plexus.[119,218,219] ω-Conotoxin GVIA markedly reduced (70%) the evoked release of [3H]-acetylcholine from the myenteric plexus of the small intestine, with an IC_{50} of 0.7 nmol/L; the potency was similar at 3 and 10 Hz stimulation. An increase in the extracellular Ca^{2+} concentration attenuated the inhibitory effect of ω-conotoxin GVIA.[119] No species difference was observed as to the channel controlling Ca^{2+} entry for transmitter release.

In the guinea pig jejunum, ω-conotoxin GVIA blocked only partially (33%) the inhibitory NANC transmission upon electrical stimulation. This was also the case at the *Taenia caecum* (20% inhibition).[219] In the proximal duodenum, the NANC transmission was insensitive to ω-conotoxin GVIA.[220]

Therefore, cholinergic transmission at this level seems to be regulated by Ca^{2+} entering through N-type Ca^{2+} channels, while NANC transmission is regulated by another Ca^{2+} entry pathway besides N channels.

39.7.9 Lower Urinary Tract

In the rat or guinea pig isolated bladder, ω-conotoxin GVIA produced a concentration and time-dependent inhibition of twitch responses to field stimulation without affecting the response to exogenous acetylcholine. In the rat bladder, the maximal effect did not exceed 25% inhibition, while a much larger fraction of the response (70%) was inhibited in the guinea pig bladder. In the rat bladder, the effects of ω-conotoxin GVIA were frequency dependent; maximal effects of ω-conotoxin GVIA were observed at 2–5 Hz. Frew and Lundy.[221] have demonstrated that neurotransmission in the rat urinary bladder is supported by both N- and Q-type Ca^{2+} channels. In their experiments, the resistant portion (non-N non-P) was sensitive to ω-conotoxin MVIIC, which in addition to N and P also blocks Q channels. Further experiments carried out by Waterman[222] in mouse bladder using Ca^{2+} channel toxins demonstrates that acetylcholine release in these parasympathetic neurons depends primarily on N-type channels, and to a lesser extent on P- and Q-type channels, whereas ATP release involves predominantly P- and Q-type channels.

In the rabbit urethra and detrusor, Zygmunt et al.[223] have studied the effects of ω-conotoxin GVIA on adrenergic, cholinergic, and NANC responses induced by electrical stimulation. The adrenergic contraction (25 Hz) and NANC relaxation (10 Hz) in the urethra, and the cholinergic and NANC contractions (10 Hz) in the detrusor, were inhibited in a concentration-dependent manner by ω-conotoxin GVIA. The adrenergic contraction of the urethra was 10 times and the cholinergic contraction in the detrusor was 3 times more sensitive to ω-conotoxin GVIA than the NANC responses. These results suggest that NANC transmission is less sensitive to ω-conotoxin GVIA than transmission mediated by adrenergic and cholinergic nerves in the rabbit lower urinary tract.

39.7.10 Vas Deferens

In rat or guinea pig isolated vas deferens ω-conotoxin GVIA (1 nM–1 μM) produced concentration and time-dependent inhibition of the response to electrical-field stimulation, while the response to K^+, norepinephrine, or ATP was unaffected. A concentration as low as 1 nM produced almost complete inhibition of twitches, but this effect took about 1 h to be completed. With higher concentrations, the time course of the inhibition was much faster.[220] In a study performed by Wright and Angus[224] in rat and mouse vas deferens, they observe that ω-conotoxin GVIA (10 nM) and ω-conotoxin MVIIC (1 μM) block the twitch responses completely when they are induced at low frequencies (0.05 Hz), but when higher frequencies are used (20 Hz), there is a ω-conotoxin GVIA–resistant component that can be blocked by 1 μM ω-agatoxin IVA or ω-conotoxin MVIIC. These results indicate that sympathetic transmission in the vas deferens is mainly controlled by Ca^{2+} entering through N channels, although when high-frequency stimulation is employed (20 Hz), P–Q-type channels are also implicated.[224]

As to the purinergic transmission in the vas deferens, Hata et al.[225] showed that the ATP-mediated component of the biphasic contraction was found to be more susceptible to ω-conotoxin GVIA than the adrenergic component. In a study performed 5 years later by Hirata and coworkers,[226] electrically induced twitch responses of the prostatic segment of the rat vas deferens, which depends mainly on ATP release, was fully blocked by nanomolar concentrations of ω-conotoxin GVIA, MVIIA, and MVIIC, most likely by inhibiting Ca^{2+} entry through presynaptic N-type Ca^{2+} channels that control ATP release. The main conclusion we can withdraw from these studies is that sympathetic and purinergic transmission in the vas deferens is predominantly controlled by N-type Ca^{2+} channels.

39.7.11 Heart

The innervation in mammalian atria is both sympathetic and parasympathetic, which regulate the heart rate and the contractile strength. The subtypes of Ca^{2+} channels involved in neurotransmitter release have been studied by various investigators. Vega et al.[25] have shown that electrically stimulated guinea pig left atria are sensitive to N-type Ca^{2+} channel blockers. Thus, ω-conotoxin GVIA and ω-conotoxin MVIIA blocked the inotropic response in a concentration-dependent fashion with IC_{50} values of 0.20 and 0.044 μM, respectively. The N–P–Q channel blocker, ω-conotoxin MVIIC showed an IC_{50} of 0.19 μM;

ω-agatoxin IVA had no effect. These results were confirmed later on by Wright and Angus[224] in the right atria of mouse and rat, where they see full inhibition of contraction with 100 nM ω-conotoxin GVIA.

Hong and Chang[227] have studied the Ca^{2+} channel subtypes mediating the cholinergic and adrenergic neurotransmission in the guinea pig atria. In the left atria paced at 2–4 Hz, the negative inotropic effect induced by electrical-field stimulation on parasympathetic nerves (in the presence of propranolol) was abolished by ω-conotoxin MVIIC. On the other hand, the inotropic response resulting from electrical-field stimulation of the sympathetic nerves (in the presence of atropine) was abolished by ω-conotoxin GVIA and ω-conotoxin MVIIC. None of the peptide toxins affected the chronotropic and the inotropic responses evoked by carbachol, isoprenaline, or norepinephrine.[25,227]

These results suggest that under physiological conditions, the release of acetylcholine from parasympathetic nerves to the heart is dominated by a P/Q subfamily of Ca^{2+} channels, while that of norepinephrine from sympathetic nerves is controlled by an N-type Ca^{2+} channel.

39.7.12 Motor Nerve Terminals

Neurotransmitter release at this level is controlled by different Ca^{2+} channels depending on the species. The electroplax of marine electric fish is highly rich in motor nerve endings; this is the reason why it has been so widely used as a model to study transmitter release from motor nerve endings. ω-Conotoxin GVIA blocks the release of acetylcholine and Ca^{2+} uptake induced by depolarization in electric organ nerve terminals of the ray; the IC_{50} values were 3 μM for blocking transmitter release and 2 μM for blocking Ca^{2+} entry.[115] Sierra et al.[117] have also shown that N-type Ca^{2+} channels mediate transmitter release at the electromotoneuron–electrocyte synapses of the weakly electric fish *Gymnotus carapo;* ω-conotoxin GVIA (2.5 μM) blocked over 95% of the end plate potential (EPP), while ω-agatoxin IVA and nifedipine had no effect. In contrast to these data, in *torpedo* synaptosomes, Fariñas et al.[116] showed that ω-conotoxin GVIA (10^{-8}–5×10^{-5} M) showed a differential effect on acetylcholine and ATP release: nucleotide release was inhibited 90% at the highest concentration tested, while acetylcholine release was only moderately decreased (30%). In the frog neuromuscular junction, Jahromi et al.[118] have demonstrated that synaptic transmission is also governed by Ca^{2+} entry through an N-type Ca^{2+} channel.

In contrast, in mammalian motor nerve terminals, Ca^{2+} entry serving to discharge acetylcholine release seems to be ruled by a P-type Ca^{2+} channel rather than an N-type Ca^{2+} channel, as in fish and amphibians. So in the rat phrenic nerve, [^{3}H]-acetylcholine release was only partially inhibited by ω-conotoxin GVIA.[119] In the mouse, EPP were almost completely abolished (>95%) with 200 nM ω-agatoxin IVA. The twitch responses of the phrenic nerve hemidiaphragm were blocked in a different manner depending on the animal species. In the mouse, ω-agatoxin IVA at 100 nM blocked 92% of the twitches, while in the rat, ω-agatoxin IVA (≤ 100 nM) and ω-conotoxin GVIA (≤ 1 μM) had little effect although ω-conotoxin MVIIC caused 57% blockade.[224] In normal human muscles, Protti et al.[17] have shown that transmitter release at the motor nerve terminals is mediated by a P-type Ca^{2+} channel.

39.7.13 Chromaffin Cells

As described earlier, different Ca^{2+} channel subtypes are found on the plasmalemmal membrane of chromaffin cells. This coexistence raises the question as to whether all of the channel types participate in the control of exocytosis and how their density and properties would condition their participation if any. Furthermore, the presence and proportion of the various Ca^{2+} channels subtypes varies widely between animal species (Figure 39.3). Therefore, catecholamine secretion from these cells will presumably be controlled differently, in accordance with the Ca^{2+} channels expressed by the cells. In this section, we will review how catecholamine secretion is controlled in different animal species and how some subtypes of Ca^{2+} channels are more directly implicated in the control of exocytosis. It is important to emphasize that, depending on the type of stimulus used (i.e., K^+ depolarization, acetylcholine, step depolarizations, action potentials), one type of channel may be more favored over another in secretion. For this reason, the type of stimulus used is indicated in each of the following sections.

39.7.13.1 Cat Chromaffin Cells

The K⁺-evoked secretion of catecholamines is effectively blocked in a concentration-dependent manner by DHPs and other drugs acting on L-type Ca^{2+} channels like verapamil and diltiazem.[228] Measuring differential secretion of epinephrine and norepinephrine, Cárdenas et al.[229] demonstrated that secretion of both amines are completely blocked when it is induced by either high K⁺ or the nicotinic agonist dimethylphenylpiperazinium (DMPP). Initially, these data indicated that an L-type channel controlled secretion in these cells. But Albillos et al.[137] showed that cat chromaffin cells also contained ω-conotoxin GVIA–sensitive channels in addition to the L-type channels. It was then demonstrated that HVA L and N Ca^{2+} channels in cat chromaffin cells were present in an approximate proportion of 50%–50% and that the increase in $[Ca^{2+}]_c$ induced by short (10 s) depolarizing pulses (70 mM K⁺) could also be reduced 44% by furnidipine and 43% by ω-conotoxin GVIA. In a perfused adrenal gland or isolated cat chromaffin cells, catecholamine release induced by 10 s pulses of 70 mM K⁺ was blocked by more than 95% with furnidipine and only 25% with ω-conotoxin GVIA. These results show that though Ca^{2+} entry through both channels (N and L type) leads to similar increments of the average $[Ca^{2+}]_c$, the control of the K⁺-evoked catecholamine release response in cat chromaffin cells is dominated by the Ca^{2+} entering through L-type Ca^{2+} channels.[230] It may be that previous experiments using cell populations or intact cat adrenal glands[228,229] and long-duration (seconds) depolarizing stimuli inactivated the N-type Ca^{2+} channels.

39.7.13.2 Bovine Chromaffin Cells

K⁺-evoked catecholamine secretion from bovine chromaffin cells is greatly potentiated in the presence of the DHP L-type channel agonist BayK8644; the rise in secretion parallels the increase in ⁴⁵Ca uptake.[231] Ceña et al.[232] showed that nitrendipine completely blocked catecholamine release ([³H]-norepinephrine) in bovine chromaffin cells stimulated with high K⁺. These results do not agree with those obtained by other authors who found that in bovine chromaffin cells, DHP did not block more than 40%–50% of the secretion.[233–235] The differences may be based on different stimulation patterns and the use of cultured chromaffin cells, fast-superfused cell populations, or the intact perfused adrenal gland.

When toxins were available to block selectively specific subtypes of Ca^{2+} channels, it was demonstrated that these cells contain other Ca^{2+} channel subtypes besides L, that is, N, and the P/Q type.[129,131–133,236] ω-Conotoxin GVIA was ineffective or just barely effective in blocking K⁺-evoked catecholamine secretion in bovine chromaffin cells.[140,141,146,234,235,237,238]

As the contribution of P-type Ca^{2+} channels to catecholamine secretion, we find different results in the literature. Thus, Granja et al.[239] showed that catecholamine secretion induced by high K⁺ is not affected by ω-agatoxin IVA (100 nM); nevertheless, when secretion was activated by nicotine, the ω-agatoxin significantly decreased catecholamine release by 50%. Thus, Granja et al.[239] conclude that ω-agatoxin IVA could also affect the nicotinic receptor. Duarte et al.[237] show that FTX decreases K⁺-evoked norepinephrine release to 25% and epinephrine release to 39% of the control levels; the combination of FTX plus nitrendipine further decreases norepinephrine and epinephrine release to 12% and 24% of the control levels. Baltazar et al.[240] showed that bovine chromaffin cells contain two types of ω-agatoxin IVA-sensitive Ca^{2+} channels and that the contribution of the P-type channels to secretion is higher at low levels of depolarization.

The L–N–P-insensitive portion of catecholamine release in bovine chromaffin cells seems to be ω-conotoxin MVIIC sensitive. López et al.[140] observed that catecholamine release from superfused bovine chromaffin cells (stimuli: 70 mM K⁺ for 10 s) was inhibited 50% by DHP furnidipine (3 μM). ω-Conotoxin MVIIC (3 μM) also reduced the secretory response by 50%. The combination of furnidipine with ω-conotoxin MVIIC completely abolished secretion. On the other hand, these authors also demonstrated that ω-conotoxin GVIA and ω-agatoxin IVA have no effect on secretion. These results strongly suggest that secretion in these cells is predominantly controlled by Ca^{2+} entering through the L- and Q-type Ca^{2+} channels.

Further studies performed by Lara et al.[241] suggest that Q-type channels are coupled more tightly to active exocytotic sites than are the L-type channels. This hypothesis was suggested by the observation that the external Ca^{2+} that enters the cell through a Ca^{2+} channel, located near chromaffin vesicles, will saturate the K^+ secretory response at both $[Ca^{2+}]_e$, that is, 0.5 and 5 mM. In contrast, Ca^{2+} ions entering through more distant channels will be sequestered by intracellular buffers and will therefore not saturate the secretory machinery at a lower $[Ca^{2+}]_e$.

Moreover, a study of distinct populations of bovine chromaffin cells established that exocytosis in norepinephrine-containing cells is dominated by L-type channels, while in epinephrine-containing cells, exocytosis was controlled by P/Q-type channels.[242]

When the correlation between VDCCs and exocytosis was evaluated at the single cell level by measuring membrane capacitance changes or by amperometric detection of catecholamine release, some reports supported the view that there is no preferential role of any VDCC subtype in eliciting exocytosis.[127,147,148,243,244] These experiments suggest an uneven distribution of calcium channels in bovine chromaffin cells.

By characterizing the preferential localization of secretion in the terminals of neurite-emitting bovine chromaffin cells in contrast with the random distribution secretion in spherical cells, Gil et al.[245] observed a preferential distribution of the P/Q subtype of Ca^{2+} channels in these neurite terminals that colocalized with vesicles present in these structures, in sharp contrast with the overall distribution of the L-subtype channels. The same immunofluorescence technique did not allow to detect N-type calcium channels in these terminals. In addition, ω-agatoxin IVA was able to block 70% of the exocytotic release occurring into the neurites, whereas L-type blockers had a weak effect.[245]

39.7.13.3 Rat Chromaffin Cells

In adult rat chromaffin cells, the whole-cell inward Ba^{2+} current through VACCs is carried 50% by L channels, 30% by N channels, and 20% by PQ channels; a T channel component is not visible.[80] The role of each Ca^{2+} channel subtype in catecholamine secretion has been studied both in intact whole adrenal glands from rats as well as in isolated rat chromaffin cells.

DHPs block secretion in perfused rat adrenal glands in a concentration-dependent manner. The magnitude of this blockade is related to the type of stimuli employed to induce secretion. The DHP isradipine can fully block secretion when the stimuli used are K^+ or nicotine. In contrast, when electrical-field stimulation is used, the DHPs can only obtain a partial blockade and the inhibition is frequency dependent.[246]

In other studies, secretion evoked by depolarizing stimuli like high K^+ was strongly inhibited (80%) by L-type Ca^{2+} channel blockers, whereas acetylcholine-evoked responses were inhibited equally by either furnidipine or ω-conotoxin MVIIC.[247] Electrical-field stimulation of intact glands releases acetylcholine and other cotransmitters from the splanchnic nerves.[248] Under these conditions, N-type Ca^{2+} channels seem to contribute to the maintenance of the secretory responses, probably by acting on presynaptic channels at the splanchnic nerve terminals.[247]

In isolated rat chromaffin cells, by measuring Ca^{2+} currents and capacitance, Kim et al.[249] have shown that ω-conotoxin GVIA (1 μM) blocks 40% and nicardipine around 60% of the total capacitance increase in rat chromaffin cells. Therefore, in these cells, secretion would be controlled by L- as well as by N-type Ca^{2+} channels. In a recent study, it has been shown that upon stimulation with K^+ depolarizing pulses, adult rat chromaffin cells respond with quantal catecholamine release responses that are triggered by the Ca^{2+} entering through L as well as PQ VDCCs.[250]

Only after their exposure to chronic hypoxia, the adult rat chromaffin cells do express T channels; under this experimental condition, the stimulation of Ca^{2+} entry through these channels is capable of triggering the so-called low-threshold exocytosis.[251] Similarly, in rat chromaffin cells treated with cAMP, a "low-threshold" exocytotic response was triggered at very low depolarizations; this unusual secretory response is associated with the α_{1H} subtype of Ca^{2+} channels.[126,127,252]

Pharmacological dissection of I_{Ba} in rat embryo chromaffin cells (RECCs) also revealed the presence of functional L, N, and PQ channels[250] at relative densities similar to those we found in adult rat chromaffin cells.[80] Furthermore, we found that the challenging of RECCs with a K^+ depolarizing pulse triggered a quantal catecholamine release response that was potentiated by L channel activator BayK8644 and nearly fully suppressed by L channel blocker nimodipine; in contrast, ω-conotoxin

MVIIC did not affect the response, suggesting that in RECCs, depolarization-elicited secretion is mostly controlled by L-type VACCs.[250]

The relative contribution of the different subtypes of VDCCs to exocytosis in RECCs triggered by depolarization or hypoxic stimuli is an unresolved problem. Thus, in a careful study, it was found that only 50% of RECCs were found to express functional T channels together with HVA VDCCs. However, a train of depolarizing pulses causing substantial Ca^{2+} entry through T channels did not evoke exocytosis; nevertheless, similar Ca^{2+} entry through HVA VDCCs produced a healthy exocytotic response.[122] In contrast, a more recent study[124] shows that the hypoxia-induced secretory response in rat neonatal slices was suppressed by 25 μM Ni^{2+}, a concentration that selectively targets T channels.[253] Because this Ni^{2+} concentration did not affect the K^+ response, Levitsky and Lopez-Barneo[124] explained this finding in the context of enhanced excitability of immature chromaffin cells expressing T channels as well as low-threshold exocytosis. However, it should be noted that these authors did not study the effects of nimodipine that, as Ni^{2+}, fully blocked the hypoxia-induced secretion, as there are major evidences suggesting its control by L-type VDCCs, as nifedipine blocks this response in cultured neonate rat chromaffin cells,[254] in neonatal adrenal slices,[255] and in ovine fetal perfused adrenals.[256]

39.7.13.4 Dog Chromaffin Cells

Kitamura et al.[136] have studied the effects of ω-conotoxin GVIA and L-type Ca^{2+} channel blockers (nifedipine and verapamil) on catecholamine release in anesthetized dogs. Catecholamine release into the blood stream was induced either by electrical stimulation of the splanchnic nerve or by intra-arterial injection of acetylcholine. Administration of 0.4 μg/mL of ω-conotoxin GVIA reduced catecholamine secretion by 30% in response to electrical stimulation; nifedipine or verapamil had no effect under these experimental conditions. However, when catecholamine release was induced by acetylcholine, ω-conotoxin GVIA blocked secretion by around 50% and nifedipine also reduced it by 50%. These results suggest that N- and L-type Ca^{2+} channels contribute to the release of catecholamines in the dog adrenal gland. To our knowledge, a patch-clamp study that determines the subtypes of Ca^{2+} channels expressed by dog chromaffin cells is not available.

39.7.13.5 Mouse Chromaffin Cells

Simultaneous recordings of I_{Ca} and ΔCm in isolated mouse chromaffin cells indicate that exocytosis is proportional to the relative density of each Ca^{2+} channel subtype: 40% L, 34% N, 14% P/Q, and 11% R.[145] This indicates that under the perforated-patch configuration, the secretory response elicited by 200 ms depolarizing pulses is a strict function of the amount of Ca^{2+} entering the cell, by whatever Ca^{2+} channel subtype, L, N, P/Q, or R. In addition, it seems that any Ca^{2+} channel type colocalizes with the secretory machinery in a similarly random manner and shows the same relative efficacy in activating exocytosis, depending on its density.[145] This conclusion differs from that obtained in another study in acutely isolated adrenal mouse slices. In this latter study,[149] the proportion of channel subtypes differs from that obtained in cultured mouse chromaffin cells,[135] that is, 27% L, 35% N, 22% P, 23% Q, and 22% R. It is curious however that the R channels (22% of total current) control as much as 55% of the rapid secretion. Thus, Albillos et al.[149] concluded that "R-type Ca^{2+} channels in mouse adrenal slice chromaffin cells are in close proximity to the exocytotic machinery and can rapidly regulate the secretory process."

Although the critical role of L-type VDCCs in triggering exocytosis in mouse chromaffin cells is well established, there are no clear indications of a possible distinct role of $Ca_v1.2$ and $Ca_v1.3$ to exocytosis, despite the different inactivation kinetics and voltage range of activation of these two isoforms of L channels. Some recent observations show that deletion of Ca_v1-3 subunits in mouse chromaffin cells lowers the amount of exocytosis at very negative potentials, suggesting that besides sustaining action potential firing, $Ca_v1.3$ preferentially contributes to exocytosis at low membrane potentials. In this way, $Ca_v1.3$ contributes to the low-threshold exocytosis similar to the T-type $Ca_v3.2$ channels.[127,251,257,258]

39.8 Contribution of Each Channel Type to Exocytosis Varies with the Stimulation Pattern and the Ca^{2+} Gradient

The efficacy of the different channels in controlling exocytosis varies with the degree of depolarization and the concentration of external Ca^{2+} used in the experiments. There are different examples in the literature that demonstrate this fact. For instance, Turner et al.[104] observed that the efficacies of ω-agatoxin IVA and ω-conotoxin GVIA to block glutamate release from rat cortical synaptosomes increased when Ca^{2+} influx was reduced by decreasing the external concentration of KCl, decreasing the extent of depolarization, decreasing of the external concentration of Ca^{2+}, or by partially blocking the Ca^{2+} influx with an antagonist or another. For example, glutamate release was inhibited by ω-conotoxin MVIIC with an IC_{50} of 200 nM when stimulation of secretion was induced with 30 mM KCl; however, the same toxin had no effect when synaptosomes were stimulated with 60 mM KCl. The same investigators also found that dopamine release from rat striatal synaptosomes[198] could be blocked by ω-agatoxin IVA and ω-conotoxin GVIA when they used mild depolarizations with KCl. In contrast, with strong depolarizations, neither toxin alone was effective, although a combination of both toxins together produced a synergistic inhibition of 60%–80% of the Ca^{2+}-dependent dopamine release.

Transmitter release in parasympathetic neurons in the mouse bladder shows a similar pattern; bladder strip contraction was stimulated by single pulses or trains of 20 pulses at 1–50 Hz. Waterman and Small[259] observed that ω-conotoxin GVIA and MVIIC inhibited contractions in a concentration-dependent manner with IC_{50} values of approximately 30 and 200 nM, at low stimulation frequencies; the same toxins had little effect at high stimulation frequencies.

Dunlap et al.[260] try to explain these puzzling findings as follows: (1) with strong depolarizations, neurotransmitter exocytosis is not affected when a single Ca^{2+} entry pathway is blocked; (2) a synergic inhibitory effect is observed when a combination of toxins is used to block two Ca^{2+} entry pathways; and (3) in synapses with several Ca^{2+} channel subtypes, when one tries to sum up the individual inhibitory effects of the toxins, the values obtained are greater than 100%. They suggest that these findings could be explained by the presence of "spare" channels. Under conditions in which the $[Ca^{2+}]_c$ is saturating for the acceptor, participation of multiple Ca^{2+} channels might increase the reliability of excitation–secretion coupling, since activation of a single channel will be sufficient to maximize the release probability. This "spare channel" model might describe excitation–secretion coupling under conditions of relatively strong stimulation, such as high-frequency trains of action potentials, or with prolonged depolarizations using increasing concentrations of K^+. Biochemical modifications (such as phosphorylation), which increase the sensitivity of the Ca^{2+} acceptor, would also predict an increased probability of release elicited by entry of Ca^{2+} through a single channel. Under these conditions, the binding affinity of the Ca^{2+} channel antagonists would be underestimated by their effect on synaptic transmission, since blockade of one of several channels at the active zone would have little or no effect on release. This would produce a rightward shift in the concentration–response relationship relative to the binding curve.

A Ca^{2+}-dependency of the blockade of different Ca^{2+} channel subtypes is also shown in the study performed by Lara et al.[241] in bovine chromaffin cells, where it was demonstrated that L and Q channels predominantly control catecholamine release. These investigators observed that blockade of secretion mediated by L-type channels is not dependent on the extracellular concentration of Ca^{2+}, while blockade of Q-type channels is. The explanation that these authors give to these findings is that Q-type channels could be more tightly coupled to exocytotic active sites in comparison to L type. The physiological meaning given to this channel distribution might be found in considering the need for regular secretory rate during normal activity of the body (L-type secretion) and explosive catecholamine secretion that occurs under stressful conditions (P/Q-type secretion). An additional effort should be done to understand further how and why the combined blockade of two channels and/or the Ca^{2+} gradient have synergic effects on secretion in chromaffin cells.

A number of studies performed in voltage-clamped bovine chromaffin cells have also produced contradictory results. For instance, Artalejo et al.[141] measured ΔCm elicited by a train of 10 depolarizing pulses of 50 ms to +10 mV separated by 500 ms (5 s of stimulation) in bovine chromaffin cells; 10 mM Ba^{2+} (or Ca^{2+}) was used as charge carrier. They found that N or P channels contributed about 20%

to exocytosis; the so-called "facilitation" Ca^{2+} channels (DHP-sensitive L-type channels), which were recruited by previous pretreatment with D1 receptor agonists or cAMP, contributed 80% of the exocytosis. The authors suggest that "facilitation Ca^{2+} channels may be closer to the docking and release sites than either of the other two channels."

Lukyanetz and Neher[147] also measured ΔCm in response to single 200 ms depolarizing pulses applied to bovine chromaffin cells under the whole-cell configuration of the patch-clamp technique, using 60 mM Ca^{2+} as charge carrier. They could not obtain the facilitation of ΔCm observed by Artalejo et al.[141] In addition, they could not observe a preferential role of any Ca^{2+} channel subtype (in eliciting exocytosis) because ΔCm was proportional to the Ca^{2+} charge, irrespective of channel type. Contrary to Artalejo et al.,[141] Lukyanetz and Neher[147] reported that "participation of N-type channels (in exocytosis) is higher than that of L-type." The P/Q channel contributed little to I_{Ca} and ΔCm; this may be due to the fact that under conditions of excess divalent cations (60 mM Ca^{2+} was used as charge carrier by Lukyanezt and Neher,[147]) ω-conotoxin MVIIC binds and blocks P/Q channels poorly.[142] Ulate et al.[148] studied voltage-clamped bovine chromaffin cells, measuring I_{Ca} and ΔCm elicited by single 100 ms depolarizing pulses in 10 mM Ca^{2+}. They found that "all Ca^{2+} channel types (20% L, 48% N, 43% P/Q) contributed to the secretory response in a manner roughly proportional to the current they allow to pass, thus implying a similar efficacy in triggering catecholamine release." Finally, Engisch and Nowycky[243] found that ΔCm evoked by single-step depolarizations "was strictly related to the integral of the voltage-clamped Ca^{2+} currents, regardless of the Ca^{2+} channel subtype."

Different views are also obtained from experiments performed using other preparations and stimulation procedures. For instance, with brief depolarizing K^+ pulses (seconds), L channels contribute more than N or P/Q channels to trigger secretion in populations of cat and bovine chromaffin cells.[140,230] Also, by changing the Ca^{2+} concentration of the superfusion medium, it was suggested that P/Q channels colocalize closer to the secretory machinery than L channels.[241] Furthermore, O'Farrell et al.[261] obtained evidence in perfused bovine adrenal glands suggesting that "N-type Ca^{2+} channels are largely responsible for catecholamine release induced by nerve stimulation."

Neither depolarizing pulses in the range of milliseconds applied to voltage-clamped cells nor pulses in the range of seconds applied to cells with their membrane potential free are representative of the physiological conditions in which chromaffin cells are being stimulated in situ. It is true that the first approach has a time resolution closer to the duration of action potentials triggered by endogenously released acetylcholine.[262] However, by holding the membrane potential at hyperpolarizing voltages, the voltage inactivation of N and P/Q, but not L channels,[150] might be prevented. The second approach has a more limited time resolution but cells keep their "physiological" membrane potential free at the moment of application of the depolarizing pulse. At their resting membrane potential,[263,264] chromaffin cells might well have partially inactivated the N and P/Q channels; thus, their role in exocytosis could be underestimated when using K^+ depolarization, giving more protagonism to L channels.[140,230]

The real sequence of events leading from stimulus to release of catecholamines at the adrenal medulla is unknown. However, several studies make the following sequence feasible. Acetylcholine depolarizes the chromaffin cell[265] and this causes the firing of action potentials.[266] This recruits Ca^{2+} channels, triggering Ca^{2+} entry and exocytosis. However, the various Ca^{2+} channel subtypes suffer different degrees of inactivation, depending on the cytosolic Ca^{2+} concentration[151] and on the membrane potential.[150] Furthermore, chromaffin cells express Ca^{2+}-dependent K^+ channels of small conductance[267] that will also contribute to the regulation of action potential firing and exocytosis.[268,269] In summary, all these factors suggest that each type of Ca^{2+} channel could exhibit different efficacies to trigger and control the secretory process. Selection of the appropriate experimental conditions might reveal these differences.

39.9 Regulation of Endocytosis by Different VDCC Subtypes

Although calcium has been suggested to regulate endocytosis and vesicle recycling in synapses and neuroendocrine cells,[270–272] a controversy still looms over the precise role of Ca^{2+} in membrane retrieval during endocytosis. The results and observations from several different laboratories can be grouped into two extremes: First, Ca^{2+} along with Ba^{2+} supports excessive membrane retrieval in bovine chromaffin cells[273–275] and second, Ca^{2+} is not required for endocytosis[276,277] or even behaves as an inhibitor.[278]

In an attempt to establish the precise relationship between Ca^{2+} entry, exocytosis, and endocytosis in bovine chromaffin cells, we found that the variations in Ca^{2+} entry induced by the application of depolarizing pulses (DPs) of increasing length (50–2000 ms) produced different patterns of exo-/endocytosis, as measured by changes in membrane capacitance (ΔCm). In this study, ΔCm changes were measured during the 8 s period that followed the DP. A linear relationship between exocytotic responses and DP duration was found; however, endocytotic responses were absent with short DPs (50–200 ms) and were present and/or were more pronounced with longer DPs (500–2000 ms).[279] These data raise a question: what is the relationship between Ca^{2+} entry, exocytosis, and endocytosis, that is, is the Ca^{2+} entry that triggers exocytosis also responsible to initiate endocytosis?

As far as specific contributions of different VDCCs in controlling endocytosis are concerned, we have recently provided evidence that L channels are much more dominant than N or PQ channels in controlling endocytosis. This was examined in voltage-clamped bovine adrenal chromaffin cells by applying single DPs of long duration.[1] In this work, specific blockers of the different subtypes of VDCCs were used and the Ca^{2+} current and exo-/endocytosis induced by a 500 ms DP were studied. We found that, despite the small contribution of L-type VDCCs to the total global Ca^{2+} current, their inhibition by the DHP nifedipine (L-channel blocker) almost completely abolished the endocytotic response without significantly affecting exocytosis. ω-Conotoxin GVIA (N-channel blocker) had a little effect on the exo-/endocytotic responses, while ω-agatoxin IVA (P/Q-channel blocker) markedly blocked those responses in a parallel manner. These data support the following hypotheses that L-type Ca^{2+} channels might have a selective action for the control of endocytosis in bovine chromaffin cells, a function that seems to depend on Ca^{2+} entry through N or P/Q types of VDCCs to a much lesser extent.[1] Similar results were obtained in a related study by using FM-dye methodology, in which we found that endocytosis was inhibited by about 50% after long stimulation with high K^+ of bovine chromaffin cells when the L-channel blocker nifedipine was present.[280]

This functional coupling between L-type channels and endocytosis has been later on corroborated at the mouse neuromuscular junction using fluorescence microscopy of FM dyes-labeled synaptic vesicles and electrophysiological recordings[281] and at *Drosophila* synapse.[282]

39.9.1 How Do L-Type VDCCs Control Endocytosis in Bovine Chromaffin Cells?

The functional coupling between L-type channels and endocytosis observed in bovine chromaffin cells could be related to the following: (1) the existence of a close colocalization between endocytosis proteins and L-type channels; (2) the total amount of Ca^{2+} entering the chromaffin cell through a given VDCC; and/or (3) the mode of Ca^{2+} entry, that is, a slow and prolonged Ca^{2+} entry through the less inactivating L-type channels.

39.9.1.1 Colocalization between L-Type Channels and Endocytosis Proteins

A direct interaction between VDCCs and endophilin, a key regulator of clathrin-mediated endocytosis has been reported in hippocampal neurons. VDCCs and endophilin form a macromolecular complex in neurons, and formation of this complex is Ca^{2+} dependent. Endophilin is thought to interact with all three main types of VDCCs (i.e., L, N, and P/Q channels).[283]

We sought to identify the possible colocalization of the different VDCC subtypes with other endocytosis-related proteins such as dynamin and/or clathrin. Immunofluorescence experiments on bovine chromaffin cells showed that the colocalization of clathrin was practically negligible with the three VDCC subtypes ($Ca_v1.3$, $Ca_v2.1$, and $Ca_v2.2$) studied. Also, only a mild colocalization rate (about 20%–30%) was observed between VDCCs and dynamin. Taken together, these experiments do not support the existence of a close colocalization of VDCC subtypes with the endocytotic proteins clathrin and dynamin in bovine chromaffin cells.[280]

39.9.1.2 Influence of Total Amount of Ca^{2+} Entry

To characterize the influence of the total amount of Ca^{2+} (Q_{Ca}) on the endocytotic process, we compared the endocytic behavior of cells treated with nifedipine with others treated with a low concentration of ω-agatoxin IVA (to block P/Q channels). The low ω-agatoxin IVA concentration decreased the calcium current about 20%, which represents an extent similar to that produced by nifedipine on L channels. We found that in the presence of 10 mM extracellular Ca^{2+}, 200 nM ω-agatoxin IVA caused a 59% reduction of total Ca^{2+} entering the bovine chromaffin cell during a 500 ms DP, a value comparable with that obtained in the presence of nifedipine (50% blockade of Q_{Ca}). Despite this effect on Q_{Ca}, 200 nM ω-agatoxin IVA reduced endocytosis only by 37%, whereas nifedipine caused 93% inhibition. Thus, it seems that more relevant than the total Ca^{2+} entry into the cell during the 500 ms depolarizing pulse is the manner used by Ca^{2+} to trigger endocytosis, that is, the slow-inactivating L-type of VDCCs.[280]

If reduction of Ca^{2+} entry through L-type channels decreases endocytosis, one could test if increasing Ca^{2+} entry through this pathway enhances this response. To test this assumption, bovine chromaffin cells were treated with the L-type VDCC activator FPL64176 (FPL). In the presence of FPL, L channels inactivated more slowly and deactivated also at a slower rate. Related to its effects on the exo-/endocytosis processes, we found that FPL caused only around 18% increase in total Ca^{2+} entry, but this augmentation of Ca^{2+} entry gave rise to an almost threefold increase in the endo-/exocytosis ratio. Additional experiments were performed with isolation of L from N/PQ channels by blocking the non-L channels with ω-conotoxin MVIIC (MVIIC). It was found that, in cells treated with MVIIC, FPL increased Ca^{2+} entry and doubled the endo-/exocytosis ratio, indicating a selective augmentation of endocytosis related to this Ca^{2+} entry through L-type channels.[280]

Similar results were obtained when exo-/endocytosis responses were monitored with immunofluorescence techniques using FM1-43 dye. Chromaffin cells were challenged with a high-K^+ solution in the presence of FM1-43; in response to this long-lasting depolarization, the dye inserts into the outer leaflet on the plasma membrane and is internalized during vesicle retrieval[284] and fluorescence tends to accumulate near the plasmalemma.[285] Under these experimental conditions, endocytosis was 30% of total fluorescence. When the effect of VDCC blockers on the FM1-43 exo-/endocytotic responses was characterized, we found that the endo-/exocytosis relationship was not affected by GVIA. However, MVIIC reduced by 40% the endo-/exocytosis ratio and a 53% reduction of endo-/exocytosis ratio was observed in the presence of nifedipine. In cells treated with MVIIC to abolish non-L-type channels, FPL increased the endo-/exocytosis ratio. Although less clearly than the data derived from patch-clamp experiments, the FM1-43 data also support the view that Ca^{2+} entering through L-type VDCCs is preferentially coupled to endocytosis.[280]

In a recent study, Bay et al.[286] have also reported the implication of L-type VDCC in the membrane excess retrieval that follows a strong Ca^{2+} entry in mouse chromaffin cells. In this study, excess retrieval (a rapid endocytosis process that retrieves more membrane than the one fused by preceding exocytosis) was monitored with FM1.43 after the application of high-K^+ or cholinergic agonists for 15 or 30 s. It was found that this excess retrieval membrane pool is associated with the generation of a non-releasable fraction of membrane colocalizing with the lysosomal compartment and is controlled by the concerted contribution of extracellular and intracellular Ca^{2+} sources. The blocking of the L-type VDCC with nitrendipine suppressed excess retrieval.[286]

39.9.1.3 Influence of Intracellular Ca^{2+} Stores

Many evidences have shown that cytosolic organelles as endoplasmic reticulum and mitochondria work together with VDCCs to orchestrate a complex mechanism that control $[Ca^{2+}]_c$ levels and vesicle release. Experimental approaches used either to release Ca^{2+} or inhibit Ca^{2+} release from intracellular stores demonstrated an activation of specific proteins that recruit or prime secretory granules for exocytosis.[287,288] In the same way that intracellular stores are modulating exocytotic responses, an endocytotic modulation may actually be caused by Ca^{2+} contribution from intracellular stores. Thus, in the recent study by Bay et al.,[286] it was shown that endocytosis could also be inhibited by preventing the release of Ca^{2+} from the endoplasmic reticulum with ryanodine or thapsigargin. This observation suggests some type of synergism between Ca^{2+} regulation through extracellular and intracellular sources. A possible explanation is the activation of the Ca^{2+}-induced Ca^{2+} release, a mechanism that has been previously found in chromaffin cells.[152,289]

39.9.1.4 Influence of the Mode of Ca^{2+} Entry

In the study by Rosa et al.,[1] upon the application of a 500 ms DP, the degree of inactivation of each Ca^{2+} channel subtype strongly conditioned the kinetics and the amount of Ca^{2+} entry. Thus, a slow-inactivating

Ca^{2+} channel such as the L type,[150,151] which contributes only by about 30% to the initial peak I_{Ca}, carried more than half of the total Ca^{2+} entry along the 500 ms depolarizing pulse. Conversely, the fast-inactivating N-type channel that also contributes by about 30% to the initial I_{Ca} peak only contributed by about 24% to the total Q_{Ca}. These data suggested that a low-rate, noninactivating Ca^{2+} entry might be more critical to trigger compensatory as well as excess endocytosis.[1]

A pharmacological approach that serves to further slow down the Ca^{2+} entry through the slow-inactivating L-type calcium channels is based on the use of L-channel activators such as FPL64176 (FPL) and BayK8644 (BayK). Both compounds act by slowing the deactivation of L channels, thereby prolonging the mean open time of this channel type. As a result, more Ca^{2+} enters the cell through activated L channels. Membrane capacitance recordings and fluorescence imaging with FM dyes in chromaffin cells have demonstrated that the endocytotic process is increased in the presence of both agonists without significantly altering exocytosis.[280,286] The effect of BayK on endocytosis was also studied in the mouse neuromuscular junction, where the vesicle loading with FM2-10 was increased in the presence of the agonist BayK.[281] This finding further supports the hypothesis that L channels are preferentially coupled to the endocytotic machinery than the exocytotic and that not all calcium that enters into the cell through VDCCs have the same function.

We also explored the possibility that a more sustained Ca^{2+} entry through non-L (N/PQ) VDCCs could also activate endocytosis. For this, we used the cyclin-dependent kinase inhibitor roscovitine. Roscovitine is known to delay N/PQ channel deactivation, thereby prolonging channel opening time[108–110,290] and thus producing a slower Ca^{2+} entry. This mimics the slow mode of Ca^{2+} entry through L channels to activate endocytosis. We found that when roscovitine was given in the presence of nifedipine, endocytosis could be recovered to near control levels[280](unpublished data). It is conceivable that a sustained Ca^{2+} entry through N/PQ channels would also be able to maintain an endocytotic response even though the Ca^{2+} entry through L channels, which is responsible to initiate the membrane retrieval, is inhibited.

39.10 Basic and Clinical Perspectives

In over three decades of ω-toxins use, at least six subtypes of HVA Ca^{2+} channels have been identified and characterized. New toxins are needed to target selectively the Q-type Ca^{2+} channel without affecting the N or P. The R- or T-type channels also need selective toxins to characterize their functions. Whether the P and Q channels are the same or separate entities in various cell types remains to be clarified. The question of how many Ca^{2+} channel subtypes remain to be discovered is also relevant. In addition, differences among tissues and cell types for a given Ca^{2+} channel are emerging; L-type Ca^{2+} channels differ from skeletal, to cardiac, to smooth muscles, and to the brain. Are the Q channels from hippocampal and chromaffin cells identical? What about the N, P, or R channels? Why are different Ca^{2+} channels required to control exocytosis of the same transmitter (i.e., acetylcholine, catecholamines) in the same cell type and in different animal species? Another important question relates to the expression of various channel subtypes in the same cell. Why does exocytosis require Ca^{2+} from different pathways? Is it a safety valve to secure the efficiency of the process? If the N channel is a part of the secretory machinery, what about the L, P, or Q channels? How close are they from exocytotic active sites? And most interesting, are the channels of a paraneuronal cell such as the chromaffin cell equally organized than those of brain synapses? Why does the release of norepinephrine controlled by N channels in sympathetic neurons and by L or Q channels in chromaffin cells? Do action potentials recruit different Ca^{2+} channel subtypes in those two catecholaminergic cell types? Furthermore, do Ca^{2+} channel subtypes that dominate secretion in cultured chromaffin cells differ in intact adrenal glands or in adrenal slices? Will a K^+ depolarizing stimulus recruit Ca^{2+} channels different to those recruited by action potentials in neurons or by acetylcholine receptors in chromaffin cells? Is the electrical pattern of different excitable cells causing different secretion patterns by simply recruiting specific Ca^{2+} channels with particular gating and kinetic properties?

Another critical question relates to the development of a pharmacology for neuronal Ca^{2+} channels. While L-type Ca^{2+} channels have a rich pharmacology that have provided novel therapeutic approaches to treat cardiovascular diseases, non-peptide molecules that block or inactivate the N, P, Q, T, or R channels are lacking. Thus, a major goal for research in this field is the search for selective blockers or modulators of specific Ca^{2+} channel subtypes that could eventually be used as therapeutic tools in disease. The recent introduction of mibefradil as a T-type Ca^{2+} channel blocker opened new possibilities to study the functions of these channels. The knowledge of the 3D structure in solution of the different toxins is very important for studying the specificity of their interactions with Ca^{2+} channel subtypes and to define active sites that can serve as models to design and synthesize non-peptide blockers. The ω-conotoxins are small peptides containing 24–29 amino acid residues. It is interesting that the amino acid sequence of ω-conotoxin MVIIA is much more similar to that of ω-conotoxin MVIIC than to ω-conotoxin GVIA; yet the pharmacology of ω-conotoxin MVIIA is much more closer to that of ω-conotoxin GVIA (blockade of N-type channels). Thus, it will be very important to define structural differences determining the toxin selectivity for N- or Q-type Ca^{2+} channels. The 3D structures of ω-conotoxin GVIA,[291–294] ω-conotoxin MVIIA,[295] and ω-conotoxin MVIIC[296,297] have been elucidated. Other new toxins will facilitate their comparisons and the definition of structural determinants for specific binding to Ca^{2+} channel subtypes, to identify a pharmacophore, and to facilitate the synthesis of non-peptide HVA Ca^{2+} channel modulators of therapeutic interest.[298]

Non-peptide blockers for neuronal Ca^{2+} channels are emerging, but they lack selectivity. For instance, the piperazine derivatives flunarizine, R56865, lubeluzole, and dotarizine are "wide-spectrum" Ca^{2+} channel blockers.[84,85,299] Fluspirilene, a member of the diphenylbutylpiperidine class of neuroleptic drugs (which also includes pimozide, clopimozide, and penfluridol) has antischizophrenic actions and blocks N-type Ca^{2+} channels in PC12 cells.[300] It may be that its neuroleptic properties are due, at least in part, to an inhibition of neuronal N-type Ca^{2+} channels. Thus, inhibition (or facilitation) of specific neurotransmitter release by selective blockers (or activators) of Ca^{2+} channels may have functional and therapeutic consequences. For instance, synthetic ω-conotoxin MVIIA protected hippocampal CA1 pyramidal neurons from damage caused by transient, global forebrain ischemia in the rat.[24]

Channelopathies are increasingly being associated to specific diseases.[301] For instance, mutations of the Cav2.1 gene that encodes the α_{1A} subunit of the P/Q Ca^{2+} channel are responsible for the human familial hemiplegic migraine, episodic ataxia type 2, and spinocerebellar ataxia type 6.[302–304] Also, natural P/Q mutations have been reported for the tottering and leaner mice, of which the homozygous rodents exhibit symptoms of ataxia and epilepsy.[305,306] Additionally, P/Q knockout mice display progressive ataxia and dystonia until they are finally unable to walk, followed by death.[307]

In patients suffering paraneoplastic Lambert–Eaton syndrome and in passive transfer animal models of the disease, due to an autoimmune reaction against the P/Q-type Ca^{2+} channel located at the presynaptic motor nerve terminal, a reduction of neurotransmitter release is observed.[308] It is interesting that L-type Ca^{2+} channels, which are normally absent at the muscle endplate, become coupled to neurotransmitter release after neuromuscular junctions were treated with immunoglobulins from either Lambert–Eaton patients[309] or amyotrophic lateral sclerosis patients[310] during reinnervation[311] and during functional recovery from botulinum toxin type-A poisoning.[312]

In hair cells, the L-type Ca^{2+} channel current is associated to a gene expressing a Cav1.3 α_1 subunit. The central role of these currents in auditory transduction was shown through deletion of the gene expressing Cav1.3, which caused complete deafness.[313]

ω-Toxin Ca^{2+} channel blockers have entered the clinic as therapeutic tools. Such is the case of ω-conotoxin MVIIA, also known as SNX-111 or ziconotide.[314] The approval of Prialt®, a synthetic version of ω-conotoxin MVIIA, by several drug regulatory agencies, for the treatment of severe chronic pain associated with cancer, AIDS, and neuropathies represents a significant advancement in analgesia. Ziconotide has shown potent efficacy in a postsurgical setting[315] as well as in patients suffering from a variety of chronic, and otherwise intractable, severe pain syndromes.[316] The drug has to be given intrathecally to prevent important side effects such as orthostatic hypotension.[317] Its potent analgesic effects, which are manifested even in patients resistant to opioids, is due to inhibition of proprioceptive neurotransmitter and neuromodulators from the central nerve terminals of primary afferent neurons in the dorsal horn of the spinal cord.[318,319]

Another target that is intensely being studied for pain treatment is the T-type Ca^{2+} channel.[314,320] So Cav1.3 knockout mice are hyperalgesic in a model of visceral pain that is likely related to a T-type Ca^{2+} channel-dependent antinociceptive mechanism operating in the thalamus.[321] On the other hand, antiepileptic ethosuximide is a selective T-type Ca^{2+} channel blocker.[322] The drug reverses tactile allodynia and thermal hyperalgesia in nerve-ligated rats.[323]

An interesting Ca^{2+} channel therapeutic target is the auxiliary subunit $\alpha_2\delta$. Gabapentin is an approved analgesic and antiepileptic drug that binds with high affinity to $\alpha_2\delta_1$ and $\alpha_2\delta_2$ subunits of HVA Ca^{2+} channels.[324,325] This causes a blockade of Ca^{2+} currents, particularly after an injury such as constriction of the sciatic nerve in rats.[326] Its antinociceptive effects in rats in the absence of tolerance[327,328] led to clinical trials showing moderate efficacy in postherpetic neuralgia, diabetic neuropathy, trigeminal neuralgia, low back pain, and cancer pain. Recently, another $\alpha_2\delta$ ligand, pregabalin, has shown higher efficacy in animal models and in diseases developing neuropathic pain. Its association with the $\alpha_2\delta_1$ subunit has been clearly demonstrated because pregabalin loses its antinociceptive effects in transgenic mice expressing $\alpha_2\delta_1$ subunit with a point mutation that prevents pregabalin binding.[329] Pregabalin is presently being used in the clinic to treat neuropathic pain of various origins (see review by Horga de la Parte and Horga[330]).

Many questions have been answered during three decades of intense research in the field of neuronal VDCCs. Most of the studies performed were possible only because particularly the group of Professor Baldomero Olivera made available to many groups of researchers potent ω-toxins to type and characterize those channels. The same is true for the patch-clamp techniques, which exploded at the same time than ω-toxins thanks to the efforts of the group of Professor Erwin Neher. We are sure that some references on this topic escaped our review; we apologize to those authors not cited here involuntarily.

Given the notable role of L-type VDCCs in controlling compensatory and excess endocytosis, the next issue is whether $Ca_V1.2$ or $Ca_V1.3$ has a preferential control on vesicle retrieval. One argument in favor of $Ca_V1.3$ is its slower and less complete time-dependent inactivation with respect to $Ca_V1.2$. The delayed inactivation of $Ca_V1.3$ could be physiologically relevant for sustaining prolonged Ca^{2+} influxes that support normal endocytosis.[258] Finally, also the coupling of $Ca_V1.2$ and $Ca_V1.3$ to calmodulin, the Ca^{2+} sensor of different forms of endocytosis could be a further molecular target of differential regulation of the endocytotic response. These issues could be answered using specific L-type KO animal models.[331]

L-type VDCCs play multiple roles in the control of neurotransmitter release. Spontaneous AP firing, low-threshold exocytosis, and compensatory/excess endocytosis are likely to be directly controlled by $Ca_V1.3$, which then turns out to be an important molecular gateway for controlling neurotransmitter release. Since $Ca_V1.3$ is also critical for the control of vital functions such as heart beating,[332] hearing,[333] and dopamine release,[334] it is evident that the availability of new DHP compounds that selectively block $Ca_V1.3$ would be beneficial for the potential therapeutic treatment of Parkinson disease, cardiac arrhythmias, chronic stress, and other neuro- and cardiovascular pathologies in which $Ca_V1.3$ is likely to be involved.[258]

ACKNOWLEDGMENTS

The work of the authors referred to in this review has been supported by grants from Ministerio de Economía y Competitividad (SAF2010-21795 to AGG; SAF2010-18837 to LG) and Instituto de Salud Carlos III (RETICS RD06/0009). We also thank the continued support of Fundación Teófilo Hernando, UAM, Madrid, Spain.

REFERENCES

1. Rosa, J. M., de Diego, A. M., Gandia, L., and Garcia, A. G., 2007. L-type calcium channels are preferentially coupled to endocytosis in bovine chromaffin cells. *Biochem Biophys Res Commun*, 357, 834–839.
2. Olivera, B. M., 2006. Conus peptides: Biodiversity-based discovery and exogenomics. *J Biol Chem*, 281, 31173–31177.
3. Olivera, B. M., Miljanich, G. P., Ramachandran, J., and Adams, M. E., 1994. Calcium channel diversity and neurotransmitter release: The omega-conotoxins and omega-agatoxins. *Annu Rev Biochem*, 63, 823–867.
4. Olivera, B. M. and Cruz, L. J., 2001. Conotoxins, in retrospect. *Toxicon*, 39, 7–14.
5. Lewis, R. J., Dutertre, S., Vetter, I., and Christie, M. J., 2012. Conus venom peptide pharmacology. *Pharmacol Rev*, 64, 259–298.
6. Nicke, A., Wonnacott, S., and Lewis, R. J., 2004. Alpha-conotoxins as tools for the elucidation of structure and function of neuronal nicotinic acetylcholine receptor subtypes. *Eur J Biochem*, 271, 2305–2319.

7. Leipold, E., Hansel, A., Olivera, B. M., Terlau, H., and Heinemann, S. H., 2005. Molecular interaction of delta-conotoxins with voltage-gated sodium channels. *FEBS Lett*, 579, 3881–3884.

8. Shon, K. J., Stocker, M., Terlau, H. et al., 1998. kappa-Conotoxin PVIIA is a peptide inhibiting the shaker K+ channel. *J Biol Chem*, 273, 33–38.

9. Li, R. A. and Tomaselli, G. F., 2004. Using the deadly mu-conotoxins as probes of voltage-gated sodium channels. *Toxicon*, 44, 117–122.

10. Terlau, H., Shon, K. J., Grilley, M., Stocker, M., Stuhmer, W., and Olivera, B. M., 1996. Strategy for rapid immobilization of prey by a fish-hunting marine snail. *Nature*, 381, 148–151.

11. Llinas, R., Sugimori, M., Hillman, D. E., and Cherksey, B., 1992. Distribution and functional significance of the P-type, voltage-dependent Ca^{2+} channels in the mammalian central nervous system. *Trends Neurosci*, 15, 351–355.

12. Adams, M. E., Bindokas, V. P., Hasegawa, L., and Venema, V. J., 1990. Omega-agatoxins: Novel calcium channel antagonists of two subtypes from funnel web spider (*Agelenopsis aperta*) venom. *J Biol Chem*, 265, 861–867.

13. Adams, M. E., 2004. Agatoxins: Ion channel specific toxins from the American funnel web spider, *Agelenopsis aperta*. *Toxicon*, 43, 509–525.

14. de Weille, J. R., Schweitz, H., Maes, P., Tartar, A., and Lazdunski, M., 1991. Calciseptine, a peptide isolated from black mamba venom, is a specific blocker of the L-type calcium channel. *Proc Natl Acad Sci USA*, 88, 2437–2440.

15. Schweitz, H., Heurteaux, C., Bois, P., Moinier, D., Romey, G., and Lazdunski, M., 1994. Calcicludine, a venom peptide of the Kunitz-type protease inhibitor family, is a potent blocker of high-threshold Ca^{2+} channels with a high affinity for L-type channels in cerebellar granule neurons. *Proc Natl Acad Sci USA*, 91, 878–882.

16. Myers, R. A., Cruz, L. J., Rivier, J. E., and Olivera, B. M., 1993. Conus peptides as chemical probes for receptors and ion channels. *Chem Rev*, 93, 1923–1936.

17. Protti, D. A., Reisin, R., Mackinley, T. A., and Uchitel, O. D., 1996. Calcium channel blockers and transmitter release at the normal human neuromuscular junction. *Neurology*, 46, 1391–1396.

18. Shon, K. J., Hasson, A., Spira, M. E., Cruz, L. J., Gray, W. R., and Olivera, B. M., 1994. Delta-conotoxin GmVIA, a novel peptide from the venom of *Conus gloriamaris*. *Biochemistry*, 33, 11420–11425.

19. Olivera, B. M., Gray, W. R., Zeikus, R. et al., 1985. Peptide neurotoxins from fish-hunting cone snails. *Science*, 230, 1338–1343.

20. Terlau, H. and Olivera, B. M., 2004. Conus venoms: A rich source of novel ion channel-targeted peptides. *Physiol Rev*, 84, 41–68.

21. Olivera, B. M., McIntosh, J. M., Cruz, L. J., Luque, F. A., and Gray, W. R., 1984. Purification and sequence of a presynaptic peptide toxin from *Conus geographus* venom. *Biochemistry*, 23, 5087–5090.

22. McIntosh, M., Cruz, L. J., Hunkapiller, M. W., Gray, W. R., and Olivera, B. M., 1982. Isolation and structure of a peptide toxin from the marine snail *Conus magus*. *Arch Biochem Biophys*, 218, 329–334.

23. Kerr, L. M. and Yoshikami, D., 1984. A venom peptide with a novel presynaptic blocking action. *Nature*, 308, 282–284.

24. Valentino, K., Newcomb, R., Gadbois, T. et al., 1993. A selective N-type calcium channel antagonist protects against neuronal loss after global cerebral ischemia. *Proc Natl Acad Sci USA*, 90, 7894–7897.

25. Vega, T., De Pascual, R., Bulbena, O., and Garcia, A. G., 1995. Effects of omega-toxins on noradrenergic neurotransmission in beating guinea pig atria. *Eur J Pharmacol*, 276, 231–238.

26. Hillyard, D. R., Monje, V. D., Mintz, I. M. et al., 1992. A new Conus peptide ligand for mammalian presynaptic Ca^{2+} channels. *Neuron*, 9, 69–77.

27. Gandia, L., Lara, B., Imperial, J. S. et al., 1997. Analogies and differences between omega-conotoxins MVIIC and MVIID: Binding sites and functions in bovine chromaffin cells. *Pflugers Arch*, 435, 55–64.

28. Adams, M. E., Herold, E. E., and Venema, V. J., 1989. Two classes of channel-specific toxins from funnel web spider venom. *J Comp Physiol [A]*, 164, 333–342.

29. Pocock, J. M., Venema, V. J., and Adams, M. E., 1992. Omega-agatoxins differentially block calcium channels in locust, chick and rat synaptosomes. *Neurochem Int*, 20, 263–270.

30. Dolphin, A. C. and Scott, R. H., 1987. Calcium channel currents and their inhibition by (-)-baclofen in rat sensory neurones: Modulation by guanine nucleotides. *J Physiol*, 386, 1–17.

31. Bindokas, V. P. and Adams, M. E., 1989. omega-Aga-I: A presynaptic calcium channel antagonist from venom of the funnel web spider, *Agelenopsis aperta*. *J Neurobiol*, 20, 171–188.

32. Mintz, I. M., Venema, V. J., Swiderek, K. M., Lee, T. D., Bean, B. P., and Adams, M. E., 1992. P-type calcium channels blocked by the spider toxin omega-Aga-IVA. *Nature*, 355, 827–829.

33. Venema, V. J., Swiderek, K. M., Lee, T. D., Hathaway, G. M., and Adams, M. E., 1992. Antagonism of synaptosomal calcium channels by subtypes of omega-agatoxins. *J Biol Chem*, 267, 2610–2615.

34. Ertel, E. A., Warren, V. A., Adams, M. E., Griffin, P. R., Cohen, C. J., and Smith, M. M., 1994. Type III omega-agatoxins: A family of probes for similar binding sites on L- and N-type calcium channels. *Biochemistry*, 33, 5098–5108.

35. Mintz, I. M., Venema, V. J., Adams, M. E., and Bean, B. P., 1991. Inhibition of N- and L-type Ca^{2+} channels by the spider venom toxin omega-Aga-IIIA. *Proc Natl Acad Sci USA*, 88, 6628–6631.

36. Mintz, I. M., 1994. Block of Ca channels in rat central neurons by the spider toxin omega-Aga-IIIA. *J Neurosci*, 14, 2844–2853.

37. Cohen, M. W., Jones, O. T., and Angelides, K. J., 1991. Distribution of Ca^{2+} channels on frog motor nerve terminals revealed by fluorescent omega-conotoxin. *J Neurosci*, 11, 1032–1039.

38. Mintz, I. M., Sabatini, B. L., and Regehr, W. G., 1995. Calcium control of transmitter release at a cerebellar synapse. *Neuron*, 15, 675–688.

39. Mintz, I. M. and Bean, B. P., 1993. Block of calcium channels in rat neurons by synthetic omega-Aga-IVA. *Neuropharmacology*, 32, 1161–1169.

40. Turner, T. J., Adams, M. E., and Dunlap, K., 1992. Calcium channels coupled to glutamate release identified by omega-Aga-IVA. *Science*, 258, 310–313.

41. Adams, M. E., Mintz, I. M., Reily, M. D., Thanabal, V., and Bean, B. P., 1993. Structure and properties of omega-agatoxin IVB, a new antagonist of P-type calcium channels. *Mol Pharmacol*, 44, 681–688.

42. Teramoto, T., Kuwada, M., Niidome, T., Sawada, K., Nishizawa, Y., and Katayama, K., 1993. A novel peptide from funnel web spider venom, omega-Aga-TK, selectively blocks, P-type calcium channels. *Biochem Biophys Res Commun*, 196, 134–140.

43. Catterall, W. A., 2000. Structure and regulation of voltage-gated Ca^{2+} channels. *Annu Rev Cell Dev Biol*, 16, 521–555.

44. Arikkath, J. and Campbell, K. P., 2003. Auxiliary subunits: Essential components of the voltage-gated calcium channel complex. *Curr Opin Neurobiol*, 13, 298–307.

45. Catterall, W. A., Perez-Reyes, E., Snutch, T. P., and Striessnig, J., 2005. International Union of Pharmacology. XLVIII. Nomenclature and structure-function relationships of voltage-gated calcium channels. *Pharmacol Rev*, 57, 411–425.

46. Catterall, W. A., 2011. Voltage-gated calcium channels. *Cold Spring Harb Perspect Biol*, 3, a003947.

47. Hofmann, F., Lacinova, L., and Klugbauer, N., 1999. Voltage-dependent calcium channels: From structure to function. *Rev Physiol Biochem Pharmacol*, 139, 33–87.

48. Klugbauer, N., Marais, E., and Hofmann, F., 2003. Calcium channel alpha2delta subunits: Differential expression, function, and drug binding. *J Bioenerg Biomembr*, 35, 639–647.

49. Kang, M. G. and Campbell, K. P., 2003. Gamma subunit of voltage-activated calcium channels. *J Biol Chem*, 278, 21315–21318.

50. Lacinova, L., 2005. Voltage-dependent calcium channels. *Gen Physiol Biophys*, 24(Suppl 1), 1–78.

51. Pragnell, M., De Waard, M., Mori, Y., Tanabe, T., Snutch, T. P., and Campbell, K. P., 1994. Calcium channel beta-subunit binds to a conserved motif in the I-II cytoplasmic linker of the alpha 1-subunit. *Nature*, 368, 67–70.

52. Van Petegem, F., Clark, K. A., Chatelain, F. C., and Minor, D. L. Jr., 2004. Structure of a complex between a voltage-gated calcium channel beta-subunit and an alpha-subunit domain. *Nature*, 429, 671–675.

53. Beguin, P., Nagashima, K., Gonoi, T. et al., 2001. Regulation of Ca^{2+} channel expression at the cell surface by the small G-protein kir/Gem. *Nature*, 411, 701–706.

54. Berggren, P. O., Yang, S. N., Murakami, M. et al., 2004. Removal of Ca^{2+} channel beta3 subunit enhances Ca^{2+} oscillation frequency and insulin exocytosis. *Cell*, 119, 273–284.

55. Hansen, J. P., Chen, R. S., Larsen, J. K. et al., 2004. Calcium channel gamma6 subunits are unique modulators of low voltage-activated (Cav3.1) calcium current. *J Mol Cell Cardiol*, 37, 1147–1158.

56. Chen, L., Chetkovich, D. M., Petralia, R. S. et al., 2000. Stargazin regulates synaptic targeting of AMPA receptors by two distinct mechanisms. *Nature*, 408, 936–943.

57. Vandenberghe, W., Nicoll, R. A., and Bredt, D. S., 2005. Stargazin is an AMPA receptor auxiliary subunit. *Proc Natl Acad Sci USA*, 102, 485–490.

58. Ertel, E. A., Campbell, K. P., Harpold, M. M. et al., 2000. Nomenclature of voltage-gated calcium channels. *Neuron*, 25, 533–535.

59. Hamill, O. P., Marty, A., Neher, E., Sakmann, B., and Sigworth, F. J., 1981. Improved patch-clamp techniques for high-resolution current recording from cells and cell-free membrane patches. *Pflugers Arch*, 391, 85–100.

60. Carbone, E. and Lux, H. D., 1984. A low voltage-activated, fully inactivating Ca channel in vertebrate sensory neurones. *Nature*, 310, 501–502.

61. Fox, A. P., Nowycky, M. C., and Tsien, R. W., 1987. Kinetic and pharmacological properties distinguishing three types of calcium currents in chick sensory neurones. *J Physiol*, 394, 149–172.

62. Fox, A. P., Nowycky, M. C., and Tsien, R. W., 1987. Single-channel recordings of three types of calcium channels in chick sensory neurones. *J Physiol*, 394, 173–200.

63. Hollywood, M. A., Woolsey, S., Walsh, I. K., Keane, P. F., McHale, N. G., and Thornbury, K. D., 2003. T- and L-type Ca^{2+} currents in freshly dispersed smooth muscle cells from the human proximal urethra. *J Physiol*, 550, 753–764.

64. Lee, J. H., Gomora, J. C., Cribbs, L. L., and Perez-Reyes, E., 1999. Nickel block of three cloned T-type calcium channels: Low concentrations selectively block alpha1H. *Biophys J*, 77, 3034–3042.

65. Hagiwara, N., Irisawa, H., and Kameyama, M., 1988. Contribution of two types of calcium currents to the pacemaker potentials of rabbit sino-atrial node cells. *J Physiol*, 395, 233–253.

66. Todorovic, S. M. and Lingle, C. J., 1998. Pharmacological properties of T-type Ca^{2+} current in adult rat sensory neurons: Effects of anticonvulsant and anesthetic agents. *J Neurophysiol*, 79, 240–252.

67. Huguenard, J. R., 1996. Low-threshold calcium currents in central nervous system neurons. *Annu Rev Physiol*, 58, 329–348.

68. Chuang, R. S., Jaffe, H., Cribbs, L., Perez-Reyes, E., and Swartz, K. J., 1998. Inhibition of T-type voltage-gated calcium channels by a new scorpion toxin. *Nat Neurosci*, 1, 668–674.

69. Sidach, S. S. and Mintz, I. M., 2002. Kurtoxin, a gating modifier of neuronal high- and low-threshold ca channels. *J Neurosci*, 22, 2023–2034.

70. Mishra, S. K. and Hermsmeyer, K., 1994. Selective inhibition of T-type Ca^{2+} channels by Ro 40-5967. *Circ Res*, 75, 144–148.

71. Okubo, K., Takahashi, T., Sekiguchi, F. et al., 2011. Inhibition of T-type calcium channels and hydrogen sulfide-forming enzyme reverses paclitaxel-evoked neuropathic hyperalgesia in rats. *Neuroscience*, 188, 148–156.

72. Fang, L. M. and Osterrieder, W., 1991. Potential-dependent inhibition of cardiac Ca^{2+} inward currents by Ro 40–5967 and verapamil: Relation to negative inotropy. *Eur J Pharmacol*, 196, 205–207.

73. Bezprozvanny, I. and Tsien, R. W., 1995. Voltage-dependent blockade of diverse types of voltage-gated Ca^{2+} channels expressed in Xenopus oocytes by the Ca^{2+} channel antagonist mibefradil (Ro 40-5967). *Mol Pharmacol*, 48, 540–549.

74. Randall, A. D. and Tsien, R. W., 1997. Contrasting biophysical and pharmacological properties of T-type and R-type calcium channels. *Neuropharmacology*, 36, 879–893.

75. Viana, F., Van den Bosch, L., Missiaen, L. et al., 1997. Mibefradil (Ro 40-5967) blocks multiple types of voltage-gated calcium channels in cultured rat spinal motoneurones. *Cell Calcium*, 22, 299–311.

76. Huang, L., Keyser, B. M., Tagmose, T. M. et al., 2004. NNC 55-0396 [(1S,2S)-2-(2-(N-[(3-benzimidazol-2-yl)propyl]-N-methylamino)ethyl)-6-fluoro-1,2, 3,4-tetrahydro-1-isopropyl-2-naphtyl cyclopropanecarboxylate dihydrochloride]: A new selective inhibitor of T-type calcium channels. *J Pharmacol Exp Ther*, 309, 193–199.

77. Li, M., Hansen, J. B., Huang, L., Keyser, B. M., and Taylor, J. T., 2005. Towards selective antagonists of T-type calcium channels: Design, characterization and potential applications of NNC 55-0396. *Cardiovasc Drug Rev*, 23, 173–196.

78. Lacinova, L., 2004. Pharmacology of recombinant low-voltage activated calcium channels. *Curr Drug Targets CNS Neurol Disord*, 3, 105–111.

79. Nowycky, M. C., Fox, A. P., and Tsien, R. W., 1985. Three types of neuronal calcium channel with different calcium agonist sensitivity. *Nature*, 316, 440–443.

80. Gandia, L., Borges, R., Albillos, A., and Garcia, A. G., 1995. Multiple calcium channel subtypes in isolated rat chromaffin cells. *Pflugers Arch*, 430, 55–63.

81. Plummer, M. R., Logothetis, D. E., and Hess, P., 1989. Elementary properties and pharmacological sensitivities of calcium channels in mammalian peripheral neurons. *Neuron*, 2, 1453–1463.

82. Fleckenstein, A., 1983. History of calcium antagonists. *Circ Res*, 52, I3–I16.

83. Spedding, M., 1985. Calcium antagonists subgroups. *Trends Pharmacol Sci*, 6, 109–114.

84. Garcez-Do-Carmo, L., Albillos, A., Artalejo, A. R. et al., 1993. R56865 inhibits catecholamine release from bovine chromaffin cells by blocking calcium channels. *Br J Pharmacol*, 110, 1149–1155.

85. Villarroya, M., Gandia, L., Lara, B., Albillos, A., Lopez, M. G., and Garcia, A. G., 1995. Dotarizine versus flunarizine as calcium antagonists in chromaffin cells. *Br J Pharmacol*, 114, 369–376.

86. Lara, B., Gandia, L., Torres, A. et al., 1997. Wide-spectrum Ca^{2+} channel antagonists: Lipophilicity, inhibition, and recovery of secretion in chromaffin cells. *Eur J Pharmacol*, 325, 109–119.

87. Villalobos, C., Fonteriz, R., Lopez, M. G., Garcia, A. G., and Garcia-Sancho, J., 1992. Inhibition of voltage-gated Ca^{2+} entry into GH3 and chromaffin cells by imidazole antimycotics and other cytochrome P450 blockers. *FASEB J*, 6, 2742–2747.

88. Artalejo, C. R., Perlman, R. L., and Fox, A. P., 1992. Omega-conotoxin GVIA blocks a Ca^{2+} current in bovine chromaffin cells that is not of the "classic" N type. *Neuron*, 8, 85–95.

89. Kasai, H., Aosaki, T., and Fukuda, J., 1987. Presynaptic Ca-antagonist omega-conotoxin irreversibly blocks N-type Ca-channels in chick sensory neurons. *Neurosci Res*, 4, 228–235.

90. Olivera, B. M., Cruz, L. J., de Santos, V. et al., 1987. Neuronal calcium channel antagonists. Discrimination between calcium channel subtypes using omega-conotoxin from *Conus magus* venom. *Biochemistry*, 26, 2086–2090.

91. Lewis, R. J., Nielsen, K. J., Craik, D. J. et al., 2000. Novel omega-conotoxins from *Conus catus* discriminate among neuronal calcium channel subtypes. *J Biol Chem*, 275, 35335–35344.

92. Berecki, G., Motin, L., Haythornthwaite, A. et al., 2010. Analgesic (omega)-conotoxins CVIE and CVIF selectively and voltage-dependently block recombinant and native N-type calcium channels. *Mol Pharmacol*, 77, 139–148.

93. Monje, V. D., Haack, J. A., Naisbitt, S. R. et al., 1993. A new Conus peptide ligand for Ca channel subtypes. *Neuropharmacology*, 32, 1141–1149.

94. Lampe, R. A., Defeo, P. A., Davison, M. D. et al., 1993. Isolation and pharmacological characterization of omega-grammotoxin SIA, a novel peptide inhibitor of neuronal voltage-sensitive calcium channel responses. *Mol Pharmacol*, 44, 451–460.

95. Piser, T. M., Lampe, R. A., Keith, R. A., and Thayer, S. A., 1994. omega-Grammotoxin blocks action-potential-induced Ca^{2+} influx and whole-cell Ca^{2+} current in rat dorsal-root ganglion neurons. *Pflugers Arch*, 426, 214–220.

96. Meunier, F. A., Feng, Z. P., Molgo, J., Zamponi, G. W., and Schiavo, G., 2002. Glycerotoxin from *Glycera convoluta* stimulates neurosecretion by up-regulating N-type Ca^{2+} channel activity. *EMBO J*, 21, 6733–6743.

97. Schenning, M., Proctor, D. T., Ragnarsson, L. et al., 2006. Glycerotoxin stimulates neurotransmitter release from N-type Ca^{2+} channel expressing neurons. *J Neurochem*, 98, 894–904.

98. Llinas, R., Sugimori, M., Lin, J. W., and Cherksey, B., 1989. Blocking and isolation of a calcium channel from neurons in mammals and cephalopods utilizing a toxin fraction (FTX) from funnel-web spider poison. *Proc Natl Acad Sci USA*, 86, 1689–1693.

99. Regan, L. J., 1991. Voltage-dependent calcium currents in Purkinje cells from rat cerebellar vermis. *J Neurosci*, 11, 2259–2269.

100. Mintz, I. M., Adams, M. E., and Bean, B. P., 1992. P-type calcium channels in rat central and peripheral neurons. *Neuron*, 9, 85–95.

101. Usowicz, M. M., Sugimori, M., Cherksey, B., and Llinas, R., 1992. P-type calcium channels in the somata and dendrites of adult cerebellar Purkinje cells. *Neuron*, 9, 1185–1199.

102. Umemiya, M. and Berger, A. J., 1995. Single-channel properties of four calcium channel types in rat motoneurons. *J Neurosci*, 15, 2218–2224.

103. Piser, T. M., Lampe, R. A., Keith, R. A., and Thayer, S. A., 1995. Omega-grammotoxin SIA blocks multiple, voltage-gated, Ca^{2+} channel subtypes in cultured rat hippocampal neurons. *Mol Pharmacol*, 48, 131–139.

104. Turner, T. J., Lampe, R. A., and Dunlap, K., 1995. Characterization of presynaptic calcium channels with omega-conotoxin MVIIC and omega-grammotoxin SIA: Role for a resistant calcium channel type in neurosecretion. *Mol Pharmacol*, 47, 348–353.

105. Randall, A. and Tsien, R. W., 1995. Pharmacological dissection of multiple types of Ca^{2+} channel currents in rat cerebellar granule neurons. *J Neurosci*, 15, 2995–3012.

106. Wheeler, D. B., Randall, A., and Tsien, R. W., 1994. Roles of N-type and Q-type Ca^{2+} channels in supporting hippocampal synaptic transmission. *Science*, 264, 107–111.

107. Nimmrich, V. and Gross, G., 2012. P/Q-type calcium channel modulators. *Br J Pharmacol*, 167, 741–759.

108. Yan, Z., Chi, P., Bibb, J. A., Ryan, T. A., and Greengard, P., 2002. Roscovitine: A novel regulator of P/Q-type calcium channels and transmitter release in central neurons. *J Physiol*, 540, 761–770.

109. Buraei, Z., Anghelescu, M., and Elmslie, K. S., 2005. Slowed N-type calcium channel (CaV2.2) deactivation by the cyclin-dependent kinase inhibitor roscovitine. *Biophys J*, 89, 1681–1691.

110. Buraei, Z., Schofield, G., and Elmslie, K. S., 2007. Roscovitine differentially affects CaV2 and Kv channels by binding to the open state. *Neuropharmacology*, 52, 883–894.

111. Tottene, A., Moretti, A., and Pietrobon, D., 1996. Functional diversity of P-type and R-type calcium channels in rat cerebellar neurons. *J Neurosci*, 16, 6353–6363.

112. Newcomb, R., Szoke, B., Palma, A. et al., 1998. Selective peptide antagonist of the class E calcium channel from the venom of the tarantula *Hysterocrates gigas*. *Biochemistry*, 37, 15353–15362.

113. Arroyo, G., Aldea, M., Fuentealba, J., Albillos, A., and Garcia, A. G., 2003. SNX482 selectively blocks P/Q Ca^{2+} channels and delays the inactivation of Na$^+$ channels of chromaffin cells. *Eur J Pharmacol*, 475, 11–18.

114. Bowman, D., Alexander, S., and Lodge, D., 1993. Pharmacological characterisation of the calcium channels coupled to the plateau phase of KCl-induced intracellular free Ca^{2+} elevation in chicken and rat synaptosomes. *Neuropharmacology*, 32, 1195–1202.

115. Ahmad, S. N. and Miljanich, G. P., 1988. The calcium channel antagonist, omega-conotoxin, and electric organ nerve terminals: Binding and inhibition of transmitter release and calcium influx. *Brain Res*, 453, 247–256.

116. Farinas, I., Solsona, C., and Marsal, J., 1992. Omega-conotoxin differentially blocks acetylcholine and adenosine triphosphate releases from Torpedo synaptosomes. *Neuroscience*, 47, 641–648.

117. Sierra, F., Lorenzo, D., Macadar, O., and Buno, W., 1995. N-type Ca^{2+} channels mediate transmitter release at the electromotoneuron-electrocyte synapses of the weakly electric fish Gymnotus carapo. *Brain Res*, 683, 215–220.

118. Jahromi, B. S., Robitaille, R., and Charlton, M. P., 1992. Transmitter release increases intracellular calcium in perisynaptic Schwann cells in situ. *Neuron*, 8, 1069–1077.

119. Wessler, I., Dooley, D. J., Werhand, J., and Schlemmer, F., 1990. Differential effects of calcium channel antagonists (omega-conotoxin GVIA, nifedipine, verapamil) on the electrically-evoked release of [3H] acetylcholine from the myenteric plexus, phrenic nerve and neocortex of rats. *Naunyn Schmiedebergs Arch Pharmacol*, 341, 288–294.

120. Garcia-Palomero, E., Cuchillo-Ibanez, I., Garcia, A. G., Renart, J., Albillos, A., and Montiel, C., 2000. Greater diversity than previously thought of chromaffin cell Ca^{2+} channels, derived from mRNA identification studies. *FEBS Lett*, 481, 235–239.

121. Diverse-Pierluissi, M., Dunlap, K., and Westhead, E. W., 1991. Multiple actions of extracellular ATP on calcium currents in cultured bovine chromaffin cells. *Proc Natl Acad Sci USA*, 88, 1261–1265.

122. Bournaud, R., Hidalgo, J., Yu, H., Jaimovich, E., and Shimahara, T., 2001. Low threshold T-type calcium current in rat embryonic chromaffin cells. *J Physiol*, 537, 35–44.

123. Hollins, B. and Ikeda, S. R., 1996. Inward currents underlying action potentials in rat adrenal chromaffin cells. *J Neurophysiol*, 76, 1195–1211.

124. Levitsky, K. L. and Lopez-Barneo, J., 2009. Developmental change of T-type Ca^{2+} channel expression and its role in rat chromaffin cell responsiveness to acute hypoxia. *J Physiol*, 587, 1917–1929.

125. Souvannakitti, D., Nanduri, J., Yuan, G., Kumar, G. K., Fox, A. P., and Prabhakar, N. R., 2010. NADPH oxidase-dependent regulation of T-type Ca^{2+} channels and ryanodine receptors mediate the augmented exocytosis of catecholamines from intermittent hypoxia-treated neonatal rat chromaffin cells. *J Neurosci*, 30, 10763–10772.

126. Novara, M., Baldelli, P., Cavallari, D., Carabelli, V., Giancippoli, A., and Carbone, E., 2004. Exposure to cAMP and beta-adrenergic stimulation recruits Ca(V)3 T-type channels in rat chromaffin cells through Epac cAMP-receptor proteins. *J Physiol*, 558, 433–449.

127. Giancippoli, A., Novara, M., de Luca, A. et al., 2006. Low-threshold exocytosis induced by cAMP-recruited CaV3.2 (alpha1H) channels in rat chromaffin cells. *Biophys J*, 90, 1830–1841.

128. Schrier, A. D., Wang, H., Talley, E. M., Perez-Reyes, E., and Barrett, P. Q., 2001. alpha1H T-type Ca^{2+} channel is the predominant subtype expressed in bovine and rat zona glomerulosa. *Am J Physiol Cell Physiol*, 280, C265–C272.

129. Albillos, A., Garcia, A. G., and Gandia, L., 1993. Omega-Agatoxin-IVA-sensitive calcium channels in bovine chromaffin cells. *FEBS Lett*, 336, 259–262.

130. Artalejo, C. R., Mogul, D. J., Perlman, R. L., and Fox, A. P., 1991. Three types of bovine chromaffin cell Ca²⁺ channels: Facilitation increases the opening probability of a 27 pS channel. *J Physiol*, 444, 213–240.

131. Bossu, J. L., De Waard, M., and Feltz, A., 1991. Two types of calcium channels are expressed in adult bovine chromaffin cells. *J Physiol*, 437, 621–634.

132. Bossu, J. L., De Waard, M., and Feltz, A., 1991. Inactivation characteristics reveal two calcium currents in adult bovine chromaffin cells. *J Physiol*, 437, 603–620.

133. Gandia, L., Albillos, A., and Garcia, A. G., 1993. Bovine chromaffin cells possess FTX-sensitive calcium channels. *Biochem Biophys Res Commun*, 194, 671–676.

134. Prakriya, M. and Lingle, C. J., 1999. BK channel activation by brief depolarizations requires Ca²⁺ influx through L- and Q-type Ca²⁺ channels in rat chromaffin cells. *J Neurophysiol*, 81, 2267–2278.

135. Hernandez-Guijo, J. M., de Pascual, R., Garcia, A. G., and Gandia, L., 1998. Separation of calcium channel current components in mouse chromaffin cells superfused with low- and high-barium solutions. *Pflugers Arch*, 436, 75–82.

136. Kitamura, N., Ohta, T., Ito, S., and Nakazato, Y., 1997. Calcium channel subtypes in porcine adrenal chromaffin cells. *Pflugers Arch*, 434, 179–187.

137. Albillos, A., Artalejo, A. R., López, M. G., Gandía, L., García, A. G., and Carbone, E., 1994. Calcium channel subtypes in cat chromaffin cells. *J Physiol*, 477, 197–213.

138. Gandia, L., Mayorgas, I., Michelena, P. et al., 1998. Human adrenal chromaffin cell calcium channels: Drastic current facilitation in cell clusters, but not in isolated cells. *Pflugers Arch*, 436, 696–704.

139. Baldelli, P., Hernandez-Guijo, J. M., Carabelli, V. et al., 2004. Direct and remote modulation of L-channels in chromaffin cells: Distinct actions on alpha1C and alpha1D subunits? *Mol Neurobiol*, 29, 73–96.

140. Lopez, M. G., Villarroya, M., Lara, B. et al., 1994. Q- and L-type Ca²⁺ channels dominate the control of secretion in bovine chromaffin cells. *FEBS Lett*, 349, 331–337.

141. Artalejo, C. R., Adams, M. E., and Fox, A. P., 1994. Three types of Ca²⁺ channel trigger secretion with different efficacies in chromaffin cells. *Nature*, 367, 72–76.

142. Albillos, A., Garcia, A. G., Olivera, B., and Gandia, L., 1996. Re-evaluation of the P/Q Ca²⁺ channel components of Ba²⁺ currents in bovine chromaffin cells superfused with solutions containing low and high Ba²⁺ concentrations. *Pflugers Arch*, 432, 1030–1038.

143. Sather, W. A., Tanabe, T., Zhang, J. F., Mori, Y., Adams, M. E., and Tsien, R. W., 1993. Distinctive biophysical and pharmacological properties of class A (BI) calcium channel alpha 1 subunits. *Neuron*, 11, 291–303.

144. McDonough, S. I., Swartz, K. J., Mintz, I. M., Boland, L. M., and Bean, B. P., 1996. Inhibition of calcium channels in rat central and peripheral neurons by omega-conotoxin MVIIC. *J Neurosci*, 16, 2612–2623.

145. Aldea, M., Jun, K., Shin, H. S. et al., 2002. A perforated patch-clamp study of calcium currents and exocytosis in chromaffin cells of wild-type and alpha(1A) knockout mice. *J Neurochem*, 81, 911–921.

146. Artalejo, C. R., Dahmer, M. K., Perlman, R. L., and Fox, A. P., 1991. Two types of Ca²⁺ currents are found in bovine chromaffin cells: Facilitation is due to the recruitment of one type. *J Physiol*, 432, 681–707.

147. Lukyanetz, E. A. and Neher, E., 1999. Different types of calcium channels and secretion from bovine chromaffin cells. *Eur J Neurosci*, 11, 2865–2873.

148. Ulate, G., Scott, S. R., Gonzalez, J., Gilabert, J. A., and Artalejo, A. R., 2000. Extracellular ATP regulates exocytosis in inhibiting multiple Ca(2+) channel types in bovine chromaffin cells. *Pflugers Arch*, 439, 304–314.

149. Albillos, A., Neher, E., and Moser, T., 2000. R-Type Ca²⁺ channels are coupled to the rapid component of secretion in mouse adrenal slice chromaffin cells. *J Neurosci*, 20, 8323–8330.

150. Villarroya, M., Olivares, R., Ruiz, A. et al., 1999. Voltage inactivation of Ca²⁺ entry and secretion associated with N- and P/Q-type but not L-type Ca²⁺ channels of bovine chromaffin cells. *J Physiol*, 516(Pt 2), 421–432.

151. Hernández-Guijo, J. M., Maneu-Flores, V. E., Ruiz-Nuno, A., Villarroya, M., García, A. G., and Gandía, L., 2001. Calcium-dependent inhibition of L, N, and P/Q Ca²⁺ channels in chromaffin cells: Role of mitochondria. *J Neurosci*, 21, 2553–2560.

152. Garcia, A. G., Garcia-De-Diego, A. M., Gandia, L., Borges, R., and Garcia-Sancho, J., 2006. Calcium signaling and exocytosis in adrenal chromaffin cells. *Physiol Rev*, 86, 1093–1131.

153. Felix, R., 2005. Molecular regulation of voltage-gated Ca²⁺ channels. *J Recept Signal Transduct Res*, 25, 57–71.

154. Doering, C. J., Kisilevsky, A. E., Feng, Z. P. et al., 2004. A single Gbeta subunit locus controls cross-talk between protein kinase C and G protein regulation of N-type calcium channels. *J Biol Chem*, 279, 29709–29717.

155. Christel, C. and Lee, A., 2012. Ca^{2+}-dependent modulation of voltage-gated Ca^{2+} channels. *Biochim Biophys Acta*, 1820, 1243–1252.

156. Budde, T., Meuth, S., and Pape, H. C., 2002. Calcium-dependent inactivation of neuronal calcium channels. *Nat Rev Neurosci*, 3, 873–883.

157. Bahler, M. and Rhoads, A., 2002. Calmodulin signaling via the IQ motif. *FEBS Lett*, 513, 107–113.

158. Lee, A., Zhou, H., Scheuer, T., and Catterall, W. A., 2003. Molecular determinants of $Ca(2+)$/calmodulin-dependent regulation of $Ca(v)2.1$ channels. *Proc Natl Acad Sci USA*, 100, 16059–16064.

159. Peterson, B. Z., DeMaria, C. D., Adelman, J. P., and Yue, D. T., 1999. Calmodulin is the Ca^{2+} sensor for Ca^{2+}-dependent inactivation of L-type calcium channels. *Neuron*, 22, 549–558.

160. Qin, N., Olcese, R., Bransby, M., Lin, T., and Birnbaumer, L., 1999. Ca^{2+}-induced inhibition of the cardiac Ca^{2+} channel depends on calmodulin. *Proc Natl Acad Sci USA*, 96, 2435–2438.

161. Lee, A., Wong, S. T., Gallagher, D. et al., 1999. Ca^{2+}/calmodulin binds to and modulates P/Q-type calcium channels. *Nature*, 399, 155–159.

162. DeMaria, C. D., Soong, T. W., Alseikhan, B. A., Alvania, R. S., and Yue, D. T., 2001. Calmodulin bifurcates the local Ca^{2+} signal that modulates P/Q-type Ca^{2+} channels. *Nature*, 411, 484–489.

163. Welsby, P. J., Wang, H., Wolfe, J. T., Colbran, R. J., Johnson, M. L., and Barrett, P. Q., 2003. A mechanism for the direct regulation of T-type calcium channels by Ca^{2+}/calmodulin-dependent kinase II. *J Neurosci*, 23, 10116–10121.

164. Wolfe, J. T., Wang, H., Perez-Reyes, E., and Barrett, P. Q., 2002. Stimulation of recombinant $Ca(v)3.2$, T-type, $Ca(2+)$ channel currents by CaMKIIgamma(C). *J Physiol*, 538, 343–355.

165. Dunlap, K. and Fischbach, G. D., 1978. Neurotransmitters decrease the calcium component of sensory neurone action potentials. *Nature*, 276, 837–839.

166. Dunlap, K. and Fischbach, G. D., 1981. Neurotransmitters decrease the calcium conductance activated by depolarization of embryonic chick sensory neurones. *J Physiol*, 317, 519–535.

167. Galvan, M. and Adams, P. R., 1982. Control of calcium current in rat sympathetic neurons by norepinephrine. *Brain Res*, 244, 135–144.

168. Deisz, R. A. and Lux, H. D., 1985. Gamma-aminobutyric acid-induced depression of calcium currents of chick sensory neurons. *Neurosci Lett*, 56, 205–210.

169. Hille, B., 1992. G protein-coupled mechanisms and nervous signaling. *Neuron*, 9, 187–195.

170. Dolphin, A. C., 1996. Facilitation of Ca^{2+} current in excitable cells. *Trends Neurosci*, 19, 35–43.

171. Carbone, E. and García, A. G., 1997. More on calcium currents. *Trends Neurosci*, 20, 448–450.

172. Garcia, A. G. and Carbone, E., 1996. Calcium-current facilitation in chromaffin cells. *Trends Neurosci*, 19, 383–385.

173. Lewis, D. L., Weight, F. F., and Luini, A., 1986. A guanine nucleotide-binding protein mediates the inhibition of voltage-dependent calcium current by somatostatin in a pituitary cell line. *Proc Natl Acad Sci USA*, 83, 9035–9039.

174. Holz, G. G., 4th., Rane, S. G., and Dunlap, K., 1986. GTP-binding proteins mediate transmitter inhibition of voltage-dependent calcium channels. *Nature*, 319, 670–672.

175. Hescheler, J., Rosenthal, W., Trautwein, W., and Schultz, G., 1987. The GTP-binding protein, Go, regulates neuronal calcium channels. *Nature*, 325, 445–447.

176. Ikeda, S. R., 1991. Double-pulse calcium channel current facilitation in adult rat sympathetic neurones. *J Physiol*, 439, 181–214.

177. Wanke, E., Ferroni, A., Malgaroli, A., Ambrosini, A., Pozzan, T., and Meldolesi, J., 1987. Activation of a muscarinic receptor selectively inhibits a rapidly inactivated Ca^{2+} current in rat sympathetic neurons. *Proc Natl Acad Sci USA*, 84, 4313–4317.

178. Marchetti, C., Carbone, E., and Lux, H. D., 1986. Effects of dopamine and noradrenaline on Ca channels of cultured sensory and sympathetic neurons of chick. *Pflugers Arch*, 406, 104–111.

179. Fenwick, E. M., Marty, A., and Neher, E., 1982. Sodium and calcium channels in bovine chromaffin cells. *J Physiol*, 331, 599–635.

180. Bean, B. P., 1989. Neurotransmitter inhibition of neuronal calcium currents by changes in channel voltage dependence. *Nature*, 340, 153–156.

181. Aicardi, G., Pollo, A., Sher, E., and Carbone, E., 1991. Noradrenergic inhibition and voltage-dependent facilitation of omega-conotoxin-sensitive Ca channels in insulin-secreting RINm5F cells. *FEBS Lett*, 281, 201–204.

182. Boland, L. M. and Bean, B. P., 1993. Modulation of N-type calcium channels in bullfrog sympathetic neurons by luteinizing hormone-releasing hormone: Kinetics and voltage dependence. *J Neurosci*, 13, 516–533.

183. Cox, D. H. and Dunlap, K., 1992. Pharmacological discrimination of N-type from L-type calcium current and its selective modulation by transmitters. *J Neurosci*, 12, 906–914.

184. Lipscombe, D., Kongsamut, S., and Tsien, R. W., 1989. Alpha-adrenergic inhibition of sympathetic neurotransmitter release mediated by modulation of N-type calcium-channel gating. *Nature*, 340, 639–642.

185. Pollo, A., Lovallo, M., Sher, E., and Carbone, E., 1992. Voltage-dependent noradrenergic modulation of omega-conotoxin-sensitive Ca^{2+} channels in human neuroblastoma IMR32 cells. *Pflugers Arch*, 422, 75–83.

186. Zamponi, G. W. and Currie, K. P., 2012. Regulation of Ca(V)2 calcium channels by G protein coupled receptors. *Biochim Biophys Acta*, 1828, 1629–1643.

187. Mehrke, G., Pereverzev, A., Grabsch, H., Hescheler, J., and Schneider, T., 1997. Receptor-mediated modulation of recombinant neuronal class E calcium channels. *FEBS Lett*, 408, 261–270.

188. Ottolia, M., Platano, D., Qin, N. et al., 1998. Functional coupling between human E-type Ca^{2+} channels and mu opioid receptors expressed in Xenopus oocytes. *FEBS Lett*, 427, 96–102.

189. Luebke, J. I. and Dunlap, K., 1994. Sensory neuron N-type calcium currents are inhibited by both voltage-dependent and -independent mechanisms. *Pflugers Arch*, 428, 499–507.

190. Swartz, K. J., 1993. Modulation of Ca^{2+} channels by protein kinase C in rat central and peripheral neurons: Disruption of G protein-mediated inhibition. *Neuron*, 11, 305–320.

191. Albillos, A., Gandia, L., Michelena, P. et al., 1996. The mechanism of calcium channel facilitation in bovine chromaffin cells. *J Physiol*, 494(Pt 3), 687–695.

192. Pollo, A., Lovallo, M., Biancardi, E., Sher, E., Socci, C., and Carbone, E., 1993. Sensitivity to dihydropyridines, omega-conotoxin and noradrenaline reveals multiple high-voltage-activated Ca^{2+} channels in rat insulinoma and human pancreatic beta-cells. *Pflugers Arch*, 423, 462–471.

193. Amico, C., Marchetti, C., Nobile, M., and Usai, C., 1995. Pharmacological types of calcium channels and their modulation by baclofen in cerebellar granules. *J Neurosci*, 15, 2839–2848.

194. Bley, K. R. and Tsien, R. W., 1990. Inhibition of Ca^{2+} and K^+ channels in sympathetic neurons by neuropeptides and other ganglionic transmitters. *Neuron*, 4, 379–391.

195. Suszkiw, J. B., Murawsky, M. M., and Fortner, R. C., 1987. Heterogeneity of presynaptic calcium channels revealed by species differences in the sensitivity of synaptosomal 45Ca entry to omega-conotoxin. *Biochem Biophys Res Commun*, 145, 1283–1286.

196. Vickroy, T. W., Schneider, C. J., and Hildreth, J. M., 1992. Pharmacological heterogeneity among calcium channels that subserve acetylcholine release in vertebrate forebrain. *Neuropharmacology*, 31, 307–309.

197. Hofmann, F. and Habermann, E., 1990. Role of omega-conotoxin-sensitive calcium channels in inositolphosphate production and noradrenaline release due to potassium depolarization or stimulation with carbachol. *Naunyn Schmiedebergs Arch Pharmacol*, 341, 200–205.

198. Turner, T. J., Adams, M. E., and Dunlap, K., 1993. Multiple Ca^{2+} channel types coexist to regulate synaptosomal neurotransmitter release. *Proc Natl Acad Sci USA*, 90, 9518–9522.

199. Turner, T. J. and Dunlap, K., 1995. Pharmacological characterization of presynaptic calcium channels using subsecond biochemical measurements of synaptosomal neurosecretion. *Neuropharmacology*, 34, 1469–1478.

200. Tanaka, Y. and Ando, S., 2001. Age-related changes in the subtypes of voltage-dependent calcium channels in rat brain cortical synapses. *Neurosci Res*, 39, 213–220.

201. Herdon, H. and Nahorski, S. R., 1989. Investigations of the roles of dihydropyridine and omega-conotoxin-sensitive calcium channels in mediating depolarisation-evoked endogenous dopamine release from striatal slices. *Naunyn Schmiedebergs Arch Pharmacol*, 340, 36–40.

202. Phillips, P. E. and Stamford, J. A., 2000. Differential recruitment of N-, P- and Q-type voltage-operated calcium channels in striatal dopamine release evoked by 'regular' and 'burst' firing. *Brain Res*, 884, 139–146.

203. Dooley, D. J., Lupp, A., and Hertting, G., 1987. Inhibition of central neurotransmitter release by omega-conotoxin GVIA, a peptide modulator of the N-type voltage-sensitive calcium channel. *Naunyn Schmiedebergs Arch Pharmacol*, 336, 467–470.

204. Luebke, J. I., Dunlap, K., and Turner, T. J., 1993. Multiple calcium channel types control glutamatergic synaptic transmission in the hippocampus. *Neuron*, 11, 895–902.

205. Takahashi, T. and Momiyama, A., 1993. Different types of calcium channels mediate central synaptic transmission. *Nature*, 366, 156–158.

206. Simmons, M. L., Terman, G. W., Gibbs, S. M., and Chavkin, C., 1995. L-type calcium channels mediate dynorphin neuropeptide release from dendrites but not axons of hippocampal granule cells. *Neuron*, 14, 1265–1272.

207. Momiyama, A. and Takahashi, T., 1994. Calcium channels responsible for potassium-induced transmitter release at rat cerebellar synapses. *J Physiol*, 476, 197–202.

208. Wang, X., Treistman, S. N., and Lemos, J. R., 1992. Two types of high-threshold calcium currents inhibited by omega-conotoxin in nerve terminals of rat neurohypophysis. *J Physiol*, 445, 181–199.

209. Lemos, J. R., Ortiz-Miranda, S. I., Cuadra, A. E. et al., 2012. Modulation/physiology of calcium channel sub-types in neurosecretory terminals. *Cell Calcium*, 51, 284–292.

210. Wang, G., Dayanithi, G., Kim, S. et al., 1997. Role of Q-type Ca^{2+} channels in vasopressin secretion from neurohypophysial terminals of the rat. *J Physiol*, 502(Pt 2), 351–363.

211. Tobin, V. A., Douglas, A. J., Leng, G., and Ludwig, M., 2011. The involvement of voltage-operated calcium channels in somato-dendritic oxytocin release. *PLoS One*, 6, e25366.

212. Hirning, L. D., Fox, A. P., McCleskey, E. W. et al., 1988. Dominant role of N-type Ca^{2+} channels in evoked release of norepinephrine from sympathetic neurons. *Science*, 239, 57–61.

213. Przywara, D. A., Bhave, S. V., Chowdhury, P. S., Wakade, T. D., and Wakade, A. R., 1993. Sites of transmitter release and relation to intracellular Ca^{2+} in cultured sympathetic neurons. *Neuroscience*, 52, 973–986.

214. Rittenhouse, A. R. and Zigmond, R. E., 1991. Omega-conotoxin inhibits the acute activation of tyrosine hydroxylase and the stimulation of norepinephrine release by potassium depolarization of sympathetic nerve endings. *J Neurochem*, 56, 615–622.

215. Uhrenholt, T. R. and Nedergaard, O. A., 2005. Involvement of different calcium channels in the depolarization-evoked release of noradrenaline from sympathetic neurones in rabbit carotid artery. *Basic Clin Pharmacol Toxicol*, 97, 109–114.

216. Taschenberger, H. and Grantyn, R., 1995. Several types of Ca^{2+} channels mediate glutamatergic synaptic responses to activation of single Thy-1-immunolabeled rat retinal ganglion neurons. *J Neurosci*, 15, 2240–2254.

217. Tamura, N., Yokotani, K., Okuma, Y., Okada, M., Ueno, H., and Osumi, Y., 1995. Properties of the voltage-gated calcium channels mediating dopamine and acetylcholine release from the isolated rat retina. *Brain Res*, 676, 363–370.

218. Lundy, P. M. and Frew, R., 1988. Evidence of omega-conotoxin GV1A-sensitive Ca^{2+} channels in mammalian peripheral nerve terminals. *Eur J Pharmacol*, 156, 325–330.

219. Lundy, P. M. and Frew, R., 1994. Effect of omega-agatoxin-IVA on autonomic neurotransmission. *Eur J Pharmacol*, 261, 79–84.

220. Maggi, C. A., Patacchini, R., Santicioli, P. et al., 1988. The effect of omega conotoxin GVIA, a peptide modulator of the N-type voltage sensitive calcium channels, on motor responses produced by activation of efferent and sensory nerves in mammalian smooth muscle. *Naunyn Schmiedebergs Arch Pharmacol*, 338, 107–113.

221. Frew, R. and Lundy, P. M., 1995. A role for Q type Ca^{2+} channels in neurotransmission in the rat urinary bladder. *Br J Pharmacol*, 116, 1595–1598.

222. Waterman, S. A., 1996. Multiple subtypes of voltage-gated calcium channel mediate transmitter release from parasympathetic neurons in the mouse bladder. *J Neurosci*, 16, 4155–4161.

223. Zygmunt, P. M., Zygmunt, P. K., Hogestatt, E. D., and Andersson, K. E., 1993. Effects of omega-conotoxin on adrenergic, cholinergic and NANC neurotransmission in the rabbit urethra and detrusor. *Br J Pharmacol*, 110, 1285–1290.

224. Wright, C. E. and Angus, J. A., 1996. Effects of N-, P- and Q-type neuronal calcium channel antagonists on mammalian peripheral neurotransmission. *Br J Pharmacol*, 119, 49–56.

225. Hata, F., Fujita, A., Saeki, K., Kishi, I., Takeuchi, T., and Yagasaki, O., 1992. Selective inhibitory effects of calcium channel antagonists on the two components of the neurogenic response of guinea pig vas deferens. *J Pharmacol Exp Ther*, 263, 214–220.

226. Hirata, H., Albillos, A., Fernandez, F., Medrano, J., Jurkiewicz, A., and Garcia, A. G., 1997. Omega-conotoxins block neurotransmission in the rat vas deferens by binding to different presynaptic sites on the N-type Ca^{2+} channel. *Eur J Pharmacol*, 321, 217–223.

227. Hong, S. J. and Chang, C. C., 1995. Inhibition of acetylcholine release from mouse motor nerve by a P-type calcium channel blocker, omega-agatoxin IVA. *J Physiol*, 482(Pt 2), 283–290.

228. Gandia, L., Lopez, M. G., Fonteriz, R. I., Artalejo, C. R., and Garcia, A. G., 1987. Relative sensitivities of chromaffin cell calcium channels to organic and inorganic calcium antagonists. *Neurosci Lett*, 77, 333–338.

229. Cardenas, A. M., Montiel, C., Esteban, C., Borges, R., and Garcia, A. G., 1988. Secretion from adrenaline- and noradrenaline-storing adrenomedullary cells is regulated by a common dihydropyridine-sensitive calcium channel. *Brain Res*, 456, 364–366.

230. Lopez, M. G., Albillos, A., de la Fuente, M. T. et al., 1994. Localized L-type calcium channels control exocytosis in cat chromaffin cells. *Pflugers Arch*, 427, 348–354.

231. García, A. G., Sala, F., Reig, J. A. et al., 1984. Dihydropyridine BAY-K-8644 activates chromaffin cell calcium channels. *Nature*, 309, 69–71.

232. Ceña, V., Nicolás, G. P., Sánchez-García, P., Kirpekar, S. M., and García, A. G., 1983. Pharmacological dissection of receptor-associated and voltage-sensitive ionic channels involved in catecholamine release. *Neuroscience*, 10, 1455–1462.

233. Gandia, L., Michelena, P., de Pascual, R., Lopez, M. G., and Garcia, A. G., 1990. Different sensitivities to dihydropyridines of catecholamine release from cat and ox adrenals. *Neuroreport*, 1, 119–122.

234. Jimenez, R. R., Lopez, M. G., Sancho, C., Maroto, R., and Garcia, A. G., 1993. A component of the catecholamine secretory response in the bovine adrenal gland is resistant to dihydropyridines and omega-conotoxin. *Biochem Biophys Res Commun*, 191, 1278–1283.

235. Owen, P. J., Marriott, D. B., and Boarder, M. R., 1989. Evidence for a dihydropyridine-sensitive and conotoxin-insensitive release of noradrenaline and uptake of calcium in adrenal chromaffin cells. *Br J Pharmacol*, 97, 133–138.

236. Ballesta, J. J., Palmero, M., Hidalgo, M. J. et al., 1989. Separate binding and functional sites for omega-conotoxin and nitrendipine suggest two types of calcium channels in bovine chromaffin cells. *J Neurochem*, 53, 1050–1056.

237. Duarte, C. B., Rosario, L. M., Sena, C. M., and Carvalho, A. P., 1993. A toxin fraction (FTX) from the funnel-web spider poison inhibits dihydropyridine-insensitive Ca^{2+} channels coupled to catecholamine release in bovine adrenal chromaffin cells. *J Neurochem*, 60, 908–913.

238. Fernandez, J. M., Granja, R., Izaguirre, V., Gonzalez-Garcia, C., and Cena, V., 1995. Omega-conotoxin GVIA blocks nicotine-induced catecholamine secretion by blocking the nicotinic receptor-activated inward currents in bovine chromaffin cells. *Neurosci Lett*, 191, 59–62.

239. Granja, R., Fernandez-Fernandez, J. M., Izaguirre, V., Gonzalez-Garcia, C., and Cena, V., 1995. Omega-agatoxin IVA blocks nicotinic receptor channels in bovine chromaffin cells. *FEBS Lett*, 362, 15–18.

240. Baltazar, G., Ladeira, I., Carvalho, A. P., and Duarte, E. P., 1997. Two types of omega-agatoxin IVA-sensitive Ca^{2+} channels are coupled to adrenaline and noradrenaline release in bovine adrenal chromaffin cells. *Pflugers Arch*, 434, 592–598.

241. Lara, B., Gandia, L., Martinez-Sierra, R., Torres, A., and Garcia, A. G., 1998. Q-type Ca^{2+} channels are located closer to secretory sites than L-type channels: Functional evidence in chromaffin cells. *Pflugers Arch*, 435, 472–478.

242. Lomax, R. B., Michelena, P., Nunez, L., Garcia-Sancho, J., Garcia, A. G., and Montiel, C., 1997. Different contributions of L- and Q-type Ca^{2+} channels to Ca^{2+} signals and secretion in chromaffin cell subtypes. *Am J Physiol*, 272, C476–C484.

243. Engisch, K. L. and Nowycky, M. C., 1996. Calcium dependence of large dense-cored vesicle exocytosis evoked by calcium influx in bovine adrenal chromaffin cells. *J Neurosci*, 16, 1359–1369.

244. Carabelli, V., D'Ascenzo, M., Carbone, E., and Grassi, C., 2002. Nitric oxide inhibits neuroendocrine Ca(V)1 L-channel gating via cGMP-dependent protein kinase in cell-attached patches of bovine chromaffin cells. *J Physiol*, 541, 351–366.

245. Gil, A., Viniegra, S., Neco, P., and Gutierrez, L. M., 2001. Co-localization of vesicles and P/Q Ca^{2+}-channels explains the preferential distribution of exocytotic active zones in neurites emitted by bovine chromaffin cells. *Eur J Cell Biol*, 80, 358–365.

246. Lopez, M. G., Shukla, R., Garcia, A. G., and Wakade, A. R., 1992. A dihydropyridine-resistant component in the rat adrenal secretory response to splanchnic nerve stimulation. *J Neurochem*, 58, 2139–2144.

247. Santana, F., Michelena, P., Jaen, R., Garcia, A. G., and Borges, R., 1999. Calcium channel subtypes and exocytosis in chromaffin cells: A different view from the intact rat adrenal. *Naunyn Schmiedebergs Arch Pharmacol*, 360, 33–37.

248. Wakade, A. R., 1981. Studies on secretion of catecholamines evoked by acetylcholine or transmural stimulation of the rat adrenal gland. *J Physiol*, 313, 463–480.

249. Kim, S. J., Lim, W., and Kim, J., 1995. Contribution of L- and N-type calcium currents to exocytosis in rat adrenal medullary chromaffin cells. *Brain Res*, 675, 289–296.

250. Fernandez-Morales, J. C., Cortes-Gil, L., Garcia, A. G., and de Diego, A. M., 2009. Differences in the quantal release of catecholamines in chromaffin cells of rat embryos and their mothers. *Am J Physiol Cell Physiol*, 297, C407–C418.

251. Carabelli, V., Marcantoni, A., Comunanza, V. et al., 2007. Chronic hypoxia up-regulates alpha1H T-type channels and low-threshold catecholamine secretion in rat chromaffin cells. *J Physiol*, 584, 149–165.

252. Carbone, E., Giancippoli, A., Marcantoni, A., Guido, D., and Carabelli, V., 2006. A new role for T-type channels in fast "low-threshold" exocytosis. *Cell Calcium*, 40, 147–154.

253. Carbone, E. and Lux, H. D., 1984. A low voltage-activated calcium conductance in embryonic chick sensory neurons. *Biophys J*, 46, 413–418.

254. Thompson, R. J., Jackson, A., and Nurse, C. A., 1997. Developmental loss of hypoxic chemosensitivity in rat adrenomedullary chromaffin cells. *J Physiol*, 498(Pt 2), 503–510.

255. Takeuchi, Y., Mochizuki-Oda, N., Yamada, H., Kurokawa, K., and Watanabe, Y., 2001. Nonneurogenic hypoxia sensitivity in rat adrenal slices. *Biochem Biophys Res Commun*, 289, 51–56.

256. Adams, M. B., Simonetta, G., and McMillen, I. C., 1996. The non-neurogenic catecholamine response of the fetal adrenal to hypoxia is dependent on activation of voltage sensitive Ca^{2+} channels. *Brain Res Dev Brain Res*, 94, 182–189.

257. Carabelli, V., Marcantoni, A., Comunanza, V., and Carbone, E., 2007. Fast exocytosis mediated by T- and L-type channels in chromaffin cells: Distinct voltage-dependence but similar Ca^{2+}-dependence. *Eur Biophys J*, 36, 753–762.

258. Comunanza, V., Marcantoni, A., Vandael, D. H. et al., 2010. CaV1.3 as pacemaker channels in adrenal chromaffin cells: Specific role on exo- and endocytosis? *Channels (Austin)*, 4, 440–446.

259. Waterman, S. R. and Small, P. L., 1996. Characterization of the acid resistance phenotype and rpoS alleles of shiga-like toxin-producing *Escherichia coli*. *Infect Immun*, 64, 2808–2811.

260. Dunlap, K., Luebke, J. I., and Turner, T. J., 1995. Exocytotic Ca^{2+} channels in mammalian central neurons. *Trends Neurosci*, 18, 89–98.

261. O'Farrell, M., Ziogas, J., and Marley, P. D., 1997. Effects of N- and L-type calcium channel antagonists and (+/-)-Bay K8644 on nerve-induced catecholamine secretion from bovine perfused adrenal glands. *Br J Pharmacol*, 121, 381–388.

262. Kidokoro, Y. and Ritchie, A. K., 1980. Chromaffin cell action potentials and their possible role in adrenaline secretion from rat adrenal medulla. *J Physiol*, 307, 199–216.

263. Fenwick, E. M., Marty, A., and Neher, E., 1982. A patch-clamp study of bovine chromaffin cells and of their sensitivity to acetylcholine. *J Physiol*, 331, 577–597.

264. Brandt, B. L., Hagiwara, S., Kidokoro, Y., and Miyazaki, S., 1976. Action potentials in the rat chromaffin cell and effects of acetylcholine. *J Physiol*, 263, 417–439.

265. Douglas, W. W., Kanno, T., and Sampson, S. R., 1967. Effects of acetylcholine and other medullary secretagogues and antagonists on the membrane potential of adrenal chromaffin cells: An analysis employing techniques of tissue culture. *J Physiol*, 188, 107–120.

266. Kidokoro, Y., Miyazaki, S., and Ozawa, S., 1982. Acetylcholine-induced membrane depolarization and potential fluctuations in the rat adrenal chromaffin cell. *J Physiol*, 324, 203–220.

267. Artalejo, A. R., Garcia, A. G., and Neher, E., 1993. Small-conductance Ca(2+)-activated K^+ channels in bovine chromaffin cells. *Pflugers Arch*, 423, 97–103.

268. Uceda, G., Artalejo, A. R., de la Fuente, M. T. et al., 1994. Modulation by L-type Ca^{2+} channels and apamin-sensitive K^+ channels of muscarinic responses in cat chromaffin cells. *Am J Physiol*, 266, C1432–C1439.

269. Michelena, P., Vega, T., Montiel, C. et al., 1995. Effects of tyramine and calcium on the kinetics of secretion in intact and electroporated chromaffin cells superfused at high speed. *Pflügers Arch*, 431, 283–296.

270. Neher, E. and Zucker, R. S., 1993. Multiple calcium-dependent processes related to secretion in bovine chromaffin cells. *Neuron*, 10, 21–30.

271. von Gersdorff, H. and Matthews, G., 1994. Inhibition of endocytosis by elevated internal calcium in a synaptic terminal. *Nature*, 370, 652–655.

272. Wang, C. and Zucker, R. S., 1998. Regulation of synaptic vesicle recycling by calcium and serotonin. *Neuron*, 21, 155–167.

273. Nucifora, P. G. and Fox, A. P., 1998. Barium triggers rapid endocytosis in calf adrenal chromaffin cells. *J Physiol*, 508(Pt 2), 483–494.

274. Artalejo, C. R., Henley, J. R., McNiven, M. A., and Palfrey, H. C., 1995. Rapid endocytosis coupled to exocytosis in adrenal chromaffin cells involves Ca^{2+}, GTP, and dynamin but not clathrin. *Proc Natl Acad Sci USA*, 92, 8328–8332.

275. Nucifora, P. G. and Fox, A. P., 1999. Tyrosine phosphorylation regulates rapid endocytosis in adrenal chromaffin cells. *J Neurosci*, 19, 9739–9746.

276. Ryan, T. A., Smith, S. J., and Reuter, H., 1996. The timing of synaptic vesicle endocytosis. *Proc Natl Acad Sci USA*, 93, 5567–5571.

277. Wu, L. G. and Betz, W. J., 1996. Nerve activity but not intracellular calcium determines the time course of endocytosis at the frog neuromuscular junction. *Neuron*, 17, 769–779.

278. Rouze, N. C. and Schwartz, E. A., 1998. Continuous and transient vesicle cycling at a ribbon synapse. *J Neurosci*, 18, 8614–8624.

279. de Diego, A. M., Arnaiz-Cot, J. J., Hernandez-Guijo, J. M., Gandia, L., and Garcia, A. G., 2008. Differential variations in Ca^{2+} entry, cytosolic Ca^{2+} and membrane capacitance upon steady or action potential depolarizing stimulation of bovine chromaffin cells. *Acta Physiol (Oxf)*, 194, 97–109.

280. Rosa, J. M., Torregrosa-Hetland, C. J., Colmena, I., Gutierrez, L. M., Garcia, A. G., and Gandia, L., 2011. Calcium entry through slow-inactivating L-type calcium channels preferentially triggers endocytosis rather than exocytosis, in bovine chromaffin cells. *Am J Physiol Cell Physiol*, 301, C86–C98.

281. Perissinotti, P. P., Giugovaz Tropper, B., and Uchitel, O. D., 2008. L-type calcium channels are involved in fast endocytosis at the mouse neuromuscular junction. *Eur J Neurosci*, 27, 1333–1344.

282. Kuromi, H., Ueno, K., and Kidokoro, Y., 2010. Two types of Ca^{2+} channel linked to two endocytic pathways coordinately maintain synaptic transmission at the Drosophila synapse. *Eur J Neurosci*, 32, 335–346.

283. Chen, Y., Deng, L., Maeno-Hikichi, Y. et al., 2003. Formation of an endophilin-Ca^{2+} channel complex is critical for clathrin-mediated synaptic vesicle endocytosis. *Cell*, 115, 37–48.

284. Smith, C. B. and Betz, W. J., 1996. Simultaneous independent measurement of endocytosis and exocytosis. *Nature*, 380, 531–534.

285. Lagnado, L., Gomis, A., and Job, C., 1996. Continuous vesicle cycling in the synaptic terminal of retinal bipolar cells. *Neuron*, 17, 957–967.

286. Bay, A. E., Belingheri, A. V., Alvarez, Y. D., and Marengo, F. D., 2012. Membrane cycling after the excess retrieval mode of rapid endocytosis in mouse chromaffin cells. *Acta Physiol (Oxf)*, 204, 403–418.

287. Giovannucci, D. R., Hlubek, M. D., and Stuenkel, E. L., 1999. Mitochondria regulate the Ca(2+)-exocytosis relationship of bovine adrenal chromaffin cells. *J Neurosci*, 19, 9261–9270.

288. Low, J. T., Shukla, A., Behrendorff, N., and Thorn, P., 2010. Exocytosis, dependent on Ca^{2+} release from Ca^{2+} stores, is regulated by Ca^{2+} microdomains. *J Cell Sci*, 123, 3201–3208.

289. Alonso, M. T., Barrero, M. J., Michelena, P. et al., 1999. Ca^{2+}-induced Ca^{2+} release in chromaffin cells seen from inside the ER with targeted aequorin. *J Cell Biol*, 144, 241–254.

290. DeStefino, N. R., Pilato, A. A., Dittrich, M. et al., 2010. (R)-roscovitine prolongs the mean open time of unitary N-type calcium channel currents. *Neuroscience*, 167, 838–849.

291. Sevilla, P., Bruix, M., Santoro, J., Gago, F., Garcia, A. G., and Rico, M., 1993. Three-dimensional structure of omega-conotoxin GVIA determined by 1H NMR. *Biochem Biophys Res Commun*, 192, 1238–1244.

292. Davis, J. H., Bradley, E. K., Miljanich, G. P., Nadasdi, L., Ramachandran, J., and Basus, V. J., 1993. Solution structure of omega-conotoxin GVIA using 2-D NMR spectroscopy and relaxation matrix analysis. *Biochemistry*, 32, 7396–7405.

293. Pallaghy, P. K., Duggan, B. M., Pennington, M. W., and Norton, R. S., 1993. Three-dimensional structure in solution of the calcium channel blocker omega-conotoxin. *J Mol Biol*, 234, 405–420.

294. Skalicky, J. J., Metzler, W. J., Ciesla, D. J., Galdes, A., and Pardi, A., 1993. Solution structure of the calcium channel antagonist omega-conotoxin GVIA. *Protein Sci*, 2, 1591–1603.

295. Kohno, T., Kim, J. I., Kobayashi, K., Kodera, Y., Maeda, T., and Sato, K., 1995. Three-dimensional structure in solution of the calcium channel blocker omega-conotoxin MVIIA. *Biochemistry*, 34, 10256–10265.

296. Nemoto, N., Kubo, S., Yoshida, T. et al., 1995. Solution structure of omega-conotoxin MVIIC determined by NMR. *Biochem Biophys Res Commun*, 207, 695–700.

297. Farr-Jones, S., Miljanich, G. P., Nadasdi, L., Ramachandran, J., and Basus, V. J., 1995. Solution structure of omega-conotoxin MVIIC, a high affinity ligand of P-type calcium channels, using 1H NMR spectroscopy and complete relaxation matrix analysis. *J Mol Biol*, 248, 106–124.

298. Nielsen, K. J., Schroeder, T., and Lewis, R., 2000. Structure-activity relationships of omega-conotoxins at N-type voltage-sensitive calcium channels. *J Mol Recognit*, 13, 55–70.

299. Hernandez-Guijo, J. M., Gandia, L., de Pascual, R., and Garcia, A. G., 1997. Differential effects of the neuroprotectant lubeluzole on bovine and mouse chromaffin cell calcium channel subtypes. *Br J Pharmacol*, 122, 275–285.

300. Grantham, C. J., Main, M. J., and Cannell, M. B., 1994. Fluspirilene block of N-type calcium current in NGF-differentiated PC12 cells. *Br J Pharmacol*, 111, 483–488.

301. Fisher, T. E. and Bourque, C. W., 2001. The function of Ca(2+) channel subtypes in exocytotic secretion: New perspectives from synaptic and non-synaptic release. *Prog Biophys Mol Biol*, 77, 269–303.

302. Hans, M., Luvisetto, S., Williams, M. E. et al., 1999. Functional consequences of mutations in the human alpha1A calcium channel subunit linked to familial hemiplegic migraine. *J Neurosci*, 19, 1610–1619.

303. Kraus, R. L., Sinnegger, M. J., Glossmann, H., Hering, S., and Striessnig, J., 1998. Familial hemiplegic migraine mutations change alpha1A Ca^{2+} channel kinetics. *J Biol Chem*, 273, 5586–5590.

304. Zhuchenko, O., Bailey, J., Bonnen, P. et al., 1997. Autosomal dominant cerebellar ataxia (SCA6) associated with small polyglutamine expansions in the alpha 1A-voltage-dependent calcium channel. *Nat Genet*, 15, 62–69.

305. Fletcher, C. F., Lutz, C. M., O'Sullivan, T. N. et al., 1996. Absence epilepsy in tottering mutant mice is associated with calcium channel defects. *Cell*, 87, 607–617.

306. Doyle, J., Ren, X., Lennon, G., and Stubbs, L., 1997. Mutations in the Cacnl1a4 calcium channel gene are associated with seizures, cerebellar degeneration, and ataxia in tottering and leaner mutant mice. *Mamm Genome*, 8, 113–120.

307. Jun, K., Piedras-Renteria, E. S., Smith, S. M. et al., 1999. Ablation of P/Q-type Ca(2+) channel currents, altered synaptic transmission, and progressive ataxia in mice lacking the alpha(1A)-subunit. *Proc Natl Acad Sci USA*, 96, 15245–15250.

308. Vincent, A., Beeson, D., and Lang, B., 2000. Molecular targets for autoimmune and genetic disorders of neuromuscular transmission. *Eur J Biochem*, 267, 6717–6728.

309. Xu, Y. F., Hewett, S. J., and Atchison, W. D., 1998. Passive transfer of Lambert-Eaton myasthenic syndrome induces dihydropyridine sensitivity of ICa in mouse motor nerve terminals. *J Neurophysiol*, 80, 1056–1069.

310. Fratantoni, S. A., Weisz, G., Pardal, A. M., Reisin, R. C., and Uchitel, O. D., 2000. Amyotrophic lateral sclerosis IgG-treated neuromuscular junctions develop sensitivity to L-type calcium channel blocker. *Muscle Nerve*, 23, 543–550.

311. Katz, E., Ferro, P. A., Weisz, G., and Uchitel, O. D., 1996. Calcium channels involved in synaptic transmission at the mature and regenerating mouse neuromuscular junction. *J Physiol*, 497(Pt 3), 687–697.

312. Santafe, M. M., Urbano, F. J., Lanuza, M. A., and Uchitel, O. D., 2000. Multiple types of calcium channels mediate transmitter release during functional recovery of botulinum toxin type A-poisoned mouse motor nerve terminals. *Neuroscience*, 95, 227–234.

313. Platzer, J., Engel, J., Schrott-Fischer, A. et al., 2000. Congenital deafness and sinoatrial node dysfunction in mice lacking class D L-type Ca^{2+} channels. *Cell*, 102, 89–97.

314. McGivern, J. G., 2006. Targeting N-type and T-type calcium channels for the treatment of pain. *Drug Discov Today*, 11, 245–253.

315. Atanassoff, P. G., Hartmannsgruber, M. W., Thrasher, J. et al., 2000. Ziconotide, a new N-type calcium channel blocker, administered intrathecally for acute postoperative pain. *Reg Anesth Pain Med*, 25, 274–278.

316. Staats, P. S., Yearwood, T., Charapata, S. G. et al., 2004. Intrathecal ziconotide in the treatment of refractory pain in patients with cancer or AIDS: A randomized controlled trial. *JAMA*, 291, 63–70.

317. Penn, R. D. and Paice, J. A., 2000. Adverse effects associated with the intrathecal administration of ziconotide. *Pain*, 85, 291–296.

318. Santicioli, P., Del Bianco, E., Tramontana, M., Geppetti, P., and Maggi, C. A., 1992. Release of calcitonin gene-related peptide like-immunoreactivity induced by electrical field stimulation from rat spinal afferents is mediated by conotoxin-sensitive calcium channels. *Neurosci Lett*, 136, 161–164.

319. Smith, M. T., Cabot, P. J., Ross, F. B., Robertson, A. D., and Lewis, R. J., 2002. The novel N-type calcium channel blocker, AM336, produces potent dose-dependent antinociception after intrathecal dosing in rats and inhibits substance P release in rat spinal cord slices. *Pain*, 96, 119–127.

320. McGivern, J. G. and McDonough, S. I., 2004. Voltage-gated calcium channels as targets for the treatment of chronic pain. *Curr Drug Targets CNS Neurol Disord*, 3, 457–478.

321. Kim, D., Park, D., Choi, S. et al., 2003. Thalamic control of visceral nociception mediated by T-type Ca^{2+} channels. *Science*, 302, 117–119.

322. Coulter, D. A., Huguenard, J. R., and Prince, D. A., 1990. Differential effects of petit mal anticonvulsants and convulsants on thalamic neurones: Calcium current reduction. *Br J Pharmacol*, 100, 800–806.

323. Dogrul, A., Gardell, L. R., Ossipov, M. H., Tulunay, F. C., Lai, J., and Porreca, F., 2003. Reversal of experimental neuropathic pain by T-type calcium channel blockers. *Pain*, 105, 159–168.

324. Marais, E., Klugbauer, N., and Hofmann, F., 2001. Calcium channel alpha(2)delta subunits-structure and Gabapentin binding. *Mol Pharmacol*, 59, 1243–1248.

325. Qin, N., Yagel, S., Momplaisir, M. L., Codd, E. E., and D'Andrea, M. R., 2002. Molecular cloning and characterization of the human voltage-gated calcium channel alpha(2)delta-4 subunit. *Mol Pharmacol*, 62, 485–496.

326. Sarantopoulos, C., McCallum, B., Kwok, W. M., and Hogan, Q., 2002. Gabapentin decreases membrane calcium currents in injured as well as in control mammalian primary afferent neurons. *Reg Anesth Pain Med*, 27, 47–57.

327. Field, M. J., Oles, R. J., Lewis, A. S., McCleary, S., Hughes, J., and Singh, L., 1997. Gabapentin (neurontin) and S-(+)-3-isobutylgaba represent a novel class of selective antihyperalgesic agents. *Br J Pharmacol*, 121, 1513–1522.

328. Christensen, D., Gautron, M., Guilbaud, G., and Kayser, V., 2001. Effect of gabapentin and lamotrigine on mechanical allodynia-like behaviour in a rat model of trigeminal neuropathic pain. *Pain*, 93, 147–153.

329. Field, M. J., Cox, P. J., Stott, E. et al., 2006. Identification of the alpha2-delta-1 subunit of voltage-dependent calcium channels as a molecular target for pain mediating the analgesic actions of pregabalin. *Proc Natl Acad Sci USA*, 103, 17537–17542.

330. Horga de la Parte, J. F. and Horga, A., 2006. Pregabalin: New therapeutic contributions of calcium channel alpha2delta protein ligands on epilepsy and neuropathic pain. *Rev Neurol*, 42, 223–237.

331. Striessnig, J. and Koschak, A., 2008. Exploring the function and pharmacotherapeutic potential of voltage-gated Ca^{2+} channels with gene knockout models. *Channels (Austin)*, 2, 233–251.

332. Mangoni, M. E., Couette, B., Bourinet, E. et al., 2003. Functional role of L-type Cav1.3 Ca^{2+} channels in cardiac pacemaker activity. *Proc Natl Acad Sci USA*, 100, 5543–5548.

333. Marcotti, W., Johnson, S. L., Rusch, A., and Kros, C. J., 2003. Sodium and calcium currents shape action potentials in immature mouse inner hair cells. *J Physiol*, 552, 743–761.

334. Olson, P. A., Tkatch, T., Hernandez-Lopez, S. et al., 2005. G-protein-coupled receptor modulation of striatal CaV1.3 L-type Ca^{2+} channels is dependent on a Shank-binding domain. *J Neurosci*, 25, 1050–1062.

335. Harvey, J., Wedley, S., Findlay, J. D., Sidell, M. R., and Pullar, I. A., 1996. Omega-Agatoxin IVA identifies a single calcium channel subtype which contributes to the potassium-induced release of acetylcholine, 5-hydroxytryptamine, dopamine, gamma-aminobutyric acid and glutamate from rat brain slices. *Neuropharmacology*, 35, 385–392.

336. Kimura, T., Takeuchi, A., and Satoh, S., 1994. Inhibition by omega-conotoxin GVIA of adrenal catecholamine release in response to endogenous and exogenous acetylcholine. *Eur J Pharmacol*, 264, 169–175.

337. Haass, M., Richardt, G., Brenn, T., Schomig, E., and Schomig, A., 1991. Nicotine-induced release of noradrenaline and neuropeptide Y in guinea-pig heart: Role of calcium channels and protein kinase C. *Naunyn Schmiedebergs Arch Pharmacol*, 344, 527–531.

338. Hong, S. J. and Chang, C. C., 1995. Calcium channel subtypes for the sympathetic and parasympathetic nerves of guinea-pig atria. *Br J Pharmacol*, 116, 1577–1582.

Part VII

Toxins as Drugs

40

Marine Compounds as a Starting Point to Drugs

Juan A. Rubiolo, Eva Alonso, and Eva Cagide

CONTENTS

40.1 Introduction

In the drug development history, several bioactive compounds have been obtained from natural sources. One of the most famous and well-known discoveries was penicillin by Dr Fleming in 1929. Since then, there have been several examples of drugs derived from natural products reaching the pharmaceutical market (e.g., morphine, digitalis glycosides, etc.). It was not until about 40 years ago when the seabed was first explored as a natural drug source for several and unknown bioactive compounds. Since then, various active compounds with unique structural and chemical characteristics have been discovered from corals, mollusks, echinoderms, bryozoans, and dinoflagellates,[1] which has started the "blue biotechnology" concept for use of these organisms and derivatives to develop new and attractive ingredients for humankind, such as drugs, cosmetics or nutraceutics. Oceans cover 70% of the Earth's surface, and depending on their location, temperature, salinity, etc, a great diversity of beings inhabits them, forming a much more extensive phylogenetic diversity than in the terrestrial environment. In fact, of the approximately 34 fundamental phyla, 17 occupy terrestrial habitats, whereas 32 inhabit marine biotopes. This points toward oceans as a unique and rich source for active compounds for the pharmaceutical industry, with the association of a great genetic diversity of marine organisms and a great ecological diversity, ranging from accessible beaches to extreme ocean depths.

Most of the compounds that have attracted the interest of the pharmaceutical industry till now are those that have antimicrobial, antitumoral, anti-inflammatory, and immunosuppressive activity. It was estimated that in 2008 there would be around 20,000 marine compounds purified and identified from different sea species all over the world.[2] Of these, up to 2012, only seven have been approved by the Food and Drug Administration (FDA), four for cancer treatment, one for pain treatment, one as an antiviral drug, and one for hyperglyceridemia.[3]

The problem with marine compounds in most cases is associated with the limited source origin and complex chemical structures, which make them difficult to synthesize. Sampling in extreme environments, studying the genetics of the organisms, compound isolation, and structure elucidation are problems that laboratories or industries need to tackle to reach a good flow into the final clinical market. For initial in vitro studies, use of analytical techniques such as high-performance liquid chromatography is needed to obtain purified compounds in very minute amounts, usually in the micromolar range, to allow studies on their mechanism of action or to investigate their therapeutic targets. Nuclear magnetic resonance studies allow to know the chemical structure and in some cases to synthesize a compound. But sometimes due to the complexity of the molecular skeletons of these marine compounds, it is not possible or it becomes too expensive and time-consuming to reach the goal. Advances in these purification and isolation techniques together with the chemical synthesis of several natural compounds have permitted to look deeper into their mechanism of action and search for therapeutic applications so as to avoid relying on natural sources.

In the following sections, areas of research focused on human health have been described in which great effort has been invested.

40.2 Anticancer Potential of Marine Compounds

Cancer is one of the most outstanding causes of death worldwide, causing 7.56 million deaths in 2008, and it is expected to continue rising, reaching a predicted figure of 13.08 million deaths by 2030.[4]

This severe impact has favored and improved efforts on attention and medical assistance, as well as scientific research needed to acquire new knowledge and for discovery of relevant factors that may assist to explain the biological processes, which are translated into medications, technological diagnoses, and better medical practices.

Several plant-derived metabolites are now leading drugs used in the treatment of different types of cancer and many of them are now being tested in various phases of clinical and preclinical trials. Over the past decades, discovery of metabolites with biological activities in marine organisms has also increased greatly, and marine compounds isolated from aquatic fungi, cyanobacteria, sponges, algae, and tunicates have been found to also exhibit various anticancer activities.[1] Many of these compounds display structural and chemical features not found in terrestrial natural products, and interesting mechanisms of action against cancer, including:

1. Anti-angiogenesis, which plays a critical role in the growth and spread of cancer, due to the formation of new blood vessels, which is induced by pro-angiogenic factors (angiogenin, vascular endothelial growth factor, fibroblast growth factor, etc). Anti-angiogenic compounds reduce the production of pro-angiogenic factors, prevent them to binding to their receptors, or block their actions.

2. Apoptosis induction: In tumor cells, the balance between pro-apoptotic and pro-survival signaling pathways is disrupted. Antiproliferative agents act through the induction of programmed cell death through multiple mechanisms.

3. Cell-cycle inhibition: Inhibitors of several proteins specifically designed to regulate the cell cycle, such as cyclin-dependent kinases, checkpoint kinases, and dual-specificity phosphatases.

4. Topoisomerase inhibition: Topoisomerases act on DNA by breaking one or both strands and joining them after turning. The most common mechanism of inhibition consists of acting as intercalating agents, preventing the action of the enzyme.

5. Microtubule stability: Microtubules are the main components of the cytoskeleton, which are formed by the aggregation of tubulin heterodimers; therefore, compounds acting on the tubulin system inhibit cell mitosis, preventing polymerization or depolymerization.

6. DNA alkylation: Alkylating agents that react with the DNA molecule, adding alkyl groups and causing breakage of the DNA strands or deforming the DNA molecule and, eventually, the death of the cells.

However, despite intense research effort and the possibilities shown, very few products with real potential have been identified or developed.

In the 1950s, C-nucleosides isolated from the Caribbean sponge *Cryptotheca crypta* provided the basis for the synthesis of cytarabine (Cytosar-U/Tarabine PFS). This is considered the first marine-derived anticancer agent developed for clinical use[5] and is currently used alone or with other chemotherapeutic drugs for routine treatment of patients with certain types of leukemia, including acute myeloid leukemia, acute lymphocytic leukemia, chronic myelogenous leukemia, and meningeal leukemia. It is also used sometimes for the treatment of certain types of non-Hodgkin's lymphoma. It is defined by the National Cancer Institute (NCI; http://www.cancer.gov) as an antimetabolite analog of cytidine with a modified sugar moiety (arabinose instead of ribose). Cytarabine is converted to the triphosphate form within the cell and then competes with cytidine for incorporation into DNA. Because the arabinose sugar sterically hinders the rotation of the molecule within the DNA, DNA replication ceases, specifically during the S phase of the cell cycle. This agent also inhibits DNA polymerase, resulting in a decrease in DNA replication and repair.[6]

Over the past decades, several new experimental anticancer compounds derived from marine sources have entered preclinical and clinical trials. Table 40.1 lists some of them (for a complete review, see Singh et al.[7] and Mahdi et al.[8]).

Trabectedin (ecteinascidin 743, Yondelis®) is a tetrahydroisoquinoline alkaloid originally extracted from the colonial tunicate *Ecteinascidia turbinata*, which is currently in clinical use. It binds to the minor groove of DNA, being a guanine-specific alkylating agent at the N2 position, and produces specific adducts. This results in a particular DNA bending, which affects various transcription factors involved in cell proliferation, gene transcription processes, and the DNA repair machinery, especially the transcription-coupled nucleotide excision repair machinery.[9,10] Trabectedin is a controversial agent, which was authorized by the European Union in 2007 for the treatment of advanced soft-tissue sarcoma after failure of anthracyclines and ifosfamide, or in patients who cannot be given these medicines, and in combination with pegylated liposomal doxorubicin for treatment of platinum-sensitive ovarian neoplasms. It has also been designated as an orphan drug by the European Commission for treatment of soft tissue sarcoma and ovarian cancer in 2001 and 2003, respectively.[11] Yondelis is marketed by PharmaMar and Ortho Biotech Products, L.P. (http://www.pharmamar.com/).

An analog of trabectedin, PM01183 (lurbinectedin), was recently reported to exert in vitro and in vivo antitumor effects, binding to the minor groove of DNA and slowing the growth of cancer.[12,13] It has been designated as an orphan drug in 2012 by the European Commission for the treatment of ovarian cancer, and clinical phase-II trials are ongoing, with promising preliminary results in patients with platinum-resistant/refractory ovarian cancer.[14]

Another promising drug is eribulin mesylate (E7389, ER-086526; Halaven®). This is the mesylate salt of a synthetic analog of halichondrin B, a substance derived from a marine sponge with antineoplastic activity. It binds to the vinca domain of tubulin and inhibits tubulin polymerization, resulting in the induction of cell-cycle arrest at the G2/M phase and tumor regression.[15,16] It was approved by the European Commission in 2011 for the treatment of locally advanced or metastatic breast cancer that continued to spread after at least two other treatments for advanced cancer. Previous treatment should include an anthracycline and a taxane unless these treatments are not suitable. Halaven is marketed by Eisai Inc. (http://www.eisai.com/).

The European Commission had also included plitidepsin (Aplidine, Aplidin®) as an orphan drug for the treatment of acute lymphoblastic leukemia in 2003; multiple myeloma in 2004; and post-essential thrombocythemia myelofibrosis, post-polycythemia vera myelofibrosis, and primary myelofibrosis in 2011. All of them were withdrawn in 2011, and it is currently designated an orphan drug just for treatment of multiple myeloma since it may act in a different way than other available medicines.[11] This compound is a cyclic depsipeptide isolated from the marine tunicate *Aplidium albicans*. It has been reported to display a broad spectrum of antitumor activities, which includes early release of cytochrome *c*, activation of caspase-3, apoptosis induction, as well as initiation of the Fas–CD95 pathways and the JNK pathway.[17] This agent also inhibits elongation factor 1-a, induces G1 arrest and G2 blockade, and exerts an antiangiogenic effect.[18] Despite this, its mode of action is still under research and shall be confirmed for marketing authorization.

Plitidepsin showed better results than its related compound, didemnin B, which was originally isolated from another tunicate, the Caribbean *Trididemnum solidum*. The bioactivity of this compound comprises marked antitumor, antiviral, and immunosuppressive activity in in vitro tests.[19,20] However, its complete mode of action still remains unclear. It has been reported to inhibit protein synthesis during

TABLE 40.1

Marine Compounds with Antineoplastic Activity in Preclinical and Clinical Trials

Compound	Source Organism	Molecular Target	Current Status
Ecteinascidin 743 (Yondelis)	*Ecteinascidia turbínata* (tunicate)	Tubulin	In clinical use
E7389 (Halaven, halichondrin B-inspired)	*Halichondria okadai* (sponge)	Tubulin	Phase III
Dehydrodidemnin B (Aplidine)	*Trididemnum solidum* (tunicate)	Ornithine decarboxylase	Phase II
Dolastatin 10, 15 (soblidotin, synthadotin, cemadotin, etc)	*Dolabella auricularia* (mollusk, sea hare)	Tubulin	Phase I, II
Bryostatin 1	*Bugula neritina* (bryozoan)	PKC	Phase II
Kahalalide F	*Elysia rufescens/Bryopsis* sp. (mollusk/green alga)	Lysosomes/ErbB pathway	Phase II
AE-941 (Neovastat)	*Squalus acanthias* (shark)	Angiogenesis	Phase II
Didemnin B	*Trididemnum solidum* (tunicate)	Elongation factor 2	Phase II (discontinued)
Discodermolide	*Discodermia dissoluta* (sponge)	Tubulin	Phase II (discontinued)
LBH589 (psammaplin derivative)	*Psammaplysilla* sp. (sponge)	HDAC	Phase I
Marizomib (Salinosporamide A, NPI-0052)	*Salinospora* sp. (bacterium)	20S proteasome	Phase I
HTI-286, E7974 (Hemiasterlin-inspired)	*Cymbastella* sp. (sponge)	Tubulin	Phase I
KRN7000	*Agelas mauritianus* (sponge)	Natural killer T cells	Phase I
Bengamides (LAF-389)	*Jaspis digonoxea* (sponge)	Methionine aminopeptidase	Phase I (discontinued)
ES-285 (spisulosine)	*Mactromeris polynyma* (mollusk)	Rho (GTP-bp)	Preclinical/phase I
Dictyostatin-1 (similar to discodermolide)	*Spongia* sp. (sponge)	Tubulin	Preclinical
Fijianolide B (laulimalide)	*Cacospongia mycofijiensis, Hyatella* sp. (sponge)	Tubulin	Preclinical
Spongistatin-1	*Hyrtios erecta* (sponge)	Tubulin	Preclinical
Desmethoxymajusculamide C	*Lyngbya majuscule* (cyanobacterium)	Tubulin	Preclinical
Laulimalide	*Cacospongia mycofijiensis* (sponge)	Tubulin	Preclinical
Aplyronine A	*Aplysia kurodai* (mollusk, sea hare)	Actin	Preclinical
Diazonamide	*Diazona angulata* (tunicate)	Tubulin	Preclinical
Eleutherobin	*Eleutherobia* sp./*Erythropodium caribaeorum* (soft corals)	Tubulin	Preclinical
Sarcodictyins	*Sarcodictyon roseum/Eleutherobia aurea/Bellonella albiflora* (soft corals)	Tubulin	Preclinical
Peloruside A	*Mycale hentscheli* (sponge)	Tubulin	Preclinical
Salicylihalamides	*Haliclona* sp. (sponge)	Vacuolar ATPase	Preclinical
Thiocoraline	*Micromonospora marina* (actinomycete bacteria)	DNA polymerase	Preclinical
Ascididemin	*Didemnum* sp. (sponge)	Caspase-2/mitochondria	Preclinical
Variolins	*Kirkpatrickia variolosa* (sponge)	CDK	Preclinical
Lamellarins	*Lamellaria* sp. (mollusk)	Topoisomerase I/P-glycoprotein 1	Preclinical
Dictyodendrins	*Dictyodendrilla verongiformis* (sponge)	Telomerase	Preclinical
Lasonolides	*Forcepia* sp. (sponge)	Chromosome condensation	Preclinical
Vitilevuamide	*Didemnum cuculiferum/Polysyncraton lithostrotum* (ascidians)	Tubulin	Preclinical

Source: Singh, R. et al., 2008, *Anticancer Agents Med. Chem.*, 8, 603; Mahdi, E. and Fariba, K., 2012, *Ann. Biol. Res.*, 3, 622.

the elongation cycle by preventing eukaryotic elongation factor 2-dependent translocation and to activate caspases, thereby inducing apoptosis.[21,22] It was the first defined marine natural product to enter clinical trials as a potential anticancer drug, reaching phase II and showing promising results.[23] Unfortunately, it was never carried into phase-III trials due to the high toxicity exhibited, and NCI withdrew the drug from clinical trials.[24,25]

Case studies demonstrate that the rate of anticancer drug discovery can be greatly increased by screening natural compounds from marine sources;[26] however, despite numerous efforts, drugs such as bryostatin 1 have failed also in phase-II clinical trials. Bryostatins are macrolide lactones isolated from the marine bryozoan *Bugula neritina*, which activate the enzyme activity of protein kinase C (PKC).[27,28] Bryostatin 1 was granted orphan designation by the European Commission for treatment of esophageal cancer, but was withdrawn from the Community Register of designated Orphan Medicinal Products in 2006. Although it failed to show significant activity against tumors either on its own or in combination with other chemotherapeutic agents, it has started to raise interest as a treatment for other diseases such as Alzheimer's disease (AD) and HIV.[29,30]

Dolastatins, such as dolastatin 10, are linear peptides extracted from sea hare, *Dolabella auricularia*, which show antimitotic activity due to binding to the β-tubulin-inhibiting microtubule assembly,[31,32] Despite reaching phase II, currently there are no active clinical trials since it has not been successful as a single agent.[33]

Kahalalide F belongs to the family of depsipeptides isolated from the Hawaiian *Elysia rufescens*. This herbivorous mollusk is able to sequester the bioactive compound by feeding on the green algae *Bryopsis* sp. from which Kahalalide F has also been isolated.[34] It has been suggested to specifically interact with membranes or proteins, inducing cytoplasmic swelling as a consequence of changes in lysosomal membranes and DNA clumping, as well as a downregulation of ErbB3 and inhibition of the phosphatidylinositol-3-kinase–Akt signaling pathway.[35–37] PM02734 (elisidepsin) is a synthetic marine-derived cyclic peptide of the kahalalide family, which has reached phase-II clinical development.[38,39]

Psammaplin is a phenolic natural product isolated from various marine sponges, which showed potent cytotoxicity against several cancer cell lines. It has been reported to have topoisomerase-II-, aminopeptidase N-, and class-I histone deacetylase-inhibitory activity,[40,41] thus with the potential to play a key role in the inhibition of tumor cell invasion and angiogenesis. LBH589 (panobinostat) is a synthetically derived compound of psammaplin with active phase I–II clinical trials, which has been granted as an orphan drug by the European Commission for treatment of cutaneous T-cell lymphoma in 2007 and multiple myeloma in 2012.[11]

It is important to emphasize that during the development of a candidate, there are different steps and areas of great complexity, and some issues must be considered, such as the supply and formulation of the compounds, since they are usually structurally complex molecules and a sustainable supply should be ensured for preclinical and clinical investigations. It is clear that the marine environment offers a huge potential for the discovery of bioactive compounds anyway, and available data report a great variety of experimental agents that are currently undergoing preclinical and early clinical evaluation.

The in vitro potential and high bioactivity of marine compounds make them excellent candidates. Among these cases, yessotoxin is a complex molecule produced by marine dinoflagellates of the genera *Protoceratium* and *Gonyaulax*. This compound can induce programmed cell death in different model systems, including apoptotic and paraptotic characteristics, which makes it a molecule of interest in the development of therapeutic methods to avoid drug resistance in cancer cells.[42,43] It is a poorly toxic compound when administered orally, but is considered a seafood toxin because it results in toxicity to mice when injected intraperitoneally. Its capability to act as a modulator of cytosolic calcium levels[42] and to decrease the levels of cyclic adenosine monophosphate through the activation of cellular phosphodiesterases[44] led it to be claimed as being capable of activating cellular phosphodiesterases for use in the treatment of human hepatocellular carcinoma due to its cytotoxic activity on cells (EP1875906—therapeutic use of yessotoxin as a human tumor cell growth inhibitor), and it has been further shown that this toxin induces apoptosis in neuroblastoma. Apoptosis is a mechanism, which involves the elimination of altered cells, without causing an inflammatory reaction.[45] It is a programmed cell death, which results from the activation of an intracellular self-destruction system induced by external stimuli or by the lack of necessary factors for maintenance of cellular life. Apoptosis is a multistep phenomenon, which is correlated with biochemical and structural changes in a cell. In this way, it has been reported that yessotoxin alters mitochondrial potential, causes DNA fragmentation, decreases the total nucleic acid content, increases the activity of caspase-3, and induces changes in membrane phospholipids (phosphatidyl serine translocation to the cell surface),[46] evidencing an apoptotic activity. This effect was further explored for the treatment of gliomas (ES1596.42), where it is demonstrated that yessotoxin causes cell-cycle arrest in G0/G1, provoking stress in the endoplasmic reticulum and autophagy.

Therefore, the marine ecosystem is not only an excellent environment to discover anticancer entities, but also a challenging tool to identify new cellular targets and modes of action for therapeutic intervention.

40.3 Marine Toxins for Treatment of Neurological Disorders

Nowadays, neurological and neurodegenerative diseases have become a growing problem in industrialized countries due to an increase in life expectancy, with important socioeconomic consequences. An important field of research related to marine products is the study of marine biotoxins and their related seafood consumption risks due to their accumulation in filter bivalves and fishes. Among these marine biotoxins, some are classified as neurotoxins. Neurotoxins are a diverse group of marine compounds highly specific for ion- and ligand-gated channels. Ciguatoxins, brevetoxins, and paralytic shellfish-poisoning toxins have voltage-gated ion channels as their main cellular targets, whereas others as imine cyclic toxins or conotoxins have ligand-gated receptors as key components in their mechanism of action. Ion channels are fundamental for proper function of excitable cells. They are involved in neurotransmission and it has been found that an incorrect function is often related with neurological diseases. The wide chemical and pharmacological variety of these compounds makes them a great candidate in the drug pursuit.

40.3.1 Marine Toxins and Voltage-Gated Channels: Implications in Neurological Disorders

Voltage-gated ion channels are very sensitive to small changes in membrane potential and are essential for normal physiology of excitable cells. Among them are sodium, calcium, and potassium channels. Participation of these voltage-gated ion channels in normal cell physiology as well as different alterations in these channels, observed in several diseases, make marine toxins potential candidate compounds to be developed as new drugs, especially for neurological disorders.

Voltage-gated sodium channels (VGSCs) selectively conduct sodium ions across cells' plasma membrane in response to variations in membrane potential; this Na^+ flux is responsible for the initiation and propagation of action potential in excitable cells.[47] They are large integral membrane proteins formed by one α-subunit and one or more β-subunits, which form a central pore. Different compounds can block these channels through the pore or through modifications in the channel gating, such as tetrotodoxin, which binds to receptor site 1 on the sodium channels, with consequent pore blocking (Table 40.2).[48] This marine biotoxin has been used to identify and classify voltage-dependent sodium channels (Na_v) subtypes with respect to tetrodotoxin (TTX) sensitivity.[49] TTX-resistant subtypes, Na_v 1.8 and Na_v 1.9 are implicated in neuropathic pain states,[50] whereas the TTX-sensitive subtypes Na_v 1.7, 1.3, 1.2, and 1.1 are implicated in inflammation, epilepsy, or neuropathic pain. The α-subunit of Na_v is the binding site for several drugs such as anti-epileptics, anti-arrhythmics, and local anesthetics.[51] Mutation in genes encoding VGSCs (known as channelopaties) is directly related to several diseases of heart, muscle, brain, and peripheral nerves, and changes in nonmutated genes are related to other diseases such as multiple sclerosis.[52–54] This turns Na_v into an important cellular target in the pharmacology research and several marine-derived compounds have been tested till now because of this relationship; some of them are TTX and conotoxins. TTX is of therapeutic interest for pain treatment and several preclinical studies have been performed. Even though some of them reached clinical trials, further research is needed.[55] Conotoxins are small peptides produced by tropical marine mollusks of the *Conus* species that have different pharmacological targets, including VGSCs. Venom from these species is used to immobilize prey or for defense. There are four conotoxin families that specifically bind to VGSC sites with different

TABLE 40.2

Relation between Different Marine
Neurotoxins and their Na-Binding Sites

Sodium Channel-Binding Site	Toxin
Site 1	Tetrodotoxin
	Saxitoxin
	μ-Conotoxin
Site 2	—
Site 3	Sea anemone toxins
Site 4	—
Site 5	Brevetoxin
	Ciguatoxins
Site 6	δ-Conotoxins

effects, namely, μ-, μO-, δ-, and ί-conotoxins. μ- and μO-conotoxins inhibit VGSCs, whereas δ- and ί-conotoxins activate the channel. As a result, this group of toxins is of interest for potential use as analgesics, thanks to their subtype selectivity.[56]

Another group of neurotoxins, which bind to Na_v, are brevetoxins. Brevetoxins bind to Na_v receptor site 5 and cause its activation.[57] Due to their ability to bind to the sodium channel, derivatives of these neurotoxins have been patented as potential drugs for the treatment of pulmonary-related diseases such as cystic fibrosis or asthma. β-Naphthoyl-PbTx-3, a synthetic PbTx-3 antagonist, shows an antagonistic effect on brevetoxin 2 Na_v activation, which can be useful for the treatment of respiratory diseases.[58] This group of neurotoxins has also been patented for the possible treatment of neurodegenerative diseases due to the enhancement of neurite growth that they can produce.[59]

Another fundamental voltage-gated channel for proper neuronal function is voltage-gated potassium channels (K_v). They have a crucial role in cell depolarization. Opening of K_v channels generates an efflux of positive charge, which hyperpolarizes or re-polarizes the cellular membrane. With 78 family members, they are the largest family of voltage-gated ion channels. Pharmacological activation of K_v plays a key role in different physiological processes such as Ca^{2+} signaling, cellular volume regulation, secretion, cellular migration, and proliferation. Modulators of K_v are usually divided as (1) metal ions, (2) organic small molecules, and (3) venom-derived peptides. These compounds regulate these channels by blocking the pore from the internal or external side, or by binding to the voltage-sensor domain.

Nowadays, K_v channels have become important cellular targets for the pharmaceutical industry due to their potential use as modulators of neurological or autoimmune diseases and also in inflammation-related pathologies. In fact, some K_v channels modulators are currently used clinically for the treatment of diseases such as epilepsy or type-2 diabetes,[60] whereas others are under study for memory impairment or cancer. K^+ blockers, such as tetraethylammonium or 4-aminopyridine, have shown beneficial effects by decreasing cell mortality in vitro in serum, staurosporine, or amyloid β treatments,[61] suggesting that K^+ modulators could be a therapeutic option for AD.[62] Gambierol, a marine polycyclic ether produced by the dinoflagellate *Gambierdiscus toxicus*, showed beneficial effects in the main hallmarks, tau and Aβ, of a triple transgenic mouse model for AD (3xTg-AD) together with a decrease in K_v 3.1 upregulation observed in this cellular model.[63,64] Full synthesis of this marine compound allowed researchers to study smaller and less toxic analogs with the same effects as gambierol,[63,65,66] as well as guarantying a source of the synthetic compound.

The last major group of voltage-gated channels is the voltage-gated calcium channels (VGCCs). VGCCs participate in cell excitability, modulate the gating of other channels, and are involved in neurotransmitter release. Due to their involvement in Ca^{2+} signaling, they are related with different diseases such as pain, stroke, epilepsy, migraine, and hypertension. It was not until the discovery of the conotoxin peptide GVIA, an inhibitor of Ca 2.2 VGCCs, that this ionic channel was recognized as an important target for pain treatment.[67] Ziconitide (Prialt®) (Figure 40.1), the synthetic ω-conotoxin MVIIA, was approved by the FDA for the management of long-term neuropathic pain and was the first conotoxin-derived

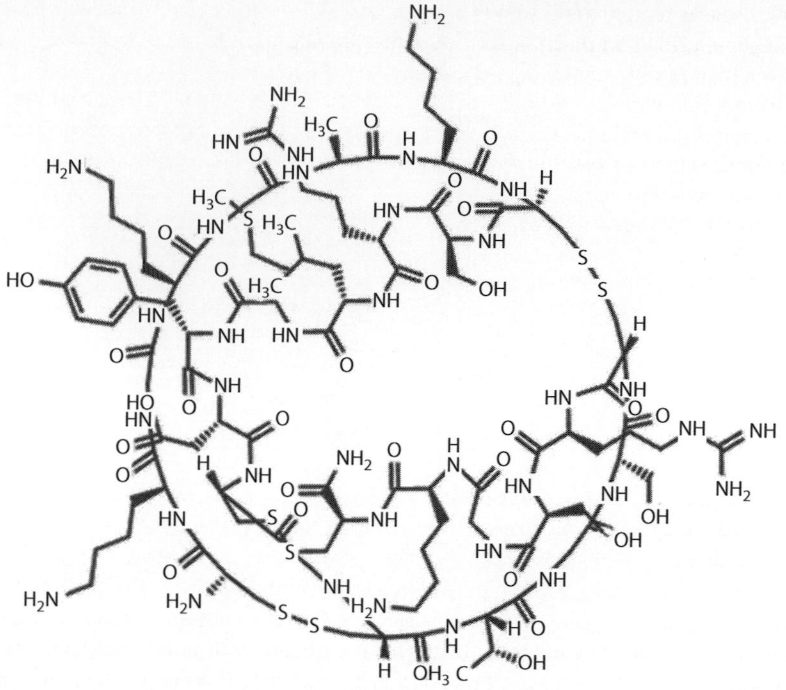

FIGURE 40.1 Structure of ω-conotoxin MVIIA (ziconitide, Prialt), the only marine compound in the market for treatment of neurological disorders.

therapeutic molecule. Since then, several other conotoxin analogs has been under study for their potential use and to improve ziconitide's side effects related with its narrow therapeutic window.[68]

40.3.2 Marine Toxins and Ligand-Gated Receptors: Implications in Neurological Disorders

Besides voltage-gated ionic channels, another important target of neurotoxins is ligand-gated receptors. Nicotinic receptors consist of five subunits that form a central channel permeable to cations, which opens due to acetylcholine neurotransmitter binding. In mammals there are 16 nicotinic receptor subtypes, five of which are neuromuscular and the remaining 11 neuronal. The most abundant in brain are the α7, α4β2, and α3β4 subtypes,[5] which are implicated in diseases such as AD, Parkinson, or schizophrenia,[69–71] whereas the others, such as α9α10, are related with chronic neuropathic pain.[72] Muscarinic receptors are transmembrane receptors coupled to protein G and to a phospholipase or adenylate cyclase, and are classified from M1 to M5. The most abundant isoforms in the central nervous system are M1[72] and M2.[73] Due to their widespread distribution, they have been studied as pharmacological targets for different diseases such as:[74]

M1 and M2 antagonists for AD

M1 and M4 agonists for schizophrenia

M4 antagonist for Parkinson disease

M5 antagonist for drug dependence

Acetylcholine receptors have been described as the target of cyclic imine toxins. 13-Desmethyl spirolide-C and gymnodimine have shown upregulation of muscarinic M1, M2, and M5 and nicotinic α2 and α4 receptors in vitro and in vivo.[75,76] Binding assays and antagonism assays showed a strong affinity of these two marine toxins for α7 and α2β4 neuronal receptors,[77] indicating these toxins and their analogs can be useful tools for cholinergic receptor function–activity studies and also for therapeutic investigations of diseases related to these receptors. In fact, 13-desmethyl spirolide-C and gymnodimine have shown beneficial effects in an in vitro model of AD, and the spirolide has been able to diminish neurodegeneration markers in vivo in 3xTg-AD mice.[78–80]

Conotoxins have demonstrated to be disulfide-rich peptides, which besides targeting VGSCs, also specifically block neuronal and muscle nicotinic receptors.[2] Thanks to their selectivity, they are considered great tools for the study of specific receptor subtype function and activity, and are really promising candidates for diseases where specific nicotinic acetylcholine receptors (nAchRs) or muscarinic acetylcholine receptors (mAchRs) are implicated, as happens with the α-conotoxin PelA[S9H,V10A,E14N], which selectively inhibits α6β2β3 nAchRs, which are widely expressed in dopaminergic neurons and are related with Parkinson disease and nicotine dependence.[81]

Another example of an nAchR-related compound is anabaseine. This alkaloid was first detected in *Amphiporus lactifloreus*[82] and later several analogs such as 3-(2,4-dimethoxybenzylidene)-anabaseine (DMBXA) were synthesized for its high antagonism over α7 nAchRs. This compound has displayed improvement of cognition and learning in mammals such as rats, rabbits, and monkeys, and is under clinical study in Taiho Pharmaceutical Company for AD treatment.[83]

N-methyl-D-aspartate (NMDA) receptors are ligand-gated receptors named for their high affinity to NMDA. They are implicated in numerous neurological processes, such as learning, memory, or neurodegeneration. NMDA receptors are formed by three different subunits (NR1–NR3), which can be linked in different combinations. A "traditional" NMDA receptor is a heterotetramer formed by two NR1 and two NR2 subunits. NR1 forms the ionic channel and bestows on the receptor the activation/inactivation properties, polyamine interaction, and pH sensitivity. Meanwhile, the NR2 subunits are involved in the regulation and definition of the receptor function. Activation of these receptors is a complex process, which requires union of various ligands and also cellular depolarization. For their activation, it is required to have glutamate binding and cellular depolarization for Mg^{2+} removal to unblock the channel.[84] Nowadays, 1-amino-3,5-dimetil-adamantano (memantine), an NMDA antagonist, is the only approved drug for the treatment of AD with acetylcholine esterase inhibitors. It is a well-tolerated drug usually employed for mild and severe AD.[85,86] One example of a marine compound that targets an NMDA receptor is the neuroactive peptide conantokin-G, which is isolated from the marine cone snail *Conus geographus* and is under preclinical study by Cognetix Company as a potential therapy for stroke and brain ischemia. It also has reached phase-I clinical trials as an effective antiepileptic drug under the name CGX-1007.[87] Another conopeptide derived from the same snail, contulakin-G (CGX-1160), has been stated by the FDA as an orphan drug for intrathecal treatment of chronic intractable pain associated with spinal cord injury. However, this peptide has the neurotensin receptor as its cellular target.[15,88]

Neurological and aging-related disorders remain as one of the major concerns in the industrialized world where the elderly people population is constantly increasing. Nowadays, there is no effective treatment for neurodegenerative diseases and the side effects of current drugs are often an additional problem. The diversity of bioactive compounds in the marine environment converts them into potential tools for prevention and cure of neurodegenerative and neuronal dysfunctions, and opens a wide window of new and promising chemical products for further investigations where the variety of cellular targets of marine compounds is a pivotal key in the successful development of new medicines.

40.4 Marine Compound and the Need for Novel Antibiotics

Infectious diseases caused by bacteria, fungi, and viruses are still a major threat to human and animal health. Antibiotic resistance, which is continuously evolving in microbial pathogens, makes obvious the need of new and effective antimicrobial compounds. In common terms, "antibiotic" describes any compound, which kills (microbicidal) or inhibits the growth (microstatic) of microorganisms. Most of the antimicrobials used for human treatment are either produced naturally or are derived from natural products. For example, as shown in Table 40.3, among the 12 antibacterial classes, 9 of the molecular structures are derived from a natural product template. Antivirals in use have also been obtained from natural sources, the antiviral acyclovir used against herpes simplex virus was derived from metabolites isolated from the sponge *Cryptotethya crypta*.[89] The synthetic purine nucleoside vidarabine (Ara-A) was

TABLE 40.3

Antibacterial Classes in Use for Human Health

Class of Compound	Antibiotics	Origin of the Molecule or Parental Molecule	Producing Genus	Mechanism of Action
β-Lactams	Penicillins, cephalosporins, carbapenems, monobactams	Naturally produced natural product template	*Penicillium Acremonium Streptomyces Chromobacterium Gluconobacter Acetobacter Pseudomonas Agrobacterium Flexibacter*	Inhibit bacterial cell wall biosynthesis, bind to transpeptidases and carboxypeptidases, and interfere with cross-linking
Polyketides	Tetracycline	Naturally produced natural product template	*Streptomyces*	Bind to the 30S subunit of microbial ribosomes and inhibit protein synthesis
Phenylpropanoid	Chloramphenicol	Naturally produced natural product template	*Streptomyces*	Bacteriostatic; prevents protein chain elongation by inhibiting the peptidyl transferase activity of the bacterial ribosome
Aminoglycosides	Streptomycin	Naturally produced natural product template	*Streptomyces*	Protein synthesis inhibitor; bind to the small 16S rRNA of the 30S subunit of the bacterial ribosome, interfering with the binding of formyl-methionyl-tRNA to the 30S subunit
Macrolides	Erythromycin	Naturally produced natural product template	*Saccharopolyspora*	Bacteriostatic; bind to the 50S subunit of the bacterial 70S rRNA complex. It interferes with aminoacyl translocation, preventing the transfer of the tRNA bound at the A site of the rRNA complex to the P site of the rRNA complex
Glycopeptides	Vancomycin	Naturally produced natural product template	*Amycolatopsis*	Inhibit cell wall synthesis in Gram-positive bacteria, inhibiting cross-linking. It forms hydrogen bond interactions with the terminal D-alanyl-D-alanine moieties of the NAM/NAG-peptides
Streptogramins	Pristinamycin	Naturally produced natural product template	*Streptomyces*	Bind to the bacterial 50S ribosomal subunit and inhibits the elongation process of protein synthesis
Lipopeptides	Daptomycin	Naturally produced natural product template	*Streptomyces*	By binding to the cell membrane they cause rapid depolarization, resulting in loss of membrane potential, leading to inhibition of protein, DNA, and RNA synthesis
Glycylcyclines	Tigecycline	Natural product template	Derived from tetracyclines	Bacteriostatic; inhibit protein synthesis by binding to the 30S ribosomal subunit of bacteria, thereby blocking the entry of aminoacyl-tRNA into the A site of the ribosome

TABLE 40.3 (continued)

Antibacterial Classes in Use for Human Health

Class of Compound	Antibiotics	Origin of the Molecule or Parental Molecule	Producing Genus	Mechanism of Action
Sulfonamides		Synthetic	—	Competitively inhibit the enzyme dihydropteroate synthetase (DHPS), preventing folate synthesis
Quinolones	Ciprofloxacin	Synthetic	—	Inhibit DNA gyrase, a type-II topoisomerase, and topoisomerase IV, inhibiting cell division
Oxazolidinones	Linezolid	Synthetic	—	Protein synthesis inhibitors. Mechanism not fully understood. Apparently, they inhibit the initiation of protein synthesis

developed from spongouridine, a nucleoside isolated from the Caribbean sponge *Tethya crypta*, and is now obtained from *Streptomyces antibioticus*. This last one was the first antibiotic of marine origin to be approved by the FDA. It was approved in 1976 and was discontinued in 2001.[90]

Most of the antimicrobial classes were discovered between 1940 and 1960. Since then, antimicrobial resistance has made it necessary to introduce new molecules to combat resistant microorganisms. To do so, modern pharmaceutical development of antimicrobials based on incremented semi-synthetic modifications of natural molecules was validated more than a century ago. As a result, 73% of the antibacterial drugs approved between 1981 and 2005 were encompassed by only three classes, the β-lactams, macrolides, and quinones. This approach generated molecules that evaded the existing mechanisms of resistance but only temporarily. Despite this, the number of approved antibiotics has decreased systematically up to now. Sixteen antibiotics were approved between 1988 and 1992, 14 between 1988 and 1992, 10 between 1993 and 1997, 6 between 1998 and 2002, and 4 between 2003 and 2007.[91] This makes obvious the need to discover new molecules with novel molecular scaffolds targeting unknown microbial targets, to address the long-term concerns of microbial resistance.

To identify pharmacological metabolites, the pharmaceutical industry in the last 60 years has focused on the terrestrial environment. Success in obtaining effective antimicrobials from terrestrial microorganisms has prompted search in the oceans, which hold the biggest and still much unknown reserve of bacterial, algal, and fungal species, with the aim of finding new leads for drug candidates. Even though the traditional medicine used products extracted from marine organisms to treat multiple diseases[92] and that it had been known for centuries that some organisms in the oceans produced poisonous substances,[93] it was only by the 1950s that scientists began to systematically investigate the oceans in the search for new active molecules.

Why do several marine organisms produce so many different antimicrobial molecules? The answer to this ecological question could be that marine sessile invertebrates such as sponges, corals, and tunicates feed by filtering seawater. This water contains high concentrations of bacteria, so these organisms produce defensive chemical weapons (secondary metabolites) for protection against potentially harmful microorganisms. The diversity of secondary metabolites produced by marine organisms has been reviewed extensively.[94–100] In addition to their diversity, is that when these compounds are released into water, they are rapidly diluted and therefore need to be highly potent to have any effect. For these reasons, it is recognized that an immense number of natural products and novel chemical entities exist in oceans, with biological activities that may be useful in the quest for finding drugs for the treatment of human diseases.[100,101]

Among the most important producers of secondary metabolites with antimicrobial effect are sponges. These organisms appeared early in evolution and over time they have developed many chemicals for auto-defense. They are sessile marine filter feeders, which produce a wide variety of pharmacologically active chemicals effective against foreign attackers such as viruses, bacteria, or eukaryotic organisms. More than 200 new metabolites are reported each year from this type of organisms and more than 5300 different secondary metabolites are known from sponges.[89,102] The production of secondary metabolites in sponges is not constitutive but regulated by environmental conditions. This fact becomes important for the pharmaceutical industry at the time of developing an antibiotic, since lack of knowledge of the conditions which induce the production of a secondary metabolite by specific species of sponges, can become an important drawback as explained later in this section.

Algae are other important producers of antimicrobials and are present in oceans, rivers, and lakes, as well as in several terrestrial environments. The potential commercial value of the metabolites produced by these organisms has been recognized by various authors.[3,103,104] Many of the secondary metabolites produced by algae are halogenated with bromide, which is more frequently present than chloride for organohalogen production.[105] Even though marine algae produce a variety of useful products, little attention has been paid to these organisms in the search for novel anti-infective compounds. On the other hand, diatoms and cyanobacteria have been shown to produce many compounds of this type with novel structures. Diatoms produce many active metabolites that constitute their chemical defense and may have potential as marine drugs or lead molecule candidates. Even though cyanobacteria share many structural features with bacteria, they are classified with algae since they contain chlorophyll and related compounds. They are capable of producing diverse chemical structures, which may serve to avoid predation by diverse types of phytoplankton-eating fish and mollusks.[3] Many cyanobacteria-produced molecules have been the focus of attention due to their biological activities and diverse structures.[106]

Table 40.4 summarizes most of the antimicrobial molecules discovered between 2000 and 2012, and illustrates the magnitude of the economical and human effort made with this aim. The table only includes isolated molecules with known structures and would have been much bigger if the antimicrobials present in the extracts of various marine organisms were included.

As shown in Table 40.4 and Figure 40.2, the main sources of antimicrobials are sponges, fungi, corals, bacteria, and algae. Many molecules with novel structures have been isolated from these organisms, several of which could be developed as antibiotics for human use or as lead molecules for this purpose. The type of molecules isolated includes terpenoids, steroids, phenolic compounds, alkaloids, polysaccharides, peptides, polyketides, and fatty acids. As stated previously in this chapter, products derived from metabolites produced by sponges are now in the market, for example, acyclovir and Ara-A, which indicates that many more could be waiting to be developed as antimicrobials for human or veterinary use.

The mechanism of action of most of the antimicrobial molecules isolated from marine organisms over the last decade remains unknown, and so a lot of work is still needed for any of these molecules to be included in the drug development pipeline of the pharmaceutical industry. Different mechanisms of toxicity have been reported among molecules with known targets or mechanisms of action. For example, there are some that permeabilize microbial cells, such as MC21A and halocidin;[107,108] some that inhibit or reverse the multidrug protein 1, such as a sterol from *Dysidea arenaria* and capisterones A and B;[109,110] and some that affect the cell actin or tubulin cytoskeleton, in the case of antifungals or antiprotozoals, such as dolostatin 10, spongistatin, and Jasplakinolide.[111–113] As for antivirals, again for many of them, the mechanism of action remains unknown. Among those with a known mechanism, molecules that inhibit DNA polymerase, that bind to integrase, and that inhibit hydrophobic interactions were reported.[114–116]

Among the new antimicrobials reported in the last decade, there are many effective against microorganisms infectious to humans some of which have shown resistance to antibiotics actually in use. Of the antibacterials included in Table 40.4, it should be noted that some were successfully tested against resistant strains of human-infecting bacteria, as for example, plicatamide (effective against methicillin-resistant *Staphylococcus aureus*), ingenamine G (effective against resistant *S. aureus*), MC21A (effective against methicillin-resistant *S. aureus*), caminoside A (effective against antibiotic-resistant *S. aureus*), halocidin (effective against antibiotic-resistant *S. aureus*), and pestalone (effective against antibiotic-resistant *S. aureus*).[107,117–120] This implies that effective molecules, against bacteria that have acquired resistance to antibiotics commonly used in clinical practice, could be obtained from marine organisms. Also, several antimicrobials have shown cytotoxic effects against a broad spectrum of microbes, being effective against bacteria and fungi (see Table 40.4).

When considering the type of structure generated by each producing organism, have been the most important contributors of alkaloids. Corals, sponges, and algae are responsible for most of the terpenoids isolated, whereas bacteria, fungi, and sponges have contributed to most of the polyketides and peptides. Tunicates have also shown to be important producers of antimicrobial peptides (Figure 40.3).

TABLE 40.4

Marine Compounds with Antibacterial, Antifungal, Anthelmintic, Antiprotozoal, and Antiviral Activities Reported between 2000 and 2012

Class[a]	Chemistry	Producing Organism	Effective Against[b]	Reference
Terpenoids				
Antibacterial	Sesterterpenoid	*Laurencia pannosa*[c]	*Proteus mirabilis*	[123]
			Chromobacterium violaceum	
			Vibrio cholera	
Antifungal	Triterpene glycoside	*Psolus patagonicus*[h]	*Cladosporium cucumerinum*	[124]
Antiparasitic	Sesterterpenoid	*Halorosellinia oceanica*[d]	*Plasmodium falciparum*	[125]
Antibacterial	Diterpene	*Pseudopterogorgia elisabethae*[f]	*Mycobacterium tuberculosis*	[126]
Antiparasitic	Sesquiterpene	*Didiscus oxeata*[e]	*Plasmodium falciparum*	[127]
Antibacterial	Diterpene	*Myrmekioderma styx*[e]	*Mycobacterium tuberculosis*	[128]
Antifungal	Terpene	*Dysidea arenaria*[e]	*Candida albicans*	[109]
Antiparasitic	Diterpene	*Briareum polyanthes*[f]	*Plasmodium falciparum*	[129]
Antibacterial	Diterpene	*Pseudopterogorgia elisabethae*[f]	*Mycobacterium tuberculosis*	[130]
Antibacterial	Diterpene	*Acanthella cavernosa*[e]	*Bacilus subtilis*	[131]
Antibacterial	Sesterterpene	*Luffariella* sp.[e]	*Staphylococcus aureus*	[132]
Antibacterial	Diterpene	*Pseudopterogorgia elisabethae*[f]	*Staphylococcus aureus*	[133]
			Enterococcus faecalis	
Antibacterial	Sesquiterpene	*Axinyssa n.* sp.[e]	*Staphylococcus aureus*	[134]
			Bacilus subtilis	
Antibacterial	Diterpene	*Dendrilla membranosa*[e]	*Staphylococcus aureus*	[135]
			Escherichia coli	
Antifungal	Diterpene	*Hippospongia communis*[e]	*Candida tropicalis*	[136]
			Fusarium oxysporum	
Antiparasitic	Diterpene	*Pseudopterogorgia kallos*[f]	*Plasmodium falciparum*	[137]
Antiparasitic	Diterpene	*Eunicea* sp.[f]	*Plasmodium falciparum*	[138]
Antiprotozoal	Sesquiterpene	*Euplotes crassus*[j]	*Leishmania major*	[139]
			Leishmania infantum	
Antibacterial	Sesterterpene	*Brachiaster* sp.[e]	*Mycobacterium tuberculosis*	[140]
Antiviral	Furanoterpene	*Lendenfeldia* sp.[e]	Reverse transcriptase	[141]
			RNA- and DNA-directed DNA polymerase	
Antiviral	Diterpene	*Dictyota menstrualis*[c]	HIV-1	[142]
Antibacterial	Sesterterpene	*Halichondria* sp.[e]	*Micrococcus luteus*	[143]
Antiparasitic	Diterpenes	*Pseudopterogorgia bipinnata*[f]	*Plasmodium falciparum*	[144]
Antiparasitic	Sesterterpenoid	*Eunicea* sp.[f]	*Plasmodium falciparum*	[145]
Antiparasitic	Diterpenes	*Leptogorgia alba*[f]	*Plasmodium falciparum*	[146]
Antiviral	Terpenoid	*Sargassum micracanthum*[c]	HCMV	[147]
			Measles	
Antiviral	Diterpene	*Dictyota menstrualis*[c]	HIV	[114]
Antiparasitic	Diterpenes	*Pseudopterogorgia* sp.[f]	*Plasmodium falciparum*	[148]
Antibacterial	Diterpenes	*Xenia novaebrittanniae*[f]	*Escherichia coli*	[149]
			Bacilus subtilis	
Antiprotozoan	Meroterpenoid	*Callyspongia* sp.[e]	*Leishmania* sp.	[150]

(continued)

TABLE 40.4 (continued)

Marine Compounds with Antibacterial, Antifungal, Anthelmintic, Antiprotozoal, and Antiviral Activities Reported between 2000 and 2012

Class[a]	Chemistry	Producing Organism	Effective Against[b]	Reference
Antibacterial	Diterpene	*Pseudopterogorgia elisabethae*[f]	*Mycobacterium tuberculosis*	[151]
Antibacterial	Sesquiterpenoid-hydroquinone	*Laurencia* sp.[c]	*Chromobacterium violaceum*	[152]
			Proteus mirabilis	[153]
			Proteus vulgaris	
			Erwinia sp.	
			Vibrio parahaemolyticus	
			Vibrioalginolyticus	—
			Staphylococcus aureus	
			Escherichia coli	
Antibacterial	Diterpene	*Aspergillus* sp.[d]	*Staphylococcus aureus*	[154]
Antibacterial Antifungal	Sesterterpenoid	*Dysidea* sp.[e]	*Candida albicans*	[155]
			Bacillus subtilis	
			Proteus vulgaris	
Antiviral	Sesterterpenoid	*Hyrtios erectus*[e]	Inhibits HIV integrase (IN) binding to viral DNA	[156]
Antiviral	Sesquiterpenoid-hydroquinone	*Dysidea arenaria*[e]	Moderate inhibitory activity on HIV reverse transcriptase	[157]
Antiparasitic	Meroterpenoid	New Caledonian deep water[e] sponge	*Plasmodium falciparum*	[158]
Antifungal	Sesquiterpene-dihydroquinone	*Hyrtios* sp.[e]	*Cryptococcus neoformans*	[159]
			Candida krusei	
Antibacterial	Diterpene	*Sargassum macrocarpum*[c]	*Propionibacterium acnes*	[160]
Antibacterial	Sesquiterpene-hydroquinone	*Peyssonnelia* sp.[c]	*Pseudoalteromonas bacteriolytica*	[161]
Antifungal			*Lindra thalassiae*	
Antiviral	Diterpene	*Dictyota pfaffi*[c] *Dictyota menstrualis*[c]	Inhibits herpes simplex type-1 (HSV-1) replication in Vero cells. Non-competitive inhibitor of HIV RT	[162] [163]
Antibacterial	Meroterpenoid	*Fasciospongia* sp.[e]	*Staphylococcus aureus*	[164]
			Bacillus subtilis	
Antibacterial Antifungal Antifouling	Diterpene	*Cymbastela hooperi*[e]	*Plasmodium falciparum* *Escherichia coli* *Vibrio harvey* *Bacillus megaterium* *Ustilago violacea* *Eurotium repens* *Mycotypha microspora* *Fusarium oxysporum* *Chlorella fusca* *Mycobacterium tuberculosis*	[165]

TABLE 40.4 (continued)

Marine Compounds with Antibacterial, Antifungal, Anthelmintic, Antiprotozoal, and Antiviral Activities
Reported between 2000 and 2012

Class[a]	Chemistry	Producing Organism	Effective Against[b]	Reference
Steroids				
Antiviral	Sulfated sterol	*Clathria* sp.[e]	HIV	[166]
Antibacterial	Steroidal glycosides	*Codium iyengarii*[c]	Gram-positive and Gram-negative marine bacteria	[167]
Antifungal	Sulfated sterol	Astroscleridae family[e]	*Saccharomyces cerevisiae*	[168]
Antifungal	Steroid	*Penicillus capitatus*[c]	*Saccharomyces cerevisiae*	[110]
Antifungal	Sulfated sterol	*Euryspongia* sp.[e]	*Candida albicans*	[169]
Antifungal	Sulfated sterol	*Topsentia* sp.[e]	*Saccharomyces cerevisiae* *Candida albicans*	[170]
Antibacterial	Bile acid derivative	*Psychrobacter* sp.[g]	*Staphylococcus aureus* *Pseudomonas aeruginosa* *Enterobacter cloacae*	[171]
Antibacterial Antifungal Antifouling	Ergosteroid	*Colletotrichum* sp.[d]	*Microbotryum violaceum* *Chlorella fusca* *Escherichia coli* *Bacillus megaterium*	[172]
Phenolic Compounds				
Antiviral	Sulfated flavones	*Thalassia testudinum*[k]	HIV	[116]
Antibacterial	Halogenated phenolic compounds	*Pseudoalteromonas phenolica*[g]	*Staphylococcus aureus*	[107]
Antibacterial	Halogenated phenolic compounds	*Rhodomela confervoides*[c]	*Staphylococcus aureus* *Staphylococcus epidermidis* *Pseudomonas aeruginosa*	[173]
Antibacterial	Halogenated phenolic compounds	*Lamellodysidea herbacea*[e]	*Bacillus subtilis*	[174]
Antibacterial Antifungal	Anthraquinone	*Monodictys* sp.[d]	*Bacillus subtilis* *Escherichia coli* *Candida albicans*	[175]
Antifungal	Halogenated phenolic compounds	*Odonthalia corymbifera*[c]	*Candida albicans* *Aspergillus fumigatus* *Trichophyton rubrum* *Trichophyton mentagrophytes*	[176]
Antibacterial	Halogenated phenolic compounds	*Dysidea* sp.[e]	*Streptomyces*	[177]
Antibacterial	Hexahydroanthrones	*Aspergillus* sp.[d]	*Staphylococcus aureus* *Escherichia coli* *Staphylococcus aureus*	[178]
Antibacterial Antifungal	Anthraquinone	*Nocardia* sp.[g]	*Escherichia coli* *Pseudomonas aeruginosa* *Bacillus subtilis* *Bacillus cereus* *Staphylococcus aureus* *Micrococcus luteus* *Mycobacterium smegmatis*	[179]

(continued)

TABLE 40.4 (continued)

Marine Compounds with Antibacterial, Antifungal, Anthelmintic, Antiprotozoal, and Antiviral Activities Reported between 2000 and 2012

Class[a]	Chemistry	Producing Organism	Effective Against[b]	Reference
Antibacterial Antifungal	Coumarin Flavonoids	*Streptomyces* sp.[g]	*Corynebacterium xerosis* *Rhodotorula acuta* *Pichia angusta* *Candida albicans* *Cryptococcus neoformans* *Aspergillus niger* *Botrytis fabae* *Bacillus subtilis* *Staphylococcus aureus* *Micrococcus luteus* *Rhodotorula minuta* *Pichia angusta* *Candida albicans* *Cryptococcus neoformans* *Aspergillus niger* *Botrytis fabae*	[180]
Antibacterial	Sulfoalkylresorcinol	*Zygosporium* sp.[d]	*Mycobcterium tuberculosis* *Mycobacterium bovis* *Mycobacterium avium* *Pseudomonas aeruginosa* *Staphylococcus aureus*	[181]
Antibacterial	Halogenated phenolic compounds	*Dysidea granulosa*[e]	*Staphylococcus aureus* *Enterococcus* sp. *Bacillus* sp.	[182]
Antibacterial	Halogenated phenolic compounds	*Pseudoalteromonas phenolica*[g]	*Staphylococcus aureus* *Bacillus subtilis* *Enterococcus serolicida*	[183]
Antibacterial	Halogenated phenolic compounds	*Pseudoalteromonas* sp.[g]	*Staphylococcus aureus*	[184]
Antibacterial	Anthraquinones	*Arpergillus versicolor*[d]	*Streptococcus pyogenes* *Staphylococcus aureus*	[185]
Alkaloids				
Antibacterial	Bromotyrosine	*Pseudoceratina purpurea*[e]	*Rhodospirillum salexigens*	[186]
Antiparasitic	Manzamine-type alkaloids	Family Petrosiidae, order Haplosclerida[e]	*Plasmodium berghei*	[187]
Antibacterial	Tetracyclic alkylpiperidine alkaloid	*Arenosclera brasiliensis*[e]	*Staphylococcus aureus*	[188]
Antiparasitic	Pyrrole alkaloid	From an α-proteobacteria[g]	*Plasmodium falciparum* *Plasmodium berghei*	[189]
Antiparasitic	Decahydroquinoline derivatives	*Didemnum* sp.[i]	*Plasmodium falciparum*	[190]
Antibacterial	β-Carbolines	*Eudistoma* sp.[i]	*Staphylococcus aureus* *Bacillus subtilis* *Escherichia coli*	[191]
Antibacterial	Bicyclic guanidine alkaloid	*Ptilocaulis speculifer*[e]	*Staphylococcus aureus*	[192]

TABLE 40.4 (continued)

Marine Compounds with Antibacterial, Antifungal, Anthelmintic, Antiprotozoal, and Antiviral Activities
Reported between 2000 and 2012

Class[a]	Chemistry	Producing Organism	Effective Against[b]	Reference
Antifungal	Bicyclic guanidine alkaloid	*Stylissa aff.* massa[e]	*Cryptococcus neoformans*	[193]
Antiparasitic	Manzamine-type alkaloids	*Haliclona* sp.[e]	*Plasmodium falciparum*	[194]
Antibacterial	Manzamine-type alkaloids	*Haliclona* sp.[e]	*Mycobacterium tuberculosis*	[194]
Antiviral	Polycyclic guanidine alkaloids	*Monanchora* sp.[e]	HIV	[195]
Antiviral	Bis-quinolizidine alkaloids	*Petrosia similis*[e]	HIV	[196]
Antibacterial	Bromotyrosine alkaloids	*Psammaplysilla purpurea*[e]	*Staphylococcus aureus* *Bacillus subtilis* *Chromobacterium violaceum*	[197]
Antibacterial	Dimeric bromopyrrole alkaloids	*Agelas* sp.[e]	*Micrococcus luteus* *Bacillus subtilis* *Escherichia coli*	[198]
Antibacterial	Imidazo[5,1-a] isoquinoline alkaloid	*Cribrochalina* sp.[e]	*Streptococcus pneumoniae*	[199]
Antifungal	Imidazole alkaloids	*Leucetta chagosensis*[e]	*Cladosporium herbarum*	[200]
Antiprotozoan	Alkaloid	*Neopetrosia* sp.[e]	*Leishmania amazonensis*	[201]
Antibacterial	Alkaloid	*Pachychalina* sp.[e]	*Staphylococcus aureus* *Escherichia coli* *Mycobacterium tuberculosis*	[117]
Antibacterial	Bis(indole) alkaloid (9)	*Spongosorites* sp.[e]	*Staphylococcus aureus*	[202]
Antibacterial	Alkylated iminosugar	*Batzella* sp.[e]	*Staphylococcus epidermidis*	[203]
Antibacterial	4,4′-Bis(7-hydroxy) indole alkaloid	*Dictyodendrilla* sp.[e]	*Bacillus subtilis* *Micrococcus luteus*	[204]
Antiparasitic	Manzamine-type alkaloids	*Acanthostrongylophora* sp.[e]	*Plasmodium falciparum*	[205]
Antibacterial	Manzamine-type alkaloid	*Acanthostrongylophora* sp.[e]	*Mycobacterium tuberculosis*	[205]
Antibacterial	Bis(indole) alkaloid	*Spongosorites* sp.[e]	*Streptococcus pyogenes* *Staphylococcus aureus*	[206]
Antibacterial	Bromopyrrole alkaloid	*Agelas oroides*[e]	*Plasmodium falciparum* *Mycobacterium tuberculosis* *Escherichia coli*	[207]
Antifungal	Bromotyrosine alkaloids	*Pseudoceratina purpurea*[e]	*Candida albicans*	[208]
Antibacterial Antiviral	1*H*-benzo[*de*] [1,6]-naphthyridine alkaloids	*Aaptos aaptos*[e]	Inhibits HSV-1 replication *Staphylococcus aureus*	[209] [210]
Antibacterial	Alkylpiperidine alkaloid	*Haliclona* sp.[e]	*Mycobacterium smegmatis* *Mycobacterium bovis* *Mycobacterium tuberculosis*	[211]
Antibacterial	Bromopyrrole alkaloid	*Streptomyces* sp.[g]	*Staphylococcus aureus*	[212]
Antibacterial	Alkylpiperidine alkaloid	*Haliclona* sp.[e]	*Mycobacterium bovis*	[213]

(continued)

TABLE 40.4 (continued)

Marine Compounds with Antibacterial, Antifungal, Anthelmintic, Antiprotozoal, and Antiviral Activities Reported between 2000 and 2012

Class[a]	Chemistry	Producing Organism	Effective Against[b]	Reference
Antibacterial	Macrocyclic diamine	*Haliclona* sp.[e]	*Staphylococcus aureus*	[118]
			Bacillus subtilis	
			Micrococcus luteus	
			Proteus vulgaris	
			Escherichia coli	
Antibacterial	Bromopyrrole alkaloids	*Agelas* sp.[e]	*Staphylococcus aureus*	[214]
			Cryptococcus neoformans	[215]
			Micrococcus luteus	[216]
			Bacillus subtilis	[217]
			Trichophyton mentagrophytes	
			Cryptococcus neoformans	
			Candida albicans	
			Aspergillus niger	
Antibacterial Antiviral Antiparasitic	Polycyclic guanidine alkaloids	*Monanchora unguifera*[e]	Significant activities against HIV	[218] [219]
			Vibrio anguillarum	
			Tripanosoma brucei brucei	
			Plasmodium falciparum	
Antibacterial	Sulfated sesterterpene alkaloids	*Fasciospongia* sp.[e]	*Streptomyces* sp.	[220] [221]
Antifungal	5-Hydroxyindole-type alkaloids	*Hyrtios* sp.[e]	*Candida albicans*	[222]
Antibacterial Antifungal	Diketopiperazine alkaloids	*Alternaria raphani*[d]	*Escherichia coli*	[223]
			Bacillus subtilis	
			Candida albicans	
Antiviral	Sulfated alkaloids	*Iotrochota baculifera*[e]	Potent inhibitors against the HIV IIIB	[224]
Antifungal	Bromotyrosine alkaloids	*Pseudoceratina* sp.[e]	*Cryptococcus neoformans*	[225]
			Candida albicans	
Antibacterial	Pyrroloiminoquinone alkaloids	*Sceptrella* sp.[e]	*Staphylococcus aureus*	[226]
Antibacterial	Isonitrile-containing indole alkaloids	*Fischerella ambigua*[g]	*Mycobacterium tuberculosis*	[227]
Polysaccharides				
Antibacterial	Lipopolysaccharide	*Caminus sphaeroconia*[e]	*Staphylococcus aureus*	[119]
Antiparasitic	Glycoside	*Streptomycete* sp.[g]	*Plasmodium falciparum*	[228]
Antiviral	Sulfated galactan	*Callophyllis variegata*[c]	HSV-1	[229]
			HSV-2	
			DENV-2	
Antiviral	Sulfated galactan	*Schizymenia binderi*[c]	HSV-1	[230]
			HSV-2	
Antibacterial	Glycolipids	*Caminus sphaeroconia*[e]	*Escherichia coli*	[231]
Antiviral	Sulfated polysaccharide	*Navicula directa* (W. Smith) Ralfs[c]	HSV-1	[232]
			HSV-2	

TABLE 40.4 (continued)

Marine Compounds with Antibacterial, Antifungal, Anthelmintic, Antiprotozoal, and Antiviral Activities
Reported between 2000 and 2012

Class[a]	Chemistry	Producing Organism	Effective Against[b]	Reference
Antiviral	Acidic polysaccharide	*Nostoc flagelliforme*[c]	Anti-HSV-1	[233]
Antifungal	Chitinase	*Streptomyces* sp.[g]	*Aspergillus niger*	[235]
			Candida albicans	
Peptides				
Antibacterial	Cationic peptide	*Bacillus* sp.[g]	*Staphylococcus aureus*	[236]
			Enterococcus sp.	
Antibacterial	Peptide	*Halocynthia aurantium*[i]	*Escherichia coli*	[237]
			Pseudomonas aeruginosa	
			Listeria monocytogenes,	
			Staphylococcus aureus	
Antibacterial	Peptide	*Halocynthia aurantium*[i]	*Staphylococcus aureus*	[238]
			Pseudomonas aeruginosa	
Antiviral	Depsipeptide	*Sidonops microspinosa*[e]	HIV	[239]
Antiparasitic	Cyclic peptide	*Jaspis johnstoni*[e]	*Plasmodium falciparum*	[112]
Antibacterial	Octapeptide	*Styela plicata*[i]	*Staphylococcus aureus*	[120]
			Escherichia coli	
			Pseudomonas aeruginosa	
			Listeria monocytogenes	
Antibacterial	33-Residue peptide	*Dolabella auricularia*[l]	*Bacillus subtilis*	[240]
			Haemophilus influenzae	
			Vibrio vulnificus	
Antibacterial	Cationic peptides	*Hippoglossoides*	*Aeromonas salmonicida*	[241]
Antifungal		*platessoides*[m]	*Salmonella typhimurium*	
			Pseudomonas aeruginosa	
			Escherichia coli	
			Staphylococcus epidermidis	
			Candida albicans	
Antiparasitic	Peptides	*Dolabella auricularia*[l]	*Plasmodium falciparum*	[111]
Antibacterial	21-Residue peptides	*Arenicola marina*[n]	*Escherichia coli*	[242]
Antifungal			*Listeria monocytogenes*	
			Candida albicans	
Antibacterial	51-Residue peptide	*Perinereis aibuhitensis*[n]	*Escherichia coli*	[243]
Antifungal			*Pseudomonas aeruginosa*	
			Proteus vulgaris	
			Staphylococcus aureus	
			Bacillus megaterium	
			Micrococcus luteus	
			Aerococcus viridans	
			Paecilomyces heliothis	
Antiprotozoan	Peptides	*Mytilus*	*Trypanosoma brucei*	[244]
		galloprovincialis[o]	*Leishmania major*	
Antiviral	Depsipeptide	*Neamphius huxleyi*[e]	HIV	[245]
Antibacterial	Amphiphilic peptide	*Grammistes sexlineatus*[m]	*Bacillus subtilis*	[246]
			Staphylococcus aureus	
			Escherichia coli	

(continued)

TABLE 40.4 (continued)

Marine Compounds with Antibacterial, Antifungal, Anthelmintic, Antiprotozoal, and Antiviral Activities Reported between 2000 and 2012

Class[a]	Chemistry	Producing Organism	Effective Against[b]	Reference
Antifungal	Glycosylated lipopeptide	*Hassallia* sp.[g]	*Candida albicans*	[247]
			Aspergillus fumigatus	
Antiviral	Protein	*Griffithsia* sp.[c]	HIV	[248]
Antibacterial	Peptide	*Aurelia aurita*[q]	*Escherichia coli*	[249]
Antifungal	Heterodimeric peptide	*Halocynthia aurantium*[i]	*Candida albicans*	[108]
Antiviral	Cyclic depsipeptides	*Siliquariaspongia*	HIV	[250]
Antibacterial		*mirabilis*[e]	*Bacillus subtilis*	
Antifungal			*Candida albicans*	
Antibacterial	Nonribosomal peptides	*Brevibacillus*	*Streptococcus mutans*	[251]
Antifungal		*laterosporus*[g]	*Staphylococcus aureus*	
			Escherichia coli	
			Pseudomonas putrefaciens	
			Candida albicans	
Antibacterial	Lipopeptide	*Brevibacillus laterosporus*[g]	*Enterococcus* sp.	[252]
Antibacterial	Depsipeptides	*Photobacterium* MBIC06485[g]	*Pseudovibrio* sp.	[253]
Antioomycete (fungus-like)	Cyclic hybrid polyketide-peptide	*Paraliomyxa miuraensis*[g]	*Phytophthora capsici*	[254]
Antibacterial	Linear hybrid polyketide-nonribosomal peptide	*Rapidithrix* sp.[g]	*Brevibacterium* sp.	[255]
			Staphylococcus aureus	
			Bacillus subtilis	
Antiviral	Cyclic depsipeptides	*Homophymia* sp.[e]	HIV	[256]
Antibacterial	Cyclic depsipeptides	*Alternaria* sp.[d]	*Bacillus subtilis*	[257]
			Staphylococcus aureus	
Antiviral	Cyclic depsipeptides	*Theonella* sp.[e]	HIV	[258]
Antibacterial	Cyclic depsipeptides	*Callyspongia aerisuza*[e]	*Staphylococcus aureus*	[259]
Antifungal			*Bacillus subtilis*	
			Escherichia coli	
			Candida albicans	
Antibacterial	Aminolipopeptides	*Trichoderma* sp.[d]	*Mycobacterium smegmatis*	[260]
			Mycobacterium bovis	
			Mycobacterium tuberculosis	
Antibacterial	Aminolipopeptides	*Aspergillus sclerotiorum*[d]	*Candida albicans*	[261]
Antifungal			*Pseudomonas aeruginosa*	[262]
Antifungal	Cyclic lipopeptides	*Bacillus marinus*[g]	*Sclerotium* sp.	[263]
			Penicillium sp	
			Colletotrichum sp.	
Antifungal	Lipopeptides	*Bacillus amyloliquefaciens*[g]	*Fusarium oxysporum* f. sp. cucumerinum	[264]
			Fusarium graminearum	
			Fusarium oxysporum f. sp. vasinfectum	
			Fusarium oxysporum f. sp. cucumis melo L.	
			Fusarium graminearum f. sp. *zea mays* L.	

TABLE 40.4 (continued)

Marine Compounds with Antibacterial, Antifungal, Anthelmintic, Antiprotozoal, and Antiviral Activities Reported between 2000 and 2012

Class[a]	Chemistry	Producing Organism	Effective Against[b]	Reference
Antibacterial	Thiopeptide	*Nocardiopsis* sp.[g]	*Staphylococcus aureus*	[265]
			Staphylococcus haemolyticus	
			Staphylococcus epidermidis	
			Enterococcus faecalis	
			Streptococcus	
			Streptococcus pneumoniae	
Antibacterial Antifungal	Nonribosomal peptides	Cyanobacterial isolates[g]	*Bacillus subtilis*	[266]
			Salmonella typhimurium	
			Candida krusei	
Polyketides				
Antiparasitic	Lactone	*Plakortis* sp.[e]	*Plasmodium falciparum*	[267]
Antibacterial	Halogenated acetogenin	*Laurencia* sp.[c]	Marine bacteria isolated from algal habitats	[268]
Antibacterial	Macrolide	*Cladosporium herbarum*[d]	*Staphylococcus aureus* *Bacillus subtilis*	[269]
Antibacterial	Macrolide	*Streptomyces* sp.[g]	*Staphylococcus aureus*	[270]
Antibacterial	Pyrrolidinone derivatives	*Zopfiella latipes*[d]	*Arthrobacter citreus,* *Bacillus brevis*	[271]
			Bacillus subtilis	
			Bacillus licheniformis Corynebacterium insidiosum	
			Micrococcus luteus	
			Mycobacterium phlei Streptomyces sp.	
			Acinetobacter calcoaceticus	
Antifungal	Polyketide	*Bacillus laterosporus*[g]	*Candida albicans*	[272]
			Aspergillus fumigatus	
Antifungal	Polyacetylenic acids	*Petrosia corticata*[e]	*Candida albicans*	[273]
			Aspergillus fumigatus	
Antifungal	Calyculin derivative	*Theonella swinhoei*[e]	*Candida albicans*	[274]
			Aspergillus fumigatus	
Antifungal	Polyketide	*Keissleriella* sp.[d]	*Candida albicans*	[275]
			Tricophyton rubrum	
			Aspergillus niger	
Antifungal	Macrolide	*Hypoxylon oceanicum*[d]	*Neurospora crassa*	[276]
Antifungal	Macrolide	*Penicillium cf. montanense*[d]	*Candida albicans*	[277]
Antiparasitic	Macrolide	*Aigialus parvus*[d]	*Plasmodium falciparum*	[278]
Antibacterial Antifungal	Cyclic tetramic acid derivatives	*Melophlus sarassinorum*[e]	*Bacillus subtilis* *Staphylococcus aureus* *Candida albicans*	[279]
Antifungal	Polyketide	*Clavelina oblonga*[i]	*Candida albicans* *Candida glabrata*	[280]

(continued)

TABLE 40.4 (continued)

Marine Compounds with Antibacterial, Antifungal, Anthelmintic, Antiprotozoal, and Antiviral Activities Reported between 2000 and 2012

Class[a]	Chemistry	Producing Organism	Effective Against[b]	Reference
Antibacterial	Nitro-tetraene spiro-β-lactone-γ-lactam	*Streptomyces nodosus*[g]	*Staphylococcus aureus* *Streptococcus pneumoniae*	[281]
Antibacterial	Quinone-related	*Streptomycete* sp.[g]	*Bacillus subtilis*	[282]
Antifungal	Brominated cyclopropyl carboxylic acid	Cyanobacteria[g]	*Candida albicans*	[283]
Antiparasitic	Poliketide	Fungal origin[d]	*Plasmodium falciparum*	[284]
Antiparasitic	Polyketide cycloperoxides	*Plakortis simplex*[e]	*Plasmodium falciparum*	[285]
Antifungal	Bromo diphenyl ethers	*Dysidea herbacea*[e]	*Candida albicans* *Aspergillus niger*	[286]
Antifungal	Macrocyclic lactone polyether	*Hyrtios erecta*[e]	Fungicidal for the majority of 74 reference strains and clinical isolates	[113]
Antibacterial	Lactone	Brown alga endophytic fungus[d]	*Bacillus subtilis* *Staphylococcus aureus* *Salmonella enteritidis*	[287]
Antibacterial	Macrolide	Proposed genus: *Marinispora*[g]	*Staphylococcus aureus* *Enterococcus faecium*	[288]
Antibacterial	Bisanthraquinone	*Streptomycete* sp.[g]	*Staphylococcus aureus*	[289]
Antifungal	Macrolide	*Negombata magnifica*[e]	*Candida albicans*	[290]
Antiparasitic	Quinone	*Xestospongia* sp.[e]	*Plasmodium falciparum*	[291]
Antiprotozoal	Cyclic peroxides	*Plakortis* sp.[e]	*Leishmania mexicana*	[292]
Antiprotozoal	Polyol compound	*Amphidinium* sp.[c]	*Trichomonas foetus*	[293]
Antibacterial Antifungal	24-Membered macrolide	*Bacillus marinus*[g]	*Pyricularia oryzae* *Alternaria solani* *Staphylococcus aureus*	[294]
Antibacterial Antifungal	Polyene δ-lactone	*Bacillus marinus*[g]	*Pyricularia oryzae* *Alternaria solani* *Staphylococcus aureus*	[295]
Antibacterial Antifungal	Macrolide	*Eupenicillium* sp.[g]	*Bacillus subtilis* *Staphylococcus aureus* *Saccharomyces cerevisiae* *Sclerotinia sclerotiorum*	[296]
Antibacterial Antifungal	Macrolide	*Penicillium* sp.[g]	*Staphylococcus aureus* *Microsporum gypseum*	[297]
Antibacterial	Macrolide	*Nigrospora* sp.[d]	*Staphylococcus aureus*	[298] [299]
Antiparasitic	Halenaquinone-type polyketides	*Xestospongia* sp.[e]	*Plasmodium falciparum*	[300]
Antifungal	Macrolide	Sponge of the family Neopeltidae[e]	*Candida albicans*	[300]
Antifungal	Tricyclic polyketides	*Trichoderma koningii*[d]	*Candida albicans*	[301]

TABLE 40.4 (continued)

Marine Compounds with Antibacterial, Antifungal, Anthelmintic, Antiprotozoal, and Antiviral Activities Reported between 2000 and 2012

Class[a]	Chemistry	Producing Organism	Effective Against[b]	Reference
Fatty Acids				
Antiviral	Sulfated ceramides	*Discodermia calyx*[e]	Neuraminidase	[302]
Antiviral	Acetylenic fatty acid	*Petrosia* sp.[e]	RNA- and DNA-dependent DNA polymerase	[115]
Antibacterial Antifungal	Ceramides	*Sinularia grandilobata* Verseveldt[f]	*Bacillus pumilus* *Escherichia coli* *Pseudomonas aeruginosa* *Aspergillus niger* *Rhizopus oryzae* *Candida albicans*	[303]
Antifungal	Sphingolipid	*Aspergillus niger*[d]	*Candida albicans*	[304]
Antibacterial	Brominated unsaturated fatty acids	Sponge collected in Papua New Guinea[e]	*Staphylococcus aureus* *Streptococcus mutans* *Streptococcus sobrinus*	[305]
Antibacterial	Monounsaturated fatty acid Polyunsaturated fatty acid	*Phaeodactylum Tricornutum*[o]	*Listonella anguillarum* *Staphylococcus aureus*	[306]
Antibacterial	Acetylenic fatty acid	*Paragrantia* cf. *waguensis*[e]	*Staphylococcus aureus* *Escherichia coli*	[307]
Antibacterial	Brominated unsaturated fatty acids	*Siliquariaspongia* sp.[e]	*Staphylococcus aureus*	[308]
Antibacterial	Eicosapentaenoic acid	*Phaeodactylum Tricornutum*[o]	*Listonella anguillarum* *Micrococcus luteus* *Photobacterium* sp. *Planococcus citreus* *Bacillus cereus* *Bacillus weihenstephanensis* *Staphylococcus epidermidis* *Staphylococcus aureus*	[309]

[a] Antimicrobial effect tested. In most cases, this does not mean that the compound is ineffective against other types of microorganisms that are not indicated in the table, but that their effect has not been tested.

[b] The organisms listed in this column include those in which growth inhibition or a microbicidal effect was observed, in the case of bacteria, fungi, and protozoans. In the case of viruses, decrease in host infection and a direct effect on the replicative capacity of the viruses was observed.

[c] Alga.

[d] Fungus.

[e] Sponge.

[f] Coral.

[g] Bacterium.

[h] Sea cucumber.

[i] Tunicate.

[j] Ciliate.

[k] Sea grass.

[l] Sea hare.

[m] Fish.

[n] Polychaete.

[o] Bivalve.

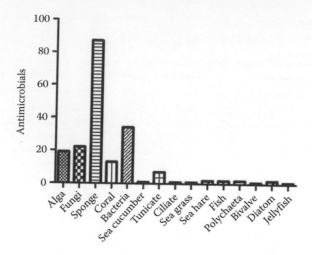

FIGURE 40.2   Number of antimicrobial molecular leads isolated from marine organisms between 2000 and 2012.

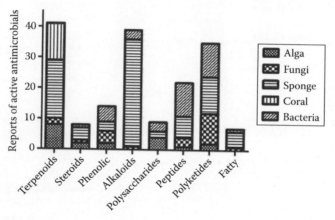

FIGURE 40.3   Molecular leads by type of compound isolated from algae, fungi, sponges, corals, and bacteria between 2000 and 2012.

40.4.1 Why Do We Need Novel Antibiotics and What Has Been Done?

Intensive use of antibiotics for human health and veterinary purposes has resulted in antimicrobial resistance; so, besides the fact that better use of existing antibiotics is advised, there is also the need to develop novel antibiotics. The development of this type of drugs is scarce since the pharmaceutical industry is not much interested in investing in research and development of novel antibiotics. These companies assume that a new antibiotic may be less profitable than drugs in other therapeutic areas, such as chronic diseases, possibly due to the low frequency of prescriptions for severe infections; the limited duration of use compared with drugs for chronic diseases; and possible appearance of resistance, with consequent shortening of clinical lifespan.

Among the three greatest threats to human health, the World Health Organization has identified anti-microbial resistance as one. Recent reports by the European Centre for Disease Prevention (ECDP) and the Infectious Diseases Society of America (IDSA) have highlighted that there are few candidate drugs in the pipeline that offer benefits over existing drugs (http://www.ecdc.europa.eu/en/healthtopics/Pages/Antimicrobial_Resistance.aspx; http://www.idsociety.org/topic_antimicrobial_resistance/). To tackle this problem, the European Union has proposed innovative incentives to keep research for new antibiotics going (http://www.consilium.europa.eu/uedocs/cms_data/docs/pressdata/en/lsa/111608.pdf). Similarly, the IDSA has developed the 10×20 initiative[121] for the development of 10 new antibiotics by 2020 (http://www.idsociety.org/10x20/).

Since most antibiotics currently in use are of terrestrial origin, and screening projects mainly focus on samples from terrestrial environments, there is a low probability of finding novel antibiotics from the same type of environments. The search for novel organisms, which have evolved novel metabolisms that produce chemical weaponry through continuous evolution in an environment polluted with infectious agents, in order to find novel antimicrobial molecules, seems reasonable. The greatest reservoirs of such organisms are the oceans, and so focusing on this environment appears to be a good approach.

40.5 Final Considerations

Even though many molecules isolated from marine organisms could be of pharmaceutical interest, as shown in this chapter, the main challenges for the pharmaceutical development of these compounds are many. Among these, availability and secure access to the marine resources; property rights and intellectual property; quality of the marine resources (identification and variability); the technology used for screening active compounds, preventing repeated rediscovery; and the structural costs of drug isolation from marine products are most important. Lack of taxonomic knowledge of marine species can lead to unnecessary recollection of particular species. It can also make it difficult to target the recollection of a particular species when it is required for further study. To increase the efficiency of marine biodiscovery, classical and DNA-based methods should be applied. As briefly mentioned earlier in the chapter, besides the taxonomy problem, the same marine organism can produce different secondary metabolites in different locations. This adds a difficulty at the time of recollecting specimens to isolate material for follow-up studies, and represents an important complication when trying to culture these organisms on a large scale to obtain a desired metabolite. This supply issue makes it necessary to intensify the development of methods to cultivate marine organisms under bioactive-producing conditions. To avoid the cultivation of bioactive-producing marine organisms, methods to find, identify, clone, and genetically manipulate complex biosynthetic pathways will have to be applied to produce the bioactives under controlled conditions and to speed up the processes. This technological advance would also provide a more stable source of the desired metabolite.

The European Science Foundation made several recommendations to improve the biodiscovery of novel marine-derived biomolecules and the development of new tools and approaches for human health; these are: simplification of access- and benefit-sharing agreements through Europe and its territories through the development of a common template agreement that should not be limited to Europe but should be addressed at the international level; resolution of the conflict between the UN Convention on Laws of the Sea and intellectual property rights; development of a legal framework to bring functional products to the market safely, quickly, and at low cost; increased focus on the taxonomy, systematics, physiology, molecular genetics, and ecology of marine species, with greater emphasis on organisms from unusual and extreme environments, to increase the chances of success in finding novel bioactives; improvement in the technical aspects of the biodiscovery pipeline so that marine derived compounds could be acceptable to the pharmaceutical industry; maintaining sustained supply, focus on integrated development of aquaculture, tissue culture, microbial isolation/culture, chemical synthesis/semi-synthesis, molecular genetics, and the availability of appropriate central resources for scale-up by these methods; and development of appropriate measures to strengthen the focus on marine environments.[122] These recommendations give an idea of the complexity that surrounds the process of isolating an active compound from a given marine organism, proving its effectiveness in several known human pathologies or pathogens, and then developing it for industrial production, which should assure sustained supply of the active molecule.

REFERENCES

1. Carté, B. K., 1996. Biomedical potential of marine natural products. *BioScience*, 46, 271–286.
2. Essack, M., Bajic, V. B., and Archer, J. A., 2012. Conotoxins that confer therapeutic possibilities. *Mar Drugs*, 10, 1244–1265.
3. Nunnery, J. K., Mevers, E., and Gerwick, W. H., 2010. Biologically active secondary metabolites from marine cyanobacteria. *Curr Opin Biotechnol*, 21, 787–793.

4. Ferlay, J., Shin, H. R., Bray, F., Forman, D., Mathers, C., and Parkin, D. M., 2010. GLOBOCAN 2008 v2.0, *Cancer Incidence and Mortality Worldwide: IARC CancerBase No. 10 [Internet]*, Lyon, France: International Agency for Research on Cancer.
5. Schwartsmann, G., Brondani da Rocha, A., Berlinck, R. G., and Jimeno, J., 2001. Marine organisms as a source of new anticancer agents. *Lancet Oncol*, 2, 221–225.
6. Prakasha Gowda, A. S., Polizzi, J. M., Eckert, K. A., and Spratt, T. E., 2010. Incorporation of gemcitabine and cytarabine into DNA by DNA polymerase beta and ligase III/XRCC1. *Biochemistry*, 49, 4833–4840.
7. Singh, R., Sharma, M., Joshi, P., and Rawat, D. S., 2008. Clinical status of anti-cancer agents derived from marine sources. *Anticancer Agents Med Chem*, 8, 603–617.
8. Mahdi, E. and Fariba, K., 2012. Cancer treatment with using cyanobacteria and suitable drug delivery system. *Ann Biol Res*, 3, 622–627.
9. Soares, D. G., Escargueil, A. E., Poindessous, V. et al., 2007. Replication and homologous recombination repair regulate DNA double-strand break formation by the antitumor alkylator ecteinascidin 743. *Proc Natl Acad Sci USA*, 104, 13062–13067.
10. Pommier, Y., Kohlhagen, G., Bailly, C., Waring, M., Mazumder, A., and Kohn, K. W., 1996. DNA sequence- and structure-selective alkylation of guanine N2 in the DNA minor groove by ecteinascidin 743, a potent antitumor compound from the Caribbean tunicate *Ecteinascidia turbinata*. *Biochemistry*, 35, 13303–13309.
11. EMA, European Medicines Agency. http://www.ema.europa.eu/ema/.
12. Leal, J. F., Martinez-Diez, M., Garcia-Hernandez, V. et al., 2010. PM01183, a new DNA minor groove covalent binder with potent *in vitro* and *in vivo* anti-tumour activity. *Br J Pharmacol*, 161, 1099–1110.
13. Soares, D. G., Machado, M. S., Rocca, C. J. et al., 2011. Trabectedin and its C subunit modified analogue PM01183 attenuate nucleotide excision repair and show activity toward platinum-resistant cells. *Mol Cancer Ther*, 10, 1481–1489.
14. Berton-Rigaud, D., Alexandre, J., Provansal, M. et al., 2012. Lurbinectedin (PM01183) activity in platinum-resistant/refractory ovarian cancer patients. Preliminary results of an ongoing two-stage phase II study, in *37th Congress of the European Society of Molecular Oncology (ESMO)*, Vienna, Austria.
15. McBride, A. and Butler, S. K., 2012. Eribulin mesylate: A novel halichondrin B analogue for the treatment of metastatic breast cancer. *Am J Health Syst Pharm*, 69, 745–755.
16. Jordan, M. A., Kamath, K., Manna, T. et al., 2005. The primary antimitotic mechanism of action of the synthetic halichondrin E7389 is suppression of microtubule growth. *Mol Cancer Ther*, 4, 1086–1095.
17. Gajate, C., An, F., and Mollinedo, F., 2003. Rapid and selective apoptosis in human leukemic cells induced by Aplidine through a Fas/CD95- and mitochondrial-mediated mechanism. *Clin Cancer Res*, 9, 1535–1545.
18. Taraboletti, G., Poli, M., Dossi, R. et al., 2004. Antiangiogenic activity of Aplidine, a new agent of marine origin. *Br J Cancer*, 90, 2418–2424.
19. Jiang, T. L., Liu, R. H., and Salmon, S. E., 1983. Antitumor activity of didemnin B in the human tumor stem cell assay. *Cancer Chemother Pharmacol*, 11, 1–4.
20. Lee, J., Currano, J. N., Carroll, P. J., and Joullie, M. M., 2012. Didemnins, tamandarins and related natural products. *Nat Prod Rep*, 29, 404–424.
21. SirDeshpande, B. V. and Toogood, P. L., 1995. Mechanism of protein synthesis inhibition by didemnin B *in vitro*. *Biochemistry*, 34, 9177–9184.
22. Johnson, K. L., Grubb, D. R., and Lawen, A., 1999. Unspecific activation of caspases during the induction of apoptosis by didemnin B in human cell lines. *J Cell Biochem*, 72, 269–278.
23. Chun, H. G., Davies, B., Hoth, D. et al., 1986. Didemnin B. The first marine compound entering clinical trials as an antineoplastic agent. *Invest New Drugs*, 4, 279–284.
24. Kucuk, O., Young, M. L., Habermann, T. M., Wolf, B. C., Jimeno, J., and Cassileth, P.A., 2000. Phase II trail of didemnin B in previously treated non-Hodgkin's lymphoma: an Eastern Cooperative Oncology Group (ECOG) Study. *Am J Clin Oncol*, 23, 273–277.
25. Sondak, V. K., Kopecky, K. J., Liu, P. Y., Fletcher, W. S., Harvey, W. H., and Laufman, L. R., 1994. Didemnin B in metastatic malignant melanoma: A phase II trial of the Southwest Oncology Group. *Anticancer Drugs*, 5, 147–150.
26. Ma, X. and Wang, Z., 2009. Anticancer drug discovery in the future: An evolutionary perspective. *Drug Discov Today*, 14, 1136–1142.

27. Kim, H., Han, S. H., Quan, H. Y. et al., 2012. Bryostatin-1 promotes long-term potentiation via activation of PKCalpha and PKCepsilon in the hippocampus. *Neuroscience*, 226, 348–355.

28. Ramsdell, J. S., Pettit, G. R., and Tashjian, A. H. Jr., 1986. Three activators of protein kinase C, bryostatins, dioleins, and phorbol esters, show differing specificities of action on GH4 pituitary cells. *J Biol Chem*, 261, 17073–17080.

29. DeChristopher, B. A., Loy, B. A., Marsden, M. D., Schrier, A. J., Zack, J. A., and Wender, P. A., 2012. Designed, synthetically accessible bryostatin analogues potently induce activation of latent HIV reservoirs *in vitro*. *Nat Chem*, 4, 705–710.

30. Sun, M. K. and Alkon, D. L., 2006. Bryostatin-1: Pharmacology and therapeutic potential as a CNS drug. *CNS Drug Rev*, 12, 1–8.

31. Bài, R., Pettit, G. R., and Hamel, E., 1990. Dolastatin 10, a powerful cytostatic peptide derived from a marine animal. Inhibition of tubulin polymerization mediated through the vinca alkaloid binding domain. *Biochem Pharmacol*, 39, 1941–1949.

32. Kavallaris, M., Verrills, N. M., and Hill, B. T., 2001. Anticancer therapy with novel tubulin-interacting drugs. *Drug Resist Updat*, 4, 392–401.

33. Vaishampayan, U., Glode, M., Du, W. et al., 2000. Phase II study of dolastatin-10 in patients with hormone-refractory metastatic prostate adenocarcinoma. *Clin Cancer Res*, 6, 4205–4208.

34. Rao, K. V., Na, M. K., Cook, J. C., Peng, J., Matsumoto, R., and Hamann, M. T., 2008. Kahalalides V-Y isolated from a Hawaiian collection of the sacoglossan mollusk *Elysia rufescens*. *J Nat Prod*, 71, 772–778.

35. Garcia-Rocha, M., Bonay, P., and Avila, J., 1996. The antitumoral compound Kahalalide F acts on cell lysosomes. *Cancer Lett*, 99, 43–50.

36. Sewell, J. M., Mayer, I., Langdon, S. P., Smyth, J. F., Jodrell, D. I., and Guichard, S. M., 2005. The mechanism of action of Kahalalide F: Variable cell permeability in human hepatoma cell lines. *Eur J Cancer*, 41, 1637–1644.

37. Janmaat, M. L., Rodriguez, J. A., Jimeno, J., Kruyt, F. A., and Giaccone, G., 2005. Kahalalide F induces necrosis-like cell death that involves depletion of ErbB3 and inhibition of Akt signaling. *Mol Pharmacol*, 68, 502–510.

38. Martin-Algarra, S., Espinosa, E., Rubio, J. et al., 2009. Phase II study of weekly Kahalalide F in patients with advanced malignant melanoma. *Eur J Cancer*, 45, 732–735.

39. Shilabin, A. G. and Hamann, M. T., 2011. *In vitro* and *in vivo* evaluation of select kahalalide F analogs with antitumor and antifungal activities. *Bioorg Med Chem*, 19, 6628–6632.

40. Kim, D., Lee, I. S., Jung, J. H., Lee, C. O., and Choi, S. U., 1999. Psammaplin A, a natural phenolic compound, has inhibitory effect on human topoisomerase II and is cytotoxic to cancer cells. *Anticancer Res*, 19, 4085–4090.

41. Shim, J. S., Lee, H. S., Shin, J., and Kwon, H. J., 2004. Psammaplin A, a marine natural product, inhibits aminopeptidase N and suppresses angiogenesis *in vitro*. *Cancer Lett*, 203, 163–169.

42. de la Rosa, L. A., Alfonso, A., Vilarino, N., Vieytes, M. R., and Botana, L. M., 2001. Modulation of cytosolic calcium levels of human lymphocytes by yessotoxin, a novel marine phycotoxin. *Biochem Pharmacol*, 61, 827–833.

43. Korsnes, M. S., 2012. Yessotoxin as a tool to study induction of multiple cell death pathways. *Toxins (Basel)*, 4, 568–579.

44. Alfonso, A., de la Rosa, L., Vieytes, M. R., Yasumoto, T., and Botana, L. M., 2003. Yessotoxin, a novel phycotoxin, activates phosphodiesterase activity. Effect of yessotoxin on cAMP levels in human lymphocytes. *Biochem Pharmacol*, 65, 193–208.

45. Elmore, S., 2007. Apoptosis: A review of programmed cell death. *Toxicol Pathol*, 35, 495–516.

46. Leira, F., Alvarez, C., Vieites, J. M., Vieytes, M. R., and Botana, L. M., 2002. Characterization of distinct apoptotic changes induced by okadaic acid and yessotoxin in the BE(2)-M17 neuroblastoma cell line. *Toxicol In Vitro*, 16, 23–31.

47. Catterall, W. A., 2000. From ionic currents to molecular mechanisms: The structure and function of voltage-gated sodium channels. *Neuron*, 26, 13–25.

48. Hille, B., 1975. The receptor for tetrodotoxin and saxitoxin. A structural hypothesis. *Biophys J*, 15, 615–619.

49. Catterall, W. A., Goldin, A. L., and Waxman, S. G., 2005. International Union of Pharmacology. XLVII. Nomenclature and structure–function relationships of voltage-gated sodium channels. *Pharmacol Rev*, 57, 397–409.

50. Wood, J. N., Boorman, J. P., Okuse, K., and Baker, M. D., 2004. Voltage-gated sodium channels and pain pathways. *J Neurobiol*, 61, 55–71.

51. Ragsdale, D. S., McPhee, J. C., Scheuer, T., and Catterall, W. A., 1996. Common molecular determinants of local anesthetic, antiarrhythmic, and anticonvulsant block of voltage-gated Na$^+$ channels. *Proc Natl Acad Sci USA*, 93, 9270–9275.

52. Amin, A. S., Asghari-Roodsari, A., and Tan, H. L., 2010. Cardiac sodium channelopathies. *Pflugers Arch*, 460, 223–237.

53. Kullmann, D. M. and Waxman, S. G., 2010. Neurological channelopathies: New insights into disease mechanisms and ion channel function. *J Physiol*, 588, 1823–1827.

54. Shi, X., Yasumoto, S., Nakagawa, E., Fukasawa, T., Uchiya, S., and Hirose, S., 2009. Missense mutation of the sodium channel gene SCN2A causes Dravet syndrome. *Brain Dev*, 31, 758–762.

55. Nieto, F. R., Cobos, E. J., Tejada, M. A., Sanchez-Fernandez, C., Gonzalez-Cano, R., and Cendan, C. M., 2012. Tetrodotoxin (TTX) as a therapeutic agent for pain. *Mar Drugs*, 10, 281–305.

56. Knapp, O., McArthur, J. R., and Adams, D. J., 2012. Conotoxins targeting neuronal voltage-gated sodium channel subtypes: Potential analgesics? *Toxins (Basel)*, 4, 1236–1260.

57. Lombet, A., Bidard, J. N., and Lazdunski, M., 1987. Ciguatoxin and brevetoxins share a common receptor site on the neuronal voltage-dependent Na$^+$ channel. *FEBS Lett*, 219, 355–359.

58. Baden, D. G., Abraham, W. M., and Bourdelais, A. J., 2005. Polyether brevetoxin derivatives as a treatment for cystic fibrosis, mucociliary dysfunction and pulmonary diseases. WO2005028482 (A1).

59. Taupin, P., 2009. Brevetoxin derivative compounds for stimulating neuronal growth: University of North Carolina at Wilmington: WO2008131411. *Expert Opin Ther Pat*, 19, 269–274.

60. Wulff, H. and Zhorov, B. S., 2008. K$^+$ channel modulators for the treatment of neurological disorders and autoimmune diseases. *Chem Rev*, 108, 1744–1773.

61. Yu, S. P., Yeh, C. H., Sensi, S. L. et al., 1997. Mediation of neuronal apoptosis by enhancement of outward potassium current. *Science*, 278, 114–117.

62. Yu, S. P., Farhangrazi, Z. S., Ying, H. S., Yeh, C. H., and Choi, D. W., 1998. Enhancement of outward potassium current may participate in beta-amyloid peptide-induced cortical neuronal death. *Neurobiol Dis*, 5, 81–88.

63. Alonso, E., Fuwa, H., Vale, C. et al., 2012. Design and synthesis of skeletal analogues of gambierol: Attenuation of amyloid-beta and tau pathology with voltage-gated potassium channel and *N*-methyl-D-aspartate receptor implications. *J Am Chem Soc*, 134, 7467–7479.

64. Botana Lopez, L. M., Alonso Lopez, E., Vale Gonzalez C., 2011. Use of gambierol for treating and/or preventing neurodegenerative diseases related to tau and beta-amyloid. WO2011/051521 A2. 05.05.2011.

65. Fuwa, H., Kainuma, N., Tachibana, K., Tsukano, C., Satake, M., and Sasaki, M., 2004. Diverted total synthesis and biological evaluation of gambierol analogues: Elucidation of crucial structural elements for potent toxicity. *Chemistry*, 10, 4894–4909.

66. Fuwa, H., Kainuma, N., Tachibana, K., and Sasaki, M., 2002. Total synthesis of (−)-gambierol. *J Am Chem Soc*, 124, 14983–14992.

67. Rivier, J., Galyean, R., Gray, W. R. et al., 1987. Neuronal calcium channel inhibitors. Synthesis of omega-conotoxin GVIA and effects on 45Ca uptake by synaptosomes. *J Biol Chem*, 262, 1194–1198.

68. Vink, S. and Alewood, P. F., 2012. Targeting voltage-gated calcium channels: Developments in peptide and small-molecule inhibitors for the treatment of neuropathic pain. *Br J Pharmacol*, 167, 970–989.

69. Buckingham, S. D., Jones, A. K., Brown, L. A., and Sattelle, D. B., 2009. Nicotinic acetylcholine receptor signalling: Roles in Alzheimer's disease and amyloid neuroprotection. *Pharmacol Rev*, 61, 39–61.

70. Quik, M., Bordia, T., Huang, L., and Perez, X., 2011. Targeting nicotinic receptors for Parkinson's disease therapy. *CNS Neurol Disord Drug Targets*, 10, 651–658.

71. Marquis, K. L., Comery, T. A., Jow, F. et al., 2011. Preclinical assessment of an adjunctive treatment approach for cognitive impairment associated with schizophrenia using the alpha7 nicotinic acetylcholine receptor agonist WYE-103914/SEN34625. *Psychopharmacology (Berl)*, 218, 635–647.

72. Vincler, M., Wittenauer, S., Parker, R., Ellison, M., Olivera, B. M., and McIntosh, J. M., 2006. Molecular mechanism for analgesia involving specific antagonism of alpha9alpha10 nicotinic acetylcholine receptors. *Proc Natl Acad Sci USA*, 103, 17880–17884.

73. Raiteri, M., Marchi, M., and Paudice, P., 1990. Presynaptic muscarinic receptors in the central nervous system. *Ann N Y Acad Sci*, 604, 113–129.

74. Langmead, C. J., Watson, J., and Reavill, C., 2008. Muscarinic acetylcholine receptors as CNS drug targets. *Pharmacol Ther*, 117, 232–243.

75. Gill, S., Murphy, M., Clausen, J. et al., 2003. Neural injury biomarkers of novel shellfish toxins, spirolides: A pilot study using immunochemical and transcriptional analysis. *Neurotoxicology*, 24, 593–604.

76. Wandscheer, C. B., Vilarino, N., Espina, B., Louzao, M. C., and Botana, L. M., 2010. Human muscarinic acetylcholine receptors are a target of the marine toxin 13-desmethyl C spirolide. *Chem Res Toxicol*, 23, 1753–1761.

77. Hauser, T. A., Hepler, C. D., Kombo, D. C. et al., 2012. Comparison of acetylcholine receptor interactions of the marine toxins, 13-desmethylspirolide C and gymnodimine. *Neuropharmacology*, 62, 2239–2250.

78. Alonso, E., Otero, P., Vale, C. et al., 2013. Benefit of 13-desmethyl spirolide C treatment in triple transgenic mouse model of Alzheimer disease: Beta-amyloid and neuronal markers improvement. *Curr Alzheimer Res*, 10, 279–289.

79. Alonso, E., Vale, C., Vieytes, M. R., Laferla, F. M., Gimenez-Llort, L., and Botana, L. M., 2011. 13-Desmethyl spirolide-C is neuroprotective and reduces intracellular Abeta and hyperphosphorylated tau *in vitro*. *Neurochem Int*, 59, 1056–1065.

80. Alonso, E., Vale, C., Vieytes, M. R., Laferla, F. M., Gimenez-Llort, L., and Botana, L. M., 2011. The cholinergic antagonist gymnodimine improves Abeta and tau neuropathology in an *in vitro* model of Alzheimer disease. *Cell Physiol Biochem*, 27, 783–794.

81. Hone, A. J., Scadden, M., Gajewiak, J., Christensen, S., Lindstrom, J., and McIntosh, J. M., 2012. Alpha-conotoxin PeIA[S9H,V10A,E14N] potently and selectively blocks alpha6beta2beta3 versus alpha6beta4 nicotinic acetylcholine receptors. *Mol Pharmacol*, 82, 972–982.

82. Kem, W. R., Scott, K. N., and Duncan, J. H., 1976. Hoplonemertine worms—A new source of pyridine neurotoxins. *Experientia*, 32, 684–686.

83. Zawieja, P., Kornprobst, J. M., and Metais, P., 2012. 3-(2,4-Dimethoxybenzylidene)-anabaseine: A promising candidate drug for Alzheimer's disease? *Geriatr Gerontol Int*, 12, 365–371.

84. Mayer, M. L., Westbrook, G. L., and Guthrie, P. B., 1984. Voltage-dependent block by Mg^{2+} of NMDA responses in spinal cord neurones. *Nature*, 309, 261–263.

85. Bakchine, S. and Loft, H., 2007. Memantine treatment in patients with mild to moderate Alzheimer's disease: Results of a randomised, double-blind, placebo-controlled 6-month study. *J Alzheimers Dis*, 11, 471–479.

86. Gauthier, S., Wirth, Y., and Mobius, H. J., 2005. Effects of memantine on behavioural symptoms in Alzheimer's disease patients: An analysis of the Neuropsychiatric Inventory (NPI) data of two randomised, controlled studies. *Int J Geriatr Psychiatry*, 20, 459–464.

87. Malmberg, A. B., Gilbert, H., McCabe, R. T., and Basbaum, A. I., 2003. Powerful antinociceptive effects of the cone snail venom-derived subtype-selective NMDA receptor antagonists conantokins G and T. *Pain*, 101, 109–116.

88. Craig, A. G., Norberg, T., Griffin, D. et al., 1999. Contulakin-G, an *O*-glycosylated invertebrate neurotensin. *J Biol Chem*, 274, 13752–13759.

89. Laport, M. S., Santos, O. C., and Muricy, G., 2009. Marine sponges: Potential sources of new antimicrobial drugs. *Curr Pharm Biotechnol*, 10, 86–105.

90. Mayer, A. M., Glaser, K. B., Cuevas, C. et al., 2010. The odyssey of marine pharmaceuticals: A current pipeline perspective. *Trends Pharmacol Sci*, 31, 255–265.

91. Demain, A. L., 2009. Antibiotics: Natural products essential to human health. *Med Res Rev*, 29, 821–842.

92. Ruggieri, G. D., 1976. Drugs from the sea. *Science*, 194, 491–497.

93. Colwell, R. R., 2002. Fulfilling the promise of biotechnology. *Biotechnol Adv*, 20, 215–228.

94. Faulkner, D. J., 2002. Marine natural products. *Nat Prod Rep*, 19, 1–48.

95. Haefner, B., 2003. Drugs from the deep: Marine natural products as drug candidates. *Drug Discov Today*, 8, 536–544.

96. Jha, R. K. and Zi-rong, X., 2004. Biomedical compounds from marine organisms. *Mar Drugs*, 2, 123–146.

97. Jimeno, J., Lopez-Martin, J. A., Ruiz-Casado, A., Izquierdo, M. A., Scheuer, P. J., and Rinehart, K., 2004. Progress in the clinical development of new marine-derived anticancer compounds. *Anticancer Drugs*, 15, 321–329.

98. Molinski, T. F., Dalisay, D. S., Lievens, S. L., and Saludes, J. P., 2009. Drug development from marine natural products. *Nat Rev Drug Discov*, 8, 69–85.

99. Munro, M. H., Blunt, J. W., Dumdei, E. J. et al., 1999. The discovery and development of marine compounds with pharmaceutical potential. *J Biotechnol*, 70, 15–25.
100. Proksch, P., Edrada, R. A., and Ebel, R., 2002. Drugs from the seas—Current status and microbiological implications. *Appl Microbiol Biotechnol*, 59, 125–134.
101. Mayer, A. M. and Lehmann, V. K. B., 2000. Marine pharmacology. *Pharmacologist*, 42, 62–69.
102. Sagar, S., Kaur, M., and Minneman, K. P., 2010. Antiviral lead compounds from marine sponges. *Mar Drugs*, 8, 2619–2638.
103. Cardozo, K. H., Guaratini, T., Barros, M. P. et al., 2007. Metabolites from algae with economical impact. *Comp Biochem Physiol C Toxicol Pharmacol*, 146, 60–78.
104. Nair, R., Chabhadiya, R., and Chanda, S., 2007. Marine algae: Screening for a potent antibacterial agent. *J Herb Pharmacother*, 7, 73–86.
105. Cabrita, M. T., Vale, C., and Rauter, A. P., 2010. Halogenated compounds from marine algae. *Mar Drugs*, 8, 2301–2317.
106. Tan, L. T., 2007. Bioactive natural products from marine cyanobacteria for drug discovery. *Phytochemistry*, 68, 954–979.
107. Isnansetyo, A. and Kamei, Y., 2003. MC21-A, a bactericidal antibiotic produced by a new marine bacterium, *Pseudoalteromonas phenolica* sp. nov. O-BC30(T), against methicillin-resistant *Staphylococcus aureus*. *Antimicrob Agents Chemother*, 47, 480–488.
108. Jang, W. S., Kim, H. K., Lee, K. Y., Kim, S. A., Han, Y. S., and Lee, I. H., 2006. Antifungal activity of synthetic peptide derived from halocidin, antimicrobial peptide from the tunicate, *Halocynthia aurantium*. *FEBS Lett*, 580, 1490–1496.
109. Jacob, M. R., Hossain, C. F., Mohammed, K. A. et al., 2003. Reversal of fluconazole resistance in multidrug efflux-resistant fungi by the *Dysidea arenaria* sponge sterol 9alpha,11alpha-epoxycholest-7-ene-3beta,5alpha,6alpha,19-tetrol 6-acetate. *J Nat Prod*, 66, 1618–1622.
110. Li, X. C., Jacob, M. R., Ding, Y. et al., 2006. Capisterones A and B, which enhance fluconazole activity in *Saccharomyces cerevisiae*, from the marine green alga *Penicillus capitatus*. *J Nat Prod*, 69, 542–546.
111. Fennell, B. J., Carolan, S., Pettit, G. R., and Bell, A., 2003. Effects of the antimitotic natural product dolastatin 10, and related peptides, on the human malarial parasite *Plasmodium falciparum*. *J Antimicrob Chemother*, 51, 833–841.
112. Mizuno, Y., Makioka, A., Kawazu, S. et al., 2002. Effect of jasplakinolide on the growth, invasion, and actin cytoskeleton of *Plasmodium falciparum*. *Parasitol Res*, 88, 844–848.
113. Pettit, R. K., Woyke, T., Pon, S., Cichacz, Z. A., Pettit, G. R., and Herald, C. L., 2005. *In vitro* and *in vivo* antifungal activities of the marine sponge constituent spongistatin. *Med Mycol*, 43, 453–463.
114. de Souza Pereira, H., Leao-Ferreira, L. R., Moussatche, N. et al., 2005. Effects of diterpenes isolated from the Brazilian marine alga *Dictyota menstrualis* on HIV-1 reverse transcriptase. *Planta Med*, 71, 1019–1024.
115. Loya, S., Rudi, A., Kashman, Y., and Hizi, A., 2002. Mode of inhibition of HIV-1 reverse transcriptase by polyacetylenetriol, a novel inhibitor of RNA- and DNA-directed DNA polymerases. *Biochem J*, 362, 685–692.
116. Rowley, D. C., Hansen, M. S., Rhodes, D. et al., 2002. Thalassiolins A–C: New marine-derived inhibitors of HIV cDNA integrase. *Bioorg Med Chem*, 10, 3619–3625.
117. de Oliveira, J. H., Grube, A., Kock, M. et al., 2004. Ingenamine G and cyclostellettamines G–I, K, and L from the new Brazilian species of marine sponge *Pachychalina* sp. *J Nat Prod*, 67, 1685–1689.
118. Jang, K. H., Kang, G. W., Jeon, J. E. et al., 2009. Haliclonin A, a new macrocyclic diamide from the sponge *Haliclona* sp. *Org Lett*, 11, 1713–1716.
119. Linington, R. G., Robertson, M., Gauthier, A., Finlay, B. B., van Soest, R., and Andersen, R. J., 2002. Caminoside A, an antimicrobial glycolipid isolated from the marine sponge *Caminus sphaeroconia*. *Org Lett*, 4, 4089–4092.
120. Tincu, J. A., Menzel, L. P., Azimov, R. et al., 2003. Plicatamide, an antimicrobial octapeptide from *Styela plicata hemocytes*. *J Biol Chem*, 278, 13546–13553.
121. Gilbert, D. N., Guidos, R. J., Boucher, H. W. et al., 2010. The 10 × '20 Initiative: Pursuing a global commitment to develop 10 new antibacterial drugs by 2020. *Clin Infect Dis*, 50, 1081–1083.
122. Querellou, J., 2010. Marine biotechnology: A new vision and strategy for Europe, in Marine Board-ESF Position Paper 15, Børresen, T., Boyen, C., Dobson, A. et al., eds., European Science Foundation, Beernem, Belgium.

123. Suzuki, M., Daitoh, M., Vairappan, C. S., Abe, T., and Masuda, M., 2001. Novel halogenated metabolites from the Malaysian *Laurencia pannosa*. *J Nat Prod*, 64, 597–602.

124. Murray, A., Muniain, C., Seldes, A., and Maier, M., 2001. Patagonicoside A: A novel antifungal disulfated triterpene glycoside from the sea cucumber *Psolus patagonicus*. *Tetrahedron*, 57, 9563–9568.

125. Chinworrungsee, M., Kittakoop, P., Isaka, M., Rungrod, A., Tanticharoen, M., and Thebtaranonth, Y., 2001. Antimalarial halorosellinic acid from the marine fungus *Halorosellinia oceanica*. *Bioorg Med Chem Lett*, 11, 1965–1969.

126. Rodriguez, A. D. and Ramirez, C., 2001. Serrulatane diterpenes with antimycobacterial activity isolated from the West Indian sea whip *Pseudopterogorgia elisabethae*. *J Nat Prod*, 64, 100–102.

127. El Sayed, K. A., Yousaf, M., Hamann, M. T., Avery, M. A., Kelly, M., and Wipf, P., 2002. Microbial and chemical transformation studies of the bioactive marine sesquiterpenes (*S*)-(+)-curcuphenol and -curcudiol isolated from a deep reef collection of the Jamaican sponge *Didiscus oxeata*. *J Nat Prod*, 65, 1547–1553.

128. Peng, J., Walsh, K., Weedman, V. et al., 2002. The new bioactive diterpenes cyanthiwigins E–AA from the Jamaican sponge *Myrmekioderma styx*. *Tetrahedron*, 58, 7809–7819.

129. Ospina, C. A., Rodriguez, A. D., Ortega-Barria, E., and Capson, T. L., 2003. Briarellins J–P and polyanthellin A: New eunicellin-based diterpenes from the gorgonian coral *Briareum polyanthes* and their antimalarial activity. *J Nat Prod*, 66, 357–363.

130. Rodriguez, II and Rodriguez, A. D., 2003. Homopseudopteroxazole, a new antimycobacterial diterpene alkaloid from *Pseudopterogorgia elisabethae*. *J Nat Prod*, 66, 855–857.

131. Bugni, T., Singh, M., Chen, L. et al., 2004. Kalihinols from two *Acanthella cavernosa* sponges: Inhibitors of bacterial folate biosynthesis. *Tetrahedron*, 60, 6981–6988.

132. Namikoshi, M., Suzuki, S., Meguro, S. et al., 2004. Manoalide derivatives from a marine sponge *Luffariella* sp collected in Palau. *Fisheries Sci*, 70, 152–158.

133. Ata, A., Win, H., Holt, D., Holloway, P., Segstro, E., and Jayatilake, G., 2004. New antibacterial diterpenes from *Pseudopterogorgia elisabethae*. *Helvetica Chimica Acta*, 87, 1090–1098.

134. Satitpatipan, V. and Suwanborirux, K., 2004. New nitrogenous germacranes from a Thai marine sponge, *Axinyssa n*.sp. *J Nat Prod*, 67, 503–505.

135. Ankisetty, S., Amsler, C. D., McClintock, J. B., and Baker, B. J., 2004. Further membranolide diterpenes from the antarctic sponge *Dendrilla membranosa*. *J Nat Prod*, 67, 1172–1174.

136. Rifai, S., Fassouane, A., Kijjoa, A., and Van Soest, R., 2004. Antimicrobial activity of Untenospongin B, a metabolite from the marine sponge *Hippospongia communis* collected from the Atlantic Coast of Morocco. *Mar Drugs*, 2, 147–153.

137. Marrero, J., Rodriguez, A. D., Baran, P. et al., 2004. Bielschowskysin, a gorgonian-derived biologically active diterpene with an unprecedented carbon skeleton. *Org Lett*, 6, 1661–1664.

138. Wei, X., Rodriguez, A., Baran, P. et al., 2004. Antiplasmodial cembradiene diterpenoids from a Southwestern Caribbean gorgonian octocoral of the genus *Eunicea*. *Tetrahedron*, 60, 11813–11819.

139. Savoia, D., Avanzini, C., Allice, T., Callone, E., Guella, G., and Dini, F., 2004. Antimicrobial activity of euplotin C, the sesquiterpene taxonomic marker from the marine ciliate *Euplotes crassus*. *Antimicrob Agents Chemother*, 48, 3828–3833.

140. Wonganuchitmeta, S. N., Yuenyongsawad, S., Keawpradub, N., and Plubrukarn, A., 2004. Antitubercular sesterterpenes from the Thai sponge *Brachiaster* sp. *J Nat Prod*, 67, 1767–1770.

141. Chill, L., Rudi, A., Aknin, M., Loya, S., Hizi, A., and Kashman, Y., 2004. New sesterterpenes from Madagascan *Lendenfeldia* sponges. *Tetrahedron*, 60, 10619–10626.

142. Pereira, H. S., Leao-Ferreira, L. R., Moussatche, N. et al., 2004. Antiviral activity of diterpenes isolated from the Brazilian marine alga *Dictyota menstrualis* against human immunodeficiency virus type 1 (HIV-1). *Antiviral Res*, 64, 69–76.

143. Ishiyama, H., Hashimoto, A., Fromont, J., Hoshino, Y., Mikami, Y., and Kobayashi, J., 2005. Halichonadins A–D, new sesquiterpenoids from a sponge *Halichondria* sp. *Tetrahedron*, 61, 1101–1105.

144. Ospina, C. A., Rodriguez, A. D., Sanchez, J. A., Ortega-Barria, E., Capson, T. L., and Mayer, A. M., 2005. Caucanolides A–F, unusual antiplasmodial constituents from a colombian collection of the gorgonian coral *Pseudopterogorgia bipinnata*. *J Nat Prod*, 68, 1519–1526.

145. Garzon, S. P., Rodriguez, A. D., Sanchez, J. A., and Ortega-Barria, E., 2005. Sesquiterpenoid metabolites with antiplasmodial activity from a Caribbean gorgonian coral, *Eunicea* sp. *J Nat Prod*, 68, 1354–1359.

146. Gutierrez, M., Capson, T. L., Guzman, H. M. et al., 2005. Leptolide, a new furanocembranolide diterpene from *Leptogorgia alba*. *J Nat Prod*, 68, 614–616.

147. Iwashima, M., Mori, J., Ting, X. et al., 2005. Antioxidant and antiviral activities of plastoquinones from the brown alga *Sargassum micracanthum*, and a new chromene derivative converted from the plastoquinones. *Biol Pharm Bull*, 28, 374–377.

148. Marrero, J., Ospina, C., Rodriguez, A. et al., 2006. New diterpenes of the pseudopterane class from two closely related *Pseudopterogorgia* species: Isolation, structural elucidation, and biological evaluation. *Tetrahedron*, 62, 6998–7008.

149. Bishara, A., Rudi, A., Goldberg, I., Benayahu, Y., and Kashman, Y., 2006. Novaxenicins A–D and xeniolides I–K, seven new diterpenes from the soft coral *Xenia novaebrittanniae*. *Tetrahedron*, 62, 12092–12097.

150. Gray, C. A., de Lira, S. P., Silva, M. et al., 2006. Sulfated meroterpenoids from the Brazilian sponge *Callyspongia* sp. are inhibitors of the antileishmaniasis target adenosine phosphoribosyl transferase. *J Org Chem*, 71, 8685–8690.

151. Rodriguez, I., Rodriguez, A., Wang, Y., and Franzblau, S., 2006. Ileabethoxazole: A novel benzoxazole alkaloid with antimycobacterial activity. *Tetrahedron Lett*, 47, 3229–3232.

152. Vairappan, C. S., Suzuki, M., Ishii, T., Okino, T., Abe, T., and Masuda, M., 2008. Antibacterial activity of halogenated sesquiterpenes from Malaysian *Laurencia* spp. *Phytochemistry*, 69, 2490–2494.

153. Ji, N. Y., Li, X. M., Li, K., Ding, L. P., Gloer, J. B., and Wang, B. G., 2007. Diterpenes, sesquiterpenes, and a C15-acetogenin from the marine red alga *Laurencia mariannensis*. *J Nat Prod*, 70, 1901–1905.

154. Nguyen, H. P., Zhang, D., Lee, U., Kang, J. S., Choi, H. D., and Son, B. W., 2007. Dehydroxychlorofusarielin B, an antibacterial polyoxygenated decalin derivative from the marine-derived fungus *Aspergillus* sp. *J Nat Prod*, 70, 1188–1190.

155. Lee, D., Shin, J., Yoon, K. M. et al., 2008. Inhibition of *Candida albicans* isocitrate lyase activity by sesterterpene sulfates from the tropical sponge *Dysidea* sp. *Bioorg Med Chem Lett*, 18, 5377–5380.

156. Du, L., Shen, L., Yu, Z. et al., 2008. Hyrtiosal, from the marine sponge *Hyrtios erectus*, inhibits HIV-1 integrase binding to viral DNA by a new inhibitor binding site. *Chem Med Chem*, 3, 173–180.

157. Qiu, Y. and Wang, X. M., 2008. A new sesquiterpenoid hydroquinone from the marine sponge *Dysidea arenaria*. *Molecules*, 13, 1275–1281.

158. Desoubzdanne, D., Marcourt, L., Raux, R. et al., 2008. Alisiaquinones and alisiaquinol, dual inhibitors of *Plasmodium falciparum* enzyme targets from a New Caledonian deep water sponge. *J Nat Prod*, 71, 1189–1192.

159. Xu, W. H., Ding, Y., Jacob, M. R. et al., 2009. Puupehanol, a sesquiterpene-dihydroquinone derivative from the marine sponge *Hyrtios* sp. *Bioorg Med Chem Lett*, 19, 6140–6143.

160. Kamei, Y., Sueyoshi, M., Hayashi, K., Terada, R., and Nozaki, H., 2009. The novel anti-*Propionibacterium acnes* compound, Sargafuran, found in the marine brown alga *Sargassum macrocarpum*. *J Antibiot (Tokyo)*, 62, 259–263.

161. Lane, A. L., Mular, L., Drenkard, E. J. et al., 2010. Ecological leads for natural product discovery: Novel sesquiterpene hydroquinones from the red macroalga *Peyssonnelia* sp. *Tetrahedron*, 66, 455–461.

162. Abrantes, J. L., Barbosa, J., Cavalcanti, D. et al., 2010. The effects of the diterpenes isolated from the Brazilian brown algae *Dictyota pfaffii* and *Dictyota menstrualis* against the herpes simplex type-1 replicative cycle. *Planta Med*, 76, 339–344.

163. Cirne-Santos, C. C., Souza, T. M., Teixeira, V. L. et al., 2008. The dolabellane diterpene Dolabelladienetriol is a typical noncompetitive inhibitor of HIV-1 reverse transcriptase enzyme. *Antiviral Res*, 77, 64–71.

164. Zhang, H., Khalil, Z., and Capon, R., 2011. Fascioquinols A–F: Bioactive meroterpenes from a deep-water Southern Australian marinesponge, *Fasciospongia* sp. *Tetrahedron*, 67, 2591–2595.

165. Wright, A. D., McCluskey, A., Robertson, M. J., MacGregor, K. A., Gordon, C. P., and Guenther, J., 2011. Anti-malarial, anti-algal, anti-tubercular, anti-bacterial, anti-photosynthetic, and anti-fouling activity of diterpene and diterpene isonitriles from the tropical marine sponge *Cymbastela hooperi*. *Org Biomol Chem*, 9, 400–407.

166. Rudi, A., Yosief, T., Loya, S., Hizi, A., Schleyer, M., and Kashman, Y., 2001. Clathsterol, a novel anti-HIV-1 RT sulfated sterol from the sponge *Clathria* species. *J Nat Prod*, 64, 1451–1453.

167. Ali, M. S., Saleem, M., Yamdagni, R., and Ali, M. A., 2002. Steroid and antibacterial steroidal glycosides from marine green alga *Codium iyengarii* Borgesen. *Nat Prod Lett*, 16, 407–413.

168. Yang, S., Chan, T., Pomponi, S. et al., 2003. Structure elucidation of a new antifungal sterol sulfate, Sch 575867, from a deep-water marine sponge (Family: Astroscleridae). *J Antibiot (Tokyo)*, 56, 186–189.

169. Boonlarppradab, C. and Faulkner, D. J., 2007. Eurysterols A and B, cytotoxic and antifungal steroidal sulfates from a marine sponge of the genus *Euryspongia*. *J Nat Prod*, 70, 846–848.

170. Digirolamo, J. A., Li, X. C., Jacob, M. R., Clark, A. M., and Ferreira, D., 2009. Reversal of fluconazole resistance by sulfated sterols from the marine sponge *Topsentia* sp. *J Nat Prod*, 72, 1524–1528.

171. Li, H., Shinde, P. B., Lee, H. J. et al., 2009. Bile acid derivatives from a sponge-associated bacterium *Psychrobacter* sp. *Arch Pharm Res*, 32, 857–862.

172. Zhang, W., Draeger, S., Schulz, B., and Krohn, K., 2009. Ring B aromatic steroids from an endophytic fungus, *Colletotrichum* sp. *Nat Prod Commun*, 4, 1449–1454.

173. Xu, N., Fan, X., Yan, X., Li, X., Niu, R., and Tseng, C. K., 2003. Antibacterial bromophenols from the marine red alga *Rhodomela confervoides*. *Phytochemistry*, 62, 1221–1224.

174. Hanif, N., Tanaka, J., Setiawan, A. et al., 2007. Polybrominated diphenyl ethers from the Indonesian sponge *Lamellodysidea herbacea*. *J Nat Prod*, 70, 432–435.

175. El-Beih, A. A., Kawabata, T., Koimaru, K., Ohta, T., and Tsukamoto, S., 2007. Monodictyquinone A: A new antimicrobial anthraquinone from a sea urchin-derived fungus *Monodictys* sp. *Chem Pharm Bull (Tokyo)*, 55, 1097–1098.

176. Oh, K. B., Lee, J. H., Chung, S. C. et al., 2008. Antimicrobial activities of the bromophenols from the red alga *Odonthalia corymbifera* and some synthetic derivatives. *Bioorg Med Chem Lett*, 18, 104–108.

177. Zhang, H., Skildum, A., Stromquist, E., Rose-Hellekant, T., and Chang, L. C., 2008. Bioactive polybrominated diphenyl ethers from the marine sponge *Dysidea* sp. *J Nat Prod*, 71, 262–264.

178. Xu, J., Nakazawa, T., Ukai, K. et al., 2008. Tetrahydrobostrycin and 1-deoxytetrahydrobostrycin, two new hexahydroanthrone derivatives, from a marine-derived fungus *Aspergillus* sp. *J Antibiot (Tokyo)*, 61, 415–419.

179. El-Gendy, M. M., Hawas, U. W., and Jaspars, M., 2008. Novel bioactive metabolites from a marine derived bacterium *Nocardia* sp. ALAA 2000. *J Antibiot (Tokyo)*, 61, 379–386.

180. El-Gendy, M. M., Shaaban, M., El-Bondkly, A. M., and Shaaban, K. A., 2008. Bioactive benzopyrone derivatives from new recombinant fusant of *marine Streptomyces*. *Appl Biochem Biotechnol*, 150, 85–96.

181. Kanoh, K., Adachi, K., Matsuda, S. et al., 2008. New sulfoalkylresorcinol from marine-derived fungus, *Zygosporium* sp. KNC52. *J Antibiot (Tokyo)*, 61, 192–194.

182. Shridhar, D. M., Mahajan, G. B., Kamat, V. P. et al., 2009. Antibacterial activity of 2-(2',4'-dibromophenoxy)-4,6-dibromophenol from *Dysidea granulosa*. *Mar Drugs*, 7, 464–471.

183. Isnansetyo, A. and Kamei, Y., 2009. Anti-methicillin-resistant *Staphylococcus aureus* (MRSA) activity of MC21-B, an antibacterial compound produced by the marine bacterium *Pseudoalteromonas phenolica* O-BC30T. *Int J Antimicrob Agents*, 34, 131–135.

184. Feher, D., Barlow, R., McAtee, J., and Hemscheidt, T. K., 2010. Highly brominated antimicrobial metabolites from a marine *Pseudoalteromonas* sp. *J Nat Prod*, 73, 1963–1966.

185. Lee, Y. M., Li, H., Hong, J. et al., 2010. Bioactive metabolites from the sponge-derived fungus *Aspergillus versicolor*. *Arch Pharm Res*, 33, 231–235.

186. Takada, N., Watanabe, R., Suenaga, K. et al., 2001. Zamamistatin, a significant antibacterial bromotyrosine derivative, from the Okinawan sponge *Pseudoceratina* purpurea. *Tetrahedron Lett*, 42, 5265–5267.

187. El Sayed, K. A., Kelly, M., Kara, U. A. et al., 2001. New manzamine alkaloids with potent activity against infectious diseases. *J Am Chem Soc*, 123, 1804–1808.

188. Torres, Y. R., Berlinck, R. G., Nascimento, G. G., Fortier, S. C., Pessoa, C., and de Moraes, M. O., 2002. Antibacterial activity against resistant bacteria and cytotoxicity of four alkaloid toxins isolated from the marine sponge *Arenosclera brasiliensis*. *Toxicon*, 40, 885–891.

189. Lazaro, J. E., Nitcheu, J., Predicala, R. Z. et al., 2002. Heptyl prodigiosin, a bacterial metabolite, is antimalarial *in vivo* and non-mutagenic *in vitro*. *J Nat Toxins*, 11, 367–377.

190. Wright, A. D., Goclik, E., Konig, G. M., and Kaminsky, R., 2002. Lepadins D–F: Antiplasmodial and antitrypanosomal decahydroquinoline derivatives from the tropical marine tunicate *Didemnum* sp. *J Med Chem*, 45, 3067–3072.

191. Schupp, P., Poehner, T., Edrada, R. et al., 2003. Eudistomins W and X, two new beta-carbolines from the micronesian tunicate *Eudistoma* sp. *J Nat Prod*, 66, 272–275.

192. Yang, S. W., Chan, T. M., Pomponi, S. A. et al., 2003. A new bicyclic guanidine alkaloid, Sch 575948, from a marine sponge, *Ptilocaulis spiculifer*. *J Antibiot (Tokyo)*, 56, 970–972.

193. Nishimura, S., Matsunaga, S., Shibazaki, M. et al., 2003. Massadine, a novel geranylgeranyltransferase type I inhibitor from the marine sponge *Stylissa aff*. massa. *Org Lett*, 5, 2255–2257.

194. Rao, K. V., Santarsiero, B. D., Mesecar, A. D., Schinazi, R. F., Tekwani, B. L., and Hamann, M. T., 2003. New manzamine alkaloids with activity against infectious and tropical parasitic diseases from an Indonesian sponge. *J Nat Prod*, 66, 823–828.

195. Chang, L., Whittaker, N. F., and Bewley, C. A., 2003. Crambescidin 826 and dehydrocrambine A: New polycyclic guanidine alkaloids from the marine sponge *Monanchora* sp. that inhibit HIV-1 fusion. *J Nat Prod*, 66, 1490–1494.

196. Venkateshwar Goud, T., Srinivasa Reddy, N., Raghavendra Swamy, N., Siva Ram, T., and Venkateswarlu, Y., 2003. Anti-HIV active petrosins from the marine sponge *Petrosia similis*. *Biol Pharm Bull*, 26, 1498–1501.

197. Goud, T. V., Srinivasulu, M., Reddy, V. L. et al., 2003. Two new bromotyrosine-derived metabolites from the sponge *Psammaplysilla purpurea*. *Chem Pharm Bull (Tokyo)*, 51, 990–993.

198. Endo, T., Tsuda, M., Okada, T. et al., 2004. Nagelamides A–H, new dimeric bromopyrrole alkaloids from marine sponge *Agelas* species. *J Nat Prod*, 67, 1262–1267.

199. Pettit, R. K., Fakoury, B. R., Knight, J. C. et al., 2004. Antibacterial activity of the marine sponge constituent cribrostatin 6. *J Med Microbiol*, 53, 61–65.

200. Hassan, W., Edrada, R., Ebel, R. et al., 2004. New imidazole alkaloids from the Indonesian sponge *Leucetta chagosensis*. *J Nat Prod*, 67, 817–822.

201. Nakao, Y., Shiroiwa, T., Murayama, S. et al., 2004. Identification of Renieramycin A as an antileishmanial substance in a marine sponge *Neopetrosia* sp. *Mar Drugs*, 2, 55–62.

202. Oh, K., Mar, W., Kim, S. et al., 2005. Bis(indole) alkaloids as sortase A inhibitors from the sponge *Spongosorites* sp. *Bioorg Med Chem Lett*, 15, 4927–4931.

203. Segraves, N. L. and Crews, P., 2005. A Madagascar sponge *Batzella* sp. as a source of alkylated iminosugars. *J Nat Prod*, 68, 118–121.

204. Tsuda, M., Takahashi, Y., Fromont, J., Mikami, Y., and Kobayashi, J., 2005. Dendridine A, a bis-indole alkaloid from a marine sponge *Dictyodendrilla* species. *J Nat Prod*, 68, 1277–1278.

205. Rao, K. V., Donia, M. S., Peng, J. et al., 2006. Manzamine B and E and ircinal A related alkaloids from an Indonesian *Acanthostrongylophora* sponge and their activity against infectious, tropical parasitic, and Alzheimer's diseases. *J Nat Prod*, 69, 1034–1040.

206. Bao, B., Sun, Q., Yao, X. et al., 2007. Bisindole alkaloids of the topsentin and hamacanthin classes from a marine sponge *Spongosorites* sp. *J Nat Prod*, 70, 2–8.

207. Tasdemir, D., Topaloglu, B., Perozzo, R. et al., 2007. Marine natural products from the Turkish sponge *Agelas oroides* that inhibit the enoyl reductases from *Plasmodium falciparum*, *Mycobacterium tuberculosis* and *Escherichia coli*. *Bioorg Med Chem*, 15, 6834–6845.

208. Jang, J. H., van Soest, R. W., Fusetani, N., and Matsunaga, S., 2007. Pseudoceratins A and B, antifungal bicyclic bromotyrosine-derived metabolites from the marine sponge *Pseudoceratina purpurea*. *J Org Chem*, 72, 1211–1217.

209. Souza, T. M., Abrantes, J. L., de, A. E. R., Leite Fontes, C. F., and Frugulhetti, I. C., 2007. The alkaloid 4-methylaaptamine isolated from the sponge *Aaptos aaptos* impairs herpes simplex virus type 1 penetration and immediate-early protein synthesis. *Planta Med*, 73, 200–205.

210. Jang, K. H., Chung, S. C., Shin, J. et al., 2007. Aaptamines as sortase A inhibitors from the tropical sponge *Aaptos aaptos*. *Bioorg Med Chem Lett*, 17, 5366–5369.

211. Arai, M., Sobou, M., Vilcheze, C. et al., 2008. Halicyclamine A, a marine spongean alkaloid as a lead for anti-tuberculosis agent. *Bioorg Med Chem*, 16, 6732–6736.

212. Hughes, C. C., Prieto-Davo, A., Jensen, P. R., and Fenical, W., 2008. The marinopyrroles, antibiotics of an unprecedented structure class from a marine *Streptomyces* sp. *Org Lett*, 10, 629–631.

213. Arai, M., Ishida, S., Setiawan, A., and Kobayashi, M., 2009. Haliclonacyclamines, tetracyclic alkylpiperidine alkaloids, as anti-dormant mycobacterial substances from a marine sponge of *Haliclona* sp. *Chem Pharm Bull (Tokyo)*, 57, 1136–1138.

214. Araki, A., Tsuda, M., Kubota, T., Mikami, Y., Fromont, J., and Kobayashi, J., 2007. Nagelamide J, a novel dimeric bromopyrrole alkaloid from a sponge *Agelas* species. *Org Lett*, 9, 2369–2371.

215. Araki, A., Kubota, T., Tsuda, M., Mikami, Y., Fromont, J., and Kobayashi, J., 2008. Nagelamides K and L, dimeric bromopyrrole alkaloids from sponge *Agelas* species. *Org Lett*, 10, 2099–2102.

216. Araki, A., Kubota, T., Aoyama, K., Mikami, Y., Fromont, J., and Kobayashi, J., 2009. Nagelamides Q and R, novel dimeric bromopyrrole alkaloids from sponges *Agelas* sp. *Org Lett*, 11, 1785–1788.

217. Kuboto, T., Araki, A., Yasuda, T. et al., 2009. Benzosceptrin C, a new dimeric bromopyrrole alkaloid from sponge *Agelas* sp. *Tetrahedron Lett*, 50, 7268–7270.

218. Hua, H., Peng, J., Dunbar, D. et al., 2007. Batzelladine alkaloids from the Caribbean sponge *Monanchora unguifera* and the significant activities against HIV-1 and AIDS opportunistics infections pathogens. *Tetrahedron*, 63, 11179–11188.

219. Takishima, S., Ishiyama, A., Iwatsuki, M. et al., 2009. Merobatzelladines A and B, anti-infective tricyclic guanidines from a marine sponge *Monanchora* sp. *Org Lett*, 11, 2655–2658.

220. Yao, G. and Chang, L. C., 2007. Novel sulfated sesterterpene alkaloids from the marine sponge *Fasciospongia* sp. *Org Lett*, 9, 3037–3040.

221. Yao, G., Kondratyuk, T. P., Tan, G. T., Pezzuto, J. M., and Chang, L. C., 2009. Bioactive sulfated sesterterpene alkaloids and sesterterpene sulfates from the marine sponge *Fasciospongia* sp. *J Nat Prod*, 72, 319–323.

222. Lee, H. S., Yoon, K. M., Han, Y. R. et al., 2009. 5-Hydroxyindole-type alkaloids, as *Candida albicans* isocitrate lyase inhibitors, from the tropical sponge *Hyrtios* sp. *Bioorg Med Chem Lett*, 19, 1051–1053.

223. Wang, W., Wang, Y., Tao, H., Peng, X., Liu, P., and Zhu, W., 2009. Cerebrosides of the halotolerant fungus *Alternaria raphani* isolated from a sea salt field. *J Nat Prod*, 72, 1695–1698.

224. Fan, G., Li, Z., Shen, S. et al., 2010. Baculiferins A–O, *O*-sulfated pyrrole alkaloids with anti-HIV-1 activity, from the Chinese marine sponge *Iotrochota baculifera*. *Bioorg Med Chem*, 18, 5466–5474.

225. Kon, Y., Kubota, T., Shibazaki, A., Gonoi, T., and Kobayashi, J., 2010. Ceratinadins A–C, new bromotyrosine alkaloids from an Okinawan marine sponge *Pseudoceratina* sp. *Bioorg Med Chem Lett*, 20, 4569–4572.

226. Jeon, J. E., Na, Z., Jung, M. et al., 2010. Discorhabdins from the Korean marine sponge *Sceptrella* sp. *J Nat Prod*, 73, 258–262.

227. Mo, S., Krunic, A., Santarsiero, B. D., Franzblau, S. G., and Orjala, J., 2010. Hapalindole-related alkaloids from the cultured cyanobacterium *Fischerella ambigua*. *Phytochemistry*, 71, 2116–2123.

228. Maskey, R. P., Helmke, E., Kayser, O. et al., 2004. Anti-cancer and antibacterial trioxacarcins with high anti-malaria activity from a marine *Streptomycete* and their absolute stereochemistry. *J Antibiot (Tokyo)*, 57, 771–779.

229. Rodriguez, M. C., Merino, E. R., Pujol, C. A., Damonte, E. B., Cerezo, A. S., and Matulewicz, M. C., 2005. Galactans from cystocarpic plants of the red seaweed *Callophyllis variegata* (Kallymeniaceae, Gigartinales). *Carbohydr Res*, 340, 2742–2751.

230. Matsuhiro, B., Conte, A. F., Damonte, E. B. et al., 2005. Structural analysis and antiviral activity of a sulfated galactan from the red seaweed *Schizymenia binderi* (Gigartinales, Rhodophyta). *Carbohydr Res*, 340, 2392–2402.

231. Linington, R. G., Robertson, M., Gauthier, A. et al., 2006. Caminosides B–D, antimicrobial glycolipids isolated from the marine sponge *Caminus sphaeroconia*. *J Nat Prod*, 69, 173–177.

232. Lee, J. B., Hayashi, K., Hirata, M. et al., 2006. Antiviral sulfated polysaccharide from *Navicula directa*, a diatom collected from deep-sea water in Toyama Bay. *Biol Pharm Bull*, 29, 2135–2139.

233. Kanekiyo, K., Hayashi, K., Takenaka, H., Lee, J. B., and Hayashi, T., 2007. Anti-herpes simplex virus target of an acidic polysaccharide, nostoflan, from the edible blue-green alga *Nostoc flagelliforme*. *Biol Pharm Bull*, 30, 1573–1575.

234. Sato, Y., Okuyama, S., and Hori, K., 2007. Primary structure and carbohydrate binding specificity of a potent anti-HIV lectin isolated from the filamentous cyanobacterium *Oscillatoria agardhii*. *J Biol Chem*, 282, 11021–11029.

235. Han, Y., Yang, B., Zhang, F., Miao, X., and Li, Z., 2009. Characterization of antifungal chitinase from marine *Streptomyces* sp. DA11 associated with South China Sea sponge *Craniella australiensis*. *Mar Biotechnol (NY)*, 11, 132–140.

236. Barsby, T., Kelly, M. T., Gagne, S. M., and Andersen, R. J., 2001. Bogorol A produced in culture by a marine *Bacillus* sp. reveals a novel template for cationic peptide antibiotics. *Org Lett*, 3, 437–440.

237. Lee, I. H., Lee, Y. S., Kim, C. H. et al., 2001. Dicynthaurin: An antimicrobial peptide from hemocytes of the solitary tunicate, *Halocynthia aurantium*. *Biochim Biophys Acta*, 1527, 141–148.

238. Jang, W. S., Kim, K. N., Lee, Y. S., Nam, M. H., and Lee, I. H., 2002. Halocidin: A new antimicrobial peptide from hemocytes of the solitary tunicate, *Halocynthia aurantium*. *FEBS Lett*, 521, 81–86.

239. Rashid, M. A., Gustafson, K. R., Cartner, L. K., Shigematsu, N., Pannell, L. K., and Boyd, M. R., 2001. Microspinosamide, a new HIV-inhibitory cyclic depsipeptide from the marine sponge *Sidonops microspinosa*. *J Nat Prod*, 64, 117–121.

240. Iijima, R., Kisugi, J., and Yamazaki, M., 2003. A novel antimicrobial peptide from the sea hare *Dolabella auricularia*. *Dev Comp Immunol*, 27, 305–311.

241. Patrzykat, A., Gallant, J. W., Seo, J. K., Pytyck, J., and Douglas, S. E., 2003. Novel antimicrobial peptides derived from flatfish genes. *Antimicrob Agents Chemother*, 47, 2464–2470.

242. Ovchinnikova, T. V., Aleshina, G. M., Balandin, S. V. et al., 2004. Purification and primary structure of two isoforms of arenicin, a novel antimicrobial peptide from marine polychaeta *Arenicola marina*. *FEBS Lett*, 577, 209–214.

243. Pan, W., Liu, X., Ge, F., Han, J., and Zheng, T., 2004. Perinerin, a novel antimicrobial peptide purified from the clamworm *Perinereis aibuhitensis* grube and its partial characterization. *J Biochem*, 135, 297–304.

244. Roch, P., Beschin, A., and Bernard, E., 2004. Antiprotozoan and antiviral activities of non-cytotoxic truncated and variant analogues of mussel defensin. *Evid Based Complement Alternat Med*, 1, 167–174.

245. Oku, N., Gustafson, K. R., Cartner, L. K. et al., 2004. Neamphamide A, a new HIV-inhibitory depsipeptide from the Papua New Guinea marine sponge *Neamphius huxleyi*. *J Nat Prod*, 67, 1407–1411.

246. Sugiyama, N., Araki, M., Ishida, M., Nagashima, Y., and Shiomi, K., 2005. Further isolation and characterization of grammistins from the skin secretion of the soapfish *Grammistes sexlineatus*. *Toxicon*, 45, 595–601.

247. Neuhof, T., Schmieder, P., Preussel, K. et al., 2005. Hassallidin A, a glycosylated lipopeptide with antifungal activity from the cyanobacterium *Hassallia* sp. *J Nat Prod*, 68, 695–700.

248. Mori, T., O'Keefe, B. R., Sowder, R. C., 2nd, et al., 2005. Isolation and characterization of griffithsin, a novel HIV-inactivating protein, from the red alga *Griffithsia* sp. *J Biol Chem*, 280, 9345–9353.

249. Ovchinnikova, T. V., Balandin, S. V., Aleshina, G. M. et al., 2006. Aurelin, a novel antimicrobial peptide from jellyfish *Aurelia aurita* with structural features of defensins and channel-blocking toxins. *Biochem Biophys Res Commun*, 348, 514–523.

250. Plaza, A., Gustchina, E., Baker, H. L., Kelly, M., and Bewley, C. A., 2007. Mirabamides A–D, depsipeptides from the sponge *Siliquariaspongia mirabilis* that inhibit HIV-1 fusion. *J Nat Prod*, 70, 1753–1760.

251. Ren, Z. Z., Zheng, Y., Sun, M., Liu, J. Z., and Wang, Y. J., 2007. [Purification and properties of an antimicrobial substance from marine *Brevibacillus laterosporus* Lh-1]. *Wei Sheng Wu Xue Bao*, 47, 997–1001.

252. Desjardine, K., Pereira, A., Wright, H., Matainaho, T., Kelly, M., and Andersen, R. J., 2007. Tauramamide, a lipopeptide antibiotic produced in culture by *Brevibacillus laterosporus* isolated from a marine habitat: Structure elucidation and synthesis. *J Nat Prod*, 70, 1850–1853.

253. Oku, N., Kawabata, K., Adachi, K., Katsuta, A., and Shizuri, Y., 2008. Unnarmicins A and C, new antibacterial depsipeptides produced by marine bacterium *Photobacterium* sp. MBIC06485. *J Antibiot (Tokyo)*, 61, 11–17.

254. Ojika, M., Inukai, Y., Kito, Y., Hirata, M., Iizuka, T., and Fudou, R., 2008. Miuraenamides: Antimicrobial cyclic depsipeptides isolated from a rare and slightly halophilic myxobacterium. *Chem Asian J*, 3, 126–133.

255. Oku, N., Adachi, K., Matsuda, S., Kasai, H., Takatsuki, A., and Shizuri, Y., 2008. Ariakemicins A and B, novel polyketide-peptide antibiotics from a marine gliding bacterium of the genus *Rapidithrix*. *Org Lett*, 10, 2481–2484.

256. Zampella, A., Sepe, V., Luciano, P. et al., 2008. Homophymine A, an anti-HIV cyclodepsipeptide from the sponge *Homophymia* sp. *J Org Chem*, 73, 5319–5327.

257. Kim, M. Y., Sohn, J. H., Ahn, J. S., and Oh, H., 2009. Alternaramide, a cyclic depsipeptide from the marine-derived fungus *Alternaria* sp. SF-5016. *J Nat Prod*, 72, 2065–2068.

258. Andavan, G. S. and Lemmens-Gruber, R., 2010. Cyclodepsipeptides from marine sponges: Natural agents for drug research. *Mar Drugs*, 8, 810–834.

259. Ibrahim, S. R., Min, C. C., Teuscher, F. et al., 2010. Callyaerins A–F and H, new cytotoxic cyclic peptides from the Indonesian marine sponge *Callyspongia aerizusa*. *Bioorg Med Chem*, 18, 4947–4956.

260. Pruksakorn, P., Arai, M., Kotoku, N. et al., 2010. Trichoderins, novel aminolipopeptides from a marine sponge-derived *Trichoderma* sp., are active against dormant mycobacteria. *Bioorg Med Chem Lett*, 20, 3658–3663.

261. Zheng, J., Zhu, H., Hong, K. et al., 2009. Novel cyclic hexapeptides from marine-derived fungus, *Aspergillus sclerotiorum* PT06-1. *Org Lett*, 11, 5262–5265.

262. Zheng, J., Xu, Z., Wang, Y., Hong, K., Liu, P., and Zhu, W., 2010. Cyclic tripeptides from the halotolerant fungus *Aspergillus sclerotiorum* PT06-1. *J Nat Prod*, 73, 1133–1137.

263. Zhang, D. J., Liu, R. F., Li, Y. G., Tao, L. M., and Tian, L., 2010. Two new antifungal cyclic lipopeptides from *Bacillus marinus* B-9987. *Chem Pharm Bull (Tokyo)*, 58, 1630–1634.

264. Chen, L., Wang, N., Wang, X., Hu, J., and Wang, S., 2010. Characterization of two anti-fungal lipopeptides produced by *Bacillus amyloliquefaciens* SH-B10. *Bioresour Technol*, 101, 8822–8827.

265. Engelhardt, K., Degnes, K. F., Kemmler, M. et al., 2010. Production of a new thiopeptide antibiotic, TP-1161, by a marine *Nocardiopsis* species. *Appl Environ Microbiol*, 76, 4969–4976.

266. Silva-Stenico, M. E., Silva, C. S., Lorenzi, A. S. et al., 2011. Non-ribosomal peptides produced by Brazilian cyanobacterial isolates with antimicrobial activity. *Microbiol Res*, 166, 161–175.

267. Gochfeld, D. J. and Hamann, M. T., 2001. Isolation and biological evaluation of filiformin, plakortide F, and plakortone G from the Caribbean sponge *Plakortis* sp. *J Nat Prod*, 64, 1477–1479.

268. Vairappan, C. S., Daitoh, M., Suzuki, M., Abe, T., and Masuda, M., 2001. Antibacterial halogenated metabolites from the Malaysian *Laurencia* species. *Phytochemistry*, 58, 291–297.

269. Jadulco, R., Proksch, P., Wray, V., Sudarsono, Berg, A., and Grafe, U., 2001. New macrolides and furan carboxylic acid derivative from the sponge-derived fungus *Cladosporium herbarum*. *J Nat Prod*, 64, 527–530.

270. Asolkar, R. N., Maskey, R. P., Helmke, E., and Laatsch, H., 2002. Chalcomycin B, a new macrolide antibiotic from the marine isolate *Streptomyces* sp. B7064. *J Antibiot (Tokyo)*, 55, 893–898.

271. Daferner, M., Anke, T., and Sterner, O., 2002. Zopfiellamides A and B, antimicrobial pyrrolidinone derivatives from the marine fungus *Zopfiella latipes*. *Tetrahedron*, 58, 7781–7784.

272. Barsby, T., Kelly, M. T., and Andersen, R. J., 2002. Tupuseleiamides and basiliskamides, new acyldipeptides and antifungal polyketides produced in culture by a *Bacillus laterosporus* isolate obtained from a tropical marine habitat. *J Nat Prod*, 65, 1447–1451.

273. Nishimura, S., Matsunaga, S., Shibazaki, M. et al., 2002. Corticatic acids D and E, polyacetylenic geranylgeranyltransferase type I inhibitors, from the marine sponge *Petrosia corticata*. *J Nat Prod*, 65, 1353–1356.

274. Edrada, R. A., Ebel, R., Supriyono, A. et al., 2002. Swinhoeiamide A, a new highly active calyculin derivative from the marine sponge *Theonella swinhoei*. *J Nat Prod*, 65, 1168–1172.

275. Liu, C. H., Meng, J. C., Zou, W. X., Huang, L. L., Tang, H. Q., and Tan, R. X., 2002. Antifungal metabolite with a new carbon skeleton from *Keissleriella* sp. YS4108, a marine filamentous fungus. *Planta Med*, 68, 363–365.

276. Schlingmann, G., Milne, L., and Carter, G., 2002. Isolation and identification of antifungal polyesters from the marine fungus *Hypoxylon oceanicum* LL-15G256. *Tetrahedron*, 58, 6825–6835.

277. Edrada, R. A., Heubes, M., Brauers, G. et al., 2002. Online analysis of xestodecalactones A–C, novel bioactive metabolites from the fungus *Penicillium* cf. montanense and their subsequent isolation from the sponge *Xestospongia exigua*. *J Nat Prod*, 65, 1598–1604.

278. Isaka, M., Suyarnsestakorn, C., Tanticharoen, M., Kongsaeree, P., and Thebtaranonth, Y., 2002. Aigialomycins A–E, new resorcylic macrolides from the marine mangrove fungus *Aigialus parvus*. *J Org Chem*, 67, 1561–1566.

279. Wang, C. Y., Wang, B. G., Wiryowidagdo, S. et al., 2003. Melophlins C–O, thirteen novel tetramic acids from the marine sponge *Melophlus sarassinorum*. *J Nat Prod*, 66, 51–56.

280. Kossuga, M. H., MacMillan, J. B., Rogers, E. W. et al., 2004. (2*S*,3*R*)-2-aminododecan-3-ol, a new antifungal agent from the ascidian *Clavelina oblonga*. *J Nat Prod*, 67, 1879–1881.

281. Manam, R. R., Teisan, S., White, D. J. et al., 2005. Lajollamycin, a nitro-tetraene spiro-beta-lactone-gamma-lactam antibiotic from the marine actinomycete *Streptomyces nodosus*. *J Nat Prod*, 68, 240–243.

282. Kock, I., Maskey, R. P., Biabani, M. A., Helmke, E., and Laatsch, H., 2005. 1-Hydroxy-1-norresistomycin and resistoflavin methyl ether: New antibiotics from marine-derived streptomycetes. *J Antibiot (Tokyo)*, 58, 530–534.

283. Macmillan, J. B. and Molinski, T. F., 2005. Majusculoic acid, a brominated cyclopropyl fatty acid from a marine cyanobacterial mat assemblage. *J Nat Prod*, 68, 604–606.

284. Wright, A. D. and Lang-Unnasch, N., 2005. Potential antimalarial lead structures from fungi of marine origin. *Planta Med*, 71, 964–966.

285. Campagnuolo, C., Fattorusso, E., Romano, A. et al., 2005. Antimalarial polyketide cycloperoxides from the marine sponge *Plakortis simplex*. *Eur J Org Chem*, 23, 5077–5083.

286. Sionov, E., Roth, D., Sandovsky-Losica, H. et al., 2005. Antifungal effect and possible mode of activity of a compound from the marine sponge *Dysidea herbacea*. *J Infect*, 50, 453–460.

287. Yang, R. Y., Li, C. Y., Lin, Y. C., Peng, G. T., She, Z. G., and Zhou, S. N., 2006. Lactones from a brown alga endophytic fungus (No. ZZF36) from the South China Sea and their antimicrobial activities. *Bioorg Med Chem Lett*, 16, 4205–4208.

288. Kwon, H. C., Kauffman, C. A., Jensen, P. R., and Fenical, W., 2006. Marinomycins A–D, antitumor-antibiotics of a new structure class from a marine actinomycete of the recently discovered genus "marinispora". *J Am Chem Soc*, 128, 1622–1632.

289. Socha, A. M., Garcia, D., Sheffer, R., and Rowley, D. C., 2006. Antibiotic bisanthraquinones produced by a streptomycete isolated from a cyanobacterium associated with *Ecteinascidia turbinata*. *J Nat Prod*, 69, 1070–1073.

290. El Sayed, K. A., Youssef, D. T., and Marchetti, D., 2006. Bioactive natural and semisynthetic latrunculins. *J Nat Prod*, 69, 219–223.

291. Laurent, D., Jullian, V., Parenty, A. et al., 2006. Antimalarial potential of xestoquinone, a protein kinase inhibitor isolated from a Vanuatu marine sponge *Xestospongia* sp. *Bioorg Med Chem*, 14, 4477–4482.

292. Lim, C., Kim, Y., Youn, H., and Park, H., 2006. Enantiomeric compounds with antileishimanial activities from a sponge, *Plakortis* sp. *Agric Chem Biotechnol*, 49, 21–23.

293. Washida, K., Koyama, T., Yamada, K., Kita, M., and Uemura, D., 2006. Karatungiols A and B, two novel antimicrobial polyol compounds, from the symbiotic marine dinoflagellate *Amphidinium* sp. *Tetrahedron Lett*, 47, 2521–2525.

294. Xue, C., Tian, L., Xu, M., Deng, Z., and Lin, W., 2008. A new 24-membered lactone and a new polyene delta-lactone from the marine bacterium *Bacillus marinus*. *J Antibiot (Tokyo)*, 61, 668–674.

295. Lu, X. L., Xu, Q., Shen, Y. H. et al., 2008. Macrolactin S, a novel macrolactin antibiotic from marine *Bacillus* sp. *Nat Prod Res*, 22, 342–347.

296. Xie, L. W., Ouyang, Y. C., Zou, K. et al., 2009. Isolation and difference in anti-*Staphylococcus aureus* bioactivity of curvularin derivates from fungus *Eupenicillium* sp. *Appl Biochem Biotechnol*, 159, 284–293.

297. Trisuwan, K., Rukachaisirikul, V., Sukpondma, Y., Phongpaichit, S., Preedanon, S., and Sakayaroj, J., 2009. Lactone derivatives from the marine-derived fungus *Penicillium* sp. PSU-F44. *Chem Pharm Bull (Tokyo)*, 57, 1100–1102.

298. Trisuwan, K., Rukachaisirikul, V., Sukpondma, Y. et al., 2008. Epoxydons and a pyrone from the marine-derived fungus *Nigrospora* sp. PSU-F5. *J Nat Prod*, 71, 1323–1326.

299. Trisuwan, K., Rukachaisirikul, V., Sukpondma, Y., Preedanon, S., Phongpaichit, S., and Sakayaroj, J., 2009. Pyrone derivatives from the marine-derived fungus *Nigrospora* sp. PSU-F18. *Phytochemistry*, 70, 554–557.

300. Longeon, A., Copp, B. R., Roue, M. et al., 2010. New bioactive halenaquinone derivatives from South Pacific marine sponges of the genus *Xestospongia*. *Bioorg Med Chem*, 18, 6006–6011.

301. Song, F., Dai, H., Tong, Y. et al., 2010. Trichodermaketones A–D and 7-*O*-methylkoninginin D from the marine fungus *Trichoderma koningii*. *J Nat Prod*, 73, 806–810.

302. Nakao, Y., Takada, K., Matsunaga, S., and Fusetani, N., 2001. Calyceramides A–C: Neuraminidase inhibitory sulfated ceramides from the marine sponge *Discodermia calyx*. *Tetrahedron*, 57, 3013–3017.

303. Dmitrenok, A., Radhika, P., Anjaneyulu, V. et al., 2003. New lipids from the soft corals of the Andaman Islands. *Russ Chem Bull*, 52, 1868–1872.

304. Zhang, Y., Wang, S., Li, X. M., Cui, C. M., Feng, C., and Wang, B. G., 2007. New sphingolipids with a previously unreported 9-methyl-C20-sphingosine moiety from a marine algous endophytic fungus *Aspergillus* niger EN-13. *Lipids*, 42, 759–764.

305. Taniguchi, M., Uchio, Y., Yasumoto, K., Kusumi, T., and Ooi, T., 2008. Brominated unsaturated fatty acids from marine sponge collected in Papua New Guinea. *Chem Pharm Bull (Tokyo)*, 56, 378–382.

306. Desbois, A. P., Lebl, T., Yan, L., and Smith, V. J., 2008. Isolation and structural characterisation of two antibacterial free fatty acids from the marine diatom, *Phaeodactylum tricornutum*. *Appl Microbiol Biotechnol*, 81, 755–764.

307. Tianero, M. D., Hanif, N., de Voogd, N. J., van Soest, R. W., and Tanaka, J., 2009. A new antimicrobial fatty acid from the calcareous sponge *Paragrantia* cf. waguensis. *Chem Biodivers*, 6, 1374–1377.

308. Keffer, J. L., Plaza, A., and Bewley, C. A., 2009. Motualevic acids A–F, antimicrobial acids from the sponge *Siliquariaspongia* sp. *Org Lett*, 11, 1087–1090.

309. Desbois, A. P., Mearns-Spragg, A., and Smith, V. J., 2009. A fatty acid from the diatom *Phaeodactylum tricornutum* is antibacterial against diverse bacteria including multi-resistant *Staphylococcus aureus* (MRSA). *Mar Biotechnol (NY)*, 11, 45–52.

Index

A

α-Amino-3-hydroxy-5-methylisoproprionic acid
   (AMPA), 876
Achatina fulica Ferussac, 881
Acute reference dose (ARfD), 200, 748
A-kinase anchoring proteins (AKAPs), 659
Albert–Post model, 749
Alkaloids
   ascidians, 90–91
   sponges, 92–93
   worms, 88–89
Alutera scripta, 743
Amnesic shellfish poisoning (ASP)
   AOAC MBA extraction method, 379
   chemical structures, 378–379
   chronic exposure, 147
   clinical features, 146–147
   epidemiology chain
      risk factors, 146
      toxin source, 144–146
      vectors, 144–145
   geographic distribution, 146
   HPLC-UV methods
      C18-SPE cleanup, 379
      development and validation, 379
      domoic acid recoveries, 380
      EURLMB-harmonized standard operating
         procedure (SOP), 380
      fluorometric methods, 380
      high-throughput analysis method, 379
      post-column derivatization method, 381
      strong anion-exchange (SAX) cleanup,
         379–380
   incidence, 144
   public health issues, 147
   seasonal variations, 146
   toxin, 144
AMPA, *see* α-Amino-3-hydroxy-5-
   methylisoproprionic acid (AMPA)
Amphidinium
   A. carterae, 578
   A. operculatum, 581, 593
Amphidinols (AMs), 865–866
Amphidoma languida
   light microscopy and electron
      microscopy, 775
   morphological features, 774
Amphiporus lactifloreus, 1149
Anatoxin
   AN-a(s), 1063
   biosynthetic pathways, 1062–1063
   chemical structures, 1062

chemistry, 1061–1063
detection
   animal bioassays, 1064
   LC-FLD analysis, 1065
   LC-MS analysis, 1065
   UV detection method, 1065
incidents, 1064
methylene analogue, 1062
sources and metabolism, 1063–1064
toxic effects, 1063
Animal-based testing, 419
9-anthryldiazomethane (ADAM), 643
Antibody techniques
   antibody structure and function
      antibody formats, 481
      detection of, 475
      generation strategies, 474
      IgG components and recombinant fragments,
         472, 473
      immunoassay formats, 482
      immunoglobulin formats, 472, 473
      monoclonal antibodies, 477–479
      polyclonal antibodies, 475–477
      recombinant antibodies, 480–481
   display techniques, 484–485
   immune response generation
      conjugate carriers, 482–483
      coupling chemistry, 483–484
      immunogen preparation, 482
      purification and characterization, 484
   immunosensors
      Abraxis and Envirologix
         QualiTube, 488
      commercial kits, 488–489
      electrochemical immunosensors,
         485–486
      Jellett MIST Alert, 488
      optical immunosensors, 487–488
      RIDASCREEN STX assay, 488
Antigen-presenting cells (APCs), 482
Aphanizomenon ovalisporum, CYN
   biosynthesis, 1037
   developmental pathways, 1040
   HPLC-PDA, LC-MS, and LC-MS/MS, 1048
   isolation, 1035
Aplidium albicans, 1143
Apoptosis, 1145–1146
Aptamers, 353
ARfD, *see* Acute reference dose (ARfD)
Ascidians
   alkaloids, 90–91
   peptides, 90

1179

Printed and bound by CPI Group (UK) Ltd, Croydon, CR0 4YY

23/10/2024

01778268-0004